New Oxford Textbook of

# Psychiatry

New Oxford Textbook of

# Psychiatry

## VOLUME 2

# New Oxford Textbook of
# Psychiatry

## SECOND EDITION

Edited by

**Michael G. Gelder**

*Emeritus Professor of Psychiatry,
Warneford Hospital, University of Oxford,
Oxford, UK*

**Nancy C. Andreasen**

*Director, Mental Health Clinical Research Centre,
University of Iowa Hospital and Clinic,
Iowa City, USA*

**Juan J. López-Ibor Jr.**

*Professor of Psychiatry,
Complutense University, Madrid, Spain*

and

**John R. Geddes**

*Professor of Epidemiological Psychiatry
University of Oxford, Warneford Hospital,
Oxford, UK*

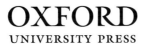

OXFORD
UNIVERSITY PRESS

# OXFORD

## UNIVERSITY PRESS

Great Clarendon Street, Oxford ox2 6DP

Oxford University Press is a department of the University of Oxford.
It furthers the University's objective of excellence in research, scholarship,
and education by publishing worldwide in

Oxford  New York

Auckland  Cape Town  Dar es Salaam  Hong Kong  Karachi
Kuala Lumpur  Madrid  Melbourne  Mexico City  Nairobi
New Delhi  Shanghai  Taipei  Toronto

With offices in

Argentina  Austria  Brazil  Chile  Czech Republic  France  Greece
Guatemala  Hungary  Italy  Japan  Poland  Portugal  Singapore
South Korea  Switzerland  Thailand  Turkey  Ukraine  Vietnam

Oxford is a registered trade mark of Oxford University Press
in the UK and in certain other countries

Published in the United States
by Oxford University Press Inc., New York

© Oxford University Press 2009

The moral rights of the author have been asserted
Database right Oxford University Press (maker)

First edition published 2000
Reprinted 2003

This edition published 2009

British Library Cataloguing in Publication Data
Data available

Library of Congress Cataloguing in Publication Data
Data available

Typeset in Cepha Imaging Pvt. Ltd., Bangalore, India
Printed in Italy on acid-free paper by Rotolito Lombarda SpA

ISBN 978-0-19-920669-8
ISBN 978-0-19-920669-8 (set)
ISBN 978-0-19-955992-3 (Volume 1)
ISBN 978-0-19-955993-0 (Volume 2)

10 9 8 7 6 5 4 3 2 1

# Preface to the second edition

This new edition, like the first, aims to present a comprehensive account of clinical psychiatry with reference to its scientific basis and to the ill person's perspective. As in the first edition, the authors are drawn from many countries, including the UK, the USA, 12 countries in continental Europe, and Australasia. The favourable reception of the first edition has led us to invite many of the original authors to revise their chapters for this second edition but 50 chapters are the work of new authors, many concerned with subjects that appeared in the first edition, while others are completely new. The forensic psychiatry section has the most new chapters, followed by the section on psychology as a scientific basis of psychiatry.

The overall plan of the book resembles that of the first edition (see preface to the 1st edition, reprinted on pages vii and viii). One important feature is that information about treatment appears in more than one place. The commonly used physical and psychological treatments are described in Section 6. Their use in the treatment of any particular disorder is considered in the chapter concerned with that disorder and the account is in two parts. The first part is a review of evidence about the effects of each of the treatments when used for that disorder. The second part, called Management, combines evidence from clinical trials with accumulated clinical experience to produce practical advice about the day to day care of people with the disorder.

Although much information can now be obtained from internet searches, textbooks are still needed to provide the comprehensive account of established knowledge into which new information can be fitted and against which recent findings can be evaluated. As well as seeking to provide an authoritative account of essential knowledge, each chapter in the new edition includes a brief list of sources of further information, including where appropriate, regularly updated web sites.

An essential component of good practice is the need to be aware of patients' perspectives, to respect their wishes, and to work with them, and often their families, as partners. The book opens with an important chapter on the experience of being a patient, and there are chapters on stigma, ethics, and the developing topic of values-based practice.

We are grateful to the following who advised us about parts of the book; Professor John Bancroft (Psychosexual Disorders), Professor Tom Burns (Social and Community Psychiatry), Professor William Fraser (Intellectual Disability), Professor Keith Hawton (Suicide and Deliberate Self Harm), Professor Susan Iversen (Psychology), Professor Robin Jacoby (Old Age Psychiatry), Professor Paul Mullen (Forensic Psychiatry), Sir Michael Rutter (Child and Adolescent Psychiatry), and Professor Gregory Stores (Sleep Disorders).

The editors

# Preface to the first edition

Three themes can be discerned in contemporary psychiatry: the growing unity of the subject, the pace of scientific advance, and the growth of practice in the community. We have sought to reflect these themes in the *New Oxford Textbook of Psychiatry* and to present the state of psychiatry at the start of the new millennium. The book is written for psychiatrists engaged in continuous education and recertification; the previous, shorter, *Oxford Textbook of Psychiatry* remains available for psychiatrists in training. The book is intended to be suitable also as a work of reference for psychiatrists of all levels of experience, and for other professionals whose work involves them in the problems of psychiatry.

## The growing unity of psychiatry

The growing unity in psychiatry is evident in several ways. Biological and psychosocial approaches have been largely reconciled with a general recognition that genetic and environmental factors interact, and that psychological processes are based in and can influence neurobiological mechanisms. At the same time, the common ground between the different psychodynamic theories has been recognized, and is widely accepted as more valuable than the differences between them.

The practice of psychiatry is increasingly similar in different countries, with the remaining variations related more to differences between national systems of health care and the resources available to clinicians, than to differences in the aims of the psychiatrists working in these countries. This unity of approach is reflected in this book whose authors practise in many different countries and yet present a common approach. In this respect this textbook differs importantly from others which present the views of authors drawn predominantly from a single country or region.

Greater agreement about diagnosis and nosology has led to a better understanding of how different treatment approaches are effective in different disorders. The relative specificity of psychopharmacological treatments is being matched increasingly by the specificity of some of the recently developed psychological treatments, so that psychological treatment should no longer be applied without reference to diagnosis, as was sometimes done in the past.

## The pace of scientific advance

Advances in genetics and in the neurosciences have already increased knowledge of the basic mechanisms of the brain and are beginning to uncover the neurobiological mechanisms involved in psychiatric disorder. Striking progress has been achieved in the understanding of Alzheimer's disease, for example, and there are indications that similar progress will follow in uncovering the causes of mood disorder, schizophrenia, and autism. Knowledge of genetics and the neurosciences is so extensive and the pace of change is so rapid that it is difficult to present a complete account within the limited space available in a textbook of clinical psychiatry. We have selected aspects of these sciences that seem, to us and the authors, to have contributed significantly to psychiatry or to be likely to do so before long.

Psychological and social sciences and epidemiology are essential methods of investigation in psychiatry. Although the pace of advance in these sciences may not be as great as in the neurosciences, the findings generally have a more direct relation to clinical phenomena. Moreover, the mechanisms by which psychological and social factors interact with genetic, biochemical, and structural ones will continue to be important however great the progress in these other sciences. Among the advances in the psychological and social sciences that are relevant to clinical phenomena, we have included accounts of memory, psychological development, research on life events, and the effects of culture. Epidemiological studies continue to be crucial for defining psychiatric disorders, following their course, and identifying their causes.

## Psychiatry in the community

In most countries, psychiatry is now practised in the community rather than in institutions, and where this change has yet be completed, it is generally recognized that it should take place. The change has done much more than transfer the locus of care; it has converted patients from passive recipients of care to active participants with individual needs and preferences. Psychiatrists are now involved in the planning, provision, and evaluation of services for whole communities, which may include members of ethnic minorities, homeless people, and refugees. Responsibility for a community has underlined the importance of the prevention as well as the treatment of mental disorder and of the role of agencies other than health services in both. Care in the community has also drawn attention to the many people with psychiatric disorder who are treated in primary care, and has led to new ways of working between psychiatrists and physicians. At the same time, psychiatrists have worked more in general hospitals, helping patients with both medical and psychiatric problems. Others have provided care for offenders.

## The organization of the book

In most ways, the organization of this book is along conventional lines. However, some matters require explanation.

Part 1 contains a variety of diverse topics brought together under the general heading of the subject matter and approach to psychiatry. Phenomenology, assessment, classification, and ethical problems are included, together with the role of the psychiatrist as educator and as manager. Public health aspects of psychiatry are considered together with public attitudes to psychiatry and to psychiatric patients. Part 1 ends with a chapter on the links between science and practice. It begins with a topic that is central to good practice—the understanding of the experience of becoming a psychiatric patient.

Part 2 is concerned with the scientific foundations of psychiatry grouped under the headings neurosciences, genetics, psychological sciences, social sciences, and epidemiology. The chapters contain general information about these sciences; findings specific to a particular disorder are described in the chapter on that disorder. Brain imaging techniques are discussed here because they link basic sciences with clinical research. As explained above, the chapters are selective and, in some, readers who wish to study the subjects in greater detail will find suggestions for further reading.

Part 3 is concerned with dynamic approaches to psychiatry. The principal schools of thought are presented as alternative ways of understanding the influence of life experience on personality and on responses to stressful events and to illness. Some reference is made to dynamic psychotherapy in these accounts, but the main account of these treatments is in Part 6. This arrangement separates the chapters on the practice of dynamic psychotherapy from those on psychodynamic theory, but we consider that this disadvantage is outweighed by the benefit of considering together the commonly used forms of psychotherapy.

Part 4 is long, with chapters on the clinical syndromes of adult psychiatry, with the exception of somatoform disorders which appear in Part 5, Psychiatry and Medicine. This latter contains more than a traditional account of psychosomatic medicine. It also includes a review of psychiatric disorders that may cause medical symptoms unexplained by physical pathology, the medical, surgical, gynaecological, and obstetric conditions most often associated with psychiatric disorder, health psychology, and the treatment of psychiatric disorder in medically ill patients.

Information about treatment appears in more than one part of the book. Part 6 contains descriptions of the physical and psychological treatments in common use in psychiatry. Dynamic psychotherapy and psychoanalysis are described alongside counselling and cognitive behavioural techniques. This part of the book contains general descriptions of the treatments; their use for a particular disorder is considered in the chapter on that disorder.

In the latter, the account is generally in two parts: a review of evidence about the efficacy of the treatment, followed by advice on management in which available evidence is supplemented, where necessary, with clinical experience. Treatment methods designed specially for children and adolescents, for people with mental retardation (learning disability), and for patients within the forensic services are considered in Parts 9, 10, and 11 respectively.

Social psychiatry and service provision are described in Part 7. Public policy issues, as well as the planning, delivery, and evaluation of services, are discussed here. Psychiatry in primary care is an important topic in this part of the book. There are chapters on the special problems of members of ethnic minorities, homeless people, and refugees, and the effects of culture on the provision and uptake of services.

Child and adolescent psychiatry, old age psychiatry, and mental retardation are described in Parts 8, 9, and 10. These accounts are less detailed than might be found in textbooks intended for specialists working exclusively in the relevant subspecialty. Rather, they are written for readers experienced in another branch of psychiatry who wish to improve their knowledge of the special subject. We are aware of the controversy surrounding our choice of the title of Part 10. We have selected the term 'mental retardation' because it is used in both ICD-10 and DSM-IV. In some countries this term has been replaced by another that is thought to be less stigmatizing and more acceptable to patients and families. For example, in the United Kingdom the preferred term is 'learning disability'. While we sympathize with the aims of those who adopt this and other alternative terms, the book is intended for an international readership and it seems best to use the term chosen by the World Health Organization as most generally understood. Thus the term mental retardation is used unless there is a special reason to use another.

In Part 11, Forensic Psychiatry, it has been especially difficult to present a general account of the subject that is not tied to practice in a single country. This is because systems of law differ between countries and the practice of forensic psychiatry has to conform with the local legal system. Although many of the examples in this part of the book may at first seem restricted in their relevance because they are described in the context of English law, we hope that readers will be able to transfer the principles described in these chapters to the legal tradition in which they work.

Finally, readers should note that the history of psychiatry is presented in more than one part of the book. The history of psychiatry as a medical specialty is described in Part 1. The history of ideas about the various psychiatric disorders appears, where relevant, in the chapters on these disorders, where they can be considered in relation to present-day concepts. The history of ideas about aetiology is considered in Part 2, which covers the scientific basis of psychiatric aetiology, while the historical development of dynamic psychiatry is described in Part 3.

Michael Gelder
Juan López-Ibor
Nancy Andreasen

# Acknowledgements from the first edition

We are grateful to the many colleagues who have advised us about certain parts of the book.

The following helped us to plan specialized parts of the book: Dr Jeremy Holmes (Section 3, Psychodynamic Contributions to Psychiatry); Professor Richard Mayou (Section 5, Psychiatry and Medicine); Professor Robin Jacoby (Section 8, Psychiatry of Old Age); Sir Michael Rutter (Section 9, Child and Adolescent Psychiatry); Professor William Fraser (Section 10, Intellectual Disablity); Professor Robert Bluglass (Section 11, Forensic Psychiatry).

The following helped us to plan certain sections within Section 4, General Psychiatry: Professor Alwyn Lishman (delirium, dementia, amnestic syndrome, and other cognitive disorders); Professor Griffith Edwards (alcohol use disorders); Dr Philip Robson (other substance use disorders); Professor Guy Goodwin (mood disorders); Professor John Bancroft (sexuality, gender identity, and their disorders); Professor Gregory Stores (sleep–wake disorders); Professor Keith Hawton (suicide and attempted suicide). In Section 6, Professor Philip Cowen advised about somatic treatments, Dr Jeremy Holmes about psychodynamic treatments, and Professor David Clark about cognitive behavioural therapy. Dr Max Marshall provided helpful advice about forensic issues for Section 7. We also thank the many other colleagues whose helpful suggestions about specific problems aided the planning of the book.

Finally, we record our special gratitude to the authors and to the staff of Oxford University Press.

# Contents
# Volume 1

Preface to the second edition *v*

Preface to the first edition *vii*

Acknowledgements from the first edition *ix*

Contributors list *xxi*

## Section 1 The Subject Matter of and Approach to Psychiatry

**1.1 The patient's perspective** *3*
Kay Redfield Jamison, Richard Jed
Wyatt, and Adam Ian Kaplin

**1.2 Public attitudes and the challenge of stigma** *5*
Graham Thornicroft, Elaine Brohan,
and Aliya Kassam

**1.3 Psychiatry as a worldwide public health problem** *10*

1.3.1 Mental disorders as a worldwide
public health issue *10*
Benedetto Saraceno

1.3.2 Transcultural psychiatry *13*
Julian Leff

**1.4 The history of psychiatry as a medical specialty** *17*
Pierre Pichot

**1.5 Ethics and values** *28*

1.5.1 Psychiatric ethics *28*
Sidney Bloch and Stephen Green

1.5.2 Values and values-based practice
in clinical psychiatry *32*
K. W. M. Fulford

**1.6 The psychiatrist as a manager** *39*
Juan J. López-Ibor Jr. and Costas Stefanis

**1.7 Descriptive phenomenology** *47*
Andrew Sims

**1.8 Assessment** *62*

1.8.1 The principles of clinical assessment in
general psychiatry *62*
John E. Cooper and Margaret Oates

1.8.2 Assessment of personality *78*
C. Robert Cloninger

1.8.3 Cognitive assessment *85*
Graham E. Powell

1.8.4 Questionnaire, rating, and behavioural methods
of assessment *94*
John N. Hall

**1.9 Diagnosis and classification** *99*
Michael B. First and Harold Alan Pincus

**1.10 From science to practice** *122*
John R. Geddes

## Section 2 The Scientific Basis of Psychiatric Aetiology

**2.1 Brain and mind** *133*
Martin Davies

**2.2 Statistics and the design of experiments and surveys** *137*
Graham Dunn

**2.3 The contribution of neurosciences** *144*

2.3.1 Neuroanatomy *144*
R. C. A. Pearson

2.3.2 Neurodevelopment *156*
Karl Zilles

2.3.3 Neuroendocrinology *160*
Charles B. Nemeroff and Gretchen N. Neigh

2.3.4 **Neurotransmitters and signalling** *168*
Trevor Sharp

2.3.5 **Neuropathology** *177*
Peter Falkai and Bernhard Bogerts

2.3.6 **Functional position emission tomography in psychiatry** *185*
P. M. Grasby

2.3.7 **Structural magnetic resonance imaging** *191*
J. Suckling and E. T. Bullmore

2.3.8 **Functional magnetic resonance imaging** *196*
E. T. Bullmore and J. Suckling

2.3.9 **Neuronal networks, epilepsy, and other brain dysfunctions** *201*
John G. R. Jefferys

2.3.10 **Psychoneuroimmunology** *205*
Robert Dantzer and Keith W. Kelley

2.4 **The contribution of genetics** *212*

2.4.1 **Quantitative genetics** *212*
Anita Thapar and Peter McGuffin

2.4.2 **Molecular genetics** *222*
Jonathan Flint

2.5 **The contribution of psychological science** *234*

2.5.1 **Development psychology through infancy, childhood, and adolescence** *234*
William Yule and Matt Woolgar

2.5.2 **Psychology of attention** *245*
Elizabeth Coulthard and Masud Husain

2.5.3 **Psychology and biology of memory** *249*
Andreas Meyer-Lindenberg and Terry E. Goldberg

2.5.4 **The anatomy of human emotion** *257*
R. J. Dolan

2.5.5 **Neuropsychological basis of neuropsychiatry** *262*
L. Clark, B. J. Sahakian, and T. W. Robbins

2.6 **The contribution of social sciences** *268*

2.6.1 **Medical sociology and issues of aetiology** *268*
George W. Brown

2.6.2 **Social and cultural anthropology: salience for psychiatry** *275*
Arthur Kleinman

2.7 **The contribution of epidemiology to psychiatric aetiology** *280*
Scott Henderson

## Section 3  Psychodynamic Contributions to Psychiatry

3.1 **Psychoanalysis: Freud's theories and their contemporary development** *293*
Otto F. Kernberg

3.2 **Object relations, attachment theory, self-psychology, and interpersonal psychoanalysis** *306*
Jeremy Holmes

3.3 **Current psychodynamic approaches to psychiatry** *313*
Glen O. Gabbard

## Section 4  Clinical Syndromes of Adult Psychiatry

4.1 **Delirium, dementia, amnesia, and other cognitive disorders** *325*

4.1.1 **Delirium** *325*
David Meagher and Paula Trzepacz

4.1.2 **Dementia: Alzheimer's disease** *333*
Simon Lovestone

4.1.3 **Frontotemporal dementias** *344*
Lars Gustafson and Arne Brun

4.1.4 **Prion disease** *351*
John Collinge

4.1.5 **Dementia with Lewy bodies** *361*
I. G. McKeith

4.1.6 **Dementia in Parkinson's disease** *368*
R. H. S. Mindham and T. A. Hughes

4.1.7 **Dementia due to Huntington's disease** *371*
Susan Folstein and Russell L. Margolis

4.1.8 **Vascular dementia** *375*
Timo Erkinjuntti

4.1.9 **Dementia due to HIV disease** *384*
Mario Maj

4.1.10 **The neuropsychiatry of head injury** *387*
Simon Fleminger

4.1.11 **Alcohol-related dementia (alcohol-induced dementia; alcohol-related brain damage)** *399*
Jane Marshall

4.1.12 **Amnesic syndromes** *403*
Michael D. Kopelman

4.1.13 **The management of dementia** *411*
John-Paul Taylor and Simon Fleminger

4.1.14 **Remediation of memory disorders** *419*
Jonathan J. Evans

**4.2 Substance use disorders** 426

4.2.1 Pharmacological and psychological aspects of drugs abuse 426
David J. Nutt and Fergus D. Law

4.2.2 Alcohol use disorders 432

4.2.2.1 Aetiology of alcohol problems 432
Juan C. Negrete and Kathryn J. Gill

4.2.2.2 Alcohol dependence and alcohol problems 437
Jane Marshall

4.2.2.3 Alcohol and psychiatric and physical disorders 442
Karl F. Mann and Falk Kiefer

4.2.2.4 Treatment of alcohol dependence 447
Jonathan Chick

4.2.2.5 Services for alcohol use disorders 459
D. Colin Drummond

4.2.2.6 Prevention of alcohol-related problems 467
Robin Room

4.2.3 Other substance use disorders 472

4.2.3.1 Opioids: heroin, methadone, and buprenorphine 473
Soraya Mayet, Adam R. Winstock, and John Strang

4.2.3.2 Disorders relating to the use of amphetamine and cocaine 482
Nicholas Seivewright and Robert Fung

4.2.3.3 Disorders relating to use of PCP and hallucinogens 486
Henry David Abraham

4.2.3.4 Misuse of benzodiazepines 490
Sarah Welch and Michael Farrell

4.2.3.5 Disorders relating to the use of ecstasy and other 'party drugs' 494
Adam R. Winstock and Fabrizio Schifano

4.2.3.6 Disorders relating to the use of volatile substances 502
Richard Ives

4.2.3.7 The mental health effects of cannabis use 507
Wayne Hall

4.2.3.8 Nicotine dependence and treatment 510
Mª Inés López-Ibor

4.2.4 Assessing need and organizing services for drug misuse problems 515
John Marsden, Colin Bradbury, and John Strang

**4.3 Schizophrenia and acute transient psychotic disorders** 521

4.3.1 Schizophrenia: a conceptual history 521
Nancy C. Andreasen

4.3.2 Descriptive clinical features of schizophrenia 526
Peter F. Liddle

4.3.3 The clinical neuropsychology of schizophrenia 531
Philip D. Harvey and Christopher R. Bowie

4.3.4 Diagnosis, classification, and differential diagnosis of schizophrenia 534
Anthony S. David

4.3.5 Epidemiology of schizophrenia 540
Assen Jablensky

4.3.6 Aetiology 553

4.3.6.1 Genetic and environmental risk factors for schizophrenia 553
R. M. Murray and D. J. Castle

4.3.6.2 The neurobiology of schizophrenia 561
Paul J. Harrison

4.3.7 Course and outcome of schizophrenia and their prediction 568
Assen Jablensky

4.3.8 Treatment and management of schizophrenia 578
D. G. Cunningham Owens and E. C. Johnstone

4.3.9 Schizoaffective and schizotypal disorders 595
Ming T. Tsuang, William S. Stone, and Stephen V. Faraone

4.3.10 Acute and transient psychotic disorders 602
J. Garrabé and F.-R. Cousin

**4.4 Persistent delusional symptoms and disorders** 609
Alistair Munro

**4.5 Mood disorders** 629

4.5.1 Introduction to mood disorders 629
John R. Geddes

4.5.2 Clinical features of mood disorders and mania 632
Per Bech

4.5.3 Diagnosis, classification, and differential diagnosis of the mood disorders 637
Gordon Parker

4.5.4 Epidemiology of mood disorders 645
Peter R. Joyce

4.5.5 Genetic aetiology of mood disorders 650
Pierre Oswald, Daniel Souery, and Julien Mendlewicz

4.5.6 Neurobiological aetiology of mood disorders 658
Guy Goodwin

4.5.7 Course and prognosis of mood disorders 665
Jules Angst

4.5.8 Treatment of mood disorders 669
E. S. Paykel and J. Scott

4.5.9 Dysthymia, cyclothymia, and hyperthymia 680
Hagop S. Akiskal

**4.6 Stress-related and adjustment disorders** 693

4.6.1 Acute stress reactions 693
Anke Ehlers, Allison G. Harvey and Richard A. Bryant

4.6.2 Post-traumatic stress disorder 700
Anke Ehlers

4.6.3 Recovered memories and false memories *713*
Chris R. Brewin

4.6.4 Adjustment disorders *716*
James J. Strain, Kimberly Klipstein, and
Jeffrey Newcorm

4.6.5 Bereavement *724*
Beverley Raphael, Sally Wooding, and Julie Dunsmore

**4.7 Anxiety disorders** *729*

4.7.1 Generalized anxiety disorders *729*
Stella Bitran, David H. Barlow, and David A. Spiegel

4.7.2 Social anxiety disorder and specific
phobias *739*
Michelle A. Blackmore, Brigette A. Erwin,
Richard G. Heimberg, Leanne Magee,
and David M. Fresco

4.7.3 Panic disorder and agoraphobia *750*
James C. Ballenger

**4.8 Obsessive–compulsive disorder** *765*
Joseph Zohar, Leah Fostick, and Elizabeth
Juven-Wetzler

**4.9 Depersonalization disorder** *774*
Nick Medford, Mauricio Sierra, and Anthony S. David

**4.10 Disorders of eating** *777*

4.10.1 Anorexia nervosa *777*
Gerald Russell

4.10.2 Bulimia nervosa *800*
Christopher G. Fairburn,
Zafra Cooper, and Rebecca Murphy

**4.11 Sexuality, gender identity, and their
disorders** *812*

4.11.1 Normal sexual function *812*
Roy J. Levin

4.11.2 The sexual dysfunctions *821*
Cynthia A. Graham and John Bancroft

4.11.3 The paraphilias *832*
J. Paul Fedoroff

4.11.4 Gender identity disorder in adults *842*
Richard Green

**4.12 Personality disorders** *847*

4.12.1 Personality disorders: an
introductory perspective *847*
Juan J. López-Ibor Jr.

4.12.2 Diagnosis and classification of
personality disorders *855*
James Reich and Giovanni de Girolamo

4.12.3 Specific types of personality disorder *861*
José Luis Carrasco and Dusica Lecic-Tosevski

4.12.4 Epidemiology of personality disorders *881*
Francesca Guzzetta and Giovanni de Girolamo

4.12.5 Neuropsychological templates for
abnormal personalities: from genes to
biodevelopmental pathways *886*
Adolf Tobeña

4.12.6 Psychotherapy for personality disorder *892*
Anthony W. Bateman and Peter Fonagy

4.12.7 Management of personality disorder *901*
Giles Newton-Howes and Kate Davidson

**4.13 Habit and impulse control disorders** *911*

4.13.1 Impulse control disorders *911*
Susan L. McElroy and Paul E. Keck Jr.

4.13.2 Special psychiatric problems
relating to gambling *919*
Emanuel Moran

**4.14 Sleep–wake disorders** *924*

4.14.1 Basic aspects of sleep–wake disorders *924*
Gregory Stores

4.14.2 Insomnias *933*
Colin A. Espie and Delwyn J. Bartlett

4.14.3 Excessive sleepiness *938*
Michel Billiard

4.14.4 Parasomnias *943*
Carlos H. Schenck and Mark W. Mahowald

**4.15 Suicide** *951*

4.15.1 Epidemiology and causes of suicide *951*
Jouko K. Lonnqvist

4.15.2 Deliberate self-harm: epidemiology
and risk factors *957*
Ella Arensman and Ad J. F. M. Kerkhof

4.15.3 Biological aspects of suicidal behaviour *963*
J. John Mann and Dianne Currier

4.15.4 Treatment of suicide attempters and prevention
of suicide and attempted suicide *969*
Keith Hawton and Tatiana Taylor

**4.16 Culture-related specific psychiatric
syndromes** *979*
Wen-Shing Tseng

**Index**

# Contents
# Volume 2

**Preface to the second edition** *v*

**Preface to the first edition** *vii*

**Acknowledgements** *ix*

**Contributors list** *xxi*

**Section 5  Psychiatry and Medicine**

**5.1 Mind–body dualism, psychiatry, and medicine** *989*
Michael Sharpe and Jane Walker

**5.2 Somatoform disorders and other causes of medically unexplained symptoms** *992*

5.2.1 Somatoform disorders and functional symptoms *992*
Richard Mayou

5.2.2 Epidemiology of somatoform disorders and other causes of unexplained medical symptoms *995*
Gregory Simon

5.2.3 Somatization disorder and related disorders *999*
Per Fink

5.2.4 Conversion and dissociation disorders *1011*
Christopher Bass

5.2.5 Hypochondriasis (health anxiety) *1021*
Russell Noyes Jr.

5.2.6 Pain disorder *1029*
Sidney Benjamin and Stella Morris

5.2.7 Chronic fatigue syndrome *1035*
Michael Sharpe and Simon Wessely

5.2.8 Body dysmorphic disorder *1043*
Katharine A. Phillips

5.2.9 Factitious disorder and malingering *1049*
Christopher Bass and David Gill

5.2.10 Neurasthenia *1059*
Felice Lieh Mak

**5.3 Medical and surgical conditions and treatments associated with psychiatric disorders** *1065*

5.3.1 Adjustment to illness and handicap *1065*
Allan House

5.3.2 Psychiatric aspects of neurological disease *1071*
Maria A. Ron

5.3.3 Epilepsy *1076*
Brian Toone

5.3.4 Medical conditions associated with psychiatric disorder *1081*
James R. Rundell

5.3.5 Psychiatric aspects of infections *1090*
José-Luis Ayuso-Mateos

5.3.6 Psychiatric aspects of surgery (including transplantation) *1096*
S. A. Hales, S. E. Abbey, and G. M. Rodin

5.3.7 Psychiatric aspects of cancer *1100*
Jimmie C. Holland and Jessica Stiles

5.3.8 Psychiatric aspects of accidents, burns, and other physical trauma *1105*
Ulrik Fredrik Malt

**5.4 Obstetric and gynaecological conditions associated with psychiatric disorder** *1114*
Ian Brockington

**5.5 Management of psychiatric disorders in medically ill patients, including emergencies** *1128*
Pier Maria Furlan and Luca Ostacoli

**5.6 Health psychology** *1135*
John Weinman and Keith J. Petrie

**5.7 The organization of psychiatric services for general hospital departments** *1144*
Frits J. Huyse, Roger G. Kathol, Wolfgang Söllner, and Lawson Wulsin

## Section 6    Treatment Methods in Psychiatry

**6.1 The evaluation of treatments** *1151*

6.1.1 **The evaluation of physical treatments** *1151*
Clive E. Adams

6.1.2 **The evaluation of psychological treatment** *1158*
Paul Crits-Christoph and Mary Beth Connolly Gibbons

**6.2 Somatic treatments** *1168*

6.2.1 **General principles of drug therapy in psychiatry** *1168*
J. K. Aronson

6.2.2 **Anxiolytics and hypnotics** *1178*
Malcolm Lader

6.2.3 **Antidepressants** *1185*
Zubin Bhagwagar and George R. Heninger

6.2.4 **Lithium and related mood stabilizers** *1198*
Robert M. Post

6.2.5 **Antipsychotic and anticholinergic drugs** *1208*
Herbert Y. Meltzer and William V. Bobo

6.2.6 **Antiepileptic drugs** *1231*
Brian P. Brennan and Harrison G. Pope Jr.

6.2.7 **Drugs for cognitive disorders** *1240*
Leslie Iversen

6.2.8 **Drugs used in the treatment of the addictions** *1242*
Fergus D. Law and David J. Nutt

6.2.9 **Complementary medicines** *1247*
Ursula Werneke

6.2.10 **Non-pharmacological somatic treatments** *1251*

6.2.10.1 **Electroconvulsive therapy** *1251*
Max Fink

6.2.10.2 **Phototherapy** *1260*
Philip J. Cowen

6.2.10.3 **Transcranial magnetic stimulation** *1263*
Declan McLoughlin and Andrew Mogg

6.2.10.4 **Neurosurgery for psychiatric disorders** *1266*
Keith Matthews and David Christmas

**6.3 Psychological treatments** *1272*

6.3.1 **Counselling** *1272*
Diana Sanders

6.3.2 **Cognitive behaviour therapy** *1285*

6.3.2.1 **Cognitive behaviour therapy for anxiety disorders** *1285*
David M. Clark

6.3.2.2 **Cognitive behaviour therapy for eating disorders** *1298*
Zafra Cooper, Rebecca Murphy, and Christopher G. Fairburn

6.3.2.3 **Cognitive behaviour therapy for depressive disorders** *1304*
Melanie J. V. Fennell

6.3.2.4 **Cognitive behaviour therapy for schizophrenia** *1313*
Max Birchwood and Elizabeth Spencer

6.3.3 **Interpersonal psychotherapy for depression and other disorders** *1318*
Carlos Blanco, John C. Markowitz, and Myrna M. Weissman

6.3.4 **Brief individual psychodynamic psychotherapy** *1327*
Amy M. Ursano and Robert J. Ursano

6.3.5 **Psychoanalysis and other long-term dynamic psychotherapies** *1337*
Peter Fonagy and Horst Kächele

6.3.6 **Group methods in adult psychiatry** *1350*
John Schlapobersky and Malcolm Pines

6.3.7 **Psychotherapy with couples** *1369*
Michael Crowe

6.3.8 **Family therapy in the adult psychiatric setting** *1380*
Sidney Bloch and Edwin Harari

6.3.9 **Therapeutic communities** *1391*
David Kennard and Rex Haigh

**6.4 Treatment by other professions** *1399*

6.4.1 **Rehabilitation techniques** *1399*
W. Rössler

6.4.2 **Psychiatric nursing techniques** *1403*
Kevin Gournay

6.4.3 **Social work approaches to mental health work: international trends** *1408*
Shulamit Ramon

6.4.4 **Art therapy** *1413*
Diane Waller

**6.5 Indigenous, folk healing practices** *1418*
Wen-Shing Tseng

## Section 7    Social Psychiatry and Service Provision

**7.1 Public policy and mental health** *1425*
Matt Muijen and Andrew McCulloch

**7.2 Service needs of individuals and populations** *1432*
Mike Slade, Michele Tansella, and Graham Thornicroft

**7.3 Cultural differences care pathways, service use, and outcome** *1438*
Jim van Os and Kwame McKenzie

**7.4 Primary prevention of mental disorders** *1446*
J. M. Bertolote

**7.5 Planning and providing mental health services for a community** *1452*
Tom Burns

**7.6 Evaluation of mental health services** *1463*
Michele Tansella and Graham Thornicroft

**7.7 Economic analysis of mental health services** *1473*
Martin Knapp and Dan Chisholm

**7.8 Psychiatry in primary care** *1480*
David Goldberg, André Tylee, and Paul Walters

**7.9 The role of the voluntary sector** *1490*
Vanessa Pinfold and Mary Teasdale

**7.10 Special problems** *1493*

7.10.1 The special psychiatric problems of refugees *1493*
Richard F. Mollica, Melissa A. Culhane, and Daniel H. Hovelson

7.10.2 Mental health services for homeless mentally ill people *1500*
Tom K. J. Craig

7.10.3 Mental health services for ethnic minorities *1502*
Tom K. J. Craig and Dinesh Bhugra

## Section 8 The Psychiatry of Old Age

**8.1 The biology of ageing** *1507*
Alan H. Bittles

**8.2 Sociology of normal ageing** *1512*
Sarah Harper

**8.3 The ageing population and the epidemiology of mental disorders among the elderly** *1517*
Scott Henderson and Laura Fratiglioni

**8.4 Assessment of mental disorder in older patients** *1524*
Robin Jacoby

**8.5 Special features of clinical syndromes in the elderly** *1530*

8.5.1 Delirium in the elderly *1530*
James Lindesay

8.5.1.1 Mild cognitive impairment *1534*
Claudia Jacova and Howard H. Feldman

8.5.2 Substance use disorders in older people *1540*
Henry O'Connell and Brian Lawlor

8.5.3 Schizophrenia and paranoid disorders in late life *1546*
Barton W. Palmer, Gauri N. Savla, and Thomas W. Meeks

8.5.4 Mood disorders in the elderly *1550*
Robert Baldwin

8.5.5 Stress-related, anxiety, and obsessional disorders in elderly people *1558*
James Lindesay

8.5.6 Personality disorders in the elderly *1561*
Suzanne Holroyd

8.5.7 Suicide and deliberate self-harm in elderly people *1564*
Robin Jacoby

8.5.8 Sex in old age *1567*
John Kellett and Catherine Oppenheimer

**8.6 Special features of psychiatric treatment for the elderly** *1571*
Catherine Oppenheimer

**8.7 The planning and organization of services for older adults** *1579*
Pamela S. Melding

## Section 9 Child and Adolescent Psychiatry

**9.1 General issues** *1589*

9.1.1 Developmental psychopathology and classification in childhood and adolescence *1589*
Stephen Scott

9.1.2 Epidemiology of psychiatric disorder in childhood and adolescence *1594*
E. Jane Costello and Adrian Angold

9.1.3 Assessment in child and adolescent psychiatry *1600*
Jeff Bostic and Andrés Martin

9.1.4 Prevention of mental disorder in childhood and other public health issues *1606*
Rhoshel Lenroot

**9.2 Clinical syndromes** *1612*

9.2.1 Neuropsychiatric disorders *1612*
James C. Harris

9.2.2 Specific developmental disorders in childhood and adolescence *1622*
Helmut Remschmidt and Gerd Schulte-Körne

9.2.3 Autism and the pervasive
developmental disorders  *1633*
Fred R. Volkmar and Ami Klin

9.2.4 Attention deficit and hyperkinetic disorders
in childhood and adolescence  *1643*
Eric Taylor

9.2.5 Conduct disorders in childhood
and adolescence  *1654*
Stephen Scott

9.2.6 Anxiety disorders in childhood
and adolescence  *1664*
Daniel S. Pine

9.2.7 Paediatric mood disorders  *1669*
David Brent and Boris Birmaher

9.2.8 Obsessive–compulsive disorder and tics
in children and adolescents  *1680*
Martine F. Flament and Philippe Robaey

9.2.9 Sleep disorders in children
and adolescents  *1693*
Gregory Stores

9.2.10 Suicide and attempted suicide in
children and adolescents  *1702*
David Shaffer, Cynthia R. Pfeffer, and
Jennifer Gutstein

9.2.11 Children's speech and
language difficulties  *1710*
Judy Clegg

9.2.12 Gender identity disorder in children
and adolescents  *1718*
Richard Green

**9.3 Situations affecting child mental health**  *1724*

9.3.1 The influence of family, school,
and the environment  *1724*
Barbara Maughan

9.3.2 Child trauma  *1728*
David Trickey and Dora Black

9.3.3 Child abuse and neglect  *1731*
David P. H. Jones

9.3.4 The relationship between physical
and mental health in children
and adolescents  *1740*
Julia Gledhill and M. Elena Garralda

9.3.5 The effects on child and adult mental
health of adoption and foster care  *1747*
June Thoburn

9.3.6 Effects of parental psychiatric
and physcial illness on
child development  *1752*
Paul Ramchandani, Alan Stein, and Lynne Murray

9.3.7 The effects of bereavement in childhood  *1758*
Dora Black and David Trickey

**9.4 The child as witness**  *1761*
Anne E. Thompson and John B. Pearce

**9.5 Treatment methods for children
and adolescents**  *1764*

9.5.1 Counselling and psychotherapy
for children  *1764*
John B. Pearce

9.5.2 Psychodynamic child psychotherapy  *1769*
Peter Fonagy and Mary Target

9.5.3 Cognitive behaviour therapies for
children and families  *1777*
Philip Graham

9.5.4 Caregiver-mediated interventions
for children and families  *1787*
Philip A. Fisher and Elizabeth A. Stormshak

9.5.5 Medication for children and
adolescents: current issues  *1793*
Paramala J. Santosh

9.5.6 Residential care for social reasons  *1799*
Leslie Hicks and Ian Sinclair

9.5.7 Organization of services for children and
adolescents with mental health problems  *1802*
Miranda Wolpert

9.5.8 The management of child and adolescent
psychiatric emergencies  *1807*
Gillian Forrest

9.5.9 The child psychiatrist as consultant
to schools and colleges  *1811*
Simon G. Gowers and Sian Thomas

## Section 10   Intellectual Disability (Mental Retardation)

**10.1 Classification, diagnosis, psychiatric
assessment, and needs assessment**  *1819*
A. J. Holland

**10.2 Prevalence of intellectual disabilities and
epidemiology of mental ill-health in
adults with intellectual disabilities**  *1825*
Sally-Ann Cooper and Elita Smiley

**10.3 Aetiology of intellectual disability:
general issues and prevention**  *1830*
Markus Kaski

**10.4 Syndromes causing intellectual disability**  *1838*
David M. Clarke and Shoumitro Deb

**10.5 Psychiatric and behaviour disorders among mentally retarded people** *1849*

10.5.1 Psychiatric and behaviour disorders among children and adolescents with intellectual disability *1849*
Bruce J. Tonge

10.5.2 Psychiatric and behaviour disorders among adult persons with intellectual disability *1854*
Anton Došen

10.5.3 Epilepsy and epilepsy-related behaviour disorders among people with intellectual disability *1860*
Matti Iivanainen

**10.6 Methods of treatment** *1871*
T. P. Berney

**10.7 Special needs of adolescents and elderly people with intellectual disability** *1878*
Jane Hubert and Sheila Hollins

**10.8 Families with a member with intellectual disability and their needs** *1883*
Ann Gath and Jane McCarthy

**10.9 The planning and provision of psychiatric services for adults with intellectual disability** *1887*
Nick Bouras and Geraldine Holt

## Section 11  Forensic Psychiatry

**11.1 General principles of law relating to people with mental disorder** *1895*
Michael Gunn and Kay Wheat

**11.2 Psychosocial causes of offending** *1908*
David P. Farrington

**11.3 Associations between psychiatric disorder and offending** *1917*

11.3.1 Associations between psychiatric disorder and offending *1917*
Lindsay Thomson and Rajan Darjee

11.3.2 Offending, substance misuse, and mental disorder *1926*
Andrew Johns

11.3.3 Cognitive disorders, epilepsy, ADHD, and offending *1928*
Norbert Nedopil

**11.4 Mental disorders among offenders in correctional settings** *1933*
James R. P. Ogloff

**11.5 Homicide offenders including mass murder and infanticide** *1937*
Nicola Swinson and Jennifer Shaw

**11.6 Fraud, deception, and thieves** *1941*
David V. James

**11.7 Juvenile delinquency and serious antisocial behaviour** *1945*
Susan Bailey

**11.8 Child molesters and other sex offenders** *1960*
Stephen Hucker

**11.9 Arson (fire-raising)** *1965*
Herschel Prins

**11.10 Stalking** *1970*
Paul E. Mullen

**11.11 Querulous behaviour: vexatious litigation, abnormally persistent complaining and petitioning** *1977*
Paul E. Mullen

**11.12 Domestic violence** *1981*
Gillian C. Mezey

**11.13 The impact of criminal victimization** *1984*
Gillian C. Mezey and Ian Robbins

**11.14 Assessing and managing the risks of violence towards others** *1991*
Paul E. Mullen and James R. P. Ogloff

**11.15 The expert witness in the Criminal Court: assessment, reports, and testimony** *2003*
John O'Grady

**11.16 Managing offenders with psychiatric disorders in general psychiatric sevices** *2009*
James R. P. Ogloff

**11.17 Management of offenders with mental disorder in specialist forensic mental health services** *2015*
Pamela J. Taylor and Emma Dunn

**Index**

# Contributors list

**S.E. Abbey** Associate Professor of Psychiatry, University of Toronto, Toronto, Canada
*Chapter 5.3.6*

**Henry David Abraham** Distinguished Life Fellow, American Psychiatric Association, USA
*Chapter 4.2.3.3*

**Clive E. Adams** Cochrane Schizophrenia Group, University of Oxford Department of Psychiatry, Warneford Hospital, Oxford, UK
*Chapter 6.1.1*

**Hagop S. Akiskal** Professor of Psychiatry and Director of the International Mood Center, University of California at San Diego, California, USA
*Chapter 4.5.9*

**Nancy C. Andreasen** Dept of Psychiatry, University of Iowa Hospitals & Clinics, Iowa City, USA
*Chapter 4.3.1*

**Adrian Angold** Associate Professor of Child and Adolescent Psychiatry, Duke University Medical Center, Durham, North Carolina, USA
*Chapter 9.1.2*

**Jules Angst** Emeritus Professor of Psychiatry, Zurich University, Switzerland
*Chapter 4.5.7*

**Ella Arensman** Director of Research, National Suicide Research Foundation, Ireland
*Chapter 4.15.2*

**J.K. Aronson** Reader in Clinical Pharmacology, University Department of Primary Health Care, Headington, Oxford, UK
*Chapter 6.2.1*

**José-Luis Ayuso-Mateos** Chairman, Department of Psychiatry, Universidad Autónoma de Madrid, Hospital Universitario de la Princesa, Spain
*Chapter 5.3.5*

**Susan Bailey** Consultant Child and Adolescent Forensic Psychiatrist, Salford NHS Trust and Maudsley NHS Trust; Senior Research Fellow, University of Manchester, UK
*Chapter 11.7*

**Robert Baldwin** Consultant, Old Age Psychiatrist, and Honorary Senior Lecturer, Manchester Royal Infirmary, UK
*Chapter 8.5.4*

**James C. Ballenger** Retired Professor and Chairman, Department of Psychiatry and Behavioral Sciences and Director, Institute of Psychiatry, Medical University of South Carolina, USA
*Chapter 4.7.3*

**John Bancroft**, The Kinsey Institute for Research in Sex, Gender, & Reproduction and Department of Psychiatry, University of Oxford, UK
*Chapter 4.11.2*

**David H. Barlow** Center for Anxiety and Related Disorders at Boston University, Massachusetts, USA
*Chapter 4.7.1*

**Delwyn J. Bartlett** Woolcock Institute of Medical Research, Sydney, Australia
*Chapter 4.14.2*

**Christopher Bass** Consultant in Liaison Psychiatry, John Radcliffe Hospital, Oxford, UK
*Chapters 5.2.4 and 5.2.9*

**Antony W. Bateman** Halliwick Psychotherapy Dept, St Ann's Hospital, London, UK
*Chapter 4.12.6*

**Per Bech** Professor of Psychiatry and Head of Psychiatric Research Unit, WHO Collaborating Centre, Frederiksborg General Hospital, Hillerød, Denmark
*Chapter 4.5.2*

**Sidney Benjamin** Senior Lecturer, University of Manchester, UK
*Chapter 5.2.6*

**Thomas P. Berney** Consultant Developmental Psychiatrist Honorary Research Associate, University of Newcastle upon Tyne, UK
*Chapter 10.6*

**Jose M. Bertolote** Chief, Mental Disorders Control Unit, World Health Organization, Geneva; Associate Professor, Department of Psychogeriatrics, University of Lausanne, Switzerland
*Chapter 7.4*

**Zubin Bhagwagar** CT Mental Health Center, Yale University, New Haven CT, USA
*Chapter 6.2.3*

**Mary Beth Connolly Gibbons** Assistant Professor of Psychology in Psychiatry Department of Psychiatry, University of Pennsylvania, Pennsylvania, USA
*Chapter 6.1.2*

**Dinesh Bhugra** Professor of Mental Health and Cultural Diversity, King's College London, Institute of Psychiatry, London, UK
*Chapter 7.10.3*

**Michel Billiard** Professor of Neurology, School of Medicine, Guide Chauliac Hospital, Montpellier, France
*Chapter 4.14.3*

**Max Birchwood** Director, Early Intervention Service, Northern Birmingham Mental Health Trust, and University of Birmingham, UK
*Chapter 6.3.2.4*

**Boris Birmaher** UPMC Western Psychiatric Institute, Pittsburgh, USA
*Chapter 9.2.7*

**Stella Bitran,** Center for Anxiety and Related Disorders, Boston University, Beacon, MA, USA
*Chapter 4.7.1*

**Alan H. Bittles** Centre for Comparative Genomics, Murdoch University, Perth, Australia
*Chapter 8.1*

**Dora Black** Honorary Consultant, Child and Adolescent Psychiatry, Traumatic Stress Clinic, London; Honorary Lecturer, University of London, UK
*Chapters 9.3.2 and 9.3.7*

**Michelle A. Blackmore,** Doctoral Student of Clinical Psychology Adult Anxiety Clinic at Temple University, Philadelphia, Pennsylvania, USA
*Chapter 4.7.2*

**Carlos Blanco** New York State Psychiatric Institute, New York, USA
*Chapter 6.3.3*

**Sidney Bloch** Professor of Psychiatry, University of Melbourne; Senior Psychiatrist, St Vincent's Hospital, Melbourne, Australia
*Chapters 1.5 and 6.3.8*

**William V. Bobo** Assistant Professor of Psychiatry, Vanderbilt University School of Medicine Nashville, Tennessee (USA)
*Chapter 6.2.5*

**Bernhard Bogerts** Department of Psychiatry, University of Magdeburg, Germany
*Chapter 2.3.5*

**Jeff Bostic** School of Psychiatry, Harvard Medical School, Cambridge MA, USA
*Chapter 9.1.3*

**Nick Bouras** Professor, Institute of Psychiatry - King's College London MHiLD - York Clinic, London, UK
*Chapter 10.9*

**Christopher R. Bowie** Department of Psychiatry, Mount Sinai School of Medicine, New York, USA
*Chapter 4.3.3*

**Colin Bradbury** Department of Psychological Medicine, Institute of Psychiatry, De Crespigny Park, London, UK
*Chapter 4.2.4*

**Brian P. Brennan** Instructor in Psychiatry, Harvard Medical School and Associate Director for Translational Neuroscience Research, Biological Psychiatry Laboratory, McLean Hospital, Belmont, MA, USA
*Chapter 6.2.6*

**David Brent** Dept of Psychiatry, University of Pittsburgh Medical School, Pittsburgh PA, USA
*Chapter 9.2.7*

**Chris R. Brewin** Research Dept of Clinical, Educational & Health Psychology, University College London, UK
*Chapter 4.6.3*

**Elaine Brohan** Institute of Psychiatry, David Goldberg Centre, De Crespigny Park, London, UK
*Chapter 1.2*

**Ian Brockington** Professor of Psychiatry, University of Birmingham, UK
Chapter 5.4

**George W. Brown** Professor of Sociology, Academic Department of Psychiatry, St Thomas's Hospital, London, UK
*Chapter 2.6.1*

**Arne Brun** Professor of Neuropathology. Department of Pathology, Lund University Hospital, Lund, Sweden
*Chapter 4.1.3*

**Richard A. Bryant** School of Psychology, University of New South Wales, Sydney NSW, Australia
*Chapter 4.6.1*

**E.T. Bullmore** Institute of Psychiatry, King's College London, UK
*Chapters 2.3.7 and 2.3.8*

**Tom Burns** Professor of social psychiatry, Dept of Psychiatry, University of Oxford, Warneford Hospital, Oxford, UK
*Chapter 7.5*

**José Luis Carrasco** Professor of Psychiatry, Hospital Fundacion Jimenez Diaz, Universidad Autonoma, Madrid, Spain
*Chapter 4.12.3*

**D.J. Castle** University of Western Australia, Fremantle, Australia
*Chapter 4.3.6.1*

**Jonathan Chick** Consultant Psychiatrist, NHS Lothian, and Senior Lecturer, Department of Psychiatry, University of Edinburgh, UK
*Chapter 4.2.2.4*

**Daniel Chisholm** Department of Health System Financing, Health Systems and Services, World Health Organization, Geneva, Switzerland
*Chapter 7.7*

**David Christmas** Dept of Psychiatry, University of Dundee, Dundee, UK
*Chapter 6.2.10.4*

**David M. Clarke** Consultant Psychiatrist, Lea Castle Centre, Kidderminster DY10 3PP, UK
*Chapters 6.3.3.1 and 10.4*

**L. Clark** Dept of Experimental Psychology, University of Cambridge, Cambridge, UK
*Chapter 2.5.5*

**Judy Clegg** Lecturer, Speech and language therapist, HPC, RCSLT Department of Human Communication Sciences University of Sheffield, UK
*Chapter 9.2.11*

**C. Robert Cloninger** Dept of Psychiatry, Washington University School of Medicine, St Louis MO, USA
*Chapter 1.8.2*

**John Collinge** Head of the Department of Neurodegenerative Disease at the Institute of Neurology, University College London and the Director of the UK Medical Research Council's Prion Unit, London, UK
*Chapter 4.1.4*

**Henry O'Connell** Consultant Psychiatrist, Co. Tipperary, Ireland
*Chapter 8.5.2*

**Melissa A. Culhane** Harvard Program in Refugee Trauma, Department of Psychiatry, Massachusetts General Hospital, Cambridge, USA
*Chapter 7.10.1*

**John E. Cooper** Emeritus Professor of Psychiatry, University of Nottingham, UK
*Chapter 1.8.1*

**Sally-Ann Cooper** Professor of Learning Disabilities, Division of Community Based Sciences, Faculty of Medicine, University of Glasgow, UK
*Chapter 10.2*

**Zafra Cooper** Principal Research Psychologist, Oxford University Department of Psychiatry, Warneford Hospital, Oxford, UK
*Chapters 4.10.2 and 6.3.2.2*

**E. Jane Costello** Department of Psychiatry and Behavioral Sciences, Duke University Medical Center, Brightleaf Square, Durham NC, USA
*Chapter 9.1.2*

**Elizabeth Coulthard** Institute of Neurology, University College London, UK
*Chapter 2.5.2*

**F.-R. Cousin** Psychiatrist, Centre Hospitalier Saint-Anne, Paris, France
*Chapter 4.3.10*

**Philip J. Cowen** Professor of Psychopharmacology, Department of Psychiatry, University of Oxford, UK
*Chapter 6.2.10.2*

**Tom K.J. Craig** Professor of Social Psychiatry, King's College London, Institute of Psychiatry, London, UK
*Chapters 7.10.2 and 7.10.3*

**Paul Crits-Christoph** Professor of Psychology in Psychiatry; Director, Center for Psychotherapy Research Department of Psychiatry, University of Pennsylvania. Pennsylvania, USA
*Chapter 6.1.2*

**Michael Crowe** Consultant Psychiatrist, South London and Maudsley NHS Trust; Honorary Senior Lecturer, Institute of Psychiatry, King's College London, UK
*Chapter 6.3.7*

**D.G. Cunningham Owens** Reader in Psychiatry, Department of Psychiatry, University of Edinburgh, UK
*Chapter 4.3.8*

**Dianne Currier** Division of Molecular Imaging & Neuropathology, Department of Psychiatry, Columbia University, USA
*Chapter 4.15.3*

**Robert Dantzer** Integrative Immunology and Behavior Program, University of Illinois at Urbana-Champaign, Edward R. Madigan Laboratory, West Gregory Drive, Urbana, IL, USA
*Chapter 2.3.10*

**Rajan Darjee** Division of Psychiatry, University of Edinburgh, Edinburgh, UK
*Chapter 11.3.1*

**Anthony S. David** Professor of Cognitive Neuropsychiatry, Institute of Psychiatry, King's College London, UK
*Chapters 4.3.4 and 4.9*

**Kate Davidson** Senior Research Psychologist, Department of Psychological Medicine, University of Glasgow, UK
*Chapter 4.12.7*

**Martin Davies** Dept of Experimental Psychology, University of Oxford, Oxford, UK
*Chapter 2.1*

**Giovanni de Girolamo** Health Care Research Agency, Emilia-Romagna Region, Bologna, Italy
*Chapters 4.12.2 and 4.12.4*

**Shoumitro Deb** Clinical Professor of Neuropsychiatry & Intellectual Disability, Division of Neuroscience, University of Birmingham, UK
*Chapter 10.4*

**R.J. Dolan** Institute of Neurology, University College London, UK
*Chapter 2.5.4*

**Anton Došen** Emeritus Professor of Psychiatric Aspects of Intellectual Disability at the Radboud University, Nijmegen, The Netherlands
*Chapter 10.5.2*

**D. Colin Drummond** Professor of Addiction Psychiatry, Section of Alcohol Research, National Addiction Centre, Division of Psychological Medicine and Psychiatry, Institute of Psychiatry, King's College London, UK
*Chapter 4.2.2.5*

**Emma Dunn** School of Medicine, Cardiff University, Cardiff, UK
*Chapter 11.17*

**Graham Dunn** Professor of Biomedical Statistics, Health Methodology Research Group, School of Community Based Medicine, University of Manchester, UK
*Chapter 2.2*

**Julie Dunsmore** Honorary Clinical Associate, SciMHA Unit, University of Western Sydney, Australia
*Chapter 4.6.5*

**Anke Ehlers** Department of Psychiatry, University of Oxford, UK
*Chapters 4.6.1 and 4.6.2*

**Timo Erkinjuntti** Professor of Neurology, Head of the University Department of Neurological Sciences, University of Helsinki and Head Physician, Department of Neurology and Memory Research Unit, Helsinki University Central Hospital, Finland
*Chapter 4.1.8*

**Brigette A. Erwin** Adult Anxiety Clinic of Temple University, Philadelphia, Pennsylvania, USA
*Chapter 4.7.2*

**Colin A. Espie** Professor of Clinical Psychology and Head of Department of Psychological Medicine, University of Glasgow, UK
*Chapter 4.14.2*

**Jonathan J. Evans** Section of Psychological Medicine, University of Glasgow, Glasgow, UK
*Chapter 4.1.14*

**Christopher G. Fairburn** Wellcome Principal Research Fellow and Professor of Psychiatry, University of Oxford, UK
*Chapters 4.10.2 and 6.3.2.2*

**Peter Falkai** Professor of Medical Psychology, Rheinische Friedrich-Wilhelms-Universität, Bonn, Germany
*Chapter 2.3.5*

**Stephen V. Faraone** Director, Medical Genetics Research, Professor of Psychiatry and of Neuroscience & Physiology, Director, Child and Adolescent Psychiatry Research, SUNY Upstate Medical University, New York, USA
*Chapter 4.3.9*

**Michael Farrell** Senior Lecturer and Consultant Psychiatrist, National Addiction Centre, South London and Maudsley NHS Trust, London, UK
*Chapter 4.2.3.4*

**David P. Farrington** Professor of Psychological Criminology, University of Cambridge, UK
*Chapter 11.2*

**J. Paul Fedoroff** Director, Sexual Behaviors Clinic Royal Ottawa Mental Health Centre and Director of Forensic Research University of Ottawa Institute of Mental Health Research, Canada
*Chapter 4.11.3*

**Howard H. Feldman** Professor and Head, Division of Neurology, Department of Medicine, University of British Columbia, Vancouver, BC, Canada
*Chapter 8.5.1.1*

**Melanie J.V. Fennell** Consultant Clinical Psychologist; Director, Oxford Diploma in Cognitive Therapy, University of Oxford Department of Psychiatry, Warneford Hospital, Oxford, UK
*Chapter 6.3.2.3*

**Max Fink** Emeritus Professor of Psychiatry and Neurology, State University of New York at Stony Brook; Professor of Psychiatry, Albert Einstein College of Medicine; Attending Psychiatrist, Long Island Jewish Medical Center, New York, USA
*Chapter 6.2.10.1*

**Michael B. First** Columbia University, New York, USA
*Chapter 1.9*

**Per Fink** Director, Research Unit for Functional Disorders, Aarhus University Hospital, Risskov, Denmark
*Chapter 5.2.3*

**Philip A. Fisher** Research Scientist, Oregon Social Learning Center, Eugene, Oregon, USA
*Chapter 9.5.4*

**Martine F. Flament** Chargée de Récherche INSERM, CNRS UMR 7593, Paris, France
*Chapter 9.2.8*

**Simon Fleminger** Consultant Neuropsychiatries, Lishman Brain Injury Unit, Maudsley Hospital, London, UK
*Chapters 4.1.10 and 4.1.13*

**Jonathan Flint** Wellcome Trust Centre for Human Genetics Roosevelt Drive, Oxford, UK
*Chapter 2.4.2*

**Susan Folstein** Professor of Psychiatry and Behavioral Sciences, Johns Hopkins School of Medicine, Baltimore, USA
*Chapter 4.1.7*

**Peter Fonagy** Freud Memorial Professor of Psychoanalysis, University College London; Director of Research, Anna Freud Centre, London, UK; Director, Child and Family Center and Clinical Protocols and Outcomes Center, Menninger Clinic, Topeka, Kansas, USA
*Chapters 4.12.6, 6.3.5 and 9.5.2*

**Gillian C. Forrest** Consultant Child and Adolescent Psychiatrist
*Chapter 9.5.8*

**Leah Fostick** Department of Psychiatry, Chaim Sheba Medical Centre, Tel Hashomer, Israel
*Chapter 4.8*

**W. Fraser** Division of Psychological Medicine, University of Wales College of Medicine, Cardiff, UK
*Introduction to Section 10*

**Laura Fratiglioni** Aging Research Centre, Karolinska Institute, Stockholm, Sweden
*Chapter 8.3*

**David M. Fresco** Adult Anxiety Clinic of Temple University, Philadelphia, Pennsylvania, USA
*Chapter 4.7.2*

**K.W.M. Fulford** Professor of Philosophy and Mental Health, University of Warwick; Honorary Consultant Psychiatrist, University of Oxford, UK
*Chapter 1.5.2*

**Robert Fung**, Specialist Registrar in Psychiatry, Sheffield Care NHS Trust, UK
*Chapter 4.2.3.2*

**Pier Maria Furlan** Director of Department of Mental Health San Luigi Gonzaga Hospital - University of Torino, Italy
*Chapter 5.5*

**Glen O. Gabbard** Bessie Walker Callaway Distinguished Professor of Psychoanalysis and Education in the Kansas School of Psychiatry, Menninger Clinic, Topeka; Clinical Professor of Psychiatry of Kansas School of Medicine, Wichita, Kansas, USA
*Chapter 3.3*

**Jean Garrabé** Honorary President of L'Evolution psychiatrique, Paris, France
*Chapter 4.3.10*

**M. Elena Garralda** Professor of Child and Adolescent Psychiatry, Imperial College of Medicine, London, UK
*Chapter 9.3.4*

**Ann Gath** Formerly of University College London, UK
*Chapter 10.8*

**John R. Geddes** Professor of Epidemiological Psychiatry, Department of Psychiatry, University of Oxford, Warneford Hospital, Oxford, UK
*Chapters 1.10 and 4.5.1*

**David Gill** Research Fellow, Department of Psychiatry, University of Oxford, UK
*Chapters 5.2.9*

**Kathryn J. Gill** MUHB Addictions Unit, McGill University, Montreal QC, Canada
*Chapter 4.2.2.1*

**Julia Gledhill** Clinical Research Fellow, Imperial College of Medicine, London, UK
*Chapter 9.3.4*

**David Goldberg** Director of Research and Development, Institute of Psychiatry, King's College London, UK
*Chapter 7.8*

**Terry E. Goldberg** The Zucker Hillside Hospital, Glen Oaks NY, USA
*Chapter 2.5.3*

**Guy Goodwin** Professor, University Department, Warneford Hospital, Oxford, UK
*Chapter 4.5.6*

**Kevin Gournay** Emeritus Professor, Institute of Psychiatry, King's College London, UK
*Chapter 6.4.2*

**Simon G. Gowers** Professor of Adolescent Psychiatry, University of Liverpool, UK
*Chapter 9.5.9*

**Cynthia A. Graham**, Oxford Doctoral Course in Clinical Psychology Warneford Hospital, Oxford and The Kinsey Institute for Research in Sex, Gender, & Reproduction, UK
*Chapter 4.11.2*

**Philip Graham** Emeritus Professor of Child Psychiatry, Institute of Child Health, London, UK
*Chapter 9.5.3*

**P.M. Grasby** Senior Lecturer, MRC Cyclotron Unit, Hammersmith Hospital, London, UK
*Chapter 2.3.6*

**Richard Green** Head, Gender Identity Clinic, and Visiting Professor of Psychiatry, Imperial College of Medicine at Charing Cross Hospital, London, UK; Emeritus Professor of Psychiatry, University of California, Los Angeles, California, USA
*Chapters 4.11.4 and 9.2.12*

**Stephen Green** Clinical Professor of Psychiatry, Georgetown University School of Medicine, Washington, D.C., USA
*Chapter 1.5.1*

**Michael Gunn** Professor of Law and Head of Department, Department of Academic Legal Studies, Nottingham Law School, Nottingham Trent University, UK
*Chapter 11.1*

**Lars Gustafson** Professor of Geriatric Psychiatry, Lund University Hospital, Lund, Sweden
*Chapter 4.1.3*

**Francesca Guzzetta** Bologna, Italy
*Chapter 4.12.4*

**Jennifer Gutstein** Department of Child Psychiatry, College of Physicians and Surgeons, Columbia University, New York, USA
*Chapter 9.2.10*

**Sarah Harper** Oxford Institute for Aging, University of Oxford, Oxford, UK
*Chapter 8.2*

**Rex Haigh** Project Lead, Community of Communities, Centre for Quality Improvement, Royal College of Psychiatrists, London; Consultant Psychiatrist, Berkshire Healthcare NHS Foundation Trust, UK
*Chapter 6.3.9*

**S.A. Hales** Psychiatry Fellow, Princess Margaret Hospital, University Health Network, Toronto, Canada
*Chapter 5.3.6*

**John N. Hall** Professor of Mental Health, School of Health and Social Care, Oxford Brookes University, Oxford, UK
*Chapter 1.8.3*

**Wayne Hall** Professor of Public Health Policy, University of Queensland, Herston, Australia
*Chapter 4.2.3.7*

**Edwin Harari** Consultant Psychiatrist, St Vincent's Hospital, Melbourne, Australia
*Chapter 6.3.8*

**Sarah Harper** Oxford Institute for Aging, University of Oxford, Oxford, UK
*Chapter 8.2*

**James C. Harris** Director Developmental Neuropsychiatry Clinic, Professor of Psychiatry and Behavioral Sciences, Pediatrics, and Mental Hygiene, The Johns Hopkins University School of Medicine, USA
*Chapter 9.2.1*

**Paul J. Harrison** Clinical Reader in Psychiatry, University of Oxford Department of Psychiatry, Warneford Hospital, Oxford, UK
*Chapter 4.3.6.2*

**Allison G. Harvey** Department of Experimental Psychology, University of Oxford, UK
*Chapter 4.6.1*

**Philip D. Harvey** Professor of Psychiatry and Behavioral Sciences, Emory University School of Medicine, Woodruff Memorial Building, Atlanta, GA, USA
*Chapter 4.3.3*

**Keith Hawton** Director, Centre for Suicide Research, University Department of Psychiatry, Warneford Hospital, Oxford, UK
*Chapter 4.15.4*

**Richard G. Heimberg** Adult Anxiety Clinic of Temple University, Philadelphia, Pennsylvania, USA
*Chapter 4.7.2*

**Scott Henderson** Emeritus Professor, The Australian National University, Canberra, Australia
*Chapters 2.7 and 8.3*

**George R. Heninger** Professor, Department of Psychiatry, Yale University School of Medicine, New Haven, Connecticut, USA
*Chapter 6.2.3*

**Leslie Hicks**, University of York, UK
*Chapter 9.5.6*

**A.J. Holland** Lecturer, Department of Psychiatry, University of Cambridge, UK
*Chapter 10.1*

**Jimmie C. Holland** Wayne E. Chapman Chair in Psychiatric Oncology, Department of Psychiatry and Behavioral Sciences, Memorial Sloan Kettering Cancer Center, New York, USA
*Chapter 5.3.7*

**Sheila Hollins** Professor of Psychiatry of Learning Disability, Department of Psychiatry and Disability, St George's Hospital Medical School, University of London, UK
*Chapter 10.7*

**Jeremy Holmes** Consultant Psychiatrist/Psychotherapist, North Devon District Hospital, Barnstaple; Senior Lecturer, University of Bristol, UK
*Chapter 3.2*

**Suzanne Holroyd** Professor, Director of Geriatric Psychiatry, Department of Psychiatry and Neurobehavioral Science, University of Virginia, Charlottesville VA, USA
*Chapter 8.5.6*

**Geraldine Holt** Honorary Senior Lecturer in Psychiatry at the Institute of Psychiatry, King's College London, UK
*Chapter 10.9*

**Allan House** Professor of Liaison Psychiatry, University of Leeds, UK
*Chapter 5.3.1*

**Daniel H. Hovelson The** Harvard program in refugee trauma, Massachusetts general hospital, Dept of psychiatry, USA
*Chapter 7.10.1*

**Jane Hubert** Senior Lecturer in Social Anthropology, Department of Psychiatry and Disability, St George's Hospital Medical School, University of London, UK
*Chapter 10.7*

**Stephen Hucker** University of Toronto, Toronto, Canada
*Chapter 11.8*

**T. A. Hughes** Consultant Psychiatrist, St Mary's Hospital, Leeds, UK
*Chapter 4.1.6*

**Masud Husain** Institute of Neurology & Institute of Cognitive Neuroscience, UCL, London and National Hospital for Neurology & Neurosurgery, London, UK
*Chapter 2.5.2*

**Frits J. Huyse** Psychiatrist, Consultant integrated care, Department of General Internal Medicine, University Medical Centre Groningen (UMCG), Groningen, The Netherlands
*Chapter 5.7*

**Matti Iivanainen** Professor, Department of Child Neurology, University of Helsinki, Finland
*Chapter 10.5.3*

**Leslie Iversen** Visting Professor, Department of Pharmacology, University of Oxford, UK
*Chapter 6.2.7*

**Richard Ives** National Children's Bureau, London, UK
*Chapter 4.2.3.6*

**Assen Jablensky** Professor of Psychiatry, University of Western Australia, Perth, Australia
*Chapters 4.3.5 and 4.3.7*

**Robin Jacoby** Clinical Reader in the Psychiatry of Old Age, University of Oxford, UK
*Chapters 8.4 and 8.5.7*

**Claudia Jacova** Assistant Professor, Division of Neurology, Department of Medicine, University of British Columbia, Vancouver, BC, Canada
*Chapter 8.5.1.1*

**David V. James** Consultant Forensic Psychiatrist, North London Forensic Service and Fixated Threat Assessment Centre, UK
*Chapter 11.6*

**Kay Redfield Jamison** Professor of Psychiatry, Johns Hopkins School of Medicine, Baltimore, Maryland, USA
*Chapter 1.1*

**John G.R. Jefferys** Department of Neurophysiology, Division of Neuroscience, University of Birmingham, UK
*Chapter 2.3.9*

**Andrew Johns** Consultant Forensic Psychiatry and Honorary Senior Lecturer, Maudsley Hospital, London, UK
*Chapter 11.3.2.*

**E.C. Johnstone** Professor of Psychiatry and Head, Department of Psychiatry, University of Edinburgh, UK
*Chapter 4.3.8*

**David P.H. Jones** Senior Clinical Lecturer in Child Psychiatry, Park Hospital for Children, University of Oxford, UK
*Chapter 9.3.3*

**Peter R. Joyce** Professor, Department of Psychological Medicine, Christchurch School of Medicine, Christchurch, New Zealand
*Chapter 4.5.4*

**Elizabeth Juven-Wetzler** Department of Psychiatry, Chaim Sheba Medical Centre, Tel Hashomer, Israel
*Chapter 4.8*

**Horst Kachele** Universitätsklinik Psychosomatische Medizin and Psychotherapie Universitätsklinik Ulm, Germany
*Chapter 6.3.5*

**Adam Ian Kaplin** Assistant Professor, Departments of Psychiatry and Neurology, Johns Hopkins University School of Medicine, Johns Hopkins Hospital, Baltimore, MD, USA
*Chapter 1.1*

**Markus Kaski** Director, Rinnekoti Research Foundation, Director and Chief Physician of Rinnekoti Foundation, Espoo, Finland
*Chapter 10.3*

**Aliya Kassam** Institute of Psychiatry, David Glodberg Centre, De Crespigny Park, London, UK
*Chapter 1.2*

**Roger G. Kathol**, Adjunct Professor of Internal Medicine and Psychiatry, University of Minnesota, President, Cartesian Solutions, Inc. Burnsville, MN, USA
*Chapter 5.7*

**Paul E. Keck Jr.** Lindner Center of HOPE, Mason, and Department of Psychiatry, University of Cincinnati College of Medicine, Cincinnati, OH, USA
*Chapter 4.13.1*

**John Kellett** St George's Hospital Medical School, London, UK
*Chapter 8.5.8*

**Keith W. Kelley** Department of Animal Sciences, University of Illinois, Urbana-Champaign, USA
*Chapter 2.3.10*

**David Kennard** Chair of the UK Network of the International Society for the Psychological Treatments of the Schizophrenias and other psychoses (ISPS UK); former Head of Psychology Services, The Retreat, York, UK
*Chapter 6.3.9*

**Ad.J.F.M. Kerkhof** Professor of Clinical Psychology, Vrije Universiteit, Amsterdam, The Netherlands
*Chapter 4.15.2*

**Otto F. Kernberg** Professor of Psychiatry, Cornell University Medical College, New York; Training and Supervising Analyst, Columbia University Center for Psychoanalytic Training and Research, New York, USA
*Chapter 3.1*

**Falk Kiefer** Professor of Addiction Research, Deputy Director, Department of Addictive Behaviour and Addiction Medicine, Central Institute of Mental Health CIMH, University of Heidelberg, Mannheim, Germany
*Chapter 4.2.2.3*

**Arthur Kleinman** Presley Professor of Anthropology and Psychiatry, Harvard University; Chair, Department of Social Medicine, Harvard Medical School, Cambridge, Massachusetts, USA
*Chapter 2.6.2*

**Ami Klin** Yale University, New Haven, Connecticut, USA
*Chapter 9.2.3*

**Kimberly Klipstein** Department of Psychiatry, Mount Sinai School of Medicine, New York, USA
*Chapter 4.6.4*

**Martin Knapp** Institute of Psychiatry, King's College London; London School of Economics and Political Science, University of London, UK
*Chapter 7.7*

**Michael D. Kopelman** Professor of Neuropsychiatry at King's College London, Institute of Psychiatry, UK
*Chapter 4.1.12*

**Malcolm Lader** Emeritus Professor of Clinical Psychopharmacology, King's College London, Institute of Psychiatry, Denmark Hill, London, UK
*Chapter 6.2.2*

**Fergus D. Law** Honorary Senior Registrar and Clinical Lecturer, Psychopharmacology Unit, University of Bristol, UK
*Chapters 4.2.1 and 6.2.8*

**Brian Lawlor** Conolly Norman Professor of Old Age Psychiatry, St. James's Hospital & Trinity College, Dublin, Ireland
*Chapter 8.5.2*

**Dusica Lecic-Tosevski** Professor of Psychiatry, Institute of Mental Health, School of Medicine, University of Belgrade, Belgrade, Serbia
*Chapter 4.12.3*

**Julian Leff** Emeritus Professor, Department of Psychological Medicine, Institute of Psychiatry, King's College London, UK
*Chapter 1.3.2*

**R.J. Levin** Department of Biomedical Science, University of Sheffield, UK
*Chapter 4.11.1*

**Rhohel Lenroot** Child Psychiatry Branch, NIMH, Bethesda MD, USA
*Chapter 9.1.4*

**Peter F. Liddle** Professor of Psychiatry, University of British Columbia, Vancouver, British Columbia, Canada
*Chapter 4.3.2*

**Felice Lieh Mak** Emeritus Professor, Department of Psychiatry, University of Hong Kong, Hong Kong
*Chapter 5.2.10*

**James Lindesay** Professor of Psychiatry for the Elderly, University of Leicester, UK
*Chapters 8.5.1 and 8.5.5*

**Jouko K. Lonnqvist** Professor, National Public Health Institute, Helsinki, Finland
*Chapter 4.15.1*

**Juan J. López-Ibor Jr.** Chairman, Department of Psychiatry, San Carlos University Hospital, Complutense University, Madrid, Spain
*Chapters 1.6 and 4.12.1*

**Mª Inés López-Ibor** San Carlos University Hospital, Complutense University, Madrid, Spain
*Chapter 4.2.3.8*

**Simon Lovestone** Professor of Old Age Psychiatry, NIHR Biomedical Research Centre for Mental Health, MRC Centre for Neurodegeneration Research, Departments of Psychological Medicine and Neuroscience, King's College London, Institute of Psychiatry, London, UK
*Chapter 4.1.2*

**Leanne Magee** Temple University, Philadelphia, Pennsylvania, USA
*Chapter 4.7.2*

**Andrew McCulloch** The Mental Health Foundation, London, UK
*Chapter 7.1*

**Jane McCarthy** Division of Mental Health, St George's Hospital, London, UK
*Chapter 10.8*

**Susan L. McElroy** Lindner Center of HOPE, Mason, and Department of Psychiatry, University of Cincinnati College of Medicine, Cincinnati, Ohio, USA
*Chapter 4.13.1*

**Peter McGuffin** Director and Professor of Psychiatric Genetics, Institute of Psychiatry, King's College London, UK
*Chapter 2.4.1*

**I.G. McKeith** Clinical Director, Institute for Ageing and Health, Newcastle University, Newcastle Upon Tyne, UK
*Chapter 4.1.5*

**Kwame McKenzie** Centre for Addictions and Mental Health, Toronto, Canada; University of Toronto, Canada; University of Central Lancashire, UK
*Chapter 7.3*

**Declan McLoughlin** Institute of Psychiatry, King's College London, UK
*Chapter 6.2.10.3*

**Mark W. Mahowald** Director, Minnesota Regional Sleep Disorders Center, Hennepin County Medical Center; Professor of Neurology, University of Minnesota Medical School, Minneapolis, Minnesota, USA
*Chapter 4.14.4*

**Mario Maj** Institute of Psychiatry, University of Naples, Italy
*Chapter 4.1.9*

**Ulrik Fredrik Malt** Professor of Psychiatry (Psychosomatic Medicine), National Hospital, University of Oslo, Norway
*Chapter 5.3.8*

**J. John Mann** Vice Chair for Research Scientific Director, Kreitchman PET Center, Columbia University and Chief, Division of Molecular Imaging & Neuropathology, New York State Psychiatric Institute, USA
*Chapter 4.15.3*

**Karl F. Mann** Professor and Chair in Addiction Research, Deputy Director Central Institute of Mental Health (CIMH), University of Heidelberg, Mannheim, Germany
*Chapter 4.2.2.3*

**Russell L. Margolis** Professor of Psychiatry and Neurology Director, Johns Hopkins Schizophrenia Program Director, Laboratory of Genetic Neurobiology Division of Neurobiology, Department of Psychiatry, Johns Hopkins University School of Medicine, Baltimore, USA
*Chapter 4.1.7*

**John C. Markowitz** Associate Professor of Psychiatry, Weill Medical College of Cornell University; Director, Psychotherapy Clinic, Payne Whitney Clinic, New York Presbyterian Hospital, New York, USA
*Chapter 6.3.3*

**John Marsden** Lecturer, Institute of Psychiatry, King's College London, UK
*Chapter 4.2.4*

**Jane Marshall** Senior Lecturer in the Addictions, National Addiction Centre, Institute of Psychiatry, King's College London, UK
*Chapters 4.1.11 and 4.2.2.2*

**Andrés Martin** Professor of Child Psychiatry, Child Study Center Yale University School of Medicine, New Haven, Connecticut, USA
*Chapter 9.1.3*

**Keith Matthews** Dept of Psychiatry, University of Dundee, Dundee, UK
*Chapter 6.2.10.4*

**Barbara Maughan** MRC Child Psychiatry Unit, Institute of Psychiatry, King's College London, UK
*Chapter 9.3.1*

**Soraya Mayet** National Addiction Centre, Institute of Psychiatry, King's College London, UK
*Chapter 4.2.3.1*

**Richard Mayou** Emeritus Professor of Psychiatry, University of Oxford, UK
*Chapter 5.2.1*

**Nick Medford** Institute of Psychiatry, King's College London, UK
*Chapter 4.9*

**David Meagher** Dept of Adult Psychiatry, Midwestern Regional Hospital, Limerick, Ireland
*Chapter 4.1.1*

**Thomas W. Meeks** Division of Geriatric Psychiatry, University of California San Diego, La Jolla CA, USA
*Chapter 8.5.3*

**Pamela S. Melding** Honorary Senior Lecturer, Department of Psychological Medicine, University of Auckland, New Zealand and Consultant in Psychiatry of Old Age, Mental Health Serviced, North Shore Hospital, Waitemata District Health Board, Takapuna, North Shore City, Auckland, New Zealand
*Chapter 8.7*

**Herbert Y. Meltzer** Bixler/May/Johnaon Professor of Psychiatry, Professor of Pharmacoloqy Vanderbilt University School of Medicine, Nashville, Tennessee, USA
*Chapter 6.2.5*

**Julien Mendlewicz** Department of Psychiatry, University Clinics of Brussels, Erasme Hospital, Brussels, Belgium
*Chapter 4.5.5*

**Andreas Meyer-Lindenberg** Dept of Psychiatry, Central Institute of Mental Health, Mannheim, Germany
*Chapter 2.5.3*

**Gillian C. Mezey** Consultant and Senior Lecturer in Forensic Psychiatry, Traumatic Stress Service, St George's Hospital Medical School, London, UK
*Chapters 11.12 and 11.13*

**R.H.S. Mindham** Emeritus Professor of Psychiatry, University of Leeds, UK
*Chapter 4.1.6*

**Andrew Mogg** Institute of Psychiatry, King's College London, UK
*Chapter 6.2.10.3*

**Richard F. Mollica** Director, Harvard Program in Refugee Trauma; Associate Professor of Psychiatry, Harvard Medical School and Harvard School of Public Health, Cambridge, Massachusetts, USA
*Chapter 7.10.1*

**Emanuel Moran** Consultant Psychiatrist, Grovelands Priory Hospital, London, UK
*Chapter 4.13.2*

**Stella Morris** Dept of Psychological Medicine, Hull Royal Infirmary, Hull, UK
*Chapter 5.2.6*

**Matt Muijen** WHO Regional Office for Europe, Copenhagen, Denmark
*Chapter 7.1*

**Paul E. Mullen** Professor of Forensic Psychiatry, Monash University; Clinical Director, Victorian Institute of Forensic Mental Health, Monash University, Melbourne, Australia
*Chapters 11.10, 11.11 and 11.14*

**Alistair Munro** Emeritus Professor of Psychiatry, Dalhousie University, Halifax, Nova Scotia, Canada
*Chapter 4.4*

**Rebecca Murphy** Research Psychologist, Oxford University Department of Psychiatry, Warneford Hospital, Oxford, UK
*Chapters 4.10.2 and 6.3.2.2*

**Lynne Murray** Winnicott Research Unit, University of Reading, Reading, UK
*Chapter 9.3.6*

**R.M. Murray** Institute of Psychiatry, King's College London, UK
*Chapter 4.3.6.1*

**Norbert Nedopil** Professor of Forensic Psychiatry, Head of the Department of Forensic Psychiatry at the Psychiatric Hospital of the University of Munich, Munich, Germany
*Chapter 11.3.3*

**Juan C. Negrete** Professor and Head, Addictions Psychiatry Program, University of Toronto, Canada
*Chapter 4.2.2.1*

**Gretchen N. Neigh** Dept of Psychiatry and Behavioral Sciences, Emory University, Atlanta GA, USA
*Chapter 2.3.3*

**Charles B. Nemeroff** Reunette W. Harris Professor and Chairman, Department of Psychiatry and Behavioral Sciences, Emory University School of Medicine, Atlanta, Georgia, USA
*Chapter 2.3.3*

**Giles Newton-Howes** Division of Neurosciences and Mental Health, Imperial College School of Medicine, London, UK
*Chapter 4.12.7*

**Jeffrey Newcorm** Mount Sinai School of Medicine, New York, USA
*Chapter 4.6.4*

**Russell Noyes Jr.** Department of Psychiatry, University of Iowa College of Medicine, Iowa City, Iowa, USA
*Chapter 5.2.5*

**David J. Nutt** Professor of Psychopharmacology and Head of Clinical Medicine, University of Bristol, UK
*Chapters 4.2.1 and 6.2.8*

**Margaret Oates** Senior Lecturer in Psychiatry, University of Nottingham, UK
*Chapter 1.8.1*

**James R.P. Ogloff** Victorian Institute of Forensic Mental Health, Thomas Embling Hospital, Fairfield VIC, Australia
*Chapters 11.4 ,11.14, and 11.16*

**John O'Grady** Knowle Hospital, Fareham, UK
*Chapter 11.15*

**Catherine Oppenheimer** Consultant Psychiatrist, Warneford Hospital, Oxford, UK
*Chapter 8.5.8 and 8.6*

**Luca Ostacoli** Liaison Psychiatry and Psychosomatic Unit, Department of Mental Health, San Luigi Gonzaga Hospital - University of Torino, Italy
*Chapter 5.5*

**Pierre Oswald** Dept of Psychiatry, ULB Erasme, Brussels, Belgium
*Chapter 4.5.5*

**Barton W. Palmer** Veterans Affairs Medical Center, University of California, San Diego CA, USA
*Chapter 8.5.3*

**Gordon Parker** Professor, University of New South Wales; and Executive Director, Black Dog Institute, Australia
*Chapter 4.5.3*

**E.S. Paykel** Emeritus Professor of Psychiatry, Department of Psychiatry, University of Cambridge, UK
*Chapter 4.5.8*

**John B. Pearce** Emeritus Professor of Child and Adolescent Psychiatry, University of Nottingham, UK
*Chapters 9.4 and 9.5.1*

**†R.C.A. Pearson** Department of Biomedical Science, University of Sheffield, UK
*Chapter 2.3.1*

**Keith J. Petrie** Associate Professor, School of Medicine,University of Auckland, New Zealand
*Chapter 5.6*

**Cynthia R. Pfeffer** Weill Medical College of Cornell University, New York Presbyterian Hospital-Westchester Division, White Plains, New York, USA
*Chapter 9.2.10*

**Katharine A. Phillips** Professor of Psychiatry and Human Behavior, The Warren Alpert Medical School of Brown University; Director, Body Dysmorphic Disorder Program, Butler Hospital, Providence, USA
*Chapter 5.2.8*

**Pierre Pichot** Académie Nationale de Médecine, Paris, France
*Chapter 1.4*

**Harold Alan Pincus** Columbia University, New York, USA
*Chapter 1.9*

**Vanessa Pinfold** 'Rethink', London, UK
*Chapter 7.9*

**Daniel S. Pine** Division of Intramural Research Programs, National Institutes of Health, Bethesda, USA
*Chapter 9.2.6*

**Malcolm Pines** Founding Member, Institute of Group Analysis, London, UK
*Chapter 6.3.6*

**Harrison G. Pope Jr.** Professor of Psychiatry, Harvard Medical School, Boston; Chief, Biological Psychiatry Laboratory, McClean Hospital, Belmont, Massachusetts, USA
*Chapter 6.2.6*

**Robert M. Post** Chief, Biological Psychiatry Branch, National Institute of Mental Health, Bethesda, Maryland, USA
*Chapter 6.2.4*

**Graham E. Powell** Psychology Services, Powell Campbell Edelmann, London, UK
*Chapter 1.8.3*

**Herschel Prins** Professor, Midlands Centre for Criminology and Criminal Justice, University of Loughborough, UK
*Chapter 11.9*

**Paul Ramchandani** Dept of Psychiatry, University of Oxford, Warneford Hospital, Oxford, UK
*Chapter 9.3.6*

**Shulamit Ramon** Professor of Interprofessional Health and Social Studies, Anglia Polytechnic University, Cambridge, UK
*Chapter 6.4.3*

**Beverley Raphael** University of Western Sydney Medical School, Sydney NSW, Australia
*Chapter 4.6.5*

**James Reich** Clinical Professor of Psychiatry, University of California, San Francisco Medical School and Adjunct Associate Professor of Psychiatry, Stanford School of Medicine, USA
*Chapter 4.12.2*

**Helmut Remschmidt** Director, Department of Child and Adolescent Psychiatry, Philipps Universität, Marburg, Germany
*Chapter 9.2.2*

**Philippe Robaey** Institute of Mental Health Research, Royal Ottawa Hospital, Ottawa, Canada
*Chapter 9.2.8*

**Ian Robbins** Consultant Clinical Psychologist, St George's Hospital, London, UK
*Chapter 11.13*

**T.W. Robbins** Section of Forensic Psychiatry, St George's Hospital Medical School, London, UK
*Chapter 2.5.5*

**G.M. Rodin** Professor of Psychiatry, University of Toronto, Toronto, Canada
*Chapter 5.3.6*

**Maria A. Ron** Professor of Neuropsychiatry, Institute of Neurology, University College London, UK
*Chapter 5.3.2*

**Robin Room** Professor, School of Population Health, University of Melbourne; and Director, AER Centre for Alcohol Policy Research, Turning Point Alcohol and Drug Centre, Fitzroy, Victoria, Australia
*Chapter 4.2.2.6*

**W. Rössler** Professor of Clinical Psychiatry and Psychology, University of Zürich, Switzerland
*Chapter 6.4.1*

**James R. Rundell** Department of Psychiatry and Psychology, Mayo Clinic Professor of Psychiatry, Mayo Clinic College of Medicine, USA
*Chapter 5.3.4*

**Gerald Russell** Emeritus Professor of Psychiatry, Director of the Eating Disorders Unit, Hayes Grove Priory Hospital, Hayes, Kent, UK
*Chapter 4.10.1*

**B.J. Sahakian** Dept of Psychiatry, University of Cambridge, Cambridge, UK
*Chapter 2.5.5*

**Diana Sanders** Chartered Counselling Psychologist, working in Psychological Medicine in Oxford, UK
*Chapter 6.3.1*

**Paramala J. Santosh** Great Ormond Street Hospital for Sick Children, London, UK
*Chapter 9.5.5*

**Benedetto Saraceno** Director of Department of Mental Health and Substance Abuse, World Health Organization WHO
*Chapter 1.3.1*

**Gauri N. Savla,** Veterans Affairs Medical Center, University of California, San Diego CA, USA
*Chapter 8.5.3*

**Carlos H. Schenck** Staff Psychiatrist, Minnesota Regional Sleep Disorders Center, Hennepin County Medical Center; Associate Professor of Psychiatry, University of Minnesota Medical School, Minneapolis, Minnesota, USA
*Chapter 4.14.4*

**John Schlapobersky** Consultant Psychotherapist, Trumatic Stress Clinic Middlesex/University College Hospital, formerly also of The Medical Foundation for the Care of Victims of Torture London, UK
*Chapter 6.3.6*

**Fabrizio Schiffano,** Chair in Clinical Pharmacology and Therapeutics Associate Dean, Postgraduate Medical School, Hon Consultant Psychiatrist Addictions, University of Hertfordshire, School of Pharmacy, College Lane Campus, Hatfield, UK
*Chapter 4.2.3.5*

**Gerd Schulte-Körne** Director of the Department of Child and Adolescent Psychiatry, Psychosomatics and Psychotherapy, University of Munich, Pettenkoferstr, München/Germany
*Chapter 9.2.2*

**J. Scott** Professor of Psychological Medicine, University of Newcastle & Honorary Professor, Psychological Treatments Research, Institute of Psychiatry, London and University Department of Psychiatry, Leazes Wing, Royal Victoria Infirmary, Newcastle upon Tyne, UK
*Chapter 4.5.8*

**Stephen Scott** Professor of Child Health & Behaviour, King's College London, Institute of Psychiatry, and Director of Research National Academy for Parenting Practitioners, London, UK
*Chapters 9.1.1 and 9.2.5*

**Nicholas Seivewright** Consultant Psychiatrist in Substance Misuse, Community Health Sheffield NHS Trust, Sheffield, UK
*Chapter 4.2.3.2*

**David Shaffer** Department of Child Psychiatry, College of Physicians and Surgeons, Columbia University, New York, USA
*Chapter 9.2.10*

**Trevor Sharp** Dept of Pharmacology, University of Oxford, Oxford, UK
*Chapter 2.3.4*

**Michael Sharpe** Professor of Psychological Medicine & Symptoms Research, University of Edinburgh, UK
*Chapters 5.1 and 5.2.7*

**Jennifer Shaw** Centre for Suicide Prevention, The School of Medicine, University of Manchester, UK
*Chapter 11.5*

**Mauricio Sierra** Institute of Psychiatry, King's College London, UK
*Chapter 4.9*

**Gregory Simon** Investigator, Center for Health Studies, Group Health Cooperative, Seattle, Washington, USA
*Chapter 5.2.2*

**Andrew Sims** Professor of Psychiatry, University of Leeds, UK
*Chapter 1.7*

**Ian Sinclair** Professor of Social Work, University of York, UK
*Chapter 9.5.6*

**Mike Slade** Health Service and Population Research Department and Institute of Psychiatry, King's College London, UK
*Chapter 7.2*

**Elita Smiley** Consultant Psychiatrist and Clinical Senior Lecturer, Division of Community Based Sciences, Faculty of Medicine, University of Glasgow, UK
*Chapter 10.2*

**Wolfgang Söllner** Department of Psychosomatic Medicine and Psychotherapy General Hospital Nuremberg, Prof.Ernst-Nathan-Str. 1, Nürnberg, Germany
*Chapter 5.7*

**Daniel Souery** Department of Psychiatry, University Clinics of Brussels, Erasme Hospital, Brussels, Belgium
*Chapter 4.5.5*

**Elizabeth Spencer** Senior Clinical Medical Officer, Early Intervention Service, Northern Birmingham Mental Health Trust, Birmingham, UK
*Chapter 6.3.2.4*

**David A. Spiegel** Center for Anxiety and Related Disorders at Boston University, Boston, Massachusetts, USA
*Chapter 4.7.1*

**Costas Stefanis** Honorary Professor of Psychiatry, University of Athens, Greece
*Chapter 1.6*

**Alan Stein** Royal Free and University College Medical School, University College London, and Tavistock Clinic, London, UK
*Chapter 9.3.6*

**Jessica Stiles** Department of Psychiatry and Behavioral Sciences, Memorial Sloan Kettering Cancer Center, New York, USA
*Chapter 5.3.7*

**William S. Stone** Assistant Professor of Psychology, Director of Neuropsychology Training and Clinical Services, Department of Psychiatry, Harvard Medical School, Massachusetts Mental Health Center Public Psychiatry, Division of the Beth Israel Deaconess Medical Center, Boston, USA
*Chapter 4.3.9*

**Gregory Stores** Emeritus Professor of Developmental Neuropsychiatry, University of Oxford, UK
*Chapters 4.14.1 and 9.2.9*

**Elizabeth A. Stormshak** Assistant Professor, University of Oregon, Eugene, Oregon, USA
*Chapter 9.5.4*

**James J. Strain** Professor/Director, Behavioral Medicine and Consultation Psychiatry, Mount Sinai School of Medicine, New York, USA
*Chapter 4.6.4*

**John Strang** National Addiction Centre, Institute of Psychiatry, King's College London, UK
*Chapters 4.2.3.1 and 4.2.4*

**J. Suckling** Brain Mapping Unit, Department of Psychiatry, University of Cambridge, Addenbrookes Hospital, Cambridge, UK
*Chapters 2.3.7 and 2.3.8*

**Nicola Swinson** Centre for Suicide Prevention, The School of Medicine, University of Manchester, UK
*Chapter 11.5*

**Michele Tansella** Professor of Psychiatry and Chairman, Department of Medicine and Public Health, Section of Psychiatry, University of Verona, Italy
*Chapters 7.2 and 7.6*

**Mary Target** Senior Lecturer in Psychoanalysis, Psychoanalysis Unit, University College London; Deputy Director of Research, Anna Freud Centre, London, UK
*Chapter 9.5.2*

**Eric Taylor** Head of Department, Child & Adolescent Psychiatry, King's College London, Institute of Psychiatry, UK
*Chapter 9.2.4*

**John-Paul Taylor** Academic Specialist Registrar, Institute for Ageing and Health Newcastle University, Campus for Ageing and Vitality, Newcastle upon Tyne, UK
*Chapter 4.1.13*

**Pamela J. Taylor** School of Medicine, Cardiff University, Cardiff, UK
*Chapter 11.17*

**Tatiana Taylor** Dept of Psychiatry, University of Oxford, Warneford Hospital, Oxford, UK
*Chapter 4.15.4*

**Mary Teasdale** 'Rethink', London, UK
*Chapter 7.9*

**Anita Thapar** Department of Psychological Medicine, School of Medicine, Cardiff University, UK
*Chapter 2.4.1*

**June Thoburn** Emeritus Professor of Social Work, University of East Anglia, Norwich, UK
*Chapter 9.3.5*

**Sian Thomas** Chester Young People's Centre, Chester, UK
*Chapter 9.5.9*

**Lindsay Thomson** Division of Psychiatry, University of Edinburgh, Edinburgh, UK
*Chapter 11.3.1*

**Anne E. Thompson** Emeritus Professor Child and Adolescent Psychiatry, University of Nottingham, UK
*Chapter 9.4*

**Graham Thornicroft** Professor of Community Psychiatry, Institute of Psychiatry, King's College London, UK
*Chapters 1.2, 7.2 and 7.6*

**Adolf Tobeña** Professor of Psychiatry, Director of the Dept. of Psychiatry and Forensic Medicine, Autonomous University of Barcelona, Bellaterra (Barcelona), Spain
*Chapter 4.12.5*

**Bruce J. Tonge** Head Monash University School of Psychology Psychiatry & Psychological Medicine, Monash Medical Centre, Clayton, Victoria, Australia
*Chapter 10.5.1*

**Brian Toone** Consultant, Maudsley Hospital; Honorary Senior Lecturer, Institute of Psychiatry, King's College London, UK
*Chapter 5.3.3*

**David Trickey** Leicester Royal Infirmary, Leicestershire Partnership NHS Trust, UK
*Chapters 9.3.2 and 9.3.7*

**Paula Trzepacz** Eli Lilly & Co, USA
*Chapter 4.1.1*

**Wen-Shing Tseng** Professor at Department of Psychiatry, University of Hawaii School of Medicine, USA
*Chapters 4.16 and 6.5*

**Ming T. Tsuang** Behavioral Genomics Endowed Chair and University Professor, University of California; Distinguished Professor of Psychiatry and Director, Center for Behavioral Genomics, Department of Psychiatry, University of California, San Diego, CA, USA
*Chapter 4.3.9*

**André Tylee** Director, Royal College of General Practitioners Unit for Mental Health Education in Primary Care, Institute of Psychiatry, King's College London, UK
*Chapter 7.8*

**Amy M. Ursano** Department of Psychiatry, University of North Carolina at Chapel Hill School of Medicine, Chapel Hill, North Carolina, USA
*Chapter 6.3.4*

**Robert J. Ursano** Professor and Chairman, Department of Psychiatry, Uniformed Services University of the Health Sciences, F. Edward Herbert School of Medicine, Bethesda, Maryland, USA
*Chapter 6.3.4*

**Jim van Os** Professor of Psychiatric Epidemiology, Maastricht University, Maastricht, The Netherlands and Visiting Professor of Psychiatric Epidemiology Institute of Psychiatry, London, UK
*Chapter 7.3*

**Fred R. Volkmar** Yale University, New Haven, Connecticut, USA
*Chapter 9.2.3*

**Jane Walker** Clinical Lecturer and Honorary Specialist Registrar in Liaison Psychiatry, Psychological Medicine & Symptoms Research Group, School of Molecular & Clinical Medicine, University of Edinburgh, UK
*Chapter 5.1*

**Diane Waller** Professor of Art Psychotherapy, Goldsmiths, University of London, UK
*Chapter 6.4.4*

**Paul Walters** MRC Fellow & Specialist Psychiatrist , Programme Leader MSc in Mental Health Services Research, Section of Primary Care Mental Health, Health Service and Population Research Department, David Goldberg Centre, Institute of Psychiatry, London, UK
*Chapter 7.8*

**John Weinmann** Professor of Psychology as applied to Medicine, Institute of Psychiatry, King's College London, UK
*Chapter 5.6*

**Myrna M. Weissman** Professor of Epidemiology in Psychiatry, College of Physicians and Surgeons of Columbia University; Chief, Division of Clinical and Genetic Epidemiology, New York State Psychiatric Institute, New York, USA
*Chapter 6.3.3*

**Sarah Welch** Gloucestershire Partnership NHS Foundation Trust, UK
*Chapter 4.2.3.4*

**Ursula Werneke** Consultant Psychiatrist, Norrkoping, Sweden
*Chapter 6.2.9*

**Simon Wessely** Professor of Epidemiological and Liaison Psychiatry, Institute of Psychiatry, King's College London, UK
*Chapter 5.2.7*

**Kay Wheat** Senior Lecturer in Law, Department of Academic Legal Studies, Nottingham Law School, Nottingham Trent University, UK
*Chapter 11.1*

**Adam R. Winstock** Senior Staff Specialist, Drug Health Services, Conjoint Senior Lecturer, National Drug and Alcohol Research Centre, UNSW, Australia
*Chapters 4.2.3.1 and 4.2.3.5*

**Sally Wooding** Senior Research Fellow, SciMHA Unit, University of Western Sydney, Australia
*Chapter 4.6.5*

**Matt Woolgar** Institute of Psychiatry, King's College London, UK
*Chapter 2.5.1*

**Miranda Wolpert** Director of Child and Adolescent Mental Health Services, Evidence Based Practice Unit, University College London and Anna Freud Centre, UK
*Chapter 9.5.7*

**Lawson Wulsin** Professor of Psychiatry and Family Medicine, University of Cincinnati, OH, USA
*Chapter 5.7*

**Richard Jed Wyatt**[†] National Institutes of Mental Health, Bethesda, Maryland, USA
*Chapter 1.1*

**William Yule** Professor of Applied Child Psychology, Institute of Psychiatry, King's College London, UK
*Chapter 2.5.1*

**Karl Zilles** Professor, Institute of Neuroscience and Biophysics, INB-3 Research Centre, Jülich and C.&O. Vogt Institute of Brain Research, University Düsseldorf, Germany
*Chapter 2.3.2*

**Joseph Zohar** Psychiatric Medical Center, Sheba Medical Center, Tel Hashomer and Sackler School of Medicine, Tel Aviv University, Israel
*Chapter 4.8*

# SECTION 5

# Psychiatry and Medicine

**5.1 Mind–body dualism, psychiatry, and medicine** 989
Michael Sharpe and Jane Walker

**5.2 Somatoform disorders and other causes of medically unexplained symptoms** 992

5.2.1 Somatoform disorders and functional symptoms 992
Richard Mayou

5.2.2 Epidemiology of somatoform disorders and other causes of unexplained medical symptoms 995
Gregory Simon

5.2.3 Somatization disorder and related disorders 999
Per Fink

5.2.4 Conversion and dissociation disorders 1011
Christopher Bass

5.2.5 Hypochondriasis (health anxiety) 1021
Russell Noyes Jr.

5.2.6 Pain disorder 1029
Sidney Benjamin and Stella Morris

5.2.7 Chronic fatigue syndrome 1035
Michael Sharpe and Simon Wessely

5.2.8 Body dysmorphic disorder 1043
Katharine A. Phillips

5.2.9 Factitious disorder and malingering 1049
Christopher Bass and David Gill

5.2.10 Neurasthenia 1059
Felice Lieh Mak

**5.3 Medical and surgical conditions and treatments associated with psychiatric disorders** 1065

5.3.1 Adjustment to illness and handicap 1065
Allan House

5.3.2 Psychiatric aspects of neurological disease 1071
Maria A. Ron

5.3.3 Epilepsy 1076
Brian Toone

5.3.4 Medical conditions associated with psychiatric disorder 1081
James R. Rundell

5.3.5 Psychiatric aspects of infections 1090
José-Luis Ayuso-Mateos

5.3.6 Psychiatric aspects of surgery (including transplantation) 1096
S. A. Hales, S. E. Abbey, and G. M. Rodin

5.3.7 Psychiatric aspects of cancer 1100
Jimmie C. Holland and Jessica Stiles

5.3.8 Psychiatric aspects of accidents, burns, and other physical trauma 1105
Ulrik Fredrik Malt

**5.4 Obstetric and gynaecological conditions associated with psychiatric disorder** 1114
Ian Brockington

**5.5 Management of psychiatric disorders in medically ill patients, including emergencies** 1128
Pier Maria Furlan and Luca Ostacoli

**5.6 Health psychology** 1135
John Weinman and Keith J. Petrie

**5.7 The organization of psychiatric services for general hospital departments** 1144
Frits J. Huyse, Roger Kathol, Wolfgang Söllner, and Lawson Wulsin

# Mind–body dualism, psychiatry, and medicine

Michael Sharpe and Jane Walker

## Introduction

Patients usually attend doctors because they are concerned about symptoms. When these symptoms are associated with persistent distress or disability we refer to the patient as having an illness. When assessing the patient's illness the doctor aims to make a diagnosis, on the basis of which management can be planned and prognosis made. The diagnoses available to doctors are conventionally defined as either 'medical' or 'psychiatric'. This division of illness into two types is such an accepted feature of current medical practice that we tend to take it for granted. But is it really the best way to think about patients' illnesses and to plan their care?

In order to answer this question we will examine what is meant by 'medical' and 'psychiatric' diagnoses and the assumptions underpinning this division. The disadvantages of this dualistic approach will be considered and solutions proposed.

## Diagnosis

### Medical diagnosis

A medical diagnosis is a label for a condition that is: (a) conventionally treated by medical doctors and (b) listed in the classifications of medical conditions such as ICD-10. Most medical diagnoses are based on identifiable bodily pathology (abnormal structure and/or function). Therefore, to make a medical diagnosis (such as cancer) doctors will seek specific bodily symptoms before confirming the presence of bodily pathology with physical signs and biological investigations (such as X-rays).

### Psychiatric diagnosis

Similarly a psychiatric diagnosis is a label for a condition that is: (a) conventionally treated by psychiatrists and (b) defined in the psychiatric diagnostic classifications of ICD and DSM. Psychiatric diagnoses are not based not on bodily pathology. They are however associated with the idea of 'psychopathology', that is proposed abnormalities of the mind. Unlike bodily pathology these abnormalities of the mind cannot be objectively identified and have to be inferred from the patient's mental symptoms and their behaviour. Investigations play little or no role in diagnosis. Psychiatric diagnoses are therefore defined on the basis of symptoms and syndromes.

## When is an illness psychiatric?

Why are some illnesses regarded as 'mental' or 'psychiatric' as opposed to 'medical'? Examination of the criteria for diagnoses listed as psychiatric reveals that readily observable factors common to most 'psychiatric' illnesses are:

◆ an absence of known bodily pathology

◆ an abnormal mental state as inferred by the patient's report

◆ a presentation with disturbed behaviour

## Mind–body dualism

The underlying assumption of this dichotomous view is that it is both valid and useful to divide human illnesses into those of the body and those of the mind.[1] This idea of mind–body dualism is commonly attributed to the writings of the philosopher Descartes. So-called Cartesian dualism has exerted a profound influence on Western medical thinking and still shapes our thinking, training, and service provision.

However, dualism is at best an oversimplification and at worst a source of serious theoretical and practical problems. It may be argued that there is no such thing as a purely 'bodily' or purely 'mental' illness and that all illnesses have mental and bodily aspects.[2] Furthermore, the assumption that bodily symptoms indicate bodily pathology and that mental symptoms indicate psychopathology gives rise to specific problems: (a) when bodily symptoms occur without bodily pathology and (b) when mental symptoms occur together with bodily pathology (see Table 5.1.1).

## Bodily symptoms with no bodily pathology: somatization

When patients present with bodily symptoms and bodily pathology is confirmed they are given a medical diagnosis. When patients have bodily symptoms but there is no evidence of bodily pathology the terms 'somatization' or 'somatoform disorder' are used to describe their illness. It is unclear, however, whether these illnesses are properly regarded as 'psychiatric' or as 'medical' as they do not clearly fulfil criteria for either. One solution to this dilemma is to allocate these illnesses to psychiatry. The assumption is made that their somatic symptoms are really explained by psychopathology. The absence of mental symptoms, from which psychopathology

**Table 5.1.1** Diagnoses symptoms and bodily pathology

| Symptoms | Bodily pathology | Diagnosis |
|---|---|---|
| Bodily symptoms | Present | Medical diagnosis |
| | Absent | Somatization |
| Mental symptoms | Present | Comorbidity |
| | Absent | Psychiatric diagnosis |

can be inferred, is explained by the idea that the psychopathology is hidden and 'converted' into bodily symptoms by a process called 'somatization' (literally making the mental somatic). Clearly these are questionable assumptions.[3]

A second solution is to assume that the patients really do have bodily pathology in some form (even though is it unknown) and to give them a medical diagnosis of a so-called 'functional disorder' such as fibromyalgia.[4] As with somatization this approach is based on questionable assumptions.

A third, and all too common solution, is for the patient to be rejected as 'not really ill' by both psychiatry and medicine. They then end up in a no-man's land between specialities. The inadequacy of all three solutions has been particularly well illustrated by the controversy and conflict surrounding the condition called Chronic Fatigue Syndrome (CFS) or Myalgic Encephalomyelitis (ME).[5]

### Mental symptoms and bodily pathology: comorbidity

When a patient has both bodily pathology and mental symptoms they are given both a medical diagnosis (based on the bodily pathology) and a psychiatric diagnosis (based on presumed psychopathology). This idea of 'comorbidity' gives rise to both theoretical and practical problems, however.

The theoretical problem concerns the psychiatric diagnosis. To make this diagnosis the doctor must identify symptoms, which are considered to be evidence of psychopathology. However, some symptoms may be considered as evidence of both psychopathology and bodily pathology. For example, a patient has mental symptoms of low mood and worthlessness, and a medical diagnosis of cancer, based on bodily pathology. Should the patient's weight loss be counted toward a psychiatric diagnosis of depression or regarded as a symptom of his cancer? There is no generally agreed answer to this conundrum (although a variety of ways of addressing it have been proposed[6]), probably because it is a manifestation of the fundamentally flawed dualistic assumption.

The main practical problem that results from making two diagnoses is a failure to adequately treat the patient. Depressive disorder comorbid with a chronic medical condition is a major cause of morbidity. However, the patient's need for psychiatric treatment often goes unmet[7] because the patient is considered to have two illnesses, each requiring diagnosis and treatment by a different speciality and the treatment of the medical condition takes precedence.

## Solutions to dualism

### Theoretical solutions

New scientific knowledge, such as the demonstration of a bodily (neural) basis to many 'mental' symptoms is increasingly rendering crude dualistic thinking theoretically untenable.[8] Mind and brain are coming to be regarded as two sides of the same coin—the mind/brain. This paradigm shift implies that 'psychiatric' illnesses are no more distinct from 'medical conditions' than the nervous system is separate from the rest of the body. Hence, there is a need for psychiatry to become less 'brain-less' and for medicine to become less 'mind-less'.[9] According to this new way of thinking, all symptoms, whether previously regarded as 'bodily' or 'mental' are in fact products of the mind/brain's integration of bodily, psychological, and social information. Therefore to speak of 'medical' and 'psychiatric' symptoms makes no sense. Symptoms are just symptoms.

If this paradigm shift is to be fully translated into clinical practice a new unified classification system is needed that would be used by both medicine and psychiatry. One way of achieving this might be to create a multi-axial system as is currently used by DSM-IV. However, rather than using separate axes for psychiatric and medical diagnoses, separate axes would be used for symptoms (not distinguishing between medical and psychiatric) and bodily pathology.[10] Other axes could be added to ensure that other important information is included. An example is shown in Table 5.1.2.

### Practical solutions

For the present we must accept that dualism continues to shape our every day thinking, practice, and service organization. It is important therefore, that the psychiatrist is aware of the practical problems that result and is equipped with ways of addressing them. In this regard the psychiatrist is especially well placed to make a major contribution to the care of all patients by ensuring that biological, psychological, and social aspects of illness are considered in every case. This so-called 'biopsychosocial' formulation was first proposed by Engel.[11] A further enhancement of this formulation is to divide the aetiological factors into those that predisposed the patient to the illness, those that precipitated or triggered it, and those that are perpetuating it. The last group of causes is a target for treatment and the first two for prevention. A useful diagram that lists factors to consider in a biopsychosocial formulation is shown in Table 5.1.3.

### Service solutions

Finally, the consequence of the professional and organizational separation of medicine and psychiatry has been a major obstacle to the integrated care of patients, especially those with comorbidity and somatoform disorders. One service solution has been the establishment of so-called liaison (linking) psychiatry services to general hospital inpatient units. Another is the increasing integration of psychological management into chronic illness management programmes.[12] However truly integrated care remains the exception rather than the rule.

**Table 5.1.2** A proposed multi-axial diagnostic system for use by both psychiatry and medicine

| | |
|---|---|
| Axis 1 | Symptoms or syndrome, e.g. chronic fatigue or depression |
| Axis 2 | Bodily pathology, e.g. cancer |
| Axis 3 | Biological factors, e.g. autonomic arousal |
| Axis 4 | Psychological factors, e.g. beliefs |
| Axis 5 | Social and situational factors, e.g. bereavement |

**Table 5.1.3** A biopsychosocial formulation

| Main factors | Subfactors | Predisposing | Precipitating | Perpetuating |
|---|---|---|---|---|
| Biological | Disease physiology | | | |
| Psychological | Cognition mood behaviour | | | |
| Social | Interpersonal social and occupational health care system | | | |

## Conclusion

It has been taken for granted that it is appropriate and desirable to separate patients' illnesses into medical and psychiatric types. Such an approach has had advantages in allowing specialization of training and service planning but has also created obstacles to effective patient care. It is important that practising psychiatrists are aware of these obstacles and ways of overcoming them. It also seems increasingly likely that in time better understanding of neuroscience will make dualism increasingly theoretically untenable and that a better understanding of chronic illness management will make it practically redundant. Only then will psychiatry become fully reintegrated with the rest of medicine.

## Further information

White, P.D. (2005). *Biopsychosocial medicine*. Oxford University Press, Oxford.

Damasio, A.R. (1994) *Descartes' error*. GP Putnam's Sons, New York.

## References

1. Miresco, M.J. and Kirmayer, L.J. (2006). The persistence of mind-brain dualism in psychiatric reasoning about clinical scenarios. *The American Journal of Psychiatry*, **163**, 913–8.
2. Wade, D.T. and Halligan, P.W. (2004). Do biomedical models of illness make for good healthcare systems? *British Medical Journal*, **329**, 1398–401.
3. DeGucht, V. and Fischler, B. (2002). Somatization: a critical review of conceptual and methodological issues. *Psychosomatics*, **43**, 1–9.
4. Wessely, S., Nimnuan, C., and Sharpe M. (1999). Functional somatic syndromes: one or many? *Lancet*, **354**, 936–9.
5. Sharpe, M. (2002). The English Chief Medical Officer's Working Parties' report on the management of CFS/ME: significant breakthrough or unsatisfactory compromise? *Journal of Psychosomatic Research*, **52**, 437–8.
6. Cohen-Cole, S.A., Brown, F.W., and McDaniel, J.S. (1993). Diagnostic assessment of depression in the medically ill. In *Psychiatric care of the medical patient* (eds. A. Stoudemire and B. Fogel), pp. 53–70. Oxford University Press, New York.
7. Moussavi, S., Chatterji, S., Verdes, E., *et al*. (2007). Depression, chronic diseases, and decrements in health: results from the World Health Surveys. *Lancet*, **370**, 851–8.
8. Kendler, K.S. (2001). A psychiatric dialogue on the mind-body problem. *The American Journal of Psychiatry*, **158**, 989–1000.
9. Eisenberg, L. (1986). Mindless and brainless in psychiatry. *British Journal of Psychiatry*, **148**, 497–508.
10. Sharpe, M., Mayou, R., and Walker, J. (2006). Bodily symptoms: new approaches to classification. *Journal of Psychosomatic Research*, **60**, 353–6.
11. Engel, G.L. (1977). The need for a new medical model: a challenge for biomedicine. *Science*, **196**, 129–96.
12. Von Korff, M., Glasgow, R.E., and Sharpe, M. (2002). Organising care for chronic illness. *British Medical Journal*, **325**, 92–4.

# Somatoform disorders and other causes of medically unexplained symptoms

## Contents

5.2.1 **Somatoform disorders and functional symptoms**
Richard Mayou

5.2.2 **Epidemiology of somatoform disorders and other causes of unexplained medical symptoms**
Gregory Simon

5.2.3 **Somatization disorder and related disorders**
Per Fink

5.2.4 **Conversion and dissociation disorders**
Christopher Bass

5.2.5 **Hypochondriasis (health anxiety)**
Russell Noyes Jr.

5.2.6 **Pain disorder**
Sidney Benjamin and Stella Morris

5.2.7 **Chronic fatigue syndrome**
Michael Sharpe and Simon Wessely

5.2.8 **Body dysmorphic disorder**
Katharine A. Phillips, M. D.

5.2.9 **Factitious disorder and malingering**
Christopher Bass and David Gill

5.2.10 **Neurasthenia**
Felice Lieh Mak

## 5.2.1 Somatoform disorders and functional symptoms

Richard Mayou

Non-specific symptoms that are not explained by organic pathology are extremely frequent in the general population[1] and in all medical settings. Most are transient, but a substantial minority is persistent, disabling, and often associated with frequent consultation. They are likely, especially when there are multiple unexplained symptoms, to be associated with psychiatric disorder (see Chapter 5.2.3). They are widely regarded as difficult to treat but only a very small proportion is seen by psychiatrists and psychologists.

This chapter covers general issues relating to functional symptoms and syndromes and their psychiatric associations. The following chapters provide more detail about the more specific forms of somatoform disorder and about functional syndromes (pain, chronic fatigue).

### Terminology of functional symptoms

The terminology is unsatisfactory.[2] These symptoms are often referred to as 'medically unexplained symptoms'. This usage has the advantage of describing the clinical problem without assumptions of aetiology, but it is unsatisfactory in that it wrongly implies that there is no medical explanation. Other generally used terms include somatization, somatoform symptoms, and functional overlay. It is perhaps most satisfactory to refer to functional symptoms and functional syndromes.

This chapter is concerned with functional symptoms whether or not they are associated with psychiatric disorder.

### Aetiology

A traditional Western dualist view of aetiology as being either physical or psychological, continues to influence clinical practice and current psychiatric classifications (see Chapter 5.1). In western countries, this view has resulted in great problems in psychiatric and lay understanding, in taxonomy, and in the treatment of 'unexplained' symptoms. It has also caused bewilderment in cultures that do not share this dualist approach.

An increasingly widely held alternative view, for which there is compelling evidence, is that functional symptoms result from the interaction of physiological, pathological, and psychosocial variables.[2] A primary bodily sensation or concern (Table 5.2.1.1) is then attributed or interpreted as being of sinister significance with resulting subjective symptoms, disability, and behavioural and emotional consequences. For example, awareness of normal heart rate increase due to excitement or anxiety can result in, on the one hand, panic and, on the other, worry about heart disease, restriction of daily activities, and repeated consultation to seek investigation

**Table 5.2.1.1** Causes of bodily sensations

Major pathology
Minor pathology
Physiological processes, for example:
    Sinus tachycardia and benign minor arrhythmias
    Effects of fatigue
    Hangover
    Effects of overeating
    Effects of prolonged inactivity
    Autonomic effects of anxiety
    Lack of sleep

and reassurance. The role of these factors may vary over time during the course of any individual clinical problem.

There is considerable evidence on the ways in which psychological processes affect the interpretation of physical symptoms, whatever the underlying (major or minor) pathology or physiological processes. Cognitive-behavioural formulations emphasize the central significance of health anxiety and suggest that feedback of the physiological, cognitive, affective, and behavioural consequences of this anxiety can reinforce the physical symptoms as well as their effects on everyday life.

The process of interpretation of a bodily sensation or fear is affected by several sets of factors:

- the individual's medical experience and beliefs
- social circumstances (Table 5.2.1.2)
- personality and mental state

Once symptoms have developed they may be maintained by behavioural and psychological factors and also by the reactions of others. As with other forms of anxiety, neurobiological mechanisms may perpetuate and complicate the initial presentation.

Simple reassurance is often ineffective especially in those who, by reason of personality, are inclined to worry about their health. Misconceptions are frequently reinforced and maintained by the lack of any medical explanation for worrying symptoms or by ambiguous or contradictory advice.

## The association with psychiatric disorder

The majority of functional symptoms in general populations are short lived and not associated with psychiatric disorder. There is now considerable evidence both from smaller local studies and international collaborative research that the more severe and

**Table 5.2.1.2** Illness experience, which may affect the interpretation of bodily sensations and concern

Childhood illness
Family illness and consultation in childhood
Childhood consultation and school absence
Physical illness in adult life
Experience and satisfaction with medical consultation
Illness in family and friends
Publicity in television, newspapers, etc.
Knowledge of illness and its treatment

disabling functional symptoms are associated with anxiety and depressive disorder, and that this relationship is strongest for those who have the greatest number of 'unexplained' symptoms. This is so for all ethnic groups and cultures studied.[1] There are also associations with the somatoform disorders as described below.

### Classification of unexplained symptoms

The classification of persistent and disabling functional symptoms has taken two parallel approaches.

#### (a) Medical descriptive syndromes

These are very numerous, clinical patterns and terms overlap and some include assumptions about aetiology. There are cultural differences in the definition and naming. There is little evidence for the validity of separate syndromes. Lay pressure groups have increasingly claimed specific syndromes, such as alleged sensitivity to dental amalgam and many 'food allergies', which are more likely to be due to their own predicaments and the apparent lack of success of conventional medicine.[3] A small number of syndromes have now received operational diagnostic criteria which have proved valuable in clinical understanding and in planning treatment, for example the criteria for chronic fatigue (Chapter 5.2.7).

#### (b) Psychiatric classification

This covers both well established categories, such as anxiety and depressive disorders, and the new concept, first introduced in DSM-III, of somatoform disorder.

#### (i) Somatoform disorder

Somatoform disorders (Table 5.2.1.3) were seen as speculative and provisional in DSM-III. The defining feature was *'physical symptoms suggesting a physical disorder for which there are no demonstrable organic findings on known physiological mechanisms, and for which there is strong evidence, or a strong presumption, that the symptoms are linked to psychological factors or conflicts'.*

The original DSM-III classification was relatively narrow but subsequent revisions of DSM and ICD-10 have incorporated non-specific categories which have turned out to be much more prevalent in all settings.

**Table 5.2.1.3** Categories of somatoform disorders in ICD-10 and DSM-IV

| ICD-10 | DSM-IV |
| --- | --- |
| Somatization disorder | Somatization disorder |
| Undifferentiated somatoform disorder | Undifferentiated somatoform disorder |
| Hypochondriacal disorder | Hypochondriasis |
| Somatoform autonomic dysfunction | — |
| Persistent pain disorder | Pain disorder associated with psychological factors (and a general medical condition) |
| Other somatoform disorders | Somatoform disorders not otherwise specified |
| — | Body dysmorphic disorder |
| — | Conversion disorders |
| Neurasthenia | — |

It is important to recall that somatoform disorder remains a provisional grouping for statistical purposes rather than a grouping of categories that satisfy the normal requirements of disease entities. It nevertheless indicates a substantial clinical problem associated with considerable use of health care provisions.[3]

### (ii) Factitious disorder

DSM-III also introduced another new category of 'factitious disorder' for self-inflicted physical problems. These are described in Chapter 5.2.9 and should be distinguished from deliberate falsification for external gain—*malingering*. It must be remembered that patients with factitious disorder may also suffer from unexplained symptoms attributable to somatoform or other psychiatric disorders and, indeed, not uncommonly also report symptoms of undoubted physical illness.

## Somatoform disorders in DSM and ICD

There are substantial differences between the use of subcategories in DSM and ICD.[4] Neurasthenia is included in ICD-10 but is not used in any section of DSM-IV; conversion disorder is a somatoform disorder in DSM-IV but not in ICD. Both classifications include both relatively specific categories (e.g. *somatization disorder* and *hypochondriasis*) and also several very vaguely defined non-specific categories. These latter include *Undifferentiated Somatoform Disorder*, *Somatoform Autonomic Dysfunction* (ICD-10 only), and *Other Somatoform Disorders*. Although these latter have attracted less clinical and research attention, they are by far the most common forms of somatoform disorder in all epidemiological studies. So broad are the criteria that it is possible to use these categories for almost all persistent unexplained physical symptoms. Epidemiological comparisons of ICD and DSM show that the use of their rather different criteria results in substantially different prevalences of somatoform disorder in community and primary care populations.

## Problems in the definition of somatoform disorder

It is widely recognized that there are serious problems[2] in the overall concept of somatoform disorders and in the definition of subcategories:

- There is no unifying theoretical basis for the whole category; it is a disparate group of problems that are not easily fitted into other parts of the classifcations.

- Comorbidity is very common, especially with anxiety disorder, depressive disorder, and personality disorder.

- Some types of somatoform disorder could be more satisfactorily reassigned to other parts of the classification (for example hypochondriasis might be renamed health anxiety and moved to anxiety disorder).

- The definitions of the less specific categories (pain disorder, Undifferentiated Somatoform Disorder) do not include any psychological criteria. Instead they rely on the description and the number of physical symptoms, the same symptoms that are used to make accompanying Axis III diagnoses. Somatization disorder has attracted disproportionate attention, but appears to be no more than an uncommon, arbitrary and unreliable extreme of the spectrum of multiple physical symptoms.

- Criteria have little meaning for cultures that do not share the western presumption of the separation of body and mind.

It has become apparent that the present classifications have no value in guiding treatment and that they are both confusing and unpopular with patients and with those who treat them.

DSM-V and ICD-11 can be expected to make large changes which will depend on the resolution of conceptual arguments and substantial further research. It is hoped that the new classification and terminology will be more reliable and valid and also be much more meaningful and acceptable.[2]

It is likely that the more specific subcategories (hypochondriasis, body dysmorphic disorder) will be reassigned to other parts of the classification and that there will be modifications in their criteria. The greatest problems relate to the much more prevalent non-specific categories. There is a consensus that a more rational operational approach is required to categorize multiple symptoms which should result in either a renamed grouping on Axis I or more logically a transfer to Axis III. It should be possible to give much greater prominence both in criteria and in accompanying text to underlying psychological and behavioural abnormalities.

## Classification in clinical practice

The following chapters in this section of the book describe syndromes that have proved to have some administrative value despite the acknowledged lack of validity. Anxiety and depression are considered fully elsewhere. The recognition of anxiety and depression is important because of the therapeutic implications.

In everyday clinical practice it is rarely necessary (or helpful) to attach a somatoform label. It is more useful to be able to provide brief descriptions of the clinical problem, since these can be used as a basis for formulating treatment:

- acute or chronic

- number of physical symptoms

- the nature and pattern of symptoms (i.e. clinical syndromes such as fatigue)

- association with anxiety disorder, depressive disorder, or other specific psychiatric disorder

- beliefs about cause

## Assessment and treatment

The majority of those presenting unexplained symptoms in primary care require no more than medically appropriate assessment and reassurance (Table 5.2.1.4). The latter should convey to the patient that the symptoms are accepted as real and provide an explanation for their origin as well as answering the patient's worries. It is also necessary to discuss the results of any negative investigations fully.

Symptoms that persist or recur despite reassurance are generally regarded as difficult to treat. Continuing symptoms without any specific medical explanation are likely to confirm and maintain worries about serious illness, which may be further exacerbated by secondary anxiety and behavioural consequences. Therefore

**Table 5.2.1.4** General principles of assessment

| **Consider psychological factors from the outset** |
| --- |
| Use appropriate physical investigation to exclude physical cause |
| Clarify psychological and physical complaints |
| Clarify previous personality and concerns about physical illness |
| Understand patient's beliefs and expectations |
| Identify depression or other psychiatric disorder |
| Identify psychosocial problems |

effective treatment depends upon sympathetic treatment that meets the needs of both the patient and the family. A multi-causal view of aetiology leads to conclusions about treatment and avoids psychiatric diagnoses that may be unacceptable to the patient. Much can be done by general practitioners or non-specialists.

The general principles of treatment (Table 5.2.1.5) are similar for all forms of unexplained symptoms, single or multiple, but individual treatment plans must take account of psychiatric diagnoses of anxiety or depression and the particular type of physical symptoms.

The treatments for particular forms of somatoform disorder are discussed in later chapters. It is important to be aware that the commonest type of somatoform disorder, Undifferentiated Somatoform Disorder is not discussed separately; treatment follows the general principles described in this and other chapters. The treatments of other functional syndromes such as irritable bowel syndrome, chronic fatigue, and atypical facial pain all depend on the therapist being familiar with these syndromes and being able to provide an appropriate combination of treatment methods. For example, the management of physical de-conditioning is central to the treatment of chronic fatigue, whereas antidepressant medication has a major role in the treatment of atypical facial pain. The chapter on chronic fatigue (Chapter 5.2.7) is an example of a functional syndrome.

Much can be achieved by components of good non-specialist care, such as the following:

◆ discussion and explanation of the aetiology

◆ treatment of any minor underlying physical problem

◆ anxiety management (including tapes and handouts)

◆ advice on diary monitoring and graded return to full activities

◆ specific self-help programmes (e.g. chronic fatigue, irritable bowel syndrome)

◆ including relatives in the assessment, discussion of the nature of the problems, and explanations of the treatment

**Table 5.2.1.5** General principles of treatment

| |
| --- |
| Emphasize that symptoms are real and familiar and that medical care is appropriate |
| Minimize and control physical care |
| Offer an explanation and discuss |
| Allow patients and families to ask questions |
| Discuss the role of psychological factors in all medical care |
| Treat any primary psychiatric disorder |
| Agree a treatment plan |

However, chronic and recurrent problems may need specialist treatment:

◆ psychotropic medication (antidepressants, anxiolytics)

◆ cognitive behavioural therapy

◆ interpretative psychotherapy (individual and group)

◆ specific psychiatric treatment for associated psychiatric and social problems

◆ programme to co-ordinate and control all medical care

There is a lot of evidence on the effectiveness of a range of treatments in specialist care,[5,6] but there is much less evidence about simple routine measures. The outlook for simpler syndromes of relatively recent onset is good, but the prognosis for very prolonged chronic, multiple, or recurrent syndromes (e.g. somatization disorder) is not as good. In these circumstances the control of medical care and the prevention of further iatrogenic disability may be more realistic than cure.

## Further information

Mayou, R., Kirmayer, L.J., Simon, G., *et al.* (2005). Somatoform disorders: time for a new approach. *American Journal of Psychiatry*, **162**, 847–55.

Maj, M., Akiskal, H.S., Mezzich, J., *et al.* (eds.) *Somatoform disorders*. Wiley, Chichester.

## References

1. Üstün, T.B. and Sartorius, N. (1995). *World health organization. Mental illness in general health care. An international study*. Wiley, Chichester.

2. Mayou, R., Kirmayer, L.J., Simon, G., *et al.* (2005). Somatoform disorders: time for a new approach. *American Journal of Psychiatry*, **162**, 847–55.

3. Barsky, A.J., Orav, E.J., and Bates, D.W. (2005). Somatization increases medical utilization and costs independent of psychiatric and medical comorbidity *Archives of General Psychiatry*, **62**, 903–10.

4. Fink, P., Hansen, M.S., and Oxhoj, M.L. (2004). The prevalence of somatoform disorders among internal medicine patients. *Journal of Psychosomatic Research*, **56**, 413–18.

5. Kroenke, K. and Swindle, R. (2000). Cognitive-behavioral therapy for somatization and symptom syndromes; a critical review of controlled clinical trials. *Psychotherapy and Psychosomatics*, **69**, 205–15.

6. O'Malley, P.G., Jackson, J.L., Santoro, J., *et al.* (2005) Antidepressant therapy for unexplained symptoms and symptom syndromes. *The Journal of Family Practice*, **48**, 980–90.

# 5.2.2 Epidemiology of somatoform disorders and other causes of unexplained medical symptoms

Gregory Simon

While nearly every psychiatric syndrome may include some somatic signs or symptoms, a specific group of syndromes has been traditionally defined as somatoform. This group of disorders is distinguished by certain key features: prominent reporting of somatic symptoms, concern about medical illness, and frequent presentation to general medical providers. As in other categories of mental disorder, the boundaries between individual syndromes are more distinct in our systems of classification than they are in nature. Understanding that various somatoform disorders often overlap, this review is organized according to the major categories of somatoform disorder described in the ICD and DSM classification systems.

## Somatization disorders

### Phenomenology

The term somatization has been used to refer to a variety of clinical phenomena. One traditional view defines somatization as an inability or unwillingness to express emotional distress,[1] so that somatic symptoms are an alternative 'idiom of distress'. An alternative view defines somatization as the presentation of somatic complaints to medical providers in the presence of an occult anxiety or depressive disorder.[2] A third view defines somatization as somatic symptoms, which have no clear medical explanation.[3] While these definitions appear closely related, they identify somewhat different groups of patients. The third definition (presentation of unexplained somatic symptoms) is used by official systems of classification and by most epidemiological studies, so this review will focus on that phenomenon.

Both the ICD and DSM classification systems define somatization disorder as a chronic condition characterized by the reporting of numerous unexplained somatic symptoms.[4, 5] Recent versions of both classification systems identify a core syndrome of somatization (a persistent tendency to report multiple unexplained somatic symptoms) using a simplified set of diagnostic criteria.

### Prevalence

The reported prevalence of well-defined somatization disorder appears to depend significantly on the method used for assessment. Community and primary care surveys have typically relied on structured interviews to assess the lifetime prevalence of unexplained somatic symptoms. Community surveys in North America[6] and Western Europe[7, 8] have found prevalence rates of less than 2 per cent with primary care surveys finding only slightly higher prevalence rates.[9] Data from the World Health Organization (**WHO**) multicentre primary care survey indicate that recall during structured interviews may significantly underestimate the lifetime prevalence of somatization symptoms.[10] More accurate recall of lifetime symptoms (by either repeated assessments or the use of medical records) might yield significantly higher prevalence rates.

### Correlates

The prevalence of somatization disorder and unexplained somatic symptoms is typically twice as high in women as in men,[11, 12] and this difference appears at time of menarche.[13] Community and primary care surveys demonstrate a substantial overlap between somatization disorder and anxiety and depressive disorders.[7, 14, 15] Anxiety and depressive disorders also predict the subsequent onset of somatization disorder.[16]

Available data show a mixed picture regarding cross-national or cross-cultural differences in the prevalence of somatization. Studies of clinical samples find that somatic symptoms are a common accompaniment of depressive and anxiety disorders worldwide.[17–19] The WHO primary care survey documented large differences in the prevalence of unexplained somatic symptoms with a markedly higher prevalence in South America than in Europe or the United States.[9] That same study, however, found that the association between unexplained symptoms and symptoms of depression or anxiety was similar across a wide range of cultures and levels of economic development.[14] One explanation for these apparently disparate findings is that the prevalence of unexplained somatic symptoms (like the prevalence of anxiety or depressive disorder) varies widely across nations and cultures, but the association between somatic and psychological distress is universal. Countries or cultures with higher rates of anxiety or depressive disorders would be expected to have higher prevalence of somatization disorder and other somatization syndromes. Given the consistent overlap between somatization disorders and other common mental disorders, some have questioned whether these conditions actually belong in a distinct category.[20, 21]

### Controversies and questions

Available data do not support a specific diagnostic threshold based on the number or distribution of unexplained somatic symptoms. An increasing number of somatic symptoms is consistently associated with increases in comorbid mood or anxiety disorder, functional impairment, and use of health services.[14,15] Mindful of this continuum, both Escobar et al.[22] and Kroenke et al.[23] have described less restrictive somatization syndromes, which, despite their higher prevalence, are strongly associated with impairment and the use of health services. Both the ICD and DSM classification systems describe subthreshold or less extreme forms of this condition characterized by a smaller number of medically unexplained symptoms.[5, 24]

Longitudinal data raise questions about the presumed stability or chronicity of somatization disorder or medically unexplained somatic symptoms. Traditional descriptions of somatization disorder emphasize its stability and chronicity. Data from the WHO primary care survey, however, suggest that individual somatization symptoms vary considerably over time.[9] While the syndrome of somatization seemed somewhat more stable than anxiety and depressive disorders (typically regarded as episodic), only half of the primary care patients, satisfying Escobar's criteria for somatization syndrome at the baseline assessment, continued to meet the criteria one year later.

## Hypochondriacal disorders

### Phenomenology

Both the ICD and DSM classification systems define hypochondriasis by the triad of disease conviction, functional impairment, and refusal to accept appropriate reassurance.

### Prevalence

Attempts to estimate the prevalence of hypochondriasis have been limited by the absence of proven standardized methods for standardized assessment. Community surveys find prevalence rates of 1 per cent or less,[25] while primary care surveys typically find rates of approximately 5 per cent,[26, 27] while the WHO multicentre primary care survey[28] found an overall prevalence of only 0.8 per cent.

In reviewing data from the WHO survey, Gureje *et al.*[28] found that a less restrictive definition more than doubled the prevalence rate (to 2.2 per cent). Cases added by this relaxed definition did not differ significantly from those satisfying CIDI/ICD criteria, suggesting that CIDI/ICD criteria may be somewhat too restrictive.

### Correlates

Despite the variation in prevalence, primary care surveys yield similar results regarding demographic correlates of hypochondriasis. The prevalence of hypochondriasis is 1.5 to 2 times as great in women as men but does not appear to vary significantly with age.[28]

### Controversies and questions

While the ICD and DSM classification systems suggest that hypochondriasis is distinct from anxiety and depressive disorders, available data suggests considerable overlap. In every sample examined, hypochondriasis is strongly associated with major depression, panic disorder, and generalized anxiety disorder.[26,28–30] Among those with hypochondriasis, clinical features do not clearly distinguish those with and without a comorbid psychiatric diagnosis.[30] In addition, changes over time in anxiety or depression are consistently associated with parallel changes in symptoms of hypochondriasis.[31] As with somatization disorders, some have recently argued that hypochondriasis be re-classified as a form of anxiety disorder.[20,21]

## Pain syndromes

### Phenomenology

While the ICD and DSM classification systems both define somatoform pain disorders, the two systems differ in their descriptions of the clinical features. In the ICD diagnostic system, somatoform pain disorder is defined as persistent pain without clear medical explanation.[5] The DSM system[4] specifies that 'psychological factors are judged to have an important role in the onset, severity, exacerbation, or maintenance of the pain'. Both definitions are somewhat problematic. Basic research on neural changes associated with persistent pain raise doubts about the distinction between pain with and without a biomedical explanation.[32] As discussed below, longitudinal research supports the view that persistent pain causes psychological disorder as much as it supports the DSM view that pain results from psychological distress. Recent epidemiological research has attempted to avoid questions of aetiology and has examined the prevalence and correlates of persistent pain.

### Prevalence

Epidemiological studies consistently find that pain syndromes are among the most common problems presented to general medical providers. Population surveys indicate that over 25 per cent of community residents suffer from recurrent or persistent pain symptoms and that 2 to 3 per cent experience disabling pain syndromes.[33] The recent WHO primary care survey[34] found that approximately 20 per cent of primary care patients suffered from persistent pain (one or more pain symptoms present for most of the last 6 months). Pain syndromes are approximately twice as prevalent in women as in men.[15]

The limited data available do not allow definite conclusions about cross-cultural or cross-national variability in pain syndromes.

Some studies have documented cross-national or cross-cultural differences based on small samples of patients treated for pain syndromes—often in specialist pain clinics.[35] The WHO primary care survey[34] included both the largest number of patients with pain syndromes as well as the broadest range of cultures and levels of economic development. In that study, both the prevalence and correlates of persistent pain varied widely across sites. No clear pattern (e.g. a higher prevalence in developing or non-Western countries) was evident.

### Correlates

All available data indicate that pain symptoms are strongly associated with anxiety and depressive disorders. This relationship has been consistently demonstrated in both community[36] and primary care[34] studies across a broad range of cultural and socioeconomic divides. Psychological distress is most strongly associated with pain occurring at multiple sites and pain associated with functional impairment.[37, 38] While epidemiological studies strongly support an association between pain complaints and psychological distress, this does not necessarily imply that pain is a consequence of psychological distress. Some studies find that the presence of psychological distress predicts the onset of pain syndromes,[39,40] while others support the opposite relationship—that persistent pain predicts subsequent psychological disorder.[41]

## Other somatoform conditions

### Specific somatoform syndromes

A number of specific somatic syndromes have been described over the last several decades. These specific syndromes are sometimes defined by the particular somatic symptoms experienced (e.g. fibromyalgia, irritable bowel syndrome, chronic fatigue syndrome) and sometimes by particular beliefs about aetiology (e.g. multiple chemical sensitivity, systemic candidiasis, electrical allergy). In every case, controversy persists about whether the somatic symptoms should be considered 'medically unexplained' (that is to say a somatoform disorder). Community surveys suggest that non-specific symptoms (such as fatigue or diffuse musculoskeletal pain) are common, but that the prevalence of strictly defined syndromes (such as fibromyalgia or chronic fatigue syndrome) varies considerably with the criteria applied.[42, 43] Most of these syndromes appear more often in women than in men.[44] Both community[43, 44] and primary care surveys[45, 46] have found several of these syndromes to be associated with anxiety and depressive symptoms. However, two studies of chronic fatigue[47] and irritable bowel[48] symptoms found that psychological distress was associated with seeking care for somatic symptoms rather than the presence or nature of the somatic symptoms themselves.

### Body dysmorphic disorder or monosymptomatic hypochondriasis

Body dysmorphic disorder has recently been identified as a distinct clinical entity. The limited epidemiological data available suggest significant overlap with anxiety and depressive disorders.[8, 50] Prevalence estimates range from less than 1 per cent among unselected primary care patients,[8] to as high as 5 to 10 per cent among patients seeking cosmetic surgery[49] or outpatients with anxiety

**Table 5.2.2.1** Summary of prevalence rates of specific somatoform disorders in community and primary care studies

| | Community studies | Primary care studies | Notes |
|---|---|---|---|
| Somatization disorder | 1% | 1–2% | Diagnostic interviews probably under-count past symptoms, records reviews tend to find higher rates |
| Multisomatoform disorder or subthreshold somatization | 5% | 8–10% | Less extreme form of somatization, but still strongly associated with disability and symptoms of depression and anxiety |
| Hypochondriasis | 1% | 1–5% | Strongly associated with anxiety disorders |
| Persistent pain syndromes | 2–3% | 15–20% | Bi-directional relationship with depressive and anxiety disorders |
| Body dysmorphic disorder | 1% | 1–5% | Significantly higher in certain medical settings (dermatology, cosmetic surgery) and in people with anxiety disorders |

disorders.[50] Some questionnaire studies find prevalence rates as high as 5 per cent among university students.[51]

### Conversion disorders

Limited epidemiological data are available concerning conversion-type somatoform disorders. As with other varieties of unexplained somatic symptoms, these disorders appear to be more common among women[52] and are associated with increased prevalence of depressive and anxiety disorders.[53] Some evidence suggests that these conditions have declined in prevalence.[52] While many sources report that these conditions are more common in non-Western or developing countries, available epidemiological data do not necessarily support this view.[9]

### Factitious disorders

No systematic data are available regarding the epidemiology of factitious disorders. The available data include numerous case reports and a small number of case series—typically drawn from medical inpatient or medical specialty settings. Because the syndrome is defined by deception, it is likely that a large proportion of cases go undetected.

## Further information

Creed, F. and Barsky, A. (2004). A systematic review of the epidemiology of somatisation disorder and hypochondriasis. *Journal of Psychosomatic Research*, **56**, 391–408.

Ustun, T.B. and Sartorius, N. (eds.). (1995). *Mental illness in general health care*. John Wiley & Sons, Chichester, England.

## References

1. Kleinman, A. (1977). Depression, somatization and the "new cross-cultural psychiatry". *Social Science & Medicine*, **11**, 3–10.
2. Goldberg, D. and Bridges, K. (1988). Somatic presentations of psychiatric illness in primary care. *Journal of Psychosomatic Research*, **32**, 137–44.
3. Barsky, A. (1992). Amplification, somatization, and the somatoform disorders. *Psychosomatics*, **33**, 28–34.
4. American Psychiatric Association. (1994). *Diagnostic and statistical manual of mental disorders* (4th edn). American Psychiatric Association, Washington, DC.
5. World Health Organization. (1992). *The ICD-10 classification of mental and behavioural disorders. Clinical descriptions and diagnostic guidelines.* World Health Organization, Geneva.
6. Swartz, M., Blazer, D., George, L., *et al.* (1986). Somatization disorder in a community population. *American Journal of Psychiatry*, **143**, 1403–8.
7. Grabe, H., Meyer, C., Hapke, U., *et al.* (2003). Specific somatoform disorders in the general population. *Psychosomatics*, **44**, 304–11.
8. Faravelli, C., Salvatori, S., Galassi, F., *et al.* (1997). Epidemiology of somatoform disorders: a community survey in Florence. *Social Psychiatry and Psychiatric Epidemiology*, **32**, 24–9.
9. Gureje, O., Simon, G., Ustun, T., *et al.* (1997). Somatization in cross-cultural perspective: a World Health Organization study in primary care. *American Journal of Psychiatry*, **154**, 989–95.
10. Simon, G. and Gureje, O. (1999). Stability of somatization disorder and somatization symptoms among primary care patients. *Archives of General Psychiatry*, **56**, 90–5.
11. Kroenke, K. and Spitzer, R. (1998). Gender differences in the reporting of physical and somatoform symptoms. *Psychosomatcic Medicine*, **60**, 150–5.
12. Ladwig, K., Marten-Mittag, B., Erazo, N., *et al.* (2001). Identifying somatization disorder in a population-based health examination survey: psychosocial burden and gender differences. *Psychosomatics*, **42**, 511–18.
13. LeResche, L., Mancl, L., Drangsholt, M., *et al.* (2005). Relationship of pain and symptoms to pubertal development in adolescents. *Pain*, **118**, 201–9.
14. Simon, G.E., VonKorff, M., Piccinelli, M., *et al.* (1999). An international study of the relation between somatic symptoms and depression. *New England Journal of Medicine*, **341**, 1329–35.
15. Kroenke, K., Spitzer, R.L., Williams, J.B.W., *et al.* (1994). Physical symptoms in primary care: predictors of psychiatric disorders and functional impairment. *Archieves of Family Medicine*, **3**, 774–9.
16. Gureje, O. and Simon, G. (1999). The natural history of somatisation in primary care. *Psychological Medicine*, **29**, 669–76.
17. Ulasahin, A., Basoglu, M., and Paykel, E. (1994). A cross-cultural comparative study of depressive symptoms in British and Turkish clinical samples. *Social Psychiatry and Psychiatric Epidemiology*, **29**, 31–9.
18. Escobar, J., Gomez, J., and Tuason, V. (1983). Depressive phenomenology in North and South American patients. *American Journal of Psychiatry*, **140**, 47–51.
19. Ebert, D. and Martus, P. (1994). Somatization as a core symptom of melancholic type depression. Evidence from a cross-cultural study. *Journal of Affective Disorder*, **32**, 253–6.
20. Creed, F. and Barsky, A. (2004). A systematic review of the epidemiology of somatisation disorder and hypochondriasis. *Journal of Psychosomatic Research*, **56**, 391–408.
21. Mayou, R., Kirmayer, L., Simon, G., *et al.* (2005). Somatoform disorder: time for a new approach in DSM-V. *American Journal of Psychiatry*, **162**, 847–55.
22. Escobar, J.I., Burnam, M.A., Karno, M., *et al.* (1987). Somatization in the community. *Archives of General Psychiatry*, **44**, 713–18.
23. Kroenke, K., Spitzer, R., deGruy, F., *et al.* (1997). Multisomatoform disorder. An alternative to undifferentiated somatoform disorder for the somatizing patient in primary care. *Archives of General Psychiatry*, **54**, 352–8.

24. American Psychiatric Association. (1995). *Diagnostic and statistical manual of mental disorders (DSM-IV)* (4th edn), *primary care version*. American Psychiatric Press, Washington.

25. Looper, K.J. and Kirmayer L.J. (2001). Hypochondriacal concerns in a community population. *Psychological Medicine*, **31**, 577–84.

26. Escobar, J., Gara, M., Waitzkin, H., *et al.* (1998). DSM-IV hypochondriasis in primary care. *General Hospital Psychiatry*, **20**, 155–9.

27. Barsky, A., Wyshak, G., Klerman, G., *et al.* (1990). The prevalence of hypochondriasis in medical outpatients. *Social Psychiatry and Psychiatric Epidemiology*, **25**, 89–94.

28. Gureje, O., Ustun, T., and Simon, G. (1997). The syndrome of hypochondriasis: a cross-national study in primary care. *Psychological Medicine*, **27**, 1001–10.

29. Noyes, R.J. (1999). The relationship of hypochondriasis to anxiety disorders. *General Hospital Psychiatry*, **21**, 8–17.

30. Barsky, A., Wyshak, G., and Klerman, G. (1992). Psychiatric comorbidity in DSM-IIIR hypochondriasis. *Archives of General Psychiatry*, **49**, 101–8.

31. Simon, G., Gureje, O., and Fullerton, C. (2001). Course of hypochondriasis in an international primary care study. *General Hospital Psychiatry*, **23**, 51–5.

32. Coderre, T., Katz, J., Vaccarine, A.L., *et al.* (1993). Contribution of central neuroplasticity to pathological pain: review of clinical and experimental evidence. *Pain*, **52**, 259–85.

33. Von Korff, M., Dworkin, S.F., and Le Resche, L. (1990). Graded chronic pain status: an epidemiologic evaluation. *Pain*, **40**(3), 279–91.

34. Gureje, O., Von Korff, M., Simon, G.E., *et al.* (1998). Persistent pain and well-being. A World Health Organization study in primary care. *Journal of American Medical Association*, **280**, 147–51.

35. Sanders, S., Brena, S., Spier, C., *et al.* (1992). Chronic low back pain patients around the world: cross-cultural similarities and differences. *Clinical Journal of Pain*, **8**, 317–23.

36. McWilliams, L., Cox, B., and Enns, M. (2003). Mood and anxiety disorders associated with chronic pain: an examination in a nationally representative sample. *Pain*, **106**, 127–33.

37. Dworkin, S.F., Von Korff, M., and LeResche, L. (1990). Multiple pains and psychiatric disturbance: an epidemiologic investigation. *Archives of General Psychiatry*, **47**, 239–44.

38. Benjamin, S., Morris, S., McBeth, J., *et al.* (2000). The association between chronic widespread pain and mental disorder: a population-based study. *Arthritis and Rheumatism*, **43**, 561–7.

39. Von Korff, M., Le Resche, L., and Dworkin, S.F. (1993). First onset of common pain symptoms: a prospective study of depression as a risk factor. *Pain*, **55**, 251–8.

40. Croft, P., Papageorgiou, A., Ferry, S., *et al.* (1995). Psychologic distress and low back pain. Evidence from a prospective study in the general population. *Spine*, **15**, 2731–7.

41. VonKorff, M. and Simon, G.E. (1996). The relationship between pain and depression. *British Journal of Psychiatry*, **168**(Suppl. 30), 101–8.

42. Wessely, S., Chalder, T., Hirsch, S., *et al.* (1997). The prevalence and morbidity of chronic fatigue and chronic fatigue syndrome: a prospective primary care study. *American Journal of Public Health*, **87**, 1449–55.

43. Wolfe, F., Ross, K., Anderson, J., *et al.* (1995). The prevalence and characteristics of fibromyalgia in the general population. *Arthritis and Rheumatism*, **38**, 19–28.

44. Pawlikowska, T., Chalder, T., Hirsch, S., *et al.* (1994). Population-based study of fatigue and psychological distress. *British Medical Journal*, **308**, 763–6.

45. Wessely, S., Chalder, T., Hirsch, S., *et al.* (1996). Psychological symptoms, somatic symptoms, and psychiatric disorder in chronic fatigue and chronic fatigue syndrome: a prospective study in the primary care setting. *American Journal of Psychiatry*, **153**, 1050–9.

46. Henningsen, P., Zimmermann, T., and Sattel, H. (2003). Medically unexplained physical symptoms, anxiety, and depression: a meta-analytic review. *Psychosomatic Medicine*, **65**, 528–33.

47. Lawrie, S., Manders, D., Geddes, J., *et al.* (1997). A population-based incidence study of chronic fatigue. *Psychological Medicine*, **27**, 343–53.

48. Whitehead, W., Bosmajian, L., Zonderman, A., *et al.* (1988). Symptoms of psychologic distress associated with irritable bowel syndrome. Comparison of community and medical clinic samples. *Gastroenterology*, **95**, 709–14.

49. Sarwer, D., Wadden, T., Pertschuk, M., *et al.* (1998). Body image dissatisfaction and body dysmorphic disorder in 100 cosmetic surgery patients. *Plastic and Reconstructive Surgery*, **101**, 1644–9.

50. Simeon, D., Hollander, E., Stein, D., *et al.* (1995). Body dysmorphic disorder in the DSM-IV field trial for obsessive-compulsive disorder. *American Journal of Psychiatry*, **152**, 1207–9.

51. Bohne, A., Wilhelm, S., Keuthen, N., *et al.* (2002). Prevalence of body dysmorphic disorder in a German college student sample. *Psychiatry Research*, **109**, 101–4.

52. Singh, S. and Lee, A. (1997). Conversion disorders in Nottingham: alive, but not kicking. *Journal of Psychosomatic Research*, **43**, 425–30.

53. Sar, V., Akyuz, G., Kundakci, T., *et al.* (2004). Childhood trauma, dissociation, and psychiatric comorbidity in patients with conversion disorder. *American Journal of Psychiatry*, **161**, 2271–6.

# 5.2.3 Somatization disorder and related disorders

Per Fink

## Introduction

The essential feature of somatization disorder and related disorders is that the patient presents multiple, medically unexplained symptoms or functional somatic symptoms. These physical complaints are not consistent with the clinical picture of known, verifiable, conventionally defined diseases, and are unsupported by clinical or paraclinical findings. The phenomenon of medically unexplained symptoms cannot simply be classified into one or a few diagnostic categories, but must be regarded as an expression of a basic mechanism by which people may respond to stressors as in the cases of depression and anxiety.[1–3] Somatization disorder and related disorders must thus be considered to possess a spectrum of severity.[3, 4] In this chapter, the focus will be on the chronic and multisymptomatic forms.

The somatization disorder diagnosis has its origin in the concept of hysteria. It was introduced in DSM-III in 1980 and was based on the criteria for 'Briquet's syndrome', a syndrome described in the early 1960s by Perley and Guze.[5] They listed 59 physical and psychological symptoms distributed in 10 groups: 25 of the symptoms from nine groups were required to qualify for the diagnosis of somatization disorder. All psychological symptoms were eliminated in the DSM-III modification to avoid overlapping with other diagnoses.

The diagnostic criteria for DSM somatization disorder varied until the introduction of the current DSM-IV. The diagnosis was included in ICD-10 in 1992, but the ICD-10 criteria list different symptoms, and require a different number of symptoms compared with the corresponding DSM criteria.

The somatization disorder diagnosis has been criticized for being too rigid for clinical use. Only the most severe cases with a specific predefined symptom profile fulfil the diagnostic criteria, and the majority of those with multiple symptoms fall into one of the residual categories of 'undifferentiated' or 'not otherwise specified' somatoform disorders.[6]

To increase the sensitivity, Escobar *et al.*[7] introduced an abridged somatization index. This required 4 symptoms for males and 6 symptoms for females out of the 37 somatic symptoms listed in the DSM-III, compared with 12 and 14 symptoms respectively for the full DSM-III somatization disorder diagnosis. Kroenke *et al.*[8] have suggested a diagnosis of 'multisomatoform disorder', defined as three or more medically unexplained physical symptoms from a 15-symptom checklist along with at least a 2-year history of medically unexplained symptoms.

However, these abridged versions share the same basic problem as the original ones, namely that the chosen number of symptoms to qualify for the individual diagnoses is arbitrary and not empirically based. Recently a new empirically based construct was introduced, and this may have solved the problem. This new 'bodily distress disorder' diagnosis is based on positive criteria and not solely on the exclusion of all organic possibilities.[3] (Table 5.2.3.1)

This chapter will not differentiate between the different subcategories of somatoform and related disorders that are present along with somatic symptoms.

**Table 5.2.3.1** Symptoms of and diagnostic criteria for bodily distress disorder

| Yes | No | Symptom groups |
|-----|-----|----------------|
| | | ≥ 3 Cardiopulmonal/autonomic arousal<br>Palpitations, heart pounding, precordial discomfort, breathlessness without exertion, hyperventilation, hot or cold sweats, trembling or shaking, dry mouth, churning in stomach, "butterflies", flushing or blushing |
| | | ≥ 3 Gastrointestinal arousal<br>Frequent loose bowel movements, abdominal pains, feeling bloated, full of gas, distended, heavy in the stomach, regurgitations, constipation, nausea, vomiting, burning sensation in chest or epigastrium |
| | | ≥ 3 Musculoskeletal tension<br>Pains in arms or legs, muscular aches or pains, feelings of paresis or localized weakness, back ache, pain moving from one place to another, unpleasant numbness or tingling sensations |
| | | ≥ 3 General symptoms<br>Concentration difficulties, impairment of memory, feeling tired, headache, memory loss, dizziness |
| | | ≥ 4 symptoms from one of the above groups |

**Diagnostic criteria:**

1–3: 'yes': Moderate 'bodily distress disorder'
4–5: 'yes': Severe 'bodily distress disorder'

# Clinical features

## Physical symptoms and complaints

Patients with somatization and related disorders may complain of any medically unexplained non-verifiable subjective physical symptoms, and the symptoms may refer to any part or system of the body.

Complaints can be divided into:

◆ *Subjective symptoms*, which are sensations and other complaints that cannot be verified by another individual or by general methods of examination (e.g. pains and paraesthesia).

◆ *Objective symptoms*, which are complaints that can be verified if present at the time of examination (e.g. haematuria, icterus, etc.).

Findings can be divided into:

◆ *Provoked findings*, i.e. symptoms or signs (such as soreness resulting from pressure or sensory impairment), which the patient is unaware of until these are provoked during the physical examination

◆ *Certain findings*, which include objective symptoms that are verified and phenomena unnoticed by the patient but found during the physical examination (such as an abdominal tumor)

The symptom complaints in patients with somatization disorder and related disorders are dominated by subjective symptoms and provoked findings, whereas objective symptoms and positive certain findings and paraclinical findings are unusual.

Subjective symptoms may be considered to be psychological phenomena arising from personal experiences, which others cannot judge or measure, despite the fact that these symptoms could be fully explained by the presence of organic pathology. This means that there are considerable inter-individual, cultural, and historical variations in the symptom presentation, which are determined by the patient's life experience and sociocultural background, and the setting in which the patient is seen also plays a role.[9] However, the patients may also present verifiable symptoms and signs due to a physical disease or defect, which they exaggerate and incorporate into their illness. Incidental inborn errors or degenerative changes, which are asymptomatic in most individuals, may tenuously be assigned clinical importance by the doctor or the patient. For instance, degenerative changes in the spinal column are seen in most individuals when they become older, and most do not have any pain, but a patient's backache may be attributed to those changes. Furthermore, over time, the patient with a chronic condition is likely to have undergone multiple tests, invasive procedures, operations, and received medications for treatment or diagnostic purposes, and this may cause not only iatrogenic harm but also physical complications.[10] Finally, the patient may have a concurrent physical disease. The presented symptoms may thus be a difficult mixture of complaints of both organic and non-organic origin.[11]

The patients typically complain of *multiple physical symptoms*, but the number of symptoms reported by the patients vary considerably from one patient to another and over time in the same individual. The patients may complain of multiple, medically unexplained symptoms in numerous bodily systems at presentation, but sometimes the complaints are concentrated on one symptom pattern at one time (e.g. a gastrointestinal illness) and on a different symptom pattern at another (e.g. a cardiopulmonary illness).[11] This single-organ illness picture may be due to physicians being inclined to focus their attention and investigation on the organ of their own specialty—especially in a multisymptomatic, complex patient, i.e. a gastroenterologist will focus on gastrointestinal symptoms and may ignore musculoskeletal symptoms. A new set of symptoms from another organ system may come to attention when diagnoses and treatment options have been ruled out for the current complaint. Iatrogenic factors may thus contribute significantly to the presented symptom pattern and changes in symptom pattern. Patients with somatization disorder are often inconsistent historians. They may supply incorrect information about previous episodes of their illness, minimizing or ignoring earlier instances of illness and exclusively focusing on the current symptom pattern. This may be because the patients find it difficult to account for their complicated medical history, or because they do not want to confuse the doctor with what they believe is irrelevant information. Therefore, the full clinical picture often only becomes evident after a full medical history has been obtained and the patient has been followed for some time.

Symptoms and findings are not idiosyncratic but need clarification or specification before becoming meaningful clinically. For instance, a patient complains of chest pain. There are multiple causes for chest pain, so for the doctor this is not very informative. A clarification or specification is needed. A retrosternal-localized pain of a pressing nature offers the doctor a very different diagnostic association than a chest pain that is described as being stabbing and located in the left side of the chest. In somatization disorder and related disorders, the patient usually presents a *vague illness picture*

with symptoms of *non-specific* character and of low diagnostic value, i.e. symptoms that are common in the general population and which are found in many different mental and physical disorders (symptoms like fatigue, nausea, headache, dizziness).

The presentation of medically unexplained symptoms is *atypical*, that is to say the symptoms lie outside what is usual in an authentic physical disease.[11] However, the patients may have 'learned' the typical symptom presentation from different sources. For example, a patient with atypical asthma-like attacks shared a room with a patient with genuine asthma during her third hospital stay; subsequently, her attacks took on a more 'authentic' appearance.[11]

Descriptions of *symptoms are usually vague, imprecise, and inconsistent*, and the patients often have difficulties giving further details about their illness and symptoms, i.e. describing the quality, intensity, and chronology. The symptoms are described as being of maximum intensity all the time, but if the patients keep a diary of symptoms or if information is gathered from other sources like relatives or the family physician, a considerable variation in the symptom intensity from day to day or from year to year often surfaces. The patients may have difficulties in the chronology of symptoms, mixing current and past symptoms and illness episodes in a disorganized and confusing manner. It is difficult for the patients to identify relieving factors or behaviour and to identify triggering events or things that make them worse, or these are multiple, or vague and unspecific. This is in contrast to patients with physical disease, who usually describe their symptoms in a consistent and precise manner (Table 5.2.3.2).

Typically, there is a marked *discrepancy* between a patient's subjective complaints and reports on his or her functioning when this is compared with the way the patient is observed to act, move

**Table 5.2.3.2** Characteristic differences in symptom description and other characteristics of well-defined somatic and related disorders including functional somatic syndromes

| | Somatization disorder and related disorders | Physical disease |
|---|---|---|
| **Symptom description** | | |
| Location | Vague, diffuse, alternating | Well-defined, constant |
| Intensity | Vague, indistinctly defined intensity, few variations, often at maximum at all times | Well-defined changes and levels of intensity |
| Periodicity | Diffuse, difficult to define, are often denied | Typically well-defined periods with aggravation or improvement |
| Relieving or aggravating factors | Vague, indistinct, numerous | Well-defined, few |
| Number of symptoms | Numerous, vague | Few, well-defined, clearly described |
| The nature of symptoms | Unspecific | Specific |
| The character of the symptoms | Uncharacteristic | Characteristic |
| Iatropic symptoms and main complaints | Vague, difficult to identify | Can be identified and delimited from comorbid symptoms |
| Description | Affective, emotional, interpreting | Clear and descriptive |
| **Other characteristics** | | |
| Treatment and medication | Difficult to assess the effect, transitory | Level of effect well-defined |
| Previous treatment | Unclear what treatment the patient has undergone. Diagnostic tests are often interpreted as treatment | The patient can account for previous treatments |
| Emotionality | Inadequate, e.g. exaggerated or marked unaffectedness ('la belle indifférence') | Adequate - empathic |

and perform during the examination, or compared with information from other sources like family. For instance, the patient moves and sits completely freely despite complaining of severe back pain or gives detailed information despite complaints of severe memory impairment.

There may be *emotional discrepancy* in which the patient shows a lack of concern about the nature and implications of the symptoms despite presenting severe symptoms that are threatening the patient's future functioning and quality of life. Other patients may in turn be very affected and emotional in their description of the symptoms and illness, describing in a colourful, dramatic, and strikingly graphic manner.

The patient's centre of attention is typically on the suffering, on the psychosocial consequences, and the restrictions that the symptoms impose on their life. On the contrary, patients with well-defined physical disease are concerned or worried about the implication of their disease for their future health, i.e. will they recover or will they die from the disease. This emotional or *psychosocial communication* among patients with somatization disorder may put pressure on the doctor to do something.

Patients with somatization disorder and related disorders usually attribute their symptoms to a physical disease, and in some cases they persistently may *refuse to accept medical reassurance* despite appropriate medical evaluations. The ICD-10 criteria for somatoform disorders include this refusal to accept medical reassurance, but recent research indicates that many patients are unsure what is wrong with them, and they do not necessarily refuse non-medical explanations if they are presented in a meaningful and understandable way.[12] Although the patients may recognize that their physical symptoms are caused by, e.g. stressful events, this does not make the symptoms disappear, and they still need treatment. The weight of the symptom (refusing to accept medical reassurance) in the medical literature therefore seems out of proportion. However, in the most severe cases, patients may be involved in patient organizations fighting for their illness to be recognized as an 'authentic' physical disease or fighting for a particular causality of their illness as, e.g. whiplash-associated disorder or hypersensitivity to electricity or chemicals (multiple chemical sensitivity). The patients may also fight for disability pension or financial compensation. This is often more a question of getting their illness recognized than receiving financial compensation. Some patients may be preoccupied with the idea that they have been mistreated or neglected by doctors, and this group will often become involved in conflicts with doctors and in legal disputes.

In some cases, there is a sudden onset of the disorder in connection with a medical condition or a trauma in a previously normal and healthy individual. It could be a whiplash trauma, a fracture, an infection, or an acute intoxication. The symptoms persist despite the original disease being cured according to a biomedical or a surgical judgement. Instead, the illness worsens and more symptoms may emerge. Our knowledge about such disorders with abrupt onset is sparse.

## Psychological symptoms and comorbidity

At examination, the patients may deny emotional symptoms or conflicts, and when they do report them, they often blame them on their physical affliction. Patients may also be reluctant to display emotional difficulties because of bad experiences of doing so. They may have experienced that doctors did not believe them or accused them of making up their symptoms and have consequently felt that their physical problems are not taken seriously. However, sooner or later, most patients will exhibit emotional difficulties, and if the patients feel understood by the physician, emotional problems may as well be presented. Patients may present many different types of emotional symptoms, often unspecific, but prominent anxiety and depressive symptoms are prevalent. Although the symptoms may be as marked as in affective and anxiety disorders, they are usually more transient, changing from one day to another and especially related to specific events. At times, the psychological symptoms may fulfil the criteria for a mood or anxiety disorder; but it is characteristic that the illness picture shows variations in both bodily and emotional symptoms.

Suicidal attempts are unusual but may occur especially among severe cases, but suicide is rare. Substance abuse is frequent, whether or not this is iatrogenic sanctioned.

The way the patients present themselves is inextricably linked to personal style and possible personality disorder. As a broad spectrum of personality disorders or traits[13] is associated with somatization disorder, the presenting style varies greatly from one patient to another. Characteristically, three broad patterns of personality style may be found in these patients, especially in chronic cases: dramatic–emotional type, paranoid–hostile type, and passive–aggressive-dependent type. The same patient may show all three patterns. In less severe cases it is often observed clinically that the patients have previously been very active and hard working, have conformed socially, and had a strong social network with many responsibilities. The patients often display perfectionist traits and prefer to be in control of a situation.

## Illness behaviour

Typically, patients with somatization disorder persistently exhibit consulting behaviour which results in an excessive use of medical services and alternative therapies. In chronic cases, they have often been subject to a large number of futile examinations, surgery, and medical/surgical attempts at treatment.[10,14,15] However, some patients realize quite early in the illness course that the doctors cannot help them, or they are well managed by their family physician, so they do not necessarily display this consultation behaviour.

Due to negative results of medical check-up and treatment attempts and the patients' persistent belief that they must have a physical disease, the patients may consult different physicians. The patients may have been, or may feel, mistreated or neglected by doctors and therefore want to get a second opinion, or they want to find a doctor who can help them. Sometimes this behaviour, together with the patients' personality, can result in disagreement and a mutual hostility between the patients and their doctors.

Furthermore, the different illness patterns at different times, combined with the patients' seductive, demanding personality style, may result in disagreements between the different health care professionals involved in their care, which may complicate their care.

In chronic cases, all aspects of the patients' social and family life may be centered around their illness, so that the whole of their family life is adjusted to the patients' demands ('illness as a way of living').[16]

## Classification

The diagnostic criteria for somatization disorder and related disorders have varied, with different permutations of the diagnostic terminology reflecting difficulties in classification and in establishing valid criteria. The distinction between the individual somatoform disorders is unclear, which means that the majority of patients will exhibit clinical characteristics from different diagnostic categories.[6]

Except for hypochondriasis or health anxiety, the somatoform disorder categories are primarily based on the number or specificity of bodily symptoms and on the duration of illness.[17] The disorders can be divided into acute and chronic forms, into a multisymptomatic form, and into a form in which the patients only present few symptoms or symptoms mainly referring to a single organ system. The somatization disorder diagnosis includes the most chronic multisymptomatic cases lasting for 2 years or more.

The ICD-10 criteria require the following:

1 at least 2 years of multiple and variable physical symptoms for which no adequate physical explanation has been found;

2 persistent refusal to accept the advice or reassurance of several doctors that there is no physical explanation for the symptoms;

3 some degree of impairment of social and family functioning attributable to the nature of the symptoms and resulting behaviour.

The ICD-10 criteria require 'multiple physical symptoms' to include at least 6 out of 14 predefined symptoms, involving at least 2 of the following: gastrointestinal, cardiovascular, urogenital, or skin or pain symptoms. In contrast, the DSM-IV criteria demand four pain symptoms, two gastrointestinal symptoms, one sexual symptom, and one pseudoneurological symptom that are not fully explained by a medical condition. No specific symptoms are listed, but examples are given. Consequently, there is only poor to moderate agreement between the DSM-IV and ICD-10 diagnostic criteria.[16] Cases lasting less than 2 years are classified as undifferentiated somatization disorder. In ICD-10, multiple symptoms are required, which is not the case in DSM-IV.

Functional or somatoform diagnoses defined mainly by the number or specificity of bodily symptoms include, besides somatization disorder (F45.0 and 300.81), undifferentiated SD (F45.1 and 300.81), persistent somatoform pain disorder (F45.4 and 307.80), and somatoform disorder unspecified/NOS (F45.9 and 300.82). In ICD-10, this also includes somatoform autonomic dysfunction.[3–5] There may be reasons for also including neurasthenia (F48.0) into the group. The somatoform disorder concept has never been accepted among non-psychiatrists, which has led to the introduction of many different functional somatic syndromes, e.g. chronic fatigue syndrome (CFS), fibromyalgia, irritable bowel syndrome (IBS), and chronic benign pain syndrome, and new syndromes are intermittently introduced.[18]

The newly introduced diagnosis of bodily distress syndrome or disorder may be a solution to this classification problem, although it has not yet been sufficiently tested in daily clinical practice.[3] The suggested diagnosis is based on an analysis of a large sample of patients from different medical settings, and it seems to encompass the various functional syndromes advanced by different medical specialties as well as somatization disorder and related diagnoses of the psychiatric classification. The disorder may have different manifestations, i.e. GI, MS, or CP syndromes as shown in Table 5.2.3.1.

## Diagnosis

A somatization disorder should be suspected in any individual with a vague or complicated medical history or unaccountable non-responsiveness to therapy. Patients with somatization disorder may not have or may deny emotional symptoms or conflicts, so the absence of significant emotional symptoms at the general psychiatric interview and history taking will not exclude the diagnosis. But the presence of a previous or current emotional disturbance does support the diagnosis, as do previous episodes of medically unexplained bodily symptoms. Taken at face value, the physical symptoms are only of modest diagnostic importance, whereas unspecific or atypical symptoms in several bodily systems, or a very unusual presentation, speak in favour of the diagnosis. Multiple fluctuating symptoms of obscure origin, and their onset before the age of 30, strongly support the diagnosis. The diagnostic criteria displayed in Table 5.2.3.1 may be used, or the criteria listed in the DSM-IV or ICD-10 diagnostic criteria for somatoform disorders may be used.

## Differential diagnosis

### Mental and somatoform disorders

In **malingering**, the patient feigns illness with a conscious motivation to avoid responsibility or to gain an advantage. In **factitious disorder**, the symptoms are intentionally produced and the patient may self-inflict or induce diseases and lesions. In contrast to malingering, there is no external incentive for producing the symptom(s), and the motive is unconscious and only understandable in a psychopathological context.[19, 20] In somatoform disorders, both the symptom-producing behaviour and the motive are believed to be unconscious. However, factitious or malingering symptoms, mixed with other non-intentional symptoms, may occur in somatization disorder and related disorders.[11]

**Hypochondriasis or health anxiety** is mainly defined in cognitive terms with the emphasis on a preoccupation with physical appearance or the fears of harbouring or developing a serious physical disease. The other categories of somatoform disorders put more emphasis on bodily symptoms. In **dissociative or conversion disorder** the patients usually present fewer symptoms, but these are almost exclusively pseudoneurological symptoms. The onset is sudden, and closely associated in time with traumatic events, insoluble and intolerable problems, or disturbed relationships. The symptoms are transient and often remit suddenly after a few days, although they may persist for longer, but seldom for more than a few months. Episodes of dissociative or conversion disorders frequently occur in patients with other somatoform disorders.

In **pain disorder**, the predominating complaints are of medically unexplained pain in one or more anatomical sites. Various aches and pains are common in somatization disorder but are more fluctuating and not so dominating in the clinical presentation since they merge with other complaints.

In **ICD-10 somatoform autonomic dysfunction**, the patients complain of symptoms associated with a specific system or organ that is largely or completely under autonomic innervation and control. For example, the patient refers the symptoms to the heart and cardiovascular system, the gastrointestinal tract, respiratory system, genitourinary system, etc.

In most **other mental disorders** physical symptoms are prominent; it is the rule, rather than the exception, that patients with mental disorders consult their family physician because of physical and not emotional symptoms.[2, 21] The symptoms may be misinterpreted by the patient and the doctor as being caused by a physical disease. However, in these cases of 'presenting' or 'facultative' somatizing, the patient will accept the diagnosis of a psychiatric disorder when it is established and will accept that the symptoms are attributable to a psychic rather than a physical affliction.[2]

Autonomic bodily symptoms are prominent in panic disorder and generalized anxiety disorders, but the emotional component of the disorders is unmistakable and the patients will not, or only temporarily, attribute their symptoms to a physical disease.

In psychoses, particular schizophrenic physical symptoms and hypochondriacal belief are common. However, the complaints are of a paranoid quality and other psychotic symptoms are prominent, except in the case of hypochondriacal paranoia. Psychotic episodes may occur in somatization disorder, but these are usually transient.[22]

In depressive disorders, the patient's complaints are mood congruent, and the symptoms will disappear if the depression is treated. In a few cases, however, a depression may be expressed in mainly bodily complaints (i.e. masked depression), and if left untreated may result in a prolonged course.

In obsessive-compulsive disorder (OCD), the patient may fear contracting a disease from an outside source (e.g. dirt, germs, viruses, etc.). The OCD disorders share many similarities with hypochondriasis, i.e. cognitive and emotional complaints are the main problem, whereas bodily symptoms seldom are dominating.

### Medical conditions

The onset of multiple physical symptoms after the age of 40, in a previously physically and mentally healthy individual, suggests a general medical condition. However, multiple vague physical complaints may be prominent in mental disorders with late onset such as mood disorders, dementia, and withdrawal states.

Only a limited number of general medical conditions present vague, non-specific, and multiple somatic symptoms (e.g. hyperparathyroidism, hyperthyroidism, acute intermittent porphyria, myasthenia gravis, AIDS, multiple sclerosis, systemic lupus erythematosus, lyme disease, and connective tissues disease). In most of these medical conditions there will be positive paraclinical findings.

In genuine physical disorders, the key symptoms will usually be characteristic from one patient to another and across illness episodes. In contrast, the constellation of symptoms in somatization disorder and related disorders will usually be incompatible with any known, authentic physical disease, and the symptom picture will be of a more fluctuating nature.

## Epidemiology

The prevalence of somatization disorder is about 1 per cent in the general population and 1 to 6 per cent in primary care and in inpatient medical settings, but it is much higher if less restrictive, abridged criteria are used.[3, 7, 8, 21, 23–28] Both among primary care patients, newly referred neurological in and outpatients, and among internal medicine inpatients, the prevalence of severe bodily distress disorder is 3.3 per cent, whereas the prevalence of modest bodily distress is 25.3 per cent.[3] Regardless of the criteria used, females predominate with a male-to-female ratio of 1:2 to 1:6, and the prevalence is rather constant as to age.[21, 24–29]

The age of onset is usually before 30 to 40 years.[14] This patient group poses a considerable financial burden to health and social service provision, a loss to industry, and a dependence on invalidity benefits for long periods.[14, 24, 30, 31]

Somatization disorder and related disorders are associated with a wide spectrum of heterogeneous psychiatric disorders, including personality disorders and mental retardation. The comorbidity rates are highest in the most chronic cases, in which rates of 50 per cent or higher are reported.[3, 13, 22, 24] Cultural and ethnic factors may affect the prevalence rate. This may be due to the influence of these factors on the likelihood of presentation to health care rather than real prevalence differences in the general population.[7, 21, 23] The typical presentation of physical complaints has varied throughout history and with the sociocultural environment of the patient.[32]

## Aetiology

The aetiology of somatization disorder is unknown, but it is most likely multifactorial including biological, physiological, psychological, social, cultural, and iatrogenic factors. Different factors may have different importance at different times in the natural course of the illness. For instance, it may be a psychological trauma that precipitates the illness—but iatrogenic factors that maintain the illness. Whether the behavioural, cognitive, and other typical disturbances in somatization disorder and related disorders develop as a consequence of a basic biological defect in interaction with the patient's life experiences, or vice versa, or whether the mentioned disturbances and other predisposing factors have an independent impact is, as yet, unresolved.

Viewing functional somatic symptoms as a common reaction of human beings to stressors, like in the case of depressed mood and anxiety, results in the conclusion that different unspecific predisposing factors common for different mental disorders are involved.[33] Relatively specific predisposing factors are physical or sexual abuse and parental complaints of poor physical health and medically unexplained symptoms during the patient's childhood, whereas neither parental nor childhood well-defined physical illnesses seem to be predisposing factors.[34, 35]

The reported family transmission in somatization disorder may be due to sociocultural learning. However, there is some support for genetic transmission in somatization disorder, although twin studies have been inconclusive.[36]

### Psychological theories

In the classical psychodynamic drive theory, medically unexplained physical symptoms are believed to develop as a reaction to the repression of unacceptable wishes or instinctual impulses and internal psychic conflicts.[37]

According to the theory of self-psychology, the anxiety connected with a threatening defragmentation or disintegration of the self is the most profound form of anxiety that a person can experience.[37] In a defence against the feeling of emptiness, the individual becomes directed on the outside world and on physical stimuli. This process has been called 'stimulus entrapment' meaning that in somatization disorder, the individual becomes addicted to stimuli to his or her body.[38]

Individuals with alexithymia have a poorly developed language of emotions, and it has been suggested that instead they might respond with bodily symptoms. It is, however, unlikely that alexithymia has a specific aetiological role in somatization disorder.

The cognitive theory endorses the importance of the patients' misinterpretation of benign symptoms and normal physical sensations that they erroneously attribute to a physical disease.[39]

### Biological factors

It is beyond doubt that an important biological component is involved, although the specific nature has still to be discovered. A neurophysiological dysfunction in the attention process has been demonstrated in somatization disorder, which may be explained by a reduced corticofugal inhibition in the diencephalon and the brainstem of afferent bodily stimuli, resulting in insufficient filtering of irrelevant bodily stimuli. A dysfunction of the secondary somatosensory area in the brain, a hypersensitivity of the limbic system towards bodily stimuli, or other dysfunctions may also be aetiologically involved.[40–42]

### Other factors

In a few cases, a simple compensation claim may be of aetiological importance.

Physicians are primarily trained in a biomedical illness model and may have insufficient knowledge about diagnosing and managing somatization disorder and related disorders. Physicians may thus have a tendency to pursue organic possibilities and feel compelled to evaluate and treat all symptoms, and consequently a considerable iatrogenic reinforcement of physical symptoms is often involved.

## Course and prognosis

Somatization disorder and related disorders have a spectrum of severity ranging from cases that may be difficult to delimit from normality to severely ill patients.[17]

In severe cases, the patients are chronically ill for most of their lives, but there may be periods of partial, but seldom full, remission. Some patients are able to work, others are severely disabled and are chair or bed bound, and their families have to provide virtually all aspects of physical care. Patients with somatization disorder and related disorders are often subjectively more functionally handicapped than patients who have a comparable, yet fully explained medical condition.[31]

## Assessment

The purposes of the initial assessment are to (a) establish the diagnosis and rule out differential diagnoses, (b) examine which specific management or treatment strategies are possible and best for the patient, and (c) engage the patient in therapy.[15]

A scheme for the initial assessment by the psychiatric specialist is given in Table 5.2.3.3. For primary care physicians and in general

**Table 5.2.3.3** Clinical assessment of patients with somatoform and related disorders including functional somatic syndromes

| Before the meeting with the patient | |
| --- | --- |
| Review medical records and other relevant material | |
| **At the examination** | |
| Attitude towards the referral and the treatment | |
| Physical complaints | Chronology, intensity, provoking / relieving factors etc. |
| Triggering factors | Physical trauma or disease |
| | Psychosocial stressors |
| Current and previous emotional and behavioural complaints | |
| Social, funtional level, strain and coping | |
| The patient's illness belief and perception of symptoms | |
| Expectations to treatment and investigation | Physical Psychiatric |
| Past medical, surgical, and psychological history | |
| Dispositions | |
| Physical examination | |
| Paraclinical tests: Obtain focused diagnostic tests if not already done | |

hospitals this may be too comprehensive, and step one in the TERM model (Table 5.2.3.5) or another more simple model may be used.[43]

### Before meeting the patient

Before meeting the patient it is important to review medical case notes and to gather information from other sources, e.g. the primary care physicians or the family, as patients with somatization disorder and related disorders may be inconsistent historians as a result of their complex medical history. The aim is to get an overview of the patient's medical history, the illness picture and complaints, examinations and diagnostic tests, and treatments and the outcome of these. It must also be assessed whether the patient is sufficiently examined for relevant differential diagnoses. The review may furthermore impart important information about psychological and social issues.

### The examination

#### (a) Attitudes towards the referral and treatment

Patients with somatization disorder and related disorders may be sceptical about seeing a psychiatrist as they believe their problem to be of a physical nature and not psychiatric. This should be addressed directly by asking the patients what they have been told by the referring doctor, their reasons for coming to see the psychiatrist, and their feelings about it. It is important that such thoughts are brought to light to avoid misunderstandings and misconceptions, and to help the patients feel understood and in safe hands. In acknowledging the patients' fears of being stigmatized, it may be helpful to discuss negative public attitudes to psychiatry.

### (b) Current physical complaints

The patients' physical complaints should be reviewed in detail for diagnostic purposes and to make the patients feel understood and taken seriously, which is a precondition for a good rapport between doctor and patient. Each symptom is explored to establish their characteristics, location, intensity, chronology and variation in intensity, onset, duration, and impact on daily life. Besides, provoking/relieving factors, previous treatments and the outcome of these are explored. It may be helpful together with the patient to write down the medical history on a time axis as patients may have difficulties with the chronology of their illness.

### (c) Triggering factors

It is explored if onset of the illness is associated with physical trauma or diseases or with exposure to psychosocial stress or trauma.

### (d) Current and previous emotional and behavioural complaints

As to a high comorbidity between somatization disorder and related disorders and other mental disorders, it is necessary to methodically clarify if the patients have a depression, anxiety disorder, or another mental illness.

### (e) Illness beliefs and perception of symptoms

The patients' illness beliefs and perception of symptoms are of paramount importance for their illness and functioning as the illness behaviour has its origin in those beliefs and in illness attitudes. To change an inappropriate behaviour, it is necessary to identify such dysfunctional beliefs. Also, the attitudes and behaviour of the family may be a crucial factor in understanding the presentation and in planning the intervention.

### (f) Expectations to treatments and investigations

The patients are questioned about wishes for and expectations to treatment and diagnostics tests and about what they believe may help them. Patients with somatization disorder and related disorders often have an unrealistic expectation to the impact of diagnostic tests and the effect of medical or surgical treatments. This may result in an intensive use of consultations. The patients must be helped to face the limits of what medicine can do and to acknowledge that continued medical consultations will be fruitless.

### (g) Past medical, surgical, and psychological history

The patients' history is reviewed and related to the information gathered during the medical case note review. Furthermore, it is attempted to elucidate the patients' premorbid psyche and personality.

### (h) Dispostions

Somatoform and related disorders often run in families and are associated with other mental disorders, and hence dispositions are explored.

### (i) Physical examination

If not already made, a clinical examination ought to be carried out. Besides excluding organic possibilities, it also has a psychological purpose in making the patients feel that their physical complaints are taken seriously and that the psychiatrist is not exclusively focusing on the psychological part of the problem.

Routine laboratory test battery may be; complete blood count, electrolytes, blood urea nitrogen, creatinine, glucose, calcium, phosphate, liver function test, total protein, thyroid-stimulation hormone, erythrocyte sedimentation rate or CPR, urinalysis, and if indicated by symptoms or history, serological tests for Epstein–Barr virus, lyme disease, and immunological function test. Other tests may be relevant depending on the patient's illness picture.

## Feedback of the results

Feedback of the psychiatric examination results to the referring doctor must be done in a way that is intelligible to a doctor who may not be psychologically minded. Statements like 'no formal psychiatric disorders are found', which unfortunately are frequent in consultation notes, may be somewhat useful when dealing with a patient referred for functional somatic symptoms. Such a statement just proves that the psychiatrist is unfamiliar with somatization disorder and related disorders.

The psychiatrist must be careful not to become involved in criticism of medical colleagues and in the divisions that these patients sometimes try to create between different therapists.

# Treatment and management

## Evidence-based treatment

Many different therapies have been used in patients with somatization disorder and related disorders like family therapy, physical therapy, biofeedback, relaxation therapies, hypnotherapy, psychodynamic psychotherapy, cognitive-behavioural therapy etc. The focus in the management varies a lot from (a) focus on the patients (organ-oriented approach or cognitive interpersonal approach, i.e. pattern of bodily and emotional symptoms over time, focus on dysfunction of central processing and context factors, interventions aimed at sensations, cognitions, affects, behaviours, and restoring overall function), (b) focus on the doctor (early recognition, communication skills, avoidance of iatrogenic harm), and (c) focus on context factors (doctor reimbursement system, patient compensation schemes, health care system, workplace characteristics, cultural belief).[44]

It must be concluded that the evidence for an effective treatment of patients with multiple functional symptoms is unsystematic. The use of multiple treatment methods and outcome measurement makes it difficult to compare studies. However, there seems to be substantial evidence that a specialized assessment with discharge letter, CBT, brief psychodynamic psychotherapy, and antidepressants have some effect on one or more outcome parameters.[44–47]

## Treatment setting

Functional somatic symptoms and functional somatic syndromes are common in all medical settings. The patients often believe that they have a physical and not a psychological problem and will primarily seek medical and not psychological care. Hence, the management of somatization disorder and related disorders is not only an issue for psychiatrists but for all settings within the health care system.

The management must follow a stepped-care model, in which it is defined at which level of specialization each patient should be treated and, for each step, who is responsible for which parts of the treatment. For example, the mild and uncomplicated cases are treated by the primary care physician, modest to severe cases mainly by the primary care physician but in collaboration with a specialist, whereas the severe and complicated cases are managed in specialized care.

Besides the severity of the disorder, defining the steps in the model includes considerations about feasibility both as to available treatment resources and what is acceptable to the patient and the skills and knowledge of the primary care physician. Patients with a chronic somatization disorder may be well cared for by their primary care physician, provided the latter has the necessary skills and knowledge.

Inpatient care may be appropriate in a few cases, but patients with somatization disorder and related disorders are difficult to treat in ordinary psychiatric wards, where they are often met with considerable resistance from the psychiatric staff. Specialized inpatient units only exist in a few places in the world, and this treatment has not been documented.

## Non-specialiszed treatment and management

### (a) General hospital departments and non-psychiatric specialists

Because of the prevalence and the risk of iatrogenic harm, it is important that non-psychiatric specialists know about somatoform and related disorders and know how to identify and diagnose them. If the assessing physician exclusively focuses on symptoms that he finds relevant for his own specialty, there is a great risk of pursuing a wrong diagnosis. The fear of overlooking a definite physical disease, as an explanation of the physical symptoms, is deeply rooted in doctors, and this may, together with a poor knowledge about somatoform disorders, result in the doctor attempting to rule out even the rarest physical causes before a somatization disorder is even considered. However, there is little evidence that important medical diagnoses are missed more often in patients with somatoform disorders than in patients with other disorders.[48–50] Unnecessary procedures and diagnostic tests are not only unpleasant and potentially risky for the patient but may also delay or hinder sufficient treatment resulting in an aggravation of the disorder or perhaps chronicity. However, it must always be borne in mind that patients with a somatoform disorder may also have or acquire a concurrent physical disease. Instead of viewing somatization disorder and related disorders as a diagnosis of exclusion, all diagnostic possibilities ought to be included in the diagnostic consideration and the examination plan from the initial contact in the same way as when it is a question about two well-defined organic diseases. Diagnostic tests should be on medical indication and not on patient demand.

The primary role of the non-psychiatric specialists in the treatment of somatization disorder and related disorders is to:

◆ Exclude physical disease or trauma that can be treated medically or surgically

◆ In an empathic way, make it clear to the patient that he or she does not have the physical disease he or she fears, and that there is no indication of any other physical disease or defect that needs medical attention.

◆ That there is no medical indication for further diagnostic tests or examinations

◆ Coordinate the management with the primary care physician and other doctors that the patient may be in contact with.

◆ Consider a referral to a psychiatrist for examination or treatment

◆ In chronic cases, follow the advice given in Table 5.2.3.4.

**Table 5.2.3.4** General advice on the non-specialized management of chronic somatization

### Physical

1. Make a brief physical examination focusing on the organ system from which the patient has (new) complaints.
   - Look for signs of disease instead of symptoms.
   - Avoid tests and procedures unless indicated by signs of disease or a well-defined (new) clinical illness picture.
2. Reduce unnecessary drugs. Do not use on demand prescriptions and avoid dependence-forming medication.

### Psychological

3. Make the diagnosis and inform the patient that the disorder is known and has a name.
4. Acknowledge the reality of the symptoms.
5. Be direct and honest with the patient about the areas you agree on, those you do not agree on, but be careful as not to make the patient feel ignorant or not respected.
6. Be stoical; do not expect rapid change or cure.
7. Reduce expectations of cure and accept the patient as being chronically ill. Aim at containment and (iatrogenic) damage limitation, i.e. use the management rather than treatment.
8. Perceive worsening of/or new symptoms as emotional communication rather than as a manifestation of a new disease.
9. Apply a specific therapeutic technique if you master it and consider referral to specialist treatment.

### Psychopharmacological treatment

10. Consider treatment with psychoactive mediation (primarily antidepressant).
11. Choose non-habit forming medication and, if possible, choose medication that can be serum monitored.
12. Start with a smaller dosage than usual and increase slowly. Be stoical about side effects.
13. Take regular serum values to compliance issued and for validating complaints of adverse effects.
14. Treat any co-existing psychiatric disorders according to usual guidelines.

### Administrative

15. Be proactive rather than reactive. Agree on a course with fixed, scheduled appointments with 2–6-weeks intervals and avoid consultations on patient demand (if needed, accept on demand a maximum of 1 phone appointment per week).
16. If the patient has a job, avoid giving him sick leave if at all possible.
17. Try to become the patient's only physician and minimize the patient's contact to other health care professionals, doctors on call, and alternative therapists.
18. Inform your colleagues of your management plans and develop contingency plans for when you are not accessible.
19. Inform the patient's nearest relative and try to co-opt a relative as a therapeutic ally.
20. If necessary, arrange support/supervision for yourself.
21. If necessary, motivate the patient to receive psychiatric treatment.

As previously mentioned, patients with somatization disorder are often resistant to psychiatric referral as they believe they have a physical and not a psychological problem. They may construe the referral as a sign that the physicians are not taking their symptoms seriously. It is important that the referring physicians avoid giving the message that the patients are not genuinely ill, that they trouble the doctors unnecessarily, or that they are 'mad'.[51] Instead, the physician must try to meet the patients' wishes about knowing the cause of their illness, being taken seriously, getting explanations, information, advice, and reassurance.[52] A close liaison with medical colleagues guiding them in making a psychiatric referral in an acceptable way is important for engaging the patient in treatment.

# Primary care

The TERM model (the extend reattribution model) is a simple cognitive-behavioural orientated treatment method to improve the primary care physicians' detection and management of patients presenting with medically unexplained symptoms. The method can effectively be taught to primary care physicians and will improve the outcome of their patients' treatment.[43] The TERM model is one of several different models that have been developed on the basis of the original reattribution model.[53,54]

The first stage of the TERM model (Table 5.2.3.5) is called 'understanding', as the important point, besides assessment of the patient, is that the patient feels understood and taken seriously by the doctor. The second stage is called 'the physician's expertise and acknowledgement of illness', in which the physician feeds back the results of his examination, but at the same time acknowledges the reality of the symptoms. The third stage is called 'reframing', in which a new model of understanding of the patient's problem is negotiated between patient and doctor. As a fourth stage, the model includes techniques for negotiating further treatment.[43]

Finally, the model includes principles for management of chronic, somatizing patients (Table 5.2.3.4). In chronic cases, damage limitation is a more realistic therapeutic goal than cure, and management is thus a more realistic aim than treatment.[51,55,56] The main aim is to stop the pathological cycle of interventions and consultations and the consequential somatic 'overtreatment' (i.e. treatment on obscure indication), and then, if possible, gradually to motivate the patient to accept specialized care if available in the area. Management according to these principles has shown to be effective in randomized controlled studies and should therefore always be implemented either solely or combined with one of the treatments described below.[57]

## Specialized treatment and management

Cognitive-behavioural therapy is the best documented and most widely used therapy and is hence the focus in this section along with pharmacotherapy. The general principles of CBT are described elsewhere, so this section concentrates on the general techniques used in somatization disorder and related disorders, and how they differ from the CBT techniques applied in other disorders.

### (a) Goal setting

Early in the therapy, the goals for the therapy are established. It is important to set up goals that are realistic in the light of the patient's illness and the framework of the therapy.

### (b) Engagement and motivation

Treatment of somatization disorder and related disorders differs from the treatment of other mental disorders on several points, one being that it is very important to work systematically by engaging the patients in therapy. As the patients believe they have a medical condition, they may have very low belief in psychological treatment. It may be helpful to discuss the idea that all illnesses have an emotional component and that a psychological treatment focusing

**Table 5.2.3.5** The TERM model

| |
|---|
| 1. **Understanding** |
| Take a full history of the symptoms |
| Explore emotional clues |
| Inquire directly about symptoms of anxiety and depression |
| Explore life events, stress, and other external factors |
| Explore functional level |
| Explore the patient's health beliefs |
| Explore the patient's expectations to treatment |
| Make a brief, focused physical examination |
| 2. **The physician's expertise and acknowledgement of illness** |
| Provide feedback on the results of the physical examination |
| Acknowledge the reality of the symptoms |
| Make it clear that there is no (or that there is indeed) indication for further examination of nonpsychiatric treatment |
| 3. **Negotiating a new model of understanding (reframing)** |
| Simple explanations |
|    Physical symptoms are common reactions to, for example, stress and strain/nervousness |
|    Depression lowers the threshold of pain |
|    Muscular tension in anxiety and nervousness causes pain |
| Demonstrations |
|    Practical (hyperventilation, muscular tension) |
|    Establish the association between physical discomfort, emotional reactions, and life events |
|    "Here and now" (nervous about consulting the physician) |
| Severe cases |
|    Known phenomenon with a name: somatization |
|    Basically the cause is unknown, but nothing indicates a hidden physical disease |
|    Biological explanation: some are bodily sensitive than others, which explains their more intense symptoms |
|    Individual symptom coping and reactions determine one's future well-being |
| 4. **Negotiating further treatment** |
| Sum up agreements made during the consultation |
| Agree on specific objectives, contents, and form for the future course |
| Acute cases: no further appointments |
| Subacute cases: therapy sessions, regular scheduled appointments |
| Chronic: consider status consultation, regular scheduled appointments |
| Consider referral to psychiatrist, psychologist, or specialist service |
| 5. **Chronic cases** |
| See Table 5.2.3.4 |

on the emotional component is often helpful in reducing suffering. The motivation and engagement should preferably be established during the assessment interview.

### (c) Psychoeducation

The patient needs to be taught about somatoform and related disorders and about the body's normal reactions to stress and how stress may be expressed in physical symptoms. It is important that the patient learns about the possible biological and physiological basis in the CNS for the symptoms. This will make the reality of the symptoms clear to the patient and emphasize that the illness is not imaginary or made up. The education may be supported by written information. Parts of the information ought to be repeated during the therapy when it, in a relevant way, can be linked to the patient's personal experience.

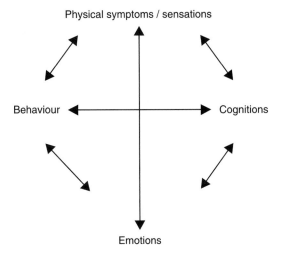

**Fig. 5.2.3.1** Basic model in cognitive behavioural therapy.

#### (d) Physical symptoms and symptom attribution

Figure 5.2.3.1 illustrates the relationship between symptoms, cognitions, emotions, and behaviour in the cognitive-behavioural model. The first step in the therapy is to clarify the patient's dysfunctional automatic thoughts and basic beliefs about illness and symptoms, i.e. cause, consequences for future health and function, treatment, etc. Those thoughts are related to feelings and illness behaviour.

In the next step, the patient's disease model and symptom attributions are challenged. The therapist asks the patient to consider alternative possibilities, in which process even the most unlikely explanations are welcome. The therapist and the patient then explore which explanation is the most likely by investigating pros and cons for each possible explanation.

Finally, it is clarified how the patient would behave and react to a particular understanding or belief and which feelings this would produce.

#### (e) Behaviour and coping

Even if the patient does not want to or cannot work with his or her illness perception and symptom attribution, it would still be possible to work with the way the patient copes with illness. Illness behaviour and coping with symptoms and illness are scrutinized, and the behaviour is linked to the underlying thoughts and feelings if possible. When an example of a behaviour or coping strategy is elucidated, it is listed with arguments for and against a particular behaviour or coping strategy. A brainstorm on alternative possibilities is advisable, and pros and cons for each of these are also scrutinized. In a negotiation with the therapist, the patient chooses an alternative possibility, which is tested by the patient as homework, and at next session the effect of this is explored.

It is important to go slowly for the patient to experience success. The therapist is obliged to make sure that the patient sets up realistic goals with a good chance of success.

#### (f) Links between symptoms and stressors

The cause of somatization disorder and related disorder may be viewed as a combination of personal vulnerability and the stress and strain an individual is exposed to. The patients are often unaware of their patterns of reaction, but this can be established by careful registration of variations in symptom intensity and then relating them to what the patients are doing or thinking at that time. Based on variation in symptom intensity and stressors, potential important stressors in everyday life may be identified. This may provide a focus for intervention.

#### (g) Family and social network

The patient's health beliefs are often shared with the family and social network. Therefore it is necessary to create an alliance with the family to make sure they support the patient and not counteract the therapy. Family members are invited to a consultation and informed about the nature of the disorder and about the planned treatment. Misunderstandings and prejudgements about somatization disorder are eliminated.

#### (h) Treatment and help seeking behaviour and the physicians' handling

For patients with somatization disorder, social and family life is often centered on their illness, and an objective of the therapy is to reduce the importance of the illness and try to build up other interests and aspects of life. The patient's consulting behaviour may result in multiple fruitless diagnostic tests, referrals, and treatment attempts, which expose the patient to iatrogenic harm. Often, the patient grows tired of the doctors responding to their questions merely by referring or prescribing medication. In therapy, the patients are taught how to present their problems to the physicians in a way that prevents referrals and medication.[58] A patient may for instance tell the doctor that he or she is worried about some new symptoms, because he or she does not know whether the symptoms are just part of his or her somatoform disorder or something else, and that the doctor's expertise is required in order to clarify this.

### Medication

Coexisting mood, anxiety, or other mental disorders are as effectively treated with psychotropic medication in patients with a somatoform disorder as in patients without.[59] Patients without coexisting mental disorders also seem to benefit from psychopharmacological treatment, antidepressants being the first choice.[44] In some cases, medication with peripheral action may be helpful as symptomatic treatment, for example in case of gastrointestinal symptoms like IBS.[44] Tricyclic antidepressants seem most effective, but due to side effects SSRI or SNRI ought to be the first choice. A useful strategy in the psychopharmacological treatment of somatizing patients is to start on a lower dosage than is usually recommended and to increase the dosage only gradually in order to avoid side effects. Antidepressants with the fewest interactions should be chosen as polypharmacy is common in these patients. The use of benzodiazepines and other dependence-producing drugs should be avoided. Stronger painkillers usually only produce a partial and temporary improvement, but they may result in misuse and should be avoided. Mild painkillers and tricyclic antidepressants are to be preferred.

In general, a degree of stoicism is required on the part of the clinician as patients may have varying symptom intensity and motivation and because patients may complain of side effects as a result of increased sensitivity to bodily sensations. Drugs that can be serum-monitored are preferred so that compliance and the likelihood of side effects can be assessed.

## Possibilities for prevention

Patients with medically unexplained symptoms are often unpopular both with general psychiatrists and other doctors. The patients are seen as neither physically nor mentally ill, but simply as individuals complaining in order to avoid normal life responsibilities. Overcoming these negative attitudes is a matter of proper training of doctors and education of medical students.

Since an early diagnosis is important for preventing physical fixation, iatrogenic harm, and chronicity, doctors must be taught to view somatization disorder and related disorders with the same seriousness as well-defined physical diseases. The dominating dualistic way of thinking in medicine must be counteracted.

## Further information

Mayou, R., Sharpe, M., and Carson, A.J. (eds.) (2004). *ABC of psychological medicine*. BMJ Books, London.

Woolfolk, R.L. and Allen, L.A. (2006). *Treating somatization. A cognitive-behavioral approach*. The Guilford Press.

Bass, C. (1990). *Somatization: physical symptoms & psychological illness* (1st edn). Blackwell Scientific Publications Oxford.

Mayou, R., Bass, C., and Sharpe, M. (1995). *Treatment of functional somatic symptoms*. Oxford University Press, Oxford.

## References

1. Goldberg, D.P. and Bridges, K. (1988). Somatic presentations of psychiatric illness in primary care setting. *Journal of Psychosomatic Research*, **32**(2), 137–44.

2. Simon, G., Gater, R., Kisely, S., *et al.* (1996). Somatic symptoms of distress: an international primary care study. *Psychosomatic Medicine*, **58**(5), 481–8.

3. Fink, P., Toft, T., Hansen, M.S., *et al.* (2007). Symptoms and syndromes of bodily distress: an exploratory study of 978 internal medical, neurological, and primary care patients. *Psychosomatic Medicine*, **69**(1), 30–9.

4. Katon, W., Lin, E., Von Korff, M., *et al.* (1991). Somatization: a spectrum of severity. *American Journal of Psychiatry*, **148**(1), 34–40.

5. Perley, M.J. and Guze, S.B. (1962). Hysteria-the stability and usefulness of clinical criteria. A quantitative study based on a follow-up period of six to eight years in 39 patients. *The New England Journal of Medicine*, **266**, 421–6.

6. Murphy, M.R. (1990). Classification of the somatoform disorders. In *Somatization: physical symptoms & psychological illness* (ed. C. Bass), pp. 10–39. Blackwell Scientific Publications, Oxford.

7. Escobar, J.I., Rubio-Stipec, M., Canino, G., *et al.* (March 1989). Somatic symptom index (SSI): a new and abridged somatization construct. Prevalence and epidemiological correlates in two large community samples. *The Journal of Nervous and Mental Disease*, **177**(3), 140–6.

8. Kroenke, K., Spitzer, R.L., deGruy, F.V., *et al.* (1997). Multisomatoform disorder. An alternative to undifferentiated somatoform disorder for the somatizing patient in primary care. *Archives of General Psychiatry*, **54**(4), 352–8.

9. Kirmayer, L.J., Groleau, D., Looper, K.J., *et al.* (2004). Explaining medically unexplained symptoms. *Canadian Journal of Psychiatry*, **49**(10), 663–72.

10. Fink, P. (1992). Surgery and medical treatment in persistent somatizing patients. *Journal of Psychosomatic Research*, **36**, 439–47.

11. Fink, P. (1992). Physical complaints and symptoms of somatizing patients. *Journal of Psychosomatic Research*, **36**, 125–36.

12. Salmon, P., Peters, S., and Stanley, I. (1999). Patients' perceptions of medical explanations for somatisation disorders: qualitative analysis. *British Medical Journal*, **318**(7180), 372–6.

13. Stern, J., Murphy, M., and Bass, C. (1993). Personality disorders in patients with somatisation disorder. A controlled study. *British Journal of Psychiatry*, **163**, 785–9.

14. Fink, P. (1992). The use of hospitalizations by persistent somatizing patients. *Psychological Medicine*, **22**, 173–80.

15. House, A. (1995). The patient with medically unexplained symptoms: making the initial psychiatric contact. In *Treatment of functional somatic symptoms* (eds. R. Mayou, C. Bass, and M. Sharpe), pp. 89–102. Oxford University Press, Oxford.

16. Yutzy, S.H., Cloninger, C.R., Guze, S.B., *et al.* (1995). DSM-IV field trial: testing a new proposal for somatization disorder. *The American Journal of Psychiatry*, **152**(1), 97–101.

17. Fink, P., Rosendal, M., and Olesen, F. (2005). Classification of somatization and functional somatic symptoms in primary care. *Australian and New Zealand Journal of Psychiatry*, **39**(9), 772–81.

18. Wiesmuller, G.A., Ebel, H., Hornberg, C., *et al.* (2003). Are syndromes in environmental medicine variants of somatoform disorders? *Medical Hypotheses*, **61**(4), 419–30.

19. Feldman, M.D. and Ford, C.V. (1994). *Patient or pretender. Inside the strange world of factitious disorders*. John Wiley & Sons, Inc, NY, USA.

20. Eisendrath, S.J. (1984). Factitious illness: A clarification. *Psychosomatics*, **25**, 110–17.

21. Üstün, T.B. and Sartorius, N. (1995). *Mental illness in general health care, an international study*. John Wiley & Sons, Chichester, UK.

22. Fink, P. (1995). Psychiatric illness in patients with persistent somatisation. *British Journal of Psychiatry*, **166**(1), 93–9.

23. Gureje, O., Simon, G.E., Ustun, T.B., *et al.* (1997). Somatization in cross-cultural perspective: a World Health Organization study in primary care. *The American Journal of Psychiatry*, **154**(7), 989–95.

24. Creed, F. and Barsky, A. (2004). A systematic review of the epidemiology of somatisation disorder and hypochondriasis. *Journal of Psychosomatic Research*, **56**(4), 391–408.

25. Fink, P., Steen, H.M., and Sondergaard, L. (2005). Somatoform disorders among first-time referrals to a neurology service. *Psychosomatics*, **46**(6), 540–8.

26. Fink, P., Hansen, M.S., and Oxhoj, M.L. (2004). The prevalence of somatoform disorders among internal medical inpatients. *Journal of Psychosomatic Research*, **56**(4), 413–18.

27. Toft, T., Fink, P., Oernboel, E., *et al.* (2005). Mental disorders in primary care: prevalence and co-morbidity among disorders. Results from the functional illness in primary care (FIP) study. *Psychological Medicine*, **35**(8), 1175–84.

28. De Waal, M.W., Arnold, I.A., Eekhof, J.A., *et al.* (2004). Somatoform disorders in general practice: prevalence, functional impairment and comorbidity with anxiety and depressive disorders. *British Journal of Psychiatry*, **184**, 470–6.

29. Kroenke, K. and Spitzer, R.L. (1998). Gender differences in the reporting of physical and somatoform symptoms. *Psychosomatic Medicine*, **60**(2), 150–5.

30. Barsky, A.J., Orav, E.J., and Bates, D.W. (2005). Somatization increases medical utilization and costs independent of psychiatric and medical comorbidity. *Archives of General Psychiatry*, **62**(8), 903–10.

31. Hansen, M.S., Fink, P., Frydenberg, M., *et al.* (2002). Use of health services, mental illness, and self-rated disability and health in medical inpatients. *Psychosomatic Medicine*, **64**(4), 668–75.

32. Shorter, E. (1992). *From paralysis to fatigue. A history of psychosomatic illness in the modern era*. The Free Press, Macmillan Inc. New York.

33. Mayou, R., Bass, C., and Sharpe, M. (1995). Overview of epidemiology, classification, and aetiology. In *Treatment of functional somatic symptoms* (eds. R. Mayou, C. Bass, and M. Sharpe), pp. 42–65. Oxford University Press, Oxford.

34. Hotopf, M., Carr, S., Mayou, R., *et al.* (1998). Why do children have chronic abdominal pain, and what happens to them when they grow

up? Population based cohort study. *British Medical Journal*, **316**(7139), 1196–200.

35. Leserman, J., Drossman, D.A., Li, Z., *et al.* (1996). Sexual and physical abuse history in gastroenterology practice: how types of abuse impact health status. *Psychosomatic Medicine*, **58**(1), 4–15.

36. Guze, S.B. (1993). Genetics of Briquet's syndrome and somatization disorder. A review of family, adoption, and twin studies. *Annals of Clinical Psychiatry*, **5**, 225–30.

37. Rodin, G.M. (1991). Somatization: a perspective from self psychology. *Journal of American Academy Psychoanalysis*, **19**, 367–84.

38. Meares, R. (1997). Stimulus entrapment: on a common basis of somatization. *Psychoanalytic Inquiry*, **17**(2), 223–34.

39. Sharpe, M. (1995). Cognitive behavioural therapies in the treatment of functional somatic symptoms. In *Treatment of functional somatic symptoms* (eds. R. Mayou, C. Bass, and M. Sharpe), pp. 122–43. Oxford University Press, Oxford.

40. Miller, L. (1984). Neuropsychological concepts of somatoform disorders. *International Journal of Psychiatry in Medicine*, **14**(1), 31–46.

41. Rief, W. and Barsky, A.J. (2005). Psychobiological perspectives on somatoform disorders. *Psychoneuroendocrinology*, **30**, (10), 996–1002.

42. Mertz, H. (2002). Role of the brain and sensory pathways in gastrointestinal sensory disorders in humans. *Gut*, **51**(Suppl. 1), i29–i33.

43. Fink, P., Rosendal, M., and Toft, T. (2002). Assessment and treatment of functional disorders in general practice: the extended reattribution and management model—an advanced educational program for nonpsychiatric doctors. *Psychosomatics*, **43**(2), 93–131.

44. Henningsen, P., Zipfel, S., and Herzog, W. (2007). Management of functional somatic syndromes. *Lancet*, **369**(9565), 946–55.

45. O'Malley, P.G., Jackson, J.L., Santoro, J., *et al.* (1999). Antidepressant therapy for unexplained symptoms and symptom syndromes. *Journal of Family Practice*, **48**(12), 980–90.

46. Kroenke, K. (2007). Efficacy of treatment for somatoform disorders. A review of randomized controlled trials. *Psychosomatic Medicine*, in press.

47. Kroenke, K. and Swindle, R. (2000). Cognitive-behavioural therapy for somatization and symptom syndromes: a critical review of controlled clinical trials. *Psychothererapy and Psychosomatics*, **69**(4), 205–15.

48. Fink, P. (1997). *Persistent somatization*. Thesis; faculty of health sciences. University of Aarhus, Denmark.

49. Crimlisk, H.L., Bhatia, K., Cope, H., *et al.* (1998). Slater revisited: 6 year follow up study of patients with medically unexplained motor symptoms. *British Medical Journal*, **316**(7131), 582–6.

50. Stone, J., Wojcik, W., Durrance, D., *et al.* (2002). What should we say to patients with symptoms unexplained by disease? The 'number needed to offend'. *British Medical Journal*, **325**(7378), 1449–50.

51. Bass, C. (1990). Assessment and management of patients with functional somatic symptoms. In *Somatization: physical symptoms & psychological illness* (ed. C. Bass), pp. 40–72. Blackwell Scientific Publications, Oxford.

52. Price, J. and Leaver, L. (2002). ABC of psychological medicine: beginning treatment. *British Medical Journal*, **325**(7354), 33–5.

53. Gask, L. (1995). Management in primary care. In *Treatment of functional somatic symptoms* (eds. R. Mayou, C. Bass, and M. Sharpe), pp. 391–409. Oxford University Press, Oxford.

54. Morriss, R., Gask, L., Ronalds, C., *et al.* (1998). Cost-effectiveness of a new treatment for somatized mental disorder taught to GPs. *Family Practice*, **15**(2), 119–25.

55. Smith, G.R. Jr. (1995). Treatment of patients with multiple symptoms. In *Treatment of functional somatic symptoms* (eds. R. Mayou, C. Bass, and M. Sharpe), pp.175–87. Oxford University Press, Oxford.

56. Bass, C., Sharpe, M., and Mayou, R. (1995). The management of patients with functional somatic symptoms in the general hospital. In *Treatment of functional somatic symptoms* (eds. R. Mayou. C. Bass, and S. Sharpe), pp. 410–27. Oxford University Press, Oxford.

57. Smith, G.R. Jr., Rost, K., and Kashner, T.M. (1995). A trial of the effect of a standardized psychiatric consultation on health outcomes and costs in somatizing patients. *Archives of General Psychiatry*, **52**(3), 238–43.

58. Salmon, P., Humphris, G.M., Ring, A., *et al.* (2006). Why do primary care physicians propose medical care to patients with medically unexplained symptoms? A new method of sequence analysis to test theories of patient pressure. *Psychosomatic Medicine*, **68**(4), 570–7.

59. Katon, W. and Sullivan, M. (1995). Antidepressant treatment of functional somatic symptoms. In *Treatment of functional somatic symptoms* (eds. R. Mayou, C. Bass, and M. Sharpe), pp. 103–21. Oxford University Press, Oxford.

# 5.2.4 Conversion and dissociation disorders

Christopher Bass

## Introduction

Of all the disorders characterized by symptoms in the absence of disease, conversion disorders are perhaps the most difficult to explain. How, for example, can one explain functional blindness or a loss of function of both legs in the absence of conspicuous organic disease? The ancient Greeks recognized that if we suffer emotional disturbance as a result of some serious stress (such as personal injury or bereavement), this causes a change in the nervous system which leads in turn to symptoms in different parts of the body according to the underlying pathophysiology. Nineteenth century neurologists made significant advances when they identified specific ideas at the root of the symptoms. In the early nineteenth century Collie[1] also observed that the significance of, and attention to, a symptom or set of symptoms may depend more on what they mean (or their value) to the individual than on the biological underpinnings of the symptom itself.

Spence has recently argued that the problem in hysterical motor disorders is not the voluntary motor system *per se*: rather, *it is in the way that the motor system is utilized in the performance (or nonperformance) of certain willed, chosen, actions.*[2] This model invokes a consciousness that acts upon the body and the world. By contrast, the psychodynamic ('conversion') model, which Freud introduced and which held sway for most of the twentieth century, invokes an unconscious mechanism 'acting' independently of consciousness, to interfere with voluntary movement. Spence has further argued that hysterical paralyses are maintained not by unconscious mechanisms, but by conscious processes. The maintenance of these symptoms requires the patient's attention, a characteristic of higher motor acts; the paralyses break down when the subject is distracted, consciousness is obtunded, or when it (the 'paralyses') is circumvented by reflexive motor routines. Hysterical paralyses, Spence avers, are quintessentially disorders of action (or inactions), which the patient disavows, when faced with some overwhelming situation, which threatens the identity of the self.[2]

One regrettable development of psychiatry's adoption of Freudian theory was the fracture in communication between the disciplines of psychiatry and neurology, which has only recently been restored by the sort of collaborative research currently being carried out by neurologists and psychiatrists.[3] In the last decade there have also been exciting advances in neuroimaging, which have stimulated research into the neurophysiology of hysteria, and these will be described later. This chapter will also emphasize contemporary approaches to management of these difficult clinical problems.

## Problems with definition

There are a number of problems with the definition of the conversion disorders (CD). First, physical disorder must be excluded, but neurological co-morbidity is known to be high in patients with CD,[4] and distinguishing which symptoms are accounted for by organic disease and which are not can be difficult. Second, it is stated that a temporal association between a psychological stressor and the onset on the disorder should be identified, but in practice this is often impossible to establish and depends to a large extent on the skill of the interviewing doctor. Finally, by definition (according to the glossaries ICD-10 and DSM-IV)[5, 6]; the process should be unconsciously mediated, but it is difficult (some would say impossible) to distinguish between symptoms that are not consciously produced and those that are intentionally manufactured. The DSM-IV provides no criteria to distinguish conscious from unconscious intent, and many authors have argued that the criteria for whether the patients are consciously aware of producing these symptoms should be dropped from the diagnosis of CD.[7]

In clinical practice it is often difficult for a physician, faced with a patient in a hospital bed unable to use his or her legs despite normal tests and clinical findings, to differentiate between conversion disorder, factitious or fabricated disorder, or frank malingering. What the clinician is being asked to do is to determine whether or not the symptoms are being produced intentionally or not; and what the motives are. Table 5.2.4.1 attempts to provide a framework, but it highlights the shortcomings of psychiatric glossaries, which in turn expose the limitations of the medical model, which forces doctors to place patients in categories without taking into account the normal moral capacity of many individuals to exercise choice and determine (at least to some extent) their actions.[8] These medical conundrums have been explored in more detail in the chapter on factitious disorders and malingering (Chapter 5.2.9).

## The role of volition

Central to recent debates about hysteria and conversion disorders is the extent to which a person's illness presentation is considered a product of free will and hence social deviance or the result of psychopathology and/or psychosocial influences beyond the volitional control of the subject.[9] The proposal that voluntary processes are involved in some way has a very long history: something prevents a specific voluntary behaviour from being executed through a 'negative', lack of movement (as in paralysis), or a 'positive', abnormality of movement (as in psychogenic tremor). If 'will' is regarded as a conscious capacity that humans possess to choose what to do or refrain from doing, then the problem in CD appears to be that the will fails to produce normal action.[10] Hence, the diagnostic

**Table 5.2.4.1** Relationships between conversion hysteria, factious disorder, and malingering

| | Subject insight | | Target of deception | | Perceived outcome | Motivation/ reason |
|---|---|---|---|---|---|---|
| | Aware | Unaware | Conscious self | Other | | |
| Hysterical conversion | | + | + | | Sick and disabled role | Care/ dependency |
| Factious disorder | + | | | + | Sick and disabled role | Care/ dependency |
| Malingering | + | | | + | Sick and disabled role | Personal benefit, e.g. financial, avoiding prison |

(Reproduced from Halligan, P. Bass, C. and Oakley, D. Wilful deception as illness behaviour. In *Malingering and illness deception* (eds. P. Halligan, C. Bass, and D. Oakley), pp. 3–28. Copyright 2003, with permission from Oxford University Press).

importance is placed on the patient's veracity: if we believe him when he says that he cannot act normally we conclude that his will is impeded pathologically; if we do not believe him we conclude instead that his will is deployed to deceive us. This is the distinction required by the diagnostic systems.

## Conversion and dissociation

The word *conversion* is conventionally applied to somatic symptoms whereas if the symptom is psychological (e.g. a loss of memory or an external hallucination) rather than bodily (e.g. a loss of power) it is regarded as dissociative. *Dissociation* has attracted considerable recent interest, and it has been argued that the available evidence is more consistent with a model that identifies at least two distinct categories of dissociative phenomena—'detachment' and 'compartmentalization'—that have different definitions, mechanisms, and treatment implications.[11] These have been referred to as Type 1 (compartmentalization) and Type 2 (detachment), respectively (see Table 5.2.4.2).

*Compartmentalization phenomena* are characterized by impairment in the ability to control processes or actions that would usually be amenable to such control and which are otherwise functioning normally. This category encompasses unexplained neurological symptoms (including dissociative amnesia) and benign phenomena such as those produced by hypnotic suggestion. By contrast, *detachment phenomena* are characterized by an altered state of consciousness associated with a sense of separation from the self, the body, or the world. Depersonalization, derealization and out-of-body experiences constitute archetypal examples of detachment in this account. Evidence suggests that these phenomena are generated by a common pathophysiological mechanism involving the top-down inhibition of limbic emotional processing by frontal brain systems. Although these two types of dissociation are typically conflated, evidence suggests that different pathological mechanisms may be operating in each case.

**Table 5.2.4.2** Classification of two types of pathological dissociation

| Type 1 dissociation (compartmentalisation) | Type 2 dissociation (detachment) |
| --- | --- |
| Conversion disorders | Depersonalization/derealization |
| Dissociative amnesia | Peri-traumatic dissociation |
| Dissociative fugue | Out of body experiences |
| Dissociative identity disorder | Autoscopy (?) |

(Reproduced with permission, from R. Brown (2002))

Support for the compartmentalization model comes from psychophysiological research, which suggests that psychogenic illness is associated with a deficit in attentional, conscious processing and the preservation of preattentive, preconscious processes. According to Brown[12] there is very little difference between 'negative' symptoms such as sensory loss, paralysis, etc. and 'positive' symptoms such as tremor, dystonia, etc. in terms of basic underlying mechanisms. By this view, all symptoms result from a loss of normal high-level attentional control over low-level processing systems; in this sense, all symptoms can be thought of as involving a form of compartmentalization.

## Pathophysiology

There has been considerable progress in cognitive neuroscience and functional imaging over the last decade, which has provided a conceptual and empirically based platform for developing a neuroscience of not only hysterical symptoms but also free will.[13,14]

Recent functional neuroimaging data suggest that neural circuits linking volition, movement, and perception are disrupted in CD.[13] There are many studies examining the role of specific prefrontal regions in action generation (particularly the dorsolateral prefrontal and supplementary motor areas) and action suppression (especially the orbitofrontal cortices). These 'higher' executive centres supervene only when a change of behaviour is required: inappropriate behaviour must be suppressed or difficult procedures attended to, as when concentration is necessary. Hence, if the problem in hysteria is one of the will, and of abnormality emerging only when subjects attend to their actions, then this suggests the hypothesis that the prefrontal cortex is pivotal to the conversion process (see Fig. 5.2.4.1).

Further evidence that the prefrontal cortices play a key role in the control of action comes from a study of a woman with a left-sided conversion disorder affecting her leg. Marshall et al.[15] demonstrated that her attempt to move her paralysed leg was associated with increased activation of orbitofrontal (inhibitory) prefrontal regions, in the absence of motor cortical activity. They argued for an inhibition of motor behaviour by higher centres. Spence and colleagues[16] demonstrated that in three men with conversion symptoms affecting their upper limbs, hypokinetic movement was associated with reduced activation of dorsolateral (action-generation) areas of prefrontal cortex. Moreover, these areas of hypoactivity differed from those exhibited by four healthy men who were asked to feign the same motor impairments (see Fig. 5.2.4.2). It is possible that the application of functional neuroimaging techniques might allow clinicians to distinguish conversion from feigning on objective, empirical grounds.

DISORDERS WITH SOMATIC PRESENTATION

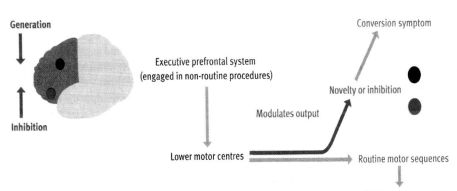

The executive supervenes on lower motor centres when there is need for novel action generation (black circle) or suppression of inappropriate action (red circle), each implicating specific prefrontal regions: the dorsolateral and orbitofrontal cortices, respectively. Under conditions where the executive may be hypothesized to be disengaged (by distraction or sedation) normal movements emerge (as would be expected of routine actions). Conversion movements seem to require attention, and hence the engagement of the executive. There are 2 mechanisms by which conversion might emerge: failure to generate new actions, consequent upon dorsolateral hypofunction (black circle) or suppression of ongoing motor action, secondary to orbitofrontal activation (red circle). Other mechanisms may also operate. Acknowledgement: Mrs Jean Woodhead.

**Fig. 5.2.4.1** Schematic diagram illustrating the role of prefrontal executive in modulating lower motor systems, and its hypothesized involvement in conversion disorder. (Reproduced with permission from Spence, S. (2006). Hysteria: a new look. In *Psychiatry*, **5**(2), pp. 56–60, Elsevier Ltd.)

**Image showing regions where those with conversion disorder exhibited hypofunction during hypokinetic hand movements**

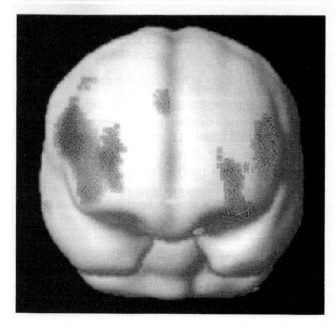

Conversion patients exhibited reduced activity in left dorsolateral and ventrolateral prefrontal cortices (red). Healthy subjects deliberately feigning disorder exhibited reduced activity in right prefrontal areas (green).

**Fig. 5.2.4.2** Image showing regions where those with conversion disorder exhibited hypofunction during hypokinetic hand movements. (Reproduced with permission (sought) from Spence, S. (2006). Hysteria: a new look. In *Psychiatry*, **5**(2), pp. 56–60, Elsevier Ltd.

In another recent case report using fMRI a patient with right-sided paralysis was asked to recall traumatic memories using a standard life event schedule: cued recall of the event was associated with regional brain activities characteristic of emotional arousal, including the amygdala and right inferior frontal lobe. Such recall was also associated with reduced motor activity in the area corresponding to the subjective paralysed limb.[17] This case study provides neuroimaging evidence for a connection between traumatic events and ongoing neurological symptoms (see Problems with definition, above).

## Epidemiology

It is ironic that these research advances have occurred at a time when social historians have confidently asserted that hysteria has disappeared from clinical practice:

> The most consequential development in the history of hysteria in the last century was the rapid decline in the medically recorded incidence of the disorder . . . . . . . .Hysteria—considered variously as a term, a theory, and a behaviour—is vanishing.[18]

It is extraordinary that this was written in 2001, at a time when symptoms considered 'functional, psychogenic, medically unexplained or hysterical' account for up to a third of new referrals to neurology outpatient departments.[3] and up to 9 per cent of admissions to a UK neurology in patient ward.[19] Akagi and House[20] concluded that the lowest prevalence figures suggested a rate of about 50 per 100 000 for cases of CD known to health services at any one time, with perhaps twice that number affected over a 1-year period. These figures suggest that hysteria is as common as other disabling conditions such as multiple sclerosis and schizophrenia. Furthermore, the burden of disability associated with chronic hysteria is far higher than a typical practising psychiatrist might expect, or than is reflected in standard textbooks of psychiatry or clinical neurology.[21]

It is regrettable therefore that it receives none of the resources or media attention that these disorders attract.

## Clinical features

### Conversion disorder: motor symptoms

The most typical motor symptoms are paralyses, functional weakness, gait disturbances, fits resembling epilepsy, and abnormal movements.

In the last decade diagnostic procedures have improved and the availability of non-invasive, accurate imaging has drastically reduced the rates of undetected organic pathology in patients with diagnoses of hysteria. Indeed, several recent studies have reported rates of misdiagnosis of between 0 and 4 per cent in regional and tertiary neurological centres,[22] which suggests that a diagnosis of CD can be made relatively confidently and accurately. In the following section the process of diagnosis will be briefly outlined through the history, examination, and investigation.

#### (a) The history

The onset, temporal sequence, and character of the presenting complaint may not be typical of a neurological disorder, and a number of other features may emerge, especially after an interview with a family member or a review of the hospital and general practitioner notes. If the patient is admitted to a general hospital bed the psychiatrist should routinely telephone the patient's primary care doctor and request a recent print out of his/her medical records (with consent). These often reveal key information about life events and/or antecedent illnesses, investigations, etc.

#### (i) Age of onset and sex

The average age of onset is the mid-30s, and patients with functional paralysis are less likely to be female than patients with pseudo seizures.

#### (ii) Mode of onset/recent life events or difficulties

An increased number of life events in the year preceding symptom onset have been recorded in small controlled studies of unexplained motor symptoms[23,24]. When patients are interviewed carefully, some report symptoms of panic just before the onset of, for example, functional weakness.[25] Judicious questions about sensations of sweating, dizziness, and difficulty breathing may reveal these somatic symptoms of anxiety, which may also be reported before the onset of sensory symptoms (see below). There is also an important literature describing unilateral somatic symptoms (which may present with sudden onset of functional weakness in a limb) following hyperventilation/panic.[26,27] These patients may present acutely in the A and E department of a general hospital, where they may be admitted to the hospital stroke unit, or be sent to the general hospital as an emergency with an accompanying letter from the patient's GP describing the patient as 'off legs-please see and investigate.' The following clinical vignette is typical:

*A 40-year-old woman was admitted as an emergency to the Stroke unit of the general hospital after collapsing at home. She had been involved in a dispute with her employers for weeks, and on the morning of the referral had an argument with her mother which made her very upset, and during the course of this she became distressed and developed paraesthesiae down the left side of her body, slurred speech, and collapsed, losing consciousness for 30 s. An ambulance was called and she was admitted to the A and E department, where she was noted to be hyperventilating and agitated, and to have weakness of the left leg, unintelligible speech, and claimed not to be able to see. All neurological investigations were normal, and after 12 days in hospital she made a gradual recovery, but was left with functional weakness in the left leg (requiring a wheelchair), and her speech was intermittently 'child-like'. History revealed a similar episode 3 years previously, a recent 2-year history of treatment for irritable bowel syndrome, and considerable work and domestic stress.*

*She was followed up by the liaison service and community mental health team, but despite the efforts of a community physiotherapist, psychologist, and nursing support her limb weakness continued and she remained disabled; 1 year after admission she was in receipt of disability benefits.*

### (iii) Previous unexplained symptoms

Evidence is accumulating that the more unexplained symptoms the patient has, the more likely the primary symptom is to be unexplained by disease.[28] In a recent study of patients with medically unexplained motor symptoms, additional unexplained symptoms including paraesthesia (65 per cent), pseudo epileptic seizures (23 per cent), and memory impairment (20 per cent) were reported.[4] It is often useful therefore, when CD is being considered as a diagnosis, to obtain a print out of the patient's past history from the primary care doctor (having obtained the patient's consent). This may reveal repeated presentations to different specialists as well as a history of repeated surgical procedures, particularly without clear evidence of pathology. It is also worth noting that patients with a diagnosis of somatization disorder (what used to be referred to as Briquet's syndrome) have high rates of conversion disorders, which punctuate their illness careers, often after a life event or physical injury/procedure.[29]

### (iv) Psychiatric co-morbidity

Rates of depression (38 to 50 per cent) and anxiety (10 to 16 per cent) have been identified in a number of studies. In a recent small prospective controlled study there was a fourfold increase in depression in comparison with matched control with similar organic disability.[30]

### (v) Neurological disease and other physical factors

A diagnosis of functional paralysis can be made in a patient who already has some paralysis from another cause, for example, the 'disproportionate disability' in a patient with multiple sclerosis. In a recent study of patients with unexplained motor symptoms 42 per cent had a co-morbid neurological disease and half of these had a peripheral origin.[4] Epilepsy is thought to coexist in a significant percentage of patients with non-epileptic attacks.[31]

It is also important for the physician or surgeon to be aware of the diverse ways in which conversion symptoms can present in the general hospital. In the last decade the author has seen many patients with conversion disorders after surgical procedures, investigations, and operations such as hysterectomy, minor injuries in the workplace, and after (often trivial) road traffic accidents. Numerous case reports implicating accidents, minor surgical procedures, and general anaesthetics as initiating factors have been described, for patients with both non-epileptic seizures and functional neurological syndromes.[32–34] These presentations are more likely to be seen in a medico legal setting, where the symptoms are shaped by the prospect of financial gain.

### (vi) Secondary gain/litigation

This is a complex issue but impending litigation has been described in a number of studies of patients with unexplained motor symptoms and tremor.[4,35] One group of patients who may develop abnormal movements are those with reflex sympathetic dystrophy (RSD) which has been renamed Complex Regional Pain Syndrome Type I (CRPS I). It has been reported that patients with CRPS I with abnormal movements typically exhibit pseudo neurological (non-organic) signs, and in some cases malingering has been documented by secret surveillance.[36] The authors concluded that abnormal movements in CRPS I are a key clinical feature that differentiates CRPS I from CRPS II. Psychiatrists will often be asked to express opinions on patients with chronic painful extremities (often labelled as 'CRPS') in which abnormal movements have developed, especially in a medico legal setting. Pearce[37] has remarked that CRPS is best construed as a reaction to injury, or to excessive, often iatrogenic, immobilization after injury; but should not be seen as an independent disease. He asserts that the diagnosis of CRPS groups together ill-defined symptoms under a convenient, but medically untestable label, and that patients, lawyers, and support groups commonly deny psychogenesis, with the sadly mistaken notion that this implies a bogus or spurious cause.

### (vii) Laterality of the symptoms

The idea that left-sided symptoms are more common than right has a long history but a recent systematic review found no evidence to support this view.[38]

### (viii) History from relative/informant

There is a considerable amount of evidence to suggest that the observations and attitudes of carers may be important in the perpetuation of medically unexplained symptoms, especially motor conversion symptoms. For example, Davison et al.[39] found carers to be ill-informed and dissatisfied with the advice they had received from doctors about their relatives' diagnosis and disabilities. The education of carers and relatives is essential and will be dealt with in the section on management.

### (b) The examination and diagnostic discrepancies

There is often a discrepancy between the patient's concept of the symptoms and the physician's knowledge of the anatomy and physiology. The way in which a patient moves or undresses may indicate a global affection that is incompatible with a specific nerve lesion or with a hemiplegia.

When considering any sign of functional weakness it is important to remember the following caveats:

1 Any sign that depends on inconsistency does not distinguish 'hysterical' from 'malingered' weakness.

2 The presence of a positive sign of functional weakness does not exclude the possibility that the patient also has an organic disease as well.

3 All physical signs, whether for organic or non-organic signs, have a limited reliability and inter-rater reliability.[22]

Another myth wedded to the concept of hysteria (I have already referred to the mistaken but common belief that it has 'disappeared' and that symptoms are more common on the left) is that the patients exhibit 'la belle indifference' or are inappropriately under concerned about their symptoms. In a recent systematic review Stone et al.[40] found that the median frequency of la belle indifference was 21 per cent (range 0–54 per cent) in 356 patients with conversion symptoms and 29 per cent (range 0–60 per cent) in 157 patients with organic disease. Indifference to symptoms is more likely to be noted in patients with factitious disorder (see Chapter 5.2.9).

Give way weakness is often used as a diagnostic test of hysterical paralyses, but it is unreliable. Unilateral functional weakness of a leg, if severe, tends to produce a characteristic gait in which the leg is dragged behind the body as a single unit, like a sack of potatoes. The hip is either held in external or internal rotation so that the foot points inwards or outwards. The most impressive quantitative discrimination to date between hysterical and neurological weakness is reported in a study of Hoover's sign—the involuntary extension of hysterically paralysed leg when the 'good leg' is flexing against resistance. Ziv and colleagues[41] demonstrated a clear difference in the pattern of response between neurological and psychogenic patient groups. It should be borne in mind however that the patient may have both a functional and organic disorder.[4]

## Individual symptoms

### (a) Paralyses

Paralyses may affect one or more limbs, or one side of the face. They may be flaccid or occur with contractures. In hysterical spasm both arm and leg are contracted on the same side of the body, the hand is closed tightly, the knee is flexed, and perhaps the leg and the foot are drawn up. Paralysis with contractures is one of the most extreme examples of disability caused by hysterical illness.

Hysterical paraplegia has been described,[42] and both spinal and orthopaedic surgeons, as well as rehabilitation specialists and neurologists, should be alert to the development of this disorder in their patients.[43] These patients have the potential to use considerable health care resources.[21]

### (b) Abnormal movements

Psychogenic movement disorders are thought to account for 1 in 30 of all patients attending a movement disorder clinic[35] and have been the subject of a recent book.[44] During the last two decades a number of case series of patients with psychogenic dystonia have been reported.[45,46] Clinical features that suggest a psychogenic movement disorder are shown in Table 5.2.4.3.

In a recent systematic study of patients with fixed dystonia Schrag et al.[47] found that 37 per cent fulfilled criteria for psychogenic dystonia and 29 per cent criteria for *somatization disorder*, which is characterized by chronic, multiple, persistent, medically unexplained symptoms. Despite the fact that many patients fulfilled strict criteria for a somatoform disorder/psychogenic dystonia, in a

**Table 5.2.4.3** Features that suggest a psychogenic movement disorder

Abrupt onset
- Inconsistent movements (changing characteristics over time)
- Incongruous movements (movements do not fit with recognized patterns or with normal physiological patterns)
- Presence of additional types of abnormal movements that are not consistent with the basic abnormal movement pattern or are not congruous with a known movement disorder, particularly:
  - Rhythmical shaking
  - Bizarre gait
  - Deliberate slowness in carrying out the requested voluntary movement
  - Bursts of verbal gibberish
  - Excessive startle (bizarre movements in response to sudden, unexpected noise or threatening movement)
- Entrainment of the psychogenic tremor to the rate of the requested rapid successive movement the patient is asked to perform
- Demonstrating exhaustion and fatigue
- Spontaneous remissions
- Movements disappear with distraction
- Response to placebo, suggestion, or psychotherapy
- Presence as a paroxysmal disorder
- Dystonia beginning as a fixed posture

(Adapted with permission, from S. Fahn (1995))

proportion of patients the diagnosis remained uncertain, and whether the disorder was primarily neurological or psychiatric remains an open question. These patients require the services of a multi-disciplinary team.

The most common form of psychogenic movement disorder however is *psychogenic tremor*.[48] Almost 75 per cent of presenting patients are female and preceding events include work-related injuries and other accidents. A positive entrainment test (see Table 5.2.4.3), absence of finger tremor, and slowness of voluntary movements are suggestive of psychogenic origin. One-third has co-morbid somatoform disorders and one-fifth is involved in litigation or compensation. Prognosis is relatively poor if the condition has persisted for over 1 year, and in the long-term 80–90 per cent of patients continue to have abnormal movements.

### (c) Seizures (psychogenic non-epileptic seizures or PNES)

It is estimated that more than 25 per cent of patients receiving a diagnosis of refractory epilepsy in a chronic epilepsy clinic do not have epilepsy.[49] Although the population incidence of PNES may be only 4 per cent that of epilepsy, PNES comprises a large share of the workload of neurologists and emergency and general physicians. Unlike patients with epilepsy however, those with PNES often do not have designated nurses or health care workers assigned to help with the management of this potentially disabling disorder.

PNES can be distinguished from epileptic seizures: PNES generally occur in the presence of an audience or when one is close at hand. They may be precipitated by stress, but more often seem to occur in response to the social setting. The fall to the ground is not usually abrupt, and movements may follow the fall with clutching, but the characteristic regular tonic–clonic sequence of epilepsy is not found. Tongue biting and incontinence of urine are rare in hysterical fits, the corneal reflexes are preserved and the plantars are flexor, unless previously abnormal. Firm handling and pressure on the supra orbital nerves to the point of pain may arouse the patient. PNES occur most often among epileptic patients or among others who have seen epileptic fits. A few epileptic patients learn how to induce ictal discharges and can produce extra fits. Although rarely available during a fit, the EEG is generally abnormal in epilepsy and normal during hysterical fits.[31]

If PNES is not diagnosed and managed early, significant iatrogenic harm may occur. The outcome is not always favourable in these patients: in one recent study carried out at a mean of 11.9 years after manifestation and 4.1 years after diagnosis of PNES, 71 per cent of patients continued to have seizures and 56 per cent were dependent on social security. Outcome was better in patients with greater educational attainments, younger onset and diagnosis, attacks with less dramatic features, and fewer additional medically unexplained complaints.[50]

It has recently been reported that patients with PNES have a consistently different psychosocial profile from patients with motor conversion symptoms. In a prospective study of consecutive neurological inpatients with either motor conversion or pseudo seizures of recent onset, patients with PNES were younger, more likely to have both an emotionally unstable personality disorder and a lower perception of parental care, to report incest, and to have reported more life events in the 12 months before symptom onset than patients with motor conversion symptoms.[24] Recently a helpful fact sheet has been produced to help patients with PNES, which explains the nature of the disorder and approaches to management.[51] Although cognitive–behavioural therapy has been shown to be helpful in an open trial of patients with PNES, these findings need replication in a controlled setting.[52]

### Sensory symptoms

#### (a) Sensory disturbance

The clinical detection and localization of sensory dysfunction is probably one of the least reliable areas of the neurological examination. Sensory loss may involve half the entire body from top to toe or from right to left. It may affect the whole of a limb, and characteristically has a glove or stocking distribution on the arms or legs, or both. The sensory loss generally fails to fit in with known anatomical boundaries but conforms more with the patient's concept of physiology and anatomy. Thus hysterical sensory loss is likely to stop sharply at the midline, while non-hysterical sensory change will only approach the midline since at this point segmental nerves overlap by one or two centimetres on each side.

Unfortunately these classical signs are often unreliable. 'Psychogenic' features on sensory examination and diminished vibration sense over the affected part of the forehead have been found in over half of patients with neurological disorders.[53, 54] Rolak also found that 'midline splitting' of sensory function was not helpful in determining whether there was an underlying neurological disorder.[54] These clinical findings should clearly be interpreted with circumspection.

Toth has recently described 34 patients with the 'hemisensory' syndrome, in which patients present with hemisensory disturbance and intermittent blurring of vision in the ipsilateral eye (asthenopia) and sometimes ipsilateral hearing problems as well.[55] Hemisensory symptoms are increasingly recognized in patients with chronic pain and in patients with reflex sympathetic dystrophy.

#### (b) Visual disturbances

Ophthalmologists have estimated that psychogenic visual disorders account for up to 5 per cent of their practice.[56] Simple observation of visually guided behaviour will sometimes reveal telling inconsistencies, particularly in the case of severe apparent visual loss. A number of reliable optometric techniques are available to support bedside tests and the diagnosis of psychogenic visual loss, field disturbance, or gaze abnormality (for more details see Stone *et al.*[23]). Disabling hysterical blindness presents more difficulties. Evoked potential studies will help to demonstrate intact visual pathways.

## The disability associated with chronic conversion disorders

This topic is under-researched, but it is worth noting that, as the prognosis of CD is often poor, (not infrequently because patients are not diagnosed promptly, and even after diagnosis there are no resources to treat the patient). In the experience of the author this clinical conundrum is not improving: with the increase in provision of psychiatric services to the community and those with 'serious mental illness', patients with CD, even if they are profoundly disabled, often do not receive the appropriate treatment. Much of the disability is iatrogenic, and these patients will, not infrequently, be referred to the psychiatric service after having become confined to a wheelchair and/or in receipt of long-term disability benefits.[21,39] By this time the patients are usually entrenched in the sick role and it is very difficult to change the status quo.

## Prognosis

The aetiological implications accruing from recent follow-up studies[4, 57] suggest that a short history and young age are held to be predictors of good outcome, while the presence of a personality disorder, chronicity of symptoms, receipt of disability benefits, and involvement with litigation predict poor recovery. As regards social circumstances, a change in marital status, good family functioning, and the elimination of a stressor has been shown to have a positive effect on outcome.[58] There is little chance of improvement once the symptoms have become chronic and enduring.

Patients with chronic motor symptoms, e.g. unilateral functional weakness, as well as those with sensory symptoms, appear to do particularly poorly. In particular, patients with unexplained motor symptoms who are referred to tertiary care centres continue to do very poorly following discharge. Despite the stability of the diagnosis, a pattern of multiple hospital referrals continues for many of these patients once they have been discharged from the tertiary care centre. Interviews of patients conducted on an average of 6 years after their original admission to a tertiary care centre revealed that many continued to be referred to neurologists and other specialists, but that subsequent psychiatric referral was rare.[59] Many changed their primary care doctor after discharge from hospital and a disproportionate number of re-referrals were made by primary care doctors who had known their patients for less than 6 months. Psychological attribution of symptoms was rare, and many patients felt dissatisfied with the treatment they had received. Many were exposed to unnecessary iatrogenic harm. These consistent findings of very poor outcome following discharge from neurological outpatient and inpatient services in patients with both unexplained motor disorders as well as PNES suggest that without appropriate treatment the prognosis is poor.

## Management

It is remarkable that a disorder as common as schizophrenia and multiple sclerosis should have attracted so little research interest or treatment resources. One reason for this is that there have been no randomized controlled treatment studies of CD, and so at the time of writing there is no good evidence about the best intervention for conversion disorder. There has been considerable interest in this topic however, which has been the subject of a recent Cochrane review.[60] All of the studies in this review were of poor methodological quality. On the credit side there is evidence that interest in CD is increasing and attracting more research funding.

### Resources

Before any discussion of treatment it is important to consider the resources available to the neurologist to manage these patients. It is anomalous that, unlike disorders such as MS and schizophrenia, which have a similar prevalence, there are no designated resources for these patients. Some neurologists may have no access whatever to mental health resources, whereas others may have close collaborative links with either clinical psychology or psychiatry services. There is no doubt that the successful management of these patients requires the co-operation of a number of clinical specialties, including psychologists, nurses, physiotherapists, and occupational therapists (OTs). Some patients may be so disturbed or disabled (or both) that they may require inpatient admission to a specialized unit with access to both, mental health care and medical nurses, as well as physiotherapists and OTs. In the opinion of this writer every neurology service should have access to a specialist liaison psychiatry service.[61]

### Management strategies for the neurologist

First, the diagnosis has to be established by a neurologist after relevant organic disease has been excluded. Second, the neurologist has to not only explain to the patient that there is no serious underlying organic disease but also provide an explanation for the symptoms that is comprehensible to the patient.

It is worth noting at this stage that patients prefer the term 'functional' rather than 'hysterical', when their unexplained weakness, fits, etc. are being referred to.[62] It is also important to avoid verbal landmines—for example using the phrase 'not sinister' instead of 'not serious'; or 'not structural' instead of 'not physical'. In patients who are generally hostile to psychological explanations it is best to use the word 'functional' instead of 'psychological'.

An example of an explanation to a patient with functional weakness and sensory disturbance may be something like: *you have what we call functional weakness. This is a common medical problem. Your nervous system is not damaged—we can see that from the examination and scans, etc. This is why why when you try and send the messages to your limbs they do not move properly. Similarly this is why the sensations from your body are not being felt properly. The most important thing about this condition is that because your nervous system is not damaged, the problem is potentially reversible. All the parts of the nervous system are there but are just not working properly, so that when you try to move your leg it doesn't do it as well as*

*it should. Sometimes stress can cause these symptoms, which are often accompanied by worry and low mood but these are not the cause of the problem. Stress is a common problem and can lead to headache and abdominal pain as well as what we call functional weakness.*

This explanation can be supplemented by giving the patient a **fact sheet** containing information about functional weakness, which contains information about how to become involved with rehabilitation[51] (Fig. 5.2.4.3).

### Further management

Ideally the neurologist and psychiatrist should interview the patient together at the bedside, but this is not always possible. At the very least however close collaboration between the two is essential before the patient is reviewed by the psychiatrist and a formulation proposed (and any potential for iatrogenic illness or diagnostic confusion eliminated).

Traditional behavioural approaches to treatment are based on the premise that the symptoms reported by the patient are interpreted as physical but are amenable to recovery. Treatment aims to bring about a gradual increase in function through a combination of physical and occupational therapies. The patient receives rewards and praise for improvement of function, and withdrawal of reinforcement for continuing signs of disability. Avoiding direct confrontation of psychological problems and providing 'face-saving' techniques are also regarded as key components.[63] More recently the approach to patients has moved from a predominantly medical one, to one in which psychological and sociocultural aspects are equally important, and the need for organized specialist rehabilitation services involving a multi-disciplinary team is recognized as essential.

## What is the evidence?

With one or two recent exceptions,[64] there are no large, randomized controlled studies of treatment in patients with CDs. Neither is there any good evidence to support the use of one specific intervention, e.g. biofeedback, hypnosis, psychotherapy. Although repeated case series have documented the effectiveness of multi-disciplinary inpatient behavioural treatment, there is little controlled research.

In the absence of good experimental evidence a possible framework for future research has been developed which is based on published evidence and described in the WHO ICIDH.[65] This is particularly useful for patients in whom there is a disability that is out of proportion to known disease and signs. The model provides opportunities for intervention, and is well suited to the kind of multi-disciplinary approach that is likely to be successful in these patients.

The model emphasizes that whatever the primary cause of an illness, many factors (both individual and systemic) will have an influence on its manifestations. *For example: a vignette here.*

*A 20-year-old woman was referred to the liaison service with functional paraplegia of 12 months duration. Onset was temporally related to a back strain caused by lifting a chair. She was confined to a wheelchair and lived with her parents and 14-year-old brother in an adapted house (specially adapted chair and stair rails) and was in receipt of benefits. A home visit was carried out and the patient denied any current problems or recent life events, although she described a long history of medically unexplained symptoms, multiple food allergies, and previous treatment in an adolescent unit for chronic*

**Functional Weakness**

This leaflet aims to explain a bit about the symptom of functional weakness and what it means.

Not all of it may apply to you and you should discuss it with the doctor who gave it to you

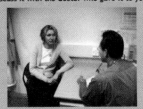

Patients with functional weakness often end up not feeling believed by doctors

It is likely that in common with other patients with functional weakness, that this is not your only symptom. This leaflet is not an attempt to cover all these symptoms but explanation of one of them.

**What is functional weakness ?**

Functional weakness refers to weakness of an arm or leg due to the nervous system not working properly. It is not caused by damage or disease of the nervous system.

Patients with functional weakness experience symptoms of limb weakness which can be disabling and frightening such as problems walking or a 'heaviness' down one side, dropping things or a feeling that a limb just doesn't feel normal or 'part of them'.

*Why are my tests normal?*

Patients with functional weakness have normal scans and other investigations. When they are examined, the doctor usually does not find any change in reflexes or other evidence of nervous system disease.

This is because in functional weakness all the parts of the nervous system are there, they are just not working properly so that when you try to move your arm or leg it doesn't do it as well as it should.

Your doctor may be able to find specific positive physical signs of functional weakness when you are examined and make the diagnosis in the same way as you would with a condition like migraine (which also does not have a 'test')

If you were a computer, it's a bit a like having a software problem rather than a hardware problem.

*Am I just imagining it then?*

One of the big problems patients with functional weakness experience is a feeling that they are not being believed. This is partly because many doctors are not trained well in physical symptoms that are not due to disease and research in these areas is very poor. Some doctors really don't believe patients with these symptoms. Others do believe them but find it hard to know how to help.

So if it's a real condition but its not a disease, what is it? Am I just imagining it?

The answer is you are not imagining or making up your symptoms and you are not 'going crazy'. You have a functional symptom or functional illness.

*What about all my other symptoms?*

These are some of the other symptoms that patients with functional weakness can experience as part of their illness. Often these symptoms are also caused by a dysfunction of the nervous system as part of one illness.

- Numbness or tingling
- Fatigue
- Arm or Leg pain
- Back or Neck pain
- Headache
- Poor concentration
- Sleep disturbance
- Word finding difficulty
- Slurred speech
- Blurred vision
- Bladder and Bowel sensitivity

- A floaty, distant feeling that things around you aren't quite real (derealisation)
- Episodes that look like epilepsy but are not
- Frustration, Anger
- Low mood
- Lack of enjoyment
- Worry
- Panic

*Why has it happened?*

Functional weakness is a complex phenomenon. It arises for different reasons in different people. Often the symptoms are accompanied by feelings of frustration, worry and low mood but these are not the *cause* of the problem.

We recognise a number of different situations in which functional weakness can arise. Your symptom may fall in to one of these categories although oftens none of these appear relevant:

1. After an injury / with pain—People seem particularly vunerable to functional weakness after a physical injury or if they have a lot of pain (particularly acute neck and back pain)
2. An illness with a lot of fatigue or bed rest— weakness can develop slowly in people who are suffering from excessive fatigue or exhaustion. In some patients too much rest can bring the symptoms on
3. Waking up from an anaesthetic—this is not due to damage from the anaesthetic but may be something to do with the transiently altered brain state when coming round. Similar things sometimes occur on normal waking

**Fig. 5.2.4.3** Fact sheet for patient with functional weakness (Reproduced from Stone, J. Carson, A. and Sharpe, M. (2005), Functional symptoms in neurology: management. *Neurology in Practice*, **71**(Suppl. 1), i13–i21. Copyright 2005, BMJ Publishing Group Ltd.)

*fatigue syndrome. She was seeing a chiropractor for her symptoms, and had been told that she had nerve damage (not confirmed). Her brother was off school with chronic fatigue and her mother had a long history of emotional problems. At interview, the family were polite but could not identify any link between recent events and her disabling symptoms. Discussion with the GP did not reveal any other relevant information and a follow-up was arranged 1 month later. Before this appointment the patient telephoned the psychiatrist to say that she had not disclosed certain facts at the initial meeting, and revealed that she had confronted her physically abusive step father and asked him to leave the house to live with his mistress (which he duly did). At follow-up there was a great deal of expressed relief, and the patient agreed with our formulation that, to some extent, she had developed weakness in the legs and become wheelchair bound in order to avoid being hit by her step father. She agreed to a brief admission to a rehabilitation unit, was encouraged to mobilize gradually and had regular sessions with a clinical psychologist. She responded well to treatment, commenced a college course, and learned to drive a car. At 3 year follow-up she was symptom free and in gainful employment. [the first vignette in this chapter].*

## Psychological treatments

Because patients with conversion disorders share features in common with patients with other medically unexplained syndromes, treatments that have been used in these latter disorders may have

potential. Most of the evidence-based treatments in this field involve cognitive–behavioural therapy (CBT,[66] or interpersonal therapy (IPT)). These usually have to be undertaken by trained clinical psychologists or other clinicians. However, increasing numbers of specialist nurses are being trained to deliver these treatments, so they should become more widely available.

CBT is concerned mainly with helping the patients overcome identified problems and ascertain specified goals. It discourages 'maintaining factors' such as repeated body self-checking and excessive bedrest, and challenges patients' negative or false beliefs about symptoms. Chalder has described specific CBT based treatment for patients with conversion disorders.[67]

## Hypnosis and intravenous sedation

In an inpatient trial of hypnosis both patients with CD and controls improved equally and no extra effect from hypnosis was found.[68] Others have found the use of intravenous sedatives, particularly propofol, helpful in persuading some patients with whom a good relationship has been established, that they can eventually make a recovery.[51]

## Pharmacological treatments

There is evidence from randomized controlled trials (RCTs) and systematic reviews that antidepressants (both tricyclics and selective serotonin reuptake inhibitors (SSRIs)) can be useful in the treatment of patients with medically unexplained symptoms (such as poor sleep and pain), whether or not depression is present.[69]

## Further information

Halligan, P., Bass, C., and Marshall, J. (eds.) (2001). *Contemporary approaches to the study of hysteria. Clinical and theoretical perspectives.* Oxford University Press, Oxford.

Hallett, M., Fahn, S., Jancovic, J., *et al.* (eds.) (2005). *Psychogenic movement disorders: psychobiology and treatment of a functional disorder.* Lippincott, Williams and Wilkins.

Trimble, M. (2004). *Somatoform disorders: a medicolegal guide.* Cambridge University Press, Cambridge.

## References

1. Collie, J. (1913). *Malingering and feigned sickness.* Edward Arnold, London.
2. Spence, S. (1999). Hysterical paralyses as disorders of action. *Cognitive Neuropsychiatry*, **4**, 203–26.
3. Carson, A., Ringbauer, B., Stone, J., *et al.* (2000). Do medically unexplained symptoms matter? A prospective cohort study of 300 new referrals to neurology outpatient clinics. *Journal of Neurology, Neurosurgery, and Psychiatry*, **68**, 207–11.
4. Crimlisk, H., Bhatia, K., Cope, H., *et al.* (1998). Slater revisited: 6 year follow up study of patients with medically unexplained motor symptoms. *British Medical Journal*, **316**, 582–6.
5. ICD-10 Classification of Mental and Behavioural Disorders (1992). WHO, Geneva.
6. American Psychiatric Association. (1994). *Diagnostic and statistical manual of mental disorders* (4th edn.). American Psychiatric Association, Washington, DC.
7. Shapiro, A. and Teasell, R.W. (2004). Behavioural interventions in the rehabilitation of acute v chronic non-organic (conversion/factitious) motor disorders. *British Journal of Psychiatry*, **185**, 140–6.
8. Bass, C. and Halligan, P. (2007). Illness related deception: social or psychiatric problem? *Journal of the Royal Society of Medicine*, **100**, 81–4.
9. Halligan, P., Bass, C., and Oakley, D. (2003). Wilful deception as illness behaviour. In *Malingering and illness deception* (eds. P. Halligan, C. Bass, and D. Oakley), pp. 3–28. Oxford University Press, Oxford.
10. Spence, S., Hunter, M., and Harpin, G. (2002). Neuroscience and the will. *Current Opinion in Psychiatry*, **15**, 519–26.
11. Holmes, E., Brown, R., Mansell, W., *et al.* (2005). Are there two qualitatively distinct forms of dissociation? A review and some clinical implications. *Clinical Psychology Review*, **25**, 1–25.
12. Brown, R.J. (2004). Psychological mechanisms of medically unexplained symptoms: an integrative conceptual model. *Psychological Bulletin*, **130**, 793–812.
13. Broome, M. (2004). A neuroscience of hysteria? *Current Opinion in Psychiatry*, **17**, 465–9.
14. Ghaffar, O., Staines, W., and Feinstein, A. (2006). Unexplained neurologic symptoms: an fMRI study of sensory conversion disorder. *Neurology*, **67**, 2036–8.
15. Marshall, J., Halligan, P., Gink, G., *et al.* (1997). The functional anatomy of a hysterical paralysis. *Cognition*, **64**, B1–8.
16. Spence, S., Crimlisk, H., Cope, H., *et al.* (2000). Discrete neurophysiological correlates in prefrontal cortex during hysterical and feigned disorder of movement. *Lancet*, **355**, 1243–4.
17. Kanaan, R.A., Wessely, S., and David, A. (2007). Imaging repressed memories in motor conversion disorder. *Psychosomatic Medicine*, **69**, 202–5.
18. Micale, M. (2001). Hysteria. In *The Oxford companion to the body* (eds. C. Blakemore and S. Jennett), pp. 382–4. Oxford University Press, Oxford.
19. Parry, A., Murray, B., Hart, Y., *et al.* (2006). Audit of resource use in patients with non-organic disorders admitted to a UK neurology unit. *Journal of Neurology, Neurosurgery and Psychiatry*, **77**, 1200–1.
20. Akagi, H. and House, A. (2002). The clinical epidemiology of hysteria: vanishingly rare, or just vanishing? *Psychological Medicine*, **32**, 191–4.
21. Allanson, J., Wade, D., and Bass, C. (2002). Characteristics of patients with persistent severe disability and medically unexplained neurological symptoms: a pilot study. *Journal of Neurology, Neurosurgery, and Psychiatry*, **73**, 307–9.
22. Stone, J. and Zeman, A. (2001). Hysterical conversion-a view from clinical neurology. In *Contemporary approaches to the science of hysteria* (eds. P. Halligan, C. Bass, and J. C Marshall) pp. 102–25, Oxford University Press, Oxford.
23. Stone, J., Sharpe, M., and Binzer, M. (2004). Motor conversion symptoms and pseudoseizures: a comparison of clinical characteristics. *Psychosomatics*, **45**, 492–9.
24. Binzer, M., Stone, J., and Sharpe, M. (2004). Recent onset pseudoseizures—clues to aetiology. *Seizure*, **13**, 146–55.
25. O'Sullivan, G., Harvey, I., Bass, C., *et al.* (1992). Psychophysiological investigations of patients with unilateral symptoms in the hyperventilation syndrome. *British Journal of Psychiatry*, **160**, 664–7.
26. Tavel, M. (1964). Hyperventilation syndrome with unilateral somatic symptoms. *Journal of the American Medical Association*, **187**, 301–3.
27. Blau, N., Wiles, M., and Solomon, F. (1989). Unilateral somatic symptoms due to hyperventilation. *British Medical Journal*, **286**, 1108.
28. Wessely, S., Nimnuan, C., and Sharpe, M. (1999). Functional somatic syndromes: one or many? *Lancet*, **354**, 36–9.
29. Bhui Hotopf, M. (1997). Somatisation disorder. *British Journal of Hospital Medicine*, **58**, 145–9.
30. Binzer, M., Andersen, P., and Kullgren, G. (1997). Clinical characteristics of patients with motor disability due to conversion disorder: a prospective control group study. *Journal of Neurology, Neurosurgery, and Psychiatry*, **63**, 83–8.
31. Reuber, M. and Elger, C. (2003). Psychogenic non epileptic seizures: review and update. *Epilepsy & Behaviour*, **4**, 205–16.
32. Letonoff, E.J., Williams, T.R., and Sidhu, K. (2002). Hysterical paralysis: a report of three cases and a review of the literature. *Spine*, **27**, E441–5.
33. Lichter, I., Goldstein, L., Toone, B., *et al.* (2004). Nonepileptic seizures following general anaesthetic: a report of 5 cases. *Epilepsy & Behaviour*, **5**, 1005–13.
34. Reuber, M., Howlett, S., Khan, A., *et al.* (2007). Non-epileptic seizures and other functional neurological symptoms: predisposing, precipitating, and perpetuating factors. *Psychosomatics*, **48**, 230–8.
35. Factor, S., Podskalny, R., and Molho, E. (1995). Psychogenic movement disorders: frequency, clinical profile and characteristics. *Journal of Neurology, Neurosurgery and Psychiatry*, **59**, 406–12.
36. Verdugo, R. and Ochoa, J. (2000). Abnormal movements in complex regional pain syndrome: assessment of their nature. *Muscle Nerve*, **23**, 198–205.
37. Pearce, J. (2005). Chronic regional pain and chronic pain syndromes. *Spinal Cord*, **43**, 263–8.
38. Stone, J., Sharpe, M., Carson, A., *et al.* (2002). Are functional motor and sensory symptoms really more frequent on the left? A systematic review. *Journal of Neurology, Neurosurgery, and Psychiatry*, **73**, 578–81.
39. Davison, P., Sharpe, M., Wade, D., *et al.* (1999). "Wheelchair" patients with non organic disease: a psychological enquiry. *Journal of Psychosomatic Research*, **47**, 93–103.
40. Stone, J., Smyth, R., Carson, A., *et al.* (2006). La belle indifference in conversion symptoms and hysteria: systematic review. *British Journal of Psychiatry*, **188**, 204–9.
41. Ziv, I., Djaldetti, R., and Zoldan, Y. (1998). Diagnosis of "non-organic" limb paresis by a novel objective motor assessment: the quantitative Hoover's test. *Journal of Neurology*, **245**, 797–802.
42. Baker, J. and Silver, J. (1987). Hysterical paraplegia. *Journal of Neurology, Neurosurgery and Psychiatry*, **50**, 375–82.

43. Heruti, R., Reznik, J., Adunski, A., *et al.* (2002). Conversion motor paralysis disorder: analysis of 34 consecutive referral. *Spinal Cord*, **430**, 335–40.

44. Hallett, M., Fahn, S., Jankovic, J., *et al.* (eds.) (2005). *Psychogenic movement disorders: psychobiology and treatment of a functional disorder*. Lippincott, Williams and Wilkins, Philadelphia.

45. Fahn, S. and Williams, D. (1988). Psychogenic dystonia. In *Advances of Neurology*, Vol. 50: *Dystonia 2* (eds. S. Fahn, *et al.*), pp. 431–55. Raven Press, New York.

46. Lang, A.E. (1995). Psychogenic dystonia: a review of 18 cases. *Canadian Journal of Neurological Sciences*, **22**, 136–43.

47. Schrag, A., Trimble, M., Quinn, N., *et al.* (2004). The syndrome of fixed dystonia: an evaluation of 103 patients. *Brain*, **127**, 2360–72.

48. Bhatia, K. and Schneider, S. (2007). Psychogenic tremor and related disorders. *Journal of Neurology*, Apr 9; [Epub ahead of print].

49. Smith, D., Defalla, B., and Chadwick, D. (1999). The misdiagnosis of epilepsy and the management of refractory epilepsy in a specialist clinic. *Quarterly Journal of Medicine*, **92**, 15–23.

50. Reuber, M., Pukrop, R., Bauer, J., *et al.* (2003). Outcome in psychogenic nonepileptic seizures: 1 to 10 year follow up in 164 patients. *Annals of Neurology*, **53**, 305–11.

51. Stone, J., Carson, A., and Sharpe, M. (2005). Functional symptoms in neurology: management. *Neurology in Practice*, **71**(Suppl. 1), i13–i21. http://www.jnnp.com.

52. Goldstein, L., Mellors, J., and Toone, B. (2004). An evaluation of cognitive behavioral therapy as a treatment for dissociative seizures: a pilot study. *Cognitive Behavioural Neurology*, **17**, 41–9.

53. Gould, R., Miller, B., Goldberg, M., *et al.* (1986). The validity of hysterical signs and symptoms. *Journal of Nervous and Mental Diseases*, **174**, 593–7.

54. Rolak, L. (1988). Psychogenic sensory loss. *Journal of Nervous and Mental Disease*, **176**, 686–7.

55. Toth, C. (2003). Hemisensory syndrome is associated with a low diagnostic yield and a nearly uniform benign prognosis. *Journal of Neurology, Neurosurgery, and Psychiatry*, **74**, 1113–6.

56. Kathol, R., Cox, T., Corbett, J., *et al.* (1983). Functional visual loss: I. A true psychiatric disorder? *Psychological Medicine*, **13**, 307–14.

57. Stone, J., Sharpe, M., Rothwell, P., *et al.* (2003). The 12-year prognosis of unilateral functional weakness and sensory disturbance. *Journal of Neurology, Neurosurgery, and Psychiatry*, **74**, 591–6.

58. Ron, M. (2001). The prognosis of hysteria/somatisation disorder. In *Contemporary approaches to the study of hysteria* (eds. P. Halligan, C. Bass, and J. Marshall), pp. 271–83, Oxford University Press, Oxford.

59. Crimlisk, H., Bhatia, K., Cope, H., *et al.* (2000). Patterns of referral in patients with medically unexplained motor symptoms. *Journal of Psychosomatic Research*, **49**, 217–9.

60. Ruddy, R. and House, A. (19 October 2005). Psychosocial interventions for conversion disorder. *Cochrane Database Systematic Review*, (4): CD005331.

61. Gotz, M. and House, A. (1998). Prognosis of symptoms that are medically unexplained. *British Medical Journal*, **317**, 536.

62. Stone, J., Wojcik, W., and Durrance, D., (2002). What should we say to patients with symptoms unexplained by disease? The number needed to offend. *British Medical Journal*, **325**, 1449–50.

63. Teasell, R. and Shapiro, A. (1993). Rehabilitation of chronic motor conversion disorder. *Critical Review of Physical and Rehabilitation Medicine*, **5**, 1–13.

64. Moene, F., Spinhoven P, *et al.* (2003). A randomized controlled clinical trial of a hypnosis-based treatment for patients with conversion disorder, motor type. *International Journal of Clinical and Experimental Hypnosis*, **51**, 29–50.

65. WHO. (2001). International classification of functioning, disability and health. World Health Organization, Geneva. http://www3.who.int/icficftemplate.cfm

66. Kroenke, K. and Swindle, R. (2001). Cognitive behavioural therapy for somatisation and symptom syndromes: a critical review of controlled clinical trials. *Psychotherapy and Psychosomatics*, **69**, 205–15.

67 Chalder, T. (2001). Cognitive behavioural therapy as a treatment for conversion disorders. In *Contemporary approaches to the study of hysteria: clinical and theoretical perspectives* (eds. P. Halligan, C. Bass, and J. Marshall), pp. 298–311. Oxford University Press, Oxford.

68. Moene, F., Spinhoven, P., Hoogduin, K., *et al.* (2002). A randomised controlled clinical trial on the additional effect of hypnosis in a comprehensive treatment programme for inpatients with conversion disorder of the motor type. *Psychotherapy and Psychosomatics*, **71**, 66–76.

69. Jackson, J., O'Malley, P., and Kroenke, K. (2006). Antidepressants and cognitive-behavioral therapy for symptom syndromes. *CNS Spectrum*, **11**, 212–22.

# 5.2.5 Hypochondriasis (health anxiety)

Russell Noyes Jr.

## Introduction

Hypochondriasis is a preoccupation with the fear that one has, or may develop, serious disease despite evidence to the contrary. So defined, the disorder affects between 2 and 7 per cent of patients attending general medical clinics and is a cause of physical dysfunction and disability.[1] It is also a reason for increased health care utilization and dissatisfaction with care received. To their physicians, patients with this disorder are an enigma and a source of frustration.

Unfortunately, relatively little is known about hypochondriasis. Primary care physicians have had little interest and psychiatrists see few patients with the condition. It is a pejorative label that, even if entertained, is rarely communicated. And, even if communicated, the diagnosis would not, until very recently, have led to effective treatment.

### History

Hypochondria was used by Hippocrates to refer to a region below the cartilage of the ribs. In the second century, Galen linked it to organs in this area as well as humours and animal spirits. The symptom picture was ill-defined and only gradually took on the characteristics recognized today. From earliest times the disorder was associated with melancholia, a temperamental disturbance caused by an excess of black bile. Burton (1621) described hypochondriacal melancholy in terms of vague physical symptoms, disturbances of mood, and fears. In the seventeenth century, Sydenham viewed hypochondria in men as the counterpart of hysteria in women, but the first modern description was published in 1799 by Sims.

By the eighteenth century, hypochondria became part of a fashionable disturbance that Cheyne attributed to the English way of life and environment. However, as notions of aetiology began to shift under the influence of Cartesian dualism, hypochondria was increasingly seen as a weakness and moral failing. Falret (1822) was

**Table 5.2.5.1** Essential and associated features of hypochondriasis

Essential features
    Fear of disease
    Disease conviction
    Bodily preoccupation
    Somatic symptoms
    Reassurance-seeking
Associated features
    Fear of aging and death
    Overvaluation of health
    Low self-esteem
    Sense of vulnerability to illness

perhaps the first to identify it as a mental disorder, one of the neuroses. Freud viewed hypochondria as an 'actual neurosis', having a physiological basis and not amenable to psychoanalysis. However, present-day descriptions began with Gillespie,[2] who in 1928 defined hypochondriasis as 'a mental preoccupation with a real or supposititious physical or mental disorder'.

## Conceptualizations

Authors disagree about how hypochondriasis should be conceptualized. Some look upon it as a personality trait; its early onset and long-term stability in many patients fit this conception. Others view it as a dimension of psychopathology. They see illness worry as a continuum with hypochondriasis falling on the severe end. For those who take a categorical approach, the issue of whether hypochondriasis is primary or secondary remains unsettled. High rates of comorbidity create doubt about its independent status. Based on existing evidence, some question whether hypochondriasis can be regarded as a discrete psychiatric disorder.[3]

## Clinical picture

### Essential features

The essential characteristics of hypochondriasis are shown in Table 5.2.5.1. These include fear of serious disease, the consequences of which may include pain, suffering, disability, and death. Such fears take the form of alarming thoughts and images of specific diseases. They also include conviction or belief that the feared disease is already present. This belief is overvalued meaning that it is strongly held despite lack of evidence; it is not delusional.

Bodily preoccupation is perhaps the most important feature.[4] This takes the form of intense interest in, and attention to, what is happening in the body. The focus is upon somatic symptoms which tend to be multiple and diffuse. Attention is also directed to bodily sensations, bodily functions, and minor abnormalities as well as related concerns such as diet, exercise, and environmental exposures. The activities and conversation of patients are dominated by medical concerns. As a consequence of their self-absorption, interest in other people and pursuits is withdrawn.

Reassurance-seeking is the main behavioural feature. Patients repeatedly check their bodies for signs of serious disease. They check their pulse, look for lumps, examine themselves in the mirror, etc. In addition, they search medical sources for the meaning of their symptoms. Such patients also ask friends, family, and medical professionals for reassurance. Their search may lead to excessive utilization of health services.

## Associated features

Associated characteristics include fears of aging and death, which appear to be an integral part of hypochondriasis. Overvaluation of health and appearance is another related feature. Hypochondriacal patients may become preoccupied with eating natural foods, achieving physical fitness, and living a healthy lifestyle, activities that reflect their idealized conception of good health.

Patients with hypochondriasis feel unworthy and unlovable.[4] As a consequence of their low self-esteem they have negative expectations of others including medical professionals. In addition, they have a sense of vulnerability to illness.[5] These characteristics have to do with fundamental aspects of the self that the hypochondriacal patient views as deficient.

## Subtypes

Hypochondriacal patients are heterogeneous and subtypes may exist. Separate dimensions of disease phobia and disease conviction have consistently been identified; in some patients fears are prominent and in others conviction dominates the picture. Others may resemble patients with obsessive-compulsive disorder or personality disorders of one kind or another.

## Classification

### Criteria

Hypochondriasis initially appeared in DSM-II as one of the neuroses. In DSM-III, it was moved to the somatoform disorders, and diagnostic criteria were provided. In a revision of the classification (DSM-III-R), a duration of 6 months was added, and patients with delusional beliefs were excluded. The DSM-IV criteria are shown in Table 5.2.5.2. They exclude patients whose symptoms are better explained by other anxiety, depressive, or somatoform disorders.[1] Also, in DSM-IV, specific phobia of illness is separated from hypochondriasis. The illness phobic is said to fear contracting an illness whereas the hypochondriac fears disease already present.

The ICD-10 criteria for hypochondriacal disorder differ from those in DSM-IV. They require a persistent belief about having one or more specifically named serious physical diseases.[6] In addition, they include body dysmorphic disorder. With respect to illness behaviour, the ICD-10 criteria state that hypochondriacal concerns cause persons to seek medical investigation or treatment. They also state that patients may accept reassurance in the short-term, but that in the long run they are not likely to respond.

**Table 5.2.5.2** Abbreviated DSM-IV diagnostic criteria for hypochondriasis

(a) Preoccupation with fears of having, or the idea that one has, a serious disease based on misinterpretation of bodily symptoms

(b) The preoccupation persists despite appropriate medical evaluation and reassurance

(c) Belief not of delusional intensity

(d) Preoccupation causes significant distress or impairment

(e) Duration of at least 6 months

(f) Not better accounted for by other anxiety, depressive, or somatoform disorders

The somatoform disorders category to which hypochondriasis belongs is controversial, and many question its inclusion in the classification.[7] They see these disorders as ill-defined, of questionable validity and based more on illness behaviour than on distinctive features. They also view them as creations of Western biomedicine that serve to devalue patients who challenge the theoretical model upon which it is based.[8] According to that model, illness is a response to disease, and the person who is ill without disease, e.g. hypochondriasis, is marginalized.

Were the somatoform disorders to be eliminated, some have proposed moving hypochondriasis to the anxiety disorders (health anxiety) or to a proposed grouping, the obsessive-compulsive spectrum disorders.

## Validity

Evidence for the validity and utility of the diagnosis of hypochondriasis remains limited. In studies aimed at demonstrating validity, Barsky et al.[9] showed that distinguishing characteristics of the disorder aggregated in some medical outpatients but were less common in others. The same patients had other features of hypochondriasis indicating external validity. Using a structured interview for hypochondriasis, these investigators and others[10,11] observed a positive correlation between interview and physician ratings (concurrent validity). Hypochondriacal patients also had more ancillary features of hypochondriasis than did control patients (external validity). Also, other clinical characteristics distinguished interview positive from interview negative patients, indicating discriminate validity. Follow-up studies have shown a degree of diagnostic stability suggesting predictive validity.[12,13]

## Measures

A variety of measures have been developed to screen for hypochondriasis and assess the severity of hypochondriacal concerns.[14] These are shown in Table 5.2.5.3. The Whiteley Index, a self-report instrument based on the observed characteristics of hypochondriacal psychiatric patients, is one of the most widely used.[15] It consists of 14 yes versus no items, but recent work suggests that a 7-item version is satisfactory for screening. The Illness Attitude Scales is a 27-item measure of psychopathology associated with hypochondriasis.[16] A principal components' analysis yielded two factors, one measuring health anxiety and the other illness

**Table 5.2.5.3** Measures for the assessment of hypochondriasis

| Self-rated questionnaires |
| --- |
| Whiteley index |
| Illness worry scale |
| Illness attitude scales |
| Health anxiety questionnaire |
| Health anxiety inventory |
| Multidimensional inventory of hypochondriacal traits |
| Psychiatric diagnostic screening questionnaire |
| Structured interviews |
| Structured diagnostic interview for hypochondriasis |
| Structured clinical interview for DSM-IV |
| Composite international diagnostic interview |
| Schedules for clinical assessment in neuropsychiatry |

behaviour. The health anxiety subscale has been used to distinguish hypochondriacal from non-hypochondriacal patients.

Recently, self-assessment measures have been developed to assess the various dimensions of health anxiety and hypochondriasis. The Health Anxiety Inventory contains 47 items covering a range of hypochondriacal features.[17] An advantage of this scale is that it distinguishes patients with high health anxiety from those with physical illness.

The Structured Clinical Interview for DSM-IV (SCID) and the Composite International Diagnostic Interview (CIDI) are comprehensive diagnostic interviews that contain somatoform disorder modules. The CIDI has been used in epidemiologic surveys. Its stem question for hypochondriasis is, 'In the past 12 months, have you had a period of 6 months or more when most of the time you worried about having a serious physical illness or deformity?'

Based on the SCID, Barsky et al.[10] developed a structured interview that focuses exclusively on hypochondriasis. It begins with a series of probe questions that, if answered affirmatively, trigger the remaining interview. It is suitable for confirming the diagnosis in a screened population.

Diagnostic assessment remains less than satisfactory because the threshold for caseness has not been established, medical and psychiatric comorbidity make diagnostic decision-making difficult, and independent medical evaluation is rarely part of the process.

## Differential diagnosis

### Physical disorders

A few hypochondriacal patients suffer from undetected physical disease. Consequently, it is important to exclude medical conditions that, in their early stages, may cause vague symptoms with few signs or laboratory abnormalities. These include neurological conditions, such as multiple sclerosis or myasthenia gravis; endocrine conditions, such as thyroid or parathyroid disorders; multisystem disease such as systemic lupus erythematosus or occult malignancies. Because of such possibilities, a physical cause warrants continuing consideration even after the initial work-up has been completed.

### Psychiatric disorders

Patients with **panic disorder** may be difficult to distinguish from those with hypochondriasis because they commonly have hypochondriacal features. A diagnosis of hypochondriasis should not be made if illness concerns are better accounted for by panic disorder. Patients with hypochondriasis tend to fear the long-term consequences of illness (such as cancer) whereas those with panic fear the immediate consequences of illness events (such as a heart attack); the former fear death, the latter dying. Also, those with hypochondriasis misinterpret a range of bodily sensations, whereas those with panic misinterpret the symptoms of autonomic arousal.

Hypochondriasis must be distinguished from **specific phobia, illness subtype**.[1] Patients with hypochondriasis are preoccupied with a disease they believe is already present, whereas illness phobics fear developing a disease they do not yet have. Illness phobic symptoms are triggered by external as well as internal cues. For instance, exposure to a person with the feared disease may elicit a fear response.

Hypochondriasis must be distinguished from **obsessive-compulsive disorder**. Patients with the latter often have intrusive thoughts about disease or contamination and rituals that involve checking or reassurance-seeking. They differ from patients with hypochondriasis in having other obsessions and compulsions. Obsessive-compulsive patients tend to regard their ideas as senseless and resist them, whereas those with hypochondriasis regard them with conviction.

Hypochondriasis must also be distinguished from **generalized anxiety disorder** which is characterized by excessive worry about a number of areas. These may include health but other areas are generally involved as well. If worry is confined to illness, then a diagnosis of GAD should not be made. Patients with GAD tend to have health worries that are general, whereas those with hypochondriasis involve specific diseases such as cancer.

Hypochondriasis that develops during an episode of **major depression** and remits with treatment of the mood disturbance may be better accounted for by the depressive disorder. In that case, the patient is likely to focus concern upon the vegetative symptoms of depression and interpret these as irreversible loss of health. On the other hand, a diagnosis of hypochondriasis may be appropriate when hypochondriacal concerns are not confined to an episode of depression and are not focused on symptoms of the mood disorder.

Hypochondriasis and **somatization disorder** are both characterized by somatic symptoms. However, patients with hypochondriasis worry about the meaning of symptoms rather than the symptoms themselves. They are concerned about the consequences of serious illnesses rather than securing the gains of illness (e.g. sick role) as are patients with somatization disorder. Patients with hypochondriasis have an equal sex distribution whereas those with somatization disorder are predominantly women.

Hypochondriacal beliefs of a delusional nature may occur in patients with psychoses, but these patients usually have other psychotic features. However, delusions of disease may be the main or only manifestation of **delusional disorder, somatic type**. Such delusions may be bizarre or unrealistic, whereas the beliefs of patients with hypochondriasis are overvalued.

# Epidemiology

## Prevalence

The prevalence of hypochondriasis in the **general population** has not been established. Major surveys of psychiatric disorders have either excluded the somatoform disorders or identified few cases. For instance, Looper and Kirmayer[18] found that 6 per cent responded affirmatively to screening for illness worry, but only 0.2 per cent met full criteria for hypochondriasis according to a structured interview. Two studies that focused exclusively on somatoform disorders obtained higher estimates (4.5 and 7.7 per cent).[19, 20] Two other surveys focusing on illness worry found that half the respondents with such worry had the illness they worried about.[18, 21] Among such people it may be difficult to distinguish excessive from normal worry.

The prevalence of hypochondriasis among **primary care outpatients** had been examined in a number of studies. In a cross-national survey, Gureje et al.[22] noted that, if the criterion of failure to respond to reassurance were set aside, 2.2 per cent of patients qualified for this diagnosis and were as impaired as those meeting full criteria. In studies based on structured interviews, prevalence estimates have ranged from 2.2 per cent to 9.4 per cent.

Hypochondriasis may be prevalent in **medical specialty populations** where patients with functional disturbances are common.

For instance, one survey found the disorder in 13 per cent of otolaryngology clinic patients. Also, hypochondriacal concerns are higher in patients with functional than with organic illnesses. For example, in one study higher hypochondriasis scores were obtained from patients with irritable bowel syndrome than from patients with organic gastrointestinal disease. Hypochondriacal concerns and health anxiety are especially high in patients with chronic pain.

High health anxiety is one of the factors shared by functional somatic syndromes in the general population.[23] However, it is not clear whether this represents a vulnerability factor or a consequence of unexplained symptoms.

## Risk factors

Risk factors for unexplained somatic symptoms include female gender, older age, non-white race, less education, and lower income. With respect to hypochondriasis, few of these demographic factors appear important although findings have been inconsistent. The risk for men appears to be equal that for women. Some studies have shown persons with illness worry and hypochondriasis to be older and to have more physical illness. Two studies found them to have less education.

## Comorbidity

Hypochondriacal patients in primary care have high levels of psychological as well as somatic symptoms. Strong positive correlations have been observed between hypochondriacal concerns and depressive ($r = 0.58$), anxiety ($r = 0.55$), and somatic symptoms ($r = 0.52$). In one study, the proportions of hypochondriacal and control patients, having one or more comorbid disorder, were 62 and 30 per cent respectively. Anxiety and depressive disorders accounted for most of the excess.

## Family and twin studies

Taylor et al.[24] used a twin study to examine the genetic and environmental contribution to excessive health anxiety. After controlling for medical morbidity, which may be a source of health anxiety, they found that genetic factors accounted for 37 per cent of the variance in fear of disease and 10 per cent in disease conviction. For both dimensions the remainder of the variance (63 and 90 per cent respectively) was accounted for by non-shared environmental factors. These and other results suggest that some dimensions of health anxiety are moderately heritable. They also suggest that such anxiety is largely a learned phenomenon.

A family study compared the first-degree relatives of probands with and without hypochondriasis obtained from a general medicine clinic.[25] No difference in the frequency of hypochondriasis was found between these groups of family members. However, certain traits and attitudes, such as hostility, low agreeableness, and dissatisfaction with care, were significantly higher among the relatives of hypochondriasis probands. Such traits and attitudes may confer vulnerability to hypochondriasis and/or other somatoform disorders.

## Morbidity and service utilization

Hypochondriasis is associated with impairment in physical functioning and work performance. Patients with this disorder view their health as worse, and experience more physical disability as well as impairment in occupational roles than patients without hypochondriasis.[10, 11] They use more medical services yet are less satisfied with them than non-hypochondriacal patients. This increased utilization includes physician visits, laboratory tests, outpatient costs, and hospitalizations. Hypochondriacal patients tend to feel that their medical problems have not been thoroughly evaluated and as a consequence consult many physicians (i.e. doctor-shopping).

Hypochondriasis and health anxiety tend to be associated with increased symptom reporting and functional impairment, although the findings from various clinical populations have been inconsistent. For instance, hypochondriacal concerns are associated with higher disability and lower quality of life among patients with irritable bowel syndrome, chronic fatigue, and fibromyalgia.[26] One study found hypochondriasis the strongest predictor of pain due to osteoarthritis, and another showed high health anxiety predictive of abdominal pain 1 year later. Hypochondriasis was also a predictor of disability in patients with coronary artery disease. Consistent with these observations, hypochondriasis is associated with increased reporting of, and distress from, medication side effects.

## Aetiology and pathogenesis

### Personality

Hypochondriacal concerns are strongly related to the major personality dimension of neuroticism or negative emotionality.[27] Positive correlations between neuroticism and hypochondriacal concerns ranging from 0.4 to 0.5 have consistently been observed in non-clinical samples. Neuroticism refers to a tendency to experience and report negative emotions and overreact to stress. Persons high on this dimension are prone to find bodily sensations noxious and interpret them as signs of serious illness. Neuroticism may represent a vulnerability factor for hypochondriasis.

Certain personality traits may have more to do with difficult patient–doctor relationships than with hypochondriasis itself. Patients with hypochondriasis have been described as angry and mistrustful. Such characteristics might reflect negative emotions belonging to the domain of neuroticism or the negative pole of agreeableness, another of the major personality dimensions. They might also reflect obsessive-compulsive or masochistic personality traits observed in some patients.

### Developmental factors

Childhood influences appear to be important in the development of hypochondriasis. Reports of **traumatic events during childhood**, including physical and sexual abuse, have been elicited more frequently from hypochondriacal than non-hypochondriacal patients. Although findings are preliminary, they are consistent with a literature linking childhood neglect and abuse to unexplained somatic symptoms in adults.

**Childhood experience of illness** may contribute to the development of hypochondriasis. For instance, Noyes et al.[28] obtained reports of serious illness or injury before age 17 from a third of adults with hypochondriasis. Similar findings from patients with hypochondriasis and somatization have been reported by others. Early illness may create a sense of physical vulnerability in susceptible individuals. Childhood exposure to serious illness or death of a family member or friend may do likewise.

**Parental attitudes** may also contribute to hypochondriasis. Excessive concern for a child's health or overprotection on the part of a parent may lead to anxiety about health as may special caretaking and rewards for illness. A child may also model exaggerated illness behaviour displayed by a parent. The importance of developmental factors—early adversity, experience of illness, over solicitous parents—suggest that hypochondriasis is in large measure learned behaviour.

### Life events

Stressful life events appear to be related to increased reporting of physical symptoms and hypochondriasis, although there have been few studies. Events involving illness and death may have a specific role as the symptoms of hypochondriacal patients sometimes resemble those of family members who have been ill or died. In addition, illness events may give rise to hypochondriacal symptoms; 'cardiac neurosis' following myocardial infarction is an example. Transient hypochondriasis has been observed following medical illness in predisposed individuals.

### Cognitive and perceptual factors

According to the cognitive-perceptual model, hypochondriasis is based on misinterpretation of bodily symptoms as signs of serious disease and on the experience of somatic sensations as intense, noxious, and disturbing.[29] In this model, the faulty attribution of innocuous sensations is the central defect. A number of studies have shown that, when symptoms are attributed to pathological processes, they become intensified. Such attribution may focus attention on symptoms thereby amplifying them. Misinterpretation of this kind may arise from cognitive schemata that were established through earlier experience with illness.

The tendency to experience bodily sensations as intense and disturbing has been termed somatosensory amplification. One study that used the Somatosensory Amplification Scale found a positive correlation of 0.56 between amplification and hypochondriasis. This finding suggests that individuals with hypochondriasis have a constitutionally lowered threshold for physical symptoms or that they have a heightened attentional focus and increased physiological arousal.

Evidence of physiological abnormalities was obtained by Gramling et al.[30] In a preliminary investigation, they observed physiological reactivity that distinguished women with hypochondriasis from those without. Hypochondriacal subjects had a higher mean heart rate and lower mean hand temperature during a cold pressor test compared to controls. These subjects terminated the test more frequently and rated it as more unpleasant than did controls.

### Interpersonal factors

According to the interpersonal model, hypochondriasis is a form of care-eliciting behaviour that finds expression in physical complaints. Through unexplained somatic symptoms and expressions of illness worry, patients with this disorder seek emotional and interpersonal support from family members and physicians. Need for support of this kind arises from insecure attachment that originated in early relationships with caregivers. In a test of this model, Noyes et al.[31] found that hypochondriacal concerns among primary care patients were associated with various insecure attachment styles. These concerns were also associated with interpersonal problems and lack of reassurance from medical care.

### Social and cultural factors

Social and cultural factors are important determinants of hypochondriasis. Throughout the world physical symptoms are common vehicles for the communication of distress. Somatic distress gains the attention of **family and community** because it signals impairment in functioning that could alter social roles. Such distress not only calls forth caretaking but also obtains the sick role for those with acute illness. This social role with its privileges and responsibilities protects society from the disruptive effects of illness and promotes the return to health and social functioning of its members. Persons who are socially isolated or lacking in social support are more likely to manifest care-eliciting behaviour such as hypochondriasis.

**Physicians** play an important role in the development of hypochondriasis. They may make alarming statements or fail to provide reassurance that is based on thorough evaluation. In addition, they may order unnecessary tests, diagnose undetected disease, or treat injudiciously. They may add to concerns by failing to diagnose the psychiatric disturbance—hypochondriasis—telling patients instead that nothing is wrong. In doing this, they challenge and reject patients thereby contributing to suffering and alienation from the health care system.

**Cultural attitudes** may contribute to hypochondriasis. The American lifestyle, which emphasizes fitness and attractiveness, fosters preoccupation with health and encourages people to see their distress in terms of physical illness. There are, for example, cultural differences in the threshold for pain, pain tolerance, patterns of arousal, and physiological and behavioural responses to pain.

## Course and outcome

### Course

Hypochondriasis may begin at any age including childhood. The onset may be associated with stressful life events that in some instances involve illness. Some individuals develop hypochondriacal concerns transiently and others lastingly in reaction to physical illness. Among family medicine patients, those who became hypochondriacal a year after initial assessment were found to have had more illness worry and unexplained symptoms and to have rated their health as worse at baseline than non-hypochondriacal patients. Ambiguous symptoms or illness events may contribute to hypochondriacal concerns in patients so predisposed. Hypochondriasis appears to follow a chronic, fluctuating course.

### Outcome

Follow-up studies show that, after their initial clinic visit, most patients with hypochondriasis improve. Still, a substantial proportion continue to meet criteria for the disorder and many more have persisting symptoms. For instance, among hypochondriacal general medicine patients, Noyes et al.[12] and Barsky et al.[13] found that, after 1 to 4 years, two-thirds continued to qualify for the diagnosis and the remaining one-third had persisting symptoms. Thus, despite improvement, the patients continued to be more hypochondriacal, more impaired, and more symptomatic than non-hypochondriacal patients.

Like patients in general, those with hypochondriacal concerns tend to seek care when they are most distressed. Their subsequent improvement may represent a natural fluctuation, a response to physician contact or to non-specific treatment. Some patients report having responded to reassurance. In a few instances, serious medical illness may relieve hypochondriacal concerns by legitimizing symptoms.

Studies indicate that greater severity and longer duration of symptoms are predictive of worse outcome. Failure to remit in one or more follow-up studies was predicted by more severe hypochondriacal concerns and somatic symptoms, longer duration of hypochondriasis, more psychiatric comorbidity, poorer perception of health, and greater neuroticism.

### Complications

There is little information concerning complications of hypochondriasis. Because some patients utilize extensive medical care, one might expect complications resulting from repeated or unnecessary evaluations, tests, procedures, or treatments. Such iatrogenic complications have been reported for somatoform disorders but there is little documentation for hypochondriasis. On the other hand, physical illness may be overlooked in patients whose problems are considered psychiatric. There is almost no information on mortality. Suicide is said to be rare in hypochondriasis unless accompanied by severe depression in which case the risk may be increased.

## Treatment

Until recently, the treatment of hypochondriasis was regarded with pessimism. It now appears that effective psychological, even pharmacological, interventions are being developed. A variety of approaches have been proposed but controlled trials of cognitive-behavioural therapy have established its efficacy, and preliminary trials of antidepressant medication have shown promise.

### Psychological therapies

Most hypochondriacal patients, referred to mental health professionals, receive **psychotherapy** although such treatment has received little study. In one controlled trial a small number of patients with hypochondriasis were randomly assigned to explanatory therapy or a waiting list. The therapy yielded significant improvement in illness behaviour and health care utilization compared to no treatment, and gains were maintained for 6 months. This form of therapy involves repeated physical examinations, reassurance concerning symptoms, and information about psychophysiologic processes. Additional controlled trials of this and other forms of psychotherapy (e.g. psychodynamic, interpersonal) are clearly needed.

Four randomized, controlled trials for patients with hypochondriasis have shown that **cognitive behavioural therapies** are superior to no therapy with benefits sustained for up to 12 months.[32–35] These trials show that psychological treatment is efficacious for referred patients. However, one study showed that behavioural stress management, a non-specific intervention, was effective as well,[33] and another showed that cognitive and behavioural procedures, by themselves, were equally effective.[34]

Cognitive procedures include identifying and challenging dysfunctional thoughts and formulating more realistic beliefs. Behavioural procedures involve exposure *in vivo* with response prevention. These techniques include exposure to feared internal and external stimuli (e.g. physical exercise, visiting sick persons, reading about feared diseases, writing one's obituary) and prevention of checking and reassurance-seeking behaviours.

These trials showed that psychological treatment is effective but leave important questions unanswered. For instance, is psychological therapy acceptable to most hypochondriacal patients in primary care? Are the techniques specific or do the benefits result from non-specific factors (e.g. therapeutic attention, therapist–patient relationship, credible procedures)? Also, are these treatments cost-effective? One trial involved up to 16 sessions over 4 months, which is expensive in terms of time and resources.

In consideration of these issues, several authors have advocated a **group approach**. For example, one study showed that group treatment is feasible. To improve acceptance, the authors referred to their intervention as a course in stress management and carried it out in a general practice setting.

### Pharmacological therapies

There is evidence that patients with secondary hypochondriasis respond to drug therapy for the primary disorder. For example, Noyes et al.[36] assessed hypochondriacal concerns in patients receiving pharmacological treatment for panic disorder and agoraphobia. At the completion of treatment, a significant reduction in concerns was observed among those whose anxiety symptoms had improved. Observations of a similar kind have been made in patients with major depression.

No randomized controlled trials of pharmacotherapy for hypochondriasis have yet been completed, but a series of open label studies suggest that medication has promise. For example, Fallon et al.[37] reported that 10 or 16 patients with primary hypochondriasis given fluoxetine were very much improved after 12 weeks. And others have reported similar results with paroxetine, fluvoxamine, and nefazodone. Of the more than 50 patients enrolled in these trials, two-thirds responded to an SSRI. In these trials, drugs were relatively well tolerated and few patients dropped out because of side effects. This is noteworthy in view of the sensitivity to adverse effects observed in such patients. Controlled trials are needed to show proof of efficacy in primary hypochondriasis.

### Management

Most hypochondriacal patients are best managed by their primary physicians. Few are successfully referred for specialty care because the focus of their concerns is, at least initially, on unexplained somatic symptoms. Although for some the ultimate goal is specific treatment, such treatment is not yet widely available.

Successful management depends upon a trusting relationship with a physician. To establish this, the physician should first **legitimize the patient's symptoms** by listening carefully and completing a thorough evaluation. Respectful treatment and statements to the effect that unexplained symptoms are nonetheless real are often helpful (see Table 5.2.5.4).

The scheduling of **regular visits** is an important strategy. Such visits serve several purposes. First, they reduce the reward for more

**Table 5.2.5.4** Management strategies for patients with hypochondriasis

| |
|---|
| Legitimize the patient's symptoms |
| Establish a regular schedule of visits |
| Base diagnostic evaluation on objective findings |
| Approach treatment of physical symptoms cautiously |
| Provide a plausible explanation for symptoms |
| Establish a goal of improved functioning |

severe or new symptoms that patients often present at unscheduled calls or visits. Next, they assure patients that the physician has an ongoing interest in their well-being. Finally, they provide reassurance through continued health monitoring.

Physicians should use **restraint in evaluating** hypochondriacal patients. New symptoms must be thoroughly evaluated, but overly aggressive diagnostic evaluation can be counterproductive. Extensive and dramatic tests can generate alarm, and when testing is repeated, it may convey physician uncertainty. Physicians should also avoid making diagnoses simply to have something to treat.

Physicians should also **approach treatment cautiously**. Medications, even when prescribed for benign indications, cause patients to worry about the conditions for which they are given. And too often they result in intolerable side effects and iatrogenic complications.

Hypochondriacal patients need an **explanation for their distress**, one that counters the notion of serious disease. Patients may be told their problem lies in the central nervous system processing of bodily sensations; this means they have a sensitive nervous system that amplifies discomforts and dysfunctions. Such an explanation gives legitimacy to the problem and avoids the stigmatizing label of hypochondriasis. Alternatively, patients may be told that they suffer from excessive health anxiety or worry. An explanation of the role of anxiety in altering attention, amplifying bodily sensations, and generating physiological symptoms may also be acceptable.

The goal of medical management is not to remove symptoms but help patients cope with them. The expectations of patients seeking elimination of symptoms may need to be modified. Reduced dependence on the technical aspects of care (namely, diagnostic testing and corrective intervention) is an important aspect of this overall objective. Patients need assistance in managing their lives so as to minimize continuing symptoms. The **aim is improved functioning**, a greater sense of control, and improved self-esteem. These objectives may accompany a gradual return to work and meaningful activity, and may be enhanced by improvements in exercise, diet, and daily routine.

Developing and **maintaining a therapeutic relationship** with the hypochondriacal patient is often challenging. The patient may be mistrustful and feel that his or her suffering is not understood. Masochistic and obsessional personality traits may contribute to a difficult doctor–patient relationship. A patient with such traits may seek mistreatment and thwart the physician's attempts to be helpful. Yet, a positive relationship is the key to successful management and can be achieved with acceptance, empathy, and understanding.[38]

### Specific treatment

Many hypochondriacal patients have psychiatric comorbidity, and treatment of comorbid anxiety and depressive disorders may yield significant improvement. If hypochondriasis has arisen during the course of an anxiety or depressive disorder, then successful treatment of the primary disorder may bring remission of hypochondriacal symptoms.

Specific treatments, to be acceptable, must be available in the primary care setting. Treating professionals must let patients know that their concerns are legitimate and their suffering understood. Beyond this, they must place a premium on engaging the patient, techniques for which have been described by a number of authors.

These patients are prone to drug side effects and often discontinue medication. For this reason, initial doses should be small, with gradual increases according to a modifiable schedule. Treating physicians should acknowledge the patient's sensitivity, and indicate that side effects are likely but may be dealt with.

Hypochondriasis is a significant medical condition for which treatment is now available.

## Further information

Asmundson, G.J.G., Taylor, S. and Cox, B.J. (eds.) (2001). *Health anxiety: clinical and research perspectives on hypochondriasis and related disorders*. John Wiley, New York.

Lipsitt, D.R. and Starcevic, V. (eds.) (2001). *Hypochondriasis: modern perspectives on an ancient malady*. Oxford University Press, New York.

Taylor, S. and Asmundson, G.J.G. (2004). *Treating health anxiety: a cognitive-behavioral approach*. Guilford Press, New York.

## References

1. American Psychiatric Association. (1994). *Diagnostic and statistical manual of mental disorders* (4th edn). American Psychiatric Association, Washington, DC.

2. Gillespie, R.D. (1928). Hypochondria: its definition, nosology, and psychopathology. *Guy's Hospital Report*, **8**, 408–60.

3. Creed, F. and Barsky, A. (2004). A systematic review of the epidemiology of somatization disorder and hypochondriasis. *Journal of Psychosomatic Research*, **56**, 391–408.

4. Starcevic, V. (2001). Clinical features and diagnosis of hypochondriasis. In *Hypochondriasis: new perspectives on an ancient malady* (eds. V. Starcevic and D.R. Lipsitt), pp. 21–60. Oxford University Press, New York.

5. Barsky, A.J., Ahern, D.K., Bailey, E.D., *et al.* (2001). Hypochondriacal patient's appraisal of health and physical risks. *American Journal of Psychiatry*, **158**, 783–7.

6. World Health Organization. (1993). The ICD-10 classification of mental and behavioural disorders: diagnostic criteria for research. World Health Organization, Geneva.

7. Mayou, R., Kirmayer, L.J., Simon, G., *et al.* (2005). Somatoform disorders: time for a new approach in DSM-V. *American Journal of Psychiatry*, **162**, 847–55.

8. Rief, W. and Sharpe, M. (2004). Somatoform disorders—new approaches to classification, conceptualization and treatment. *Journal of Psychosomatic Research*, **56**, 387–90.

9. Barsky, A.J., Wyshak, G., and Klerman, G.L. (1986). Hypochondriasis: an evaluation of the DSM-III criteria in medical outpatients. *Archives of General Psychiatry*, **43**, 493–500.

10. Barsky, A.J., Cleary, P.D., Wyshak, G., *et al.* (1992). A structured diagnostic interview for hypochondriasis: a proposed criterion standard. *Journal of Nervous and Mental Disease*, **180**, 20–7.

11. Noyes, R., Kathol, R.G., Fisher, M.M., *et al.* (1993). The validity of DSM-III-R hypochondriasis. *Archives of General Psychiatry*, **50**, 961–70.

12. Noyes, R., Kathol, R.G., Fisher, M.M., *et al.* (1994). One-year follow-up of medical outpatients with hypochondriasis. *Psychosomatics*, **35**, 533–45.

13. Barsky, A.J., Fama, J.M., Bailey, D., *et al.* (1998). A prospective 4- to 5-year study of DSM-III-R hypochondriasis. *Archives of General Psychiatry*, **55**, 737–44.

14. Speckens, A.E.M. (2001). Assessment of hypochondriasis. In *Hypochondriasis: new perspectives on an ancient malady* (eds. V. Starcevic and D.R. Lipsitt), pp. 61–88. Oxford University Press, New York.

15. Pilowsky, I. and Spence, N.D. (1983). *Manual for the illness behavioural questionnaire (IBQ)* (2nd edn.). Department of Psychiatry, University of Adelaide, Adelaide, South Australia.

16. Kellner, R. (1986). *Somatization and hypochondriasis*. Praeger, New York.

17. Salkovskis, P.M., Rimes, K.A., Warwick, H.M.C., *et al.* (2002). The health anxiety inventory: development and validation of scales for the measurement of health anxiety and hypochondriasis. *Psychological Medicine*, **32**, 843–53.

18. Looper, K. and Kirmayer, L.J. (2001). Hypochondriacal concerns in a community population. *Psychological Medicine*, **31**, 577–84.

19. Faravelli, C., Salvatori, S., Galassi, F., *et al.* (1999). Epidemiology of somatoform disorders: a community survey in Florence. *Social Psychiatry and Psychiatric Epidemiology*, **32**, 24–9.

20. Noyes, R., Happel, R.L., and Yagla, S.J. (1999). Correlates of hypochondriasis in a nonclinical population. *Psychosomatics*, **40**, 461–78.

21. Noyes, R., Carney, C.P., Hillis, S.L., *et al.* (2005). Prevalence and correlates of illness worry in the general population. *Psychosomatics*, **46**, 529–39.

22. Gureje, O., Üstün, T.B., and Simon, G.E. (1997). The syndrome of hypochondriasis: a cross-national study in primary care. *Psychological Medicine*, **27**, 1001–10.

23. Aggarwal, V.R., McBeth, J., Zakrzewska, J.M., *et al.* (2006). The epidemiology of chronic syndromes that are frequently unexplained: do they have common associated factors? *International Journal of Epidemiology*, **35**, 468–76.

24. Taylor, S., Thordarson, D.S., Jang, K.L., *et al.* (2006). Genetic and environmental origins of health anxiety: a twin study. *World Psychiatry*, **5**, 47–50.

25. Noyes, R., Holt, C.S., Happel, R.L., *et al.* (1997). A family study of hypochondriasis. *Journal of Nervous and Mental Disease*, **185**, 223–32.

26. Robbins, J.M., Kirmayer, L.J., and Kapusta, M.A. (1990). Illness worry and disability in fibromyalgia syndrome. *International Journal of Psychiatry in Medicine*, **20**, 49–63.

27. McClure, E.B. and Lilienfeld, S.O. (2001). Personality traits and health anxiety. In *Health anxiety: clinical and research perspectives on hypochondriasis and related conditions* (eds. G.J.G. Asmundson, S. Taylor, and B.J. Cox), pp. 65–91. John Wiley, New York.

28. Noyes, R., Stuart, S., Langbehn, D.R., *et al.* (2002). Childhood antecedents of hypochondriasis. *Psychosomatics*, **43**, 282–9.

29. Salkovskis, P.J. and Warwick, H.M.C. (2001). Meaning, misinterpretations, and medicine: a cognitive-behavioural approach to understanding health anxiety and hypochondriasis. In: *Hypochondriasis: modern perspectives on an ancient malady* (eds. V. Starcevic and D.R. Lipsitt), pp. 202–22. Oxford University Press, New York.

30. Gramling, S.E., Clawson, E.P., and McDonald, M.K. (1996). Perceptual and cognitive abnormality model of hypochondriasis: amplification and physiological reactivity in women. *Psychosomatic Medicine*, **58**, 423–31.

31. Noyes, R., Stuart, S. Langbehn, *et al.* (2003). Test of an interpersonal model of hypochondriasis. *Psychosomatic Medicine*, **65**, 292–300.

32. Warwick, H.M.C., Clark, D.M., Cobb, A.M., *et al.* (1996). A controlled trial of cognitive behavioral treatment of hypochondriasis. *British Journal of Psychiatry*, **169**, 189–95.

33. Clark, D.M., Salkovskis, P.M., Hackman, A., *et al.* (1998). Two psychological treatments for hypochondriasis: a randomized controlled trial. *British Journal of Psychiatry*, **173**, 218–25.

34. Visser, S. and Bouman, T.K. (2001). The treatment of hypochondriasis: a randomized controlled trial. *Behavior Research and Therapy*, **39**, 423–42.

35. Barsky, A.J. and Ahern, D.K. (2004). Cognitive behavioral therapy for hypochondriasis: a randomized controlled trial. *Journal of the American Medical Association*, **291**, 1464–70.

36. Noyes, R., Reich, J., Clancy, J., *et al.* (1986). Reduction in hypochondriasis with treatment of panic disorder. *British Journal of Psychiatry*, **149**, 631–5.

37. Fallon, B.A., Liebowitz, M.R., Salman, E., *et al.* (1993). Fluoxetine for hypochondriacal patients without major depression. *Journal of Clinical Psychopharmacology*, **13**, 438–41.

38. Starcevic, V. (2002). Overcoming therapeutic pessimism in hypochondriasis, *American Journal of Psychotherapy*, **56**, 167–77.

# 5.2.6. Pain disorder

Sidney Benjamin and Stella Morris

## Introduction

**Persistent somatoform pain** disorder is an ICD-10 diagnosis, which is included in the group of somatoform disorders. The term **pain disorder** is used in DSM-IV, and for convenience that is the term used here to refer to both classifications, unless a distinction needs to be made. This chapter aims to clarify the relationship of pain to mental disorders, the diagnosis of pain disorder and its differential diagnosis, and then considers how psychosocial factors contribute to pain, the treatments that stem from them, and the psychiatrist's potential contribution.

Pain has been defined by the International Association for the Study of Pain (**IASP**) as 'an unpleasant sensory and emotional experience associated with actual or potential tissue damage or described in terms of such damage'. 'Pain' is used here in this sense; it is not used primarily to indicate mental distress or anguish. As a perception, pain is essentially a subjective experience, and is directly accessible only to the patient. By contrast, tissue damage can be assessed by others, and its relationship with the subjective characteristics of pain have been shown to be variable, modulated by social and cultural experience, as well as within the central and peripheral nervous system.

## Pain and the psychiatrist

Psychiatrists are likely to see patients with pain in psychiatric, general hospital, and community settings. Pain is associated with a wide range of mental disorders, and there are different ways in which this relationship may arise.

Pain may contribute to the cause of a mental disorder; for example, when a patient with cancer has pain, which is unrelieved by analgesics, and becomes depressed. This can result in additional distress and disability, and subsequently an exacerbation of pain. Treatment of depression may contribute to the relief from pain and improve the quality of life.

In a general hospital psychiatrists may see patients with **acute pain**, like the patient described above, but more often will see patients with **chronic pain**. Whatever the initial cause, the longer pain persists the more likely is it to result in the development of inappropriate patterns of illness behaviour and to have a profound effect on relationships with the family and other carers, presenting more complex challenges for management and poorer prognosis.

## Pain disorder

### Diagnostic and clinical features

**Persistent somatoform pain disorder** in **ICD-10** is the only somatoform disorder that is essentially characterized by pain. The **diagnostic requirements** are as follows:

1 'persistent, severe, and distressing pain';

2 pain 'cannot be explained fully by a physiological process or a physical disorder';

3 'pain occurs in association with emotional conflict or psychosocial problems that are sufficient to allow the conclusion that they are the main causative influences'.

There are also likely to be many of the features that occur in the other somatoform disorders, which have been described in previous chapters. The pain can be localized, as in low back pain, or generalized, as in fibromyalgia.

In **ICD-10**, the diagnosis is excluded if pain, presumed to be mainly psychological in origin, occurs in the course of schizophrenia or depressive disorder, or is believed to be due to psychophysiological mechanisms such as muscle tension. The main **differential diagnosis**, according to ICD-10, is the histrionic elaboration of pain primarily due to organic causes, particularly if this has not yet been diagnosed. In practice, it is uncommon for pain that has been properly investigated, and has persisted for more than 6 months, to be found subsequently to have a specific organic cause.

The **DSM-IV** diagnosis of 'pain disorder' also needs to be considered because the requirements for diagnosis and the underlying rationale are rather different. This diagnosis is divided into three **subtypes**:

1 '**Pain disorder associated with psychological factors**', in which psychological factors are judged to play the major role, and physical disorders play either no part or only a minor part in its onset or maintenance.

2 '**Pain disorder associated with both psychological factors and a general medical condition**', in which both psychological processes and an organic disorder are judged to make important contributions to causation.

3 '**Pain disorder associated with a general medical condition**', due to an organic disorder and in which psychological factors are judged to make no contribution or to play only a minor role. This subtype is not regarded as a mental disorder but is coded on Axis III.

For the first two subtypes the diagnostic criteria, all of which must be satisfied, are summarized as follows:

(a) Pain, localized or more general, is the predominant symptom and its severity warrants clinical attention

(b) Pain results in distress, and impairment in social, occupational, or other areas of functioning.

(c) Psychological factors are judged to have an important role in the onset, severity, exacerbation, or maintenance of pain.

(d) It is not intentionally produced or feigned (factitious disorder and malingering are specifically excluded).

(e) Pain is not better accounted for by a mood, anxiety, or psychotic disorder and does not meet criteria for dyspareunia.

Pain disorder can also be coded according to whether it is acute or chronic (less or more than 6 months duration).

## Comparison of ICD-10 and DSM-IV

The diagnoses of pain disorder in ICD-10 and DSM-IV share a number of characteristics. Pain disorder should be diagnosed as a mental disorder if psychological factors are thought to make a significant contribution to predisposition, precipitation, or maintenance, or to the severity of pain. In ICD-10, there should be evidence that emotional conflict or psychosocial problems are the main 'causative influences', whereas in DSM-IV psychological factors are judged to play either the 'major role' or 'an important role'. In both, the diagnosis can be made even though there may be possible or definite evidence of an organic disorder that contributes to pain (for instance, a prolapsed intervertebral disc), provided that this is judged to be insufficient to account fully for the features of pain. Both classifications stress the severity of pain and the distress caused by it, but only DSM-IV specifically requires a degree of disability as a diagnostic feature. The implication is that diagnosis requires detailed physical and psychiatric evaluation, including an assessment of the family and social context, as well as of disability.

## Differential diagnosis of pain disorder

Pain can occur in the setting of virtually any mental disorder. Table 5.2.6.1 lists the ICD-10 diagnoses and their DSM-IV equivalents in which pain may be a predominant feature. The general description of most of these disorders is provided in other chapters of this book and the following account focuses only on aspects relevant to pain.

### (a) Organic disorders

Many painful disorders have a well-recognized organic pathology that accounts for the occurrence of pain (for example, angina, sickle cell arthropathy), but psychosocial processes tend to modify the severity of pain and associated disability. Thus, psychological and social interventions may make an important contribution to management, and as pain becomes more chronic, or fails to respond to usually effective physical treatments, psychosocial interventions assume greater significance. These disorders can be diagnosed in ICD-10 within the diagnoses headed 'Psychological interactions with physical disorders' in Table 5.2.6.1.

### (b) Pain syndromes of uncertain origin

There are many disorders characterized by pain, which are essentially syndromes with no known consistent organic pathology (Table 5.2.6.2). Psychological and social factors are thought to contribute to the development and maintenance in many cases,[1] but psychological causes specific to these different syndromes have not been identified. Patients with these pain syndromes tend to have a greater prevalence of non-psychotic mental disorders than is found in the general population. The pain itself can usually be accommodated in ICD-10 within the categories of **somatoform autonomic dysfunction** or **somatoform pain disorder** (see below). The 'diagnoses' listed in Table 5.2.6.2 tend to be used by non-psychiatrists to describe clusters of medically unexplained symptoms and are terms which are likely to be acceptable to patients. Treatments for these disorders generally include physical approaches, often of limited efficacy, as well as a range of psychosocial interventions, which are described below.

### (c) Pain and mental disorders

#### (i) Psychoses

At the beginning of the twentieth century, French psychiatrists described **coenestopathic states** as disorders characterized by unpleasant sensations, particularly pains, thought to be of central origin, but unrelated to organic brain disease.[2] Such disorders were a daily occurrence in psychiatric clinics, commonly associated with the psychoses, and in this setting were related to **somatic hallucinations** and **systematized delusional states**. Such presentations are now described infrequently in Europe and North America.

Patients with any psychosis may complain of pain, sometimes with bizarre descriptions of quality and **delusional attribution**. In practice, it is difficult to differentiate between a **somatic hallucination** and an illusion (arising from physiological or pathological processes). Complaints of pain in psychotic disorders have no psychiatric diagnostic specificity. Pain has been described particularly in association with schizophrenia and depressive psychoses, but may occur in any psychotic disorder. In the course of a psychotic disorder, illusions and delusional interpretations of pain may arise from unrelated organic disorders and therefore require careful **physical assessment**.

#### (ii) Mood- and anxiety-related disorders

These are by far the most common mental disorders associated with pain in most settings. In the general population, 12 per cent of adults have experienced **chronic widespread pain** (defined according to the criteria of the American College of Rheumatologists) in the previous 3 months and their prevalence of mental disorders is three times that of the pain-free population.[3] Most of these diagnoses are mood and anxiety disorders, with the former being more common in those with chronic pain. In **pain clinic settings**, the prevalence of mental disorders varies according to referral patterns, but about 30 to 40 per cent of patients have depressive disorders, and this is similar in those with and those without a relevant physical disorder.[4] Those without organic disorders tend to have lower ratings for both mood disorders and pain severity. Those with mood disorders report more severe pain.

Diagnosis of mood and anxiety disorders is based on the usual standardized criteria, but may be missed due to the process of **somatization**, particularly where patients attribute their depressed mood to pain and an underlying physical condition (whether present or not) and invite their doctors to share this belief.[5] In the past, pain has been thought of as a proxy for depression, giving rise to the concept of a '**depressive equivalent**' or '**masked depression**'. This has been based mainly on evidence for the psychogenicity of chronic pain rather than a specific relationship to depressive disorders, has received widespread criticism, and has not advanced theoretical knowledge or clinical practice.

#### (iii) Post-traumatic stress disorder

Many patients with post-traumatic stress disorder (PTSD) have been subjected to actual or threatened physical injury, so it is not surprising that pain is one of the commonest symptoms that they report, the prevalence ranging from 20 to 80 per cent. Further, 10 to 50 per cent of patients with chronic pain satisfy criteria for PTSD, and patients with musculoskeletal pain are four times more likely to develop PTSD than those without it.[6] **Pain disorder and PTSD** can be diagnosed jointly, if criteria for both are satisfied. Mechanisms including shared vulnerability, fear-avoidance, and

**Table 5.2.6.1** Mental disorders included in the differential diagnosis of pain disorder

| ICD-10 | | DSM-IV | |
|---|---|---|---|
| *Psychotic disorders* | | | |
| F00–09 | Organic mental disorders | 290 | Dementia 293 Delirium |
| F20–29 | Schizophrenia, schizotypal, and delusional disorders | 273 | Schizophrenia and other psychotic disorders |
| *Mood- and anxiety-related disorders* | | | |
| F32/33 | Depressive episode | 296.2/3 | Major depressive disorder |
| F34.1 | Dysthymia | 300.4 | Dysthymic disorder |
| F41 | Anxiety disorders | 300.02 | Generalized anxiety disorder |
| F43.1 | Post-traumatic stress disorder | 309.81 | Post-traumatic stress disorder |
| F43.2 | Adjustment disorders | 309 | Adjustment disorders |
| *Somatoform disorders* | | | |
| F44.4 | Dissociative (conversion) disorders | 300.11 | Conversion disorder |
| F45.0 | Somatization disorder | 300.81 | Somatization disorder |
| F45.1 | Undifferentiated somatoform disorder | 300.81 | Undifferentiated somatoform disorder |
| F45.2 | Hypochondriacal disorder | 300.7 | Hypochondriasis |
| F45.3 | Somatoform autonomic dysfunction | 300.8 | Pain disorder |
| F45.4 | Somatoform pain disorder | 300.81 | Somatoform disorder NOS |
| F45.8 | Other somatoform disorders | | |
| F45.9 | Somatoform disorder, unspecified | | |
| *Other neurotic disorders* | | | |
| F48.0 | Neurasthenia | | |
| F48.8 | Other specified neurotic disorders (occupational neurosis, e.g. writer's cramp) | | |
| *Sexual disorders* | | | |
| F52.5 | Non-organic vaginismus | 306.51 | Vaginismus |
| F52.6 | Non-organic dyspareunia | 302.76 | Dyspareunia |
| *Psychological interactions with physical disorders* | | | |
| F54 | Pyschological or behavioural factors associated with disorders or diseases classified elsewhere | 316 | Psychological factors affecting medical condition |
| F68.0 | Elaboration of physical symptoms for psychological reasons | | |
| *Disorders of behaviour* | | | |
| F68.1 | Intentional production or feigning of symptoms | 300.19 | Factitious disorder |
| | | V65.2 | Malingering |
| **Comorbidity of pain disorder** | | | |
| Any of the above except psychoses and other somatoform disorders | | | |
| *Substance abuse* | | | |
| F10 | Disorders due to alcohol | 291 & 303.9 | Alcohol-induced disorders and dependence |
| F11–13 | Disorders due to psychoactive substance abuse | 292 & 304 | Other substance-induced disorders and dependence |
| F55 | Abuse of non-dependence-producing substances | | |
| *Personality disorders* | | | |
| F60–62 | Personality disorders and changes | 301 | Personality disorders |

mutual maintenance have been postulated to account for this comorbidity.[7] This has implications for assessment (described below), and treatment programmes may need to be modified accordingly.

### (iv) Somatoform disorders

Somatoform disorders are uncommon in people with chronic pain in the general population.[3] Prevalence varies considerably in clinical samples, but somatoform disorders have been reported in 12 to 52 per cent of patients,[4] so they include highly selected samples.

Complaints of pain occur commonly in each of the somatoform disorders and may be the predominant symptom. Multiple physical complaints, often including pains at different sites, fluctuate from time to time usually for many years, providing a characteristic feature of **somatization disorder**. In **hypochondriacal disorder** pain is a common complaint, and forms the focus for concern and overvalued beliefs about unidentified disease.

The diagnosis of **somatoform autonomic disorder** is based on autonomic arousal (palpitation, sweating, tremor), which must be a prominent feature of the clinical picture, together with physical complaints, often pain, referred to specific organs, systems, or parts of the body. As with other somatoform disorders, the patient will be distressed about the possibility of underlying physical disease and is not reassured by negative findings on appropriate assessment and explanation. This diagnosis is sometimes appropriate for syndromes listed in Table 5.2.6.2.

Pain, as a form of **conversion**, has a traditional place in the literature on **hysteria**, based on the concepts of psychogenicity, the

**Table 5.2.6.2** Disorders of uncertain origin, presenting primarily with pain, in which psychosocial factors are thought to contribute to predisposition, precipitation, or course

| Generalized |
| --- |
| Fibromyalgia |

| **Relatively localized** |
| --- |
| Tension headache—acute or chronic |
| Temporomandibular pain and dysfunction syndrome |
| Atypical facial pain |
| Atypical (non-cardiac) chest pain |
| Abdominal pain of psychological origin |
| Non-ulcer dyspepsia |
| Irritable bowel syndrome |
| Chronic pelvic pain |
| Irritable bladder syndrome |
| Procatalgia fugax |

contribution of stressful experiences with dissociation, and primary gain. In recent years, however, research has focused on other psychological processes, and the concept of conversion as a primary mechanism now seems to be of limited interest. The category of **dissociative (conversion) disorder** in ICD-10 specifically includes sensory loss but excludes pain (sensory amplification), which therefore should not be diagnosed as a dissociative disorder. DSM-IV also excludes pain from the diagnosis of conversion disorder, unless other diagnostic criteria are satisfied.

The uncertain relationship and limited value of the different diagnoses included within the group of somatoform disorders in ICD-10 have been discussed in Chapter 5.2.1, and are well illustrated by the fact that pain may be a prominent feature of each category. Somatoform disorders presenting with pain are usually diagnosed as **somatization disorder or pain disorder**, with the former taking precedence if the diagnostic criteria are satisfied.

## Comorbidity

Any physical or mental disorder may be diagnosed in addition to pain disorder. Anxiety and depression are common, and an additional diagnosis of **anxiety disorder** or **mood disorder** can be made if the criteria are satisfied. This dual diagnosis can be useful if, for example, a depressive disorder develops in the presence of a long-standing pain disorder. Any temporal relationship can occur, however, with pain onset preceding, developing simultaneously with, or following the onset of a mood disorder.

Other common comorbid diagnoses include **substance abuse** and dependence, sometimes of iatrogenic origin, and their management is an important component of pain-treatment programmes.[8] **Personality disorders** are an additional category of comorbidity. No single disorder predominates but histrionic, narcissistic, anxious (avoidant), and dependent features are all common in clinical practice, and anankastic traits may feed an inflexible focus on physical illness.

## Epidemiology

Although the association of psychiatric symptoms with chronic pain has been studied in the general population, the prevalence of pain disorder, and other mental disorders presenting with pain, is uncertain because large-scale surveys of mental disorders do not include an assessment of pain and of related physical conditions.

## Assessment of pain

### Clinical assessment

The psychiatric assessment requires a full **psychiatric history** and **mental state examination**, with particular attention to those additional features relevant to pain. **The pain history** should include total duration (often underestimated by the patient), a detailed inquiry about the location and distribution of pain, including direct questions aimed at a total body survey, and the timing of first onset, subsequent periods of relapses and remissions, and their relationship to life events and difficulties. The **family history** should include assessment of severe, chronic or disabling physical disorders, and the patient's involvement with them. The **personal history** should include adverse childhood experiences (discussed below) and the **past history** of physical disorders and disability is particularly important.

Patients who **somatize** will tend to deny concurrent psychosocial events and their significance. For example, one of our patients was consistently unable to recall any distressing events in the year prior to the onset of severe, persistent, and disabling headache. His wife gave an account of the deaths of his father, brother, and closest friend during that year, and moreover described him as so distressed by these bereavements that he felt unable to attend any of the funerals. It is essential to take a **history from other informants**, and this can also provide an opportunity to assess the attitudes, knowledge, and beliefs of carers, and their interaction with the patient.

The patient's **pain beliefs and behaviours** (described below) are key aspects of the **mental state examination**. Patients often attribute chronic pain to an organic disorder and offer diagnoses; it is essential to review their **medical records** to assess the clinical findings and investigations, and the extent to which they support any diagnosis which is offered. Chronic pain associated with an underlying organic disorder may be exacerbated when the patient suffers a stressful life event, so it is important to **avoid assumptions of a dichotomy** of either 'organic' or 'psychogenic' pain.

### Standardized psychometric assessments

Many standardized questionnaires have been developed for the assessment of patients with chronic pain. They can be valuable for identifying mechanisms that contribute to pain, planning treatment, and monitoring changes during and after treatment. The evaluation of pain and associated beliefs and behaviours requires measures developed specifically for this purpose, and these are described below.

Other assessments, for example of **mood, illness behaviour**, and **social dysfunction**, have been developed within the field of pain research. Some measures are rather idiosyncratic, with uncertain psychometric properties, aimed at restricted diagnostic groups and clinical settings. This undermines the need to use consistent methods that allow comparison of different groups of patients, with physical, mental, and mixed disorders, at different places and times.

### (a) Pain

The **severity** of pain can be assessed[9] using standardized **visual analogue scales** and **numeric analogue scales**. Such scales may have anchor points ranging from 'no pain' to 'the worst possible pain'.

The **quality** of pain can be assessed with **verbal descriptor scales**.[9] Factor analysis has resulted in the emergence of two that have best survived the test of time: an '**affective' dimension** (represented by words such as exhausting, terrifying, vicious), and a '**sensory' dimension** (e.g. stabbing, crushing, burning). They have been found consistently when administered in different languages and to different cultural groups. Ratings on both these scales are positively correlated with pain severity and mood ratings and, in the presence of mental disorders, contribute little to diagnosis.

The **topographical distribution of pain** can be assessed by using outline drawings of the body (front, back, and sometimes sides), which the patient is asked to shade to indicate the distribution of pain. These can help to identify pain that does not conform to physiological distributions and also widespread pain. Measures of pain intensity, quality, and distribution can be used toget her to capture the rather elusive and entirely subjective experience of pain.

### (b) Pain behaviours

Although the experience of pain is entirely personal, it may be communicated to others by a range of verbal and non-verbal behaviours, which in some cases may be maladaptive, and which in turn influence the responses of others. Using a **learning theory model**, Fordyce[10] classified all pain into '**operant' and 'non-operant' pain**. The former includes all pain that is modified by positive or negative reinforcement, whether or not organic pathology is present. Standardized **structured assessments** are available to measure a range of well-defined **behaviours**.[11] These may include complaints of pain, requests for medication, groaning, facial expression, restricted mobility and the use of aids, time spent resting, and postures such as guarding and bracing. Such behaviours have been shown to fluctuate in response to changes in the environment, including different **attitudes and responses of carers**. This has led to the assessment of pain behaviours and their **environmental reinforcers**, and the development of pain-treatment programmes that originally focused on behavioural change by modifying reinforcement. Recent interest has focused on **pain-related fears** (e.g. of exacerbating pain by injury) and the management of consequent **avoidance**.[12]

### (c) Pain beliefs

The belief that chronic as well as acute pain signals an underlying physical disease, which requires and should respond to physical intervention, whilst avoiding usual activities and functions, contributes to the development and maintenance of chronic pain and non-adherence to treatment, and the widespread dissatisfaction often expressed by patients and their doctors. Inappropriate beliefs that are relevant to pain assessment fall into three groups[13]:

1 beliefs about the nature of reality—for example, 'life should be pain-free';

2 beliefs in response to challenging circumstances, such as pain—including **locus of control**, **attributional style**, **cognitive errors**, and **coping strategies**;

3 specific ideas about the cause of a pain, appropriate management, and outcome.

The questionnaire assessment of pain-related beliefs has assumed increasing importance in the field of pain research,[13] with the recognition that pain beliefs interact with pain, cognitions, behaviours, affects and disability, and contribute to the prediction of outcome. Thus cognitive approaches to treatment are often integrated with behavioural management.

## Psychosocial contributions to the development of pain

The origins of chronic pain are, in several respects, similar to those of somatization and other somatoform disorders. Current models of causation involve the interaction of biological, psychological, and social factors, each contributing to predisposition, precipitation, and maintenance.

The **family and personal histories** of patients with chronic pain include an excess of mood disorders, pain and disability, substance abuse, and personality disorders. Engel[14] described the dynamics of '**the pain prone patient**' involving abusive childhood experiences, and noted how pain can become a pathway for the expression of guilt and expiation. Recent research[15] has reconsidered the significance of reports of **physical and sexual abuse** and other **adverse childhood experiences**. The relationship between chronic pain in adults and these childhood experiences appears, at least to some extent, to be determined by **selective reporting**, particularly in those with associated mental disorders,[16] but these experiences may make a significant contribution to pain in some individuals.

Precipitation of chronic pain is, in effect, **transition from acute to chronic pain**, and factors associated with this transition[17,18] include current mood and anxiety disorders, negative life events including physical illnesses and trauma, the social support network and dissatisfaction with work. A population based prospective study[19] found that new episodes of chronic widespread pain were predicted by the number of previous non-pain somatic symptoms and by a measure of illness behaviour which assessed numbers of consultations, treatments and perceived disability, and these two measures had an additive effect. Recent research has indicated the potential value of interventions designed to prevent the progression from acute to chronic pain.[17,18]

## The psychiatric and psychological management of pain

### Treatment of mental disorders

The treatment of chronic pain has presented a challenge to the ingenuity of health professionals, particularly because no single specialty or profession has the range of skills that is required. The treatment of mental disorders,[5] such as depressive or anxiety disorders,[20] is similar in most respects, whether or not pain is a prominent feature. In the presence of pain, however, mental disorders tend to be missed, and when recognized are treated inadequately. Depressive disorders with features indicating a good response to **antidepressants** should be treated with full therapeutic doses, but not with **narcotics**. **Anxiolytic drugs** including **benzodiazepines**, which result in dependence, should not be used in the treatment of these chronic disorders.

### The use of antidepressants for pain relief

Antidepressant drugs are often used for the treatment of pain in patients who are not depressed. Randomized controlled trials[21] indicate that antidepressants, in doses within the usual therapeutic range, provide more effective **analgesia** than placebo preparations in the treatment of diabetic neuropathy, postherpetic neuralgia, and atypical facial pain, as well as chronic non-malignant pain. Different **tricyclic antidepressants** (TCAs) appear to be equally effective and are more effective than **selective serotonin-reuptake inhibitors**. Data on **seretonin noradrenaline-reuptake inhibitors** are increasing and suggest that they may be effective, and preferable to TCAs because of a superior side effect profile.[22] The analgesic effect of antidepressants occurs in patients who are not depressed and is independent of any antidepressant effect.

## Psychological treatments

Psychological treatments[5,23] are derived from different theoretical formulations of the aetiology of chronic pain. These include behavioural, cognitive, and psychodynamic approaches. Reviews of randomized controlled trials of **behavioural and cognitive approaches**[24] that have been developed specifically for the treatment of chronic pain illustrate the problems in assessing outcome due to different sampling methods, different types of control groups, non-standardized treatment components, and the different assessments that are included. Despite these limitations, the best studies demonstrate that these treatments are more effective than 'usual' medical treatment, remaining on a waiting list, or exercise programmes, and improvements can be sustained during lengthy follow-up periods.

Other approaches include various forms of 'stress management' including **relaxation techniques**, **biofeedback**, and **hypnosis**. Their value is uncertain; although pain ratings tend to be reduced, this is not a consistent finding on all measures.

Psychological treatments are rarely used in isolation, either from each other or from additional interventions, and integrating different approaches may enhance their effects.[23]

## Multi-disciplinary pain management clinics

**Pain-treatment centres**[25] have been established in many countries and provide a diverse range of professional skills, treatments, and models of service delivery. In some, management is based mainly on anaesthetic techniques and medication, but psychological approaches are provided in others by **clinical psychologists** and **nurse therapists**. The management of problems due to inappropriate medication and **substance abuse** is an essential component of treatment.[8] Many clinics offer **structured programmes** of education and rehabilitation, with increments of **exercise**, to overcome **disability**, rather than aiming primarily at pain relief, and to which **physiotherapists or occupational therapists** may contribute. There is often an emphasis on the patient assuming increasing responsibility, rather than maintaining **dependence on medical services**.

Direct input from **psychiatrists** is variable and some centres specifically exclude the treatment of patients with serious mental disorders because their response to treatment is less certain. Although it is well recognized that social and environmental factors contribute to chronic pain problems, and can undermine progress following treatment, few specialized centres involve **carers** routinely in treatment or offer **family therapy**.

A range of physical, psychological, and social approaches should be offered, based on an **individual structured assessment** of needs. Members of the multi-disciplinary team require specific **training** in the management of pain. The work of the team has to be carefully coordinated, both within the team and with other health professionals, to avoid any ambiguity concerning the methods and goals of treatment.

Many pain clinics provide a treatment package in which cognitive therapy and graded exercise are predominant features. A similar approach is used for a number of other conditions, including **somatization disorder**, **hypochondriacal disorder**, **fibromyalgia**, and **chronic fatigue**, but the extent to which they may have similar origins and outcomes is uncertain.

## Effects of treatment

The **outcome of psychological and psychiatric treatment** has been studied extensively,[5,24] but is difficult to evaluate because reports differ with regard to the characteristics of patients and disorders, inclusion criteria, assessments, and treatments as well as details of treatment delivery, attrition rates, choice of control groups, and the duration of follow-up. Many patients with chronic pain are unwilling to accept treatment and others are considered unsuitable. Nevertheless, psychological and rehabilitation treatments can have a sustained effect, based on the range of assessments that have been described. In addition, they can result in reductions in **sickness and benefit payments**,[26] **return to work**[27] and reduced **use and costs of medical services**.[28]

The outcome for patients with different mental disorders has not been assessed systematically. Patients involved in seeking **compensation** tend to have a poorer outcome, even after **litigation** has been concluded, but they can also benefit from treatment. There is some evidence that **secondary prevention** programmes may help to avoid the transition from acute to chronic pain in those who are particularly vulnerable.

# Further information

For more information on the topic of this chapter, we have marked with an asterisk (*) those references, which will be of particular interest to the reader.

# References

1. *Kellner, R. (1991). *Psychosomatic syndromes and somatic symptoms*. American Psychiatric Press, Washington, DC.

2. Dupré, E. (1913). *Les cénestopathies*. Reprinted as: Coenestopathic states. In *Themes and variations in European psychiatry* (eds. S.R. Hirsch and M. Shepherd), pp. 385–94. John Wright, Bristol, 1974.

3. Benjamin, S., Morris, S., McBeth, J., *et al.* (2000). The association between chronic widespread pain and mental disorder. *Arthritis and Rheumatism*, **43**, 561–7.

4. Benjamin, S., Barnes, D., Berger, S., *et al.* (1988). The relationship of chronic pain, mental illness and organic disorders. *Pain*, **32**, 185–95.

5. Benjamin, S. and Main, C.J. (1995). Psychiatric and psychological approaches to the treatment of chronic pain: concepts and individual treatments. In *Treatment of functional somatic symptoms* (eds. R. Mayou, C. Bass, and M. Sharpe), pp. 188–213. Oxford University Press.

6. Asmundson, J.G., Coons, M.J., Taylor, S., *et al.* (2002). PTSD and the experience of pain; research and clinical implications of shared vulnerability and mutual maintenance models. *Canadian Journal of Psychiatry*, **47**, 930–7.

7. *Otis, J.D., Keane, T.M., and Kerns, R.D. (2003). An examination of the relationship between chronic pain and post-traumatic stress disorder. *Journal of Rehabilitation Research and Development*, **40**, 397–406.

8. British Pain Society. (2006). *Pain and substance misuse: improving the patient experience*. British Pain Society, London.

9. *Williams, A.C.deC. (2004). Assessing chronic pain and its impact. In *Psychosocial aspects of pain: a handbook for healthcare professionals, progress in pain research and management*, Vol. 27 (eds. R.H. Dworkin and W.S. Breitbart). IASP Press, Seattle.

10. Fordyce, W.E. (1985). The behavioural management of chronic pain: a response to critics. *Pain*, 22, 113–25.

11. Keefe, F.J. and Williams, D.A. (1992). Assessment of pain behaviours. In *Handbook of pain assessment* (eds. D.C. Turk and R. Melzack), pp. 277–92. Guilford Press, New York.

12. De Jong, J.R., Vlaeyen, J.W.S., Onghena, P., *et al.* (2005). Reduction of pain-related fear in complex regional pain syndrome type I: the application of graded exposure in vivo. *Pain*, 116, 264–75.

13. *DeGood, D.E. and Shutty, M.S. (1992). Assessment of pain beliefs, coping and self-efficacy. In *Handbook of pain assessment* (eds. D.C. Turk and R. Melzack), pp. 214–34. Guilford Press, New York.

14. Engel, G. (1959). 'Psychogenic' pain and the pain prone patient. *The American Journal of Medicine*, 26, 899–918.

15. Morley, S. (2004). What impact does childhood experience have on the childhood development of chronic pain? In *Psychosocial aspects of pain: a handbook for healthcare professionals, progress in pain research and management*, Vol. 27 (eds. R.H. Dworkin and W.S. Breitbart). IASP Press, Seattle.

16. McBeth, J., Morris, S., Benjamin, S., *et al.* (2001). Associations between adverse events in childhood and chronic widespread pain in adulthood: are they explained by differential recall? *The Journal of Rheumatology*, 28, 2305–9.

17. *Poleshuck, E.L. and Dworkin, R.H. (2004). Risk factors for chronic pain in patients with acute pain and their implications for prevention. In *Psychosocial aspects of pain: a handbook for healthcare providers, progress in pain research and management*, Vol. 27 (eds. R.H. Dworkin and W.S. Breitbart). IASP Press, Seattle.

18. *Linton, S.J. (2004). Environment and learning factors in the development of chronic pain and disability. In *Psychological methods of pain control: basic science and clinical perspectives, progress in pain research and management*, Vol. 29 (eds. D.D. Price and E.M. Bushnell). IASP Press, Seattle.

19. McBeth, J., Macfarlane, G.J., Benjamin, S., *et al.* (2001). Features of somatization predict the onset of chronic widespread pain. Results of a large population based study. *Arthritis and Rheumatism*, 44, 940–6.

20. *Gallagher, R.M. and Verma, S. (2004). Mood and anxiety disorders in chronic pain. In *Psychosocial aspects of pain: a handbook for healthcare professionals, progress in pain research and management*, Vol. 27 (eds. R.H. Dworkin and W.S. Breitbart). IASP Press, Seattle.

21. Atkinson, J.H., Meyer, J.M., and Slater, M.A. (2004). Principles of psychopharmacology in pain treatment In *Psychosocial aspects of pain: a handbook for health care professionals, progress in pain research and management*, Vol. 27 (eds. R.H. Dworkin and W.S. Breitbart). IASP Press, Seattle.

22. Sindrup, S., Otto, M., Finnerup, N., *et al.* (2005). Antidepressants in the treatment of neuropathic pain. *Basic and Clinical Pharmacology and Toxicology*, 96, 399–409.

23. *Waters, S.J, Campbell, L.C., Keefe, F.J., *et al.* (2004). The essence of cognitive-behavioral pain management. In *Psychosocial aspects of pain: a handbook for healthcare professionals, progress in pain research and management*, Vol. 27 (eds. R.H. Dworkin and W.S. Breitbart). IASP Press, Seattle.

24. Morley, S., Eccleston, C., and Williams, A. (1999). Systematic review and meta-analysis of randomised controlled trials of cognitive behaviour therapy and behaviour therapy for chronic pain in adults, excluding headache. *Pain*, 80, 1–13.

25. Cohen, M.J.M. and Campbell, J.N. (eds.) (1996). *Pain treatment centers at a crossroads: a practical and conceptual reappraisal*. IASP Press, Seattle.

26. Thomsen, A.B., Sorensen, J., and Sjogren, P. (2002). Chronic non-malignant pain patients and health economic consequences. *European Journal of Pain*, 6, 341–52.

27. Haldorsen, E.M.H., Grasdal, A.L., Skouen, J.S., *et al.* (2002). Is there a right treatment for a particular patient group? Comparison of ordinary treatment, light multidisciplinary treatment, and extensive multidisciplinary treatment for long-term sick-listed employees with musculoskeletal pain. *Pain*, 95, 49–63.

28. Peters, L., Simon, E.P., Folen, R.A., *et al.* (2000). The COPE program: treatment efficacy and medical utilisation outcome of a chronic pain management program at a major military hospital. *Military Medicine*, 165, 954–60.

# 5.2.7 Chronic fatigue syndrome

## Michael Sharpe and Simon Wessely

## Introduction

Chronic fatigue syndrome is a controversial condition, conflicts about which have frequently burst out of the medical literature into the popular media. Whilst these controversies may initially seem to be of limited interest to those who do not routinely treat such patients, they also exemplify important current issues in medicine. These issues include the nature of symptom-defined illness; patient power versus medical authority; and the uncomfortable but important issues of psychological iatrogenesis.[1,2] The subject is therefore of relevance to all doctors.

### Fatigue as a symptom

Fatigue is a subjective feeling of weariness, lack of energy, and exhaustion. Approximately 20 per cent of the general population report significant and persistent fatigue, although relatively few of these people regard themselves as ill and only a small minority seek a medical opinion. Even so, fatigue is a common clinical presentation in primary care.[2]

### Fatigue as an illness: chronic fatigue syndrome

When fatigue becomes chronic and associated with disability it is regarded as an illness. Such a syndrome has been recognized at least since the latter half of the last century. Whilst during the Victorian era patients who went to see doctors with this illness often received a diagnosis of neurasthenia, a condition ascribed to the effect of the stresses of modern life on the human nervous system the popularity of this diagnosis waned and by the mid-twentieth century it was rarely diagnosed (although the diagnosis subsequently became popular in the Far East—see Chapter 5.2.1). Although it is possible that the prevalence of chronic fatigue had waned in the population, it is more likely that patients who presented in this way were being given alternative diagnoses. These were mainly the new psychiatric syndromes of depression and anxiety, but also other labels indicating more direct physical explanations, such as chronic brucellosis, spontaneous hypoglycaemia, and latterly chronic Epstein–Barr virus infection.[2]

As well as these sporadic cases of fatiguing illness, epidemics of similar illnesses have been occasionally reported. One which occurred among staff at the Royal Free Hospital, London in 1955 gave rise to the term myalgic encephalomyelitis (ME), although it should be emphasized that the nature and symptoms of that outbreak are dissimilar to the majority of those now presenting to general practitioners under the same label.

A group of virologists and immunologists proposed the term chronic fatigue syndrome in the late 1980s.[3] This new and aetiologically neutral term was chosen because it was increasingly recognized that many cases of fatigue were often not readily explained either by medical conditions such as Epstein–Barr virus infection or by obvious depression and anxiety disorders. Chronic fatigue syndrome has remained the most commonly used term by researchers. The issue of the name is still not completely resolved however: Neurasthenia remains in the ICD-10 psychiatric classification as a fatigue syndrome unexplained by depressive or anxiety disorder, whilst the equivalent in DSM-IV is undifferentiated somatoform disorder. Myalgic encephalomyelitis or (encephalopathy) is in the neurological section of ICD-10 and is used by some to imply that the illness is neurological as opposed to a psychiatric one. Unfortunately the case descriptions under these different labels make it clear that they all reflect similar symptomatic presentations, adding to confusion. Official UK documents have increasingly adopted the uneasy and probably ultimately unsatisfactory compromise term CFS/ME.[4] In this chapter, we will use the simple term chronic fatigue syndrome (CFS).

## Clinical features

### Symptoms

Chronic mental and physical fatigue, tiredness, or exhaustion that is typically exacerbated by activity is the core symptom of CFS. Commonly associated symptoms include impaired memory and concentration, muscular and joint pain, unrefreshing sleep, dizziness and breathlessness, headache, tender lymph glands, and sore throat. Patients often describe day-to-day fluctuations in symptoms, irrespective of activity. Periods of almost complete recovery may be followed by relapse, often described as sufficiently severe to make normal daily activity impossible. Depression and anxiety are common, and a proportion of patients suffer panic attacks.

### Physical signs

Physical examination is typically unremarkable. Complaints of fever and lymphadenopathy are not confirmed on examination. The presence of definite physical signs (such as objectively measured fever) should not be ascribed to the syndrome and alternative diagnoses should be sought.

### Other common characteristics

As well as the symptoms described above patients with CFS commonly have additional clinical characteristics. These are listed in Table 5.2.7.1.

Patients are often worried that remaining active despite fatigue will harm them and consequently avoid activity or oscillate between rest and bursts of activity, which produces fatigue, leading to a return to rest and so on.

Some patients feel strongly that their illness is 'medical' rather than 'psychiatric' and are particularly concerned that a psychiatric diagnosis implies that the illness is their fault, an indication of personal

**Table 5.2.7.1** Common characteristics of patients with CFS

| | |
|---|---|
| Thoughts beliefs and attitudes | Thought that symptoms indicate harm<br>Belief that the illness is purely 'medical'<br>Perfectionist attitudes |
| Coping behaviours | Avoidance of activities associated with symptoms<br>Reduced activity level<br>Oscillation in overall activity level |
| Physiology | Poor sleep<br>Physiological deconditioning<br>Effects of inactivity |
| Interpersonal and social | Dependence on carer<br>Psychological iatrogenesis<br>Occupational difficulties |

weakness or even an accusation of malingering. Perfectionist and high achieving lifestyles often with low underlying self-esteem are commonly observed in patients referred to hospital clinics.

Although there are no physical signs there may be measurable effects of reduced activity with so-called physiological deconditioning leading to poor tolerance of activity, and in cases where rest has been prolonged other physiological changes such as postural hypotension. Sleep is often unrefreshing and fragmented.

Some patients can become markedly dependent on a carer. Occupational stresses and difficulties are common and it can be difficult to determine if these were contributors to, or are consequence of their illness. Finally many patients have received unhelpful medical attention. Such psychological iatrogenesis includes, on the one hand dismissal of their complaints and on the other over investigation.[5]

## Case study

A typical patient is found in the infectious disease department of the general hospital. She is a 30-years-old nurse and her principal complaints are of fatigue, poor concentration, and muscle pain. Her symptoms fluctuate and are made worse by physical and mental exertion. She is no longer able to work and has substantially reduced her daily activities. The history is of an acute onset of symptoms after a 'viral illness'. Enquiry reveals symptoms suggestive of depression or anxiety, but without obvious mood change. The patient strongly believes the illness to be 'medical' rather than 'psychiatric'.

## Classification and diagnosis

There are several published case definitions for CFS. The currently most widely used definition is based on an international consensus of researchers is shown in Table 5.2.7.2.[6] A guide on its application has also been published.[7] It should be remembered that this definition represents nothing more than a working definition of a clinical problem, pending further understanding, and as with most psychiatric diagnoses, does not delineate a single disease.

### Issues for a definition of chronic fatigue syndrome

The case definition shown in Table 5.2.7.2 has been useful in unifying the field and providing a widely used operational definition. However, it also has significant limitations.

**Table 5.2.7.2** International consensus definition of chronic fatigue syndrome

| |
|---|
| 1 Complaint of fatigue |
|   Of new onset |
|   Not relieved by rest |
|   Duration at least 6 months |
| 2 At least four of the following additional symptoms |
|   Subjective memory impairment |
|   Sore throat |
|   Tender lymph nodes |
|   Muscle pain and joint pain |
|   Headache |
|   Unrefreshing sleep |
|   Post-exertional malaise lasting more than 24 h |
| 3 Impairment of functioning |
| 4 Other conditions that might explain fatigue excluded |

(Reproduced from Fukuda, K. Straus, S.E. Hickie, I.B. *et al.* Chronic fatigue syndrome: a comprehensive approach to its definition and management, *Annals of Internal Medicine,* **121**, 953–9. Copyright 1994, The American College of Physicians.)

- It excludes fatigue associated with known organic disease.

- It overlaps with other functional medical diagnoses.

- It overlaps with psychiatric diagnosis.

- The homogeneity of the patient group it identifies is doubtful.

### (a) Differentiation from fatigue associated with organic disease

Fatigue is a common symptom of most medical and psychiatric conditions. CFS refers only to fatigue where there is no clear alternative diagnosis (but does not exclude depression and anxiety unless the depression is of melancholic type or a manifestation of a bipolar disorder). It therefore only refers to idiopathic fatigue. This means that the definition highlights an important clinical problem but also means that the interesting equally important and probably informative phenomenon of fatigue in patients with diseases such as multiple sclerosis is excluded from this definition.

### (b) Overlap with other medically unexplained syndromes

A number of medical diagnoses are defined only by symptoms. These functional syndromes are medical diagnoses where there is no identifiable pathology. They include chronic pain, fibromyalgia, and irritable bowel syndrome. Although chronic pain syndromes are principally characterized by pain, fibromyalgia by tender points, and irritable bowel syndrome by symptoms of bowel disturbance, all these syndromes are also associated with chronic fatigue, and patients diagnosed with one of these syndromes often meet the diagnostic criteria for CFS.[8]

### (c) Overlap with psychiatric syndromes

Most patients who meet criteria for CFS also fulfil criteria for a psychiatric diagnosis. Many meet criteria for anxiety and depressive disorders and others merit diagnoses of somatoform disorder or neurasthenia. This issue is discussed further below.

#### (i) Depression

If patients with a depressive disorder are asked about a wide range of somatic symptoms including fatigue and/or muscle pain (which they are usually not) they often report these. If the diagnostic criteria for depressive disorders are applied to patients with fatigue a high proportion meet these.[9] Furthermore the prevalence of major depressive disorder in patients referred to hospital with CFS is substantially higher than in patients with chronic disabling medical diseases suggesting that depression is not simply a reaction to disability.[10] In practice, the diagnosis of depression can be difficult in patients presenting with fatigue: depressed mood is often not prominent and anhedonia can be hard to distinguish from the inability to pursue previously enjoyed activities because of fatigue. Finally, whilst there is a strong association between major depressive disorder and CFS, for as many as half of the patients seen in hospital clinics the symptoms cannot be readily given that diagnosis.

#### (ii) Anxiety disorders

Although less attention has been given to the association between fatigue and anxiety, an examination of diagnostic criteria for anxiety disorders reveals that the typical somatic symptoms of anxiety include fatigue and other symptoms listed as typical of CFS. If sought, generalized anxiety disorder can often be diagnosed in patients with CFS and panic can often be diagnosed in patients with severe episodic symptoms.[11] As with depression, however, anxious mood is rarely obvious and may be hard to distinguish from reasonable concern about consequences of being ill. Likewise, true phobic avoidance may be hard to distinguish from the consequences of fatigue and/or weakness.

#### (iii) Neurasthenia

ICD-10 differs from DSM-IV in including this diagnosis. It requires that the patient suffers from fatigue which is exacerbated by exertion, as well as several other somatic symptoms, and does not meet the criteria for a depressive or anxiety disorder (see Chapter 5.2.10). One study found that almost all of the referrals to a medical CFS clinic met the criteria for neurasthenia as defined by ICD-10.[12]

#### (iv) Somatoform disorders

According to DSM-IV patients with severe persistent fatigue who do not meet criteria for anxiety or depressive disorders are assigned to a somatoform disorder diagnosis. These are a controversial group of psychiatric syndromes characterized by medically unexplained symptoms and of presumed psychological origin.[13] There are a number of subcategories:

- Somatization disorder (Briquet's syndrome) is used to describe patients who report multiple, recurrent, medically unexplained symptoms; a minority of patients with CFS will meet the criteria for this disorder.

- Hypochondriasis describes a syndrome in which the patient's main concern is with the possibility that they are suffering from an organic disease. Whilst this diagnosis would seem to be applicable to many patients with CFS, it is problematic when the cause of the illness in question, which is regarded as uncertain by doctors as well as patients.

- Almost all patients with CFS not meeting the criteria for any of the above DSM disorders are likely to fall into the undemanding residual category in DSM-IV of 'undifferentiated somatoform disorder'. This diagnosis is of dubious practical use, and in effect merely confirms that the patient has multiple physical symptoms of unclear aetiology.

### (v) Conclusion

Many patients with CFS meet the diagnostic criteria for a depressive or anxiety disorder, although in practice the presentation is often 'atypical'. It is likely that patients who do not meet the criteria for either of these could be diagnosed as having either neurasthenia (ICD-10) or undifferentiated somatoform disorder (DSM-IV).

### Should we use the diagnosis of CFS?

From the psychiatrist's perspective it is parsimonious to ask whether a diagnosis of CFS is ever necessary or appropriate when the symptoms can always be described by a psychiatric diagnosis? This unsatisfactory situation is an artefact of parallel medical and psychiatric diagnostic systems for patients with somatic symptoms unexplained by disease. Consequently whether one uses a 'medical' diagnosis of CFS or a 'psychiatric' diagnosis of somatoform disorder is merely a matter of choice. When making that choice the following must be considered:

- A diagnosis of CFS only describes a presenting clinical syndrome, rather than a specific disorder or disease process.

- Pragmatically the relative acceptability of the alternative diagnosis to the patient is important. There is no point in giving a diagnosis that is rejected by the patient and impedes any therapeutic relationship and chances of treatment.

- One approach to overcoming the issue of parallel classification systems is to combine the medical diagnosis of CFS and the psychiatric diagnoses: According to such a scheme CFS would be subclassified into CFS/depression, CFS/anxiety, and CFS without depression or anxiety disorder (i.e. CFS/somatoform or CFS/neurasthenia). Psychiatric diagnoses that have important clinical utility such as major depressive disorder should obviously be made if present. The usefulness of diagnoses such as undifferentiated somatoform disorder is less clear.

- Finally rather than becoming side-tracked by the unanswerable question of whether the patients symptoms are ultimately 'medical' or 'psychiatric' in nature an open-minded and pragmatic approach is required.

## Epidemiology

### Prevalence

Fatigue is common but CFS is rare. As it can be difficult to differentiate CFS from depressive and anxiety disorders estimates that have attempted to exclude these diagnoses are lower than those that have not. Population studies in the United Kingdom and United States suggest that only approximately 0.5 per cent of the population can be regarded as having CFS.[1] Most of these persons are aged between 20 and 40 with a predominance of females. The syndrome is also seen in children and adolescents but less commonly.

### Epidemics

Epidemics of a chronic fatigue-like syndrome have been described from various parts of the globe. This observation is compatible with, but does not establish, an infective cause. It remains unclear whether these were true epidemics and also whether the clinical picture reported is similar to that of cases of sporadic chronic fatigue syndrome.

## Aetiology

### Limitations in the available data

Although a considerable amount of research has been devoted to investigating the nature and causes of CFS there are few firm conclusions that can be drawn. This partly because many of the studies have had major methodological shortcomings:

- Patients have often been recruited from tertiary care clinics, using various diagnostic criteria inconsistently applied.

- Only a minority of studies have included comparison groups of patients with diagnoses of depression or anxiety disorders.

- Because most studies have used a case–control design, it is often impossible to know whether the findings they report are causes or consequences of the illness (for instance, as the result of reduced activity or sleep disturbance).

- CFS is almost certainly heterogeneous.

Considering these caveats there are a number of areas where positive findings have been reported.

### Pathophysiology

Clinical observations of patients with CFS have led to the investigation of a number of hypotheses about the underlying pathophysiological mechanisms.

#### (a) Genetics

Twin studies suggest that CFS is moderately heritable.[1] Preliminary studies suggesting the involvement of specific genes require replication. Gene expression studies are likewise in their infancy—one problem being that the number of genes studied usually exceeds by several orders of magnitude the numbers of patients studied. Another problem is confounders—a large Swedish twin registry study for example suggested that genetic factors contributed to the risk of CFS both directly and via personality type.[14]

#### (b) Cardiovascular and respiratory abnormalities

Several investigators have reported abnormalities in the cardio-respiratory systems that may underpin the exercise intolerance. Hyperventilation has been suggested as a mechanism of symptom production, but only a minority of patients have biochemically confirmed hyperventilation. Low blood pressure has long been associated with the symptom of fatigue, and in some parts of Europe unexplained fatigue is confidently ascribed to this. Postural hypotension has been noted in some patients and whilst this may be a cause of fatigue it may also be a consequence of inactivity. Finally, various abnormalities in cardiac function have also been reported but are of uncertain significance.

#### (c) Infection

Perhaps because patients commonly describe their illness as beginning with 'flu-like symptoms' and because of the apparent epidemics, many investigators have sought objective evidence of an initiating or ongoing viral infection. Viral infection can probably initiate CFS. A prospective follow-up of people with positive evidence of acute Epstein–Barr infection did find that some patients went on to develop a fatigue syndrome.[15] Other infectious agents that may trigger CFS include Q fever and viral meningitis. If viruses do play a role in precipitating CFS, it would appear that it is only when certain types of viruses infect vulnerable persons. If CFS can be precipitated by viral infection does persistence of the virus cause the ongoing symptoms? On current evidence the answer to this question seems to be no.

### (d) Immune dysfunction

The evidence for an association between immunological abnormalities and CFS is more consistent than that for infective agents, with several studies suggesting abnormalities in lymphocyte numbers and function. However, similar changes can be found in patients with depressive disorders, and, although some studies have attempted to control for emotional disorder, both the specificity and causal importance of these observations remain unclear.[16]

### (e) Sleep

Unrefreshing sleep is an almost ubiquitous complaint of people suffering from CFS. While studies have identified major sleep disorders such as sleep apnoea and narcolepsy as alternative diagnoses for small number of patients with daytime fatigue, simple disruption of slow-wave sleep is a much more common observation. While inefficient sleep could contribute to the daytime fatigue reported in both conditions, its specificity and aetiological role are uncertain.[16]

### (f) Neuroendocrine and neurotransmitter abnormalities

The prominent fatigue of Addison's disease has led to the hypothesis that adrenal function is impaired in patients with CFS. In support of this suggestion there is reasonable evidence that patients with chronic fatigue and fibromyalgia have both low levels of cortisol, a point of difference from major depression. However it remains unclear if this apparent abnormality is cause or effect of the illness and associated inactivity. Patients with CFS also have evidence of abnormal functioning of cerebral serotonergic systems, which differ from those found in patients with depression. Like the abnormalities in adrenal function these findings are preliminary but of potential interest.[17]

### (g) Brain imaging

Finally, a variety of techniques have been used to examine both the function and structure of the brain in patients with CFS. Cerebral perfusion studies have shown abnormalities, although similar, if not identical, abnormalities are also found in patients with depression. Possible white-matter changes reported on magnetic resonance scans are more controversial, and harder to interpret.[1,16]

### (h) Conclusions

Despite a considerable research effort, so far no single pathophysiological process has been conclusively identified as causal of CFS. There is some evidence for a loss of physical fitness and possibly for abnormalities of neuroendocrine function. Viral infection can play a role as precipitating agent, although its importance as a perpetuating factor is less certain. Immunological abnormalities are common but of uncertain specificity, and appear not to be related to chronic symptoms. The current attention on neuroendocrine function takes the focus of investigation closer to those features known to be associated with depressive states. However, the evidence suggests that the changes in neurotransmitter and neuroendocrine function in patients with CFS may differ from those commonly observed in patients diagnosed with depressive disorder. Further studies are needed to confirm all these abnormalities and to clarify whether they are causal or merely epiphenomena.

## Psychopathology

If there are no substantial biological abnormalities are there psychological ones? The initial psychiatric explanation of CFS was that it was misdiagnosed depressive disorder. However, whilst such misdiagnosis does occur, more complex explanations are required to adequately explain many cases of CFS.

### (a) Somatization

It has been hypothesized that depression may still be 'behind' CFS even if not apparent. It is argued that a process referred to as 'somatization' (making the mental physical) is responsible. Whist the idea that the somatic symptoms of CFS are readily understandable as part of an emotional disturbance is a parsimonious alternative to some of the more elaborate mechanisms outlined above, as there is no 'marker' for somatization this hypothesis is hard to prove.

### (b) Attribution

Patients attending specialist clinics with CFS typically attribute their illness to organic disease even when no evidence of this can be found by their physicians. Perhaps more importantly, some strongly resist psychological explanations for their illness, although most take a more mixed view. Whether these patients are biased in their views about illness or simply wiser than their physicians is unclear. However, strong and exclusively physical disease attributions may be a marker for an important illness-perpetuating process in CFS as they predict a poorer clinical outcome.

### (c) Perceptual processes

Patients with CFS report a greater sense of effort in response to both psychological and physical demands than is explicable from objectively measured impairments. This observation raises the possibility that they are especially sensitive to bodily sensations such as effort, that is they 'amplify' or focus on them. Thus, one may hypothesize that as in panic disorder, the patients' beliefs about their symptoms may lead them to focus attention on to bodily sensations. Although plausible there is so far only limited evidence that this process is important in patients with CFS.[1]

### (d) Coping behaviour

A tendency to avoid activities that exacerbate symptoms has been shown to occur in patients with CFS. The avoidance may be persistent or episodic in response to exacerbations of symptoms resulting in a 'boom and bust' pattern. Avoidance is associated with persistent disability, and has been suggested as the mechanism by which disease attributions for symptoms predicts poor outcome.[1]

### (e) Personality characteristics

Both research studies and clinical experience suggest that many persons with CFS have a tendency towards hard driving, perfectionist, or obsessive–compulsive personalities, and associated overactive lifestyles. Evidence from the UK 1946 birth cohort for example indicates that ratings of physical activity in early life predict later CFS. In a large prospective Swedish twin registry measure of stress and emotionality are consistently associated with subsequent CFS. Those CFS sufferers may be predisposed to becoming physically and emotionally exhausted, and biased towards presenting emotional distress in a somatic form.[14]

### (f) Stigma, misinformation, and iatrogenesis

Psychiatric diagnoses are stigmatized in the popular mind as indicating weakness or even unreal illness. Patients with CFS may be susceptible to those social pressures and consequently prefer a medical diagnosis for their distress and inability to function. It has also been suggested that CFS may serve as culturally defined function of social communication, allowing a socially acceptable and hence 'non-psychiatric' expression of distress and protest about intolerable occupational and personal pressures. Much the same was said of neurasthenia in the People's Republic of China (see Chapter 5.2.1).

Another potentially important social factor is the controversy and the often misleading information about the illness that patients are exposed to. Self-help books the media and some doctors have frequently given the impression that the medial profession is more divided than it actually is in its understanding of CFS and have emphasized 'medical' explanations such as myalgic encephalopathy (ME) as the only appropriate diagnosis.

### (g) Conclusions

Psychological and social factors are important perpetuating factors and include focusing of attention on symptoms avoidance of activity and a strong and exclusive medical disease attribution.

## A comprehensive view of the cause of CFS

It now seems clear that rather than regarding pathophysiological and psychopathological studies as separate and competing approaches to the problem, it is more useful to consider a formulation of CFS that combines these factors. Table 5.2.7.3 summarizes relevant aetiological factors.

According to this integrated scheme causal factors are divided into those that may predispose to the illness, those that precipitate it, and those that perpetuate an established illness. Predisposing factors include previous episodes of major depressive disorder, and perhaps also certain personality characteristics, particularly achievement orientation and perfectionism associated with chronic stress, especially occupational stress. The precipitation of CFS by a viral infection is clinically plausible and proven in certain circumstances, whilst life stresses also seem to be important. Perpetuating factors may include neuroendocrine dysfunction, emotional disorder, and physical disease attributions, as well as coping by avoidance, chronic unresolved personal difficulties, and misinformation about the illness. They may be effectively combined in a cognitive–behavioural model of the illness that provides a basis for treatment with CBT.[1,18]

## Course and prognosis of CFS

Anecdotal reports of the prognosis of CFS make gloomy reading. What is more, systematic studies are hardly more encouraging, suggesting that the commonest outcome of those attending a specialist CFS clinic is continuing ill health, up to and beyond 5 years.[19] However, these observations need elaboration. The rather dispiriting prognostic studies all refer to patients seen in specialist centres. Nearly all had several years of illness prior to referral, and it is unsurprising to find that chronicity predicts chronicity. Patients seen in specialist clinics often have strong views about illness aetiology and illness management that may negatively influence their acceptance of and adherence to potentially effective treatment. Primary care and community samples and patients appear to have a better outcome, as do children and adolescents. Finally, the current generation of outcome studies refer to the situation

**Table 5.2.7.3** An aetiological formulation of CFS

|  | Predisposing | Precipitating | Perpetuating |
|---|---|---|---|
| Biological | Genetics<br><br>Previous depression | Infection | Effects of inactivity<br>CNS dysfunction<br>Reduced HPA activity |
| Psychological | Personality (perfectionism) | Response to stressor | Focus on symptoms<br>Disease attribution<br>Avoidant coping |
| Social | Chronic stress | Social/occupation stress | Life conflicts<br><br>Psychological iatrogenesis |

without treatment as potentially effective treatment was rarely given. Later sections of this chapter suggest that this view requires revision.

## Evidence for treatments

### Drug treatment

Many pharmacological treatments have been suggested for CFS. To date, none are of proven efficacy and several are potentially harmful.[4, 20] The evidence for antidepressant agents is mixed. Of available agents none is clearly superior for this patient group, although clinical experience suggests that the selective serotonin-reuptake inhibitor antidepressants may be better tolerated.

### Graded activity (exercise) therapy

Well-conducted randomized controlled trials suggest that graded increases in physical activity is helpful in improving function and relieving symptoms.[4, 20]

### Cognitive behaviour therapy

Systematic reviews have concluded that the strongest evidence for efficacy is for a rehabilitative type of cognitive–behaviour therapy (CBT).[4, 20]

## Practical management

### Assessment

Both a medical and psychiatric assessment is required in every case of suspected CFS.[21]

### (a) Excluding organic disease

A small minority of those patients who present with severe chronic fatigue will be found to have occult organic disease. How frequently organic disease is found will depend on how thorough an assessment the patient has already received. The differential diagnosis is listed in Table 5.2.7.4.

There are no specific diagnostic tests and no characteristic abnormalities on laboratory investigations in CFS. Tests are conducted purely to exclude other diseases. All patients should have a full blood count, erythrocyte sedimentation rate or C-reactive

**Table 5.2.7.4** Conditions to be considered in the differential diagnosis of chronic fatigue syndrome

| Nature of symptoms | Possible condition |
|---|---|
| General | Occult malignancy |
| | Autoimmune disease |
| | Endocrine disease |
| | Cardiac, respiratory, or renal failure |
| Gastroenterological | Malabsorption including celiac disease |
| Neurological | Disseminated sclerosis |
| | Myasthenia gravis |
| | Parkinson's disease |
| | Early dementia |
| | Cerebrovascular disease |
| Infectious disease | Chronic active hepatitis (B or C) |
| | Lyme borreliosis |
| | HIV |
| | Tuberculosis |
| Respiratory disease | Nocturnal asthma |
| | Obstructive sleep apnoea |
| Chronic toxicity | Alcohol |
| | Solvents |
| | Heavy metals |
| | Irradiation |
| Psychiatric | Major depressive disorder |
| | Dysthymia |
| | Anxiety and panic disorder |
| | Somatoform disorder |

protein, basic biochemistry screen, creatine kinase, random blood glucose, urine analysis, thyroid function, and possibly antinuclear antibody tests. Further investigation depends on the clinical findings and differential diagnoses under consideration. In our clinical experience unusual clinical features, such as weight loss, an absence of mental fatigue/fatigability, or a history of recent foreign travel, should all increases suspicion of alternative diagnoses.

### (b) Excluding psychiatric diagnoses

All patients should have a psychiatric history taken and their mental state examined. The assessment should seek evidence of major depression, anxiety, and panic disorder, and also evaluate any suicidal intent. The psychiatric assessment should be systematic, as hidden distress is common and casual estimates of the patient's degree of distress may be misleading.

### Making the diagnosis

As explained above the choice of diagnosis should be pragmatic; there is little merit in giving a diagnosis of CFS if the patient's symptoms are clearly those of depression or anxiety. In other cases, a diagnosis of CFS may be the most appropriate and useful; it offers the patient a coherent label for their symptoms and will therefore lessen the risk that they will embark on a fruitless search for a 'better' explanation. Above all, it is most important that neither the physician nor the patient stops at this diagnosis, but goes on to explain what it does and does not mean.

### Making a formulation

An adequate individual patient assessment must identify all the important obstacles to recovery. It often needs to go beyond diagnosis to include a systematic individualized description of the aetiological factors in each case. These should include those factors listed in Table 5.2.7.1.

### (a) Case formulation

A multidimensional description of the patient's illness provides a comprehensive picture of the factors that may be relevant to the patient's illness and is an important supplement to diagnosis. Its use can be illustrated by returning to the case example described above.

---

*Case Study*

Assessment of the patient described earlier revealed that she believed that her symptoms were by an ongoing virus infection and associated immune disturbance and that she should beware of exacerbating them. She consequently avoided activity and had been profoundly inactive for over a year, often lying in bed and sleeping for long periods. Therefore she had become physiologically deconditioned. She was frustrated with her inability to do things and sometimes felt low in mood about her predicament. Her previous job had been very stressful, but since becoming ill she had been unable to work. She had now lost her job and was cared for by her mother who also believed she had a permanent disability. Her doctor said that the best thing was rest. She had rejected a psychiatric consultation but was paying to see an alternative medicine therapist.

---

The findings can be summarized in an individualized form of Table 5.2.7.3 with an emphasis on the perpetuating factors, which can be seen as reversible barriers to recovery.

### General management

The five basic steps essential to the care of patients with CFS are listed in Table 5.2.7.5.

The doctor should listen to the patient's story and ask about his or her own understanding of the illness. It is usually also worth seeing the partner or relevant family members. It is important to address misunderstandings about the nature of the illness and especially to make clear that it is not progressive or life threatening. A positive explanation of CFS as a 'dysfunction of the central nervous system' emphasizing reversibility is often helpful. Anxiety and depression can be explained as understandable consequences of illness and treatment given for them. The adverse physiological and psychological effects of prolonged bed rest should be explained, and the patient encouraged to avoid extremes of both inactivity

**Table 5.2.7.5** Principles of management of CFS

1 Acknowledge the reality of the patient's symptoms and disability
2 Provide appropriate education about the nature of the syndrome
3 Treat identifiable depression and anxiety disorder
4 Encourage a very gradual return to normal functioning
5 Help the patient overcome occupational and interpersonal obstacles to normal functioning

and exertion. Finally there are often problem in relationships and with employers than the patient may need help to address.

An initial hospital appointment that achieves all the above usually requires at least 45 min. An evidence-based self-help book may be recommended.[22]

### (a) Pharmacological treatments

Patients are often reluctant to take antidepressants and careful explanation and follow-up are required. Other pharmacological agents should only be used with care and preferably only as part of randomized controlled trials.

### (b) Graded activity and exercise therapy

This should be considered for patients who are physically inactive. However, they need to be slowly graded and tailored to the patients' ability and progress; a simplistic application of fixed exercise regimens, particularly if given without adequate explanation is unlikely to be helpful, and may exacerbate symptoms and damage confidence.

### (c) CBT

Whilst CBT is currently the mainstay of management it is not effective in all patients and requires both careful explanation and therapists skilled in its delivery to patients with CFS. It is particularly important that patients do not interpret referral for a behavioural treatment as the doctor implying that their illness is imaginary. It can be explained that the most likely cause of fatigue in CFS is changes in brain and neuroendocrine function and that these can be reversed by these therapies. It is also both useful and true to draw attention to studies showing the effective of CBT in improving symptoms, quality of life and outcome in conditions such as diabetes, cancer, and rheumatoid arthritis. General physical rehabilitation services may be useful for patients with chronic severe disability.

### Potential management problems

Several issues may complicate the management of patients with CFS. These include:

### (a) Strong illness beliefs

Difficulties are most likely to arise when patient and physician hold differing beliefs about the nature and best management of the illness. This problem can often be overcome by the physician acknowledging the patient's beliefs without either agreeing with them or arguing about them. If the patient's family, friends, or acquaintances suggest or encourage views that the physician regards as unhelpful the problem is more difficult and a meeting with the other parties may be necessary.

### (b) Alternative therapies

Patients with CFS often turn to alternative and complementary medicine. Whilst some of these therapies may be easily continued in parallel with rehabilitative management, others may interfere either by the explanation of the illness they offer or by their practical requirements. In such cases it can be helpful to explain the need to pursue one approach at a time in order to learn what helps.

### (c) Official reports and financial benefits

Perhaps the greatest difficulty is when patients ask the physician to write reports on their behalf, confirming that they suffer from permanent disability. The physician wants to help the patient and ensure that they get appropriate benefits but also to avoid a self-fulfilling prophecy. This dilemma has no easy solution, but it seems important not to confirm a negative prognosis until potentially effective treatment has been tried.

### (d) Poor prognosis patients

For patients who have been identified as having a poor prognosis because of a long history of severely impaired functioning, or poor response to treatment, regular (albeit infrequent) long-term follow-up is, at the least, likely to limit iatrogenic harm from unnecessary investigations and ineffective treatments. Often in such cases the best strategy is simply to tell the patient how well they are managing in difficult circumstances.

## Possibilities for prevention

We do not know how to prevent CFS, but its development can probably be modified.

The most important place for such intervention may be the transition from an acute fatigue state to chronic disability. For example, although most of us have been exposed to Epstein–Barr virus infection by the time we reach 30 years of age, few go on to develop CFS. Encouraging modest amounts of activity in the weeks after an acute infection has been shown to be effective in reducing the duration of symptoms. Intervention that maintain activity and prevent a slide into a vicious circle of symptoms, reduced activity, demoralization, disability, and depression might therefore offer an opportunity for prevention. The second area for intervention is in achieving better attitudes to symptoms and distress. Simplistic depictions of illness as either physical or psychological and the corresponding division in medical services are clearly unhelpful. The third area is in employment practice. CFS is often associated with work stress and dissatisfaction and only a minority of employers allow a flexible return to work. Finally, a doctor–patient relationship that both allows the patient to be ill and encourages recovery is probably the most important preventive strategy.

## Conclusions and future directions

Chronic fatigue syndrome is best regarded as a descriptive term for a clinical presentation, rather than as a discrete condition. The group of patients it defines is almost certainly aetiologically heterogeneous. While psychiatric diagnosis provides one approach to subclassification of CFS, both the medical and psychiatric current diagnostic systems have significant limitations, and a multidimensional description of the patient's characteristics may be more clinically useful.[23]

The illness defined by the term chronic fatigue syndrome is important because it represents potentially treatable disability and suffering. It is also important because the clinical problems it gives rise to highlight shortcomings in our present approach to illness. Whatever is ultimately discovered about the causes of CFS, the attention it is receiving offers a golden opportunity to reappraise our understanding and classification of human illness and to re-examine our current organization of medical care.

## Further information

Wessely, S., Sharpe, M., and Hotopf, M. (1998). *Chronic fatigue and its syndromes*. Oxford University Press, Oxford.

National Institute for Health and Clinical Excellence Guideline number 53. Chronic fatigue syndrome/ myalgic encephalomyelitis (or encephalopathy); diagnosis and management. http://guidance.nice.org.uk/CG53

## References

1. Prins, J.B., Van der Meer, J.W., and Bleijenberg, G. (2006). Chronic fatigue syndrome. *Lancet*, **367**, 346–55.
2. Wessely, S., Hotopf, M.H., and Sharpe, M. (1998). *Chronic fatigue and its syndromes*. Oxford University Press, Oxford.
3. Holmes, G.P., Kaplan, J.E., Gantz, N.M., *et al.* (1988). Chronic fatigue syndrome: a working case definition. *Annals of Internal Medicine*, **108**, 387–9.
4. Baker, R. and Shaw, E.J. (2007). Diagnosis and management of chronic fatigue syndrome or myalgic encephalomyelitis (or encephalopathy): summary of NICE guidance. *British Medical Journal*, **335**, 446–8.
5. Sharpe, M. (1998). Doctors' diagnoses and patients' perceptions: lessons from chronic fatigue syndrome. *General Hospital Psychiatry*, **20**, 335–8.
6. Fukuda, K., Straus, S.E., Hickie, I.B., *et al.* (1994). Chronic fatigue syndrome: a comprehensive approach to its definition and management. *Annals of Internal Medicine*, **121**, 953–9.
7. Reeves, W.C., Lloyd, A., Vernon, S.D., *et al.* (2003). Identification of ambiguities in the 1994 chronic fatigue syndrome research case definition and recommendations for resolution. *BMC Health Services Research*, **3**, 25.
8. Wessely, S., Nimnuan, C., and Sharpe, M. (1999). Functional somatic syndromes: one or many? *Lancet*, **354**, 936–9.
9. Skapinakis, P., Lewis, G., and Meltzer, H. (2000). Clarifying the relationship between unexplained chronic fatigue and psychiatric morbidity: results from a community survey in Great Britain. *The American Journal of Psychiatry*, **157**, 1492–8.
10. Katon, W., Buchwald, D.S., Simon, G.E., *et al.* (1991). Psychiatric illness in patients with chronic fatigue and rheumatoid arthritis. *Journal of General Internal Medicine*, **6**, 277–85.
11. Fischler, B., Cluydts, R., De Gucht, Y., *et al.* (1997). Generalized anxiety disorder in chronic fatigue syndrome. *Acta Psychiatrica Scandinavica*, **95**, 405–13.
12. Farmer, A., Jones, I., Hillier, J., *et al.* (1995). Neurasthenia revisited. *British Journal of Psychiatry*, **167**, 496–502.
13. Mayou, R., Kirmayer, L.J., Simon, G., *et al.* (2005). Somatoform disorders: time for a new approach in DSM-V. *American Journal of Psychiatry*, **162**, 847–55.
14. Kato, K., Sullivan, P.F., Evengard, B., *et al.* (2006). Premorbid predictors of chronic fatigue. *Archives of General Psychiatry*, **63**, 1267–72.
15. White, P.D., Thomas, J.M., Amess, J., *et al.* (1995). The existence of a fatigue syndrome after glandular fever. *Psychological Medicine*, **25**, 907–16.
16. Afari, N. and Buchwald, D. (2003). Chronic fatigue syndrome: a review. *American Journal of Psychiatry*, **160**, 221–36.
17. Cho, H.J., Skowera, A., Cleare, A., *et al.* (2006). Chronic fatigue syndrome: an update focusing on phenomenology and pathophysiology. *Current Opinion in Psychiatry*, **19**, 67–73.
18. Surawy, C., Hackmann, A., Hawton, K.E., *et al.* (1995). Chronic fatigue syndrome: a cognitive approach. *Behaviour Research and Therapy*, **33**, 535–44.
19. Cairns, R. and Hotopf, M. (2005). A systematic review describing the prognosis of chronic fatigue syndrome. *Occupational Medicine (London)*, **55**, 20–31.
20. Chambers, D., Bagnall, A.M., Hempel, S., *et al.* (2006). Interventions for the treatment, management and rehabilitation of patients with chronic fatigue syndrome/myalgic encephalomyelitis: an updated systematic review. *Journal of the Royal Society of Medicine*, **99**, 506–20.
21. Sharpe, M., Chalder, T., Palmer, I., *et al.* (1997). Chronic fatigue syndrome. A practical guide to assessment and management. *General Hospital Psychiatry*, **19**, 185–99.
22. Campling, F. and Sharpe, M. (2000). *Chronic fatigue syndrome: the facts*. Oxford University Press, Oxford.
23. Sharpe, M., Mayou, R., and Walker, J. (2006). Bodily symptoms: new approaches to classification. *Journal of Psychosomatic Research*, **60**, 353–6.

## 5.2.8 Body dysmorphic disorder

Katharine A. Phillips

*The dysmorphophobic patient is really miserable; in the middle of his daily routines, talks, while reading, during meals, everywhere and at any time, he is caught by the doubt of deformity.... Enrico Morselli, 1891*[1]

### Introduction

Body dysmorphic disorder (BDD), also known as dysmorphophobia, is a relatively common, severe, and sometimes difficult-to-treat condition that has been described for more than a century.[1–3] BDD consists of a distressing or impairing preoccupation with an imagined or slight defect in one's physical appearance. BDD is classified as a separate disorder in DSM-IV and a type of hypochondriasis in ICD-10. This disorder can cause severe distress and notably impaired functioning. In addition, risk behaviours—suicidality, violence, problematic substance use, and compulsive tanning—appear common in BDD. Despite its severity, BDD is underrecognized in clinical settings.

### Clinical features

#### Demographic characteristics

BDD occurs in all age groups.[3–5] It appears about equally common in females and males or may be somewhat more common in females.[3] Most individuals with BDD have never been married, and a high proportion is unemployed, often because of their psychopathology.[3–7]

#### Bodily preoccupations

People with BDD are preoccupied with the idea that some aspect of their appearance is ugly, unattractive, deformed, flawed, or defective in some way.[1–6, 8–10] Concerns usually focus on the face or head but can involve any body area.[3–6, 8–10] Skin (e.g. acne, scars, lines, or pale skin), hair (e.g. thinning or excessive body or facial hair), and nose (e.g. size or shape) concerns are most common. Most patients are preoccupied with several body areas. The preoccupation usually focuses on specific areas but may involve overall appearance.

BDD preoccupations are distressing, time consuming (occurring for an average of 3–8 h a day), and usually difficult to resist or control.[3] They are often associated with low self-esteem, shame, rejection sensitivity, and high levels of neuroticism, introversion, depressed mood, anxiety, anger-hostility, and perceived stress.[3] Patients often believe that they are unacceptable—e.g. worthless, inadequate, unlovable, and an object of ridicule and rejection.[3,9]

### Insight/delusionality

Insight is usually poor or absent; 27–39 per cent of patients are currently delusional (completely convinced that their belief is accurate and undistorted).[3,11,12] Most do not recognize that their belief is due to a mental illness or has a psychological/psychiatric cause.[3,12] In addition, a majority have ideas or delusions of reference, believing that others take special notice of the supposed appearance defects—for example, stare at them or mock the person because of how they look.[3,12] Referential thinking can fuel feelings of anger and rejection as well as social isolation.

### Compulsive and safety behaviours

Nearly all patients perform BDD-related compulsive or safety behaviours (Table 5.2.8.1), which are time consuming (occurring for hours a day) and difficult to resist or control.[3–6,10] The behaviours usually aim to examine, improve, hide, or obtain reassurance about the perceived defects. These behaviours typically do not alleviate distress and may even worsen it.

Compulsive skin picking, which 27–45 per cent of BDD patients do to try and improve their appearance, can cause considerable skin damage.[3,5] Emergency surgery is sometimes required—for example when sharp implements used for picking rupture major blood vessels. Compulsive tanning to darken 'pale' skin or minimize perceived acne, scarring, or 'marks' can cause skin damage and may increase cancer risk.[3]

### Psychosocial functioning and quality of life

Functioning and quality of life are usually very poor.[3,4,7] Some people, with effort, function adequately despite their distress, although usually below their potential. Those with severe BDD

**Table 5.2.8.1** Common compulsive and safety behaviors in body dysmorphic disorder

- Comparing one's appearance 'defects' with the same body areas of other people
- Checking the perceived defects directly, in mirrors, or in other reflecting surfaces
- Excessive grooming—for example, applying make-up, shaving, hair cutting or removal, hair styling
- Camouflaging—for example with a hat, clothes, sunglasses, hair, body position, hand, or make-up
- Seeking reassurance from others or trying to convince others of the 'defect's' ugliness
- Skin picking
- Excessive exercising or weightlifting
- Tanning
- Frequent clothes changing
- Touching the perceived defect
- Dieting
- Body measuring
- Compulsive shopping for beauty products, remedies, or clothes
- Seeking surgical, dermatologic, and other cosmetic treatment for the perceived deformity

may be profoundly impaired by their symptoms—for example, housebound for years, unemployed and socially isolated, and chronically suicidal.

Social impairment is nearly universal.[3,7] People with BDD feel embarrassed and ashamed of their 'ugliness', are anxious around others as a result, and fear being rejected because of how they look. Thus, they may have few or no friends; avoid dating, physical intimacy, and other social interactions; or get divorced. Impairment in academic or occupational functioning is common, due to the time consuming and distracting nature of BDD symptoms and a desire to avoid interactions with others.[3,7] In a broadly ascertained BDD sample ($n = 200$), 36 per cent of individuals were not currently working and 32 per cent were not able to be in school or do school work because of psychopathology (BDD was the primary diagnosis for most).[7] In two BDD series, more than a quarter of individuals had been completely housebound for at least 1 week because of BDD symptoms, and more than 40 per cent had been psychiatrically hospitalized.[5,13] Mental health related quality of life is markedly poorer than for the general population and even poorer than for patients with diabetes, a recent myocardial infarction, or clinical depression.[7]

### Suicidality

Suicidal ideation and attempts appear very common. Reported lifetime rates of suicidal ideation and suicide attempts are 78–81 and 24–28 per cent, respectively.[9,13,14] Among adolescent inpatients, those with BDD have significantly greater suicidality than those without BDD. The rate of completed suicide, while preliminary, appears markedly high. In a prospective study, the annual suicide rate was 0.35 per cent, which is approximately 45 times higher than for the US population (adjusted for age, gender, and geographic region) and higher than for most other mental disorders.[15] A study of dermatology patients who committed suicide found that most had acne or BDD.[16] Indeed, individuals with BDD have many suicide risk factors.[3,14]

### Aggression and violence

In several BDD studies, 36–38 per cent of patients reported lifetime aggression/violence due specifically to BDD symptoms.[3,10] Such behaviour may be fuelled by anger about looking 'deformed', an inability to fix the perceived defect, and misperceptions of being rejected, ridiculed, or mocked because of the appearance 'defects'. Individuals with BDD tend to misinterpret self-referent facial expressions as contemptuous and angry,[17] misinterpret ambiguous social (and other) situations as threatening,[18] and have high levels of anger/hostility.[3] Surgeons and dermatologists may be victims of violence—even murder—fuelled by dissatisfaction with the outcome of cosmetic procedures.[3] In a survey of 265 plastic surgeons, 12 per cent reported that a BDD patient had physically threatened them.[19]

### Comorbidity

Major depressive disorder is the most frequently comorbid disorder, occurring in about 75 per cent of individuals with BDD.[5,13] Social phobia, OCD, and substance use disorders are also common.[5,8,13] Of note, one study found that 49 per cent of 200 BDD subjects had a lifetime substance use disorder, 70 per cent of whom reported that BDD contributed to their substance use.[5] Muscle dysmorphia, a preoccupation with the idea that one's body is insufficiently lean or muscular, may lead to anabolic steroid abuse.[3]

## Gender

Men and women appear to have largely similar clinical features.[10, 13, 20] However, in two United States studies ($n = 200$ and $n = 188$[13, 20]) males were more likely to be single, have a substance use disorder, and be preoccupied with thinning hair and small body build. Females were more likely to be preoccupied with weight, hips, and excessive body hair, and were more likely to pick their skin and use their hands or make-up for camouflage. One of these two studies, and a study from Italy ($n = 58$[10]), found that females were more likely to be preoccupied with their breasts/chest and legs, check mirrors, and use camouflaging. In all three studies, a concern with genitals was more common in males, and a comorbid eating disorder more common in females.

## BDD in children and adolescents

BDD usually begins during early adolescence and can occur in childhood.[4, 5, 10] While data are limited, BDD's clinical features in youth appear largely similar to those in adults. Of note, children and adolescents appear to have lifetime rates of functional impairment similar to those in adults, despite having had fewer years over which to have developed these problems.[3] In the one study that directly compared adolescents to adults, adolescents were more likely to have delusional BDD beliefs and had a significantly higher lifetime suicide attempt rate (44 per cent versus 24 per cent), underscoring the importance of recognizing BDD in this age group.

## Cross-cultural aspects of BDD

Case reports and series from around the world suggest that BDD's clinical features are generally similar across cultures but that cultural factors may produce nuances and accents on a basically invariant, or universal, expression of BDD.[3] It is unclear whether koro (a belief that one's penis is shrinking, which occurs primarily in Southeast Asia) is a form of BDD.

## Classification and relationship to other disorders

A clinically important classification controversy is whether delusional and non-delusional BDD are the same or different disorders. Whereas BDD is classified as a somatoform disorder, its delusional variant is classified as a psychotic disorder—a type of delusional disorder. DSM-IV, however, allows delusional patients to be diagnosed with both BDD and delusional disorder, reflecting data suggesting that its delusional and non-delusional variants may constitute the same disorder, which spans a spectrum of insight. Indeed, delusional and non-delusional BDD appear more similar than different, although delusional BDD appears more severe.[11,12] Of clinical significance, delusional and non-delusional patients both appear to respond to serotonin-reuptake inhibitors (SRIs) as monotherapy but not to antipsychotic monotherapy.[21]

Another important question is whether BDD is related to OCD, social phobia, major depressive disorder, or eating disorders.[3] BDD is widely conceptualized as an OCD-spectrum disorder. Supporting this conceptualization, OCD often co-occurs with BDD, and BDD appears more common in first-degree relatives of OCD probands than control probands.[3] Data from a variety of domains suggest that BDD and OCD have many similarities.[3] However, BDD and OCD have some differences and do not appear to be identical disorders.[3] Although BDD's relationship to other disorders has received less investigation, preliminary data suggest that BDD may also be related to major depressive disorder. However, BDD does not appear to simply be a symptom of depression.[3] Although ICD-10 classifies BDD as a type of hypochondriasis, no studies have examined their relationship.

## Diagnosis

BDD can be diagnosed using questions at the top of Table 5.2.8.2, which follow DSM-IV's diagnostic criteria. Clinicians should adequately probe for examples of clinically significant distress and impairment in social, occupational, and other aspects of functioning. BDD is diagnosed if the person is excessively preoccupied with a non-existent or slight physical flaw (for example, thinks about it for at least an hour a day), and the concern causes clinically significant distress or impairment in functioning. The appearance concerns should not be better accounted for by an eating disorder. However, BDD and eating disorders may co-occur, in which case both disorders should be diagnosed.

The bottom of Table 5.2.8.2 includes questions that are **not** recommended for screening for or diagnosing BDD. The word 'imagined' is problematic, because most patients have poor or absent insight and do not think their appearance problem is imagined. Terms such as 'deformed' or 'disfigured' are too extreme for some patients to endorse. Asking if there is something wrong with one's body is too broad, as patients may interpret this to refer to bodily functioning.

ICD-10's criteria require that patients persistently refuse to accept the advice and reassurance of several different doctors that they do not have an abnormality. However, many people with BDD do not disclose their appearance concerns to doctors or even seek medical care because they are housebound, ashamed, believe they cannot be helped, lack medical insurance, or do not have access to

**Table 5.2.8.2** Questions to diagnose BDD

---

*Recommended questions for diagnosing BDD:*

1 Are you very worried about your appearance in any way? *OR:* Are you unhappy with how you look? *If yes:* Can you tell me more about your concern?

2 Does this concern preoccupy you? Do you think about it a lot and wish you could worry about it less? How much time would you estimate you spend each day thinking about how you look, if you were to add up all the time you spend?

3 What effect does this preoccupation with your appearance have on your life? Has it caused you a lot of distress (for example, anxiety or depression)? Has it significantly interfered with your social life, relationships, school work, job, or any other activities? Has it affected your family or friends?

*Questions that are **not** recommended when screening for or diagnosing BDD:*

1 It is recommended that patients **not** be asked if they are concerned with an 'imagined' defect in their appearance, whether they think they are 'deformed' or 'disfigured', or whether there is something 'wrong with (their) body'

2 To diagnose BDD, it should not be required that patients refuse to accept the advice and reassurance of doctors that they do not have an abnormality

health care for other reasons. Using this diagnostic criterion will underdiagnose BDD. BDD is also underidentified in many mental health databases because its ICD-9 diagnostic code identifies it as hypochondriasis.

BDD usually goes undiagnosed in clinical settings.[3,4,22] Sufferers often conceal their symptoms due to embarrassment and shame.[3,4,22] They may volunteer only depression, anxiety, or discomfort in social situations. The compulsive and safety behaviours in Table 5.2.8.1 may be clues to BDD's presence. BDD may be misdiagnosed as another disorder[3]: social phobia or agoraphobia (due to secondary social anxiety and isolation), panic disorder (because panic attacks may occur after looking in the mirror or when feeling scrutinized by others), trichotillomania (when hair is cut or plucked to improve perceived flaws, such as uneven eyebrows), or OCD (due to obsessional preoccupations and compulsive behaviours). Delusional patients are sometimes misdiagnosed with schizophrenia, psychotic depression, or psychotic disorder NOS. To diagnose BDD, patients must usually be asked directly about BDD symptoms.

## Epidemiology

BDD has been reported in 0.7–1.7 per cent of community samples.[3] In the largest study, a nationwide survey in Germany ($n = 2552$), BDD was present in 1.9 per cent of women and 1.4 per cent of men.[23] In smaller non-clinical student samples, BDD's prevalence has ranged from 2.3–13 per cent.[3] A prevalence of 9–12 per cent has been reported in dermatology settings, 3–15 per cent in cosmetic surgery or plastic surgery settings, 8–37 per cent in patients with OCD, 11–13 per cent in social phobia, 26 per cent in trichotillomania, and 14–42 per cent in atypical major depression.[3] In a study of 122 general psychiatric inpatients, 13 per cent had BDD's, which was higher than for schizophrenia, OCD, PTSD, and eating disorders.[22]

## Pathogenesis

BDD's pathogenesis is likely to be complex and multifactorial.[3] Aetiologic factors likely involve a complex interplay of genetic and environmental risk factors.[3] Preliminary data indicate an association of the GABA$_A$-γ2 gene with BDD. Environmental risk factors may include perceived childhood neglect and/or abuse, teasing, and low parental warmth. A role is also likely for socio-cultural and evolutionary pressures (e.g. symmetrical features may signal reproductive health).

Neuropsychological studies indicate a tendency to focus on isolated details of visual and verbal stimuli rather than more global, configurational attributes[24]—consistent with clinical observations that patients selectively attend to specific aspects of their appearance or minor flaws. Cognitive processing studies indicate that BDD patients tend to misinterpret ambiguous social (and other) situations as threatening and misinterpret self-referent facial expressions as contemptuous and angry.[17,18] These interpretive biases may combine with rejection sensitivity, perfectionism, and a focus on aesthetics to contribute to BDD's development.[3] High neuroticism and low extroversion may also play a role.[3] Many potential risk factors (e.g. neuroticism) are not specific to BDD, but the overall combination of risk factors may be. BDD's neurocircuitry is unknown but likely involves a complex interplay of

dysfunction in several neural systems,[3,25] including circuitry involved in OCD (orbitofrontal cortex, anterior cingulate cortex, caudate, thalamus). BDD's shared features with other anxiety disorders and depression points to possible dysfunction in amygdala, prefrontal cortex, and anterior cingulate cortex. Brain regions involved in body image and facial emotion perception (e.g. right parietal cortex, amygdala, occipitotemporal cortex [e.g. fusiform face and extrastriate body areas]) may also be involved.

## Course and prognosis

Prospective and retrospective studies indicate that BDD is usually chronic.[5,13,26] More severe BDD, a longer duration of BDD, and the presence of a personality disorder predict a lower probability of remission. However, when BDD is accurately identified and its treatment optimized, the prognosis appears much more favourable.

## Treatment

BDD's treatment is described in more detail elsewhere, including in a guideline from the United Kingdom's National Institute of Clinical Excellence (NICE).[3,21,27,28] Serotonin-reuptake inhibitors (SRIs, or SSRIs) and cognitive–behavioural therapy (CBT) are currently recommended as the first-line treatments.[3,21,27,29] Treatment studies are limited, and more research is needed. However, available data consistently indicate that a majority of patients improve with these treatments.

## Evaluation of treatments

### Surgical, dermatologic, and other cosmetic treatment

A majority of BDD patients seek often-costly cosmetic treatment.[3,8,9,13,30] Dermatologists and surgeons are most often consulted, but any type of physician may be seen. It appears that most BDD patients are dissatisfied with such treatment.[3,9,13,30] Occasionally, dissatisfied patients sue, or are violent towards, the physician. Some patients perform their own surgery[3,6]—e.g. cutting open one's nose with a razor blade and trying to replace nose cartilage with chicken cartilage in the desired shape.

### Pharmacotherapy and other somatic treatments

All SRI studies to date indicate that SRIs are often efficacious for BDD.[3,21] These studies include a placebo-controlled fluoxetine study ($n = 67$), a controlled and blinded cross-over study comparing the SRI clomipramine to the non-SRI antidepressant desipramine ($n = 29$), and open-label trials of fluvoxamine, citalopram, and escitalopram ($n = 15–30$). In these studies, 53 per cent to 73 per cent of patients responded to the SRI. The cross-over trial found greater efficacy for clomipramine than desipramine, suggesting that SRIs may be more efficacious than non-SRI antidepressants for BDD. This important finding is consistent with clinical series and retrospective data suggesting that SRIs are more efficacious than a broad range of non-SRI medications for BDD.[3,21]

Response to an SRI usually develops gradually and may require up to 12–14 weeks of treatment (while reaching a relatively high dose) to be evident.[3,21] Although dose-finding studies are lacking, relatively high SRI doses (higher than typically used for depression) appear to often be needed.[3,21] Response to medication usually includes a decrease in appearance preoccupations, distress, and compulsive/safety behaviours, as well as improved functioning. Suicidality, depressive symptoms, anxiety, and anger-hostility often improve.[3] Of note, delusional patients often improve with SRI monotherapy, whereas limited data suggest that antipsychotic monotherapy is usually ineffective for delusional BDD.[3,21]

Patients who do not improve with one SRI may improve with another SRI.[3, 21] Regarding SRI augmentation, a small double-blind randomized controlled trial found that pimozide was not more efficacious than placebo as a fluoxetine augmenter.[3,21] Clinical series suggest that augmentation of an SSRI with buspirone, lithium, or clomipramine may be helpful.[3,21] (SSRIs may increase clomipramine blood levels, however, which may cause toxicity; thus, if this approach is tried, clomipramine should be started at a very low dose with monitoring of levels.) Clinical observations suggest that SSRI augmentation with venlafaxine, atypical neuroleptics, or bupropion may be helpful for some patients.[3,21]

Monotherapy with agents other than SRIs has not been well studied.[3, 21] A small open-label trial ($n = 11$) suggests that venlafaxine may be efficacious.[3] For severe and treatment-refractory cases an MAO inhibitor may be worth trying (but should never be combined with an SRI). Available case series and reports, while very limited, suggest that ECT is generally ineffective for BDD and secondary depressive symptoms.[3,21]

Clinical experience suggests that many patients relapse after SRI discontinuation and that long-term treatment may be needed, with efficacy usually sustained over time.[3,21] For patients who appear at high risk of suicide or violence, lifelong treatment with an effective SRI is recommended, as suicides have been known to occur after SRI discontinuation.

### Cognitive behavioural therapy (CBT)

Preliminary data suggest that CBT is often efficacious for BDD.[3,27,29] CBT typically includes:[3,27–29]

1 *Cognitive restructuring* to identify cognitive errors and develop more accurate and helpful BDD-related thoughts and beliefs

2 *Behavioural experiments* to test the accuracy of BDD beliefs

3 *Exposure* to avoided situations (e.g. leaving the house, attending social gatherings)

4 *Response prevention* to decrease or stop compulsive behaviours (e.g. stopping excessive mirror checking, limiting grooming time)

In two randomized studies ($n = 54$ and $19$), patients improved more with CBT than on a waiting list.[3,29] Several case series ($n = 5$–$13$) found that CBT was efficacious for BDD.[3,29] The number of sessions in these reports ranged from twelve 60-min sessions to sixty 90-min sessions.

Data on exposure and response prevention alone—without a cognitive element—is limited to a retrospective study and small case series with up to 10 subjects.[3,29] These reports note favourable outcomes, although in the author's experience cognitive approaches are a helpful, even necessary, component of treatment for most patients. It can be particularly helpful to work on core beliefs, which typically involve feelings of inadequacy and being unwanted by others.[3, 9] Clinical experience additionally suggests that the following are beneficial components of CBT:[3, 28]

1 *Mirror retraining*, which involves learning to see one's entire body in a non-judgemental and 'holistic' way (rather than focusing on disliked areas), while refraining from excessive mirror checking

2 *Habit reversal* for skin picking and repetitive hair pulling or plucking

3 *Mindfulness skills*

4 *Activity scheduling* and *scheduling pleasant activities* for more severely ill, depressed, and inactive patients

5 *Motivational interviewing*, which may be needed to engage and keep patients in treatment

Future studies (e.g. dismantling studies) are needed to determine which specific components of CBT are necessary and effective.

Other types of psychotherapy have not been well studied and are not currently recommended as first-line treatments.[3] Nonetheless, clinical experience suggests that insight-oriented or supportive therapy—in addition to an SRI and/or CBT—may help some patients cope with their illness or with co-occurring problems or disorders.[3]

## Management

Management approaches are described in more detail elsewhere.[3, 21, 27, 28]

1 First try to engage the patient and establish an alliance so they are willing to try treatment. This can be difficult to accomplish, as many patients are delusional, prefer cosmetic treatment, are rejection sensitive, and do not want other people (including a clinician) to see them.

2 Empathize with the patient's suffering.

3 Take patients' appearance concerns seriously, neither dismissing their concerns about how they look nor agreeing that there is something wrong with their appearance. Trying to convince patients (especially delusional patients) that their beliefs are irrational or that they look normal is usually not helpful.

4 Instead, focus on the potential for psychiatric treatment to diminish their distress and preoccupation and improve their functioning and quality of life.

5 Provide psychoeducation about BDD and recommend reading.

6 For patients who wish to pursue cosmetic treatments, explain that such treatment appears ineffective for BDD.

7 Provide education about recommended treatments. It can be helpful to explain, for example, that SRIs are usually well tolerated, are not habit forming, appear to normalize the brain (and do not cause brain damage), and often diminish suicidal thinking in people with BDD. CBT is a practical 'here-and-now' treatment in which patients actively collaborate with the therapist and learn helpful skills by attending sessions and doing homework.

Treatment should be initiated with an SRI and/or CBT. SRIs are also the first-line medication for delusional BDD. All severely ill patients, especially those who are highly suicidal, should, in the author's opinion, receive an SRI. Patients with severe comorbid depression also warrant SRI treatment. Other comorbidity may warrant additional medication.

Before concluding that an SRI is ineffective, it should be tried for 12–16 weeks, reaching the highest dose recommended by the manufacturer or tolerated by the patient (if necessary) for at least 2–3 of those 12–16 weeks. If tolerated, higher doses than those recommended by the manufacturer can be cautiously tried to obtain or optimize a response (excluding clomipramine). If this is not effective, an augmentation strategy or switching to another SRI is indicated. For patients who refuse or are ambivalent about treatment motivational techniques should be tried. Patients who are not improving with CBT may need more frequent sessions, longer sessions, or a change in the current CBT focus. At least 4–6 months of weekly or more frequent CBT sessions, plus daily homework, is generally recommended. More severely ill and delusional patients may require much longer or more intensive treatment. Maintenance/booster sessions following CBT may reduce relapse risk. It may be helpful to add CBT to an SRI, or vice versa, if either treatment alone is insufficient.

For certain patients, adjunctive individual supportive therapy or family therapy may be helpful.[3] Families can be an invaluable support and facilitate treatment.[3] Mental health professionals may need to interface with dermatologists, plastic surgeons, and other physicians from whom patients have requested or are receiving cosmetic treatment.

## Prevention

Because little is known about BDD's pathogenesis and risk factors, the disorder cannot currently be prevented. However, BDD should be treated in its early stages, before it causes substantial morbidity or interferes with a child's, adolescent's, or young adult's development.

## Conclusions

Although this disorder has received far less investigation than many other serious mental illnesses, BDD research is rapidly advancing. It is important that clinicians screen patients for this often-secret disorder and be aware that it typically goes unrecognized in clinical settings, causing significant morbidity. While much more research is needed, available treatments are often very helpful for this distressing and often-disabling disorder.

## Further information

Further information about BDD and its treatment is provided in references 3, 27, and 28 below and at www.bodyimageprogram.com.

## References

1. Morselli, E. (1891). Sulla dismorphophobia e sulla tafefobia. *Bolletinno della R accademia di Genova*, **6**, 110–9.
2. Phillips, K.A. (1991). Body dysmorphic disorder: the distress of imagined ugliness. *The American Journal of Psychiatry*, **148**, 1138–49.
3. Phillips, K.A. (1996, 2005). *The broken mirror: understanding and treating body dysmorphic disorder*. Oxford University Press, New York. Revised and Expanded Edition, 2005.
4. Phillips, K.A., McElroy, S.L., Keck, P.E. Jr., *et al.* (1993). Body dysmorphic disorder: 30 cases of imagined ugliness. *The American Journal of Psychiatry*, **150**, 302–8.
5. Phillips, K.A., Menard, W., Fay, C., *et al.* (2005). Demographic characteristics, phenomenology, comorbidity, and family history in 200 individuals with body dysmorphic disorder. *Psychosomatics*, **46**, 317–32.
6. Fontanelle, L.F., Telles, L.L., Nazar, B.P., *et al.* (2006). A sociodemographic, phenomenological, and long-term follow-up study of patients with body dysmorphic disorder in Brazil. *International Journal of Psychiatry in Medicine*, **36**, 243–59.
7. Phillips, K.A., Menard, W., Fay, C., *et al.* (2005). Psychosocial functioning and quality of life in body dysmorphic disorder. *Comprehensive Psychiatry*, **46**, 254–60.
8. Hollander, E., Cohen, L.J., and Simeon, D. (1993). Body dysmorphic disorder. *Psychiatric Annals*, **23**, 359–64.
9. Veale, D., Gourney, K., Dryden, W., *et al.* (1996). Body dysmorphic disorder: a survey of fifty cases. *The British Journal of Psychiatry*, **169**, 196–201.
10. Perugi, G., Akiskal, H.S., Giannotti, D., *et al.* (1997). Gender-related differences in body dysmorphic disorder (dysmorphophobia). *The Journal of Nervous and Mental Disease*, **185**, 578–82.
11. Phillips, K.A., Menard, W., Pagano, M., *et al.* (2006). Delusional versus nondelusional body dysmorphic disorder: clinical features and course of illness. *Journal of Psychiatric Research*, **40**, 95–104.
12. Phillips, K.A. (2004). Psychosis in body dysmorphic disorder. *Journal of Psychiatric Research*, **38**, 63–72.
13. Phillips, K.A. and Diaz, S. (1997). Gender differences in body dysmorphic disorder. *The Journal of Nervous and Mental Disease*, **185**, 570–7.
14. Phillips, K.A., Coles, M., Menard, W., *et al.* (2005). Suicidal ideation and suicide attempts in body dysmorphic disorder. *The Journal of Clinical Psychiatry*, **66**, 717–25.
15. Phillips, K.A. and Menard, W. (2006). Suicidality in body dysmorphic disorder: a prospective study. *The American Journal of Psychiatry*, **163**, 1280–2.
16. Cotterill, J.A. and Cunliffe, W.J. (1997). Suicide in dermatological patients. *The British Journal of Dermatology*, **137**, 246–50.
17. Buhlmann, U., Etcoff, N.L., and Wilhelm, S. (2006). Emotion recognition bias for contempt and anger in body dysmorphic disorder. *Journal of Psychiatric Research*, **40**, 105–11.
18. Buhlmann, U., Wilhelm, S., McNally, R.J., *et al.* (2002). Interpretive biases for ambiguous information in body dysmorphic disorder. *CNS Spectrums*, **7**, 435–6, 441–3.
19. Sarwer, D.B. (2002). Awareness and identification of body dysmorphic disorder by aesthetic surgeons: results of a survey of American Society for Aesthetic Plastic Surgery members. *Aesthetic Surgery Journal*, **22**, 531–5.
20. Phillips, K.A., Menard, W., and Fay, C. (2006). Gender similarities and differences in 200 individuals with body dysmorphic disorder. *Comprehensive Psychiatry*, **47**, 77–87.
21. Phillips, K.A. and Hollander, E. (in press). Treating body dysmorphic disorder with medication: Evidence, misconceptions, and a suggested approach. *Body Image: An International Journal of Research*.
22. Grant, J.E., Kim, S.W., and Crow, S.J. (2001). Prevalence and clinical features of body dysmorphic disorder in adolescent and adult psychiatric inpatients. *Journal of Clinical Psychiatry*, **62**, 517–22.
23. Rief, W., Buhlmann, U., Wilhelm, S., *et al.* (2006). The prevalence of body dysmorphic disorder: a population-based survey. *Psychological Medicine*, **36**, 877–85.
24. Deckersbach, T., Savage, C.R., Phillips, K.A., *et al.* (2000). Characteristics of memory dysfunction in body dysmorphic disorder. *Journal of the International Neuropsychological Society*, **6**, 673–81.
25. Saxena, S. and Feusner, J.D. (2006). Toward a neurobiology of body dysmorphic disorder. *Primary Psychiatry*, **13**, 41–8.
26. Phillips, K.A., Pagano, M.E., Menard, W., *et al.* (2006). A 12-month follow-up study of the course of body disorder. *The American Journal of Psychiatry*, **163**, 907–12.
27. National Collaborating Centre for Mental Health. (2006). Core interventions in the treatment of obsessive compulsive disorder and body dysmorphic disorder (a guideline from the National Institute

for Health and Clinical Excellence, National Health Service). British Psychiatric Society and Royal College of Psychiatrists, London. http://www.nice.org.uk/page.aspx?o=289817

28. Wilhelm, S., Phillips, K.A., and Steketee, G (in press). *Cognitive-behavioral therapy for body dysmorphic disorder: a modular treatment manual*. Guilford Publications Inc., New York.

29. Neziroglu, F. and Khemlani-Patel, S. (2002). A review of cognitive and behavioral treatment for body dysmorphic disorder. *CNS Spectrums*, **7**, 464–71.

30. Crerand, C.E., Franklin, M.E., and Sarwer, D.B. (2006). Body dysmorphic disorder and cosmetic surgery. *Plastic and Reconstructive Surgery*, **118**, 167e–80e.

# 5.2.9 Factitious disorder and malingering

Christopher Bass and David Gill

## Factitious disorder

### Introduction

Patients with factitious disorder feign or simulate illness, are considered not to be aware of the motives that drive them to carry out this behaviour, and keep their simulation or induction of illness secret. In official psychiatric nomenclature, factitious disorder has replaced the eponym Munchausen syndrome, introduced by Asher[1] to describe patients with chronic factitious behaviour. Asher borrowed the term from Raspe's 1785 fictional German cavalry officer, Baron Karl von Munchausen, who always lied, albeit harmlessly, about his extraordinary military exploits.

The criteria for factitious disorder in DSM-IV[2] are (a) the intentional production or feigning of physical or psychological signs or symptoms; (b) motivation to assume the sick role; and (c) lack of external incentives for the behaviour (e.g. economic gain, avoidance of legal responsibility, or improved physical well-being, as in malingering) and lack of a better classification for the disorders.

In the last 10 years there has been increased interest in deception in medical practice, with specific focus on pathological lying and the diagnostic dilemmas in this field: specifically, how to differentiate between hysteria, factitious disorders, and malingering. Some of these topics will be discussed in the next section.

This chapter concentrates on factitious physical complaints; fabricated psychological symptoms are considered under malingering.

### Diagnostic problems

The DSM-IV criteria have recently come under attack. Turner[3] has argued that criterion B (motivation to assume the sick role) has no empirical content and fulfils no diagnostic function. He also argues that criterion A, the intentional production of physical or psychological signs or symptoms, emphasizes symptoms and cannot accommodate pseudologia fantastica (PF), voluntary false confessions, and impersonations. He concludes that the two criteria need reformulating in terms of lies and self-harm, respectively. Bass and Halligan[4] have also suggested that because the conceptual

justification for factitious disorders is 'empirically unsubstantiated' and the motivation for diagnostic purposes (conscious versus unconscious; voluntary versus involuntary) essentially unknowable, it seems reasonable to question the clinical status and legitimacy of factitious disorder. More recently there has been a resurgence of interest in **pathological lying**, because this is often easier to identify than, for example, the degree of 'voluntariness' or 'motivation' to attain the sick role (however that is defined).

### Pathological lying (pseudologia fantastica): a key component of factitious disorder

It is possible to identify pathological lying if the clinician has sufficient information at his disposal (most often the medical notes). If the patient reports, for example, that they are being treated for leukaemia, and when there is evidence that contradicts this, then this suggests dissimulation. On some occasions the patient will admit to lying, but this is rare.

Because pathological lying is often a key component in factitious disorders, evidence for it should be actively sought by the clinician. But what distinguishes the pathological liar from the person who just lies a lot? Dike *et al.*[5] suggest that the diagnosis is made when lying is persistent, pervasive, disproportionate, and not motivated primarily by reward or other external factors. They also suggest, however, that a key characteristic of pathological lying may be its compulsive nature, with pathological liars 'unable to control their lying'. Psychiatric conditions that have been traditionally associated with deception in one form or another include malingering, confabulation, Ganser's syndrome, factitious disorder, borderline personality disorder and antisocial personality disorder. Lying may also occur in histrionic and narcissistic personality disorders. It is important to note however that pathological lying can occur in the absence of a psychiatric disorder, and that there may be different types of pathological lying, e.g. the benefit fraudster and the stereotypical wandering Munchausen patient describe different subgroups. Furthermore, it has been reported that up to 40 per cent of cases of pseudologia fantastica have a history of central nervous system abnormalities, which suggests that brain dysfunction in these patients requires closer study.[6]

In recent years, functional neuroimaging techniques (especially functional magnetic resonance imaging) have been used to study deception. Attempted deception is associated with activation of executive brain regions (particularly prefrontal and anterior cingulate cortices), while truthful responding has not been shown to be associated with any areas of increased activation (relative to deception).[7] Furthermore, Yang *et al.*[8] reported that pathological liars showed a 22–26 per cent increase in prefrontal white matter and a 36–42 per cent reduction in prefrontal grey/white ratios compared with both antisocial controls and normal controls. These findings suggest that increased prefrontal white matter developmentally provides a person with the cognitive capacity to lie, although Spence[9] has urged caution in the interpretation of these results.

### Clinical features of factitious disorder

Clinical features are diverse, and attempts to subtype patients have not always been helpful. The majority of patients with factitious disorders are non-wandering, socially conformist young women (often nurses) with relatively stable social networks.[10-12] These patients are likely to enact their deceptions in general hospitals, especially accident and emergency departments, and the liaison psychiatrist should be alert to these clinical problems, which can be referred from a variety of different medical and surgical specialties.

Factitious disorders typically begin before the age of 30 years;[13,14] there are often prodromal behaviours in childhood and adolescence (see below). These individuals often report an unexpectedly large number of childhood illnesses and operations, and many have some association with the health care field.[10] High rates of substance abuse, mood disorder, and borderline personality disorder have been reported.[10,12] Approximately four-fifths of factitious disorder patients are women, and 20–70 per cent work in medically related occupations.[12]

Clinicians should be alert to the presentation of more exotic forms of factitious presentation. For example, some women present themselves to family cancer or genetic-counselling clinics and provide a false family history of breast cancer to their medical attendants.[15] Another recent example is 'electronic' factitious disorder,[16] used to describe patients who falsify their electronic medical records to create a factitious report (e.g. of cancer). Another important group is encountered in pregnancy, and this will clearly have important implications for child protection.[17]

In medico-legal practice factitious disorders have been described in patients with a diagnosis of reflex sympathetic dystrophy (RSD), specially involving the forearm,[18] and others have reported that the abnormal movements commonly associated with RSD (CPRS Type I) are consistently of somatoform or malingered origin.[19] Cases have been described where patients involved in litigation have died of factors directly related to factitious physical disorder.[20]

It is being increasingly recognized that these disorders can occur in childhood and adolescence, and child psychiatrists need to be alert to factitious presentations, especially in departments of infectious diseases.[21] Unlike adult patients, many of these children admit to their deceptions when confronted, and some have positive outcomes at follow-up. The descriptions of some of these children as bland, depressed, and fascinated with health care are remarkably similar however to adults with factitious disorders.[22]

## Classification

Four main subtypes are distinguished in DSM-IV.[2]

1 Factitious disorder with predominantly psychological signs and symptoms. This is more difficult to diagnose than factitious disorder with physical complaints, because there is no way of excluding a 'true' psychiatric disorder by physical examination or laboratory investigation: see below under malingering.

2 Factitious disorders with predominantly physical signs and symptoms. Almost every illness has been produced factitiously. However, four subgroups describe most cases[23]:

(a) self-induced infections

(b) simulated illnesses, for example adding blood to urine

(c) interference with pre-existing lesions or wounds

(d) surreptitious self-medication, for example self-injection of insulin

These categories are not mutually exclusive or jointly exhaustive.

3 Factitious disorders with combined psychological and physical symptoms

4 Factitious disorders not otherwise specified. This includes factitious disorder by proxy (see below and Chapter 9.3.3).

## Diagnosis

Clinicians should become suspicious that a patient may be fabricating symptoms if the following features are noted:

◆ The course of the illness is atypical and does not follow the natural history of the presumed disease, e.g. a wound infection does not respond to appropriate antibiotics (self-induced skin lesions often fall into this category, when 'atypical' organisms in the wound may alert the physician).

◆ Physical evidence of a factitious cause may be discovered during the course of treatment, e.g. a concealed catheter, a ligature applied to a limb to induce oedema.

◆ The patient may eagerly agree to or request invasive medical procedures or surgery.

◆ There is a history of numerous previous admissions with poor outcome or failure to respond to surgery (these patients may overlap with the chronic somatoform patient with 'surgery prone behaviour').[24]

◆ Many physicians have been consulted and have been unable to find a relevant cause for the symptoms.

Additional clues include the patient being socially isolated on the ward and having few visitors, or the patient being prescribed (or obtaining) opiate medication, often pethidine, when this drug is not indicated. When these findings occur in someone who has either worked in or is related to someone who has worked in the health field, the caregivers should have a high index of suspicion for a factitious disorder. Obtaining collateral information from family members, prior physicians, and hospitals is crucial.

## Differential diagnosis

Factitious disorder must be distinguished from authentic medical conditions. It is not uncommon in clinical practice however to find patients with **both** factitious disorder and coexisting physical illness. For example, patients with brittle diabetes are usually young females who deliberately interfere with their treatment, causing unstable diabetic control.[25] A syndrome of severely unstable asthma ('brittle asthma') which also affects young females has also been described;[26] this can occur (especially in A and E departments) with paradoxical adduction of the vocal cords during inspiration.[27] Such patients can neglect to take medication at appropriate times and then ignore adequate management of the potentially dangerous consequences. This may lead to repeated admissions to hospital with medical emergencies such as diabetic ketoacidosis, status asthmaticus, or even pseudo status (simulated status epilepticus).

Factitious disorders are differentiated from somatoform disorders, where physical symptoms, although not caused by physical disease, are deemed not to be intentionally produced. Patients with factitious disorder, although they may state that they are not aware of the motives that drive them, voluntarily produce their physical or psychological symptoms. The disorders may overlap, however, and non-wandering female patients with factitious physical disorders may have more in common with those females who have somatoform disorders than with men with factitious disorder or with malingerers. Fink[28] found that 20 per cent of patients with persistent somatization (i.e. patients with more than six admissions to the general hospital with medically unexplained symptoms) also had a factitious illness. One of the authors (Christopher Bass) has also found coexisting chronic somatoform and factitious disorders in the female perpetrators of factitious or induced illness.[29]

A more difficult distinction is between factitious disorder and malingering. Malingerers, described below, have clear-cut goals, often personal profit, and lack a history of hazardous, unnecessary invasive procedures. In our opinion the boundaries between the two disorders are more porous than the glossaries would have us believe, and we have stated above that the differentiation between conversion disorders, factitious disorders and malingering is extremely difficult in clinical practice. Case reviews have demonstrated how behaviour may shift from somatization to factitious to malingering when patients are followed longitudinally.[30] In our opinion the clinical status and diagnostic legitimacy of factitious disorder as a selective medical disorder is questionable, because it fails to take account of a morally questionable but volitional-based choice to deceive others by feigning illness. Considered as an act of wilful deception, illness deception can be meaningfully conceptualized within a socio-legal or moral model of human nature that recognizes the capacity for choice and the potential for pursuing benefits associated with the sick role. This model, which recognizes the human capacity to exercise free will, is shown diagrammatically in Fig. 5.2.9.1.

## Epidemiology

Factitious disorders are relatively uncommon but probably underdiagnosed. Prevalence depends on clinical setting and the investigators' index of suspicion. Factitious disorder (probably underreported) is probably more common than full-blown Munchausen syndrome (probably overreported). In a recent survey of physicians from Germany, frequency estimates of factious disorder among their patients averaged 1.3 per cent, with dermatologists and neurologists giving the highest estimations.[31]

Of 1288 liaison psychiatric consecutive referrals, seen in a North American general hospital, 0.8 per cent had factitious disorder.[13] Similar figures have been reported by Dutch investigators.[14]

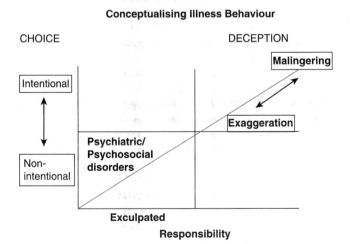

**Conceptualising Illness Behaviour**

CHOICE                          DECEPTION

**Fig. 5.2.9.1** Model of illness deception incorporating patient choice, free will and intentionality. (Reproduced from Bass, C. and Halligan, P. Illness related deception: social or psychiatric problem? *Journal of the Royal Society of Medicine*, **100**, 81–4. Copyright 2007, The Royal Society of Medicine Press.)

Prevalence rates for factitious disorder with psychological symptoms in patients under the age of 65 in a psychiatric hospital are approximately 0.4 per cent.[32]

## Aetiology

There is little aetiological information, as large studies are lacking and the self-reported histories of many patients are fallacious. However, a number of themes are apparent[13]:

Developmental

◆ Parental abuse, neglect, or abandonment: Many factitious disorder patients experienced significant deprivation in childhood that left them with unfulfilled cravings for attention and care. These patients then seek to gratify these dependency needs by creating illness to obtain the 'attention and care' of the medical system

◆ early experiences of chronic illness or hospitalization

Medically related

◆ a significant relationship with a physician in the past

◆ experiences of medical mismanagement leading to a grudge against doctors

◆ paramedical employment

Physical

◆ Organic brain disorder: There is increasing evidence that neurobiological factors have a role in some patients, and it has been recommended that screening for evidence of brain dysfunction be carried out in these patients.[33] It is thought however that it is the pseudologia fantastica, and not the factitious disorder per se, that is associated with brain dysfunction (see previous section on Pathological Lying), though such a distinction may be difficult to support in clinical practice.

The authors have found it useful to conceptualize the problem using a cognitive behavioural formulation suggested by Fehnel and Brewer.[34] This allows the assessors to examine for relevant developmental factors and recent life events (especially losses or threatened losses and separations; see Fig. 5.2.9.2).

## Course and prognosis

Factitious disorder may be limited to one or more brief episodes, but is usually chronic. For example, of 10 patients identified in a general hospital setting and followed up, at least one was known to have died as a result of factitious behaviour 4 months after the index admission.[13] Only one of the remaining nine patients accepted psychiatric treatment after discharge from hospital. Other authors have, however, reported a less gloomy outcome.[10] Outcome may be determined by how patients are managed, once their deceptions become manifest. Regrettably, the unmasking of the disorder is often the end of the story. Psychological support following hospital discharge may be associated with improved outcome.[10] Non-wanderers with more stable social networks may have a better prognosis than wanderers.[14] Engaging a patient with factitious disorder in long-term psychological treatment occurs so rarely that it often becomes the subject of a case report. One such report, of a 20-year follow-up of a patient with factious disorder with a favourable outcome is, in the opinion of the authors, the exception to the rule.[35]

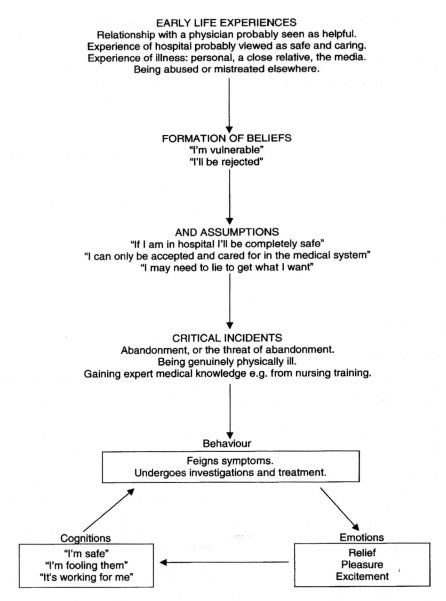

**EARLY LIFE EXPERIENCES**
Relationship with a physician probably seen as helpful.
Experience of hospital probably viewed as safe and caring.
Experience of illness: personal, a close relative, the media.
Being abused or mistreated elsewhere.

**FORMATION OF BELIEFS**
"I'm vulnerable"
"I'll be rejected"

**AND ASSUMPTIONS**
"If I am in hospital I'll be completely safe"
"I can only be accepted and cared for in the medical system"
"I may need to lie to get what I want"

**CRITICAL INCIDENTS**
Abandonment, or the threat of abandonment.
Being genuinely physically ill.
Gaining expert medical knowledge e.g. from nursing training.

Behaviour
Feigns symptoms.
Undergoes investigations and treatment.

Cognitions
"I'm safe"
"I'm fooling them"
"It's working for me"

Emotions
Relief
Pleasure
Excitement

**Fig. 5.2.9.2** A cognitive behavioural conceptualization of factitious disorder. Reproduced from Kinsella, P. Factitious disorder: a cognitive behavioural perspective, *Behavioural Cognitive Psychotherapy*; **29**: 195–202, copyright 2001, with permission from Cambridge University Press

## Treatment

There are no systematic or controlled treatment studies on patients with factitious disorders. This is hardly surprising, as the patient's primary motive is deception, and the doctor's is to understand or unmask these motives, usually leading to rapid discharge from hospital after the deception has been exposed.

## Management

Once the diagnosis is established, the doctor–patient relationship may have become irreparably damaged: negative emotions in the doctor may need to be dealt with before any consideration can be given to 'engaging' the patient in any therapeutic endeavour. Ethical and legal issues may also intrude (see below) and affect management. Although psychotropic medications have been used, the main treatment is psychological, using either confrontational or non-confrontational strategies.

Before treatment takes place however, it is important to establish the diagnosis, which is nearly always initially made by a non-psychiatrist, e.g. A and E physician, infectious disease specialist. A meeting should take place between the physician/surgeon and the psychiatrist and a strategy worked out before any confrontation or other approach is embarked on. These preliminary procedures are important and preparation before the joint interview is crucial (Table 5.2.9.1).

### (a) Confrontational approaches

This process is easier if the physician has tangible evidence of fabrication, for example catheters, or medication used in the patient's deception. It is also desirable to have the psychiatrist present when

**Table 5.2.9.1** Supportive confrontation: preparation and process (for non-psychiatrists)

- Collect firm evidence of fabrication, e.g. catheter, syringe, medication
- Discuss with psychiatrist (or hospital legal team if no psychiatrist available)
- Arrange meeting to marshall the facts; discuss strategy. Discuss with GP
- CONFRONTATION with patient should be non-judgemental, non-punitive, with . . .
- Proposal of ongoing support/follow-up
- If patient is a health care worker, the doctor should discuss with his/her medical defence organization
- Discuss the outcome of the confrontation with the patient's GP
- Document full record of the meeting and proposed outcome in patient's notes

the physician confronts the patient. The approach during confrontation and thereafter should be non-punitive and supportive, stressing continuity of care, and that the patient is a sick person who needs help. This approach was adopted in perhaps the largest published series of patients with factitious disorder treated systematically.[10] Thirty-three patients were 'confronted' with objects found in their room or with clinical data showing that their conditions were factitious. Only 12 (36 per cent) patients acknowledged the truth; the remaining 21 continued to deny that they played any role in creating their disorders. No confronted patient developed serious psychological disturbance or became suicidal, or discharged themselves against medical advice. Four of the most chronic cases became asymptomatic. Most, however, greeted the idea with either overt hostility or passivity and covert negativism.

More recently Krahn et al.[12] replicated these findings, but found that only one in six of their patients acknowledged their factitious behaviour. Many patients will experience confrontation as humiliating and seek care from a different hospital. Others will refuse to see the psychiatrist with the treating clinician to discuss the deception, and discharge themselves against clinical advice.

### (b) Non-confrontational strategies

These approaches, advocated by Eisendrath and Feder,[36] are less concerned with the origin of the illness and more with shaping future behaviours. Face-saving is a key element, and it is important for the patient to subsequently explain their 'recoveries' without admitting that their original problems were psychiatric.

One strategy is the therapeutic 'double-bind'. In this approach the patient is presented with two choices: prove that his or her disorder is not factitious by responding to a relatively minor and benign medical intervention, or prove that the disorder is factitious by failing to respond. For example, a woman was offered the double-bind for a wound that had failed to heal in 4 years despite numerous surgical closures. Following this strategy the plastic surgeon told her that her wound should respond to a skin grafting procedure. If it did not, it would mean that her disorder was factitious in origin. The graft took place, and there was no recurrence of infection at 2-year follow-up.[36] This approach has also been used with some success in the rehabilitation of three patients with factitious motor disorders.[37] The strategy was successful in providing patients with a face-saving legitimization of both their illnesses and recoveries.

Another face-saving approach uses 'inexact interpretations', i.e. suggesting a relationship between certain events or stressors, for

example being abandoned, and emergence of factitious symptoms. It involves presenting a brief formulation of the problem to the patient, stopping short of overtly identifying the factitious origin. By avoiding confrontation the doctor makes it safe for the patient to relinquish the symptom with a feeling of control. Regrettably, none of these non-confrontational techniques have been evaluated in a systematic fashion.

### (c) Systemic interventions

Patients with factitious disorders can create havoc on medical and surgical wards. They often elicit negative and hostile emotions in general hospital staff, especially after the deception has been exposed. The psychiatrist can help staff members to vent and reduce the anger they experience when a factitious diagnosis is confirmed, and also help the staff to understand the likely mechanisms underlying the factitious behaviour. These issues are often best addressed at a multi-disciplinary staff meeting. The major task of this group, which should include a member of the hospital medico-legal department as well as the patient's family doctor, is to develop practical treatment guidelines and to discuss the complex legal and ethical issues raised with factitious physical disorders. Some of these issues are discussed in the next section.

## Ethical and legal issues

Patients with factitious disorders create unique ethical and medico-legal issues, some of which will be described below.

### (a) Confidentiality

If no meaningful doctor–patient relationship exists or can be established, it has been argued that the physician is not bound by ethical codes, and that drastic solutions such as keeping 'blacklists' and the use of a central register can therefore be justified.[38] Objections to these approaches include breach of doctor–patient confidentiality and possible denial of treatment for genuine illness. Anyway, the use of aliases and poor record-keeping reduces the effectiveness of blacklists. Furthermore, physicians who disclose information without patient consent may have to justify the decision to their licensing body. In the United States, there is a consensus that disclosure should only occur where there is a specific risk to the patient and/or another party. In such situations, a multi-disciplinary staff meeting can help to develop treatment policy, and share responsibility for difficult decisions (see above).

### (b) Invasion of privacy

The medical literature contains many descriptions of how the diagnosis of factitious disorder was established following a search of the patient's room or belongings. Some physicians, however, consider that such behaviour infringes patients' rights, and that no search should be undertaken without the patient's knowledge and consent. One way of avoiding this dilemma is to make it clear to the patient that factitious disorder is among the differential diagnoses, and then request permission for a room search. If needles or syringes are discovered during the course of treating the patient, the ethical issue of invasion of privacy does not arise.

### (c) Involuntary hospitalization or treatment

Because the patient with factitious disorder may engage in behaviour that leads to permanent maiming or even death, it has been argued that in such cases a compulsory order may be used to protect the patient from himself or herself. This will provide time for not only a more in-depth psychiatric assessment but also the development of a more trusting relationship with a therapist. This is a contentious subject, but some case reports do indicate that extended involuntary hospitalization may result in therapeutic progress.[39]

### Induced factitious illness (Munchausen syndrome by proxy)

Meadow[40] first described this disorder as 'the deliberate production or feigning of physical or psychological symptoms or signs in another person who is under that individual's care', which has recently been renamed fabricated or induced illness or FII.[29] The perpetrator is usually the mother and the victim her child: the syndrome is considered to be a form of child abuse. The parent's aim is to have the child considered seriously ill: this may involve providing false histories, poisoning, or persuading doctors to carry out invasive and potentially dangerous procedures.

Factitious disorder and FII can be interrelated. Psychiatrists (and general practitioners) should be aware of the implications of a diagnosis of factitious disorder for any children of the index patient. For example, 75 per cent of mothers of these children have a history of a factitious or somatoform disorder, and most meet criteria for personality disorder.[41] With the birth of a child some mothers with pre-existing factitious disorder abandon dissimulation themselves, only to extend it to the next generation through factitious disorder by proxy. Because factitious disorder and FII can co-occur, the finding of one should always trigger judicious efforts to establish, or hopefully disconfirm, the other.

Long-term outcome in factitious disorder by proxy is poor, so active early intervention is recommended, with child protection agencies working closely with paediatric and psychiatric services (see also Chapter 9.3.3).

### Factitious disorder in health care workers

If factitious disorder is diagnosed in a health care worker, the investigating psychiatrist should consider whether their continuing clinical work would pose risks to either patients (often children) with whom that person comes into contact (i.e. of factitious disorder by proxy), and/or the health of the factitious disorder patient himself or herself. These issues have been thrown into sharp focus by some highly publicized cases in both the United States and the United Kingdom.[42,43] Any employee who manufactures crises, for example multiple cardiac arrests and resuscitations, is obviously of great concern. The British commission that investigated the 1993 case made several stringent recommendations, for example 'We recommend that no candidate for nursing in whom there is evidence of major personality disorder should be employed in the profession'.[44] Nevertheless, psychiatrists should seek medico-legal advice before communicating concerns about such patients to any third party, including the employing hospital.

## Malingering and exaggeration

### Introduction

Malingering is the deliberate simulation or exaggeration of physical or psychiatric symptoms for obvious and understandable gain (e.g. financial compensation, disabled status and benefits, avoidance of criminal prosecution or conscription).

Treating doctors have been understandably reluctant to diagnose malingering lest it adversely affect the patient. However, recent research indicates that it may not be uncommon, especially where financial rewards attach to disability status, such as benefits for sickness or compensation for injury. We here describe some types of malingering seen in psychiatry, and discuss newer specialist psychological tools, especially *symptom validity testing*, which are emerging as useful additions to the overall assessment.

### Definition

Malingering is not coded as a mental disorder in either ICD-10 or DSM-IV, although in the latter it is denoted as an 'additional condition that may be the focus of clinical attention'.

DSM-IV[2] suggests that malingering should be 'strongly suspected' when two or more of the following factors apply:

1 medico-legal context

2 antisocial personality disorder

3 discrepancy between complaints and objective findings

4 lack of co-operation with the assessment

This actually sets a very low bar: in effect, DSM advises it should be 'strongly suspected' in any disputed medico-legal case (where points 1 and 3 apply), but does not give guidance as to how this 'suspicion' should be followed up. The ICD-10 definition ('the intentional production or feigning of either physical or psychological symptoms or disabilities, motivated by external stresses or incentives') is broad, but again does not give practical suggestions regarding assessment.

Malingering includes:

1 Pure malingering: complete fabrication of symptoms

2 Partial malingering: exaggerating real symptoms or saying that past symptoms are continuing

3 False attribution: falsely saying that real health problems are due to a compensable accident or other circumstance

### Epidemiology

Until recently, there has been little systematic information on prevalence, although it has generally been agreed that exaggeration of real symptoms is more common than outright faking expect them to dissimulate. Exaggeration, dissimulation, or feigning can be considered one of several rational/economic/adaptive options open to patients when seeking health care and/or limited social and welfare resources.

Using the 'Composite Disability Malingering Index' Griffin et al.[45] suggested that 19 per cent of disability claimants in the United States malingered to some degree. A recent study of 131 practicing members of the American Board of Clinical Neuropsychology provided estimates of the prevalence of malingering and symptom exaggeration for a variety of different clinical conditions.[46] In this study, estimates of the base rate of malingering/symptom exaggeration were calculated using over 33 000 annual cases seen by a group of clinical neuropsychologists. The reported base rates (when statistically adjusted to remove for the influence of referral source) were 29 per cent for personal injury, 30 per cent in the case of disability or workers compensation, 19 per cent in criminal cases, and 8 per cent in medical or psychiatric cases. The same rates broken down by diagnosis revealed 39 per cent in the case of mild head injury, 35 per cent in fibromyalgia and chronic fatigue, 31 per cent in chronic pain, 15 per cent for depressive disorders, and 11 per cent in the case of dissociative disorders. In a separate review of 1363 compensation-seeking cases, Larrabee[47] found similar figures for mild head injury of 40 per cent. The use of symptom validity testing has confirmed these high rates of exaggeration (see under 'Psychological tests'). For example, about 42 per cent in the Canadian series of Richman et al.[48] and about 60 per cent in the United Kingdom in a series studied by one of the authors (Gill et al. submitted for publication).

## Clinical features

### (a) Malingered neurosis: post-traumatic stress disorder

The archetypal disorder after trauma is post-traumatic stress disorder. Malingering of other disorders seen after trauma, notably depression is less frequent, confirming malingerers' preference for dramatic positive symptoms such as nightmares and flashbacks.

In 1983 Sparr and Pankratz[49] described five men who claimed to have been 'traumatized' in the Vietnam War; three claimed to have been PoWs. It turned out that none had been PoWs, four had never been in Vietnam and two had never been in the services. The patients were seeking the generous benefits, which the United States accords to ex-service (Veterans' Administration) personnel. The key point in this paper was that the authors *supplemented their clinical assessment by seeking external data*, in this case service records; relying on clinical assessment alone would have led to wrong diagnosis. Seeking corroboration is vital in the assessment of possible malingering.

Rosen, in another classic paper, documented malingered PTSD in the case of the *Aleutian Enterprise*, a fish-processing ship, which sank in the Bering Sea in 1990.[50] Of the 31 on board, 9 were lost, 2 went back to sea, and the remaining 20 sued. Nineteen (86 per cent) of these 22 survivors consulted psychiatrists or psychologists with the key features of PTSD. But this is much higher than the expected rates: most individuals exposed to a traumatic event do not develop PTSD. Even if they do, it resolves over a few weeks or months in many cases, whereas here the claimants' symptoms did not show any tendency to resolve. Furthermore, they all had almost all of the classic features of the condition, in other words, they did not display the case to case variability, which would be expected in real individuals. Rosen documented that the patients had in fact 'shared symptoms' and had been 'coached' by their attorneys, some of whom had advanced the claimants money so they would not have to settle.

Most cases of suspected malingered post-traumatic stress disorder involve less dramatic civilian trauma, most commonly road accidents. Again, exaggeration of genuine symptoms is much more common than outright fabrication. For example, a person involved in a car accident, with apparently genuine phobic travel anxiety, may report that they have nightmares and 'flashbacks', but their description of these experiences lacks vividness on close enquiry. Holistic assessment is vital; if a minor accident is to be accepted as causing a severe psychiatric condition such as PTSD, there must be some evidence of pre-existing vulnerability. Otherwise, the apparent result will be disproportionate to the cause, and the possible influence of external incentives on symptom presentation will need to be considered.

### (b) Malingered psychosis

This disorder can occur in various circumstances, for example in homeless persons wishing to obtain shelter in hospital, in previously psychotic inpatients whose discharge is imminent, in illegal migrants seeking to avoid deportation or in criminal defendants trying to avoid standing trial or to influence sentencing.

A (perhaps somewhat academic) distinction can be made between malingered and factitious psychosis, in that malingerers are conscious of their motivation, and their goal is not merely confined to gaining patient status. However, the following description covers both. It is 'positive' symptoms, which are usually mimicked (e.g. hallucinations). They are often dramatic or bizarre. Patients are keen to describe them at interviews, unlike, for example, most patients with schizophrenia. Symptoms are obvious during assessments, less so when the patient is unobserved. More subtle features of genuine psychosis, such as thought disorder and negative symptoms, are absent. Florid hallucinations may be unaccompanied by delusions, which would be unusual in genuine psychosis.

For example, Jaffe and Sharma[51] described nine defendants on serious criminal charges that developed uncommon symptoms such as coprophagia and 'seeing little green men'. Eight were judged to be malingering, and fit to plead, based on evidence such as the association between visual hallucinations and organic brain syndromes, of which there was no evidence on investigation. Malingering in forensic settings also includes feigned memory deficits, when isolated amnesia for an alleged crime would place malingering in the differential diagnosis. Forensic psychiatry is dealt with elsewhere in this book.

*Ganser syndrome* does not appear in current classifications. It was originally described in prisoners, as comprising confusion and so-called 'approximate answers' (or Vorbereiden: *Question*: for example: how many legs has a horse? *Answer*: three). If true confusion (diminished level of consciousness) is present, the diagnosis is the cause of this. Approximate answers may be seen in several conditions, including mental retardation, organic brain disorders, and malingering; again, the diagnosis will be the underlying condition. The term Ganser syndrome has now largely and rightly been dropped.

### (c) Malingered cognitive deficit

Study of cognitive deficits following brain injury has recently led to advances in understanding of malingering, through the development of special neuropsychological tests, especially *effort testing*, to gauge the effort the patient brings to cognitive testing. These tests seem likely to have broader application than just brain injury assessment.

Discussion of the question of malingering post head injury has until recent years been rich in opinion, though comparatively light on facts. Miller's view,[52] long influential, was that many patients malingered their memory and other cognitive symptoms and that symptoms were in inverse proportion to injury severity and were only resolved with receipt of compensation. He used the term 'accident neurosis'. Mendelson, by contrast,[53] found that disability continued after settlement in many patients, and inferred from this that disability was generally not malingered.

The question is obviously not capable of being resolved scientifically without data. But such data is now becoming available. Recent findings however have supported Miller's original observations that embellishment rises as injury severity decreases in a compensable context.[54] Moving forward from mere debate, the American Academy of Neuropsychologists recently published a consensus statement which concluded that 'Symptom exaggeration or fabrication occurs in a sizeable minority of neuropsychological examinees, with greater prevalence in forensic contexts', and that the use of effort testing is mandatory in neuropsychological assessments.[55]

In clinical assessment, immediate recall (e.g. digit span) is important, as even organic amnesic patients (e.g. Korsakoff's syndrome) perform normally; poor performance suggests that poor motivation or malingering should be among the differential diagnoses. Claims of being unable to remember personal information (e.g. name and birthday, also preserved in organic amnesia), yet having been able to come to the assessment independently, are highly suggestive of malingering, but seen only in gross cases. However, these 'bedside' tests are only a guide: psychiatric assessment of brain injury patients is not complete without quantitative assessment of cognitive function, including effort testing (see below).

### (d) Malingered physical disease

This usually presents either as a referral to a liaison psychiatrist, or in a medico-legal context. A frequent example is a patient with post-injury back or neck pain who is involved in litigation or seeking disability payments. Often, some form of accident has undoubtedly occurred, so the potential for initial physical injury is not in doubt; but the length and severity of symptoms, disability, and distress may seem out of proportion, and raise the possibility of malingering.

In a seminal paper, Richman[48] administered effort testing to 106 people claiming injury or sickness benefits. Forty-five (42 per cent) failed. On one easy subtest, those who failed the effort test overall had a similar score on average to patients with dementia tested previously, even though none of them had a clinical diagnosis of dementia. Schmand et al.[56] found that 61 per cent of litigants after whiplash neck injury had evidence of underperformance on memory testing compared with 29 per cent of outpatient controls. The underperforming litigants scored as low as controls with definite evidence of closed head injury.

## Classification

Malingering should be distinguished from factitious disorder, and from other syndromes such as hypochondriasis, other somatoform disorders, and conversion/dissociation disorder. These distinctions may involve difficult judgements such as how 'intentional' is the production of a symptom, or how 'genuine' it is. As an alternative, it has been suggested that such patients lie on a continuum between those in whom the production of symptoms is assumed to be wholly unconscious (conversion/dissociation disorder) and those in whom it is wholly conscious (malingering, factitious disorder).

However, use of the concept of the unconscious has to be very cautious when there are external incentives. It stretches credulity to think that a claimant would be conscious of there having been an accident so as to pursue litigation, and conscious that the outcome could include financial compensation, but somehow unconscious that presentation of symptoms could form a desired link between the two.

It is possible that the emergence of effort testing may cast new light on the area of unexplained physical symptoms. For example, the concept of somatoform disorders assumes that the symptoms are not consciously produced. However, if large-scale studies reveal that a substantial proportion of somatoform patients turn out to fail effort tests, or in other words to display evidence of conscious symptom exaggeration, then the concept of somatoform disorders may need to be re-examined.

## Diagnosis and differential diagnosis

Doctors' training and culture rightly encourage the treating physician towards a generally trusting relationship with his patients. However, assumptions that patients' accounts are generally trustworthy and that malingering is rare are not appropriate if the main responsibility of the doctor lies elsewhere, for example, to the Court, if he is preparing an expert report.

Identifying ungenuine cases requires an enquiring approach, and the methodical use of all sources of information:

♦ awareness of the possibility of exaggeration or faking of symptoms

♦ neutral attitude

♦ open questions initially; use closed questions with caution

♦ unlikely questions (see below)

♦ mental state—changes appropriately as sensitive topics discussed?

♦ informants (but they may also have vested interests)

♦ observation—overt (e.g. in a ward) or covert (e.g. video surveillance)

♦ medical records (and legal documents if applicable)

♦ look for consistency of accounts

♦ standard psychometric tests—consistency of results across measures

♦ specialist instruments: symptom validity tests

The medical notes should be read, ideally before interview, especially the general practice records, and any discrepancies noted for specific enquiry. Legal assessments, case papers and previous reports should be studied.

In the clinical interview, a neutral attitude is essential; a confrontational approach, even if malingering is strongly suspected, may cause further exaggeration of symptoms. Open questions should be used at first. Closed questions should be avoided (e.g. 'Do you ever get nightmares where you seem to re-experience the accident?'). The careful use of unlikely questions can be useful. For example, in suspected malingered post-traumatic stress disorder the answer 'Yes' to the question 'Have you had any problems with colour vision since the accident?' would be suggestive, but would still need clarification with open questions. 'I am now colour-blind' might suggest malingering, but 'Red makes me nervous—it was a red car which crashed into me' might not.

Questions must be appropriate to the case, ideally prepared beforehand and introduced tactfully to prevent the patient feeling that the interviewer is attempting to 'catch him out'. The interviewer should look for the clinical characteristics of the particular malingered disorder in question.

Surveillance by video or other means may be used by lawyers or insurers, although is seldom initiated by clinicians, for ethical reasons (except perhaps in suspected factitious disorder by proxy—see Chapter 9.3.3).

## Psychological tests

Since the last edition of this book, consensus has developed that symptom validity testing is essential in neuropsychology, that is, in the field primarily concerned with memory problems and brain injury. The tests in practical use are in fact specialized memory tests, and it is likely that their use will be extended from head injury cases to other cases in which memory complaints occur (such complaints are in fact very common in patients with pain or distress for any reason). We are about to discuss what currently appear to be the leading symptom validity tests in UK neuropsychology, the Word Memory Test[57] and the ToMM,[58] but first we mention some other tests by way of historical background.

Inconsistent patterns of response on standard instruments (e.g. high scores on one measure of depression and low on another) might be suggestive. However, this should not be overinterpreted, because there is substantial test–retest variation on many tests, and there is also variation between subscales on the same occasion. Certain subscales of the Minnesota Multiphasic Personality Index have been proposed as measures of tendency to malinger. Specialist instruments have been developed, for example the Structured Inventory of Malingered Symptoms,[59] which identifies features associated with malingering such as endorsement of rare symptoms, which occur only infrequently in clinical populations. However, consensus on such tests remains some way off and they are not in general use in the United Kingdom.

Tests for malingered memory deficits present memory tasks, which appear difficult but are in fact easy. For example, 50/50 psychiatric and 10/16 mentally retarded inpatients were able to recall nine of the 15 items on the Rey 15-item.[60] Forced choice testing (e.g. Portland Digit Recognition Test) is another approach. A sequence of digits is presented. Subjects must identify it among two further sequences, one identical and the other different. By chance alone, they must score around 50 per cent on a large number of items, and so below chance scores (below 50 per cent) strongly suggest malingering.[61] However, this is very gross, and will miss many cases where the degree of exaggeration is less. Again, these tests are not in general use in the United Kingdom.

In the United Kingdom, the Word Memory Test and the ToMM have become established as leading symptom validity tests in neuropsychology. They are regarded as having the best research support and are administered in standard formats.

TOMM stands for *Test Of Malingered Memory*.[58] It is a pictorial test, not computerized, and is mainly used by psychologists. Word Memory Test (WMT) (Green: wordmemorytest.com) is available either on paper or on computer. It is mainly used by psychologists as part of a 'battery' of neuropsychological tests. An abbreviated form for physicians, the Medical Symptom Validity Test, is available.[57] The key point is that patients are given a test of memory, which looks difficult, but is in fact known to be easy from previous administration to control subjects.

Someone making a **good effort:**

♦ scores well on tests which are in fact easy (even though they may look hard)

♦ scores lower on more difficult tests

Someone making an **inconsistent or poor effort:**

♦ may score low on tests which look hard (though they are in fact easy)

♦ may not score lower on more difficult tests

If the patient's scores are low, where even say primary school children score almost perfectly, it would suggest that he might not have been making a full effort on the test. If at the end of the test he said that he had made a full effort, this would be evidence that his self-report of effort brought to cognitive testing is not accurate. This would be consistent with the proposition that he might have been exaggerating at least the memory aspects of his complaints, and by extension, possibly other symptom areas also.

## Aetiology

Malingering is not a mental disorder, so complex general theories about causation are unlikely to be helpful. It has been suggested for example that[62] 'adaptation' is the simplest model for malingering: ' . . . malingering is more likely to occur when the evaluation is perceived as adversarial, when the personal stakes are very high, and when no alternatives appear to be viable'. However, this really just restates the problem in different terms. Nor do the 'response styles' described by psychologists seem to offer fundamental insights. It is more helpful to consider each case in a common sense way, bearing in mind the presence or absence of external incentives, and the results of the holistic assessment process outlined above, in combination with the results of symptom validity testing.

## Course and prognosis

Malingerers are so heterogeneous that it is impossible to state prognosis in general. There are few adequate follow-up studies.

*In forensic and inpatient settings*, malingering is usually episodic, associated with particular circumstances such as impending discharge, trial, or change in conditions of imprisonment (e.g. transfer to a single cell or hospital wing). The behaviour often stops when the circumstances no longer remain, although they may recur. Similar situations occur in persons facing conscription, or in migrants at risk of repatriation.

The prognosis of malingering *in personal injury litigants* is unknown. Studies indicating poor outcome of many compensated litigants cannot be extrapolated, as the number of malingerers in these samples is unknown. Clinical experience suggests that patients with long-standing disability, even if partly or wholly non-organic, often fail to recover fully in any event.

## Treatment

There is very little evidence on management, which will largely be dictated by whether the clinician has clinical responsibility, or whether he or she has been asked to give an opinion to a third party. Even if the diagnosis of malingering is clear, it may be appropriate to inform the referrer, rather than the patient directly, as the patient may become very angry. If there is a psychiatric disorder present when, as it were, the dust has settled, then this should be treated in standard fashion.

Clinical experience is that patients for whom the exercise of attempted malingering seems worthwhile do often have substantial pre-existing psychosocial problems, including lack of skills or employment; there is a tendency towards a regionality of such claims, with areas of deprivation ('rust-belt') overrepresented.

Efforts at retraining and vocational rehabilitation may be more likely to be of assistance in the long-term than specialist psychiatric care.

## Possibilities for prevention

These seem mainly confined to malingering after injury. First, systems of litigation should be expedited. Prolonged cases certainly make for exaggeration of symptoms and disability. Second, some patients with chronic disability, irrespective of cause, do respond to rehabilitative treatment (e.g. programmes assisting in return to work or in the management of chronic pain), even at a late stage. If such programmes were easily and generally available at an earlier stage in the evolution of the disorder, symptoms and subsequent disability could certainly be ameliorated or even prevented in some patients.

## Ethical legal and personal issues

As previously indicated, malingering poses a number of particular challenges to the doctor himself and to the doctor–patient relationship, including amongst others the following.

There is no doubt that seeing substantial numbers of likely ungenuine patients has the potential to affect the practitioner himself. Appropriate 'supervision', as in psychotherapy, may be appropriate.

If the doctor has a treatment responsibility to the patient, he naturally tends to give the patient the benefit of doubt, for example in respect of disability payments. But he will be wise to be cautious: if, for example, he signs a form saying that the patient cannot undertake certain activities of daily living, but without direct observation of that, he could potentially be considered to be an accessory if the claim was subsequently found to be fraudulent.

The use of the word 'malingering' itself in reports must usually be avoided, as it is tantamount to an accusation of a criminal offence such as deception. The medical duty is to present the evidence to the Court, which can then decide the question itself.

Finally, it must not be forgotten that the Data Protection Act gives patients the right to see personal information about themselves such as medical reports. Any suggestion of ungenuine presentation in reports must therefore be well-founded on evidence and properly argued.

## Further information

Malleson, A. (2002). *Whiplash and other useful illnesses*. Magill-Queens University Press.
Halligan, P., Bass, C., and Oakley, D. (2003). Willful deception as illness behaviour. In: *Malingering and illness deception* (eds. P. Halligan, C. Bass, and D. Oakley). Oxford University Press.
Vrij, A. (2001). *Detecting lies and deceit*. Wiley.

## References

1. Asher, R. (1951). Munchausen's syndrome. *Lancet*, **1**, 339–41.
2. American Psychiatric Association. (1994). *Diagnostic and statistical manual of mental disorders* (4th edn). American Psychiatric Association, Washington, DC.
3. Turner, M. (2006). Factitious disorders. Reformulating the DSM-IV criteria. *Psychosomatics*, **47**, 23–32.
4. Bass, C. and Halligan, P. (2007). Illness related deception: social or psychiatric problem? *Journal of the Royal Society of Medicine*, **100**, 81–4.
5. Dike, C., Baranoski, M., and Griffith, E. (2005). Pathological lying revisited. *The Journal of the American Academy of Psychiatry and the Law*, **33**, 342–9.
6. King, B. and Ford, C. (1988). Pseudologia fantastica. *Acta Psychiatrica Scandinavica*, **77**, 1–6.
7. Spence, S., Hunter, M., Farrow, T., *et al.* (2004). A cognitive neurobiological account of deception: evidence from functional neuroimaging. *Philosophical Transactions of the Royal Society of London*, **359**, 1755–62.
8. Yang, Y., Raine, A., Lencz, T., *et al.* (2005). Prefrontal white matter in pathological liars. *The British Journal of Psychiatry*, **187**, 320–5.
9. Spence, S. (2005). Letter in *The British Journal of Psychiatry*, **187**, 326–7.
10. Reich, P. and Gottfried, L.A. (1983). Factitious disorders in a teaching hospital. *Annals of Internal Medicine*, **99**, 240–7.
11. Eisendrath, S.J. (1996). Current overview of factitious physical disorders. In *The spectrum of factitious disorders* (eds. M. Feldman and S. Eisendrath), pp. 21–36. American Psychiatric Press, Washington, DC.
12. Krahn, L., Honghzhe, L., and O'Connor, K. (2003). Patients who strive to be ill: factitious disorder with physical symptoms. *The American Journal of Psychiatry*, **160**, 1163–8.
13. Sutherland, A.J. and Rodin, G.M. (1990). Factitious disorders in a general hospital setting: clinical features and review of the literature. *Psychosomatics*, **31**, 392–9.
14. Hengeveld, M.W. (1992). Factitious disorders: what can the psychiatrist do? In *Practical problems in clinical psychiatry* (eds. K. Hawton and P. Cowen), pp. 118–29. Oxford University Press, Oxford.
15. Kerr, B., Foulkes, W., Cade, D., *et al.* (1998). False family history of breast cancer in the family cancer clinic. *European Journal of Surgical Oncology*, **24**, 275–9.
16. Hadeed, V., Trump, D.L., and Mies, C. (1998). Electronic cancer Munchausen syndrome. *Annals of Internal Medicine*, **129**, 73.
17. Feldman, M and Hamilton, J. (2006). Serial factitious disorder and Munchausen by proxy in pregnancy. *International Journal of Clinical Practice*, **60**, 1675–8.
18. Taskaynatan, M.A., Balaban, M., Karlidere, T., *et al.* (2005) Factitious disorders encountered in patients with the diagnosis of reflex sympathetic dystrophy. *Clinical Rheumatology*, **24**, 521–6.
19. Verdugo, R. and Ochoa, J. (2000). Abnormal movements in complex regional pain syndrome: assessment of their nature. *Muscle & Nerve*, **23**, 198–205.
20. Eisendrath, S. and McNeil, D. (2004). Factitious physical disorders, litigation, and mortality. *Psychosomatics*, **45**, 350–3.
21. Peebles, R., Sabella, C., Franco, K., *et al.* (2005). Factitious disorder and malingering in adolescent girls: case series and literature review. *Clinical Pediatrics*, **44**, 237–43.
22. Libow, J. (2000). Child and adolescent illness falsification. *Pediatrics*, **105**, 336–41.
23. Parker, P. (1996). Factitious psychological disorders. In *The spectrum of factitious disorders* (eds. M. Feldman and S. Eisendrath), pp. 37–49. American Psychiatric Press, Washington, DC.
24. DeVaul, R.A. and Faillance, L.A. (1978). Persistent pain and illness insistence. A medical profile of proneness to surgery. *American Journal of Surgery*, **135**, 828–33.
25. Kent, L., Gill, G., and Williams, G. (1994). Mortality and outcome of patients with brittle diabetes and recurrent keto-acidosis. *Lancet*, **344**, 778–81.
26. Barnes, P. and Cheung, K. (1998). Difficult asthma. *British Medical Journal*, **299**, 695–8.
27. Renz, V., Hern, J., Tostevin, T., *et al.* (2000). Functional laryngeal dyskinesia: an important cause of stridor. *The Journal of Laryngology and Otology*, **114**, 790–2.
28. Fink, P. (1992). The use of hospitalisations by persistent somatizing patients. *Psychological Medicine*, **22**, 173–80.
29. Bass, C. and Adshead, G. (2007). Fabrication of illness in children: the psychopathology of abuse. *Advances in Psychiatric treatment*, in press.
30. Eisendrath, S and McNeil, D. (2002). Factitious disorders in civil litigation: twenty cases illustrating the spectrum of abnormal illness-affirming behaviour. *The Journal of the American Academy of Psychiatry and the Law*, **30**, 391–9.

31. Fliege, H., Grimm, A., Eckhardt–Henn, A., *et al.* (2007). Frequency of ICD-10 factitious disorder: survey of senior hospital consultants and physicians in private practice. *Psychosomatics*, **48**, 60–4.

32. Bhugra, D. (1988). Psychiatric Munchausen's syndrome. Literature review with case reports. *Acta Psychiatrica Scandinavica*, **77**, 497–503.

33. Diefenbacher, A. and Heim, S. (1997). Neuropsychiatric aspects in Munchausen syndrome. *General Hospital Psychiatry*, **19**, 281–5.

34. Fehnel, C. and Brewer, E. (2006). Munchausen's syndrome with 20 year follow up. *The American Journal of Psychiatry*, **163**, 547.

35. Kinsella, P. (2001). Factitious disorder: a cognitive behavioural perspective. *Behavioural and Cognitive Psychotherapy*, **29**, 195–202.

36. Eisendrath, S.J. and Feder, A. (1996). Management of factitious disorders. In *The spectrum of factitious disorders* (eds. M. Feldman and S. Eisendrath). American Psychiatric Press, Washington, DC.

37. Teasell, R.W. and Shapiro, A.P. (1994). Strategic–behavioral intervention in the treatment of chronic non-organic motor disorders. *American Journal of Physical Medicine Rehabilitation*, **73**, 44–50.

38. Powell, R. and Boast, N. (1993). The million dollar man: resource implications for chronic Munchausen's syndrome. *The British Journal of Psychiatry*, **162**, 253–6.

39. O'Shea, B., McGennis, A., Cahill, M., *et al.* (1984). Munchausen's syndrome. *British Journal of Hospital Medicine*, **35**, 269–74.

40. Meadow, R. (1977). Munchausen syndrome by proxy: the hinterland of child abuse. *Lancet*, **2**, 343–5.

41. Bools, C., Neale, B., and Meadow, R. (1994). Munchausen syndrome by proxy: a study of psychopathology. *Child Abuse & Neglect*, **18**, 773–84.

42. Elkind, P. (1989). *The death shift: the true story of nurse Genene Jones and the Texas baby murders*. Viking Penguin, New York.

43. Davies, N. (1993). *Murder on ward four*. Chatto and Windus, London.

44. *The Allitt enquiry.* (1994). HMSO, London.

45. Griffin, G. (1996). Assessing dissimulation among social security disability income claimants. *Journal of Consulting and Clinical Psychology*, **64**, 1425–30.

46. Mittenberg, W., Patton, C., Vanyock, E., *et al.* (2002). Base rates of malingering and symptom exaggeration. *Journal of Clinical and Experimental Neuropsychology*, **24**, 1094–102.

47. Larrabee, G. (2003). Detection of malingering using atypical performance patterns on standard neuropsychological tests. *The Clinical Neuropsychologist*, **17**, 410–25.

48. Richman, J., Green, P., Gervais, R., *et al.* Objective tests of symptom exaggeration in independent medical examinations. *Journal of Occupational and Environmental Medicine*, **48**, 303–311.

49. Sparr, L.D. and Pankratz, L. (1983). Factitious post traumatic stress disorder. *The American Journal of Psychiatry*, **140**, 1016–9.

50. Rosen, G. (1995). The Aleutian Enterprise sinking and post-traumatic stress disorder: misdiagnosis in clinical and forensic practice. *Professional Psychology: Research and Practice*, **26**, 82–7.

51. Jaffe, M.E. and Sharma, K.K. (1998). Malingering uncommon psychiatric symptoms among defendants charged under California's 'three strikes and you're out' law. *Journal of Forensic Science*, **43**, 549–55.

52. Miller, H. (1961). Accident neurosis. *British Medical Journal*, **1**, 919–25.

53. Mendelson, G. (1995). Compensation neurosis revisited: outcome studies of the effects of litigation. *Journal of Psychosomatic Research*, **39**, 695–706.

54. Grieffenstein, M. and Baker, J. (2005). Miller was (mostly) right: head injury severity inversely related to simulation. *Legal and Criminological Psychology*, **10**, 1–16.

55. Bush S., Ruff, R.M., Tröster, A.I., *et al.* (2005). Symptom validity assessment: Practice issues and medical necessity, NAN Policy & Planning Committee. *Archives of Clinical Neuropsychology*, **20**, 419–26, NAN position paper.

56. Schmand, B., Lindeboom, J., Schagen, S., *et al.* (1998). Cognitive complaints in patients after whiplash injury: the impact of malingering. *Journal of Neurology, Neurosurgery and Psychiatry*, **64**, 339–43.

57. Word Memory Test (WMT) (Green: wordmemorytest.com)

58. Tombaugh, T.N. (1996). The test of memory malingering. Multi-Health Systems, Toronto, Canada.

59. Smith, G.P. and Burger, G.K. (1997). Detection of malingering: validation of the SIMS. *Journal of the American Academy of Science and the Law*, **25**, 183–9.

60. Goldberg, J.O. and Miller, H.R. (1986). Performance of psychiatric inpatients and intellectually deficient individuals on a task that assesses the validity of memory complaints. *Journal of Clinical Psychology*, **42**, 792–5.

61. Binder, L.M. and Willis, S.C. (1991). Assessment of motivation after financially compensable minor head trauma. *Psychological Assessment*, **3**, 175–81.

62. Rogers, R. (1997). *Clinical assessment of malingering and deception*. Guilford Press, New York.

## 5.2.10 **Neurasthenia**

Felice Lieh Mak

### Introduction

The term neurasthenia has had a variegated history, and although retained as a diagnostic entity in the ICD-10 it does not appear in the DSM-IV. In cultures where neurasthenia still enjoys popular professional and lay acceptance it has a variety of usages:

◆ a nosological entity

◆ an idiom for expressing distress

◆ a culturally sanctioned illness behaviour

◆ an explanatory model for a constellation of somatic symptoms

◆ an euphemism for avoiding the stigma of mental disorder.

Therefore, in diagnosing, understanding, and managing neurasthenia the clinician has to be aware of the context in which the term is used.

### Concept and diagnostic entity

The concepts of nervous weakness and asthenia (debility, lack of strength) have existed throughout the history of medicine. Hippocrates described the illness of the Scythians as a general asthenia linked to damage to the genitalia caused by horseback riding. In France, Bouchut (1764) described a syndrome similar to the latter-day neurasthenia, which he called 'neuropathie'. Cullen (1772) conceived muscles and nerves as a unitary nervous force and all diseases as movements against the nature of that nervous force. He coined the word neuroses for this process and postulated that diseases were due to the various alternations of excitement and atony in the nervous system. A few years later, his pupil Brown (1780) elaborated on the hypothesis by dividing diseases into sthenic diseases, which were due to excessive excitement, and asthenic diseases, which were due to deficient excitement. These views on the polarity of the nervous system as a cause of mental illness set the scene for neurasthenia to become a disease entity.

By the beginning of nineteenth century the term neurasthenia was already in use. In 1869, Van Deusen in Holland published a monograph on neurasthenia. This was quickly followed by the publication of a paper, which Beard[1] had presented to the New York Medical Journal Association. Beard based his description of the disorder on a series of 30 cases. In reorganizing the subjective nature of the complaints and the unique clustering of symptoms in each patient, Beard had difficulties in attempting to limit the number of symptoms that constituted the syndrome; he started with 50 symptoms and expanded it to 75 in later publications.

Eventually it became clear that the expanding kaleidoscope of symptoms should be managed in a way that made some sense. Beard approached this problem by organizing the symptoms into subtypes of neurasthenia: cerebrasthenia (cerebral exhaustion) characterized by symptoms that were directly or indirectly connected with the head; myelasthenia (spinal exhaustion) was defined by symptoms related to the involvement of the spinal cord; digestive asthenia was characterized by dyspepsia, constipation, and flatulence. As time went on more subtypes were added by other investigators and specific treatment approaches were developed.

Despite the over inclusiveness of the term, Beard maintained that neurasthenia belonged to one family with a common pathology, prognosis, history, and treatment. As more cases were reported, he felt able to claim that neurasthenia was predominantly an American illness.[2] He attributed the increase in prevalence to the pressures of modern civilization.

Notwithstanding its vagueness, or perhaps because of its vagueness, neurasthenia gained popular acceptance not only by the medical profession but also by the general public. Although by the turn of the century it had become practically a household word, its popularity did not preclude dissent. Most of the criticisms focused on the disorder's over inclusiveness and lack of precision; for instance, Brill called it 'the newest garbage can' in medicine.

The first two decades of the twentieth century witnessed an increasing number of discoveries of more specific causes of disease. This period also saw greater attention being paid to the taxonomy of neuroses. These forces combined to bring about the decline of neurasthenia as a diagnostic entity.

In 1895, Freud published two seminal papers in which he drew up the blueprint for reconfiguring the various neurotic disturbances that were grouped together under the term neurasthenia. In the paper entitled 'On the grounds for detaching a particular syndrome from neurasthenia under the description of 'anxiety neurosis'[3] he questioned the validity of continuing to allow neurasthenia to cover all the symptoms described by Beard. He saw the need to classify different categories of neuroses based on the following:

- collection of symptoms that were more closely related to one another
- common aetiology
- common psychical mechanism.

In the paper 'Obsessions and phobias: their psychical mechanism and their aetiology',[4] Freud removed obsessions and phobias from neurasthenia. As a result of these two papers, neurasthenia ceased to be an amorphous concept and was differentiated into the following categories:

- neurasthenia proper
- anxiety neuroses

- obsessions
- phobias
- pseudoneurasthenias due to cachexia, arteriosclerosis, early stages of the general paralysis of the insane, and psychoses.

Intermittent and periodic types of neurasthenia were to be included under melancholia.

The first list of symptoms Freud proposed for neurasthenia proper included headache, spinal irritation, dyspepsia with flatulence, and constipation. Later, he added sexual weakness and fatigue.

The possibility of including some neurasthenic symptoms under melancholia was mentioned but not expanded on by Freud. This task was taken up by Kraepelin.[5] He distinguished three major types of depression: manic–depressive disorder, involutional melancholia, and a milder form of neurasthenic depression. He asserted that all these types of depression were due to an underlying disordered brain function.

Having been so denuded, the use of the term neurasthenia as a diagnostic entity by the medical professions had declined in the United States by the time of the First World War. The first edition of the DSM-I published in 1952 gave no formal recognition to neurasthenia. Instead, it was replaced by the category of 'Psychophysiological nervous system reaction', the predominant symptom of which was general fatigue. In an effort to make DSM-II congruent with ICD-8, neurasthenia reappeared in American psychiatry as neurasthenic neurosis.

In DSM-III neurasthenia disappeared as an entity and appeared only in the index where readers were asked to refer to 'Dysthymic disorder'. However, unlike the DSM classification, neurasthenia consistently remained a subtype of neurosis throughout the many versions of the ICD. ICD-9 defined neurasthenia as follows.

A neurotic disorder characterized by fatigue, irritability, headache, depression, insomnia, difficulty in concentration, and lack of capacity for enjoyment (anhedonia). It may follow or accompany an infection or exhaustion or arise from continued emotional stress.

The following categories were included:

- fatigue neurosis
- nervous disability
- psychogenic asthenia
- general fatigue.

## Spread to other countries

One of the most fascinating aspects of the history of neurasthenia is its ready acceptance by countries other than the United States where it was originally conceived as a peculiarly American phenomenon. The diagnostic entity took firmer root in some countries than in others. In many countries the concept was indigenized and took on local cultural colour.

The reasons for its spread can be summarized as follows:

- The all-embracing nature of the entity provided a foothold for almost everyone involved.
- The concept provided a blend of scientific theory, thus lending legitimacy to a cluster of symptoms, which are mostly subjective.
- It is considered to be a disease resulting from overwork, which affects the upper social class.

## Asia and Australia

In all probability neurasthenia was introduced into China in the 1920s by American psychiatrists and returning Chinese doctors who were trained in the United States. Up to the end of the Second World War, Chinese physicians accepted and used the diagnostic concept of neurosis and neurasthenia from the United States. With the firm establishment of communism in 1949, Pavlovian theory was adopted as the sole model on which Chinese psychiatrists practice, teach, and research.[6] In China, as in the former USSR, neuroses were divided into neurasthenia, psychasthenia, and hysteria. The cause of neurasthenia, as indeed of neuroses, followed the Pavlovian theory of overstrain in the excitation and inhibition processes and mobility of the higher nervous system.

The concept of neurasthenia or *shenjing shuairuo* (nerve weakness), as translated by the Chinese, was not an entirely alien idea. The symptoms associated with neurasthenia (fatigue, loss of memory, poor attention span, headache, tension, insomnia, and all varieties of vague pains) are similar to those in patients suffering from a deficiency in *qi* (vital essence), that is weakness of the kidney, spleen, or heart in traditional Chinese medicine. In addition, the theory of nerve weakness and depletion of nervous energy as causes of neurasthenia fits in with the traditional Chinese medicine concept of organ weakness and *yin–yang* deficiency. Thus in no time at all neurasthenia was incorporated into the body of the practice of traditional Chinese medicine and the vocabulary of the lay public.

In the 1950s, the number of patients suffering from neurasthenia increased enormously. Medical or neurology clinics reported that 80 to 90 per cent of their outpatients were suffering from neurasthenia. It was particularly rampant among the 'brain or mind workers'. The Chinese government regarded it as a serious public health problem, so much so that in its First Five Year Plan (1958–1962) a large-scale national campaign was initiated to eradicate neurasthenia. Research on neurasthenia carried out during this period focused on the role of stress as the external factor, and on heredity and personality as endogenous factors. Treatment included intensive group re-education, herbal medicine, and tranquillizers. Lin[7] postulated that the marked increase in neurasthenia was due to the presence of a deep-seated tension in the revolutionary development of China during the 1950s. Neurasthenia became the vehicle to express political, social, and physical stresses.

About a decade after China's 'open-door policy', an epidemiological survey was conducted in 12 districts in China. The instrument used was the Present State Examination. The results showed that neurasthenia affected 12.59 per cent of persons aged from 15 to 59 years, accounting for 56.7 per cent of all neurotic disorders.[8] In 1982, Kleinman[9] conducted a study of 100 patients diagnosed with neurasthenia in the Psychiatric Outpatient Clinic of the Hunan Medical College. He found that 89 patients satisfied the DSM-III diagnostic criteria for 'Major depressive disorder', 70 per cent of whom responded substantially to antidepressant medication. Despite their improvement, few experienced decreased help-seeking behaviour. This led him to conclude that neurasthenia should be regarded as a special form of somatization related to culturally sanctioned idioms of distress.

In Taiwan, neurasthenia attracted little interest among western-trained doctors. However, it became enormously popular among traditional Chinese doctors, and consequently neurasthenia established itself as a major disease in the minds of the Taiwan public during the 1940s and 1950s.[10]

The mostly British-trained doctors in Hong Kong largely ignored neurasthenia as a diagnostic entity. As in Taiwan, neurasthenia became the domain of traditional Chinese doctors.[11]

In the late nineteenth century psychiatry in Japan was essentially German in orientation. Psychiatrists applied the diagnosis of neurasthenia to patients who presented with weakness, headaches, mental distraction, fatigue, and reduced psychic productivity.[12] The diagnostic entity became a popular term until Morita[13] supplanted it with the term *shinkeishitsu* (nervous or nervous disposition). He described this disorder as basically a psychological reaction to anxiety in predisposed personalities—the personality type being characterized by introversion, perfectionism, hypochondria, hypersensitivity, and self-consciousness. He developed a specific treatment aimed at breaking up the vicious cycle of sensitivity and anxiety, the initial phase of which consisted of isolated bed rest followed by a second phase of work therapy.

Doctors in Malaysia, Singapore, India, Pakistan, Burma, and Sri Lanka are mostly trained in the British tradition. After the First World War neurasthenia lost its popularity in Britain. Standard British textbooks regarded the disorder as rare and outmoded. As a result psychiatrists in these countries tended not to diagnose neurasthenia. However, neurasthenia is used in the Chinese communities where traditional Chinese medicine maintains a stronghold. In India and countries where Ayurvedic medicine is practised, neurasthenia was not added on to the more traditional ways of explaining fatigue, pain, dizziness, and headaches. Instead, concepts such as *dhàtu* loss (loss of semen) and *vàta roga* (wind disease) remained the preferred explanation.

In Australia, Paterson[14] reported that over a 15-year period from 1950 to 1965 neurasthenia was one of the 10 major illness categories reported by a large Sydney-based industry. He claimed that, since he had a fairly representative sample, the 10 categories of illness could very well apply to the rest of Australia.

## Europe

From 1880 to 1920 neurasthenia was one of the diseases most frequently discussed. From an 'American nervousness' it rapidly evolved into a western European bourgeois illness. Practically every academic neurologist and psychiatrist wrote a major piece on neurasthenia (see Drinka[15]).

In England, neurasthenia was described in Osler's *The Principles and Practice of Medicine* published in 1900.[16] During the First World War it was a common diagnosis used for invaliding out many soldiers. In order to cope with its diagnosis, treatment, and disposal, the Army instituted a short course of training for medical officers who graduated with the title of 'neurasthenic expert' (see Sims[17]).

Russian psychiatry is largely based on Pavlovian psychophysiological theories. The Pavlovian classification of the principle of neuroses was adopted by all countries that came under the influence of the former USSR. Opinions on the subdivisions of neurasthenia were divided in Russia. One school of thought based its classification on the course of the illness, and the other was based on aetiology.[18] Neurasthenia as a cause of inefficiency and low productivity in the workplace was a recurrent theme in both Russia and Eastern Europe.

## Current usage

In ICD-10,[19] neurasthenia is classified as a neurotic disorder in which two main, but overlapping, types of neurasthenia are described:

◆ the predominant symptom is increased fatigue after mental effort

◆ predominant feelings of bodily or physical weakness and exhaustion after only minimal efforts.

For a definite diagnosis ICD-10 requires the following:

(a) either persistent and distressing complaints of increased fatigue after mental effort, or persistent and distressing complaints of bodily weakness and exhaustion after minimal effort;

(b) at least two of the following:

  ◆ feelings of muscular aches and pains

  ◆ dizziness

  ◆ tension headaches

  ◆ sleep disturbances

  ◆ inability to relax

  ◆ irritability

  ◆ dyspepsia;

(c) any autonomic or depressive symptoms present are not sufficiently persistent and severe to fulfil the criteria for any of the more specific disorders in this classification.

The following are excluded:

◆ asthenia not otherwise specified

◆ burn-out

◆ malaise and fatigue

◆ postviral fatigue syndrome

◆ psychasthenia.

DSM-IV does not include neurasthenia as a nosological entity. Instead, it is replaced by 'Undifferentiated somatoform disorder'.

In the third edition of the *Chinese Classification of Mental Disorders*[20] neurasthenia is classified under 'Neurotic disorder'. The criteria for diagnosis have been made more stringent, requiring three symptoms out of five non-hierarchical groups of symptoms, which include weakness, emotionality, excitement, nervous pain, and sleep disturbance. The duration of the symptoms should be at least 3 months. Other psychiatric disorders have to be excluded. Because of the different connotations of fatigue and weakness in Chinese culture, fatigue is not included in the list of symptoms.[21]

## Differential diagnosis

Fatigue is a ubiquitous symptom. It can occur in many psychiatric illnesses and in a wide range of physical illnesses. In cultures where the term neurasthenia is loosely used, many of the cases would probably meet the ICD-10 or DSM-IV diagnostic criteria for depressive disorder or anxiety disorder. Physical illness is a common cause of fatigue. In this respect, a detailed history and judicious investigation will be necessary.

## Epidemiology

Merikangas and Angst[22] studied a cohort of young adults from a community sample in Zurich, Switzerland, and reported the prevalence of neurasthenia, defined according to the ICD-10 criteria, as 1 per cent across 10 years. The sex ratio across the 10 years of follow-up revealed an equal prevalence among males and females during the initial stages of the study, but females exhibited an l.6-fold greater rate than males during the later stages.

The World Health Organization (WHO) international study[23] of patients with psychological problems seen in primary-care settings reported a prevalence of 1.7 per cent of pure neurasthenia. The prevalence rate increased to 5.4 per cent when the syndrome was diagnosed comorbid with depression or anxiety. The prevalence rate in each centre is shown in Table 5.2.10.1.

The differences in the prevalence rate can be due to many factors, including perception of what health services can treat and the existence of alternative sources of care.

The results of an epidemiological study conducted in 1998 in seven areas in China showed a prevalence rate of 2 per cent.[24]

In a national survey by the Australian Bureau of Statistics Hickie *et al.*[25] reported that 1.5 per cent of the general population met the ICD-10 criteria for neurasthenia in the past year.

All the studies were consistent in demonstrating that the syndrome tended to affect patients below the age of 45 and the absence of significant gender differences.

## Aetiology

Although theories abound, the predisposing, precipitating, and perpetuating causes of the syndrome remain unclear.

**Table 5.2.10.1** Prevalence of neurasthenic syndrome among patients contacting general health care facilities

| Centre | Overall prevalence (%) | Males (%) | Females (%) |
|---|---|---|---|
| Ankara | 4.1 | 1.0 | 5.6 |
| Athens | 4.6 | 3.3 | 5.2 |
| Bangalore | 2.7 | 1.7 | 3.7 |
| Berlin | 7.4 | 4.0 | 9.7 |
| Mainz | 7.7 | 7.4 | 8.0 |
| Groningen | 10.5 | 7.1 | 12.8 |
| Ibadan | 1.1 | 3.4 | 0.2 |
| Manchester | 9.7 | 6.1 | 11.3 |
| Nagasaki | 3.4 | 3.8 | 3.0 |
| Paris | 9.3 | 5.0 | 14.2 |
| Rio de Janiero | 4.5 | 2.3 | 5.3 |
| Santiago | 10.5 | 6.4 | 12.1 |
| Seattle | 2.1 | 2.3 | 2.0 |
| Shanghai | 2.0 | 1.5 | 2.2 |
| Verona | 2.1 | 1.8 | 2.3 |

## Course and prognosis

The 10-year follow-up study conducted by Merikangas and Angst[22] revealed that approximately 50 per cent of patients continued to exhibit symptoms. The WHO study[23] reported that patients with a diagnosis of neurasthenia had, on average, been disabled for 8 to 7 days during the month preceding the examination. Hickie et al.[25] confirmed the chronicity of the condition. They reported that 80 per cent of people who met the ICD-10 criteria in the past 12 months were also current cases.

## Comorbidity

In the Australian study Hickie et al.[25] showed that there was more comorbidity with major depression, panic disorder, and generalized anxiety disorder than could be expected by chance after adjustment for the prevalence of the comorbid disorder and the average level of comorbidity of that disorder.

## Treatment

Although there are reports that antidepressants can be effective these are not supported by published data on randomized double-blind controlled trials. Indeed, no such trials have been carried out on any form of psychiatric treatment for neurasthenia. In the absence of such data the clinician will have to rely on the adage of 'When not able to do any good, avoid doing any harm'. Thus aggressive treatment and investigations should be avoided. Patients are best managed in a supportive relationship with due regard given to their psychological and psychosocial needs.

General and non-specific strategies may also be used. These can include regular graded increase in exercise, promotion of sleep hygiene, cognitive techniques to break the cycle of symptoms leading to decreased activities, and improving social support.

Clinicians working in an environment where people with mental illnesses are stigmatized might find it easier to accede to social demands. Clinicians work at two levels in these situations. At one level he or she will have made a diagnosis of a psychiatric disorder and have prescribed the appropriate treatment. At another level the practitioner will be using neurasthenia as a euphemism for mental illness. Therefore, until stigmatization can be reduced or abolished, this unenviable state of affairs will continue.

### Complementary medicine

The extracts of leaves from the Ginkgo biloba tree contain ginkgo-flavone glycosides and trepenoids. Ginkgo is widely used as a cognitive enhancer. The roots of the Panax ginseng contain several triterpine glycosides, which are believed to have physical performance enhancing properties. This root is used in traditional Chinese medicine to treat a large variety of diseases including neurasthenia. Wesnes et al.[26] evaluated the effects of a Ginkgo biloba/ginseng combination on 64 healthy volunteers who fulfilled the ICD-10 criteria for neurasthenia. This was a 90-day, double-blind, placebo-controlled, parallel group study. They reported that the combined dose of 120 mg Ginkgo extract and 300 mg of ginseng extract was significantly better than placebo in reducing the symptoms of neurasthenia by day 90. Adverse effects were nausea and abdominal pain.

The mushroom, Ganoderma lucidum, known as lingzhi in China has been widely used to treat cancer, diabetes, and neurasthenia. It is the only known source of ganoderic acid, which has a molecular structure similar to steroid hormones and is a source of biologically active polysaccharide. Ganoderma is one of the most highly ranked herbal medicines by Asian people. Tang et al.[27] conducted a randomized, double-blind, placebo-controlled parallel study to investigate its efficacy and safety in the treatment of Chinese patients who fulfilled the ICD-10 diagnostic criteria for neurasthenia. Their findings indicated that Ganoderma was significantly superior to placebo with respect to the clinical improvement of symptoms in neurasthenic. Adverse effects were mild consisting of nausea, dry mouth, and vomiting.

Complementary medicine is increasingly being used either as an alternative or in addition to conventional psychotropic medications. Refer to Chapter 6.2.9 for further information.

## Future directions

As to whether neurasthenia will be replaced by chronic fatigue syndrome (Chapter 5.2.7) or subsumed under somatoform disorders (Chapter 5.2.1), and thus be relegated to a footnote in the history of medicine, or will enjoy resurgence with a new set diagnostic criteria will be determined by future research and clinical data.

## Further information

Starcevic, V. (1999). Neurasthenia: cross-cultural and conceptual issues in relation to chronic fatigue syndrome. *General Hospital Psychiatry*, **21**, 249–55.

Tang, W., Gao, Y., Chen, G., et al. (2005). A randomized, double-blind and placebo-controlled study of a *Ganoderma lucidum* polysaccharide extract in neurasthenia. *Journal of Medicinal Food*, **8**, 53–8.

Web pages: www.kosmix.com/health Type in neurasthenia to search

## References

1. Beard, G.M. (1869). Neurasthenia or nervous exhaustion. *Boston Medical and Surgical Journal*, **3**, 217–20.

2. Beard, G. (1881). *American nervousness: its causes and consequences.* Putnam, New York.

3. Freud, S. (1895). On the grounds for detaching a particular syndrome from neurasthenia under the description of 'anxiety neurosis'. In *Standard edition of the complete psychological works of Sigmund Freud*, Vol. 1 (ed. J. Strachey), p. 139. Hogarth Press, London.

4. Freud, S. (1895). Obsessions and phobias: their psychical mechanism and their etiology. In *Standard edition of the complete psychological works of Sigmund Freud*, Vol. 3 (ed. J. Strachey), pp. 74–82. Hogarth Press, London.

5. Kraepelin, E. (1902). *Clinical psychiatry* (trans. A.R. Defendorf), pp. 96–104. Macmillan, New York.

6. Lin, T.S. (1989). Neurasthenia revisited: its place in modern psychiatry. *Culture, Medicine and Psychiatry*, **13**, 105–29.

7. Lin, T.S. (1985). The shaping of Chinese psychiatry in the context of politics and public health. In *Mental health planning for one billion people* (eds. T.S. Lin and L. Eisenberg), pp. 13–14. University of British Columbia Press, Vancouver.

8. Li, C.P. and Zhang, W.H. (1985). Neurasthenia. In *Psychiatry* (ed. Y.C. Shen), pp. 407–12. People's Health Press, Beijing (in Chinese).

9. Kleinman, E.A. (1982). Neurasthenia and depression: a study of somatization and culture in China. *Culture, Medicine and Psychiatry*, **6**, 117–90.

10. Rin, H. and Huang, M.G. (1989). Neurasthenia as a nosological dilemma. *Culture, Medicine and Psychiatry*, **13**, 215–26.

11. Cheung, F. (1989). The indigenization of neurasthenia in Hong Kong. *Culture, Medicine and Psychiatry*, **13**, 227–41.

12. Suzuki, T. (1989). The concept of neurasthenia and its treatment in Japan. *Culture, Medicine and Psychiatry*, **13**, 203–13.

13. Morita, M., Kondo, A. and LeVine, P. (1998). Morita therapy and the true nature of anxiety-based disorders (Shinkeishitsu) translated by Kondo, A. pp. 55–62. SUNY Press, New York..

14. Paterson, G.O. (1969). The economics of illness: an employee sickness study. *The Medical Journal of Australia*, **2**, 249–52.

15. Drinka, G.F. (1984). *The birth of neurosis: myth, malady and the Victorians*. Simon and Schuster, New York.

16. Osler, W. (1900). *The principles and practice of medicine* (7th edn), pp. 166–7. Appleton, New York.

17. Sims, M. (1968). *Guide to psychiatry*, p. 444. Livingstone, Edinburgh.

18. Chatel, J.C. and Peele, R. (1970). A centennial review of neurasthenia. *The American Journal of Psychiatry*, **126**, 1404–13.

19. World Health Organization. (1992). *The ICD–10 classification of mental and behavioural disorders: clinical descriptions and diagnostic guidelines*. WHO, Geneva.

20. Chinese Psychiatric Society. (2001). *The Chinese classification of mental disorders (CCMD-3)*. Shandong Publishing House of Science and Technology, Shandong (in English and Chinese).

21. Lee, S. (1996). Cultures in psychiatric nosology: the CCMD–2–R and the International classification of mental disorders. *Culture, Medicine and Psychiatry*, **20**, 421–73.

22. Merikangas, K. and Angst, J. (1994). Neurasthenia in a longitudinal cohort study of young adults. *Psychological Medicine*, **24**, 1013–24.

23. Üstün, T.B. and Sartorius, N. (1995). *Mental illness in general health care: an international study*. Wiley, Chichester.

24. Zhang, W.X., Shen, Y.C., and Li, S.R. (1998). Epidemiological investigations on mental disorders in 7 areas of China. *Chinese Journal of Psychiatry*, **31**, 69–71.

25. Hickie, I., Davenport, I., Issakidis, C., *et al.* (2002). Neurasthenia: prevalence, disability and health care characteristics in the Australian community. *The British Journal of Psychiatry*, **181**, 56–61.

26. Wesnes, K.A., Faleni, R.A., Hefting, N.R., *et al.* (1997). The subjective, cognitive and physical effects of a *Ginkgo biloba/Panax ginseng* combination in healthy volunteers with neurasthenic complaints. *Psychopharmacology Bulletin*, **33**, 677–83.

27. Tang, W., Gao, Y., Chen, G., *et al.* (2005). A randomized, double-blind and placebo-controlled study of a *Ganoderma lucidum* polysaccharide extract in neurasthenia. *Journal of Medicinal Food*, **8**, 53–8.

# 5.3

# Medical and surgical conditions and treatments associated with psychiatric disorders

5.3.1 Adjustment to illness and handicap
Allan House

5.3.2 Psychiatric aspects of neurological disease
Maria A. Ron

5.3.3 Epilepsy
Brian Toone

5.3.4 Medical conditions associated with psychiatric disorder
James R. Rundell

5.3.5 Psychiatric aspects of infections
José Luis Ayuso-Mateos

5.3.6 Psychiatric aspects of surgery (including transplantation)
S. A. Hales, S. E. Abbey, and G. M. Rodin

5.3.7 Psychiatric aspects of cancer
Jimmie C. Holland and Jessica Stiles

5.3.8 Psychiatric aspects of accidents, burns, and other physical trauma
Ulrik Fredrik Malt

## 5.3.1 Adjustment to illness and handicap

Allan House

### Introduction

Not everybody who develops a serious physical illness will have psychiatric problems as a consequence. To understand why, it is useful to have a model of the normal process of adjustment to stress; psychiatric disorder can then be seen as arising when that process, often called coping, is either maladaptive or is adaptive but only partially successful. This chapter will start with an outline of one theory of stress and coping as it applies to physical illness, followed by a review of disorders of adjustment to illness. A distinction will be drawn between recent-onset illness, which provokes an acute response, and long-standing illness, where the challenge is more often to adjust to chronic disability.

### Adjustment to illness and handicap

A number of diseases are reviewed in later chapters, and therefore this chapter will deal with general principles. For more details on particular diseases, the reader should consult specialist textbooks of psychiatry or health psychology.

#### Illness as a stress

Stress is a word that is used in different ways. Sometimes it refers to an environmental stimulus—a threat or demand from the outside world. This definition lies behind various measures, such as the Social Readjustment Rating Scale[1] or the Bedford College Life Events and Difficulties Schedule[2] which characterize life experiences and produce standardized measures of their severity. According to this view, experiences have properties—as losses, or challenges, or dilemmas—that can be identified by knowing something of the social circumstances of the subject of those experiences but without knowing about the meaning given to them by the person experiencing them.

Another meaning of stress is that it is a bodily state, so that events are only regarded as stressful if they produce changes in the individual. The best-known example of this usage comes from physiology.[3] Stress as a psychological state is also a common lay meaning; when people describe themselves as 'stressed' they are usually referring to a state of tension or autonomic arousal.

Yet another way to understand stress, which is useful in considering physical illness, is that it arises out of an interaction between environmental demands and the resources available to deal with them. This view is articulated in the transactional model of Lazarus and Folkman.[4] According to the theory, when faced with a new experience individuals assesses its likely impact (the primary appraisal) and assess their resources (the secondary appraisal). Stress arises when this double appraisal identifies a mismatch between demands and resources that cannot be narrowed by coping manoeuvres.

## (a) Illness as a demand or threat (the primary appraisal)

There are a number of characteristics of an experience that increase the chances of it being appraised as threatening. These include immediacy, ambiguity, uncontrollability, or undesirability. The probability that many people will share an interpretation of a particular episode explains the similarity of people's responses to certain illnesses. The possibility of individual, even idiosyncratic, interpretations can explain sharp differences between people with apparently the same disorder.

A useful way to construe individual appraisals of illness is outlined by Leventhal *et al.*[5] in their theory of internal illness representations. The common elements of the illness representation can be identified from a simple self-report questionnaire[6].

Illness beliefs cannot be assumed solely on the basis of the illness from which a person is suffering, or from his or her social context.[7] Individuals may hold unpredictable beliefs—that an illness is inherited from a family member, or that it is a punishment for a misdemeanour, or that it may be curable by adopting an unusual diet. For some, the representation of illness overlaps with the representation of self, so that sufferers see themselves as living their illness rather than suffering from it.[8] (see Box 5.3.1.1)

The characteristics of a particular disease are not the only component of the illness that can make it threatening. Illness occurs in a social and interpersonal context, and while the responses of other people may be helpful, they may in some cases contribute to the demands of the situation. For example, a partner may withdraw or become depressed, or family members may become intrusive or overcontrolling. Being ill confers a special status, the so-called sick role, but it is a status acquired at a cost in the loss of independence and certain rights. While disability may arise largely from the impairments caused by a disease, much handicap is socially determined.

## (b) Resources for responding to illness (the secondary appraisal)

The focus of secondary appraisal is twofold: the person's personal resources, and the resources external to them, mainly in the immediate social network.

Personal resources may be defined in a number of ways, for example cognitive attributes, personal characteristics, or personality traits.

The other resource for the individual is social support. There are many approaches to understanding support, but a useful one[9] is to regard it as having four components:

1 emotional support, conveying a sense of being cared about or loved

2 esteem support, conveying a sense of being valued or respected

3 instrumental support, conveying practical help

---

**Box 5.3.1.1** Components of the illness representation

- identity (label and associated symptoms)
- causal ideas
- consequences (severity and likely impact)
- time-line (natural history)
- curability or controllability

---

4 informational support, conveying knowledge relevant to tackling the problem

The family's reaction to illness has an important impact on the type of support available. If they are rejecting, intolerant of dependence, or unsympathetic to the needs of the patient—for example, to change their diet, or stop smoking, or take more (or less) exercise—then they may offer too little support. On the other hand, they may be overprotective, refusing to allow the patient a reasonable degree of autonomy and discouraging active coping. Sometimes, members of a family will hold different views about the nature of an illness, leading to conflict, which is not always revealed to doctors. More often, they share views. If such views are inaccurate (so-called family myths) and yet strongly held, then they can be a powerful barrier to the patient accepting medical advice. It is a common observation that patients with chronic illness who are depressed often have a carer who is depressed, and this tendency to share (often dysfunctional) beliefs and coping styles is one reason for that.

## (c) Coping with illness

Coping refers to efforts to reduce the gap between demands and resources. Coping is described according to its aims, the techniques used to achieve those aims, and according to the overall coping style adopted.

The *aims* of coping are either problem focused, designed to modify the demands of the situation, or emotion focused, designed to modify how one feels about a situation.[4] Emotion focused coping generally works well but only transiently. It is best reserved for brief stresses, such as unpleasant medical procedures, or for situations in which nothing can realistically be done to modify the stress.

The *techniques* for coping serve to mobilize available resources. Vocabularies differ for describing them. Cognitive coping techniques include information seeking, downplaying, or adopting a defiant or overoptimistic attitude. In psychodynamic terms, the two most commonly used techniques are probably denial and regression. In common usage, the techniques referred to by these vocabularies overlap. Behavioural coping may involve changing ones lifestyle, such as exercising more or excessive drinking of alcohol. Social coping is a particular form of behavioural coping, and may involve increasing contacts or accepting help from professional agencies. In chronic illness, successful coping may be accompanied by a slower process of reappraisal—in which the patient comes to a different understanding of the illness, from that apparent at initial diagnosis—through for example *benefit-finding* and *downward comparison* (with others who have worse disability, pain, or whatever).

Coping *styles* are more general approaches to coping. Two contrasted styles are active/engaged (sometimes called 'approach') coping and passive/disengaged (sometimes called 'avoid') coping.[10] While it is appealing to characterize people as having a particular coping style, and while it is possible to think of typical examples from personal experience, in fact most people do not have a sufficiently unchangeable repertoire of coping techniques to merit the label of a style.

## Adjustment disorders

### (a) Definition and classification

The emphasis in ICD-10[11] is on emotional disturbance as the characteristic feature of adjustment disorders—some disturbance of behaviour is acknowledged, particularly in adolescence.

However, it is common to encounter cognitive or behavioural changes that interfere with social functioning and quality of life, and yet which are not attributable to the consequences of mood disorder. DSM-IV[12] acknowledges this possibility more directly, including a category of 'Adjustment disorder, unspecified', which covers 'maladaptive reactions (e.g. physical complaints, social withdrawal, or work or academic inhibition)'.

Examples of cognitive problems are extreme helplessness, denial of the existence of illness, or of the handicap associated with it. Behavioural problems may include marked social withdrawal or lack of self-care, or irrational non-adherence to treatment. Emotional problems are typically thought of as anxiety or depression, but irritability is also common.

### (b) Diagnosis and differential diagnosis

The diagnostic features of adjustment disorders are relatively non-specific, comprising mood symptoms and behaviour disturbances, which do not meet the criteria for a diagnosis of another disorder, and yet which are sufficient to amount to a mental disorder. The two main diagnostic questions are as follows.

- Does the patient have a diagnosable mental disorder?

- If there is a mental disorder, should it be given another more specific label than 'adjustment disorder'?

What distinguishes normal adjustment from a disorder? The first criterion is whether the symptoms are persisting beyond the time when they might be attributable to the stressor. This judgement is relatively straightforward when the stressor is a single event. However, if illness is more persistent or intermittent—such as cancer followed by intensive treatment, or multiple sclerosis—then it is less easy to judge.

The second criterion is whether the response is causing avoidable social dysfunction. For example, in many cultures illness is followed by a period of convalescence, during which activity is reduced and a return to full social responsibilities is deferred. This may be a healthy avoidance of activity, if it allows full recovery from illness, but prolonged avoidance of activity may lead to secondary physical problems as well as social isolation and loss of role.

When adjustment disorders are associated with chronic illness and handicap, the duration criterion cannot apply. An individual may present symptoms because his or her response is outside the culturally acceptable range; for example, he or she may be too demanding or uncooperative, or too passive and dependent. It is unwise to regard a presentation as disordered simply on these grounds. The best indicator is whether the individual is achieving the highest level of function and the lowest level of distress of which they are capable under the circumstances. This means that each person must be diagnosed according to his or her own context, and that a standardized set of criteria cannot be applied.

The differentiation of adjustment disorders from other psychiatric disorders is more straightforward, and depends on the presence or absence of key symptoms. The main conditions found in association with physical illness are depressive disorders, anxiety disorders, and occasionally post-traumatic stress disorder.

### (c) Epidemiology

Little is known about the epidemiology of adjustment disorders other than those involving mood disturbance, because of the absence of standardized diagnostic criteria.

Psychiatric symptoms are distributed in the general population, with a positive skew to the distribution. In the physically ill, the same pattern of distribution is seen, but the curve is shifted to the right. The increase in psychiatric symptoms is contributed to by a general increase in all the common symptoms. The usual way to identify cases is to select those who cross an accepted threshold for symptom levels—as determined, for example, by one of the standardized self-report questionnaires—and then to apply diagnostic criteria. Adopting this approach, rates of diagnosable mood disorder among the physically ill are about double what they are in the general population. That is, 30 to 50 per cent (depending on the population studied and the diagnostic criteria employed) of the physically ill have a mental disorder. Approximately two-thirds of these cases are adjustment disorders, the rest meeting criteria for another disorder (usually depressive).

The elderly report lower rates of psychiatric disturbance. This may be a cultural effect, with the elderly disposed to report fewer symptoms of distress as a result of stoicism learned through experience of adversity earlier in life. Alternatively, the elderly may genuinely respond differently to physical illness.

Mood symptoms and adjustment disorders are commoner in response to acute illness than they are in chronic illness.

### (d) Aetiology

There are several reasons why coping might fail.

First, demands may be overwhelming. The news that one has a terminal illness takes time to assimilate—to understand all its meanings, grasp all the threats and losses involved. While that process of appraisal is going on, it is difficult to marshal resources and use them effectively. This explains, in part, why mood disorder is more commonly associated with acute than chronic illness.

Second, resources may be inadequate or missing. One problem associated with physical illness is that it may impair personal resources as a primary effect of the disease process—most importantly when the illness has effects on the central nervous system by virtue of the direct involvement of the brain or through the neurological effects of systemic disturbance.

Third, coping responses may be ineffective. There are few rules about what makes effective coping. In general, a broad and flexible repertoire is desirable, with a strong element of active problem-focused techniques. However not all illnesses, nor all aspects of a particular illness, are likely to be amenable to problem-focused coping. Probably the most effective coping is matched to the situation. That is, the coping matches the demands, so that heavy reliance is not placed on problem-focused coping when little in the situation can change, nor excessive use made of emotion-focused coping when active involvement in illness management is needed.

A common problem of failure to match coping to the situation is found in patients with chronic illness, who are responding to their circumstances as if they none the less have an acute illness. In acute illness, problem-focused coping often involves seeking reversal or even cure of the illness process, while emotion-focused coping involves dealing with the anxiety of uncertainty, or grieving if the prognosis is clearly poor. On the other hand, in chronic illness, problem-focused coping involves symptom management and maximizing function, while emotion-focused coping requires a degree of acceptance.

It is not easy to predict who will develop an adjustment disorder. Certainly the risk is not strongly linked to physical diagnosis, or within a particular diagnostic group to physical disability. The most robust finding is that a previous history of psychiatric problems increases the risk of psychiatric problems associated with physical illness.

### (e) Course and prognosis

By definition, adjustment disorders arise shortly after diagnosis. In practice, there is variation; some people respond immediately and develop symptoms within days, while others develop symptoms weeks or even months after diagnosis. The losses associated with illness may only become apparent when a person leaves hospital and faces functional impairment at home. Carers and others in the social network respond differently to acute and chronic illness, and it may take time for that to become clear. The greater the delay from the onset of illness to the emergence of symptoms, the harder it is to make a diagnosis of adjustment disorder. In clinical practice, it is reasonable to set an upper limit of a year.

Most adjustment disorders provoked by a newly onset illness, resolve within weeks. Slower recovery takes place over 12 or 18 months. If recovery has not occurred by then, the patient has usually developed another mental disorder, such as a depressive disorder. Accurate data are few, but probably no more than 10 per cent of patients develop a prolonged adjustment disorder.

The psychiatric symptoms of adjustment disorder impair quality of life, so much so that all standardized quality-of-life measures include mood symptoms in their profile. Psychiatric morbidity associated with physical illness is also a risk factor for self-harm and for completed suicide. Adjustment disorders are likely to have an effect on the outcomes of treatment for physical disease.[13] Health service costs are greater for patients with physical illness and psychiatric co-morbidity; lengths of stay are longer for hospital inpatients; the functional outcomes of rehabilitation may be poorer, and there is some evidence that there may also be an increased mortality. The mechanism for these effects may be broadly behavioural or physiological. Examples of the former are increased rates of smoking, lack of exercise, and poor adherence to treatment regimes among people with mental disorders. Examples of the latter include activation of the hypothalamic–pituitary–adrenal axis or increased cytokine production associated with chronic emotional disorder.

### (f) Treatment
#### (i) Drug treatments

Antidepressants can be effective in the presence of physical illness.[14] There is no good evidence to support claims for a great superiority in efficacy of serotonin-reuptake inhibitors. Although their long-term tolerability may be greater than older drugs in patients with physical disease, they are not without toxicity—for example they have been associated with increased falls and gastrointestinal haemorrhage. Tricyclic antidepressants have advantages in treating patients with insomnia or chronic pain. Cost differences are substantial.

#### (ii) Psychological treatments

A number of brief psychological therapies have been shown to be effective in treating depression; namely cognitive-behaviour therapy, problem-solving therapy, interpersonal therapy, and brief dynamic therapy. Such therapies may also be effective in treating adjustment disorder in the physically ill,[15,16] although they may have disappointingly weak effects upon physical outcomes. Therapy may need to be modified to allow for fatigue or concentration problems, and sessions need to be arranged flexibly to accommodate hospital appointments and other treatment needs.

### (g) Management
#### (i) Identifying cases

A major difficulty in delivering treatment to people with adjustment disorders is the difficulty in identifying cases. There are several self-report questionnaires, which may be used to screen for patients with mood disorder. In certain settings such questionnaires can be delivered routinely to all patients, for example by means of computers with touch screen technology, and they are useful for alerting staff to the presence of mood symptoms—but their positive predictive value is too low to allow for accurate use in identifying those who need referral to specialist services. Their use is also difficult to integrate into routine clinical practice, and response rates outside research studies are usually low.[17] Their use is best restricted to specialist services where the clinical staff are clear about what response they will make to a high score, since this is where there is some evidence for the benefits of case-finding. There are no useful standardized instruments for the detection of other problems with adjustment.

Instead, clinicians should be encouraged to consider the possibility of psychiatric disorder when there is a gap between impairment and handicap so that the patient is doing worse in rehabilitation than the severity of their disease would suggest they should be, when there are multiple complaints that are difficult to explain, or when multiple drug treatments are being administered without conspicuous benefit. The clinical interview is the mainstay of diagnosis.

There are a number of common reasons for failing to recognize adjustment disorders. First, the questions simply are not asked, or attempts by the patient to introduce the topic of psychological problems are blocked or sidestepped. Second, questions may be asked, but in circumstances where it is difficult for the patient to answer honestly—when there is no privacy, or the person asking is obviously too busy to listen to any but a conventional answer. Third, expressions of distress may be normalized, and thus dismissed: 'Of course it's natural you will feel like that' means to the patient 'So please don't mention it again'.

#### (ii) Broadening the repertoire of psychological responses

No single intervention is going to be effective for all patients with psychological problems arising from difficulties with adjustment to illness. Realistic management therefore involves offering what has been called a 'menu of interventions'.[18] A currently favoured model is a so-called **stepped care** model in which intervention is organized in a hierarchy according to intensity of treatment and the expertize needed to deliver it e.g. see Box 5.3.1.2. While unfocused 'support' is of limited value (because it does not encourage active secondary appraisal and experiments with different coping strategies) there are now many brief and flexible psychological therapies available, some of which may be deliverable by staff in the primary care or physical healthcare service (see Box 5.3.1.3). In **collaborative care** such first line psychological treatments, along with medication management and simple social care, are delivered by non-mental health staff and monitored by a case manager, with a mental health professional providing supervision and back-up consultation. Successful trials have been conducted in (for example) heat disease[19] and diabetes.[20]

**Box 5.3.1.2** Stepped care in the treatment of depression (NICE clinical guideline 2004)

| | Who is responsible for care? | What is the focus? | What do they do? |
|---|---|---|---|
| Step 5 | Inpatient care, crisis teams | Risk to life, severe neglect | Medication, combined treatments, ECT |
| Step 4 | Mental health specialists including crisis teams | Treatment-resistant, recurrent, atypical and psychotic depression, and those at significant risk | Medication, complex psychological interventions, combined treatments |
| Step 3 | Primary care team, primary care mental health worker | Moderate or severe depression | Medication, psychological interventions, social support |
| Step 2 | Primary care team, primary care mental health worker | Mild depression | Watchful waiting, guided self-help, computerized CBT, exercise brief psychological interventions |
| Step 1 | GP, practice nurse | Recognition | Assessment |

National Institute for Health and Clinical Excellence (NICE) (2005). CG22 Anxiety: quick reference guide. London: NICE. Available from http://www.nice.org.uk/nicemedia/pdf/CGO22quickrefguideamended.pdf. Reproduced with permission.

---

**Box 5.3.1.3** Brief psychological treatment of use in the medically ill

♦ **Motivational interviewing** is an approach developed to encourage people to attempt change in addictive behaviours. It may be useful in engaging people in demanding treatments, or in improving adherence to treatment regimes.

♦ **Graded activity** has been used to treat negative symptoms in mental illness like schizophrenia or depressive disorder. It is effective in improving function in chronic fatigue syndrome, and is worth using in other conditions where inactivity and passivity is out of proportion to physical disability.

♦ **Anger management** is a modification of cognitive-behaviour therapy, which may be useful where irritability or aggressive behaviour is complicating adjustment.

♦ **Interpersonal therapy**[21] was initially developed for the treatment of depression, but it has obvious applications in the field of physical illness. In the terminology of interpersonal therapy, illness represents a role transition, and the focus in therapy is therefore on negotiating that transition with key others in the patient's life.

♦ **Family therapy and couples therapy** are rarely considered (or available) for adults with physical illness, and yet many of the external resources needed for coping are in the family.

For more severe or persistent problems, referral to specialist services is appropriate—ideally liaison services that operate in the primary or secondary care settings where patients receive their main care. Psychiatric treatment of the physically ill, especially in hospital, requires a number of modifications to routine clinical practice, which are sometimes overlooked.

First, an extra effort has to be made to meet the family and carers. They may be reluctant to attend if there is hostility in the family, or if missed time from work is creating financial pressures, but failure to interview others makes it near impossible to come to a full and accurate formulation of the problem.

Second, personal contact with the referrer is highly desirable. The 'real' question may not be that posed in the referral, and can only be identified by probing. Advice is much more likely to be followed if it is delivered face to face, and followed up with a later visit to check on compliance! This direct contact with non-psychiatric colleagues is one of the defining characteristics of liaison psychiatry, and its importance cannot be overemphasized.

Third, it must be recognized that the course of psychiatric treatment needs to be modified. Appointments will be missed, or interrupted, by the demands of physical treatment. And psychological issues may well not be resolved by a single clinical encounter; a relapse of illness may provoke a further episode with new features, and patients often have to return repeatedly to work through themes in therapy, as they are re-challenged with new physical problems.

### (h) Prevention

There are two broad approaches to prevention, namely education and support.

Education and the provision of information and advice about the illness and its management is desirable as an informed patient is more likely to be an effective partner in treatment, and because it is popular with patients. Disappointingly, however, it is not an effective means of preventing psychiatric problems. This is probably because, while it facilitates primary appraisal, it does nothing to facilitate secondary appraisal or the use of effective coping strategies.

Provision of support is also popular. It takes a number of forms, including self-help groups, volunteer visiting, and professional support workers—usually with knowledge of a particular disease such as AIDS or a stroke. Again, there is little evidence that it prevents psychiatric problems. Perhaps this is because it usually provides emotional support; which in itself may be worthwhile but which is insufficient if not combined with a more problem-focused approach.

In conclusion, there are no clear indications that we can prevent the development of adjustment disorders. The mainstay of current management is therefore to identify existing cases and to offer specialist care to those who are most symptomatic or handicapped, and to those who are not improving spontaneously.

## Adjustment to terminal illness: care of the dying

Adjustment to terminal illness has much in common with adjustment to other severe illness, and is not specifically the province of psychiatrists. For a detailed discussion of the care of the dying, the reader is referred to a more specialized text.[22] Here we will discuss two issues that are commonly presented to the psychiatrist in this setting: the diagnosis of depression and other adjustment disorders, and the issue of suicide.

## Diagnosis of depression and adjustment disorders in the terminally ill

As with physical illness, somatic complaints are common in the dying and thus, individually, lose their diagnostic or predictive usefulness in the major depressive syndrome. Even psychologically, a degree of hopelessness may be appropriate. Anxiety is a common symptom in the dying, but it is not necessarily pathological. Like depression, it may result from physical disability, uncontrolled pain, or pre-existing anxiety disorders. In these circumstances a more detailed examination of the attitudes of the patient is necessary. Pervasive global hopelessness, feelings that life has had no meaning, strong feelings of guilt or punishment, and suicidal thoughts are pointers towards depressive illness in the terminally ill.

## Assessing suicidal thoughts in the terminally ill

Several studies have shown that the prevalence of suicidal thoughts among patients with terminal cancer is less than 10 per cent.[23] However, this contradicts the clinical impression that most patients admit to either suicidal thoughts or thoughts of assisted suicide as an escape from the imaged consequences of losing control. In some patients, having a belief in a 'way out' can be positive in offering a sense of control.

Completed suicide is an important complication in patients with a terminal illness. General predictors of suicide apply, with the addition of severity of functional impairment, isolation, and delirium. The two most important factors to watch out for are uncontrolled pain and depression. These two factors greatly increase suicide risk but are nevertheless treatable in the terminal illness setting.[24]

People who express a desire to die are nearly always ambivalent. The expression of suicidal ideas should never be accepted as rational without a searching enquiry for evidence of subtle external pressures, fear of terminal symptoms or of being a burden on others, and treatable depression.

## Pharmacological management of psychiatric disorders in the dying

Alleviation of distress rather than cure is the guiding principle of the management of the terminally ill. Caution is needed in the selection and prescription of psychotropic drugs.

Anxiolytic medication is usually well tolerated and the concern over dependence and tolerance is less of an issue. Terminal metabolite benzodiazepines, such as lorazepam and oxazapam, can provide symptomatic relief for a variety of conditions even in patients with hepatic impairment. Occasionally, opiates are used in this role where first-line treatments are unsuccessful.

Antidepressant use in the dying may be more problematic due to the adverse effects of sedation, seizures, hypotension, and constipation and urinary retention. For this reason, the choice of drug needs to be individually tailored. Dosage has to be carefully adjusted, beginning at low doses and increasing gradually. The use of psychostimulants (dextroamphetamine, methylphenidate) is worth considering. These drugs are used infrequently in general psychiatry because of the risks of dependence, but in the terminally ill they may have advantageous 'energizing' properties, including increased energy, improved concentration, increased appetite, and possibly, a faster onset of action.

## Further information

Sharpe, L. and Curran, L. (2006). Understanding the process of adjustment to illness. *Social Science & Medicine*, **62**, 1153–66.

Fletcher, J., Bower, P., Gask, L., *et al.* (2006). *Primary care services for depression: a guide to best practice care services improvement partnership.* National Institute for mental Health in England, Department of Health, London.

## References

1. Holmes, T.H. and Rahe, R.H. (1967). The social readjustment rating scale. *Journal of Psychosomatic Research*, **11**, 213–18.
2. Brown, G. and Harris, T. (1978). *Social origins of depression.* Tavistock Publications, London.
3. Selye, H. (1956). *The stress of life.* McGraw–Hill, New York.
4. Lazarus, R.S. and Folkman, S. (1984). *Stress, appraisal and coping.* Springer, New York.
5. Leventhal, H., Nerenz, D., and Steele, D. (1984). Illness representations and coping with health threats. In *Handbook of psychology and health* (4th edn) (eds. A. Baum, S.E. Taylor, and J.E. Singer), pp. 219–52. Erlbaum, Hillsdale, NJ.
6. Weinman, J., Petrie, K., Moss–Morris, R., *et al.* (1996). The illness perception questionnaire: a new method for assessing the cognitive representations of illness. *Psychology and Health*, **11**, 431–45.
7. Petrie, K. and Weinman, J. (eds.) (1997). *Perceptions of health and illness.* Harwood, Amsterdam.
8. Kleinman, A. (1988). *The illness narratives: suffering, healing and the human condition.* Basic Books, New York.
9. Cohen, S. and Wills, T.A. (1985). Stress, social support and the buffering hypothesis. *Psychological Bulletin*, **98**, 310–57.
10. Carver, C.S., Weintraub, J.K., and Scheier, M.F. (1989). Assessing coping strategies: a theoretically based approach. *Journal of Personality and Social Psychology*, **56**, 267–83.
11. World Health Organization. (1992). *International statistical classification of diseases and related health problems,* 10th revision. WHO, Geneva.
12. American Psychiatric Association. (1994). *Diagnostic and statistical manual of mental disorders* (4th edn). American Psychiatric Association, Washington, DC.
13. Saravay, S.M. and Lavin, M. (1994). Psychiatric comorbidity and length of stay in the general hospital–a critical review of outcome studies. *Psychosomatics*, **35**, 233–52.
14. Gill, D. and Hatcher, S. (2000). Antidepressants for depression in medical illness. *Cochrane Library*, **4**.
15. MacHale, S. (2002). Managing depression in physical illness. *Advances in Psychiatric Treatment*, **8**, 297—305.
16. Winkley, K., Landau, S., Eisler, I., *et al.* (2006). Psychological interventions to improve glycaemic control in patients with Type I diabetes: systematic review and meta-analysis of randomized controlled trials. *British Medical Journal*, **333**, 65–8.
17. House, A. (1988). Mood disorders in the physically ill: problems of definition and measurement. *Journal of Psychosomatic Research*, **32**, 345–53.
18. Goodheart, C.D. and Lansing, M.H. (1997). *Treating people with chronic disease: a psychological guide.* American Psychological Association, Washington, DC.
19. Schrader, G., Cheok, F., Holdacre, *et al.* (2003). Effect of psychiatry liaison with general practitioners on depression severity in recently hospitalized cardiac patients: a randomized controlled trial. *JAMA: The Journal of the American Medical Association*, **288**, 2836–45.
20. Williams, J.W., Katon, W., Lin, E.H.B., *et al.* (2004). The effectiveness of depression care management on diabetes-related outcomes in older patients. *Annals of Internal Medicine*, **140**(12), 1015—24.
21. Klerman, G.L. and Weissman, M.M. (1993). *New applications of interpersonal psychotherapy.* American Psychiatric Press, Washington, DC.

22. Wiener, I., Breitbart, W., and Holland, J. (1996). Psychiatric issues in the care of dying patients. In *Textbook of consultation–liaison psychiatry* (eds. J.R. Rundell and M.G. Wise), pp. 804–31. American Psychiatric Press, Washington, DC.

23. Brown, J.H., Henteleff, P., Baratat, S., *et al.* (1986). Is it normal for terminally ill patients to desire death? *The American Journal of Psychiatry*, **143**, 208–11.

24. Bolund, C. (1985). Suicide and cancer II: medical and care factors in suicide by cancer patients in Sweden. *Journal of Psychosocial Oncology*, **3**, 17–30.

# 5.3.2 Psychiatric aspects of neurological disease

Maria A. Ron

Psychiatric abnormalities are an integral part of neurological disease and their study can improve our understanding of the neural basis of psychiatric illness. This chapter deals with common neurological diseases where psychiatric symptoms are prominent.

## Stroke

Stroke is defined as the sudden loss of blood supply to an area of the brain resulting in permanent tissue damage and is the commonest neurological disorder. The incidence of stroke for those aged between 35 and 65 is between 90 and 330 per 100 000. It is commoner in men and the incidence increases with advancing age. Ischaemic stroke is commoner than haemorrhagic stroke and accounts for 80 to 85 per cent of all cases.

### Depression

Its prevalence is around 30 per cent in the first few weeks after a stroke—two-thirds of the patients fit the criteria for major depression and the rest for minor depression. Survivors remain at an elevated risk for depression for many years.

#### (a) Clinical features

◆ Diurnal variation of mood, weight loss, anergia, insomnia, and loss of libido are prominent in the early stages.

◆ Anhedonia, suicidal ideation, loss of self-esteem, and feelings of guilt become evident later.

◆ Irritability and aggressive behaviour are common, especially in those with cognitive impairment.[1]

◆ The onset of depression may occur acutely in the early post-stroke period or be delayed for 6 months or more.

#### (b) Factors associated with post-stroke depression

Early after stroke, anterior left-sided lesions involving the cortex and subcortical regions, especially the basal ganglia, and right posterior lesions are more frequently associated with depression.[2] In time these associations become less marked.[3] Cognitive impairment is closely associated with depression early after stroke,[4] and is present in 70 per cent of those with major and 43 per cent of those with minor depression. Old age, a past or family history of depression, and negative life events in the preceding 6 months substantially increase the incidence of post-stroke depression.

Disruption of fronto-subcortical circuits, directly or as a distant effect of stroke, plays a central role in the causation of depression. Decreased metabolism in orbitofrontal, anterior cingulate, and inferior temporal regions has been reported using PET.[5] Serotonergic mechanisms have been implicated, with a reduction of 5-hydroxytryptamine-2 receptor binding in the temporal cortex, especially in left hemisphere stroke.

#### (c) Course and prognosis

The average duration of major depression is around 1 year, with spontaneous remission in many patients. Symptoms of minor depression may persist for 2 years or more. The presence of depression and other psychiatric diagnosis in the first 3 years after a stroke substantially increases the risk of death after controlling for cardiovascular and other risk factors.

### Anxiety

◆ About a quarter of patients fulfil criteria for generalized anxiety disorder during the acute post-stroke phase.

◆ Rates are lower in community studies (5 per cent)[6] and 1 or 2 years after stroke (4 to 18 per cent). Half of those with anxiety disorder also satisfy criteria for depression.

◆ Right-sided subcortical lesions may be more common in anxiety disorder, while left-sided pathology, usually involving cortical regions, is more likely when anxiety and depression coexist.[2] Serotonergic abnormalities are also likely to be relevant.

#### (a) Course and prognosis

Anxiety in the acute post-stroke phase is associated with high mortality rates, comparable to those in depressed patients.

### Emotionalism (abnormal crying or laughing)

Emotionalism is usually mood-congruent and is triggered by sad or emotional events. Most patients have some degree of voluntary control.

Emotionalism occurs in a quarter of patients during the first year post-stroke, with a peak in the first month and decreasing gradually thereafter.[7] It is associated with the severity of depression and with left-anterior lesions disrupting serotonergic pathways.

### Management

The first step in treating the psychiatric manifestations of stroke is for these to be recognized, and patients need to be routinely assessed for the presence of psychiatric symptoms.

### Treatment

Double-blind placebo-controlled trials using nortriptyline, trazodone, and selective serotonin reuptake inhibitors (SSRIs) have shown these drugs to be effective.[4] Improvement in depression also results in lasting improvement in cognition and physical activity. Treatment within 3 months of stroke may be followed by the best outcome.

The treatment of anxiety symptoms has been less well documented. Short-acting benzodiazepines, buspirone, and SSRIs are the main pharmacological approaches. The usefulness of psychotherapeutic or behavioural interventions has not been established and may depend on the severity of symptoms and cognitive impairment.

Emotionalism responds well to treatment with SSRIs and tricyclic antidepressants, even in those without associated depression.

# Parkinson's disease

The neurological and cognitive features of Parkinson's disease are dealt with in Chapter 4.1.6 and only commonly encountered psychiatric symptoms will be considered here.

## Depression

Its overall prevalence is approximately 40 per cent.[8] Depressive symptoms are more common early in the disease (50 per cent) and in those with onset before the age of 55. For many people, adaptation to the disease results in a return to normal mood. Depression becomes more frequent again in the advanced stages of the disease, particularly in those with rapidly progressive disability.

Major depression is commoner in those with akinetic Parkinson's disease (38 per cent) than in those with classical forms of the disease (15 per cent), but dysthymia is equally common in both. Depression, severe in some patients, has also been reported in the first few weeks after bilateral subthalamic stimulation, a successful treatment for the motor symptoms of Parkinson's disease,[9] but mood changes were less commonly observed a year after surgery.

### (a) Clinical features

◆ Anxiety, agitation, and depressed mood are prominent.

◆ Depressive symptoms are not closely associated with the severity of motor signs, but may be more severe during 'off' periods and are commoner in those with cognitive impairment.

◆ Early awakening, motor retardation, and apathy in the absence of mood abnormalities may not be indicative of depression.

◆ Major depression is associated with functional deterioration at 1-year follow-up.[10]

◆ Three-quarters of patients with depression also fulfil criteria for anxiety disorder, but only 10 per cent have symptoms of anxiety in isolation.[11]

### (b) Mechanisms underlying depression

Studies using PET have suggested that depression and anxiety in Parkinson's disease are associated with a specific loss of dopamine and noradrenaline innervation in the limbic system.[12] Postmortem studies have also described loss of dopaminergic neurones in the ventral tegmental area.[13] Degeneration of these neurones leads to dysfunction of the orbitofrontal cortex with secondary effects on the serotonergic cell bodies of the dorsal raphe.[5]

### (c) Management

Optimal control of neurological symptoms may lead to improvement in depression and should be a management aim. Repeated assessment may be needed to differentiate features of the disease, such as apathy, from the symptoms of depression.

### (d) Treatment

There are few studies describing the treatment of depression in Parkinson's disease. When antidepressants are clinically indicated because of the severity or persistence of symptoms, the antidepressant profile of side-effects should be considered. Antidepressants with strong anticholinergic effects, such as amitriptyline, may increase cognitive impairment and SSRIs may be preferable. Electroconvulsive treatment is also effective for Parkinson's disease patients with depression and may also transiently improve motor symptoms.

## Psychotic symptoms

### (a) Clinical features

◆ Up to 40 per cent of patients on long-term treatment experience visual hallucinations.

◆ Long duration of illness, age, cognitive impairment, and depression are associated with visual hallucinations.

◆ Visual hallucinations in clear consciousness are usually fully formed images of people or animals, non-threatening, fleeting, and stereotyped. They are recurrent and tend to occur at night, more commonly in the 'on' periods.

◆ Sleep disturbances (fragmented sleep, alteration of sleep rhythms, and vivid dreams) often precede daytime hallucinations and may be part of a continuum.

◆ Delusions are less frequent than hallucinations but are more stressful and difficult to manage. They are usually paranoid, with conspiracy and infidelity themes.

◆ Severe psychosis is associated with institutional placement, progressive dementia, and increased risk of death (over a quarter of patients within 2 years).

### (b) Mechanisms

Psychotic symptoms may represent intrusion of REM sleep imagery into wakefulness. They may be more frequent in those receiving anticholinergics and dopamine agonists, but there is no clear association with dosage or duration of treatment. Stimulation of hypersensitive dopaminergic receptors in the nigrostriatal system by dopaminergic drugs may explain psychosis early in the disease, but it is unlikely to explain late psychosis. The therapeutic efficacy of atypical neuroleptics suggests a role for mesolimbic dopaminergic and serotonergic pathways. Cholinergic deficiency may also be relevant, in patients with dementia and atrophy of the nucleus basalis.

### (c) Management

In patients with clouded consciousness, infection, cerebrovascular accidents, and other relevant pathologies need to be excluded. Revision of dopaminergic medication should come next, with reduction of polypharmacy and dose tapering. Anticholinergics, selegiline, amantadine, and dopamine agonists may need to be discontinued, as they are more likely to trigger psychosis.

### (d) Treatment

In most patients antipsychotic drugs are needed, as dopaminergic medication is needed to preserve acceptable motor function. Atypical neuroleptics such as clozapine, with its low D2 receptor affinity and few extrapyramidal side-effects, are preferable to typical neuroleptics. Clozapine is effective at doses of less than 100 mg per day. Initial recommended doses of 6.25 to 12.5 mg daily should be gradually increased until the symptoms are controlled. The danger of agranulocytosis and the need to monitor the blood picture are the main drawbacks, and other atypical neuroleptics (particularly quietiapine) may be preferable. Cholinesterase inhibitors may also be helpful in treating psychotic symptoms in patients with cognitive impairment.

## Dopamine dysregulation syndrome

The syndrome is characterized by the compulsive use of dopaminergic medication beyond that needed to control motor symptoms. It is commoner in males with young onset and may affect 4 per cent of patients. Drug-hoarding and drug-seeking behaviour, impaired social functioning, aggression, and reluctance to reduce medication despite severe dyskinesias are common features. Hypomania and frank psychosis may follow.[14]

### (a) Management

Reduction of medication resolves symptoms, but a withdrawal state characterized by dysphoria and irritability follows. Treatment is difficult and often unsuccessful, and primary prevention is preferable.

## Tourette syndrome

The syndrome is characterized by motor and phonic tics of fluctuating severity.

- Motor tics appear early, between the ages of 3 and 8 years. Simple tics, e.g. eye blinking, are followed by complex stereotypies (i.e. touching, licking). Phonictics (sniffing, throat clearing) appear later.

- Severity of tics peaks by the age of 20 and may lessen thereafter, but total recovery is rare. Severe cases may start in adulthood.

- Tics, preceded by premonitory urges, occur many times a day and are exacerbated by anxiety, boredom, fatigue, and excitement and lessened by alcohol, relaxation, and sleep. Patients may be able to suppress tics for long periods at the expense of a build-up of tension.

- Coprolalia (utterance of obscenities), copropraxia (obscene gestures), echolalia and echopraxia (repetition of words and actions), and self-harm are also common.

Tourette syndrome is part of a spectrum that includes transient childhood tic disorders. Secondary tic disorders following trauma, encephalitis, rheumatic fever, and metabolic and toxic encephalopathies, and those present in inherited degenerative conditions such as Huntington's disease and neuroacanthocytosis, need to be considered in the differential diagnosis.

### Epidemiology

Tourette syndrome is more frequent in males (4:1). Its prevalence in male adolescents is around 4 per 10 000, but it may be higher (49 per 10 000) in children with behavioural disturbances[15] and is as high as 1 to 3 per cent in school children if a broad definition of chronic motor and phonic tics is used.

### Aetiology

Major gene effects with an autosomal mode of inheritance seem likely. Monozygotic twins have a concordance rate between 50 and 70 per cent for the syndrome compared with 10 to 20 per cent for dizygotic twins, and a third of relatives may have features of the syndrome. Several candidate genes have been assessed including

dopamine receptors, the dopamine transporter, and various noradrenergic and serotonergic genes, and although isolated changes in a single locus are unlikely to lead to the syndrome, these alleles could have a significant cumulative effect. Gestational and perinatal risk factors may also play a role. Multiple streptococcal infections in the months preceding symptom onset are commoner in Tourette patients than in controls, suggesting that the paediatric autoimmune neuropsychiatric disorder associated with streptococcal infection (PANDAS) may be the cause of Tourette syndrome in vulnerable patients.

The efficacy of dopamine antagonists and SSRIs in the treatment of tics and obsessive–compulsive symptoms has implicated dopaminergic and serotonergic pathways and the regions where dopaminergic and serotonergic neurons interact (i.e. striatum, substantia nigra, and prefrontal cortex). The beneficial effects of basal ganglia deep brain stimulation also point to basal ganglia dysfunction. PET studies have suggested decreased metabolism and blood flow in basal ganglia–thalamo-cortical projection systems.[16] Post-mortem studies have not shown consistent abnormalities in D1/D2 receptors, and *in vivo* receptor-binding studies have been conflicting, as have structural brain-imaging studies.

### Psychiatric comorbidity

#### (a) Clinical features

- About half of the patients meet criteria for other psychiatric disorders,[17] but it is uncertain whether they should be considered part of the phenotype.

- Depression and anxiety occur in about 25 per cent of patients.

- Personality disorder is present in two-thirds of patients. Borderline, obsessive–compulsive, and paranoid types are the commonest types.

- Attention-deficit hyperactivity disorder may be more common in males and may have educational and behavioural implications. Wide variations in prevalence have been reported (8 to 80 per cent).

- Obsessive–compulsive disorder may be more common in females, reaching its peak in late adolescence. Concern for symmetry, violent and sexual thoughts, forced touching, fear of harming self and others, and a need to do things 'just right' are common features.

- Intellectual ability tends to be normal, but poor performance in complex attentional tasks is associated with attention-deficit hyperactivity disorder.

#### (b) Management

Explanation and reassurance are often enough in mild cases; for the rest, drug treatment or cognitive-behaviour therapy may be indicated.

#### (c) Treatment

Neuroleptics are useful in treating tics. Haloperidol, pimozide, and sulpiride are commonly prescribed and atypical neuroleptics (e.g. risperidone, zipresidone, and olanzapine) are also useful, although few controlled trials are available. Clonidine, a α2 adrenergic agonist, is useful, with less severe side-effects. Behavioural interventions (e.g. habit reversal training and bio-feedback techniques) may also suppress tics. Deep brain stimulation of the centromedian-parafascicular complex of the thalamus or the internal segment of the globus pallidus is reported to ameliorate tics and self-harm.

Variable success has been achieved with behavioural techniques, SSRIs (fluoxetine), and risperidone in the treatment of obsessive–compulsive disorder. The treatment of attention-deficit hyperactivity disorder is more controversial, but benefits may follow the use of clonidine and stimulants such as methylphenidate, pemoline, and dextroamphetamine without increasing tic severity. (See also Chapter 9.2.4.)

# Multiple sclerosis

Multiple sclerosis is a common neurological disease, with a prevalence of 50 to 60 per 100 000; it is more common in women. It usually starts between the ages of 20 to 40 and is characterized by multiple demyelinating lesions with a predilection for the optic nerves, cerebellum, brainstem, and spinal cord. In most cases the disease initially follows a relapsing–remitting course, entering a secondary, progressive phase after some years. For a few patients the disease is progressive from the outset.

Purely psychiatric presentations of multiple sclerosis other than dementia are rare, but psychiatric symptoms are common in the course of the illness.

## Depression

- Depressive symptoms occur in about 50 per cent of patients in cross-sectional studies[18] and their lifetime prevalence is also around 50 per cent.

- The rates of suicide are more than twice those of the general population, and young males and those socially isolated or with drinking problems are at a greater risk.

- Low mood, negative thoughts, anhedonia, and suicidal ideation are common features of depression.

- Fatigue and poor concentration may be features of multiple sclerosis and have less diagnostic value.

## Euphoria

- It is only present in about 10 per cent of patients and is characterized by mild, continuous elation.

- It is best considered as an organic type of personality change.

## Emotional lability

- It is as frequent as euphoria.

- Excessive crying is more frequent than laughter.

- It tends to be more severe in those with significant depression.[19]

## Psychosis

- It is uncommon, but brief affective or schizophrenia-like psychoses may occur in patients with well-established multiple sclerosis, sometimes coinciding with a relapse.[20]

- Persecutory delusions and lack of insight are common.

- In most patients these are single episodes lasting 4 to 6 weeks that respond well to symptomatic treatment.

### (a) Mechanisms of psychotic symptoms

**Severity of brain disease**, as measured by magnetic resonance imaging (**MRI**), and duration of illness are not closely correlated with **depression**, but they are a risk factor. The personal and social limitations imposed by the disease are an important risk factor for depression.[18] A **genetic predisposition** has been reported in multiple sclerosis patients with bipolar illness.

**Euphoria** and **emotional lability** tend to occur in patients with advanced disease and cognitive impairment and are more closely related to MRI indices of brain damage. MRI lesions tend to cluster around the temporal lobes in patients with **psychotic symptoms**.

### (b) Management of psychotic symptoms

All patients should be assessed for the presence of depression. Fatigue and poor concentration have limited diagnostic value, as they may be features of multiple sclerosis. Although disease-modifying treatments do not increase the overall risk of depression, they may do so in the first 6 months of treatment in those with a previous history of depression.[21] Regular psychiatric assessment in the early stages of treatment is, therefore, important.

### (c) Treatment of psychotic symptoms

Few studies have assessed the effect of antidepressants in patients with multiple sclerosis, but SSRIs and other antidepressants appear to be effective. Their side-effects need to be carefully considered for their potential to aggravate or improve neurological symptoms. Cognitive-behaviour therapy aimed at improving coping strategies is also useful. **Emotional lability** responds well to small doses of SSRIs or tricyclic antidepressants but tends to recur when these drugs are discontinued.

Psychotic episodes may require the use of neuroleptics for brief periods, but the long-term use of these drugs is rarely required.

## Cognitive impairment

Cognitive impairment is present in about 40 per cent of multiple sclerosis patients[22] and contributes significantly to the overall disability. The pattern of impairment is characterized by the following:

- Attention deficits and slowing of information processing speed are often the first manifestations and may be present early in the disease.[23]

- Memory disturbances, with greater impairment of recall over recognition, appear later.

- Executive function deficits, with poor working memory, abstract reasoning, and use of strategy, are common.

- Language skills and visuospatial functions tend to be preserved.

Cognitive impairment is greater in those with progressive, severe disease, although cases presented as dementia have also been described.[24] Depression worsens cognitive impairment by slowing down information processing and interfering with learning and working memory. Cognitive impairment correlates with MRI markers of disease severity, in particular brain atrophy.

### (a) Management of cognitive impairment

Disease-modifying treatments may slow down cognitive impairment, but evidence is insufficient. The same applies to cholinesterase inhibitors. Cognitive rehabilitation has so far been disappointing.

# Space-occupying lesions

## Brain tumours

Their clinical manifestations are determined by location and by the effects of raised intracranial pressure. Psychiatric symptoms occur in 50 per cent of patients[25] and are of three main types:

- Confusional states and/or progressive cognitive deterioration occur in a third of patients. Disorientation with clouding of consciousness, euphoria, apathy, and loss of insight are prominent in those with confusional states. Progressive memory impairment, loss of initiative, and bradyphrenia occur in patients with a more protracted course and may coexist with signs of raised intracranial pressure.

- Behavioural and mood disturbances occur in 20 per cent of patients. Irritability, euphoria, depression, and, less frequently, psychosis are part of the picture.

- Paroxysmal disturbances such as poorly formed visual hallucinations and automatisms, indicating temporal lobe involvement, are less common.

Fast-growing tumours are more likely to cause psychiatric symptoms (60 per cent in patients with gliomas and 42 per cent in those with meningiomas). Frontal lobe tumours may present with psychiatric symptoms in the absence of other neurological abnormalities.[26] Medial and orbitofrontal tumours lead to emotional symptoms while disinhibition and irritability or marked apathy occurs when the anterior cingulate is involved. Tumours involving the dorsolateral prefrontal regions are more likely to produce abnormalities of executive function (planning, goal-directed behaviour, ability to monitor effective performance). Disturbances of micturition are specifically associated with frontal tumours.

### (a) Management

Brain tumours should be suspected in patients with the above syndromes or when psychiatric symptoms are accompanied by neurological abnormalities or appear *de novo* late in life. Imaging usually confirms the diagnosis.

## Neurofibromatosis

There are two types of neurofibromatosis, both inherited as autosomal dominant disorders.

*Neurofibromatosis 1* is the commonest (incidence 1/3000) and is characterized by cutaneous manifestations (café-au-lait pigmentation) and neurofibromas, which are benign nerve sheath tumours. Gliomas and hamartomas, especially in the eye and optic pathways, and bone dysplasia are also features. Severe learning disability occurs in 4 per cent of patients, but milder cognitive impairment is commoner (80 per cent of cases). Attentional difficulties are common and a third of patients fulfil criteria for attention-deficit hyperactivity disorder. Perceptual and executive functions are worse than memory functions.[27, 28] Epilepsy is twice as common as in the general population. Ventricular enlargement and $T_2$ MRI hyperintensities in the basal ganglia, internal capsule, thalamus, brainstem, and cerebellum not closely related to the severity of the learning disability are often present.

*Neurofibromatosis 2* is much less common (incidence 1/40 000) and is characterized by bilateral vestibular schwannomas, which may also occur in other peripheral nerves. Meningiomas and ependymomas also occur. Hearing loss, vestibular disturbances, and cataracts are the commonest clinical presentations. Cognition is normal.

The loci for neurofibromatosis 1 and 2 have been located to 17q 11.2 and 22q 12.2 respectively. The rate of spontaneous mutations is high and both genes may have tumour-suppressant roles.

*Management* is aimed at dealing with attention-deficit hyperactivity disorder, learning disability, and epilepsy.

## Tuberous sclerosis

Tuberous sclerosis is a rare autosomal dominant disorder with a prevalence of 1/27 000, variable expressivity, and a high spontaneous mutation rate. There is genetic heterogeneity, with loci described in chromosomes 9 and 16. It is characterized by the presence of skin lesions (adenoma sebaceum), calcified subependymal nodules (tubers), and cortical dysplasias. Hamartomas and other neoplasms of the brain, heart, kidney, and liver are part of the picture.

- **Epilepsy** occurs in 60 to 80 per cent of patients, and infantile spasms, a type of epilepsy, with onset in the first 6 months of life, are particularly common.

- Moderate to severe **learning disability** is present in over 50 per cent of patients and is associated with the presence of infantile spasms and poorly controlled epilepsy.[29]

- **Autism** is 200 times more common in tuberous sclerosis than in the general population and tuberous sclerosis occurs in 1 per cent of autistic patients.[30]

- The number of cortical tubers detected by MRI is a marker of disease severity and is related to the degree of learning disability.[31] The presence of tubers in the temporal lobes has been reported to be associated with autism in patients with tuberous sclerosis.

*Management* is aimed at control of epilepsy and learning disability.

## Further information

Lishman, W.A. (1997). *Organic psychiatry: psychological consequences of cerebral disorder* (3rd edn). Blackwell, London.

Mitchell, A.J. (2003). *Neuropsychiatry and behavioural neurology explained*. WB Saunders, Edinburgh.

Rickards, H. (2005). Depression in neurological disorders: Parkinson's disease, multiple sclerosis, and stroke. *Journal of Neurology, Neurosurgery, and Psychiatry*, **76**(Suppl. 1), 48–52.

Burn, D.J. and Tröster, A.I. (2004). Neuropsychiatric complications of medical and surgical therapies for Parkinson's disease. *Journal of Geriatric Psychiatry and Neurology*, **17**, 172–80.

Siegert, R.J. and Abernethy, D.A. (2005). Depression in multiple sclerosis: a review. *Journal of Neurology, Neurosurgery and Psychiatry*, **76**, 469–75.

Amato, M.P., Zipoli, V., and Portaccio, E. (2006). Multiple sclerosis-related cognitive changes: a review of cross-sectional and longitudinal studies. *Journal of the Neurological Sciences*, **245**, 41–6.

Albin, R.L. and Mink, J.W. (2006). Recent advances in Tourette syndrome research. *Trends in Neurosciences*, **29**, 175–82.

Prather, P. and de Vries, P.J. (2004). Behavioral and cognitive aspects of tuberous sclerosis complex. *Journal of Child Neurology*, **19**, 666–74.

## References

1. Chan, K.-L., Campayo, A., Moser, D.J., *et al.* (2006). Aggressive behavior in patients with stroke: association with psychopathology and results of antidepressant treatment on aggression. *Archives of Physical Medicine and Rehabilitation*, **87**, 793–8.

2. Robinson, R.G. (1998). Relationship of depression to lesion location. In *The clinical neuropsychiatry of stroke: cognitive, behavioural and emotional disorders following vascular brain injury*, pp. 94–124. Cambridge University Press.

3. Sharpe, M., Hawton, K., Seagroatt, V., *et al.* (1994). Depressive disorders in long-term survivors of stroke: associations with demographic and social factors, functional status, and brain lesion volume. *The British Journal of Psychiatry*, **164**, 380–6.

4. Narushima, K., Chan, K.-L., Kosier, J.T., *et al.* (2003). The effect of early versus late antidepressant treatment on physical impairment associated with poststroke depression: is there a time-related therapeutic window? *The Journal of Nervous and Mental Disease*, **191**, 645–52.

5. Mayberg, H.S. and Solomon, D.H. (1995). Depression in Parkinson's disease: a biochemical and organic viewpoint. *Advances in Neurology*, **65**, 49–60.

6. House, A., Dennis, M., Mogridge, L., *et al.* (1991). Mood disorders in the year after stroke. *British Journal of Psychiatry*, **158**, 83–92.

7. House, A., Dennis, M., Molyneau, A., *et al.* (1989). Emotionalism after stroke. *British Medical Journal*, **198**, 991–4.

8. Brown, R. and Jahanshahi, M. (1995). Depression and Parkinson's disease: a psychosocial viewpoint. *Advances in Neurology*, **65**, 61–84.

9. Berney, A., Vingerhoets, F., Perrin, A., *et al.* (2002). Effect on mood of subthalamic DBS for Parkinson's disease: a consecutive series of 24 patients. *Neurology*, **59**, 1427–9.

10. Starkstein, S.E., Mayberg, H.S., Leiguarda, R., *et al.* (1992). A prospective longitudinal study of depression in patients with Parkinson's disease. *Journal of Neurology, Neurosurgery and Psychiatry*, **55**, 377–82.

11. Menza, M.A., Robertson–Hoffman, D.E., and Bonapace, A.S. (1993). Parkinson's disease and anxiety: comorbidity with depression. *Biological Psychiatry*, **34**, 465–70.

12. Remy, P., Doder, M., Lees, A., *et al.* (2005). Depression in Parkinson's disease: loss of dopamine and noradrenaline innervation in the limbic system. *Brain: a Journal of Neurology*, **128**, 1314–22.

13. Paulus, W. and Jellinger, K. (1991). The neuropathologic basis of different clinical subgroups of Parkinson's disease. *Journal of Neuropathology and Experimental Neurology*, **50**, 743–55.

14. Giovannoni, G., O'Sullivan, J.D., Turner, K., *et al.* (2000). Hedonistic homeostatic dysregulation in patients with Parkinson's disease on dopamine replacement therapies. *Journal of Neurology, Neurosurgery, and Psychiatry*, **68**, 423–8.

15. Robertson, M.M. and Stern, J.S. (1997). The Gilles de la Tourette syndrome. *Critical Reviews in Neurobiology*, **11**, 1–19.

16. Tanner, C.M. and Goldman, S.M. (1997). Epidemiology of Tourette syndrome. *Neurologic Clinics*, **15**, 395–402.

17. Eidelberg, D., Moeller, J.R., Antonini, A., *et al.* (1997). The metabolic anatomy of Tourette's syndrome. *Neurology*, **48**, 927–34.

18. Ron, M.A. and Logsdail, S.J. (1989). Psychiatric morbidity in multiple sclerosis. A clinical and MRI study. *Psychological Medicine*, **19**, 887–95.

19. Dark, F.L., McGrath, J.J., and Ron, M.A. (1996). Pathological laughing and crying. *The Australian and New Zealand Journal of Psychiatry*, **30**, 472–9.

20. Feinstein, A., du Boulay, G., and Ron, M.A. (1992). Psychotic illness in multiple sclerosis. A clinical and magnetic resonance imaging study. *British Journal of Psychiatry*, **161**, 680–5.

21. Goldman Consensus Group. (2005). The Goldman consensus statement on depression in multiple sclerosis. *Multiple Sclerosis*, **11**, 328–37.

22. Rao, S.M., Leo, G.J., Ellington, L., *et al.* (1991). Cognitive dysfunction in multiple sclerosis. II: impact on employment and social functioning. *Neurology*, **41**, 692–6.

23. Feinstein, A., Youl, B., and Ron, M. (1992). Acute optic neuritis: a cognitive and magnetic resonance imaging study. *Brain: a Journal of Neurology*, **115**, 1403–15.

24. Hotopf, M.H., Pollock, S., and Lishman, W.A. (1994). An unusual presentation of multiple sclerosis. Case report. *Psychological Medicine*, **24**, 525–8.

25. Hecaen, H. and Ajuriaguerra, J. (1956). *Troubles mentaux au cours des tumeurs intracraniennes*. Masson, Paris.

26. Ron, M.A. (1989). Psychiatric manifestations of frontal lobe tumours. *British Journal of Psychiatry*, **155**, 735–8.

27. Hyman, S.L., Shores, A., and North, K.N. (2003). The nature and frequency of cognitive deficits in children with neurofibromatosis type 1. *Neurology*, **65**, 1037–44.

28. Yohay, K. (2006). Neurofibromatosis types 1 and 2. *The Neurologist*, **12**, 86–93.

29. Jozwiak, S., Goodman, M., and Lamm, S.H. (1998). Poor mental development in patients with tuberous sclerosis complex: clinical risk factors. *Archives of Neurology*, **55**, 379–84.

30. Fombonne, E., Du Mazaubrun, C., Cans, C., *et al.* (1997). Autism and associated medical disorders in a French epidemiological survey. *Journal of the American Academy of Child and Adolescent Psychiatry*, **36**, 1561–9.

31. Joinson, C., O'Callaghan, F.J., Osborne, J.P., *et al.* (2003). Learning disability and epilepsy in an epidemiological sample of individuals with tuberous sclerosis complex. *Psychological Medicine*, **33**, 335–44.

## 5.3.3 Epilepsy

Brian Toone

### Introduction

An epileptic seizure has been defined as 'a clinical manifestation presumed to result from an abnormal and excessive discharge of a set of neurones in the brain'.[1] A diagnosis of epilepsy applies with the recurrence of two or more discrete and unprovoked seizures (febrile and neonatal seizures are excluded from this definition).

Epilepsy is one of the more common neurological disorders. It carries with it a greater psychiatric morbidity than is to be found in other neurological disorders of comparable severity. Many of its manifestations resemble and may be confused with psychiatric phenomenology. It is often associated with learning difficulties; it may be a manifestation of acquired brain damage or disease; seizures may occur in the course of substance abuse or be caused by psychiatric treatment. For these and for many other reasons psychiatrists should be familiar with epilepsy, its manifold aetiologies, presentations, and treatment.

### Classification: epileptic seizures and epilepsy

A comprehensive taxonomy should embrace classifications of both seizure semiology (i.e. the manifestations of abnormal discharge activity) and of epilepsy syndromes. The position of each seizure type in a seizure classification system is determined by its clinical manifestations, by electroencephalographic changes during the seizure, and by the interictal electroencephalographic abnormalities. A classification of epilepsy syndromes takes into account seizure subtype, and also anatomical substrate, aetiology, age of onset, and other characteristics. Seizure classification is dependent upon entities that are immediately ascertainable; epilepsy syndrome classification depends upon entities (e.g. neuroanatomical substrate) that are more speculative. The International League Against Epilepsy

(ILAE) has chosen to give the former priority, while recognizing the importance of the latter.

A familiarity with terminology, with the more common seizure subtypes, and the more commonly encountered epileptic syndromes, will assist in an understanding of the psychiatric disorders that occur in patients with epilepsy. The aura is a simple partial seizure, i.e. a seizure of focal onset in which consciousness is retained. It may progress to a complex partial seizure in which consciousness is disturbed, or into a generalized tonic, clonic, or tonic–clonic seizure. It may subside without further development. It rarely lasts for more than a few seconds, although patients often find time estimation difficult. It is to be distinguished from the epileptic prodrome, a period characterized by dysphoria, impaired memory and concentration, and minor motor manifestations, which precede the seizure and may last for hours or even days. An automatism may be defined as 'a state of clouding of consciousness which occurs during or after a seizure, and during which the individual retains the control of posture and muscle tone and performs simple or complex movements without being aware of what is happening'.[2] The initial phase, consisting of staring or simple chewing movements, may progress to more complex, stereotyped, and repetitive movements such as fumbling or picking. Automatisms rarely last more than a few minutes and are often very brief. They usually arise from temporal lobe discharges, but may be associated with orbital and mesial frontal lesions. The ictus refers to the period of manifest seizure activity. If this persists for 30 min or more it is described as status epilepticus and constitutes a medical emergency (Table 5.3.3.1).

## Seizure types

### Partial seizures

Partial seizures have a focal onset and may or may not generalize. They may be simple or complex, depending upon whether or not consciousness remains undisturbed. For this purpose, consciousness is defined as the ability to remain aware or to respond.

### (a) Simple partial seizures

The content of the simple partial seizure depends upon the site of the focus. One that arises from motor territory may present as a Jacksonian 'march' or as a versive turning of the head. Speech arrest may be present. A focus in the primary sensory cortex may give rise to poorly formed sensations. The more elaborate sensations and the psychic symptoms that arise, respectively, from the association

**Table 5.3.3.1** Classification of seizures

| |
|---|
| **1 Localization (partial, focal) seizures** |
|   (a) Simple partial seizures |
|   (b) Complex partial seizures |
|   (c) Partial seizures evolving to secondary generalized seizures |
| **2 Generalized seizures** |
|   (a) Absence seizures |
|   (b) Myoclonic jerks |
|   (c) Clonic seizures |
|   (d) Tonic seizures |
|   (e) Tonic–clonic seizures |
|   (f) Atonic seizures |

cortex and from the mesial frontotemporal structures are more likely to progress to complex partial seizures.

### (b) Complex partial seizures

These may begin as a simple partial seizure or 'aura', or consciousness may be impaired from the beginning. Characteristic auras include epigastric sensations rising into the thorax and olfactory and gustatory hallucinations, elaborated auditory and visual hallucinations, complex changes in perception (e.g. micropsia, depersonalization), and psychic phenomena such as *déjà vu*. As discharge activity spreads, automatic behaviour may supervene or a secondary generalized seizure may ensue. Complex partial seizures commonly arise from temporal, particularly mesial temporal, structures. Hence the obsolete term 'temporal lobe epilepsy'. They may also arise from the orbital and mesial frontal cortices. Complex partial status, previously known as temporal lobe status, is uncommon. It may present as an organic confusional state and may be mistaken for a florid psychosis. Electroencephalography will usually confirm the diagnosis.

### Generalized seizures

Both hemispheres are initially and simultaneously involved, the ictal electroencephalographic pattern and motor manifestations are bilateral and consciousness may be impaired from the onset.

### Tonic–clonic seizures

This is the common 'major' seizure formerly referred to as 'grand mal'. A brief tonic phase leads into clonic activity, the entire seizure lasting about 2 min. Generalized seizures may be primary, arising from both hemispheres simultaneously, or they may be due to secondary generalization from a focal onset.

### Absence seizures

An absence attack is characterized by abrupt cessation of ongoing activity, a vacant stare, and a period of unresponsiveness lasting from a few seconds to half a minute. The absence may be accompanied by brief clonic movements, especially of the eyelids, a reduction in tone causing the body to slump, or automatic movements. Absence seizures occur more commonly during childhood. The absence must be distinguished from the complex partial seizure, which it may resemble. Absence status is not uncommon in childhood and may be mistaken for inattention.

### Myoclonic seizures

These are brief shock-like contractions of groups of muscles.

## The epilepsy syndromes

The ILAE, in order to embrace a wider range of clinical features than is possible in a classification based on seizure types, introduced a classification of seizures and epilepsy syndromes. In this classification the broad division lies between the localization-related or partial epilepsies, the great majority of which, in adults, is made up of symptomatic epilepsies (i.e. epilepsy arising from a known or suspected cause) and the generalized epilepsies. The characteristics of the partial epilepsies are determined by the function of the cortical site from which the seizure emanates. The more common generalized epilepsies are age-related. Though admirable in concept, the classification has proved unwieldy and the terminology clumsy: as such it seems unlikely to displace the seizure-type classification.

## Epidemiology

The cumulative incidence (i.e. lifetime risk) is 3.4 per cent for males, 2.8 per cent for females, but the prevalence is only 7 per 1000. This is because prevalence represents the balance between newly diagnosed cases and permanent remission or death, and epilepsy has a good prognosis with 76 per cent of newly diagnosed cases entering long-term remission.[3] Approximately half can be classified as partial seizures and 40 per cent as generalized. Prognosis varies according to the epilepsy subtype, with partial epilepsy having a poorer outcome. Consequently, people who attend a hospital clinic are unrepresentative, in that they are more likely to have treatment-refractory partial seizures along with the other adverse prognostic factors such as mental handicap, neurological dysfunction, or psychiatric disorders.

## Aetiology

Aetiology varies according to the age of onset. In childhood- and adolescence-inherited disorders of metabolism, ante- and perinatal complications, infection, migrational errors, and the consequences of febrile convulsions predominate, in middle life trauma and tumour are most common, and in advanced years cerebrovascular disease and degenerative disorders are predominant.

Only one-quarter to one-third of cases of epilepsy are due to known causes. Many others fall into recognizable syndromes about which much is understood. The partial epilepsies are, by definition, due to focal areas of damage and dysfunction usually involving the cortex. However, although the site may be suggested by the seizure semiology, comprehensive investigation may fail to identify any abnormality. Even when it does so, the radiological appearance may lack aetiological specificity. Some generalized seizures may be identified as primary generalized epilepsy syndromes; for example, juvenile myoclonic epilepsy. These are of uncertain aetiology, though genetic factors are considered important; onset is in childhood or adolescence and the prognosis favourable.

In psychiatric practice seizures may arise iatrogenically; they are usually due to pharmacotherapy, less commonly to electroconvulsive therapy. They may result from the overhasty withdrawal of benzodiazepines or to the use of antidepressant or antipsychotic drugs, most of which are epileptogenic. Such seizures are thought to be provoked and do not form grounds for a diagnosis of epilepsy. Adjustment of drug dosage is usually all that is required. Provoked seizures may also occur during alcohol intoxication ('rum fits') or withdrawal; a genetic predisposition may play a part.

## Diagnosis

The diagnosis of epilepsy depends first and foremost on historical information; the patient's own account of the seizure and the observations of a reliable informant are of tantamount importance. A family history of epilepsy should be sought; age of onset should be determined when possible. A history of birth complications, febrile fits, early head injury, or cerebral infection is of particular importance in seizures starting in childhood, adolescence, or early adult life. In middle life symptoms suggestive of developing intracranial pathology and in later life cerebrovascular and degenerative

disorders should be sought. The clinician should be aware of specific circumstances and situations that may provoke seizures: alcohol or substance abuse, prescribed drugs that have epileptogenic properties, and intermittent photic stimulation. Physical examination will detect not only gross congenital abnormalities such as tuberosclerosis, but also more subtle features, for example facial or skull asymmetries. The differential diagnosis varies according to age group, but will include vasovagal attacks and pseudoseizures, particularly in the young, vertigo and transient ischaemic attacks in the elderly, and cardiogenic syncope, hypoglycaemic episodes, and migraine at any age.

The role of physical investigation is to confirm the diagnosis of epilepsy when this is in doubt and to identify the cause; it may also help to determine the type of epilepsy and, in the partial epilepsies, the site of seizure onset. Magnetic resonance scanning is now widely available and all new cases of adult-onset epilepsy and patients of any age with partial epilepsy should have the benefit of this technology. A sleep electroencephalograph is still mandatory and may be invaluable not only in differential diagnosis, but in determining the epilepsy subtype and seizure localization. Video-telemetry is invaluable when there is continuing diagnostic uncertainty, and in those cases in which precise localization is necessary for presurgical assessment. Functional neuroimaging may also aid localization.

In psychiatric practice epileptic seizures must be distinguished from psychogenic pseudoseizures, panic attacks, and aggressive episodes. The pseudoseizure may take different forms: the patient may fall or slump to the ground and remain still as in a syncopal attack; or there may be jerking or thrashing of limbs resembling a major tonic–clonic seizure. The absence of tongue-biting, incontinence, or significant injury is often said to distinguish the pseudoseizure from the epileptic seizure, but such guides are frequently unreliable. A history of other conversion disorders or illness behaviour may be obtained, but pseudoseizures also occur in individuals with epilepsy. A detailed description of the attack from the patient and from a witness will be of the greatest assistance in diagnosis, but when in serious doubt video-telemetry may offer a definitive answer. Other useful investigations include serum prolactin levels, which rise postictally to reach a peak between 20 and 30 min after a major epileptic seizure. Episodes of panic are sometimes mistaken for epileptic seizures. Extreme anxiety, especially when accompanied by hyperventilation, may lead to a subjective diminution in awareness, altered perception, and other features suggestive of complex partial seizures. The context in which the attack occurs, a description of initial autonomic arousal, and other symptoms of anxiety should lead to the correct diagnosis. Sudden outbursts of aggressive behaviour, particularly when out of character and context, often give rise to suspicions of epilepsy. Aggression, especially directed aggression, is extremely unusual as a feature of the epileptic seizure, though it may occasionally be seen during the phase of postictal confusion or postictal psychosis.

## The psychiatric consequences of epilepsy

The prevalence of psychiatric morbidity among persons with epilepsy is greater than in the general population, but the increase in prevalence will vary according to the type of epilepsy, the presence and extent of brain damage, and the presence of cognitive and physical disability. The more reliable studies are drawn from community samples. Of children between the ages of 5 and 14 years, 29 per cent showed some psychiatric disorder compared with 6.8 per cent of the general population. The figure rose to 58 per cent when brain damage was present.[4] Pond and Bidwell[5] surveyed 14 general practices and reported a prevalence of 29 per cent in adults, increasing to over 50 per cent in patients with temporal lobe epilepsy. Neurotic disability accounted for the great majority of cases. Psychiatric morbidity is over-represented in clinic attenders and in patients with partial epilepsy.[6]

## Personality disorder and social development

Notions of an epileptic personality arising out of a hereditary 'taint' persisted well into the present century. The person with epilepsy was said to be explosively aggressive, rigid, egocentric, and irritable. These beliefs were formed by observations of often oversedated inmates of epileptic institutions. The concept of a specific epileptic personality has now largely been abandoned, though it is acknowledged that some features associated with, but not specific to, epilepsy may exercise a powerful influence on personality development. Many of these are consequences of brain damage rather than epilepsy as such. Thus learning difficulties, leading to limited educational opportunity, adult unemployment, and socioeconomic disadvantage may be significant personality determinants. But even in the epileptic individual without brain damage the sedative actions of anticonvulsant medication, the continuing stigma of seizure activity, and the social and occupational constraints are not without their effects on the developing personality.

A particular link between temporal epilepsy and abnormalities of personality has long been debated[7] and certain exaggerated traits (e.g. hypergraphia) are consistently reported,[8] but many of the personality difficulties may be explained by the refractory nature of temporal lobe seizures and the need for increased medication.

## Psychoses

### (a) Chronic interictal psychoses

Throughout the first half of this century the relationship between epilepsy and schizophrenia was debated at length, usually in terms of whether the presence of one condition encouraged or discouraged the development of the other—the affinity and antagonism hypotheses, respectively. In recent years, particularly following the publication of Slater's seminal studies,[9] informed opinion has moved firmly behind the first view. Epidemiological studies based on national registers[10,11] find a higher prevalence of chronic psychosis in epileptic subjects than in the general population. A neurology outpatient clinic study[12] reported schizophrenia to be nine times more common in epilepsy than in a migraine control group. The onset, cause, and clinical characteristics are, to a very large extent, indistinguishable from those of more usual forms of schizophrenia, although negative symptoms occur less frequently, thought disorder is rarely encountered and the outcome may be more benign. Psychosis usually develops 11–15 years following the onset of epilepsy. The aetiology remains uncertain. Cases in which the epilepsy takes the form of complex partial seizures arising from the mesial temporal or frontal lobes are over-represented; there may be a slight left-sided predominance. A family history of schizophrenia was thought to be unusual, but some recent studies have cast doubt on this assumption. Neuropathological examination, more readily available with the increasing practice of epilepsy

surgery, has proved less informative than had been hoped, but subjects undergoing temporal lobectomy for resection of small neurodevelopmental lesions, e.g. ganglioglioma, dysembryoplastic neuroepithelioma (DNET)[13] appear at greater risk of developing a post-operative chronic interictal psychosis. The results of structural neuroimaging studies have been inconclusive with reports of both reduction and increase in amygdala size. The risk of bipolar illness or affective psychosis does not appear to be increased in epilepsy.

### (b) Postictal psychosis

The other common form of epileptic psychosis develops following an exacerbation of seizure activity. Because of this close temporal relationship the instrumental role of epilepsy in the aetiology of the psychosis is not open to question. The salient characteristics have been described.[14] The psychosis usually occurs following a cluster of complex partial seizures usually followed by secondary generalization. Characteristically, the subject appears to make a complete recovery, but 1 to 2 days later, the so-called lucid interval, becomes floridly psychotic. Affective, schizophrenic, and confusional elements may be present. An electroencephalogram recorded at the time shows increased focal discharge activity, though less than would be seen in partial status. Spontaneous recovery is to be expected, usually within a week of onset. The first episode is usually delayed until early adult life, a decade and a half after the first seizure. Half of those affected will have further similar episodes. Fifteen to 20 per cent will progress to develop a chronic interictal psychosis. Bilateral EEG discharges are seen more commonly in those patients who develop postictal psychosis. Functional neuroimaging at the time of the psychosis demonstrates relative mesial temporal hyperperfusion suggestive of an active process, either continuous seizure discharge or seizure inhibition.

Rarely, the introduction of certain anticonvulsant drugs may seem to precipitate psychotic episodes. This may be associated with rapid seizure control and give rise to the term 'forced normalization'.[15] In recent years vigabatrin has seemed to be the drug most responsible.

## Sexual function

A diminution in sexual interest, a decrease in activity, and impaired performance are the most common aspects of sexual dysfunction in epilepsy. Men have been studied more thoroughly than women. In patients receiving antiepilepsy drugs libido may be diminished and erectile potency impaired. Levels of free testosterone, the biologically active hormone, may be diminished. Sperm concentrations may be reduced, morphological abnormalities may occur more commonly and mobility may be reduced. Menstrual irregularities are increased in women with epilepsy and are related to seizure frequency, polytherapy with antiepilepsy drugs, and the use of sodium valproate. Infertility, ovulation, and the polycystic ovarian syndrome occur more commonly. Hyposexuality may be more pronounced in patients with partial epilepsy, but this may simply reflect the refractory nature of partial epilepsy and the greater amount of drugs prescribed.[16,17]

## Epilepsy and crime

There is an association between epilepsy and criminal activity. Male epileptics are three times more likely to receive a criminal conviction,[18] in England and Wales between 0.7 and 0.8 per cent of the prison population suffers from epilepsy, a figure considerably higher than in the general population,[19] but the pattern of offence does not differ. The reasons for this are unclear. Low intelligence and low socioeconomic class are common to both epilepsy and prison populations; the role of brain damage as distinct from epilepsy has not been fully evaluated. Crimes of violence in the context of disturbed ictal or postictal behaviour do occur, but are extremely rare.[20]

## Neurotic illness

Neurotic illness, more especially anxiety and depression, largely account for the increased psychiatric morbidity that is to be found in patients with epilepsy. These disorders have few distinctive characteristics. They may be explained by the adverse social, educational, and economic disadvantages that confront people with epilepsy. A phobic anxiety akin to agoraphobia may be seen in some individuals who fear the onset of a seizure in public places. Obsessive–compulsive disorder does not seem to occur more commonly in epilepsy.

## Epilepsy and suicide

Suicide is increased fivefold among patients with epilepsy, but is considerably higher among those with temporal lobe epilepsy.[21] Among patients presenting with self-harm, epileptic subjects are over-represented from five- to sevenfold.[22]

## Treatment

Seizure control is most effectively achieved through the appropriate use of anticonvulsant drugs. The use of behavioural techniques to inhibit seizure activity holds promise, but is still in its infancy. Surgical treatment is increasingly available, but should only be considered for those patients who have failed repeatedly to respond to drug therapy and who have resectable lesions. Drug treatment should aim to achieve seizure control through the use of a single anticonvulsant drug, thus minimizing unwanted side-effects. This should be possible in the great majority of patients. If a first-choice drug fails, a second-choice drug should be substituted. Polytherapy may be necessary, notably in the management of partial seizures, but should be avoided wherever possible. Most first-line drugs, except phenytoin, are described in Chapter 6.2.6. Phenytoin, although relatively toxic, especially to the cerebellum, is an effective anticonvulsant and still widely prescribed. Serum monitoring is particularly important. More recently introduced drugs include topiramate and levetiracetam. The benzodiazepines, clobazam and clonazepam, may be used in adjunctive therapy. Lamotrigine and levetiracetam appear to be as efficacious as the longer established drugs and have less side-effects. There is little place for either phenobarbitone, which is unduly sedative and may cause depression and behavioural disturbance especially in children and adolescents, or vigabatrin, which may cause visual field constrictions. Vigabatrin, and to a lesser extent topiramate may cause psychotic episodes. The need for continuing anticonvulsant therapy should be reviewed by a specialist neurologist once the patient has been free of seizures for 2 years. For a more detailed account of the management of epilepsy and of status epilepticus the reader is referred to Shorvon et al.[23]

The treatment and outcome for psychogenic seizures have received increasing attention. The importance of early diagnosis is emphasized.[24] Psychological treatment, particularly cognitive–behavioural therapy, can be effective. Reduction or cessation of symptoms can be achieved in at least half of the cases within a 6–12 month period.

## Further information

Asbury, A.K., McKhann, G.M., et al. (eds.) (1992). *Diseases of the nervous system* (2nd edn). W.B. Saunders, Philadelphia, PA.

Hopkins, A., Shorvon, S., and Cascino, G. (eds.) (1995). *Epilepsy* (2nd edn). Chapman & Hall Medical, London.

Lishman, W.A. (1998). *Organic psychiatry* (3rd edn). Blackwell Science, Oxford.

Trimble, M.R. (1991). *The psychoses of epilepsy*. Raven Press, New York.

## References

1. Hopkins, A. and Shorvon, S. (1995). Definitions and epidemiology of epilepsy. In *Epilepsy* (2nd edn) (eds. A. Hopkins, S. Shorvon, and G. Cascino), pp. 1–25. Chapman & Hall Medical, London.

2. Fenton, G.W. (1981). Psychiatric disorder of epilepsy: classification and phenomenology. In *Epilepsy and psychiatry* (eds. E.H. Reynolds and M.R. Trimble), pp. 12–26. Churchill Livingstone, Edinburgh.

3. Annegers, J.F., Hauser, W.A., and Elveback, L.R. (1979). Remission of seizures and relapse in patients with epilepsy. *Epilepsia*, 20, 729–37.

4. Graham, P. and Rutter, M. (1968). Organic brain dysfunction and child psychiatric disorder. *British Medical Journal*, 3, 695–700.

5. Pond, D.A. and Bidwell, B.H. (1960). A survey of epilepsy in fourteen general practices. II. Social and psychological aspects. *Epilepsia*, 1, 285–99.

6. Edeh, J., Toone, B.K., and Corney, R.H. (1990). Epilepsy, psychiatric morbidity, and social dysfunction in general practice. *Neuropsychiatry, Neuropsychology and Behavioural Neurology*, 3, 180–92.

7. Bear, D.M. and Fedio, P. (1977). Quantitative analysis of inter-ictal behaviour in temporal lobe epilepsy. *Archives of Neurology*, 34, 454–67.

8. Waxman, S.G. and Geschwind, N. (1974). Hypergraphia in temporal lobe epilepsy. *Neurology*, 24, 629–36.

9. Slater, E., Beard, A.W., and Glithero, E. (1963). The schizophrenia-like psychoses of epilepsy. *British Journal of Psychiatry*, 109, 95–150.

10. Bredkjaer, S.R., Mortensen, P.B., and Parnas, J. (1998). Epilepsy and non-organic non-affective psychosis. National epidemiological study. *British Journal of Psychiatry*, 172, 235–9.

11. Stefansson, S.B., Olafsson, E., and Hauser, W.A. (1998). Psychiatric morbidity in epilepsy: a case control study of adults receiving disability benefit. *Journal of Neurology, Neurosurgery and Psychiatry*, 64, 238–41.

12. Mendez, M.F., Grau, R., Doss, R.C., et al. (1993). Schizophrenia in epilepsy: seizure and psychosis variables. *Neurology*, 43, 1073–7.

13. Andermann, L.F., Savard, G., Meencke, H.J., et al. (1999). Psychosis after resection of ganglioglioma or DNET: evidence for an association. *Epilepsia*, 40, 83–7.

14. Logsdail, S.J. and Toone, B.K. (1988). Post-ictal psychoses. *British Journal of Psychiatry*, 152, 246–52.

15. Landolt, H. (1953). Some clinical EEG correlations in epileptic psychoses (twilight states). *EEG and Clinical Neurophysiology*, 5, 121.

16. Toone, B.K. (1995). Epilepsy and sexual life. In *Epilepsy* (2nd edn) (eds. A. Hopkins, S. Shorvon, and G. Cascino), pp. 555–65. Chapman & Hall Medical, London.

17. Hertzog, A.G. and Fowler, K.M. (2005). Sexual hormones and epilepsy: threat and opportunities. *Current Opinion in Neurology*, 18, 167–172.

18. Gudmundsson, G. (1966). Epilepsy in Iceland. A clinical and epidemiological investigation. *Acta Neurologica Scandinavica*, 25, 7–124.

19. Gunn, J. and Fenton, G.W. (1971). Epilepsy, automatism and crime. *Lancet*, i, 1173–6.

20. Delgado-Escueta, A.V., Mattson, R.H., King, L., *et al.* (1981). The nature of aggression during epileptic seizures. *New England Journal of Medicine*, **305**, 7110–16.

21. Barraclough, B. (1981). Suicide and epilepsy. In *Epilepsy and psychiatry* (eds. E.H. Reynolds and M.R. Trimble), pp. 72–6. Churchill Livingstone, Edinburgh.

22. Hawton, K., Fagg, J., and Marsack, P. (1980). Association between epilepsy and attempted suicide. *Journal of Neurology, Neurosurgery and Psychiatry*, **43**, 168–70.

23. Shorvon, S., Dreifuss, F., Fish, D., *et al.* (eds.) (1996). *The treatment of epilepsy*. Blackwell Science, Oxford.

24. Reuber, M., Fernandéz, G. Bauer, J., *et al.* (2002). Diagnostic delay in psychogenic non-epileptic seizures. *Neurology*, **58**, 493–5.

# 5.3.4 Medical conditions associated with psychiatric disorder

James R. Rundell

## Introduction

Seven out of 10 office visits to a primary care practitioner are related to a chronic illness.[1] There are high levels of association of many of these chronic conditions with psychiatric disorders.[1] Comorbid medical and psychiatric conditions increase use of medical resources and costs, as well as amplify functional impairment.[2] For example, depression is associated with an approximately 50 per cent increase in medical costs of chronic medical illness, even after controlling for severity of physical illness.[2, 3] Dementia is associated with hospital costs up to 75 per cent higher than for non-demented patients.[4]

As important as a comprehensive knowledge of psychiatric diagnosis and psychosocial formulation is to a consulting psychiatrist, it is also vital to understand the pathophysiology and clinical characteristics of the medical and surgical conditions that frequently coexist with psychiatric disorders. It is also important to know the behavioural and psychiatric side effects of medications and substances. Lacking this data permits only a partial and inadequate approach to diagnosis and treatment.

This section describes general medical disorders associated with psychiatric syndromes. The pathophysiology and clinical characteristics of the medical disorder are described first, followed by psychiatric syndromes often seen with that diagnosis.

## Cardiovascular disorders

### Ventricular dysrhythmias

Sudden cardiac death is responsible for 300 000 deaths annually in the United States.[5,6] Sympathetic nervous system activity increases the likelihood of ventricular dysrhythmias[6] especially when there is prior ischaemic damage. Sympathetic nervous system stimulation, which increases heart rate, can trigger ectopic sites in the myocardium, which override normal conductive pathways, producing potentially fatal dysrhythmias. Either the peripheral sympathetic nervous system or the central nervous system can generate stimuli leading to this phenomenon. Therefore, anxiety and stress may increase the risk of dysrhythmia.[7] Among individuals with pre-existing heart disease or dysrhythmias, activities which precipitate adrenergic discharge may produce ventricular dysrhythmias—for example, public speaking, road rage, and recall of emotionally charged events.[8] In one series of patients, psychological stressors were more reliable triggers of dysrhythmias than physical manoeuvres such as carotid sinus massage, hyperventilation, and the Valsalva manoeuvre.[8] Simple and inexpensive non-pharmacological techniques such as relaxation training, hypnosis, and medication have been shown to improve ventricular dysrhythmias.[8, 9]

Depression has also been associated with lower threshold for ventricular dysrhythmias.[10] Patients with depression exhibit dysregulation of the sympathoadrenal system—hypothalamic corticotropin releasing factor-containing neurons appear to stimulate several autonomic centres involved in regulating sympathetic activity.[11] Smith *et al.*[8] found that deaths within 18 months of a myocardial infarction were concentrated among depressed patients with 10 or more premature ventricular contractions per hour. In this group of patients, 83 per cent of mortality was due to 'arrhythmic deaths'.

### Hypertension

More than 60 million Americans have hypertension. The prevalence among whites is about 15 per cent, but is over 25 per cent in the African–American population. 95 per cent of people with hypertension have primary, or idiopathic, hypertension. The remaining 5 per cent have secondary hypertension, due to conditions or substances such as renal disease, steroids, or oral contraceptives. Managing hypertension reduces the morbidity and mortality of the condition. Constitutional and stress-related factors contribute to hypertension. Patients with hypertension, in general, have a more prolonged vasoconstrictive response to psychological stress than patients with normotension,[12] which may result in both short-term and long-term blood pressure elevation due to this interplay of environmental and constitutional factors.[13]

### Myocardial infarction

Myocardial ischaemia often leads to myocardial infarction. Acute myocardial infarction can develop at rest or with normal activity. Deaths associated with acute myocardial infarction occur during the first few hours after the onset of symptoms, and are the result of ventricular fibrillation. It is important that patients know the warning signs and seek care promptly when symptoms develop. Unfortunately, as many as 20 per cent of myocardial infarctions are unrecognized. Denial of acute myocardial infarction symptoms and warning signs by individuals, particularly men, are a frequent source of mortality and morbidity. The roles of gender-specific differences in terms of establishing predictors for clinical outcomes is understudied.[14]

The most common precipitant of myocardial ischaemia among patients with pre-existing coronary artery disease is stress.[15] Stress-induced ischaemia is more common than ischaemia induced by physical stressors. Recovery from a myocardial infarction is also highly dependent on psychosocial factors. Ruberman *et al.*[16] demonstrated that postmyocardial infarction patients, who are socially isolated and have high stress levels, have at least four times the risk of death, compared to their counterparts who have lower levels of stress and isolation. Particularly, lack of a close confidant predicts negative outcomes after myocardial infarction, including further cardiac events.[17] In addition, emotional distress after myocardial infarction is associated with poorer outcomes in terms of quality of life and psychological adjustment.[18]

Depression may occur in 31 per cent of patients admitted for acute myocardial infarction.[19] Presence of major depressive disorder in a patient with cardiac disease has a significant association with morbidity and mortality. Carney *et al.*[20] found that major depressive disorder was the best single predictor of myocardial infarction, angioplasty, and death during the 12 months following cardiac catheterization. Patients with a history of myocardial infarction and major depressive disorder are up to three to five times more likely to die within 6 months of discharge than non-depressed patients following infarction.[19] As to how depression increases risk include hypothalamic–pituitary–adrenocortical and/or sympathoadrenal hyperactivity, diminished heart rate responsivity, ventricular instability, myocardial ischaemia due to stress, and alterations in platelet receptors and reactivity.[21, 22] The data are limited, antidepressant treatment, stress management, and relaxation training in patients with coronary artery disease or myocardial infarction and major depression probably reduces mortality.[23]

### Type A and type D personality

Assessment of the patient's personality and behavioural style is important because type A behavioural patterns increase the risk of a myocardial infarction.[24] The type A behaviour pattern includes ambitiousness, aggressiveness, competitiveness, impatience, muscle tenseness, alertness, rapid and emphatic vocal style, irritation, cynicism, hostility, and an increased potential for anger. Very frequently, such individuals are also hard-working 'workaholics' who deny physical or emotional vulnerability. Their self-esteem is often dependent on constant achievement. Unstable cardiac function poses an immediate and ongoing threat to them, and challenges their need to be in control of their environment and bodies. Many clinicians believe that modifying a type A behaviour pattern is an integral part of preventing future myocardial infarctions.[24] Group or individual psychotherapy that reduces type A behaviour and other behavioural risks has been shown to lower the incidence of recurrent infarction and cardiac death in patients with a previous myocardial infarction.[25]

There has been recent attention to the type D personality construct.[26, 27] D behaviour is characterized by inhibition of negative emotions and avoiding social contacts with others. D personality patients may be at increased risk for cardiovascular morbidity and mortality.[26] Cortisol may be a mediating factor for this increased risk. D personality predicts cardiac events after controlling for concurrent stress and anxiety.[27] Studies are needed to validate this personality construct, further define associations with cardiac outcome, and develop treatment approaches for patients with this personality style.

## Respiratory disorders

### Asthma

Asthma affects between 3 and 5 per cent of the population of the United States. The three hallmarks of the disease are airway inflammation, airway hyperresponsiveness, and a partially reversible airway

obstruction. It is one of the classic 'psychosomatic diseases'. Emotional arousal causes changes in airway tone. The severity of an asthma attack is highly correlated with presence of major depressive disorder, panic attacks, general anxiety, and level of fear among children, adolescents, and adults.[28] Asthma patients with psychiatric disorders have worse asthma control, more frequent exacerbations, and worse quality of life than asthma patients without psychiatric disorders.[29] Education, relaxation, biofeedback, and family therapy have each shown efficacy in the management of asthma.[30] Important in the management of asthma is education about the adverse effects of antiasthma medications, which include jitteriness, palpitations, and insomnia. These side effects may require treatment with behavioural and/or psychopharmacological therapies.

### Chronic obstructive pulmonary disease

Patients with chronic obstructive pulmonary disease (COPD) have slowly progressive airway obstruction. The course of the disease is punctuated by exacerbations due to pulmonary infection, heart failure, and poor compliance with prescribed therapy. Generally affects middle-aged and older patients. They present with dyspnoea, exercise intolerance, cough, and sputum production. Physical examination reveals lung overinflation, prominent use of accessory muscles to augment respiration, diminished breath sounds, and diffuse wheezing. As with asthma, pharmacological treatments for COPD can cause psychiatric symptoms, especially higher doses of steroid medications. Patients with COPD must stop smoking; pulmonary function declines faster in smokers who develop COPD than non-smokers who develop COPD.

The chronic hypoxia caused by COPD compromises cognition and mood, which, in turn, can produce delirium, mood lability, mood disorders, and restriction in daily activities. Depression is present in 20–60 per cent of COPD patients.[31] Depression adversely affects treatment adherence and may increase risk for poor outcomes. There is considerable evidence that supplemental oxygen improves cognitive function and quality of life.[30] Unfortunately, mood improvement with supplemental oxygen has not been conclusively demonstrated.

Panic attacks are reported in up to 38 per cent of patients with COPD.[32] Benzodiazepines, which are highly effective for controlling panic attacks, have limited usefulness in patients with COPD because they can suppress respiratory function and if used chronically result in tolerance and dependence. Carbon dioxide likely plays a role in promoting panic attacks; carbon dioxide levels increase with COPD disease progression. Antidepressants are useful in patients with COPD who develop panic attacks. Low-dose neuroleptic medications (e.g. 0.5–1.0 mg risperidone orally two to three times daily) are also sometimes used for severe fear and panic, especially in intensive care unit settings (e.g. when weaning the patient from a respirator). Neuroleptics do not directly suppress respiration, though caution must be exercised so that the sedation induced by neuroleptics—potentially combined with other sedating agents—does not reduce respiratory effort beyond that required to maintain adequate oxygenation. Function must also be monitored to ensure that neuroleptic use does not affect cardiac conduction or cause dysrhythmias.

### Pulmonary embolism

Patients with psychiatric disorders, including bipolar disorder, anxiety disorder, and schizophrenia, are at increased risk for pulmonary embolism.[33] Embolism may account for a portion of the excess risk of death among people with schizophrenia, even after controlling for blood pressure, cholesterol, body mass index, smoking, exercise, alcohol intake, and education level.[34] Most thromboemboli originate in the deep veins of the thigh. The diagnosis of pulmonary embolus is often missed because the clinical findings are non-specific. They include dyspnoea, pleuritic chest pain, haemoptysis, tachypnoea, and wheezing or crackles on pulmonary examination. Number of factors predispose to pulmonary thromboemboli: cancer, stroke, myocardial infarction, congestive heart failure, sepsis, pregnancy, lower extremity fractures, major surgical procedures, polycythaemia vera, and paroxysmal nocturnal haemoglobinuria. Pulmonary emboli are treated with heparin and warfarin. Fibrinolytic drugs and acute embolectomy are used in certain situations. The differential diagnosis of sudden anxiety or a panic attack includes pulmonary embolus.

### Sleep apnoea

Apnoea is defined as the complete cessation of respiratory airflow for 10 or more seconds.[35] Apnoea can occur during any sleep stage, but is particularly likely to occur during the period of rapid eye movement sleep. It is important to remember that normal people have apnoeic episodes during sleep. When apnoeic events are frequent and prolonged, they lead to chronically disrupted sleep and excessive daytime somnolence. This defines the condition known as sleep apnoea. Sleep apnoea can be central, obstructive, or a mixture of the two. Central sleep apnoea is caused by an abnormal central drive to the respiratory muscles. Congestive heart failure is the most common cause, followed by neurological disorders involving the brainstem and respiratory centres. Obstructive sleep apnoea is more common; obesity is a major risk factor, but is not always present. Aside from disrupted sleep and daytime somnolence, associated symptoms include an inability to concentrate, depressed mood, irritability, and personality changes. The sleeping partner often sleeps in another room because of the individual's very loud snoring, snorting, gasping, and restlessness. Treatment with continuous positive airway pressure is often effective. Patients should avoid sedatives and alcohol. If obese, they should lose weight.

## Gastrointestinal disorders

### Oesophageal dysmotility

Oesophageal dysmotility can be demonstrated in 30 per cent of patients with non-cardiac chest pain;[36] a significant number of non-cardiac chest pain patients lack any evidence of oesophageal reflux and have reduced perception thresholds for pain. Cases of oesophageal dysmotility often lead to psychiatric consultation. Situational stress has not been conclusively linked to oesophageal dysmotility, but major psychiatric illness has.[37] The majority of patients with oesophageal motility disorders have an Axis I psychiatric illness, especially major depressive disorder (52 per cent), generalized anxiety disorder (36 per cent), somatization disorder (20 per cent), and substance-related disorders (20 per cent).[38] Smooth muscle relaxants, such as calcium-channel blockers, are superior to psychiatric treatments in improving physiological measures (such as oesophageal motility testing), antidepressants, and behavioural therapies produce more impressive changes in patients' subjective oesophageal complaints and level of psychological well-being.[39]

### Irritable bowel syndrome

Irritable bowel syndrome (IBS) ranks second only to the common cold as a cause of absenteeism from work,[40, 41] affecting between 8 and 17 per cent of the general population in the United States.[40] Symptoms include abdominal pain (relieved by defecation), and various forms of disturbed defecation such as altered stool frequency, altered stool form, altered stool passage, passage of mucus, and bloating. Symptoms must be continuous or recur within 3 months to meet the criteria for a diagnosis of irritable bowel syndrome. The severity of this syndrome frequently correlates with periods of emotional stress; the sympathetic nervous system inhibits gastric motility.

The enteric nervous system contains approximately 100 million neurons, close to the same number found in the spinal cord,[41] and more than those distributed to any other organ or physiological system. It therefore, makes sense that the gastrointestinal tract is uniquely sensitive to the neurophysiological aspects of the stress response. With IBS who seek medical care exhibit high rates of psychiatric disorders. The most frequently occurring are panic disorder (26 per cent), generalized anxiety disorder (26 per cent), social phobia (26 per cent), and major depressive disorder (23 per cent).[42] Patients with irritable bowel syndrome who are depressed and complain of diarrhoea may benefit from tricyclic antidepressant treatment, at least partially because of their anticholinergic effects. Anxious patients may also benefit from, and well-tolerate buspirone. At least one in eight IBS patients are offered an antidepressant,[43] though data suggest that antidepressants are more consistent in improving global measures than specific gastrointestinal symptoms. A group of patients with treatment-refractory irritable bowel syndrome—nearly half had no psychiatric disorder—more than 90 per cent benefited from low-dose antidepressant or antianxiety medications: 92 per cent of patients improved, and 56 per cent experienced complete remission of irritable bowel symptoms.

### Inflammatory bowel disease

Inflammatory bowel disease is the collective term for patients who have ulcerative colitis or Crohn's disease. The aetiology of inflammatory bowel disease is unknown, but it may involve immunological, infectious, or environmental factors.[44] The primary manifestations of acute ulcerative colitis are rectal bleeding, diarrhoea, urgency, fever, weight loss, and, sometimes, abdominal pain. Crohn's disease presents with malaise, fever, abdominal pain, and frequently rectal bleeding. Surgical treatment (colectomy) cures ulcerative colitis but not Crohn's disease. However, surgery is usually a last resort in ulcerative colitis.

Despite the strong beliefs of early psychosomatic theorists, there is no objective evidence that psychiatric disorders cause inflammatory bowel disease. However, patients with this disease and who have psychiatric disorders are more likely to have unexplained physical symptoms in other organ systems, more disability than patients with similar disease severity and no psychiatric disorder, and prior histories of physical and sexual abuse.[45] Exacerbations of inflammatory bowel disease symptoms are positively associated with major life events and major stressors.[41,46] Stress-induced alterations in gastrointestinal inflammation may be mediated through changes in hypothalamic–pituitary–adrenal axis function and alterations in bacterial-mucosal interactions, and via mucosal mast cells and mediators such as corticotrophin releasing factor.[47] Treatment focuses on the identification and treatment of psychiatric disorders, if found, and on stress management and quality of life issues. Walker et al.[44] treated inflammatory bowel disease patients who had major depression with an antidepressant and found marked improvement in depression and ability to function. Relaxation, stress management,[45, 48] and hypnotherapy were found to reduce abdominal pain and diarrhoea.

### Gastroesophageal reflux and peptic ulcer disease

Acid reflux and peptic ulcer disease are common causes of non-cardiac chest pain.[49] Ulcer disease occurs when the balance between stomach acid and mucosal defence factors is disrupted. Gastric acid, *Helicobacter pylori*, and non-steroidal antiinflammatory drugs are the most important risk factors in the development of peptic ulcers.[50] The majority of patients with peptic ulcer disease are present with epigastric pain that begins 1 to 3 h after eating. Treatment is aimed at reducing gastric acid (e.g. using cimetidine and ranitidine), improving mucosal defences (with, for instance, sucralfate), and/or eradicating *H. pylori* (antibiotics).

On examination, at least half of the patients initially suspected of having peptic ulcer disease do not have evidence of an ulcer.[51] Among patients with non-ulcer dyspepsia, psychiatric comorbidity is high. Magni reported that 87 per cent of patients with non-ulcer dyspepsia have one or more anxiety disorders compared with 25 per cent of those with dyspepsia where there is endoscopic evidence of ulcer.[52] Ang et al. reported that a majority of patients who have typical symptoms of gastroesophageal reflux do not have erosions on examination; those patients with non-erosive reflux disease have a higher prevalence of psychiatric morbidity.[53]

# Metabolic disorders

## Obesity

Obesity is becoming an epidemic throughout the developed world. Existing standard treatments in university settings, only 20 per cent of obese patients lose around 9 kg (about 20 lbs) at 2-year follow-up and only 5 per cent of patients lose about 18 kg (40 lbs).[54] The majority of people who lose weight on a diet gain it all back. Weight loss and weight maintenance after loss is associated with more initial weight loss, reaching a self-determined goal weight, having a physically active lifestyle, a regular meal rhythm including breakfast and healthier eating, control of overeating, and self-monitoring of behaviours.[55] Associated with weight regain after significant weight loss include a history of weight cycling, disinhibited eating, binge eating, more hunger, eating in response to negative emotions and stress, and more passive reactions to problems.

There is no ideal treatment for weight loss. Weight-loss programmes vary considerably in terms of risk, cost, and efficacy. For most patients with mild to moderate obesity, a multidimensional approach is best, combining diet, exercise, behaviour modification, and social support. Motivated patients with morbid obesity (more than 100 per cent overdesired body weight) may be considered for very low calorie diets, with the emphasis on long-term diet, behavioural change, exercise, and social support. Increasingly, surgical approaches are being used; patient selection procedures have been developed to address motivations, psychological resilience, dietary education, potentially complicating psychiatric or substance-related factors, and ensuring patients are aware these procedures are not without risk—there are many structural and metabolic complications, including death. It is important to treat comorbid psychiatric

illnesses. It is associated with excessive intake of carbohydrate-rich foods and with resistance to engaging in physical activity.[56] With mood disorders and schizophrenia have a high prevalence of risk factors for cardiovascular disease, diabetes, and obesity, which are on the order of 1.5 to 2.5 times higher than in the general population.[56] On the other hand, it is also important to be mindful of metabolic effects of psychopharmacological agents, especially second generation antidepressants. The latter are associated with weight gain, dyslipidemia, and abnormal glucose homeostasis, especially with olanzapine.[56]

### Wilson's disease

Wilson's disease, or hepatolenticular degeneration, is an autosomal recessive disorder affecting between one and three persons per 100 000 of the population. The abnormality in Wilson's disease is defective hepatic excretion of copper. The consequence is copper deposition and injury to many organs, particularly the liver and the brain, including diffuse white matter lesions seen on MRI in many patients.[57] The genetic defect occurs on chromosome 13, and the gene product is probably a transmembrane copper transporter.[58] Because copper accumulation is slow, signs and symptoms do not appear before the age of 6 years. Most patients present with manifestations of organ damage between the ages of 8 and 20. Prolonged extrahepatic release of copper not bound to ceruloplasmin causes basal ganglion destruction, and sometimes cerebral cortex destruction. Prominent neuropsychiatric symptoms include irritability, aggression, disinhibition, and recklessness. Depressive features are also common. The severity of psychiatric symptoms correlates with the severity of neurological symptoms, especially dystonic and bulbar manifestations.[58]

### Disorders of lipid metabolism

Intervention studies have shown that cholesterol reduction using diet, drugs, or surgery reduces the risk of developing or worsening coronary disease. In general, a 1 per cent reduction in low-density lipoprotein-cholesterol has been associated with roughly a 2 per cent reduction in disease end-points.[59] General agreement exists that eating less saturated fat and cholesterol, and adopting a diet and exercise habits to reduce obesity will benefit the health of most people. Exercise has a much greater effect in reducing triglyceride levels than in reducing low-density lipoprotein-cholesterol concentrations. Triglyceride levels are reduced after even a single exercise session. The efficacy of regular aerobic exercise in mild to moderate hypertriglyceridaemia has been repeatedly demonstrated.[60]

### Hepatic encephalopathy

The pathogenesis of hepatic encephalopathy is related to widespread hepatic necrosis, commonly due to an acute viral infection, such as hepatitis B, or exposure to hepatotoxins. Common hepatotoxins that lead to liver failure include acetaminophen, isoniazid, halothane, valproic acid, mushroom toxin, and carbon tetrachloride. Hepatic encephalopathy that accompanies acute fulminant liver failure is frequently associated with cerebral oedema, which might be reversible and a treatable factor. Oedema is the leading cause of death in acute hepatic failure. It may respond to the administration of mannitol and measures to control agitation.[61] For patients with acute hepatic failure who have significant hepatic encephalopathy, liver transplantation increases survival from 20 to 80 per cent, making rapid and accurate diagnosis vital. Survival of liver transplant patients with neuropsychiatric involvement is significantly lower if there is liver disease alone.[61] There is also an increased incidence of liver disease among patients with primary psychiatric disorders, including substance use disorders.[62] B virus carriers are almost three times more likely to have psychiatric disorders than comparison subjects.[63]

# Endocrine disorders

## Diabetes mellitus

Type I diabetes (insulin-dependent diabetes mellitus) occurs when the pancreas' ability to secrete insulin is clinically impaired. Hyperglycaemic symptoms emerge when 80 to 90 per cent of islet cells fail to produce insulin. Around 90 per cent of diabetics have type II diabetes (non-insulin-dependent diabetes mellitus). Type II diabetes is characterized by peripheral resistance to the action of insulin and decreased insulin secretion, in spite of the presence of elevated serum glucose levels. Patients with type II diabetes can often avoid or postpone the need for insulin treatment with appropriate diet and exercise. Both type I and II diabetes are associated with a genetic predisposition.[64]

The most frequent psychiatric disorders in patients with diabetes are anxiety and depressive disorders. Among general populations of diabetics, anxiety disorders occurred in up to 45 per cent and depressive disorders in up to 33 per cent.[65] Rosenthal et al.[66] in a 3-year prospective study of hospitalizations and mortality in older patients with diabetes, found that the combined presence of retinopathy and a high depression score on the Geriatric Depression scale had the strongest relationship with mortality. Patients with diabetes are twice as likely to experience depression as those without diabetes; this holds true for both type I and II diabetes.[66] Patients with schizophrenia are at increased risk for developing type II diabetes[67] is growing interest in the possibility that there are shared inherited risk factors for the two disorders,[68] though the evidence is weak and largely circumstantial. In addition, second generation antipsychotic medications, especially olanzapine, are associated with type II diabetes mellitus and abnormal glucose metabolism.

Diabetic patients who have psychiatric disorders can have less disease morbidity when their psychiatric disorders are appropriately treated, highlighting the importance of monitoring diabetic patients for psychiatric disorders and monitoring psychiatric patients for excess weight and diabetes.[69] Independent of the level of physical illness present in type I or II diabetes, the presence of anxiety and/or depression is important in determining the quality of a patient's life.[70] Treatment adherence problems complicate care, particularly in children and adolescents with type I diabetes. A great deal of patience, family support, and education is necessary to minimize passive and active non-compliance.

## Hypothyroidism

Hypothyroidism is usually the result of primary failure or ablation of the thyroid gland, hypothalamic dysfunction, pituitary dysfunction, autoimmune thyroiditis, or lithium therapy. Clinical manifestations of hypothyroidism include fatigue, cold intolerance, lethargy, weakness, weight gain, constipation, menstrual irregularities, hair loss, slow reaction time, oedema, delayed reflexes, and bradycardia. Hypothyroidism occurs in as many as 10 per cent of patients taking lithium; lithium-induced hypothyroidism is more likely to occur in women.[70]

The association between clinical hypothyroidism and depression is well known. Gold et al.[71] found that 5 per cent of a series of 250 patients with major depressive syndromes had at least subclinical hypothyroidism. In many patients with hypothyroidism, the depression responds to thyroid hormone replacement alone,[72] but the response may take a long time. When that is the case, antidepressants are indicated and efficacious.[71]

## Hyperthyroidism

The most frequent clinical manifestations of hyperthyroidism are nervousness, diaphoresis, hypersensitivity to heat, palpitations, fatigue, weight loss, tachycardia, dyspnoea, and weakness. The most common causes include Graves' disease, toxic adenoma, and toxic multinodular goitre. Less common causes include Hashimoto's thyroiditis, postpartum hyperthyroidism, and factitious hyperthyroid state.

As with hypothyroidism, depressive and anxiety syndromes are the most common psychiatric conditions seen among patients with hyperthyroid states; there is a three-fold increased risk for development of mood disorder following hospitalization with hyperthyroidism.[73,74] When patients have depressive or anxiety syndromes in the context of hyperthyroidism, and have no past histories of psychiatric disorders, the psychiatric symptoms resolve more than 90 per cent of the time when the hyperthyroidism resolves. This obviates the need for other psychiatric interventions unless antithyroid medication, radioactive iodine, or thyroid surgery has not been successful.[74] Anxiety symptoms will disappear in direct relation to the reduction of thyroid hormone levels. Depressive symptoms are not quite so linearly related and may resolve at a slower pace as thyroid hormone level normalize.

## Hypoparathyroidism

Parathyroid hormone mobilizes calcium from bone, induces renal reabsorption of calcium, increases renal clearance of inorganic phosphate, and promotes intestinal reabsorption of calcium. Hypoparathyroidism would be expected to result in hypocalcaemia, which can cause delirium. Hypoparathyroidism can result from autoimmune destruction of the parathyroid glands, removal of the parathyroids, disruption of the glands' blood supply, tumour, or neck irradiation. Medical and neuropsychiatric symptoms and signs are related to the level of serum calcium and the rate at which hypocalcaemia develops. Faster the hypocalcaemia develops, the more likely delirium and other neuropsychiatric symptoms are to occur. The most frequent symptoms are caused by neuromuscular irritability and include paraesthesias, carpal pedal spasm, laryngospasm, blepharospasm, and bronchospasm.[75] Cardiovascular manifestations include prolonged Q–T interval, heart block, and congestive heart failure. The most common neuropsychiatric symptoms and signs are seizures, EEG abnormalities, increased intracranial pressure, disorientation, confusion, and extrapyramidal symptoms. The mainstays of treatment are calcium and vitamin D. Neuropsychiatric syndromes should resolve with the normalization of serum calcium.

## Hyperparathyroidism

Typically, hypercalcaemia is discovered by routine laboratory testing in patients without obvious illness. Primary hyperparathyroidism is the most common cause of hypercalcaemia among adult patients; among hospitalized patients, malignancy is the most common cause.[75] Reversible hyperparathyroidism and hypercalcaemia are also associated with lithium therapy.[76] In primary hyperparathyroidism, parathyroid hormone is secreted inappropriately, despite an elevation in the ionized calcium level. Signs and symptoms of hyperparathyroidism include nausea, vomiting, anorexia, constipation, proximal muscle weakness, polyuria, polydipsia, impaired renal function, hypertension, short Q–T interval, bradycardia, and a number of neuropsychiatric symptoms. The latter include lethargy, drowsiness, impaired concentration ability, and confusion. In severe cases, there may be stupor or coma, psychosis, and cognitive impairment are common in patients who have serum calcium levels above 16 mg/dl. Depressive symptoms, but not cognitive symptoms, tend to resolve with treatment.[77] Cognitive symptoms may improve, but residual symptoms usually remain.

### Cushing's syndrome

Hypersecretion of cortisol by the adrenal gland can result in Cushing's syndrome. Cushing's syndrome can also be due to exogenous ACTH or glucocorticoid administration, or endogenous hyperproduction of these hormones. Because a physiological release of cortisol occurs during periods of stress or duress, it is common to see elevations of serum cortisol during the courses of many psychiatric disorders, including major depressive disorder, alcoholism, anorexia nervosa, panic disorder, and psychoactive substance-withdrawal syndromes. The more common clinical signs and symptoms of Cushing's syndrome, whether endogenous or exogenous, include fat redistribution, menstrual irregularities, dysphoria, thin skin, moon facies, increased appetite, sleep disturbances, hypertension, hypercholesterolaemia, hypertriglyceridaemia, poor concentration, impaired memory, euphoria, glucose intolerance, striae, and hirsutism.

At least half of all patients with Cushing's syndrome will experience depressive or manic symptoms[78]; the symptoms will be moderate to severe in half of these patients. Many will also experience psychotic symptoms. Symptoms are dose-related when due to exogenous steroids. Depression or mania due to Cushing's syndrome will eventually remit when the hypercortisolaemia is corrected, the return to euthymia is usually gradual. When depression or mania is slow to remit, treatment with antidepressants or mood stabilizers is warranted.

### Addison's disease

Addison's disease is the result of an autoimmune process that destroys the adrenal glands; it is the most common cause of primary adrenal insufficiency in the industrialized world, accounting for about 65 per cent of cases.[70] Both glucocorticoid and mineralocorticoid secretion are diminished in this condition. Clinical manifestations of adrenal insufficiency include weight loss, fatigue, vomiting, diarrhoea, anorexia, and salt-craving. Patients with Addison's disease will require lifelong replacement of both glucocorticoids and mineralocorticoids. Patients may be misdiagnosed with major depressive disorder, personality disorder, dementia, or somatoform disorders. It is not uncommon for the diagnosis to be delayed for many months; Addison's disease is a disorder to be continually mindful about in a patient with treatment-resistant depression.

### Hyperprolactinaemia

Prolactin is synthesized in the pituitary gland; its secretion is increased during pregnancy, enhancing breast development. Prolactin secretion is inhibited by glucocorticoids and thyroid hormone, it is predominantly under the inhibitory control of dopamine.[70] Dopamine is, in fact, prolactin inhibiting factor. This is why dopamine blocking medications such as neuroleptics can cause hyperprolactinaemia. Symptoms of hyperprolactinaemia include breast development and lactation. These bothersome side effects of neuroleptics, particularly in men, can be modulated by changing to a more favourable neuroleptic medication, such as a second generation antipsychotic.

### Hypopituitarism

Hypopituitarism occurs when multiple pituitary hormones exhibit decreased secretion. It can be due to either gland destruction or inadequate stimulation by factors that regulate pituitary functioning. Common causes of hypopituitarism are pituitary adenomas, hypothalamic tumours, metastatic carcinoma (especially breast and bronchus), and cerebral trauma and haemorrhage.[70] Other causes include vascular disorders, immunological conditions, and a variety of congenital anomalies. Clinical manifestations depend on which hormones are deficient; signs and symptoms are those of the individual deficiency states. Other signs that may be present when there is hypopituitarism include headache, visual loss, and radiographically discovered sella enlargement. Treatment of patients with hypopituitarism involves hormone replacement therapy and surgery when accessible lesions are present.[70]

## Autoimmune disorders

### Systemic lupus erythematosus

Systemic lupus erythematosus is characterized by the production of autoantibodies that injure tissue in several organ systems, most frequently the skin, central nervous system, kidney, and lungs. In addition, non-specific symptoms occur in a large majority of patients, including fatigue, fever, weight loss, arthralgias, and myalgias.[79] The most common presenting symptoms are fever, arthralgias, butterfly rash, photosensitivity, Raynaud's phenomenon, and mucous ulcers. The laboratory diagnostic hallmark of systemic lupus erythematosus is the production of high-titre autoantibodies directed against a variety of cell nucleus components (antinuclear antibodies). Systemic lupus erythematosus has no known cure, so treatment is based on symptom relief, suppression of inflammation, and preventing future pathology.

The most common psychiatric presentations of active systemic lupus erythematosus are psychosis, delirium, seizures, and cognitive dysfunction.[80] Autoantibodies to neuronal membranes, which interfere with the ability of neurones to respond to stimuli, may account for most neuropsychiatric deficits and symptoms,[81] though CNS vasculitis during the course of this disease may also play a role in some patients. Symptoms in lupus patients are likely to be related to unique sets of autoantigens,[82] and are related to antibodies against N-methyl-D-aspartate (NMDA) receptors.[83] Antibodies may be partially responsible for depression, short-term memory problems, and new learning difficulties in lupus patients. Significantly associated with declining cognitive function are consistently positive antiphospholipid antibodies, consistent steroid use, diabetes, and higher depression scores.[83] Mood syndromes are probably the most common psychiatric presentation of patients with systemic lupus erythematosus,[84] but mood change is not always due to involvement of the central nervous system. Patients are frequently treated with steroids, which raise the possibility of steroid-induced neuropsychiatric syndromes. However, in many cases, addition of steroids to treatment may improve psychiatric syndromes.

## Renal disorders

### Acute renal failure

Acute renal failure is an abrupt decrease in renal function sufficient to result in azotaemia—retention of nitrogenous waste in the body.[85] Acute renal failure can result from a decrease of renal blood flow (prerenal azotaemia), intrinsic renal disease (renal azotaemia), or obstruction of urine flow (postrenal azotaemia). Prerenal azotaemia can be caused by renal arterial occlusion or a decrease in the effective blood volume (e.g. haemorrhage, congestive heart failure, diarrhoea). Intrinsic renal azotaemia is most commonly caused by acute tubular necrosis due to an acute ischaemic or nephrotoxic insult. Azotaemia is due to obstruction of the urine collecting system; this may occur when there is bladder outlet obstruction or ureteral obstruction.

Medical complications of acute renal failure include hyperkalaemia, hyperuricaemia, arrhythmias, anaemia, coagulopathies, vomiting, nausea, and urinary tract infections. Metabolic perturbations can lead to delirium. Neuropsychiatric manifestations include somnolence, asterixis (flapping tremor), neuromuscular irritability, and seizures. Mental status abnormalities in acute (but not chronic) renal failure begin to occur for most adults when the serum creatinine level acutely rises to about 4.0 mg/dl. In oliguric renal failure, serum blood urea nitrogen levels can be expected to rise by about 10 to 20 mg/dl per day. Serum creatinine levels can be expected to rise by about 1 mg/dl per day. Neuropsychiatric complications of acute renal failure are best treated by correcting the underlying cause of the renal failure. Dialysis may be used to manage acute manifestations. While awaiting reversal of neuropsychiatric manifestations, symptomatic management with antiseizure medications and neuroleptics may be necessary.

### Chronic renal failure and end stage renal disease

Chronic renal failure is a progressive and irreversible loss of renal function.[86] The most common aetiologies of renal insufficiency ultimately leading to end stage renal disease are diabetes, hypertension, and glomerulonephritis. Loss of up to 75 per cent of glomerular filtration rate does not usually result in pronounced clinical symptoms, as the remaining glomeruli adapt with hyperfiltration. Serum creatinine is a sensitive indicator of early, subclinical, chronic renal failure. For example, the doubling of serum creatinine from 0.7 to 1.4 mg/dl signifies a loss of approximately 50 per cent of glomerular filtration rate, emphasizing the importance of early detection and prevention.

Patients with chronic renal failure usually become symptomatic when glomerular filtration rate is less than 10 ml/min. Uraemia affects every organ system, including the central nervous system. Neuropsychiatric manifestations of chronic renal failure include irritability, insomnia, lethargy, anorexia, seizures, and restless legs syndrome.[86] In contrast to acute renal failure—where neuropsychiatric signs and symptoms may appear with a creatinine level as low as 4 mg/dl—in chronic renal failure, patients may have a normal mental status examination with a serum creatinine level as high as 9 to 10 mg/dl. Symptomatic treatments with low-dose neuroleptics, antiseizure medications, or benzodiazepines are sometimes necessary in chronic renal failure.

Kimmel et al.[86] studied the prevalence of hospitalizations for psychiatric illness in patients with end stage renal disease and compared that rate with four other chronic medical conditions (diabetes, ischaemic heart disease, cerebrovascular disease, and peptic ulcer disease). Hospitalizations for mental disorders were 1.5 to 3.0 times higher in these patients than in patients with the four other chronic diseases. Dementias and depression were the most common reasons for hospitalization. With end stage renal disease are almost twice as likely to die by suicides as the general populations, after controlling for other potential demographic and clinical contributors to suicide risk.[87]

Sexual dysfunction is very common in patients with end stage renal disease. Abrams et al.[88] found that 75 per cent of his sample of men with this disease reported a decrease in frequency of sexual intercourse of at least 50 per cent. Disruptions in sexual function, which may be physiological (e.g. vascular complications of diabetes, fatigue following dialysis treatments) or psychological or both, account for at least a portion of the dysphoria experienced by patients with end stage renal disease.

The definitive treatments for most patients with chronic renal failure are transplantation or haemodialysis. In general, transplantation is encouraged because of a better quality of life and a greater chance for rehabilitation and symptom resolution. Researchers in three separate prospective studies found that patients who received renal transplants experienced better physical and psychological outcomes than patients who remained on dialysis.[89] Neuropsychiatric signs and symptoms resolve much more completely with transplantation than with haemodialysis. Psychiatric aspects of organ transplantation are discussed later. The psychiatric aspects of haemodialysis are discussed next.

### Haemodialysis

The average patient on haemodialysis requires 3.5 h of dialysis three times per week to achieve adequate creatinine clearance.[86] Haemodialysis has enabled the survival of countless thousands of patients with chronic renal failure and provides a temporary management tool for patients on transplantation waiting lists. However, it is not a benign procedure, and has a number of potential neuropsychiatric complications. Patients on haemodialysis are at high risk for developing volume overload, pulmonary oedema, hyperkalaemia, hyperphosphataemia, and metabolic bone disease if compliance with restricted diet and fluid intake is not optimal. Patient adherence to these diet and fluid-intake protocols are used as one of the criteria for making decisions about appropriateness for transplantation. Psychiatric reasons for non-adherence should be addressed and are usually reversible, with the exception of personality disorders. These include mood disorders, phobias, panic disorder, substance-related disorders, adjustment disorder, and cognitive disorders.

## Haematological disorders

### Anaemia due to vitamin deficiency

Both folic acid and cobalamin (vitamin B12) are necessary for the production of DNA; in their absence, the nucleus of the cell cannot undergo normal mitosis. The main cause of folic acid deficiency is dietary insufficiency.[90] This commonly occurs in severe alcoholics. The main cause of cobalamin deficiency is malabsorption. The major clinical manifestations of folate or vitamin B12 deficiency include fatigue, pallor, and for cobalamin deficiency, neuropsychiatric manifestations. The latter include loss of proprioception in the lower extremities, loss of vibratory perception, anosmial, forgetfulness, and even dementia. Diagnosis is based on measurement of serum levels of vitamin B12 and folate. Treatment is replacement of folate (1 mg/day or improved diet) and vitamin B12 (administered parenterally).

In cobalamin deficiency, neuropsychiatric findings can occur even when megaloblasts and anaemia are absent.[91] Patients with cobalamin levels between 100 and 200 pg/ml, and especially those with levels less than 100 pg/ml, may have cobalamin-reversible neuropsychiatric deficits.[138] Even dementia due to chronic cobalamin deficiency may be partially reversible when diagnosed and aggressively treated. It is also associated with a higher risk of depression, especially in older adults; anaemia severity and depression severity scores are highly correlated.[92] Treatment of the anaemia may result in resolution of depressive symptoms; in some cases depressive symptoms are slower to resolve and may require extended treatment with antidepressant medication, particularly for patients predisposed to mood disorders.

### Iron-deficiency anaemia

When erythrocyte-cytoplasm production is abnormally low due to the reduced production or availability of one of the three components of haemoglobin (iron, globin, or haem), the ratio of cytoplasm to the contents of the rest of the cell declines. This results in a microcytic anaemia. In most cases, microcytic anaemia is due to iron-deficient haemopoiesis.[92] Deficiency is usually due to an iron-poor diet or defective iron utilization by the body. Clinical manifestations of iron-deficiency anaemia are related to the severity of the iron deficiency and include severe fatigue, pallor, changes in nail curvature ('spoon nails'), and, at times, pica and cheilosis at the corners of the mouth. A diminished haematocrit and mean corpuscular volume, and low serum iron are the cornerstones of the diagnosis. The severe fatigue associated with iron deficiency can be misdiagnosed as major depressive disorder; treatment with an antidepressant will not help unless there is also clinical major depression apart from the iron deficiency. Iron replenishment to correct the underlying deficiency is the specific. With iron replenishment, the haemoglobin should correct to normal, and symptoms should resolve, within 4 to 6 weeks.

## Conclusions

There is increasing recognition that patients with psychiatric signs and symptoms frequently have associated medical disorders. Interactions between the disorders can be quite complex and may involve neuropsychiatric manifestations of medical illness, medical effects of psychiatric treatments, psychiatric effects of medical treatment, increased medical illness related to factors inherent in the psychiatric condition, and maladaptive personality styles or disorders that affect outcomes of medical and psychiatric illness. Psychiatric disorders in patients with other medical illnesses increase mortality, morbidity, health care costs, and decrease adherence to medical therapies. Appropriate and cost-effective management must integrate knowledge from psychiatry and primary care to assure maximal therapeutic gains for the patient. Those involved in consultation to primary care providers must understand both the basic pathophysiology and clinical characteristics of the medical disorders and their treatments, as well as possess the psychiatric knowledge necessary to ensure that the patient with medical illness is adequately managed.

## Further information

Robinson, M.J. and Owen, J.A. (2005). Psychopharmacology. In *Textbook of psychosomatic medicine* (ed. J.L. Levenson), pp. 871–3. American Psychiatric Publishing, Inc., Washington, DC.

Saha, S., Chant, D., and McGrath, J. (2007). A systematic review of mortality in schizophrenia. *Archives of General Psychiatry*, **64**, 1123–31.

Schmitz, N., Thefeld, W., and Kruse, J. (2006). Mental disorders and hypertension: factors associated with awareness and treatment of hypertension in the general population of Germany. *Psychosomatic Medicine*, **68**, 246–52.

## References

1. Chapman, D.P., Perry, G.S., and Strine, T.W. (2005). The vital link between chronic disease and depressive disorder. *Preventing Chronic Disease*, **2**, 1–12.

2. Barsky, A.J., Orav, J., and Bates, D.W. (2005). Somatization increases medical utilization and costs independent of psychiatric and medical comorbidity. *Archives of General Psychiatry*, **62**, 903–10.

3. Brod, J. (1970). Circulatory changes underlying blood pressure elevation during acute emotional stress (mental arithmetic) in normotensive and hypertensive subjects. *Clinical Scientist*, **18**, 269–78.

4. Torian, L., Davidson, E., Fulop, G., *et al.* (1992). The effect of dementia on acute care in a geriatric medical unit. *International Psychogeriatrics*, **4**, 231–9.

5. Thomas, S.A., Friedmann, E., and Kelley, F.J. (2001). Living with an implantable cardioverter-defibrillator: a review of the current literature related to psychosocial factors. *The Journal of Cardiovascular Nursing*, **12**, 156–63.

6. Lown, B., DeSilva, R.A., and Reich, P. (1980). Psychophysiologic factors in sudden cardiac death. *The American Journal of Psychiatry*, **137**, 1325–35.

7. Tennant, C. (1999). Life stress, social support and coronary heart disease. *The Australian and New Zealand Journal of Psychiatry*, **33**, 636.

8. Frasure-Smith, N., Lesperance, F., and Talajic, M. (1995). Depression and 18-month prognosis after myocardial infarction. *Circulation*, **91**, 999–1005.

9. Benson, H., Alexander, S., and Feldman, C.L. (1975). Decreased premature ventricular contractions through the use of relaxation response in patients with stable ischaemic heart disease. *Lancet*, **2**, 380–2.

10. Grippo, A.J., Santos, C.M., Johnson, R.F., *et al.* (2004). Increased susceptibility to ventricular arrhythmias in a rodent model of experimental depression. *American Journal of Physiology—Heart and Circulatory Physiology*, **286**, H619–26.

11. Musselman, D.L., Evans, D.L., and Nemeroff, C.B. (1998). The relationship of depression to cardiovascular disease: epidemiology, biology, and treatment. *Archives of General Psychiatry*, **55**, 580–92.

12. Brod, J. (1970). Circulatory changes underlying blood pressure elevation during acute emotional stress (mental arithmetic) in normotensive and hypertensive subjects. *Clinical Scientist*, **18**, 269–78.

13. Harburg, E., Erfurt, J.C., and Hauenstein, L.S. (1973). Socio-ecological stress, suppressed hostility, skin color, and black-white male blood pressure: Detroit. *Psychosomatic Medicine*, **35**, 276–96.

14. Bankier, B. and Littman, A.B. (2002). Psychiatric disorders and coronary heart disease in women—a still neglected topic: review of the literature from 1971 to 2000. *Psychotherapy and Psychosomatics*, **71**, 133–40.

15. Rozanski, A., Bairey, C.N., and Krantz, D.S. (1988). Mental stress and the induction of silent myocardial ischemia in patients with coronary artery disease. *The New England Journal of Medicine*, **318**, 1005–11.

16. Ruberman, W., Weinblatt, A.B., Goldberg, J.D., *et al.* (1984). Psychosocial influences on mortality after myocardial infarction. *The New England Journal of Medicine*, **311**, 552–9.

17. Dickens, C.M., McGowan, L., Percival, C., *et al.* (2004). Lack of a close confidant, but not depression, predicts further cardiac events after myocardial infarction. *Heart*, **90**, 518–22.

18. Mayou, R.A., Gill, D., Thompson, D.R., *et al.* (2000). Depression and anxiety as predictors of outcome after myocardial infarction. *Psychosomatic Medicine*, **62**, 212–19.

19. Lesperance, F., Frasure-Smith, N., and Talajic, M. (1996). Major depression before and after myocardial infarction: its nature and consequences. *Psychosomatic Medicine*, **58**, 99–110.

20. Carney, R.M., Rich, M.W., and Freedland, K.E. (1988). Major depressive disorder predicts cardiac events in patients with coronary artery disease. *Psychosomatic Medicine*, **50**, 627–33.

21. Plotsky, P.M., Owens, M.J., and Nemeroff, C.B. (1998). Psychoneuroendocrinology of depression the Hypothalamic-Pituitary-Adrenal Axis. *The Psychiatric Clinics of North America*, **21**, 293–307.

22. Musselman, D.L., Evans, D.L., and Nemeroff, C.B. (1998). The relationship of depression to cardiovascular disease. *Archives of General Psychiatry*, **55**, 580–92.

23. Langosch, W., Seer, P., Brodner, G., *et al.* (1982). Behavior therapy with coronary heart disease patients: results of a comparative study. *Journal of Psychosomatic Research*, **26**, 475–84.

24. Preckel, D., von Kanel, R., Kudielka, B.M., *et al.* (2005). Over commitment to work is associated with vital exhaustion. *International Archives of Occupational and Environmental Health*, **78**, 117–22.

25. Friedman, M. and Thoresen, C.E. (1986). Alteration of type A behavior and its effect on cardiac recurrences in post-myocardial infarction patients: summary results of the recurrent coronary prevention project. *American Heart Journal*, **112**, 653–65.

26. Sher, L. (2005). Type D personality: the heart, stress, and cortisol. *Quarterly Journal of Medicine*, **98**, 323–9.

27. Denollet, J., Pedersen, S.S., Vrints, C.J., *et al.* (2006). Usefulness of type D personality in predicting five-year cardiac events above and beyond concurrent symptoms of stress in patients with coronary heart disease. *The American Journal of Cardiology*, **97**, 970–3.

28. Katon, W.J., Richardson, L., Lozano, P., *et al.* (2004). The relationship of asthma and anxiety disorders. *Psychosomatic Medicine*, **66**, 349–55.

29. Ten Brinke, A., Sterk, P.J., Masclee, A.A.M., *et al.* (2005). Risk factors of frequent exacerbations in difficult-to-treat asthma. *The European Respiratory Journal*, **26**, 812–18.

30. Greenberg, D.B., Halperin, P., Kradin, R.L., *et al.* (2000). Internal medicine and medical subspecialties. In *American psychiatric publishing textbook of consultation–liaison psychiatry* (2nd edn) (eds. M. Wise and J.R. Rundell), pp. 548–608. American Psychiatric Publishing, Washington, DC.

31. Norwood, R. (2006). Prevalence and impacts of depression in chronic obstructive pulmonary disease. *Current Opinion in Pulmonary Medicine*, **12**, 113–17.

32. Porzelius, J., Vest, M., and Nochomovitz, M. (1992). Respiratory function, cognitions, and panic in chronic obstructive pulmonary patients. *Behavioural Research and Therapy*, **30**, 75–7.

33. Strudsholm, U., Johannessen, L., Foldager, L., *et al.* (2005). Increased risk for pulmonary embolism in patients with bipolar disorder. *Bipolar Disorders*, **7**, 77–81.

34. Joukamaa, M., Heliovaara, M., Knekt, P., *et al.* (2006). Schizophrenia, neuroleptic medication, and mortality. *The British Journal of Psychiatry*, **188**, 122–7.

35. Clouse, R.E. and Lustman, P.J. (1989). Value of recent psychological symptoms in identifying patients with esophageal contraction abnormalities. *Psychosomatic Medicine*, **51**, 570–6.

36. Van Handel, D. and Fass, R. (2005). The pathophysiology of non-cardiac chest pain. *Journal of Gastroenterology and Hepatology*, **20**, S6–11.

37. Clouse, R.E. and Lustman, P.J. (1983). Psychiatric illness and contraction abnormalities of the esophagus. *The New England Journal of Medicine*, **309**, 1337–42.

38. Castell, D.O. and Richter, J.E. (1987). Edrophonium testing for esophageal pain: concurrence and discord. *Digestive Disease Scientist*, **32**, 897–9.

39. Cybulska, E.M. (1997). Globus hystericus: a somatic symptom of depression? *Psychosomatic Medicine*, **59**, 67–9.

40. Drossman, D.A., Sandler, R.S., and McKee, D.C. (1982). Bowel patterns among subjects not seeking health care. *Gastroenterology*, **83**, 529–34.

41. Bhatia, V. and Tandon, R.K. (2005). Stress and the gastrointestinal tract. *Journal of Gastroenterology and Hepatology*, **20**, 332–44.

42. Clouse, R.E., Richter, J.E., Heading, R.C., *et al.* Functional esophageal disorders. *Gut*, **45**, 31–6.

43. Clouse, R.E. and Lustman, P.J. (2005). Use of psychopharmacological agents for functional gastrointestinal disorders. *Gut*, **54**, 1332–41.

44. Walker, E.A., Gelfand, M.D., Gelfand, A.N., *et al.* (1996). The relationship of current psychiatric disorders to functional disability and distress in patients with inflammatory bowel disease. *General Hospital Psychiatry*, **18**, 220–9.

45. Bennett, P. and Wilkinson, S. (1985). A comparison of psychological and medical treatment of the irritable bowel syndrome. *The British Journal of Clinical Psychology*, **24**, 215–16.

46. Maunder, R. (2005). Evidence that stress contributes to inflammatory bowel disease: evaluation, synthesis, and future directions. *Inflammatory Bowel Diseases*, **11**, 600–8.

47. Mawdsley, J.E. and Rampton, D.S. (2005). Psychological stressing IBD: new insights into pathogenic and therapeutic implications. *Gut*, **54**, 1481–91.

48. Whorell, P.J., Prior, A., and Faragher, E.B. (1984). Controlled trial of hypnotherapy in the treatment of severe refractory irritable bowel syndrome. *Lancet*, **2**, 1232–4.

49. Cremonini, F., Wise, J., Moayyedi, P., *et al.* (2005). Diagnostic and therapeutic use of proton pump inhibitors in non-cardiac chest pain: a meta-analysis. *The American Journal of Gastroenterology*, **100**, 1226–9.

50. Littman, A.B. and Ketterer, M.W. (2000). Behavioural medicine. In *American psychiatric publishing textbook of consultation–liaison psychiatry* (2nd edn) (eds. M. Wise and J.R. Rundell), pp. 1080–95. American Psychiatric Publishing, Washington, DC.

51. Magni, G. (1987). On the relationship between chronic pain and depression when there is no organic lesion. *Pain*, **31**, 1–21.

52. Whitehead, W.E. (1992). Behavioural medicine approaches to gastrointestinal disorders. *Journal of Consulting and Clinical Psychology*, **60**, 605–12.

53. Ang, T.L., Fock, K.M., Ng, T.M., *et al.* (2005). A comparison of the clinical, demographic and psychiatric profiles among patients with erosive and non-erosive reflux disease in a multi-ethnic Asian country. *World Journal of Gastroenterology*, **11**, 3558–61.

54. Elfhag, K. and Rossner, S. (2005). Who succeeds in maintaining weight loss? A conceptual review of factors associated with weight loss maintenance and weight regain. *Obesity Reviews*, **6**, 67–86.

55. Morriss, R. and Mohammed, F.A. (2005). Metabolism, lifestyle and bipolar disorder. *Journal of Psychopharmacology*, **19**, 94–101.

56. Casey, D.E. (2005). Metabolic issues and cardiovascular disease in patients with psychiatric disorders. *The American Journal of Medicine*, **118**(Suppl. 2), 15S–22S.

57. Prashanth, L.K., Sinha, T.S., Ravishankar, S., *et al.* (2005). Prognostic factors in patients presenting with severe neurological forms of Wilson's disease. *Quarterly Journal of Medicine*, **98**, 557–63.

58. Dening, D.C. and Berrios, G.E. (1989). Wilson's disease: psychiatric symptoms in 195 cases. *Archives of General Psychiatry*, **46**, 1126–34.

59. National Cholesterol Education Program. (1993). Summary of the second report of the National Cholesterol Education Program (NCEP) expert panel on detection, evaluation and treatment of high blood

cholesterol in adults. (Adult Treatment Panel 11). *The Journal of the American Medical Association*, **264**, 3015–23.

60. Freedman, D.S., Byers, T., Barrett, D.H., *et al.* (1995). Plasma lipid levels and psychological characteristic in men. *American Journal of Epidemiology*, **141**, 507–17.

61. Medici, V., Mirante, V.G., Fassati, L.R., *et al.* (2005). Liver transplantation for Wilson's disease: the burden of neurological and psychiatric disorders. *Liver Transplantation*, **11**, 1056–63.

62. Crone, C.C., Gabriel, G.M., and DiMartini, A. (2006). An overview of psychiatric issues in liver disease for the consultation-liaison psychiatrist. *Psychosomatics*, **47**, 188–205.

63. Atesci, F.C., Cetin, B.C., Oguzhanoglu, N.K., *et al.* (2005). Psychiatric disorders and functioning in Hepatitis B virus carriers. *Psychosomatics*, **46**, 142–7.

64. Lustman, P.J., Griffith, L.S., Clouse, R.E., *et al.* (1986). Psychiatric illness in diabetes mellitus: relationship to symptoms and glucose control. *The Journal of Nervous and Mental Disease*, **174**, 736–42.

65. Kathol, R. (2000). In *American psychiatric publishing textbook of consultation–liaison psychiatry* (2nd edn) (eds. M. Wise and J.R. Rundell), pp. 579–84. American Psychiatric Publishing, Washington, DC.

66. Rosenthal, M.J., Morley, J.E., Fajardo, M., *et al.* (1998). Hospitalization and mortality of diabetes in older adults. *Diabetes Care*, **21**, 231–5.

67. Chafetz, L., White, M.C., Collins-Bride, G., *et al.* (2005). The poor general health of the severely mentally ill: impact of schizophrenic diagnosis. *Community Mental Health Journal*, **41**, 169–84.

68. Gough, S.C.L. and O'Donovan, M.C. (2005). Clustering of metabolic comorbidity in schizophrenia: a genetic contribution? *Journal of Psychopharmacology*, **19**, 47–55.

69. McIntyre, R.S., Mancini, D.A., Pearce, M.M., *et al.* (2005). Mood and psychotic disorders and type 2 diabetes: a metabolic trial. *Canadian Journal of Diabetes*, **29**, 122–32.

70. Goldman, M.B. (2002). Neuropsychiatric features of endocrine disorders. In *The American psychiatric publishing textbook of neuropsychiatry* (4th edn) (eds. S. Yudofsky and R. Hales), pp. 519–40. American Psychiatric Publishing, Washington, DC.

71. Gold, M.S., Pottash, A.L.C., and Extein, I. (1981). Hypothyroidism and depression. *The Journal of the American Medical Association*, **245**, 1919–22.

72. Rouchell, A.M., Pounds, R., and Tierney, J.G. (2000). Depression. In *American psychiatric publishing textbook of consultation–liaison psychiatry* (2nd edn) (eds. M. Wise and J.R. Rundell), pp. 310–45. American Psychiatric Publishing, Washington, DC.

73. Williams, R.H. (1946). Thiouracil treatment of thyrotoxicosis. *The Journal of Clinical Endocrinology and Metabolism*, **6**, 1–22.

74. Thomsen, A.F., Kvist, T.K., Andersen, P.K., *et al.* (2005). Increased risk of affective disorder following hospitalization with hyperthyroidism—a register based study. *European Journal of Endocrinology*, **152**, 535–43.

75. Brown, G.G., Preisman, R.C., and Kleerekoper, M. (1987). Neurobehavioural symptoms in mild primary hyperparathyroidism: related to hypercalcemia but not improved by parathyroidectomy. *Henry Ford Hospital Medical Journal*, **35**, 211–15.

76. Khandwala, H.M. and Van Uum, S. (2006). Reversible hypercalcemia and hyperparathyroidism associated with lithium therapy: case report and review of the literature. *Endocrine Practice*, **12**, 54–8.

77. Allerheiligen, D.A., Schoeber, J., Houston, R.E., *et al.* (1998). Hyperparathyroidism. *American Family Physician*, **57**, 1795–802.

78. Thompson, J.M., Gallagher, P., Hughes, J.H., *et al.* (2005). Neurocognitive impairment in euthymic patients with bipolar affective disorder. *The British Journal of Psychiatry*, **186**, 32–40.

79. Yagniak, P.M. and Cohen, M.M. (1988). Systemic lupus erythematosus nervous system involvement. In *Diagnosis and management of rheumatic diseases* (2nd edn) (ed. W. Katz), pp. 220–3. J.B. Lippincott, Philadelphia, PA.

80. Greenberg, D.B. (2000). Systemic lupus erythematosus. In *American psychiatric publishing textbook of consultation–liaison psychiatry* (2nd edn) (eds. M. Wise and J.R. Rundell), p. 585. American Psychiatric Publishing, Washington, DC.

81. Baker, M. (1973). Psychopathology in SLE: psychiatric observations. *Seminars in Arthritis and Rheumatology*, **3**, 95–110.

82. Margutti, P., Sorice, M., Conti, F., *et al.* (2005). Screening of an endothelial cDNA library identifies the C-terminal region of Nedd5 as a novel autoantigen in systemic lupus erythematosus with psychiatric manifestations. *Arthritis Research & Therapy*, **7**, R896–903.

83. Omdal, R., Brokstad, K., Waterloo, K., *et al.* (2005). Neuropsychiatric disturbances in systemic lupus erythematosus are associated with antibodies against NMDA receptors. *European Journal of Neurology*, **12**, 392–400.

84. McLaurin, E.Y., Holliday, S.L., Williams, P., *et al.* (2005). Predictors of cognitive dysfunction in patients with systemic lupus erythematosus. *Neurology*, **64**, 297–303.

85. Cohen, L.M. (2000). Renal disease. In *American psychiatric publishing textbook of consultation–liaison psychiatry* (2nd edn) (eds. M. Wise and J.R. Rundell), pp. 573–8. American Psychiatric Publishing, Washington, DC.

86. Kimmel, P.L., Thamer, M., Richard, C.M., *et al.* (1998). Psychiatric illness in patients with end-stage renal disease. *The American Journal of Medicine*, **105**, 214–21.

87. Kurella, M., Kimmel, P.L., Young, B.S., *et al.* (2005). Suicide in the United States end-stage renal disease program. *Journal of the American Society of Nephrology*, **16**, 774–81.

88. Abrams, H.S., Hester, L.R., and Sheridan, W.F. (1975). Sexual functioning in patients with chronic renal failure. *The Journal of Nervous and Mental Diseases*, **160**, 220–6.

89. Russell, J.D., Beecroft, M.L., Ludlow, D., *et al.* (1992). The quality of life in renal transplantation—a prospective study. *Transplantation*, **54**, 656–60.

90. Stabler, S.P. and Allen, R.H. (1990). Clinical spectrum and diagnosis of cobalamin deficiency. *Blood*, **76**, 871–81.

91. Greenberg, D.B. (2000). Cobalamin deficiency. In *American psychiatric publishing textbook of consultation–liaison psychiatry* (2nd edn) (eds. M. Wise and J.R. Rundell), p. 586. American Psychiatric Publishing, Washington, DC.

92. Onder, G., Penninx, B.W., Cesari, M., *et al.* (2005). Anemia is correlated with depression in older adults: results from the InCHIANTI study. *Gerontology*, **60**, 1168–72.

93. Badminton, M.N. and Elder, G.H. (2005). *Journal of Inherited Metabolic Disease*, **28**, 277–86.

# 5.3.5 **Psychiatric aspects of infections**

José Luis Ayuso-Mateos

Neuropsychiatric disturbances stemming from infectious diseases are widespread in both the industrialized world and developing countries. Such neuropsychiatric syndromes are not necessarily the result of infectious processes directly involving the central nervous system, they may also be complications of systemic infections. There are many microbial, viral, and parasitic agents, as well as other types of infectious substances, which can affect the central nervous system, leading to the appearance of neurological and psychiatric symptoms that may cause suffering to the patient, and even be disabling.

When considering the psychiatric manifestations of infectious illness, it is important to consider clinical manifestations derived from a possible systemic infection, which can be less obvious than a direct involvement of the central nervous system. Acute organic reactions may accompany many systemic infections, especially at the extremes of life. A clear example is the delirium that frequently occurs with pneumonia in the elderly. In these clinical syndromes, several factors could be responsible for the alterations in cerebral metabolism. The mere fact of having a fever could be involved. Cerebral anoxia often appears to be responsible, or the influence of toxins derived from the infecting micro-organism. More complex metabolic disturbances or the accumulation of toxic intermediate products can also be implicated.

Likewise, infections that course as chronic or subacute illnesses are frequently accompanied by the onset of depressive syndromes. One of the factors implied in clinical depression that occurs within the context of systemic infectious illnesses (e.g. tuberculosis and infectious mononucleosis), is a sense of physical vulnerability, possibly heightened by a loss of strength and negative changes in the patient's appearance. Patients are often afraid of losing their earning capacity or even their jobs, as well as other social and occupational problems associated with the illness.

Another very important factor, above all with the human immunodeficiency virus (**HIV**) and other sexually transmitted disease (**STD**), is the social stigma that these patients may suffer.[1] Sexually transmitted disease infection implies sexual activity that historically carries connotations of illicit, casual, sexual encounters, and acquiring an STD is frequently associated with embarrassment and social stigma.

In addition to the disease itself, the medications commonly used to treat infectious illnesses can have side-effects that alter patients' behaviour, as well as their cognitive and affective functioning (Table 5.3.5.1).

In this chapter we consider infections of clinical interest in the practice of psychiatry. These conditions will be dealt with briefly, and textbooks of general medicine should be consulted for further details. Prion diseases and chronic fatigue syndromes, which are also related to the subject of the present chapter, are discussed in Chapters 4.1.4 and 5.2.7, respectively.

## HIV infection

Patients infected with HIV are at an increased risk for a variety of mental disorders. Those encountered most frequently in psychiatric practice are discussed below. HIV dementia is discussed in Chapter 4.1.9.

### Nature of neuropsychiatric disorders in HIV-infected patients

Neuropsychiatric disorders are common in HIV-infected patients, and they can be either primary or secondary. **Primary** complications are those that can be attributed directly to the infection of the central nervous system by the virus, or to immunopathological events precipitated by HIV infection. Primary HIV-related brain disorders include HIV-related dementia and minor cognitive disorder.[2] Immune suppression can lead to a variety of secondary complications affecting the brain, including opportunistic infections (e.g. cerebral toxoplasmosis and progressive multifocal leucoencephalopathy) and tumours (e.g. cerebral lymphoma). **Secondary** complications in the form of acute and subacute syndromes (e.g.

**Table 5.3.5.1** Neuropsychiatric adverse effects of drugs frequently used in the treatment of infectious diseases

| Drug | Adverse effect |
| --- | --- |
| Aciclovir | Headache, somnolence, tremor, confusion, lethargy, seizures, agitation, major depression with psychotic symptoms |
| Amphotericin B | Delirium |
| Chloramphenicol | Memory impairment, confusion, depersonalization, hallucinations |
| Cycloserine | Depression, anxiety, confusion, hallucinations, paranoia, agoraphobia |
| Didanosine (ddI) | Headache, asthenia, polyneuropathy |
| Efavirenz | Dizziness, headache, insomnia, inappropriate behaviour, depression, concentration impairment, agitation, abnormal dreaming, and somnolence |
| Foscarnet | Asthenia |
| Gentamicin | Confusion, hallucinations |
| Interferon | Depression, anxiety, irritability, delirium |
| Isoniazid (INH) | Headaches, vertigo, hyper-reflexia, neuritis, convulsions, ataxia, toxic, encephalopathy, confusion, psychosis, antidepressant effect |
| Ketoconazole | Somnolence, delirium |
| Para-aminosalicylate (PAS) | Toxic psychosis |
| Penicillin G (procaine) | Hallucinations, seizures, agitation, confusion |
| Rifampicin (rifampin) | Myopathy, headache if hypersensitivity |
| Streptomycin | Toxic effects on cranial nerve VIII (vestibular), vertigo, nystagmus, ataxia, neuromuscular junction blockade |
| Sulphonamide | Anxiety, depression, insomnia, hallucinations |
| Trimethoprim-sulphamethoxazole | Vertigo and confusion |
| Zalcitabine (ddC) | Polyneuropathy |
| Zidovudine (AZT) | Headache, myalgia, insomnia, asthenia, somnolence, anxiety, depression, mania, restlessness |

delirium) often occur as a result of cerebrovascular complications and toxic states induced by various therapeutic agents.

### HIV-associated acute stress reaction

This transitory syndrome appears in some individuals after they are notified of their seropositivity. It is equally frequent among those who, after a period as an asymptomatic carrier, are informed that the infection has progressed towards full-blown AIDS. The appearance of these symptoms is closely linked in time to the stressful circumstance, and generally remits in hours or days.

The symptoms are highly varied. Some patients suffer from intrusive thoughts or brooding related to their uncertainties regarding health, the future, the risk of contagion to others (especially loved ones), and the idea of death. The vegetative symptoms of panic attacks are also usually present. In more severe cases, the patient may also present social isolation, verbal expressions of rage or feelings of desperation, and other forms of altered behaviour.

## Depression

### (a) Clinical features

Depression is one of the most common psychiatric disorders found among HIV-infected individuals. Symptomatic stages of HIV infection are associated with an increased prevalence of depressive symptoms and a syndromal diagnosis of major depression.[3]

There are several factors behind the increased morbidity for affective disorders found in this population. First of all, the patient's discovery of the infection has a dramatic **psychological impact**, as does the disease's relentless progression. Second, the **neurotropism of the virus** itself produces neuropathological changes in deep grey structures whose dysfunction is known to cause mood disturbances and changes in the neurotransmission systems, which may contribute to the development of depression. Finally, the groups that in Western countries are at the highest risk for HIV infection (intravenous drug users and male homosexuals/bisexuals) are also known to be at a **high risk for depressive syndromes**, independently of having the virus. The risk factors for depression appear to be similar to those for HIV-seronegative patients and include, besides advanced HIV infection: loss of social support; personal and family history of depression; drug use; and lack of confidants.

When severe physical disease is present the diagnosis of major depression can be difficult to make, because the disease itself may be the real source of many depressive symptoms, for example insomnia, loss of appetite and weight, fatigue, lack of energy, retardation, and concentration difficulties. To avoid misdiagnosing depression, it is important to focus on the more psychological, as opposed to somatic, symptoms associated with low mood. These include **persistent low mood**, **loss of enjoyment** of usually pleasurable activities, **suicidal thoughts** and marked **feelings of hopelessness, guilt,** and **self-reproach**. Suicidal ideation may not be expressed directly, but may be expressed more passively, for example poor adherence to medical treatment. Assessment of depressed mood also requires evaluation of the probable contributing factors.

### (b) Management

#### (i) Pharmacological treatment

Antidepressants are the treatment of choice in major depression, as well as in less severe depressive syndromes that are unresponsive to psychological and social intervention. Tricyclic antidepressants have been shown to be effective in treating depressed HIV-positive patients.[4] AIDS patients can respond to lower dosages of tricyclics (25–100 mg), but they may also suffer severe anticholinergic effects at reduced dosages. Therefore, the choice of an antidepressant for these patients should be guided by its side-effect profile.

Several studies have been published showing therapeutic response to selective serotonin reuptake inhibitors in seropositive patients with major depression.[5] Many clinicians prefer the newer drugs in the medically ill, not only because of their higher acceptance among patients, but also because of their greater overdose safety margin.

#### (ii) Psychotherapy

Psychosocial interventions derived from a wide variety of theoretical orientations are effective in treating depression among individuals infected with HIV. There is good evidence for the value of psychological intervention in the management of HIV patients. Both interpersonal psychotherapy[6] and cognitive–behavioural group therapy[7] may be particularly beneficial for HIV patients with depressive symptoms.

## Psychosis

Psychotic disorders sometimes occur in people with HIV infection. While their prevalence is not high, such a development can lead to complicated diagnostic and management problems. The fact that psychosis can be related to HIV infection does not imply that a new disease entity or diagnostic category has been identified. When seropositive individuals present with psychotic symptoms, efforts should be made to clarify the clinical features and to establish their aetiology, which could well be unrelated to HIV. While in some cases the psychotic symptoms may be the result of subtle or gross brain pathology associated with HIV infection, in others it may be iatrogenic or secondary to substance misuse. Psychiatric patients per se may be considered a group at risk for contracting HIV infection.[8]

Neuroleptics are the treatment of choice for controlling psychotic symptoms. The risk of developing antipsychotic-induced extrapyramidal symptoms is higher in psychotic patients with AIDS than in psychotic patients without AIDS. AIDS patients may have an increased risk of developing tardive dyskinesia, neuroleptic malignant syndrome, and severe dystonic reactions.[9] The presence of organic cerebral deterioration, in particular HIV-associated dementia, is a risk factor for the development of neuroleptic malignant syndrome. In general, when using neuroleptics in this population, the best course is to start off with low doses, and increase the dosage slowly and progressively. The new antipsychotic risperidone has been associated with fewer extrapyramidal side-effects and used successfully in this group of patients.[10]

## Mania

HIV seems to increase the risk of manic episodes, and mania is a frequent reason for psychiatric hospitalization among people with the virus.[11] In some cases illicit drug use or iatrogenic causes are implicated, for example the chance association of HIV infection and bipolar affective disorders, but generally no obvious aetiological factors can be identified. Mania has been found to be a side-effect of medication frequently used for HIV/AIDS, including **didanosine (ddI), ganciclovir, procarbazine, estavudine** (d4T), steroids, and **zidovudine (AZT)**. Most cases of new-onset mania occur in advanced HIV disease and they are often associated with the presence of substantial cognitive impairment. New-onset mania in severe symptomatic disease is predictive of reduced survival.

Standard pharmacotherapy with neuroleptics and lithium are effective, but the usefulness of these drugs may be restricted by the development of severe adverse effects in immunosuppressed HIV-infected patients. Most psychiatrists choose atypical neuroleptics for HIV. However, these agents are not without risk for extrapyramidal side-effects in HIV patients, including the risk for metabolic inhibition of some agents by protease inhibitors. Potent antiretroviral therapy has been documented to protect against the development of HIV-associated mania.[12]

## Delirium

Delirium is one of the organic mental disorders observed most frequently in hospitalized HIV-infected patients. The exact prevalence of delirium or acute organic brain syndrome in HIV is unknown.

**Table 5.3.5.2** Aetiology of delirium in HIV-infected patients

| Infections | Encephalitis due to HIV, syphilis, toxoplasmosis, cryptococcosis, coccidioidomycosis, progressive multifocal leucoencephalopathy, herpesvirus |
|---|---|
| Abstinence | Alcohol, opiates |
| Metabolic | Depletion of volume, hydro-electrolytic alterations, transfusions |
| Hypoxia | Pneumonia with respiratory, compromise |
| Deficiencies | B-complex vitamins |
| Cerebral vascular event | |
| Medication | Anticholinergics, central nervous system depressors |
| Intracranial mass | Haematoma, neoplasias |
| Toxic | Drugs of abuse |

Patients with advanced systemic disease and dementia are at a high risk for delirium, the cause of which is often multifactorial. The precipitant organic factors involved are listed in Table 5.3.5.2.

A conservative attitude has been recommended for the management of these conditions, with the use of low oral or intramuscular doses of neuroleptics, and correction of the organic disorders responsible for the development of disturbances in the level of consciousness.[13] However, other authors have postulated that patients suffering from delirium and agitation should be given high doses of neuroleptics—alone or in combination with lorazepam—in cases where quick control of the symptoms is vital.[14] The efficacy of pharmacological interventions in patients with delirium is heightened if treatment is begun as soon as the first symptoms appear.

### Other central nervous infections in HIV-related illness

In the advanced phases of AIDS, opportunistic infections are highly varied, as are the neoplasias that can develop in immunodepressed individuals, which affect the central nervous system. The more frequents are:

- **Progressive multifocal leucoencephalopathy.** This is a grave neurological complication, linked to papovavirus infection. Dementia can develop rapidly, with focal neurological alterations such as blindness, ataxia, and hemiparesis. Death follows very quickly thereafter, and there is no known treatment. Computerized brain images taken from these patients show a characteristic involvement of the white matter.

- **Cerebral toxoplasmosis.** It is linked to the reactivation of a latent cerebral infection by *Toxoplasma gondii*, an opportunistic intracellular protozoan. The clinical presentation can vary greatly, but it is characterized by the rapid development of a marked alteration in the mental state. The focal involvement can produce headache and lateralized neurological effects. The lesions tend to be located in basal ganglia. Diagnosis is based on structural neuroimaging tests, and treatment is with pyrimethamine and sulphadiazine.

- **Cryptococcal meningitis (torulosis).** This form of meningitis, caused by infestation with the yeast-like fungus *Cryptococcus neoformans,* is characterized by headache, meningism (although it sometimes courses without this symptom), photophobia, nausea, fever, and delirium. The diagnosis is made after a lumbar puncture, and analysis of the culture and antibodies.

## Syphilis

A century ago, patients with general paresis due to cerebral syphilitic infections constituted a high proportion of mental hospital admissions, and accounted for an appreciable part of the chronic population of such institutions. With the identification in the early twentieth century of the causative agent, *Treponema pallidum*, and the development of effective methods of treating syphilis, this condition has become relatively rare. Historically, the study of syphilis of the central nervous system has been of great interest to psychiatrists due to the light it sheds on the nature of the relationship between cerebral and mental disease. It was one of the first mental disorders for which a specific organic aetiology was demonstrated, and the first to respond to a medical treatment.

Syphilis remains a major problem in certain areas of the world. Because during its early stages it is a genital ulcerative disease, syphilis facilitates the transmission of HIV and may be particularly important in contributing to HIV transmission in those regions where the rates of both infections are high.

### Clinical features

Syphilis is a complex STD with an extremely variable clinical course. Neurosyphilis presents 5 years or more after the initial infection. It affects 10 per cent of non-treated cases, and can take several clinical forms.[15]

- **Asymptomatic neurosyphilis.** Infected subjects have abnormalities in the cerebrospinal fluid (pleocytosis, elevated protein, and reactive VDRL score), but no symptoms or signs of central nervous system disorder. It can evolve into a symptomatic form or remit on its own.

- **Meningovascular syphilis.** Appears within 1 to 5 years of primary infection, although it can occur as early as 6 months and as late as 12 years.[16] In the clinical picture, the patient may develop stroke syndromes of subacute onset with a preceding encephalic picture, including psychiatric disturbances such as lability or personality changes. The patient may complain of headache, lethargy, and malaise, and may experience difficulty in concentration and exhibit faulty judgement. Emotional instability and irritability are common. Mental deterioration may progress to dementia, which can be accompanied by delusional symptomatology and episodes of excitation.[16]

- **General paresis.** This form of parenchymal neurosyphilis is also known as *dementia paralytica* or *general paralysis of the insane.* It usually first appears some 20 years after the initial infection. Its initial symptoms are memory disturbance, dysarthria, and hyper-reflexia, which may be accompanied by personality changes and irritability—in many cases the latter are the presenting abnormalities. The symptoms progress to dementia with abnormal motor function and psychotic symptoms. These organic psychoses were frequent in the pre-penicillin era and are known for their florid clinical picture—prominent euphoric mood, expansive demeanour, and delusions of power, wealth, or social position. Other cases may resemble depressive psychosis with somatic delusions.

- **Tabes dorsalis.** This condition is a degeneration of the ascending fibres from the dorsal root ganglia, resulting in atrophy of the dorsal roots and demyelinization in the posterior columns of the cord. It can develop from 3 to 20 years after the initial infection. Main symptoms are the loss of position reflexes, ataxia, vibration sense, incontinence, and lacinating pains involving many areas of the body.

### Diagnosis and management

The clinical picture of neurosyphilis is so variable that routine serological testing upon admission to psychiatric inpatient units has been recommended. In clinical practice, a rise in atypical syndromes with minor symptomatology has been attributed to partial suppression of the infection during its early stages by antibiotics taken for other reasons.[16] The diagnosis of neurosyphilis should be considered on the basis of the patient's symptoms and clinical signs, and confirmed by serology and analysis of the cerebrospinal fluid.

Penicillin is the drug of choice for *T. pallidum* infections, and in the treatment of neurosyphilis, but the dosage must achieve treponemicidal levels within the cerebrospinal fluid. In untreated cases, death usually occurs within 4 to 5 years. If treatment is given early, the condition usually remits; in already established cases, the progression of the disease can be halted. Antipsychotics are indicated for the symptomatic management of the excitement and psychotic symptoms that these patients may present. Clinicians should have in mind that all patients who have syphilis should be tested for HIV.

## Other sexually transmitted diseases

A diverse range of psychological symptomatology is associated with STDs, in which maladaptive or pathological responses to infection (or fear of infection) may occur. Most of the studies that evaluated the psychological effects of having a STD have been carried out in patients attending genitourinary clinics, and focused on genital herpes, a common, recurrent, and painful infection. The response to diagnosis of a STD can include depression, anxiety, anger, social withdrawal, feelings of loneliness, and sexual dysfunction.[17,18] Also, high rates of hypochondriasis and veneroneurosis (a strong but unfounded conviction of having a venereal disease) are found in STD clinics and are frequently associated with psychiatric morbidity. Psychological interventions can effectively reduce the distress associated with STDs, contribute to the control of the infection, increase compliance with medication regimens, and reduce somatic symptoms misattributed to a STD.

## Tuberculosis

### Clinical picture

In spite of pharmacological advances, tuberculosis continues to be a serious public health problem in many parts of the world, especially due to the increased tuberculosis rate in HIV-infected patients and the appearance of multidrug-resistant tuberculosis.

Tuberculosis patients may present with vegetative signs suggestive of depression, especially the elderly and those in the symptomatic stages of HIV infection. The initial depressive symptoms are weight loss, lethargy, lack of interest, and mental confusion. They may also develop sleep disturbances due to night sweats and nocturnal coughing.

Tuberculosis patients quite frequently present with neuropsychiatric symptoms, which can be related to very different circumstances.

First, clinicians should bear in mind that tuberculosis infection often develops in patients who previously had a severe psychiatric pathology, such as alcoholism or intravenous drug abuse, or in the chronic mentally ill. Also, the most common psychiatric symptoms, such as emotional lability and depression, could be related, among other factors, to the feeling of invalidity that accompanies the illness, and its social stigma. In addition, the preventive treatment of those in contact with the patient can trigger feelings of guilt. In some cases, tuberculosis leads to chronic respiratory disease, which is also associated with depressive symptoms, suicidal ideation, and cognitive impairment, particularly in debilitated patients.

Neuropsychiatric disorders in patients with tuberculosis can also be related to cerebral infections: tuberculous meningitis, potentially a very serious complication, develops in 5 per cent of all cases. Since these patients frequently present with mental symptoms that can figure prominently from the outset and even precede overt signs of meningeal infection, the correct diagnosis should be established urgently, in order to institute specific therapy as soon as possible.

### Diagnosis and management

Sputum tests, cultures, and chest radiographs, as well as a tuberculin skin test, are standard diagnostic tools. In cases of suspected tuberculous meningitis, a spinal puncture is necessary to determine whether the patient has lymphocytosis and a moderate increase in protein. The diagnosis is confirmed when tubercle bacilli can be identified or cultured from the fluid; however, since irreversible brain damage may result from waiting for cultural confirmation, it is often necessary to begin therapy on the basis of a presumptive clinical diagnosis. The brain scan may show hydrocephalus, focal infarcts, and exudate in basal brain cisterns.[19]

It is important in psychiatric settings that suspected tuberculosis patients receive a proper diagnostic evaluation, not only for the sake of their own health but also for that of other patients who may be exposed to the infection in the unit. It may be necessary to transfer psychiatric inpatients with tuberculosis to a ward where isolation can be assured. The Centres for Disease Control recommend routine tuberculosis screening for patients in HIV risk groups, and for residents of mental health facilities.[20]

The most commonly used drugs for the treatment of tuberculosis are isoniazid, rifampicin, pyrazinamide, ethambutol, and streptomycin. Compliance is vital to achieve effective treatment.

## Lyme disease

First described in the United States in 1975, this infection has also been reported in Europe, Australia, and other parts of the world. It is caused by the spirochaete *Borrelia burgdorferi*, which is carried and transmitted by the deer tick. The somatic symptomatology features a characteristic skin lesion, an expanding erythematous annular lesion which usually first appears 3 to 32 days after the initial transmission and may last for several weeks. In 15 per cent of the patients, the disease progresses to a secondary phase marked by neurological symptoms, for example meningoencephalitis, radiculitis, central and peripheral neuropathy, and myelitis.

The neuropsychiatric symptomatology consists in difficulties involving memory, orientation, and calculation. Even years after the first infection, patients can present with violent and impulsive behaviour, labile affect, and depression. Cases of psychotic or catatonic syndromes and chronic dementia have been described. Many patients with Lyme disease, who suffer from neurological symptoms, present with signs of encephalopathy with alterations in their sleep, affect, and memory. The diagnosis can be established from a serological analysis.

## Encephalitis

Encephalitis may be caused primarily by a viral disease affecting the brain or can be a complication of bacterial meningitis, septicaemia, or brain abscesses. It can occur after influenza, herpes simplex, measles, rubella infections, and also after vaccination. In the acute stage, the patient may present with headache, vomiting, and seizures. Patients may develop a confusional syndrome. In rare cases, the encephalitis may present with predominantly psychiatric symptoms. That is the case of herpesvirus encephalitis, which due to its damage to temporal lobes can cause a serious amnestic syndrome.

In clinical practice, the psychiatrist is more likely to see the complications that appear after the acute episode in the form of anxiety and depressive syndromes, personality change, and dementia. In the early years of life, encephalitis may be followed by behavioural disorders.[16]

## Infectious mononucleosis

The Epstein–Barr virus causes 90 per cent of all cases of infectious mononucleosis. It can appear at any age, but the illness tends to manifest itself clinically in adolescents and young adults.

The most important symptoms are fever, general malaise, diffuse lymphadenopathies, and laryngitis. However, complications can lead to encephalitis and paralysis of the cranial nerves. In the case of encephalitic compromise, delirium can result. Depressive syndromes have also been observed after an acute infectious episode, accompanied by fatigue.

## Brucellosis

This infection is produced by micro-organisms of the genus *Brucella*, and is transmitted by exposure to or ingestion of contaminated animal products, especially unpasteurized milk products, or contact with infected animal tissues. Onset can be insidious, since it mimics other more common illnesses, with low fever, fatigue, and sweating, but 10 to 20 per cent of cases present with splenomegaly. The psychiatric manifestations of the disease can include depressive or anxious syndromes. Diagnosis can be confirmed by blood or lymph cultures or bone marrow biopsy, although the majority of diagnoses are made serologically.

## Further information

Fernandez, F. and Ruiz, P. (eds.) (2006). *Psychiatric aspects of HIV/AIDS*. Lippincott Williams & Wilkins, Philadelphia, PA.

APA AIDS resource center: www.psych.org/AIDS

CDC resource center: www.cdc.gov/std

## References

1. Forstein, M. (1988). Understanding the psychological impact of AIDS: the other epidemic. *New England Journal of Public Policy*, **4**, 159–73.
2. Catalan, J., Burgess, A., and Klimes, I. (1995). *Psychological medicine of HIV infection*. Oxford Medical Publications, Oxford.
3. Ciesla, J.A. and Roberts, J.E. (2001). Meta-analysis of the relationship between HIV infection and risk for depressive disorders. *The American Journal of Psychiatry*, **158**, 725–30.
4. Markowitz, J.C., Rabkin, J.G., and Perry, S.W. (1994). Treating depression in HIV-positive patients. *AIDS*, **8**, 403–12.
5. Rabkin, J.G., Wagner, G.J., and Rabkin, R. (1999). Fluoxetine treatment for depression in patients with HIV and AIDS: a randomized, placebo-controlled trial. *The American Journal of Psychiatry*, **156**, 101–7.
6. Markowitz, J., Kocsis, J.H., Fishman, B., *et al.* (1998). Treatment of depressive symptoms in human immunodeficiency virus-positive patients. *Archives of General Psychiatry*, **55**, 452–7.
7. Blanch, J., Rousaud, A., Hautzinger, M., *et al.* (2002). Assessment of the efficacy of a cognitive-behavioral group psychotherapy programme for HIV infected patients referred to a consultation-liaison psychiatry department. *Psychotherapy and Psychosomatics*, **71**, 77–84.
8. Ayuso-Mateos, J.L., Montañes, F., Lastra, I., *et al.* (1997). HIV infection in psychiatric inpatients: an unlinked anonymous study. *British Journal of Psychiatry*, **170**, 181–5.
9. Ayuso, J.L. (1994). Use of psychotropic drugs in patients with HIV infection. *Drugs*, **4**, 599–610.
10. Singh, A.N., Golledge, H., and Catalan, J. (1997). Treatment of HIV related psychotic disorders with risperidone: a series of 21 cases. *Journal of Psychosomatic Research*, **42**, 489–93.
11. Kierburz, K., Zettelmaier, A., Ketonen, L., *et al.* (1991). Manic syndrome in AIDS. *The American Journal of Psychiatry*, **148**, 1068–70.
12. Mijch, A.M., Judd, F.K., Lyketsos, C.G., *et al.* (1999). Secondary mania in patients with HIV infection: are antiretrovirals protective? *Journal of Neuropsychiatry and Clinical Neurosciences*, **11**, 475–80.
13. Breitbart, W., Marotta, R., Platt, M.M., *et al.* (1996). A double-blind trial of haloperidol, chlorpromazine and lorazepam in the treatment of delirium in hospitalised AIDS patients. *The American Journal of Psychiatry*, **153**, 231–7.
14. Fernandez, F., Levy, J.K., and Mansell, P.W. (1989). Management of delirium in terminally ill AIDS patients. *International Journal Psychiatry in Medicine*, **19**, 165–72.
15. Simon, R.P. (1985). Neurosyphilis. *Archives of Neurology*, **42**, 606–13.
16. Lishman, W.A. (1998). *Organic psychiatry* (3rd edn). Blackwell Science, Oxford.
17. Catalan, J., Bradley, M., Gallwey, J., *et al.* (1981). Sexual dysfunction and psychiatric morbidity in patients attending a clinic for sexually transmitted diseases. *British Journal of Psychiatry*, **138**, 292–6.
18. Hedge, B. (1997). Sexually transmitted diseases. In *Cambridge handbook of psychology, health and medicine* (eds. A. Baum, S. Newman, J. Weinman, R. West, and C. McManus), pp. 584–5. Cambridge University Press, Cambridge.
19. Rovira, M., Romero, F., and Torrent, O. (1980). Study of tuberculosis meningitis by CT. *Neuroradiology*, **19**, 137–41.
20. Dooley, S.W., Castro, K.G., Hutton, M.D., *et al.* (1990). Guidelines for preventing the transmission of tuberculosis in health-care settings, with special focus on HIV-related issues. *Morbidity and Mortality Weekly Report*, **39** (RR-17), 1–29.

## 5.3.6 Psychiatric aspects of surgery (including transplantation)

S. A. Hales, S. E. Abbey, and G. M. Rodin

Attention to psychiatric disturbances and to emotional distress is important in the surgical setting, from the time of the initial diagnostic assessment, to the perioperative period and the phase of subsequent recovery and rehabilitation. Psychiatric illness and psychological factors, which are not taken into account prior to surgery, may contribute to inaccurate diagnoses, unrealistic assessment of the surgical risk, unnecessary surgery, and complications that could have been avoided or minimized. This chapter will address these factors and provide an approach to the consideration of psychiatric factors and interventions in this setting.

## Preoperative assessment and intervention

The assessment of all patients being considered for surgery should include a brief evaluation of their current emotional state, cognitive functioning, personal circumstances, present or past history of psychiatric illness, and personality and coping style, as these factors may affect their adjustment to surgery. Psychiatric consultation may be indicated for a number of specific reasons discussed below.

### Psychological contributors to the patient's physical symptoms

The most common psychological factor that complicates the surgical assessment is a low pain threshold and a tendency to somatize, i.e. to experience and communicate emotional distress in physical terms. When emotional factors amplify somatic symptoms, it is more difficult to distinguish organic from functional disorders on the basis of the clinical history. At the extreme end of the continuum of somatization is the dramatic presentation of physical symptoms, which may mimic a surgical condition, in the absence of organic disease. This syndrome may fulfil criteria for a somatoform disorder, such as a somatization disorder, conversion disorder, or somatoform pain disorder.[1] In such cases, careful attention to the objective indications for surgery is required. Individuals with a body dysmorphic disorder, a syndrome of perceived or imagined ugliness, may present with repeated requests for cosmetic surgery.[2] However, cosmetic surgery is unlikely to relieve the body dissatisfaction of such patients, whose condition has much in common with obsessive–compulsive disorder. Dissatisfaction with the results of surgery is common in patients with body dysmorphic disorder, and litigiousness and threats towards the treating surgeon may occur in a small proportion of cases. In general, the failure of clinicians to consider the contribution of somatization to the clinical presentation may lead to unnecessary or inappropriate surgery. When this occurs, postsurgical complications may interfere with the subsequent evaluation of persistent physical symptoms. Somatoform disorders are discussed further in Chapter 5.2.2.

Although physicians commonly consider that emotional factors may amplify physical symptoms, the possibility that disease has been intentionally simulated or fabricated is usually not entertained.

Factitious disorder refers to a syndrome in which such behaviour is enacted for no apparent reason, other than to assume the patient role. This is in contrast with malingering, in which there may be reports of physical symptoms motivated by the desire for some specific secondary gain, which may be financial or compensation-related. While relatively rare, factitious disorder poses particular challenges, in both detection and treatment, to psychiatric and surgical teams. Individuals with this disorder may produce or simulate disease in various ways, such as by self-inflicting wounds that require surgical intervention or by surreptitiously contaminating themselves to produce infection. Patients with this condition may also communicate plausible symptoms of a surgical condition. Such patients are at risk to receive unnecessary surgery and should be regarded as suffering from a serious and potentially life-threatening condition. The majority of such patients are unwilling to accept psychological or psychiatric assistance, but an ongoing, supportive relationship with a medical caregiver may diminish this symptom pattern. Factitious disorder is discussed further in Chapter 5.2.9.

### Capacity to consent to surgery

Providing information and obtaining informed consent are routine and essential aspects of preoperative care provided by the surgical team. Informed consent to a surgical procedure requires disclosure of pertinent information by the treating physician, and understanding of the information, decisional capacity, and voluntary choice on the part of the patient.[3] The decisional capacity of patients depends on their ability not only to understand information relevant to the decision, but also to apply it to their own situation and to express a consistent voluntary choice.[4] Information required by patients to make an informed surgical decision includes the rationale, risks, and benefits of the surgery, the potential alternative treatments, and the risk of not proceeding with surgery. In most jurisdictions, the emergency treatment of incapable persons is permitted, when substitute consent is not available, unless the clinician has reason to believe that the person would refuse such treatment if he or she were capable.[3] When it is not an emergency, substitute consent must be obtained on behalf of individuals who are incapable of providing informed consent. The legal requirements for substitute consent vary in different jurisdictions.

The capacity to provide informed consent may be impaired by cognitive dysfunction, by psychiatric illness, or by contextual factors, such as the clarity and relevance of the information disclosed or the manner of disclosure. If screening by the treating surgeon indicates that the patient may be incapable, a psychiatric consultation may be requested to evaluate the patient's decisional capacity.[5] Patients with cognitive impairment or a major psychiatric disorder, such as schizophrenia, are not necessarily incapable of making treatment decisions, unless these conditions affect their understanding and appreciation of information relevant to the decision. Numerous tools have been developed to assess decisional capacity but there is no current gold standard.[6]

Obtaining informed consent for surgery is not only a legal and ethical requirement, but also a crucial dimension of the surgeon–patient relationship. In some cases, treatment refusal reflects a breakdown in the relationship between the surgeon and the patient more than it does an informed decision of the patient to reject a recommendation for surgery. When this occurs, attention to the physician–patient relationship, and the provision of additional information, may help to relieve the impasse so that an informed decision can be made. In other cases, treatment of a major psychiatric illness, such as a psychotic episode in a patient with schizophrenia, is necessary to restore the patient's capacity to provide consent.

## Assessment of the response to surgery

Surgical patients face numerous stressors, including the fear of pain, disfigurement, and the loss of control, as well as the possibility of major medical complications and death. The response to these stressors may be affected by the nature of the illness and the surgical procedure, its personal meaning, the prior history of trauma, the support which is anticipated and perceived from medical caregivers and significant others, and the prior experience of the individual with medical or surgical procedures. The age and life stage of the individual, the risk associated with the procedure, and the prognosis of the underlying or associated medical conditions may also affect the psychological response in the perioperative period. Apprehension and mistrust are more common in those who have previously suffered from the adverse effects of missed or delayed diagnosis or treatment. Attitudinal factors, including positive expectations and the desire to participate actively in the recovery process, may also affect clinical outcomes. The desire to maintain a sense of control may be adaptive during the preparation and rehabilitation phases but may be associated with greater distress immediately following surgery, when there is an inescapable and predominant requirement to depend on others.[7] Those with more attachment anxiety, i.e. concern about the availability of support from others, may benefit from predictability and reliability in relation to caregivers, whereas those who tend to be more self-sufficient may benefit most from strategies which promote self-reliance and self-care.[8, 9]

There has been particular interest in psychosocial issues in the setting of transplantation surgery. This occurred, in part, because of the desire of transplant programmes to select optimal candidates for organ transplants, which were experimental and/or in scarce supply. However, the psychiatric and psychosocial selection criteria for transplant surgery have become less stringent, as the transplantation of particular organs has become more routine.[10] At present, psychosocial evaluation of transplant candidates by a multidisciplinary team allows for the identification, treatment, and monitoring of factors that may affect compliance, morbidity, and psychosocial outcomes. Organ transplants from living donors, such as for bone marrow, kidney, and liver transplantation, are unlike most other surgical interventions in that they necessitate surgery for individuals without pre-existing disease. Psychosocial evaluation of such donors includes consideration of the process of decision-making and informed consent, the adaptive capacities of the individual, the degree of social support, and the relationship of the donor to the recipient.[11] Although there has been concern about the psychological consequences of such surgery, the available evidence suggests that organ donation is usually well tolerated and experienced in positive terms by the donor, particularly when the surgical and medical outcomes are favourable.[12]

There is now increasing evidence that the systematic preoperative education of patients and their family caregivers in a therapeutic context may enhance adjustment to surgical procedures.[13] Postoperative education may also improve subsequent rehabilitation following surgical procedures. Such approaches are consistent with modern Western trends towards consumerism and patient empowerment, in which greater emphasis is placed on assisting patients to assume more responsibility for their medical course and treatment outcome. This approach has also been necessitated by the trend towards earlier hospital discharge of surgical patients into the community where much more self-care is required.

## Anxiety

Preoperative anxiety is common and may be particularly problematic in patients awaiting procedures such as transplantation, which usually occur in the course of a life-threatening condition, and are associated with long and unpredictable waiting periods for surgery. Anxiety has been reported to be more common in younger patients, in females, and in those who are unmarried or who have less perceived social support.[14] Research suggests that preoperative anxiety may complicate postoperative recovery through behavioural and physiological mechanisms.[15] Symptoms of anxiety can usually be managed with education and reassurance, but when they are persistent and problematic, interventions such as progressive relaxation and guided imagery may be helpful both to reduce symptoms of anxiety and to enhance feelings of self-control.[16] Some patients benefit from a benzodiazepine to reduce preoperative anxiety, but those with antecedent anxiety disorders may require more intensive intervention, as outlined in Chapter 4.6.1. Prior to elective procedures, patients with specific blood or needle phobias may benefit from systematic desensitization. Those with comorbid panic disorder may require a higher dose of anxiolytic medication in the preoperative period. The surgical team should be aware of such treatment so that the medication can be restarted promptly after surgery, to avoid symptoms of withdrawal and anxiety. If oral medications cannot be reinstituted for a prolonged period of time after surgery, intramuscular lorazepam or intravenous lorazepam or diazepam may be used.

## Mood disorders

It is important to detect and treat mood disorders prior to surgery because they are associated with increased surgical morbidity and mortality, and with reduced treatment compliance in the postoperative period.[17] Anaesthetists must be aware of any drugs taken to treat and prevent bipolar and depressive disorders, because some can significantly prolong muscle paralysis secondary to neuromuscular blockade. Furthermore, attention should be paid to serum lithium levels and signs of lithium toxicity since they may be affected by the patient's fluid and volume status. Conventional heterocyclic antidepressants and selective serotonin reuptake inhibitors can be continued until the time of surgery, and then restarted postoperatively, when oral medications can be tolerated. Selective serotonin reuptake inhibitors are known to affect platelet serotonin levels and platelet aggregation and to be occasionally associated with prolonged bleeding times, increased perioperative blood loss, and an increased subsequent need for transfusion.[18] Patients receiving monoamine oxidase inhibitors (MAOIs) are usually advised to discontinue this medication for 1 to 2 weeks prior to their surgery, although this recommendation must be weighed against the risk of withdrawal symptoms and of precipitating a current depression. The medical charts of patients receiving MAOIs should be clearly labelled to advise that all drugs administered should be screened for their interactions with these drugs and that pethidine (meperidine) and dextromethorphan in particular should not be prescribed due to risk of a serotonin syndrome, which is associated with gastrointestinal, neurological, cardiovascular, and psychiatric symptoms. In addition, hospital charts of patients taking MAOIs should be clearly marked to indicate that they must avoid foods containing tyramine. Patients with bipolar disorder should be monitored for mood alterations since they may be at risk of developing hypomania or mania when steroid medications are used following transplantation surgery.

## Psychotic disorders

These disorders, most commonly related to schizophrenia or bipolar disorder, pose challenges which vary depending upon the requirements of the surgery and the patient's mental status. Patients with schizophrenia may be at increased perioperative risk for hypotension, hypothermia, confusion, infection, and for ileus, in those who undergo abdominal surgery. These complications may occur due both to pathology of the endocrine, immune, and cardiovascular systems associated with schizophrenia and to the effects of antipsychotic medications.[19] Those who are being treated with a low-potency antipsychotic may be switched to a high-potency agent to decrease the risk of hypotension, particularly with cardiovascular surgery in the postoperative period. For their own comfort and for that of others, individuals who are actively psychotic may require special arrangements, such as a single room, close or constant observation, and, when feasible, greater family involvement. Such patients require closer monitoring for many reasons, including the increased likelihood that they may misinterpret common ward events as threatening and because they may be at increased risk for exacerbation of their underlying condition and for the occurrence of delirium.

## Cognitive disorders

The capacity of patients to understand information and to provide a coherent account of their symptoms is fundamental to the process of diagnosis, informed consent, and assessment of the indications for surgery and the risk of specific postoperative complications. Cognitive impairment prior to surgery may complicate these processes and may be associated with an increased risk of delirium or dementia in the postoperative period. In such cases, neuropsychological testing may be indicated prior to elective surgery to establish a baseline, to assist in the evaluation of decisional capacity, and, to aid in the prediction of postoperative delirium or worsening of dementia.

## Personality disorders

Patients with personality disorders are more likely to have greater difficulty than others adapting to the multiple and unpredictable stresses associated with surgery. Those with impulsivity may have difficulty adhering to the preoperative and postoperative regimen and those who are suspicious and mistrustful may be more limited in their ability to form effective treatment relationships and to make treatment decisions, in which an enormous degree of trust is required. Those with a borderline personality disorder may be highly sensitive to feelings of personal injury or neglect and may tend to idealize some caregivers and to denigrate others. These responses may create problematic divisions amongst the treatment team and may adversely affect the care of the patient. A psychiatric consultant may be of help to provide patient support and to educate staff about the underlying psychiatric disorder in such individuals, who may otherwise be viewed negatively by staff who regard their behaviour as simply wilful or manipulative.

## Substance abuse disorders

The preoperative assessment should include enquiry about substance use, in order to adjust current medication appropriately and to prevent the occurrence of postoperative withdrawal syndromes. Consultation psychiatrists may play a role in continuing medical education about the value of routine, non-judgemental screening for substance use in medical patients, and about the importance of recording these details in the medical record.

## Assessment of psychotropic medications

The pharmacological effects of psychotropic medications must be taken into account in the perioperative period. Important factors that affect the risks and benefits associated with psychotropic medication use perioperatively include:

1 End-organ sensitivity to side effects based on medical comorbidity and organ dysfunction;

2 direct effects of psychotropic medications and their potential interactions with anaesthetic and analgesic agents likely to be prescribed;

3 route of access available (oral, suppository, subcutaneous, intramuscular, intravenous);

4 risk of withdrawal symptoms and recurrence or relapse of a psychiatric disorder if psychotropic medications are to be discontinued.[20]

Information on drug–drug interactions is constantly being updated and current information can be obtained from internet sites such as http://www.drugdigest.org/DD/Home or http://search.medscape.com/drug-reference-search.

# Postoperative complications and interventions

## Agitation and delirium

Agitation is a common postoperative problem, the frequency of which depends upon the characteristics of the disease, the nature of the surgery and its complications, and the pre-existing vulnerability of the patient. A concerted effort should be made to identify the source of the agitation, which may be a worsening of the medical condition, inadequately controlled pain, or delirium. Delirium, which is described in more detail in Chapter 4.1.1, is a common complication, which develops in more than one-third of cases following surgery.[21] Higher rates of delirium are found following longer procedures, due to intraoperative hypoxemia, following cardiac surgeries, due to hypoperfusion and microemboli formation, following orthopaedic procedures, due to fat emboli, and following cataract surgery, due to the impact of vision loss and of ophthalmic drugs with anticholinergic side effects.[22]

Measures to prevent and ameliorate delirium include the identification and treatment of predisposing risk factors and reversible causes, symptomatic treatment, and environmental interventions to reduce distress and agitation. The latter may include measures to prevent sensory deprivation and disorientation, to monitor safety, and to educate patients and family members about the condition. When distress or agitation associated with delirium threaten the safety and care of the patient, pharmacologic interventions may be necessary. There have been trials of cholinesterase inhibitors[23] and of atypical antipsychotics in those patients who can take oral medications, but haloperidol remains the first-choice medication for management of delirium-associated agitation. It is preferred because it has fewer active metabolites and fewer anticholinergic and sedative effects than other antipsychotic medication and because it can be administered intravenously. This route of administration is usually safe, although arrhythmias with its intravenous use have been reported in patients with histories of alcohol abuse or with cardiomyopathy.[24] Benzodiazepines should be used to treat withdrawal from alcohol and sedative-hypnotics using standard protocols.

Delirium may be highly distressing for both patients and family caregivers.[25] Some patients subsequently retain disturbing memories of their experience during a delirium. Such traumatic recall may also occur, in rare instances, when there has been inadequate anaesthesia. In these cases, patients and their family caregivers typically appreciate a discussion of their concerns and the opportunity to review these events with the surgeon and the anaesthetist. A small number of patients with these disturbing experiences develop symptoms of post-traumatic stress disorder and may benefit from a brief course of psychotherapy or pharmacotherapy to alleviate their symptoms.

### Ventilator weaning

Some patients experience difficulty being weaned from the ventilator due to anxiety, depression, delirium, or other psychological factors related to their disease or to the ICU environment. Behavioural approaches to facilitate weaning may include relaxation techniques that do not depend on observation or manipulation of breathing, guided imagery, and/or biofeedback.[26] Weaning problems due to anxiety typically respond to benzodiazepines or to haloperidol, administered in a single dose prior to weaning. Apathetic or depressed patients who have difficulty being weaned may benefit from a psychostimulant.[27] When delirium is the cause of weaning problems, its underlying cause should be identified and treated.

### Pain management

Effective pain management is a fundamental aspect of postoperative treatment and may reduce distress, agitation, sleep disturbance, anxiety, mood symptoms, and behavioural disorders. Suboptimal pain management may occur due to inadequate assessment of this symptom, insufficient knowledge of the pharmacokinetic and pharmacodynamic properties of analgesic medication, and unfounded concerns about 'addiction'. Further, some patients refuse to accept adequate analgesia because of misconceptions or personal beliefs regarding the importance of stoicism, vigilance, or personal control. Consultant psychiatrists may help patients to address their concerns about analgesic medication and analgesic adjuvants and may act also as advocates or intermediaries for patients to ensure adequate analgesia.

### Sleep disturbance

Sleep disturbances, including reduced total sleep time, fragmentation of sleep, frequent arousals and awakenings, and reduced slow-wave sleep, are common in the immediate postoperative period. These disturbances may be caused by multiple factors, including the noise, temperature and light of the hospital environment, neuroimmunological and other changes associated with the surgical insult, and anaesthetic and analgesic medications.[28] Daytime sleeping, related to prolonged bed rest, lack of intellectual and social stimulation, and reduced circadian cues, may disrupt normal sleep chronobiology and increase difficulty with night-time sleep.

Treatment of sleep disturbances should be directed to the identified cause. In those patients in whom anxiety or the intrusiveness of the hospital environment is the main cause of the sleep disturbance, benzodiazepines may be temporarily used. When there are concerns about substance abuse, newer non-benzodiazepine hypnotics may be preferable, due to the lower risk of tolerance associated with their use.[28] Caution should be exercised with patients for whom benzodiazepine-induced nocturnal respiratory compromise may be problematic or with elderly patients who are susceptible to cognitive compromise or to falls.

### Cognitive impairment

Cognitive impairment is a common short-term and long-term complication of major surgery, particularly in those with more advanced age. Gradual recovery of cognitive functions occurs in most patients within 3 months after surgery, although it may take as long as 6 to 12 months.[29] Delirium that is slow to resolve may be an early sign of an associated dementing illness or of a cerebral insult that has occurred during or after surgery. Cognitive impairment may be permanent when there has been irreversible brain damage due to neurosurgery or perioperative complications, such as hypoxia or stroke. Neuropsychological testing may be helpful to document or track changes in cognitive functioning. Education of primary caregivers about the risk and manifestations of cognitive impairment is essential, and institution of home supports and respite care for patients and families facing this complication may be necessary. Some patients with cognitive impairment may also benefit from neurorehabilitation interventions.

### Adjustment issues

Longer-term problems in adjustment may occur, particularly following disfiguring surgeries, such as facial surgery, amputations, ostomies, or following procedures such as organ transplantation, which impose complicated postoperative regimens. Sexual difficulties that result from procedures that compromise the neural input or functional integrity of genital structures, or that negatively affect body image or feelings of attractiveness, may be disturbing to patients and spouses who may benefit from specific enquiry and assistance. Patients and their families should be informed about the possibility of adjustment problems with such surgeries and should be given information about available resources. A minority of patients develop clinically significant mood or anxiety disorders or significant compliance problems during the rehabilitation phase which may necessitate psychiatric consultation and intervention.

## Prolonged dysfunction

Prolonged and disproportionate pain and disability occur in a subset of patients. In some of these cases, the surgery was undertaken to relieve refractory symptoms that subsequently proved to be functional or medically unexplained. This may occur with hysterectomies performed to relieve pelvic pain and in surgery to relieve chronic back pain. In other cases, persistent disproportionate symptoms may be perpetuated by secondary gain of a financial or social nature, or by opiate dependence. Undiagnosed and untreated mood, anxiety, and somatoform disorders may also contribute to persistent symptoms. The consultation psychiatrist may be called upon to identify these factors and to help distinguish them from undetected medical/surgical pathology or from the effects of inadequate pain regimens.

## Further information

Levenson, J.L. (ed.) (2005). *American psychiatry publishing textbook of psychosomatic medicine.* American Psychiatric Press, Washington, DC.

Lloyd, G. and Guthrie, E. (eds.) (2007). *Handbook of liaison psychiatry.* Cambridge University Press, Cambridge.

## References

1. Abbey, S.E. (2002). Somatization and somatoform disorders. In: *The American psychiatric publishing textbook of consultation-liaison psychiatry* (2nd edn) (ed. M.G. Wise and J.R. Rundell), pp. 361–92. American Psychiatric Press, Washington, DC.
2. Phillips, K.A., McElroy, S.L., Keck, P.E. Jr., *et al.* (1993). Body dysmorphic disorder: 30 cases of imagined ugliness. *The American Journal of Psychiatry*, **150**, 302–8.
3. Etchells, E., Sharpe, G., Walsh, P., *et al.* (1996). Bioethics for clinicians: 1. consent. *CMAJ: Canadian Medical Association Journal*, **155**, 177–80.
4. Grisso, L.B. and Appelbaum, P.S. (1998). *Assessing competence to consent to treatment: a guide for physicians and other health professionals.* Oxford University Press, New York.
5. Etchells, E., Sharpe, G., Elliott, C., *et al.* (1996). Bioethics for clinicians: 3. Capacity. *CMAJ: Canadian Medical Association Journal*, **155**, 657–61.
6. Dunn, L.B., Nowrangi, M.A., Palmer, B.W., *et al.* (2006). Assessing decisional capacity for clinical research or treatment: a review of instruments. *The American Journal of Psychiatry*, **163**, 1323–34.
7. Rosenberger, P.H., Jokl, P., and Ickovics, J. (2006). Psychosocial factors and surgical outcomes: an evidence-based literature review. *The Journal of the American Academy of Orthopaedic Surgeons*, **14**, 397–405.
8. Hunter, J.J. and Maunder, R.G. (2002). Using attachment theory to understand illness behavior. *General Hospital Psychiatry*, **23**, 177–82.
9. Tan, A., Zimmermann, C., and Rodin, G. (2005). Interpersonal processes in palliative care: an attachment perspective on the patient–clinician relationship. *Palliative Medicine*, **19**, 143–50.
10. Olbrisch, M.E., Benedict, S.M., Ashe, K., *et al.* (2002). Psychological assessment and care of organ transplant patients. *Journal of Consulting and Clinical Psychology*, **3**, 771–83.
11. Olbrisch, M.E., Benedict, S.M., Haller, D.L., *et al.* (2001). Psychosocial assessment of living organ donors: clinical and ethical considerations. *Progress in Transplantation*, **11**, 40–9.
12. Shrestha, R. (2003). Psychosocial assessment of adult living donors. *Liver Transplantation*, **9**, S8–11.
13. Walker, J. (2002). Emotional and psychological preoperative preparation in adults. *British Journal of Nursing*, **11**, 567–75.
14. Karanci, A.N. and Dirik, G. (2003). Predictors of pre- and postoperative anxiety in emergency surgery patients. *Journal of Psychosomatic Research*, **55**, 363–9.
15. Kiecolt-Glaser, J.K., Page, G.G., Marucha, P.T., *et al.* (1998). Psychological influences on surgical recovery: perspectives from psychoneuroimmunology. *The American Psychologist*, **53**, 1209–18.
16. Horne, D. (1994). Preparing patients for invasive medical and surgical procedures. 2: using psychological interventions with adults and children. *Behavioral Medicine*, **20**, 15–21.
17. Rodin, G., Craven, J., and Littlefield, C. (1991). *Depression in the medically ill: an integrated approach.* Brunner–Mazel, New York.
18. Movig, K.L., Janssen, M.W.H.E., de Waal Malefijt, J., *et al.* (2003). Relationship of serotonergic antidepressants and need for blood transfusion in orthopedic surgical patients. *Archives of Internal Medicine*, **163**, 2354–8.
19. Kudoh, A. (2005). Perioperative management for chronic schizophrenic patients. *Anesthesia and Analgesia*, **101**, 1867–72.
20. Huyse, F.J., Touw, D.J., van Schijndel, R.S., *et al.* (2006). Psychotropic drugs and the perioperative period: a proposal for a guideline in elective surgery. *Psychosomatics*, **47**, 8–22.
21. Dyer, C.B., Ashton, C.M., and Teasdale, T.A. (1995). Postoperative delirium. A review of 80 primary data-collection studies. *Archives of Internal Medicine*, **155**, 461–5.
22. Winawer, N. (2001). Postoperative delirium. *The Medical Clinics of North America*, **85**, 1229–39.
23. Overshott, R., Burns, A., and Karim, S. (2005). Cholinesterase inhibitors for delirium. (Protocol) Cochrane Database of Syst Rev [serial online] [cited 2005 Apr 20] Issue 2. Art. No.: CD005317. DOI: 10.1002/14651858.CD005317. Available from: URL:http://www.mrw.interscience.wiley.com/cochrane/clsysrev/articles/CD005317/frame.html
24. Schwartz, T. and Masand, P. (2002). The role of atypical antipsychotics in the treatment of delirium. *Psychosomatics*, **43**, 171–4.
25. Breitbart, W., Gibson, C., and Tremblay, A. (2001). The delirium experience: delirium recall and delirium-related distress in hospitalized patients with cancer, their spouses/caregivers, and their nurses. *Psychosomatics*, **43**, 183–94.
26. Hannich, H.J., Hartmann, U., Lehmann, C., *et al.* (2004). Biofeedback as a supportive method in weaning long-term ventilated critically ill patients. *Medical Hypotheses*, **63**, 21–5.
27. Johnson, C.J., Auger, W.R., Fedullo, P.F., *et al.* (1995). Methylphenidate in the 'hard to wean' patient. *Journal of Psychosomatic Research*, **39**, 63–8.
28. Morin, A.K., Jarvis, C.I., and Lynch, A.M. (2007). Therapeutic options for sleep-maintenance and sleep-onset insomnia. *Pharmacotherapy*, **27**, 89–110.
29. Dijkstra, J.B. and Jolles, J. (2002). Postoperative cognitive dysfunction versus complaints: a discrepancy in long-term findings. *Neuropsychology Review*, **12**, 1–14.

## 5.3.7 **Psychiatric aspects of cancer**

Jimmie C. Holland and Jessica Stiles

## Introduction

Psycho-oncology addresses the two major psychiatric and psychological dimensions of cancer: first, the responses of patients and their families at all stages of disease and the psychological stresses on health professionals delivering their care. The patient and physician relationship, dependent on effective communication, impacts the care of all patients, at every visit, at all sites and stages of cancer, and during all treatments. The second dimension addresses the psychological, behavioural, and social factors that influence cancer risk, detection, and survival.

Many cancer centres and hospitals now have multi-disciplinary psychosocial teams consisting of clinicians and clinical investigators from psychology, psychiatry, social work, nursing, and clergy. These teams provide consultation for patients and their caregivers, psychosocial education for oncology staff, and collaboration in studies in which quality of life is important. In addition, active research in brain, immune, and endocrine links is occurring, particularly in the mechanism of cytokines in producing 'sickness behaviour' that may provide a biological basis for common symptoms of fatigue, depression, anxiety, weakness, and cognitive chances in cancer patients.[1,2]

Despite the fact that many cancer centres and oncology divisions now have a psycho-oncology or psychosocial unit, only a few centres have programmes that include both research and training.

This chapter describes the common psychiatric disorders and psychosocial challenges experienced by cancer patients and the range of interventions available.

## Psychiatric disorders

A key challenge for the oncologist is the differentiation of expected, tolerable, transient distress associated with cancer, such as fear, worry, and sadness, from excessive, disabling, persistent distress requiring therapeutic intervention. Most psychiatric disturbances in patients with cancer relate to their illness or treatment side effects.[3] One-third of patients will experience distress that requires evaluation and treatment.[3–6] The percentage is greater among younger patients, those with sites of cancer with poorer prognosis, for example, brain, pancreas, lung, and those who are hospitalized with greater level of illness causing confusional states and greater anxiety and depression.[7,8]

### Anxiety

Anxiety is the most common form of distress experienced by patients in the oncology setting (Table 5.3.7.1). It occurs with abnormal metabolic states: hypoxia, pulmonary embolus, sepsis, delirium, bleeding, cardiac arrhythmia, and hypoglycemia. Hormone-secreting neoplasms that produce psychiatric symptoms consistent with mood or anxiety disorder are pheochromocytoma, thyroid tumour, carcinoid, parathyroid adenoma, adrenocorticotropic hormone-producing tumour, insulinoma, and paraneoplastic syndrome, an immunologic non-metastatic central nervous system complications of several tumours (particularly, lung and ovary) that may present with mood or cognitive changes.

Numerous medications produce symptoms of anxiety: corticosteroids, neuroleptics, bronchodilators, thyroxine, and psychostimulants. The antiemetics, including metoclopramide and prochlorperazine, which are widely used for chemotherapy-related nausea and vomiting, produce restlessness, akathisias, and dystonias. Benzodiazepines promptly reduce the restless movements, anxiety, and agitation. Withdrawal states from alcohol, benzodiazepines, sedative-hypnotics, and opioids produce anxiety as prominent symptoms.

Some patients undergoing cyclic chemotherapy receiving highly emetogenic regimens develop anticipatory anxiety, nausea, and vomiting days to hours in advance of receiving the next cycle of

**Table 5.3.7.1** Causes of anxiety in patients with cancer

Situational
  Diagnosis of cancer, prognosis discussion
  Crisis, illness/treatment
  Conflicts with family or staff
  Anticipating a frightening procedure
  Awaiting results of tests
  Fears of recurrence <u>after</u> completing treatment
Disease-related
  Poorly controlled pain
  Abnormal metabolic states
  Hormone secreting tumors
  Paraneoplastic syndromes (remote CNS effects)
Treatment-related
  Frightening or painful procedures (MRI, scans, wound debridement)
  Anxiety-producing drugs (antiemetic neuroleptics, bronchodilators)
  Withdrawal states (opioids, benzodiazepines, alcohol)
  Conditioned (anticipatory) anxiety, nausea, and vomiting with cyclic chemotherapy
Exacerbation of preexisting anxiety disorder
  Phobias (needles, claustrophobia)
  Panic or generalized anxiety disorder
  Posttraumatic stress disorder (Holocaust survivors, Vietnam veterans, recall of the death of a relative with cancer)
  Obsessive compulsive disorder

treatment.[9–11] More effective antiemetic regimens have significantly reduced the frequency and severity of this problem. However, behavioural interventions paired with antianxiety medications continue to assist in providing relief from this distress.

Patients who have pre-existing phobias, panic attacks, generalized anxiety disorder, or obsessive–compulsive disorder are at risk of experiencing symptom exacerbations during treatment (Table 5.3.7.1).[12] Phobias of needles, blood, hospitals, magnetic resonance imaging machines, or radiation simulators complicate a patient's ability to tolerate hospital procedures or adhere to recommended treatments. Panic attacks superimposed on physical symptoms of dyspnea and tachycardia may be partially alarming to patients.[3,13] Patients with previous traumatic experiences may suffer a recurrence of intrusive re-experiences of painful memories, maladaptive avoidant behaviour or withdrawal, and hypervigilance.[14,15]

Cancer patients with OCD may have increased difficulty during treatment. Intrusive fears may lead to indecisiveness regarding treatment options and reluctance to accept interventions with known therapeutic efficacy. Excessively time-consuming rituals may interfere with a patient's adherence to medical appointments. Inflexibility of thought, hostility, overwhelming distress, and occasionally poor insight contribute to the challenge of engaging these patients and assisting them in accepting interventions.

*Management.* Anticipatory anxiety prior to medical interventions responds to empathic validation of the fear, adequate preparation to set realistic expectations for the encounter, and rehearsal of the dreaded event.

Significant disabling anxiety symptoms are frequently treated pharmacologically with benzodiazepines, selective serotonin-reuptake inhibitors (SSRIs), mirtazapine, venlafaxine, buspirone, antihistamines, beta-blockers, or neuroleptics. Table 5.3.7.2 outlines the benzodiazepines commonly used and their initial and

**Table 5.3.7.2** Common anxiolytic agents

| Drug | Brand name | Starting dose/day | Theraputic dose/day |
|---|---|---|---|
| SSRIs | | | |
| Sertraline | Zoloft | 25–50 mg AM | 50–150 mg |
| Fluoxetine | Prozac | 10–20 mg AM | 20–60 mg |
| Paroxetine | Paxil | 10–20 mg | 20–60 mg |
| Citalopram | Celexa | 10–20 mg | 20–60 mg |
| Escitalopram | Lexapro | 5–10 mg | 10–30 mg |
| Benzodiazepines | | | |
| Alprazolam, XR | Xanax | 0.25–0.5 mg | 0.5–2.0 mg |
| Clonazepam, wafers | Klonopin | 0.25–0.5 mg | 0.5–2.0 mg |
| *Lorazepam | Ativan | 0.25–0.5 mg | 0.5–2.0 mg |
| *Diazepam | Valium | 2 mg | 5–20 mg |
| Hypnotics | | | |
| Temazepam | Restoril | 15 mg | 15–45 mg |
| Zolpidem | Ambien | 5 mg | 5–20 mg |
| Zaleplon | Sonata | 5 mg | 5–20 mg |
| Eszopiclone | Lunesta | 2 mg | 2–3 mg |

* Also IV, IM

**Table 5.3.7.3** Medical-related risk factors for depression in patients with cancer

Poorly controlled pain
Other chronic disease/disability; advanced stage
Medications
    Corticosteroids
        Prednisone, dexamethasone
    Inteferon and Interleukin-2
    Chemotherapeutic agents
        Vincristine, vinblastine, procarbazine, L-asparaginase
Other medications
    Cimetidine
    Indomethacin
    Levodopa
    Methyldopa
    Pentazocine
    Phenmetrazine
    Phenobarbital
    Propranolol
    Rauwolfia alkaloids
    Tamoxifen
    Antibiotics
    (Amphotericin B)
Other medical conditions
    Metabolic (anemia; hypercalcemia)
    Nutritional ($B_{12}$ or folate)
    Endocrine (hyper-hypothyroidism; adrenal insufficiency)
    Neurologic (paraneoplastic syndrome)
Sites of cancer
    Pancreatic, small cell lung, breast cancer, lymphoma (producing remote CNS effects)

therapeutic doses. A shorter half-life enhances control during the upward titration process and decreases the risk of accumulation and intoxications.

# Mood disorders

Depression in cancer patients requires early recognition and therapeutic intervention. Depression is more challenging to diagnose in patients with cancer because illness produces many neurovegetative symptoms: sleep disturbances, appetite reduction and weight loss, psychomotor retardation, fatigue, apathy, and poor concentration.[16] Focusing the assessment on the psychological symptoms of dysphoria, anhedonia, hopelessness, worthlessness, excessive guilt, and suicidal ideation helps distinguish depression in the context of medical illness.[17]

Table 5.3.7.3 outlines the medically related risk factors for developing depression: increasing levels of debilitation, advanced disease, and concurrent presence of other chronic illnesses or disabilities. Medications frequently encountered in the oncology setting that contribute to depressive symptoms are corticosteroids (dexamethasone and prednisone), chemotherapeutics (interferon, interleukin-2, vincristine, procarbazine, l-asparaginase), and supportive care medications.[17] Depression may relate to organ failure or nutritional, endocrine, and neurologic complications of cancer. Depression is a common symptom of pancreatic cancer, which led to speculation about a tumour-induced mood disturbance mediated by alteration of brain serotonergic function through the effect of proinflammatory cytokines.[18–21]

*Management.* Psychotropic medications are effective in reducing depressive symptoms present in cancer patients.[22] Table 5.3.7.4 lists the most frequently used antidepressant medications in patients with cancer and their initial and maintenance doses. The antidepressants commonly used today are SSRIs, mirtazapine, venlafaxine, or buproprion. Tricyclic antidepressants and duloxetine are beneficial for patients with depressive symptoms and neuropathic pain. Psychostimulants treat depressive symptoms, and counter fatigue related to advanced illness and the somnolence associated with opioids. For depressed cancer patients not expected to survive weeks to months, psychostimulants provide more rapid relief from distressing depressive symptoms. Initiating antidepressants at low doses for elderly and debilitated patients and titration upward as tolerated provides similar benefits, but over a longer period of time.

# Suicide and cancer

The incidence of suicide is increased in patients with cancer compared with the general population, but it is not as high as is often assumed. Suicide is more likely to occur in advanced disease as depression, hopelessness, and the presence of poorly controlled symptoms (especially pain) escalate.

Evaluation of suicidal thoughts should take into account disease stage and prognosis. Almost all patients who receive a diagnosis of cancer, even if the prognosis is optimistic, consider or contemplate suicide in the event of developing unbearable or intolerable distress. Some patients maintain supplies of medications for this purpose. This practice allows the patient to maintain a perception of control over progressive disease and feared intolerable pain and inevitable distress. Maintaining this option sometimes allows patients to tolerate difficult treatments.

Morbid preoccupation with suicide or ruminative plans to commit suicide in cancer patients for whom the disease is in remission or in whom a good prognosis exists require careful evaluation.[23] Patients with a poor prognosis, advanced disease, and poorly controlled symptoms often have thoughts of suicide that are more

**Table 5.3.7.4** Commonly used antidepressants in cancer

| Drug | Brand name | Starting daily dosage PO (mg) | Therapeutic daily dosage PO (mg) |
|---|---|---|---|
| Selective serotonin-reuptake inhibitors | | | |
| Sertraline | (Zoloft) | 25–50 mg AM | 50–150 mg |
| Fluoxetine | (Prozac) | 10–20 mg AM | 20–60 mg |
| Paroxetine | (Paxil) | 10–20 mg AM | 20–60 mg |
| Citalopram | (Celexa) | 10–20 mg AM | 20–60 mg |
| Escitalopram | (Lexapro) | 5–10 mg | 10–20 mg |
| Tricyclics (neuropathic pain management primarily) | | | |
| Nortriptyline | (Pamelor) | 25–50 mg | 50–200 mg |
| Amitriptyline | (Elavil) | 25–50 mg | 50–200 mg |
| Desipramine | (Norpramin) | 25–50 mg | 50–200 mg |
| Other agents | | | |
| Venlafaxine | (Effexor) | 18.75–37.5 mg | 75–225 mg |
| Trazodone | (Desyrel) | 50–100 mg | 100–200 mg |
| Bupropion (XL, SR) | (Wellbutrin, Zyban) | 50–75 mg | 150–400 mg |
| Mirtazapine | (Remeron) | 15 mg HS | 15–45 mg |
| Psychostimulants | | | |
| Methylphenidate | (Ritalin) | 5–10 mg (8AM & Noon) | 10–30 mg |
| Modafinil | (Provigil) | 50–100 mg (8AM & Noon) | 100–400 mg |
| Dextroamphetamine | (Dexedrine) | 5–10 mg (8AM &Noon) | 10–20 mg |

Lithium and mood stabilizers only for bipolar disorder;

MAOIs not recommended.

likely to be viewed as rational by physicians.[24] These patients may request assistance from a physician in obtaining a prescription for medications to use to commit suicide. A treatable major depressive episode may precipitate their suicidal ideation, so it is particularly important to evaluate for the presence of hopelessness, which is a better predictor of suicidal risk than depression itself.[23]

*Management.* Attentiveness to uncontrolled physical symptoms, especially pain, is crucial. Adequate pain control may have a dual effect of hastening death, while ameliorating suffering. Most physicians feel comfortable providing comfort and relieving distress. Increasing numbers of physicians do not consider this practice to be assisted suicide but as best medical care geared to maximal comfort.[25]

Poorly controlled pain in patients with organ failure and metabolic encephalopathy may result in poor judgement and impulse control leading to unpredictable suicide attempts.[26] These patients benefit from a 24 h companion, nurse, or family member who understands the patient's compromised state and treatment for delirium.

## Delirium

Delirium is a global cerebral dysfunction characterized by a fluctuating level of arousal and cognitive disturbances. Symptoms include disorientation and confusion, inattention and poor concentration, perceptual disturbances, disordered thought process, psychomotor agitation or retardation, and an altered sleep–wake cycle. Delirium is distinguished from dementia in part by its reversibility. However, in advanced cancer, as organ failure progresses and results in refractory metabolic derangements, delirium may be irreversible. The primary goal is ensuring the safety of the patient and caregivers. Protecting others from aggressive or combative behaviour is essential. Family members should be told that the cause of the behaviour

is brain dysfunction, not a mental aberration, and a given guidance in understanding the patient's states.

In patients with cancer, especially those in advanced stages, an abrupt shift in mood or behaviour is most often related to a change in neurologic, vascular, or metabolic status; a psychological basis is far less likely. In fact, up to three-fourths of terminally ill patients may develop a delirium before death. Common causes of delirium in cancer are outlined in Table 5.3.7.5.

*Management* begins with attention to the patient's safety. It is important to have constant 1:1 observation, preferably by a person who can correct the patient's misinterpretations of reality. Providing

**Table 5.3.7.5** Common causes of delirium in cancer

| Causes | Examples |
|---|---|
| Metabolic encephalopathy because of vital organ failure | Liver, kidney, lung (hypoxia), thyroid, adrenal |
| Electrolyte imbalance | Sodium, potassium, calcium, glucose |
| Treatment side effects | Narcotic/analgesics |
| | Anticholinergics |
| | Phenothiazines |
| | Antihistamines |
| | Chemotherapuetic agents |
| | Steroids |
| | Radiation therapy to brain |
| Infection | Septicemia |
| Hematologic abnormalities | Microcytic and macrocytic anemias, coagulopathies |
| Nutritional | General malnutrition, thiamine, folic acid, vitamin B$_{12}$ |
| Paraneoplastic syndromes | Remote effects of tumors |
| Metastatic or primary brain tumor | Glioblastoma multiforme, primary CNS lymphoma |

**Table 5.3.7.6** Behavioral symptoms of delirium in patients with cancer

| State | Symptom |
|---|---|
| Early, mild | Alteration of sleep-wake cycle, transient periods of disorientation<br>Unexplained anxiety and sense of dread<br>Increased irritability, anger, temper outbursts<br>Withdrawal, refusal to talk to staff or relatives<br>New onset of forgetfulness |
| Late, severe with behavioral changes | Refusal to cooperate with reasonable requests; pulling out tubes and lines<br>Angry, swearing, shouting, abusive<br>Demanding to go home, pacing corridor<br>Illusions (misidentifies staff, visual and sensory clues)<br>Delusions (misinterprets events, usually paranoid, fears of being harmed)<br>Hallucinations (visual and auditory) |

consistent caregivers, structured interactions with others, and frequent reorientation may limit the distress experienced by the patient. Elderly patients are more vulnerable to developing delirium, and those with cognitive impairment or dementia are at even higher risk. It is preferable to avoid physical restraints. However, containment of severe agitation may temporarily require restraints to prevent removal of endotracheal tubes, intravenous access, and loss of indwelling catheters, and also to avert falls. Behavioural symptoms of delirium in patients with cancer are outlined in Table 5.3.7.6.

Medications commonly used in managing delirium are summarized in Table 5.3.7.7. Identification and corrections of the underlying aetiology of the delirium is not always possible and in these circumstances, neuroleptics providing relief for the patient from distressing symptoms should be the primary intervention. While haloperidol and lorazepam administered in conjunction provide additional sedative effects for patients with sever agitation,[27] patients with hypoactive subtype of delirium will benefit from the administration of neuroleptics for symptomatic relief.[26,28] In the terminal stage of cancer, delirium may be irreversible and refractory to neuroleptics. Additional sedation with alternative agents may be required to provide comfort and safety for the patient and family.

**Table 5.3.7.7** Medications for managing delirium in cancer patients

| Drug | Brand name | Approximate daily dosage |
|---|---|---|
| Neuroleptics | | |
| Haloperidol | Haldol | 0.5–5 mg every 2–12 h, PO, IV, SC, IM |
| Chlorpromazine | Thorazine | 12.5–50 mg every 4–12 h, PO, IV, IM |
| Risperidone | Risperdal | 1–3 mg every 12 h, PO |
| Olanzapine | Zyprexa | 2.5–5 mg every 6–8 h, PO |
| Quetiapine | Seroquel | 12.5–50 mg every 12 h, PO |
| Benzodiazepines | | |
| Lorazepam | Ativan | 0.5–2.0 mg every 1–4 h, PO, IV, IM |
| Midazolam* | | 30–100 mg every 24 h, IV, SC |
| Anesthetics | | |
| Propofol* | | 10–50 mg every h, IV |

PO, orally; IV, intravenously; SC, subcutaneously; IM, intramuscularly.

* Usually IV continuous infusion in intensive care setting.

## Further information

www.apos-society.org

Free online education program for multidisciplinary training in Psycho-Oncology. Website contains fifteen web-cast lectures in the five following tracks: Introduction to oncology, program administration, symptom detection and management (eight web-casts), interventions (four web-casts), and population-specific issues.

Direct link: http://www.apos-society.org/professionals/meetings-ed/webcasts/webcasts-multidisciplinary.aspx

www.ipos-society.org

Free online lectures: Multilingual core curriculum in psycho-oncology. Five web-cast lectures translated into English, French, German, Hungarian, Italian, and Spanish.

Direct link: http://www.ipos-society.org/professionals/meetings-ed/core-curriculum/core-curriculum-pres.htm

Holland, J.C. (2002). History of psycho-oncology: overcoming attitudinal and conceptual barriers. *Psychosomatic Medicine*, **64**, 206–21.

Holland, J.C., (ed.) (2006). *Quick reference for oncology clinicians: the psychiatric and psychological dimensions of symptom management*. IPOS Press, Charlottesville.

*Psycho-oncology: Journal of the American Psychosocial Oncology Society, Behavioral and Ethical Aspects of Cancer*. Published monthly in hard copy and online by John Wiley & Sons, Ltd.

## References

1. Cleeland, C.S., Bennett, G.J., and Dantzen, R. (2003). Are the symptoms of cancer and cancer treatment due to a shared biologic mechanism? *Cancer*, **97**, 2919–25.

2. Musselman, D.L., Miller, A.H., Parter, M.R., *et al.* (2001). Higher than normal interleukin-6 concentrations in cancer patients with depression: preliminary findings. *The American Journal of Psychiatry*, **158**, 1252–7.

3. Strain, J. (1998). Adjustment disorders. In *Psycho-oncology* (ed. J.C. Holland), pp. 509–17. Oxford University Press, New York.

4. Hewitt, M., Herdman, R., and Holland, J. (eds.) (2004). *Meeting psychosocial needs of women with breast cancer*. Institute of Medicine, National Academies Press, Washington, DC.

5. Barg, F.K., Cooley, M., Pasacreta, J., *et al.* (1994). Development of a self-administered psychosocial cancer screening tool. *Cancer Practice*, **2**, 288–96.

6. Farber, D.M., Wienerman, B.H., and Kuypers, J.A. (1984). Psychosocial distress in oncology outpatients. *Journal of Psychosocial Oncology*, **2**, 109.

7. Zabora, J. (2001). The prevalence of psychological distress by cancer site. *Psycho-oncology*, **10**, 19–28.

8. Bukberg, J., Penman, D., and Holland, J.C. (1984). Depression in hospitalized cancer patients *Psychosomatic Medicine*, **46**, 199.

9. Jacobsen, P.B., Bovbjerg, D.H., Schwartz, M., *et al.* (1995). Conditioned emotional distress in women receiving chemotherapy for breast cancer. *Journal of Consulting and Clinical Psychology*, **63**, 108–14.

10. Andrykowski, M.A. and Redd, W.H. (1987). Longitudinal analysis of the development of anticipatory nausea. *Journal of Consulting and Clinical Psychology*, **55**, 36.

11. Redd, W.H., Jacobsen, P.B., Die-Trill, M., *et al.* (1987). Cognitive/attentional distraction in the control of conditioned nausea in pediatric oncology patients receiving chemotherapy. *Journal of Consulting and Clinical Psychology*, **55**, 391.

12. Payne, D. and Massie, M. (2000). Anxiety in palliative care. In *Handbook of psychiatry in palliative medicine* (eds. H. Chochinov and W. Breitbart). pp. 63–74. Oxford University Press, New York.

13. Noyes, R. Jr., Holt, C., and Massie, M. (1998). Anxiety disorders. In *Psycho-oncology* (ed. J.C. Holland), pp. 548–63. Oxford University, New York.

14. Rowland, J.H. (1989). Intrapersonal resources: developmental stage of adaptation: adult model. In *Handbook of psycho-oncology: psychological care of the patient with cancer* (eds. J.C. Holland and J.H. Rowland), pp. 25–43. Oxford University Press, New York.

15. Peretz, T., Baider, L., Ever-Hadani, P., *et al.* (1994). Psychological distress in female cancer patients with holocaust experience. *General Hospital Psychiatry*, **16**, 413–18.

16. Roth, A.J. and Holland, J.C. (1994). Treatment of depression in cancer patients. *Primary Care in Cancer*, **14**, 23–9.

17. Coups, E., Winell, J., and Holland, J. (2005). Depression in the context of cancer. In *Biology of depression: from novel insights to therapeutic strategies*, Vol. 1 (eds. J. Lucinio and W. Ma-LeWong), pp. 365–85. Wiley, Weinheim, Germany.

18. Ebrahimi, B., Tucker, S.L., Li, D., *et al.* (2004). Cytokines in pancreatic carcinoma. *Cancer*, **101**, 2727–36.

19. McDaniel, J.S., Musselman, D.L., and Porter, M.R. (1995). Depression in cancer: diagnosis, biology and treatment. *The Journal of General Psychology*, **52**, 89–99.

20. Lerner, D.M., Stoudemire, A., and Rosenstein, D.L. (2001). Cytokine-induced neuropsychiatric toxicity. In *Cytokine therapeutics in infectious diseases* (ed. S.M. Holland), pp. 323–32. Lippincott Williams & Wilkins, Philadelphia, PA.

21. Mussleman, D.L., Lawson, D.H., Gumnick, J.F., *et al.* (2001). Paroxetine for the prevention of depression induced by high-dose interferon alpha. *The New England Journal of Medicine*, **344**, 961–6.

22. Wilson, K., Chochinov, H., de Faye, B., *et al.* (2000). Diagnosis and management of depression in palliative care. In *Handbook of psychiatry in palliative medicine* (eds. H. Chochinov and W. Breitbart), pp. 25–51. Oxford University Press, New York.

23. Rosenfeld, B., Krevo, S., Breitbart, W., *et al.* (2000). Suicide, assisted suicide, and euthanasia in the terminally ill. In *Handbook of psychiatry in palliative medicine* (eds. H. Chochinov and W. Breitbart), pp. 51–63. Oxford University Press, New York.

24. Conwell, Y. and Caine, E.D. (1991). Rational suicide and the right to die: reality and myth. *The New England Journal of Medicine*, **325**, 1100.

25. Chochinov, H.M. (2002). Dignity-conserving care- a new model for palliative care: helping the patient feel valued. *The Journal of the American Medical Association*, **287**, 2253–60.

26. Breitbart, W. and Cohen, K. (1998). Delirium. In *Psycho-oncology* (ed. J.C. Holland), pp. 564–75. Oxford University Press, New York.

27. Breitbart, W., Marotta, R., Platt, M., *et al.* (1996). A double-blind trial of haloperidol, chlorpromazine and lorazepam in treatment of delirium in hospitalized AIDS patients. *The American Journal of Psychiatry*, **153**, 231–7.

28. Breitbart, W. (2002). Spirituality and meaning- centered group psychotherapy interventions in advanced cancer. *Support Care in Cancer*, **10**, 272–80.

# 5.3.8 **Psychiatric aspects of accidents, burns, and other physical trauma**

Ulrik Fredrik Malt

## **Epidemiology of accidents and injury**

The one-year prevalence of accidents is about 15–20 per cent with highest prevalence in the younger age groups. About 80 per cent of accidents cause personal injury, and 1/3 to 1/2 of these injuries result in medical attention. About 10 per cent of medically attended injured victims require hospitalization.[1] In the UK (population about 60 million) 31 845 people were killed or seriously injured in 2006 due to road accidents and there were 2 58 404 road casualties.

## **Accident occurrence and psychiatric disorders**

On a group basis, lower social classes, subjects with less education and lower intelligence tend to sustain more accidents and injuries (and have higher morbidity and mortality in general). The ratio of males to females for both fatal and non-fatal accidents is about 2:1 in subjects below 60 years of age. Individual variables associated with increased liability of being involved in an accident include antisocial tendencies, aggressiveness, impulsiveness, thrill and adventure-seeking behaviour. Conscious or unconscious intention is not an important explanation of the overall prevalence of accidents or injuries in the society.

Patients with significant psychological problems (psychopathology including substance abuse) sustain more severe injuries than healthy subjects and the prevalence of psychiatric disorders is increased among hospitalized injured adults compared to surgical patients admitted for other reasons. At least 15–20 per cent of persons brought to hospital emergency rooms due to accidental injury have clinical significant blood concentrations of alcohol. Furthermore, patients with schizophrenia, affective illness and post-traumatic stress disorder have more accidental *deaths* (and suicides) compared to the general population.

## **Physical injuries**

Most non-fatal injuries treated in hospitals are minor head concussion and lacerations, strains/sprains, contusions/abrasions and fractures to body parts such as limbs. More severe injuries are mostly related to high energy accidents (e.g. motor vehicle accidents) and often involve both the head and limbs. Injuries to the inner organs are less frequent, but mostly more severe. The anatomical based Abbreviated Injury Scale (AIS) and Injury Severity Score (ISS) are the most widely used classification system of physical injury. Other classification systems based on physiological impact of trauma (e.g. Revised Trauma Score, Glasgow Coma Score) and combinations of anatomical injury and physiological impact (e.g. Trauma and Injury Severity Score) exist as well. See: http://www.trauma.org/archive/scores/ais.html;

## **Physical injury as psychological trauma**

Accidental injury implies several important sources of threat, loss or conflict which may cause psychological distress or psychiatric disorders. The most important accident related variables associated with subsequent psychological problems include,

- Severity of the accident (e.g. real degree of threat to life of one self and others)
- Degree of helplessness
- Duration of the stressor
- Presence and type of actual physical injury
- Exposure to dead and mutilated bodies.

Nevertheless, pre-accident adjustment, personality and the personal meaning of the accident or injury are the strongest predictors of both acute psychological responses and long-term psychiatric outcome. This observation holds even in the presence of a severe injury,[2] although the type of injury *per se* may influence the short- and long-term outcome. The relative contribution of 'objective' accident related compared to 'subjective' appraisal related variables in shaping the acute response varies. A rule of thumb is that the less severe the accident, the more important are variables not directly related to the accident *per se* (i.e. the personal meaning of the accident and its consequences for the individual.[3] Important individual variables include,[4–6]

◆ Pre-injury mental health and adjustment problems

◆ Personality traits (e.g. neuroticism, quality of attachment)

◆ Trauma history

The accident *per se* may represent a blow to the person's feeling of invulnerability (narcissistic loss). In some, the accident situation may provoke conflictual feelings (e.g. self-blame, survivor guilt) or shame (e.g. own actions or fantasies prior to the situation). Injury to the body may threaten self-esteem and body image; or represent a loss of function. In some cases, the injury may even serve as a primary gain in a psychodynamic sense. The immediate responses will also be influenced by psychological issues like fear of losing control, or the effect of that phenomenon if it occurs. Conflicts related to secondary gains may also influence the clinical response observed by others.

## Clinical features and assessment of trauma at the accident scene

The ABC rule of assessment (Airway, Blood pressure, Circulation) should always be the first step in any medical assessment of acute injury followed by physical examination of the thorax, abdomen, head and finally the extremities. However, except for head injuries associated with impaired cognitive function and injuries that significantly interfere with ventilation or cardiovascular function (e.g. agitation due to hypoxia or apathy due to cardiovascular hypotension), the injury it self plays a minor role for the immediate *psychological* responses to trauma.

Early and marked psychophysiological arousal symptoms like (in decreasing frequency) heartbeat, tremor, dry mouth, restlessness, shaking/trembling, weakness in legs, and sweating are common responses to an acute accident. However, the majority of accident victims appear reasonably calm[5] although many have some degree of inner turmoil that may impair the ability to receive, retrieve, and handle information. If behavioural disturbances are seen during the first seconds to minutes, they mimic phylogenetic responses known from all mammals exposed to acute and severe stressful events: flight, freeze, or fight.

### (a)  Flight response (anxiety, panic)

The patient appears frightened, may scream or cry. Clear cut panic (e.g. overt confusion, bewildered or aimless behaviour or running away), is rather infrequent even during disasters (<1 per cent). Although lowering of blood pressure is not part of the clinical features of panic, panic is often included in the concept of 'shock' used by lay people and media.

Physiological response to physical injury may be misunderstood as flight response. Patients with injury to the thorax hyperventilate and may appear anxious and scared. Cyanosis is not a sign of emotional distress in adults, and hyperventilation should always be considered as sign of respiratory problems needing urgent medical attention (e.g. pneumothorax). Patients with head injury may be confused and bewildered, but they seldom display the open anxiety seen in patients who panic.

Panic with severe behavioural disturbances may threaten the safety of the subject and provoke anxiety in bystanders and other victims who may themselves be afraid to lose control. Thus, whenever possible, patients with strong anxiety or panic should be offered immediate psychological support. Establishing physical (e.g. hand around the shoulder) and verbal contact is important to reduce panic and provide a sense of security and control. Verbal contact may also reveal the subject's real or imagined fears and provide the subject with an alternative way to express their inner turmoil and despair and thus pave the way for more optimal coping and subsequent behavioural control. The subject should be removed from the accident scene, but not left alone. These subjects need to move around and should not be forcefully immobilized. A helper may walk with the patient until he calms down. The exception to this rule is rare instances where the subject's behaviour is completely out of control representing an immediate threat to the physical safety of self or others.

Reuniting family members may reduce anxiety and worries.

Hyperventilation is treated as usual (breathing into a bag to increase the $CO_2$-level) combined with physical and verbal contact as described above. It is crucial that somatic causes (e.g. pneumothorax, intoxication) have been ruled out.

### (b)  Freeze response (apathy)

Freeze responses include halted surprise or in more extreme cases emotional numbness (apathy). Apathy causing lack of appropriate lifesaving activities occur rather infrequently among random samples of accidentally injured adults (less than 10 per cent). In less than 1 per cent, significant parasympathetic (vagus) responses with lowering of blood pressure occurs ('emotional shock'). These patients appear pale and silent. The look of their eyes gives an impression of detached distance, if they were looking onto their own personal world somewhere far away from the actual accident scene. Rarely, an atypical freeze response characterized by blank denial of having sustained an injury when one, in fact, exists may be seen. These subjects may continue to behave as if nothing had happened and not take appropriate precautions at the accident scene.

Several physical injuries may mimic freeze-response. Patients with internal bleedings (e.g. liver, spleen) may appear pale and silent as if in emotional shock ('freeze response'). The pulse is weak and fast (tachycardia), however, in contrast to the vagus tonus induced bradycardia of the freeze response.

If there is a risk of further injury associated with remaining at the accident scene, patients with freeze responses must be removed to a safe place. They should not be left alone, but covered with a jacket or a blanket over their shoulders and attended to in a calm and gentle way, encouraging them to express some of their thoughts and emotions. If the freeze response is severe and prolonged, the patient should be brought to an emergency room for renewed and extended medical evaluation and basic psychological care. Cases of complete denial of having sustained an injury despite evidence for the opposite, should clinically be handled as a freeze response.

### (c)  Dissociative symptoms

Dissociative symptoms occur in about 15 per cent during the 1st second to minutes after an accident and may be associated with flight or freeze responses. Brief symptoms of derealization are most common, even in relatively minor accidents (e.g. 'unreal', like a 'dream' or 'slow movie'). Symptoms of depersonalization (e.g. 'I watched my body burn from a distance') are less common and usually signal a more severe psychological response. Brief symptoms of dissociation do not predict later psychiatric problems,[5,7,8] but marked and prolonged dissociative symptoms still present weeks after the accident.[7]

#### (d) Fight response (aggression)

Fight responses include irritability, anger and more rarely, open aggression. This response is most often seen among bystanders or helpers who feel threatened by the exposure of dead and mutilated bodies. They may quarrel with the rescue team, and sometimes even interfere with the work of police or helpers. Open aggression is rare among victims themselves with the exception of intoxicated victims with severe personality disorders and a few who have sustained severe head injuries (e.g. subdural hematoma, frontal brain contusion).

Irritability and aggressive comments should not be taken personally by the helpers, but interpreted a symptom of helplessness. In most cases, this response is psychological, but impaired behavioural control due to drug or alcohol may be contributing factors. The patient should be treated as being extremely anxious and under high emotional distress. Reuniting with family or significant others if possible may be helpful. Physical activity may reduce aggression. If suitable, simple tasks which require physical movements may be therapeutic ('Can you give me a hand with . . . . .'), but subjects under stress should never be involved in important rescue tasks due to their impaired judgement ability and tendency to act irrationally.

#### (e) Acute stress reaction

Marked or severe flight, freeze or fight reponses are included in the ICD-10 (F43.0) definition of acute stress reaction (ASR). ASR is defined as immediate onset of marked psychological symptoms (within 1 hour) following exposure to an exceptional mental or physical stressor. The symptoms must begin to decrease after 8 hours if the stressor is transient (e.g. accident). If exposure to the stress continues (e.g. combat zone, hostage situation) the symptoms must begin to diminish after 48 hours. In contrast, the DSM-IV concept 'acute stress disorder' (ASD) describes development of symptoms not earlier than 2 days after the trauma but within one month after exposure.

Psychotropic drugs are seldom needed to treat acute psychological responses at the accident scene if proper medical care including emotional contact from skilled, empathic helpers is offered. Violence towards victims having lost behavioural control may increase the anxiety among other victims and bystanders, and in fact, increase the risk for more behavioural disturbance within the group, and should thus be avoided.

#### (f) Acute pain

Some injured persons do not report pain complaints during the 1st second to minutes after even severe physical injury, and some may even continue to perform tasks as usual. This response occurs particularly in situations with continous threat to others or own life (e.g. wounded soldiers). This is part of a brief dissociative response which may be life saving and does not reflect psychopathology. However, a few accident victims respond differently.

They may report the most painful physical sensations ever experienced. In the absence of severe physical injury, this response most often reflects catastrophic cognitions associated with severe anxiety[5] and should be treated accordingly. Most injured patients report some degree of pain as minutes pass, however.

Severe pain should be treated at the accident scene and will contribute to psychological and physical recovery from the injury.[9] Anxiety and fear may lead to increased pain complaints, so may imagined (!) severe injuries. For those reasons, it is important not only to examine the presence of actual injury, but also explicitly ask the victim if he or she *believes* or *fears* having sustained serious or life-threatening injuries not detected by the medical personnel. If yes, factual information combined with additional proper medical examination if needed, should be provided to reduce the subject's fears and worries. Faced with true life-threatening injuries, the helper should admit facts if asked, but nevertheless provide some hope and cautioned optimism. It is often hard to evaluate true prognosis at the accident scene and advanced trauma surgery may save the life of many severely injured subjects who would have died a few decades ago.

### Responses seen in the emergency room

In urban areas, most subjects will be brought to emergency rooms within less than an hour. At that time most victims have started the process of working through the accident, the injury and its implications. This process is reflected in a characteristic cluster of emotions, cognitions and physiological symptoms observed in humans exposed to all types of stressful situations.[10–12]

◆ Intrusion includes images of the accident popping into the victims mind, and thinking about the accident even when the person do not want to do so. The main load of intrusive symptoms are related to the severity of the accident and the personal meaning. Intrusive symptoms are common both in post-traumatic depression and anxiety.[5]

◆ Avoidance includes trying not to talk about the accident or avoiding any cognitive or behavioural activities which reminds the person about the accident. Such symptoms and signs are strongly related to accident-independent variables such as personality traits (e.g. coping style) and more often associated with anxiety than depression.[5]

◆ Hyperarousal includes startle response, strongly increased heart rate, shivering and trembling, irritability, difficulty in concentrating, hypervigilance and disturbed sleep. With the exception of difficulty to sleep, clinically significant hyperarousal is rather infrequent in randomly selected accidentally injured subjects (less than 10 per cent). However, severe hyperarousal signifies a strong physiological and emotional response and is increased among injured compared to non-injured accident victims and is in some studies associated with later post-traumatic distress problems.[13]

The three most common types of behavioural problems seen in the emergency room are,

◆ Uncontrolled crying or screaming

◆ Strong anxiety which may include excessive pain complaints

◆ Aggression and dyssocial behaviour

Crying and anxiety are associated with high levels of intrusion and avoidance, and may be part of ASR. Systematic and carefully conducted medical examinations accompanied by supporting questions about the patients emotions, thoughts, and fantasies are the most effective way to put the patient at ease. Sedating drugs are seldom needed if the necessary psychological support is provided. Separation from family members or significant others may increase anxiety and despair, and family reunion may be helpful. If symptoms of high arousal persist, prazosin, a central nervous system (CNS) active alpha-1 adrenoreceptor antagonist or a beta-blocker (e.g. 40–60 mg propranolol) or alfa—may be given to attenuate extreme adrenergic tonus.[14]

Aggressive behaviour occurs in about 5 per cent of injured persons brought to hospital, mostly among intoxicated subjects. The presence of head injury must be ruled out. Most cases can be brought under control with the help of significant others and firm, but calm attitude, addressing the fear or helplessness. In a few cases, acute administration of benzodiazepines or a sedating neuroleptic may be necessary. If the patient is intoxicated or suffer from respiration difficulties, neuroleptics may be the safest option. In cases of armed patients, the necessary precautions must be taken.

Psychotic forms of ASR are seldom seen in injured adults and even patients with schizophrenia or other psychotic disorder prior to the accident appear remarkably calm and collected upon arrival in the hospital. If psychosis is present at arrival in the emergency room, influence of psychoactive substances, severe injury (e.g. brain injury, respiratory failure) or a concurrent psychotic disorder must be ruled out.

### (a) Whiplash injury

Rear end collision may cause a whiplash like movement of the neck. Biomechanical studies suggest overstretch of cervical facet-joint capsules as a possible source of pain. Neck pain, stiffness or tenderness may occur minutes to hours after the accident. A medical examination including an X-ray of the cervical columna seldom reveals pathological findings (Quebec classification grade I). In more severe cases, distortion and minor bleeding in capsules, ligaments, tendons or muscles (grade II) may lead to additional musculoskeletal signs such as decreased range of motion and point tenderness. In severe injuries, neurological findings (impaired myostatic reflexes, pareses, loss of sensibility, grade III) or even fractures (grade IV) may be present. In patients with whiplash related injury grade I or II, acute psychological distress and associated neck pain is the most important predictor of long-term outcome.

In the emergency room, treatment should aim at providing the subject with adequate information about the good prognosis. Pain after whiplash-injury usually lasts for four-to-six weeks (!), but gradually disappears. In cases of pain without somatic findings, pain killers or antiflogistic medication have uncertain effect and should not be prescribed for more than a week. Sick leave should be avoided or be as short as possible. Mobilization and early return to work is recommended. Overtreatment by physicians or physiotherapists (e.g. application of stiff collar despite no findings of injury to the cervical columna) may lead to permanent illness behaviour and pain-fixation.[15] The optimal physical treatment of whiplash injury is still unsettled,[16] but premorbid pain and psychiatric disorders represent a risk for development of chronic disabling symptoms and should be treated.

### (b) Significant others' needs

Relatives or survivors may want to see dead significant others brought to hospital, and touch them. This process helps the relatives to work through the traumatic event and should be encouraged. If the dead body is grotesquely disfigured, the most horrifying parts should be covered prior to exposure. In any case, a physician or a skilled nurse should accompany the relatives during exposure. Small childrens' emotional response to dead bodies mirror the adults' response. Accordingly, reducing the anxiety and fear of the adults is the best way to help children cope with dead ones. Correspondingly, in cases of severe anxiety in accompanying small children, addressing the helplessness and anxiety of the parents is important. If dead bodies are stored in hospital chapels, care must be taken to cover the presence of religious symbols incongruent to the religious status of the dead one and his family (e.g. Christian crosses should be covered in case of a Jew or a Muslim). The reader is referred to chapter 4.16 for more information on culture specific responses to stress and trauma.

In disaster situations, the need for information varies among relatives, depending on whether their loved ones are missing, injured, or dead (survivor status). Those who have lost loved ones often want to talk to rescuers or get information with regard to any hint about the emotional status of the dead one at the time of death. Accordingly, in situations with several hundred relatives come to the hospital, information is provided in separate groups according to the significant other survivor status. The logistics of such procedures should be outlined in the hospital's disaster plan.

## Psychiatric treatment during hospital stay

Most studies indicate that risk factors, emotional, and behavioural responses correspond to that of medically ill patients and identifying those who are at increased risk can follow the same guidelines as for medicine in general.[17] Some patients may complain about physical symptoms suggesting undetected injury. Such complaints may in fact be true. If not addressed and attended to, psychological distress presented by means of somatic complaints or symptoms is the rule.

Clinical syndromes requiring psychiatric attention during hospital stay are listed in Table 5.3.8.1. Complete denial of severity of injury or avoidant coping is maladaptive and should be counteracted.[18] Relatives or significant others should be contacted. They may convey unrealistic fears—or hopes (e.g. 'you will be able to walk'—attitudes in patients with permanent paralysis of legs)—which strongly influence the behaviour and emotional well-being of the patient. They may also provide information which may be helpful to understand current behaviour (e.g. previous dysfunction, 'silent' delirium undetected by staff).

### (a) Anxiety and acute stress reaction

Worrying and compulsive thoughts about the accident or the injury (intrusion) is seen both in anxiety and depression. Extreme anxiety may infrequently lead to cardiovascular complications (e.g. pulmonary embolia) in subjects with cardiovascular risk factors (e.g. elderly subjects often smokers with hypertension and arterosclerosis).

Sleep problems may be present or related to physical pain and treatment procedures. The aetiology of nightmares following traumatic injury is complex.[19] They mostly emerge a couple of days after the accident and disappear gradually. Persisting nightmares for more than two weeks without any signs of mastery in the dream content, suggest development of post-traumatic stress disorder and should thus be treated.

**Table 5.3.8.1** The most frequently seen psychiatric syndromes during hospital stay following accidental injury

| Type of syndrome or clinical problem | Clinical symptoms and signs | Comment |
|---|---|---|
| Delirium | Confused, strange behaviour; episodic disorientation; irritability; episodic fearful look | May occur without obvious signs of agitation if sedated; Relatives may detect it and be upset. Diagnosis: 'Draw a clock test' helpful |
| Abstinence from drug or alcohol | increased pulse; sweating; tremor; insomnia; agitation; anxiety; nausea; abdominal pain; dysphoric. | May be interpreted falsely as accident-provoked anxiety |
| Antisocial personality, histrionic or borderline personality disorder | Aggressive behaviour; poor compliance with treatment; abusive language; high demand for analgesics | Undetected brain dysfunction must be ruled out; Relatives may provide important pre-injury information |
| Hypomanic or manic responses | Elated mood; emotions do not correspond to the situation; uncritical behaviour | Undetected brain dysfunction; bipolar disorder or hypomanic response as a defence against survivor guilt |
| Anxiety | Tense, anxious, restless, worrying, increased startle reflexes; insomnia; dissociative symptoms may occur. | Prolonged or delayed stress response or disorder; imagined or real threat from accident or injury; physical complication (e.g. hypoxia, delirium); abstinent or side effects of drug. Obsessive-compulsive traits and high inner tension with fear of losing emotional control. If unexplained, consult relatives for psychological clues. |
| Depression | Withdrawn, loss of appetite; inability to feel; sad; worrying; passive; lassitude; anxiety symptoms frequent | Grief; survivor guilt; psychological response to disfigurement or loss (real or imagined) of function or self-esteem; reactivating of previous painful memories |
| Medically unexplained physiological events including delayed healing of wounds | Rare phenomena; typical senior physicians statement 'I've never seen something like it before' | Secondary gain by extended hospital stay (e.g. alternative prison); factitious disorder; extreme stress (psychophysiological activation) |
| Excessive pain | Complaints of pain; poor sleep and appetite; poor performance; do not reveal emotions. | Undetected physical complication; insufficient pain treatment; anxiety or depression response in past with obsessive-compulsive traits; withdrawal syndrome; drug abuser. |
| Partial or complete denial of actual injury | As-if-nothing-has-happened behaviour; refuse treatment; request early dismissal from hospital | Undetected brain dysfunction; psychotic disorder. If male and partial denial, consider obsessive-compulsive traits and high inner tension with fear of passivity |

Psychological interventions should be based on clear indication and be brief, distress focused and time limited. Symptoms of intrusion including nightmares may be treated by simple psychological techniques. If one specific traumatic event which can be delineated (e.g. visual image of a traumatic moment), psychological video replay techniques (VRT) may be useful. The subject is taught how to relax. Subsequently, the subject reviews the pre-accident and accident situation on an imagined (i.e. mental) video screen. When the anxiety rises to unacceptable levels, the subject is asked to push the (imagined) stop button and press fast replay until a pre-accident situation where the subjects is at ease is reached. When calm, the procedure is repeated, until the subject can view the whole accident without strong anxiety.

If the anxiety level is high or the traumatic event is more complex, more comprehensive interventions are needed, e.g. Eye Movement Desensitization and Reprocessing (EMDR) or Trauma-Focused Cognitive Behavioural Therapy (TF-CBT).[20] If strong anxiety is not brought under control by means of psychotherapy or other behavioural techniques (e.g. applied relaxation), psychoactive drugs can be added. In injured patients with childhood trauma or other traumatic events in the past, a selective serotonin reuptake inhibitor (SSRI) probably should be the first choice. Sleep problems are best dealt with by environmental adjustment whenever possible, or by optimal pain control if appropiate. Sedative drugs are secondary option. Mianserin or mirtazapine combine sedative and antidepressant effects and may be alternative to benzodiazepines.

Acute stress disorder (ASD) may be conceptualized as an acute form of PTSD and may predict chronic PTSD.[21] The main treatment is psychotherapy (i.e. EMDR, TF-CBT). In PTSD, prazosin reduces nightmares and sleep disturbance in placebo-controlled studies, and may thus be an option also during the first days to weeks after trauma. Some studies have reported propranolol given within days following a traumatic event to be useful for mitigating PTSD symptoms or perhaps even preventing the development of PTSD. The mechanism is thought to be explained by reduced consolidation of emotional memory. Small doses of glucocorticoids may reduce traumatic memories in ASD as well,[22] but larger controlled studies are needed to verify this finding. Benzodiazepines may also reduce acute distress, but may not reduce the risk of 6-month psychiatric anxiety problems. In conclusion, all psychopharmacological treatments must be provided together with psychological interventions addressing the key psychological sources of distress and worry.

### (b) Depression

Depressed mood during the first days to weeks following an accident are mostly due to guilt, shame, or grief due to real or imagined losses. The key to understanding the response is the meaning of the accident or the injury for the patient. Guilt, shame or rumination over real or imagined losses is associated with long-term problems[23] and may require specific therapy.[24] Premorbid causes of depression (e.g. bereavement, mood disorder at the time of the accident), must be kept in mind. In patients with immobilizing injuries staying in hospital for an extended period, some degree of depressive symptoms is the rule. If the symptomatology is severe and persistent, antidepressants are indicated.

Persisting depression has been found to be highly predictive of a long-term psychiatric consequence, and moderate to severe depression predicts less likeliness of returning to preaccident functional level. Thus, depression should always be taken seriously. If marked depression presist for more then 2–3 weeks, an antidepressant should be given. Due to lower incidence of side effects, the newer low-toxic antidepressants are preferred. Delirinm and abstinence are treated as usual. Detailed presentations of the psychopharmacology of the injured or medically ill are available.[34–36]

### (c) Pain

Both the injury itself (e.g. burn injuries, injuries to the pelvis, penetrating traumas) or medical treatment (e.g. physiotherapy to prevent contractures, ICU) may be associated with psychological distress and pain.[25,26] Pre-accident psychopathology increases the prevalence and severity of pain complaints. Pain or fear of bringing about pain leads to diminished movement, which can engender contractures, muscle atrophy, and bed ulcers. Traumatic amputation may be associated with phantom pain and exacerbation of pain in response to imagined movements has been reported in subjects with spinal cord injury.[27] Poorly treated pain can be demoralizing to patients and provoke psychological regression, giving-up responses and long-term psychiatric problems[28] including increased risk for suicide.[29] Thus active pain control is crucial and may reduce the prevalence of long-term suffering.[30] Comprehensive reviews of the psychological care of burned subjects are available.[31]

Concerns that trauma patients with injury related pain will become addicted if treated properly with analgesics is neither supported by clinical experience nor by empirical data.[32] However, co-morbid psychiatric disoders must be taken into account when treating injury-associated pain. Patients with a history of substance abuse may have greater tolerance to analgesics and will have to be titrated to higher doses.[33]

### (d) Confusion and psychoses

In civilian life situations, confusion or psychotic responses appearing for the first time days after being admitted to hospital are almost exclusively due to a central nervous system dysfunction. Risk factors are severe injuries (ISS >15; third degree burn injury) and major head injuries (e.g. contusion). Impaired cognitive functions or drug or alcohol abuse prior to accident and age >50 increase the risk of organic mental dysfunction.

In a few cases, psychotic-like confusional and agitated responses occurring during the hospital stay may be due to abrupt disruption of intake of psychotropic medication taken for long periods prior to the accident. If in doubt about the aetiology of a psychotic response seen during the first days to weeks (including severe manic episodes), the psychiatrist should consider the response to be of organic origin and explore the pathophysiological processes as

done in cases of delirium. Asking the patient to draw a clock, may be a simple and effective way of detecting organic dysfunction.[37]

### (e) Alcohol and drug abuse

A significant number of accident victims brought to hospital have an alcohol or drug problem, and symptoms of abstinence may be misinterpreted as psychological anxiety.[38] In cases of grossly deviant behaviour, the presence of co-morbid severe personality disorder should be considered. Alternative explanations include delirium or side effects to drugs (e.g. steroids).

### (f) Psychological needs of rescue personnel and staff

Debriefing is a psychological treatment intended to reduce the psychological morbidity that may arise after exposure to accident or injury. Debriefing involves promoting emotional processing/catharsis or ventilation by systematically encouraging recollection/ventilation/reworking of the traumatic event. There is no evidence that this method reduces the incidence of post-accident problems in civilian life.[20,39] Accordingly, psychiatric intervention in the emergency room should be limited to those who display acute and severe psychiatric disorders.

Rescue personnel and medical staff may be psychologically affected by sudden exposure to grotesquely mutilated bodies.[40] The same individual vulnerability found in injured subjects apply. Group debriefing has been recommended if the rescue operation was extremely difficult; there were many dead or there was explicit harsh critique of the rescue operation from the media. Debriefing offered and conducted by a respected senior member of the rescue team is probably more appropriate than debriefing offered by psychologists or psychiatrists. However, empirical data regarding efficacy of emotionally focused group debriefing is scarce.

## Long-term behavioural and psychiatric consequences of physical trauma

Physical injury may cause permanent physical change including neurological dysfunction,[41] impaired physical function, changes in perceived somatic health including pain,[30] decreased capacity to work (in children: play), decreased social contact and decreased leisure pleasure.[42] In an unselected population of hospitalized accidentally injured adults, about half will report some complaints three years later. Among those with most severe injuries (ISS >15), only 1/3 will have made full recovery after three years, and about half will report at least moderate disabilities.[43]

The prevalence of non-organic mental disorders among hospitalized adults is about 20 per cent after six months and 10 per cent after two years.[29, 44–49] Depressive symptoms and disorder are most frequently seen followed by specific accident-related phobia and PTSD. Subsyndromal PTSD-cases must be added to these numbers. PTSD is associated with several physical health problems including cardiovascular diseases, respiratory diseases, chronic pain conditions, gastrointestinal illnesses, and cancer.[12] The prevalence of alcohol and drug abuse is increased as well.

The prevalence of long-term psychiatric is increased in injuries associated with visual disfigurement, loss of body parts or physical function (e.g. spinal cord injury), neck injuries and injuries to the pelvis and genital areas.[42] Chronic pain following accidental injury is often associated with concommittant mental disorders, in particular mood disorders or PTSD.[50] Man-made accidental injury (e.g. assault, combat, rape, terrorism) cause more long-term mental problems than other types of accidental injury (e.g. natural disasters). Studies comparing outcomes in *men versus women* have been mixed. Current evidence suggests that women are at higher risk for anxiety and depression, and men are more at risk for substance abuse and antisocial behaviour.

Following extreme psychological and physical trauma (e.g. torture, concentration camp survivors, hostage situations), permanent change in the person's pattern of perceiving, relating to, and thinking about the environment and the self may occur (ICD-10 F62.0: Enduring personality change after catastrophic experience). The changes should not fully be explained by the presence of PTSD. This diagnostic category does not exist in the DSM-IV.

## Assessment of long-term psychiatric consequences of traumatic injury

The following key-points need to be explored when evaluating long-term effects of traumatic injury

- Social and cognitive resources (including social support)
- History of mental disorder, social dysfunction or trauma in the past
- Overlooked physical injury (increased risk if high energy accident or severe injury, e.g. undetected frontal brain damage or other neurological injury)
- Deviant behaviour or accident-related psychiatric disorders following the accident (including ASR or ASD)
- Painful treatment procedures
- Accident-independent traumatic life-events during the post-injury period
- Current psychiatric disorders

Patients, relatives and physicians may evaluate long-term problems differently[51] and psychiatric co-morbidity is prevalent. Thus the clinical assessment should be supplemented by a systematic screening for the most common psychiatric disorders (e.g. MINI neuropsychiatric interview) and cognitive, behavioural and quality-of-life issues (e.g. Impact of Event scale, General Health Questionnaire). Questionnaires specifically designed to address physical, emotional and social outcome of accidental injury are available.[42] A proper, complaint-focused medical examination is often necessary as well.[52] The psychiatrist may improve the quality of the medical examination by providing the examining physician with specific diagnostic questions based on information of the patient's trauma history and symptom complaints.

## Treatment of long-term problems

Psychiatric disorders occurring in the aftermath of injury are treated according to general treatment guidelines of mental disorders with some modifications. EMDR and TF-CBT are the best validated psychotherapeutic interventions for trauma related PTSD.[20] If the psychological themes are related to conflicts, family issues or secondary events, short-term psychotherapy as outlined by Horowitz and his group[10] may be conducted. Body-focused treatments may be helpful in some subjects with chronic pain problems after trauma.[53] Randomized controlled treatment trials

of accidentally injured adults with post-injury psychosomatic and psychiatric problems are few, however. Comprehensive treatment of patients may provide better results than intervention performed by one single professional only.[54]

Antidepressants should be given in cases of mood disorders or PTSD not responding to psychotherapeutic interventions alone. SSRIs and related drugs are first choice. Drugs acting on nor-adrenalin reuptake alone (e.g. atomoxetine, reboxetin) may increase anxiety and should be avoided. Psychopharmacological treatment of somatoform pain disorders should target both serotonin and nor-adrenalin (e.g. amitryptyline, chlomipramine, duloxetine, venlafaxine). In cases of chronic PTSD with high level of intrusive symptoms, prazosin or propranolol may be added. Betablockers may be valuable as a supplement to anxiety provoking exposure therapy. Benzodiazepines may reduce PTSD-related anxiety, but differences in modulation of skin conductance compared to patients with panic disorder support clinical experience that drug treatment should be supplemented with psychological interventions in order to achieve optimal results. Guidelines for psychopharmacological treatment in patients with co-morbid physical disorders exist (e.g.[36]).

## Compensation claims and litigation

Most accidentally injured subjects do not exaggerate their loss,[55] and in non-litigant situations malingering is an unlikely explanation in most cases of chronic disturbances after accidents. Neither is economical settlement followed by significant change in clinical situation in most cases. However, in litigation situations, the patient's problem report may sometimes be exaggerated or even invalid. Studies of personal injury plaintiffs indicate that a significant number report pre-injury functioning superior to that of controls, and malingering has been estimated to 20–30 per cent.

Studies consistently show that delayed-onset PTSD in the absence of any prior symptoms is rare, whereas delayed onsets that represent exacerbations or reactivations of prior symptoms may occur.[56] Untrained subjects are able to endorse symptoms on checklists to meet criteria for diagnoses of major depression, PTSD and GAD, and PTSD self-report measures cannot be used for diagnosis.[57] Furthermore, intrusive symptoms are not PTSD-specific and may be significant in depression as well.[5] This fact is often neglected which explains why some expert testimonies misinterpret depression as being PTSD.

The physician should always try to get patient-independent information from reliable sources (e.g. medical records, general practitioners) also related to pre-injury function[58] before concluding about long-term problems due to physical injury. The possibility that clinically significant brain injury or non-injury related illnesses or psychiatric disorders occurring after the injury, have been overlooked during the medical evaluation part of litigation and compensation cases must be kept in mind.

There is no evidence that physical injury provoke *de novo* bipolar disorder or disorganized schizophrenia, even among severely maltreated subjects.[59] However, permanent injury to frontal and temporal lobes of the brain may provoke manic episodes, paranoid psychoses with schizophrenic-like symptomatology and chronic depression. Both in clinical and court settings, such brain dysfunctions may be overlooked due to lack of classical neurological signs.

Expert testimony should be based on the best available evidence and standards of care, which requires that experts stay current in their field of expertise, and revise old opinions as new information is published. Personal experience alone is rarely sufficient. The psychological difficulties and challenges faced by an expert witness is discussed elsewhere.[60]

# Further information

## Web links

### Physical injury scoring systems

This web link provides access to description and on-line calculation of physical injury trauma scores and links to other resources about physical trauma.

http://www.trauma.org/archive/scores/ais.html

### Psychiatric treatment

Several databases providing information about treatment in medicine, including psychiatry and psychosomatic medicine are available. These databases include systematic reviews metaanalysis, clinical trials, and more, including both psychological and biological interventions.

The Cochrane Library

http://www3.interscience.wiley.com/cgi-bin/mrwhome/106568753/HOME

NICE (National Institute for Health and Clinical Excellence):

http://www.nice.org.uk/).

The limitation of such databases is infrequent updates. In areas with limited research, the conclusions reported may be outdated even shortly after they are published. Thus these databases cannot replace continuous updates from databases of original research like:

PubMed http://www.ncbi.nlm.nih.gov/sites/entrez

PsychInfo.http://www.apa.org/psycinfo/

or National center for post-traumatic stress disorder database with information about treatment of PTSD and traumatic stress for Mental Health Care Providers. http://www.ncptsd.va.gov/ncmain/index.jsp

### Other useful web links

Practice guidelines for psychiatric consultation in the general medical settings provided by the

Academy of Psychosomatic Medicine: http://www.apm.org/prac-gui/psy 39-s8.shtml

The European association for consultation-liaison psychiatry and psychosomatics publishes power-point presentations about different aspects of psychiatry in the medical ill or injured: http://www.eaclpp.org/

# References

1. Zatzick, D.F., Rivara, F.P., Nathens, A.B., *et al.* (2007). A nationwide US study of post-traumatic stress after hospitalization for physical injury. *Psychological Medicine,* **37**(10), 1469–80.

2. Zatzick, D.F., Grossman, D.C., Russo, J., *et al.* (2006). Predicting posttraumatic stress symptoms longitudinally in a representative sample of hospitalized injured adolescents. *Journal of the American Academy of Child and Adolescent Psychiatry* **45**(10), 1188–95.

3. O'Donnell, M.L., Elliott, P., Wolfgang, B.J., *et al.* (2007). Posttraumatic appraisals in the development and persistence of posttraumatic stress symptoms. *Journal of Traumatic Stress,* **20**(2), 173–82.

4. Krupnick, J.L. and Horowitz, M.J. (1981). Stress response syndromes. Recurrent themes. *Archives of General Psychiatry,* **38**(4), 428–35.

5. Schnyder, U. and Malt, U.F. (1998). Acute stress response patterns to accidental injuries. *Journal of Psychosomatic Research,* **45**(5), 419–24.

6. Creamer, M., McFarlane, A.C., Burgess, P., *et al.* (2005). Psychopathology following trauma: the role of subjective experience. *Journal of affective disorders,* **86**(2–3), 175–82.

7. Murray, J., Ehlers, A., Mayou, R.A., *et al.* (2002). Dissociation and post-traumatic stress disorder: two prospective studies of road traffic accident survivors. *The British Journal of Psychiatry,* **180**, 363–8.

8. Wittmann, L., Moergeli, H., Schnyder, U., *et al.* (2006). Low predictive power of peritraumatic dissociation for PTSD symptoms in accident survivors. *Journal of Traumatic Stress,* **19**(5), 639–51.

9. Saxe, G., Stoddard, F., Courtney, D., *et al.* (2001). Relationship between acute morphine and the course of PTSD in children with burns. *Journal of the American Academy of Child and Adolescent Psychiatry,* **40**(8),915–21.

10. Horowitz, M.J. (1997). *Stress response syndromes: PTSD, grief and adjustment disorders* (3rd edn.). Jason Aronson, Northvale, New Jersey.

11. Skari, H., Malt, U.F., Bjornland, K., *et al.* (2006). Prenatal diagnosis of congenital malformations and parental psychological distress–a prospective longitudinal cohort study. *Prenatal Diagnosis,* **26**(11), 1001–9.

12. Sareen, J., Cox, B.J., Stein, M.B., *et al.* (2007). Physical and mental comorbidity, disability, and suicidal behavior associated with posttraumatic stress disorder in a large community sample. *Psychosomatic Medicine ,* **69**(3), 242–8.

13. O'Donnell, M.L., Creamer, M., Elliott, P., *et al.* (2007). Tonic and phasic heart rate as predictors of posttraumatic stress disorder. *Psychosomatic Medicine,* **69**(3), 256–61.

14. Schelling, G. (2007). Post-traumatic stress disorder in somatic disease: lessons from critically ill patients. *Prog Brain Res,* **167**, 229–37.

15. Malleson, A. (2002). *Whiplash and other useful illnesses.* McGill-Queens University Press, Montreal.

16. Verhagen, A.P., Scholten-Peeters, G.G., van, W.S., *et al.* (2007). Conservative treatments for whiplash. *Cochrane database of systematic reviews,* (2):CD003338.

17. Huyse, F.J., and Stiefel, F.C. (2006). Integrated care for the complex medically ill. pp. 1-767. Philadelphia, Saunders. *Medical Clinics of North America.*

18. Dougall, A.L., Ursano, R.J., Posluszny, D.M., *et al.* (2001). Predictors of posttraumatic stress among victims of motor vehicle accidents. *Psychosomatic Medicine,* **63**(3), 402–11.

19. Phelps, A.J., Forbes, D., Creamer, M., *et al.* (2007). Understanding posttraumatic nightmares: An empirical and conceptual review. *Clinical psychology review.*

20. Bisson, J.I., Ehlers, A., Matthews, R., *et al.* (2007). Psychological treatments for chronic post-traumatic stress disorder. Systematic review and meta-analysis. *British Journal of Psychiatry,* **190**, 97–104.

21. Meiser-Stedman, R., Yule, W., Smith, P., *et al.* (2005). Acute stress disorder and posttraumatic stress disorder in children and adolescents involved in assaults or motor vehicle accidents. *American Journal of Psychiatry,* **162**(7), 1381–3.

22. de Quervain, D.J.F. (2008). Glucocorticoid-induced reduction of traumatic memories: implications for the treatment of PTSD. In *Progress in Brain Research* (eds. E.R. de Kloet, M.S. Oitzl, E. Vermetten), pp. 239–47. Elsevier.

23. Kleim, B., Ehlers, A., Glucksman, E., *et al.* (2007). Early predictors of chronicpost-traumatic stress disorder in assault survivors. *Psychological Medicine ,* **37**(10), 1457–67.

24. Speckens, A.E., Ehlers, A., Hackmann, A., *et al.* (2007). Intrusive memories and rumination in patients with post-traumatic stress disorder: a phenomenological comparison. *Memory,* **15**(3), 249–57.

25. Richter, J.C., Waydhas, C., Pajonk, F.G., *et al.* (2006). Incidence of posttraumatic stress disorder after prolonged surgical intensive care unit treatment. *Psychosomatics,* **47**(3), 223–30.

26. Berben, S.A., Meijs, T.H., van Dongen, R.T., *et al.* (2007). Pain prevalence and pain relief in trauma patients in the Accident & Emergency department. *Injury.*

27. Gustin, S.M., Wrigley, P.J., Gandevia, S.C., *et al.* (2008). Movement imagery increases pain in people with neuropathic pain following complete thoracic spinal cord injury. *Pain.* 137 (2), 237–24.

28. Norman, S.B., Stein, M.B., Dimsdale, J.E., *et al.* (2007). Pain in the aftermath of trauma is a risk factor for post-traumatic stress disorder. *Psychological Medicine* , **10**, 1–10.

29. Edwards, R.R., Magyar-Russell, G., Thombs, B., *et al.* (2007). Acute pain at discharge from hospitalization is a prospective predictor of long-term suicidal ideation after burn injury. *Archives of Physical Medicine and Rehabilitation,* **88**(12 Suppl 2), S36–S42.

30. Castillo, R.C., Mackenzie, E.J., Wegener, S.T., *et al.* (2006). Prevalence of chronic pain seven years following limb threatening lower extremity trauma. *Pain,* **124**(3), 321–9.

31. Van Loey, N.E., and Van Son, M.J. (2003). Psychopathology and psychological problems in patients with burn scars: epidemiology and management. *American Journal of Clinical Dermatology,* **4**(4), 245–72.

32. Abdi, S., and Zhou, Y. (2002). Management of pain after burn injury. *Current Opinions in Anaesthesiology,* **15**(5), 563–7.

33. Alford, D.P., Compton, P., Samet, J.H., *et al.* (2006). Acute pain management for patients receiving maintenance methadone or buprenorphine therapy. *Annals of Internal Medicine,* **144**(2), 127–34.

34. Simon, A., and Gorman, J. (2004). Psychopharmacological possibilities in the acute disaster setting. *The Psychiatric clinics of North America,* **27**(3), 425–58.

35. Fleminger, S., Greenwood, R.J., Oliver, D.L., *et al.* (2006). Pharmacological management for agitation and aggression in people with acquired brain injury. *Cochrane Database of Systematic Reviews,* **4**: CD003299.

36. Malt, U.F., Llody, G.G. (2007). Psychopharmacological treatment in liaison psychiatry. In (eds. G.G. Lloyd, E. Guthrie), pp. 763–94. Cambridge University Press, Cambridge.

37. Royall, D.R., Cordes, J.A., Polk, M., *et al.* (2006). CLOX: an executive clock drawing task. *Journal of Neurology, Neurosurgery, and Psychiatry,* **64**(5), 588–94.

38. Moss, M., and Burnham, E.L. (2006). Alcohol abuse in the critically ill patient. *Lancet,* **368**(9554), 2231–42.

39. Rose, S., Bisson, J., Wessely, S., *et al.* (2003). A systematic review of single-session psychological interventions ('debriefing') following trauma. *Psychotherapy and Psychosomatics,* **72**(4), 176–84.

40. Benedek, D.M., Fullerton, C., Ursano, R.J., *et al.* (2007). First responders: mental health consequences of natural and human-made disasters for public health and public safety workers. *Annual review of public health,* **28**, 55–68.

41. Gurvits, T.V., Gilbertson, M.W., Lasko, N.B., *et al.* (1997). Neurological status of combat veterans and adult survivors of sexual abuse PTSD. *Annals of the New York Academy of Sciences* , **821**, 468–71.

42. Malt, U.F. (1994). Traumatic effects of accidents. In: *Individual and community responses to trauma and disaster.* (eds. R.J. Ursano, B.G. McCaughey, and C.S. Fullerton), pp. 103–35. Cambridge University Press, Cambridge.

43. Schnyder, U., Moergeli, H., Klaghofer, R., *et al.* (2001). Incidence and prediction of posttraumatic stress disorder symptoms in severely injured accident victims. *American Journal of Psychiatry,* **158**(4), 594–9.

44. Bryant, B., Mayou, R., Wiggs, L., *et al.* (2004). Psychological consequences of road traffi c accidents for children and their mothers. *Psychological Medicine,* **34**(2), 335–46.

45. Creamer, M., O'Donnell, M.L., Pattison, P., *et al.* (2004). The relationship between acute stress disorder and posttraumatic stress disorder in severely injured trauma survivors. *Behaviour Research and Therapy,* **42**(3), 315–28.

46. Fann, J.R., Burington, B., Leonetti, A., *et al.* (2004). Psychiatric illness following traumatic brain injury in an adult health maintenance organization population. *Archives of General Psychiatry,* **61**(1), 53–61.

47. Grieger, T.A., Cozza, S.J., Ursano, R.J., *et al.* (2006). Posttraumatic stress disorder and depression in battle-injured soldiers. *American Journal of Psychiatry* , **163**(10), 1777–83.

48. Glynn, S.M., Shetty, V., Elliot-Brown, K., *et al.* (2007). Chronic posttraumatic stress disorder after facial injury: a 1-year prospective cohort study. *Journal of Trauma* , **62**(2), 410–8.

49. Hoge, C.W., Terhakopian, A., Castro, C.A., *et al.* (2007). Association of posttraumatic stress disorder with somatic symptoms, health care visits, and absenteeism among Iraq war veterans. *American Journal of Psychiatry,* **164**(1), 150–3.

50. Geisser, M.E., Roth, R.S., Bachman, J.E., *et al.* (1996). The relationship between symptoms of post-traumatic stress disorder and pain, affective disturbance and disability among patients with accident and non-accident related pain. *Pain,* **66**(2–3), 207–14.

51. Biddle, D., Elliott, P., Creamer, M., *et al.* (2002). Self-reported problems: a comparison between PTSD-diagnosed veterans, their spouses, and clinicians. *Behaviour Research and Therapy,* **40**(7), 853-65.

52. Frenisy, M.C., Benony, H., Chahraoui, K., *et al.* (2006). Brain injured patients versus multiple trauma patients: some neurobehavioral and psychopathological aspects. *Journal of Trauma,* **60**(5), 1018–26.

53. Haugstad, G.K., Haugstad, T.S., Kirste, U.M., *et al.* (2006). Mensendieck somatocognitive therapy as treatment approach to chronic pelvic pain: results of a randomized controlled intervention study. *American Journal of Obstetrics and Gynecology,* **194**(5), 1303–10.

54. Zatzick, D., Roy-Byrne, P., Russo, J., *et al.* (2004). A randomized effectiveness trial of stepped collaborative care for acutely injured trauma survivors. *Archives of General Psychiatry,* **61**(5), 498–506.

55. Bryant, B., Mayou, R., Lloyd-Bostock, S., *et al.* (1997). Compensation claims following road accidents: a six-year follow-up study. *Medicine, Science, and the Law,* **37**(4), 326–36.

56. Andrews, B., Brewin, C.R., Philpott, R., *et al.* (2007). Delayed-onset posttraumatic stress disorder: a systematic review of the evidence. *American Journal of Psychiatry* , **164**(9), 1319–26.

57. Sumpter, R.E., and McMillan, T.M. (2005). Misdiagnosis of post-traumatic stress disorder following severe traumatic brain injury. *British Journal of Psychiatry,* **186**, 423–6.

58. Duckworth, M.P., and Iezzi, T. (2005). Chronic pain and posttraumatic stress symptoms in litigating motor vehicle accident victims. *Clinical Journal of Pain,* **21**(3), 251–61.

59. Eitinger, L., and Strøm, A. (1973). Mortality and morbidity after excessive stress. Humanities press, New York.

60. Gutheil, T.G., and Simon, R.I. (2005).Narcissistic dimensions of expert witness practice. *Journal of the American Academy of Psychiatry and the Law,* **33**(1), 55–8.

# Obstetric and gynaecological conditions associated with psychiatric disorder

Ian Brockington

## Introduction

This chapter covers the psychiatry of menstruation, various manifestations of the desire for children (such as surrogate pregnancy and pseudocyesis), pregnancy and mental health, the psychopathology of parturition, infant loss, postpartum psychiatric disorders, the mother–infant relationship and infanticide.

## The psychiatry of menstruation

It has long been realized that menstruation and mental illness are linked. As early as 1827 menstrual mood disorder was used as a defence in filicide.[1] In the 1850s, Brière de Boismont[2] and Schlager[3] carried out the first surveys showing that 20–30 per cent of women suffered a mood disorder before or during the menses—usually irritability or depression, occasionally euphoria. There are descriptions of a wide variety of deviant behaviours, including nymphomania, food cravings, binge drinking, pathological lying, shoplifting, and fire-setting, as well as suicide, violence, homicide, and morbid jealousy. There are other nervous diseases associated with menstruation, including epilepsy, migraine, and hypersomnia.

Recently, there has been much research into the biological basis and treatment of 'premenstrual tension' (or its synonyms). A number of daily rating schedules have been published, but self-devised rating scales, tailored to an individual patient's symptoms, can be used, provided that they are carefully completed every day. Scientific studies are bedevilled by difficulties in defining the disorders.[4] It is not known whether this is one syndrome or many. Irritability is striking, but otherwise the symptoms are common to many other disorders.

Although little is known about the aetiology, progress has been made in treatment. There may be a response to serotonin-reuptake-inhibiting antidepressants (e.g. fluoxetine, chlomipramine). In so far as a luteal-phase defect may be a factor, ovulation-promoting drugs such as clomiphene can be tried. The synthetic steroid danazol, and the gonadorelin agonists (which suppress menstruation), are draconian treatments for severe cases. All interventions should be prescribed in the context of a long-term study using daily ratings.

Rarely, menstruation is linked to a psychosis with acute onset, brief duration, and full recovery. Premenstrual, catamenial, paramenstrual, mid-cycle, and 'epochal' variants have been described.[5]

Menstrual psychosis is rare, but perhaps not excessively so. There is a clustering of episodes around puberty and after childbirth, although only a small proportion of menstrual cycles are involved. There are sufficient case reports from Japan, India, and Islamic countries to suggest a worldwide disorder. This is not a specific entity, and most typical examples manifest non-menstrual bipolar disorder at another stage of life. Clinically, it resembles puerperal psychosis. The close relationship between these two psychoses is emphasized by women who develop puerperal and menstrual psychosis at different times.[6] A Japanese investigation showed an association with anovulatory cycles.[7] Pregnancy has a beneficial effect, and there are claims of successful treatment with oral contraceptives, progesterone, clomiphene, danazol, and gonadorelins. The basis for intervention is a long-term study, with a good baseline and exact timing of events in relation to the menstrual cycle.

## Infertility

Motherhood is among the strongest and most universal of motivations. For many infertile women, childlessness is the most upsetting experience of their lives, and the yearning for children dominates everything. Infertility is stigmatizing, especially in some cultures. Infertile couples often suffer from self-reproach over sexual indiscretions, abortions, or contraception. They envy fertile couples, and contacts with other people's children, family celebrations, and friends' pregnancies are problematic. The security of the marriage may be threatened by the fear that the spouse will desert to a fertile partner; nevertheless, the marriages themselves are often happy.

Infertility differs from other stresses in its duration. The psychological reaction unfolds over years. When treatment begins, there is a cycle of optimism and hope, with a build-up of tension towards the end of the cycle, followed by disappointment and despair. Sexual functioning comes under strain during the investigation, and the discovery of azoospermia is especially stressful. There is some evidence that stress affects conception, though more prospective studies are needed.

### Assisted reproduction

Artificial insemination (using the husband's or partner's semen) has been available from the late eighteenth century, and donor insemination since 1884. Its psychological effects on marriage seem minimal; husbands or partners rarely react with jealousy to the baby, any more than to an adopted child. The proof that the experience is acceptable is that it is often repeated. One of the principles is privacy, ensuring that donor and couple never meet and remain ignorant of each other's identity. It is felt that violating anonymity might compromise the marriage, since donor and mother are too deeply involved in procreation to regard their relationship with detachment; but times may be changing. The interests of the children have to be considered; donor insemination obscures the genetic lineage, and the child cannot benefit from advances in genetics.

*In vitro* fertilization (IVF) was first performed in 1978, and was achieved with a donated oocyte in 1984; it is now widely used—in Holland, 1/60 babies are born by IVF. The procedure is harrowing, and counselling is mandatory. There is an increase in multiple births, which are more stressful. But the quality of parenting may be superior to that of families with naturally conceived children.

### Surrogate motherhood

This has two meanings:

- A woman is inseminated (artificially or naturally) with the husband's or partner's semen, and surrenders the child to the genetic father and adoptive mother. The surrogate provides oocyte and womb, and is a substitute spouse.

- The wife donates a fertilized oocyte to the surrogate gestational mother. This method, involving *in vitro* fertilization and embryo transfer, is the only way a woman without a uterus can have a child that is genetically her own.

A considerable number of women apply to become surrogate mothers, for motives of financial gain, altruism, pleasure in being pregnant, or atonement.[8] A child can now have 3 mothers—genetic, gestational, and rearing.

Surrogate pregnancy has stirred up an ethical debate. Apart from religious objections, there is concern about the physical and psychological consequences for the gestational mother, and there are endless opportunities for custody disputes and other legal complications. It has been found that the gestational mother does not bond strongly to the foetus, and most surrogate and commissioning mothers do not suffer from psychological problems.

## Pseudocyesis

When a woman believes herself to be pregnant and develops symptoms and signs of pregnancy, this is called pseudocyesis. In a classic monograph, Bivin and Klinger[9] collected 444 cases from the literature. Many sufferers were parous, including women with as many as 10 children, and as many as six episodes of pseudocyesis.

The differential diagnosis includes delusions of pregnancy, in which there are no somatic changes. This is a common delusion and can also occur in men. There is also pregnancy simulated for social, mercenary, or legal purposes (e.g. to escape the death penalty).

The clinical features include:

- a firm belief in the pregnancy, usually lasting until the onset of a false labour at 9 months, after which the disorder usually resolves

- amenorrhoea

- morning sickness and/or pica

- enlargement of the breasts and nipples, and even a discharge of colostrum

- abdominal enlargement, caused by muscular contraction, tympanites, fat, or pathological lesions, but without effacement of the navel

- an illusion of foetal movements

- enlargement of the uterus to the size of a 6-week pregnancy.

Modern diagnostic tests have greatly reduced the frequency. The diagnosis should be made on ultrasound examination. Where radiology or ultrasound are unavailable, an examination under anaesthetic is recommended—in the presence of a family member to avoid accusations of abortion.

The psychological basis is usually an intense desire for children, especially in older childless women. In some cases, however, a guilty fear of pregnancy has been the background; this has occasionally led to dangerous attempts at abortion by non-pregnant women. Pseudocyesis is a demonstration of the influence of psyche over soma, mediated by hormonal secretion. It occurs in dogs, cattle, and rodents. Persistence of the corpus luteum would explain breast changes, moderate uterine enlargement, and secretory endometrium; but it is not the only basis: hormonal measurements have been made in at least 30 patients, some of whom had chronic anovulatory states, hyperprolactinaemia, or androgen excess.

These women require psychotherapy. Simply revealing the diagnosis is unsatisfactory because the patient may consult another doctor with the same symptoms, or develop a recurrence. The underlying conflicts must be explored, helping the patient to accept that she is not pregnant.

## Sterilization

Women can be prevented from bearing children by various operations on the uterus and Fallopian tubes, indications for which are contraceptive, medical, eugenic, or psychiatric. Sterilization is the most effective and widespread contraceptive method. A large number of studies have looked at its effect on mental health, but many had methodological weaknesses. Ekblad, however, published two thorough studies in 1950s—a general study of 225 women, of whom 99 per cent were interviewed 5 to 6 years later, and a unique study of 60 sterilized women with no living children.[10]

There have been two modern prospective studies. Cooper and colleagues in Oxford[11] interviewed 201 women 4 weeks before non-puerperal tubal sterilization for contraceptive reasons; 190 were re-interviewed 6 months later, and 193 at 18 months after sterilization: the number with psychiatric illness fell from 21 before the operation to 9 at 6 months, and rose to 18 at 18 months. Not surprisingly, the presence of psychiatric disorder before the operation was a predictor of its continued presence; only two who were in good psychological health before the operation developed psychiatric illness 6 months later. A WHO collaborative study, involving five countries (India, Colombia, Nigeria, Philippines, and England), compared 926 sterilized women with 924 who used other methods of contraception: those who chose sterilization had more preoperative psychiatric disorder. The results from the Nottingham field centre[12] were published separately, and found that 9/138 sterilized women had psychiatric disorder before the operation; after surgery there were only three new cases at 6 weeks, and four more at 6 months, less than the control group.

A small minority of sterilized women are troubled by frigidity or severe regret. The most concrete evidence is a request for reversal, several studies of which have been published. Regret is more common in the following groups of women:

- Younger women or those with fewer children: Ekblad[10] found that none of his 60 childless women required hospitalization for depression, but 16 were seriously distressed and 29 expressed a longing for children of their own.

- Those in whom sterilization was the condition for a termination—a barbaric and punitive practice that used to be the rule in some countries.

- Those sterilized at a time of crisis—after parturition, or during a psychiatric illness—when it is difficult to make a balanced judgement.

- Those under external pressure.

- Those with learning difficulties: the issue of sterilization, which has from time to time been practised in various countries, is becoming more important. With a policy of community care and a greater tolerance of sexual activity, there is an increased risk of pregnancy in women with severe learning difficulties, with the spectre of inherited disorders and problems in mothering. Yet these women greatly desire children, and do not have the same resources to compensate for their lack.

- Those sterilized for medical reasons such as inherited disorders, for which medical advances have later provided alternative solutions (e.g. amniocentesis).

- Those who seek sterilization in a context of marital disharmony: after the marriage has failed, the wife may remarry and change her mind about further children.

- Those with religious scruples.

## Hysterectomy

This is one of the commonest operations, and is performed in about 10 per cent of women. There have been claims that it leads to 'post-hysterectomy depression'. But this idea has been thoroughly and systematically refuted. Several prospective investigations have shown that mental health improves after hysterectomy. Three comparable Oxford studies, conducted between 1975 and 1990, have addressed this problem: all showed that psychiatric morbidity fell below its preoperative level, or remained low.[13] The ranks of women with 'post-hysterectomy' depression are swollen by those seeking a surgical remedy for psychosomatic complaints.

In younger women, infertility can be a source of discontent. It would not be surprising if the loss of the womb affected feminine identity and libido; but this is probably also a myth. Prospective studies from Oxford,[13] St Louis,[14] and Aberdeen showed an increase in the frequency of intercourse, and of enjoyment. Concomitant oöphorectomy does not adversely affect psychiatric well-being.[15]

## The psychiatry of pregnancy

### Pregnancy adjustment

The psychopathology of pregnancy needs to be understood in terms of the adjustment all women must make when they conceive.

Pregnancy is not only a biological event, but also an adaptive process.[16] A pregnant woman must carry the baby safely through to delivery, and adjust to the sacrifices that motherhood demands. She must ensure the acceptance of the child by the family, develop an attachment to the baby within, and prepare for the birth. She must adjust to the alteration in her physical appearance, and develop a somewhat different relationship with the child's father.

Many pregnancies are unplanned and not initially welcomed. Many women react to conception with grief and anger. A random sample of English mothers showed that 44 per cent of pregnancies were unintentional, including 17 per cent that ended by legal abortion. In married women aged 25 to 29 years with one child, 80 to 84 per cent of pregnancies were planned, compared with 26 per cent in the unmarried.[17] The planning of pregnancy and its acceptance are two different things. The fact of planning does not guarantee acceptance; 6 to 12 per cent of those who plan their pregnancies subsequently regret them. Most unplanned pregnancies are immediately accepted; even if the initial response is negative, gradual acceptance usually follows. In a small proportion of cases, rejection continues to the end of the pregnancy.

Pregnancy has a profound effect on the relationship with the child's father. At every stage this relationship is of the highest importance. A pregnant woman needs increased attention and care and is sensitive to perceived rejection. Pregnancy alters other relationships as well—with the wider family and friends. Many women become closer to their families-of-origin and in-laws.

The change in appearance and shape is sometimes distressing. Some take pride and pleasure in these changes, enjoy the extra attention, and feel an enhanced sense of womanliness. Others are concerned about their loss of figure and facial bloom, weight gain, and stretch marks. Dysmorphophobia, with ideas of reference and social avoidance can ensue.

Pregnancy may be accompanied by medical disorders, and in all there is an interaction between physical and psychological factors. Pica is common, especially geophagia (eating earth or clay), which can lead to iron deficiency anaemia, bowel obstruction, and roundworm infection; other forms of pica can lead to lead poisoning or hypokalaemia. Rarely, hyperemesis can cause Wernicke's encephalopathy, and delirium can complicate chorea gravidarum.[18]

### Denial of pregnancy

In women who do not realize they are pregnant, one must distinguish between three different phenomena: unnoticed pregnancy, deliberate concealment, and dissociative denial. A German survey of 29 000 births found 62 women who failed to recognize pregnancy until the 20th week (1/475 births); 12 were not diagnosed until they were in labour with a viable infant (1/2455).[19] A Welsh study obtained similar figures.[20]

The late discovery of an unwelcome pregnancy carries a small risk of suicide. The mother is also at risk of all those complications of delivery that, with modern antenatal care, have become rare. For the child there are increased hazards, including prematurity and neonaticide.

### Prenatal attachment

The mother 'bonds' or 'affiliates' to the unborn child in a way analogous to the formation of the mother–infant relationship after birth. Prepartum bonding is catalysed by quickening and probably by ultrasound examination. The mother begins to have fantasies about the baby and talks affectionately to it. She may engage the husband or partner and other children in 'playing' with the baby. At the same time she prepares for the birth and motherhood ('nesting behaviour').

There is a pathology of the affiliative stage. In some mothers there is minimal attachment even at term. The foetus is viewed as an intrusion, whose movements annoy the mother and disturb her sleep. A poor mother–foetus relationship is one of the predictors of impaired mother–infant bonding. When the mother's attitude to the pregnancy is obstinately rejecting, therapists can direct her attention to the relationship with the child within. Stroking the abdomen and identifying foetal body parts, or telling stories about the baby's future life, have been suggested.

### Foetal abuse

When a mother deeply resents her pregnancy, she may try to harm the foetus. This occurs, with determined intent, in self-induced abortion. It may also occur as a manifestation of rage against the baby;[21] a pregnant woman may pound on her abdomen, even to the point of causing bruising.

It is not only the mother who may 'batter' the foetus. Domestic violence is common and may increase during pregnancy, when kicks and blows are directed at the abdomen, rather than the face. The main factors are sexual frustration, substance abuse, jealousy, the mother's irritability, and unreadiness for fatherhood.

The foetus is cushioned from external violence by the amniotic fluid, but can still be damaged by severe abdominal or pelvic injuries. Domestic violence can lead to miscarriage, foetal death, and premature birth. Infants can be damaged by penetrating wounds, and there are over 100 instances of gunshot wounds to the gravid uterus—the result of murderous assaults, attempts to induce a late abortion, or suicide attempts.

### Mental illness during pregnancy

#### (a) Anxiety

For many mothers, pregnancy is a time of considerable anxiety. The first trimester may involve an anguished decision whether to continue or terminate the pregnancy. Those who have previously suffered from prolonged infertility, multiple miscarriages or foetal loss are especially prone to prepartum anxiety. In the third trimester anxiety is centred on three main themes: fears of parturition (tocophobia), of foetal abnormality, and of failure to cope with motherhood.

These anxieties will usually be managed by ventilation and support, but anxiolytic medication can be used cautiously. Of the anxiolytic agents, phenothiazines are relatively safe. Benzodiazepines are contraindicated in the last stages of pregnancy because of foetal intoxication ('the floppy infant syndrome'). Propranolol is best avoided, because of reports of intrauterine growth retardation, and neonatal cardiac and respiratory symptoms.

#### (b) Depression

Although prepartum depression has not aroused the same interest as postpartum depression, it is no less common. Depression is common in all women in the reproductive age group, and pregnancy is not protective. Depression can be recurrent, and there is an association with puerperal mania.

The frequency of suicide is a vexed question. There are problems about the accuracy of the data since not all suicides are reported to the coroner, not all have necropsies, and not all necropsies include an examination of the uterus. In addition, both suicide and pregnancy are often concealed. One must therefore treat with scepticism those enquiries which do not scrutinize the primary records. Nevertheless, there is evidence that the suicide rate has declined throughout this century; in the first quarter, about 13 per cent of women who committed suicide were pregnant—a rather high figure, suggesting that pregnancy was a risk factor at a time when illegitimate pregnancy was stigmatized. This was confirmed by the thorough mid-twentieth century study of Weir.[22] More recent studies show rates below those in the general population.

Severe prepartum depression is sometimes left untreated, because of fears about the effect of drugs on the foetus. These fears have been exaggerated. No antidepressive drug is known to have teratogenic effects. Most have no effect on the foetus, though fluoxetine may reduce uterine blood flow and paroxetine may cause neonatal pulmonary hypertension. There are reports of toxic effects or withdrawal symptoms in neonates, so that medication is more to be avoided during the last trimester. Electroconvulsive therapy is safe, provided that the mother is competently oxygenated during anaesthesia; pregnant women should be screened for rare syndromes of pseudocholinesterase deficiency before receiving this treatment.

#### (c) Alcoholism

Pregnancy has a beneficial effect on alcohol addiction, but, if heavy abuse continues, there are severe effects on the foetus. The main effect is retardation of intrauterine growth[23]; although ethanol shortens gestation, the low birth weight is not explained by prematurity, rather the infants are small for gestational age. The infant becomes addicted and may suffer neonatal withdrawal symptoms. Ethanol is also teratogenic, causing 'the foetal alcohol syndrome' (or 'spectrum disorder'), first described in France in 1968.[24] The features include facial dysmorphism due to maxillary hypoplasia, and brain damage, resulting in long-term cognitive impairment and behavioural disorders (see also Chapters 9.2.7 and 10.4). In the detection of these severe complications, systematic prenatal screening for alcohol abuse is useful.

#### (d) Other addictions

**Cannabis** is commonly abused by pregnant women; it affects foetal growth, and may lead to long-term neurobehavioural and cognitive deficits. **Lysergic acid diethylamide** may have teratogenic or mutagenic effects. **Phencyclidine** addiction leads to withdrawal symptoms.

**Narcotic addicts**, like alcoholics, have multiple emotional and social problems, and many do not seek antenatal care. The infants may be affected by maternal malnutrition and infections such as venereal disease, hepatitis, endocarditis, and AIDS. Narcotics are not teratogenic, but a high proportion of the infants are of low birth weight, partly explained by prematurity, and partly by intrauterine growth retardation. A withdrawal syndrome develops in most babies. The perinatal mortality rate and frequency of sudden infant death, are increased. There is an increased incidence of microcephaly, and there may be impaired mental development, although other factors in the maternal life style may account for this. Methadone maintenance reduces the effect on birth weight; but it may depress respiration in the newborn, and lead to a more severe and prolonged withdrawal syndrome, with a greater frequency of seizures. Buprenorphine may be a more suitable maintenance therapy, with milder withdrawal effects. If it is decided to withdraw heroin, this should be done in the second trimester, replacing it by methadone. Naloxone, which can be given by implant, has been used, although there are concerns about foetal abstinence syndromes. After birth, the infants should be kept in hospital for at least 14 days. Respiratory depression can be treated by naloxone, and seizures and withdrawal symptoms by sedatives such as diazepam, or by tincture of opium.

**Cocaine** may be teratogenic, causing genitourinary and cardiac abnormalities, but the evidence is conflicting. Its main effects are cardiovascular: it causes uterine vasoconstriction, and this can lead to placental abruption. The infants may suffer cerebral infarction. There is intrauterine growth reduction and an increased incidence of microcephaly. Premature labour is common. There is a withdrawal syndrome, but this is less severe than with narcotics. There is some evidence of an increased risk of sudden infant death. Long-term effects on language development and behaviour are controversial, and may be due to confounding factors such as maternal depression, other drugs, and the environment.

All these mothers should receive close psychiatric supervision and social casework. Hair and meconium analysis improves the diagnosis of opiate and cocaine abuse in mothers who present unexpectedly in labour.

### (e) Eating disorders

There are psychological and somatic reasons for an antagonism between pregnancy and anorexia nervosa; nonetheless, most anorexic women recover, and menstruate when their weight reaches about 80 per cent of the standard weight. Ovulation can be induced by clomiphene or menopausal gonadotrophin in those who fail to menstruate. There are numerous case reports and several long-term studies showing that many women with a history of anorexia nervosa give birth to children in the normal way. The overall effect on fertility has been quantified by a 12-year Danish study; the average number of children (0.6) was about one-third the usual figure.[25] The desire for children is shown by the frequency of infertility treatment, planned pregnancy, and breast feeding.

A minority become pregnant while in the throes of the disease. Anorexic amenorrhoea may delay the diagnosis. Pregnancy usually has a beneficial effect; but if the mother continues to restrict her diet, the foetus may suffer from malnutrition. Occasionally it has been necessary to rescue the infant by elective Caesarean section. There is a tendency to relapse in the puerperium. When mothers are actively anorexic, there is often conflict at mealtimes; occasionally children may become involved in their mother's asceticism, and suffer stunted growth.

Bulimia nervosa is often improved by pregnancy. The pressure of the enlarging uterus on the stomach makes bingeing more difficult. About half relapse after delivery.[26] Pregnancy is not much affected by bulimia, but low birth weight has been reported. Bulimic mothers sometimes show deviant mothering, ignoring or excluding their children while overeating or vomiting, or restricting food supplies.

### (f) Obstetric factitious disorder

Self-induced illness behaviour can extend into the obstetric domain.[27] Women may induce bleeding to simulate threatened miscarriage, placenta praevia, or postpartum haemorrhage. They may stimulate rupture of the membranes to precipitate an early delivery. Others have been caught manipulating instruments, for example an external tachodynamometer. Two patients even attempted to simulate hydatidiform mole, by adding human chorionic gonadotrophin to blood samples.

### (g) Psychosis

Numerous asylum surveys have testified to the lower frequency of psychosis during pregnancy than after delivery. This was confirmed by Kendell and colleagues, in their linkage of Edinburgh obstetric and psychiatric case registers[28]: in a study of 54 087 births, they found rates of 2.1 per month before conception and 2.0 per month during pregnancy, much lower than after childbirth (51 in the first month).

Pregnancy probably has no effect on chronic delusional states, but it does have a beneficial effect on menstrual, bipolar, and possibly cycloid (acute polymorphic) psychoses.[29] Nonetheless, acute manic and cycloid episodes occur during pregnancy, and some seem remarkably similar to puerperal psychosis. They would be regarded as sporadic or random, except that they have been observed in women with a history of puerperal psychosis (at least 13 in the literature).[30] There is an association with multiparity, with the postpartum episode occurring first.

Neuroleptic agents appear to be safe during pregnancy. Phenothiazines and butyrophenones are not teratogenic. The main (but infrequent) hazard is sedation and extrapyramidal symptoms in the newborn. Lithium is relatively dangerous; at least 12 cases of the rare Ebstein's anomaly have been reported. As delivery approaches, reduced renal clearance can result in toxicity with normal doses; eight cases of alarming blood levels (up to 5 mmol/l) have been reported, with coma and convulsions in the mother. Even at normal blood levels, babies exposed to lithium have suffered lethargy, hypotonicity, and other effects. Carbamazepine has been associated with rather high rates of congenital abnormality, and sodium valproate is particularly dangerous, with major abnormalities especially spina bifida, and a foetal valproate syndrome.

### (h) Obstetric liaison services

In view of the complexity of the psychological response to pregnancy, and the frequency of anxiety, depression, and other psychiatric disorders, there should be good liaison between obstetric and psychiatric services. In addition to the need to diagnose and treat prepartum psychiatric disorders, the high level of supervision in the antenatal clinics offers an opportunity for preventive psychiatry, by screening for vulnerable women, including those with unwanted pregnancies, severe social problems, or a history of psychosis, addictions, or depression.

## The psychopathology of parturition

Childbirth can be one of the severest of human ordeals, and in spite of its brevity, is a time of risk for psychopathology.[18] In advanced countries, all these complications are rare, but may still be common where obstetrics is primitive, or pregnancy denied. Acts of desperation, such as auto-Caesarean section or suicide, and rage attacks, endangering the foetus, are fully described in the older literature. Delirium is well documented; in most cases, it lasts a few hours, starting shortly before delivery and disappearing after the birth, with amnesia for the event; but it can continue into the puerperium, or start immediately after the birth. Engelhard[31] gave the best estimate of its frequency: in a 10-year survey, there were five cases of transitory confusional states in 19 910 births. The existence of this phenomenon aggravates the jurisprudential problem of neonaticide, because, in an unattended delivery, it is impossible to know whether or not the mother was temporarily confused. Unexplained stupor or coma has also been described during and immediately after delivery.

### Infant loss

The child may be lost for a variety of reasons:

◆ termination of pregnancy at the behest of the mother

◆ miscarriage, ectopic pregnancy, and late termination of a wanted child for medical reasons

◆ foetal death *in utero*, stillbirth, neonatal death, and sudden infant death ('cot death', SIDS)

◆ relinquishment to adoption.

#### (a) Termination of pregnancy

The indications for abortion include the following:

◆ medical—to preserve the health and life of the mother

◆ humanitarian—when pregnancy has resulted from rape or incest

◆ eugenic—where there is a risk of congenital abnormality

◆ psychiatric

◆ social—because pregnancy is untimely and disruptive

◆ on demand—in the belief that women should be free to decide when to have children.

There has been a debate on the validity of the psychiatric indications; this turns on the psychiatric consequences of a refusal to terminate. Suicide threats are common, but are rarely carried out; nevertheless there can be no doubt that unwanted pregnancy is a factor in completed suicide. A history of puerperal psychosis is not an indication, because it is equally likely to follow abortion; but there are other, arguably more serious, puerperal complications such as mother–infant relationship disorders, which are more common and severe after unwanted pregnancy. These can be avoided by adoption, but the psychological effects of relinquishment are not negligible.

The psychological effects of termination have been thoroughly explored. Most who voluntarily abort suffer no adverse effects, either in the short or long-term. There is often relief, even euphoria, and a reduction in anxiety, depression, anger, guilt, and shame. A minority experience regret and self-reproach over the 'murder' of the baby. Some feel like criminals and worry about punishment, a nemesis of sterility or future congenital malformations. A few develop clinical depression. A Finnish study showed that the suicide rate was increased from $11/10^5$ to $35/10^5$.[32]

There is a literature on 'postabortion psychosis', but both parts of the term have multiple meanings; 'abortion' refers to miscarriage, termination, criminal abortion, and even stillbirth after short gestation, and 'psychosis' includes delirium, Wernicke–Korsakow syndrome, melancholia, and psychogenic paranoid disorders. Manic or cycloid episodes, similar to puerperal psychosis, occur after abortion: apart from epidemiological evidence[33] and individual cases, the association of postabortion and postpartum psychosis in the same woman has been reported on at least 14 occasions.[30] Some episodes occurred after miscarriage, but several followed termination, in most cases performed to prevent a recurrence of puerperal psychosis.

To minimize the psychological risk, prudent decision taking is of the essence, and counselling has a valuable role. The most difficult part of the experience is the loneliness and isolation. Many do not inform their parents, and, when they do, face censure and unwelcome pressure. The attitude of the child's father is crucial. Attempts should be made to involve him in all aspects of the experience; unfortunately his reaction is often unhelpful. It is axiomatic that a woman should make her own decision—one of the most difficult she will ever take. It often has to be taken hastily, in an atmosphere of conflict and turmoil. The best outcomes are found when a woman makes her decision in a context of respect and support from partner, parents, friends, or counsellor.

#### (b) Miscarriage

This is a common event, perhaps 40 per cent of all conceptions, but only 10 per cent occur after pregnancy is recognized by amenorrhoea or other signs. An ectopic pregnancy is gynaecologically more serious, but has the same psychological effects. The emotional consequences of miscarriage are not trivial, and can be compared to perinatal death—less severe, because there has been little time for attachment to the newly conceived, but still the loss of a greatly desired child. The event itself, with foetal tissue passed suddenly and painfully, may be disturbing. Some of the psychological symptoms may resemble post-traumatic stress disorder, with intrusive re-experiencing ('flashbacks') and nightmares. There is a sense of failure, guilt, and anger. The incidence of depression is four times the rate found in the general population. There may be depressive episodes at the time of the expected delivery, anniversary reactions, and an increased risk of postpartum emotional disorder after a later normal delivery.

Helping a mother who has suffered a miscarriage is a variant of grief therapy, in which her intense distress is shared, and sadness, guilt, and anger ventilated.

Late termination for medical reasons, although a deliberate intervention, is psychologically similar to miscarriage and to foetal death *in utero*. Some wish to continue the pregnancy in the full knowledge that the baby will be abnormal. Depression is common, and grief long-lasting. All these women require counselling, before and after the termination.

#### (c) Foetal death *in utero*, stillbirth, neonatal death, and sudden infant death

Reactions to these events are generally more severe than to miscarriage, and each has its special characteristics. When the baby dies in late pregnancy, the mother carries a corpse within her, and must undergo a futile labour. If it dies during labour, the loss is sudden and shock pronounced, with a strong sense of unreality. When the child dies in the first week, the parents have to endure great anxiety, with dwindling hope; they may be involved in the decision to switch off the respirator, and witness the child dying. The later death of an infant, when the maternal emotional response is fully developed, especially sudden infant death, is at the very top of the catalogue of calamities; there is no warning or preparation, and the death is followed by a forensic investigation.

#### (d) Grief after infant loss

This is similar to other grieving, but has its own special character. There is shock, followed by emotional numbness and emptiness, then long-lasting and agonizing sadness. Grief hallucinations (of foetal movements, the baby's face, the infant crying or playing in the cot) may be experienced. There is guilt, anger, and recrimination. There are various crises, especially the disposal of toys, baby clothes, and nursery furniture, as well as meeting friends and relatives; some, floundering in their embarrassment, are evasive and unable to comfort or sympathize ('wall of silence'). Especially after SIDS, there may be shame, stigma, and even ostracism or malicious speculation. Envy of successful mothers is a problem; there may even be a temptation to steal babies. Surviving children may be confused by their parents' grief, upset by family turmoil, and deprived of attention and care; they are also grieving and preoccupied with their own search for the meaning of death.[34]

When helping the parents,[35] the principles are as follows:

- **Honesty and openness in communication**. The admission of errors is delicate, but the parents' guilt should not be reinforced by the obstetric team's refusal to accept responsibility. Recrimination, litigation, or querulant reactions are common. Staff should accept this as normal, and try not to be defensive. After a stillbirth, most mothers prefer to be segregated, and discharged early. One or more interviews with the consultant obstetrician are indicated. It is essential that the mother is visited by a member of the primary care team. A lactating mother may need bromocriptine, or to donate milk to a milk bank. Hypnotics may help mothers troubled by insomnia. The doctor should be alert for secondary depression.

- **All parents want to know why the baby died**. The necropsy can help, but parents should be warned that often no explanation is found. Necropsies in SIDS are specialized; the pathologist can play a vital psychological role, and should be available for discussion.

- **Mementoes** should be kept, including a photograph. The dignity of naming and a burial ceremony is helpful. The value of seeing and holding the dead baby has been challenged.[36]

- **The bereaved mother needs to share her distress**. A sensitive and sympathetic person, with the time and interest to listen, can help her grieve and accept her loss. This support will often come from the husband or partner, family, or friends. If not, professionals, especially chaplains or nurses, should step in. Self-help groups and voluntary agencies are invaluable for some mothers.

- **The next pregnancy**. No doctrinaire advice can be given about the timing of the next pregnancy. Increased anxiety during pregnancy and the puerperium can be expected.

- **The grieving sibling**. The routine and rhythm of family life should be disturbed as little as possible. The parents should not be afraid to show their emotions—it is best to acknowledge their sadness, and how much they will miss the baby. They should try to give a factual account of what happened, avoiding euphemisms. It is important to reassure the children: they are not responsible and will not lose the love of the parents; neither they nor their parents are in imminent danger of death. The child can be helped to grieve by looking at pictures of the dead sibling, attending the funeral, and visiting the graveyard. (see Chapter 9.3.7 for further information about bereavement in childhood.)

### (e) Relinquishment

Adoption used to be the main way to satisfy the longing to rear children and to handle accidental pregnancy, but there has been a great social change in Europe and North America. Since 1950, the number of children born to single mothers has climbed steeply, and is still climbing, but, despite this increase, the number of adoptions is falling steadily. This is not due to spectacular improvements in the infertility treatment, reducing the demand, nor to the relaxation in the abortion laws, reducing the supply, but a new tolerance of single motherhood. In partial compensation for the scarcity of relinquished babies, the practice of adopting foreign-born children has arisen.

Although adoption is on the wane, attention has been focused on the psychological effects of relinquishment.[37] For some relinquishing mothers, giving up the child is a painful, loving act of selfless courage. In others it is the enforced loss of a living child, with a charade of informed consent. Relinquishment is among the most stressful of events. Instead of understanding and support, there is often loneliness and ostracism. Time is no healer; the child continues to exist and can be seen again, and there is often a fantasy of reunion or restitution. As time goes on, there is a new component; the adult child may seek its biological mother, and there is the hope that this event, which she cannot influence, may happen. There has been a growth in the number of organizations to help relinquishing parents find their offspring. Many countries are grappling with the problems of legislating for reunions.

To avoid these severe and prolonged psychological effects, a relinquishing mother needs counselling during the pregnancy. The aim is to emerge from the experience with self-respect and dignity. After delivery the mother should be encouraged to see the infant and photographs should be filed. Follow-up counselling should be continued for at least 6 months. The mother may wish to join a society for relinquishing parents. There is also the relationship with the adopting family to consider. Adoptive parents should accept any gift or token of the natural mother's love. Information on the outcome of the child should be available. Some birth-mothers wish to provide up-to-date information, so that the child knows they are now respected citizens. A recent innovation is the practice of 'open adoption', in which both sets of parents meet. There is even 'continuing open adoption', which means that they remain in contact over the course of the child's development.

## The psychiatry of the postpartum period

### The normal puerperium

For many or most mothers, giving birth is a supreme moment, and euphoria or elation is common. Some may be too excited to sleep. These feelings of peace, fulfilment, and accomplishment help to sustain mothers during the weeks of strain that follow. Prolonged euphoric reactions, lasting a week or more, are probably mild puerperal mania, and are often followed by depression.

Newly delivered mothers have to face a number of challenges, including the following.

- **Physical exhaustion**. This can be coupled with the painful sequelae of pelvic trauma.

- **Breast feeding**. Although this has many advantages, it is often difficult to establish.

- **Insomnia**. Sleep deprivation, especially during the first month, is a cause of irritability, and should be borne in mind when mothers present 'at the end of their tether'.

- **Recovery of normal figure and attractiveness**. This may be threatened by weight gain and stretch marks. Mothers may occasionally develop a state similar to dysmorphophobia.[38]

◆ **Loss of libido**. Episiotomy and vaginal trauma often cause dyspareunia; fatigue may depress sexual activity. Nevertheless sexual relations are usually resumed within 1 to 3 months, though reduced in frequency, and with a delayed return of orgasm. For this and other reasons (e.g. jealousy) the marriage may come under strain.

◆ **Social privation**. The loss of employment, income, and leisure, as well as confinement to the house, are all contributory factors.

With this background of rapid biological, social, and emotional transition, it is not surprising that a wide variety of psychiatric disorders occur; indeed the psychiatric complications of childbirth are more numerous and complex than in any other human situation.

The **maternity 'blues'** is so common as to be almost normal. Usually between the third and fifth days, many mothers experience a sudden, fleeting, and unexpected period of sensitivity and uncharacteristic weeping. In the great majority this passes off within a few hours, or a day or two. There is some evidence for an association between this brief dysphoric reaction and postpartum depression.

## Reactions to severe labours

### (a) Post-traumatic stress disorder

After excessively painful labours, some women suffer nightmares, and repetitive daytime intrusion of images and memories, similar to those that occur after the harrowing experiences of war and natural disaster. Since the original description,[39] over 40 papers have been published on this subject, including 10 quantitative studies showing rates of up to 5.9 per cent of deliveries. Many of these women avoid further pregnancy (secondary tocophobia), and those who become pregnant again may experience a return of symptoms, especially in the last trimester.

This disorder can be treated by counselling and by specific psychological therapies. Tocophobia is an indication for elective Caesarean section.

### (b) Querulant reactions

Another reaction to a severe labour experience is pathological complaining (*Querulantenwahn*). These women complain bitterly about perceived mismanagement, and their angry rumination may continue for weeks or months, interfering with infant care. Some confine themselves to vengeful fantasies and verbal or written criticism, but others proceed to litigation. Careful assessment is needed to distinguish these reactions from reasonable complaining.

This disorder can be treated by a psychotherapeutic approach, which distracts the mother from her grievances and reinforces productive child-centred activity.

## Postpartum anxiety disorders

Recent research has shown that postpartum anxiety disorders are just as common as postpartum depression.[38,40] A review of eight studies of 'panic disorder' showed that 44 per cent of anxious women had an exacerbation, and 10 per cent a new onset, in the puerperium.[41] It is important to identify the focus, as well as the form, of anxiety, because there are several themes that indicate specific psychological therapies. Benzodiazepines should be used with caution in lactating mothers. They are well absorbed from the gut, and more slowly metabolized in the neonatal liver, and occasionally cause lethargy and weight loss in breast-fed infants.

### (a) Puerperal panic, and phobic avoidance of the infant

Some mothers, especially *primiparae* in isolated 'nuclear' families, are overwhelmed by the responsibility of caring for the newborn.[42] The panic and agitation seen in extreme examples is an exaggeration of the anxiety that many women experience when they first confront this awesome task. If no help is available, a mother can develop a phobic avoidance of the infant,[43] and risks losing her mothering role.

These disorders can often be handled by the wider family, without invoking professional help. The mother needs sedation, especially at night. During waking hours, she should remain with the baby, but must be supported at all times. Treatment is by desensitization. Gradually the mother takes over, at her own pace, undertaking the easiest tasks first, and involved in all decisions. In severe cases, conjoint admission may be the only way to rescue the situation. With correct diagnosis and management the prognosis is excellent.

### (b) Anxieties about infant health and survival

The care of an infant involves ceaseless vigilance. In women prone to anxiety and excessive worrying, or in those who have suffered years of infertility or recurrent miscarriage, motherhood can lead to excessive solicitude about banal tasks that put the baby at risk (e.g. bathing) and sensitivity to the slightest indication of illness. In some, the anxiety is focused on the possibility of sudden infant death.[44] These mothers lie awake listening to the baby's breathing; sleep with their hand on the infant's chest, check the infant many times each night, or even wake the baby to ensure that he or she is still alive. This results in excruciating tension, insomnia, and exhaustion.

These mothers require anxiety management. Day-hospital attendance, with relaxation therapy and group support is ideal. A mother with 'fear of cot death syndrome' may be helped by explanations about the rarity of SIDS, and the infant's resistance to asphyxia, as well as devices to monitor the infant's breathing. The vicious cycle of insomnia and hypervigilance can be interrupted periodically by involving relatives or friends, so that she can sleep under sedation. Ventilation, and the support of mothers who have recovered from similar problems, is helpful. However, these are only palliatives, because the underlying cause is an event, which, albeit uncommon, remains possible during a period of several months.

## Puerperal obsessional disorders

There is evidence that the puerperium is one of the main precipitants of obsessive–compulsive disorders.[45,46] In addition to obsessional rituals, the disorder may present with thoughts, images, or impulses of child harm. These impulses to attack the child must be distinguished from the pathological anger that precedes child abuse. The mother is gentle and devoted. She experiences extravagant infanticidal images, such as stabbing, decapitation, or strangulation. She fears being left alone with her infant, and may take extraordinary precautions.[47] The obsessional content may be of child sexual abuse, for instance masturbating or castrating their sons.

Ventilation, explanation, and psychotropic medication are part of the treatment, but are rarely sufficient. It is important to discourage avoidance of the child, and encourage cuddling and play, thus strengthening positive maternal feelings. Cognitive–behavioural treatment can help her to achieve mastery over irrational impulses. (For the treatment of obsessive–compulsive disorder, see Chapter 6.3.2.1.)

## Depression

Puerperal melancholia was one of the first postpartum psychiatric disorders to be identified. During the asylum era, only the most severe cases were admitted, and the occurrence was underestimated when compared with 'puerperal mania'. When, in the 1950s, attention turned to milder disorders, postpartum depression was found to be common in the general population. The pioneering work of the Gordons in New Jersey[48] was soon widely confirmed. In the last 10 years there has been a flood of papers from all over the world. Surveys have shown rates of at least 10–20 per cent, or even higher in the 'Third-World'.[49] 'Postnatal depression' has become a household word. It is an important lay concept, which has legitimized maternal depression in the minds of the public, providing a valid explanation for role failure, diminishing stigma, enabling mothers to accept that they are ill, and to come forward for treatment. It is a slogan that can be wielded in the political struggle to obtain better services for mothers of young families. There is a need for such concepts, which have social influence.

However, one must examine the scientific value of this concept with scepticism. Depression after childbirth is clinically similar to any other depression, and the association of depression with the puerperium is not striking. Whatever the prevalence in surveys, only about 5 per cent consult their general practitioners. The epidemiological evidence is weak. The suicide rate in the first postpartum year is below the female rate.[32] Depression is common in women during the reproductive years, whether they are infertile, pregnant, puerperal, menopausal, or involved in child rearing. The term 'postnatal depression' has the danger of introducing into the minds of the unwary the mirage of a homogeneous disorder with a single cause. Rather, it is a rubric for a heterogeneous group of disorders. Many mothers with anxiety, obsessional, or post-traumatic disorders, or with a disturbed infant relationship, are depressed, but the setting, causes, and treatment are different. Not surprisingly, research into its causes has found that they are the same as those that cause depression at all ages—heredity, a history of previous or prepartum depression, 'neuroticism', adverse events or social conditions, difficult relationships, and social isolation. It has been suggested that the burden of child rearing, rather than child bearing, is a factor, but this has been challenged by a Swedish twin study[50] and a Norwegian suicide study[51] showing that parous women have a lower risk of depression than nulliparous women. In mothers with recurrent puerperal depression one would expect to find specific factors. Adjustment to motherhood has received much less emphasis than it deserves; unwanted pregnancy has been found to be a predictor of antepartum and postpartum depression.

Whatever its frequency, the effects of depression on family life, and the emotional climate in which children are reared, is of great concern. A growing child needs emotional support, attention, approbation, and stimulation. The mother is the child's primary environment, and her mood dominates his or her world. Even very young infants are disturbed by deviant social behaviour in the mother. Although deficits are not universal,[52] her depression can lead to inattention through anergia or brooding, reduced quantity, quality, and variety of interaction, and loss of the reinforcement of the mother's gaiety and tenderness. Her anger may be misdirected at the children. Frequent irritability, impatience, and criticism induce social withdrawal, anxiety, and reciprocal anger. There may be educational deficits. These effects depend on the degree and duration of maternal depression, and the extent to which it involves interactions with the child. (See Chapter 9.3.6 for further information on the effects of maternal depression on child development.) In extreme cases, maternal depression can lead to the tragedy of combined suicide and filicide.

Treatment begins with effective diagnosis. Many more mothers are depressed than ever make their way to the surgery. The reasons for the failure to seek help are not fully understood: some recover early, some do not realize they are ill, and some are ashamed of confessing their symptoms, suffering in silence because of ignorance, stigma, and fears of losing their baby. Screening procedures help the primary care services to identify cases; an example is the Edinburgh Postnatal Depression Scale,[53] which has high sensitivity and specificity. Patients identified by screening, or self-referral, require a full psychiatric examination, in order to identify vulnerability factors and the specific components of postpartum disorders. This initial interview is best held at home, because clinic attendance is an obstacle for mothers fettered with the care of young children, and because domiciliary assessment has a quality that cannot be achieved in the office. The interview should explore the symptoms and course of the illness, study its context in the mother's life history, personality, and circumstances, review the events of this pregnancy, explore the mother's relationships with her spouse, baby, other children, and family of origin, and establish the available supports.

Treatment is focused on depression and any underlying vulnerability. It will always involve psychotherapy, if only in the form of a single interview; it will usually include medication or other specific treatments; a few require electroconvulsive therapy. Working with the baby's father, potentially the main supporter, is important; fathers can come under strain, either because their wife's intimacy with the baby disturbs conjugal dynamics, or because her depression has a domino effect on him. Home visits by community nurses are an ideal method of delivering continuing care and psychotherapy. An extensive literature has accumulated demonstrating the efficacy of psychological treatments by double-blind randomized controlled trials. As for drug treatment, there is no evidence that any drug is superior to others. There are at least 50 reviews of drug treatment in lactating mothers. The suckling infant has little body fat, less plasma protein-binding, an immature liver and kidney and an undeveloped blood-brain barrier. But the risks are minor. Only a minute dose is delivered to the infant: Epperson and colleagues demonstrated that serotonin re-uptake blocking agents do not affect serotonin levels in breast fed infants.[54] Occasionally, babies have been over sedated. It is not recommended that antidepressant agents be withheld, or that breast-feeding be stopped; but it is wise to use these drugs cautiously, and it may be helpful to take the drug after breast feeding (see also Chapter 6.2.3).

Prevention is important in mothers with a history of severe or prolonged postpartum depression. They often present during the next pregnancy, requesting advice or prophylaxis. If they are already symptomatic, or have obvious risk factors such as marital friction or social isolation, they need support from community psychiatric nurses, voluntary agencies, or other groups. If they are well, it is only necessary to establish contact, so that a recurrence is diagnosed and treated promptly. Prophylactic antidepressant medication can be considered.

## Mother–infant relationship disorders

Just as the emerging relationship with the foetus is important during pregnancy, so also the growth of the mother–infant relationship is the key psychological process in the puerperium. 'Bonding' is a popular lay term; some professionals prefer 'attachment', but one must not confuse this with infant–mother attachment. The mother–infant relationship consists essentially of ideas and emotions aroused by the infant, which find their expression in affectionate and protective behaviour. Its immense power is revealed in self-sacrifice, and the pains of separation. Its inner presence is betrayed by external signs—touching and fondling, kissing, cuddling and comforting, prolonged gazing and smiling, baby talk and cooing, recognizing signals, tolerating demands, and resisting separation; but it is hard to select a single activity that lies at the core. Particular behaviours wax and wane, but the relationship endures, even when the child is absent, even when it is gone for ever. This emotional response enables the mother to maintain the never ending vigilance, and endure the exhausting toil of the nurture of the newborn.

There is no 'critical period' in the development of the maternal response. Close proximity from the start ('rooming-in') gives confidence in mothering skills, and breast-feeding may help. The infant plays an important part. At an early stage, it can discriminate speech, and reacts preferentially to the human face and voice. Eye-to-eye contact mediates the interaction, and gazing becomes an absorbing activity on both sides. The baby's smile is another catalyst. Videotape studies have shown the infant contributing to a dialogue with its caregiver. Sometimes the maternal response is immediate, primed by affiliation to the foetus, but sometimes there is a worrying delay. For the first 3 to 4 weeks many mothers feel bruised, tired, and insecure, and their babies seem strange and distanced. As the baby begins to respond socially, a normal relationship develops rapidly.

The term 'mother–infant relationship (or bonding) disorders' covers a spectrum of clinical states, which has two main dimensions:

◆ An absent or negative emotional response. In severe cases, the mother regrets the pregnancy and expresses dislike or hatred of her baby. She may try to persuade her own mother, or another relative to take over, and may demand that the infant be fostered or adopted. The most poignant manifestation is a secret wish that the baby 'disappear'—be stolen, or die.

◆ Pathological anger. The infant's demands anger the mother and provoke aggressive impulses, which may lead to shouting, cursing, screaming, or assaults.

There is at present little data on the frequency of these disorders in the general community. At the level of 'threatened rejection'— where the mother has an aversion to her child and seeks temporary escape from child care (the threshold for active intervention)— the frequency of these disorders in the general community is probably about 1 per cent. It is much higher in mothers who seek help for 'postnatal depression'—about 10 per cent at the level of established rejection, and another 15 per cent for threatened rejection.[55]

These disorders are usually accompanied by depression, but there are many reasons to reject the euphemism 'postpartum depression with impaired mother–infant interaction'.

◆ A disturbed relationship is different from a mood disorder.

◆ When depression is associated with phobias, obsessions, or deviant behaviour, these co-morbid phenomena are still considered worthy of study and treatment in their own right.

◆ Impaired interaction, although it can be recorded and measured, is not the essence of the phenomenon, but merely its behavioural manifestation; it has other causes, especially infant-centred anxiety.

◆ Aversion to the infant is not confined to depressed mothers;[56,57]

◆ When they coexist, their severity and course often differ.

◆ Only a minority of depressed mothers have this problem. It is important to select them for treatment and not to stigmatize the others.

◆ The risks—including child abuse and neglect—are higher. It is these disorders, rather than uncomplicated depression, that have serious and long-term effects on the child's development.[58] These mothers are a high-risk group that can contribute to the vital task of preventing child abuse and neglect.

◆ The treatment is different and specific (see below). Assessment and treatment of this relationship forms an important part of the work of mother–infant mental health teams.

◆ Management must be aware of the need for training and service provision.

◆ The aetiology is different, with more emphasis on unwanted pregnancy and challenging infant behaviour.

The diagnosis can be facilitated by self-rating questionnaires, but the main clinical resource is an interview probing the mother's emotional response and behaviour. In severe cases and in research, the 'gold standard' is direct observation, preferably over a substantial length of time.

The treatment proceeds in stages:

◆ Where there is a delay in the maternal emotional response, explanation and reassurance are usually sufficient.

◆ When hostility, rejection, and anger are prominent, the primary decision is whether to attempt treatment or not. The mother must be given freedom of choice; it is dangerous for her to feel trapped in unwelcome motherhood. At the same time, the father has his rights. The option of relinquishing the infant must be openly acknowledged, and fully discussed with both parents.

◆ If it is decided to embark on treatment (as in most cases), depression should be treated with psychotherapy, drugs, or (occasionally) electroconvulsive therapy.

◆ The specific element of therapy is working on the dyadic relationship. This relationship, like others, grows through shared pleasure. The baby alone has the power to awaken its mother's feelings, so the aim is to create circumstances in which mother and child can enjoy each other. It is a mistake to separate the mother and baby completely, which merely compounds the problem by adding an element of avoidance. If there is any hint of abuse or aggressive impulses, the mother must never be left alone with her infant. She must be relieved of irksome burdens of infant care. When mother and baby are calm, she is encouraged and helped to interact with him—to cuddle, talk, play, and bring out his smile and laughter. Participant play therapy and baby massage may assist.

Treatment can take place in various settings. Home treatment can be successful, provided there is enough support to relieve the mother of night care and stressful duties: the maternal grandmother, an understanding husband or partner or a family group can sometimes achieve this. Day-hospital treatment provides individual support and group discussion, as well as specific therapies. In the most severe and refractory cases, the proper setting is an inpatient mother-and-baby unit, where an experienced team of psychiatric and nursery nurses, available 24 h a day and 7 days a week, can provide full support. Even in the most severe cases, one can feel optimistic about a successful outcome. (For further information about child abuse see Chapter 9.3.3.)

### Postpartum psychoses

These fall into two main groups—organic psychoses and bipolar disorders; a third group—reactive or psychogenic psychosis—is most convincingly seen in adoptive mothers and fathers. There are many causes of delirium after childbirth.[18] Organic psychoses are hardly ever seen in Europe or North America, but may still be important in Africa,[59] India, South-East Asia, and Latin America, where the majority of children are born. Historically the most important causes have been infection and eclampsia psychosis, but cerebral venous thrombosis is common in India.[60]

The form of psychosis still seen in Europe and North America was described by Osiander,[61] and illuminated by the case studies of Esquirol.[62] The long-standing controversy about its nosology has been resolved in favour of a relationship with the bipolar group; but there is also a connection with acute polymorphic (cycloid) psychosis, which may also belong to the bipolar rubric. These are biological brain disorders, with high heritability and an inborn tendency to develop episodes throughout life. The problem of causation can be broken down into three subsidiary questions: the nature of the diathesis, the determinants of clinical polarity (mania, depression, or cycloid), and the trigger that provokes the episode. The first two questions belong to the wider study of bipolar disorder. The third is specific to puerperal psychosis. The clinical facts suggest not one, but several triggers related to the female reproductive process—abortion, pregnancy itself (especially the last trimester), the early puerperium (especially the first 10 days), postpartum menstruation, menstruation in general (see menstrual psychosis above), and weaning. These triggers can be added to the list of other biological events that trigger bipolar episodes, including surgery, adrenocortical steroid treatment, and seasonal climatic changes. Instances can be given of the combination of all these triggers in the life history of individual women, and there may be a shared pathway in these diverse precipitants. The incidence is somewhat less than 1 in 1000 pregnancies.[28,63] The Edinburgh study showed no link with twin pregnancies, breast feeding, single parenthood, or stillbirth. The miscarriage rate has been low in two studies. This psychosis has high heritability—not just for bipolar disorder, but also the puerperal trigger.[64]

Postpartum bipolar psychoses are acute, rapidly reaching a climax of severity. The onset is usually between 2 and 14 days after delivery. Mania is severe, often with 'schizoaffective' symptoms or extreme excitement. Almost every psychotic symptom may be seen—the whole gamut of delusions, verbal hallucinations, disorders of the will and self, and catatonic features. There is often an apparent confusion or perplexity. Since the advent of electroconvulsive therapy and neuroleptic medication, the duration has fallen to a few weeks. A minority of patients show a tendency to relapse in rhythm with menstruation. Puerperal recurrences occur after 20 to 25 per cent of subsequent pregnancies. Non-puerperal recurrences are also common.

There are no specific treatments. The first resource is sedation by neuroleptic agents, but these should be used with caution because of the risk of severe extrapyramidal side effects, which include neuroleptic malignant syndrome. It is usual to stop breast-feeding, although this may not be necessary, because the infant receives only a minute dose of the neuroleptic and adverse effects have not been noted; Clozapine may, however, accumulate in breast milk. Lithium has been used increasingly since the link with manic-depressive psychosis was recognized. There is also evidence for its prophylactic value in women at high-risk. However, it may have adverse effects on breast-fed infants. Electroconvulsive therapy is highly effective in all varieties of puerperal psychosis, including puerperal mania. The location of treatment is an important issue. Since hospitalization can be disruptive to the family, this disorder should for preference be treated at home, where the patient can maintain her role as wife, homemaker, and mother, and her relationship with the newborn; but its severity and the lack of community resources make this a counsel of perfection. If hospital admission is necessary, there are great advantages in conjoint mother and baby admission.

### Services for mothers with mental illness

An outline of the services required for this area of psychiatry is slowly emerging. Its aims are prevention in those who are vulnerable, early and accurate diagnosis, and rapid effective intervention, with minimal disruption of family life. These aims require the following:

- **A multi-disciplinary specialist team** This team, a key resource whatever the cultural background, should consist of psychiatrists, nursing staff of various kinds, psychologists and social workers; it can serve a population of several million inhabitants, handle severe and intractable illness, train all staff, develop services, and conduct research.

- **A community service** Domiciliary assessment and home treatment are appropriate for mothers.

- **Day care** A day hospital can provide a full range of interventions, including groups, play therapy, motherhood classes, anxiety management, and occupational therapy, with minimal family disruption. The presence of mothers with similar disorders is an additional support. The children are cared for in a crèche.

- **Inpatient facilities** Conjoint admission of mother and infant is superior to the admission of the mother alone.[65] Wards dedicated to conjoint admission also have advantages over admissions to general psychiatric wards, although they are more expensive.

- **An obstetric liaison service** Apart from treating prepartum mental illness, this provides an opportunity for preventive psychiatry, by detecting vulnerability during pregnancy.

- **Links with other agencies providing services for mothers** The social services have a key role. Their family centres fulfil a similar function to mother-and-baby day hospitals. They can relieve the burden on the mother, and safeguard the child, by providing emergency foster care. Other agencies include the National Society for the Prevention of Cruelty to Children (in the United Kingdom), midwifery services, primary care teams, and child psychiatry services.

◆ **A network of voluntary organizations** These are independent organizations, but can have close cordial ties with the professional service. There is no one better suited to support a depressed mother than another mother who has suffered a similar problem and is now well—she knows the stratagems or words of comfort that were helpful, and is living proof of the hope of recovery. For each disorder, a panel of recovered mothers is an important resource.

◆ **Medico-legal expertise** Expert advice is often required in cases of child abuse or infanticide, and where a mother with mental illness is seeking custody of, or access to, her children.

## The psychiatry of parental children-killing

The term 'infanticide' covers the killing of infants and children by their mother or father in a wide variety of circumstances, broadly divided into 'neonaticide' (killing the newborn) and 'filicide' (the later murder of a child).

### Neonaticide

Killing neonates (especially female infants) has been customary in certain societies as an official policy or 'grass-roots' custom for controlling population growth. This is completely different from criminal neonaticide, in which a mother, who has concealed her pregnancy and given birth in secret, kills the infant immediately after parturition. This was a major public health problem in Europe during the nineteenth century. Its frequency has dwindled as a result of contraception, a relaxation of the abortion laws, and changed attitudes to single motherhood; but it still occurs.

The mental state of mothers who kill the newborn can be deduced from the methods used. Suffocation is by far the most common,[66] and this testifies to the mother's panic, faced by a crying baby. In a minority, brutal head injuries, stabbing, or decapitation testify to rage and hatred.

In Europe, starting in Russia in 1647, the public has gradually taken a humane view of this felony. By 1881, all European states, with the exception of England and Wales, made a distinction between infanticide and other forms of murder, and assigned a more lenient penalty. England and Wales at last came into line with the Infanticide Act 1922. In some American states no distinction is made between this and other forms of murder.

There has been much debate whether the defence of insanity can be invoked. Most of these babies die when the mother is in the grip of an emotional crisis—seized by fear or fury. This is not generally acceptable in law as evidence of insanity, which is defined as a defect of reason. However, impairment of consciousness undoubtedly occurs during labour (see above); it is rare in hospital practice, but may be more common in clandestine deliveries, and is hard to exclude. If the defence is burdened with the proof of insanity, there can be no valid evidence in unwitnessed deliveries; but there is the possibility of a miscarriage of justice—that a mother, who killed her baby when her consciousness was clouded, is wrongly condemned.

### Filicide

The majority of murdered children are killed by their parents, and the majority of female murderers kill their own child. A survey in Queensland gave an estimate of the frequency: of 49 infanticides between 1969 and 1978, there were 11 neonaticides and 38 filicides; this is about 3 in 100 000 per year of children under 5 years of age.[67] In Sweden, between 1971 and 1980, there were 79 cases involving 96 children—an annual rate of 2 in 100 000 children under the age of 5 years.[68] There are a variety of causes.

◆ **Depression** This is the most common cause. Studies of convicted mothers underestimate the frequency of depressive filicide, because many complete suicide. Melancholic filicide is committed in the belief that the child's best interests are being served (delusional mercy-killing). Mothers surviving depressive filicide usually make no attempt to conceal the crime; they confess and seek punishment. Mothers may kill more than one child, but family murder seems more common in men.

◆ **Child abuse** This is the other relatively common cause. Death results from ill-tempered assaults or overzealous punishment, without homicidal intent. Fathers are often involved.

◆ **Psychosis** In non-affective psychosis, filicide may occur if delusions involve the child, or as a result of command hallucinations.

◆ **Trance states** A few filicides have occurred during epileptic automatism or somnambulism.

Not all parental child killing occurs as a complication of mental illness. Unwanted infants are occasionally murdered in cold blood. Euthanasia of an incurably ill and suffering child can also occur.

## Further information

The only modern texts that cover most of this subject are *Motherhood and Mental Health* (reference 30), and *Psychological Aspects of Women's Health Care* (2002), editors D. E. Stewart & N. L. Stotland, Washington, American Psychiatric Press.

## References

1. Hitzig, J.E. (1827). Mord in einem durch Eintreten des Monatsflusses herbeigeführten unfreien Zustande. *Zeitschrift für Criminal-rechts-pflege*, **6**, 237–331.
2. Brière de Boismont, A. (1851). Recherches bibliographiques et cliniques sur la folie puerpérale, précédées d'un aperçu sur les rapports de la menstruation et de l'aliénation mentale. *Annales Médico–psychologiques*, **3**, 574–610.
3. Schlager, L. (1858). Die Bedeutung des Menstrualprocesses und seiner Anomalieen für die Entwicklung und den Verlauf der psychischen Störungen. *Zeitschrift für Psychiatrie*, **15**, 459–98.
4. Bancroft, J. (1993). The premenstrual syndrome—a reappraisal of the concept and the evidence. *Psychological Medicine*, (Suppl. 24), 1–47.
5. von Krafft-Ebing, R. (1902). *Psychosis Menstrualis. Eine klinisch–forensische Studie*. Enke, Stuttgart.
6. Brockington, I.F. (2005). Menstrual psychosis. *World Psychiatry*, **4**, 9–17.
7. Kitayama, I., Yamaguchi, T., Harada, M., *et al.* (1984). Periodic psychoses and hypothalamo-pituitary function. *Mie Medical Journal*, **34**, 127–38.
8. Parker, P.J. (1983). Motivation of surrogate mothers: initial findings. *The American Journal of Psychiatry*, **140**, 117–18.
9. Bivin, G.D. and Klinger, M.P. (1937). *Pseudocyesis*. Principia Press, Bloomington.
10. Ekblad, M. (1963). Social-psychiatric prognosis after sterilisation of women without children. *Acta Psychiatrica Scandinavica*, **39**, 481–514.
11. Cooper, P., Gath, D., Rose, N., *et al.* (1982). Psychological sequelae to elective sterilisation: a prospective study. *British Medical Journal*, **284**, 461–4.
12. Bledin, K.D., Cooper, J.E., MacKenzie, S., *et al.* (1984). Psychological sequelae of female sterilisation: short-term outcome in a prospective controlled study. *Psychological Medicine*, **14**, 379–90.

13. Gath, D., Rose, N., Bond, A., *et al.* (1995). Hysterectomy and psychiatric disorder: are the levels of psychiatric morbidity falling? *Psychological Medicine*, **25**, 277–83.

14. Martin, R.L., Roberts, W.V., and Clayton, P.J. (1980). Psychiatric status after hysterectomy. A one-year prospective follow-up. *The Journal of the American Medical Association*, **244**, 350–3.

15. Aziz, A., Bergquist, C., Nordholm, L., *et al.* (2005). Prophylactic oöphorectomy at elective hysterectomy. Effects on psychological well-being at 1-year follow-up and its correlations to sexuality. *Maturitas*, **16**, 349–57.

16. Cohen, R.L. (1988). *Psychiatric consultation in childbirth settings.* Plenum, New York.

17. Cartwright, A. (1988). Unintended pregnancies that lead to babies. *Social Science and Medicine*, **27**, 249–54.

18. Brockington, I.F. (2006). *Eileithyia's mischief: the organic psychoses of pregnancy, parturition and the puerperium.* Eyry Press, Bredenbury.

19. Wessel, J. and Buscher, U. (2002). Denial of pregnancy: a population based study. *British Medical Journal*, **324**, 458.

20. Nirmal, D., Thijs, I., Bethel, J., *et al.* (2006). The incidence and outcome of concealed pregnancies among hospital deliveries: an 11-year population-based study in South Glamorgan. *The Journal of Obstetrics and Gynaecology Research*, **26**, 118–21.

21. Condon, J.T. (1987). The battered foetus syndrome. *The Journal of Nervous and Mental Disease*, **175**, 722–5.

22. Weir, J.G. (1984). Suicide during pregnancy in London 1943–1962. In *Suicide in pregnancy* (eds. G.J. Kleiner and W.M. Greston), pp. 59–62. Wright, Boston.

23. Ulleland, C.N. (1972). The offspring of alcoholic mothers. *Annals of the New York Academy of Sciences*, **197**, 167–9.

24. Lemoine, P., Harousseau, H., Borteyru, J.P., *et al.* (1968). Les enfants de parents alcooliques: anomalies observées. *Ouest-Médical*, **25**, 476–82.

25. Brinch, M., Isager, T., and Tolstrup, K. (1988). Anorexia nervosa and motherhood: reproduction pattern and mothering behaviour of 50 women. *Acta Psychiatrica Scandinavica*, **77**, 611–17.

26. Morgan, J.F., Lacey, J.H., and Sedgwick, P.M. (1999). Impact of pregnancy on bulimia nervosa. *The British Journal of Psychiatry*, **174**, 135–40.

27. Jureidini, J. (1993). Obstetric factitious disorder and munchausen syndrome by proxy. *The Journal of Nervous and Mental Disease*, **181**, 135–7.

28. Kendell, R.E., Chalmers, J.C., and Platz, C. (1987). Epidemiology of puerperal psychoses. *The British Journal of Psychiatry*, **150**, 662–73.

29. Grof, P., Robbins, W., Alda, M., *et al.* (2000). Protective effect of pregnancy in women with lithium-responsive bipolar disorder. *Journal of Affective Disorders*, **61**, 31–9.

30. Brockington, I.F. (1996). *Motherhood and mental health*, pp. 92, 111–12. Oxford University Press, Oxford.

31. Engelhard, J.L.B. (1912). Über Generationspsychosen und der Einflus des Gestationsperiode auf schon bestehende psychische und neurologische Krankheiten. *Zeitschrift für Geburtshülfe und Gynäkologie*, **70**, 727–812.

32. Gissler, M., Hemminki, E., and Lönnqvist, J. (1996). Suicides after pregnancy in Finland, 1987–1994: register linkage study. *British Medical Journal*, **313**, 1431–4.

33. David, H.P. (1985). Post-abortion and post-partum psychiatric hospitalization. *CIBA Foundation Symposium*, **115**, 150–64.

34. Nagy, M. (1948). The child's theories concerning death. *The Journal of Genetic Psychology*, **73**, 3–27.

35. Smialek, Z. (1978). Observations on immediate reactions of families to sudden infant death. *Pediatrics*, **62**, 160–5.

36. Hughes, P., Turton, P., Hopper, E., *et al.* (2002). Assessment of guidelines for good practice in psychosocial care of mothers after stillbirth: a cohort study. *Lancet*, **360**, 114–48.

37. Condon, J. T. (1986). Psychological disability in women who relinquish a baby for adoption. *The Medical Journal of Australia*, **144**, 117–19.

38. Brockington, I.F., Macdonald, E., and Wainscott, G. (2006). Anxiety, obsessions and morbid preoccupations in pregnancy and the puerperium. *Archives of Women's Mental Health*, **9**, 253–64.

39. Bydlowski, M. and Raoul-Duval, A. (1978). Un avatar psychique méconnu de la puerpéralité: la nevrose traumatique post-obstétricale. *Perspectives Psychiatriques*, **4**, 321–8.

40. Wenzel, A., Haugen, E.N., Jackson, L.C., *et al.* (2005). Anxiety symptoms and disorders at eight weeks postpartum. *Journal of Anxiety Disorders*, **19**, 295–311.

41. Hertzberg, T. and Wahlbeck, K. (1999). The impact of pregnancy and puerperium on panic disorder: a review. *Journal of Psychosomatic Obstetrics and Gynaecology*, **20**, 59–64.

42. De Armond, M. (1954). A type of post partum anxiety reaction. *Diseases of the Nervous System*, **15**, 26–9.

43. Sved-Williams, A.E. (1992). Phobic reactions of mothers to their own babies. *The Australian and New Zealand Journal of Psychiatry*, **26**, 631–8.

44. Weightman, J., Dalal, B.M., and Brockington, I.F. (1999). Pathological fear of cot death. *Psychopathology*, **167**, 246–9.

45. Maina, G., Vaschetto, P., Ziero, S., *et al.* (2001). Il postpartum come fattore di rischio specifico per l'esordio del disturbo ossessivo-compulsivo: studio clinico controllato. *Epidemiologia e Psichiatria Sociale*, **10**, 90–5.

46. Labad, J., Menchon, J.M., Alonso, P., *et al.* (2005). Female reproductive cycle and obsessive-compulsive disorder. *The Journal of Clinical Psychiatry*, **66**, 428–35.

47. Jennings, K.D., Ross, S., Popper, S., *et al.* (1999). Thoughts of harming infants in depressed and non-depressed mothers. *Journal of Affective Disorders*, **54**, 21–8.

48. Gordon, R.E. and Gordon, K.K. (1959). Social factors in the prediction and treatment of emotional disorders of pregnancy. *American Journal of Obstetrics and Gynecology*, **77**, 1074–83.

49. Affonso, D.D., De, A.K., Horowitz, J.A., *et al.* (2000). An international study exploring levels of postpartum depressive symptomatology. *Journal of Psychosomatic Research*, **49**, 207–16.

50. Malmquist, A. and Kaij, L. (1971). Motherhood and childlessness in monozygotic twins. Part II. The influence of motherhood on health. *The British Journal of Psychiatry*, **118**, 22–8.

51. Høyer, G. and Lund, E. (1993). Suicide among women related to number of children in marriage. *Archives of General Psychiatry*, **50**, 134–7.

52. Pound, A., Puckering, C., Cox, A., *et al.* (1988). The impact of maternal depression on young children. *British Journal of Psychotherapy*, **4**, 240–52.

53. Cox, J.L., Holden, J.M., and Sagovsky, R. (1987). Detection of postnatal depression: development of the 10-item Edinburgh Postnatal Depression Scale. *The British Journal of Psychiatry*, **150**, 782–6.

54. Epperson, C.N., Czarkowski, K.A., Ward-O'Brien, D., *et al.* (2001). Maternal sertraline treatment and serotonin transport in breast-feeding mother-infant pairs. *The American Journal of Psychiatry*, **158**, 1631–7.

55. Brockington, I.F., Aucamp, H.M., and Fraser, C. (2006). Severe disorders of the mother-infant relationship: definitions and frequency. *Archives of Women's Mental Health*, **9**, 243–52.

56. Righetti-Veltema, M., Conne-Perréard, E., Bousquet, A., *et al.* (2002). Postpartum depression and mother-infant relationship at 3 months. *Journal of Affective Disorders*, **70**, 291–306.

57. Bernazzani, O., Marks, M.N., Bifulco, A., *et al.* (2005). Assessing psychosocial risk in pregnant/postpartum women using the contextual assessment of maternity experience (CAME). *Social Psychiatry and Psychiatric Epidemiology*, **40**, 497–508.

58. Murray, L., Hipwell, A., and Hooper, R. (1996). The cognitive development of 5-year-old children of postnatally depressed mothers. *Journal of Child Psychology and Psychiatry, and Allied Disciplines*, **37**, 927–35.

59. Ndosi, N.K. and Mtawali, M.L. (2002). The nature of puerperal psychosis at Muhimbili national hospital: its co-morbidity, and associated main obstetric and social factors. *African Journal of Reproductive Health*, **6**, 41–9.

60. Srinavasan, K. (1983). Cerebral venous and arterial thrombosis in pregnancy and the puerperium: a study of 135 patients. *Angiology*, **34**, 731–46.

61. Osiander, F.B. (1797). *Neue Denkwürdigkeiten für Aerzte und Geburtshelfer*, pp. 52–128. Rosenbusch, Göttingen.

62. Esquirol, J.E.D. (1818). Observations sur l'aliénation mentale à la suite de couches. *Journal Général de Médecine, de Chirurgie et de Pharmacie Françaises et Étrangères* (Series 2), **1**, 148–64.

63. Terp, I.M. and Mortensen, P.B. (1998). Post-partum psychoses: clinical diagnoses and relative risk of admission after parturition. *The British Journal of Psychiatry*, **172**, 521–6.

64. Jones, I. and Craddock, N. (2001). Familiarity of the puerperal trigger in bipolar disorder: results of a family study. *The American Journal of Psychiatry*, **158**, 913–17.

65. Main, T.F. (1958). Mothers with children in a psychiatric hospital. *Lancet*, **ii**, 845–7.

66. Tardieu, A. (1868). *Étude Médico–Légale sur l'Infanticide*. Baillière, Paris.

67. Wilkey, I., Pearn, J., Petrie, G., *et al.* (1982). Neonaticide, infanticide and child homicide. *Medicine, Science and the Law*, **22**, 31–4.

68. Somander, L.K.H. and Rammer, L.M. (1991). Intra- and extrafamilial child homicide in Sweden 1971–1980. *Child Abuse & Neglect*, **15**, 45–55.

## 5.5

# Management of psychiatric disorders in medically ill patients, including emergencies

Pier Maria Furlan and Luca Ostacoli

The coexistence of psychiatric disorders in patients with medical illnesses may influence both the diagnosis and the course of the illness by their effects on pathophysiological, diagnostic, and therapeutic processes. There may also be effects on patients' collaboration with treatment and on their relationships with health care staff. Several factors change the management of, medical illnesses and psychiatric disorders, and their inter-relation

- increased life-expectancy and increasing survival of people with severe illness alter the risk of other medical and psychiatric disorders;

- social changes affecting family structure can affect care giving. Other social factors include changes in the role of women (work, delayed maternity); increased immigration with consequent cultural diversity including different concepts of medical and psychiatric disorders (see Chapter 1.3.2);

- increased use of medication in medical and in psychiatric treatment, and changes in the organization of health care and social assistance from hospital-based to community-based.

This chapter describes how to recognize, treat and manage psychiatric disorders in medical illnesses.

## The frequency of psychiatric disorders among the medically ill

The prevalence of psychiatric disorders in medical illnesses ranges from 16–60 per cent depending on the research methodology (self-reports or interviews; inclusion or exclusion of somatic items), the setting (out-patient or hospitalized), and the sample. In general, the frequency of psychiatric disorders in patients with heart disease[1] (coronary disease, heart failure), gastrointestinal diseases (irritable bowel syndrome), lung diseases (asthma, chronic bronchitis), and diabetes is 15–20 per cent. In patients with cancer and chronic pain it is 30–40 per cent; and in neurological diseases (Parkinson's, multiple sclerosis, epilepsy) and dialysis it is 50 per cent. Ten to 20 per cent of patients have sub-threshold symptoms that nevertheless influence psychosocial functioning. The prevalence of psychiatric disorders among family members of people

with chronic disabling conditions is only slightly lower. The most frequent are organic mental disorders (5–44 per cent), followed by substance abuse (10–25 per cent), anxiety disorders (10–30 per cent), mood disorders (9–13 per cent), personality disorders (6–9 per cent), somatoform disorders (5–9 per cent), mania and psychosis (1 per cent). Recognition by medical doctors is below 50 per cent and the referral rate to liaison services is approximately 1–3 per cent.

## The frequency of medical illnesses among psychiatric patients

The most severe psychiatric disorders are frequently associated with social isolation, difficult relations with health-care providers, poor adherence to treatment, unhealthy lifestyle[2] (nutrition, smoking, hygiene), side-effects of medication and substance dependence. The presence of psychiatric symptoms can also lead to failure to recognize physical symptoms. And yet some medical illnesses are more frequent in people with schizophrenia than in the general population.[3] These conditions are cardiovascular risk (9.4 per cent in men, 7 per cent in women), diabetes (13 per cent), hypertension (27 per cent) and chronic conditions in general (41 per cent).[4]

**Table 5.5.1** Prevalence of medical illnesses in patients with mood disorders

| Disease | % |
|---|---|
| Hypertension | 18.1–34.8 |
| Stroke | 1.7–1.9 |
| Headache | 19.3 |
| Chronic pulmonary disease | 10.6–12.9 |
| Hypothyroidism | 9.6 |
| Obesity | 4.6 |
| Alcohol abuse | 12.2–24.7 |
| Nicotine | 9.1–12.6 |
| Illicit drug abuse | 9.7 |

## The diagnosis of psychiatric disorder in medically-ill patients

Anxiety, fear, demoralization, a sense of loss, decreased pleasure, and thoughts of death are frequent in advanced debilitating physical disease even when there is no coexisting anxiety or depressive disorder.

Physical disease and its treatment may cause somatic symptoms similar to those of psychiatric disorders. And the 'aetiological' criterion of the DSM-IV-TR that requires exclusion of a physical cause is often difficult to apply in advanced medical illness, as are the criteria for depression. Endicott[5] proposed replacing the four somatic items for depression (fatigue, insomnia, weight-loss, and difficulty in concentrating) with four psychological symptoms: depressed appearance, social withdrawal, brooding, non-reactive mood. However, this proposal risks excluding somatic symptoms which are a core manifestation of more severe forms of depressive disorder. In doubtful cases, an inclusive approach to somatic symptoms is preferable, and the risk of severe psychiatric disorders should not be underestimated.

Self-abasement and guilt are less frequent in medically ill patients. In assessing guilt, ethnic and cultural factors must be taken into account, for example, feelings of guilt are uncommon in depressed Arabs, whereas somatization is common.

Some syndromes in medically ill patients do not correspond to standard diagnostic categories but nevertheless influence functioning and the course of disease. The Diagnostic Criteria for Psychosomatic Research[6] mention illness denial, thanatophobia, demoralization, and alexithymia. In medical illness, psychiatric disorders may manifest with somatic symptoms (see Chapter 5.2.3).

Table 5.5.2 gives some broad indications for the differential diagnosis of psychiatric disorders in the presence of medical illness.[7]

To be classed as a psychological reaction, the psychiatric disorder must develop at the same time as the onset of the medical illness or the treatment. In some conditions such as, pancreatic cancer, multiple sclerosis, the onset of psychiatric disorder may precede the recognition of the medical illness (e.g. Multidimensional evaluation of the care requirements is essential and codified approaches exist).[8]

Atypical symptoms occur in psychiatric disorders due to medical conditions. Drium is often complex with auditory hallucinations prevailing, whereas tactile, olfactory, and gustatory hallucinations are rare.

## Causes of psychiatric illness among medical patients

These are both psychological (see Chapter 5.6). and medical (see Chapter 5.3. 4.

## Course and prognosis

If properly treated, psychiatric disorders in medically ill patients have the same prognosis as those occurring without medical illness, except in some very advanced and debilitating cases, and in these, the few reported studies give contrasting results. Psychiatric disorders may significantly influence the outcome of the medical condition. Depression is associated with an increased risk for subsequent development of ischaemic heart disease, Parkinson's disease, Alzheimer's disease (and other dementias) and medical diseases in general. It is an independent predictor of severe complications in diabetes and of mortality in ischaemic heart disease, heart failure,[9] stroke, dementia, cancer and HIV. Anxiety may exacerbate angina, arrhythmia, asthma, movement disorders, hypertension and irritable bowel syndrome and is associated with increased health-seeking behaviour and prescription of inappropriate drugs.

Delirium is reversible in 70–80 per cent of cases, but in terminally ill patients may be progressive and intractable, and is associated with increased short-term mortality.[10] Mania and psychosis may worsen the medical outcome due to behavioural alterations, poor adherence and increased drug adverse effects.

**Table 5.5.2** Differential diagnosis among psychiatric disorders (PD) in medical illnesses (MI)

| | Comorbidity (MI – PD) | Latent (PD) | Psychological Reaction | Psychoorganic PD |
|---|---|---|---|---|
| Onset with mi | - | + | + | +/- |
| Medical aetiology | - | -/+ | - | + |
| Life events | - | +/- | + | - |
| Personal/family medical history | + | + | - | - |
| Cognitive disorders | - | - | - | + |
| Altered awareness | - | - | - | + |
| Fluctuation in severity of psychic symptoms | - | - | + | + |
| Atypical psychic symptoms | - | - | - | + |
| Self-abasement | + | +/- | - | - |
| Family history for psychic symptoms | + | +/- | - | - |
| Empathy of doctor | -/+ | +/- | + | |
| Response to psychiatric treatment | +/- | + | + | - |

## Treatment

In specific populations of patients such as those with diabetes, asthma, myocardial infarction, irritable bowel syndrome, cancer, Parkinson's disease, multiple sclerosis, and rheumatic diseases, psychosocial interventions and a variety of psychological treatments have a positive effect on psychiatric disorders, and the quality of life and relationships.[11] In medical conditions requiring active patient participation, psychological treatments improve adherence to the therapeutic programmes. In diabetes they reduce glycosylated haemoglobin, in Parkinson's they produce cognitive and motor improvement. Such treatments can reduce physical symptoms including pain, nausea, dyspnoea and disability. For other indices such as mortality in heart attack, longevity in cancer, severity of hypertension and peptic ulcer, and inflammatory activity in rheumatoid arthritis, there are psychological benefits and improvements in quality of life but poor effects on medical outcome. Indeed, in the more severe psychiatric disorders, combined treatment with psychopharmacological drugs is more effective. Studies of cost-effectiveness and length of hospitalization have reported conflicting results.[12]

## Management

### The consultation process

#### (a) Forming an alliance with the medical team

The psychiatrist should initially aim to work with medical staff on their clinical rounds, and interview patients who have no psychiatric disorder to learn what it means to have the medical condition and to undergo its treatment. The psychiatrist should be present at informal discussions, such as those during coffee breaks, and share the clinical team's emotional experiences.

#### (b) Interview with medical team

The aim is to evaluate the clinical situation, review the medical records; identify the most significant reason for referral and why the consultation has been made at this time; identify the team's approach to the patient, clarify whether the patient has been informed of the consultation and in what way. If the referral seems inappropriate for the patient, does this reflect a problem within the medical team such as burn out?

#### (c) Interview with the patient

The interview should move dynamically between the 'objective' position (clinical data, psychosocial information) and the 'subjective' position. Feelings evoked in the psychiatrist frequently mirror perceptions of the patient and the medical team. To recognize them helps empathetic relations and emotional containment. A protocol for the interview is shown below. [13]

#### (d) Reporting back to the medical team

Reporting should be clear and concise with both a verbal and a written report. The focus should be on the reason for referral. Risk factors and points of strength should be identified. A verbal report of an 'image' such as an episode fom the patient's experience, a memory or even a dream can sometimes aid empathetic understanding by the medical team. Practical advice on management should be provided.

#### (e) Psychopharmacological treatment

The psychopharmacological treatment of medically ill patients may be difficult for several reasons including the stigma associated with psychiatric disorders, weariness with the many medical treatments already undergone, increased sensitivity to side-effects due to pharmacokinetic changes produced by interactions with medical drugs and any underlying liver or renal disease.[14] However when adherence is adequate, the therapeutic response is similar to that of patients without medical illnesses. Nevertheless, the prescription of medication must not replace receptiveness to the patients problems and emotional support, which are frequently the most effective intervention.

It is often useful to offer the patient a drug not for symptoms such as depression when these arise in a discouraging physical situation because this may be seen as disparaging—but for other

| Goal | Approach |
|---|---|
| Overcome stigma | The medical team: present the psychiatrist to the patient as a team member and motivate consultation<br>The psychiatrist: explores any ambivalence or negative feelings empathetically (it may not be clear to the patient why a psychiatrist is discussing his/her disorder) |
| Open questions: background and information | Why is the patient hospitalized? What does he/she think of the illness? |
| Principal emotions and fears | What does the patient feel? What is he/she most afraid of? |
| Consider constructive ways of coping; and discuss dysfunction | What and who most help the patient to overcome difficulties; who is important, what other resources are available |
| Completing the information | Medical history and current quality of life |
| Develop a shared understanding of the situation in which medical and psychological aspects are linked and not viewed as alternatives. | "Normalize" emotional disorders as reactions to illness that may amplify symptoms and influence course.<br><br>Describe physical mechanisms of symptom production such as muscular contraction, vasodilation/constriction, hyperventilation, asthenia, inactivity, immune defences.<br>Use clear, descriptive language with imagery: e.g. tension is like a tight shoe. |
| Defining goals and reducing unrealistic expectations | Discuss the main problems<br>Aim to improve problems, not solve them.<br>Set realistic goals |
| Propose a treatment plan | What interventions, "first steps"<br>Practical advice about day-to-day matters such as interpersonal relations, how to reduce tension |

realistic goals. The specific contribution that the drug can make to achieving these goals should be explained and a clear description provided of its somatic effects. The psychiatrist should also:

♦ Aim to simplify treatment as far as possible. The distinction between 'psychiatric' and 'medical' drugs is arbitrary since many drugs have both physical and psychological effects.

♦ Rationalize treatment using the fewest possible drugs. First choice should be drugs that act on more than one symptom, psychological or medical (e.g. reduce agitation and nausea, insomnia and hyporexia, depression and headache, pain and anxiety).

♦ Consider side-effects and interactions before deciding treatment including their time of onset. Thus, SSRI should be prescribed at least one week apart from any treatment with significant gastrointestinal side-effects. Investigate complementary drug use: e.g. 20–40 per cent of oncology patients take herbal remedies, many of which have significant pharmacological interactions (see Chapter 6.2.9).

♦ Prefer drugs that were effective for the patient in the past; starting with low doses and increasing them gradually.

♦ Sometimes the best action is to discontinue a drug.

## Psychosocial treatments
### Differences from traditional psychotherapy

The major aims are to control distress, maintain self-respect, maintain significant relations and doctor-patient communication, work through information, and develop adaptive coping mechanisms.

**Timing**: At times of crisis (e.g. immediately after the communication of a serious diagnosis), the need for control is paramount. At the onset of complex diseases, short cycles of interviews may prevent subsequent psychiatric disorder.

**Flexibility**: This is needed due to variations over time in the conditions of treatment (in hospital, or as a day patient or outpatient), the symptoms, and the motivation of the patient, who may alternate between the need for emotional sharing and moments of self-withdrawal. Existential uncertainty is reflected in relations with the psychiatrist and each interview is an entity in itself.

**Eclecticism**: The complexity of the situation often requires integration of different approaches at different times: expressive, cognitive, body-mediated or psycho educational. The intervention may focus on the patient, on family members or on the medical team. Flexibility and eclecticism must originate from the integration of the patient's needs and the psychiatrist's empathic and comprehensive evaluation of these needs.

**Regression**: Illness, hospitalization, fear, and the 'invalid role' may make a patient, who would otherwise refuse it, become receptive to the psychiatrist's intervention. During medical illness, emotional defences are more fluid, the relationship with the psychiatrist may form more rapidly and short interventions can be effective. After discharge the psychiatrist must be ready to change approach.

**Existential context**: A severe disease often casts doubt on the meaning of existence. Patients may fall into despair or ask themselves what really matters. They may want to reorganize their lives around new priorities. In these circumstances, interviews should focus on the present, abandoning the 'past-future' approach, and define the psychiatric disorder as an accentuation of natural human emotions. Fear should be dealt with directly, including fear of dying, and the patient's relatives, including their doctors, should be helped to provide support since fear is greater when experienced alone.

**Physical contact**: Faced with severe disease, some patients 'speak' only after having been touched. Sometimes bodily contact, for example through simple massage, may keep open communication with family members and staff, even without the use of words. A glance, a voice, the sense of touch, or other bodily sensations may form an intense dialogue between patient and therapist and be the most effective way to understand how aware the patient is of his/her condition.

## Treatment of urgent situations
### Prevention

♦ Medical treatment should address the overall quality of life, including the gap between expectations and reality. Many medical interviews target practical matters but place less emphasis on working through expectations. A doctor-patient relationship capable of offering relief while gradually reducing the gap between hope and reality is fundamental.

♦ The patient's chief supports are family members and caregivers. Improving their psychological skills through simple psychoeducational programmes may be more cost-effective than generally increasing psychiatric consultations.

♦ Psychosocial and biological risk factors should be identified early, including both current factors and those in the medical history.

### Acute anxiety

Treatment of acute anxiety should maximize the beneficial effects of the doctor-patient relationship as well as providing specific psychosocial and pharmacological interventions. At times of crisis, one-on-one companionship is useful, sometimes with simple relaxation or massage that family members can provide. When a serious medical diagnosis is communicated, it is helpful to listen, and for medical staff to be receptive to emotional reactions in the subsequent 24 hours; solitude should be alleviated, if necessary with the help of voluntary workers. Benzodiazepines should be prescribed only when really necessary and for short periods to reduce the risk of tolerance and addiction. Benzodiazepines may reduce respiratory function further in patients who retain $CO_2$, thereby worsening their asthenia. If prolonged pharmacological therapy is necessary, sedative antidepressants may be an alternative to benzodiazepines.

**Panic attacks**: Somatic symptoms of a panic attack may be confused with an exacerbation of medical conditions such as chest pain, irritable bowel syndrome, and asthma. Treatment with a selective serotonin reuptake inhibitor is usually effective but half of these patients require long-term treatment since relapse is common after discontinuation. Psychological treatment[15] (see Chapter 4.7.3) can be effective.

**Post-traumatic stress disorder**: Stress factors in medical contexts may cause and prolong this disorder. Such factors include acute medical events, intensive care, post-confusional reactions, communication of a serious diagnosis, and presence at unexpected deaths. Pharmacological therapy has limited results but psychological treatments may be effective (see Chapter 4.6.2), Risk prevention is important.

## Depression

Treatment should be based on prevention, and psycho education, psychosocial and pharmacological interventions.

**Antidepressants:** The choice of drug should be based on the side-effect profile and interactions (see Chapter 6.2.3). The somatic effect of treating depression can be important. Cognitive and motor functions can improve in stroke patients, glycaemic control can improve in diabetics, as can chronic pain, and dyspnoea in lung-disease. SSRIs may produce gastrointestinal side effects, bleeding due to platelet dysfunction, so that monitoring is essential in patients on anticoagulants. Venlafaxine in high doses may increase blood pressure. Mirtazapine has no sexual side-effects, has anti-nausea activity and stimulates the appetite, but may cause weight gain and sedation. TCAs, being anticholinergic, affecting heart conduction and the peripheral autonomic nervous system, are contraindicated in heart disease, cognitive impairment, orthostatic hypotension, hypertrophic prostate, glaucoma and epilepsy. Secondary amines, such as nortriptyline and desipramine, are preferable.

Methylphenidate may be useful in particular medical situations, such as palliative care or advanced cancer, to alleviate fatigue, increase appetite, and reduce opiate-induced sedation. It may elevate mood and has rapid onset. Agitation and insomnia are the main problems.

## Personality disorders

Personality disorders, particularly antisocial and borderline disorders, may create emergencies due either to aggressive behaviour towards self or others or to conflict within the team. Screening for substance abuse and depression is necessary since these increase impulsiveness. Patients can become aggressive when their demands are not met, e.g. for increased painkillers, or interviews with their doctors. Staff require support to manage conflicts and frustration, and to maintain a caring approach.[16]

Staff must be empathetic but at the same time act as a team. Limits and rules should be established at admission treatment to prevent escalation of aggression. Interviews must be in conditions of safety; if necessary with other staff or even police present. The agreed plan must be respected by all staff, avoiding the extremes of excessive permissiveness and excessive rigidity, which may be induced by the patient's disorder. Patients with personality disorders often use truth-based observations pathologically to exploit the therapist's and institution's weak points. Recognizing what is true in their criticisms may improve patient management.

## Delirium and dementia (see Chapters 4.1.1 and 4.1.13)

## Mania

A manic crisis affects the care of the medical condition dramatically both through excessive activity, weight-loss, reduction of sleep, and through non-compliance with treatment and conflict with staff. The medical history should be evaluated for disease-related stress factors which may trigger crises. Manic symptoms recognized early together with possible causes of insomnia such as pain, nocturia, dyspnoea, or environmental factors including noise, unsuitable temperature, frequent entrance of night-staff for other patients. Where possible, precipitating factors should be removed. When this is impossible (e.g. a requirement for high-dose cortisone), treatment is as that of mania in other situations (see Chapter 4.5.8) taking medication side-effects into account (see Chapter 6.2.4). Antipsychotic drugs are generally faster acting at lower doses than in primary mania. More potent antipsychotics are preferable since they have lower anticholinergic and alpha-blocking effects. It is useful to focus on symptoms the patient finds disturbing rather than ego-syntonic symptoms. Restraint or hospitalization in a psychiatric ward is necessary when hyperactivity could compromise physical safety or the underlying condition.

## Psychosis

Close collaboration between the psychiatrist and the medical team is necessary, with the most appropriate environment for treatment, medical or psychiatric unit, being decided case-by-case. Medical investigations and interviews should be simplified and clear basic information provided. Continuity of care among medical professionals is important. The psychological effect of medical treatment should be assessed. When there are hallucinations, medical staff should be educated about their nature and supported, so that they do not criticize any content expressed by the patient, but are able to empathize with the patient's distress. Management may require constant observation and in some cases restraint and involuntary treatment. Medically ill patients are especially sensitive to the side-effects of antipsychotic drugs but generally respond to lower doses. The choice of drug and dose are based on the side-effects and the underlying disease (see Chapter 6.2.2)). Cardiac pathology and QTc enlargement require ECG monitoring and ziprasidone, haloperidol, chlorpromazine, and thioridazine are contraindicated. Caution is also necessary in alcoholics, and patients with hypokalemia and hypomagnesemia.[17]

Extra-pyramidal effects of high doses of typical neuroleptics may cause laryngospasm and affect the diaphragm, worsening any respiratory insufficiency. For chronic treatment, newer drugs are preferable. Caution is required in hepatic and renal diseases and where there is a risk of epileptic fits. Fluid intake should be monitored carefully because dehydration increases the risk of neuroleptic malignant syndrome. In secondary psychosis, the family should be informed and supported and, after the psychotic episode has been resolved, the patient must be helped to work through the disorientating experience.

# Aggression and restraint

Aggression should be assessed, thoroughly defining the sequence of events that preceded it and the role of medical and psychiatric factors, stressful events and environmental factors. Major predictors related to the patient include a history of violence, difficulty in communication, and the psychological condition. Predictors related to the environment include: crowding, and a medical team unreceptive to the patient's discomfort. The best strategy is prevention through providing information in a clear and empathetic way, recognizing risk situations and early signs of agitation, and using de-escalation techniques if necessary with pharmacological support (see also Chapter 11.14).

Environmental measures to limit psychomotor agitation include: making the patient as comfortable as possible, reducing background noise, removing potentially harmful objects, and identifying situations of which the patients is intolerant. Patients can be distracted by walking or occupational activities, avoiding a forced stay in bed and making the timetable flexible. If possible, family members can be asked to collaboration.

Where permitted under national law, restraint may become necessary during unmanageable agitation and aggression in the course of an acute psychiatric disorder, in confusional states, especially in the elderly and aftersurgery, with metabolic diseases or during abstinence from alcohol and drugs (seen especially during the first few days of hospitalization).

If restraint is permissible, staff training is necessary because improper use may cause injury to patients or staff. Restraint should be used only when strictly necessary and for the shortest possible time, with constant monitoring of its continuing necessity and the patient's condition.

In medically ill patients restraint may increase the risk of thromboembolism, reduce respiratory function with increased risk of infection, increase cognitive deficit, pressure ulcers, urinary and intestinal incontinence. When restraint is removed there is an increased risk of falls.

## Deliberate self-harm and suicidality (see also

Chapter 4.15.4)

In advanced medical illness, suicidal ideation is frequent as an expression of the wish for release from suffering, to regain control over a condition that is perceived as unstoppable, and is wearing the patient down. The actual risk of suicide is slightly above that of the general population. Specific risk factors are: chronic disease, uncontrolled physical symptoms such as pain or dyspnoea, disfiguring surgery, unrecognized psychiatric disorder (delirium, depression, personality disorder), substance abuse, and lack of social support. The most frequent form of self-harm is drug overdose, particularly of analgesics and psychopharmacological drugs. Most lethal suicidal acts are of the impulsive type, in particular jumping. [18] The doctor-patient relationship is often the best help against loss of hope. Safety of the environment is crucial since medical contexts facilitate access to potentially lethal objects and to the possibility of jumping. In cancer, the risk is higher in the first year, decreasing with time after diagnosis. In the end stage of illness e.g. in renal failure, treatment withdrawal may have to be considered, with the: clinical and ethical problems of distinguishing a rational decision by the patient from one affected by a psychiatric disorder or another potentially modifiable factor.

## Patients refusing treatment (see also Chapter 1.5.1)

Background culture should be taken into account as some 'overall rejections' are actually related to this rather than to factors in the individual. An alliance with family members is necessary. Factors in the doctor-patient relationship should be evaluated, together with the information that the patient has received. In some cases refusal relates to fear, anger or despair. If it seems that the patient would feel belittled by a psychiatric consultation it is better to support medical staff who are receptive to the patient's emotional sate. This is done patients often then accept psychiatric support more readily. In complex cases, the history of the patient's attitude to treatment should be evaluated on admission to treatment. Aa history of interrupted treatment, changes of doctor or diffidence towards caregivers, may indicate a need for greater efforts to develop good doctor-patient relationships. When obtaining items of medical history from family members, it is important to identify whom the patient trusts most. In relations with the medical team, the most appropriate figure for dialogue should be identified. In some cases, informal conversations, for example in the evening, are more useful than formal medical interviews.

## Further information

Levenson, J.L., (2005). *Textbook of psychosomatic medicine*. American Psychiatric Publishing, Washington, DC.

Wise, M.G. and Rundell, J.R., (2005). *Clinical manual of Psychosomatic medicine: A Guide to Consultation–Liaison Psychiatry*. American Psychiatric Press, Washington, DC.

Guthrie, E. and Creed, F. (1996). *Seminars in Liaison Psychiatry*. College seminars series. Royal College of Psychiatrists, London.

### Web sites

The European Association for Consultation Liaison Psychiatry and Psychosomatics. http://www.eaclpp.org

International Organization for Consultation- Liaison Psychiatry. http://www. med.monash.edu.au/psychmed/ioclp.

The International College of Psychosomatic Medicine. http://www. icpm.org

## References

1. Rutledge, T., Reis, V.A., Linke, S.E., *et al.* (2006). Depression in heart failure a meta-analytic review of prevalence, intervention effects, and associations with clinical outcomes. *Journal of American College of Cardiology,* **48**(8), 1527–37.

2. Michael, T., Compton, M.T., Daumit, G.L., *et al.* (2006). Cigarette Smoking and Overweight/Obesity Among Individuals with Serious Mental Illnesses: A Preventive Perspective. *Harvard Review of Psychiatry,* **14**(4), 212–22.

3. Carney, C.P. and Jones, L., (2006). Medical Comorbidity in women and men with bipolar disorders: a population – based controlled study. *Psychosomatic Medicine,* **68**, 684–91.

4. Goff, D.C., Sullivan, L.M., McEvoy, J.P., *et al.* (2005). A comparison of ten-year cardiac risk estimates in schizophrenia patients from the CATIE study and matched controls. *Schizophrenia Research,* **80**, 45– 53.

5. Endicott, J., (1984). Measurement of depression in patients with cancer. *Cancer,* **53**(Suppl 10), 2243–9.

6. Fava, G.A., Freyberger, H.J., Bech, P., *et al.* (1995). Diagnostic criteria for use in psychosomatic research. *Psychotherapy Psychosomatic,* **63**(1), 1–8.

7. Lipowski, Z.J., (1967) Review of consultation psychiatry and psychosomatic medicine, II: clinical aspects. *Psychosomatic Medicine,* **29**, 201–24.

8. Huyse, F.J., Lyons, J.S., Stiefel, F.C., *et al,* (1999). INTERMED: a method to assess health service needs. I. Development and reliability. *General Hospital Psychiatry,* **21**, 39–48.

9. Barth, J., Schumacher, M. and Lingen, C.H. (2004). Depression as a Risk Factor for Mortality in Patients With Coronary Heart Disease: A Meta-analysis, *Psychosomatic Medicine,* **66**, 802–13.

10. Breitbart, W., Gibson, C. and Tremblay, A., (2002). The delirium experience: delirium recall and delirium-related distress in hospitalized patients with cancer, their spouses/caregivers, and their nurses. *Psychosomatis,* **43**, 183–94.

11. Guthrie, E. and Creed, F. (1996). Treatment methods and their effectiveness. In *Seminars in Liaison Psychiatry* (eds. E., Guthrie, and F., Creed), pp. 238-73. College seminars series. Royal College of Psychiatrists, London.

12. Andreoli, P.B., Citero, Vde A. and Mari Jde, J., (2003). A systematic review of studies of the cost-effectiveness of mental health consultation-liaison interventions in general hospitals. *Psychosomatics,* **44**(6), 499–507.

13. Stuart, M.R. and Lieberman, J.A., (2002). *The fifteen minute hour. Practical therapeutic interventions in Primary care.* Saunders, Elsevier (USA). 14 Levenson JL, (2005). Psychopharmacology. In: Levenson JL, ed. *Textbook of psychosomatic medicine,* American Psychiatric Publishing, Washington, DC.

15. Shapiro, F. (2001). *Eye Movement Desensitization and Reprocessing: Basic Principles, Protocols and Procedures.* Guilford Press, New York.

16. Hay, J.L. and PassiK, S.D. (2000). The cancer patient with borderline personality disorder: suggestions for symptom-focused management in the medical setting. *Psychooncology,* **9**(2), 91–100.

17. Gasper, J.J. and Tsai, C. (2006). Community Behavioral Health Sciences, Community Health Network of San Francisco, San Francisco General Hospital, Revised: *Guidelines for the use of atypical antipsychotics in adults.*

18. Druss, B. and Pincus, H. (2000). Suicidal ideation and suicide attempts in general medical illnesses, *Arch Intern Med,* **160**(10), 1522–6.

# Health psychology

John Weinman and Keith J. Petrie

## Introduction

Health psychology is concerned with understanding human behaviour in the context of health, illness, and health care. It is the study of the psychological factors, which determine how people stay healthy, why they become ill, and how they respond to illness and health care.

Health psychology has emerged as a separate discipline in the past 30 years and there are many reasons for its rapid development. An important background factor is the major change in the nature of health problems in industrialized societies during the twentieth century. Chronic illnesses such as heart disease and cancer have become the leading causes of death, and behavioural factors such as smoking, diet, and stress are now recognized as playing a major role in the aetiology and progression of these diseases.[1] The provision of health care has grown enormously and there is an increased awareness of good communication as a central ingredient of medical care and of the importance of such factors as patient satisfaction and quality of life as key outcomes in evaluating the efficacy of medical interventions.

Although health psychology has developed over a similar time period to general hospital/liaison psychiatry and shares some common areas of interest, there are some clear differences between these two fields. Liaison psychiatry has a primary focus on hospital patients, particularly those experiencing psychological difficulties in the face of a physical health problem. In contrast, health psychology has a much broader focus on both healthy and ill populations and on the psychological processes that influence their level of health or their degree of adaptation to disease. Whereas health psychology has been mainly concerned with developing explanations based on theory, for health-related[2] and illness-related behaviour,[3] liaison psychiatry has concentrated on the diagnosis and treatment of either unexplained symptoms or psychiatric disorders occurring in people with medical conditions (see the other chapters in Part 5 of this volume).

In this chapter we provide an overview of the main themes and areas in health psychology. Four broad areas of behaviour will be reviewed, namely behavioural factors influencing health, symptom and illness behaviour, health care behaviour, and treatment behaviour. Inevitably such an overview is selective and the interested reader should seek out a more comprehensive introductory text[4,5] or more in-depth accounts of specific areas.[2,3]

## Behavioural factors influencing health

A wide range of behavioural factors can influence health. In the following section there is a focus on stress, personality, and the main theories that have been developed to explain the variation in health-related behaviours.

### Stress and health

The term 'stress' is usually used to describe situations, in which individuals are faced with demands that exceed their immediate ability to cope. Stressful situations are typically those that are novel, unpredictable, and uncontrollable as well as those involving change or negative events such as a loss. These situations can give rise to adverse psychological and physiological changes which, in turn, may result in disease.[6]

Stress may have indirect effects on health by increasing levels of risk behaviour (e.g. smoking, alcohol consumption), or may have direct effects on specific physiological mechanisms (e.g. increase in blood pressure) as well as affecting the individual's resistance to disease through suppression of the immune system, or by exacerbating or triggering a disease process in an already vulnerable individual.

A range of behavioural and emotional responses are shown by individuals as they attempt to cope with stressful situations and these are accompanied by autonomic, neuroendocrine, and immunological changes. During stressful episodes, releasing factors from the brain cause the pituitary to release ACTH which gives rise to the release of corticosteroids from the cortex of the adrenal glands. In addition to producing a number of well-known changes associated with the mobilization of both short- and longer-term physical resources (e.g. release of adrenaline (epinephrine) or noradrenaline (norepinephrine), release of glucose, activation of endorphins/encephalins, etc.), these steroids can also have effects on the immune system.[7]

The effects of stress on immunity have sparked the development of the new multi-disciplinary field of psychoneuroimmunology which focuses on the links between psychological, endocrine, and immunological processes (see Chapter 2.3.10). A large amount of work in this area has concentrated on the links between stress and immune function, but less work has focused on impaired immunity and the later development of disease. Acute stressors, such as examinations, or more chronic stressors, such as caring for a dependent elderly relative, have been shown to lead to deleterious immunological changes. Work has also associated stress with a greater susceptibility to viral infection[8] as well as longer healing times for experimental puncture wounds[9] and wounds from surgical operations.[10] A recent meta-analysis of studies of stress and immunity shows substantial evidence for a relationship between stress and impaired immune system effectiveness, particularly for chronic uncontrollable sources of stress.[7]

## Personality and health

Although there is no consistent empirical support for the older idea that different diseases are linked with specific personality types, there is evidence from different, more credible sources that personality factors can influence health and play a role in determining illness in other ways.[11]

Probably the best known work in this area concerns the link between the so-called 'type A' personality and coronary heart disease. The *type A personality* was originally characterized by competitiveness, time urgency, hostility, and related behavioural factors, which were associated with a significantly increased risk of coronary heart disease (CHD). However, it is now thought that only certain components (e.g. anger and hostility) of the original type A formulation are 'pathogenic'.[12]

Type A individuals show a greater physiological reactivity (e.g. in blood pressure and heart rate) to environmental demands and may even generate more demands by their style of behaviour. The more frequent elevations in blood pressure and higher levels of hormonal change, characteristic of this behavioural style, may eventually cause adverse physical changes to the heart and blood vessels. Also, type A individuals are more likely to engage in unhealthy behaviours since they drink more alcohol than type B individuals and, if they smoke, they inhale their cigarette smoke for a longer time.

Type A behaviour is probably the most extensively investigated personality factor in current health psychology research, and there have been interventions developed to change the behaviour pattern, with positive health outcomes.[13] More recently the concept of the *type D personality* has been described as another major psychological risk factor for CHD. Type D refers to the tendency to experience negative emotional states and to inhibit the expression of these emotions in social settings. Type D patients with CHD have been found to have a significantly higher risk of further cardiac morbidity in the short- and longer-term.[14]

More generally, patterns of positive or negative emotional responses, associated with personality, can influence various aspects of health.[11,15] Individuals who are high in negative affect (i.e. experience more negative emotions, particularly anxiety) do not seem to be more prone to disease, but they are more likely to notice bodily changes and symptoms and consequently seek medical help more frequently (see Wiebe and Smith[15] for a more detailed account of negative affect and the links between personality and health).

Another aspect of personality which has been shown to be health protective is optimism, which describes a tendency towards positive expectations in life and which enables individuals to cope better with stressors and engage in healthier lifestyles. There is emerging evidence that optimistic individuals not only cope more effectively with illness and other life crises but also show better health outcomes than those with lower levels of optimism.[16]

## Lifestyle and health

The effects on health of behaviours such as smoking and high alcohol use are well documented.[1] There is overwhelming evidence that smokers not only are much more likely to die from lung cancer and other cancers but also have much higher rates of cardiovascular disease and chronic respiratory disorders, particularly emphysema and chronic bronchitis. Moreover, the disease risk is dose related in that higher levels of smoking are more strongly associated with all these diseases. With sustained high levels of alcohol use a different but equally unpleasant spectrum of health problems can be seen. Drinking is a major cause of accidents particularly motoring accidents and can cause liver damage as well as having detrimental effects on brain functioning.[1]

For health psychologists, the key questions about health-risk behaviours concern their origin, their maintenance, and their prevention or treatment. There are diverse determinants of these behaviours since they may start as ways of coping with stress, in response to peer pressure, for pleasure or for a number of other reasons. Similarly, they will be maintained by a variety of psychological, social, and biological factors.

There are many other risky behaviours that cannot be discussed in detail in an overview; these include drug abuse, poor diet, and accidents, and the health effects of all these are also well documented.[1] Although health psychology has an important role to play in describing, explaining, and intervening in all risk behaviours, these problems should not be conceptualized exclusively in individual behavioural terms since they often reflect adverse social circumstances or particular cultural contexts.[17]

The same caveats about the influence of social and cultural factors must also be applied to the understanding of health-protective or health-enhancing behaviours. Prospective cohort studies have confirmed that various daily behaviours (e.g. patterns of eating, sleeping, and exercise) can have significant long-term effects on health.[18] For example, there is now a growing body of evidence to indicate that regular exercise has a beneficial effect on both physical and psychological health.[19] Exercise can reduce the incidence of physical health problems in elderly people and facilitate recovery from heart attack. However, there can be significant problems in ensuring that exercise and other health-promoting activities are adhered to. Interventions need to be planned carefully, because it has been shown that it is usually very difficult to make and maintain changes in health-related behaviour. Information provision is rarely sufficient to promote behaviour change since it is also necessary to elicit and modify beliefs (see below) as well as influencing social networks in order to ensure success.

## Beliefs and health-related behaviour

Even though health psychologists acknowledge the importance of situational, dispositional, and socio-cultural factors as determinants of health-related behaviour, most current research has a primary focus on the role of beliefs in explaining variance in health-related behaviour. The most widely used explanatory approaches have been described generically as 'social cognition models' (see Conner and Norman[2] for an excellent overview of these models). These models are based on the premise that, when a person is faced with having to make a decision about a particular health behaviour (e.g. attend for a screening test; wear a seat belt, etc.), their decision-making and behaviour can best be understood in terms of their perceptions or beliefs about the health issue and the behaviour in question. The best known models here are the Health Belief Model, Theory of Reasoned Action/Theory of Planned Behaviour, and Protection-Motivation Theory. Broadly these models locate the strength of certain beliefs or evaluations of the health threat (e.g. 'is it serious? Is it likely to affect me?') and/or the associated health behaviour ('Is it an acceptable or worthwhile thing for me to do?') as the key determinants of an individual's motivation or intention to carry out the behaviour. More recent models incorporate other beliefs, such as self-efficacy, which reflect the individual's belief about their ability to implement or carry out the health-related behaviour.

For habitual and addictive health-related behaviours (e.g. dietary behaviour; substance abuse) there have also been attempts to develop stage-based models, such as the Precaution Adoption model and the Transtheoretical model[2] as ways of describing the stages which people may go through in evaluating the health issue through to thinking about, planning, and maintaining behaviour change. Although these stage models provide a framework for identifying the patient's state of readiness for a health behaviour change intervention as well as an immediate target for an intervention, the evidence for them is weak and there are now a number of serious critiques of their validity and applicability.[20]

## Symptoms and illness behaviour

### The psychology of physical symptoms

Understanding how symptoms are perceived is critical to explaining variation in illness behaviour. Psychological factors play an important role in the appraisal of symptoms. There is considerable evidence that bodily symptoms and functions are not perceived with a high degree of accuracy and individuals vary widely in what symptoms are noticed and whether medical help is sought for symptoms.[21]

The probability that individuals will attend to somatic information will depend on the competition for attention from other sources of available stimuli. When the environment is lacking in stimulation individuals tend to pay more attention to bodily symptoms. Conversely, when an individual's attention is drawn to the external environment, bodily symptoms are less likely to be noticed. This finding has wide day-to-day applications ranging from why people cough in the boring parts of movies and lectures to explaining demographic differences in symptoms reports, such as increased symptom reporting among the socially isolated and the unemployed. It also has clinical applications in chronic pain and other chronic medical conditions where patients' isolation may exacerbate the condition by increasing preoccupation with symptoms.

Cognitive schemas can also strongly influence the reporting of physical symptoms by guiding the way individuals pay attention to their body. Schemas determine the organization of incoming information and guide health directed behaviour. There is a strong tendency for individuals to search for information that is consistent with existing schemas and disregard information that does not fit. Individuals also attach more importance to symptoms consistent with a current cognitive schema than other symptoms. Schemas may develop through personal experience with the condition or by having come across the illness through family, friends, or in the media. Illness schemas can vary from vague ideas about the types of symptoms that represent an illness to more elaborate and detailed conceptions of individual illnesses. Medical students'

disease, where students studying a particular illness notice they also have the symptoms of the condition, and episodes of mass psychogenic illness are more dramatic demonstrations of this phenomenon, but the process is seen on a more subtle level with response to placebos (see below). Here, following treatment, a new cognitive schema may shift attention towards symptoms that indicate recovery rather than those of the illness.

### Patient delay

There is growing research to suggest that patients' interpretation of their symptoms can influence help-seeking behaviour.[22] One medical condition where delay can have serious consequences is myocardial infarction, as early arrival at hospital is strongly associated with improved chances of survival. There is a large variation in how long patients delay before seeking help, and a strong predictor of early arrival at hospital is the belief that the symptoms are a heart attack.[23] Heart attacks are generally seen as sudden and dramatic events that involve severe chest pain and collapse. In the case of myocardial infarction patients, the mismatch between these expectations and the symptoms experienced gives rise to patient delay.

Research investigating the stages of patient delay for medical conditions has generally found three main stages prior to entering treatment, with each stage influenced by a different set of factors and decisional processes. The first interval is generally referred to as appraisal delay, which is the time period from when the individual first detects symptoms to when an illness is inferred. The main influences on this period are factors related to interpretation of symptoms. The second interval is called illness delay—the period from the time the individual decides he or she is ill until the decision is made to seek medical help. The final period called utilization delay is the time until the individual enters hospital or has contact with medical personnel. This first period of appraisal delay has been generally found to cause the largest contribution to overall delay.[24]

### High health service users

A large percentage of medical consultations are made for non-medical complaints. This is particularly so for primary health care services. A number of studies have found that a small percentage of individuals without significant medical illness use a disproportionately large amount of medical services and at considerable cost.[25] These individuals have been variously labelled as somatizers, hypochondriacs, the worried well, patients with medically unexplained symptoms, and multiple attenders.

Research on high health service users suggests they are higher in trait anxiety. This is consistent with research showing a strong relationship between the somatic complaints and high levels of psychological distress or neuroticism. Individuals high in anxiety tend to be more introspective, watchful for any unusual symptoms, and develop more negative interpretations of symptoms they experience.[26] Symptoms of anxiety, such as tachycardia, can also be misinterpreted as signs of a physical illness by some patients.

Some individuals also seem to have a tendency to make catastrophic interpretations about physical symptoms and this may influence frequency of presentation to medical services and recovery from illness. Catastrophizing in pain patients has been associated with disability, and drop-out from pain-management programmes.[27] It has also been associated with higher levels of fatigue and disability in chronic fatigue syndrome patients.

Catastrophizing is also seen in 'cardiac invalidism'. Here patients adopt an extremely passive, dependent, and helpless role in the belief that any form of overly vigorous activity will bring on another myocardial infarction. A hypersensitivity to bodily symptoms means that normal sensations may be misconstrued to indicate overexertion or an impending fatal myocardial infarction. This pattern often results in a cycle of inactivity and loss of physical condition, which in turn can support these beliefs when patients exert themselves. Many patients who develop highly negative illness beliefs overuse medical services mainly for reassurance about symptoms.

The issue of reassurance in medical consultations is relevant here. One of the common patient expectations in primary care consultations is to have a better understanding of current symptoms. For many patients, being told there is no serious medical problem underlying their symptoms is effective in reducing concern about their condition, but for a significant number there remains worry about their health status. Continued anxiety in this group often results in further needless consultations and investigations. Evidence suggests that patients' existing beliefs about their condition are predictive of reassurance failure and that for reassurance to be effective, patients' concerns need to be elicited and appropriate information provided to explain either the patient's symptoms or why serious pathology has been ruled out.[28]

Recent work on improving reassurance following medical testing has suggested providing information to patients about the meaning of normal test results before testing, may weaken patients' preconceived beliefs about their condition and provide a context to help understand the test result. In this study, providing patients with information about normal test results prior to testing, improved their reassurance, reduced their symptoms, and lessened their use of unnecessary medication.[29]

If patients' ideas and beliefs about their symptoms are not addressed when symptoms persist or recur it is likely that health worry will also be reactivated as the patient still lacks a satisfactory cognitive model or explanation that enables them to interpret their symptoms as benign. A practical consequence of these findings is the need for clinicians to elicit the patient's own attributions and concerns about their symptoms and to use these as the basis for dealing with misconceptions and providing the patient with a more benign explanation of their symptoms.[29]

### Cognitive models of illness

Research suggests patients cluster their ideas about an illness around five coherent themes or components, which health psychologists have called illness perceptions.[30] These provide a framework for patients to make sense of their symptoms, assess health risk, and direct action in the recovery phase. The major cognitive components are as follows.

- Identity: the label of the illness and the symptoms the patient views as being part of the disease.

- Cause: personal ideas about aetiology, which may include simple single causes or more complex multiple causal models.

- Time-line: the patient's belief about the likely time course of the illness (e.g. acute, chronic, or episodic).

- Consequences: expected impact of the illness on the patient's life.

- Cure/control: the patient's beliefs about the extent to which the illness is amenable to cure or control either through personal actions or by treatment.

These components show logical interrelationships. For example, a strong belief that the illness can be cured or controlled is typically associated with short perceived illness duration and relatively minor consequences.

The theoretical framework for this research is derived from the self-regulatory model developed by Leventhal et al.[30] This model views illness perceptions as critical in guiding the patient's coping efforts to deal with symptoms, illness, and threats to health. It consists of four components: the cognitive representation of the illness, the emotional response to the illness and treatment, the coping directed by the illness representation, and the individual's appraisal of the coping outcome.

Patient cognitive models of their illness are, by their nature, private. Patients' are often reluctant to discuss their beliefs about their illness in medical consultations because they fear being seen as ignorant or misinformed. Until recently, assessment of illness perceptions has been by open-ended interviews designed to encourage patients to elaborate their own ideas on the illness. However, questionnaires have been developed to measure illness perceptions in a variety of illnesses[31,32] as well as specific beliefs about medication.[33]

The illness perception approach has recently been applied to a large number of health conditions (see Hagger and Orbell[34] for a meta-analysis). Current research in this area is building on these findings to develop cognitive–behavioural interventions designed to modify dysfunctional illness perceptions and provide better recovery. A good example of this is a study showing that the early elicitation and modification of dysfunctional illness beliefs can improve recovery and return to function in patients with a recent myocardial infarction.[35]

## Health care behaviour

In this section we examine the role of psychological processes in the delivery of health care by focusing on two broad areas: doctor–patient communication and health care in hospital.

### Doctor–patient communication

There is now considerable evidence not only of patient dissatisfaction with medical communication but also of widespread noncompliance with subsequent treatment recommendations. Early research revealed that patient dissatisfaction was often associated with receiving insufficient information, poor understanding of the medical advice, and subsequent reluctance or inability to follow recommended treatment or advice. Another source of patients' dissatisfaction is the perception that the doctor lacks interest and empathy, and is unwilling to involve them in decision-making during the consultation. Thus, an overview of research in this area[36] revealed that patient satisfaction was higher following consultations in which the doctor engaged in more social conversation, positive verbal and non-verbal behaviour, and partnership building.

A range of frameworks have been developed for describing the process of the consultation. Similarly various methods have been devised for analysing the interactional processes which occur during the consultation[36] and Roter et al.[37] have used these analyses to propose five distinct patterns of communication in doctors:

◆ narrowly biomedical, characterized by closed-ended medical questions and biomedical talk

◆ expanded biomedical, similar to the narrowly biomedical but with moderate levels of psychosocial discussion

◆ biopsychosocial, reflecting a balance of psychosocial and biomedical topics

◆ psychosocial, characterized by psychosocial exchange

◆ consumerist, characterized by patient questions and information giving by the doctor.

The highest levels of patient satisfaction were found with those who had seen doctors using the psychosocial communication pattern, whereas the lowest satisfaction scores were recorded in those who had experienced either of the two biomedical patterns.

An alternative and broader distinction has been made between consultations which are described as patient centred and those which are doctor centred, reflecting the extent to which the doctor or patient determines what is discussed. Doctor-centred consultations are ones in which closed questions are used more often and the direction is determined by the doctor, typically with a primary focus on medical problems. In contrast, patient-centred encounters involve more open-ended questions with greater scope for patients to raise their own concerns and agendas.

Patient satisfaction and understanding of their illness following the medical consultation can play a major role in influencing adherence with treatment or advice as well as other outcomes including health and well-being. A number of studies have demonstrated beneficial effects on patients' health and well-being arising from positive experiences in medical consultations.[38] These have focused on psychological states such as anxiety as well as changes in specific physical variables such as blood pressure and blood glucose control. Some of the most impressive findings here have been found in the patient-intervention studies, which are described below.

One important spin-off from the findings in this area has been the development of communication skills training packages for medical undergraduates and for experienced clinicians, particularly for improving skills in difficult areas of communication such as giving 'bad news'. There have also been a number of specific interventions aimed at patients. Generally, these have involved interventions for patients prior to a consultation in order to increase their level of participation, particularly to ensure that their own concerns are dealt with and that information provided by the doctor is clearly understood.

### Health care in hospital

Patients experience many stressors in hospital and these arise from a range of factors including enforced lifestyle changes and the demands involved in developing good relations with hospital staff.[39] Other hospital stressors include worries about aspects of communication with staff, as well as concerns about investigations and treatment. Even such factors as the layout and colour of the ward, and the view from the patient's bed have been found to affect recovery. Not surprisingly, studies that have compared home-treated and hospitalized patients with the same condition have shown less psychosocial distress in those remaining at home.

In addition to these general psychological impacts of hospitalization, there may be specific problems or demands which occur either as a result of the particular health problem or the type of treatment which the patient has to undergo. An example of the way in which patients' health problems may influence their experience of hospital care can be seen in some of the studies of patients with HIV/AIDS who may experience negative or blaming attitudes from staff or other patients. For example, with AIDS patients being treated in either special care units or integrated in more general hospital settings, the latter group reported higher levels of stress associated with feelings of abandonment, and impersonal or discriminatory treatment. Where staff perceive patients as instrumental in having brought about their own condition through their own behaviour or neglect, they may be less committed, motivated, and sympathetic towards them.

A number of studies have been made of the psychological effects of specific treatment settings such as intensive care units (ICU) and haemodialysis units. Studies of patients in intensive care reveal high levels of psychological distress both during and for some time after their stay.[40] A range of factors seem to be involved, including being intubated and not being able to communicate. Even physical aspects of the ICU can have significant effects. Thus comparisons of patients in intensive care units with and without windows found that those in the windowless units were less well oriented during their stay and had a less accurate recall of their length of stay afterwards. In addition to these general problems associated with the intensive care units, other studies have assessed the degree of stress experienced by staff and visitors. For patients' relatives there is evidence that they find the time spent by the patient on life support in the intensive care unit particularly worrying. During this time they experience considerable fear and uncertainty but this can be improved by seeking information and the use of other resources.

In contrast with the acute psychological restrictions and demands of intensive care, some patients such as those on renal dialysis are subject to much more chronic restrictions. Dialysis can have major effects on an individual's psychological and social functioning, particularly giving rise to vocational impairment, reduced sexual activity, and mood changes.[41] In addition to the physical limitations and demands of dialysis, patients are also faced with the need to adhere to strict recommendations regarding diet and fluid consumption, as well as complex medication regimens. A number of aspects of dialysis can give rise to psychological distress, including the constant threat of death, dependence on the dialysis machine and medical staff. The stringent dietary and liquid restrictions are also important factors in patients' feelings of helplessness and lack of control. The ways in which patients cope can have important influences on their well-being and outcome. For example, problem-focused types of coping have been shown to be associated with better adherence to fluid intake restrictions, when these coping strategies were used in response to stressors arising from a relatively controllable aspect of dialysis. For those stressors, which patients perceived as less controllable, emotion-focused coping strategies provide better levels of adherence.

Many medical procedures in hospital can give rise to considerable discomfort and anxiety. These include certain treatments such as surgery, and specific investigative procedures such as barium radiography, endoscopy, and cardiac catheterization, which may not only be uncomfortable and sometimes physically distressing but which also carry the threat of uncovering a serious medical condition.[42] Consequently a number of psychological interventions have been developed to prepare patients for surgery or other stressful procedures in the hospital setting. In broad terms they can help by providing the patient with information to reduce the uncertainty of the event, or with specific behavioural or cognitive skills to help with some of the discomfort or pain.[43]

These interventions have been found to improve a range of post-surgical outcomes, including anxiety, pain and use of pain medication, length of stay in hospital, and various indicators of recovery. All the interventions have been found to be successful in improving at least one aspect of outcome, and the majority of them have a positive impact on many of the outcomes. A meta-analysis by Johnston and Vogele[43] revealed that the largest recovery effects were obtained for pain, negative affect, and physiological indices of recovery but there was considerable variation in the magnitude of these effects. Smaller but more consistent advantages of psychological preparation were found on pain medication and length of hospital stay. The interventions, which had the most widespread overall effects on all the outcomes, were found to be procedural information provision and behavioural instructions. In addition to these specific psychological preparations, there is now evidence that the pre- and post-surgical social setting can have a significant effect on recovery. Studies have also revealed clear beneficial effects of sharing a room with someone who was recovering from surgery. Patients who had post-surgical room-mates, who had undergone the same type of surgery, have been shown to be less anxious prior to surgery, engaged in more post-surgical physical activity, and were discharged home sooner.

## Treatment behaviour

Patients respond to their treatment in a range of ways and these can have very significant effects on clinical outcomes. Two major areas of patient behavioural variation are seen in the extent to which patients adhere to their prescribed treatment and in the non-specific or placebo effects of the treatment on clinical outcome. An overview of research on these two areas is now presented.

### Adherence

The extent to which the patient adheres to the advice or treatment offered in health care consultations has been widely studied. Most medical consultations result in the prescription of treatment or advice, and the use of medicines is a key aspect to the self-management of most chronic illnesses. However, many patients fail to do this and low rates of adherence to recommended treatment are seen as problematic in chronic physical and psychiatric illnesses.[44]

The incidence of reported medication non-adherence varies greatly from 4 to 92 per cent across studies, converging at 30 to 50 per cent in chronic illness. In primary prevention studies, it has been found that many participants drop out of lifestyle change programmes, designed to improve diet or reduce health-risk behaviours. Even patients who have experienced major health problems, such as heart attacks, may show low levels of uptake of rehabilitation programmes as well as considerable variation in the adoption of recommended lifestyle change. In the area of mental health, there is also evidence of significant rates of non-adherence to various recommendations from health care providers.

Non-adherence behaviours may be categorized as either intentional or unintentional. Intentional non-adherence arises when the patient makes a strategic decision not to take the treatment as instructed. An example of this type of behaviour has been found among hypertensive patients who believed that they could judge when their blood pressure was high by the presence of symptoms such as stress or headache and thus took antihypertensive medication only when these symptoms were experienced. From a self-regulatory perspective, the level of treatment adherence may be indicative of a strategic coping response, which is entirely consistent with the patient's view of their problem. Thus, patients who believe that their problem will not last for long have been found to be less likely than those with a more chronic time-line representation to adhere to their medication over a long period of time.

Non-adherence may be unintentional when the patient's intentions to follow treatment recommendations are thwarted by barriers such as forgetting, and inability to follow treatment instructions because of a lack of understanding or physical problems such as poor eyesight or impaired manual dexterity. Thus, if the quality of communication is poor and patients receive information, which is difficult to understand or recall, as has been outlined above, then this makes it less likely that treatment will be adhered to.

### The determinants of non-adherence

One very obvious explanation for non-adherence arises from poor understanding and recall of information presented in the medical consultation. Many patients lack basic knowledge about their medication but there is no simple relationship between this and their adherence. Reviews of adherence research fail to demonstrate a consistent positive association between knowledge and adherence. Moreover, interventions that enhance knowledge do not necessarily improve adherence. Patient satisfaction can act as a mediator between information provision, recall, and adherence since patient surveys reveal that many patients wanted more information than they were given. Dissatisfaction with attributes of the practitioner or the amount of information and explanation provided may act as a barrier to adherence by making the patient less motivated towards treatment.

The emphasis of adherence research over the last decade or so has moved away from attempts to identify stable trait factors which characterize the non-adherent patient to achieving a greater understanding of how and why patients decide to take some treatments and not others. Much of this research is informed by psychological theories, which conceptualize behaviour as the product of cognition which occurs within a social framework.

The application of the social cognition models, described earlier in this chapter, indicates that medication non-adherence may arise from a rational decision on the part of the patient and identifies some of the cognitions which are salient to these decisions. The types of beliefs and attitudes specified by such theories as the Health Belief Model, the Theory of Planned Behaviour and the Self-Regulatory Model (SRM) have all been used to explain aspects of treatment adherence. The SRM also acknowledges the importance of symptom perception in influencing illness representations and adherence as a coping behaviour. Confirmatory evidence for this is provided by findings from studies of patients with hypertension and with diabetes, both of whom commonly use perceived symptoms to indicate their blood pressure and glucose levels respectively, and to guide self-treatment. However, patients' beliefs about their symptoms and estimations of their own blood pressure and glucose levels are often erroneous, and this can result in poor control of symptoms and illness.

More recent research has begun to focus on the role of people's beliefs about medicines and the ways in which these could influence adherence.[45] This research has revealed two broad factors describing people's beliefs about their prescribed medicines: their perceived necessity for maintaining health (specific-necessity) and concerns based on beliefs about the potential for dependence or harmful long-term effects and that medication taking is disruptive (specific-concerns). Two factors were also found to describe people's beliefs about medicines in general. The first relates to the intrinsic properties of medicines and the extent to which they are harmful addictive substances (general-harm) and the second factor comprises concerns that medicines are overused by doctors (general-overuse).

People's views about the specific medication regimen prescribed for them were found to be much more strongly related to adherence reports than are more general views about medicines as a whole. Moreover, interplay was found between concerns and necessity beliefs, which suggests that people engage in a risk–benefit analysis and consequently attempt to moderate the perceived potential for harm by taking less. Patients with stronger concerns based on beliefs about the potential for long-term effects and dependence reported lower adherence rates, whilst those with stronger beliefs in the necessity of their medication reported greater adherence to medication regimen.[45] This work points to the importance of accessing patients' beliefs as a prerequisite of any intervention designed to increase medication adherence. In particular, it would seem important to identify specific concerns about treatment and to allay these in ways which make sense to the patient.

## The placebo response

The term 'placebo' is used to describe a treatment that gains a response due to its therapeutic intent rather than the specific ingredients of the treatment itself. Placebo responses have been shown for a wide variety of medical treatments including surgery, psychotherapy, medication, therapeutic ultrasound, injections, and aerosol sprays. Placebos have also been demonstrated to have effects in countless medical conditions and also on a number of physiological functions such as blood pressure, heart rate, gastric motility, lung function, and postoperative swelling. Adverse effects from placebos or so-called 'nocebo' effects have also been noted in the literature.

Characteristics of the treatment itself and the setting it is administered in can have a strong influence on the magnitude of the placebo response. In general, treatments that involve more serious rituals and sophisticated equipment such as surgery have stronger placebo effects. Likewise, other treatments imparting a powerful impression to the patient such as foul- or strong-tasting medicine, injections, and precise instructions also enhance the placebo response. The colour of medication has been shown to have some effect depending on the condition, and known brand names seem to have an edge in placebo response over unknown drug companies.

A similar theme runs through the clinician characteristics that increase the placebo response. Clinicians and clinics seen as having high status and having high levels of credibility have an improved placebo response. At the same time, the doctor–patient interaction

is also important. If the doctor shows high levels of concern and empathy for the patient then the response increased. High confidence shown by the doctor in the treatment administered to the patient along with a clear indication of the expected response of the treatment is also likely to improve the likelihood of placebo response.

In contrast, isolating characteristics of patients who are placebo responders has yielded inconclusive results. Much of the evidence for the role of demographic, intellectual, or personality characteristics of patients likely to respond to placebos is mixed and inconsistent. Studies have found individuals who responded to placebos in one setting to be unresponsive in another. Likewise, conditioning studies have shown individuals who have been unresponsive can later respond. These findings point to the fact that individual characteristics probably play a less significant role than situational factors and the doctor–patient interaction in influencing the placebo response.

Treatment response has been divided into specific and non-specific components, with the non-specific component encompassing factors such as clinician attention, expectation, reputation, treatment setting, etc. Determining the magnitude of the specific and non-specific components of medical treatment is a difficult and probably impossible task. In an attempt to determine how powerful non-specific effects are under ideal circumstances, Roberts et al.[46] chose to look at the effect of a number of medical treatments later shown to be ineffective but where clinician faith in the treatment was initially positive. Pooling the data from diverse treatments such as gastric freezing for duodenal ulcer and glomectomy for asthma, this study found 40 per cent of patients had an excellent response to the treatments, 30 per cent good, and 30 per cent poor. This suggests that under ideal circumstances where clinician and patient expectations are high and the treatment is administered in a credible way, non-specific factors can by themselves exert a powerful effect.

The role of compliance with placebos also appears to be important. In a review of five placebo-controlled studies measuring both compliance with medication and outcome, Epstein[47] found that subjects who were more compliant did better on outcome measures, regardless of whether they were on placebo or active treatment. Outcomes included prevention of relapse in schizophrenia, reduction of fever or infection in cancer patients, alcohol abstinence, reduction of weight, and prevention of mortality in patients with heart disease. In a later study, Horwitz et al.[48] also found the risk of death was substantially less in patients who took more than 75 per cent of their medication regardless of whether the medication was placebo or β-blocker. This suggests the act of compliance may have some effects of other health-promoting behaviours or cause cognitive or emotional changes that may influence health in the long-term.

There have been a number of theories proposed to explain the placebo response but no one theory yet provides an adequate integrated theoretical framework. The reduction of anxiety following treatment and consequent effect on symptoms has been proposed as one mechanism by which the placebo effect may operate, but changes in anxiety states have not reliably been associated with placebo responses. The role of the medical situation and its accoutrements being associated through classical conditioning with symptom relief is likely to play some role. There is, however, little direct research on this proposed mechanism, although classical conditioning of drug responses has been shown in certain situations.

Two other theories proposed have been the role of cognitive dissonance and patient expectations. The cognitive dissonance argument proposes that the placebo effect may be due to the pressure on individuals to show consistency in their views and actions. Therefore, for some individuals, having treatment is inconsistent with not showing any change in symptoms and this may encourage the person to reduce this inconsistency. The role of patient expectations and placebo effects is an area that has not received a great deal of systematic research. It is suggested that patient expectations may cause changes in cognitive schemas that influence the types and nature of symptoms that patients pay attention to following treatment. New developments in research on illness perception and beliefs about treatment, outlined above, as well as in the fields of neurobiology and neuroimaging[49] hold considerable promise for increasing our understanding of the nature of the placebo effect and its determinants.

## Conclusions

This selective overview of health psychology has demonstrated the range of psychological processes in health, illness, and health care. At the present time it is primarily a disciplinary area of psychology with an emphasis on research into health and illness behaviour. However, many interventions have been developed for healthy individuals, patients, and health care staff. This practitioner aspect of health psychology is now being accompanied by specific professional developments, and formal postgraduate training in health psychology is now available in many countries.[50]

Health psychology has established itself rapidly but it is still very much an emerging discipline. Greater insights are needed into the ways in which psychological processes can influence health and illness, and more comprehensive models are required for explaining all aspects of health and illness behaviour. In the long term this will result in the increasing use of psychological interventions for preventing and managing health problems and for the effective delivery of health care.

## Further information

Weinman, J., Johnston, M., and Molloy, G. (eds.) (2007). *Health psychology, 4 volume set*. Sage, London.

http://www.health-psych.org/

Ayers, S., Baum, A. McManus, I.C. (eds.), *et al.* (2007). *Cambridge handbook of psychology, health and medicine* (2nd edn). Cambridge University Press, Cambridge.

Johnston, M., Weinman, J., and Wright, S. (1995). *Health psychology: an assessment portfolio*. NFER Nelson, Windsor.

## References

1. Mokdad, A.H., Marks, J.S., Stroup, D.F., *et al.* (2004). Actual causes of death in the United States, 2000. *JAMA*, **291**, 1238–45.
2. Conner, M. and Norman, P. (eds.) (2005). *Predicting health behaviour*. Open University Press, Buckingham.
3. Petrie, K.J. and Weinman, J. (eds.) (1997). *Perceptions of health and illness: current research and applications*. Harwood Academic, London.
4. Ayers, S., Baum, A., Newman, S. (eds.), *et al.* (2007). *Cambridge handbook of psychology, health and medicine* (2nd edn). Cambridge University Press, Cambridge.
5. Ogden, J. (2007). *Health psychology: a textbook* (4th edn). Open University Press, Buckingham.
6. McEwen, B.S. (1998). Protective and damaging effects of stress mediators. *New England Journal of Medicine*, **338**(3), 171–9.
7. Segerstrom, S.C. and Miller, G.E. (2004). Psychological stress and the human immune system: a meta-analytic study of 30 years of inquiry. *Psychological Bulletin*, **130**(4), 601–30.
8. Cohen, S., Tyrell, D.A., and Smith, A.P. (1993). Psychological stress and susceptibility to the common cold. *New England Journal of Medicine*, 325, 606–12.
9. Kiecolt-Glaser, J.K., Marucha, P.T., Malarkey, W.B., *et al.* (1995). Slowing of wound healing by psychological stress. *Lancet*, **346**, 1194–6.
10. Broadbent, E., Petrie, K.J., Booth, R., *et al.* (2003). Psychological stress impairs early wound repair following surgery. *Psychosomatic Medicine*, **65**, 865–9.
11. Friedman, H.S. and Booth-Kewley, S. (1987). The "disease-prone personality": a meta-analytic view of the construct. *The American Psychologist*, **42**(6), 539–55.
12. Hecker, M.H.L., Chesney, M.A., Black, G.W., *et al.* (1988). Coronary-prone behaviors in the western collaborative group study. *Psychosomatic Medicine*, **50**, 153–64.
13. Thoresen, C., Friedman, M., Powell, L.H., *et al.* (1985). Altering the Type A behavior pattern in postinfarction patients. *Journal of Cardiopulmonary Rehabilitation*, **5**, 258–66.
14. Denollet, J., Pedersen, S.S., Vrints, C.J., *et al.* (2006). Usefulness of type D personality in predicting five-year cardiac events above and beyond concurrent symptoms of stress in patients with coronary heart disease. *The American Journal of Cardiology*, **97**(7), 970–3.
15. Wiebe, D. and Smith, T.W. (1997). Personality and health. In *Handbook of personality psychology* (eds. R. Hogan and J.A. Johnson), pp. 891–918. Academic Press, San Diego, CA.
16. Carver, C.S., Smith, R.G., Antoni, M.H., *et al.* (2005). Optimistic personality and psychosocial well-being during treatment predict psychosocial well-being among long-term survivors of breast cancer. *Health Psychology*, **24**(5), 508–16.
17. Adler, N.E., Boyce, T., Chesney, M.A., *et al.* (1994). Socioeconomic status and health: the challenge of the gradient. *The American Psychologist*, **49**(1), 15–24.
18. Schoenborn, C.A. (1993). The Alameda Study—25 years later. In *International review of health psychology*, Vol.2 (eds. S. Maes, H. Leventhal, and M. Johnston), pp. 81–116. John Wiley & Sons Ltd., Chichester.
19. Warburton, D.E.R., Nicol, C., and Bredin, S.D.S. (2006). Health benefits of exercise: the evidence. *CMAJ: Canadian Medical Association Journal*, **174**, 801–9.
20. West, R.J. (2005). Time for a change: putting the transtheoretical (stages of change) model to rest. *Addiction*, **100**(8), 1036–9.
21. Pennebaker, J.W. (1982). *The psychology of physical symptoms*. Springer-Verlag, New York.
22. Cameron, L., Leventhal, E.A., and Leventhal, H. (1995). Seeking medical care in response to symptoms and life stress. *Psychosomatic Medicine*, **57**, 37–47.
23. Horne, R., James, D., Petrie, K.J., *et al.* (2000). Patients' interpretation of symptoms as a cause of delay in reaching hospital during acute myocardial infarction. *Heart*, **83**, 388–93.
24. Andersen, B.L. and Cacioppo, J.T. (1995). Delay in seeking a cancer diagnosis: delay stages and psychophysiological comparison processes. Special issue: social psychology and health. *The British Journal of Social Psychology*, **34**, 33–52.
25. Verhaak, P.F.M., Meijer, S.A., Visser, A.P., *et al.* (2006). Persistent presentation of medically unexplained symptoms in general practice. *Family Practice*, **23**, 414–20.
26. Sensky, T., Macleod, A.K., and Rigby, A.F. (1996). Causal attributions about common somatic sensations among frequent general practice attenders. *Psychological Medicine*, **26**, 641–6.

27. Sullivan, M.J.L., Thorn, B., Haythornthwaite, J.A., *et al.* (2001). Theoretical perspectives on the relation between catastrophising and pain. *The Clinical Journal of Pain*, **17**, 52–64.

28. Donkin L, Ellis, C.J., Powell, R., *et al.* (2006). Illness perceptions predict reassurance following negative exercise testing result. *Psychology and Health*, **21**, 421–30.

29. Petrie, K.J., Müller, J.T., Schirmbeck, F., *et al.* (2007). Effect of providing information about normal test results on patients' reassurance: randomized controlled trial. *British Medical Journal*, **334**, 352–5.

30. Leventhal, H., Nerenz, D.R., and Steele, D.J. (1984). Illness representations and coping with health threats. In *A handbook of psychology and health*, Vol. 4 (eds. A. Baum and J. Singer), pp. 219–52. Erlbaum, Hillsdale, NJ.

31. Weinman, J., Petrie, K.J., Moss-Morris, R., *et al.* (1996). The illness perception questionnaire: a new method for assessing illness perceptions. *Psychology and Health*, **11**, 431–46.

32. Broadbent, E., Petrie, K.J., Main, J., *et al.* (2006). The brief illness perception questionnaire (BIPQ). *Journal of Psychosomatic Research*, **60**, 631–7.

33. Horne, R., Weinman, J., and Hankins, M. (1999). The beliefs about medicines questionnaire: a new method for assessing cognitive representations of medication. *Psychology and Health*, **14**, 1–24.

34. Hagger, M.S. and Orbell, S. (2003). A meta-analytic review of the common-sense model of illness representations. *Psychology and Health*, **18**, 141–84.

35. Petrie, K.J., Cameron, L.D., Ellis, C.J., *et al.* (2002). Changing illness perceptions after myocardial infarction: an early intervention randomized controlled trial. *Psychosomatic Medicine*, **64**, 580–6.

36. Roter, D. and Hall, J.A. (1989). Studies of doctor patient interaction. *Annual Review of Public Health*, **10**, 163–80.

37. Roter, D., Stewart, M., Putnam, S.M., *et al.* (1997). The patient-physician relationship: communication patterns of primary care physicians. *The Journal of the American Medical Association*, **277**, 350–6.

38. Stewart, M.A. (1995). Effective physician–patient communication and health outcomes: a review. *Canadian Medical Association Journal*, **152**, 1423–33.

39. Koenig, H.G., George, L.K., Stangl, D., *et al.* (1995). Hospital stressors experienced by elderly medical in-patients: developing a hospital stress index. *International Journal of Psychiatry in Medicine*, **25**, 103–22.

40. Andrews, P., Azoulay, E., Antonelli, M., *et al.* (2005). Year in review in intensive care medicine, 2004. III. Outcome, ICU organization, scoring, quality of life, ethics, psychological problems and communication in the ICU, immunity and hemodynamics during sepsis, pediatric and neonatal critical care, experimental studies. *Intensive Care Medicine*, **31**, 356–72.

41. Kimmel, P. (2000). Psychosocial factors in end-stage renal disease patients treated with hemodialysis: correlates and outcomes. *American Journal of Kidney Diseases*, **35**, S132–40.

42. Weinman, J. and Johnston, M. (1988). Stressful medical procedures: an analysis of the effects of psychological interventions and of the stressfulness of the procedure. In *Topics in health psychology* (eds. S. Maes, P. Defares, I.G. Sarason, and C.D. Speilberger), pp. 205–17. Wiley, Chichester.

43. Johnston, M. and Vogele, C. (1993). Benefits of psychological preparation for surgery: a meta-analysis. *Annals of Behavioral Medicine*, **15**, 245–56.

44. Osterberg, L. and Blaschke, T. (2005). Adherence to medication. *The New England Journal of Medicine*, **353**, 487–97.

45. Horne, R. and Weinman, J. (1999). Patients' beliefs about prescribed medicines and their role in adherence to treatment in chronic physical illness. *Journal of Psychosomatic Research*, **47**, 555–67.

46. Roberts, A.H., Kewman, D.G., Mercier, L., *et al.* (1993). The power of non-specific effects in healing: implications of psychosocial and biological treatments. *Clinical Psychology Review*, **13**, 375–91.

47. Epstein, L.H. (1984). The direct effects of compliance on health outcome. *Health Psychology*, **3**, 385–93.

48. Horwitz, R.I., Viscoli, C.M., Berkman, L., *et al.* (1990). Treatment adherence and risk of death after a myocardial infarction. *Lancet*, **336**, 542–5.

49. Benedetti, F., Mayberg, H.S., Wager, T.D., *et al.* (2005). Neurobiological mechanisms of the placebo effect. *The Journal of Neuroscience*, **24**(45), 10390–402.

50. Jansen, M. and Weinman, J. (eds.) (1991). *The international development of health psychology*. Harwood Academic, London.

## 5.7

# The organization of psychiatric services for general hospital departments

Frits J. Huyse, Roger G. Kathol,
Wolfgang Söllner, and Lawson Wulsin

## Introduction

The organization of psychiatric services for general hospital departments might change in far-reaching ways in the coming decades. Whereas the focus was primarily on reactive services for inpatients on medical and surgical wards, the future should focus on more proactive integrated service delivery for the complex medically ill. The essential difference from other psychiatric services is that the population served is taken care of by medical specialists in the general health setting. Consequently services are delivered in the context of the medical-psychiatric interface. Consult requests are always formulated in this perspective: the patient is treated for a medical illness or physical complaints and there are signs of an interfering psychiatric disorder.[1] Nowadays these patients are referred to as the 'complex medically ill'.[1] Therefore triage and treatment integrated in the medical context is the area of expertise of consultation-liaison (CL) psychiatrists.

The development of this area of psychiatry has been hampered by dysfunctional splits in health care, such as between general and mental health care, both on the level of its organization as well as its reimbursement.[2, 3] Recent reports, such as the report of the joint working group of the United Kingdom Royal College of Physicians and the Royal College of Psychiatrists, which describe the psychological needs of the medically and surgically ill, provide guidance to counteract these dysfunctional splits.[4] As the delivery of care-trajectories for comorbid patients becomes more and more an issue on the health care agenda, CL psychiatrists should seize this opportunity and become advocates for integrated service delivery for the complex medically ill.

---

[1] Whereas in mental health comorbidity refers to making more than one criteria based psychiatric diagnosis, in the CL literature the term 'comorbidity' is generally used to describe the combination of physical diseases and psychiatric disorders.

## Current levels of service delivery

Around 1990 the extent of inpatient CL psychiatric service delivery was evaluated, based on the records of a representative national sample of hospitals (United States)[5] and based on a prospective multicentred study (Europe).[6] Both studies reported an average consult rate of 1 per cent, ranging up to 4–5 per cent in some university settings. This rate is much lower than the prevalence of psychiatric disorders in medical populations.[6] Taking this under-utilization into account, the most striking finding was still the large variation in departments served and types of patients seen. The European Consultation-Liaison Workgroup's (ECLW) Collaborative Study made clear that CL psychiatric service delivery is primarily an emergency service. Most referrals were late, as reflected by an average time of 11 days after admission before patients were referred. In addition one-third was emergency referrals: 'See the patient the same day'.[6, 7] Exceptions were the German psychosomatic services driven by their primary interest in patients with unexplained physical complaints and problems of coping with somatic illness using a more integrated liaison approach. These services showed higher consultation rates (between 2 and 4 per cent), provided more follow-up visits, and communication with aftercare providers.[6, 7–9]

It is now evident that mental disorders and physical diseases cluster in vulnerable patients. The prevalence of mental disorders in the general hospital population is on average twice as high compared to that of the general population. However, when focusing on specific populations such as cardiac, diabetes, or transplantation, the rates of major depression may reach up to 30 per cent[10, 11] (see other chapters of this section). Patients in the general hospital setting are primarily treated for their physical diseases. However, the multiple interactions between the comorbid medical and psychiatric disorders make them complex. This justifies an integrated approach and requires individualized multimodal and multidisciplinary care.[12,13] These complex patients are the target population for CL psychiatrists. They are in need of integrated services.

**Table 5.7.1** Types of service delivery

---

1 Emergency services
  • Attempted suicide
  • Acute behavioural disturbances and their prevention
    • Deliria
    • Withdrawal

---

2 Regular consults for patients with possible interfering psychiatric complications, such as anorexia, factitious disorder, anxiety- or depressive disorders, adjustment disorders, somatization and organic mental disorders.

---

3 Integrated services
  • Participation in multidisciplinary clinics, such as pain, memory, or transplant
  • Participation in multi-disciplinary rounds on 'liaison-wards' or of disease management programmes, such as for patients with Parkinson disease, diabetes, cancer, or chronic heart failure
  • Screening for depression or complexity in at risk populations, including the development of related care trajectories
  • Clinical services for highly complex patients with both medical and psychiatric acuity, such as the medical psychiatric unit

---

## Types of service delivery

Here several models of service delivery are described (Table 5.7.1). The models have an increasing level of sophistication determined by their level of integration and the related procedural collaborative activities. Service delivery requires by definition, negotiations with health plans for their reimbursement. This is especially true for the integrated models of service delivery.[7,13,14]

### Consultations

Consultations are the classical mechanism for doctors to involve other medical specialists in the treatment of patients with additional medical problems. Patients are referred if the treating physician recognizes psychiatric comorbidity or a psychological problem and if he or she thinks that psychiatric evaluation and/or intervention may be helpful. The problem linked with this type of service delivery is that physicians often do not recognize psychiatric disturbance in medical patients.[15] In some cases, this problem is avoided by organizing a 'contract type' of consultation where every patient with a defined clinical problem is referred, for instance patients with attempted suicide.

### Liaison[2]

Whereas in the consultation function psychiatrists wait for the referral, the liaison function is proactive. A preventive approach is implemented through weekly multidisciplinary rounds. In orderto establish such a role the consultant and a departmental head formulate a liaison arrangement for the provision of psychiatric services for a certain population, clinic or ward. An important additional aspect of the liaison model is its educational focus. Though every consult offers an educational opportunity, in the liaison function the consultant is better equipped to enhance the skills of the teams through weekly attendance of clinical rounds. Currently,

---

[2] Here the term 'liaison' is only used to describe the specific 'liaison function' in addition to the basic consultation function.

the liaison model is restricted to tertiary care hospitals with more extensive CL psychiatric services. In the European collaborative study only 5 per cent of the consults came from a liaison arrangement.[6, 8]

## Psychiatric-medical, medical-psychiatric units, or psychosomatic units

The 'Psych-Med unit' is an integrated clinical service for high complex patients with unstable medical disease, such as diabetes, and psychiatric disorders. Due to their mutual interactions such patients require not sequential but integrated assessment and treatment, including both intensive medical and psychiatric nursing. Depending on the required acuity levels of physical and psychiatric nursing, different types of Psych-Med units can be described.[14] Dual-trained or combined staffs are selected to provide these levels of integrated care. Organizational prototypes of this function are the US-initiated psychiatric-medical clinics and the Germfan psychosomatic wards, which focus on adjustment disorders in medical patients and complex somatization.[14] During the last years, the efforts to improve integration between inpatient and outpatient care for complex patients led to the implementation of multidisciplinary, and specialized integrated treatment programmes for specific patient groups in day hospitals (e.g. for chronic pain patients and geriatric patients).

## Screening

As the selection criteria for patients in the liaison function are not operationalized, referrals are intuitively generated on the basis of clinical expertise.[15] Nowadays instruments are available to support both clinical work and research. The liaison function can be seen as a precursor of screening. It will gradually merge into more structured preventive functions, defined by the needs of a target population and guided by screening.[16] Currently, two lines of screening are in its development. First of all there is a model with a primary focus on psychopathology and primarily depression, using the patient health questionnaire (PHQ) as an indicator of psychiatric comorbidity. It is used in (elderly) patients with physical disorders, such diabetes, or physical complaints of unknown origin.[11, 17] Until now this is mainly used in an outpatient setting. The other approach taken is screening for 'complexity'. A European group has taken the approach to operationalize complexity and to develop a screener and an assessment tool to detect and analyse the complex medically ill.[12,16] The Complexity Prediction Instrument (COMPRI)—the screener—is to be applied at admission on an internal medicine ward to detect patients at risk for negative outcomes of care. At the same time a comparable instrument has been developed for the elderly population to detect patients who are frail and are or have an increased risk of becoming complex.[18] Other indicators of complexity such as administrative and clinical are discussed elsewhere.[12] The INTERMED-method has been developed for complexity assessment and the design of related integrated interventions.[19] It starts with a structured interview evaluating 16 health risk variables (Table 5.7.2). The fitting of these 16 risks with 4 prognostic variables in a biopsychosocial schema and the uniform-scoring system providing different levels of action visualized in different colours, supports decision-making and facilitates interdisciplinary communication. The integrated multidisciplinary interventions designed might require case-management.

**Table 5.7.2** Health risks evaluated for complexity assessment with INTERMED-method

| | |
|---|---|
| Chronicity | Is patient known with physical illness/disease |
| Diagnostic dilemma | Were physical symptoms clarified |
| Severity of symptoms | Physical functioning |
| Diagnostic challenge | Complexity of current medical problem |
| Restrictions in coping | Interferences of coping with medical problems |
| Psychiatric dysfunctioning | Psychiatric history |
| Resistance to treatment | Capacity to collaborate with treatment |
| Psychiatric symptoms | Severity of symptoms |
| Restrictions in integration | Social integration reflected by work and leisure |
| Social dysfunctioning | Quality of relations |
| Residential instability | Stability of housing |
| Restrictions of network | Availability of help |
| Intensity of treatment | Utilization |
| Treatment experience | Trust in health professionals |
| Organization of care | Participating health professionals |
| Appropriateness of referral | Capacity to deliver appropriate care |

Until now this is an area of health care in which mental health care is not formally integrated. It is to be expected that screening for psychopathology or complexity in the chronically ill will be become important future tools to initiate integrated care and allow CL psychiatric teams to actively contribute to the care of complex patients.

# The organization of a consultation-liaison psychiatric service

It is unrealistic to assume that in the future the needs of general hospital patients with psychiatric morbidity can be met simply by increasing staff. To see all patients with psychiatric comorbidity would require many times the present staffing levels. Consequently, CL psychiatrists should plan their services carefully together with their medical colleagues. The following points should be considered.

## The population to be seen

Every consultant working in a general hospital, in primary care, or in a nursing-home setting needs to define what patients have to be seen and what services are to be delivered. In a general hospital, emergency services will be required for patients who attend for psychological reasons, including attempted suicide, and for patients with substance abuse withdrawal and acute deliria (Table 5.7.1). In addition consults should be done for patients with unexplained physical problems and other complex illness behaviour. The consult capacity beyond these two consult categories should be used for the development of more preventive consults integrated in existing forms of multidisciplinary service delivery. Selection of areas of interest depends on several factors, such as service delivery or research priorities of the hospital (for instance transplant or oncology) or an own research agenda. In primary care the target population in addition to the chronically ill will be patients with somatization problems including affective and anxiety disorders (see Chapter 5.2.3).

## Psychiatric assessment

As in other settings, the formal psychiatric assessment is a crucial part of the services delivered. Specific to the setting is the differential diagnosis with physical disorders, the role and the meaning of physical deregulations, effects of pharmaca, the effects of the psychiatric disturbance on compliance with the treatment of the physical disease, the consequences of the assessment for the integrated prognosis, and the subsequent long-term integrated management of the patient. As the outcome of psychiatric disorders is clearly related to the interfering problems, which contribute to the complexity of patients, inclusion of the assessment of potential risks for such problems should be considered.[19]

## Disciplines and staffing

The size and composition of the CL team needs to be defined depending on the size and type of the hospital and of the target group of patients (Table 5.7.1) as well on the financial possibilities and other available services. For the basic function, the assessment and treatment of patients seen for attempted suicide, one is referred to Chapter 4.15.4. In a European study (ECLW Collaborative Study) it became clear that there was a variation in team composition from monodisciplinary (medical model) to multidisciplinary (mental health model) depending on the size of the service as well as the country.[8] In addition to individual psychotherapeutic treatment, mutual adjustment with and instructions of other caretakers is a key aspect of CL work. Consequently, nowadays CL psychiatry cannot provide optimal care without team members focusing on psychological treatment and the organization of case-management required for long-term individualized care-trajectories. Good evidence is becoming available that psychological interventions (cognitive–behavioural, problem solving, and interpersonal psychotherapies) are effective in patients with physical illness and depression as well as unexplained physical complaints;[20,21] (see also Chapter 5.2.3). The effectiveness of interventions of CL psychiatric nurses depends on their roles. For the effectiveness of case-management in these patients is less evidence according to a recent systematic review.[22] Turning it another way around, as CL psychiatric nurses will often work in the chronic medically ill, a recent review has provided an overview to assess the effective elements of chronic disease management (Table 5.7.3).[23] To be able to contribute to integrated care programmes, such as for diabetes or for haemodialysis, tertiary care hospitals should have teams with, on average, one full-time equivalent of psychiatric staff per 300 beds and a secretary, in addition to psychiatric residents, nurses, and psychologists.[24] Both psychiatric and complexity screening functions need to be supported by manpower to translate the findings into clinical action, such as the design and implementation of a long-term individualized care trajectory and prevent decompensation in those who are vulnerable.

## Relationship between medical staff, hospital board, and regional mental health facilities

For the development of more integrated services beyond emergency consultations good working relationships are required. The psychiatrist should be a formal member of the medical staff. Negotiations on the size and focus of CL psychiatric service delivery

**Table 5.7.3** Evidence for effective chronic care management

There is evidence to support the following initiatives

◆ Broad chronic care management models
◆ Integrated community and hospital care
◆ Greater reliance on primary care
◆ Identifying people at greatest risk of complications and hospitalizations
◆ Involving people with long-term conditions in decision-making
◆ Providing accessible structured information for people with long-term conditions and their families
◆ Self-management education
◆ Self-monitoring and referral systems
◆ Electronic monitoring and telemonitoring
◆ Using nurse-led strategies, where appropriate

There is less evidence to support the following initiatives

◆ Case-management
◆ Evidence-based care pathways
◆ Shared learning among health professionals

There is limited information about

◆ New models of commissioning services
◆ Appropriate data collection and monitoring
◆ Linking health services with voluntary and community services

(From D. Singh (2006), *Transforming chronic care*, NHS Surrey and Suffolk UK. © Crown copyright.)

should be organized with representatives of the general hospital board, the regional mental health provider, and the health plan. They should decide on functions, budgets, and facilities. The lack of medical facilities in mental health institutions is a good reason to include the need to develop a psychiatric medical unit in the general hospital to serve the more serious medically ill from mental health institutions. Wards with both a psychiatric and medical function can solve the problems created by the artificial division between general and mental health care.

## Audit

Both for financial purposes as well as for strategic planning practice audit is required. It does not make much sense to have an extensive audit system such as used in studies, unless this is used for projects. Otherwise an audit system integrated in the hospital mainframe seems the most appropriate, including the basic patient documentation, the reason for referral, the referring department, their diagnoses, and treatment.[25]

## Training

In the 'western' world CL psychiatry is becoming more and more an area of special interest, which is reflected in a subspecialty-status in several countries, such as the United States, the United Kingdom, and Australia. Training should include specific medicopsychiatric aspects of the work, including psychopharmacology in the medically ill. Guidelines have been formulated by several associations and have been published.[26, 27]

## Further information

Associations for consultation-liaison psychiatry exist, which organizational format differs by country. Since the first decade of the twenty-first century there is an increasing international exchange between leading organizations as well as among leaders in the field. Leading associations are

◆ The Academy of Psychosomatic Medicine in the USA: www.apm.org. This organization has an international membership and focus and

◆ The European Association of Consultation and Liaison Psychiatry and Psychosomatics: www.eaclpp.org

## References

1. Huyse, F.J. and Stiefel, F.C. (eds.) (July 2006). *Integrated care for the complex medically ill.* Medical Clinics of North America, Elsevier.
2. Institute of Medicine. (2001). *Crossing the quality chasm: a new health system for the 21st century. Committee on quality of health care in America.* National Academy Press, Washington, DC.
3. Institute of Medicine. (2005). *Improving the quality of health care for mental and substance-use conditions: quality chasm series.* National Academy Press, Washington, DC.
4. Royal College of Physicians and Royal College of Psychiatrists. (1995). *The psychological care of medical patients. Recognition of need and service provision. Council report CR35.* Royal College of Physicians and Royal College of Psychiatrists, London.
5. Wallen, J., Pincus, H.A., Goldman, H.H., *et al.* (1987). Psychiatric consultations in short-term general hospitals. *Archives of General Psychiatry*, **44**, 163–8.
6. Huyse, F.J., Herzog, T., Lobo, A., *et al.* (2001). Consultation-liaison psychiatric service delivery: results from a European study. *General Hospital Psychiatry*, **23**(3), 124–32.
7. Huyse, F.J., Herzog, T., Lobo, A., *et al.* (2000). European consultation-liaison psychiatric services: the ECLW collaborative study. *Acta Psychiatrica Scandinavica*, **101**, 360—6.
8. Herzog, T., Creed, F., and Huyse, F.J., *et al.* (1994). Psychosomatic medicine in the general hospital. In *Psychiatry in Europe: directions and developments* (eds. C. Katona, S. Montgomery, and T. Sensky), pp. 143–51. Gaskell, London.
9. de Cruppe, W., Hennch, C., and Buchholz, C., *et al.* (2005). Communication between psychosomatic C-L consultants and general practitioners in a German health care system. *General Hospital Psychiatry*, **27**(1), 63–72.
10. Kathol, R., Saravay, S.M., Lobo, A., *et al.* (2006). Epidemiologic trends and costs of fragmentation. *The Medical Clinics of North America*, **90**, 549–72.
11. Egede, L.E. (2006). Disease-focussed or integrated treatment: diabetes and depression. *The Medical Clinics of North America*, **90**, 627–46.
12. De Jonge, P., Huyse, F.J., and Stiefel, F.C. (2006). Case and care complexity in the medically ill. *The Medical Clinics of North America*, **90**, 679–92.
13. Smith, G.C. and Clarke, D. (2006). Assessing the effectiveness of integrated interventions: terminology and approach. *The Medical Clinics of North America*, **90**, 533–48.
14. Wulsin, L.R., Söllner, W., and Pincus, H.A. (2006). Models of integrated care. *The Medical Clinics of North America*, **90**, 647–77.
15. Söllner, W., DeVries, A., and Steixner, E., *et al.* (2001). How successful are oncologists in identifying patient distress, perceived social support, and need for psychosocial counselling? *British Journal of Cancer*, **84**, 179–85.
16. Huyse, F.J., Stiefel, F.C., and de Jonge, P. (2006). Identifiers, or "red flags" of complexity and need for integrated care. *The Medical Clinics of North America*, **90**, 703–12.
17. Kroenke, K. and Rosmalen, J.G.M. (2006). Symptoms, syndromes, and the value of psychiatric diagnostics in patients who have functional somatic disorders. *The Medical Clinics of North America*, **90**, 603–26.
18. Slaets, J.P.J. (2006). Vulnerability in the elderly: frailty. *The Medical Clinics of North America*, **90**, 593–601.

19. Stiefel, F.C., Huyse, F.J., Söllner, W., *et al.* (2006). Operationalizing integrated care on a clinical level: the INTERMED project. *The Medical Clinics of North America*, **90**, 713–58.

20. Katon, W.J., Von Korff, M., Lin, E.H., *et al.* (2004). The pathways study: a randomized trial of collaborative care in patients with diabetes and depression. *Archives of General Psychiatry*, **61**(10), 1042–9.

21. Unutzer, J., Katon, W., and Callahan, C.M., (2002). Collaborative care management of late-life depression in the primary care setting: a randomized controlled trial. *The Journal of the American Medical Association*, **288**(22), 2836–45.

22. Latour, C.H., van der Windt, D.A., de Jonge, P., *et al.* (2007). Nurse-led case management for ambulatory complex patients in general health care: a systematic review. *Journal of Psychosomatic Research*, **62**(3), 385–95.

23. Singh, D. (2006). *Transforming chronic care*. NHS Surrey and Suffolk, UK.

24. Herzog, T., Stein, B., Söllner, W., *et al.* (2002). *Practice guidelines for consultation-liaison psychosomatics*. Schattauer, Stuttgart.

25. Söllner, W., Stein, B., and Hendrischke, A., *et al.* (2005). A documentation form for the consultation-liaison services: development of the CL-BaDo. *Zeitschrift fur Psychosomatische Medizin und Psychotherapie*, **51**, 310–22.

26. Gitlin, D.F., Schindler, B.A., Stern, T.A., *et al.* (1996). Recommended guidelines for CL psychiatric training in psychiatry residency programs: a report from the academy of psychosomatic medicine task force on psychiatric training in CL psychiatry. *Psychosomatics*, **37**, 3–11.

27. Söllner, W., Creed, F. and the EACLPP Workgroup on training in CL. (2007). European guidelines for training in CL psychiatry and psychosomatics. *Journal of Psychosomatic Research*, **62**(4), 501–09.

# SECTION 6

# Treatment Methods in Psychiatry

**6.1 The evaluation of treatments** *1151*

  6.1.1 The evaluation of physical treatments *1151*
    Clive E. Adams

  6.1.2 The evaluation of psychological treatment *1158*
    Paul Crits-Christoph and
    Mary Beth Connolly Gibbons

**6.2 Somatic treatments** *1168*

  6.2.1 General principles of drug
    therapy in psychiatry *1168*
    J. K. Aronson

  6.2.2 Anxiolytics and hypnotics *1178*
    Malcolm Lader

  6.2.3 Antidepressants *1185*
    Zubin Bhagwagar and George R. Heninger

  6.2.4 Lithium and related mood stabilizers *1198*
    Robert M. Post

  6.2.5 Antipsychotic and anticholinergic drugs *1208*
    Herbert Y. Meltzer and William V. Bobo

  6.2.6 Antiepileptic drugs *1231*
    Brian P. Brennan and Harrison G. Pope Jr.

  6.2.7 Drugs for cognitive disorders *1240*
    Leslie Iversen

  6.2.8 Drugs used in the treatment
    of the addictions *1242*
    Fergus D. Law and David J. Nutt

  6.2.9 Complementary medicines *1247*
    Ursula Werneke

  6.2.10 Non-pharmacological somatic treatments *1251*
    6.2.10.1 Electroconvulsive therapy *1251*
      Max Fink

    6.2.10.2 Phototherapy *1260*
      Philip J. Cowen

    6.2.10.3 Transcranial magnetic stimulation *1263*
      Declan McLoughlin and Andrew Mogg

    6.2.10.4 Neurosurgery for psychiatric disorders *1266*
      Keith Matthews and David Christmas

**6.3 Psychological treatments** *1272*

  6.3.1 Counselling *1272*
    Diana Sanders

  6.3.2 Cognitive behaviour therapy *1285*
    6.3.2.1 Cognitive behaviour therapy for
      anxiety disorders *1285*
      David M. Clark

    6.3.2.2 Cognitive behaviour therapy for
      eating disorders *1298*
      Zafra Cooper, Rebecca Murphy, and
      Christopher G. Fairburn

    6.3.2.3 Cognitive behaviour therapy for
      depressive disorders *1304*
      Melanie J. V. Fennell

    6.3.2.4 Cognitive behaviour therapy
      for schizophrenia *1313*
      Max Birchwood and Elizabeth Spencer

  6.3.3 Interpersonal psychotherapy for
    depression and other disorders *1318*
    Carlos Blanco, John C. Markowitz,
    and Myrna M. Weissman

  6.3.4 Brief individual psychodynamic
    psychotherapy *1327*
    Amy M. Ursano and Robert J. Ursano

  6.3.5 Psychoanalysis and other long-term
    dynamic psychotherapies *1337*
    Peter Fonagy and Horst Kächele

  6.3.6 Group methods in adult psychiatry *1350*
    John Schlapobersky and Malcolm Pines

  6.3.7 Psychotherapy with couples *1369*
    Michael Crowe

6.3.8 **Family therapy in the adult psychiatric setting** *1380*
Sidney Bloch and Edwin Harari

6.3.9 **Therapeutic communities** *1391*
David Kennard and Rex Haigh

6.4 **Treatment by other professions** *1399*

6.4.1 **Rehabilitation techniques** *1399*
W. Rössler

6.4.2 **Psychiatric nursing techniques** *1403*
Kevin Gournay

6.4.3 **Social work approaches to mental health work: international trends** *1408*
Shulamit Ramon

6.4.4 **Art therapy** *1413*
Diane Waller

6.5 **Indigenous, folk healing practices** *1418*
Wen-Shing Tseng

# 6.1

# The evaluation of treatments

## Contents

6.1.1 **The evaluation of physical treatments**
Clive E. Adams

6.12 **The evaluation of psychological treatment**
Paul Crits-Christoph and Mary Beth Connolly Gibbons

## 6.1.1 The evaluation of physical treatments

Clive E. Adams

### The strengths and weakness of the single trial

#### Strengths

New treatments, or variations of older therapies, rarely represent a revolutionary departure from what has gone before. As progress is usually made in modest steps, evaluation in prospective randomized trials is needed. These studies, comparing a new treatment with a relevant control, may be able to highlight and quantify relatively subtle but important differences in outcome.

Randomization controls for selection biases. If undertaken carefully, it should ensure that both known and unknown confounding variables, such as age, sex, and additional medications, are evenly distributed between groups. Any differences in outcome should then be due to the treatment, or the intention to give the treatment (see below). In 1991, the World Health Organization stated that the randomized controlled trial, if ethical and feasible, is the most objective means of evaluating mental health interventions.[1]

Certainly, large well-conducted trials, with participants, interventions, and outcomes recognizable to those working in health services, are potent guides to clinical practice. Nevertheless, even when such trials exist, it is important to view them alongside all other comparable evidence. Should the large study affirm the findings of smaller trials the clinician can proceed with confidence.

If there is a discrepancy then debate will be generated, which should clarify important issues relating to the participants, interventions, or outcomes measured or to the methods by which the trial was conducted.[2]

#### Power

As numbers within a study increase so does the precision of results, enabling important but subtle differences to be detected, if they do indeed exist. Should a new treatment be considerably better than its predecessors few people would have to be randomized in order to demonstrate clearly the advantage of the innovative approach. As the advantage expected of new treatments is usually modest, reasonably large studies are often needed.

The power calculation is an important prerequisite for any randomized trial. For example, if clinical observation suggests that a new treatment can help 20 per cent more people avoid admission than the standard care, this can form the basis for a power calculation for a trial. Using a simple formula[3] the trialist can work out how many people would have to be randomized in order to have a known probability of highlighting such a difference, should one really exist. In this case, about 150 people would have to be allocated to each arm of the trial to be reasonably confident of detecting a true 20 per cent difference ($\alpha = 0.05$, $\beta = 0.8$). Most mental health trials are far too small to show up anything but very gross differences between treatments. For example, the average number of participants in schizophrenia trials is about 100 with only a slow increase over time.[4]

A single small trial should not greatly influence the clinician, but the combined results of several studies may begin to have the power to inform practice.

#### Biases

Randomization attempts to control for the biases that would influence treatment allocation (selection biases). Blinding at outcome attempts to control for biases that would result from participants or raters knowing which treatment had been allocated to whom (observer bias). Inadequate randomization leads to an overestimate of effect in the region of 31 to 40 per cent, and poor blinding at outcome to that of about 17 per cent.[5] Further overestimate results from the use of unpublished or modified scales, commonly seen in mental health studies, and a financial or academic investment in the therapy by the trialists.[6,7]

There are many threats to the validity of a single trial. Viewing all relevant studies, each of which was subject to different degrees of bias, should give a more balanced picture. Of course, the reader of a review should be vigilant for the systematic bias, across all trials, that may consistently sway results one particular direction.

## Generalizability

Even if a study is adequately powered and undertaken with due regard for bias, a single trial may be difficult to apply to everyday practice.

### (a) Participants

Most studies involve unusual participants. Frequently those eligible for trials have to give informed consent, their problems are well defined and do not involve multiple pathologies, and they are expected to tolerate the demands of a study.

### (b) Interventions

Applying the results of a single study is made even more difficult because study interventions are often impractical. For example, drug trials may use rigid dose regimens impossible to apply to routine care. Psychosocial therapies tested within a trial are often of such high quality that they bear little resemblance to what an overstretched clinical service can provide.

### (c) Outcomes

Measurement of outcome may also limit the value of a single trial. In a survey of 2000 schizophrenia trials, 640 different scales were used to record outcomes such as mental state, behaviour, global impression, and adverse effects.[4] Specific subspecialties within psychiatry may have an even greater propensity to create scales for trials.[8] Even within poorly powered trials, these sensitive tools may be able to detect real differences between treatments that may be statistically if not clinically significant. However, few clinicians use such scales in everyday practice and interpreting results becomes a matter of conjecture.

Trials that involve carefully defined groups of participants receiving meticulously controlled treatments and having outcomes measured on sensitive scales are called 'explanatory' studies.[9] Such trials dominate the literature, although calls for more pragmatic or 'real world' methodology are increasing[4,10] and there are now examples of this broader approach.[11,12,13,14] Currently, generalizing from the results of a single trial to day-to-day practice is inadvisable. If, however, several explanatory studies, all undertaken with constrained, but different, methodologies are giving a similar result, the clinician can feel a little more comfortable when acting on their findings.

## The rogue result

Even the well-conducted generalizable trial can produce a rogue result. Currently, the acceptable level of chance is one in 20. A statistically significant result, often denoted as $p<0.05$, suggests that the finding, if the experiment was to be replicated, should occur 19 out of 20 times. One time in 20, however, a different result will appear simply because of chance. This can lead to an interesting paradox. A single trial may not provide the best evidence of how to manage people, even in the locality that the study was undertaken. The play of chance may result in an erroneous result and unless that trial is viewed in the company of all relevant evidence, clinicians will be mislead.

## Time

It is inadvisable to act on the results of a single trial because of issues of power, biases, generalizability, and the possibility of chance erroneous results. There is, however, also the issue of time. Clinicians may often prefer to read the results of a single review rather than spending time assimilating information from several similar trials. Most practitioners have very little time to keep up with research relevant to their practice. Clinicians admit to having half an hour of reading time per week,[15] and much of that may not be retained.[16] Reading reviews is time efficient.

# Reviews

There are two main approaches to the reviewing process—the traditional and the systematic.

## The traditional review

The traditional review is often undertaken by a person well respected in the relevant field who uses knowledge and acumen, supplemented by research, to produce a synopsis of the literature. This approach still dominates the current texts, journals, and lecture tours. For example, in 1987 in four major North American medical journals, 86 per cent of review articles depended on qualitative synthesis and contained no 'methods' section whatsoever.[17] In only 6 per cent of the reviews was quantification attempted in order to support opinion and the situation did not improve much across the next decade.[18] Therefore, the clinician is left in a situation where it is difficult not to operate under a double standard. On the one hand, a large relevant trial providing objective evaluation would be desirable, but frequently, a traditional subjective review is all that is available.

## Systematic reviews

The form of a systematic review encourages the introduction of basic epidemiological principles and quantification into the process of reviewing. Gene Glass, an educational psychologist, was the first to add the results of similar studies in the hope of quantifying the effects of a treatment.[19] Glass defined 'meta-analysis' as 'the statistical analysis of a large collection of analyses results from individual studies for the purpose of integrating the findings'.[20] Unsurprisingly, in the sensitive area of the psychotherapies, their first and flawed attempts in the new discipline generated controversy.[21] Critics were quick to point out that drawing conclusions from summation of very different types of therapies, undertaken by practitioners of varied experience, was likely to be inadvisable. These pioneers, who even years later are still being criticized for adding 'apples and oranges',[22] are nevertheless owed a great debt by the rest of medicine. After all, it depends on the question being asked. It is fine to mix apples and oranges, if your question is about fruit.[23]

Systematic reviews attempt to minimize bias in the identification, extraction, and summation of relevant data by applying good survey methods to the process of literature reviewing. An analogy may help. In a community survey of the prevalence of mental disorders, a researcher stands on the doorstep of the hospital and suggests that 5 per cent of the population suffers from serious mental illness. By chance, the final estimate may even be correct, but the work could not be seen as methodologically rigorous. The researcher should have written a study protocol, clearly defined an unbiased sample of individuals to interview, and specified *a priori* the analyses to be undertaken. A systematic review should do this for a survey of a 'population' of relevant literature. Within such a review, the objectives, criteria for selection of relevant studies, search strategy, methods of study selection, data extraction, and assimilation are all made explicit.

## The advantages of the systematic approach

As is suggested above, a systematic review may, by adding the results of similar studies together, at least begin to address the issue of the underpowered study, single trials of biased methodology, poor generalizability, and idiosyncratic results. Although often longer than most traditional reviews, the systematic review is still a time-efficient way to appraise research. Additional advantages are both intuitive and practical.

### (a) Objectivity

Medicine remains a scientific discipline and the attempt at objective quantification must be an integral part of this approach. However, the systematic review and meta-analysis should never become a source of clinical tyranny. Individual clinicians will always have to use wisdom and judgement in their day-to-day decision-making, but to exclude objective appraisal from this process is foolhardy.

### (b) Clinical empowerment

Systematic reviews can provide clear information to clinicians, policy makers, and recipients of care, and so help inform the decision-making process. For example, a systematic review of family therapy suggests that this educational, psychosocial package can help those with schizophrenia avoid or postpone relapse.[24] This finding is very much in line with the suggestions of traditional reviews.[25] However, the systematic review is able to illustrate how seven families have to undergo regular therapy, for up to a year, in order for a single relapse to be postponed. Such data, of course, mean different things to different people. Clinicians may find this an acceptable degree of effort, whereas managers of services, or even families of those with schizophrenia, may not. Although the findings may not decrease controversy, at least debate can be informed.

The quantification of trial data can sometimes provide information quite at odds with the advice of traditional reviewers. The best example comes from outside mental health care. In 1992, Antman *et al.* undertook a meta-analysis of randomized trials evaluating the care of those with acute myocardial infarction.[26] As the reviewers added trial data, they found that by 1973 enough studies existed to show clearly that thrombolytic treatment saved lives. Subsequent trials added precision to the result but did not change the finding. Antman and colleagues also showed how traditional reviews continued to fail to mention thrombolytic therapy up to 15 years after the summated trial data could have shown its value.[26] These traditional reviews recommended treatments for myocardial infarction that were positively harmful. Examples have emerged from mental health. Sometimes, traditional reviews make bold claims or recommendations which are not supported by the evidence in quantitative, systematic reviews. For example, some claims made for cognitive therapy for schizophrenia[27] go well beyond objectively summarized evidence.[28,29] Conversely, even when evidence is of high quality and readily accessible, traditional reviewers can be blind. For example, both the strengths and the limitations of new generation antipsychotic drugs have been evident for years[30,31,32] but traditional

reviews and texts have encouraged uncritical enthusiasm for their use[33,34] and even guilt for failing to prescribe.[35]

### (c) Gaps in research

Often a systematic review will highlight unsuspected gaps in research. The trial-base of much routine practice is not strong, and systematic reviews can help shape questions to be tested in well-planned and conducted trials.[36] Certainly, some research funders are now requiring that a systematic review be undertaken before a randomized trial is funded. This also avoids wasting resources on questions that have already been answered.

## The limitations of the systematic approach

### (a) Qualitative information

Systematic reviews focusing on the value of treatments given to those with mental health problems usually involves quantitative synthesis of data from randomized trials. Incorporating the great wealth of information from more qualitative approaches in an unbiased way is problematic.

### (b) Trial content and quality

Systematic reviews are limited by trial content and quality. For example, it is feasible that, on average, those taking a new drug may have a statistically significant 10-point-greater decrease in a modified Brief Psychiatric Rating Scale[37] score than those taking the comparison treatment. First, this finding is difficult to put into clinically meaningful terms. Second, most scales do not provide 'interval' data. A 10-point change for someone who started with a very high score may not mean the same as the same change for a person entering the study with a lower rating. Third, more problems stem from the modification of the scale. This may well not be published and so validity is questionable. The use of such data is associated with an overestimate of effect.

Undertaking a systematic review of poor-quality trials is an important prerequisite for the design of good studies, but clinical interpretation can be problematic.[38]

### (c) Rare outcomes

Randomized trials are not a powerful means of identifying rare but important outcomes. For example, large cohorts of those taking the 'atypical' antipsychotic drug, clozapine, suggest a rate of about 1 per cent for agranulocytosis, a serious adverse effect.[39] However, a systematic review of all relevant randomized trials finds a much lower incidence.[40] As the most vulnerable period for the occurrence of agranulocytosis is from weeks 6 to 18 of treatment,[39] and most studies in the systematic review were of shorter duration, the incidence was underestimated.

Trials have limited power to identify rare outcomes and, although systematic reviews may increase this power, reviews of studies of different methodologies may be needed to quantify these important effects.

### (d) Limited statistical methods

The statistics used to summate data within meta-analyses are still evolving. For example, much of the continuous scale data, seen so frequently in mental health trials, is not normally distributed. How robust the commonly used methods of meta-analysis are for these non-parametric data is not clear. In addition, as mental health begins to evaluate preventive interventions then cluster randomization, where communities or institutions are randomized rather than individuals, will become more common. The statistics for a meta-analysis of these studies is still a matter of debate.[41] Frequently, a systematic review of mental health trials must present, but not summate, relevant data.

# The methods of systematic reviews

## Setting the question

Clinical questions regarding the effects of treatments have three parts: the participants (who are the people of interest to the questioner?), the interventions (what are the specific treatments that are to be the focus of the review?), and the outcomes (what are the outcomes of interest to the reviewers?) . Although the reviewers may have knowledge of existing trials and their limitations, it is important that the questions set are relevant to the review's readership. If the review is to service clinicians then clinically relevant outcomes must be a priority and not necessarily those anticipated by foreknowledge of the trials. If all studies then provide data on mean change in the Brief Psychiatric Rating Scale and fail to mention the outcome of 'clinically important improvement', the review can highlight this important gap in knowledge.

Developing an answerable question. The next stage for formulating the question is to decide on the type of study that is best suited to answering the question. For questions related to the efficacy of treatments this is usually the randomized trial. At first glance, this may seem straightforward, but it is important to state a priori whether studies that implied, but did not state, randomization should be included. No other methodological parameter is so consistently linked with exaggerated estimations of effect than poor description of randomization.[5] Studies that describe themselves as 'prospective, double-blind, evaluative controlled trials' would be excluded from a review if the entry criteria demanded an explicit description of randomization.

## Identifying studies

Studies are usually identified by searching bibliographic databases such as EMBASE, MEDLINE, or PsycINFO. Hand-searching relevant journals, conference proceedings, and references is also often undertaken.

A systematic review would be a misnomer if the researchers did not make the means of identification of studies clear and reproducible. The exact source of trials, and the search strategies, must be explicit. It is at this poin`t that the advice of an information specialist is important. The coverage of mental health journals in many bibliographic databases is poor and often limited by region or language[42] so that searching several sources is advisable. For example, the last decade China has become highly productive of mental health trials[43] but few are reported in mainstream bibliographic databases.[44]

In recent years, however, the situation for those wishing to identify all treatment trials relevant to a particular topic has become easier. The Cochrane Controlled Trials Register within the Cochrane Library,[45] is the largest and most comprehensive bibliographic database of published and unpublished randomized trials, and controlled clinical studies, in existence. For citations of trials, this specialist register has eclipsed databases such as EMBASE, Medline, and PsycINFO. Searching the Cochrane Controlled Trials Register also avoids the problem of the numerous 'false' positive citations produced by searches of unspecialized biomedical databases.

Identifying every possible study is important. Potent biases operate in this area. Trials that have statistically significant results are more likely to be published than those reporting equivocal findings,[46] and they are more likely to be published in English.[47] Systematic reviews incorporating only Anglophone published data or trials from one region are likely to produce, at best, imprecise, and at worse, overoptimistic views of efficacy.

## Selecting studies

Once a search is completed, relevant studies must then be selected without bias. Reviewers usually work independently and document the outcome of all disputed decisions. Some feel that those selecting the trials should be blind to the study's author, source (usually a journal), and the institution where the trial was undertaken. All have potential to bias the study selection. However, such blinding would often involve prohibitive effort. In any event, a systematic review should make explicit the degree of effort made to avoid selection bias at this crucial stage.

## Quality assessment of trials

Once studies are identified and prespecified entry criteria met, a last set of quality criteria may be applied. Scales are available, but essentially they rate selection and observation bias (see above). The description of concealment of allocation is central, as this methodological parameter has consistently been shown to be linked with an estimate of effect. If this is poorly reported, the trial is likely to overestimate the effect of the experimental intervention.[5] For trials that describe allocation with nothing more than 'randomized', this single parameter may not be a sensitive measure of quality. A scale addressing both selection and observation bias by rating the description of randomization, blinding, and reasons for people withdrawing, may be more appropriate.[48]

A systematic review should prestate the level of quality that is acceptable, or, at the very least, how the data from poor-quality studies are to be managed.

## Data extraction

Reliable data extraction is important. Just as studies must be selected with due regard for the inclusion of bias, so data must be extracted carefully and reproducibly. Often reviewers ensure maximum reliability by organizing double data extraction by an independent reviewer.

## Data management

### (a) A priori primary analysis

As with any quantitative research, a systematic review will generate the potential for multiple analyses. As one in 20 will be statistically significant by chance, it is important to state a priori the primary analyses to be undertaken. Although multiple secondary analysis are often undertaken, these are only hypothesis-generating as data have been multiply tested.

### (b) Unacceptable loss to follow-up

In every study, there must be a certain attrition that renders data meaningless. For example, in a trial of tacrine for those with Alzheimer's disease 68 per cent of people taking the experimental compound were withdrawn or lost to follow-up.[49] Drawing conclusions from the data provided by the 32 per cent of 'completers' is problematic as selection bias, originally addressed by randomization, is likely to be great. Trial attrition may not be immediately apparent from first glance. For example, a meta-analysis of studies comparing the antipsychotic quetiapine with chlorpromazine and haloperidol for schizophrenia shows considerable loss to follow-up at only a few weeks.[50] The last observation of those leaving was carried forward to the results, so that data presented in the trials were on the numbers originally randomized. The trialists made an assumption that data collected just before leaving the study would reflect the situation at the end of the trial. These assumptions by the trialists may or may not be justified[51] but reviewers must also make judgements. It is crucial to make these important decisions explicit and to make them before seeing the data.

The limit at which data become meaningless may differ depending on the question addressed. For example, in the situation of trialling a new oral drug for schizophrenia, clearly a loss of nearly 60 per cent of people at 6 weeks is clinically untenable. The reviewer may judge that the unfortunate clinician may lose up to 30 per cent of people by 6 weeks but that any greater loss would reflect more than misfortune and render data of little use. In different circumstances, such as the acute care of very disturbed people in closed wards, the loss of even 10 per cent of participants could be seen as a threat to the value of the data presented.

### (c) Intention-to-treat analysis

Interventions are not randomized in trials — it is the *intention* to give treatments that is randomly allocated. Once people are lost to follow-up, the property of the randomization to distribute known and unknown confounding variables is under threat. The randomization has, in effect, been broken. The real threat of an introduction of selection bias has led to the phrase — once randomized, always analyze.[3]

Once a limit to trial attrition has been set, reviewers must, before seeing trial data, exercise more judgement in what outcome is to be attributed to those who were lost. It is impossible to avoid assumptions, but these should be based on common sense if not evidence. For example, when presenting data for the outcome of 'clinically improved', reviewers could assume, unless contrary information is provided in the trials, that those who left early did not have an important recovery. If good quality sources of information are available, this assumption can become more evidence-based. Perhaps an exemplary trial within a systematic review managed 100 per cent follow-up even on those who left the study early. If this trial found that 90 per cent of those who had not complied with the study protocol were not 'clinically improved', it would provide a rationale for applying this figure to the other trials in the meta-analysis. Unless individual patient data are available, this process is impossible for continuous outcomes and only 'completer' data must be presented.

### (d) Continuous data

Data on continuous outcomes are frequently skewed, with the mean not being the centre of the distribution. The statistics for meta-analysis are thought to be able to cope with some skew, but were formulated for parametric normally distributed data. Reviewers may wish to build in simple rules to avoid the potential pitfall of applying parametric tests to very skewed data. For example, in scale data where a mean endpoint score is provided with a standard deviation, when the latter is multiplied by 2 and is then greater than the mean, data could be stated to be too skewed to summate.[52] This rule cannot be applied for scale data reporting change, rather than endpoint, scores.

A wide range of rating scales are available to measure outcomes in mental health trials. These scales vary in quality and many are poorly validated. It is generally accepted that measuring instruments should have the properties of reliability (the extent to which a test effectively measures anything at all) and validity (the extent to which a test measures that which it is supposed to measure). Before publication of an instrument, most scientific journals insist that both reliability and validity be demonstrated to the satisfaction of referees. Reviewers may well decide, as a minimum standard, to exclude data from unpublished rating scales.[38]

### (e) Individual patient data

Most mental health meta-analyses are of aggregate data from published reports. Other specialities have set a 'gold standard' for systematic reviews by acquiring, checking, and reanalyzing each person's data from the original trialists.[53] Collecting individual patient data allows reviewers to undertake time-to-event analyses and subgroup analyses, to ensure the quality of the randomization and data through detailed checking and correction of errors by communication with triallists, and finally to update follow-up information through patient record systems (such as mortality registers).

Limited empirical evidence exists for some of the advantages of individual patient data reviews over other types of review. The former does help to control publication bias, to ensure use of the intention-to-treat principle in the analysis, and to obtain a fuller picture of the effects of different treatments over time. Undertaking individual patient data reviews requires considerable additional skills, time, and effort on the part of the reviewers when compared to meta-analyses of published aggregate data.[54]

## Statistics

### (a) Inappropriate meta-analyses

Systematic reviews may, or may not, contain meta-analyses. Where participants, interventions, or outcomes are clearly too different to summate, reviewers must resist the temptation to use powerful statistics on inappropriate data.[41]

### (b) Summary measures

Much has been written about the statistics for meta-analysis,[55] but if their meaning is not conveyed to the user of the review, they are of little value. Summary measures such as odds ratios or relative risk are frequently employed for dichotomous outcomes and weighted and standard mean difference for continuous data. Where continuous data are presented from different scales measuring similar phenomena then standard mean difference is often calculated and called the effect size. This estimate has statistical integrity, but is even more problematic to interpret clinically than weighted mean difference. In each of these summary measures, an individual trial contributes to the final statistic, inversely proportional to the precision of its result.

Currently, in this new discipline, statistics for meta-analysis are powerful and evolving. In recent years, there has been a much better understanding of how best to summate data from cluster randomized trials and crossover studies. Techniques for these types of analyses are now widely accessible. Further statistical flexibility is available through use of generic inverse variance. This statistical technique facilitates analyses of properly analyzed cross-over trials, cluster randomized trials and non-randomized studies, as well as outcome data that are ordinal, time-to-event or rates. Better methods for managing non-parametric data can confidently be expected in the next few years.[41]

### (c) Sensitivity analyses

This is where an analysis is used to determine how sensitive the results of the review are to changes in how it was undertaken. For example, the reviewers may state, again *a priori*, that they wish to compare the size of effect of industry-sponsored trials versus those undertaken independently of the manufacturer of the experimental drug.[7] The sensitivity of the final result to adding and subtracting sets of trials is then tested. Sensitivity analyses can be proposed on many variables, such as severity of illness, age of participant, means of diagnosis, subtype of intervention, and quality of trial. This can easily lead to the problems of multiple testing, although for meta-analyses of published data the quality and extent of trial reporting severely restricts the numbers of sensitivity analyses that are possible.

### (d) Heterogeneity

In systematic reviews heterogeneity refers to variability or differences between studies' estimates of effects and is a function of clinical and/or methodological diversity among the studies. Despite rigorous definition and application of inclusion criteria, the trials eventually selected may not be homogeneous enough to summate. Heterogeneity should be considered, sought, and measured, and, if present, investigated. Statistical tests of heterogeneity are used to assess whether the observed variability in study results (effect sizes) is greater than that expected to occur by chance. These tests, however, have low statistical power and careful inspection of results for outlying findings is just as valuable. Recently, partly because it is more intuitive than previous measures, the $I^2$ has become widely used. This quantifies inconsistency across studies, moves the focus away from testing whether heterogeneity is present to assessing whether the heterogeneity, that many argue is inevitable, will impact on the meta-analysis. A value greater than 50 per cent is often considered to indicate substantial heterogeneity.[41]

Heterogeneity can be caused by various factors, and its presence generates debate about differences in study design (methodological diversity) and differences between studies in key characteristics of the participants, interventions, or outcome measures (clinical diversity). Heterogeneity can be explored by undertaking subgroup analyses or employing meta-regression. In subgroup analyses, the results of one group of studies with a characteristic thought to be causing heterogeneity is compared to those of another group of trials without that characteristic. For example, trials of a new interpersonal therapy for depression may be heterogeneous. The reviewers may have stated, *a priori*, that the new therapy, targeted at young people, may not be effective for those over 30 years of age. Overall, although the trials may have heterogeneous results, if the two subgroups of studies involving people over and under the age of 30 have homogeneous results, it is feasible that the original hypothesis of the reviews regarding age was correct. Meta-regression, is an extension to subgroup analyses that allows the effect of variables, even several simultaneously, to be investigated. Again these variables should be pre-stated and this technique necessitates much high quality data to be meaningful. Even then, the regression

is essentially an observational study with all the dangers of unexplained or residual confounding. In mental health reviews, investigation of heterogeneity often generates valuable debate, rather than providing definitive answers.

### (e) Reporting bias

There are several ways to assess whether reporting (publication) bias (see above) is operating within a review. The reviews may use a funnel plot technique[56] where the results of a trial are plotted against its size. Large studies with any result, positive or negative, tend to be published. Small positive studies are also usually easily identified, but it quickly becomes apparent if small 'negative' studies have not been found. This could be due to a variety of reasons, but one of which is a selective reporting of positive outcomes.

## Sources of systematic reviews

### Journals

Systematic reviews are increasingly seen in major journals. These can be identified by simple or comprehensive methodology-specific searches of bibliographic databases such as EMBASE, Medline, or PsycINFO. Examples of these searches can be readily identified[57] but need to be updated periodically to reflect changes in notation or indexing. These search phrases would then be linked to a subject-specific phrase such as 'depression' or 'cognitive therapy', by the word 'and' to limit and focus the number of identified citations.

### DARE database

The Database of Abstracts of Reviews of Effectiveness (DARE) is a specialist database containing thousands of citations of systematic reviews of health care. These reviews are assessed according to explicit criteria, and structured abstracts describing methodology and results, and commenting on quality and clinical implications, are also included.

### Cochrane reviews

The Cochrane Database of Systematic Reviews is an electronic publication increasingly favoured by clinicians, researchers and those compiling guidelines. It contains the full text and data of reviews undertaken to the most rigorous systematic standards[58] and is updated quarterly. There is often a considerable lag time for traditional journal publication and this can result in the publication of good-quality but misleading systematic reviews. For example, an important systematic review on the effects of family intervention for schizophrenia was published in August 1994.[59] Just 2 weeks later, the same authors re-summated relevant data in an electronic version and the results were much less favourable than had been previously reported.[60] In the considerable period between completion of the paper version and its publication, less favourable trials appeared. Further updates of this review suggest that the trend is continuing. By using electronic publishing, the Cochrane Database of Systematic Reviews allows trends over time to be highlighted and reviews to be maintained.

The Cochrane Library is a collection of databases supplying high-quality evidence to inform all those interested in the evaluation of health care.[45] It is published quarterly on CD-ROM and the Internet, and includes the Cochrane Database of Systematic Reviews, the source of many of the reviews quoted in this chapter, the DARE abstracts, and The Cochrane Controlled Trials Register.

## Summary publications

There are now several periodically updated, systematically compiled, publications designed primarily for busy clinicians. For example, one such publication, Clinical Evidence,[61] now has a comprehensive mental health subset, and is available in short or very short versions, providing clinical 'bottom lines' of relevant systematic reviews or randomized trials.

# Further information

The Cochrane Handbook - http://www.cochrane-handbook.org/ contains up-to-date methodological details of systematic reviews and meta-analysis

Clinical Evidence - http://clinicalevidence.bmj.com/ceweb/index.jsp an on-line, regularly updated compendium of systematic evidence summaries

# References

1. WHO Scientific Group on Treatment of Psychiatric Disorders (1991). Evaluation of methods for the treatment of mental disorders. *World Health Organization Technical Report Series*, **812**, 1–75.

2. Egger, M. and Davey-Smith, G. (1995). Misleading meta-analysis. *British Medical Journal*, **311**, 753–4.

3. Pocock, S. (1989) *Clinical trials: a practical approach*. Wiley, Chichester.

4. Thornley, B. and Adams, C. (1998). Content and quality of 2000 randomised controlled trials in schizophrenia over 50 years. *British Medical Journal*, 1181–4.

5. Juni, P., Altman, D. and Egger, M. (2001). Systematic reviews in health care: Assessing the quality of controlled clinical trials. *British Medical Journal*, **323**, 42–6.

6. Heres, S., Davis, J., Maino, K., *et al.* (2006). Why olanzapine beats risperidone, risperidone beats quetiapine, and quetiapine beats olanzapine: an exploratory analysis of headto- head comparison studies of second-generation antipsychotics. *American Journal of Psychiatry*, **163**, 185–94.

7. Montgomery, J., Byerly, M., Carmody, T., *et al.* (2004). An analysis of the effect of funding source in randomized clinical trials of second generation antipsychotics for the treatment of schizophrenia. *Controlled Clinical Trials*, **25**, 598–612.

8. Cure, S., Chua, W., Duggan, L. *et al.* (2005). Randomised controlled trials relevant to aggressive and violent people, 1955-2000: a survey. *British Journal of Psychiatry*, **186**, 185–9.

9. Roland, M. and Torgerson, D. (1998). What are pragmatic trials? *British Medical Journal*, **316**, 285.

10. Simon, G., Wagner, E. and Vonkorff, M. (1995). Cost-effectiveness comparisons using «real world» randomized trials: the case of new antidepressant drugs. *Journal of Clinical Epidemiology*, **48**, 363–73.

11. Lieberman, J., Stroup, T., McEvoy, J., *et al.* (2005). Effectiveness of antipsychotic drugs in patients with chronic schizophrenia. *New England Journal of Medicine*, **353**, 1209–23.

12. Lewis, S., Davies, L., Jones, P., *et al.* (2006). Randomised controlled trials of conventional antipsychotic versus new atypical drugs, and new atypical drugs versus clozapine, in people with schizophrenia responding poorly to, or intolerant of, current drug treatment. *Health Technology Assessment*, **10**, iii-iv, ix-xi, 1–165.

13. TREC Collaborative Group (2003). Rapid tranquillisation for agitated patients in emergency psychiatric rooms: a randomised trial of midazolam versus haloperidol plus promethazine. *British Medical Journal*, **327**, 708–13.

14. Alexander, J., Tharyan, P., Adams, C., *et al.* (2004). Rapid tranquillisation of violent or agitated patients in a psychiatric emergency setting. Pragmatic randomised trial of intramuscular lorazepam v. haloperidol plus promethazine. *British Journal of Psychiatry*, **185**, 63–9.

15. Sackett, D., Richardson, W., Rosenberg, W. *et al.* (1997). *Evidence based medicine: how to practice and teach EBM*. Churchill Livingstone, London.

16. Kellett, C., Hart, A., Price, C., *et al.* (1996). Poor recall performance of journal-browsing doctors. *Lancet*, **348**, 479.

17. Mulrow, C. (1987). The medical review article: state of the science. *Annals of Internal Medicine*, **106**, 485–8.

18. McAlister, F., Clark, H., van, W.C., *et al.* (1999). The medical review article revisited: has the science improved? *Annals of Internal Medicine*, **131**, 947–51.

19. Smith, M. and Glass, G. (1977). Meta-analysis of psychotherapy outcome studies. *American Psychologist*, **32**, 752–60.

20. Glass, G. (1976). Primary, secondary and meta-analysis of research. *Education Research*, 3–8.

21. Eysenck, H. (1978). An exercise in mega-silliness. *American Psychologist*, **33**, 517.

22. Eysenck, H. (1994). Meta-analysis and its problems. *British Medical Journal*, **309**, 789–92.

23. Higgins, J. and Green, S. (2005). *Cochrane Handbook for Systematic Reviews of Interventions 4.2.5 [updated May 2005]*, Chichester, UK, John Wiley & Sons, Ltd.

24. Pharoah, F., Mari, J., Rathbone, J. *et al.* (2006). Family intervention for schizophrenia. *Cochrane Database of Systematic Reviews*, CD000088.

25. Leff, J. (1994). Working with the families of schizophrenic patients. *British Journal of Psychiatry. Supplement*, 71–6.

26. Antman, E., Lau, J., Kupelnick, B., *et al.* (1992). A comparison of results of meta-analyses of randomized control trials and recommendations of clinical experts. Treatments for myocardial infarction. *Journal of American Medical Association*, **268**, 240–8.

27. Kingdon, D. (2006). Psychological and social interventions for schizophrenia. *British Medical Journal*, **333**, 212–3.

28. McKenna, P. (2006). What works in schizophrenia: cognitive behaviour therapy is not effective. *British Medical Journal*, **333**, 353.

29. Jones, C., Cormac, I., Silveira, D.M.N.J. *et al.* (2004). Cognitive behaviour therapy for schizophrenia. *Cochrane Database of Systematic Reviews*, CD000524.

30. Srisurapanont, M., Disayavanish, C. and Taimkaew, K. (2000). Quetiapine for schizophrenia. *Cochrane Database of Systematic Reviews*, CD000967.

31. Duggan, L., Fenton, M., Dardennes, R., *et al.* (2000). Olanzapine for schizophrenia. *Cochrane Database of Systematic Reviews*, CD001359.

32. Kennedy, E., Song, F., Hunter, R., *et al.* (2000). Risperidone versus typical antipsychotic medication for schizophrenia. *Cochrane Database of Systematic Reviews*, CD000440.

33. Adams, C. and Jayaram, M. (2007). Do findings from new trials for schizophrenia fit with existing evidence: not duped ........ just beguiled? *Epidemiologia e Psichiatria Sociale*, **16**, 199–202.

34. Vedantam, S. (Oct 3, 2006). In antipsychotics, newer isn't better – drug find shocks researchers. *Washington Post* A01.

35. Adams, C., Tharyan, P., Coutinho, E. *et al.* (2006). The schizophrenia drug-treatment paradox: pharmacological treatment based on best possible evidence may be hardest to practise in high-income countries. *British Journal of Psychiatry*, **189**, 391–2.

36. Brown, P., Brunnhuber, K., Chalkidou, K., *et al.* (2006). How to formulate research recommendations. *British Medical Journal*, **333**, 804–6.

37. Overall, J. and Gorham, D. (1962). The Brief Psychiatric Rating Scale. *Psychological Reports*, **10**, 799–812.

38. Marshall, M., Lockwood, A., Bradley, C., *et al.* (2000). Unpublished rating scales: a major source of bias in randomised controlled

trials of treatments for schizophrenia. *British Journal of Psychiatry*, **176**, 249–52.

39. Atkin, K., Kendall, F., Gould, D., *et al.* (1996). Neutropenia and agranulocytosis in patients receiving clozapine in the UK and Ireland. *British Journal of Psychiatry*, **169**, 483–8.

40. Wahlbeck, K., Cheine, M. and Essali, M. (2000). Clozapine versus typical neuroleptic medication for schizophrenia. *Cochrane Database of Systematic Reviews*, CD000059.

41. Deeks, J., Higgins, J. and Altman, D. (2005). Analysing and presenting results. In: Higgins, J. and Green, S., (Eds.) *Cochrane Handbook for Systematic Reviews of Interventions 4.2.5 [updated May 2005] Section 8. In: The Cochrane Library*, John Wiley & Sons, Ltd., Chichester, UK.

42. McDonald, S., Taylor, L. and Adams, C. (1999). Searching the right database. A comparison of four databases for psychiatry journals. *Health Libraries Review*, **16**, 151–6.

43. Chakrabarti, A., Adams, C., Rathbone, J., *et al.* (2007). Schizophrenia trials in China: a survey. *Acta Psychiatrica Scandinavica*, (in press).

44. Xia, J., Wright, J. and Adams, C. (2007). Five large Chinese biomedical bibliographic databases: accessibility and coverage. *Health Infomation Libraries Journal*, (in press).

45. Cochrane Collaboration (2007). *The Cochrane Library*, (3rd edn.). John Wiley & Sons, Ltd., Chichester, UK.

46. Easterbrook, P., Berlin, J., Gopalan, R. *et al.* (1991). Publication bias in clinical research. *Lancet*, **337**, 867–72.

47. Egger, M., Zellweger-Zahner, T., Schneider, M., *et al.* (1997). Language bias in randomised controlled trials published in English and German. *Lancet*, **350**, 326–9.

48. Jadad, A., Moore, R., Carroll, D., *et al.* (1996). Assessing the quality of reports of randomized clinical trials: is blinding necessary? *Controlled Clinical Trials*, **17**, 1–12.

49. Knapp, M., Knopman, D., Solomon, P., *et al.* (1994). A 30-week randomized controlled trial of high-dose tacrine in patients with Alzheimer's disease. The Tacrine Study Group. *Journal of American Medical Association*, **271**, 985–91.

50. Srisurapanont, M., Maneeton, B. and Maneeton, N. (2004). Quetiapine for schizophrenia. *Cochrane Database of Systematic Reviews*, CD000967.

51. Leucht, S., Engel, R., Bauml, J. (2007). Is the superior efficacy of new generation antipsychotics an artifact of LOCF? *Schizophrenia Bulletin*, **33**, 183–91.

52. Altman, D. and Bland, J. (1996). Detecting skewness from summary information. *British Medical Journal*, **313**, 1200.

53. Early Breast Cancer Trialist's Collaborative Group (1992). Systematic treatment of early breast cancer by hormonal, cytoxic, or immune therapy: 133 randomised trials involving 31 000 recurrences and 24 000 deaths among 75 000 women. *Lancet*, **1-15**, 71–85.

54. Stewart, L. and Clarke, M. (1995). Practical methodology of meta-analyses (overviews) using updated individual patient data. Cochrane Working Group. *Statistics in Medicine*, **14**, 2057–79.

55. Petitti, D. (1994). *Meta-analysis, decision analysis and cost-effectiveness analysis. Methods for quantitative synthesis in medicine.* Oxford University Press, Oxford.

56. Egger, M., Davey-Smith, G., Schneider, M. *et al.* (1997). Bias in meta-analysis detected by a simple, graphical test. *British Medical Journal*, **315**, 629–34.

57. Shojania, K. and Bero, L. (2001). Taking advantage of the explosion of systematic reviews: an efficient MEDLINE search strategy. *Effective Clinical Practice*, **4**, 157–62.

58. Jadad, A., Cook, D., Jones, A., *et al.* (1998). Methodology and reports of systematic reviews and meta-analyses: a comparison of Cochrane reviews with articles published in paper-based journals. *Journal of American Medical Association*, **280**, 278–80.

59. Mari, J. and Streiner, D. (1994). An overview of family interventions and relapse on schizophrenia: meta-analysis of research findings. *Psychological Medicine*, **24**, 565–78.

60. Mari, J. and, S.D. Family intervention for schizophrenia. *The Cochrane Library*.

61. Tovey, D. (2007). *BMJ Clinical Evidence*, BMJ Publishing Group Ltd., London.

## 6.1.2 The evaluation of psychological treatment

Paul Crits-Christoph and
Mary Beth Connolly Gibbons

### Introduction

Psychotherapy continues to be a widely practised treatment for psychiatric disorders and other problems in living. Since publication in 1952 of the well-known article by Hans Eysenck,[1] in which he claimed that there was no evidence that psychotherapy was effective, there has been an accelerating literature concerned with methodologies for evaluating psychotherapy, as well as specific studies demonstrating the efficacy, or lack thereof, of various psychotherapies. In more recent years, pressures from the government agencies and insurance companies that bear much of the cost of mental health treatments have added to the call for accountability regarding psychotherapeutic treatment.

Despite a vast literature of over 1000 outcome studies of the effects of psychotherapy, questions remain about the role of psychotherapy as a treatment for mental disorders. Extensive meta-analytical reviews of the psychotherapy outcome literature provided evidence that, generally speaking, psychotherapy appears to be efficacious.[2] While encouraging, this information was not particularly useful. As with any medical problem or disorder, the relevant public health clinical question is whether a treatment is beneficial for the presenting problem or psychiatric disorder for which help is sought. Along these lines, a number of efforts have been made at summarizing the results of the psychotherapy outcome literature in terms of what works for different disorders or problems.[3, 4] For example, these efforts have arrived at conclusions such as 'cognitive therapy is efficacious in the treatment of major depressive disorder'.

The simplicity and clinical appeal of such conclusions, about which psychotherapy treatments work for which patient problems, belies a host of more complex issues regarding how one evaluates psychotherapy and makes a decision about whether treatment 'works' or not. Other treatments within psychiatry, such as pharmacotherapy, lend themselves to rather straightforward designs (namely placebo-controlled randomized clinical trials) that permit clear inferences about the efficacy of a treatment approach. In contrast, research on psychotherapy as a verbal interchange between two or more participants does not have the luxury of such straightforward pharmacotherapy research designs. Instead, psychotherapy outcome research is characterized by the use of a variety of research designs and methods that, while often not without limitations to strong scientific inferences about treatment efficacy, can provide incremental scientific advance in the understanding of the usefulness of psychotherapeutic treatments. The aim of the current chapter is to provide an overview of approaches to the evaluation of psychological treatments. We begin with a discussion of specific research designs employed in psychotherapy outcome research, with a discussion of some of the broad issues that currently guide the selection among these different experimental designs. This is followed by a selective review of assessment strategies for outcome evaluation, with discussion of examples of instruments.

## Issues in planning research evaluating psychotherapy

A number of other sources provide a detailed discussion of issues involved in planning a study on psychotherapy, as well as explication of various research designs. In particular, our presentation draws heavily from Kazdin,[5] supplemented with writings that illustrate more recent trends in both design and methodology.

There are, of course, a wide range of decisions to be made in designing an evaluation study of psychotherapy. These decisions affect the choice of patients, therapists, control groups, data analytical strategies, etc. Table 6.1.2.1 presents a list of the types of questions that need to be asked in designing or evaluating a study of psychotherapy outcome. A discussion of some of the key methodological issues that cut across many of the questions raised in Table 6.1.2.1 follows.

## Internal versus external validity

An initial important decision in planning an evaluation of psychotherapy outcome, or any intervention, is the relative emphasis on internal versus external validity of the inferences from the investigation. Internal validity refers to the extent to which inferences can be attributed to the intervention *per se*, as opposed to other factors. In order to maximize internal validity, the investigator attempts to control as many of the extraneous factors as possible through a variety of procedures including, among others, random assignment, the use of control groups, assessing subjects in the same ways and at the same point in time, and careful selection of a relatively homogeneous subject sample. With as many factors as possible held constant across treatment groups except for the nature of the intervention, an outcome difference detected between the experimental and control group(s) can be attributed to the intervention, rather than other factors.

External validity, in contrast, refers to the extent to which the results of a study can be generalized to other subjects, settings, treatment durations, and treatment providers other than those used within the specific study. In regard to the evaluation of psychotherapy outcomes, external validity is often invoked to raise the question of whether study results pertain to the 'real world' in which psychotherapy is practiced—the diverse set of patients, therapists, and settings occurring in the community that may be quite different from the conditions of an investigation conducted in a research setting.

Clearly, both internal and external validity are important, but it is difficult to maximize each within the context of the same study. Studies of homogeneous patient samples, for example, may have high internal validity, but generalize poorly to the mix of heterogeneous patients seen in clinical practice. The relative merits of studies with high internal versus external validity have been a source of ongoing debate among psychotherapy outcome researchers.

Different research designs are more or less appropriate depending upon the scientific question of interest. For example, the process of developing and testing new treatments generally proceeds stepwise, beginning with individual case reports and then progressing to an 'open-label' (a term derived from pharmacotherapy research) trial involving the application of a single treatment to a relatively small group of patients. Following an open-label trial, a promising treatment would then be tested within the context of a controlled, efficacy trial. In this efficacy trial, the treatment would be tested under ideal circumstances (for instance, by highly trained clinicians). If an effect is found in the controlled efficacy trial, a controlled, effectiveness trial is the next step. In this effectiveness trial, the treatment would now be tested under more 'real world' conditions. This line of research is oriented towards understanding whether the treatment *per se* is responsible for change (efficacy trial) and whether the effect generalizes (effectiveness trial).

Naturalistic studies represent an alternative type of effectiveness trial in which the scientific question is usually not a focus of type of treatment. Instead, such studies might examine the relationship of patient characteristics, therapist factors, or length (dose) of treatment to outcome.

## Selection criteria for psychotherapy outcome studies

The choice of selection criteria for a psychotherapy outcome study depends, of course, on the nature of the research question to be asked. From a public health perspective, samples are usually chosen based upon the presence of a discrete disorder or problem that has significance to society. The selection of the target disorder, however, is only the beginning of the selection process. For studies of DSM Axis I non-psychotic disorders, it is typical that other major psychotic disorders such as schizophrenia and bipolar disorder are excluded from the study. However, there is wide variability across research studies in the extent to which other Axis I and Axis II disorders are included in a study or not.

This aspect of selection criteria relates primarily to the internal versus external validity distinction discussed above. Studies that emphasize internal validity will probably exclude many comorbid diagnoses, while studies that maximize external validity will tend to be more inclusive. As the comorbidities among Axis I diagnoses can be high, the impact on the nature of the patient sample selected can be considerable.

Naturalistic studies that focus on psychotherapy *per se*, rather than public health concerns, are oriented towards external validity and typically do not have restrictive selection criteria. For these studies, the question is 'how effective is psychotherapy for the types of patients that end up in psychotherapeutic treatment in the community?' Thus, few, if any, selection criteria are specified.

One particular selection problem that affects any type of psychotherapy outcome study is whether or not patients currently treated with psychotropic medication are included in the evaluation study. Once again, from the point of view of internal validity—attempting to attribute the treatment outcome to the psychotherapy treatment *per se*—patients on concurrent medication treatment are usually excluded. In contrast, external validity concerns would lead to the inclusion of patients on medications, since increasing numbers of patients in the community with anxiety and affective

**Table 6.1.2.1** Selected questions to raise in planning a study of psychotherapy

**Sample characteristics**

1  Who are the subjects and how many of them are there in this study?
2  Why was this sample selected in light of the research goals?
3  How was this sample obtained, recruited, and selected?
4  What are the subject and demographic characteristics of the sample (e.g. sex, age, ethnicity, race, socio-economic status)?
5  What, if any, inclusion and exclusion criteria were invoked (i.e. selection rules to obtain participants)?
6  How many of those subjects eligible or recruited actually were selected and participated in the study?
7  With regard to clinical dysfunction or subject and demographic characteristics, is this a relatively homogeneous or heterogeneous sample?

**Design**

1  How were subjects assigned to groups or conditions?
2  How many groups were included in the design?
3  How are the groups similar and different in how they are treated in the study?
4  Why are these groups critical for addressing the questions of interest?

**Procedures**

1  Where was the study conducted (setting)?
2  What measures, materials, equipment, and/or apparatus were used in the study?
3  What is the chronological sequence of events to which subjects were exposed?
4  What intervals elapsed between different aspects of the study (assessment, treatment, follow-up)?
5  What variation in administration of conditions emerged over the course of the study that may introduce variation within and between conditions?
6  What procedural checks were completed to avert potential sources of bias in implementing the manipulation and assessment of dependent measures?
7  What checks were made to ensure that the conditions were carried out as intended?
8  What other information does the reader need to know to understand how subjects were treated and what conditions were provided?

**Therapists**

1  Who are the therapists, and why are these individuals selected?
2  Can the influence of the therapist be evaluated in the design as a 'factor' (as in a factorial design) or can therapist efforts be evaluated within a condition?
3  Are the therapists adequately trained? By what criteria?
4  Can the quantity and quality of their training and implementation of treatment be measured?

**Treatment**

1  What characteristics of the clinical problem or cases make this particular treatment a reasonable approach?
2  Does the version of treatment represent the treatment as it is usually carried out?
3  Does the investigation provide a strong test of treatment? On what basis has one decided that this is a strong test?
4  Has treatment been specified in manual form or have explicit guidelines been provided?
5  Has the treatment been carried out as intended? (Integrity is examined during the study but evaluated after it is completed.)
6  Can the degree of adherence of therapists to the treatment manual be codified?
7  What defines a completed case (e.g. completion of so many sessions)?

**Assessment**

1  If specific processes in the clients or their interpersonal environment are hypothesized to change with treatment, are these to be assessed?
2  If therapy is having the intended effect on these processes, how would performance be evident on the measure? How would groups differ on this measure?
3  Are there additional processes in therapy that are essential or facilitative to this treatment, and are these being assessed?
4  Does the outcome assessment battery include a diverse range of measures to reflect different perspectives, methods, and domains of functioning?
5  What data can be brought to bear regarding pertinent types of reliability and validity for these measures?
6  Are treatment effects evident in measures of daily functioning (e.g. work, social activities)?
7  Are outcomes being assessed at different times after treatment?

**Data evaluation**

1  What are the primary measures and data upon which the predictions depend?
2  What statistical analyses are to be used and how specifically do these address the original hypotheses and purposes?
3  Are the assumptions of the data analyses met?
4  What is the likely effect size that will be found based on other treatment studies or meta-analyses?
5  Given the likely effect size, how large a sample is needed to provide a strong powerful test of treatment (e.g. power $\geq 0.80$)?
6  Are there subdivisions of the sample that will be made to reduce the power of tests of interest to the investigator?
7  What is the likely rate of attrition over the course of treatment, and post-treatment and follow-up assessments?
8  With the anticipated loss of cases, is the test likely to be sufficiently powerful to demonstrate differences between groups if all cases complete treatment?
9  If multiple tests are used, what means are provided to control error rates?
10  Prior to the experimental conditions, were groups similar on variables that might otherwise explain the results (e.g. diagnosis, age)?
11  Are data missing due to incomplete measures (not filled out completely by the subject(s) or loss of subjects)? If so, how are these handled in the data analyses?
12  Will the clinical significance of client improvement be evaluated and if so by what method(s)?
13  Are there ancillary analyses that might further inform the primary analyses or exploratory analyses that might stimulate further work?

Reproduced with permission from A. Kazdin. Methodology, design and evaluation in psychotherapy research. In *Handbook of Psychotherapy and Behavior Change* (eds. A.E. Bergin and S.L. Garfield), pp. 19–71. Copyright 1994, John Wiley & Sons, Inc.

disorders are receiving psychotropic medications for their problems. Often, a compromise is struck: patients on medications are eligible for the psychotherapy study as long as they (and their prescribing doctor) agree to maintain a stable dosage of the medication for the duration of the psychotherapy study.

## Treatment standardization

Psychotherapy efficacy research, like pharmacotherapy research, requires that the treatment be standardized. Such standardization serves two related purposes. First, from a clinical point of view, it is necessary that the treatment be clearly specified, so that any conclusions about differential treatment efficacy can be translated into clear treatment recommendations. From a research point of view, treatment standardization allows studies to be replicated. In addition, by making the delivery of a treatment more standardized, differences between therapists and the statistical problems that result from the non-independence that 'therapist effects' introduce can be avoided.[6]

Standardization of pharmacological interventions is relatively straightforward—a per-day dosage (or range of dosages) is set in advance. But for psychotherapy, how can something so complex as patient–therapist dialogue be standardized? The central ingredient in standardization of a psychosocial treatment is a treatment manual. A psychotherapy manual describes the treatment in detail, with case examples and instruments for psychotherapists. Some treatment manuals, particularly those coming from a cognitive behavioural perspective, present a highly systematized step-by-step programme which therapists follow over the course of therapy. The relative success of treatment manuals in standardizing psychotherapy has been supported by a meta-analysis,[7] which documented that studies employing treatment manuals had fewer outcome differences between therapists compared with studies that did not employ treatment manuals. Thus, when a treatment manual is used, therapists appear to produce relatively more uniform outcomes. In contrast, when no treatment manual is used, therapists differ considerably in their typical outcomes with patients; suggesting that different therapists are likely to be conducting sessions in discrepant ways, with some therapists producing more favourable outcomes and other therapists producing less favourable outcomes.

Treatment standardization, however, does not simply translate to the use of a treatment manual. A variety of steps are needed to ensure that therapists are delivering the intended treatment (Table 6.1.2.2), including: the careful selection of therapists; training of therapists in the intended modality using a treatment manual; certification of therapists based upon their adherence to the treatment model during training; and continuing adherence and competence monitoring of therapists during a clinical trial.

Concerns have been raised about the 'treatment manual' concept applied to less directive treatments such as psychodynamic therapy. The belief is that session-by-session manuals would remove the essence of good psychotherapy, and good dynamic therapy in particular, by making treatment artificially rigid and taking away the necessary clinical flexibility and creativity. Psychodynamic treatment manuals, however, are perhaps better described as 'guides', which specify the principles of treatment but do not overly constrain the necessary clinical flexibility and creativity. The flexibility of treatment is fully retained through the principle of

**Table 6.1.2.2** Steps involved in the standardization of psychotherapy for outcome research

| Selection of therapists |
| --- |
| Training of therapists using a treatment manual |
| Certification of therapists based upon adherence to the treatment model |
| Continued assessment of therapist adherence and competence during a clinical trial |

tailoring the treatment intervention to the specific idiosyncratic issues that are salient for each patient. The actual learning of the practice of treatment is accomplished through supervision in the application of the treatment manual. Because dynamic treatment manuals are less like 'cookbooks', there may be a greater reliance on the supervision process compared with perhaps more straightforward behavioural treatments.

## Research designs

Unlike pharmacological research where a single form of research design (placebo-controlled study) dominates the literature, psychotherapy researchers have employed a host of different research designs to understand the effects of psychotherapy. Some of the more common designs are listed in Table 6.1.2.3 and are explicated in the next section.

### Single-case designs

Clinical evaluation of the effects of psychotherapy dates back to Freud's descriptions of individual cases in treatment. However, methods to systematically examine the effects of interventions with individual patients were developed by behaviour therapists.[8] These single-case experiments rely on comparing patient responses to differing experimental conditions over time. Typically, such single-case studies begin with an extended baseline period where patient behaviours or symptoms are recorded without any intervention. Then, different intervention phases are introduced, usually followed by more baseline (no intervention) assessment phases.

While experimental, single-case designs lend themselves well to the investigation of behavioural treatments that include a focus on immediate overt behaviour, such designs have rarely been employed with other verbal psychotherapies that emphasize longer term processes such as patient psychological growth and functioning. The generalizability of findings from single-case research is another limitation to this form of research.

**Table 6.1.2.3** Common research designs for the evaluation of psychotherapy

| Single-case designs |
| --- |
| Randomized controlled trials with non-specific or psychological 'placebo' control |
| Comparative designs |
| Dismantling or additive designs |
| Comparisons with medication and pill placebos |
| Naturalistic designs |

## Randomized controlled trials

Random assignment of subjects to treatment and control conditions is generally viewed as the preferred method of evaluating the effects of interventions in psychiatry, and in medicine in general. However, perhaps the single most vexing problem in research of psychotherapy outcome is the design of control groups. In pharmacotherapy research, a pill placebo (with 'double blinding', i.e. the patient and the doctor are unaware of treatment assignment) serves to control for all elements of treatment except for the chemical ingredient of interest. Thus, the overall effects of treatment are the sum of the specific effect of the chemical agent plus the effects of 'extraneous' or non-specific factors such as patient expectancy, hope, and aspects of the doctor-patient relationship. With psychotherapeutic treatments, it is less clear which aspects of treatment are specific and which are non-specific. Furthermore, designing a credible control treatment that contains only the non-specific elements of the treatment package is inherently difficult.

### (a) Types of control groups

A variety of types of control conditions have been implemented in psychotherapy efficacy studies. One common form of control group is the 'waiting-list' control. Patients are randomly assigned to either the experimental group or to delayed treatment. While such a control condition appears to control for the passage of time (i.e. patients generally improve over time even without treatment), assignment to a waiting-list control condition is likely to immediately change patient hope and expectations about relief of their problem. Patients in the waiting-list condition will not expect to improve until they actually receive treatment, while patients assigned to the experimental condition will likely be more hopeful about change. Thus, the treatment and control conditions are not balanced with regard to expectancy or other non-specific factors such as regular meetings with a competent caring professional. The potential superiority of the experimental condition over the control condition cannot be attributed to the hypothesized active ingredients in the experimental condition. Nevertheless, such waiting-list controls can serve as a useful initial step in evaluating a treatment.

A scientifically stronger type of control group for psychotherapy evaluation studies is one that involves regular meetings with a psychotherapist, but does not contain certain important hypothesized active elements. Some forms of supportive psychotherapy have been used as a control group in this regard. For example, in evaluating the efficacy of cognitive behavioural therapy for posttraumatic stress reactions, a supportive therapy control condition has been successfully used.[9] With some psychotherapy treatments, however, the supportive elements are an important part of the overall treatment model and are hypothesized to be curative in their own right. In this case, a supportive psychotherapy control condition is not appropriate for evaluating the efficacy of the overall package. In fact, sometimes supportive therapy has been found to be superior to other therapies.[10]

## Comparative designs

An alternative to attempting to create an adequate psychological 'placebo' control is to only compare active treatments rather than comparing active treatments to 'placebo' control groups. However, rather than solve the problem of how to evaluate the efficacy of a psychotherapeutic intervention, comparative designs simply change the scientific question from 'Is this treatment efficacious?' to 'Which treatment works best?' Comparative designs are generally only informative if one active treatment proves to be more effective than another. If, as is commonly the case in psychotherapy studies, both active treatments produce equivalent results, the investigator is left not knowing whether both treatments are effective, or whether both treatments are non-effective (beyond the effects of non-specific elements).

## Dismantling designs

Dismantling designs are an alternative to psychological placebos, waiting lists, or comparative designs. In a dismantling design, the full clinical treatment package is compared with the full package minus one element in order to establish which elements are necessary and sufficient for change. Variations on this theme include 'additive' or constructive designs that examine whether adding a new element enhances the efficacy of a treatment package.

As an example, dismantling designs have been usefully applied in the evaluation of the behavioural treatment of obsessive-compulsive disorder. The full treatment package involving exposure and response prevention techniques has been compared with each of the individual components of the package.[11] Patients were randomly assigned to either the full exposure and response prevention package, exposure alone, or response prevention alone. Those receiving the full package improved significantly more than did the patients in either of the control treatments. At follow-up assessments, 80 per cent of patients receiving the full package remained improved at follow-up, whereas only 27 per cent of those in the single components groups remained 'improved'.

The advantage of dismantling strategies in psychotherapy research is clear. Causal statements about differences in improvement between treatment conditions can be made, since all factors (including non-specific elements) except one are held constant, and the problems involved in other types of control groups are avoided. These designs, in general, should probably be used more often than they are. Some psychotherapies, however, may not easily lend themselves to such dismantling strategies. Moreover, it may be premature to attempt to dismantle a treatment package when questions about the efficacy of the whole package need to be resolved first.

## Comparisons with medication

One type of design for the evaluation of psychotherapy that has increased in importance consists of comparisons to medication treatments. An example of this type of study is a recent investigation comparing cognitive therapy, medication (paroxetine), and pill placebo in the treatment of moderate to severe major depressive disorder.[12] The rationale for this design is that the medication group provides the standard reference condition with established efficacy. The pill-placebo group allows for establishing that the particular sample in the study showed the typical medication-placebo difference that would be expected (in other words, the sample was not unusual), and controls for some of the non-specific effects of the psychotherapy (for example, regular visits to a professional, positive expectancies for change). While the pill placebo is clearly not a perfect control condition for psychotherapy, it serves as a practical function—i.e. if a specific psychotherapy is not better than a pill placebo, should the psychotherapy be pursued as a treatment option?

## Attribute by treatment interactions

An emerging emphasis in psychotherapy outcome research is the investigation of attribute by treatment interactions. Partly influenced by the common finding of no differences between psychotherapies, as well as the desire to make more specific clinical recommendations, investigators have hypothesized that certain matches of client characteristics and treatment modalities produce superior outcomes. One initial problem with pursuing potential matches of patient characteristics with the type of treatment is that there are a large number of potential variables (for instance, various combinations of diagnosis, therapist, treatment, patient's problem, setting).

The investigation of patient-treatment matches has intuitive clinical appeal, as most therapists believe that some patients seem to 'fit' a form of treatment better than others. Research on patient-treatment matching, however, is inherently difficult, particularly because large sample sizes are generally needed to adequately test interaction effects. Two of the largest randomized clinical trials ever performed with psychotherapeutic treatments have failed to find much support for specified patient-treatment interactions.[13,14] Thus, it remains to be seen whether aptitude by treatment-interaction designs will provide useful information about psychotherapy outcome.

## Naturalistic studies

Naturalistic designs are used to examine issues such as the effectiveness of treatments in real-world setting with the types of patients that typically seek treatment. For example, the effectiveness of cognitive behavioural therapy for panic disorder and agoraphobia has been examined in a naturalistic study.[15] The authors report that outcomes were better for patients receiving naturalistic cognitive behaviour therapy, compared to a non-randomized wait-list control group. However, the overall outcomes for cognitive behavioural therapy were not as robust as previously seen in controlled clinical trials. While this form of naturalistic study has several advantages, including the fact that the data are drawn from actual clinical services in the real world, such data do not add to an understanding of which forms of psychotherapy work and which do not, and they do not provide strong causal statements. Hypotheses generated from naturalistic studies can inform the planning of experiments that can make stronger statements about causality. In addition, naturalistic studies provide useful descriptive information about the service delivery system.

## Strategies for assessing psychotherapy outcome

Once a particular experimental design has been decided upon, the next crucial question in evaluating psychotherapy pertains to the selection of instruments for the study. Instruments include those needed to adequately select a patient population, such as measures of psychiatric diagnoses and initial symptomatology. Therapeutic change is often evaluated on a broad range of measures including dimensional measures of symptoms, personality, self-esteem, quality of life, and functioning in a variety of areas (for example, social and occupational functioning). In addition, the impact of treatment on specific theoretical constructs (mediators) can be examined. Discussion of each of these domains follows.

## Patient selection

### (a) Diagnosis

Because the identification of effective therapies for specific disorders is an important research priority from a public health point of view, an accurate and thorough assessment of these disorders is central to the evaluation process. The most widely used instrument for assessing the major DSM-IV Axis I diagnoses in research settings is the Structured Clinical Interview for DSM-IV.[16] The format of this semi-structured interview, with questions grouped by criteria and by diagnosis, allows an experienced clinical evaluator to assign diagnosis as the interview progresses. It is most commonly used to select subjects according to study inclusion or exclusion criteria or to characterize a study population. It can also be used to document change in diagnostic status post-treatment or over the course of a longitudinal study.

### (b) Symptom measures

Whereas categorical measures are critical for the selection of a relatively homogeneous patient sample at intake, the evaluation of patient improvement requires the measurement of symptoms and functioning on a continuum. These continuous measures of the amount, timing, and nature of change are typically the primary outcomes of intervention studies. They include ratings of a single construct representing a core feature of the disorder, scales which cover the range of symptoms present in a general diagnostic category (e.g. rating scales of 'depression' or 'anxiety'), and measures that cut across many diagnoses and are indicative of overall psychopathology or symptomatology. At each of these levels of assessment, one can find both clinician-rated and self-report tools; for practical reasons, the self-report method predominates.

## Measures of therapeutic change

### (a) Dimensional assessment of core symptoms

In general, the more circumscribed and behavioural the problem, the simpler the assessment method. For some disorders, investigators have found that single-item measures of target symptoms suffice. For example, treatment studies of panic disorder and bulimia rely on self-reporting the number of 'episodes' that occur in a well-defined interval, such as the past week or the past month. Daily diaries are often used to facilitate recall and to enhance accuracy. Obsessive-compulsive symptoms can be assessed by Likert-type ratings of the severity of compulsions and obsessions, and the improvement of specific phobias by ratings of fear and avoidance. Severity ratings can be completed by both the patient and an independent evaluator.

For most disorders, core symptom measures of greater psychometric sophistication are needed to supplement simpler methods. The Penn State Worry Questionnaire,[17] for example, assesses the central feature of generalized anxiety disorder, and the Yale-Brown Obsessive-Compulsive Scale[18] measures the various symptoms that occur with obsessive compulsive disorder. In eating disorder research, the self-report EDI-2[19] and the Eating Disorder Examination[20] are commonly used.

In depression research, the Inventory of Depressive Symptomatology[21] is the result of efforts to develop a continuous measure of the nine DSM symptoms for major depressive episode. Other widely used scales include the interview-based Hamilton Rating Scale for Depression[22] and the self-report Beck Depression

Inventory,[23] although these instruments do not map directly on to DSM criteria. The severity of specific manic symptoms can be assessed with either the Bech-Rafaelsen Mania Scale[24] or the Young Mania Rating Scale.[25]

### (b) General measures of anxiety, depression, and other symptoms

The Hamilton Rating Scale for Depression and the Beck Depression Inventory are often administered concurrently to provide clinician and patient perspectives on the level of depression, and are used both as primary outcome measures in studies of depression, and as secondary measures in treatment studies of other disorders. Because of the comorbidity of Axis I disorders in general, and the interrelatedness of anxiety and depression in particular, it is useful to include assessments of both depression and anxiety. General measures of anxiety include the Hamilton Anxiety Rating Scale[26] and the Beck Anxiety Inventory.[27] These general measures are used with a variety of diagnostic groups, but it is important to remember that they have varying relevance to different disorders within a given diagnostic group. For example, a score on the Beck Anxiety Inventory might be a good index of the severity of the generalized anxiety disorder, but be less informative about specific phobias or obsessive-compulsive behaviour.

#### (i) Psychotic symptoms

In psychological treatment studies of severe depression, mania, and psychotic disorders, it is often necessary to assess the level of psychotic symptomatology. The Brief Psychiatric Rating Scale[28] is recommended for this purpose. It has items covering five symptom clusters: thinking disturbance, anxious depression, withdrawal/retardation, hostile/suspiciousness, and agitation/excitement. As with other clinician-rated scales, it should be administered by an experienced clinician who has received standardized training on this instrument.

#### (ii) Substance use problems

Because of the frequent comorbidity of substance use problems with other Axis I disorders, it is important to evaluate the level of drug and alcohol use when screening patients for study enrollment or when characterizing a sample. The substance use modules of the DSM-IV Structured Clinical Interview are frequently used for this purpose. The Addiction Severity Index[29] has the advantage of providing more comprehensive and detailed information on problem areas associated with abuse, and yields scores that can be compared across patients, and from the beginning to the end of treatment. Because it is a rather time-consuming interview, it is recommended only in instances when the rates of substance use and related problems are expected to be high and their measurement is a research priority.

### (c) Measure of global psychological functioning/ psychopathology

The rationale for using measures that cover a broad range of psychopathology is that they characterize the sample in terms of associated symptoms (i.e. symptoms other than those of primary interest) and provide a global measure of subjective distress. They have also proved to be quite useful in detecting treatment-related changes in evaluations of diverse psychotherapies. A popular self-report measure of general psychopathology is the SCL-90-R (and its abbreviated version, the Brief Symptom Inventory).[30] The SCL-90-R is a 90-item scale; the Brief Symptom Inventory is composed of 53 items. Both yield nine symptom dimensions and three global indices of distress. Because correlations between the two instruments are very high, it is recommended that the latter be

used when time is an issue or when this measure is included as part of a larger core battery of assessment.

### (d) Measures of self

Many psychotherapies explicitly attempt to improve self-esteem, self-concept, and self-confidence, and therefore it is relevant to examine the extent to which treatment successfully impacts on these domains. One of the oldest and most widely used measures of self-esteem is the Rosenberg Self-Esteem Scale,[31] an easily administered 10-item Likert-type scale yielding a uni-dimensional indicator of global self-esteem. More recent work in this area aims to distinguish other self-related constructs (such as self-concept) from self-esteem, develop more theoretically based multifactorial models, and improve upon the psychometrics of earlier measures. Some resulting scales, such as the Beck Self-Concept Test[32] or the Selves Questionnaire,[33] are appropriate for patients with a fairly wide range of psychiatric diagnoses.

### (e) Personality assessment

Personality variables typically appear in evaluations of psychological treatment as either primary outcomes (as in the study of psychotherapy for personality pathology), or as prognostic indicators in studies of other Axis I disorders. They might also be included as part of a larger effort to thoroughly describe the patient sample. There are two ways to approach the evaluation of personality within these contexts: determination of the presence or absence of a DSM personality disorder, and dimensional ratings of personality features.

#### (i) Categorical: DSM-IV Axis II

Treatments that target specific personality disorders tend to rely on the first approach to assessment, namely the use of interviewer-administered instruments which assess criteria for the 10 specific personality disorders listed in the DSM-IV. The Structured Clinical Interview for DSM-IV Axis II[34] was designed for this purpose. A positive feature of this assessment is its efficiency in eliciting the information required to assign Axis II diagnoses, especially when used in conjunction with the self-report Personality Disorder Questionnaire.

#### (ii) Dimensional

Dimensional methods of assessing personality arise from either theoretical or factor-analytical models of the essential elements of personality structure. The Five Factor Model[35] proposes that personality, in both patient and non-patient samples, can be measured along five dimensions: neuroticism, extraversion, openness to experience, agreeable, and conscientiousness. Extremes of these traits define personality pathology. This model and several instruments used to generate scores on these factors, including the self-report NEO Personality Inventory and NEO-PI-R[36] and a semistructured interview (the Structured Interview of the Five-Factor Model of Personality[37]), have received considerable empirical support in both clinical and non-clinical samples.

Another dimensional measure of personality is the SWAP-200.[38] This instrument consists of a set of 200 personality-descriptive statements designed to be used by a clinician who knows a given patient well. The clinician arranges the 200 statements into eight categories, from those that are not descriptive to those that are highly descriptive of the patient. These scores are then used to generate both individualized, ideographic case descriptions as well as dimensional scores for the 10 personality disorders included in DSM–IV.

The categorical and dimensional methods are not entirely mutually exclusive and both are valuable in ongoing research into the phenomenology, aetiology, correlates, and treatment of personality disorder.

### (f) Measures of functioning and quality of life

In recent years, the definition of mental health has been broadened to encompass its more positive, and somewhat paradoxically, its more negative aspects. Mental health is now viewed as more than the absence of illness, but the illness itself is increasingly seen as chronic and quite disabling. This has prompted investigators to turn their attention to outcomes other than symptom change—to evaluate fully the effectiveness of a psychotherapeutic intervention means to document its broad effect on a number of relevant domains including social/interpersonal functioning, work functioning, and quality of life.

#### (i) Overall functioning

Incorporated into the DSM system as a separate axis (Axis V), the Global Assessment of Functioning scale[39] (GAF) is the most widely used measure of psychosocial impairment. Clinicians rate on a scale of 1 to 100 the current level of functioning, or if desired, the highest or lowest level of functioning within some designated time period. General well being and functioning are also assessed with scales that have been developed for the routine outcome assessment in clinical practice, rather than for efficacy trials. An example is the OQ-45,[40] a self-report measure consisting of three subscales representing broad content areas: (1) symptom distress, (2) interpersonal relations, and (3) social role (dissatisfaction and distress in tasks related to work, family roles, and leisure life).

#### (ii) Social and occupational functioning

The assessment of role performance has a fairly long history in psychotherapy research. The Social Adjustment Scale (SAS)[41] was developed to document the level in functioning in six areas: work as worker, 'housewife', or student; social activities; relationship with family; relationship with spouse; parental responsibilities; member of a family unit. There is much documentation of its psychometric properties and clinical utility, and it has been used with a wide range of adult outpatients. A unique feature of the Longitudinal Interval Follow-up Evaluation (LIFE)[42] is that it was designed to collect information on psychosocial functioning (as well as on diagnosis and symptoms) over longer periods of time. In the hands of trained evaluators, it is a structured interview that has been shown to have good reliability.

The concern among both scientists and health-care managers about the cost-effectiveness of specific treatments has generated interest in more comprehensive assessments of work functioning and productivity. Endicott and Nee developed the Endicott Work Productivity Scale,[43] a self-report instrument containing 25 items designed to be sensitive to more subtle differences among patients in work attitudes and behaviour.

Two self-report instruments measuring interpersonal difficulties have been used in studies of psychotherapy: The Inventory of Interpersonal Problems[44] and the Dyadic Adjustment Scale.[45] The Inventory of Interpersonal Problems is a 127-item self-report measure with high internal consistency and test-retest reliability of each of the six subscales: assertive, social, intimate, submissive, responsible, and controlling. The Dyadic Adjustment Scale is a 32-item scale designed to assess the severity of relationship discord in married and unmarried cohabiting couples, with higher scores indicating better adjustment. Responses on the Dyadic Adjustment Scale discriminate between distressed and non-distressed couples and yield a total score based on the factors of dyadic consensus, dyadic cohesion, dyadic satisfaction, and affectional expression.

#### (iii) Quality of life

The most promising of the quality-of-life measures for mental health outcome research are those based on a broad definition of quality of life—covering role functioning and social-material conditions as well as life satisfaction or well being—and which can be applied across disorders and across treatments. However, more widespread use and testing of quality-of-life instruments is needed to establish their utility and to help resolve a number of important measurement issues, including the value of more 'objective' indices of quality of life and the relationship between symptoms and quality-of-life judgments.

### (g) Utilization of treatment services

The impact of a treatment on usage of other health-related services is a factor to be considered in determining the cost-effectiveness of that treatment. One broad instrument designed to assess changes in service usage over the course of treatment is the Treatment Services Review.[46] This is a 5-minute interview that documents the number and types of treatment services received during rehabilitation from substance abuse, but it also can be adapted for use with other clinical populations.

### (h) Theory-based measures

Evaluation of the hypothesized important psychological constructs of a particular psychotherapy can serve as outcome measures in their own right or as mediators of change in symptoms and functioning. For example, the cognitive model of depression holds that distorted cognitions about the self and world are responsible for generating and maintaining negative emotions. Measures of depressogenic cognitions are therefore included as outcomes and mediators of symptom change in studies of cognitive therapy for depression. The Hopelessness Scale[47] is a 20-item self-report scale that assesses the hopelessness and pessimism associated with suicidal ideation and intent. The Dysfunctional Attitudes Scale[48] is a 40-item index of general attitudes and beliefs hypothesized by Beck and colleagues to underlie a propensity for depressive thinking, whereas the Automatic Thoughts Questionnaire[49] covers 30 negative thoughts proposed to occur during a symptomatic depressed state.

In regard to psychodynamic psychotherapy, theory-specific mediators include measures of core conflicts[50] and self-understanding.[51]

## Conclusions

Of all the treatments in medicine and psychiatry in particular, the evaluation of psychotherapy offers some of the greatest challenges to researchers. A wide variety of research designs and instruments have been employed, with distinct advantages and disadvantages to each. No one study of psychotherapy can answer all the important questions that need to be asked. Given the complexity of research on psychotherapy, knowledge accumulates slowly. Despite the problems, complexities, and slow pace of scientific advance, psychotherapy outcome research now has the tools and emerging findings to begin to influence the practice of psychotherapy and mental health treatments in general. We expect that in the next decade methodological advances in the evaluation of psychotherapy will lead to a stronger link between research and practice.

## Further informaion

Lambert, M. (2004). *Bergin and Garfield's handbook of psychotherapy and behavior change* (5th edn). John Wiley and Sons, New York.

Society for Psychotherapy Research. http://www.psychotherapyresearch.org

Rush, A.J. (2007). *Handbook of psychiatric measures* (2nd edn). American Psychiatric Publishing, Washington, DC.

## References

1. Eysenck, H.J. (1952). The effects of psychotherapy: an evaluation. *Journal of Consulting Psychology*, **16**, 319–24.

2. Smith, M.L., Glass, G.V., and Miller, T.I. (1980). *The benefits of psychotherapy*. Johns Hopkins University Press, Baltimore, MD.

3. Castonguay, L.G., and Beutler, L.E. (2006). (eds). *Principles of therapeutic change that work*. Oxford University Press, New York.

4. Nathan, P., and Gorman, J. (in press) (eds.). *Treatments that Work*, Oxford Unversity Press (3rd edn.), New York.

5. Kazdin, A. (1994). Methodology, design, and evaluation in psychotherapy research. In *Handbook of psychotherapy and behavior change* (ed. A.E. Bergin and S.L. Garfield), pp. 19–71. Wiley, New York.

6. Crits-Christoph, P. and Gallop, R. (2006). Therapist effects in the TDCRP and other psychotherapy studies. *Psychotherapy Research*, **16**, 178–81.

7. Crits–Christoph, P., Baramackie, K., Kurcias, J., et al. (1991). Meta-analysis of therapist effects in psychotherapy outcome studies. *Psychotherapy Research*, **1**, 81–91.

8. Kazdin, A. (1982). *Single–case research designs: methods for clinical and applied settings*. Oxford University Press, New York.

9. Blanchard, E.B., Hickling, E.J., Devineni, T., et al. (2003). A controlled evaluation of cognitive behavioral therapy for posttraumatic stress in motor vehicle accident survivors. *Behaviour Research and Therapy* **41**, 79–96.

10. McIntosh, V.V., Jordan, J., Carter, FA., et al. (2005). Three psychotherapies for anorexia nervosa: a randomized, controlled trial. *American Journal of Psychiatry*, **162**, 741–7.

11. Foa, E., Steketee, G., Grayson, J., et al. (1984). Deliberate exposure and blocking of obsessive–compulsive rituals: immediate and long-term effects. *Behavior Therapy*, **15**, 450–72.

12. DeRubeis, R.J., Hollon, S.D., Amsterdam, J.D., et al. *(2005)*. Cognitive therapy vs medications in the treatment of moderate to severe depression. *Archives of General Psychiatry*, **62**, 409–16.

13. Project MATCH Research Group (1997). Matching Alcoholism Treatments to Client Heterogeneity: Project MATCH posttreatment drinking outcomes. *Journal of Studies on Alcohol*, **58**, 7–29.

14. Crits–Christoph, P., Sigueland, L., Blaine, J., et al. (1999). Psychosocial treatments for cocaine dependence: National Institute on Drug Abuse Collaborative Cocaine Treatment Study. *Archives of General Psychiatry*, **56**, 493–502.

15. Rosenberg, N.K., and Hougaard E. (2005). Cognitive behavioural group treatment of panic disorder and agoraphobia in a psychiatric setting: A naturalistic study of effectiveness. *Nordic Journal of Psychiatry*. **59**, 198–204.

16. First, M.B., Spitzer, R.L., Gibbon, M., et al. (1994). *Structured Clinical Interview for Axis–I DSM–IV Disorders. Patient edition (SCID-II, version 2.0)*. Biometrics Research Department, New York State Psychiatric Institute.

17. Meyer, T.J., Miller, M.L., Metzger, R.L., et al. (1990). Development and validation of the Penn State Worry Questionnaire. *Behavior Research and Therapy*, **28**, 487–95.

18. Goodman, W.M., Price, L.H., Rasmussen, C.A., et al. (1989). The Yale–Brown Obsessive–Compulsive Scale. I: development, use, and reliability. *Archives of General Psychiatry*, **46**, 1006–11.

19. Garner, D.M. (1991). *Eating Disorder Inventory–2 manual*. Psychological Assessment Resources, Odessa, FL.

20. Fairburn, C. G., and Cooper, Z. (1993).The Eating Disorder Examination (12th edn.). In *Binge eating: Nature, assessment, and treatment* (eds. C.G.Fairburn and G.T. Wilson) pp. 317–60. Guilford Press, New York.

21. Rush, A.J., Carmody, T.J., Ibrahim, H.M., et al. (2006). Comparison of self-report and clinician ratings on two inventories of depressive symptomatology. *Psychiatric Services*, **57**, 829–37.

22. Hamilton, M. (1960). A rating scale for depression. *Journal of Neurological and Neurosurgical Psychiatry*, **23**, 56–62.

23. Beck, A.T., Steer, R.A., and Brown, G.K. (1996). *BDI-II manual* (2nd edn). Psychological Corporation, San Antonio, TX.

24. Bech P. (2002). The Bech-Rafaelsen Mania Scale in clinical trials of therapies for bipolar disorder: a 20-year review of its use as an outcome measure. *CNS Drugs*, **16**, 47–63.

25. Young, R.C., Biggs, J.T., Ziegler, V.E., et al. (1978). A rating scale for mania: reliability, validity and sensitivity. *British Journal of Psychiatry*, **133**, 429–35.

26. Hamilton, M. (1959). The assessment of anxiety states by rating. *British Journal of Medical Psychology*, **32**, 50–5.

27. Steer, R.A., Beck, A.T. (1997). In *Evaluating stress: A book of resources* (eds. C.P. Zalaquett and R.J Wood), pp. 23–40. Scarecrow Education, Lanham, MD.

28. Thomas, A., Donnell, A.J., and Young, T.R. (2004). Factor structure and differential validity of the expanded Brief Psychiatric Rating Scale. *Assessment*, **11**, 177–87.

29. McLellan, A.T., Kushner, H., Metzger, D. et al. (1992). The fifth edition of the addiction severity index: historical critique and normative data, *Journal of Substance Abuse Treament*, **9**, 199–213.

30. Derogatis, L.R., and Fitzpatrick, M. (2004). The SCL-90-R, the Brief Symptom Inventory (BSI), and the BSI-18 In *The use of psychological testing for treatment planning and outcomes assessment: Volume 3: Instruments for adults* (3rd edn.) (ed. M.E. Maruish). (pp. 1–41). Lawrence Erlbaum Associates Publishers, Mahwah, NJ.

31. Rosenberg, M. (1965). *Society and the adolescent self-image*. Princeton University Press.

32. Beck, A.T., Steer, R.A., Brown, G., et al. (1990). The Beck Self-Concept Test. *Psychological Assessment: A Journal of Consulting and Clinical Psychology*, **2**, 191–7.

33. Higgins, E.T., Bond, R.N., Klein, R., et al. (1986). Self-discrepancies and emotional vulnerability: how magnitude, accessibility, and type of discrepancy influence affect. *Journal of Personality and Social Psychology*, **51**, 5–15.

34. First, M.B., Spitzer, R.L., Gibbon, M., et al. (1994). *Structured Clinical Interview for DSM-IV Axis-II Personality Disorders (SCID-II, version 2.0)*. Biometrics Research Department, New York State Psychiatric Institute.

35. McCrae, R.R., and Costa, P.T. (2003). *Personality in adulthood: A five-factor theory perspective* (2nd edn.) Guilford Press, New York, NY.

36. McCrae, R.R., and Costa, P. T. (2005). The NEO-PI-3: A More Readable Revised NEO Personality Inventory. *Journal of Personality Assessment*, **84**, 261–70.

37. Trull, T.J., and Widiger, T.A. (2002). The structured interview for the five factor model of personality (SIFFM) In *Big five assessment* (eds. B. de Raad & M. Perugini). (pp. 148–66). Ashland, OH: Hogrefe & Huber Publishers.

38. Westen, D., and Muderrisoglu, S. (2006). Clinical assessment of pathological personality traits. *American Journal of Psychiatry*, **163**, 1285–7.

39. American Psychiatric Association (1994). *Diagnostic and statistical manual of mental disorders* (4th edn). American Psychiatric Association, Washington, DC.

40. Lambert., M.J., Gregersen A.T., and Burlingame, G.M. (2004). The Outcome Questionnaire-45. In *The use of psychological testing for treatment planning and outcomes assessment: Volume 3: Instruments for adults* (3rd edn) (ed. M.E. Maruish), pp. 191–234. Mahwah, NJ: Lawrence Erlbaum Associates Publishers.

41. Weissman, M.M., Klerman, G.L., Paykel, E.S., *et al.* (1974). Treatment effects in the social adjustment of depressed patients. *Archives of General Psychiatry*, **30**, 771–8.

42. Keller, M.B., Lavori, P.W., Friedman, B., *et al.* (1987). The longitudinal interval follow-up evaluation: a comprehensive method for assessing outcome in prospective longitudinal studies. *Archives of General Psychiatry*, **44**, 540–8.

43. Endicott, J. and Nee, J. (1997). Endicott Work Productivity Scale (EWPS): a new measure to assess treatment effects. *Psychopharmacology Bulletin*, **33**, 13–16.

44. Horowitz, L.M., Rosenberg, S.E., Baer, B.A, *et al.* (1988). Inventory of Interpersonal Problems: psychometric properties and clinical applications. *Journal of Consulting and Clinical Psychology*, **56**, 885–92.

45. Spanier, G.B. (1976). Measuring dyadic adjustment: new scales for assessing the quality of marriage and similar dyads. *Journal of Marital and Family Therapy*, **38**, 15–38.

46. McLellan, A.T., Alterman, A.I., Cacciola, J., *et al.* (1992). A new measure of substance abuse treatment. Initial studies of the treatment services review. *Journal of Nervous and Mental Disease*, **180**, 101–10.

47. Beck, A.T. and Steer, R.A. (1988). *Manual for Beck Hopelessness Scale*. Psychological Corporation, San Antonio, TX.

48. Weissman, A.N. (1979).The dysfunctional attitudes scale: a validation study. *Dissertation Abstracts International*, **40**, 1389–90.

49. Hollon, S.D. and Kendall, P.C. (1980). Cognitive self-statements in depression: development of an automatic thoughts questionnaire. *Cognitive Therapy and Research*, **4**, 88–100.

50. Luborsky, L. and Crits–Christoph, P. (1998). *Understanding transference: the core conflictual relationship theme method*. American Psychological Association, Washington, DC.

51. Connolly, M.B., Crits–Christoph, P., Shelton, R.C., *et al.* (1999). The reliability and validity of a measure of self–understanding of interpersonal patterns. *Journal of Counseling Psychology*, **46**, 472–82.

**6.2**

# Somatic treatments

## Contents

6.2.1 General principles of drug therapy in psychiatry
J. K. Aronson

6.2.2 Anxiolytics and hypnotics
Malcolm Lader

6.2.3 Antidepressants
Zubin Bhagwagar and George R. Heninger

6.2.4 Lithium and related mood stabilizers
Robert M. Post

6.2.5 Antipsychotic and anticholinergic drugs
Herbert Y. Meltzer and William V. Bobo

6.2.6 Antiepileptic drugs
Brian P. Brennan and Harrison G. Pope, Jr

6.2.7 Drugs for cognitive disorders
Leslie Iversen

6.2.8 Drugs used in the treatment of the addictions
Fergus D. Law and David J. Nutt

6.2.9 Complementary medicines
Ursula Werneke

6.2.10 Non-pharmacological somatic treatments
  6.2.10.1 Electroconvulsive therapy
    Max Fink
  6.2.10.2 Phototherapy
    Philip J. Cowen
  6.2.10.3 Transcranial magnetic stimulation
    Declan McLoughlin and Andrew Mogg
  6.2.10.4 Neurosurgery for psychiatric disorders
    Keith Matthews and David Christmas

## 6.2.1 General principles of drug therapy in psychiatry

J. K. Aronson

The successful use of psychotropic drugs demands an understanding of their pharmaceutical, pharmacokinetic, and pharmacodynamic properties.

- *Pharmaceutical properties*: Pharmaceutical formulations can be manipulated to produce different durations of action, for example the use of oily emulsions of antipsychotic drugs in depot formulations.

- *Pharmacokinetic properties*: Pharmacokinetics is the mathematical description of the disposition of drugs in the body by absorption, distribution (to plasma proteins and tissues), and elimination (usually by hepatic metabolism and renal excretion). Differences in drug disposition determine differences in dosage regimens and are important for drug interactions.

- *Pharmacodynamic properties*: Pharmacodynamics is the study of the pharmacological actions of drugs and how actions at the molecular level are translated, via actions at cellular, tissue, and organ levels, into therapeutic or adverse effects. The known pharmacological actions of psychotropic drugs are not necessarily the actions that produce their therapeutic or adverse effects.

### Dosage regimens

A drug dosage regimen is a recipe for drug administration, intended to produce the desired therapeutic effect with a minimum of unwanted effects. It is described in terms of the pharmaceutical formulation, the dose, and the frequency and route of administration used. The duration of administration is also important.

In treating any condition, it is best to learn initially to use a few drugs, preferably well-established ones, and to expand one's repertoire with increasing experience.

The choice of drug depends firstly on the indication—obviously an antidepressant will be the drug of choice for a patient with depression, if drug therapy is thought to be required. The choice of antidepressant will depend on features of the disease and other factors. For example, some antidepressants are more sedative and anxiolytic than others, and can be helpful in patients who are agitated. The avoidance of adverse effects or interactions can also dictate the choice; for example, tricyclic antidepressants should be avoided in men with prostatic hyperplasia and selective serotonin reuptake inhibitors (SSRIs) should not be used in children, because of the increased risk of suicidal ideation.

It is usual to start therapy with published dosage recommendations, generally beginning at the lower end of the recommended dosage range and monitoring for a therapeutic effect. A common error is to give a starting dose of a drug and then to add or substitute another drug if the first does not work. This is usually bad practice. If the desired effect does not occur with the initial dosage, increase the dose gradually until the effect occurs or the upper limit of the recommended range is reached (although adverse effects may limit this process). Only then should another drug be tried. Sometimes a poor response is due to poor adherence to therapy; careful explanation of the condition and the need for therapy helps.

Psychotropic drugs can be given orally or parenterally, and as immediate-release or modified-release formulations. Most drug administration is oral, but parenteral therapy can be useful to guarantee administration (e.g. depot formulations in schizophrenia) and for a quicker onset of action (e.g. in the treatment of acute mania). Modified-release products are used for long-term therapy. They can be given less often and produce a smoother profile of blood concentrations (Fig. 6.2.1.1).[1] The advantage of intramuscular modified-release (depot) formulations of antipsychotic drugs is that drug delivery can be ensured by supervised infrequent administration (say every 2 weeks). Different modified-release formulations of the same compounds have different release characteristics and are not interchangeable; for example, when prescribing a modified-release oral formulation of lithium always give the patient the same formulation and specify the brand name on the prescription.

Combination formulations (e.g. a phenothiazine plus a tricyclic antidepressant in a single tablet) do not allow flexibility of prescribing and should generally be avoided. Important exceptions include combination analgesic formulations (e.g. co-codamol, which contains paracetamol plus codeine) and combinations of levodopa with a dopa decarboxylase inhibitor (benserazide or carbidopa).

## Treatment of children

There are no uniform rules for determining dosage regimens in children. Pharmacokinetics and pharmacodynamics are different for some drugs but not others.

- Absorption is not greatly different from absorption in adults.
- The distribution of water-soluble drugs is different, but psychotropic drugs are lipid-soluble.
- Protein binding is reduced in neonates; phenytoin is affected.
- Hepatic oxidative metabolism and glucuronide conjugation are deficient in neonates, and mature at variable rates; this is important for psychotropic drugs.
- Glomerular and renal tubular functions are immature in neonates and take about 6 months to reach adult values.

If a child needs a psychotropic drug, consult the manufacturer's literature and always start with a low dosage.

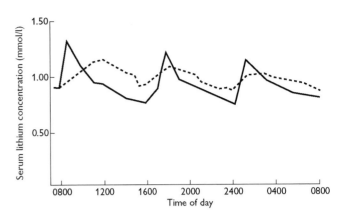

**Fig. 6.2.1.1** Administration of lithium in immediate-release and modified-release oral formulations. The immediate-release formulation (solid line) produces rapid peaks of serum concentration and large fluctuations during a dosage interval. In contrast, the modified-release formulation (dotted line) is more slowly absorbed but produces much less fluctuation in serum concentrations. Note also that the apparent half-life of lithium is longer after administration of the modified-release formulation; this is not the true half-life of lithium, but the half-life of its release from the modified-release formulation. (Adapted from A. Amdisen, Variation of serum lithium concentration during the day in relation to treatment control, absorptive side effects and the use of slow-release tablets, *Acta Psychiatrica Scandinavica*, **207**, 55–7, copyright 1969, John Wiley & Sons, Inc.)

## Treatment of elderly people

Pharmacokinetic differences in old age are more predictable than in children, but pharmacodynamic changes are variable.

- Absorption is not greatly affected.
- Elderly people have less body fat, and so lipid-soluble drugs may be more highly concentrated in the brain; however, this effect varies unpredictably from drug to drug (e.g. the apparent volume of distribution of diazepam is increased while that of nitrazepam is not).
- Protein binding is reduced in elderly people; phenytoin is affected.
- Hepatic metabolism is reduced in frail but not in fit old people; this effect is proportional to liver size.
- Renal function is impaired with age; use creatinine clearance, measured or estimated (not eGFR), as a guide.
- Inappropriate polypharmacy is common in old people, increasing the risk of drug interactions.

When treating an elderly person with a psychotropic drug always start with a low dosage and increase dosages more slowly.

## Pregnancy and breast feeding

Anticonvulsants are teratogenic.[2] For example, sodium valproate has been associated with spina bifida, cardiac malformations, hypospadias, anomalies of the brain and face, coarctation of the aorta, and limb reduction defects.[3]

Few other psychoactive drugs are teratogenic. However, most of them cross the placenta and some can cause withdrawal symptoms in the neonate. The teratogenicity of lithium has been overstated in the past; the main risk is cardiovascular teratogenicity, but although the risk of Ebstein's anomaly is increased, the absolute risk (0.05–0.1 per cent) is still very small;[4] nevertheless, some advise that it should be avoided or used with caution in the first trimester of pregnancy,[5] and fetal sonography is recommended at 18–20 weeks after first-trimester exposure.[3]

Although most psychoactive drugs are lipid-soluble and therefore enter the breast milk, few do so in high enough amounts to trouble the neonate; if a neonate becomes drowsy while breast feeding, reduce the mother's dosage or stop breast feeding. Lithium appears in the breast milk and can be found in the serum of breast-fed babies in variable concentrations, up to half of those in the mother. Because neonates have immature renal function, some recommend avoiding breast feeding.[6] However, others consider that the benefits of breast feeding to mother and child outweigh the small risk of lithium toxicity.[4] The following advice has been given:[3]

- Educate the mother about the manifestations of toxicity.

- Explain the risks of dehydration.

- Consider partial or total formula supplements during episodes of illness or dehydration.

- Suspend breast feeding if toxicity is suspected.

- Check infant and maternal serum concentrations.

## Pharmacokinetics—drug disposition

Most psychotropic drugs are rapidly and well absorbed after oral administration. However, drugs can be removed by various processes before they reach the systemic circulation. The fraction of drug that reaches the systemic circulation is called its systemic availability (or, more commonly, bioavailability).

After oral administration a formulation will generally disintegrate in the stomach and the drug it contains will dissolve in gastric contents. However, drugs are not generally absorbed in the stomach. After gastric emptying they are for the most part absorbed in the jejunum and ileum, and some are absorbed from the colon as well. During transit across the gut wall they may be metabolized by an oxidative isozyme of cytochrome P450, CYP3A4, and can be secreted back into the gut lumen by P glycoprotein. When they enter the portal circulation they may be eliminated by the liver. If hepatic metabolism is extensive, a large amount of drug will be removed during this first passage through the liver. For example, clomethiazole has extensive first-pass metabolism in the liver and its systemic availability is low (about 40 per cent); thus, intravenous doses are considerably lower than oral doses. In severe liver disease, such as cirrhosis, or when there is arteriovenous shunting, this presystemic metabolism is reduced and the systemic availability increases up to 90 per cent; oral doses of clomethiazole should be reduced in liver disease.[7]

In the systemic circulation drugs are bound to plasma proteins and distributed to the tissues. Protein binding is important for drugs that are highly bound (over 90 per cent) and not widely distributed to the body tissues; in those cases protein-binding displacement can result in a large rise in the amount of unbound drug available to the target tissue. This is important for phenytoin, which is 90 per cent bound to plasma albumin and has a low volume of distribution. The binding of phenytoin is reduced when the serum albumin concentration falls (in chronic liver disease, the nephrotic syndrome, protein malnutrition, or the third trimester of pregnancy), when binding to the protein is abnormal (in chronic renal insufficiency), or when another drug (e.g. sodium valproate) causes displacement. Acute displacement causes phenytoin toxicity, but only

transiently, because in the case of phenytoin an increase in unbound concentration causes it to be more rapidly eliminated. When measuring plasma phenytoin concentrations in patients in whom protein binding is reduced, the target concentration (and the laboratory will measure total drug, i.e. bound plus unbound) is reduced (see Fig. 6.2.1.2).

In chronic renal insufficiency the protein binding of phenytoin is reduced. This leads to an increase in the unbound plasma (or serum) concentration relative to the total concentration; the target total concentration therefore falls. The shaded area shows the range of plasma phenytoin concentrations that one would generally aim to achieve (the target concentration range) in treating a patient with epilepsy. As renal function deteriorates (indicated here by an increase in serum creatinine concentration), the target range for plasma phenytoin concentration falls from 40–80 µmol/l when renal function is normal to 10–30 µmol/l in severe renal insufficiency.

After absorption and distribution most psychoactive drugs are cleared from the body by hepatic metabolism;[8] impaired liver function, if severe (for the liver has a large capacity), reduces their elimination, and dosages should be reduced.

Lithium is cleared solely by renal elimination and therefore the dosage should be reduced in proportion to the creatinine clearance. Since renal function falls with age, lithium dosages should be lower in older people.[9]

The half-life of a drug is a function of its clearance and its distribution volume: the slower the rate of clearance or the more extensive the distribution the longer the half-life. If a drug is given in a regular maintenance dose, the amount of drug in the body will gradually accumulate; however, as the amount in the body increases, the rate at which it is eliminated also rises, and eventually a plateau (or steady state) is reached when the amount eliminated during a dosage interval equals the dose (the maintenance dose). The time it takes to reach this steady state depends on the half-life

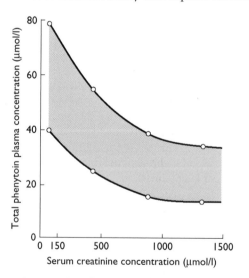

**Fig. 6.2.1.2** In chronic renal insufficiency the protein binding of phenytoin is reduced. This leads to an increase in the unbound plasma (or serum) concentration relative to the total concentration; the target total concentration therefore falls. The shaded area shows the range of plasma phenytoin concentrations that one would generally aim to achieve (the target concentration range) in treating a patient with epilepsy. As renal function deteriorates (indicated here by an increase in serum creatinine concentration) the target range for plasma phenytoin concentration falls, from 40–80 µmol/l when renal function is normal to 10–30 µmol/l in severe renal insufficiency (I. Odar-Cederlöf, unpublished data.)

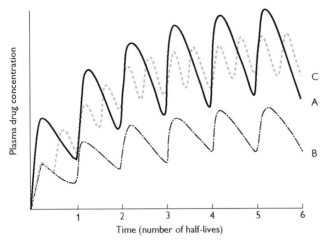

**Fig. 6.2.1.3** Curve A—during the regular administration of a maintenance dose of a drug the amount of drug in the body rises after a dose, reaches a peak, and then falls as the drug is distributed to the tissues and eliminated. If another dose is given soon after the first, the plasma concentration will rise by the same amount as before but will fall faster after peaking, since most drugs obey first-order kinetics and the plasma concentration falls exponentially. Thus, when a drug is given repeatedly the mean plasma concentration rises more slowly with each successive dose, until eventually a steady state is reached, when the amount eliminated in a dosage interval is equal to the dose itself. This takes about four half-lives of the drug. Curve B represents the concentrations during administration of half the dose given at the same frequency. The time taken to reach steady state is the same in both cases, but the eventual steady-state concentration in case B is half that in case A, being proportional to the dose. Curve C represents the concentrations during administration of half the dose given twice as often (i.e. the total dose is unchanged). Neither the time taken to reach steady state nor the eventual mean steady-state concentration is affected. However, the fluctuations in plasma concentration during a dosage interval are reduced (cf. Fig. 6.2.1.1). (Adapted from Amdisen, A. Variation of serum lithium concentration during the day in relation to treatment control, absorptive side effects and the use of slow-release tablets, *Acta Psychiatrica Scandinavica*, **207**, 55–57. Copyright 1969, John Wiley & Sons, Inc.)

of the drug; about 94 per cent of the steady-state value will be reached after four half-lives (Fig. 6.2.1.3, curve A). For example, lithium has a half-life of about 24 h; after 4 days of maintenance therapy with the same regular dose a steady state will be reached; this does not depend on the dose or frequency of administration (Fig. 6.2.1.3, curves B and C). If a modified-release formulation is used and the half-life of absorption of the drug from the formulation is longer than the drug's own half-life, the longer (apparent) half-life will determine the time to steady state; for example, the apparent half-life of flupentixol after the administration of flupentixol decanoate is 17 days, compared with 36 h for flupentixol after oral administration. When using depot antipsychotic drugs, which have long half-lives of absorption, steady-state therapy should first be established with an ordinary formulation.

Curve A shows that during the regular administration of a maintenance dose of a drug the amount of drug in the body rises after a dose, reaches a peak, and then falls as the drug is distributed to the tissues and eliminated. If another dose is given soon after the first, the plasma concentration will rise by the same amount as before but will fall faster after peaking, since most drugs obey first-order kinetics and the plasma concentration falls exponentially. Thus, when a drug is given repeatedly the mean plasma concentration rises more slowly with each successive dose, until eventually a steady state is reached, when the amount eliminated in a dosage

interval is equal to the dose itself. This takes about four half-lives of the drug. Curve B represents the concentrations during administration of half the dose given at the same frequency. The time taken to reach steady state is the same in both cases, but the eventual steady-state concentration in case B is half that in case A, being proportional to the dose. Curve C represents the concentrations during administration of half the dose given twice as often (i.e. the total dose is unchanged). Neither the time taken to reach steady state nor the eventual mean steady-state concentration is affected. However, the fluctuations in plasma concentration during a dosage interval are reduced (cf. Fig. 6.2.1.1). Kinetic characteristics of some psychotropic drugs are shown in Table 6.2.1.1.

## Pharmacological actions of drugs

Psychotropic drugs interfere with neurotransmitter functions in several ways—via actions on neurotransmitter receptors, storage, release, reuptake, and metabolism. Transmembrane neurotransmitter receptors are broadly speaking of two types—ionotropic and metabotropic receptors. Ionotropic receptors (e.g. nicotinic acetylcholine, glycine, GABA, and NMDA, AMPA, and kainate receptors) incorporate ion channels in their structures and mediate rapid responses. Metabotropic receptors (e.g. G protein-coupled receptors such as adrenaline, noradrenaline, cannabinoid, dopamine, opioid, and serotonin receptors other than $5HT_3$ receptors) produce their effects via signal transduction systems, which activate second messengers or ion channels, and produce longer lasting responses.

### Agonist action at a receptor

Agonists are substances that act by stimulating the action of a receptor.

Benzodiazepines bind to benzodiazepine receptors in the spinal cord, brainstem, cerebellum, limbic system, and cerebral cortex. These receptors are associated with receptors for the inhibitory neurotransmitter γ-aminobutyric acid (GABA), linked to a chloride channel.[10] The benzodiazepines enhance the action of GABA through its chloride channel, the presumed mechanism whereby they are anxiolytic and hypnotic. Some other hypnotics that have non-benzodiazepine structures also act via benzodiazepine receptors: zopiclone binds to the GABA–benzodiazepine receptor complex, but at a site different from that of benzodiazepines;[11] clomethiazole binds to a binding site distinct from those of benzodiazepines and barbiturates;[12] zolpidem binds to a subtype of binding site called $BZ_1$, found on GABA neurones in the sensorimotor cortex and extrapyramidal tracts.[10]

The triptans (such as sumatriptan, naratriptan, zolmitriptan), which are used to treat migraine, are agonists at 5-hydroxytryptamine ($5\text{-HT}_{1B/D}$) receptors, causing vasoconstriction. They are therefore contraindicated in patients with cardiovascular disease and in those with hemiplegic or basilar migraine because of the fear of stroke.[13]

### Antagonist action at a receptor

Antagonists are substances that have no actions of their own at receptors and act by preventing the action of an agonist, usually an endogenous one.

The antipsychotic (neuroleptic) drugs are all antagonists at receptors for the endogenous neurotransmitter dopamine; this is thought to be the basis of their antipsychotic actions in the mesolimbic system (via $D_1$ and $D_4$ receptors) and undoubtedly produces their

**Table 6.2.1.1** Pharmacokinetic information about some psychotropic drugs

| Drug | Systemic availability (%) | Half-life (h) | Route of hepatic elimination[a] |
|---|---|---|---|
| **Benzodiazepines** | | | |
| Alprazolam | 90 | 12 | CYP3A |
| Chlordiazepoxide[b] | 95 | 15 | |
| Clobazam[b] | 90 | 20 | |
| Diazepam[b] | 100 | 30 | CYP2E1/2C19 |
| Flurazepam[b] | 30 | 3 | CYP2E1 |
| Lorazepam | 90 | 15 | |
| Nitrazepam | 75 | 24 | |
| Oxazepam | 100 | 9 | |
| Temazepam | 95 | 10 | |
| **Antidepressants** | | | |
| Lithium | 100 | 24 | (Renally excreted) |
| *Tricyclics* | | | |
| Amitriptyline | 50 | 20 | CYP1A2/2D6 |
| Clomipramine | 50 | 20 | CYP1A2/2D6/2C19 |
| Desipramine | 40 | 24 | CYP2D6 |
| Imipramine[b] | 50 | 14 | CYP1A2/2D6 |
| Nortriptyline | 60 | 36 | CYP2D6 |
| *Tetracyclics* | | | |
| Maprotiline | 95 | 40 | |
| Mianserin | 25 | 16 | CYP2D6 |
| *Triazolopyridines* | | | |
| Trazodone | 100 | 10 | |
| *Selective serotonin reuptake inhibitors* | | | |
| Fluoxetine | 95 | 48 | CYP2D6/3A4 |
| Fluvoxamine | 90 | 20 | CYP1A2/2C19/3A4 |
| Paroxetine | Variable | 24 | CYP2D6 |
| Sertraline | Low | 24 | CYP2D6 |
| *Monoamine oxidase inhibitors* | | | |
| Phenelzine | High | 1 | Polymorphically acetylated |
| Tranylcypromine | Moderate | 2 | |
| Moclobemide | 40 | 2 | CYP2C19 |
| **Antipsychotic drugs** | | | |
| *Phenothiazines* | | | |
| Chlorpromazine[b] | 10 | 12 | |
| Thioridazine | 60 | 10 | CYP2D6 |
| Trifluoperazine | Low | 14 | |
| *Butyrophenones* | | | |
| Haloperidol | 60 | 20 | CYP2D6 |
| Droperidol | 75 | 2 | |
| *Thioxanthenes* | | | |
| Flupentixol | 40 | 36 | |
| Zuclopenthixol | 50 | 20 | CYP2D6 |
| *Others* | | | |
| Clozapine | 50 | 12 | |
| Risperidone | 75 | 3/20[c] | CYP2D6 |

[a] CYP refers to isozymes of the cytochrome P-450 family of enzymes.

[b] All these drugs are partly metabolized to active metabolites, Some of the metabolites have long half-lives (e.g. diazepam is metabolized to desmethyldiazepam). Some benzodiazepines (e.g. clorazepate and prazepam) are completely metabolized to active metabolites with long half-lives.

[c] Extensive and poor metabolizers respectively.

adverse effects in the extrapyramidal tracts (via $D_2$ receptors). The so-called atypical antipsychotic drugs (including clozapine and risperidone) have little effect on $D_2$ receptors and less commonly cause extrapyramidal adverse effects.[14]

Flumazenil is a competitive antagonist of benzodiazepines at benzodiazepine receptors and is used to reverse their effects.[15]

## Partial agonist action at a receptor

Partial agonists are substances that can be agonists or antagonists at receptors, depending on the endogenous tone of the system upon which they are acting. If the degree of endogenous stimulation of the receptor is low, a partial agonist will tend to act as an agonist; if high, it will end to act as an antagonist.

The anxiolytic buspirone is a partial agonist at $5\text{-HT}_{1A}$ autoreceptors and reduces the firing of 5-hydroxytryptamine (5-HT) neurones by stimulating the auto-receptors.[16]

## Actions via second messengers and ion channels

Some drugs act directly on second messenger systems and ion channels, without actions at receptors.

Lithium inhibits enzymes involved in the metabolism of inositol phosphates and may deplete cells of phosphoinositides, which are important as second messengers in neurotransmission.[17] However, other mechanisms have been proposed, including effects on the synthesis, turnover, and functional activity of brain 5-HT and effects on neuronal membrane function by effects on sodium and potassium fluxes via the sodium/potassium pump enzyme.[18]

## Altered neurotransmitter storage

Reserpine, which causes depression, inhibits the incorporation of neurotransmitters into presynaptic storage vesicles and thus causes depletion of neurotransmitter stores.

## Increased neurotransmitter release

Amphetamines cause increased release of noradrenaline (norepinephrine) and dopamine and have mood-enhancing effects.[19]

## Inhibition of neurotransmitter reuptake

Most antidepressants inhibit the reuptake of monoamines into the presynaptic nerve ending after their release.[20] The effects of different antidepressants on monoamine reuptake are listed in Table 6.2.1.2. Reduced reuptake of monoamines occurs immediately, but the full therapeutic effects of antidepressants take some weeks to occur. This is explained by the occurrence of adaptive changes in presynaptic and postsynaptic receptors, including down-regulation of β-adrenoceptors, reduced sensitivity of β- and $\alpha_2$-adrenoceptors, and increased sensitivity of $\alpha_1$-adrenoceptors and 5-HT receptors. However, it is not known how these actions are translated into the therapeutic effect. The last of these effects has led to the use of 5-HT autoreceptor antagonists, in the hope of producing a quicker onset of antidepressant action by enhancing 5-HT neurotransmission.[21,22] For example, the partial β-adrenoceptor agonist and $5\text{-HT}_{1A}$ receptor antagonist pindolol hastens the response to SSRIs, although it does not affect the extent of the response.[23] Another strategy involves drugs with several actions, which inhibit more than one reuptake system and are antagonists at neurotransmitter receptors.[24]

**Table 6.2.1.2** Effects of antidepressants on monoamine reuptake

| Drug | Inhibition of uptake | | |
|------|---------------|------|----------|
| | Noradrenaline | 5-HT | Dopamine |
| *Tricyclics* | | | |
| Amitriptyline | +++ | ++ | — |
| Clomipramine | +++ | +++ | — |
| Desipramine | +++ | ++ | — |
| Imipramine[a] | ++[a] | + | — |
| Nortriptyline | ++ | + | — |
| *Tetracyclics* | | | |
| Maprotiline | ++ | — | — |
| Mianserin | ++ | — | — |
| *Phenylethylamines* | | | |
| Venlafaxine | ++ | ++++ | — |
| *Triazolopyridines* | | | |
| Trazodone | — | + | — |
| *Specific serotonin reuptake inhibitors* | | | |
| Fluoxetine | — | +++ | — |
| Fluvoxamine | + | ++ | — |
| Paroxetine | — | +++ | — |
| Sertraline | + | ++++ | + |

[a] Through its metabolite desipramine.

## Altered neurotransmitter metabolism

Inhibitors of monoamine oxidase (MAO) enhance monoamine neurotransmission by irreversibly and non-selectively inhibiting the breakdown of monoamines after their release. Moclobemide[25] is a RIMA, a reversible inhibitor of MAO type A, which metabolizes 5-HT and noradrenaline. Moclobemide is therefore less likely to cause hypertension when taken in combination with amine-containing foods, such as cheese, since this reaction requires inhibition of both MAO type A and MAO type B.

Valproate partly acts by inhibiting GABA transaminase, thus enhancing GABA inhibitory transmission. However, it has other actions: it inhibits GABA reuptake, increases the sensitivity of GABA receptors to GABA, reduces the concentrations of the excitatory neurotransmitter aspartate, and may open potassium channels, thus stabilizing neuronal cell membranes.

## Adverse effects of drugs

Unwanted effects of drugs are commonly referred to as toxic effects or side effects. However, these are ambiguous terms, for several reasons:

♦ Toxic effects occur through exaggeration of the desired pharmacological action of the drug, and therefore occur at doses that are above those usually associated with a therapeutic effect. For example, antipsychotic drugs produce some toxic effects by antagonism at dopamine receptors in the extrapyramidal tracts.

♦ Toxic effects can also occur through exaggeration of actions other than those that are thought to produce the therapeutic action. Paracetamol toxicity occurs because an active metabolite binds covalently to liver proteins, damaging them.

♦ Side effects occur either through actions that are unrelated to the desired pharmacological effect or through actions that are related

to the desired pharmacological effect but occur in another tissue. Tricyclic antidepressants cause dry mouth, glaucoma, and urinary retention by anticholinergic action. Sildenafil causes colour vision disturbances by inhibiting phosphodiesterase type V in the eye, the action by which it has its therapeutic effect in erectile dysfunction. True side effects are more properly called collateral effects.[26]

It is therefore better to use the terms 'unwanted effects' or 'adverse effects/reactions'. Adverse reactions and adverse effects are identical—the former are seen from the point of view of the patient, the latter from the point of view of the drug.

Adverse drug effects are classified according to the scheme known as DoTS (Dose, Time, and Susceptibility).[26]

### Classification according to dose-relatedness

1 *Hypersusceptibility reactions*: Here the dose–response curve for harm is far to the left of the dose–response curve for benefit; hypersusceptibility adverse reactions therefore occur at doses below those that are normally beneficial. Penicillin allergy is an example.

2 *Collateral reactions*: Here the dose–response curve for harm is in a region that is bounded by a curve that is just to the left of the dose–response curve for benefit and one that is just to the right; collateral adverse reactions therefore occur at doses within the range of those that are normally beneficial. They can occur (i) through a pharmacological effect that is distinct from that involved in the beneficial effect (for example an anticholinergic effect of a tricyclic antidepressant) or (ii) through the same pharmacological effect as that associated with the beneficial effect, but in a different tissue (for example colour vision disturbance due to sildenafil).

3 *Toxic reactions*: Here the harm occurs through the same mechanism as benefit (i.e. is on the same dose–response curve) but at doses that are above those that are normally beneficial. An example is serotonin syndrome due to fluoxetine.

### Classification according to time-relatedness

Adverse drug reactions can be either time-dependent or time-independent (Table 6.2.1.3).

1 Time-independent reactions can occur at any time during therapy and are generally toxic reactions. They occur when the actual concentration of the drug increases or dose response curve shifts to the left, for whatever reason. An example is digoxin toxicity, which can occur for pharmaceutical reasons (for example administration of the wrong tablets), pharmacokinetic reasons (for example renal insufficiency), or pharmacodynamic reasons (for example hypokalemia). In the first two cases the concentration at the site of action increases and in the last the dose–response curve is shifted to the left.

2 Time-dependent adverse drug reactions are of six types; examples are given in Table 6.2.1.3.

♦ Immediate or rapid reactions occur when a drug is given too quickly.

♦ First-dose reactions occur only after the first dose of a course.

♦ Early reactions occur soon after the first administration; they either wear off with time (early tolerant effects) or persist (early persistent effects).

**Table 6.2.1.3**  Time-related classification of adverse drug reactions in the DoTS method. (Reproduced from *British Medical Journal*, Aronson, J.K. and Ferner, R.E. (2005), **327**, 1222–5, with permission from BMJ Publishing Group Ltd.)

| Type of reaction | Examples | Implications |
|---|---|---|
| *Time independent* | | |
| Due to a change in dose or concentration (pharmaceutical effects) | Toxicity due to increased systemic availability | Beware of changing formulations of some drugs (e.g. modified-release formulations of lithium) |
| Due to a change in dose or concentration (pharmacokinetic effects) | Lithium toxicity due to renal insufficiency | Forewarn the patient; monitor carefully throughout treatment; alter dosage when pharmacokinetics change (e.g. renal insufficiency); avoid interacting drugs |
| Occurs without a change in dose (pharmacodynamic effects) | Digitalis toxicity due to hypokalaemia | Forewarn the patient; monitor carefully throughout treatment; avoid precipitating (pharmacodynamic) factors; avoid interacting drugs |
| Time dependent | | |
| Immediate (due to rapid administration) | Red man syndrome (vancomycin)<br>Hypertension (digitalis)<br>Hypotension (iodipamide) | Administer slowly |
| First dose [of a course] | Hypotension (Ð1 adrenoceptor antagonists and angiotensin converting enzyme inhibitors)<br>Type I hypersensitivity reactions | Take special precautions for the first dose<br>Careful history taking; if a reaction occurs, avoid re-exposure; counsel the patient |
| Early tolerant | Adverse reactions that involve tolerance (e.g. nitrate-induced headache) | Monitor during the early stages; give appropriate reassurance; expect adverse effects if strategies to avoid tolerance are adopted |
| Early persistent | Glucocorticoid-induced diabetes mellitus | Monitor during the early stages and treat appropriately or withhold |
| Intermediate (risk increases at first, then diminishes) | Venous thromboembolism (classical antipsychotic drugs)<br>Neutropenia (clozapine)<br>Hypersensitivity reactions types II, III, and IV | Monitoring not needed after the high-risk period unless susceptibility changes; withdraw drug if a reaction develops |
| Late (risk increases with time) | Osteoporosis (glucocorticosteroids)<br>Tardive dyskinesia (dopamine receptor antagonists)<br>Retinopathy (chloroquine)<br>Tissue phospholipid deposition (amiodarone) | Assess baseline function; forewarn the patient; monitor periodically during prolonged treatment |
| | Withdrawal syndromes: opiates, benzodiazepines, hypertension (clonidine and methyldopa), myocardial infarction (beta-blockers) | Withdraw slowly; forewarn the patient; replace with a longer acting drug if withdrawal is not possible |
| Delayed | Carcinogenesis (ciclosporin, diethylstilbestrol)<br>Teratogenesis (thalidomide) | Avoid or screen; counsel or forewarn the patient |

◆ Intermediate reactions occur within the first few weeks or months of administration but not thereafter; those who are susceptible will suffer the reaction and those who are not will not (healthy survivors); for example, clozapine causes neutropenia predominantly during the first 24 weeks of therapy—thereafter the risk is small.

◆ Late reactions occur late in the course of administration, the risk increasing with time; this group includes withdrawal reactions.

◆ Delayed reactions are seen at some distant time after the initial exposure, even if the drug is withdrawn before the reaction appears.

### Classification according to susceptibility factors

The risk of an adverse drug reaction differs among members of an exposed population. For some reactions some individuals are susceptible, others are not—for example, prolonged muscle relaxation due to suxamethonium in people with pseudocholinesterase deficiency. In other cases susceptibility follows a continuous distribution—for example, increasing susceptibility with increasing impairment of renal function. Although reasons for increased susceptibility may be unknown, several types are recognized (Table 6.2.1.4).[27–34] These include:

◆ genetic variation;

◆ age;

◆ sex;

◆ physiological variation (for example pregnancy, body weight);

◆ exogenous factors (for example drugs and food);

◆ diseases (for example renal or hepatic impairment).

More than one susceptibility factor can be present in an individual.

**Table 6.2.1.4** Sources of susceptibility to adverse drug reactions

| Source of susceptibility* | Examples | Implications |
|---|---|---|
| Genetic | Porphyria<br>Suxamethonium sensitivity<br>Malignant hyperthermia<br>CYP isozyme polymorphisms | Screen for abnormalities; avoid specific drugs |
| Age | Neonates (chloramphenicol[27])<br>Elderly people (hypnotics[28]) | Adjust dosages according to age |
| Sex | Alcohol intoxication<br>Mefloquine, neuropsychiatric effects[29]<br>Lupus-like syndrome[30] | Use different doses in men and women |
| Physiology altered | Phenytoin in pregnancy[31] | Alter dosage or avoid |
| Exogenous factors | Drug interactions<br>Interactions with food (e.g. grapefruit juice with drugs cleared by CYP3A4[32]; see Table 6.1) | Alter dosage or avoid co-administration |
| Diseases | Renal insufficiency (e.g. lithium[33])<br>Hepatic cirrhosis (e.g. morphine[34]) | Screen for abnormalities; avoid specific drugs; use reduced dosages |

*Mnemonic GASPED

## Factors that increase the risk of an adverse effect

### (a) Pharmaceutical factors

Adverse effects can arise from changes in the pharmaceutical formulation. There is a risk of lithium toxicity or loss of action when one modified-release formulation of lithium is replaced by another.

### (b) Pharmacokinetic factors

Changes in the pharmacokinetics of a drug can result in toxic or collateral adverse effects. This most commonly occurs through impaired liver function (Table 6.2.1.1) or renal insufficiency (lithium).

### (c) Pharmacodynamic factors

Changes in the sensitivity of a tissue to a drug occur during long-term therapy and can result in adverse effects. Tardive dyskinesia with dopamine receptor antagonists may be related to altered sensitivity of dopamine receptors,[35] although there are problems with this hypothesis, and complex interactions with other neurotransmitters may be involved.[36]

When adaptive changes occur during long-term therapy, sudden withdrawal of the drug can result in rebound reactions. Examples include the typical syndromes that occur after the sudden withdrawal of narcotic analgesics[37,38] or of alcohol (delirium tremens).[39] Sudden withdrawal of barbiturates can cause restlessness, sleeplessness, mental confusion, and convulsions; a similar syndrome, in which anxiety features prominently, can occur after the sudden withdrawal of benzodiazepines.[24,40]

## Drug interactions

In a drug interaction one drug alters the effects of another, resulting in increased or decreased effects. Fluvoxamine inhibits the hepatic metabolism of warfarin and increases its anticoagulant effect,[41] whereas carbamazepine reduces the anticoagulant effect of warfarin by increasing its metabolism.[42]

1  Pharmaceutical interactions occur when there is a physicochemical interaction between two compounds in solution. Lists of such incompatibilities are too long to remember. To avoid pharmaceutical interactions, do not combine drugs in an infusion solution and use only sodium chloride 0.9% or glucose 5% in drug infusions.

2  Pharmacokinetic interactions occur when one drug interferes with the disposition of another during absorption, distribution, or elimination. Here are examples that are relevant to psychotropic drugs.

  ◆ Sucralfate reduces the absorption of amitriptyline by about 50 per cent;[43] this might be of clinical importance, but drug absorption interactions are not usually important.

  ◆ Phenytoin is displaced from protein-binding sites by valproate (which also inhibits its metabolism).[44]

  ◆ The metabolism of psychotropic drugs can theoretically be inhibited by drugs that inhibit metabolism via cytochrome P450 in the liver (Table 6.2.1.1). Reports of such interactions appear frequently. Inhibitory drugs include cimetidine, antifungal imidazoles (such as fluconazole), and macrolides (such as erythromycin).

  ◆ Non-selective MAO inhibitors, such as tranylcypromine, inhibit the metabolism (by MAO type A) of dietary amines in the gut and metabolism (by MAO type B) of the noradrenaline that they release, resulting in hypertension. Avoid this combination.

  ◆ Diuretics inhibit the renal excretion of lithium; alter the dosage of lithium and monitor the serum concentration when starting a diuretic or changing the diuretic dosage.

3  Pharmacodynamic interactions occur when two drugs interact at the same site of action. Alcohol potentiates the actions of all psychotropic drugs; patients taking psychotropic drugs should be warned that even one alcoholic drink can impair their ability to drive or operate machinery. The combination of reuptake inhibitors with non-selective irreversible monoamine oxidase inhibitors can cause the serotonin syndrome,[45] which is

sometimes fatal.[46] The combination of lithium with either SSRIs[47] or the SNRI venlafaxine[48] can also cause the serotonin syndrome. Flumazenil reverses the effects of benzodiazepines—a beneficial pharmacodynamic interaction.

## Monitoring drug therapy

If possible, monitor drug therapy by observing the clinical outcome. In psychiatric disorders this is difficult, but it can be done by asking patients or their carers to keep diaries of symptoms.

Next best is to monitor some pharmacological effect of the drug, in the way that one measures the international normalized ratio (INR) in patients taking warfarin (thus measuring the effect of the drug on the blood, being unable to monitor its clinical effect of preventing pulmonary embolism). However, there are no comparable routine tests available for monitoring the pharmacological effects of psychotropic drugs.

Because of these difficulties one falls back on measurements of serum concentrations of some drugs. The assumptions in doing this are that the serum concentration reflects the concentration at the site of action and that there is a concentration–effect relationship. Few psychoactive drugs can be monitored in this way, the principal ones being lithium and phenytoin. Some advocate monitoring treatment with some tricyclic antidepressants,[49] but this use is controversial.

Serum concentration measurement can be used to individualize therapy in the early stages of treatment or when the dosage is being changed, to check adherence to therapy, to help diagnose toxicity, and to monitor the effects of drug interactions.

### Carbamazepine

The target plasma carbamazepine concentration range is 17–42 mmol/l, but plasma concentrations do not correlate well with effect, since it has an active metabolite, oxcarbazepine; higher concentrations are associated with an increased risk of toxicity.[50] Carbamazepine induces its own metabolism, and its half-life is therefore shortened during long-term therapy. So, after an initial apparent steady state has been reached 3 or 4 days after starting therapy, a new steady state occurs at a lower concentration a few weeks later, and the dose may need to be increased at that time. Blood samples should be taken immediately before a dose.

### Lithium

The target serum lithium concentration is 0.4–1.0 mmol/l. Concentrations above 1 mmol/l are associated with an increased risk of toxicity. Take blood samples at a standard time—12 h after the last dose. In my view, routine monitoring is unnecessary, and the serum lithium concentration should be measured at times when toxicity is most likely, for example in patients with changing renal function or with acute alterations in electrolyte balance.[51,52] Many psychiatrists prefer to measure the serum lithium concentration routinely at, say, 3- or 6-monthly intervals. However, although regular monitoring may emphasize the dangers to the patient and give an opportunity for a consultation, it is no substitute for proper monitoring at the appropriate times.

### Valproate

The target serum valproate concentration range is 40–80 μmol/1, although this range is based on its use in epilepsy rather than bipolar

affective disorder;[53] higher concentrations are associated with an increased risk of toxicity. The blood sample can be taken at any time after the last dose.

## Further information

Aronson, J.K. (ed.) (2006). *Meyler's side effects of drugs. The international encyclopedia of adverse drug reactions and interactions* (15th edn). Elsevier, New York.

Aronson, J.K., Hardman, M., and Reynolds, D.J.M. (1993). *ABC of monitoring drug therapy.* BMJ Publishing, London.

Association of British Pharmaceutical Industries. *ABPI compendium of data sheets and summaries of product characteristics.* Datapharm Publications, London (published annually).

Baxter, K. (ed.) (2006). *Stockley's drug interactions: a source book of interactions, their mechanisms, clinical importance and management* (7th edn). Pharmaceutical Press, London.

Bennett, P.N. (ed.) (1996). *Drugs and human lactation* (2nd edn). Elsevier, Amsterdam.

Denham, M.J. and George, C.F. (eds.) (1990). Drugs in old age. *British Medical Bulletin,* **46.**

Dollery, C. (ed.) (1999). *Therapeutic drugs* (2nd edn). Churchill Livingstone, Edinburgh.

Grahame-Smith, D.G. and Aronson, J.K. (2002). *Oxford textbook of clinical pharmacology* (3rd edn). Oxford University Press, Oxford.

Gilstrap, L.C. and Little, B.B. (eds.) (1998). *Drugs and pregnancy* (2nd edn). Chapman & Hall, New York.

Joint Formulary Committee. *British national formulary.* British Medical Association and The Pharmaceutical Society of Great Britain, London (published every 6 months).

Paediatric Formulary Committee. *British national formulary for children.* British Medical Association and The Pharmaceutical Society of Great Britain, London (published annually).

## References

1. Amdisen, A. (1969). Variation of serum lithium concentration during the day in relation to treatment control, absorptive side effects and the use of slow-release tablets. *Acta Psychiatrica Scandinavica,* **207,** 55–7.

2. Malone, F.D. and D'Alton, M.E. (1997). Drugs in pregnancy: anticonvulsants. *Seminars in Perinatology,* **21,** 114–23.

3. Rodriguez-Pinilla, E., Arroyo, I., Fondevila, J., et al. (2000). Prenatal exposure to valproic acid during pregnancy and limb deficiencies: a case-control study. *American Journal of Medical Genetics,* **90,** 376–81.

4. Jefferson, J.W. (2006). Lithium. In *Meyler's side effects of drugs. The international encyclopedia of adverse drug reactions and interactions* (15th edn) (ed. J.K. Aronson), pp. 2073–116. Elsevier, Amsterdam.

5. Anonymous (1999). Lithium. In *Therapeutic drugs* (2nd edn), Vol. 2 (ed. C. Dollery), pp. L71–5. Churchill Livingstone, Edinburgh.

6. Chisholm, C.A. and Kuller, J.A. (1997). A guide to the safety of CNS–active agents during breastfeeding. *Drug Safety,* **17,** 127–42.

7. Pentikainen, P.J., Neuvonen, P.J., and Jostell, K.G. (1980). Pharmacokinetics of chlormethiazole in healthy volunteers and patients with cirrhosis of the liver. *European Journal of Clinical Pharmacology,* **17,** 275–84.

8. Caccia, S. (1998). Metabolism of the newer antidepressants. An overview of the pharmacological and pharmacokinetic implications. *Clinical Pharmacokinetics,* **34,** 281–302.

9. Norman, T.R., Walker, R.G., and Burrows, G.D. (1984). Renal function related changes in lithium kinetics. *Clinical Pharmacokinetics,* **9,** 349–53.

10. Korpi, E.R., Mattila, M.J., Wisden, W., *et al.* (1997). GABA(A) receptor subtypes: clinical efficacy and selectivity of benzodiazepine site ligands. *Annals of Medicine*, **29**, 275–82.

11. Wagner, J., Wagner, M.L., and Hening, W.A. (1998). Beyond benzodiazepines: alternative pharmacologic agents for the treatment of insomnia. *Annals of Pharmacotherapy*, **32**, 680–91.

12. Cross, A.J., Stirling, J.M., Robinson, T.N., *et al.* (1989). The modulation by chlormethiazole of the GABA$_A$-receptor complex in rat brain. *British Journal of Pharmacology*, **98**, 284–90.

13. Evans, R.W. and Lipton R.B. (2001). Topics in migraine management: a survey of headache specialists highlights some controversies. *Neurologic Clinics*, **19**, 1–21.

14. Seeman, P. and Tallerico, T. (1998). Antipsychotic drugs which elicit little or no parkinsonism bind more loosely than dopamine to brain D$_2$ receptors, yet occupy high levels of these receptors. *Molecular Psychiatry*, **3**, 123–34.

15. Weinbroum, A.A., Flaishon, R., Sorkine, P., *et al.* (1997). A risk benefit assessment of flumazenil in the management of benzodiazepine overdose. *Drug Safety*, **17**, 181–96.

16. Gardner, C.R. (1988). Potential use of drugs modulating 5HT activity in the treatment of anxiety. *General Pharmacology*, **19**, 347–56.

17. Harwood, A.J. (2005). Lithium and bipolar mood disorder: the inositol-depletion hypothesis revisited. *Molecular Psychiatry*, **10**, 117–26.

18. Marmol, F. (2006). Litio: 55 anos de historia en el tratamiento del trastorno bipolar. *Medica Clinica (Barcelona)*, **127**, 189–95.

19. Fleckenstein, A.E., Volz, T.J., Riddle. E.L., *et al.* (2007). New insights into the mechanism of action of amphetamines. *Annual Reviews of Pharmacology and Toxicology*, **47**, 681–98.

20. Stahl, S.M. (1998). Basic psychopharmacology of antidepressants, part 1: antidepressants have seven distinct mechanisms of action. *The Journal of Clinical Psychiatry*, **59**(Suppl. 4), 5–14.

21. Blier, P. and Bergeron, R. (1997). Early onset of therapeutic action in depression and greater efficacy of antidepressant treatments: are they related? *International Clinical Psychopharmacology*, **12**(Suppl. 3), S21–8.

22. Sussman, N. and Joffe, R.T. (1998). Antidepressant augmentation: conclusions and recommendations. *The Journal of Clinical Psychiatry*, **59**(Suppl. 5), 70–3.

23. Artigas, F., Adell, A., and Celada, P. (2006). Pindolol augmentation of antidepressant response. *Current Drug Targets*, **7**, 139–47.

24. Sambunaris, A., Hesselink, J.K., Pinder, R., *et al.* (1997). Development of new antidepressants. *The Journal of Clinical Psychiatry*, **58**(Suppl. 6), 40–53.

25. Fulton, B. and Benfield, P. (1996). Moclobemide. An update of its pharmacological properties and therapeutic use. *Drugs*, **52**, 450–74 (erratum 869).

26. Aronson, J.K. and Ferner, R.E. (2003). Joining the DoTS. New approach to classifying adverse drug reactions. *British Medical Journal*, **327**, 1222–5.

27. Mulhall, A., de Louvois, J., and Hurley, R. (1983). Chloramphenicol toxicity in neonates: its incidence and prevention. *British Medical Journal*, **287**, 1424–7.

28. Greenblatt, D.J., Divoll, M., Harmatz, J.S., *et al.* (1981). Kinetics and clinical effects of flurazepam in young and elderly noninsomniacs. *Clinical Pharmacology and Therapeutics*, **30**, 475–86.

29. Schwartz, E., Potasman, I., Rotenberg, M., *et al.* (2001). Serious adverse events of mefloquine in relation to blood level and gender. *American Journal of Tropical Medicine and Hygiene*, **65**, 189–92.

30. Batchelor, J.R., Welsh, K.I., Tinoco, R.M., *et al.* (1980). Hydralazine-induced systemic lupus erythematosus: influence of HLA-DR and sex on susceptibility. *Lancet*, **1**, 1107–9.

31. Dickinson, R.G., Hooper, W.D., Wood, B., *et al.* (1989). The effect of pregnancy in humans on the pharmacokinetics of stable isotope labelled phenytoin. *British Journal of Clinical Pharmacology*, **28**, 17–27.

32. Aronson, J.K. (2001). Forbidden fruit. *Nature Medicine*, **7**, 7–8.

33. Clericetti, N. and Beretta-Piccoli, C. (1991). Lithium clearance in patients with chronic renal diseases. *Clinical Nephrology*, **36**, 281–9.

34. Hasselstrom, J., Eriksson, S., Persson, A., *et al.* (1990). The metabolism and bioavailability of morphine in patients with severe liver cirrhosis. *British Journal of Clinical Pharmacology*, **29**, 289–97.

35. Jenner, P. and Marsden, C.D. (1987). Chronic pharmacological manipulation of dopamine receptors in brain. *Neuropharmacology*, **26**, 931–40.

36. Gill, H.S., DeVane, C.L., and Risch, S.C. (1997). Extrapyramidal symptoms associated with cyclic antidepressant treatment: a review of the literature and consolidating hypotheses. *Journal of Clinical Psychopharmacology*, **17**, 377–89.

37. Puntillo, K., Casella, V., and Reid, M. (1997). Opioid and benzodiazepine tolerance and dependence: application of theory to critical care practice. *Heart & Lung*, **26**, 317–24.

38. O'Connor, P.G. and Kosten, T.R. (1998). Rapid and ultrarapid opioid detoxification techniques. *The Journal of the American Medical Association*, **279**, 229–34.

39. Miller, N.S. (1995). Pharmacotherapy in alcoholism. *Journal of Addictive Diseases*, **14**, 23–46.

40. Ashton, H. (1994). The treatment of benzodiazepine dependence. *Addiction*, **89**, 1535–41.

41. Perucca, E., Gatti, G., and Spina, E. (1994). Clinical pharmacokinetics of fluvoxamine. *Clinical Pharmacokinetics*, **27**, 175–90.

42. Cropp, J.S. and Bussey, H.I. (1997). A review of enzyme induction of warfarin metabolism with recommendations for patient management. *Pharmacotherapy*, **17**, 917–28.

43. Ryan, R., Carlson, J., and Farris, F. (1986). Effect of sucralfate on the absorption and disposition of amitriptyline in humans. *Federation Proceedings*, **45**, 205.

44. Suzuki, Y., Nagai, T., Mano, T., *et al.* (1995). Interaction between valproate formulation and phenytoin concentrations. *European Journal of Clinical Pharmacology*, **48**, 61–3.

45. Hilton, S.E., Maradit, H., and Moller, H.J. (1997). Serotonin syndrome and drug combinations: focus on MAOI and RIMA. *European Archives of Psychiatry and Clinical Neuroscience*, **247**, 113–9.

46. Keltner, N. and Harris, C.P. (1994). Serotonin syndrome: a case of fatal SSRI/MAOI interaction. *Perspectives in Psychiatric Care*, **30**, 26–31.

47. Sobanski, T., Bagli, M., Laux, G., *et al.* (1997). Serotonin syndrome after lithium add-on medication to paroxetine. *Pharmacopsychiatry*, **30**, 106–7.

48. Adan-Manes, J., Novalbos, J., Lopez-Rodriguez, R., *et al.* (2006). Lithium and venlafaxine interaction: a case of serotonin syndrome. *Journal of Clinical Pharmacy and Therapy*, **31**, 397–400.

49. Isacson, G., Bergman, U., Wasserman, D., *et al.* (1996). The use of antidepressants and therapeutic drug monitoring by general practitioners and psychiatrists: findings from a questionnaire survey in two Swedish areas. *Annals of Clinical Psychiatry*, **8**, 153–60.

50. Vasudev, K., Goswami, U., and Kohli, K. (2000). Carbamazepine and valproate monotherapy: feasibility, relative safety and efficacy, and therapeutic drug monitoring in manic disorder. *Psychopharmacology (Berlin)*, **150**, 15–23.

51. Aronson, J.K. and Reynolds, D.J. (1992). ABC of monitoring drug therapy. Lithium. *British Medical Journal*, **305**, 1273–4.

52. Glasziou, P. and Aronson, J.K. (2008). An introduction to monitoring therapeutic interventions in clinical practice. In *Evidence-based medical monitoring: from principles to practice* (eds. P.P. Glasziou, L. Irwig, and J.K. Aronson), Chap. 1. Wiley-Blackwell Publications, Oxford.

53. Fleming, J. and Chetty, M. (2006). Therapeutic monitoring of valproate in psychiatry: how far have we progressed? *Clinical Neuropharmacology*, **29**, 350–60.

# 6.2.2 **Anxiolytics and hypnotics**

Malcolm Lader

## Introduction

Anxiety is a commonly experienced emotion that becomes a clinical disorder when it is too severe, too protracted, or too pervasive for the subject to bear. Insomnia is a failure to experience satisfying sleep, together with a feeling of tiredness during the day. Many compounds, the anxiolytics and hypnotics, are used to treat these conditions, but the two groups of drugs overlap.

The classical antianxiety drugs (anxiolytics) are alcohol, the opioids, and the barbiturates. For the past 45 years, the benzodiazepines, such as diazepam and lorazepam, have dominated the field. They are effective anxiolytics in the short term but their long-term efficacy remains in dispute. Their disadvantages include cognitive and psychomotor impairment, paradoxical reactions, tolerance, and dependence, and they are major drugs of abuse.

Other anxiolytics act on the 5-hydroxytryptamine (5-HT; serotonin) systems of the brain and include buspirone and the selective serotonin reuptake inhibitors (SSRIs). Newer compounds are still being introduced that lie outside these groups.

The use of benzodiazepine and benzodiazepine-like hypnotics, by contrast, continues apace. Some switching to the shorter-acting benzodiazepines has occurred, together with the introduction of the 'z-compounds', zopiclone, zolpidem, and zaleplon. These drugs tend to have fewer residual effects the next day than the benzodiazepines, and are claimed to be less likely to induce rebound and dependence than equivalent benzodiazepines. Particular care is needed in prescribing such hypnotics to the elderly.

The rational use of both anxiolytics and hypnotics requires minimal dosage, short durations of use, and simultaneous exploitation of non-pharmacological methods.

## Definitions

'Sedative' originally meant a substance that has the property of allaying anxiety. However, it has now come to denote feelings of drowsiness or torpor. This state was originally called 'oversedation', and was often noted with the barbiturates and other older drugs such as chloral. Next, the term 'tranquillizer' was introduced 40 or more years ago in an attempt to distinguish between the older sedatives and the newer drugs, supposedly non-sedative, such as the benzodiazepines. But this distinction is artificial as, apart from safety in overdosage, the benzodiazepines closely resemble the barbiturates in pharmacological and clinical properties. The term 'anxiolytic' is now generally favoured.

## Anxiolytic drugs

Anxiety-allaying drugs have been used for thousands of years, dating back to the discovery that, among its psychotropic properties, alcohol could induce sedation. The nineteenth century saw the development of inorganic and, later, organic chemical compounds. Bromides were introduced as sedatives and became widely used despite their poor effectiveness, toxicity, and potential abuse.

Organic chemists in the second half of the nineteenth century introduced sedatives such as chloral and paraldehyde.

The first barbiturate was introduced over a 100 years ago. This group of drugs is divisible into the ultrashort-acting (e.g. anaesthetic-induction agents such as thiopentone and methohexital), short-acting (e.g. secobarbital), medium-acting (e.g. butobarbital), and long-acting (e.g. phenobarbital) barbiturates. Most of the rest are of medium duration with half-lives of 16 h or so. The disadvantages of the barbiturates include drowsiness, tolerance to their effects, dangers of overdose, and possible physical and psychological dependence with severe withdrawal syndromes.[1] Meprobamate was introduced as the first of the 'tranquillizers', but its advantages over the barbiturates proved minimal.

The benzodiazepines were first synthesized in the 1930s, but not developed until 2 years later. The prototype, chlordiazepoxide, was evaluated in the clinic, found effective, and soon introduced into medical practice. More than 1000 benzodiazepines and related compounds have been synthesized, including diazepam, the most widely used of all. Anxiolytic and hypnotic, as well as muscle-relaxant and anticonvulsant properties are licensed indications. However, the distinction between anxiolytic and hypnotic uses often seems to owe more to commercial expediency than to scientific rationale; some compounds, such as lorazepam, are marketed for both indications.

### The benzodiazepines

The main reason for the original popularity of the benzodiazepines was the perceived safety in overdose compared with the quite marked toxicity of the barbiturates. In turn, concern has mounted concerning the benzodiazepines.[2] These drugs are widely prescribed by many physicians for patients with emotional problems, circulatory disorders, tension headaches, and pains in the chest and back as well as digestive disorders, all with the common symptom of anxiety. This widespread use, even overuse and the induction of dependence even at normal therapeutic dose has led to official injunctions for greater caution in prescribing.

### Pharmacokinetics

Two aspects of the pharmacokinetics of the benzodiazepines are relevant to the prescriber—speed of onset of action and the duration of that action. The speed of onset depends on the mode of administration and the penetration time to the brain. Given by mouth, most benzodiazepines are rapidly absorbed and exert a prompt anxiolytic effect, for instance in panic states. Diazepam and lorazepam are prime examples. Although temazepam enters the brain more rapidly than, say, oxazepam, it still takes an appreciable time to induce sleep. The redistribution phase can be pronounced and will then largely determine the duration of effect of single doses of benzodiazepines such as diazepam and flunitrazepam.

The metabolic half-lives of the benzodiazepines also vary greatly. *N*-desmethyldiazepam (nordiazepam) is the major and active metabolite of diazepam and several other benzodiazepines. It has a long half-life, about 60 h, and accumulates over the first month of treatment. Metabolism of these drugs is even slower in the elderly and in patients with liver damage.

Benzodiazepines with a 3-hydroxyl grouping, such as lorazepam, oxazepam, and temazepam, have half-lives averaging 12 h or less. Liver damage has to be severe before the metabolism of these drugs is affected. Alprazolam is a triazolobenzodiazepine with a half-life of 9 to 16 h, and with hydroxy metabolites of low biological activity. Both chlordiazepoxide and diazepam are absorbed erratically after intramuscular injection. Lorazepam, however, is well absorbed after intramuscular injection.

### Basic pharmacology

The benzodiazepines potentiate the widespread inhibitory neurotransmitter γ-amino butyric acid (GABA). Benzodiazepines do not act directly on GABA receptors but have their own receptors. Because of this widespread inhibitory effect, benzodiazepines alter the turnover of neurotransmitters such as norepinephrine and serotonin. The main sites of action of the benzodiazepines are in the spinal cord where muscle-relaxant effects are mediated, the brainstem (perhaps accounting for their anticonvulsant properties), the cerebellum (causing ataxia), and the limbic and cortical areas involved in the organization of emotional experience and behaviour.

### Clinical pharmacology

The depressant effects of single therapeutic doses of a benzodiazepine can usually be readily detected. However, lower doses may fail to impair psychological functioning and subjective effects are usually absent. In the clinical context with anxious patients and with repeated higher doses, sustained impairment of functioning is more difficult to demonstrate. Some studies have shown decrements in performance after the first dose, but improvements in functioning, in comparison to predrug levels, may become apparent by the end of a week of repeated usage. This suggests that the well-known impairment of performance produced by pathologically high levels of anxiety is first worsened by the sedative effects. Then as the antianxiety effects build-up, the patient's psychological functions may improve.

A second mechanism concerns tolerance, which reflects several biochemical mechanisms including alteration in benzodiazepine-receptor type. Patients who have a high alcohol intake are tolerant to benzodiazepines.

The benzodiazepines have marked and selective effects on memory by interfering with episodic memory, that is to say the system concerned with remembering personal experiences.[3] This effect seems independent of any sedation or attentional impairment. Alcohol adds to the cognitive impairment induced by the benzodiazepines but does not necessarily potentiate it.

The dependence potential of benzodiazepines is seen in drug-preference studies, but these drugs are much less preferred than say the amphetamines. Differences among benzodiazepines have been documented; for example, oxazepam seems to have less abuse liability than diazepam.

The largest gap in our knowledge of these drugs is on their long-term usage, which has been evaluated in relatively few studies.[4] Thus, it is still largely unclear whether therapeutic effects are maintained in most patients for longer than a few weeks and when dependence supervenes in the minority of patients who encounter problems on protracted usage.

## Hypnotic drugs

The main groups of drugs used in the modern treatment of insomnia are the benzodiazepines, and the newer compounds, zopiclone, eszopiclone, zolpidem, and zaleplon. The pharmacology of these benzodiazepines is essentially the same as that of the anxiolytic compounds.

Nitrazepam is a long-acting benzodiazepine with an elimination half-life ranging between 25 and 35 h, but it is longer in the elderly. Because of this, it is likely to produce residual effects and to accumulate. Flunitrazepam is more potent, but is somewhat shorter acting with a half-life of 10 to 20 h. It has a rapid redistribution phase, which can result in a short duration of intense action. It has earned an undeserved reputation as the 'date-rape' drug. Flurazepam is still widely used in the United States. It has a very long-acting metabolite, which can produce psychological impairment on regular dosage, especially in the elderly. Of the intermediate-acting compounds, temazepam has a half-life of 10 to 15 h, without active metabolites. At modest dose (10–15 mg daily), it results in few residual effects and is fairly well tolerated by the elderly. Major problems with abuse have limited its popularity, but it is still widely prescribed worldwide. Lormetazepam is slightly shorter acting, loprazolam has a fairly short half-life, but its absorption may be slow and erratic.

Triazolam is the archetypal short-acting benzodiazepine, with a mean half-life of around 3 to 4 h, and no clinically significant metabolites. Daytime sedation is seen after high doses (0.5 mg daily), but not usually with lower ones. These higher doses have also been associated with an increased incidence of anterograde amnesia and unusual behaviours, including depressive reactions and hostility.

Zopiclone is a cyclopyrrolone derivative believed to bind close to, but not exactly at, the benzodiazepine receptor. It has a half-life of about 5 h in younger subjects and about 8 h in the elderly. Its sedative and hypnotic effects are similar to those of the benzodiazepines, but its side effect profile is generally superior with fewer central nervous system effects such as oversedation, confusion, and memory impairment. Rebound and withdrawal problems also seem to be less.

Eszopiclone is the S-enantiomer of zopiclone, which is a racemic mixture. It is licensed for the long-term treatment of insomnia in the United States, following successful clinical trials.

Zolpidem is an imidazopyridine compound that binds selectively to one subtype of the benzodiazepine receptor. It is rapidly absorbed and has a short elimination half-life of 0.7 to 3.5 h (mean 2.4 h). It decreases sleep-onset latency but has less consistent effects on total sleep time.[5] Residual effects are minimal, as are memory disturbances. Rebound and withdrawal are uncommon but have been documented.

Zaleplon is also a selective compound with a very short half-life averaging only 1 h. It shortens sleep onset without usually prolonging total sleep time. Residual effects are absent, and memory is minimally disturbed.

## Clinical effects of anxiolytics

Although the usual licensed indications are generalized anxiety and panic disorder,[6,7] the main practical application of the benzodiazepines is to aid in the symptomatic management of anxiety and stress-related conditions.[8] These indications are often so wide as to be difficult to define in terms of recognized disorders. Instead the symptoms of anxiety, in whatever context, are the main indication.

Thousands of comparative trials among the benzodiazepines have been carried out, but few differences with respect to risk–benefit ratios have been found.

Antianxiety medications are difficult to assess. Anxiety disorders are very varied in their natural history; some resolve over a few weeks, whereas others become chronic for no apparent reason, with subsequent acute-on-chronic exacerbations. The patients with chronic, severe unresponsive illnesses tend to be referred to psychiatric outpatient departments. Uncontrolled observations on family practice patients will give a more encouraging impression of antianxiety drugs than will assessment of the more chronic patients attending psychiatric clinics. Even in the latter type of patient, useful symptomatic relief is often obtained without complete resolution of the illness.

Drugs such as diazepam have a long elimination half-life so that once daily or nightly dosage is sufficient. Nevertheless, many patients prefer to take a divided dosage during the day, often claiming that they can detect further antianxiety activity after each dose and are thereby reassured. For episodic anxiety, shorter-acting compounds such as lorazepam can be used, taken 30 min or so before entering the anxiety-provoking situation. If the panic has already started, lorazepam can still be given and will exert a fairly prompt action. Lorazepam is also invaluable in the emergency management of the acutely anxious and disturbed psychotic patient.

Antipanic actions have been claimed for the benzodiazepines, in particular alprazolam, acting to prevent the episodes rather than aborting them. However, although suppression of the panic attack is often quite effective, relapse, and even rebound may occur when the benzodiazepine is discontinued, even if it is tapered off.[9] Because of this SSRI antidepressants are generally preferred.[7]

The short-acting benzodiazepines are also used as adjuncts to relaxation therapy, preoperative medication, and deep sedation for minor operative procedures such as dentistry. The drugs render the patient calm, conscious, and cooperative, with often total anterograde amnesia for the operation.

### Unwanted effects

The commonest unwanted effects of the anxiolytic benzodiazepines are tiredness, drowsiness, and torpor, features of 'oversedation'. The effects are dose and time related, being maximal within the first 2 h after large doses. Drowsiness is most noticeable during the first week of treatment, after which it largely disappears probably due to a true tolerance effect. Patients should be warned of the potential side effects of any prescribed benzodiazepine and the initial dosage should be cautious. Both psychomotor skills and intellectual and cognitive skills are affected. In particular, patients should be advised not to drive during the initial adjustment of dosage. Important decisions should be deferred during this period because judgement may be clouded.

Benzodiazepines have major effects on cognitive function in long-term users. A meta-analysis of 13 research studies revealed impairments across all cognitive categories examined.[4] The drugs differ in their ability to produce memory deficits, with lorazepam being especially powerful.[3] However, most benzodiazepines can cause problems, especially in higher dose and in the elderly.

Psychomotor performance is also affected, with elderly drivers particularly at risk. As with other depressant drugs, potentiation of the effects of alcohol can occur. Patients must be warned not to drink alcohol when taking benzodiazepines, either chronically or intermittently. Patients taking benzodiazepines may develop paradoxical behavioural responses such as uncontrollable weeping, increased aggression and hostility, and acute rage reactions or uncharacteristic criminal behaviour such as shoplifting.[10] This phenomenon is by no means confined to the benzodiazepines; alcohol is a cardinal example of a drug whose use may lead to excessive violence or criminal behaviour. Paradoxical reactions, including the release of anxiety or hostility, are most common during the initial week of treatment, and usually resolve spontaneously or respond to dose adjustment. Reports of the induction of depression by the benzodiazepines in patients with apparent generalized anxiety disorder are probably the result of an initial misdiagnosis and a failure to detect the underlying depression.

Other unwanted effects include respiratory depression, excessive weight gain, skin rash, impairment of sexual function, menstrual irregularities, and rarely, blood dyscrasias. The use of benzodiazepines in pregnancy is generally regarded as reasonably safe. However, benzodiazepines pass readily into the foetus and can produce respiratory depression in the neonate. Finally, benzodiazepines pass into the mother's milk and can over sedate the baby, so breastfeeding should be discouraged if benzodiazepines are prescribed, especially in high dose.

### Overdosage

Overdosage with benzodiazepines is common; deaths are not. Although fatal-overdose statistics contain deaths ascribed to benzodiazepines alone,[11] many such attributions are suspect. Only in children and the physically frail, especially those with respiratory illness, are the benzodiazepines on their own hazardous. However, they can markedly potentiate other central nervous system depressant drugs such as alcohol. Typically, the person falls into a deep sleep but can be roused the administration of the benzodiazepine antagonist, flumazenil.

### Tolerance and dependence

If tolerance occurred regularly, then escalation of dosage would be the norm. This does occur with the benzodiazepines, but is fairly uncommon. Escalation of dose is often stepwise, with each increment following a temporary deterioration in psychosocial circumstances. Most patients later reduce the dose as the stress resolves, but others continue the higher dose to which they presumably have developed some tolerance.

Tolerance to the clinical effects in patients maintaining moderate doses of benzodiazepines is now generally accepted.[12] Few controlled observations concern the long-term efficacy of antianxiety compounds in chronically anxious patients. If medication is withdrawn, the original symptoms may reappear. This is taken as evidence that therapeutic benefit still continues. However, it may reflect 'rebound' rather than long-term clinical benefit. Undoubtedly, many chronically anxious patients are helped by their treatment with benzodiazepines, but this raises the question as to the frequency of psychological and physical dependence on these drugs. Dependence is easily demonstrable in those patients who have attained high doses. Rebound and withdrawal symptoms after the long-acting benzodiazepine diazepam are not usually apparent until about 5 to 10 days after discontinuation. It is much shorter in patients discontinuing the shorter-acting benzodiazepines (2–4 days). The mildest symptoms and signs are anxiety, tension, apprehension, dizziness, tremulousness, insomnia, and anorexia. More severe physical dependence is shown by the withdrawal symptoms of nausea and vomiting, severe tremor, muscle weakness, postural hypotension, and tachycardia. Occasionally, hyperthermia, muscle twitches, convulsions, and confusional psychoses may develop.

After normal dose usage, perceptual changes can be particularly troublesome.[13] The proportion of patients taking benzodiazepines chronically who experience withdrawal symptoms on discontinuing medication ranges between 27 and 45 per cent, depending on the criteria used. Sometimes the withdrawal reactions seem very prolonged[14] or depression may supervene.

### Management of withdrawal

It is widely accepted that the most appropriate way to manage patients withdrawing from benzodiazepines is to taper the dose gradually, because the severe symptoms of withdrawal, such as epileptic fits and confusional episodes, are more likely to follow abrupt than gradual withdrawal. Views differ as to the rate of withdrawal. Detailed guidelines,[15,16] based on a consensus view in the United Kingdom, recommend minimal intervention first, usually by a general practitioner (Fig. 6.2.2.1). This may comprise

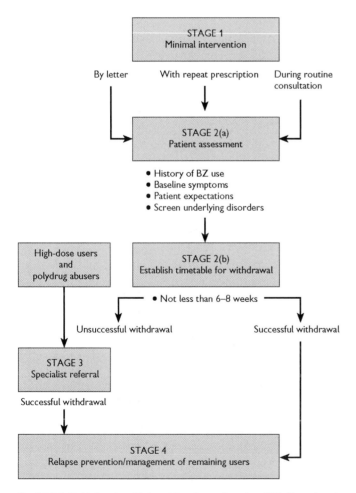

**Fig. 6.2.2.1** Guidelines for withdrawal from benzodiazepines (BZ). (Reproduced with permission from J. Russell and M. Lader (eds.), *Guidelines for the prevention and treatment of benzodiazepine dependence*, Mental Health Foundation, London. Copyright 1993, Mental Health Foundation, London.)

a letter to the long-term user, or an interview on a routine visit, with advice to taper the medication. More active intervention involves careful assessment, education, and then the adoption, with the patient's agreement, of a timetable of about 6 to 8 weeks for withdrawal. Some agencies suggest a month of tapering for every year of benzodiazepine use, but this may result in patients becoming preoccupied with their symptoms. One strategy is to try a fairly brisk withdrawal, say over 6 to 8 weeks, and only resort to more gradual tapering if the symptoms become intolerable. Another ploy is first to substitute a long-acting for a short-acting benzodiazepine, say 10 mg of diazepam for 1 mg of lorazepam, and then to taper off the diazepam later.

Patients must be carefully followed up as a depressive illness is not uncommon and may need vigorous treatment. Such an illness may be reactive to the stress of withdrawal or be a recurrence of an earlier affective episode.

Other drugs have been advocated, but most patients are loath to substitute yet another medication. Depressed patients should have the depression treated before attempting withdrawal. Based on evidence from animal studies, fairly large single doses of flumazenil have been tried with some success.

Psychological support is essential, with the doctor or a practice nurse maintaining close contact with the patient during withdrawal. The physician should show clearly that he understands the problems of withdrawal in order to capture the confidence of the patient. He or she must recognize that patients frequently incubate numerous misconceptions and negative expectations about tranquillizers and withdrawal. These must be elicited, identified, discussed, and corrected.

Cognitive behavioural treatment is currently favoured and is often effective if administered by an experienced professional. Relaxation treatment and training in anxiety management skills in the framework of group therapy can boast of only moderate effectiveness.

## Other anxiolytics

### Benzodiazepine-receptor partial agonists

The disadvantages of the benzodiazepines include sedation, psychomotor and cognitive impairment, and withdrawal symptoms after long-term use. Increased understanding of benzodiazepine-receptor mechanisms suggested that compounds might be developed which are partial agonists and/or selective to some subtypes of receptor.[17] Such compounds would be less efficacious than full agonists but might have better adverse-effect profiles and less dependence potential, that is superior risk–benefit ratios. Their promise has not been fulfilled, as the risk–benefit ratios of these compounds do not seem superior to those of the full agonists.

### 5-HT$_{1A}$ partial agonists

These drugs have a complex pharmacology. The first, buspirone, was licensed in many countries some years ago. These drugs suppress activity in presynaptic serotonergic neurones, diminishing serotonin activity, and leading on to down-regulation of 5-HT$_2$ and perhaps other 5-HT receptors. Buspirone is much less sedative than the benzodiazepines and causes little or no psychomotor or cognitive impairment, nor does it potentiate the effects of alcohol. In formal clinical trials, buspirone was equi-effective and equipotent to diazepam, but patients taking buspirone improve more slowly.[18] The side effects of buspirone include headache, dizziness, and nausea. Discontinuation is not accompanied by either rebound or withdrawal.

Other 5-HT$_{1A}$ partial agonists have been developed mainly as potential antidepressants and antianxiety agents, but few have been marketed, mainly because of disappointing efficacy.

### Pregabalin

This compound is a structural analogue of GABA although it is not active at GABA receptors.[19] It binds with high affinity to an auxiliary $\alpha_2$-$\delta$ subunit protein of voltage-gated calcium channels in the CNS: it acts as a presynaptic modulator of the excessive release of neurotransmitters in hyperexcited neurones. It is predominantly excreted unchanged in the urine. It was initially developed for use as an adjunctive treatment in epilepsy and neuropathic pain. Several clinical trials in GAD have shown it to have efficacy akin to those for benzodiazepines and venlafaxine.[20] It has a rapid onset of action and was effective in preventing relapse over 34 weeks. Tolerance was good during dosage escalation to the usual dose of 150–600 mg/day, mild dizziness and somnolence being the usual adverse effects. No clinically significant withdrawal was seen after tapering. It is approved for the treatment of GAD in Europe, and is a significant introduction.

### Antiepileptic drugs

There is a long history of the use of many of these compounds in anxiety disorders,[21] but they are not routine choices.

### Antipsychotic drugs

Phenothiazines, such as chlorpromazine and trifluoperazine, and a range of other antipsychotic drugs have been advocated for treating anxiety. The dosage recommended is quite low, typically less than half the initial antipsychotic dose used in psychotic patients. Sometimes, even at this dosage, the antipsychotic drug is not well tolerated by the anxious patient because unwanted autonomic effects, such as dry mouth and dizziness, too closely resemble the symptoms of anxiety. Even more unwelcome are extrapyramidal symptoms such as restlessness (mild akathisia) and parkinsonism, although at the low doses advocated such unwanted effects are uncommon. There may even be a risk of tardive dyskinesia. The chief advantage of this medication is that dependence is virtually unknown, so the main indication for their use is in patients with histories of dependence on other central nervous system depressant drugs such as alcohol or barbiturates.

### Antidepressants

Several of these drugs, such as amitriptyline, doxepin, and trazodone, have useful secondary sedative properties. They are widely prescribed for depressed patients with anxiety or agitation. More recently, several SSRI antidepressants such as paroxetine and escitalopram have been evaluated in the treatment of various anxiety disorders. SSRIs are now the treatment of choice in chronic anxiety disorders.[22,23]

MAOIs have been used for many years to treat phobic states, but the well-known range of unwanted effects, including hypotension, limb oedema, and dietary and drug interactions, preclude their routine use.

### β-adrenoceptor antagonists

Beta-adrenoceptor antagonists may help patients with anxiety, but usually only those complaining of somatic symptoms. They are still favoured by some primary care doctors.

### Antihistamines

The older compounds penetrate the brain readily and are quite sedative. Hydroxyzine has been evaluated in at least two placebo-controlled trials in doses of 50 mg/day: it proved to be significantly better than placebo. The advantages are that paradoxical reactions are rare, cognitive function including memory is largely unaffected, and rebound and withdrawal seem rare.

## Clinical effects of hypnotics

Insomnia is a common symptom,[24] especially in the elderly.[25] Nonetheless, many complaints of insomnia are unfounded as the patient has unreal expectations concerning sleep. Elderly people fail to appreciate that it is normal to sleep less and less deeply as they age. Napping during the day also decreases the need for sleep at night. Some people can manage on 5 to 6 h a night indefinitely, and yet worry that this is insufficient. Explanation and reassurance relieve their worries.

In many patients complaining of more severe insomnia, the cause is a physical complaint such as pain, breathlessness, or pruritus. The treatment is for that of the primary complaint. In many other cases, the insomnia is either a symptom of psychiatric distress, anxiety, or depression, or it is iatrogenic, caused by the very drugs prescribed to relieve the insomnia. In the first instance, treatment is directed towards the primary condition; in the second, a careful regimen of drug withdrawal, or substitution and subsequent withdrawal, should be instigated, as discussed earlier for anxiolytic medication. Some drugs, of which caffeine is the most common, induce insomnia. Alcohol may also disrupt sleep, particularly during the latter half of the night.

Despite this, a substantial number of patients cannot be placed into these categories and yet they persistently complain of insomnia (primary insomnia). Careful evaluation of the issues may yet reveal some relationship to stresses, both transient and persistent. It can be established that these patients are responding to unusual or protracted pressures of life: a man worries over possible redundancy, his wife is concerned about their delinquent son, their daughter is lovelorn, and grandmother is anxious over her increasing frailness. Giving drugs may set in train a long-term process culminating in drug-related insomnia without solving the basic problems.

Short-term symptomatic relief is acceptable when the stress is undoubtedly severe but transient. Even so, the hypnotic agent must be chosen carefully. The elimination half-life is the most important consideration. Those with half-lives over 12 h, such as nitrazepam, are only appropriate where an anxiolytic effect is required during the day as well as sleep induction at night. Even here, diazepam 5 to 15 mg, one dose at night, may be preferred. Temazepam with its shorter half-life will encourage sleep onset without leaving the patient with too many residual sedative effects the next day. Unfortunately, it has been extensively abused.

The management of chronic insomnia is much more problematic.[26] The newer compounds zopiclone and zolpidem are also short-acting agents and can help assure a good night's

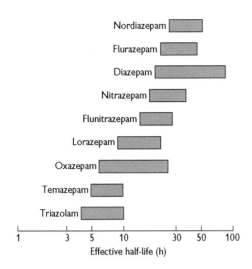

**Fig. 6.2.2.2** Table of half-lives.

sleep without much risk of residual sedative effects the next day.[27] This is dependent on the dosage being kept modest, especially in the elderly. Eszopiclone is licensed in the United States for long-term use in chronic insomnia and is already used extensively there.

Zolpidem and zaleplon can be used in a different strategic ways from other longer-acting drugs. Hypnotics are traditionally taken every night before going to bed to induce or maintain sleep. However, the severity of insomnia usually varies from night to night. Consequently, regular usage may be partly, or even largely, unnecessary, and increases the risk of habituation and dependence. Very-short-acting compounds are unlikely to leave residual effects the next day, even taken up to 5 h or so before the expected time of wakening. Consequently, the insomniac can refrain from regular hypnotic usage but, instead, wait up to an hour or so after going to bed to see if natural sleep supervenes before resorting to medication. This changes the regular prophylactic use of hypnotics to 'as needed', and lessens the risk of habituation and dependence. Furthermore, the patient is gratified to feel that he or she has control of the medication instead of vice versa.

### Residual effects

Residual effects can be a problem especially when long-acting drugs are used repeatedly. Dosage is important here, since residual effects increase in both magnitude and duration as the dose is increased. It should be remembered that hypnotics are the only class of drugs in which the main therapeutic effect (drowsiness) is identical with the main unwanted effect; the two are merely separated by 8 h in time. A short-acting hypnotic compound will be devoid of residual effects the next day, but the patient may wake early. After taking a longer-acting compound, sleep may be prolonged but hangover effects pronounced.

### Idiosyncratic effects

Adverse effects with triazolam alerted prescribers and regulators to possible major adverse effects of short-acting benzodiazepines. The adverse reactions in question include daytime anxiety, amnesic effects, and episodes, and morbid affects such as depression and hostility. In summary, the evidence suggests that these are class effects common to the benzodiazepines, although more likely to

occur the shorter the duration of action of the drug and the higher the dose. Alcohol is also capable of producing these effects.

### Rebound

Discontinuation of many hypnotics is often followed by worsening of sleep compared with pretreatment levels. In practical terms, insomniac patients find that their sleep is disturbed for a night or two after abrupt discontinuation of what appeared to be effective medication. Some of this rebound is subjective as patients taking sleeping pills tend to overestimate their sleeping time (compared with sleep laboratory recordings); on withdrawal, they underestimate their sleep. The intensity of rebound insomnia is strongly related to dose but less clearly to the duration of use, and marked individual differences exist. The risk of rebound is greater with short-half-life compared with the long-half-life compounds. Tapering off medication lessens the likelihood of rebound. However, despite clinical impressions that rebound insomnia might lead to the resumption of medication, there is little evidence for this.[28]

### Dependence

Dependence may supervene on the longer-term use of hypnotics; giving a long-acting benzodiazepine drug only once in 24 h does not protect against such an eventuality. The management of the withdrawal syndrome that may occur is largely the same as with the anxiolytic benzodiazepines.

### Abuse

A growing problem with these drugs is abuse—non-medical use, on a regular or sporadic basis, often in a polydrug context. Worldwide, flunitrazepam is the main problem and can be taken orally, by injection, or by sniffing. In the United Kingdom, temazepam is widely abused by injection. The injected drug has a marked sedative and/or disinhibiting effect, resulting in chaotic behaviour, carelessness, and an enhanced risk of the transmission of communicable diseases such as HIV infection and hepatitis.

## Other hypnotics

Gaboxadol is a GABA agonist. Preliminary data suggest useful hypnotic properties.

## Melatonin preparations

A series of compounds are being developed based on melatonin. This hormone is important in the regulation of sleep and is secreted at night. Some elderly insomniacs seem to be deficient in melatonin. Preparations include Circadin®, licensed in the UK for short-term use in insomnia in over 55s. Ramelteon is a melatonin$_1$ and melatonin$_2$ agonist. It is licensed in the United States for insomnia, and is effective in inducing sleep: it has a favourable safety profile.[29]

## Conclusions

In many countries the drug treatment of both anxiety and insomnia still largely revolves around the use of the benzodiazepines. Nevertheless, controversy and disagreement still rage about the risk–benefit ratio of compounds in this area. Short-term use in both indications is well established, with a favourable database as a rationale for this approach. However, long-term use is still only researched in a limited way. While both the efficacy and safety of long-term use remain unclear, acceptance of current guidelines limiting the use of benzodiazepines seems wise.

The advent of the SSRIs as anxiolytics has driven a wedge between the treatment methods for anxiety and insomnia. Anxiety can be treated just as effectively with an SSRI (and probably, pregabalin) as with a benzodiazepine, and more safely. The treatment of insomnia still relies on the benzodiazepines until the risk–benefit ratio of newer drugs such as the melatonin-related compounds becomes clear.

Nevertheless, in the author's opinion the most important outstanding issue is the relationship between drug and non-drug treatments.[30] The management of anxiety disorders and of insomnia is complex and is hampered by a dearth of information concerning the relative merits of various treatment modalities. Much research is also needed on the optimum strategies for combining all the therapies available to us, and on identifying predictors of response.

Developments in the neuropharmacology of insomnia hold out the promise of new compounds with novel and perhaps more effective modes of action.[31] With respect to anxiety disorders, a major shift of emphasis has followed the demonstration of the efficacy of the SSRIs.[32]

## Further information

Taylor, D., Kerwin, R., and Paton, C. (2005). *The Maudsley prescribing guidelines* (8th edn). South London and Maudsley NHS Trust.
Nutt, D. and Ballenger, J. (eds.) (2003). *Anxiety disorders*. Blackwell Science, Oxford.

## References

1. Allgulander, C. (1986). History and current status of sedative-hypnotic drug use and abuse. *Acta Psychiatrica Scandinavica*, **73**, 465–78.
2. Lader, M. (1994). Benzodiazepines. A risk–benefit profile. *CNS Drugs*, **1**, 377–87.
3. Curran, H.V. (1991). Benzodiazepines, memory and mood: a review. *Psychopharmacology*, **105**, 1–8.
4. Barker, M.J., Greenwood, K.M., Jackson, M., et al. (2004). Cognitive effects of long-term benzodiazepine use. *CNS Drugs*, **18**, 38–45.
5. Langtry, H.D. and Benfield, P. (1990). Zolpidem. A review of its pharmacodynamic and pharmacokinetic properties and therapeutic potential. *Drugs*, **40**, 291–313.
6. Sramek, J.J., Zarotsky, V., and Cutler, N.R. (2002). Generalised anxiety disorder. Treatment options. *Drugs*, **62**, 1635–45.
7. Taylor, C.B. (2006). Panic disorder. *British Medical Journal*, **332**, 951–5.
8. Hoehn–Saric, R. (1998). Generalised anxiety disorders. Guidelines for diagnosis and treatment. *CNS Drugs*, **9**, 85–98.
9. Otto, M.W., Pollack, M.H., and Sachs, G.S. (1993). Discontinuation of benzodiazepine treatment: efficacy of cognitive–behavioral therapy for patients with panic disorder. *The American Journal of Psychiatry*, **150**, 1485–90.
10. Dietch, J.T. and Jennings, R.K. (1988). Aggressive dyscontrol in patients treated with benzodiazepines. *The Journal of Clinical Psychiatry*, **49**, 184–7.
11. Serfaty, M. and Masterton, G. (1993). Fatal poisonings attributed to benzodiazepines in Britain during the 1980s. *The British Journal of Psychiatry*, **163**, 386–93.
12. Michelini, S., Cassano, G.B., Frare, F., et al. (1996). Long-term use of benzodiazepines: tolerance, dependence and clinical problems in anxiety and mood disorders. *Pharmacopsychiatry*, **29**, 127–34.
13. Petursson, H. and Lader, M.H. (1981). Withdrawal from long–term benzodiazepine treatment. *British Medical Journal*, **283**, 643–5.
14. Tyrer, P. (1991). The benzodiazepine post-withdrawal syndrome. *Stress Medicine*, **7**, 1–2.
15. Russell, J. and Lader, M. (eds.) (1993). *Guidelines for the prevention and treatment of benzodiazepine dependence*. Mental Health Foundation, London.
16. Voshaar, R.C., Couvee, J.E., van Balkom, A.J., et al. (2006). Strategies for discontinuing long-term benzodiazepine use: meta-analysis. *The British Journal of Psychiatry*, **189**, 213–20.
17. Potokar, J. and Nutt, D.J. (1994). Anxiolytic potential of benzodiazepine receptor partial agonists. *CNS Drugs*, **1**, 305–15.
18. Fulton, B. and Brogden, R.N. (1997). Buspirone. An updated review of its clinical pharmacology and therapeutic applications. *CNS Drugs*, **7**, 68–88.
19. Kavoussi, R. (2006). Pregabalin: from molecule to medicine. *European Neuropsychopharmacology*, **16**, S128–33.
20. Frampton, J.E. and Foster, R.H. (2006). Pregabalin in the treatment of generalised anxiety disorder. *CNS Drugs*, **20**, 685–93.
21. Van Ameringen, M., Mancini, C., Pipe B., et al. (2004). Antiepileptic drugs in the treatment of anxiety disorders. Role in therapy. *Drugs*, **64**, 2199–220.
22. Stein, D.J. (2006). Evidence-based treatment of anxiety disorders. *International Journal of Psychiatry in Clinical Practice*, **10**(Suppl. 1), 16–21.
23. Baldwin, D.S., Anderson, I.M., Nutt, D.J., et al. (2005). Evidence-based guidelines for the pharmacological treatment of anxiety disorders: recommendations from the British Association for Psychopharmacology. *Journal of Psychopharmacology*, **19**, 567–96.
24. Üstün, T.B., Privett, M., Lecrubier, Y., et al. (1996). Form, frequency and burden of sleep problems in general health care: a report from the WHO collaborative study on psychological problems in general health care. *European Psychiatry*, **11**(Suppl. 1), 5S–10S.
25. Kamel, N. and Gammack, J.K. (2006). Insomnia in the elderly: cause, approach, and treatment. *The American Journal of Medicine*, **119**, 463–9.
26. Kupfer, D.J. and Reynolds, C.F. (1997). Management of insomnia. *The New England Journal of Medicine*, **336**, 341–6.
27. Nowell, P.D., Mazumdar, S., Buysse, D.J., et al. (1997). Benzodiazepines and zolpidem for chronic insomnia. A meta-analysis of treatment efficacy. *The Journal of the American Medical Association*, **278**, 2170–7.
28. Roehrs, T., Merlotti, L., Zorick, F., et al. (1992). Rebound insomnia and hypnotic self administration. *Psychopharmacology*, **107**, 480–4.
29. Johnson, M.W., Suess, P.E., and Griffiths, R.R. (2006). Ramelteon: a novel hypnotic lacking abuse liability and sedative adverse effects. *Archives of General Psychiatry*, **63**, 1149–57.
30. Fineberg, N. and Drummond, L.M. (1995). Anxiety disorders. Drug treatment or behavioural cognitive psychotherapy? *CNS Drugs*, **3**, 448–66.
31. Szabadi, E. (2006). Drugs for sleep disorders: mechanisms and therapeutic prospects. *British Journal of Clinical Pharmacology*, **61**, 761–6.
32. Tyrer, P. and Baldwin, D. (2006). Generalised anxiety disorder. *Lancet*, **368**, 2156–66.

# 6.2.3 **Antidepressants**

Zubin Bhagwagar and George R. Heninger

## Introduction

Major depressive disorder is a serious, recurrent illness which levies a crippling toll on individuals, families, and society in general. The importance of depression as a major public health problem is emphasized by findings from the World Health Organization Global Burden of Disease survey in showing that in 1990 it was the fourth largest cause of burden of disease (i.e. years of life lost due either to premature mortality or to years lived with a disability). It has been estimated that by the year 2020 it is expected to be the second largest cause of burden of disease.[1] Depression is under-diagnosed and frequently under-treated, and depressed individuals have a much higher risk for suicide. The primary treatment for depression involves the use of antidepressant drugs, and it is therefore important that clinicians become familiar with and adept in utilizing this important group of compounds. Although primarily used for the treatment of depression, drugs within this category also have a number of other important uses. A thorough understanding of the pharmacology of antidepressants will aid the clinician in the selective use of these drugs for patients with depression as well as patients with a number of other disorders.

## A brief history of antidepressant discovery and theories of action

Table 6.2.3.1 gives a brief chronology of antidepressant drug discoveries and theories of drug action. It is a comment on our understanding of the illness that some of the major advances in the pharmacotherapy of depression have been serendipitous. Prior to 1954, except for the use of electroconvulsive therapy, there were few effective drug treatments for depression. In 1954, the antidepressant era was initiated with the observation that some patients with tuberculosis displayed mood elevations following treatment with the antituberculosis agent iproniazid.[2] Following this initial serendipitous observation, the antidepressant effect of iproniazid was confirmed[3] and its action of inhibiting monoamine oxidase was reported. Iproniazid had significant toxicity and other monoamine oxidase inhibitors (MAOIs) were subsequently introduced. Independent from the work on MAOIs, imipramine, which has a chemical structure similar to the phenothiazines, was assessed as an agent to treat agitation in psychotic patients where it was found to be ineffective. However, it was noticed (again serendipitously) that imipramine produced an improvement of mood in the subset of patients who had symptoms of depression. Kuhn then reported in 1958 that imipramine was an effective antidepressant.[4]

One of the earliest theories of antidepressant drug action was that the antidepressant effect was produced by an increase of serotonin (5-hydroxytryptamine (**5-HT**)) in brain. This was supported by an initial study showing that an MAOI plus tryptophan, the precursor of 5-HT, was a more effective antidepressant treatment than an MAOI alone.[5] Subsequently, the discovery that imipramine and desipramine had effects in inhibiting the reuptake of noradrenaline (norepinephrine) and adrenaline (epinephrine) into the synapse led to the catecholamine theory of depression, which proposed that antidepressant treatments act by increasing the level of catecholamines at brain synapses.[6,7] Ten years later, it was reported that in laboratory animals most antidepressant treatments lead to downregulation of β-adrenergic receptors. This supported the proposal that antidepressants act by reducing β-adrenergic receptor sensitivity.[8] However, the reduction in β-adrenergic receptor sensitivity occurred within hours and antidepressant effect requires 1 to 3 weeks and futher not all effective antidepressant treatments produce reductions in β-adrenergic receptor sensitivity.

In the 1970s and 1980s, a large number of studies on antidepressants were conducted in laboratory animals which demonstrated that they produced a number of changes in monoamine receptor sensitivity.[9] In the late 1980s, a number of neurophysiological

**Table 6.2.3.1** History of discovery of antidepressants and pharmacological theories of antidepressant drug action

| Year | Discovery or theory | Reference |
|------|---------------------|-----------|
| 1954 | Discovery that MAOIs have antidepressant effects | 2, 3 |
| 1958 | Discovery that the tricyclic drug imipramine is an effective antidepressant | 4 |
| 1963 | *Serotonin theory of depression*: MAOIs act by increasing serotonin and tryptamine in brain | 5 |
| 1965 | *Catecholamine theory of depression*: ADTs act by increasing cathecolamines in brain | 6, 7 |
| 1975 | *β-Adrenergic receptor theory of depression*: ADTs act by altering the sensitivity of several monoamine receptor subtypes in brain | 8 |
| 1981 | *Monoamine receptor sensitivity theory of depression*: ADTs act by altering the sensitivity of several monoamine receptor subtypes in brain | 9 |
| 1987 | *Serotonergic augmentation theory of depression*: ADTs act by decreasing sensitivity of presynaptic serotonergic autoreceptors and increasing sensitivity of serotonergic postsynaptic receptors to increase overall efficacy in serotonergic transmission | 10 |
| 1996 | *A molecular and cellular theory of depression*: ADTs act by producing a sustained activation of the cAMP system which increases brain levels of neurotrophic factors that reverse the effects of stres in certain brain areas | 14 |
| 1998 | Discovery that a substance P antagonist that does not interact with monoamine systems is as effective an antidepressant as an SSRI (paroxetine) | 16 |
| 2000/2006 | Demonstration of antidepressant properties of ketamine implicating the glutamatergic system in the pathophysiology of depression | 19, 20 |

ADT, antidepressant treatment.

studies provided evidence that the delay in onset of antidepressant effects could be accounted for by a slow decrease in sensitivity at presynaptic serotonergic autoreceptors which has the overall result of increasing serotonergic function after days and weeks of treatment.[10] An elaboration on the receptor sensitivity theory was the discovery that most antidepressants produce alterations in the sensitivity of a specific glycine-sensitive site on the N-methyl-d-aspartate (NMDA) receptor.[11] A subsequent study showed that an NMDA antagonist may have antidepressant actions[12] and this line of thought has borne fruit recently in a possible novel mechanism of action for antidepressant treatment. An additional receptor sensitivity change thought to be important in the mechanism of action of antidepressants involved changes in the sensitivity of receptors for glucocorticoids. It was found that antidepressants produce an overall improvement of inhibitory feedback on the hypothalamic-pituitary-adrenal axis[13] and that specific corticotrophin releasing hormone (CRH) antagonists have antidepressant properties.[14]

A more recent theory of antidepressant drug action involves findings that antidepressant treatments affect intracellular pathways and neurotrophins. It was found that many antidepressants, in spite of β-adrenergic receptor downregulation, continue to produce sustained activation of the cAMP system and that this is related to increases of neurotrophic factors in brain.[15] Neurotrophins reverse the effects of stress in some brain areas and this raise the possibility that antidepressants act by increasing neurotrophins which reverse the effects of stress in important brain areas of depressed patients.

Throughout the 1980s, and 1990s a number of compounds that do not fit the standard monoamine theories of depression have been found to be effective clinical antidepressants. One of these drugs, tianeptine, actually increases the uptake of 5-HT into nerve endings, an effect that is opposite to the standard selective serotonin reuptake inhibitors (**SSRIs**).[16] Similarly, while there was intense interest in a report of possible antidepressant efficacy of a substance P receptor antagonist,[17] which does not interact with monoamine systems, clinical trials for this specific compound were disappointing.

Although no single mechanism has been discovered that will account for the antidepressant effects of all effective antidepressant treatments, it is clear that initial effects on monoamine metabolism with subsequent effects of intracellular pathways is important. While clinical wisdom and data suggest that there is a lag of 7–21 days to antidepressant action, recent reports question this notion of delayed onset of efficacy.[18] Recently ketamine, an NMDA antagonist has been shown to have an onset of action much faster than that traditionally seen with conventional antidepressants[19,20] suggesting that the pursuit of novel mechanisms may indeed result in advances in the pharmacotherapy of depression. Using preclinical models, it has been suggested that both nonselective NMDA antagonists as well as NR2B selective antagonists exert their antidepressant effects by regulating the functional interplay between AMPA and NMDA throughput.[21]

## Pharmacology and types of compounds available

Antidepressant drugs fall into a wide variety of chemical classes and they have a wide range of neuropharmacological effects. They are grouped in Tables 6.2.3.2, 6.2.3.3, and 6.2.3.4 based on the presumed primary action that leads to an antidepressant effect. Table 6.2.3.2 lists the drugs that inhibit the uptake of the monoamines noradrenaline, 5-HT, and dopamine into nerve endings which in turn is thought to increase the function of the respective monoamine systems in brain. Table 6.2.3.3 lists the drugs that inhibit monoamine oxidase and thereby increase the concentration of many amines in brain. Table 6.2.3.4 lists the drugs with other primary actions that do not primarily involve inhibition of monoamine uptake or monoamine oxidase inhibition.

In Table 6.2.3.2, the first 12 compounds are inhibitors of noradrenaline uptake with a variable potency of inhibiting 5-HT uptake. The drugs with secondary amine structures, desipramine, nortriptyline, protriptyline, amoxapine, and maprotiline are predominantly noradrenaline uptake inhibitors with little effect on 5-HT uptake.[22] It can be seen in Table 6.2.3.2 that clomipramine, in addition to inhibiting noradrenaline uptake, is also a strong 5-HT uptake inhibitor. There are currently three selective serotonin and noradrenaline reuptake inhibitor (SNRI) drugs available; milnacipran (not licensed in the US), venlafaxine and duloxetine. Venlafaxine, inhibits both 5-HT and noradrenaline and 5-HT reuptake,[23] as do milnacipran and duloxetine though in varying proportions. While affinities vary depending on the system studied, milnacipran blocks 5-HT and norepinephrine reuptake with relatively equal affinity, while duloxetine has been suggested to have a slightly greater selectivity for 5-HT and venlafaxine a much greater selectivity for 5-HT.[24] Reboxetine (not licensed in the US) is a highly selective and potent inhibitor of noradrenaline reuptake.[25] It has only a weak effect on the 5-HT reuptake and does not affect the uptake of dopamine.

A key issue in the pharmacology of all antidepressant drugs is the relative specificity of their action. Drugs with a tertiary amine structure tend to produce more antagonism of $\alpha_1$-adrenergic receptors which can produce hypotension, histamine receptors which can produce sedation, and muscarinic cholinergic receptors which can produce blurred vision, dry mouth, and urinary retention. This leads to more side-effects for these compounds than the drugs with a secondary amine structure. Venlafaxine has relatively less effect on these receptors and thus fewer side-effects[23] (see Table 6.2.3.6).

SSRIs are probably the most widely prescribed antidepressants and represent a class of drugs that selectively inhibit 5-HT reuptake from the synapse. Unlike the tricyclics, they each have different chemical structures. The drugs listed in Table 6.2.3.2 have a relatively specific effect in inhibiting 5-HT uptake,[22] and because of their relatively specific effect on this monoamine system and the lack of antagonism of many other receptors, they have been found to have fewer side-effects. Escitalopram was introduced following the discovery that all of the inhibitory activity of citalopram on 5-HT reuptake resides in the S-(+)-enantiomer (S-citalopram),[26] with S-citalopram being 167 times more potent than R-citalopram at inhibiting 5-HT reuptake into rat brain synaptosomes.

MAOIs are listed in Table 6.2.3.3. Two isozymes, monoamine oxidases A and B, are present in many discrete cell populations within the central nervous system, and glial cells also express monoamine oxidases A and B. The main substrates for monoamine oxidase A include adrenaline, noradrenaline, and 5-HT. The breakdown of dopamine in striatal regions of the brain is preferentially by monoamine oxidase B, but it can also be broken down by monoamine oxidase A. Since monoamine oxidase is located on the

**Table 6.2.3.2** Pharmacological actions of antidepressants: drugs that inhibit monoamine reuptake at the synapse

| Drug | Chemical class | Relative reuptake inhibition | | |
|------|----------------|------------------------------|--|--|
| | | Noradrenaline | 5-Hydroxytryptamine | Dopamine |
| Imipramine | Tricyclic | ++ | + | 0 |
| Desipramine[a] | Tricyclic | ++++ | 0 | 0 |
| Amitriptyline[a] | Tricyclic | ++ | + | 0 |
| Nortriptyline[a] | Tricyclic | +++ | 0/+ | 0 |
| Trimipramine | Tricyclic | + | 0 | 0 |
| Clomipramine | Tricyclic | + | +++ | 0 |
| Protriptyline[a] | Tricyclic | ++++ | 0 | 0 |
| Doxepin | Tricyclic | ++ | 0/+ | 0 |
| Amoxapine[a] | Tricyclic | +++ | 0 | + |
| Maprotiline[a] | Tetracyclic | +++ | 0 | 0 |
| Venlafaxine | Bicyclic | + | ++ | 0/+ |
| Milnacipran | SNRI | +++ | +++ | 0/+ |
| Duloxetine | SNRI | +++ | ++ | 0/+ |
| Reboxetine | NARI | ++++ | 0 | + |
| Fluoxetine | SSRI | 0 | +++ | 0 |
| Sertraline | SSRI | 0 | ++++ | + |
| Fluvoxamine | SSRI | 0 | +++ | 0 |
| Paroxetine | SSRI | + | ++++ | 0 |
| Citalopram | SSRI | 0 | ++++ | 0 |
| Escitalopram | SSRI | 0 | ++++ | 0 |

0, None; 0/+, minimal; +, low; ++, moderate; +++, High; ++++, very high.

[a]Secondary amine.

outside of the plasma membrane of the mitochondria in neurones, it is not able to eliminate amines that are stored inside vesicles. MAOI produces an increase in monoamines in the cytoplasm. It is thought that the increase in monoamine content is the primary mechanism of action of MAOIs, and other secondary changes including β-adrenergic receptor downregulation and other receptor changes are secondary to the increased amine levels.[27]

Four of the six drugs listed in Table 6.2.3.3 are irreversible inhibitors. The two reversible inhibitors are essentially inert substrate analogues, and there is usually a correlation between their plasma

**Table 6.2.3.3** Pharmacological actions of antidepressants: drugs that inhibit monoamine oxidase

| Drug | Chemical class | MAO A | MAO B | Reversible |
|------|----------------|-------|-------|------------|
| Isocarboxazid | Hydrazine | Yes | Yes | No |
| Phenelzine | Hydrazine | Yes | Yes | No |
| Tranylcypromine | Amphetamine | Yes | Yes | No |
| Moclobemide | Morpholine | Yes | No | Yes |
| Brofaromine | Piperidine | Yes | No | Yes |
| Selegiline | Phenethylamine | No | Yes[a] | No |

MAO, Monoamine oxidase.

[a]Selective at lower doses; becomes non-selective at higher doses.

concentration and the reversible inhibition of monoamine oxidase A. Since isocarboxazid, phenelzine, and tranylcypromine are irreversible inhibitors of monoamine oxidases A and B, there can be serious side-effects when foods that are high in tyramine or other amines are ingested. In addition, these three drugs have strong interactions with other drugs that alter monoamine

**Table 6.2.3.4** Pharmacological actions of antidepressants: drugs that do not act by strong inhibition of monoamine uptake or inhibition of monoamine oxidase

| Drug | Chemical class | Possible pharmacological action |
|------|----------------|--------------------------------|
| Trazodone | Triazolopyridine | Mixed 5-HT agonist/antagonist |
| Nefazodone | Phenylpiperazine | Mixed 5-HT agonist/antagonist, weak monoamine uptake inhibitor |
| Bupropion | Unicyclic amino ketone | Weak noradrenaline and dopamine uptake inhibitor |
| Mianserin | Tetracyclic | Antagonist $\alpha_2$-adrenergic auto- and heteroreceptors, increased 5-HT and noradrenaline release |
| Mirtazapine | Tetracyclic | Antagonist $\alpha_2$-adrenergic auto and heteroreceptors, increased 5-HT and noradrenaline release |

metabolism and therefore their use as antidepressants is much more limited than the tricyclics, SSRIs, or other antidepressant compounds. Tranylcypromine, which has a structure similar to amfetamine in addition to being an MAOI, is also thought to have a stimulant-type action of rapid onset. With the reversible MAOIs moclobemide and brofaromine, the recovery of monoamine oxidase back to normal levels after the drug is stopped is much shorter than with the irreversible MAOIs. These drugs increase concentrations of 5-HT, noradrenaline, and adrenaline that are short and parallel the time course of the monoamine oxidase A inhibition. These two drugs are more easily displaced by the pressor amines such as tyramine, and therefore, are thought to be safer than the irreversible inhibitors.

Selegiline, which has recently become available as a transdermal patch,[28] is selective at lower doses for monoamine oxidase B but at higher doses it becomes non-selective.[29] It has been primarily used for the treatment of Parkinson's disease and the doses for treating depression need to be much higher (note: selegiline is not licensed in the UK for depression). Since monoamine oxidase B is not involved in the intestinal tyramine interaction, selegiline interactions with ingested monoamines have been minimal.

In addition to inhibiting monoamine oxidase, these compounds have other effects on monoamine systems that can produce side-effects. However, the major concerns are the interactions with dietary amines and other drugs that influence amine function. The combination of dietary interactions and slow recovery of monoamine oxidase following with the irreversible inhibitors makes these drugs one of the more difficult treatments to administer. They are generally reserved for patients not otherwise responding to the other less toxic antidepressants.

In Table 6.2.3.4, compounds that are effective antidepressants but do not inhibit monoamine oxidase or have strong monoamine uptake inhibition are listed. Trazodone has shown receptor antagonist activity at several 5-HT receptor subtypes although its active metabolite *m*-chlorophenylpiperazine (mCPP) is a potent direct serotonin agonist. It is a weak but relatively selective inhibitor of 5-HT reuptake, is an antagonist at 5-HT1A and 5-HT2 receptors in addition to its active metabolite mCPP being a potent 5-HT agonist.[30] This leads to trazodone being classified as a mixed 5-HT agonist/antagonist. It also has relatively weak 5-HT uptake inhibiting properties but with no effect on noradrenaline or dopamine uptake. Trazodone is virtually devoid of anticholingeric activity and therefore it has few side-effects in this area. However, it does produce considerable sedation and hypotension secondary to antagonism of α1-adrenergic receptors and histamine receptors.

Nefazodone is an analogue of trazodone that was developed to overcome the orthostatic hypotension and sedation caused by the latter. Like trazodone it is a 5-HT receptor antagonist with weak monoamine uptake inhibition activity.[31] It has less affinity for the α-adrenergic receptors and is inactive on many other receptors. It too is metabolized to *m*-chlorophenylpiperazine which is an active serotonergic agonist. Although the initial effects of nefazodone involve alterations of 5-HT neurotransmission, these effects are complex and depend on the biological test used.

Bupropion resulted from focussed research to find antidepressant compounds that would have fewer side-effects than traditional tricyclics (note: buproprion is not licensed in the UK for depression). Bupropion is a mild inhibitor of noradrenaline uptake, has some effects on inhibiting dopamine uptake but has no effect on 5-HT

uptake.[32] These effects are not associated with β-adrenergic receptor downregulation as is seen with many other antidepressants. One of the active metabolites is hydroxybupropion which also has an antidepressant profile in laboratory animals. It is of interest that bupropion is one of the few drugs that reduce REM latency since most other treatments increase it. Although the specific mechanisms of bupropions antidepressant effects are not known, its unique profile has led to its use in the treatment of bipolar disorder[33] as well as its use in the treatment of smoking cessation.[34]

Mianserin and mirtazapine both have potent effects on antagonizing α2-adrenergic auto- and heteroreceptors.[35] They also antagonize other 5-HT receptors but have minimal effects on monoamine uptake or monoamine oxidase activity. Since α2 receptors inhibit noradrenaline release, their antagonism leads to an increase in noradrenaline release in many brain areas. In addition, antagonism of α2-adrenergic heteroreceptors located on serotonergic neurones results in an enhanced 5-HT release. With mirtazapine, since 5-HT2 and 5-HT3 receptors are blocked, this could result in selective enhancement of 5-HT1-receptor-mediated neurotransmission. These drugs have low affinity for muscarinic, cholinergic, and dopamine receptors and this is related to a reduced side-effect profile. The combination of increased noradrenaline release and increased 5-HT release resulting from the α2-antagonism on auto- and heteroreceptors is hypothesized to be the central mechanism of action.

## Pharmacokinetics

Data on the pharmacokinetics of antidepressants are listed in Table 6.2.3.5. The tricyclic antidepressants are by and large well absorbed although time to peak plasma concentration can vary from 1 to 12 h depending on the drug and the individual. In general, these drugs are metabolized in the liver to a variety of metabolites, some of which are active. For instance, desipramine is a metabolite of imipramine and nortriptyline is a metabolite of amitriptyline. Most of these compounds have a long half-life (close to 24 h) that will allow for once-daily dosing. All the compounds are highly bound to plasma protein except for venlafaxine and milnacipran. Although many of the compounds have active metabolites, the exact percentage of each metabolite in patients and in their clinical effects is still largely unknown.

There is considerable individual variation in the metabolism of tricyclics, and a large component of this may be genetic. Up to 7 to 9 per cent of the Caucasian population have been classified as slow metabolizers (slow hydroxylators) which can be measured by the rate of hydroxylation of debrisoquin. The slow hydoxylation has been determined to be caused by a polymorphism in a cytochrome P-450 macrosomal enzyme (CYP2D6). It is of interest that many SSRIs are inhibitors of P-450 isoenzymes which can considerably influence the metabolism of tricyclic antidepressants.[36] In general, the increased renal clearance in children and a decreased renal clearance with age need to be taken into account with dosing.

The SSRIs are rapidly absorbed, although there is variability within the drug half-lives. The metabolism into active metabolites can vary the pharmacodynamic effects considerably. For example, fluoxetine is metabolized to norfluoxetine which has similar activity on 5-HT reuptake as fluoxetine. The elimination half-life of norfluoxetine is longer (4–16 days) than that of fluoxetine (4–6 days). The desmethyl metabolite of sertraline although not nearly as potent as the parent compound, also has a much longer half life. The desmethyl metabolite of citalopram or escitalopram, although a potent noradrenaline uptake inhibitor, is much lower in concentration than citalopram and it weakly crosses the blood-brain barrier. Fluvoxamine, paroxetine, duloxetine or milnacipran do not have any active metabolites. The relatively long half-lives of some of the SSRIs, particularly fluoxetine, require longer drug-free periods before switching to other classes of compounds especially before starting an MAOI.

The MAOIs are all rapidly absorbed. For the irreversible MAOIs, the elimination half-life and protein binding patterns are not as relevant because of the irreversible effects on monoamine oxidase. The reversible MAOIs have shorter half-lives and require multiple daily dosing.[29] With the irreversible MAOIs, once the drug is stopped, there needs to be time for new synthesis of monoamine oxidase. This requires a minimum of 5 to 7 days and the safest recommendation is to wait 2 weeks before starting other drugs that may interact with the MAOIs.

The five other antidepressants listed in Table 6.2.3.5 are rapidly absorbed but there is some variation in their elimination half-life. In general, the half-lives are short enough that multiple daily dosing is required. They are generally bound to plasma protein at a high level. The metabolites of trazodone and nefazodone have mixed effects on 5-HT receptors which results in a complex overall effect. Trazodone and nefazodone undergo extensive hepatic metabolism and one major metabolite is m-chlorophenylpiperazine which stimulates 5-HT receptors. Many metabolites have biological activity with half-lives different to the parent compounds.

Bupropion is metabolized in the liver and its metabolites can be at higher concentration than the parent compound. The relationship between plasma bupropion and clinical response has been poor.

**Table 6.2.3.5** Pharmacokinetics of antidepressants

| Drug | Absorption time to peak plasma concentration (h) | Elimination half-life (h) | Percentage plasma protein binding | Important metabolite |
|---|---|---|---|---|
| *Monoamine reuptake inhibitors* | | | | |
| Imipramine | 1.5–3 | 11–25 | 92 | Desipramine |
| Desipramine | 3–6 | 11–31 | 90 | 2-OH-desipramine |
| Amitriptyline | 1–5 | 10–26 | 94 | Nortriptyline |
| Nortrityline | 3–12 | 18–44 | 92 | 10-OH-nortriptylene |
| Trimipramine | 3 | 9–11 | 95 | None |
| Clomipramine | 2–6 | 21–31 | 97 | Desmethylclomipramine |
| Protriptyline | 6–12 | 67–89 | 93 | None |
| Doxepin | 1–4 | 11–23 | 80 | Desmethyldoxepin |
| Amoxapine | 1–2 | 8–30 | 90 | 8-OH-amoxapine |
| Maprotiline | 4–12 | 28–58 | 88 | Desmethylmaprotiline |
| Venlafaxine | 2 | 5 | 30 | O-desmethylvenlafaxine |
| Milnacipran | 0.5–4 | 8 | 13 | None |
| Duloxetine | 6–10 | 8–17 | 95 | None |
| Reboxetine | 1.5–2.4 | 12–14 | 97 | NA |
| *SSRIs* | | | | |
| Fluoxetine | 4–8 | 24–120 | 94 | Norfluoxetine |
| Sertraline | 6–8 | 27 | 99 | n-Desmethylsertraline |
| Fluvoxamine | 2–8 | 15–26 | 77 | None |
| Paroxetine | 5–7 | 24–31 | 95 | None |
| Citalopram | 1–6 | 33 | 80 | NA (monodesmethylcitalopram) |
| Escitalopram | 3–6 | 22–32 | 56 | S-desmethylcitalopram |
| *MAOIs* | | | | |
| Isocarboxazid | 3–5 | NA | NA | NA |
| Phenelzine | 2–4 | NA | NA | NA |
| Tranylcypromine | 1.5–3 | 1.5–3.5 | NA | NA |
| Moclobemide | 1–1.5 | 1.4 | NA | Numerous |
| Brofaromine | 1–2 | 12–15 | NA | n-Desmethylbrofaromine |
| Selegiline | 1–3 | 2–10 | NA | n-Desmethylselegiline |
| *Other antidepressants* | | | | |
| Trazodone | 1–2 | 6–11 | 92 | m-Chlor ophenylpiperazine |
| Nefazodone | 1 | 2–4 | 99 | m-Chlorophenylpiperazine |
| Bupropion | 3 | 10–21 | 85 | Bupropion threoamino alcohol |
| Mianserin | 2–3 | 15–22 | NA | NA |
| Mirtazapine | 2–3 | 20–40 | 85 | None |

NA, data not available

## Side-effects

The history of new drugs becoming available for the treatment of depression reflects the efforts by the pharmaceutical industry to find compounds with reduced side-effects. This is in particularly important in the treatment of patients with medical illness because some of the side-effects can have considerable negative medical consequences. In Table 6.2.3.6, the propensity of the different drugs to produce some of the side-effects caused by antidepressants can be compared. The drugs that have high affinity for the $\alpha_1$-adrenergic receptors can produce hypotension. Antagonism of histamine receptors has been associated with sedation and there is a long list of anticholinergic effects associated with antagonism of muscarinic cholinergic receptors.

For the tricyclics, it can be seen that drugs with a tertiary amine structure produce increased sedation. There is also an increase in the frequency of side-effects associated with antagonism of muscarinic cholinergic receptors such as dry mouth, constipation, blurred vision, urinary retention, dizziness, tachycardia, memory impairment, and at high and toxic doses, delirium. There is also an increased tendency for these same compounds to produce hypotension and to have unwanted cardiac effects that can lead to serious complications. In addition, the tertiary amines have a tendency to produce more weight gain than the secondary amines. The adverse effects have a particular impact on the tolerance of the patients to taking the medication. Most importantly the anticholinergic and cardiac effects can produce difficult complications in the elderly even leading to delirium when too high a dose is given. Amoxapine can cause extrapyramidal symptoms which are thought to be secondary to blocking dopamine receptors.[37] The most common adverse effects in patients taking reboxetine during clinical trials were insomnia, sweating, constipation, dry mouth, and urinary hesitancy compared with placebo, and the rates of nausea, diarrhea, and somnolence were lower compared with fluoxetine.[38] Nausea, dry mouth, dizziness, headache, somnolence, constipation, and fatigue were reported most frequently with duloxetine.[39]

The propensity to produce orthostatic hypotension is also a serious side-effect, particularly in the elderly. With the increased risk of falls and subsequent fractures in the elderly, this can be a serious health risk. A number of methods such as teaching patients to rise slowly from a supine position, tilting the bed upward, and maintenance of fluid uptake could help prevent this. However, other equally effective newer antidepressants produce much less of many of these side-effects, and they can be more safely used in the elderly.

Many of the drugs that are monoamine uptake inhibitors can cause cardiac conduction delays which may even lead to heart block in patients with pre-existing conditions. Severe overdose of these compounds can produce major and life-threatening cardiac arrhythmias. The secondary amines are generally thought to produce less cardiac effects than the tertiary amines. One of the characteristics of the SSRIs which has led to their widespread use is their low rate of side-effects. The pharmacological specificity of these compounds which bind to the 5-HT transporter, while not binding to the other neurotransmitter receptor types, results in their producing a therapeutic effect without many of the unwanted side-effects. In placebo-controlled trials the incidence of early discontinuation of SSRIs because of adverse events is intermediate between patients treated with placebo and patients treated with tricyclic antidepressants. Some of the symptoms reported with these compounds include agitation, anxiety, headache, sleep disturbance, and tremor. One of the more troublesome side-effects is sexual dysfunction especially anorgasmia. Less frequently, there are changes in appetite with nausea, dry mouth, sweating, and weight change. In general, these effects are less than those observed with the non-SSRI monoamine uptake inhibitors. The interaction of SSRIs with MAOIs to produce the serotonin syndrome is discussed under toxic effects below. Fluoxetine and sertraline induced higher rates of sedation as dosages are increased but in contrast, paroxetine produces a dose-dependent increase in arousal.

In contrast with the fewer side-effects produced by SSRIs and the other antidepressants that are not monoamine inhibitors, the MAOIs tend to produce frequent and often much more serious side-effects. Frequent side-effects include dizziness, headache, insomnia, dry mouth, blurred vision, nausea, constipation, forgetfulness, difficulty with urination, and weakness. There is also sexual dysfunction, including anorgasmia, impotence, delayed ejaculation, and decreased desire. Insomnia has also been reported. The original MAOIs iproniazid and isocarboxazid had a higher frequency of impairing liver function, but this is less with the other drugs. Pyridoxine deficiency has been reported and should be considered in evaluating side-effects. The largest problem with the MAOIs is the interactions with foods and with other drugs. Food interaction is much less of a problem with the reversible MAOIs moclobemide and brofaromine.[37–39]

Trazodone and nefazodone lack the anticholergic side-effects of many of the tricyclic drugs. This makes them useful compounds in many medical conditions where this effect would be problematic. Trazodone has an acute sedative effect which is useful in the treatment of agitation, anxiety, and insomnia. However, this can be a troublesome side-effect when the patient performs tasks that require full alertness. Trazodone appears to have more propensity to produce orthostatic hypotension than nefazodone, possibility related to the degree of $\alpha_1$-adrenergic receptor antagonism. Both trazodone and nefazodone, because of their lack of anticholinergic effects, have a low probability of producing difficulties in patients with cardiac illness. There is a slight tendency for weight gain but not nearly as strong as for some of the other antidepressants.[40] A relatively rare but important side-effect with trazodone is priapism. The risk for this side-effect is greatest during the early phase of treatment and the reporting of abnormal erectile function, including inappropriate or prolonged erections, should prompt quick discontinuation of trazodone treatment. Sexual side-effects have also been reported in women.

Bupropion has a very different side-effect profile than the conventional tricyclic antidepressants. It has no anticholinergic effects, is not sedating, and instead of weight gain, it suppresses appetite in some patients. In comparison to the SSRIs and trazodone and nefazodone, it also does not cause sexual dysfunction. There is no orthostatic hypotension, and bupropion does not produce cardiac side-effects. The possible stimulation of dopaminergic systems by bupropion can be related to its activating effects. This may be useful in patients with retardation but may exacerbate patients with agitation and insomnia. Bupropion can make tics in attention-deficit hyperactivity disorder and Tourette's disorder worse.[41] Patients have been described with bupropion-related

**Table 6.2.3.6** Side-effects of antidepressants

| Drug | Sedation | Anticholinergic effects | Hypotension | Cardiac effects | Weight gain |
|---|---|---|---|---|---|
| *Monoamine reuptake inhibitors* | | | | | |
| Imipramine | +++ | ++ | ++ | +++ | ++ |
| Desipramine | + | + | + | ++ | + |
| Amitriptyline | +++ | ++++ | +++ | +++ | +++ |
| Nortriptyline | + | + | + | ++ | + |
| Trimipramine | +++ | +++ | ++ | +++ | ++ |
| Clomipramine | ++ | +++ | ++ | +++ | + |
| Protriptyline | 0/+ | ++ | + | +++ | + |
| Doxepin | +++ | ++ | +++ | ++ | ++ |
| Amoxapine | + | ++ | + | ++ | + |
| Maprotiline | ++ | ++ | ++ | ++ | + |
| Venlafaxine | 0/+ | 0/+ | 0 | + | 0 |
| Milnacipran | 0/+ | +/++ | 0/+ | + | 0 |
| Duloxetine | + | ++ | 0/+ | 0/+ | + |
| Reboxetine | 0 | +/++ | 0/+ | 0/+ | 0 |
| *SSRIs* | | | | | |
| Fluoxetine | 0/+ | 0 | 0 | 0 | 0 |
| Sertraline | 0 | 0 | 0 | 0 | 0 |
| Fluvoxamine | 0 | 0 | 0 | 0 | 0 |
| Paroxetine | + | + | 0 | 0 | 0 |
| Citalopram | + | + | 0/+ | 0/+ | 0 |
| Escitalopram | + | + | 0/+ | 0/+ | 0/+ |
| *MAOIs* | | | | | |
| Isocarboxazid | + | + | +++ | 0 | + |
| Phenelzine | + | 0 | +++ | 0 | ++ |
| Tranylcypromine | + | 0 | ++ | 0 | 0/+ |
| Moclobemide | 0 | 0 | 0 | 0 | 0 |
| Brofaromine | 0 | 0/+ | 0/+ | 0 | 0 |
| Selegiline | 0 | 0 | + | 0 | 0 |
| *Other antidepressants* | | | | | |
| Trazodone | +++ | 0 | ++ | 0/+ | + |
| Nefazodone | + | 0 | + | 0/+ | 0/+ |
| Bupropion | 0 | 0 | 0 | + | 0 |
| Mianserin | +++ | 0/+ | 0/+ | + | + |
| Mirtazapine | +++ | + | 0/+ | + | + |

0, None; 0/+, 0ccasional; +, law; ++, moderate; +++, veryhigh.

psychosis which includes hallucinations and delusions. Psychotropic drugs also modulate seizure threshold and this needs to be carefully evaluated.[42] For example, a serious side-effect of bupropion that is rare but clinically important is the propensity to induce seizures in doses over 450 mg/day. Thus, bupropion should not be used at a dose higher than this and careful evaluation of history of seizures and other medical conditions or treatments that might lower seizure threshold should be evaluated in each patient.

Mianserin often produces drowsiness during the first weeks of treatment but has much less anticholinergic side-effects than other tricyclic antidepressants. It has less effects on producing hypotension and cardiac effects and there is only a low propensity for weight gain. Mirtazapine also has an increased amount of drowsiness and sedation. These side-effects are usually mild and transient. Mirtazapine has a low propensity to produce orthostatic

hypotension or cardiac effects. There is a tendency for increased appetite and weight gain, however, which does not appear to be as severe as with tricyclics such as amitriptyline. Mianserin and mirtazapine have not been shown to produce high rates of sexual dysfunction as has been seen with trazodone and there is little evidence of lowering of the seizure threshold.

The side-effect profiles of the antidepressants are thought to relate to their respective effects on a variety of neurotransmitter systems. Clinicians should be aware of the profile of side-effects for each of the antidepressants they prescribe. The dose and duration of treatment interact with the intensity and type of side-effect and should be considered relative to antidepressant effects when evaluating, switching or stopping treatment. Although all antidepressant treatments can provoke switches into mania in vulnerable patients with bipolar disorder, it would appear that the MAOIs have a somewhat higher propensity to do this than the other compounds.

It is important that the nature of somatic and behavioural symptoms be carefully recorded before the onset of treatment so that the emergence of side-effects can be documented for the individual patient.

## Toxic effects

There is ongoing concern recently regarding the issue of antidepressant use and suicide. The field has been grapplling with two inter-related issues: the possible risk of suicidal behaviour attributable to antidepressant treatment versus the potential decrease in suicidal behaviour afforded by antidepressant therapy. In 2004, there was an 18 per cent increase in adolescent suicides over the previous year.[43] This coincided with increased publicity about the relationship between antidepressant treatment and suicide risk in children and adolescents and a subsequent decline in antidepressant prescriptions. The Food and Drug Administration (FDA) has issued a black box warning to warn the public about the increased risk of suicidal thoughts and behaviour ('suicidality') in children and adolescents being treated with antidepressant medications.[44]

Often the most serious toxic effects are the result of overdose. Since depressed patients are at increased risk of suicide there is always the possibility that suicidally depressed patients will overdose on their antidepressants. This is a very serious consideration and should be carefully evaluated when prescribing antidepressants. The symptoms and course of events following acute antidepressant overdose are complex and can be confusing unless a clear history of overdose is obtained. With tricyclic antidepressants, restlessness and excitement are initially seen with possible myoclonus, and dystonia and seizures leading to the development of coma. Seriously compromized patients can have depressed respiration with hypoxia, depressed reflexes, hypertension, and hypothermia. With the antidepressants that have antimuscarinic activity, there can be strong anticholinergic effects with mydriasis, flushed skin, dry membranes, and tachycardia.

Antidepressant overdose can be life-threatening and patients should receive immediate emergency medical evaluation. The local poison control centre should be contacted in any case of suspected antidepressant overdose. Appropriate follow-up can include the use of activated charcoal to absorb the drug as well as other medical supportive measures. Different compounds have different probability of serious complications following an overdose and this is related to the amount ingested. However, drugs are often taken in combination, and it is difficult to know the exact composition and amount of the overdose.

Another serious toxic side-effect is the interaction of MAOIs and foods that are high in tyramine and other monoamines. Tyramine has both direct and indirect sympathomimetic actions, has a pressor action, and is present in a number of foodstuffs. It is normally broken down by the MAO enzymes and in the presence of a MAOI will increase in concentration. Some of the foods that should be restricted in the diet of patients taking MAOIs are listed in Table 6.2.3.7. The reaction usually develops 20 min to 1 h following ingestion of food and is characterized by nausea, apprehension, occasional chills, sweating, restlessness and hypotension with occipital headache, palpitations, and possibly vomiting. Neck stiffness, piloerection, dilated pupils, fever, and motor agitation are seen on examination. In severe forms, the reaction can lead to delirium,

hyperpyrexia, cerebral hemorrhage, and death. The interaction of the irreversible MAOIs with certain dietary components leading to the hypertensive reaction is one of the most serious drawbacks to the use of these types of compounds. The reversible MAOIs moclobemide and brofaromine have not been found to interact with tyramine in the same fashion as the irreversible MAOIs. Thus, they have much less liability in terms of producing the hypertensive crisis seen with the irreversible MAOIs.[29] Phentolamine (5 mg) administered intravenously or nifedipine (onset of action 5 minutes), a calcium channel blocker, have been shown to be useful in the treatment of hypertensive reactions.

Serotonin syndrome is most often encountered when a MAOI is combined with an SSRI and there is an excess of 5-HT which overstimulates serotonin receptors.[45] This syndrome can manifest itself with sweating, diarrhoea, abdominal pain, fever, tachycardia, elevated blood pressure, myoclonus, hyper-reflexia, and with irritability and agitation. In its severe form, there can be severe hyperpyrexia, motor irritability, cardiovascular shock, and death. This toxic effect can result from the use of irreversible MAOIs and the addition of high amounts of tryptophan or other drugs that release serotonin in the brain. In addition, a common cause of this syndrome can result from the use of SSRIs and irreversible MAOIs concomitantly. Thus, it is strongly recommended that when MAOIs or SSRIs are utilized in sequence that the switch of treatment from one drug to the other has a minimum of a 14-day washout drug-free period before the second drug is started. In the case of discontinuing drugs with long half-lives such as fluoxetine an even longer period of up to 3 to 5 weeks may be necessary to safely avoid any possibility of producing the serotonin syndrome as a possible reaction to the drug combination.

The use of antidepressants during pregnancy is controversial and as always clinicians need to balance up the risks and benefits of treatments for individuals in this situation. Some recent studies have suggested that the use of SSRI medication in the perinatal period may be associated with adverse events like low birth weight and respiratory distress in the new born.[46, 47] However, this needs to be balanced against the fact that women at risk for depression may be at risk if not treated with antidepressants during pregnancy[48] and both these risks need to be balanced against each other.

**Table 6.2.3.7** Dietary restrictions for patients on MAOIs

| | | |
|---|---|---|
| Aged cheeses | Liver | Raisins |
| American cheese[a] | Aged meats | Soy Sauce |
| Cottage cheese[a] | Canned meats | Ripe avocado |
| Yogurt[a] | Processed meats | Sauerkraut |
| Sour cream[a] | Meat extract | Licorice |
| Wine | Fermented foods | Chocolate[a] |
| Beer | Snails | Coffee[a] |
| Yeast extract | Anchovies | |
| Herring | Canned figs | |
| Sardines | Fava beans | |

[a] Not over 50g daily.

The elderly are much more susceptible to toxic effects of antidepressants than younger individuals. In elderly patients, there may be other illnesses and the compensatory biological systems are not as resistant as in younger individuals. Mild toxic effects can be life threatening in the elderly. The newer antidepressants with fewer side-effects are the best drugs to use in the elderly.

There are a number of other toxic events that occur with less regularity. Isocarboxizid and phenelzine, since they are hydrazines, have some propensity to produce liver toxicity. Other much less frequent toxic events have occurred following antidepressants such as idiosyncratic individualized allergic reactions to the drug, suppression of the haematopoietic system, unusual dermatological reactions and hyponatremia.[49] There are reports of death in children receiving desipramine[50] though the cause of these deaths is unknown. Similarly, there is literature documenting increased incidence of gastric bleeding in association with SSRI treatment though there is a confounding effect of concomitant non-steroidal anti-inflammatory medication.[51]

## Indications

Table 6.2.3.8 lists conditions where some antidepressant drugs have been found to be effective. Not all drugs are equally effective in each condition and very few clinical trials of the different compounds in each of the conditions have been conducted. Since the efficacy of antidepressant drugs is in part related to the dose administered and/or blood levels, it is difficult to be certain of the relative efficacy of one compound versus another when only single fixed doses are used. The expense and difficulty of multidose designs in comparing two treatments are extremely large and this is the main factor limiting comparisons of different drugs across the conditions listed in Table 6.2.3.8. In addition, the large number of compounds available would make this a very difficult task indeed. Another issue is that many of the drugs are only officially approved by the American Food and Drug Administration for use in depressed patients. Many of the indications listed in Table 6.2.3.8 are 'off-label' use of the medication. Since depression is the most prevalent illness, pharmaceutical companies have developed and brought forward drugs with depression as the primary indication. The expense of clinical trials to gain approval for other indications is high. Thus, for many of the conditions listed in Table 6.2.3.8, there is only fragmentary evidence for efficacy of some antidepressants and almost no data or comparable efficacy across drugs.

There are a number of different diagnostic approaches to depression as listed in Table 6.2.3.8. By and large, all of the drugs listed in Table 6.2.3.5 have been shown to be effective in the treatment of major depression. Most drugs have been studied in outpatient samples of patients with major depression. Their relative efficacy in the treatment of more severe conditions such as melancholia, psychotic depression, or bipolar depression remains limited. In addition, the relative efficacy of the different compounds as treatments for the depressive subtype, such as atypical depression, dysthymia, or secondary depression, has not been fully studied. There have been some reports that the MAOIs may be more effective in atypical depression[52] but not all studies have validated this. When depression in the elderly is under consideration, the side-effect profile for each drug becomes a much more relevant consideration when choosing a specific drug.

Anxiety disorders have considerable comorbidity with depression. Imipramine was initially found to be effective in the treatment of panic disorder and since then SSRIs have also been effective as well as MAOIs.[53] Clomipramine was found to be effective in obsessive-compulsive disorder though more recently SSRIs tend to be favoured as they generally have fewer side-effects. Depending on the studies, both SSRIs and MAOIs have been effective treatments in social phobia as well as some tricyclic drugs. In general anxiety disorder and post-traumatic stress disorder, antidepressants have also shown efficacy but not to the same extent as seen in panic disorder.[54]

It is of interest that some antidepressants have been effective in treating eating disorders. They are effective in bulimia nervosa[55] but not in anorexia nervosa.[56] The dose of fluoxetine to treat

**Table 6.2.3.8** Clinical indications for antidepressant treatments

| **Clinical condition** |
| --- |
| Depression |
| Major depression |
| Melancholia |
| Psychotic depression |
| Bipolar depression |
| Atypical depression |
| Secondary depression |
| Dysthymia |
| Depression in elderly (pseudodementia) |
| Prevention of depression relapse |
| **Anxiety disorders** |
| Panic disorder |
| Obsessive–compulsive disorder |
| Social phobia |
| Generalized anxiety disorder |
| Post-traumatic stress disorder |
| **Eating disorders** |
| Bulimia nervosa |
| Obesity |
| Nausea with chemotherapy |
| **Sleep disorders** |
| Insomnia |
| Narcolepsy |
| Sleep apnea |
| **Pain** |
| Migraine headache |
| Atypical facial pain |
| Chronic pain syndromes |
| Diabetic neuropathy |
| **Other disorders** |
| Substance abuse |
| Alcoholism |
| Smoking cessation |
| Borderline personality disorder |
| Neurological disorders |
| Enuresis |
| Attention-deficit disorder |
| Premenstrual dysphoric disorder |
| Peptic ulcer |
| Urticaria pruritus |
| Premature ejaculation |

bulimia nervosa is higher than the treatment of depression. The increase of weight seen following many antidepressants contrasts with some reports of the usefulness of SSRIs in the treatment of obesity.

In clinical practice, many clinicians have used trazodone as a night-time sedative. In the treatment of depression, sleep is one of the first symptoms to show improvement following initiation of most antidepressant treatments. Various reports of use of anti-depressants in the treatment of narcolepsy and sleep apnoea have also been published.

Antidepressants have been effective in various pain syndromes. Since there is a wide range of the medical conditions producing pain, the results have been quite variable. In general the antidepres-sants have been able to reduce many of the painful symptoms as well as be effective in treating the secondary depression associated with chronic pain. However, they do not demonstrate the clear analgesic effect of drugs such as opioids.

Antidepressants have been reported to be effective in many other disorders including substance abuse, alcoholism, and smoking cessation.[57] In children with enuresis a dose of imipramine as low as 25 mg has been seen to be safe and effective. In both children and adults, imipramine, desipramine, bupropion, and nortriptyline have been effective in the treatment of attention-deficient disorder.[58] Antidepressants have found use in the treatment of premenstrual disorders,[59] and they are also useful in the treatment of several neurological disorders.

In general the indications and uses of a specific antidepressant in part depend on their side-effect profile and on the previously demonstrated efficacy. A major issue in the use of drugs to treat the large number of depressed patients with a comorbid medical con-dition is the careful choice of drug to minimize possible negative interactions with the medical disease.

## Contraindications

The major contraindications in the use of antidepressants arise from the interaction of the pharmacological effects of antidepres-sant treatment with a comorbid condition of the patient or with diet or drug interactions. As mentioned above, the most serious contraindications arise from the use of irreversible MAOIs in patients taking other drugs or a diet that interacts and potentiates monoamine function resulting in a hypertensive crisis. A major contraindication is the use of MAOI in patients who receive anaesthesia.[59] Patients on MAOIs should carry a card for medical emergencies warning of drug interactions. Drugs that potentiate serotonin can interact with SSRIs to give the serotonin syndrome. The more relative contraindications involve the interaction of the side-effect profile of the antidepressant treatment with either the primary medical disease or with other medications that the patient may be taking. Another relative contraindication is the use of antidepressants during pregnancy and breast feeding though clearly there needs to be a risk benefit analysis of the use of the medication.

## Drug interactions

Many patients may be taking other medications and many are prescribed more than one psychotrophic drug at a time. Because of this, it is important that clinicians are aware of drug-drug interactions. Drugs that impair the cytochrome P-450 microsomal enzyme system in the liver can interact with other drugs that are dependent on hepatic metabolism. For example, barbiturates and carbamazepine which induce hepatic enzymes can accelerate tricyclic metabolism and reduce steady state blood levels. Another anticonvulsant increasingly prescribed in the control of affective disorders, valproate, can reduce tricyclic drug clearance. Neuroleptics can elevate tricyclic blood levels which may be related to the impairment of the hydroxylation pathway for tricyclic metabolism. One of the more important drug-drug interactions involves the use of SSRIs and tricyclic drugs. This is related to the competitive inhibition of cytochrome by all of the SSRIs except fluvoxamine. This can result in clear elevations of steady state plasma concentrations. If combinations like this are utilized, the tricyclic doses need to be reduced. The utilization of a drug where plasma concentrations can be monitored (see Table 6.2.3.10) would help in the adjustment of dose if the tricyclic is combined with an SSRI.

One of the more serious drug-drug interactions previously mentioned is the interaction of tricyclic drugs with MAOIs. This can lead to hypertensive reactions and possibly stroke as well as possible induction of the serotonin syndrome.[45] Often antide-pressants are combined with phenothiazines. There is some evidence that chlorpromazine can block the metabolism of tricy-clics and thus when these two treatments are combined a possible reduction in the tricyclic treatment may be required. Other drugs that have been shown to increase tricyclic levels through blocking their metabolism include cimetidine, methylphenidate, and haloperidol. Tricyclic drugs can reduce the effects of clonidine and guanethidine in reducing blood pressure; an anticonvulsant, phenytoin, may be elevated; and the drug warfarin may be increased following tricyclic drugs. With the SSRIs, since there is a narrow pharmacological effect, interactions with anticholinergic agents or antihistaminics or alcohol are generally less than the tricyclics. The one major interaction is through the cytochrome P-450 family of enzymes which are inhibited by most SSRIs and interact with the metabolism of other drugs.

Some of the more serious drug interactions occur with the MAOIs. In addition to the dietary interactions, the MAOIs can interact with many of the 'over-the-counter' medications such as cough syrups and decongestants. Table 6.2.3.9 lists a number of compounds that have adverse drug interactions with MAOIs. Certainly many of the drugs that are direct or indirect adrenergic and dopaminergic agonists can produce overstimulation of the sympathetic nervous system. This can result in increased blood pressure and possibly adverse effects on the central nervous system. These drugs include all of the sympathomimetics, amphetamines, methylphenidate, and other stimulants. This can also occur with drugs such as other MAOIs and tricyclics or SSRIs that increase monoamine levels. MAOIs may worsen hypoglycaemia and require readjustment of the dosage of hypoglycaemic agents. Major con-cerns arise when patients on MAOIs need surgery because of the interaction with a number of compounds used in anaesthesia. This is more likely to occur with the use of pethidine. Careful considera-tion should be given to using a minimal 2-week washout for patients on MAOIs under going elective surgery.

The mixed 5-HT agonist drugs also have important drug-drug interactions. Trazodone can potentiate barbiturate and alcohol and it can increase drowsiness and sedation in patients taking these

**Table 6.2.3.9** Adverse drug interactions with MAOIs

| | |
|---|---|
| Other antidepressants | Other MAOIs |
| Buspirone | Carbamazepine |
| Stimulants | L-Dopa |
| Sympathomimetics | Methyldopa |
| Dopamine | Guanethidine |
| Amphetamines | Dextromethorphan |
| Methylphenidate | Pethidine |
| Adrenaline | Cocaine |
| Asthma inhalants | Reserpine |
| Decongestants | Tryptophan |
| Appetite suppressants | Fenfluramine |

agents. It has also been reported to produce the serotonin syndrome at times when combined with an SSRI and possibly buspirone. Trazodone has altered the kinetics of benzodiazepines including alprazolam and triazolam. Trazodone interacts with cytochrome P-450 enzymes and has been shown to increase plasma levels of digoxin. Unlike trazodone, nefazodone does not appear to potentiate the sedative effects of alcohol.

Bupropion undergoes hepatic metabolism and its levels can be altered by other drugs effecting this metabolic route. There is some dopaminergic activation with bupropion and it has had adverse interactions with MAOIs. Because of the dopaminergic activity, there have been interactions with anti-parkinsonian medication. Because bupropion lowers the seizure threshold at higher dosages it can interact and with other medications that would have similar effects to produce seizures. A combination of bupropion and lithium may increase the likelihood of seizures. There are some reports that carbamazepine may decrease bupropion drug levels.

Mirtazapine is metabolized by cytochrome P-450 enzyme systems. There is the potential for interaction with other drugs via this system. The extent of use of mirtazapine is not as great as the older drugs and the drug-drug interactions are not as extensively reported.

In general, a large number of drug-drug interactions have been reported for the antidepressants. The drug-drug interactions can be quite variable depending on the patient and the dosage and duration of treatments. Thus, the adverse drug-drug interactions are one of the main reasons for the recommendations to use monotherapy rather than more than one drug. The use of drug combinations should, on average, be restricted to patients who have a poor response to a single treatment because of the possibility of adverse drug-drug interactions.

## Drug withdrawal

Long-term administration of a drug can produce adaptive changes in many aspects of the human biology. When the drug is abruptly discontinued, 'rebound' drug withdrawal symptoms can be observed. This is most clearly seen with longer-term opiate, benzodiazepine, or barbiturate use. Antidepressants are not addictive and dependence does not develop. With the antidepressants some degree of tolerance to the sedative and autonomic effects tends to

develop and on abrupt withdrawal patients can have emerging symptoms consisting of malaise, dizziness, nausea, diarrhoea, chills, insomnia, restlessness, and muscle aches. Symptoms emerging during drug withdrawal have been seen following treatment with tricyclics as well as SSRIs.[60] They have been described on occasion for MAOIs and the other non-monoamine uptake antidepressants. One main factor is the drug elimination half-life. Abrupt discontinuation of drugs with a short elimination half-life will produce more emergent side-effects than drugs with a long half-life. Thus, it has been found that patients taking shorter half-life drugs such as paroxetine and sertraline have more of an emergent symptom increase than patients taking the longer elimination half-life drug fluoxetine. Therefore, the dose of drugs with a shorter elimination half-life should generally be tapered over a 2- to 3-week period when being discontinued rather than being stopped abruptly. Drugs with a longer elimination half-life can be stopped abruptly since the parent drug and metabolite may last for many days. Clinicians must be aware that slow elimination means that parent drug and active metabolites remain in the body for up to several weeks.

With the irreversible MAOI inhibitors, since there is a 1- or 2-week period during with monoamine oxidase must recover following discontinuation of the MAOI, emergent side-effects have not been as regularly observed. In general with the other antidepressants the withdrawal syndromes have not been permanent. Clinicians must make special efforts to discriminate between the return of symptoms and the emergence of new symptoms related to drug withdrawal.

## Dosages and administration

In Table 6.2.3.10 some of the suggested optimal plasma concentrations for different antidepressant drugs are listed. For nortriptyline, desipramine, imipramine, and amitriptyline there is some evidence for a minimal plasma and concentration necessary for clinical response. An established therapeutic range is available for nortriptyline. Thus, patients with nortriptyline concentrations between 50 and 150 mg/ml seem to do much better. With the other drugs, it is generally thought that the plasma levels reflect a minimal threshold of plasma concentration for clinical response. Below this level patients are less likely to respond and the upper limit indicates that there is increased possibility of the systemic or cardiac toxicity. Bupropion levels between 50 and 100 ng/ml may possibly be the best range. However, it is important that the dose be kept below 450 mg/day because of the possibility of seizures.

Except for nortriptyline and the use of plasma concentrations to obtain a minimal effective level, it is generally the patient's clinical response that dictates dosage adjustments. One difficulty is that some patients with plasma concentrations outside the therapeutic range do respond and many patients with concentrations within the therapeutic range do not. Thus, the dosage needs to be adjusted depending on the individual patient's response. Clearly plasma concentration monitoring can be helpful in many situations such as evaluating plasma levels when higher than standard doses are used, assessing toxicity, use in elderly patients or patients with comorbid conditions to evaluate possible drug interactions, or where compliance is questioned. Blood for drug levels is usually obtained for plasma levels during elimination phase which is usually in the morning 12 h after the last dose.

**Table 6.2.3.10** Dosage and administration of antidepressant drugs. Doses in brackets refer to doses recommended for elderly patients

| Drug | Initial dose (mg/day) | Theraupeutic dose range (mg/day) | Recommended optimal plasma concentration (ng/ml) |
|---|---|---|---|
| *Monoamine reuptake inhibitors* | | | |
| Imipramine | 25–75 (10) | 150–300 (30–50) | 200–300[d] |
| Desipramine | 50–75 | 100–300 (25–150) | 125–300[d] |
| Amitriptyline | 75 (30–75) | 150–200 | 120–250[d] |
| Nortriptyline | 25 | 75–150 | 50–150 |
| Trimipramine | 50–75 (30–75) | 150–300 (75–150) | NA |
| Clomipramine | 10 | 30–250 (30–75) | NA |
| Protriptyline | 20–40 (15) | 20–60 | 70–240 |
| Doxepin | 75 (10–50) | 30–300 (30–50) | 110–250[d] |
| Amoxapine | 100–150 (50–75) | 100–600 (150–300) | 200–400[e] |
| Maprotiline | 25–75 (25) | 25–225 (50–75) | 200–300[d] |
| Venlafaxine | 75 | 150–375 | NA |
| Milnacipran | 50 | 50–100 | NA |
| Duloxetine | 60 | 60 | NA |
| Reboxetine | 8 | 10–12 | NA |
| *SSRIs* | | | |
| Fluoxetine | 20 | 20–60 | NA |
| Sertraline | 50 | 50–200 | NA |
| Fluvoxamine | 50–100 | 100–300 | NA |
| Paroxetine | 20 | 50 (40) | NA |
| Citalopram | 20 | 20–60 (20–40) | NA |
| Escitalopram | 10 (5) | 10–20 (10–20) | NA |
| *MAOIs* | | | |
| Isocarboxazid | 30 | 10–60 (5–10) | NA |
| Phenelzine | 45 | 15–90 | NA |
| Tranylcypromine | 20 | 10–30 | NA |
| Moclobemide | 300 | 150–600 | NA |
| Brofaromine | 50 | 50–150 | NA |
| Selegiline | 6[a] | 6–12[a] | NA |
| *Other antidepressants* | | | |
| Trazodone | 100 (150) | 150–600 | NA |
| Nefazodone | 200 (100)[b] | 200–600[b] | NA |
| Buproprion | 200[c] | 300–450[c] | 50–100 |
| Mianserin | 30–40 (30) | 30–90 | NA |
| Mirtazapine | 15 | 45 | NA |

NA, data not available.

[a] Selegiline not licensed in UK for depression. Doses quoted refer to transdermal patches marketed in the US.

[b] Nefazodone not licensed in UK.

[c] Buproprion not licensed in Uk for depression.

[d] Parent drug plus demethylated metabolite.

[e] Parent drug plus hydroxymetabolite.

These doses should not be used for patient prescriptions; clinicians should consult manufacturer's literature for recommendation of doses and frequency of administration.

## Acknowledgement

The authors would like to thank Aybala Saricicek MD for her assistance in the preparation of the chapter.

## Further information

*Biological Psychiatry* (Elsevier)—the journal of the Society of Biological Psychiatry http://www.sobp.org/

*Neuropsychopharmacology* (Nature Publishing group)—the journal of the American College of Neuropsychopharmacology http://www.acnp.org/

Schatzberg, A.F. and Nemeroff, C. B. (eds). (2004). *American Psychiatric Publishing Textbook of Psychopharmacology* (3rd edn.) American Psychiatric Publishing, Arlington, VA.

## References

1. Lopez, A.D., Murray, C.C.J.L. (1998). The global burden of disease, 1990-2020. *Nature Medicine*, **4**, 1241–3.

2. Bloch, R.G., Doonief, A.S., Buchberg, A.S., *et al.* (1954). The clinical effect of isoniazid and iproniazid in the treatment of pulmonary tuberculosis. *Annals of Internal Medicine*, **40**, 881–900.

3. Crane, G.E. (1957). Iproniazid (marsilid) phosphate, a therapeutic agent for mental disorders and debilitating diseases. *Psychiatric research reports*, **135**, 142–52.

4. Kuhn, R. (1958). The treatment of depressive states with G 22355 (imipramine hydrochloride). *American Journal of Psychiatry*, **15**, 459–64.

5. Coppen, A., Shaw, D.M., Farrell, J.P. (1963). Potentiation of the antidepressive effect of a monoamine-oxidase inhibitor by tryptophan. *Lancet*, **1**, 79–81.

6. Schildkraut, J.J. (1965). The catecholamine hypothesis of affective disorders: a review of supporting evidence. *American Journal of Psychiatry*, **122**, 509–22.

7. Bunney, W.E., Jr., Davis, J.M. (1965). Norepinephrine in depressive reactions. A review. *Archives of General Psychiatry*, **13**, 483–94.

8. Vetulani, J., Sulser, F. (1975). Action of various antidepressant treatments reduces reactivity of noradrenergic cyclic AMP-generating system in limbic forebrain. *Nature*, **257**, 495–6.

9. Charney, D.S., Menkes, D.B., Heninger, G.R. (1981). Receptor sensitivity and the mechanism of action of antidepressant treatment. Implications for the etiology and therapy of depression. *Archives of General Psychiatry*, **38**, 1160–80.

10. Blier, P., de Montigny, C., Chaput, Y. (1987). Modifications of the serotonin system by antidepressant treatments: implications for the therapeutic response in major depression. *Journal of Clinical Psychopharmacology*, **7**, 24S–35S.

11. Paul, I.A., Nowak, G., Layer, R.T., et al. (1994). Adaptation of the N-methyl-D-aspartate receptor complex following chronic antidepressant treatments. *Journal of Pharmacology and Experimental Therapeutics*, **269**, 95–102.

12. Layer, R.T., Popik, P., Olds, T., et al. (1995). Antidepressant-like actions of the polyamine site NMDA antagonist, eliprodil (SL-82.0715). *Pharmacology, Biochemistry, and Behaviour*, **52**, 621–7.

13. Holsboer, F., Barden, N. (1996). Antidepressants and hypothalamic-pituitaryadrenocortical regulation. *Endocrine Reviews*, **17**, 187–205.

14. Griebel, G., Perrault, G., Sanger, D.J. (1998). Characterization of the behavioural profile of the non-peptide CRF receptor antagonist CP-154,526 in anxiety models in rodents. Comparison with diazepam and buspirone. *Psychopharmacology (Berl)*, **138**, 55–66.

15. Duman, R.S., Heninger, G.R., Nestler, E.J. (1997). A molecular and cellular theory of depression. *Archives of General Psychiatry*, **54**, 597–606.

16. Wilde, M.I., Benfi eld, P. Tianeptine. (1995). A review of its pharmacodynamic and pharmacokinetic properties, and therapeutic effi cacy in depression and coexisting anxiety and depression. *Drugs*, **49**, 411–39.

17. Kramer, M.S., Cutler, N., Feighner, J., et al. (1998). Distinct mechanism for antidepressant activity by blockade of central substance P receptors. *Science*, **281**, 1640–5.

18. Taylor, M.J., Freemantle, N., Geddes, J.R., et al. (2006). Early Onset of Selective Serotonin Reuptake Inhibitor Antidepressant Action: Systematic Review and Meta-analysis. *Archives of General Psychiatry*, **63**, 1217–23.

19. Berman, R.M., Cappiello, A., Anand, A. et al. (2000). Antidepressant effects of ketamine in depressed patients. *Biological Psychiatry*, **47**, 351–4.

20. Zarate, C.A., Jr., Singh, J.B., Carlson, P.J. et al. (2006). A Randomized Trial of an N-methyl-D-aspartate Antagonist in Treatment-Resistant Major Depression. *Archives of General Psychiatry*, **63**, 856–64.

21. Maeng, S., Zarate, C.A., Jr., Du, J. et al. (207). Cellular Mechanisms Underlying the Antidepressant Effects of Ketamine: Role of alpha-Amino-3-Hydroxy-5-Methylisoxazole-4-Propionic Acid Receptors. *Biological Psychiatry*, **63**, 349–52.

22. Richelson, E. (2003). Interactions of antidepressants with neurotransmitter transporters and receptors and their clinical relevance. *Journal of Clinical Psychiatry*, **64** Suppl 13, 5–12.

23. Gutierrez, M.A., Stimmel, G.L., Aiso, J.Y. (2003). Venlafaxine: a 2003 update. *Clinical Therapeutics*, **25**, 2138–54.

24. Stahl, S.M., Grady, M.M., Moret, C., et al. (2005). SNRIs: their pharmacology, clinical efficacy, and tolerability in comparison with other classes of antidepressants. *CNS Spectrums*, **10**, 732–47.

25. Preskorn, S.H. (2004). Reboxetine: a norepinephrine selective reuptake pump inhibitor. *Journal of Psychiatric Practice*, **10**, 57–63.

26. Hyttel, J., Bogeso, K.P., Perregaard, J., et al. (1992). The pharmacological effect of citalopram residues in the (S)-(+)-enantiomer. *Journal of Neural Transmission. General Section*, **88**, 157–60.

27. Kennedy, S.H. (1997). Continuation and maintenance treatments in major depression: the neglected role of monoamine oxidase inhibitors. *Journal of Psychiatry & Neuroscience*, **22**, 127–31.

28. Patkar, A.A., Pae, C.U., Masand, P.S. (2006). Transdermal selegiline: the new generation of monoamine oxidase inhibitors. *CNS Spectrums*, **11**, 363–75.

29. Robinson, D.S. (2002). Monoamine oxidase inhibitors: a new generation. *Psychopharmacology Bulletin*, **36**, 124–38.

30. Haria, M., Fitton, A., McTavish, D. (1994). Trazodone: A review of its pharmacology, therapeutic use in depression and therapeutic potential in other disorders. *Drugs & Aging*, **4**, 331–55.

31. Dunner, D.L., Laird, L.K., Zajecka, J., et al. (2002). Six-year perspectives on the safety and tolerability of nefazodone. *Journal of Clinical Psychiatry*, **63** Suppl 1, 32–41.

32. Ascher, J.A., Cole, J.O., Colin, J.N. et al. (1995). Bupropion: a review of its mechanism of antidepressant activity. *Journal of Clinical Psychiatry*, **56**, 395–401.

33. Leverich, G.S., Altshuler, L.L., Frye, M.A. et al. (2006). Risk of Switch in Mood Polarity to Hypomania or Mania in Patients With Bipolar Depression During Acute and Continuation Trials of Venlafaxine, Sertraline, and Bupropion as Adjuncts to Mood Stabilizers. *American Journal of Psychiatry*, **163**, 232–9.

34. Hurt, R.D., Sachs, D.P., Glover, E.D. et al. (1997). A comparison of sustained-release bupropion and placebo for smoking cessation. *New England Journal of Medicine*, **337**, 1195–202.

35. Szegedi, A., Schwertfeger, N. (2005). Mirtazapine: a review of its clinical efficacy and tolerability. *Expert Opinion on Pharmacotheraphy*, **6**, 631–41.

36. Hemeryck, A., Belpaire, F.M. (2002). Selective serotonin reuptake inhibitors and cytochrome P-450 mediated drug-drug interactions: an update. *Current Drug Metabolism*, **3**,13–37.

37. Kapur, S., Cho, R., Jones, C., et al. (1999). Is amoxapine an atypical antipsychotic? Positron-emission tomography investigation of its dopamine2 and serotonin2 occupancy. *Biological Psychiatry*, **45**, 1217–20.

38. Scates, A.C., Doraiswamy, P.M. (2000). Reboxetine: a selective norepinephrine reuptake inhibitor for the treatment of depression. *Annals of Pharmacotheraphy*, **34**, 1302–12.

39. Detke, M.J., Lu, Y., Goldstein, D.J., et al. (2002). Duloxetine, 60 mg once daily, for major depressive disorder: a randomized double-blind placebo-controlled trial. *Journal of Clinical Psychiatry*, **63**, 308–15.

40. Sussman, N., Ginsberg, D.L., Bikoff, J. (2001). Effects of nefazodone on body weight: a pooled analysis of selective serotonin reuptake inhibitor- and imipramine-controlled trials. *Journal of Clinical Psychiatry*, **62**, 256–60.

41. Spencer, T., Biederman, J., Steingard, R., et al. (1993). Bupropion exacerbates tics in children with attention-deficit hyperactivity disorder and Tourette's syndrome. *Journal of the American Academy of Child Adolescent Psychiatry*, **32**, 211–4.

42. Alper, K., Schwartz, K.A., Kolts, R.L., et al. (2007). Seizure Incidence in Psychopharmacological Clinical Trials: An Analysis of Food and Drug Administration (FDA) Summary Basis of Approval Reports. *Biological Psychiatry*, **62**, 345–54.

43. Hamilton, B.E., Minino, A.M., Martin, et al. (2007). Annual summary of vital statistics: 2005. *Pediatrics*, **119**, 345–60.

44. Hammad, T.A., Laughren, T., Racoosin, J. (2006). Suicidality in Pediatric Patients Treated With Antidepressant Drugs. *Archives of General Psychiatry*, **63**, 332–9.

45. Boyer, E.W., Shannon, M. (2005). The serotonin syndrome. *New England Journal of Medicine*, **352**, 1112–20.

46. Chambers, C.D., Hernandez-Diaz, S., Van Marter, L.J. et al. (2006). Selective serotonin-reuptake inhibitors and risk of persistent pulmonary hypertension of the newborn. *New England Journal of Medicine*, **354**, 579–87.

47. Oberlander, T.F., Warburton, W., Misri, S., *et al.* (2006). Neonatal Outcomes After Prenatal Exposure to Selective Serotonin Reuptake Inhibitor Antidepressants and Maternal Depression Using Population-Based Linked Health Data. *Archives of General Psychiatry*, **63**, 898–906.

48. Cohen, L.S., Altshuler, L.L., Harlow, B.L. *et al.* (2006). Relapse of Major Depression During Pregnancy in Women Who Maintain or Discontinue Antidepressant Treatment. *Journal of the American Medical Association*, **295**: 499–507.

49. Madhusoodanan, S., Bogunovic, O.J., Moise, D., *et al.* (2002). Hyponatraemia associated with psychotropic medications. A review of the literature and spontaneous reports. *Adverse Drug Reactions and Toxicological Reviews*, **21**, 17–29.

50. Amitai, Y., Frischer, H. (2006). Excess fatality from desipramine in children and adolescents. *Journal of the American Academy of Child and Adolescent Psychiatry*, **45**, 54–60.

51. Yuan, Y., Tsoi, K., Hunt, R.H. (2006). Selective serotonin reuptake inhibitors and risk of upper GI bleeding: confusion or confounding? *American Journal of Medicine*, **119**, 719–27.

52. Quitkin, F.M., Stewart, J.W., McGrath, P.J., *et al.* (1993). Columbia atypical depression. A subgroup of depressives with better response to MAOI than to tricyclic antidepressants or placebo. *British Journal Psychiatry Supplement*, 30–4.

53. Otto, M.W., Tuby, K.S., Gould, R.A., *et al.* (2001). An effect-size analysis of the relative efficacy and tolerability of serotonin selective reuptake inhibitors for panic disorder. *American Journal of Psychiatry*, **158**, 1989–92.

54. Ball, S.G., Kuhn, A., Wall, D., *et al.* (2005). Selective serotonin reuptake inhibitor treatment for generalized anxiety disorder: a double-blind, prospective comparison between paroxetine and sertraline. *Journal of Clinical Psychiatry*, **66**, 94–9.

55. Group FBNCS. (1992). Fluoxetine in the treatment of bulimia nervosa. A multicenter, placebo-controlled, double-blind trial. Fluoxetine Bulimia Nervosa Collaborative Study Group. *Archives of General Psychiatry*, **49**, 139–47.

56. Attia, E., Haiman, C., Walsh, B.T., *et al.* (1998). Does fluoxetine augment the inpatient treatment of anorexia nervosa? *American Journal of Psychiatry*, **155**, 548–51.

57. Nunes, E.V., Levin, F.R. (2004). Treatment of depression in patients with alcohol or other drug dependence: a meta-analysis. *Journal of the American Medical Association*, **291**, 1887–96.

58. Culpepper, L. (2006). Primary care treatment of attention-deficit/hyperactivity disorder. *Journal of Clinical Psychiatry*, **67 Suppl 8**, 51–8.

59. Yonkers, K.A. (2004). Management strategies for PMS/PMDD. *Journal of Family Practice*, Suppl: S15–20.

60. Ditto, K.E. (2003). SSRI discontinuation syndrome. Awareness as an approach to prevention. *Postgraduate Medicine*, **114**, 79–84.

# 6.2.4 **Lithium and related mood stabilizers**

Robert M. Post

## Introduction

### Global categorization of the mood stabilizers

Lithium is the paradigmatic mood stabilizer. It is effective in the acute and prophylactic treatment of both mania and, to a lesser magnitude, depression. These characteristics are generally paralleled by the widely accepted anticonvulsant mood stabilizers valproate, carbamazepine (Table 6.2.4.1), and potentially by the less well studied putative mood stabilizers oxcarbazepine, zonisamide, and the dihydropyridine L-type calcium channel blocker nimodipine. In contrast, lamotrigine has a profile of better antidepressant effects acutely and prophylactically than antimanic effects.

### Differential responsivity among individual patients

Having grouped lithium, valproate, and carbamazepine together, it is important to note they have subtle differences in their therapeutic profiles and differential clinical predictors of response (Table 6.2.4.1). **Response to one of these agents is not predictive of either a positive or negative response to the others.**[1,2] Thus, clinicians are left with only rough estimates and guesses about which drug may be preferentially effective in which patients. Only sequential clinical trials of agents either alone or in combination can verify responsivity in an individual patient.[3] **Individual response trumps FDA-approval.**

### Requirements for method of longitudinal assessment

Given this clinical conundrum, it is advisable that patients, family members, clinicians, or others carefully rate patients on a longitudinal scale in order to most carefully assess responses and side effects. These are available from the Depression Bipolar Support Alliance (DBSA), the STEP-BD NIMH Network, or www.bipolar-networknews.org and are highly recommended.

### Increasing need for complex combination treatment

The importance of careful longitudinal documentation of symptoms and side effects is highlighted by the increasing use of multiple drugs in combination.[2] This is often required because patients may delay treatment-seeking until after many episodes, and very different patterns and frequencies of depressions, manias, mixed states, as well as multiple comorbidities may be present. Treating patients to the new accepted **goal of remission** of their mood and other anxillary symptoms usually requires use of several medications. If each component of the regimen is kept below an individual's side-effects threshold, judicious use of multiple agents can reduce rather than increase the overall side-effect burden.

### Patients and family education is a must

There is increasing evidence of reliable abnormalities of biochemistry, function, and anatomy in the brains of patients with bipolar disorder, and some of these are directly related to either duration of illness or number of episodes.[4,5] Therefore, as treatment resistance to most therapeutic agents is related to number of prior episodes, and brain abnormalities may also increase as well, it behooves the patient to begin and sustain acute and **long-term treatment as early as possible.**

### Early age of onset and treatment delay are related to an adverse outcome in adulthood

Despite the above academic, personal, and public health recommendations, bipolar disorder often takes ten years or more to diagnose and, hence, treat properly. In fact, a **younger age** of onset is highly related to presence of a **longer delay** from illness onset to **first treatment, and** as well, to **a poorer outcome** assessed both retrospectively and prospectively.[6]

**Table 6.2.4.1** Neuroprotective effects of lithium in cultured cells and animal models of diseases

| I. Therapeutic Spectrum | Lithium | Carbamazepine | Valproate | Lamotrigine | Nimodipine |
|---|---|---|---|---|---|
| A Acute Mania | ++++ | ++++ | ++++ | 0 | (++) |
| B. Mania Prophylaxis | ++++ | +++ | ++++ | + | (++) |
| C. Acute Depression | ++ | ++ | ++ | +++ | (+) |
| D. Depression Prophylaxis | ++++ | ++++ | +++ | ++++ | (++) |
| **II. Correlates of Response** | | | | | |
| A. Family History + = positive − = negative | + Mania −Depression | − Bipolar Disorder | ND | + Anxiety Disorder | ND |
| B. Bipolar Type (BP) | I | II | I,II | I,II | I,II,NOS |
| Manic Type:  Pattern: | Euphoric Intermittent | Dysphoric Continuous | Dysphoric Non-accelerating | Continuous | Euphoric Ultradian |
| C. Comorbidities | | | | | |
| Anxiety Disorder | None | ++ | +++ | +++ | (+) |
| Substance Use | None | ++ | +++ | +/− | (+) |
| D. PTSD Utility | 0 | ++ | ++ | ++ | 0 |
| E. Other Unique Targets | M-D-I vs. D-M-I Antisuicidal AntimedicalMortality | Alcohol Withdrawal Tigeminal Neuralgia | Alcohol Abstinence Migraine Prophylaxis | | (Alzheimer's Dementia) (Migraine Prophylaxis) Subarachnoid Hemorrhage |
| F. Baseline PET Activity | ? | Hyper- metabolism | ? | Hypo-metabolism | Hypo-metabolism |
| G. CSF SRIF (Somatostatin) | | | | | |
| Predicts Response: | ? | No Prediction | ? | ? | Low SRIF |
| Effect of Drug: | ? | Decreases SRIF | | | Increases SRIF |
| **III. Neurotropic Effects** | | | | | |
| A. Increase BDNF | Yes | Yes | Yes | ? | ? |
| B. Increase Neurogenesis | Yes | ? | Yes | ? | ? |
| C. Neuroprotective | Yes | Yes | Yes | Yes | (Yes) |

Legend: ++++ = very marked; +++ = marked; ++ = moderate; + = mild or some effect; +/− = equivocal; () = ambiguous data; 0 = no effect; − = worse.

## BDNF: A role in vulnerability, onset, progression, and treatment

New data indicate that the brain growth factor BDNF (brain-derived neurotrophic factor) which is initially important to synaptogenesis and neural development, and later neuroplasticity and long-term memory in the adult is involved in all phases of bipolar disorder and its treatment.[7]

It appears to be: 1) both a genetic (the val-66-val allele of BDNF) and environmental (low BDNF from childhood adversity) *risk factor*; 2) *episode-related* (serum BDNF decreasing with each episode of depression or mania in proportion to symptom severity; 3) related to some *substance abuse* comorbidity (BDNF increases in the VTA with defeat stress and cocaine self-administration); and 4) related to *treatment*. **Lithium, valproate, and carbamazepine increase BDNF and quetiapine and ziprasidone block the decreases in hippocampal BDNF that occur with stress (as do antidepressants).**

## More episodes convey more problems

A greater number of prior episodes is related to increased likelihood of: 1) a rapid cycling course; 2) more severe depressive symptoms; 3) more disability; 4) more cognitive dysfunction; and 5) even the incidence of late life dementia.[4,8,9,10]

## Early effective treatment may protect the brain

Taken together, the new data suggest a new view not only of bipolar disorder, but its treatment. Adequate effective **treatment may** not only (a) prevent affective episodes (with their accompanying risk of morbidity, dysfunction, and even death by suicide or the increased medical mortality associated with depression), but may also (b) **reverse or prevent some of the biological abnormalities associated with the illness from progressing**.

Thus, patients should be given timely information pertinent to their stage of illness and recovery that emphasizes not only the risk of treatments, but also their potential, figuratively and literally, life-saving benefits. Long-term treatment and education and targeted psychotherapies are critical to a good outcome.

## Therapeutic strategy

We next highlight several attributes of each mood stabilizer, but recognize that the choice of each agent itself is based on inadequate information from the literature, and sequencing of treatments and their combinations is currently more an art than an evidence-based science. We look forward to these informational and clinical trial deficits being reduced in the near future and the development of single nucleotide polymorphism (SNP) and other neurobiological predictors of individual clinical response to individual drugs.

In the meantime, patients and clinicians must struggle with treatment choice based on: 1) the most appropriate targetting of the predominant symptom picture with the most likely effective agent (Table 6.2.4.1 and 6.2.4.2) the best side-effects profile for that patient (Table 6.2.4.2 and 6.2.4.3) using combinations of drugs with different therapeutic targets and mechanisms of action

**Table 6.2.4.2** Global putative mechanisms of action

| | Li | CBZ | VPA | LTG | NIMOD |
|---|---|---|---|---|---|
| Antiglutamineric: | + | + | + | + | ? |
| Via: | | | | | |
| Glutamate Uptake | + | | | | |
| Sodium Blockade | | + | (+) | + | |
| ↑ Brain GABA | + | +/− | ++ | — | 0 |
| ↑ GABA-B R in hippocampus (with chronic administration) | + | + | + | | |
| ↓ Calcium Influx | + | + | + | + | ++ |
| Via: | | | | | |
| Weak NMDA Receptor Inhibition | + | + | + | + | 0 |
| Inhibition of Calcium-Channel Type | — | (L) | T | (N,P) | L |
| ↓ DA Turnover | + | + | + | | |
| Second Messenger System | | | | | |
| ↓ c-AMP, G proteins | ++ | ++ | — | — | — |
| PI Turnover | ↓ | (↑) | N.C. | ? | +/− |
| PKC Inhibition | ++ | | ++ | | |
| ↓ ras, MEK, Erk Pathway | ++ | | ++ | | |
| ↓ Inositol Transport | + | + | + | ? | ? |
| ↑ BDNF | + | + | + | | |
| ↑ Bcl-2 | + | | + | | |
| Histone Deacetylase Inhibition | — | + | ++ | ? | ? |

**Table 6.2.4.3** Global assessment of relative side-effects

| | Li | CBZ | VPA | LTG | NIMOD |
|---|---|---|---|---|---|
| Weight Gain | ++ | + | ++ | 0 | 0 |
| Tremor | ++ | +/− | ++ | +/− | 0 |
| GI Upset | ++ | + | ++ | +/− | 0 |
| Memory Disturbance | + | + | + | + | − |
| Rash | 0[a] | ++ | +/− | ++ | 0 |
| ↓WBC | — | ++ | 0 | 0 | 0 |
| Agranulocytosis | 0 | + | 0 | 0 | 0 |
| ↓Platelets | − | 0[b] | ++ | 0 | 0 |
| ↑ Liver Enzymes | 0 | ++ | ++ | (+) | 0 |
| Hepatitis | 0 | + | + | ? | 0 |
| Dizziness Ataxia Diplopia | +/− | ++ | + | + | +/− |
| Hyponatremia | − | ++ | 0 | 0 | 0 |
| Alopecia | +/− | 0 | ++ | ? | 0 |
| Thyroid Decrements | ++ | +/− | +/− | +/− | 0 |
| Teratogenic | + | ++ | ++ | 0 | 0 |
| Malformations | Epstein's Anomaly | Spina Bifida | Spina Bifida | | |
| Developmental Delay | 0 | +/− | ++ | +/− | 0 |

Legend: a = psoriasis; b=with aplastic anemia; ++ = moderate to substantial or common; + = mild to less frequent; +/− = equivocal or rare; 0 = not present or no change; − = opposite effect; () = ambiguous findings

(Table 6.2.4.3 and 6.2.4.4) careful consideration of potential advantageous pharmacodynamic interactions and disadvantageous pharmacokinetic drug-drug interactions that need to be avoided or anticipated.

# Mood stabilizers

## Lithium

In the late 1960s and early 1970s, open and double-blind randomized treatment and discontinuation studies revealed **highly significant effects of lithium in long-term prophylaxis**. These studies followed shortly after a series of studies demonstrating lithium's acute antimanic effects in comparison with both placebo and the existing neuroleptic treatments. High rates of response were touted and lithium clinics were established with the hope that the 60 to 80 per cent response rates revealed in the controlled clinical trials would be mirrored by clinical practice.[11]

However, over the past two decades there has been increasing recognition of the inadequacy of lithium both in acute treatment and long-term prophylaxis, even when used with adjunctive treatments such as antipsychotics, benzodiazepines, and antidepressants.[12,13,14] Given this increasing cognizance of lithium's less than dramatic efficacy in many patients with bipolar illness, alternative and adjunctive treatments were sought.

## The anticonvulsants carbamazepine, valproate, and lamotrigine

Carbamazepine and valproate are now well recognized as potential mood-stabilizing anticonvulsants, and initial promising data are emerging for lamotrigine as well. The data are more equivocal for oxcarbazepine and minimal for zonisamide. Importantly, **the GABA-active anticonvulsants gabapentin, tiagabine, and topiramate** are **not effective in acute mania** and thus cannot be considered mood stabilizers. Nonetheless, topiramate may be useful in some common comorbidities of bipolar illness including alcohol and cocaine abuse, bulimia, overweight, migraine, and PTSD. Similarly, gabapentin (which increases brain GABA and acts at the alpha$_2$ delta subunit of the L-type calcium channel) and its close relative pregabalin may have secondary utility in comorbid panic anxiety and social phobia, sleep disorder, alcohol withdrawal, and chronic pain syndromes.

## L-type calcium-channel blockers

The dihydropyridine L-type calcium channel blockers became a focus of possible interest for lithium-intolerant and lithium-unresponsive patients based on a variety of clinical and theoretical rationales. Dubovsky et al.[15] found increased intracellular calcium in blood elements of patients with bipolar illness, a finding that has been replicated more than a dozen times. Dubovsky et al.[16] proceeded to demonstrate the potential antimanic efficacy of the L-type calcium channel blocker verapamil. Many other small controlled studies were also positive, although less than dramatic results have recently been reported by two groups.[17,18] In addition, one controlled study found that verapamil was not an effective acute antidepressant, even though it appeared to have good antimanic properties.[19] Verapamil was never widely used in clinical practice.

Given these ambiguities with verapamil, Pazzaglia et al.[20] and Post et al.[21] at the NIMH in the U.S. chose to explore the potential antimanic and antidepressant effects of the dihydropyridine L-type calcium channel blocker nimodipine which has a very different biophysical and pharmacological profile from verapamil.[22] In contrast to the phenylalkylamine verapamil, the dihydropyridine nimodipine is a more potent anticonvulsant that blocks cocaine-induced hyperactivity, sensitization, and dopamine overflow; is positive in animal models of depression; and it improves rather than impairs cognition.

## Pharmacology

### Lithium

A series of sequential decade-related candidate mechanisms for lithium's psychotropic (mood-stabilizing) actions have been suggested over the last 50 years. These included:

- Effects on enzymes and biosynthetic aminergic neurotransmitter pathways (1950s)

- Effects on presynaptic adrenergic release and reuptake mechanisms (1960s)

- Effects on postsynaptic receptor modulation and impact on receptor supersensitivity (1970s)

- Effects on second messenger systems, adenylate cyclase and G-proteins (1980s)[23]

- Effects on phosphoinositol turnover, protein kinases (PKC and GSK-36), and other signal transduction pathways (1990s)[24,25]

- Most recently, effects on the nuclear level of DNA binding and gene transcription have been found that increase neurotrophic and other factors regulating neuroprotection versus apoptosis and cell death (2000s)[26,27]

Several of these candidate mechanisms are summarized in Figs 6.2.4.1 and 6.2.4.2, and are compared with the mechanisms of some of the other mood-stabilizing anticonvulsants such as carbamazepine and valproate. Lithium's effects on G proteins[20] are conceptually intriguing in relation to lithium's ability to modulate overactive systems, and preliminary support for its adenylate cyclase effects being important for acute mania are based on the finding that novel adenylate cyclase inhibitors are also effective in acute mania.[21] Similarly, recent studies implicating the ability of lithium and valproate to inhibit protein kinase C has been preliminarily validated with the demonstration of antimanic effects of the protein kinase C inhibitor tamoxifen in two double-blind studies.[28,29]

Most recently, lithium has emerged as a possible **neurotrophic and neuroprotective drug** via multiple potential pathways. It inhibits calcium influx through the N-methyl-$_D$-aspartate glutamate receptor;[23] it inhibits GSK-3B; and it increases the ratio of neurotrophic to cell death factors. For example, it increases Bcl-2 and brain-derived neuotrophic factor (BDNF) while decreasing the apoptotic factor BAX and P-53.[25,26] Much work remains to be done to implicate or rule out these changes in the wide array of psychotrophic actions of lithium. Lithium also increases white blood cell count and platelets by increasing granulocyte-macrophage colony-stimulating factor.[30] This effect is sufficient to overcome the benign white count suppression of carbamazepine.[31,32]

The potential clinical relevance of this finding is also evidenced by the data that pretreatment with lithium can decrease the size of a cerebral infarct following middle cerebral artery ligation and decrease the amount of neurological deficit.[33] Given the new findings of altered size of crucial structures involved in emotion regulation in the affective disorders, including amygdale,[34,35] hippocampus,[36] and prefrontal cortex,[4] one can only wonder whether lithium's neuroprotective effects could alter some of these putative neuronal- or glial-based deficits in central nervous system structure and function. The preliminary evidence supports this proposition because lithium increases patients' NAA, a marker of neuronal integrity and, grey matter volume as well.[37,38]

### Carbamazepine, valproate, and lamotrigine

As seen in Table 6.2.4.2, since lithium, carbamazepine, and valproate share a group of effects in common, one wonders if they are related to their global antimanic/antidepressant effects. Notable differences among these agents are also present, perhaps also related to some of the differences in therapeutic targets and comorbidities seen in Table 6.2.4.1.

Given the shared effects of carbamazepine and lamotrigine in potent sodium channel blockade and subsequent decreased release of glutamate, one wonders about mechanisms that account for their difference in the epilepsies (carbamazepine exacerbates while lamotrigine improves absence seizures) and bipolar disorder (lamotrigine is a better antidepressant than antimanic). Potential candidates are the effects on different calcium channel subtypes (N,P) and ability to inhibit GABA release, but factors critical to lamotrigine's antidepressant effects remain to be elucidated.[39]

### L-type calcium channel blockers

There are several subtypes of voltage-dependent blockers of calcium influx which modulate the L-type channel, i.e. one with relatively long (L) opening times. These subtypes include the widely recognized phenylalkylamines typified by verapamil, the benzodiazepines typified by diltiazem, the diphenylpiperazines typified by flunarizine, and the 1,4-dihydropyridines typified by nifedipine, nimodipine, isradipine, amlodipine, nicardipine, and nitrendipine. Remarkably, even though these agents all potently bind to this voltage-dependent calcium channel and act to inhibit calcium influx, their biochemical and physiological effects are very different, as noted above.

Verapamil and the phenylalkylamines are charged and bind at the outer portion of the calcium channel, while the dihydropyridines, which are uncharged (except amlodipine), bind deeper inside the calcium channel. These different membrane properties and binding characteristics result in a different profile of effects for the dihydropyridines compared with the phenylalkylamines, including increased lipid solubility. It is possible that these differences relate to the increased effectiveness of the dihydropyridines on depression[40] and ultra rapid cycling seen in a small subgroup of lithium-refractory bipolar patients.

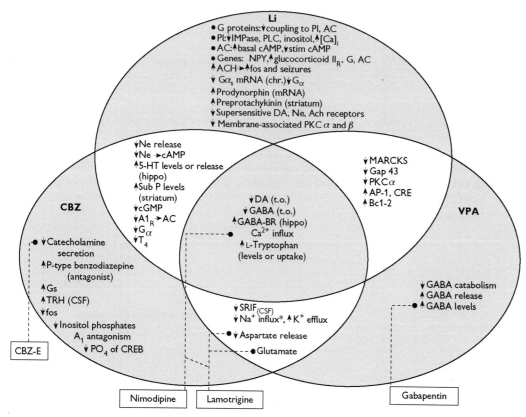

**Fig. 6.2.4.1** Common and differential mechanism of mood stabilizers: Pl, phosphoinositol; AC, adenylate cyclase; IMPase, inosital monophosphatase; PLC, phospholipase C; cAMP, cyclic adenosine monophosphate; NPY, neuropeptide Y; ACH, acetylcholine; $G\alpha_s$, G protein alpha (s) subunit; DA, dopaminergic; Ne, noradrenergic; PKC, protein kinase C; $A1_R$, adenosine A1 receptors; $T_4$, thyroxine; Gap 43, growth-associated protein 43; CRE, cyclic response element; CBZ, carbamazepine; TRH, throtrophin-releasing hormone; CREB, cyclic response element binding protein; VPA, valproate; SRIF, somatosatin; t.o., turnover.

# Pharmacokinetics, dosage, and administration

## Lithium

Lithium blood levels are conventionally described as being therapeutic from 0.5 to 1.2 mmol/l. Within this range, there is a wide agreement that higher doses are associated with increasing numbers of side-effects, but there is disagreement as to whether this is uniformly accompanied by a better therapeutic effect. Gelenberg et al.[12] reported that higher doses of lithium in the 0.8 to 1.0 mmol/l range averaging 0.83 mmol/l were 2.6 times as effective as doses achieving blood levels in the lower therapeutic range of 0.4 to 0.6, averaging 0.54 mmol/l. **This increased efficacy** (i.e. lower risk of relapse) **was achieved at the cost of a greater frequency of side effects**. Three times as many patients given doses in the high range withdrew from the study due to side effects. A series of other studies suggest that low to moderate doses of lithium may be just as effective as those in the higher range.[13]

Data of Kleindeinst et al.[41] further suggest a differential dose/effect relationship for lithium in mania versus depression prophylaxis. They found higher doses/blood levels more effective in preventing manic episodes while, **paradoxically, lower doses/levels were more effective in preventing depressions**. There is a considerable time lag before lithium reaches steady-state levels and some

attempts at lithium loading with large doses from the outset have not been successful. A certain amount of time is needed for lithium to gain access into the central nervous system compartment and steady-state levels are not typically achieved until five half-lives or approximately six days. With the advent of magnetic resonance spectroscopy it has been found that lithium levels in the brain are half those in serum and, based on one small study, may be better correlated with the degree of clinical response than serum levels. **Older individuals have higher intracellular lithium levels**, which may account for the observations of **toxicity at apparently therapeutic blood levels**.

While lithium has traditionally been administered in two, three, or four times daily dosing regimens in attempts to achieve the most consistent and stable blood levels possible, several findings have led to changes in this pattern of dosing. Extended-release preparations are now available and suitable for twice-daily dosing. Even with the original preparations of lithium carbonate many clinicians and investigators have administered lithium in single nighttime doses in order to achieve the highest blood levels (and the potential for side effects) during sleep, and utilize the much lower trough levels at a time when the kidney, for example, can be relatively spared from continuously high lithium levels. Some investigators feel that this might be associated with lower long-term renal side effects, and preliminary data suggest that this paradigm may not be associated with any loss of clinical efficacy. Given lithium's unique anti-suicide

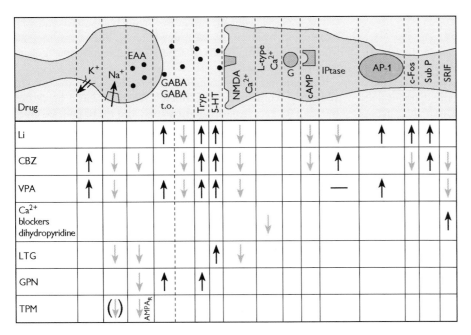

| Drug | K⁺ | Na⁺ | EAA | GABA | GABA t.o. | Tryp | 5-HT | NMDA Ca²⁺ | L-type Ca²⁺ | G | cAMP | IPtase | AP-1 | c-Fos | Sub P | SRIF |
|---|---|---|---|---|---|---|---|---|---|---|---|---|---|---|---|---|
| Li | | | | ↑ | ↓ | ↑ | ↑ | ↓ | | | ↓ | ↓ | ↑ | | ↑ | ↑ |
| CBZ | ↑ | ↓ | ↓ | | | ↑ | ↑ | ↓ | | ↓ | | ↑ | | ↓ | ↑ | ↓ |
| VPA | ↑ | ↓ | | ↑ | | ↑ | ↑ | ↓ | | — | | ↑ | | | | ↓ |
| Ca²⁺ blockers dihydropyridine | | | | | | | | | ↓ | | | | | | | ↑ |
| LTG | | ↓ | ↓ | | | | ↑ | ↓ | | | | | | | | |
| GPN | | | | ↓ | ↑ | | ↑ | | | | | | | | | |
| TPM | | (↓) | ↓ AMPAᵣ | | | | | | | | | | | | | |

**Fig. 6.2.4.2** Mechanisms of mood Stabilization. Depicted schematically at the top of the figure is a synapse with various types of channels, neurotransmitters, and proteins associated with the mechanisms of action of the mood stabilizers listed in the table below. **Row headings**: Li, lithium; CBZ, carbamazepine; VPA, valproate; LTG, lamotrigine; GPN, gabapentin; TPM, topiramate. **Column headings**; K⁺ efflux; Na⁺ influx; EAA, excitatory amino acids; GABA, γ-aminobutyric acid; GABA t.o., GABA turnover; Tryp, tryptophan; 5-HT, serotonin; NMDA Ca²⁺; L-type Ca²⁺; G, G protein; cAMP, cyclic adenosine monophosphate; IPtase, inositol phosphatase; AP-1, activator protein 1; Sub P, substance P; SRIF, somatostatin. Arrows indicate increases or deceases in substance/activity.

effects and strong evidence of neurotrophic and neuroprotective effects in animals at clinically relevant blood levels of 0.5 mmol/l, *administering lithium at whatever doses/blood levels are not associated with side effects would appear to have considerable merit.*

### Carbamazepine, valproate, lamotrigine

**Carbamazepine**, in contrast to oxcarbazepine, is a **potent inducer of CYP 3A4** hepatic enzymes, accounting for **auto-induction after one to three weeks of treatment.**[8] With immediate release preparations, B.I.D or T.I.D. dosing is required, but with long-acting preparations such as Equetro®(Tegretol Retard®), all H.S. dosing should be considered. The dose and blood level to side-effects relationships are highly variable and individual. In non-emergency situations, 200 mg H.S. may be considered as a starting dose with slow upward titration to avoid or accommodate to side effects. In manic inpatients initial dosing of 600 mg to 800 mg on day one may be tolerated.

While blood levels of 4–12 µg/ml are touted as therapeutic in epilepsy, there is no relation of blood level to degree of clinical response across either seizure disorder or affectively ill patients. Therefore, **individualized titration to good clinical effect and minimal side-effects** burden is more appropriate than compulsive blood level monitoring.

Valproate may be given in loading doses of 10 to 15 mg/kg. Efficacy is usually observed between 50–120 mg/ml with a target of 80 mg/ml or more in mania. *Single nighttime doses can be employed with both immediate release and extended release preparations,* which may be better tolerated.

**Lamotrigine must be dosed and titrated very slowly** in an attempt to avoid the occurrence of a **serious rash**. A typical procedure is to start with 25 mg/day for two weeks and then 50 mg/day for two weeks, and then increase by 25 mg (preferably) to 50 mg/week thereafter. A target dose is about 200 mg/day, but increases to 400 mg/day in those showing partial responses is often tolerated. The rate of titration and target dose of lamotrigine should be halved on **valproate** (which **doubles lamotrigine levels**) and can be doubled on carbamazepine and related potent enzyme inducers.

### L-type calcium channel blockers

The pharmacokinetics of the dihydropyridine L-type calcium channel blockers differ markedly. Nimodipine has a T½ of 1–2 h requiring T.I.D. dosing to peak total doses of 240 to 480 mg/day. Isradipine's T½ is 8 h, allowing B.I.D. dosing to a peak dose of 15 mg/day. Notably, amlodipine has a longer half-life and is suitable for single nighttime or twice-daily dosing in comparison with the better psychiatrically studied drugs nimodipine and isradipine. However, as long-acting preparations of these compounds become available, the importance of this half-life dissociation among the different compounds may dissipate. In our patient cohort at the NIMH, the pharmacokinetics of nimodipine (Bay e 9736) and its several metabolites (Bay o 1762, Bay m 5397, and Bay m 8922) were characterized by a rapid peaking (in 30–45 min) and decline in the second hour in response to a 60 mg challenge dose at steady-state blood levels after an overnight fast. Additional small secondary peaks occurred when usual dosing of four-times-a-day was resumed. There were no notable differences between capsule and tablet preparations. The phenylalkylamine verapamil has a 5–8 h half-life, also requiring T.I.D. dosing to a target peak daily dose of 480 mg/day.

# Side effects

## Lithium

Since lithium has been in use for much of the latter half of the twentieth century, its side-effects profile has been well described. Tremor and gastrointestinal distress, particularly diarrhoea, are generally dose-related, but some patients can have idiosyncratic sensitivity to these side effects, even at relatively low doses. Lithium-induced tremor can be countered with the beta-blocker propranolol in doses of 10 mg four times/day.

Side effects most likely to be associated with non-compliance or discontinuation of the drug include a sense of psychomotor slowing, cognitive dulling, acne or psoriasis, and weight gain. There is preliminary evidence that the anticonvulsants topiramate or zonisamide may help to reverse or stabilize lithium-related weight gain. Cognitive dulling could be treated with dose lowering, assessment of thyroid function, and $T_3$ (25–50 μg) augmentation even with normal thyroid indices, folate augmentation, and, potentially, an acetylcholinesterase inhibitor such as donepezil (Aricept®).

Lithium interferes with the actions of ADH (i.e. vasopressin) because of its ability to block vasopressin-induced adenylate cyclase. A syndrome of **reversible diabetes insipidus** is thus induced which, in most patients, is not problematic, although in a small percentage of patients, excretion of large volumes of urine can be extreme, inconvenient, and disruptive of normal social routines and sleep. This can be countered with amiloride or the thiazide diuretics (however, the latter also increase lithium levels).

Lithium is clearly able to induce thyroid dysfunction with increases in thyroid-stimulating hormone, sometimes proceeding to more full-blown evidence of chemical hypothyroidism. The threshold for treating lithium-related increases in thyroid-stimulating hormone has not been definitively identified, but with some evidence of lower levels of free thyroxine being associated with increased levels of depression and other low thyroid indices being associated with increased cognitive dysfunction, **replacement of thyroid hormones would appear indicated as thyroid-stimulating hormone begins to exceed normal levels**. Whether thyroid supplementation can reverse or prevent these lithium-related abnormalities remains to be directly assessed in prospective studies.

Some investigators suggest that long-term lithium may be associated with **slowly increasing creatinine levels** and a decrease in creatinine clearance.[40] The incidence of these glomerular filtration abnormalities in lithium-treated patients compared with age- and gender-matched controls remains controversial, as does the mode of treatment in the face of progressive changes in these indices. Given the availability of other potential mood-stabilizing agents, a reduction in lithium levels and supplementation or switching to other agents would be a conservative measure, if tolerated. However, others recommend careful monitoring of continued lithium therapy because the effects of lithium discontinuation on creatinine levels are highly inconsistent.

Severe episodes of lithium intoxication are to be avoided since they can be associated with a syndrome of irreversible cerebellar dysfunction.[42] The use of lithium with very high dose neuroleptic treatment is also to be avoided since occasional idiosyncratic and irreversible organic brain syndromes have resulted on rare occasions. Marked EEG changes and tonic-clonic seizures were also observed with the combination of lithium and clozapine. Lithium can be associated with alterations in calcium homeostasis and frant hyperparathyroidism. As mentioned above, lithium can increase white cells and platelets via its action on granulocyte-macrophage colony stimulating factor.

Valproate has many lithium-like side effects which may also be additive in combination treatment. **Valproate has a black box warning for rare hepatitis/pancreatitis and should not be given to children below two years of age.** It can also cause low platelets, and signs of bleeding tendency should be attended to. Because **valproate increases homocysteine, routine supplementation with folate (and possibly also B6 and B12 in women of child bearing age) would appear prudent**. Valproate can cause asymptomatic to symptomatic hyperammoniumemis; treatment with l-carnitine may be helpful. Zinc and selenium are anecdotally touted as preventing alopecia, but systematic evidence is lacking. Data are mixed as to whether valproate increases testosterone and causes the polycystic ovary syndrome (PCOS). Hirsutism is rarely seen in affectively ill patients and birth control pills will prevent PCOS. Valproate does increase the already high rates of menstrual irregularities seen in women with bipolar disorder.

Carbamazepine has less weight-gain liability than lithium or valproate, but has greater potential for rash and rare but serious hematological problems. **Carbamazepine** routinely causes a benign **drop in white blood cells via its effects on colony stimulating factor; this can be countered by lithium**. More problematic are agranulocytosis and aplastic anemia, estimated to occur in 1 in 20 000 to 50 000 patients. **Patients should be warned to consult their physician** if they develop a fever, sore throat, or other infection that could emanate from a low white blood count, or bleeding gums or petechiae that could reflect low platelets. **Hyponatremia is more common with oxcarbazepine** than carbamazepine, but the hyponatremia of carbamazepine can be treated or prevented with lithium or demeclocycline. Low $T_4$ on carbamazepine is usually not reflective of hypothyroidism because TSH is not increased, BMR is not decreased, and the degree of drop in $T_4$ and free $T_4$ may even be correlated with degree of antidepressive effect.

The **major side-effects concern of lamotrigine is that of a severe rash**, estimated to occur in 1 of 5 000 adults and 1 of 2 500 children. Even a benign rash should lead to drug discontinuation because there is no way to predict when a rash may progress to a Stevens-Johnson syndrome or Toxic Epidermal Necrolysis. Otherwise, the side-effects profile of lamotrigine fits well with bipolar depression treatment because the drug is weight-neutral, non-sedating, and without sexual dysfunction or endocrine dysregulation.

## L-type calcium channel blockers

The side-effects profile of nimodipine and related dihydropyridine L-type calcium channel blockers differs considerably from that of lithium. These drugs are primarily used in cardiology for their anti-hypertensive and anti-arrhythmogenic effects. As such, they may cause **side effects related to hypotension including dizziness and tightness in the chest**. Unlike lithium, they are not typically associated with gastrointestinal distress and tend to be slightly constipating rather than associated with diarrhea. Therefore, they might be able to replace some component of lithium's therapeutic action, as noted below, potentially without exacerbating some of lithium's related side-effects. Although these agents are often used in migraine prophylaxis, they can also be associated with headache on rare occasions. Redness and erythema with excessive warmth in the pretibial areas is also an occasional side effect of these agents, as is, more rarely, edema itself.

Nimodipine and related dihydropyridine L-type calcium channel blockers do not appear to share lithium's ability to induce cognitive slowing and, in fact, these agents have been reported to improve performance in some preclinical models of learning and memory deficits as well as in some clinical studies of patients with Alzheimer's disease. This might be related to nimodipine's ability to increase somatostatin upon chronic administration,[43] although other mechanisms remain to be explored.

Also, in contrast to lithium, which is associated with a small incidence of Epstein's anomaly, verapamil is not teratogenic. While systematic data are not available for the other dihydropyridine L-type calcium channel blockers, it is hoped that they will prove to be as safe as verapamil appears to be.

## Indications and contraindications

### Lithium

The double-blind controlled studies of lithium in acute mania were positive several decades ago, and in the largest randomized study comparing lithium with placebo in a study primarily designed to evaluate the acute antimanic efficacy of valproate, lithium and valproate appeared to show approximately equal efficacy and both were superior to placebo.[44] However, there appear to be a number of subtypes of illness with consistently higher or lower rates of response. As summarized in Table 6.2.4.1, a useful rule of thumb is that lithium is relatively less effective, with a low effectiveness rate of around 30 per cent in acute manic syndrome characterized by anxiety and dysphoria, comorbid substance abuse, comorbid medical conditions, the pattern of illness of depression-mania-well intervals as opposed to mania-depression-well intervals, in those with a negative family history of bipolar illness in first-degree relatives, in those with evidence of **EEG and neurological dysfunction, and in those with a pattern of rapid cycling or multiple prior episodes.**[2]

Lithium used to be considered contraindicated in pregnancy, but with the recognition that major cardiac malformations such as Epstein's anomaly are rare (1 in 1 200 births), many clinicians and patients are deciding to continue lithium when it appears important to continued mood stability.

### L-type calcium channel blockers

As discussed earlier, the evidence of verapamil's acute antimanic efficacy is derived from a considerable series of small double-blind studies. While the initial studies were unequivocally positive, more recent studies have not been as positive comparing either verapamil with placebo or verapamil with lithium. Only very preliminary evidence is available for the acute antimanic efficacy of nimodipine, with the open study of Brunet et al.[45] being positive in six of six individuals.[18,63] In placebo-controlled studies using an off-on-off-on design, 10 of 30 patients with refractory recurrent affective disorder responded and, in may instances, the antimanic efficacy was demonstrated both in the on-phase and with symptom exacerbation in the off-phase.[46] However, many of these individuals had ultra-rapid or ultra-ultra-rapid (ultradian) cycling patterns and most of the efficacy data reflected effective pharmacoprophylaxis of mania rather than acute antimanic efficacy per se.

Dubovsky[47] observed that a prior history of lithium response appears to be associated with a good response to verapamil. However, with the dihydropyridines we have observed some instances of response in those who were previously non-responders to lithium.[46] Among those responsive to the drug were patients with ultra-rapid and ultradian cycling and those with a pattern of recurrent brief depression. As indicated above, a number of these individuals were rechallenged and **responsiveness was confirmed in an off-on-off-on design**. Whether those bipolar patients with increased intracellular calcium would be among those responsive to the L-type calcium channel blockers also awaits completion of such a study, which is now under way.

A promising area of investigation is work using brain imaging, which has found that depressed patients with the classical pattern of relative frontal hypometabolism, and especially in the left insula, were among those who responded best to nimodipine, while equally depressed patients with left insula hypermetabolism responded to carbamazepine.[48] These data raise the possibility that regional topographies of blood flow or metabolism might ultimately help identify a subgroup of patients more responsive to the calcium-channel blocking agents. Also potentially helpful are data showing that nimodipine increases somatostatin in the CSF, and in one small study, that those with lower baseline CSF somatostatin were better responders to the drug.[49]

## Interactions

### Lithium

Owing to its renal excretion, lithium has renally-mediated rather than hepatically-mediated drug-drug interactions. Lithium excretion is decreased by medications such as thiazides, non-steroidal anti-inflammatory drugs, angiotensin-converting enzyme inhibitors, and, to a lesser extent, furosemide, and by physiological states such as dehydration, advanced age, and renal disease.[50] Owing to lithium's poor therapeutic index, these interactions can result in clinical lithium toxicity unless appropriate dosage adjustment is made. In contrast, lithium clearance is less consistently affected by amiloride, aspirin, and sulindac, and increased with other medications with diuretic effects such as acetazolamide, mannitol, aminophylline, caffeine, and theophylline, as well as during pregnancy.

### Valproate, carbamazepine, lamotrigine

Valproate is FDA-approved for migraine prevention and treatment of acute mania. However, it is **widely considered a mood stabilizer and used in long-term prophylaxis of both mood phases**. A modicum of data support acute and prophylactic efficacy in depression. **Valproate decreases alcohol intake** in bipolar patients[51] with this comorbidity and is useful in a wide range of anxiety syndromes.

**Valproate is contraindicated in pregnancy** because of a several percentage risk of neural tube defects (spina bifida) and, more recently noted, a substantial (20 per cent) incidence of other adverse events,[52] as well as moderate to severe developmental delay in a sizeable number of children.

**Carbamazepine** is approved for trigeminal neuralgia and the long-acting preparation of carbamazepine (Equetro®/Tegretol Retard®) is approved only in acute mania, but can be considered in long-term prophylaxis for those not responsive to lithium or valproate.

**Its profile of effectiveness is almost the converse of that of lithium**, with better effects in those with bipolar II illness, anxiety, and substance abuse comorbidity, mood incongruent delusions,[53] and a negative family history of bipolar disorder in first-degree relatives. Carbamazepine should not be used in pregnancy because it carries about a 0.5 per cent risk of neural tube defects.

Lamotrigine is unique because it is approved for only **prevention of depressed episodes** and to a lesser extent, manic and mixed episodes. Robust efficacy in acute depression has been seen in three studies, but not in four others, although the meta analysis remains significantly positive. A small series of patients studied in Canada identified correlates of positive response, including continuous cycling pattern and a **personal and positive family history of anxiety disorders**.[54,55] Only one of five pregnancy case registries showed a significance for the increased occurrence of cleft lip and palate, and this agent clearly appears safer than valproate or carbamazepine. Its overall serious adverse event percentage of 1 per cent does not appear to be different from that of the general population.

### L-type calcium channel blockers

Different calcium-channel blockers differentially affect carbamazepine levels. While verapamil and diltiazem increase carbamazepine levels substantially, potentially causing toxicity, this is not the case with nimodipine, isradipine, or amlodipine. Preliminary data from our group and others suggest that carbamazepine decreases nimodipine levels after a 60 mg challenge dose. In our study, group mean peak nimodipine levels during treatment with carbamazepine were about one-half those observed during treatment with nimodipine alone, although this finding showed only a trend level of significance, probably due to small sample size.

When calcium channel blockers are added to ß-adrenergic blocking agents, depression of ventricular function, cardiac slowing, and atrioventricular block can result. Combining calcium channel blockers with ß-adrenergic blocking agents may produce hypotension. Verapamil and nitrendipine increase plasma concentrations of digoxin and produce bradycardia, hypotension, or atrioventricular block.

## Effects of withdrawal

### Lithium

In addition to the variety of predictors of relative lithium nonresponsiveness from the outset, two relatively new and different mechanisms for the development of treatment resistance or loss of efficacy have been uncovered during long-term follow up in patients who are initially responsive. The first of these is the apparent development of tolerance characterized by an increasing frequency and/or severity of breakthrough episodes despite good compliance and consistent maintenance of lithium blood levels. In a group of 66 patients referred to the NIMH because of lithium nonresponsiveness, 23 patients (**34.8 per cent**) **displayed this apparent tolerance pattern**.[55] Although it has not been systematically studied, the initial therapeutic manoeuvres in the face of such loss of efficacy at maximum tolerated doses would appear to be augmenting lithium's effects with other putative mood-stabilizing agents with different mechanisms of action, and if lithium should

be discontinued, a consideration of its reinstitution with a hope for renewal of responsivity.

In contrast with this tolerance pattern in which patients suffer breakthrough episodes despite remaining under treatment, the phenomenon of lithium-discontinuation-related refractoriness refers to a small group of patients who have done extremely well on their long-term lithium, discontinue the drug, suffer additional relapses, and then fail to re-respond once lithium is reinstituted. This phenomenon accounted for nine of the 66 patients (13.6 per cent) who presented to us as lithium-refractory.[56] The average time well on lithium was 6.6 years, substantially greater than the average well interval of 1.5 years prior to instituting lithium therapy, strongly suggesting that lithium had been effective in these individuals, and if they had remained on the drug, they might have remained well. Sadly, for each of these individuals, this did not prove to be the case.

One patient had been well on lithium for more than 16 years and tapered lithium slowly, suggesting that neither the duration of time well nor the use of a slow taper would necessarily prevent the development of discontinuation-induced refractoriness. A number of other investigative groups have observed such a phenomenon.[57] In these studies, discontinuation-induced refractoriness occurred in anywhere from 3.6 per cent to 18.6 per cent of patients, with a total of 39 of 321 (12.1 per cent), and 12 of 92 (13 per cent) in studies that tracked responders only. Even if it only occurs in about 10 per cent of patients who discontinue their lithium, it would nevertheless appear to be of considerable clinical import and should be included in the informed consent process so that the patient has all of the available data when making decisions of whether or not to continue treatment. That is, in considering the risk-benefit of stopping lithium, **a patient should not only know the very high risk of relapse** (50 per cent in the first five months after discontinuing lithium, 80–90 per cent after 1.5 years,[58] but also that there is **no guarantee that responsivity would be as rapid, robust, or complete** as previously experienced, and that a small subgroup of individuals, perhaps as many as 10 per cent, will not achieve the same good response that they had previously.

### Valproate, carbamazepine, lamotrigine

Valproate will displace carbamazepine from its protein binding and inhibit the epoxide hydrolase from converting the active epoxide to the inactive diole. Thus, **carbamazepine dose will need to be decreased when used in combination with valproate. Valproate will double lamotrigine levels** such that dosing should be one-half that of normal.

**Carbamazepine as a potent 3A4 inducer has many drug-drug interactions**. It will decrease levels of oestrogen such that **high dosage forms need to be used with birth control pills**. It will lower levels of lamotrigine, haloperidol, aripiprazole, and many other compounds.

**Inhibition of 3A4 will notably increase carbamazepine levels** and potentially cause toxicity if a patient is at or near their side-effects threshold. **Erythromycin** and its analogues, **verapamil, and diltiazem** are such examples, and patients should be warned to check with their pharmacists about its many other interactions. Side effects can be avoided with lower carbamazepine doses in advance of such drugs being administered.

Each of these drugs can be discontinued rapidly without a major withdrawal syndrome. Tolerance to the efficacy of each of these agents has been observed in isolated cases or small series. Increasing doses and/or switching to or adding other agents without cross-tolerance (mechanistically different) are typically used clinically [8] In instances of tolerance development a period of time off the new ineffective drug may be associated with transient renewal of efficacy. Theoretical, but unproven ways of slowing or minimizing tolerance development include: using more maximally tolerated doses, rather than minimally effective ones; holding doses stable and not decreasing them unnecessarily; using combination of drugs; and treating earlier as opposed to later in the course of illness.

### L-type calcium channel blockers

Because so few patients have been studied with the L-type calcium channel blockers in long-term prophylaxis, it is uncertain to what extent patients may become tolerant to these agents. However, since tolerance has been observed to virtually every other putative mood-stabilizing agent, it is likely that this will also occur with nimodipine and related agents. Similarly, it is uncertain whether the phenomenon of discontinuation-related refractoriness observed with lithium would extend to the class of L-type calcium channel blockers; while we have not observed this phenomenon in our cohort of nimodipine responders (63), only a small group of patients has been studied to date.

## Further information

Post, R.M., and Leverich, G.S. (2008). *Treatment of Bipolar Illness: A Case Book for Clinicians and Patients*. WW Norton, Inc. (in press).

Post, R.M., Altshuler, L.L. (2005). Mood disorders: treatment of bipolar disorders. In: *Comprehensive Textbook of Psychiatry*. (eds. B.J. Sadock and V.A. Sadock), pp. 1661–707. Lippincott Williams & Williams, New York.

Post, R.M., Speer, A., Leverich, G.S. (2006).Complex combination therapy: the evolution toward rational polypharmacy in lithium-resistant bipolar illness. In *Bipolar Psychopharmacotherapy: Caring for the Patient*. (eds. H. Akiskal and M. Tohen), pp. 135–67. John Wiley & Sons.

## References

1. Post, R.M., and Leverich, G.S. (2007). *Treatment of Bipolar Illness: A Case Book for Clinicians and Patients*. WW Norton, Inc. (in press).

2. Post, R.M., Speer, A., Leverich, G.S., *et al.* (2006).Complex combination therapy: the evolution toward rational polypharmacy in lithium-resistant bipolar illness. In *Bipolar Psychopharmacotherapy: Caring for the Patient*. (eds. H. Akiskal and M. Tohen), pp. 135–67. John Wiley & Sons.

3. Post, R.M. and Luckenbaugh, D.A. (2003). Unique design issues in clinical trials of patients with bipolar affective disorder. *Journal of Psychiatric Research*, **37**(1), 61–73.

4. Post, R.M., Leverich, G.S., Weiss, S.R., *et al.* (2003). Psychosocial stressors as predisposing factors to affective illness and PTSD: potential neurobiological mechanisms and theoretical implications. In: *Neurodevelopmental Mechanisms in Psychopathology*. (eds. D. Cicchetti and E. Wilker). pp. 491–525. Cambridge University Press, New York.

5. Post, R.M. (2007a). Kindling and sensitization as models for affective episode recurrence, cyclicity, and tolerance phenomena. *Neuroscience and Biobehavioral Reviews*, **31**(6), 858–73.

6. Leverich, G.S., Post, R.M., Keck, P.E. Jr., *et al.* (2007). The poor prognosis of childhood-onset bipolar disorder. *Journal of Pediatrics*,**150**(5), 485–90.

7. Post, R.M. (2007b). Role of BDNF in bipolar and unipolar disorder: clinical and theoretical implications. *Journal of Psychiatric Research*, **41**, 979–90.

8. Post, R.M., Ketter, T.A., Uhde, T., *et al.* (2007). Thirty years of clinical experience with carbamazepine in the treatment of bipolar illness: principles and practice. *CNS Drugs*, **21**(1), 47–71.

9. Post, R.M. (2004). The status of the sensitization/kindling hypothesis of bipolar disorder. *Current Psychosis and Therapeutics Reports*, **2**, 135–41.

10. Kessing, L.V., and Andersen, P.K. (2004). Does the risk of developing dementia increase with the number of episodes in patients with depressive disorder and in patients with bipolar disorder? *Journal of Neurology, Neurosurgery, and Psychiatry*, **75**(12),1662–66.

11. Schou, M. (1997). Forty years of lithium treatment. *Archives of General Psychiatry*, **54**, 9–15.

12. Gelenberg, A.J., Kane, J.M., Keller, M.B., *et al.* (1989). Comparison of standard and low serum levels of lithium for maintenance treatment of bipolar disorder. *New England Journal of Medicine*, **321**, 1489–93.

13. Vestergaard, P., Licht, R.W., Brodersen, A., *et al.* (1998). Outcome of lithium prophylaxis: a prospective follow-up of affective disorder patients assigned to high and low serum lithium levels. *Acta Psychiatrica Scandinavica*, **98**, 310–15.

14. Gitlin, M.J., and Altshuler, L.L. (1997). Unanswered questions, unknown future for one of our oldest medications. *Archive General of Psychiatry*, **54**(1), 21–3.

15. Dubovsky, S.L., Murphy, J., Thomas, M. *et al.* (1992). Abnormal intracellular calcium ion concentration in platelets and lymphocytes of bipolar patients. *American Journal of Psychiatry*, **149**, 118–20.

16. Dubovsky, S.L., Franks, R.D., Allen, S. *et al.* (1986). Calcium antagonists in mania: a double-blind study of verapamil. *Psychiatry Research*, **18**, 309–20.

17. Janicak, P.G., Sharma, R.P., Pandey, G., *et al.* (1998). Verapamil for the treatment of acute mania: a double-blind, placebo controlled trial. *American Journal of Psychiatry*, **155**, 972–3.

18. Walton, S.A., Berk, M., and Brook S. (1996). Superiority of lithium over verapamil in mania: a randomized, controlled, single-blind trial. *Journal of Clinical Psychiatry*, **57**, 543–6.

19. Hoschl, C. and Kozeny, J. (1989). Verapamil in affective disorders: a controlled, double-blind study. *Biological Psychiatry*, **25**, 128–40.

20. Pazzaglia, P.J., Post, R.M., Ketter T.A., *et al.* (1993). Preliminary controlled trial of nimodipine in ultra-rapid cycling affective dysregulation. *Psychiatry Research*, **49**, 257–72.

21. Post, R.M., Pazzaglia, P.J., Ketter, T.A., *et al.* (2000). Carbamazepine and nimodipine in affective illness: efficacy, mechanisms of action, and interactions. In *Pharmacotherapy for mood, anxiety, and cognitive disorders* (eds. S. Montgomery and U. Halbreich), American Psychiatric Press, Washington, DC.

22. Triggle, D.J. (2007). Calcium Channel Antagonists: Clinical uses-past, present, and future. *Biochemical Pharmacology*, **74**, 1–9.

23. Belmaker, R.H., Avissar, S., and Schreiber, G. (1991). Effect of lithium on human neurotransmitter receptor systems and G proteins. In *Lithium and the cell: pharmacology and biochemistry* (ed. N.J. Birch), pp. 113–19. Academic Press, London.

24. Manji, H.K., Potter, W.Z., and Lenox, R.H. (1995). Signal transduction pathways. Molecular targets for lithium's actions. *Archives of General Psychiatry*, **52**, 531–43.

25. Bebchuk, J.M., Arfken, C.L., Dolan-Manji, S., *et al.* (2000). A preliminary investigation of a protein kinase C inhibitor in the treatment of acute mania. *Archives of General Psychiatry*, **57**, 95–7.

26. Nonaka, S., Hough, C.J., and Chuang, D.M. (1998). Chronic lithium treatment robustly protects neurons in the central nervous system against excitotoxicity by inhibiting $N$-methyl-$D$-aspartate receptormediated calcium influx. *Proceedings of the National Academy of Sciences of the United States of America*, **95**, 2642–7.

27. Chen G., Zeng, W.Z., Yuan, P.X., *et al.* (1998). The mood-stabilizing agents lithium and valproate dramatically increase the levels of the neuroprotective protein BCL-2 in the CNS. *Journal of Neurochemistry*, **72**, 879–82.

28. Zarate, C.A. Jr., Singh, J.B., Carlson, P.J., *et al.* (2007). Efficacy of a protein kinase C inhibitor (tamoxifen) in the treatment of acutemania: a pilot study. *Bipolar Disorders*, **9**(6), 561–70. 29. Einat, H., Yuan, P., Szabo, S.T., *et al.* (2007). Protein kinase C inhibition by tamoxifen antagonizes manic-like behavior in rats: implications for the development of novel therapeutics for bipolar disorder. *Neuropsychobiology*, **55**(3–4), 123–31.

30. Gallicchio, V.S., Chen, M.G., and Watts, T.D. (1984). Specificity of lithium (Li+) to enhance the production of colony stimulating factor (GM-CSF) from mitogen-stimulated lymphocytes *in vitro*. *Cellular Immunology*, **85**, 58–66.

31. Joffe, R.T., Post, R.M., Roy-Byrne, P.P., *et al.* (1985). Hematological effects of carbamazepine in patients with affective illness. *American Journal of Psychiatry*, **142**, 1196–9.

32. Kramlinger, K.G. and Post, R.M. (1990). Addition of lithium carbonate to carbamazepine: hematological and thyroid effects. *American Journal of Psychiatry*, **147**, 615–20.

33. Chuang, D.M., Chen, R.W., Chalecka-Franaszek, E., *et al.* (2002). Neuroprotective effects of lithium in cultured cells and animal models of diseases. *Bipolar Disorders*, **4**(2):129–36.

34. Wignall, E.L., Dickson, J.M., Vaughan, P., *et al.* (2004). Smaller hippocampal volume in patients with recent-onset posttraumatic stress disorder. *Biological Psychiatry*, **56**(11), 832–6.

35. Blumberg, H.P., Fredericks, C., Wang, F., *et al.* (2005). Preliminary evidence for persistent abnormalities in amygdala volumes in adolescents and young adults with bipolar disorder. *Bipolar Disorders*, **7**(6), 570–6.

36. Sheline, YI., Sanghavi, M., Mintun, M.A., *et al.* (1999). Depression duration but not age predicts hippocampal volume loss in medically healthy women with recurrent major depression. *Journal of Neuroscience*, **19**(12), 5034–43.

37. Moore, G.J., Bebchuk, J.M., Wilds, I.B., *et al.* (2000). Lithium-induced increase in human brain grey matter. *Lancet*, **356**(9237): 1241–2.

38. Bearden, C.E., Thompson, P.M., Dalwani, M., *et al.* (2007). Greater cortical gray matter density in lithium-treated patients with bipolar disorder. *Biological Psychiatry*, **62**(1), 7–16.

39. Ketter, T.A., Wang, P.W., Becker, O.V., *et al.* (2003). The diverse roles of anticonvulsants in bipolar disorders. *Annals of Clinical Psychiatry*, **15**(2), 95–108.

40. Taragano, F.E., Bagnatti, P., Allergri, F., *et al.* (2005). A double-blind, randomized clinical trial to assess the augmentation with nimodipine of antidepressant therapy in the treatment of 'vascular depression'. *International Psychogeriatrics*, **17**, 487–498.

41. Kleindienst, N., Engel, R., Greil, W., *et al.* (2005). Which clinical factors predict response to prophylactic lithium? A systematic review for bipolar disorders. *Bipolar Disorders*, **7**(5), 404–17.

42. Kores, B. and Lader, M.H. (1997). Irreversible lithium neurotoxicity: an overview. *Clinical Neuropharmacology*, **20**, 283–99.

43. Pazzaglia, P.J., George, M.S., Post, R.M., *et al.* (1995). Nimodipine increases CSF somatostatin in affectively ill patients. *Neuropsychopharmacology*, **13**, 75–83.

44. Bowden, C.L., Brugger, A.M., Swann, A.C., *et al.* (1994). Efficacy of divalproex vs. lithium and placebo in the treatment of mania. The Depakote Mania Study Group. *Journal of the American Medical Association*, **271**, 918–24.

45. Brunet, G., Cerlich, B., Robert, P., *et al.* (1990). Open trial of a calcium antagonist, nimodipine, in acute mania. *Clinical Neuropharmacology*, **13**, 224–8.

46. Pazzaglia, P.J., Post, R.M., Ketter, T.A., *et al.* (1998). Nimodipine monotherapy and carbamazepine augmentation in patients with refractory recurrent affective illness. *Journal of Clinical Psychopharmacology*, **18**, 404–13.

47. Dubovsky, S.L. (1995). Calcium channel antagonists as novel agents for manic-depressive disorder. In *Textbook of psychopharmacology* (eds. A.E. Schatzberg and C.B. Nemeroff), pp. 377–88. American Psychiatric Press, Washington, DC.

48. Ketter, T.A., Kimbrell, T.A., George, M.S., *et al.* (1999). Baseline cerebral hypermetabolism associated with carbamazepine response and hypometabolism with nimodipine response in mood disorders. *Biological Psychiatry*, **46**, 1364–74.

49. Frye, M.A., Pazzaglia, P.J., George, M.S., *et al.* (2003). Low CSFsomatostatin associated with response to nimodipine in patents with affective illness. *Biological Psychiatry*, **53**(2), 180–3.

50. Muller-Oerlinghausen, B. (1999). Drug interactions with lithium: aguide for clinicians. *CNS Drugs*, **11**, 41–8.

51. Salloum, I.M., Cornelius, J.R., Daley, D.C., *et al.* (2005). Efficacy of valproate maintenance in patients with bipolar disorder and alcoholism: a double-blind placebo-controlled study. *Archives of General Psychiatry*, **62**(1), 37–45.

52. Meador, K.J., Baker, G.A., Finnell, R.H., *et al.* (2006). In utero antiepileptic drug exposure: fetal death and malformations. *Neurology*, **67**(3), 407–12.

53. Greil, W., Kleindienst, N., Erazo, N., *et al.* (1998). Differential response to lithium and carbamazepine in the prophylaxis of bipolar disorder. *Journal of Clinical Psychopharmacology*, **18**(6), 455–60.

54. Passmore, M.J., Garnham, J., Duffy, A., *et al.* (2003). Phenotypic spectra of bipolar disorder in responders to lithium versus lamotrigine. *Bipolar Disorders*,**5**(2), 110–4.

55. Grof, P. (2003). Selecting effective long-term treatment for bipolar patients: monotherapy and combinations. *Journal of Clinical Psychiatry*, **64** Suppl 5, 53–61.

56. Post, R.M., Leverich G.S., Altshuler, L., *et al.* (1992). Lithium-discontinuation-induced refractoriness: preliminary observations. *American Journal of Psychiatry*, **149**, 1727–9.

57. Koukopoulos, A., Reginaldi, D., Minnai, G., *et al.* (1995). The long term prophylaxis of affective disorders. *Advances in Biochemical Psychopharmacology*, Gessa, Fratta, Pani & Serra (eds)., *Depression and Mania: From Neurobiology to Treatment*, Vol 49.

58. Suppes, T., Baldessarini, R.J., Faedda, G.L., *et al.* (1991). Risk of recurrence following discontinuation of lithium treatment in bipolar disorder. *Archives of General Psychiatry*, **48**, 1082–4.

# 6.2.5 **Antipsychotic and anticholinergic drugs**

Herbert Y. Meltzer and  William V. Bobo

## Introduction

The discovery by Delay and Denicker in 1953 that chlorpromazine was highly effective in alleviating delusions, hallucinations, and disorganized thinking, was the seminal breakthrough in the treatment of schizophrenia, the first agent to produce sufficient relief of core psychotic symptoms to permit life outside of institutions for many patients with schizophrenia, and even a return to a semblance of function within normal limits. Chlorpromazine and the other related typical antipsychotic drugs which were introduced over the next 30 years have proven to be of immense benefit to vast numbers of people who experience psychotic symptoms as a component of a diverse group of neuropsychiatric and medical disorders, as well as drug-induced psychoses. These drugs have been invaluable in providing clues to the aetiology of schizophrenia and other forms of mental illness with psychotic features and as tools in understanding fundamental neural processes, especially those involving dopamine, a key neurotransmitter involved in psychosis. This class of drugs has now been supplanted by the so-called atypical antipsychotic drugs, of which clozapine is the prototype. This chapter will describe the various classes of antipsychotic agents, with emphasis on the atypical antipsychotic drugs, their benefits and adverse effects, recommendations for use in clinical practice, and mechanism of action. The drugs used to treat the extrapyramidal side-effects (EPS) produced mainly by the typical antipsychotic drugs are also considered.

## The classes of antipsychotic drugs

Antipsychotic drugs have been classified into two broad categories: typical and atypical.[1] Typical antipsychotic drugs are those which (typically) produce EPS at clinically effective doses, including parkinsonism (muscle rigidity, tremor, bradykinesia), acute dystonic reactions, dyskinesias, akathisia (restlessness), and tardive dyskinesia. They are also called neuroleptics because of their inhibitory effect upon locomotion activity. They are sometimes referred to as first generation antipsychotic drugs, but this has multiple problems as a class designation. The prototype of the atyipcal class of agents is clozapine which was first discovered during the early stages of the development of the drugs called first generation agents. The major mode of action of typical neuroleptics is to block dopamine $D_2$ receptors in the limbic system, which includes the nucleus accumbens, stria terminalis, and amygdala.

The typical antipsychotic drugs are members of a variety of chemical families (Table 6.2.5.1). They vary in affinity for the $D_2$ receptor, with low affinity drugs such as chlorpromazine, which require high doses for clinical efficacy, to high affinity such as haloperidol, which are effective at lower doses (Table 6.2.5.1). Kapur and Seeman[3] have proposed that the rate of dissociation of all antipsychotic drugs from the $D_2$ receptor provides the basis for the distinction between typical and atypical antipsychotic drugs, with atypical antipsychotic drugs dissociating more rapidly. While this is true for clozapine and quetiapine, the atypical drugs risperidone, sertindole, olanzapine and asenapine dissociate no more rapidly or even slower than haloperidol. As such, 'fast dissociation' cannot provide the pharmacological basis for atypicality for most of the drugs that are considered atypical.

Low-potency typical neuroleptic agents are those in which the usual dose range in schizophrenia is equal to or greater than 200 mg/day, while mid- to high-potency agents are those in which the dose range is between 2 and 175 mg/day. In general, the low-potency drugs are more sedative and more hypotensive than the high-potency agents but also have less of a tendency to produce extrapyramidal side-effects. The typical antipsychotic drugs differ from one another with regard to potential for other side-effects, e.g. weight gain and hypotension, but have comparable efficacy as antipsychotic agents.[4]

Atypical antipsychotic drugs are those antipsychotic agents with a significantly lower propensity to produce EPS at clinically effective doses.[1] They are also characterized by a more diverse and complex pattern of pharmacological activity, including serotonin $(5\text{-hydroxytryptamine})_{2A}$ and dopamine $D_2$ antagonism as well as a variety of activities at other receptors whose contribution to their mode of action is still being elucidated.[2] Substituted benzamides, e.g. amisulpride, also have low EPS at clinically effective doses and may constitute another class of atypical agents. New classes of atypical antipsychotic drugs are emerging from research with considerable frequency at the current time.

The prototypical atypical antipsychotic drug is clozapine, a dibenzodiazepine (Table 6.2.5.1).[5] Others include aripiprazole,[6] olanzapine, quetiapine, paliperidone, risperidone, sertindole, ziprasidone and zotepine, while iloperidone,[7] asenapine,[8] and laurasidone[9] are in development and have a similar pharmacology to that of risperidone. These drugs are all more potent $5\text{-HT}_{2A}$ than $D_2$ receptor antagonists as well as multireceptor antagonists[9, 10] except for aripiprazole, which is a dopamine $D_2$ receptor partial agonist. Bifeprunox is also a partial $D_2$ agonist. It lacks $5\text{-HT}_{2A}$ receptor blocking properties, relying instead on $5\text{-HT}_{1A}$ partial agonism to reduce serotonergic tone. Amisulpride and remoxipride are substituted benzamides. Both are selective $D_2/D_3$ antagonists.[2]

**Table 6.2.5.1** Selected antipsychotic drugs and classification schemes

| Drug name | Trade name | Chemical class | General class | D2 potency* |
|---|---|---|---|---|
| Aripiprazole | Abilify | Dihydrocarbostyril | Atypical | |
| Chlorpromazine | Thorazine | Phenothiazine | Typical | Low |
| Clozapine | Clozaril | Dibenzazepine | Atypical | |
| Droperidol | Inapsine | Butyrophenone | Typical | Mid |
| Fluphenazine | Prolixin | Phenothiazine | Typical | High |
| Haloperidol | Haldol | Butyrophenone | Typical | High |
| Loxapine | Loxitane | Dibenzazepine | Typical | Mid |
| Mesoridazine | Serentil | Phenothiazine | Typical | Low |
| Molindone | Moban | Dihydroindolone | Typical | Mid |
| Olanzapine | Zyprexa | Thiobenzodiazepine | Atypical | |
| Paliperidone | Invega | 9-hydroxy metabolite of risperidone | Atypical | |
| Perphenazine | Trilafon | Phenothiazine | Typical | Mid |
| Pimozide | Orap | Butyrophenone | Typical | Mid |
| Promazine | | Phenothiazine | Typical | Mid |
| Quetiapine | Seroquel | Dibenzothiazepine | Atypical | |
| Risperidone | Risperdal, Risperdal CONSTA | Benzisoxazole | Atypical | |
| Thioridazine | Mellaril | Phenothiazine | Typical | Low |
| Tiotixene | Navane | Thioxanthene | Typical | High |
| Trifluoperazine | Stelazine | Phenothiazine | Typical | Mid |
| Ziprasidone | Geodon | Benzisothiazole | Atypical | |

* Classification on the basis of potency of D2 receptor binding for typical antipsychotic drugs only

Remoxipride was withdrawn shortly after its introduction because of a high rate of aplastic anaemia.

As will be discussed, the atypical antipsychotic drugs differ not only with regard to side-effects but also with regard to efficacy.[11,12] Atypical antipsychotic agents have been shown to have advantages, albeit modest, in treating negative mood symptoms[13–15] and to improve cognitive dysfunction in schizophrenia and perhaps other psychiatric disorders.[16–18]

## Pharmacology

There is abundant evidence that dopamine plays a key role in the aetiology of psychosis and the action of antipsychotic drugs.[19] The antipsychotic action of the typical antipsychotic drugs is highly correlated with their affinities for $D_2$ receptors. Amphetamine and methamphetamine, which increase synaptic concentrations of dopamine, have been found to exacerbate delusions and hallucinations in some patients with schizophrenia This effect is believed to be due to stimulation of a subgroup of $D_2$ receptors in mesolimbic nuclei.[19,20] The cell bodies of mesolimbic dopamine neurones reside in the ventral tegmentum, the so-called A10 area, and have terminals in the nucleus accumbens, stria terminalis, and olfactory tubercle. The outflow of these regions to the thalamus and the cortex is believed to mediate psychotic symptoms. The firing rate of the mesolimbic dopaminergic neurones is subject to multiple influences, including stimulatory serotonergic input from the median raphe.[21] The origin of the dopamine neurones that terminate on cholinergic neurones in the basal ganglia is the substantia nigra, the so-called A9 region.[20] Blockade of striatal $D_2$ receptors in this pathway leads to the extrapyramidal side-effects produced by antipsychotic agents. A group of ventral tegmental dopamine neurones project to various regions of the cortex and comprise the mesocortical dopamine system. There is extensive evidence that these neurones are important for cognition, especially working memory,[22] as well as negative symptoms.[23] Neuroleptic drugs occupy 80 to 95 per cent of striatal $D_2$ receptors in patients with schizophrenia at clinically effective doses, though a lower blockade threshold of 60 per cent for improving positive symptoms has been identified.[24] Extrapyramidal side-effects occur above 80 per cent occupancy of these receptors. Blockade of $D_2$ receptors in the anterior pituitary gland is the basis for their ability to stimulate prolactin secretion.[25]

The prefrontal cortex has relatively low concentrations of $D_2$ receptors and has a higher density of $D_1$, $D_3$ and $D_4$ dopamine receptors.[20] The activation of $D_1$ receptors in prefrontal cortex may be especially critical for normal working memory and other executive type functions subserved by this brain region. However, no D1 agonists are available for treatment at the current time, although several are in development. Drugs which selectively block $D_4$ receptors have not been found to have an antipsychotic effect.[26] There are only limited data regarding the aetiologic or pharmacological significance of $D_3$ receptors in schizophrenia.

The typical antipsychotic drugs vary in their *in vitro* and *in vivo* affinities for receptors such as the dopamine $D_1$, histamine $H_1$, muscarinic, $\alpha$-1 and $\alpha$-2 adrenergic, and serotonergic receptors (Table 6.2.5.2), which mediate effects on arousal, extrapyramidal, cognitive, cardiovascular, gastrointestinal, and genitourinary function (Table 6.2.5.3).[27]

Thioridazine is a relatively potent antimuscarinic agent. Most of the low-potency antipsychotic agents are potent $\alpha_1$ and $H_1$ antagonists. These affinities contribute to hypotension and weight gain, respectively. While some typical antipsychotic drugs have a high affinity for $5\text{-HT}_{2A}$ receptors, their affinities for $D_2$ receptors are even higher, which diminishes the beneficial effects of the $5\text{-HT}_{2A}$ receptor blockade. The specific receptor profile of each atypical antipsychotic is of special interest because it may account for critical differences among these compounds, especially in terms of side effect burden (Table 6.2.5.4).

The affinities of the atypical antipsychotic drug have been related to their efficacy and side effect profiles. As noted above, the most important determinant of atypicality for most of the currently available agents of this type is that they are more potent $5\text{-HT}_{2A}$ than $D_2$ receptor antagonists. An exception is aripiprazole, which combines potent $5\text{-HT}_{2A}$ antagonism and $5\text{-HT}_{1A}$ agonism, with partial $D_2$ receptor agonism. Another exception is amisulpiride, which is a selective $D_{2/3}$ antagonist with little pharmacological activity at $5\text{-HT}_{2A}$ receptors. Combined $5\text{-HT}_{2A}$ with less potent D2 antagnoism is the most consistent principle yet discovered to produce a separation between antipsychotic action and interference with motor function. This hypothesis arose from showing that it could distinguish clozapine, the prototypical atypical antipsychotic drug, and a series of other atypical antipsychotic compounds from those which have typical properties.[28] These studies suggested that the low potential for extrapyramidal side-effects of clozapine, and subsequently, olanzapine, quetiapine, risperidone, iloperidone, ziprasidone, paliperidone and asenapine are due, in part, to their relatively stronger $5\text{-HT}_2$ antagonist and weak $D_2$ antagonist properties. The serotonin-dopamine interaction in the nigrostriatal and mesolimbico-cortical pathways appears to be mediated by stimulation of $5\text{-HT}_{2A}$ receptors, which are located on dopaminergic cell bodies, whereas antagonism of these receptors may release these neurones from tonic inhibition.

The atypical antipsychotic agents have the ability to increase prefrontal cortical dopaminergic activity compared with subcortical dopaminergic activity.[29] The ability to increase the release of dopamine in the prefrontal cortex may be important for atypical antipsychotic agents to improve cognition and negative symptoms. It may also contribute to decreasing the release of dopamine in the mesolimbic region, because prefrontal dopamine neurones modulate the activity of corticolimbic glutamatergic neurones that influence the release of dopamine from nerve terminals in the limbic region.[22] Typical neuroleptic drugs do not share this ability to increase dopamine efflux in prefrontal cortex. Clozapine and some of the other atypical antipsychotic drugs that are also potent $5\text{-HT}_{2A}$ antagonists, but not typical neuroleptics, also produce marked increases in prefrontal cortical and hippocampal acetylcholine efflux.[30] These atypical agents also produce marked increases in noradrenaline efflux in the prefrontal cortex which is correlated in time and magnitude with the increase in extracellular dopamine.[31] It is of interest that in rodents, combining ritanserin (a mixed 5-HT2a/2B/2C antagonist) or M-100907 (a selective $5\text{-HT}_{2A}$ antagonist) with a selective $D_{2/3}$ antagonist resulted in increased prefrontal dopamine release.[32,33] The combination of haloperidol and M-100907 also increased prefrontal dopamine release, with the greatest effects observed when lower doses of haloperidol were used.[34] Because reduced noradrenergic and dopaminergic function in prefrontal cortex and hippocampus has been

**Table 6.2.5.2** Affinities of selected antipsychotic drugs at various neuroreceptors

| Drug name | D2 | 5-HT$_{1A}$ | 5-HT$_{2A}$ | 5-HT$_{2C}$ | α-1 | α-2 | H-1 | M-1 |
|---|---|---|---|---|---|---|---|---|
| Aripiprazole | 0.95 | 5.6 | 4.6 | 181.0 | 25.0 | 74.0 | 29.0 | >6K |
| Chlorpromazine | 2.0 | >3K | 3.2 | 26.0 | 0.28 | 184.0 | 0.18 | 47.0 |
| Clozapine | 431.0 | 105.0 | 13.0 | 29.0 | l.6 | 142.0 | 2.0 | 14.0 |
| Droperidol | 0.25 [173] | NA | NA | NA | NA | NA | NA | NA |
| Fluphenazine | 0.54 | 145.0 | 7.4 | 418.0 | 6.4 | 314.0 | 7.3 | >1K |
| Haloperidol | 2.0 | >1K | 73.0 | >10K | 12.0 | >1K | >3K | >10K |
| Loxapine | 10.0 | >2K | 3.9 | 21.0 | 31.0 | 151.0 | 2.8 | 175.0 |
| Molindone | 63.0 [43] | >3K [43] | 320.0 [43] | >10K [43] | >2K [43] | >1K [43] | >2K [43] | NA |
| Olanzapine | 72.0 | >2K | 3.0 | 24.0 | 109.0 | 314.0 | 4.9 | 24.0 |
| 9-OH risperidone* | 9.4 | 637.8 | 1.9 | 100.3 | 2.5 | 4.7 | 5.6 | >10K |
| Perphenazine | 1.4 [43] | 421.0 [43] | 5.6 [43] | 132.0 [43] | 10.0 [43] | 810.5 [43] | 8.0 [43] | NA |
| Pimozide | 0.65 [43] | 650.0 [43] | 19.0 [43] | >3K [43] | 197.7 [43] | >1K [43] | 692.0 [43] | 800.0 [174] |
| Quetiapine | 567.0 | 431.0 | 366.0 | >1K | 22.0 | >3K | 7.5 | 858.0 |
| Risperidone | 4.9 | 427.0 | 0.19 | 94.9 | 5.0 | 151.0 | 5.2 | >10K |
| Thioridazine | 10.0 | 108.0 | 11.0 | 69.0 | 1.3 | 134.0 | 14.0 | 33.0 |
| Tiotixene | 1.4 | 410.0 | 111.0 | >1K | 12.0 | 80.0 | 12.0 | >10K |
| Trifluoperazine | 1.3 [43] | 950.0 [43] | 13.0 [43] | 378.0 [43] | 24.0 [43] | 653.7 [43] | 63.0 [43] | NA |
| Ziprasidone | 4.0 | 76.0 | 2.8 | 68.0 | 18.0 | 160.0 | 130.0 | >10K |

All receptor binding affinities are reported as K$_i$ (nM) using National Institutes of Mental Health (NIMH) Psychoactive Drug Screening Program (PDSP) certified data, available online at http://pdsp.cwru.edu/pdsp.php, unless otherwise specified. In general, the lower the K$_i$ (nM) value, the higher the binding affinity for the drug at a given receptor site.

NA = human cloned receptor data not available

* 9-hydroxy (9-OH) risperidone is marketed as paliperidone

**Table 6.2.5.3** Hypothesized therapeutic and adverse effects of receptor occupancy by antipsychotic drugs

| Target receptor | Pharmacological activity | Therapeutic effect(s) | Adverse effect(s) |
|---|---|---|---|
| Dopamine D2 | Antagonism or partial agonist effects | Reduction of positive symptoms | Extrapyramidal effects (EPS) Hyperprolactinemia |
| Serotonin (5-HT)$_{1A}$ | Full or partial agonist effects | Cognitive enhancement Reduction of mood and anxiety symptoms | |
| 5-HT$_{2A}$ | Antagonism | Reduction of negative symptoms Reduction of EPS Reduction of mood and anxiety symptoms Increased deep sleep | |
| 5-HT$_{2C}$ | Antagonism | Reduced anxiety symptoms | Weight gain |
| Adrenergic α-1 | Antagonism | | Orthostatic hypotension Dizziness |
| Adrenergic α-2 | Antagonism | | Reflex tachycardia |
| Histamine H-1 | Sedation | Sedation Drowsiness Weight gain | |
| Muscarinic (cholinergic) M-1 | Antagonism | Reduction of EPS | Blurry vision Exacerbation of acute angle closure glaucoma Sinus tachycardia Constipation Urinary retention Memory dysfunction |

Adapted from Kelly, D.L. and Love, R.C. Ziprasidone and the QTC interval: pharmacokinetic and pharmacodynamic considerations, Psychopharmacology Bulletin, **35**, 66–79, copyright 2001, MedWorks Media Global, LLC.

**Table 6.2.5.4** Adverse effects of selected antipsychotic drugs

**Typical antipsychotic drugs**

| | EPS | Tardive dyskinesia | Prolactin elevation | Sedation | Weight gain | Orthostasis | Anti-cholinergic | Diabetes exacerbation & dyslipidemia |
|---|---|---|---|---|---|---|---|---|
| Chlorpromazine Fluphenazine Haloperidol Loxapine Mesoridazine Molindone Perphenazine Thioridazine Tiotixene Trifluoperazine | Some (for low potency* drugs) - +++ (for high-potency* drugs) | ++ - +++ | ++ - +++ (risk higher for high-potency drugs) | Some (for high potency drugs) - +++ (for low-potency drugs); ? least for molindone | Some (for high potency drugs) - +++ (for low-potency drugs); ? least for molindone | Some (for high potency drugs) - +++ (for low-potency drugs) | Some (for high potency drugs) - +++ (for low-potency drugs) | + - ++ |

* See Table 6.2.5.1 for list of low-, mid-, and high-potency (with respect to dopamine D2 receptor blockade) antipsychotic drugs

Adapted from the International Psychopharmacology Algorithm Project (IPAP) algorithm for the treatment of schizophrenia, available at www.ipap.org, copyright 2008 International Psychopharmacology Algorithm Project (IPAP)

**Atypical antipsychotic drugs**

| | EPS | Tardive dyskinesia | Prolactin elevation | Sedation | Weight gain | Orthostasis | Anti-cholinergic | Glucose dysregulation & dyslipidemia |
|---|---|---|---|---|---|---|---|---|
| Amisulpride | + | Rare | +++ | + | 0 - + | + | 0 | 0 |
| Aripiprazole | 0 - + | 0 - + | 0 | 0 - + | 0 - + | + - ++ | 0 | 0 |
| Clozapine | 0 | 0 | Transient | +++ | +++ | +++ | +++ | +++ |
| Olanzapine | 0 - + (if < 10 mg/day) | Rare | + (if < 20 mg/day) | ++ | +++ | + | + | +++ |
| Quetiapine | 0 | Rare | 0 | ++ | + - ++ | ++ | 0 - + | ++ |
| Risperidone | + (less if < 4 mg/day) | Rare | +++ | + | + - ++ | ++ | 0 | + |
| Ziprasidone | 0 - + | Rare | 0 - + | 0 - ++ | 0 | + - ++ | 0 | 0 |

Sufficient data for paliperidone, iloperidone and asenapine are not yet available for inclusion in this table.

Adapted from the International Psychopharmacology Algorithm Project (IPAP) algorithm for the treatment of schizophrenia, available at www.ipap.org, copyright 2008 International Psychopharmacology Algorithm Project (IPAP)

associated with negative symptoms and cognitive impairment in schizophrenia,[22,35] the cortical release of these two neurotransmitters, and possibly also acetylcholine, may provide a pharmacological basis for the advantages of atypical antipsychotics over typical neuroleptic drugs in the treatment of these critical symptom domains. In patients with schizophrenia who were stabilized on typical neuroleptics, the addition of mianserin, a 5-HT$_{2A/C}$ and adrenergic $\alpha$-2 antagonist, was associated with improved neurocognitive performance,[36] adding further support to a role of 5-HT$_{2A}$ receptors in the treatment of cognitive dysfunction in schizophrenia.

The importance of serotonin receptors other than 5-HT$_{2A}$ for the action of antipsychotic drugs has received considerable attention. Activation of 5-HT$_{1A}$ receptors are believed to have a dopamine modulating effect similar to that of 5-HT$_{2A}$ antagonism.[37] Under experimental conditions, 5-HT$_{1A}$ agonists have been shown to stimulate cortical dopamine release[38,39] and, in schizophrenic patients who were stabilized on haloperidol, the addition of tandospirone, a 5-HT$_{1A}$ partial agonist, resulted in improved neurocognitive performance.[40] This effect has also been demonstrated more recently for buspirone, another 5-HT$_{1A}$ partial agonist.[41] Serotonin-1A receptors may be important for cognitive

effects of at least some of the atypical antipsychotic drugs that are active at this receptor site. Activity at 5-HT$_{1A}$ receptors is not shared by all antipsychotic drugs (Table 6.2.5.2), however. Antagonism of 5-HT$_{2C}$ receptors also appears to result in cortical dopamine and norepinephrine release, as well as in the nucleus accumbens.[42] The cognitive effects of selective 5-HT$_{2C}$ antagonists added to typical neuroleptic drugs in patients with schizophrenia have not been examined. As is the case with 5-HT$_{1A}$ activity, not all atypical antipsychotic drugs are active at 5-HT$_{2C}$ receptors (Table 6.2.5.2). Like antagonism at histamine H$_1$ receptors,[43] 5-HT$_{2C}$ antagonist activity may be related to antipsychotic induced weight gain.[44]

Atypical antipsychotics may display regional selectivity in terms of their dopaminergic activity, relative to typical neuroleptics. For instance, atypical antipsychotic drugs appear to preferentially block cortical D$_2$ receptors, relative to those located in the striatum.[45,46] Haloperidol results in proportionally equivalent D$_2$ blockade in both brain regions.[47] The atypical antipsychotics also increase the expression of the early intermediate gene c-fos, in the prefrontal cortex and the shell of the nucleus accumbens, while sparing the core of the latter region and the striatum. Typical neuroleptic drugs have the opposite effect on c-fos expression. Sparing the dorsal striatum is believed to be related to the low potential for extrapyramidal side-effects of these agents.[2,21]

Clozapine, olanzapine, risperidone, and quetiapine are able to block the interference in prepulse inhibition produced by d-amphetamine, apomorphine, or phencyclidine at doses that do not interfere with locomotor function. Clozapine and M100907 are able to block the effects of phencyclidine, an N-methyl-D-aspartate receptor antagonist, on locomotor activity in rodents. This suggests the ability of rat $5\text{-HT}_{2A}$-receptor blockade to block some of the effects of phencyclidine which is one of the more important models for schizophrenia.[2,21] In a recent single photon emission tomography (SPECT) study, patients with schizophrenia who received treatment with clozapine evidenced reduced NMDA-active radiotracer binding compared with healthy controls, drug free patients with schizophrenia, and patients with schizophrenia who were treated with typical neuroleptics.[48] The extent of involvement of other atypical antipsychotic drugs relative to typical antipsychotics at NMDA receptors and other glutamatergic targets is an area of active interest. Other receptor targets that are of special interest in terms of improving cognitive functioning and selected psychotic symptoms include M1 muscarinic, $\alpha$-7 nicotinic, and $\alpha$-1 and $\alpha$-2 adrenergic receptors.

# Administration, pharmacokinetics, and dosage

## Administration

### (a) Typical antipsychotic drugs

The major uses of the antipsychotic drugs are for the treatment of schizophrenia, mood disorders typically with psychotic features, and senile psychoses.[4,49] Other indications are discussed elsewhere in this book in the consideration of the management of specific disorders, such as Tourette's syndrome, and aggression. The major advantage of the typical neuroleptic drugs is their ability to improve positive symptoms, i.e. delusions and hallucinations. Administration of typical neuroleptic drugs leads to the complete or nearly complete elimination of positive symptoms and disorganization of thought and affect in about 60 to 70 per cent of patients with schizophrenia and an even higher proportion of those with psychotic mania and psychotic depression.[49] The antipsychotic response in schizophrenia and mania is sometimes apparent within a few days in many patients but usually takes up to several weeks or months. A reasonable duration for a therapeutic trial with one of these agents is 4 to 6 weeks. It is not appropriate to switch medications after 1 or 2 weeks, even if a response is not apparent, unless side-effects pose a serious problem. Positive symptoms (delusions and hallucinations) do not respond to typical neuroleptic drugs in about 10 per cent of schizophrenic patients even during the first episode.[50] Another 20 per cent of patients with schizophrenia develop resistance to these agents during the subsequent course of their illnesses.[51] Development of resistance to typical neuroleptic drugs may occur at any time during the course of treatment, even after many years of control of positive symptoms. Such patients are more likely to respond to clozapine[51] or one of the other atypical antipsychotics.[50,51]

The average doses of the typical neuroleptic drugs are given in Table 6.2.5.5. The best results with these drugs in terms of efficacy and side-effects may be expected with the lowest dose needed to produce control of positive symptoms with the fewest extrapyramidal side-effects.[4,49]

There are some patients for whom higher doses are indicated, but most controlled studies have failed to find benefits from high-dose strategies of combining two or more of these agents. Increasing the dose of these agents when patients fail to respond rapidly, for example within days, is not recommended. Augmentation with a benzodiazepine may be useful to decrease anxiety until the lower doses of neuroleptic drugs produce adequate control of positive symptoms.[4,49] Patients who may require higher doses of neuroleptic drugs to respond adequately are at greater risk of hyperprolactinaemic effects, EPS, and tardive dyskinesia and are generally better treated with an atypical antipsychotic drug.

However, the improvement in positive symptoms which is often achievable with the typical antipsychotic drug is only one element in the treatment of schizophrenia and is not sufficient grounds for judging response to be adequate. Additional efficacy factors of major importance are summarized in Table 6.2.5.6.

Tolerability and safety factors, such as compliance, tardive dyskinesia, weight gain, and medical morbidity are also major elements in outcome and are influenced by the choice of a typical or atypical antipsychotic drug. Typical neuroleptic drugs are not as effective for improving primary negative symptoms of schizophrenia in the majority of patients.[52,53] There is a consensus that typical neuroleptic drugs can improve negative symptoms that are secondary to positive symptoms and depression while at the same time possibly causing secondary negative symptoms due to their ability to produce extrapyramidal side-effects.[52] Abnormalities in specific domains of cognition (Table 6.2.5.6) are present in first-episode schizophrenic patients at a moderate to severe level and show slight to moderate, rarely severe, deterioration during the course of illness.[54,55] Approximately 85 per cent of patients with schizophrenia are clinically impaired in one or more domains of cognition.[55,56] Cognition has been shown to be perhaps the most critical determinant of functional capacity among patients with schizophrenia, even more so than positive symptoms.[57] Typical neuroleptic drugs usually do not improve cognitive function.[58] Those typical neuroleptic drugs such as thioridazine and mesoridazine, which have strong antimuscarinic properties, may produce further impairment in some memory functions.[58]

All of the typical neuroleptic drugs are likely to be equally effective in treating either the initial presentation or recurrent psychosis due to breakthrough of symptoms, despite compliance, or because of having stopped medication[4,49,51] First-episode patients with schizophrenia usually require much lower doses than patients with two or more episodes, suggesting some progression of the disease process or development of tolerance to the mechanism of action of these drugs.[59] Doses for more chronic patients should be in the range of 5 to 10 mg haloperidol equivalents per day (Table 6.2.5.5) for up to 4 to 6 weeks unless there is a major need for chemical means to prevent harm to self or others, to decrease excitement, or induce sleep.[60] Auxiliary medications for anxiety and sleeplessness, for example benzodiazepines, may supplement these low doses of antipsychotics.[61]

Parenteral injections of haloperidol, chlorpromazine, or other neuroleptics may be needed for patients who refuse oral medication or where very rapid onset of action is needed to control acutely dangerous behaviours if less restrictive means either fail or cannot be utilized safely. Commonly, haloperidol (2–10 mg) with or without lorazepam (2–4 mg) is delivered intramuscularly every 30

**Table 6.2.5.5** Oral dosing of antipsychotic drugs

**Typical antipsychotic drugs**

| | Equivalent doses (mg/day) | Starting dose | Titration schedule | Dose range (mg/day) |
|---|---|---|---|---|
| Chlorpromazine[a] | 100 | 15–50 mg BID-QID | As clinically indicated | 300–1000 (divided QD-QID) |
| Fluphenazine[b] | 2 | 0.5–10 mg/day (divided Q6–8 hours) | As clinically indicated | 5–20 |
| Haloperidol[c] | 2 | 0.5–5 mg BID | As clinically indicated | 5–20 |
| Loxapine | 10 | 10 mg BID | As clinically indicated | 30–100 |
| Mesoridazine | 50 | | | 150–400 |
| Molindone | 10 | 50–75 mg/day divided TID-QID | As clinically indicated | 30–100 |
| Perphenazine[d] | 10 | 4–8 mg TID (8–16 mg BID-QID if hospitalized) | As clinically indicated | 16–64 |
| Thioridazine | 100 | 50–100 mg TID | As clinically indicated | 300–800 |
| Tiotixene | 5 | 2 mg TID | As clinically indicated | 15–50 |
| Trifluoperazine | 5 | 2–5 mg BID | As clinically indicated | 15–50 |

For elderly patients, or those with renal or hepatic problems, doses of drug may need to be reduced by one-half or more

[a] Short-acting IM formulation may be given 25–50 mg (may repeat after 1–4 hrs as required); may gradually increase dose up to 400 mg IM Q 4-6 hrs (maximum of 2000 mg/day) may be needed for severe cases

[b] Short-acting IM formulation may be given 2.5–10 mg/day in Q6–8 hr intervals; Depot IM formulation may be given 12.5–25 mg Q 3 weeks

[c] Short-acting IM formulation may be given 2–5 mg Q 1–4 hrs; Depot IM formulation may be given at approximately 10–20 times the stable oral dose Q 4 weeks

[d] Short-acting IM formulation may be given 5–10 mg Q 6 hrs (maximum of 30 mg/day)

**Atypical antipsychotic drugs**

| | Starting dose | Titration schedule | Dose range (mg/day) |
|---|---|---|---|
| Aripiprazole[a] | 10–15 mg daily | As clinically indicated, every 2 weeks | 10–30 |
| Clozapine | 12.5 mg QD-BID | Increase by 25–50 mg/day until usual effective dose of 300–450 mg/day after 2–4 weeks | 150–600 |
| Olanzapine[b] | 5–10 mg daily | As clinically indicated, by 5 mg/day every 7 days | 10–30 |
| Paliperidone | 6 mg/day | As clinically indicated, by 3 mg/day Q 2–4 week increments, up to 12 mg daily | 6–12 |
| Quetiapine | 25 mg BID | Increase by 25–50 mg BID-TID on days 2 and 3, to target dose of 300–400 mg daily (QD – TID) by day 4. Further increases as clinically indicated by 25–50 mg BID every 2 days. | 300– 800 |
| Risperidone[c] | 0.5–1 mg BID | Increase by 0.5–1 mg BID on days 2 and 3, with further dose increases thereafter by 0.5–1 mg increments Q 7 days as required | 2–8 |
| Ziprasidone[d] | 20 mg BID with food | Increase by 20–40 mg BID every 2 days to target dose of 80 mg (all doses with food) | 120–200 |

For elderly patients, or those with renal or hepatic problems, doses of drug may need to be reduced by one-half or more, and titration may be slower

[a] Short-acting IM formulation may be given at 9.75 mg, though the lower 5.25 mg dose may be indicated in some situations.

[b] Short-acting IM formulation may be given 10 mg as required (may be repeated after 2 hrs, up to 30 mg/day).

[c] Long-acting IM formulation may be initiated at 25 mg Q 2 weeks (continue oral risperidone dose for 3 weeks), with increases as clinically indicated every 4 weeks up to a dose of 50 mg Q 2 weeks

[d] Short-acting IM formulation may be given 10–20 mg as required (may be repeated Q 2–4 hrs as needed, up to 40 mg/day)

to 60 minutes as required, up to three doses. Doses of haloperidol given intramuscularly in such situations generally should not exceed 18 mg per day. Oral medication should be substituted as soon as feasible. If positive symptoms fail to respond to a single trial of a typical neuroleptic drug at adequate doses in patients with schizophrenia, there is evidence that switching to another typical antipsychotic, even of a different chemical class, is unlikely to produce greater control.[4,49,51] This is likely to be true for other indications for the use of antipsychotic agents as well.

In cases of repeated illness relapse due to poor compliance or when patients prefer it, the use of long acting (e.g. depot) injectable antipsychotic medications, typically administered once every 2–4 weeks, may be used. The use of injectable antipsychotic medication has been associated with lower rates of relapse and rehospitalization and greater global improvement compared with oral typical neuroleptics,[62] possibly as a result of ensured drug delivery. Long acting injectable drugs should not be given to ameliorate acute behavioural disturbances.

### (b) Atypical antipsychotic drugs

As implied above, there are major advantages for many patients to be treated with the atypical antipsychotic drugs and it is generally

**Table 6.2.5.6** Target signs and symptoms for the pharmacological management of schizophrenia

| Target | Description | |
|---|---|---|
| Positive syndrome | Hallucinations<br>Delusions | ◆ Typically the most amenable to treatment with all antipsychotic drugs |
| Negative syndrome | Avolition<br>Apathy<br>Anhedonia<br>Lack of responsiveness<br>Poor rapport with others<br>Passive social withdrawal<br>Poverty of speech<br>Affective flattening | ◆ Robustly correlated with functional impairment in schizohrenia<br>◆ More difficult to treat pharmacologically, and may required longer to respond than positive signs and symptoms<br>◆ Pharmacological adjuncts may be needed, though under-studied<br>◆ Atypical antipsychotic drugs are believed to be more efficacious than typical neuroleptics |
| Hostility/excitement | Verbal or physical aggression | ◆ Typically amenable to treatment with all antipsychotic drugs<br>◆ Use of parenteral formulation may be required |
| Mood and anxiety symptoms | Depressed mood<br>Anxious mood<br>Nervousness<br>Panic symptoms<br>Suicidal ideation | ◆ Believed to be more responsive to treatment with atypical antipsychotic drugs<br>◆ Clozapine has demonstrated superiority for treating chronic suicidality in schizophrenia |
| Cognitive impairment (psychopathological definition) | Disorientation<br>Problems with abstraction<br>Attentional problems<br>Preoccupations<br>Disorganized thought processes | ◆ Some domains respond favourably to antipsychotic drug treatment, though response is often incomplete |
| Cognitive impairment (neuropsychological testing definition) | Working memory<br>Attention/vigilance<br>Verbal learning/memory<br>Visual learning/memory<br>Problem solving<br>Processing speed | ◆ Neuropsychological deficits, like negative signs and symptoms, are robustly correlated with functional outcome in schizophrenia<br>◆ Very difficult to treat with medication alone<br>◆ Atypical antipsychotic drugs are believed to be superior to typical neuroleptics, though effect sizes are only mild to moderate for the former |

recommended that, where possible, these agents be considered as the first-line treatment.[63,64] The atypical antipsychotic drugs are the dominant antipsychotic treatment for schizophrenia, mania, and psychotic depression in clinical practice in many parts of the world. However, there is considerable international variation in their usage. Cost factors may explain part of the variance in the use of these agents within and between countries. The typical neuroleptic drugs are no longer covered by patent protection and are available in inexpensive generic forms. There are a number of patients whose psychosis is adequately controlled by these agents and they (and their families and prescribers) are content to continue them even when informed of the potential advantages of the newer antipsychotic agents. When only the cost of medication is considered, it may seem that fiscal reasons argue for continuation of typical neuroleptic drug treatment since the atypical agents can cost up to 100 times more. In addition, the widely accepted notion of greater overall benefit from treatment with atypical antipsychotic drugs, as opposed to typical neuroleptics, was recently challenged by results from two effectiveness studies. The first of these demonstrated no significant difference in all-cause discontinuation from the study as the primary endpoint, as well as discontinuation for lack of efficacy, between atypical drugs, with the exception of olanzapine, and the typical neuroleptic perphenazine.[65] The latter study reported a lack of significant differences in quality of life between patients who received naturalistic treatment with typical or atypical antipsychotic drugs.[66] Methodological limitations, detailed discussion of

which is beyond the scope of this chapter, limit the conclusions that can be drawn from these reports about the relative merits of one class of antipsychotics versus another, both of which are in disagreement with the majority of the clinical literature that documents differences between these broad classes of antipsychotic drugs across a wide range of outcomes. Because medication costs account for, at most, 5 per cent of the total costs of schizophrenia, with the major costs being hospitalization and indirect costs such as lost income and disability income to support patients in the community, more effective and tolerable medications may offset their greater cost.[67,68] As such, atypical antipsychotic drugs are recommended as first line treatments of schizophrenia and related psychotic disorders. Each will be discussed separately.

### (i) Clozapine

Clozapine was synthesized in 1959 as part of a project to discover antipsychotic drugs with low potential for extrapyramidal side-effects. It proved to be one of the most interesting and clinically important compounds ever discovered. It was labelled as atypical because of its ability to block amphetamine-induced locomotor activity, one of the most widely accepted models for antipsychotic activity, without producing catalepsy in rodents, the leading model for causation of extrapyramidal side-effects in humans. Subsequent clinical studies showed it to have the lowest extrapyramidal side-effects of any antipsychotic drug known.[5,69] Clinical trials in the 1960s and 1970s suggested it was also superior in efficacy with regard to control of positive symptoms, but given the standards of clinical trials of that era, these conclusions could not be relied upon.[70] In 1975, 6 years after its introduction in Europe, clozapine's ability to cause granulocytopenia or agranulocytosis was first reported. Six deaths occurred in clozapine-treated patients in a geographically restricted area of Finland over a short period of time. The role of clozapine in these deaths is still uncertain because no other such clustering has ever occurred in Finland, or elsewhere. Nevertheless, clozapine was withdrawn from general use, although it remained available for humanitarian use in patients who had previously received it, for individual cases where it seemed indicated because of its low potential for extrapyramidal side-effects, and for research purposes.[69]

Clozapine was reintroduced in 1989 after it was demonstrated to be superior to chlorpromazine to improve positive and negative symptoms in 300 patients who were resistant to the action of at least three typical neuroleptics.[71] Thirty per cent of the patients treated with clozapine responded after 6 weeks of treatment compared to 4 per cent of the chlorpromazine-treated patients. Subsequent studies have shown that up to 60 to 70 per cent of patients will respond within 6 months of treatment. Patients with shorter duration of illness tend to respond better. Some predictors of response include weight gain and absence of atrophy in the prefrontal cortex.[52] Clozapine has been reported in several studies to reduce the risk of suicide.[52,72] It has been shown in a large number of studies to improve some aspects of cognitive function, especially verbal fluency, immediate and delayed verbal learning and memory, and attention.[16–18]

Because of the side-effect profile of clozapine, it is not generally used as a first-line drug. On the other hand, monitoring the white blood count for the development of agranulocytosis or granulocytopenia, as well as improved methods of treating agranulocytosis, have made it much safer to use. Clozapine is still probably underutilized in many parts of the world. Any patient with an unsatisfactory response to the typical neuroleptics and at least one atypical antipsychotic should be considered for clozapine treatment. This amounts to at least 20 per cent of schizophrenics. Clozapine use may also be considered for patients with schizophrenia who are at high risk for suicide, even if the aforementioned threshold of inadequate response to other drugs has not yet been met.

Clozapine is usually given twice daily, but sometimes more than half of the dose or the entire dose is given at sleep time to minimize daytime sedation. The daily dosage is gradually titrated to the target range described in Table 6.2.5.5. Patients who are treatment resistant may require higher doses. Typical or non-clozapine atypical antipsychotic drugs should be discontinued either before beginning clozapine or by eliminating them over a 1- to 2-week period as the dose of clozapine is increased. Because clozapine produces only about 40 to 50 per cent occupancy of striatal $D_2$-receptors,[73] and some of its key advantages are believed to be related to its low $D_2$-receptor blockade, concomitant administration of typical neuroleptic drugs would be predicted to interfere with some of the benefits of clozapine and, thus, should not ordinarily be prescribed with clozapine. However, some patients with persistent positive symptoms despite an adequate trial of clozapine monotherapy might be expected to benefit from the addition of low-dose haloperidol, or its equivalent, to provide additional low level $D_2$-receptor blockade.

Determination of clozapine plasma levels is useful whenever patients are not responding adequately. If response is inadequate, various approaches to augment response have also been utilized. In addition to adding a low dose of a typical neuroleptic, as mentioned above, it may be useful to augment clozapine treatment with valproic acid or other mood stabilizer (such as lithium, carbamazepine, lamotrigine or topiramate), anxiolytic drugs, or an antidepressant.[52] The choice of augmenting agent is largely driven by symptomatic considerations, or pharmacokinetic interactions in the case of fluvoxamine. However, none of these strategies have strong empiric support. One exception may be the addition of sulpiride, which may result in a significant reduction in symptom burden when added to clozapine.[74] Electroconvulsive therapy (ECT) also resulted in a modest further reduction in symptoms when used in conjunction with clozapine, and appears to be well tolerated.[75] It is difficult to postulate a rationale for adding another atypical antipsychotic, with the exception of amisulpride, because of their similarity in pharmacology to clozapine. It should be discontinued if side-effects are intolerable, or if there is no apparent response after a 6-month trial of clozapine alone and subsequent trials with augmentation therapy. Clearly, further studies involving clozapine partial- or non-responders are urgently needed. It should be noted that discontinuation of clozapine can precipitate a severe relapse even when clozapine is slowly tapered.[76]

### (ii) Risperidone

Risperidone is useful as a first-line drug for the treatment of all forms of schizophrenia, including residual schizophrenia.[77–79] Definitive data are lacking for its efficacy in patients who are neuroleptic resistant or who have failed to respond to other atypical antipsychotics, including clozapine.[80] Clinical experience is not supportive of widespread efficacy in these groups but there may be some responders. However, risperidone may be useful in patients who fail to tolerate other antipsychotic agents because of side-effects not shared by risperidone, such as anticholinergic effects. Risperidone is well-tolerated in low doses by the elderly and has been widely used in the United States for the treatment of a variety of senile psychoses.[81,82] Its efficacy against haloperidol was established in a series of multicentre trials which demonstrated advantages for risperidone in overall psychopathology in mainly chronic schizophrenic patients in an acute exacerbation at doses in the 6 to 8 mg/day range.[11,77] However, these doses have proven to be higher than is needed for most patients in clinical practice, possibly reflecting some of the problems in generalizing from controlled clinical trials. The doses for schizophrenia most often used in non-elderly adults are now 4 to 6 mg/day. First-episode patients may not tolerate higher doses (e.g. above 5 mg per day), and some may respond to as little as 1 to 2 mg/day. Some treatment-resistant patients may need doses higher than 6 mg/day; however, the results of clinical studies in this population have been mixed. Whether prolonged trials, i.e. up to 6 months, are useful in such patients, as they are in clozapine patients, is not yet known.

Beyond treatment of acute symptoms, the position occupied by risperidone as a first line treatment option is also supported by long term maintenance phase and relapse prevention studies. For instance, relative to haloperidol, risperidone has also been associated with a lower risk of relapse (34 vs. 60 per cent) over a minimum of 12 months of treatment.[83] In another study that retrospectively compared rates of rehospitalization for patients who received treatment with risperidone, olanzapine, or typical neuroleptics, rehospitalization rates for risperidone and olanzapine were similar, and both were significantly less than those of patients treated with typical neuroleptics.[84]

Risperidone is usually initiated at low doses (e.g. 1–2 mg daily) and is titrated into the dosage range provided in Table 6.2.5.5. The medication is often initiated in twice daily dosing; however, because its primary active metabolite, 9-OH risperidone, is pharmacologically equivalent to its parent drug and because it has a longer elimination half-life, once daily dosing is also possible. Risperidone is available in soluble wafer and liquid forms, which may be advantageous for patients who have swallowing difficulties or require taking their medication in a non-pill form for other reasons, including their own preference.

For patients who have a history of poor compliance leading to frequently relapsing illness, or for those who prefer it, a long acting injectable form of risperidone is available (Table 6.2.5.1) for administration typically every two weeks. For treatment responsive patients, response may be expected to occur in the 25–50 mg (per every two week dose) range,[85] however, oral risperidone must be continued through at least the first 3 weeks of treatment with the long acting injectable form before being slowly tapered. Supplementation with oral medication may be required when the dose of the long-acting drug is upwardly adjusted due to breakthrough psychotic symptoms. As is the case with long-acting injectable typical antipsychotics, long-acting injectable risperidone should not be used acutely to control dangerous behaviours.

Risperidone has more of a tendency to produce extrapyramidal side-effects than any of the other atypical antipsychotics but this can be minimized by using the lowest dose which controls positive symptoms and adding an anticholinergic drug, if necessary.[82] Addition of a typical neuroleptic to risperidone will increase the risk of extrapyramidal side-effects. Risperidone is not well tolerated by patients with Parkinson's disease because of extrapyramidal side-effects. There are some data suggesting the risk of tardive dyskinesia in patients with schizophrenia, and especially the elderly, with risperidone is less than that of the typical neuroleptic drugs.[86]

Among atypical antipsychotic drugs, risperidone and paliperidone appear to be the most liable in terms of increasing prolactin release. As is the case with EPS, the effect of risperidone on prolactin concentration appears to positively correlate with dose.[25] The changes may occur in both men and women; however, the greatest elevations appear to occur among women. Elevations in prolactin levels as a result of treatment with risperidone do not always translate into clinical symptoms such as sexual dysfunction or gynaecomastia in men and menstrual changes and breast discharge in women; however, patients should be monitored clinically for these effects, and prolactin concentrations measured if these symptoms occur.

The issue of whether the improvement in negative symptoms by risperidone and other atypical antipsychotic drugs is due to an effect on so-called primary negative symptoms versus secondary negative symptoms has been much debated. Data from large multicentre trials of risperidone versus clozapine show an effect on primary negative symptoms as residual change left after adjusting for improvement due to decreases in positive or depressive symptoms and extrapyramidal side-effects.[87] In addition, results from a meta-analysis of 6 studies comparing risperidone to typical neuroleptic treatment indicated greater response rate for negative symptoms (defined as achieving >20 per cent reduction in negative symptom burden) as well as greater reduction in anxious/depressive symptoms among risperidone treated patients.[88] Risperidone has a greater ability to improve cognition in schizophrenia than the typical neuroleptic drugs.[17] Improvement in working memory has been the strongest finding, while improvements in attention, executive function, and verbal learning and memory have also been reported. Risperidone has been shown to be a cost-effective treatment for schizophrenia,[89] especially in its long-acting injectable form,[90] and to improve quality of life,[91] firm conclusions about relative cost-effectiveness between atypical antipsychotic drugs for non-treatment-resistant schizophrenia are difficult to draw at this time. Further research in this important area is needed.

In summary, risperidone is a first line pharmacological treatment of schizophrenia and other forms of psychosis. It may produce significant advantages over typical neuroleptic drugs with regard to negative symptoms, cognition, and extrapyramidal side-effects, but it does produce dose dependent increases in EPS risk, and increases in serum prolactin levels resembling those of typical antipsychotic drugs. It should be used at the lower doses where possible. A long-acting injectable form of this medication should be considered a first line treatment option in cases of frequent relapse due to poor medication compliance.

### (iii) Olanzapine

Olanzapine is indicated as a first-line treatment for all forms of schizophrenia[63,92] with the caveat that it has not been shown to be as effective as clozapine in neuroleptic-resistant patients at conventional doses.[8,60] However, some patients of this type do respond to olanzapine,[93] perhaps at high doses.[94,95] There are no means yet to determine which of this group of patients will respond to olanzapine (or risperidone) so some clinicians may elect a trial with either of these agents before considering clozapine.

The efficacy of olanzapine in treating psychosis and negative symptoms in patients with an acute exacerbation of schizophrenia has been firmly established in a variety of large-scale, multicentre trials.[92] In these trials, olanzapine at doses of 10 to 20 mg/day has been superior to placebo and equivalent or superior to haloperidol in some measures of total psychopathology, positive, or negative symptoms. For example, in the North American multicentre trial, high-dose olanzapine (15 ± 5 mg/day) was superior to haloperidol (15 ± 5 mg/day) in the treatment of negative symptoms.[96] The effect of olanzapine to improve negative symptoms was found to be on primary rather than secondary negative symptoms.[97]

Olanzapine has also been found to be effective as a maintenance treatment of schizophrenia.[98] The estimated relapse rates, defined as the need for hospitalization, during a 1-year period in three studies of patients receiving olanzapine for maintenance treatment were 19.6 to 28.6 per cent. These rates were significantly lower than those in patients receiving placebo, ineffective doses of olanzapine, or haloperidol.[98] Olanzapine has some efficacy in treating anxious and depressive symptoms,[99] as well as cognitive dysfunction,[17,18] associated with schizophrenia or schizoaffective disorder. Pharmacoeconomic studies and investigations of medication effects on quality of life measures indicate that olanzapine has a beneficial cost-outcome profile. For instance, in one investigation, the higher cost of olanzapine relative to haloperidol was offset by olanzapine-treatment associated reductions in rehospitalization and overall treatment costs.[100] Olanzapine treatment has also been associated with better outcomes as assessed by overall and health-related quality of life relative to haloperidol.[101] As mentioned above, olanzapine was found to be the most effective antipsychotic drug in the recent Clinical Antipsychotic Trials of Intervention Effectiveness (CATIE) phase I study.[65]

The average clinical dose of olanzapine is 12.5 to 20 mg/day but many patients may be expected to respond to lower doses (e.g. 10 mg daily).[102] A principle advantage of olanzapine is its once daily dosing and the feasibility of starting the medication at a dose that is clinically effective for most patients. Doses higher than 20 mg/day are rarely more effective than lower doses, especially for non-refractory cases. Augmentation of olanzapine with typical neuroleptic drugs or risperidone should be done sparingly to avoid extrapyramidal side-effects and possibly compromising efficacy. Olanzapine is also available in a soluble wafer form that may be preferred to the pill form by some patients, especially those with swallowing difficulties and related problems.

For acute situations where rapid control of agitation, hostility or other dangerous behaviours is required, olanzapine is available as a short-acting injectable medication (Table 6.2.5.1).[103] Similar to short-acting typical neuroleptic drugs, the medication is delivered intramuscularly. Doses of 5 to 10 mg per injection may be given, depending on the severity of the target behaviours. A long-acting formulation is in clinical testing.

In summary, olanzapine has found wide acceptance as an atypical antipsychotic drug because of its once-a-day administration, efficacy for negative symptoms, improvement in cognitive function, and low extrapyramidal side-effect profile. Significant weight gain and other metabolic effects may be a problem for some patients, as will be discussed below.

### (iv) Quetiapine

Quetiapine has been shown to be as effective as typical antipsychotics, with fewer extrapyramidal side-effects and no effect on serum prolactin levels.[104,105] Part of the reason for this may be that quetiapine and clozapine both appear to bind more loosely to striatal D2 receptors than other antipsychotic drugs, and that both drugs show antipsychotic activity at D2 receptor occupancies that are well below the 60 per cent threshold identified for most other antipsychotic drugs.[106] In spite of this similarity with clozapine, quetiapine does not appear to have efficacy comparable to clozapine for treatment-resistant patients.

The efficacy of quetiapine for acute phase schizophrenia is supported by results from several randomized, controlled trials that documented superiority of quetiapine relative to placebo across several doses, with some patients with some patients responding to 150 mg/day and others requiring 750 mg/day.[104] For instance, in one high- (750 mg/day) versus low-dosage (250 mg/day) study, both dosage groups evidenced greater reduction in positive symptoms relative to placebo; however, the differences were significant only for the high-dose group.[105] In another study that assessed multiple fixed doses of quetiapine (75 to 750 mg/day) compared with haloperidol and placebo, significant differences in improvement over placebo for quetiapine were observed in the dosage range of 150 to 750 mg/day.[104]

Quetiapine's effect on negative symptoms continue to be investigated. One placebo controlled comparison documented improvements in negative symptoms with quetiapine treatment across a wide range of doses, with the greatest improvement reported at 300 mg daily.[104] In the high- vs. low- dose study reviewed above, the high-dose group also experienced greater improvement in negative symptoms relative to placebo.[105] Like risperidone and olanzapine, quetiapine appears to improve depressive symptoms[107] and certain cognitive deficits[17,18] associated with schizophrenia or schizoaffective disorder. The improvements in cognition with quetiapine appear to be superior to those of haloperidol.[108]

These results suggest that, overall, the greatest improvement in positive and negative symptoms may occur when quetiapine is used at the higher end of its dosage range. The average clinical dose appears to be between 300 and 500 mg/day, usually given twice daily though some benefit from the medication when given only once daily. The effects of using higher doses for patients who do not respond adequately to these doses are uncertain. A titration of the dosage is required after initiating the medication. From the viewpoint of EPS and hyperprolactinaemic effects, quetiapine appears to confer only low risk. As such, it, like clozapine, appears to be well tolerated even among patients with idiopathic Parkinson's disease.[109] Sedation may be a limiting side effect for some, especially during dosage titration. Weight related, metabolic, and other adverse effects will be discussed in greater detail below.

In summary, quetiapine also appears to be effective for a wide range of schizophrenia-associated symptoms and confers a lower level of risk in terms of antidopaminergic adverse effects. The dosage range of this medication may be quite wide, though patients may have a greater chance of benefiting from the medication at the higher end of this range.

### (v) Ziprasidone

Ziprasidone has a varied receptor occupancy profile. Like most atypical antipsychotic drugs, it displays high affinity 5-HT2A binding coupled with relatively lower affinity D2 receptor binding. Ziprasidone is also a 5-HT1A agonist, as well as both a serotonin and norepinephrine reuptake pump inhibitor.[110] This profile predicts a wide range of pharmacological activity against core psychotic symptoms, negative and affective symptoms, as well as neurocognition.

Ziprasidone, like quetiapine, has been shown to be superior to placebo for the reduction of total psychopathology and positive and negative symptoms.[111,112] There is limited evidence to suggest superiority over typical neuroleptics with regard to improvement in positive and negative symptoms.[111,113] Studies of multiple fixed doses of ziprasidone vs. haloperidol at conventional doses indicate that ziprasidone yields similar efficacy to haloperidol for reducing positive symptoms and global psychopathology at a dose of 160 mg/day.[113] Doses greater than 160 mg/day have not been systematically investigated.

Ziprasidone significantly improved negative symptoms and reduced the risk of relapse compared to placebo in a 1-year maintenance study in stable hospitalized chronic schizophrenic patients.[114] These maintenance phase effects were not dependent on the daily dose of ziprasidone. In a 28-week comparison with haloperidol, the two groups evidenced similar overall effects for positive symptoms; however, between groups differences were documented favouring ziprasidone for negative symptoms and EPS.[115] Ziprasidone was effective against depressive symptoms associated with schizophrenia in one study at a dose of 160 mg/day.[116] Significant improvements in multiple cognitive domains have been reported among ziprasidone treated patients in a variety of treatment contexts.[117] Such changes appear to be unrelated to improvements in other symptoms of schizophrenia. Ziprasidone treatment has been associated with significant improvement in quality of life measures in one post hoc data analysis.[118] Further investigation of the effect of ziprasidone on health related quality of life and similar outcomes are warranted. Ziprasidone treatment of schizophrenia appears to be cost-effective relative to no treatment.[119] Further cost-benefit studies are needed.

The dose range of ziprasidone for acute treatment appears to be between 80 and 160 mg/day, higher doses within this range may be more effective (Table 6.2.5.5). Doses greater than 120 mg/day appear to be required to achieve >60 per cent dopamine D2 receptor blockade,[120] the D2 receptor occupancy threshold that appears to coincide with efficacy against positive symptoms, as presented earlier. The medication is usually given twice daily, although some may take the medication once daily at night time. A titration of the total daily dose into the recommended range is required after initiating the medication. One critical aspect of medication administration for ziprasidone is the requirement that the medication be taken with food. There appear to be profound differences in bioavailability at equivalent doses between the fed and unfed state.[121] A full meal, as opposed to a light snack, appears to be required. Therefore, patients are encouraged to take their medication with meals.

A short-acting intramuscular formulation of ziprasidone has been developed which should be useful in situations where more rapid action is needed. This formulation is available in two doses (10 and 20 mg), the preferred dosage being 20 mg due to significantly greater reduction in agitation relative to lower dose.[122] The use of the short-acting injectable form can facilitate a transition to oral medication, and may reduce that time required to titrate the daily dose of ziprasidone to one that is likely to be effective.

Ziprasidone appears to be well tolerated. Treatment-emergent EPS burden is low.[112,113] Initial problems with somnolence or behavioural activation are usually self limited, although temporary use of clonazepam or other benzodiazepine at low doses may improve tolerability, especially during the titration phase, should the latter occur. Importantly, data from both short- and long-term studies indicated that ziprasidone is not associated with clinically significant changes in weight, glycaemic measures, or markers of lipid homeostasis.[123]

Ziprasidone can result in partial blockade of the slow potassium rectifier current in the cardiac conduction system, which may result in prolongation of the QTc interval (discussed in greater detail below).[124] On the other hand, there is only one case report of ziprasidone induced *torsades de pointes*, the risk of which is believed to be increased if the QTc interval is >500 msec.[125] There have also been no reported deaths in the context of overdose with the medication. Under routine circumstances, screening electrocardiograms are not required. Nevertheless, caution may be warranted for individuals who are at risk for significant prolongation of the QTc, including patients who take medications other than ziprasidone that prolong the QTc. Concomitant use of CYP-450 3A4 inhibitors does not appear to pose a significant risk.[126]

In summary, ziprasidone appears to be a useful additional atypical antipsychotic agent because of its favourable side-effect profile, including no weight gain—a major problem with olanzapine and clozapine-and no prolactin elevation, which is a less serious side-effect of risperidone. Patients should be instructed to take the medication with food. Ziprasidone treatment may result in an increase in the QTc interval; however, in a great majority of cases, this is not clinically significant.

### (vi) Aripiprazole

Among the atypical antipsychotics, aripiprazole is pharmacologically unique in that it combines partial D2 receptor agonism with high potency 5-HT2A antagonism. Because it is a partial D2 receptor agonist, it binds to the receptor with full affinity, but exerts only a fraction of the intrinsic activity at that site that would be expected of endogenous dopamine. As such, in states of relative dopamine excess, as is believed to be the case in the ventral striatum among schizophrenic patients who experience positive symptoms, aripiprazole is believed to exert relative antagonist activity at D2 receptors.[127] Conversely, it is believed to act primarily as an agonist in cases of relative hypo-dopaminergia, as may be the case in the prefrontal cortex in patients with schizophrenia.[22] For this reason, aripiprazole and other D2 partial agonists in development are sometimes referred to as 'dopamine stabilizers.' Aripiprazole also functions as a potent 5-HT1A partial agonist.[128]

The efficacy of aripiprazole in the treatment of acute schizophrenia at doses ranging between 10 and 30 mg (taken once daily) was established on the basis of four short-term randomized controlled studies.[129] Relative to placebo, efficacy against negative symptoms was also demonstrated.[130] Long term superiority of aripiprazole (vs. placebo) for relapse over 26 weeks[131] and medication compliance and symptom response (vs. haloperidol) for up to 52 weeks has also been established.[133] One study reported on the effectiveness of flexibly dosed aripiprazole (15–30 mg daily) among patients with schizophrenia with a history of resistance to treatment with olanzapine or risperidone.[133] The utility of aripiprazole in the setting of well defined treatment refractory schizophrenia requires further systematic investigation.

The overall effectivenss of aripiprazole has been evaluated in two recent studies. One study reported the effectivenss of flexibly dosed aripiprazole over 8 weeks of treatment (53 per cent response rate at mean endpoint dose = 19.9 mg/day) among a cohort of patients with chronic schizophrenia and schizoaffective disorder under routine treatment conditions in a community healthcare setting.[134] The second study documented comparable effectiveness with olanzapine over 52 weeks of treatment, with more favourable effects for aripiprazole for several metabolic adverse effects.[135] As is the case with other atypical antipsychotic drugs, early evidence indicates that aripiprazole may also have beneficial effects on neurocognitive performance in patients with schizophrenia at recommended doses.[136] Further study of the effects of this medication on cognition is indicated. Clinically relevant improvement in quality of life has been documented in one study.[137] More cost-outcome studies of aripiprazole are needed.

Treatment with aripiprazole is usually initiated with 10 to 15 mg daily, although some patients may not be able to tolerate these doses due to agitation, nausea or vomiting. The dose can be increased up to 30 mg if needed, and tolerated. An oral solution form is also available. Aripiprazole is also available in a soluble wafer as well as an acute intramuscular form. The acute injectable form appears to be effective in the dosage range of 5.25 to 15 mg.[138] The recommended dose is 9.75 mg.

Aripiprazole is generally well tolerated, with an adverse effect profile similar to placebo in short-term studies involving patients with acute schizophrenia and in longer-term studies of chronic, stable patients.[129] As is the case with all atypical antipsychotic drugs, the EPS burden is lower than that of typical neuroleptics. Some patients, however, may encounter this effect if the dose is started too high or if the titration is too aggressive. Aripiprazole treatment does not appear to significantly increase, and may cause a slight decrease, in prolactin levels.[25] Importantly, short- and longer-term studies indicated that, similar to ziprasidone, aripiprazole is not associated with a high risk of significant changes in weight, glycaemic measures, or markers of lipid metabolism.[123]

In summary, aripiprazole appears to be effective as an acute and long-term maintenance treatment for schizophrenia and related psychotic disorders at recommended doses, though some patients may require higher doses. Aripiprazole was initiated in most studies at doses of 10 to 15 mg once daily; however, some patients may require a slower titration following a lower starting dose. This medication is available in many dosing forms, all of which appear to be very well tolerated. Important benefits from a tolerability viewpoint include very low rates of prolactin elevation, and low risk of weight gain and metabolic adverse effects.

### (vii) Paliperidone

Paliperidone is the most recent antipsychotic drug to gain approval for use in the US. It is the 9-OH metabolite of risperidone, which has a longer elimination half-life than the parent compound, as reviewed above. Additionally, paliperidone, which is pharmacologically similar with regard to receptor occupancy profile to risperidone, is available commercially in an extended release form.

The short-term efficacy of paliperidone has been established on the basis of three randomized, placebo controlled studies, two of which have been published,[139,140] that investigated the clinical efficacy of 5 fixed doses (3, 6, 9, 12, and 15 mg) given once daily relative to placebo. In each of these studies, all doses of paliperidone were superior to placebo for reducing global psychopathology and positive symptoms, as well as negative symptoms, anxious/depressive symptoms associated with schizophrenia, and hostility/excitement. In addition, all doses of paliperidone were superior to placebo for improving measures of functional capacity. Paliperidone has not been investigated in the context of treatment refractory schizophrenia. Paliperidone appears to be effective for the prevention of relapse on the basis of one published study.[141]

The recommended starting dose of paliperidone in its extended release form is 6 mg, given once daily. Even though there is a suggestion of greater improvement in terms of symptom reduction from the paliperidone registration studies at higher doses, the adverse effect burden may also be greater (discussed below). Doses may be upwardly adjusted at 3 mg/day increments, up to 12 mg daily. Investigatons of doses greater than 6 mg daily for patients who do not respond adequately have not been performed. A long acting injectable form of paliperidone is currently in development.

Pooled analysis of data from the three short-term, acute phase studies indicate that paliperidone appears to be well tolerated, and that the recommended starting dose (6 mg once daily) was associated with a placebo-like overall adverse effect profile.[142] At doses higher than 6 mg, there appeared to be an increase in the reported incidence of EPS, though not to the degree at any of the doses tested that would be expected with typical neuroleptic treatment. Elevations in prolactin levels appear to be consistent with those observed with risperidone treatment, and appear to be greater in magnitude at higher doses. This effect appears to be especially pronounced among female patients. There were no significant changes from baseline in weight or measures of lipid or glucose handling. Data from long term investigations will provide a more comprehensive picture of paliperidone's tolerability profile.

In summary, paliperidone, the newest atypical antipsychotic drug, appears to be safe and effective for both short- and long-term treatment of schizophrenia. The EPS and prolactinemic adverse effect burden may resemble that of risperidone, but this notion requires prospective investigation. Paliperidone in its extended release form can be started at a clinically effective dose. A long-acting injectable form is currently in development.

### (viii) Amisulpride

The efficacy of amisulpride for the treatment of positive symptoms has been established over a wide dosage range (200 to 1200 mg daily) in treatment studies of up to 12 months duration.[143] In general, it appears that higher doses (above 400 mg/day) are effective for treating patients with predominately positive symptoms, although efficacy against negative symptoms has also been demonstrated in this dosing range.[144,145] Low-dose amisulpride ($\leq$ 300 mg/day) has been shown to be effective in treating negative symptoms in schizophrenics with predominantly negative symptoms.[146–148] Evaluation of the effect of amisulpride in patients with minimal extrapyramidal side-effects and positive symptoms suggests amisulpride is able to improve primary negative symptoms, even in patients with deficit syndrome schizophrenia.[146–148] At both dose ranges, amisulpride produces minimal extrapyramidal side-effects, but may result in increased prolactin levels. Amisulpride has been directly compared with haloperidol, and with both risperidone and olanzapine. In general, amisulpride appears to be as clinically effective as all three drugs for treating positive symptoms. Improvement in negative symptoms is superior to haloperidol and appear equivalent to olanzapine and risperidone. Improvement in depressive symptoms related to schizophrenia were also equivalent between amisulpride and olanzapine; however, in a meta-analysis of three studies, amisulpride was shown to be superior to high dose risperidone (8 mg daily) and haloperidol.[149] It is unknown if it is effective in neuroleptic-resistant patients. Because its pharmacology is quite distinct from that of the 5-HT$_{2A}$-based receptor antagonists previously discussed, amisulpride may be useful in patients who fail to tolerate that class of drugs. Amisulpride has also been demonstrated as being superior to haloperidol on quality of life measures and global functioning.[150] Pharmacoeconomic analyses indicate that amisulpride has a beneficial cost-outcome profile.[151]

## (c) Iloperidone and asenapine

Clinical trials are currently taking place with both of these atypical agent to determine its efficacy and side-effect profile compared with typical and other atypical antipsychotic drugs. Like most other atypical antipsychotic drugs, both asenapine and iloperidone combine potent 5-HT2A antagonism with less potent D2 receptor antagonism. Asenapine is currently undergoing investigation in phase 3 clinical trials. Short-term, acute phase efficacy of iloperidone for symptom reduction relative to placebo has been demonstrated at daily doses of 20 to 24 mg daily, with less certain effects at lower doses.[152] Long-term investigations thus far indicate a low incidence of EPS, lack of effect on prolactin release, and minimal effect on body weight.[152] It has the potential to be made into a long-acting form, which would be of great value.

## Pharmacokinetics, metabolism, and drug interactions

### (a) Typical neuroleptics

The typical neuroleptics are well absorbed when administered orally or parenterally. Intramuscular injection leads to more rapid and higher plasma levels. Peak plasma levels are reached in 30 min after intramuscular injection and 1 to 4 h after oral injection. Steady state is achieved in 3 to 5 days. The half-life for elimination is in the range of 10 to 30 h. Substantial amounts of the antipsychotics are stored in lipids, including in the brain. There is controversy about how long these drugs persist in the system after discontinuation. By the criterion of elevations of plasma prolactin levels, the concentrations are too low to be biologically active within 48 h after discontinuing oral medication. On the other hand, some rodent and human positron emission tomography studies suggest that long-acting forms of haloperidol or fluphenazine may persist for 1 to 3 months. Metabolism of the typical and atypical antipsychotic drugs occurs in the liver for the most part, via conjugation with glucuronic acid, hydroxylation, oxidation, demethylation and sulphoxide formation. Much of this metabolism occurs via the hepatic cytochrome (CYP)-450 enzymes, particularly the 2D6 and 3A4 sub-families for most drugs. Some metabolites have significant biological activity, for example mesoridazine, and 7-hydroxyloxapine. Dosing of typical neuroleptic medications are determined by clinical effects, less by pharmacokinetic factors.

Pharmacokinetic drug-drug interactions at the level of protein binding are expected to be minimal, even though most typical neuroleptics are tightly bound to plasma proteins. Even so, appropriate therapeutic monitoring of drugs that are also tightly bound to plasma proteins but have a narrow therapeutic index (e.g. warfarin, digoxin, phenytoin) when used in conjunction with typical neuroleptics is warranted. Interactions at the level of the CYP-450 system are also thought to be minimal for most agents. Because smoking is so common among patients with schizophrenia and because smoking can be associated with potent induction of CYP-450 1A2 isoenzymatic activity, dosage adjustments may be needed for selected antipsychotic drugs during any changes in smoking status. Other combinations with typical neuroleptics may be worth avoiding for other reasons, such as increased central nervous system affects (e.g. anxiolytics, other central nervous system depressants, anticholinergics, certain antihypertensive drugs), increased EPS (e.g. metoclopramide, D2 blocking anti-nausea drugs, caffeine), impaired cardiac conduction (certain drugs combined with typical neuroleptics known to prolong the QTc interval), and neurotoxicity (lithium), especially among individuals who are more advanced in age.

### (b) Atypical antipsychotic drugs

#### (i) Clozapine

There are wide variations in the pharmacokinetics of clozapine in patients. The average half-life is 6 to 12 h. Plasma concentrations are higher in Chinese patients than in Caucasian patients, in non-smokers than smokers, and in females than males. The bioavailability is not affected by food intake, metabolism occurs mainly in the liver. The chief metabolite is N-desmethylclozapine, which has some biological activity. Clozapine is metabolized by CYP1A2, and several potential drug-drug interactions are thus possible. When agents that induce CYP-1A2 are prescribed or ingested, close monitoring of patients for a worsening of symptoms is warranted. Plasma levels of clozapine of approximately 350 ng/ml are more often associated with good response than lower levels,[153] and should be checked in such cases. Upward adjustment of the clozapine daily dosage will typically correct the problem. On the other hand, if a CYP1A2 inducer is discontinued or a potent inhibitor is added, this may result in a rise in clozapine concentration, and an increase in adverse effect risk.[154] Caution may also be warranted for drugs that are potent inhibitors of CYP 2C19 and CYP3A4.[155] In addition, caution is warranted when considering concomitant use of drugs which can also cause bone marrow suppression (e.g. carbamazepine) or precipitously drop seizure threshold.

#### (ii) Risperidone

Risperidone is well absorbed from the gut and is extensively metabolized in the liver by CYP2D6 to 9-hydroxyrisperidone in approximately 92 to 94 per cent of Caucasians.[156] Thus, 9-0H risperidone is an active species in the majority of patients. About 6 to 8 per cent of Caucasians and a small proportion of Asians have a polymorphism of the CYP2D6 gene, which leads to poor metabolism of risperidone. For poor metabolizers of risperidone, the active moiety is mainly the parent compound. The half-life of the 9-hydroxy metabolite is about 21 h whereas the half-life of risperidone is about 3 h. Thus, risperidone can be used on a once-a-day schedule for normal metabolizers whereas multiple doses are needed for those who are poor metabolizers. Risperidone should be titrated from 2 to 5 mg/day over at least a 3-day period to minimize hypotensive and neuro muscular side-effects. Drugs known to induce or inhibit CYP2D6 and 3A4 may alter plasma levels of risperidone; thus, close monitoring is advised when such agents are added to ongoing risperidone treatment.

#### (iii) Olanzapine

Olanzapine has a half-life of 24 to 30 h, which indicates that single daily administration is adequate.[92] The metabolic pathways of olanzapine involves CYP2D6, CYP1A2 and flavin-containing mono-oxygenases, as well as N-glucuronidation. It has a low potential for drug-drug interactions and requires extremely high concentrations not likely to be achieved under clinical conditions to inhibit cytochrome P-450 systems. Plasma levels of approximately 9.3 mg/ml have been reported to predict better clinical response to olanzapine in inpatients with an acute exacerbation.[157] Drugs that are known inducers or inhibitors of CYP1A2 may significantly affect plasma levels of olanzapine and alter its clinical effects at a given dosage; thus, active monitoring of symptoms and adverse effects is indicated if such agents are added. As is the case with clozapine, gender and smoking status may influence olanzapine levels leading to adjustment in dosage.[153]

#### (iv) Quetiapine

Quetiapine is well absorbed and is approximately 83 per cent protein bound.[158] Quetiapine is absorbed better after eating.[158] It has a half-life of 6 h. It is metabolized in the liver by CYP3A4 to inactive metabolites. Quetiapine has significant interactions with several inducers and inhibitors of CYP3A4. Co-administration with these agents may require dosage adjustment. Thioridazine may also significantly increase the clearance of quetiapine,[159] thus necessitating dosage adjustment. Despite the short half-life, a clinical trial compared three dosing regimens (450 mg/day given in two or three divided doses, and 50 mg/day given twice daily). Both of the higher-dose groups were superior to the low-dose group and there were no differences between the two high-dose schedules. Once daily dosing, which is also a common dosing strategy for quetiapine, is also supported in the literature.[160] The feasibility of such a dosing schedule, which does not seem to be predicted by peripheral pharmacokinetic parameters, is possible because quetiapine appears to interact centrally with both D2 and 5-HT2A receptors much longer than its 6 h elimination half-life.[161]

#### (v) Ziprasidone

Ziprasidone has a half-life of 4 to 10 h. Twice-daily administration is possible despite this relatively short half-life. Clinically, many patients are prescribed this medication only once daily. Regardless, ziprasidone should always be taken after eating in order to facilitate absorption. About two-thirds of ziprasidone is metabolized by aldehyde oxidase into inactive metabolites. The remainder is metabolized by CYP3A4 and CYP1A2 into inactive metabolites. At the current time, there are no known drug interactions with ziprasidone at the level of aldehyde oxidase, since enzymatic activity does not appear to be altered by coadministered drugs. Although CYP3A4 appears to play only a minor role in the metabolism of ziprasidone, potent inhibitors or inducers of CYP3A4 may significantly alter plasma concentrations of ziprasidone,[162] and may thus necessitate an adjustment in dosage. The use of concomitant medications that may prolong the QTc interval should be avoided. Ziprasidone is contraindicated for patients with a history of known QT prolongation, recent acute myocardial infarction, or uncompromised heart failure.

#### (vi) Aripiprazole

Aripiprazole is well absorbed from the gut, and has an elimination half-life of 75 hours. It is metabolized primarily by CYP3A4 and 2D6 isoenzymes into an active metabolite, dehydro-aripiprazole, which has a half-life of 94 hours. This pharmacokinetic pattern supports once daily dosing. Because aripiprazole is metabolized by CYP3A4 and 2D6, known inhibitors or inducers of these isoenzymes may result in increased or decreased clearance of aripiprazole and dehydro-aripiprazole.[163]

#### (vi) Paliperidone, Iloperidone, and Amisulpride

Paliperidone is currently marketed in the US and abroad only in an osmotically controlled extended release formulation, which results in steady release of active drug over a 24 hr period. Hepatic metabolism is not considered a major route of clearance. Paliperidone is converted into metabolites that are not believed to contribute significantly to its overall pharmacological activity. Few significant drug-drug interactions at the level of the CYP450 system are therefore anticipated. Even so, the plasma concentration of paliperidone may be altered by drug interactions at CYP3A4.[164]

Iloperidone has a half-life of 12 to 15 h. Its absorption is not affected by food. It should be titrated slowly because of orthostatic hypotension, and close monitoring is warranted when it is combined with antihypertensive drugs or drugs that are associated with orthostatic effects. The optimal dose has not yet been established but is likely to be in the 5 to 10 mg/day range. Amisulpride has a half-life of 10 to 15 h. It is well tolerated. As yet, there are no known drug interactions. More information regarding the metabolic handling and potential for drug-drug interactions for both of these medications is anticipated as they continue to be further developed.

## Side-effects

### Typical neuroleptics

The adverse effects that are most routinely concerning for antipsychotic drug treatment are extrapyramidal adverse effects (EPS), especially for typical neuroleptic mediations. For typical neuroleptics, high-potency drugs such as haloperidol and fluphenazine are more likely to produce EPS than low-potency agents such as chlorpromazine and thioridazine. The latter may have lower potential for extrapyramidal side-effects than other typical neuroleptics because of its relatively higher affinity for muscarinic receptors. Atypical antipsychotic drugs are less likely to cause EPS during acute and long term tretment. There are a wide range of extrapyramidal side-effects produced by the typical neuroleptics, including dystonic reactions when first administered, akathisia during the first 2–3 weeks, parkinsonism during the first several weeks with variable persistence, neuroleptic malignant syndrome at any time point but usually in the initial weeks, and tardive dyskinesia.

**Dystonic reactions** due to neuroleptic drugs can be treated with parenteral anticholinergic agents or diphenhydramine, an antihistamine with some anticholinergic properties. The use of anticholinergic and other agents to manage parkinsonism due to typical neuroleptic drugs will be discussed subsequently.

**Akathisia** may be the most common of the EPS effects, occurring in up to 70 per cent of patients treated long term with haloperidol.[165] The term refers to a subjective uncomfortable experience of motor restlessness which is relieved by movement. As such, patients will complain of discomfort, and manifest increases in psychomotor behaviour. These symptoms can be so distressing as to increase the risk of agitation or even suicidal behaviours.[166] Although patient age does not seem to influence risk of developing akathisia, women are believed to be at higher risk. Accurate diagnosis of this condition is necessary in order to prevent inadvertent increases in neuroleptic dose from a belief that the patient's discomfort from akathisia is due instead to worsening psychosis. This effect may be managed by reduction in dosage or switching medications to an atypical antipsychotic drug or a drug that is less likely to cause akathisia. When these strategies are not feasible, the symptoms may respond to anticholinergic medications, usually within 3–7 days. Other options include low doses of benzodiazepines or beta-adrenergic blockers, assuming no contraindications to either.

**Parkinsonism** caused by antipsychotic drugs resembles idiopathic parkinsonism. Diagnostically, severe neuroleptic induced parkinsonism may resemble depression or negative symptoms of schizophrenia; however, the associated motor signs and time course of symptoms in relation to starting antipsychotic treatment distinguish the former. Like akathisia, the onset and severity of antipsychotic induced parkinsonism is related to medication dosage; thus, a lowering of the dose or switching to a medication that is less likely to cause this effect may provide significant relief, or ameliorate the parkinsonian signs and symptoms altogether. When this is not feasible, anticholinergic medications may provide relief, typically within 3–7 days. The response to anticholinergic medication is quite variable, however.

**Tardive dyskinesia** emerges at various rates depending upon age, sex, and diagnosis.[167,168] The rate in younger patients is between 3 and 5 per cent per year. It is higher in bipolar than schizophrenic patients and much higher in people above the age of 60. It is related to dose and will be less likely with lower doses of typical neuroleptics. Tardive dyskinesia is ordinarily reversible, although irreversible and/or extremely severe and rarely life-threatening forms can occur. The best way to minimize its occurrence is to use an atypical antipsychotic drug in lieu of a typical agent, since these drugs as a class are associated with a much lower risk of tardive dyskinesia.[167] Patients with mood disorders should generally not receive maintenance treatment with typical antipsychotic drugs unless mood stabilizers alone prove insufficient because they are at greater risk for tardive dyskinesia. There are no definitive treatments for tardive dyskinesia. Generally, the best strategy is prevention through the use of atypical antipsychotic drugs, and periodic screening with a structured assessment tool such as the Abnormal Involuntary Movement Scale (AIMS). There is some suggestion in the literature that continuation of antipsychotic treatment does not worsen tardive dyskinesia, and may eventually result in a stabilization and improvement of tardive symptoms. Switching to clozapine appears to be helpful, although such an effect is not invariable.

**Neuroleptic malignant syndrome** is a rare life-threatening side-effect related to an apparent compromise of the neuromuscular and sympathetic nervous systems.[169] It usually occurs at the initiation of treatment with a high-potency agent but may occur with any of the typical (or atypical agents) at any point. Immediate discontinuation of the medication is essential. The condition is characterized by muscle rigidity, breakdown of muscle fibres leading to large increases in plasma creatine kinase activity, fever, autonomic instability, changing levels of consciousness, and sometimes death. It may be treated by discontinuing all antipsychotic drug treatment, applying external hypothermia, supporting blood pressure, and administering a direct-acting dopamine agonist such as bromocriptine or pergolide, and dantrolene sodium, which blocks the release of intracellular stored calcium ions. After its successful treatment, an atypical antipsychotic should be used even though these agents, including clozapine, may also induce neuroleptic malignant syndrome.

The typical neuroleptic drugs produce a wide variety of **other side-effects**, including weight gain, seizures (especially pimozide), sedation, hypotension, elevated liver enzymes, retinitis pigmentosa (thioridazine), orthostatic hypotension, prolongation of the QTc interval (low potency phenothiazines, pimozide) and anticholinergic effects (mesoridazine, chlorpromazine, thioridazine). All the typical neuroleptic drugs produce marked increases in serum prolactin levels, with the increases being greater in females than males.[25] Prolactin elevations may affect sexual function in both males and females, with difficulty achieving erection or orgasm among the most common side-effects.[25]

## Atypical antipsychotic drugs

### (a) Clozapine

#### (i) Agranulocytosis

It has now been reliably established that clozapine produces agranulocytosis in slightly less than 1 per 100 patients.[170, 171] This is 15 to 30 times the rate associated with the phenothiazines and possibly higher than that for the butyrophenones. The peak of agranulocytosis with clozapine occurs between 4 and 18 weeks, and then falls off sharply. Weekly monitoring of the white cell or absolute neutrophil count is required for 26 weeks in most countries, with the frequency decreasing to biweekly or monthly thereafter, sometimes on a voluntary basis. In the US, monthly monitoring is required assuming no hematological abnormalities after one year of treatment. The cost-effectiveness of monitoring after a year has not been studied but it is probably in the range that would lead to its abandonment by current standards. With monitoring, agranulocytosis can usually be detected before infection sets in or becomes overwhelming. Discontinuation of clozapine, beginning treatment with colony cell stimulating factors, and the usual procedures for treating an infection are usually effective in restoring the white cell line.

#### (ii) Other side-effects

Clozapine produces a wide range of side-effects.[171] These can generally be managed by dose adjustment and concomitant medications. Clozapine produces hypotension because of its potent $\alpha_1$-adrenoceptor antagonism and must be slowly titrated in most patients. Low-dose glucocorticoid treatment may be helpful in some patients with severe hypotension. Clozapine rarely if ever produces significant extrapyramidal side-effects, although some cases of akathisia and neuroleptic malignant syndrome have been reported.

Major motor seizures are another important side-effect of clozapine. They are dose related, with the incidence being about 2 per cent in patients at low doses and 6 per cent at doses greater than 600 mg/day. They are sometimes preceded by myoclonic jerks. Valproic acid and dose reductions are usually effective in preventing the progression of myoclonic jerks or treating major motor seizures. Other anticonvulsants can be combined with clozapine if needed, though caution would be clearly warranted with the use of carbamazepine due to its potential for bone marrow suppression.

Hypersalivation is another side-effect. It usually responds to anticholinergic therapy or to clonidine. Exacerbation of obsessive-compulsive symptoms has been reported with clozapine. Augmentation with an SSRI or lithium carbonate is usually effective.

Weight gain is a frequent side-effect of clozapine, with about 30 per cent of patients gaining more than 7 per cent of body weight.[171] Diet and exercise are useful in minimizing this effect. A related problem is the emergence of insulin resistance or type II diabetes, or exacerbation of existing diabetes, with or without atherogenic changes in serum lipid profile. There have also been reports of diabetic ketoacidosis that emerged in the context of clozapine treatment. Of the atypical antipsychotic drugs, clozapine and olanzapine are associated with the highest risk for clinically significant weight gain, as well as abnormalities in glycaemic control and lipid homeostasis.[123]

Somnolence, tachycardia, hypertension, constipation and stuttering are also produced by clozapine. Tachycardia is treated only when the pulse is greater than 100 beats/minute. β-Blockers are effective to reduce the heart rate, but may also result in synergism of hypotensive effects.[171]

There have been reports of clozapine-associated myocarditis and cardiomyopathy.[172] The presence of eosinophilia accompanied by cardiotoxic signs such as tachycardia, fatigue, orthostasis, or respiratory problems (many of which are adverse effects of clozapine) should alert the clinician to the possibility of myocarditis and the need for medical evaluation.

Finally, treatment with clozapine may not uncommonly result in an asymptomatic mild elevation in hepatic transaminase levels; however, there have also been reports of hepatotoxicity in the setting of clozapine treatment. Polypharmacy appears to be a risk factor. Cases of fulminant hepatotoxicity leading to liver failure are rare.

### (iii) Risperidone

Risperidone is associated with moderate weight gain, comparable to that of typical neuroleptic drugs in most cases, and less than that of clozapine and olanzapine.[123,173] Risperidone also produces some postural hypotension because of its $\alpha_1$-adrenoceptor blocking properties. Risperidone produces greater increases in serum prolactin secretion than any of the other atypical antipsychotic drugs.[25] The increases appear to be at least comparable to those of typical neuroleptics.[173] At higher doses, particularly above 6 mg daily in most adults, the incidence of EPS also increases,[77] though typically not to the degree observed when using typical neuroleptic drugs in clinical practice. Risperidone, like clozapine and other agents of this type, can sometimes exacerbate or induce symptoms of obsessive-compulsive disorder and tics, probably due to its antiserotonergic properties. This can be counteracted in some patients by the addition of an SSRI. Risperidone is not associated with agranulocytosis or increased risk of seizures. Because of its low affinity for muscarinic receptors, risperidone treatment is not associated with significant anticholinergic effects.

### (iv) Olanzapine

Olanzapine also produces dose-dependent extrapyramidal side-effects, including some dystonic reactions in patients with schizophrenia, but these are less frequent and severe than those produced by typical neuroleptic drugs or risperidone.[173] Olanzapine is less well tolerated than clozapine in patients with Parkinson's disease. Olanzapine, like other atypical antipsychotic drugs, is associated with a lower risk of tardive dyskinesia than typical neuroleptics.

The major side-effect of olanzapine is weight gain.[173] Large weight gains due to increased appetite occur in 10 to 15 per cent of olanzapine-treated patients during the first 6 months of treatment. Another 20 to 35 per cent gain between 7 and 10 per cent of body weight. These gains tend to become permanent for as long as patients continue the medication. Like clozapine, olanzapine is also associated with higher risk of insulin resistance, glycaemic changes, and development of atherogenic changes in lipid profile.[123] Cases of diabetic ketoacidosis associated with olanzapine treatment have been reported.

Olanzapine is also associated with some increase in liver enzymes, orthostatic hypotension, anticholinergic side-effects, and sedation.

Many of these adverse effects are time limited and reduce in intensity or resolve over the first few weeks of treatment with continuous use. Olanzapine produces transient increases in serum prolactin levels, which are smaller in magnitude than those produced by typical neuroleptic drugs or risperidone.[25, 173]

Olanzapine, like other agents of this type, can occasionally exacerbate or induce symptoms of obsessive-compulsive disorder and tics, probably due to its antiserotonergic properties. This can be counteracted in some patients by the addition of an SSRI. Olanzapine is not associated with agranulocytosis or increased risk of seizures.

### (v) Quetiapine

Quetiapine appears to have fewer extrapyramidal side-effects than either risperidone or olanzapine.[158,173] Quetiapine is tolerated in patients with Parkinson's disease to a much greater extent than risperidone or olanzapine. The incidence of extrapyramidal side-effects with quetiapine in schizophrenic patients appears to be comparable to placebo. The major side-effects with quetiapine are headache, agitation, dry mouth, dizziness, weight gain, and postural hypotension.[173]

With regard to weight gain and other metabolic effects, quetiapine treatment appears to confer moderate risk—similar to that of risperidone, but less than that associated with clozapine or olanzapine treatment.[123] Far less is known about the long term effects of quetiapine on markers of glycaemic and lipid homeostasis. Nevertheless, clinically significant changes in serum lipids have been reported.

Decreased serum thyroid hormone levels, increased hepatic transaminases and elevated serum lipids have been reported. Decreases in total and free thyroxine, when they occur, are mild, non-progressive, and are not believed to be clinically signficiant. The effect may be dose dependent. Similar to clozapine, asymptomatic elevations in hepatic transaminases may be encountered early in the course of treatment, followed by a return to baseline values. Animal studies suggest an increased risk of cataracts.[173] Periodic ophthalmological screening for lenticular opacities is recommended by the manufacturer, though no causal relationship between the use of quetiapine and the development of cataracts has been demonstrated to date.

### (vi) Ziprasidone

Ziprasidone does not increase serum prolactin levels and is virtually devoid of extrapyramidal side-effects, weight gain, and changes in markers of glucose handling and lipid metabolism. Its major side-effects are nasal congestion and somnolence,[173] the latter of which is usually transient. There has been some concern of cardiovascular side-effects, for example increased QTc interval; however, perusal of the available data does not reveal a significant problem in this regard. However, caution is warranted when considering the coadministration of ziprasidone with other drugs that are known to prolong the QTc interval, since ziprasidone has been associated with a significant increase in the QTc interval of 16.6 msec, which was greater than that of other atypical antipsychotics and haloperidol, but less than thioridazine.[174] Screening for electrolyte abnormalities and cardiac disease (including recent myocardial infarction, congestive heart failure symptoms and arrythmias with or without syncope) may be indicated prior to starting ziprasidone.

### (vii) *Aripiprazole and paliperidone*

Aripiprazole is well tolerated, and does not appear to routinely cause EPS or hyperprolactinaemic changes at recommended dosages. This also appears to be the case for higher than recommended doses. Aripiprazole is also not associated with clinically significant increases in weight, or changes in markers of glucose handling or lipid homeostasis. Both aripiprazole and ziprasidone are therefore believed to be the atypical antipsychotic drugs with the most advantageous metabolic risk profile.

Paliperidone in its extended release form also appears to be well tolerated during short term, acute phase treatment. In these studies, the most common side effect was tachycardia. Rates of discontinuation due to adverse effect burden were also very low. The risk of hyperprolactinaemic changes with paliperidone appears to resemble those of risperidone, although no head-to-head comparisons have been carried out. The changes in prolactin levels may be dose related. The EPS burden associated with paliperidone during the short term studies was low for the 6 mg dose; however, at higher doses, the incidence of EPS appears to be higher. Measures of weight and metabolic effects during 6 week treatment with paliperidone showed no significant changes from baseline. Similar results were found for paliperidone during medium-term treatment.[141] Future long term studies will add greatly to our understanding of paliperidone's adverse effect profile.

## Indications and contraindications

The main indication for the antipsychotic drugs is the treatment of all phases of schizophrenia, including acute, florid symptoms of psychosis, prevention of relapse, and deficit symptoms. Important other uses include the psychotic phase and prophylaxis of mania, depression with psychotic features, the psychosis, agitation, and aggression of various dementias, the treatment of psychoses due to l-dopa or other dopamine agonists in Parkinson's disease, Tourette's syndrome, treatment-resistant obsessive-compulsive disorder, self-injurious behaviour, porphyria, antiemesis, intractable hiccoughs, and as antipruritics. Some current research has suggested that the antipsychotic drugs may be of use to prevent the onset of schizophrenia by administering them to individuals who are in the prodromal phase of the illness. The atypical antipsychotics may be effective for augmenting antidepressants in patients with treatment-resistant non-psychotic depression, and are being tried on an experimental basis for various character disorders such as borderline, schizoid, and schizotypal personality disorders. Clozapine, which has the lowest incidence of extrapyramidal side-effects of any of the antipsychotic drugs, has some special applications in neurological conditions such as essential tremor and the treatment of the water intoxication syndrome in schizophrenic patients. The uses of the classical antipsychotics such as chlorpromazine and haloperidol have been limited by their side-effects, especially parkinsonism and tardive dyskinesia, a slowly developing, sometimes irreversible series of abnormal involuntary movements involving facial, limb, and girdle muscles. As has been discussed, the atypical antipsychotic drugs such as clozapine, olanzapine, quetiapine, and risperidone, as well as iloperidone and ziprasidone, which are in development, have significant advantages with regard to parkinsonism. Clozapine definitely has a vastly reduced risk of tardive dyskinesia and the other atypical agents most likely have a risk that is less than that of the typical neuroleptic drugs but more

than clozapine. Uses in other psychiatric and neurological conditions may be expected to emerge as the safety profile of these agents is better described.

## Antiparkinsonian agents

### Anticholinergic drugs

Antiparkinsonian medications, including anticholinergic, antihistaminic, benzodiazepines, dopamine agonists, and β-blockers are of importance in the management of extrapyramidal side-effects. They are usually needed with the typical neuroleptic drugs but some patients will require antiparkinsonian treatment with olanzapine, risperidone, or quetiapine. The anticholinergics and the antihistaminics (e.g. diphenhydramine) are used to treat acute dyskinesias and dystonias, pseudoparkinsonian symptoms (tremor, rigidity, bradykinesia, shuffling gait), and akathisia. These agents act centrally in the basal ganglia to block the effects of increased acetylcholine release due to $D_2$-receptor blockade. The most widely used anticholinergic drugs are benztropine, biperiden, procyclidine, and trihexyphenidyl. Benztropine is given in doses of 1 to 6mg/day usually in divided doses. Biperiden is given in doses of 2 to 16 mg/day in two or three doses. Procyclidine is given in divided doses of 5 to 30 mg/day. Trihexylphenidyl is given in doses of 1 to 15 mg/day, in a single or divided dose.

These agents are competitive antagonists of the five subtypes of muscarinic receptors that have been identified and which are labelled $M_1$ to $M_5$. They have minimal antagonist effect at nicotinic cholinergic receptors. Blockade of cholinergic receptors on intrastriatal neurones by these agents restores the cholinergic balance, which is disrupted by blockade of $D_2$ dopamine receptors by some antipsychotic agents. Other central effects include impairment of various forms of memory. Elderly patients in particular may develop anticholinergic-induced agitation, irritability, disorientation, hallucinations and delirium because of the natural loss of cholinergic neurones with aging.

## Side-effects

These agents have some preference for the central nervous system but some peripheral anticholinergic effects are to be expected. Blockade of vagal tone in the heart produces tachycardia. Other adverse effects include decreased bladder function and urinary retention and decreased bowel motility leading to constipation and impaction. Decreased saliva and bronchial secretion contribute to dry mouth and increased dental caries while decreased sweating increases the risk of heat stroke. Blockade of muscarinic receptors in the eye cause pupillary dilation and inhibition of accommodation, leading to photophobia and blurred vision. Rarely, narrow-angle glaucoma may ensue. The muscarinic receptors in the basal ganglia are predominantly $M_2$ whereas those in the periphery are $M_1$. The rank order of the anticholinergic drugs for relative selectivity for the $M_2$ receptor is biperiden, procyclidine, trihexylphenidyl, and benztropine. All these agents can cause dry mouth, blurred vision, urinary retention, constipation, and increased intraocular pressure. They may cause anticholinergic delirium in elderly patients or after taking high doses. Biperiden is less likely to cause peripheral anticholinergic effects. Benztropine, biperiden, and trihexyphenidyl may cause euphoria because of their ability to inhibit dopamine reuptake and may be subject to abuse.

## Indications

The anticholinergic drugs or the antihistamine diphenhydramine are given intramuscularly for the treatment of acute dystonic reactions. They are usually effective within minutes and may have to be repeated. It is usually not necessary to prescibe an oral anticholinergic following a dystonic reaction, though some may require their brief use depending on which anipsychotic is prescribed. These agent should not be given prophylactically unless the patient is at established risk for EPS at the dose of antipsychotic which is being started. If akathisia or parkinsonism develops following treatment with a typical neuroleptic drug, the first consideration should be whether to continue to use the offending agent and drop the dosage or to substitute an atypical antipsychotic drug. If decreasing the dose of antipsychotic drugs does not suffice or is not clinically feasible, substituting an atypical agent is the clearly the recommended choice since it avoids all the unpleasant side-effects of the anticholinergic agents.

## Other drugs

Amantadine, which also has antiviral actions, is able to increase the release of dopamine in the basal ganglia, which diminishes the release of acetylcholine. It may improve acute dystonias, akathisia, akinesia, parkinsonism, and tardive dyskinesia. It has also been reported to improve sexual function and decrease weight gain due to neuroleptic drugs. It may cause increased arousal, agitation, and indigestion, however. The usual oral dose is 100 to 400 mg/day.

β-Blockers such as propranolol, atenolol, and pindolol are useful for treating akathisia and tremor. They may cause bradycardia, and particularly immediate-release forms should not be stopped abruptly due to rebound tachycardia.

Benzodiazepines, such as clonazepam, lorazepam, and diazepam, are useful for treating akathisia, acute dystonias, and acute dyskinesias. They can cause drowsiness and lethargy, and have abuse potential.

# Conclusions

Antipsychotic drugs are invaluable tools in treating a large variety of patients with schizophrenia and other conditions. Their main benefits are, in fact, to treat psychotic symptoms, but the newer agents in particular may improve negative symptoms, cognition, mood, anxiety, and aggression as well. The evidence for atypical antipsychotic drugs to improve cognition is steadily increasing and this should be one of the driving forces behind the substitution of these agents for the typical antipsychotic drugs. Recent evidence of volumetric increases in cerebral cortical gray matter associated with atypical, but not typical, antipsychotic drugs may be related to improvement in such symptoms.[175] As such, atypical antipsychotic drugs may produce 'disease modifying' rather than just 'symptomatic' effects, a matter that is of considerable current interest.

Antipsychotic drugs are useful as both acute and maintenance treatments to prevent the recurrence of psychotic symptoms. The extrapyramidal side-effects and greater tardive dyskinesia risk of the typical antipsychotics, coupled with their lesser efficacy to improve negative symptoms and cognition suggest that newer agents are preferred. Clozapine, despite its risk of agranulocytosis, is the treatment of choice for patients who fail to respond to other typical or atypical antipsychotic agents. Risperidone, olanzapine, quetiapine, ziprasidone, aripiprazole and paliperidone have somewhat different pharmacologic profiles. It is not clear which of these agents should be tried in a given patient but on going research may clarify that. These agents, and clozapine, appear to differ significantly in their propensity for causing clinically significant changes in weight and markers of metabolic status. Amisulpride has a mechanism of action different from that of the other atypical agents, with some preference for treating negative symptoms. These compounds, as well as others expected to be approved for use in the near future, for example iloperidone and asenapine, will need to be compared with each other to determine if differential indications exist. Side-effect differences among these drugs as well as the availability of long-acting preparations may help clinicians choose among them. Cost-effective analyses currently favour use of the atypical antipsychotic drugs because of better compliance leading to less frequent relapses and shorter hospital stays. They also facilitate retention of work skills and return to work which decreases the indirect costs of illness in patients still young enough to be able to work. As long as the typical antipsychotics remain in use, and for some patients who receive atypical agents, anticholinergic and other antiparkinsonian drugs will continue to be necessary to treat extrapyramidal side-effects.

Because of the compliance problem, which is less with the atypical than the typical antipsychotics, it is important to develop more long acting atypical drugs. Risperidone is currently available in such a form, and paliperidone and olanzapine will also be in the near future. While the current group of atypical antipsychotic drugs is predominantly characterized by relatively more potent $5\text{-HT}_{2A}$ than $D_2$ receptor antagonism, it is likely that a number of different strategies will emerge for compounds which produce fewer extrapyramidal side-effects than the typical neuroleptics. Because these compounds are so effective in that regard, the real challenge is to develop agents which address other key features of schizophrenia, especially cognitive impairment and negative symptoms, without the side-effect burden of this group of compounds.

# Further information

Davis, K.L., Charney, D., Coyle, J., *et al.* (eds.) (2001). *Neuropsychopharmacology: A Fifth Generation of Progress*. New York: Raven Press.

Breier, A., Tran, P.V., Herrera, J.M., *et al.* (2001). *Current Issues in the Pharmacology of Schizophrenia*. Philadelphia: Lippincott Williams & Wilkins.

# References

1. Meltzer, H. (1995). The concept of atypical antipsychotics. In: *Advances in the neurobiology of schizophrenia* (eds. J.A. den Boer, H.G.M. Westenberg, and H.M. van Praag), pp. 265–73. Wiley, Chichester.

2. Arndt, J. and Skarsfeldt, T. (1998). Do novel antipsychotics have similar pharmacological characteristics? A review of the evidence. *Neuropsychopharmacology*, **181**, 63–101.

3. Kapur, S. and Seeman, P. (2001). Does fast dissociation from the dopamine D(2) receptor explain the action of atypical antipsychotics? A new hypothesis. *American Journal of Psychiatry*, **158**, 360–9.

4. Dixon, L., Lehman, A., and Levine, J. (1995). Conventional antipsychotic medications for schizophrenia. *Schizophrenia Bulletin*, **21**, 567–78.

5. Fitton, A. and Heel, R. (1990). Clozapine: a review of its pharmacological properties, and therapeutic use in schizophrenia. *Drugs*, **40**, 722–47.

6. Burris, K.D., Molski, T.F., Xu, C., *et al.* (2002). Aripiprazole, a novel antipsychotic, is a highaffi nity partial agonist at human dopamine D2 receptors. *Journal of Pharmacology & Experimental Therapeutics*, **302**(1), 381–9.

7. Szewezak, M., Corbett, R., Rusk, D., *et al.* (1995). The pharmacological profi le of iloperidone, a novel atypical antipsychotic agent. *Journal of Pharmacology and Experimental Therapeutics*, **274**, 1404–13.

8. Alphs, L., Panagides, J., Lancaster, S. (2007). Asenapine in the treatment of negative symptoms of schizophrenia: clinical trial design and rationale. *Psychopharmacology Bulletin*, **40**, 41–53.

9. Schotte, A., Janssen, P.F., Gommeren, W., *et al.* (1996). Risperidone compared with new and reference antipsychotic drugs: in vitro and in vivo receptor binding. *Psychopharmacology*, **124**(1–2), 57–73

10. Meltzer, H. and Fatemi, S. (1996). The role of serotonin in schizophrenia and the mechanism of action of anti–psychotic drugs. In *Serotonergic mechanisms in antipsychotic treatment* (eds. J.M. Kane., H.–J. Moller, and F. Awouters), pp. 77–107. Dekker, New York.

11. Anonymous (1998). Adverse effects of the atypical antipsychotics. Collaborative Working Group on Clinical Trial Evaluations. *Journal of Clinical Psychiatry*, **59**, 17–22.

12. Luft, B., Taylor, D. (2006). A review of atypical antipsychotic drugs versus conventional medication in schizophrenia. *Expert Opinion on Pharmacotherapy*. **7**(13), 1739–48.

13. The Collaborative Working Group (1998). Atypical antipsychotics for treatment of depression in schizophrenia and affective disorders. *Journal of Clinical Psychiatry*, **12**, 41–6.

14. McElroy, S.L., Fry, M., Denicoff, K., *et al.* (1998). Olanzapine in treatment–resistant bipolar disorder. *Affective Disorders*, **49**, 119–22.

15. Calabrese, J., Kimmel, S., Woyshville, M., *et al.* (1996). Clozapine in treatment–refractory mania. *American Journal of Psychiatry*, **153**, 759–64.

16. Keefe, R.S., Silva, S.G., Perkins, D.O., *et al.* (1999). The effects of atypical antipsychotic drugs on neurocognitive impairment in schizophrenia: a review and meta-analysis *Schizohrenia Bulletin*, **25**, 201–22.

17. Woodward, N.D., Purdon, S.E., Meltzer, H.Y., *et al.* (2005). Meta-analysis of neuropsychological change to clozapine, olanzapine, quetiapine, and risperidone in schizophrenia. *International Journal of Neuropsychopharmacology*, **8**, 457–72.

18. Keefe, R., Silva, S., Perkins, D., *et al.* (1999). The effects of atypical antipsychotic drugs on neurocognitive impairment in schizohprenia. *Schizophrenia Bulletin*, **25**, 201–32.

19. Meltzer HY. and Stahl, S.M (1976). The dopamine hypothesis of schizophrenia: A review. *Schizophrenia Bulletin* **2**, 19–76.

20. Davis, K., Kahn, R., Ko, G., *et al.* (1992). Dopamine in schizophrenia: a review and reconceptualization. *American Journal of Psychiatry*, **148**, 1474–86.

21. Meltzer, H. (1999). The role of serotonin in antipsychotic drug action. *Neuropsychopharmacology*, **21**, 106–15.

22. Goldman–Rakic, P. and Selemon, L. (1997). Functional and anatomical aspects of prefrontal pathology in schizophrenia. *Schizophrenia Bulletin*, **23**, 437–58.

23. Abi-Dargham, A., Moore, H. (2003). Prefrontal DA transmission at D1 receptors and the pathology of schizophrenia. *Neuroscientist*, **9**, 404–16.

24. Farde, L., Nordstrom, A., Wiesel, F., *et al.* (1992). Positron emission tomographic analysis of central D1 and D2 dopamine receptor occupancy in patients treated with classical neuroleptics and clozapine. Relation to extrapyramidal side effects. *Archives of General Psychiatry*, **49**, 538–44.

25. Haddad, P.M., Wieck, A. (2004). Antipsychotic-induced hyperprolactinemia: mechanisms, clinical features and management. *Drugs*, **64**, 2291–314.

26. Kramer, M., Last, B., *et al.*, and the D4 Dopamine Antagonist Group (1997). The effects of a selective D4 dopamine receptor antagonism. (L–745, 870) in acutely psychotic inpatients with schizophrenia. *Archives of General Psychiatry*, **54**, 567–72.

27. Richelson, E. (1988). Neuroleptic binding to human brain receptors: relation to clinical effects. *Annals of the New York Academy of Sciences*, **537**, 435–42.

28. Meltzer, H.Y., Matsubara, S., and Lee, M. (1989). Classification of typical and atypical antipsychotic drugs on the basis of dopamine D-1, D-2 and serotonin 2 pKi values. *Journal of Pharmacology and Experimental Therapeutics*, **251**, 238–46.

29. Kuroki, T., Meltzer, H., and Ichikawa, J. (1998). Effects of antipsychotic drugs on extracellular dopamine levels in rat medial prefrontal cortex and nucleus accumbens. *Journal of Pharmacology and Experimental Therapeutics*, **288**, 774–81.

30. Parada, M., Hernande, L., Puig de Parada, M., *et al.* (1997). Selection action of acute systemic clozapine on acetylcholine release in the rat prefrontal cortex by reference to the nucleus accumbens and striatum. *Journal of Pharmacology and Experimental Therapeutics*, **281**, 582–8.

31. Li, X., Perry, K., Wong, D., *et al.* (1998). Olanzapine increases *in vivo* dopamine and norepinephrine release in rat prefrontal cortex, nucleus accumbens and striatum. *Psychopharmacology*, **136**, 153–61.

32. Andersson, J.L., Nomikos, G.G., Marcus, M., *et al.* (1995). Ritanserin potentiates the stimulatory effects of raclopride on neuronal activity and dopamine release selectivity in the mesolimbic dopaminergic system. *Naunyn- Schmiedeberg's Archives of Pharmacology*, **352**, 374–85.

33. Westerink, B.H., Kawahara, Y., De Boer, P., *et al.* (2001). Antipsychotic drugs classified by their effects on the release of dopamine and noradrenaline in the prefrontal cortex and striatum. *European Journal of Pharmacology*, **412**, 127–38.

34. Liegois, J.F., Ichikawa, J., Meltzer, H.Y. (2002). 5HT2A receptor antagonism potentiates haloperidol-induced dopamine release in rat medial prefrontal cortex and inhibits that in the nucleus accumbens in a dose-dependent manner. *Brain Research*, **947**, 1547–65.

35. Armsten, A.F. (2004). Adrenergic targets for the treatment of cognitive deficits in schizophrenia. *Psychopharmacology (Berl)*, **174**, 25–31.

36. Poyurovsky, M., Koren, D., Gonopolsky, I., *et al.* (2003). Effects of the 5-HT2 antagonist mianserin on cognitive dysfunction in chronic schizophrenia patients: an add-on, double-blind, placebo-controlled study. *European Neuropsychopharmacology*, **13**, 123–8.

37. Araneda, R. and Andrade, R. (1991). 5-Hydroxytryptamine2 and 5-hydroxitryptamine1A receptors mediate opposing responses on membrane excitability in rat association cortex. *Neuroscience*, **40**, 399–412.

38. Ichikawa, J., Meltzer, H.Y. (1999). R(+)-8-OH-DPAT, a serotonin1A receptor agonist, potentiated S(-) sulpiride-induced dopamine release in rat medial prefrontal cortex and nucleus accumbens but not striatum. *Journal of Pharmacology and Experimental Therapeutics*, **291**, 1227–32.

39. Sakaue, M., Somboonthum, P., Nishihara, B., *et al.* (2000). Postsynaptic 5-hydroxytryptamine(1A) receptor activation increases in vivo dopamine release in rat prefrontal cortex. *British Journal of Pharmacology*, **129**, 1028–34.

40. Sumiyoshi, T., Matsui, M., Yamashita, I., *et al.* (2001). Enhancement of cognitive performance in schizophrenia by addition of tandospirone to neuroleptic treatment. *American Journal of Psychiatry*, **158**, 1722–5.

41. Sumiyoshi, T., Jayathilake, K., Roy, A., *et al.* (2006). Effect of buspirone, a serotonin(1A) partial agonist, on cognitive function in schizophrenia. [abstract]. *International Journal of Neuropsychopharmacology*, **9** (suppl 1), S248.

42. Bonaccorso, S., Meltzer, H.Y., Li, Z., *et al.* (2002). SR46349-B, a 5-HT(2A/2C) receptor antagonist, potentiates haloperidol-induced dopamine release in rat medial prefrontal cortex and nucleus accumbens. *Neuropsychopharmacology*, **27**, 430–41.

43. Kroeze, W.K., Hufeisen, S.J., Popadak, B.A., *et al.* (2003). H1-histamine receptor affinity predicts short-term weight gain for typical and atypical antipsychotic drugs. *Neuropsychopharmacology*, **28**, 519–26.

44. Reynolds, G.P., Templeman, L.A., Zhang, Z.J. (2005). The role of 5-HT2C receptor polymorphisms in the pharmacogenetics of antipsychotic drug treatment. *Progress in Neuropsychopharmacology and Biological Psychiatry*, **29**, 1021–8.

45. Bigliani, V., Mulligan, R.S., Acton, P.D., *et al.* (2000). Striatal and temporal cortical D2/D3 receptor occupancy by olanzapine and sertindole in vivo: a [123I] epidepride single photon emission tomography (SPET) study. *Psychopharmacologia*, **150**, 132–40.

46. Stephenson, C.M., Bigliani, V., Jones, H.M., *et al.* (2000). Striatal and extra-striatal D(2)/D(3) dopamine receptor occupancy by quetiapine in vivo. *British Journal of Psychiatry*, **177**, 408–15.

47. Xiberas, X., Martinot, J.L., Mallet, L., *et al.* (2001). Extrastriatal and striatal D(2) dopamine receptor blockade with haloperidol or new antipsychotic drugs in patients with schizophrenia. *British Journal of Psychiatry*, **179**, 503–8.

48. Bressan, R.A., Erlandsson, K., Stone, J.M., *et al.* (2005). Impact of schizophrenia and chronic antipsychotic treatment on [123I] CNS-1261 binding to N-methyl-Daspartate receptors in vivo. *Biological Psychiatry*, **58**, 41–6.

49. Kane, J. and Marder, S. (1993). Psychopharmacologic treatment of schizophrenia. *Schizophrenia Bulletin*, **19**, 287–302.

50. Lieberman, J., Jody, D., Geisler, S., *et al.* (1993). Time course and biologic correlates of treatment response in first–episode schizophrenia. *Archives of General Psychiatry*, **50**, 369–76.

51. Meltzer, H., Lee, M., and Colal, P. (1998). The evolution of treatment resistance. Biological implications. *Journal of Clinical Psychopharmacology*, **18**, 5–11.

52. Meltzer, H. (1997). Treatment-resistant schizophrenia: the role of clozapine. *Current Medical Research Opinion*, **14**, 1–20.

53. Tandon, R., Ribeiro, S., DeQuardo, J., *et al.* (1993). Covariance of positive and negative symptoms during neuroleptic treatment in schizophrenia: a replication. *Biological Psychiatry*, **34**, 495–7.

54. The Collaborative Working Group (1998). Assessing the effects of a typical antipsychotics on negative symptoms. *Journal of Clinical Psychiatry*, **12**, 28–35.

55. Saykin, A., Shtasel, D., Gur, R., *et al.* (1994). Neuropsychological deficits in neuroleptic naïve patients with first–episode schizophrenia. *Archives of General Psychiatry*, **51**, 124–31.

56. Palmer, B., Heaton, R., Paulsen, J., *et al.* (1997). Is it possible to be schizophrenic yet neuropsychologically normal? *Neuropsychology*, **11**, 437–46.

57. Green, M. (1996). What are the functional consequences of neurocognitive deficits in schizophrenia? *American Journal of Psychiatry*, **153**, 321–30.

58. Meltzer, H.Y., and McGurk, S. (1999). The effect of clozapine, risperidone and olanzapine on cognitive function in schizophrenia. *Schizophrenia Bulletin*, **25**, 233–56.

59. Sheitman, B., Lee, H., Strauss, R., *et al.* (1997). The evaluation and treatment of first–episode psychosis. *Schizophrenia Bulletin*, **23**, 653–61.

60. McEvoy, J., Hogarty, G., and Steingard, S. (1991). Optimal dose of neuroleptic in acute schizophrenia. A controlled study of the neuroleptic threshold and higher haloperidol dose. *Archives of General Psychiatry*, **48**, 739–45.

61. Carpenter, W., Buchanan, R., Kirkpatrick, B., *et al.* (1999). Diazepam treatment of early signs of exacerbation in schizophrenia. *American Journal of Psychiatry*, **156**, 299–303.

62. Schooler, N.R. (2003). Relapse and rehospitalization: comparing oral and depot antipsychotics. *Journal of Clinical Psychiatry*, **64** (suppl 16), 14–7.

63. Lehman, A.F., Kreyenbuhl, J., Buchanan, R.W., *et al.* (2004). The Schizophrenia Patient Outcomes Research Team (PORT): updated treatment recommendations 2003. *Schizophrenia Bulletin*, **30**, 193–217.

64. Lehman, A.F., *et al.* American Psychiatric Association; Steering Committee on Practice Guidelines. (2004). Practice guideline for the treatment of patients with schizophrenia, second edition. *American Journal of Psychiatry*, **161** (2 suppl), 1–56.

65. Lieberman, J.A., Stroup, T.S., *et al.* Clinical Antipsychotic Trials of Intervention Effectiveness (CATIE) Investigators. (2005). Effectiveness of antipsychotic drugs in patients with chronic schizophrenia. *New England Journal of Medicine*, **353**, 1209–23.

66. Jones, P.B., Barnes, T.R., Davies, L., *et al.* (2006). Randomized controlled trial of the effect on Quality of Life of second- vs first generation antipsychotic drugs in schizophrenia: Cost Utility of the Latest Antipsychotic Drugs in Schizophrenia Study (CUtLASS 1). *Archives of General Psychiatry*, **63**, 1079–87.

67. Revicki, D. (1999). Pharmacoeconomic studies of atypical antipsychotic drugs for the treatment of schizophrenia. *Schizophrenia Research*, **35**, 101–9.

68. Bobes, J., Canas, F., Rejas, J., *et al.* (2004). Economic consequences of the adverse reactions related with antipsychotics: an economic model comparing tolerability of ziprasidone, olanzapine, risperidone, and haloperidol in Spain. *Progress in Neuropsychopharmacology and Biological Psychiatry*, **28**, 1287–97.

69. Meltzer, H. (1979). The clozapine story. In: *The handbook of psychopharmacology trials* (eds. M. Hertzman and D. Feltner), pp. 137–56. New York University Press.

70. Baldessarini, R. and Frankenberg, F. (1991). Clozapine: a novel antipsychotic agent. *New England Journal of Medicine*, **324**, 746–54.

71. Kane, J., Honigfeld, G., *et al.* Clozaril Collaborative Study Group (1988). Clozapine for the treatmentresistant schizophrenic: a double–blind comparison with chlorpromazine. *Archives of General Psychiatry*, **45**, 789–96.

72. Meltzer, H.Y., Alphs, L., *et al.* International Suicide Prevention Trial Study Group. (2003). Clozapine treatment for suicidality in schizophrenia: International Suicide Prevention Trial (InterSePT). *Archives of General Psychiatry*, **60**, 82–91.

73. Nordstrom, A., Farde, L., Nyber, S., *et al.* (1995). D1, D2, and 5-HT2 receptor occupancy in relation to clozapine serum concentration: a PET study of schizophrenic patients. *American Journal of Psychiatry*, **152**, 1444–9.

74. Shiloh, R., Zemishlany, Z., Aizenberg, D., *et al.* (1997). Sulpiride augmentation in people with schizophrenia partially responsive to clozapine. A double-blind, placebo-controlled study. *British Journal of Psychiatry*, **171**, 569–73.

75. Havaki-Kontaxaki, B.J., Ferentinos, P.P., Kontaxakis, V.P., *et al.* (2006). Concurrent administration of clozapine and electroconvulsive therapy in clozapine-resistant schizophrenia. *Clinical Neuropharmacology*, **29**, 52–6.

76. Meltzer, H., Lee, M., Ranjan, R., *et al.* (1996). Relapse following clozapine withdrawal: effect of cyproheptadine plus neuroleptic. *Psychopharmacology*, **124**, 176–87.

77. Marder, S. and Meibach, R. (1994). Risperidone in the treatment of schizophrenia. *American Journal of Psychiatry*, **151**, 825–35.

78. Pajonk, F.G. (2004). Risperidone in acute and long-term therapy of schizophrenia—a clinical profile. *Progress in Neuropsychopharmacology and Biological Psychiatry*, **28**, 15–23.

79. Leucht, S., Pitschel–Walz, G., Abraham, D., *et al.* (1999). Efficacy and extrapyramidal side–effects of the new antispychotics olanzapine, quetiapine, risperidone, and sertindole compared to conventional antipsychotics and placebo. A meta–analysis of randomized controlled trials. *Schizophrenia Research*, **35**, 51–68.

80. Citrome, L., Bilder, R.M., Volavka, J. (2002). Managing treatmentresistant schizophrenia: evidence from randomized controlled trials. *Journal of Psychiatric Practice*, **8**, 205–15.

81. Kumar, V. and Brecher, M. (1999). Psychopharmacology of atypical antipsychotics and clinical outcomes in elderly patients. *Journal of Clinical Psychiatry*, **60**, 10–16.

82. Simpson, G. and Lindenmayer, J. (1997). Extrapyramidal symptoms in patients treated with risperidone. *Journal of Clinical Psychopharmacology*, **17**, 194–201.

83. Csernansky, J.G., Mahmoud, R., Brenner, R. (2002). A comparison of risperidone and haloperidol for the prevention of relapse in patients with schizophrenia. *New England Journal of Medicine*, **346**, 16–22.

84. Rabinowitz, J., Lichtenberg, P., Kaplan, Z., et al. (2001). Rehospitalization rates of chronically ill schizohprenic patients discharged on a regimen of risperidone, olanzapine, or conventional antipsychotics. *American Journal of Psychiatry*, **158**, 266–9.

85. Ehret, M.J., Fuller, M.A. (2004). Long-acting injectable risperidone. *Annals of Pharmacotherapy*, **38**, 2122–7.

86. Jeste, D., Lacro, J., Bailey, A., et al. (1999). Lower incidence of tardive dyskinesia with risperidone compared with haloperidol in older patients. *Journal of the American Geriatrics Society*, **47**, 716–19.

87. Moller, H., Muller, H., Borison, R., et al. (1995). A path-analytical approach to differentiate between direct and indirect drug effects on negative symptoms in schizophrenic patients (a re–evaluation of the North American risperidone study). *European Archives of Psychiatry Clinical Neuroscience*, **245**, 45–9.

88. Carman, J., Peuskens, J., Vangeneugden, A. (1995). Risperidone in the treatment of negative symptoms of schizophrenia: a meta-analysis. *International Clinical Psychopharmacology*, **10**, 207–13.

89. Glennie, J. (1997). Technology overview: pharmaceuticals: pharmacoeconomic evaluations of clozapine in treatment-resistant schizophrenia and risperidone in chronic schizophrenia. Ottawa (ON): Canadian Coordinating Office for Health Technology Assessment (CCOHTA).

90. Laux, G., Heeg, B., van Hout, B.A., et al. (2005). Costs and effects of long-acting risperidone compared with oral atypical and conventional depot formulations in Germany. *Pharmacoeconomics*, **23** (suppl 1), 49–61.

91. Awad, A.G. and Voruganti, L.N.P. (2004). Impact of atypical antipsychotics on quality of life in patients with schizophrenia. *CNS Drugs*, **18**, 877–93.

92. Tollefson, G. and Kuntz, A. (1999). Review of recent clinical studies with olanzapine. *British Journal of Psychiatry*, **37**, 30–35.

93. Conley, R., Kelly, D., and Gale, E. (1998). Olanzapine response in treatment-refractory schizophrenic patients with a history of substance abuse. *Schizophrenia Research*, **33**, 95–101.

94. Tollefson, G.D., Birkett, M.A., et al., Lilly Resistant Schizophrenia Study Group. (2001). Double-blind comparison of olanzapine versus clozapine in schizophrenic patients clinically eligible for treatment with clozapine. *Biological Psychiatry*, **49**, 52–63.

95. Dinakar, H.S., Sobel, R.N., Bopp, J.H., et al. (2002). Efficacy of olanzapine and risperidone for treatment-resistant schizophrenia among long-stay state hospital patients. *Psychiatric Services*, **53**, 755–7.

96. Beasley, C., Tollefson, G., Tran, P., et al. (1996). Olanzapine versus placebo and haloperidol acute phase results of the North American double-blind olanzapine trial. *Neuropsychopharmacology*, **14**, 111–23.

97. Tollefson, G. and Sanger, T. (1997). Negative symptoms, a path analytic approach to a double-blind, placebo- and haloperidol-controlled clinical trial with olanzapine. *American Journal of Psychiatry*, **54**, 466–74.

98. Tran, P., Dellva, M., Tollefson, G., et al. (1998). Oral olanzapine versus oral haloperidol in the maintenance treatment of schizophrenia and related psychoses. *British Journal of Psychiatry*, **172**, 499–505.

99. Tollefson, G., Sanger, T., Lu, Y., et al. (1998). Depressive signs and symptoms in schizophrenia: a prospective blinded trial of olanzapine and haloperidol. *Archives of General Psychiatry*, **55**, 250–8.

100. Almond, S., O'Donnell, O. (1998). Cost analysis of the treatment of schizophrenia in the UK: a comparison of olanzapine and haloperidol. *Pharmacogenomics*, **13**, 575–88.

101. Hamilton, S.H., Revicki, D.A., Edgell, E.T., et al. (1999). Clinical and economic outcomes of olanzapine compared with haloperidol for schizophrenia: results from a randomized clinical trial. *Pharmacoeconomics*, **15**, 469–80.

102. Kinon, B.J., Ahl, J., Stauffer, V.L., et al. (2004). Dose response and atypical antipsychotics in schizophrenia. *CNS Drugs*, **18**, 597–616.

103. Wagstaff, A.J., Easton, J. and Scott, L.J. (2005). Intramuscular olanzapine: a review of its use in the management of acute agitation. *CNS Drugs*, **19**, 147–64.

104. Arvanitis, L. and Miller, B. (1997). Multiple fixed dose of 'Seroquel' (quetiapine) in patients with acute exacerbation of schizophrenia: a comparison with haloperidol and placebo. The Seroquel Trial 13 Study Group. *Biological Psychiatry*, **42**, 233–46.

105. Small, J., Hirsch, S., et al. and the Seroquel Study Group (1997). Quetiapine in patients with schizophrenia: a high- and low-dose double-blind comparison with placebo. *Archives of General Psychiatry*, **54**, 549–57.

106. Gefvert, O., Lundberg, T., Wieselgren, I.M., et al. (2001). D(2) and 5HT(2A) receptor occupancy of different doses of quetiapine in schizophrenia: a PET study. *European Neuropsychopharmacology*, **11**, 105–10.

107. Emsley, R.A., Buckley, P., Jones, A.M., et al. (2003). Differential effect of quetiapine on depressive symptoms in patients with partially responsive schizophrenia. *Journal of Psychopharmacology*, **17**, 210–15.

108. Velligan, D.I., Newcomer, J., Pultz, J., et al. (2002). Does cognitive function improve with quetiapine in comparison to haloperidol? *Schizophrenia Research*, **53**, 239–48.

109. Fernandez, H.H., Trieschmann, M.E., Friedman, J.H. (2003). Treatment of psychosis in Parkinson's disease: safety considerations. *Drug Safety*, **26**, 643–59.

110. Stahl, S.M. and Shayegan, D.K. (2003). The psychopharmacology of ziprasidone: receptor-binding properties and real-world psychiatric practice. *Journal of Clinical Psychiatry*, **64** (Suppl 19), 6–12.

111. Davis, R. and Markham, A. (1997). Ziprasidone. *CNS Drugs*, **8**, 153–9.

112. Tandon, R., Harrigan, E., and Zorn, S. (1997). Ziprasidone: a novel antipsychotic with unique pharmacology and therapeutic potential. *Journal of Serotonin Research*, **4**, 159–77.

113. Swainston, H.T. and Scott, L.J. (2006). Ziprasidone: a review of its use in schizophrenia and schizoaffective disorder. *CNS Drugs*, **20**, 1027–52.

114. Arato, M., O'Connor, R., and Meltzer, H. The Ziprasidone Extended Use in Schizophrenia (Zeus) study: a prospective, double-blind, placebo-controlled, 1-year clinical trial. Submitted for publication.

115. Hirsch, S.R., Kissling, W., Bauml, J., et al. (2002). A 28-week comparison of ziprasidone and haloperidol in outpatients with stable schizophrenia. *Journal of Clinical Psychiatry*, **63**, 516–23.

116. Daniel, D.G., Zimbroff, D.L., Potkin, S.G., et al. (1999). Ziprasidone 80 mg/day and 160 mg/day in the acute exacerbation of schizophrenia and schizoaffective disorder: a 6-week placebo-controlled trial. Ziprasidone Study Group. *Neuropsychopharmacology*, **20**, 491–505.

117. Harvey, P.D. (2003). Ziprasidone and cognition: the evolving story. *Journal of Clinical Psychiatry*, **64** (suppl 19), 33–9.

118. Phillips, G.A., Van Brunt, D.L., Roychowdhury, S.M., et al. (2006). The relationship between quality of life and clinical efficacy from a randomized trial comparing olanzapine and ziprasidone. *Journal of Clinical Psychiatry*, **67**, 1397–403.

119. Bernardo, M., Ramon Azanza, J., Rubio-Terres, C., et al. (2006). Cost-effectiveness analysis of schizophrenia relapse prevention: an economic evaluation of the ZEUS (Ziprasidone-Extended-Use-In-Schizophrenia) study in Spain. *Clinical Drug Investigation*, **26**, 447–57.

120. Mamo, D., Kapur, S., Shammi, C.M., *et al.* (2004). A PET study of dopamine D2 and serotonin 5-HT1 receptor occupancy in patients with schizophrenia treated with therapeutic doses of ziprasidone. *American Journal of Psychiatry*, **161**, 818–25.

121. Hamelin, B.A., Allard, S., Laplante, L., *et al.* The effect of timing of a standard meal on the pharmacokinetics and pharmacodynamics of the novel atypical antipsychotic agent ziprasidone. *Pharmacotherapy*, **18**, 9–15.

122. Daniel, D.G., Potkin, S.G., Reeves, K.R., *et al.* (2001). Intramuscular (IM) ziprasidone 20 mg is effective in reducing acute agitation associated with psychosis: a double-bline, randomized trial. *Psychopharmacology*, **155**, 128–34.

123. Newcomer, J.W. and Haupt, D.W. (2006). The metabolic effects of antipsychotic medications. *Canadian Journal of Psychiatry*, **51**, 480–91.

124. Haddad, P.M. and Anderson, I.M. (2002). Antipsychotic-related QTc prolongation, torsade de pointes and sudden death. *Drugs*, **62**, 1649–71.

125. Heinrich, T.W., Biblo, L.A. and Schneider, J. (2006). Torsades de pointes associated with ziprasidone. *Psychosomatics*, **47**, 264–8.

126. Harrigan, E.P., Miceli, J.J., Anziano, R., *et al.* (2004). A randomized evaluation of the effects of six antipsychotic agents on QTc, in the absence and presence of metabolic inhibition. *Journal of Clinical Psychopharmacology*, **24**, 62–9.

127. Burris, K.D., Molski, T.F., Xu, C., *et al.* (2002). Aripiprazole, a novel antipsychotic, is a high-affinity partial agonist at human dopamine D2 receptors. *Journal of Pharmacology and Experimental Therapeutics*, **302**, 381–9.

128. Jordan, S., Koprivica, V., Chen, R., *et al.* (2002). The antipsychotic aripiprazole is a potent, partial agonist at the human 5-HT1A receptor. *European Journal of Pharmacology*, **441**, 137–40.

129. El-Sayeh, H.G., Morganti, C. and Adams, C.E. (2006). Aripiprazole for schizophrenia. Systematic review. *British Journal of Psychiatry*, **189**, 102–8.

130. Potkin, S.G., Saha, A.R., Kujawa, M.J., *et al.* (2003). Aripiprazole, an antipsychotic with a novel mechanism of action, and risperidone vs placebo in patients with schizophrenia and schizoaffective disorder. *Archives of General Psychiatry*, **60**, 681–90.

131. Piggott, T.A., Carson, W.H., *et al.*, Aripiprazole Study Group. (2003). Aripiprazole for the prevention of relapse in stabilized patients with chronic schizophrenia: a placebo-controlled 26-week study. *Journal of Clinical Psychiatry*, **64**, 1048–56.

132. Kasper, S., Lerman, M.N., McQuade, R.D., *et al.* (2003). Efficacy and safety of aripiprazole vs. haloperidol for long-term maintenance treatment following acute relapse of schizophrenia. *International Journal of Neuropsychopharmacology*, **6**, 325–37.

133. Kane, J.M., Meltzer, H.Y., *et al.* Aripiprazole Study Group. (2007). Aripiprazole for treatment-resistant schizophrenia: results of a multicenter, randomized, double-blind, comparison study versus perphenazine. *Journal of Clinical Psychiatry*, **68**, 213–23.

134. Tandon, R., Marcus, R.N., Stock, E.G., *et al.* (2006). A prospective, multicenter, randomized, parallel-group, openlabel study of aripiprazole in the management of patients with schizophrenia or schizoaffective disorder in general psychiatric practice: Broad Effectiveness Trial With Aripiprazole (BETA). *Schizophrenia Research*, **84**, 77–89.

135. Chrzanowski, W.K., Marcus, R.N., Torbeyns, A., *et al.* (2006). Effectiveness of long-term aripiprazole therapy in patients with acutely relapsing or chronic, stable schizophrenia: a 52-week, open-label comparison with olanzapine. *Psychopharmacology*, **189**, 259–66.

136. Kern, R.S., Green, M.F., Cornblatt, B.A., *et al.* (2006). The neurocognitive effects of aripiprazole: an open-label comparison with olanzapine. *Psychopharmacology*, **187**, 312–20.

137. Kerwin, R., Millet, B., Herman, E., *et al.* (2007). A multicentre, randomized, naturalistic, open-label study between aripiprazole and standard of care in the management of community treated schizophrenic patients Schizohprenia Trial of Aripiprazole: (STAR) study. *European Psychiatry*, in press.

138. Tran-Johnson, T.K., Stack, D.A., Marcus, R.N., *et al.* (2007). Efficacy and safety of intramuscular aripiprazole in patients with acute agitation: a randomized, double-blind, placebo-controlled trial. *Journal of Clinical Psychiatry*, **68**, 111–9.

139. Kane, J., Canas, F., Kramer, M., *et al.* (2007). Treatment of schizophrenia with paliperidone extended-release tablets: a 6-week placebo-controlled trial. *Schizophrenia Research*, **90**, 147–61.

140. Davidson, M., Emsley, R., Kramer, M., *et al.* (2007). Efficacy, safety and early response of paliperidone extended-release tablets (paliperidone ER): Results of a 6-week, randomized, placebo-controlled study. *Schizophrenia Research*, **93**, 117–30.

141. Kramer, M., Simpson, G., Maciulis, V., *et al.* (2007). Paliperidone extended-release tablets for prevention of symptom recurrence in patients with schizophrenia: a randomized, double-blind, placebo-controlled study. *Journal of Clinical Psychopharmacology*, **27**, 6–14.

142. Meltzer, H.Y., Bobo, W.V., Nuamah, I.F., *et al.* (2008). Efficacy and tolerability of oral paliperidone extended-release tablets in the treatment of acute schizophrenia: pooled data from three 6-week, placebo-controlled studies. *Journal of Clinical Psychiatry*, **69**, 817–29.

143. McKeage, K., Plosker, G.L. (2004). Amisulpride: a review of its use in the management of schizophrenia. *CNS Drugs*, **18**, 933–56.

144. Möller, J., Boyer, P., *et al.* and the PROD–ASLP Study Group. (1997). Improvement of acute exacerbations of schizophrenia with amisulpride: a comparison with haloperidol. *Psychopharmacology*, **132**, 396–401.

145. Freeman, H. (1997). Amisulpride compared with standard neuroleptics in acute exacerbations of schizophrenia: three efficacy studies. *International Clinical Psychopharmacology*, **12**, 11–17.

146. Paillere–Martinot, M., Lecrubier, Y., Martinot, J., *et al.* (1995). Improvement of some schizophrenic defi cit symptoms with low doses of amisulpride. *American Journal of Psychiatry*, **152**, 130–4.

147. Boyer, P., Lecrubier, Y., Pucch, A., *et al.* (1995). Treatment of negative symptoms in schizophrenia with amisulpride. *British Journal of Psychiatry*, **166**, 68–72.

148. Perry, P., Miller, D., Arndt, S., *et al.* (1992). Clozapine and norclozapine plasma concentrations and clinical response of treatment–refractory schizophrenic patients. *American Journal of Psychiatry*, **148**, 231–5.

149. Peuskens, J., Moller H.J. and Puech, A. (2002). Amisulpride improves depressive symptoms in acute exacerbations of schizophrenia: comparison with haloperidol and risperidone. *European Neuropsychopharmacology*, **12**, 305–10.

150. Colonna, L., Saleem, P., Dondey-Nouvel, L., *et al.* (2000). Long-term safety and effi cacy of amisulpride in subchronic or chronic schizophrenia. Amisulpride Study Group. *International Clinical Psychopharmacology*, **15**, 13–22.

151. Surguladze, S., Patel, A., Kerwin, R.W., *et al.* (2005). Cost analysis of treating schizophrenia with amisulpride: naturalistic mirror image study. *Progress in Neuropsychopharmacology and Biological Psychiatry*, **29**, 517–22.

152. Kelleher, J.P., Centorrino, F., Albert, M.J., *et al.* (2002). Advances in atypical antipsychotics for the treatment of schizophrenia: new formulations and new agents. *CNS Drugs*, **16**, 249–61.

153. Bell, R., McLaren, A., Glanos, J., *et al.* (1998). The clinical use of plasma clozapine levels. *Australian and New Zealand Journal of Psychiatry*, **32**, 567–74.

154. Prior, T.I., Chue, P.S., Tibbo, P., *et al.* (1999). Drug metabolism and atypical antipsychotics. *European Neuropsychopharmacology*, **9**, 301–9.

155. Olesen, O.V., Linnet, K. (2001). Contributions of five human cytochrome P450 isoforms to the N-demethylation of clozapine in vitro at low and high concentrations. *Journal of Clinical Pharmacology*, **41**, 823–32.

156. He, H. and Richardson, J. (1995). A pharmacological, pharmacokinetic and clinical overview of risperidone, a new antipsychotic that blocks serotonin 5–HT2 and dopamine D2 receptors. *International Clinical Psychopharmacology*, **10**, 19–30.

157. Aravagiri, M., Ames, D., Wirshing, W., *et al.* (1997). Plasma level monitoring of olanzapine in patients with schizophrenia: determination by high–performance liquid chromatography with electrochemical detection. *Therapeutic Drug Monitoring*, **19**, 307–13.

158. Casey, D. (1996). 'Seroquel'(quetiapine): preclinical and clinical findings of a new atypical antipsychotic. *Experimentation, Opinion and Investigation of Drugs*, **5**, 939–57.

159. Potkin, S.G., Thyrum, P.T., Alva, G., *et al.* (2002). The safety and pharmacokinetics of quetiapine when coadministered with haloperidol, risperidone, or thioridazine. *Journal of Clinical Psychopharmacology*, **22**, 121–30.

160. Chengappa, K.N., Parepally, H., Brar, J.S., *et al.* (2003). A random-assigment, double-blind, clinical trial of once- vs twice-daily administration of quetiapine fumarate in patients with schizophrenia or schizoaffective disorder: a pilot study. *Canadian Journal of Psychiatry*, **48**, 198–94.

161. Gefvert, O., Bergstrom, M., Langstrom, B., *et al.* (1998). Time course of central nervous dopamine-D2 and 5-HT2 receptor blockade and plasma drug concentrations after discontinuation of quetiapine (Seroquel) in patients with schizophrenia. *Psychopharmacology*, **135**, 119–26.

162. Beedham, C., Miceli, J.J., Obach, R.S. (2003). Ziprasidone metabolism, aldehyde oxidase, and clinical implications. *Journal of Clinical Psychopharmacology*, **23**, 229–32.

163. Swainston, H.T. and Perry, C.M. (2004). Aripiprazole: a review of its use in schizophrenia and schizoaffective disorder. *Drugs*, **64**, 1715–36.

164. Jung, S.M., Kim, K.A., Cho, H.K., *et al.* (2005). Cytochrome P450 3A inhibitor itraconazole affects plasma concentrations of risperidone and 9-hydroxyrisperidone in schizophrenic patients. *Clinical Pharmacology and Therapeutics*, **78**, 520–8.

165. Sachdev, P. (1995). The epidemiology of drug-induced akathisia: Part I. Acute akathisia. *Schizophrenia Bulletin*, **21**, 431–49.

166. Atbasoglu, E.C., Schultz, S.K. and Andreasen, N.C. (2001). The relationship of akathisia with suicidality and depresonalization among patients with schizophrenia. *Journal of Neuropsychiatry and Clinical Neuroscience*, **13**, 336–41.

167. Cavallaro, R. and Smeraldi, E. (1995). Antipsychotic–induced tardive dyskinesia. *CNS Drugs*, **4**, 278–93.

168. Kane, J.M. (2004). Tardive dyskinesia rates with atypical antipsychotics in adults: prevalence and incidence. *Journal of Clinical Psychiatry*, **65** (suppl 9), 16–20.

169. Velamoor, V. (1998). Neuroleptic malignant syndrome. Recognition, prevention and management. *Drug Safety*, **19**, 73–81.

170. Alvir, J., Lieberman, J., Safferman, A., *et al.* (1993). Clozapine–induced agranulocytosis: incidence and risk factors in the United States. *New England Journal of Medicine*, **329**, 162–7.

171. Lieberman, J. and Safferman, A. (1992). Clinical profile of clozapine: adverse reactions and agranulocytosis. *Psychiatric Quarterly*, **63**, 51–70.

172. Merrill, D.B., Dec, G.W. and Goff, D.C. (2005). Adverse cardiac effects associated with clozapine. *Journal of Clinical Psychopharmacology*, **25**, 32–41.

173. Collaborative Working Group. (1998). Adverse effects of the atypical antipsychotics. *Journal of Clinical Psychiatry*, **12**, 17–22.

174. Kelly, D.L., Love, R.C. (2001). Ziprasidone and the QTc interval: pharmacokinetic and pharmacodynamic considerations. *Psychopharmacology Bulletin*, 35, 66–79.

175. Garver, D.L., Holcomb, J.A. and Christensen, J.D. (2005). Cerebral cortical gray expansion associated with two second-generation antipsychotics. *Biological Psychiatry*, **58**, 62–6.

176. Marder, S.R., Kramer, M., Ford, L., *et al.* (2007). Efficacy and safety of paliperidone extended-release tablets: results of a 6-week, randomized, placebo-controlled study. *Biological Psychiatry*, **62**, 1363–70.

177. Papakostas, G.I., Shelton, R.C., Smith, J., *et al.* (2007). Augmentation of antidepressants with atypical antipsychotic medication for treatment-resistant major depressive disorder: a meta-analysis. *Journal of Clinical Psychiatry*, **68**, 826–31.

# 6.2.6 Antiepileptic drugs

Brian P. Brennan and Harrison G. Pope Jr.

## Introduction

Several drugs originally developed to treat epilepsy have been found effective in certain psychiatric disorders. This chapter reviews the antiepileptic drugs most extensively studied in psychiatric disorders: valproate, carbamazepine, lamotrigine, and topiramate. We then briefly mention six other antiepileptics currently under investigation in various psychiatric disorders, but not yet extensively studied: gabapentin, oxcarbazepine, levetiracetam, tiagabine, zonisamide, and pregabalin. The antiepileptic drug phenytoin is rarely used in psychiatric disorders, and is therefore not included in this chapter. The benzodiazepines, which have antiepileptic properties, are also omitted here, as they are discussed in Chapter 6.2.2. We briefly list studies documenting the efficacy of these various agents in psychiatric disorders, but the reader is referred to the individual chapters on specific disorders for a more detailed discussion of treatment strategies.

## Valproate[1]

### Introduction

Valproate (valproic acid) is a simple branched-chain carboxylic acid, first used as an organic solvent in the late 1800s (see Fig. 6.2.6.1). Its antiepileptic properties were discovered serendipitously in 1963, and its clinical use as an antiepileptic drug began in 1964. As early as 1966, valpromide (the amide precursor of valproate) was reported to be effective in the treatment of bipolar disorder.[1] Since then, valproate has been used effectively in the treatment of numerous psychiatric and neurologic conditions, and is now widely used as a mood stabilizer in the treatment of bipolar disorder.

Valproate is currently available as five different preparations: valproate (Depakene), sodium valproate (Depakene syrup), divalproex sodium (Depakote) (which is an equal proportion of sodium valproate and valproic acid), divalproex sodium sprinkle capsules (Depakote sprinkle capsules), and valpromide (the amide precursor of valproate, which is available in Europe, but not in the United States).

### Pharmacology

The mechanism of action of valproate in the treatment of epilepsy is unclear, but appears to be related to increased levels of gamma-aminobutyric acid (GABA) in the brain. It inhibits the breakdown and turnover of GABA, increases its release, and increases the density of the GABA-$\beta\beta$ receptor subtype.[2] Its mechanism of action in treating psychiatric disorders is unknown.

---

[1] Valproate is marketed in the British Commonwealth as 'valproic acid' and as 'sodium valproate' in the US, but these are effectively interchangeable as they both yield valproate in the bloodstream.

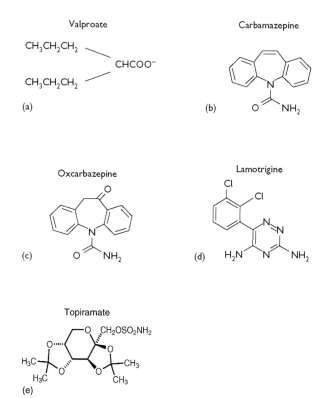

**Fig. 6.2.6.1** Molecular structures of selected antiepileptic drugs. (a) Valproate, (b) Carbamazepine, (c) Oxcarbazepine, (d) Lamotrigine, and (e) Topiramate.

## Pharmacokinetics

All preparations of valproate are completely absorbed after oral administration. The rate of absorption varies slightly with the different preparations, but these differences are probably not clinically significant. Co-administration with food can delay absorption. Valproate is approximately 90 per cent protein-bound. Only the unbound drug crosses the blood brain barrier and is pharmacologically active in the CNS. As total serum valproate concentration increases, the unbound portion of valproate is disproportionately increased, presumably due to saturation of the protein-binding sites. Therefore, at higher serum concentrations, small increases in dose may result in significant changes in efficacy and side effects. Valproate is metabolized by the liver to a glucuronide conjugate or one of several metabolites, some having antiepileptic activity. The half-life of valproate ranges from 6 to 17 h. Enzyme-inducing antiepileptic drugs, such as carbamazepine and phenytoin, shorten the half-life of valproate (see Interactions).[3]

## Side effects

Valproate is often associated with minor side effects, but can rarely cause life-threatening, idiosyncratic reactions. Common side effects include gastrointestinal symptoms, such as nausea, vomiting, abdominal pain, and diarrhoea; and neurological symptoms, such as tremor, somnolence, and dizziness. Weight gain is also common. Hair loss occurs in some patients, but is often transient and reversible upon discontinuation of the drug. Rare, but potentially fatal, idiosyncratic reactions include hepatic failure, acute haemorrhagic pancreatitis, and agranulocytosis.[2,4] Known risk factors for irreversible hepatic failure include young age (especially less than 2 years old), developmental delay, a metabolic disorder, or concomitant administration of other antiepileptic drugs.[5]

Because of this risk, liver function tests are recommended prior to initiation of therapy and periodically thereafter (see Dosage and Administration).

## Toxic effects

### (a) Overdose

Overdose with valproate can result in heart block, coma, and death. Haemodialysis may be useful in clearing the drug rapidly, and naloxone may reverse the CNS depressant effects.[3]

### (b) Pregnancy

Valproate increases the risk of neural tube defects (such as spina bifida) to approximately 1–2 per cent of pregnancies when administered in the first trimester. Other reported congenital anomalies include craniofacial defects and cardiovascular malformations. Valproate is found in human breast milk, at approximately 1–10 per cent of serum concentrations, but its effects on the nursing child are unknown.[6]

## Indications and contraindications

Controlled trials confirm that valproate is effective in the treatment of multiple seizure types, including complex partial, simple and complex absence, generalized tonic–clonic, and myoclonic seizures.[3] Several controlled studies indicate efficacy in the treatment of acute mania,[7–13] mixed episodes,[12,14] and in the prophylaxis of recurrent mood episodes.[13,15,16] One small controlled study has offered limited evidence for the efficacy of valproate in the treatment of bipolar depression.[17] There is growing support from controlled studies for the efficacy of valproate, combined with both typical and atypical antipsychotics, in the treatment of acute exacerbations of schizophrenia[18,19]; particularly when the presentation includes agitation and hostility.[20] There are also several small controlled studies demonstrating the benefit of valproate in the treatment of mood instability and impulsivity associated with borderline personality disorder.[21–23] Other conditions for which valproate may sometimes be useful include pain syndromes, anxiety disorders, alcohol and sedative withdrawal syndrome, impulse control disorders, and behavioural and affective disturbances associated with intellectual disability and dementia.[2]

Valproate is contraindicated in patients with known hypersensitivity to the drug. It should be used cautiously in patients with significant hepatic disease.

## Interactions

In general, valproate can be combined safely with other psychotropic medications and antiepileptic drugs. However, given that valproate is highly protein-bound and can inhibit hepatic enzymes, some drug–drug interactions have been identified.[3] **Aspirin**, which is highly protein-bound, elevates the free fraction of valproate, resulting in increased effects of valproate on the CNS. Valproate can displace **diazepam, phenytoin, carbamazepine**, and **warfarin** from protein-binding sites, resulting in increased activity of these drugs. Co-administration of valproate with **lamotrigine** significantly increases the half-life of the latter and can increase the risk of lamotrigine-induced rashes. When administered with **carbamazepine**, three potential interactions may occur: (1) valproate can increase the concentration of carbamazepine's metabolite, carbamazepine-10,11-epoxide, by inhibiting its further metabolism; (2) carbamazepine may lower the valproate level; and (3) valproate may increase the carbamazepine level.[24] Therefore, close monitoring of serum concentrations of both drugs is important when they are combined. **Amitriptyline** and **fluoxetine** may increase serum valproate concentrations, possibly by inhibition of valproate metabolism.

### Effects of withdrawal

As with other antiepileptic drugs, valproate should be tapered gradually over several weeks to minimize the risk of rebound seizures.

### Dosage and administration

Before initiating treatment with valproate, it is advisable to obtain a baseline complete blood count (CBC), liver function tests (LFTs), and if appropriate, a pregnancy test. CBC and liver function tests should be performed monthly for the first 3 months, and, if no abnormalities are found, every 6 to 12 months thereafter. If hepatic transaminase levels increase to more than three times normal, valproate should be discontinued. If the transaminase levels eventually return to baseline and the patient responded to valproate previously, re-challenge can be considered. If hepatic transaminase levels increase, but are less than three times normal, monitoring should be increased to once every 1–2 weeks until transaminase levels stabilize, and then monthly thereafter.[2]

The initial starting dose of valproate in adults is 250 to 1000 mg per day, given in two or three divided doses (see Table 6.2.6.1 for dosage forms). The dose may be increased every 1–3 days depending on the patient's response and tolerance. The usual therapeutic concentration is between 50–100 μg/ml (drawn 12 h after the last dose) for both psychiatric and neurological disorders. Some clinicians give the entire daily dose of valproate at bedtime. In patients with seizure disorders or acute mania, an oral loading strategy can be used.[25] In this situation, the patient receives 20 mg/kg as a bolus on the first day, resulting in rapid achievement of therapeutic levels. However, psychiatric patients who are not acutely manic usually have difficulty tolerating the oral loading strategy.

## Carbamazepine

### Introduction

Carbamazepine (Tegretol®) is an iminostilbene derivative with a structure similar to the tricyclic antidepressant imipramine (see Fig. 6.2.6.1). It was initially developed as a potential antidepressant in the 1950s, but was found to have antiepileptic and analgesic properties, and has been marketed for the treatment of seizures and pain syndromes since 1963. For many clinicians, it has been the preferred treatment for partial and generalized tonic–clonic seizures, as well as neuropathic pain. Its clinical use in affective disorders began in the early 1970s; since then, it has become widely used in psychiatry.

### Pharmacology

Carbamazepine's mechanism of action in the treatment of seizures and pain syndromes is controversial, but probably results from blockade of voltage-sensitive sodium channels or enhancement of gamma-aminobutyric acid (GABA) activity. Its mechanism of action in psychiatric disorders is unknown, and may be different, given that it affects numerous neurotransmitter systems.[26,27]

### Pharmacokinetics

Carbamazepine is absorbed slowly, with peak plasma levels occurring 4–5 h after administration of the tablets. Absorption is

**Table 6.2.6.1** Available dosage forms of antiepileptic drugs

| Drug (proprietary name) | Preparation |
|---|---|
| Valproate | |
| Valproate (Depakene) | 250 mg capsule |
| Valproate syrup (Depakene syrup) | 250 mg/5 ml |
| Divalproex sodium (Depakote) | 125, 250, and 500 mg tablets |
| Divalproex sodium extended release (Depakote ER) | 250, 500 mg tablets |
| Divlaproex sodium sprinkle capsules | 125 mg capsule |
| Carbamazepine | |
| Carbamazepine (Tegretol®) | 100, 200 mg tablets; 100 mg chewable tablets; suspension of 100 mg/5 ml |
| Carbamazepine extended-release tablets | |
| (Tegretol XR®) | 100, 200, and 400 mg tablets |
| (Carbatrol®) | 100, 200, and 300 mg capsules |
| (Equetro®) | 100, 200, and 300 mg capsules |
| Oxcarbazepine (Trileptal®) | 150, 300 and 600 mg tablets; suspension of 300 mg/5 ml |
| Lamotrigine (Lamictal®) | 25, 100, 150, and 200 mg tablets; 2, 5, and 25 mg chewable tablets |

faster for the carbamazepine liquid, and slower for carbamazepine extended-release tablets. Oral bioavailability is about 80 per cent; plasma protein binding is approximately 75 per cent. The half-life of carbamazepine is variable, as it induces its own metabolism with chronic administration (autoinduction). Initially, the half-life ranges from 18–65 h, but after autoinduction is complete (usually 3–5 weeks), it is decreased to 5–25 h. Children metabolize carbamazepine more rapidly than adults, and therefore require higher doses to achieve similar levels. Carbamazepine is metabolized in the liver by the cytochrome $P_{450}$ system to a wide variety of metabolites, some with antiepileptic activity. The predominant metabolite, carbamazepine-10, 11-epoxide (CBZ-E), is further metabolized by epoxide hydrolase to an inactive form. Most of carbamazepine's metabolites are excreted as glucuronide conjugates in the urine.[28,29]

### Side effects

Carbamazepine is generally well tolerated, with less than 5 per cent of patients discontinuing the medication because of adverse effects. Common side effects seen during initiation of treatment include dizziness, ataxia, sedation, nausea, and diplopia. These are often mild in severity, and frequently resolve with continued treatment.

#### (a) Haematological side effects

Carbamazepine commonly causes a benign suppression of white blood cell count, but in rare cases may cause severe and potentially fatal blood dyscrasias, including agranulocytosis, pancytopenia, and aplastic anaemia. The incidence of these non-dose-related, idiosyncratic reactions has been estimated to range between 1 in 10 000 to 1 in 300 000.[4]

#### (b) Hepatic toxicity

Carbamazepine is frequently associated with benign transaminase elevations. Very rarely, a non-dose-related, idiosyncratic reaction causes hepatic failure, which can be fatal.

### (c) Cardiovascular effects

Carbamazepine slows intracardiac conduction, and is relatively contraindicated in patients with heart block.

### (d) Dermatologic effects

Rashes occur in 5–15 per cent of patients. These are usually benign, but rarely lead to exfoliative dermatitis, Stevens–Johnson syndrome, or toxic epidermal necrolysis. Therefore, it is usually recommended that the drug be discontinued if any rash develops.

### (e) Endocrine effects

Carbamazepine can exert antidiuretic effects, which result in hyponatremia in 5–40 per cent of patients.[30] Usually, this effect is clinically insignificant.

Carbamazepine can result in decrease in free $T_3$ and $T_4$, but clinical hypothyroidism is extremely rare.

## Toxic effects

### (a) Overdose

Carbamazepine overdose can be fatal. Common symptoms include nystagmus, tremor, ophthalmoplegia, and myoclonus. Life-threatening effects include atrioventricular block, coma, seizures, and respiratory depression.[31]

### (b) Pregnancy

Carbamazepine exposure in the first trimester results in neural tube defects in approximately 1 per cent of infants. Craniofacial abnormalities and developmental delay have been reported as well. Carbamazepine is found in breast milk, but its effects on the nursing infant are unknown.[6,32]

## Indications and contraindications

Carbamazepine is indicated for the treatment of simple partial, complex partial, and generalized tonic–clonic seizures. It is ineffective against absence seizures, and may even exacerbate them. Carbamazepine is also indicated in the treatment of trigeminal neuralgia and other neuropathic pain syndromes. Several double-blind, placebo-controlled trials confirm carbamazepine's efficacy in treating both the manic and mixed phase of bipolar disorder.[33,34] There is limited evidence demonstrating efficacy in the treatment of either bipolar or unipolar depression. Uncontrolled reports also suggest that carbamazepine may be useful in the treatment of personality disorders, impulse control disorders, and alcohol/sedative withdrawal syndrome.

Carbamazepine is contraindicated in patients with a history of previous bone marrow depression, hypersensitivity to the drug, or hypersensitivity to any of the tricyclic antidepressants (given its structural similarity to imipramine). Its use with monoamine oxidase inhibitors is not recommended, and carbamazepine should be used with caution in patients with cardiac disease.

## Interactions

Given that carbamazepine is extensively metabolized by the liver and induces hepatic enzymes, it produces many significant drug–drug interactions (Table 6.2.6.2).[35–37] Many drug levels are reduced by carbamazepine and can become subtherapeutic. Therefore, it is important to monitor concomitantly administered medications, as dosage adjustments may be necessary.

**Table 6.2.6.2** Carbamazepine (CBZ)-drug interactions

| CBZ decreases drug levels | Drugs that increase CBZ levels |
|---|---|
| Alprazolam | Acetazolamide |
| Clobazam | Cimetidine |
| Clonazepam | Clarithromycin |
| Clozapine | Danazol |
| Dicoumarol | Dextropropoxyphene |
| Doxycycline | Diltiazem |
| Ethosuximide | Fluoxetine |
| Fentanyl | Gemfibrozil |
| Haloperidol | Isoniazid |
| Imipramine | Itraconazole |
| Lamotrigine | Ketaconazole |
| Mesuximide | Loratadine |
| Methadone | Macrolide antibiotics |
| Methylprednisolone | Metronidazole |
| Oral contraceptives (can result in contraceptive failure) | Nicotinamide |
| | Nicotinic acid |
| Pancuronium | Propoxyphene |
| Paracetamol | Remacemide |
| Phensuximide | Rifampicin |
| Phenytoin (can either increase or decrease) | Stiripentol |
| | Terfenadine |
| Prednisolone | Valproate |
| Primidone | Verapamil |
| Remacemide | Viloxazine |
| Theophylline | |
| Tiagabine | |
| Topiramate | |
| Valproate | |
| Vecuronium | |
| Warfarin | |

| CBZ increases drug levels | Drugs that decrease CBZ levels |
|---|---|
| Clomipramine (possibly) | Cisplatin |
| Phenytoin (can either increase or decrease) | Doxorubicin |
| | Felbamate |
| Primidone | Rifampicin |
| | Phenobarbital |
| | Phenytoin |
| | Primidone |
| | Theophylline |

## Effects of withdrawal

As with other antiepileptic drugs, carbamazepine should be gradually tapered over several weeks in order to avoid rebound seizures.

## Dosage and administration

Carbamazepine is generally initiated at a starting dose of 100–400 mg, taken either as a single dose or two divided doses (see Table 6.2.6.1 for dosage forms). The dose is gradually increased by 100 or 200 mg every 2 weeks as the patient tolerates. The usual therapeutic serum concentration is 4–12 mg/l (20–50 μmol/l), which is measured before the first morning dose. The half-life of carbamazepine will decrease with chronic administration due to autoinduction, necessitating frequent monitoring of the serum carbamazepine concentrations and continued dosage adjustment in the first 2 months of therapy.

### Laboratory screening

Given the risk of severe blood dyscrasias and hepatic failure, some authorities recommend obtaining a CBC and LFTs at the initiation of treatment. These tests are often repeated every 2 weeks for the first few months of treatment, and then every 3 to 6 months thereafter. However, some authorities argue that testing is unnecessary, since idiosyncratic reactions are rare and may occur too rapidly to be detected by routine laboratory monitoring.

## Lamotrigine

### Introduction

Lamotrigine (Lamictal®) is a phenyltriazine compound, structurally unrelated to other antiepileptic drugs (see Fig. 6.2.6.1). It was introduced in Ireland in 1993 and in the United Kingdom and the United States in 1994.

### Pharmacology

Lamotrigine is thought to act by blocking voltage-sensitive sodium channels, and by inhibiting the release of glutamate. In experimental animal seizure models, it has an antiepileptic profile similar to that of phenytoin and carbamazepine.[38]

### Pharmacokinetics

The oral bioavailability of lamotrigine approaches 100 per cent, and absorption is unaffected by food. Peak plasma concentrations are reached 2–3 h after an oral dose. The half-life of lamotrigine is approximately 30 h, but is altered by the presence of other antiepileptic drugs (see Interactions). Plasma protein binding is approximately 55 per cent. Lamotrigine is metabolized by the liver to an inactive glucuronide conjugate, and then excreted in the urine. The clearance of lamotrigine may be reduced in patients with renal impairment and Gilbert's syndrome, and these individuals may benefit from dosage reduction.[39]

### Side effects

In general, lamotrigine has few side effects and is better tolerated than other antiepileptic drugs. The most common side effects include dizziness, headache, diplopia, ataxia, blurred vision, nausea, somnolence, and rash. The most concerning side effect is skin rash, which can be life-threatening. Approximately 10 per cent of adults develop a rash while taking lamotrigine, but the majority of these are benign. However, about 1 in 1000 will develop a life-threatening rash, such as Stevens–Johnson syndrome or toxic epidermal necrolysis. The incidence of rash is much higher in paediatric patients, occurring in 1 in 50 to 1 in 100 patients; therefore, lamotrigine should be used with caution in patients less than 16 years of age. Starting at a low dose and slowly increasing it can minimize the risk of rash. Co-administration of valproate can increase the risk of rash. Given the difficulty in predicting who will develop a life-threatening rash, lamotrigine is usually discontinued at the first sign of any rash.

There are a few reports of possible idiosyncratic reactions in patients taking lamotrigine. These include disseminated intravascular coagulation, multiorgan failure, and acute hepatic necrosis.[40] It is unclear, however, if these conditions were actually caused by the drug itself.

### Toxic effects

#### (a) Overdose

The few reported cases of overdose on lamotrigine (at doses up to 4000 mg) were not fatal, but resulted in symptoms such as excessive sedation, dizziness, and headache.

#### (b) Pregnancy

The effects of lamotrigine on human pregnancy and breast-fed infants are unknown.

### Indications and contraindications

Several double-blind, placebo-controlled, add-on trials confirm lamotrigine's efficacy in treating some patients with partial or generalized tonic–clonic seizures.[39] Clinical trials also suggest efficacy against absence, atypical absence, and myoclonic seizures, as well as seizures associated with the Lennox–Gastaut syndrome.[41] Lamotrigine demonstrated efficacy in the treatment of bipolar depression in a large placebo-controlled trial.[42] However, it does not appear to be beneficial in the treatment of acute mania, largely due to the drug's long titration schedule. Several controlled studies have also demonstrated efficacy in the maintenance treatment of bipolar disorder.[39,43–45] and in the rapid-cycling subtype of bipolar disorder.[46] In addition to bipolar depression, lamotrigine has shown some benefit in two small placebo-controlled studies when added to selective serotonin reuptake inhibitors (SSRIs) as an augmentation strategy in the treatment of unipolar depression.[47,48] Preliminary evidence from two small placebo-controlled studies also indicates that lamotrigine may have benefit as an augmentation therapy with conventional and atypical antipsychotics in treatment-resistant schizophrenia.[49,50]

### Interactions

Lamotrigine does not appear to affect the kinetics of other antiepileptic drugs or oral contraceptives, but its own kinetics are markedly affected by the concomitant administration of other antiepileptic drugs. Valproate inhibits the metabolism of lamotrigine, resulting in a doubling of the half-life to almost 60 h. The enzyme-inducing antiepileptic drugs, such as carbamazepine and phenytoin, decrease the half-life to approximately 15 h. These interactions necessitate dosage adjustments when starting lamotrigine (see Dosage and Administration).[38]

### Effects of withdrawal

As with other antiepileptic drugs, lamotrigine should be tapered gradually over several weeks in order to avoid rebound seizures.

### Dosage and administration

Lamotrigine must be started at a low dose and increased with caution to a therapeutic dosage in order to minimize the risk of rash. The patient should be informed of the risk of developing a rash, and instructed to contact the physician immediately if one appears. The starting dose depends upon the concomitant administration of other antiepileptic drugs. See Tables 6.2.6.3–6.2.6.5 for the appropriate lamotrigine titration schedules. Table 6.2.6.1 shows dosage forms.

**Table 6.2.6.3** Suggested lamotrigine titration schedule for patients taking carbamazepine, phenytoin, phenobarbital, primidone, or rifampicin and not taking valproate

| | |
|---|---|
| Week 1 | 25 mg daily |
| Week 2 | 50 mg daily |
| Week 3 | 100 mg daily, in divided doses |
| Week 4 | 100 mg daily, in divided doses |
| Week 5 | 200 mg daily, in divided doses |
| Week 6 | 300 mg daily, in divided doses |
| Week 7 | Up to 400 mg daily, in divided doses |

**Table 6.2.6.4** Suggested lamotrigine monotherapy for patients not taking carbamazepine, phenytoin, phenobarbital, primidone, or rifampicin and not taking valproate

| | |
|---|---|
| Week 1 | 12.5 mg daily |
| Week 2 | 25 mg daily |
| Week 3 | 50 mg daily |
| Week 4 | 50 mg daily |
| Week 5 | 100 mg daily |
| Week 6 | 150 mg daily |
| Week 7 | 200 mg daily |

**Table 6.2.6.5** Suggested lamotrigine titration schedule for patients taking valproate

| | |
|---|---|
| Week 1 | 12.5 mg every *other* day |
| Week 2 | 25 mg every *other* day |
| Week 3 | 25 mg daily |
| Week 4 | 25 mg daily |
| Week 5 | 50 mg daily |
| Week 6 | 75 mg daily |
| Week 7 | 100 mg daily |

# Topiramate

## Introduction

Topiramate (Topamax®) is a sulfamate-substituted monosaccharide originally developed as an oral hypoglycemic agent. It was subsequently found to have antiepileptic effects. It is currently approved for epilepsy in over 60 countries and for migraine prophylaxis in more than 20 countries.

## Pharmacology

Topiramate is believed to act through several different mechanisms including: (1) inhibition of sodium channel conductance; (2) inhibition of L-type calcium channels; (3) increase in GABA release through an unknown mechanism; (4) decrease in glutamate-mediated excitation through blockade of kainate receptors; and (5) inhibition of carbonic anhydrase.[51]

## Pharmacokinetics

There is almost complete, linear, and rapid absorption of topiramate across dose ranges.[52] The absorption of topiramate is not affected by food. It is not significantly protein-bound. Hepatic metabolism (~20 per cent) is less important than renal clearance (~80 per cent) and inactive metabolites comprise less than 5 per cent the administered dose.[52] The normal half-life of topiramate is 19–23 h; this is not influenced by the administration of hepatic enzyme-inducing medications such as carbamazepine or phenytoin.[52]

## Side effects

The most common side effects of topiramate are memory and concentration difficulties, paresthesias, somnolence, dizziness, anorexia, and weight loss. In clinical trials with topiramate, kidney stones are reported 2–4 times more frequently than in the general population, probably as a result of the drug's inhibition of carbonic anhydrase. Patients predisposed to developing kidney stones should maintain good hydration during topiramate therapy to minimize the risk of renal stone formation. Rarely, topiramate has been associated with acute myopia precipitating secondary angle closure glaucoma and with oligohidrosis leading to hyperthermia.

## Toxic effects

### (a) Overdose

Several cases of topiramate overdose have been recorded, with signs and symptoms including severe metabolic acidosis, convulsions, drowsiness, speech disturbance, blurred vision, diplopia, lethargy, tupor, hypotension, abdominal pain, agitation, and dizziness. The clinical consequences in most cases were not severe. However, deaths have occurred after poly-drug overdoses involving topiramate.

### (b) Pregnancy

The effects of topiramate on human pregnancy and breast-fed infants are unknown.

## Indications and contraindications

Topiramate has confirmed efficacy as monotherapy for partial-onset seizures or primary generalized tonic–clonic seizures for patients 10 years and older and as adjunctive therapy for the same seizure types, including seizures associated with Lennox–Gastault syndrome, in patients of age 2 and older.[52] In addition, several large controlled studies have demonstrated benefit in the prophylaxis of migraines.[53–55] It may also be helpful in the treatment of essential tremor and chronic pain syndromes. There are no large placebo-controlled studies investigating the use of topiramate as monotherapy for bipolar disorder. However, there is limited evidence from several small open-label studies for topiramate as an adjunctive treatment for both the depressive[56] and manic[57,58] phases of bipolar disorder. Controlled studies have demonstrated efficacy in eating disorders including binge eating disorder[52] and bulimia nervosa.[59] Given its ability to reduce weight, the utility of topiramate may be greatest as an adjunctive treatment in bipolar disorder with comorbid obesity. Several small placebo-controlled studies have also suggested that topiramate may have benefit in the treatment of alcohol dependence,[60] impulse control disorders such as pathological gambling,[61] and borderline personality disorder.[62]

## Interactions

Topiramate does not typically alter the metabolism of any other drugs. One important exception to this is that the effectiveness of the ethinylestradiol component of oral contraceptives is reduced when more than 200 mg of topiramate is prescribed daily.[52] Topiramate occasionally leads to a modest increase in phenytoin concentrations (0–25 per cent) and to modest increases in the clearance of risperidone, pioglitazone, and lithium.[52] Hydrochlorothiazide can lead to modest increases in serum concentration of topiramate.[52] Concomitant administration of topiramate and valproate has been associated with hyperammonemia with or without encephalopathy in patients who have previously tolerated either drug alone.

### Effects of withdrawal

As with other antiepileptic drugs, topiramate should be tapered gradually over several weeks in order to avoid rebound seizures.

### Dosage and administration

The recommended dose for monotherapy treatment of epilepsy in adults and children 10 years of age or older is 400 mg/day in two divided doses. It is recommended that therapy be initiated at 25–50 mg/day followed by titration to an effective dose in increments of 25–50 mg/week. The recommended total daily dose for migraine prophylaxis is 100 mg/day administered in two divided doses. In patients with renal impairment one-half of the usual adult dose is recommended.

## Other antiepileptics

Several other drugs with antiepileptic activity are currently under investigation in various psychiatric disorders, but have not as yet shown well-documented efficacy. Gabapentin (Neurontin®), a structural analog of gamma-aminobutyric acid (GABA), has been marketed for use as adjunctive therapy in the treatment of epilepsy since 1993 and also carries a clinical indication for postherpetic neuralgia. It displays a pharmacological profile similar to phenytoin and carbamazepine in animal seizure models.[63]

Several placebo-controlled trials confirm gabapentin's efficacy as adjunctive therapy in some patients with partial seizures, especially complex partial seizures and partial seizures with secondary generalization.[42] Additionally, several controlled studies have demonstrated benefit in the treatment of various pain syndromes, particularly neuropathic pain.[64,65] In a large, multicentre, controlled study gabapentin failed as an adjunctive treatment with lithium and/or valproate in the treatment of acute manic or mixed episodes, and actually performed significantly more poorly than placebo.[66] Since that time, however, a small controlled study has suggested that gabapentin may have efficacy as an adjunctive maintenance treatment for bipolar disorder.[67] Two small controlled studies have also demonstrated efficacy for gabapentin in the treatment of panic disorder[68] and social anxiety[69] respectively.

Oxcarbazepine (Trileptal®), the 10-keto analog of carbamazepine, has an antiepileptic effect similar to carbamazepine, but has fewer side effects, and has not been associated with severe blood dyscrasias. The drug also has fewer effects on hepatic enzyme activity, and hence causes fewer drug interactions. Given its similarity to carbamazepine, oxcarbazepine might be expected to be effective for the manic phase of bipolar disorder. However, despite some promising uncontrolled observations, there are as yet no large controlled trials of oxcarbazepine as monotherapy in adult bipolar

disorder. A large double-blind study of oxcarbazepine in children with manic or mixed episodes did not demonstrate efficacy.[70] Preliminary evidence from one small open-label study suggests that oxcarbazepine may also reduce the risk of relapse prevention in alcohol abuse.[71]

Zonisamide (Zonegran®) is an antiepileptic that causes carbonic anhydrase inhibition; it is somewhat similar in its pharmacologic profile to topiramate. Like topiramate, it frequently causes weight loss, and has been shown effective for weight loss in a controlled study of obese individuals with binge eating disorder.[72] It also increases the risk of kidney stones to at least the same degree as topiramate. Small open-label studies have suggested that zonisamide may be effective in the treatment of both the manic and depressed phases of bipolar disorder.[73,74]

Tiagabine (Gabitril®) is believed to exert its anticonvulsant effects by enhancing the effects of GABA. This is thought to occur through blockade of reuptake of GABA into presynaptic neurones. Tiagabine showed efficacy in the treatment of generalized anxiety disorder in a large double-blind study.[75] In addition, several small open-label studies have demonstrated preliminary evidence benefit in the treatment of posttraumatic stress disorder,[76] major depressive disorder with comorbid anxiety,[77] and as an augmentation therapy for generalized anxiety disorder.[78] Tiagabine demonstrated limited efficacy as an add-on treatment for treatment-refractory bipolar disorder in one small clinical case series.[79]

Levetiracetam (Keppra®) is a novel anticonvulsant with an unclear mechanism of action. It has demonstrated benefit in the treatment of social anxiety disorder in one small controlled study, warranting further investigation into this potential use.[80]

Pregabalin (Lyrica®) is a structural derivative of GABA. However, it does not act by altering GABA levels or by binding to the GABA receptor. The exact mechanism of action of pregabalin is unknown, although it is most likely related to its high affinity for the alpha$_2$-delta site on voltage-gated calcium channels. Pregabalin has shown promise as an anxiolytic. Three separate large placebo-controlled studies have demonstrated benefit with pregabalin in the treatment of generalized anxiety disorder.[81–83] Pregabalin also demonstrated efficacy in the treatment of social anxiety disorder in one large controlled study.[84]

It is important to note that soon after the completion of this text, the United States Food and Drug Administration released an alert recommending that patients taking antiepileptic drugs be closely monitored for changes in behavior that could indicate worsening of depression or the emergence of suicidal thoughts or behavior. This warning was based on a meta-analysis of placebo-controlled trials involving eleven antiepileptic medications, including both trials in epilepsy and trials in psychiatric disorders. This meta-analysis revealed that patients receiving antiepileptic drugs had approximately twice the risk of suicidal behavior or ideation (0.43%) compared to patients receiving placebo (0.22%).[85] Further investigation and analyses of this possible association are ongoing.

## Further information

McElroy, S.L. and Pope, H.G. Jr. (1988). *Use of anticonvulsants in psychiatry: recent advances.* Oxford Health Care, Clifton, NJ.

Muzina, D.J., El-Sayegh, S., and Calabrese, J.R. (2002). Antiepileptic drugs in psychiatry: focus on randomized controlled trials. *Epilepsy Research*, **50**(1–2), 195–202.

Weisler, R.H., Cutler, A.J., Ballenger, J.C., *et al.* (2006). The use of antiepileptic drugs in bipolar disorders: a review based on evidence from controlled trials. *CNS Spectrums*, **11**(10), 788–99.

Ovsiew, F. (2004). Antiepileptic drugs in psychiatry. *Journal of Neurology, Neurosurgery, and Psychiatry*, **75**(12), 1655–8.

# References

1. Lambert, P.A., Carraz, G., Borselli, S., *et al.* (1966). Action neuropsychotrope d'un nouvel anti-épileptique: le dépamide. *Annales Medico-psychologiques*, **124**, 707–10.

2. Pope, H.G. Jr. and McElroy, S.L. (1995). Valproate. In *Comprehensive textbook of psychiatry/VI* (6th edn) (eds. H. Kaplan and B. Sadock), pp. 2112–20. Williams & Wilkins, Baltimore.

3. Davis, R., Peters, D.H., and McTavish, D. (1994). Valproate. A reappraisal of its pharmacological properties and clinical efficacy in epilepsy. *Drugs*, **47**, 332–72.

4. Tohen, M., Castillo, J., Baldessarini, R.J., *et al.* (1995). Blood dyscrasias with carbamazepine and valproate: a pharmacoepidemiological study of 2,228 patients at risk. *The American Journal of Psychiatry*, **152**, 413–18.

5. Bryant, A.E. III and Dreifuss, F.E. (1996). Valproate hepatic fatalities. III. U.S. experience since 1986. *Neurology*, **46**, 465–9.

6. Chang, S.I. and McAuley, J.W. (1998). Pharmacotherapeutic issues for women of childbearing age with epilepsy. *The Annals of Pharmacotherapy*, **32**, 794–804.

7. American Psychiatric Association. (2002). Practice guideline for the treatment of patients with bipolar disorder. *The American Journal of Psychiatry*, **159**(Suppl. 4), 1–50.

8. Pope, H.G. Jr, McElroy, S.L., Keck, P.E. Jr., *et al.* (1991). Valproate in the treatment of acute mania. A placebo-controlled study. *Archives of General Psychiatry*, **48**, 62–8.

9. Kravitz, H. M. and Fawcett, J. (1994). Efficacy of divalproex vs lithium and placebo in mania. *The Journal of the American Medical Association*, **272**, 1005–6.

10. Bowden, C.L., Brugger, A.M., Swann, A.C., *et al.* (1994). Efficacy of divalproex vs lithium and placebo in the treatment of mania. The Depakote mania study group. *The Journal of the American Medical Association*, **271**, 918–24.

11. McElroy, S.L., Keck, P.E., Stanton, S.P., *et al.* (1996). A randomized comparison of divalproex oral loading versus haloperidol in the initial treatment of acute psychotic mania. *The Journal of Clinical Psychiatry*, **57**, 142–6.

12. Freeman, T.W., Clothier, J.L., Pazzaglia, P., *et al.* (1992). A double-blind comparison of valproate and lithium in the treatment of acute mania. *The American Journal of Psychiatry*, **149**, 108–11.

13. Tohen, M., Ketter, T.A., Zarate, C.A., *et al.* (2003). Olanzapine versus divalproex sodium for the treatment of acute mania and maintenance of remission: a 47-week study. *The American Journal of Psychiatry*, **160**(7), 1263–71.

14. Swann, A.C., Bowden, C.L., Morris, D., *et al.* (1997). Depression during mania. Treatment response to lithium or divalproex. *Archives of General Psychiatry*, **54**(1), 37–42.

15. Bowden, C.L., Calabrese, J.R., McElroy, S.L., *et al.* (2000). A randomized, placebo-controlled 12-month trial of divalproex and lithium in treatment of outpatients with bipolar I disorder. Divalproex Maintenance Study Group. *Archives of General Psychiatry*, **57**(5), 481–9.

16. Gyulai, L., Bowden, C.L., McElroy, S.L., *et al.* (2003). Maintenance efficacy of divalproex in the prevention of bipolar depression. *Neuropsychopharmacology*, **28**(7), 1374–82.

17. Davis, L.L., Bartolucci, A., and Petty, F. (2005). Divalproex in the treatment of bipolar depression: a placebo-controlled study. *Journal of Affective Disorders*, **85**(3), 259–66.

18. Casey, D.E., Daniel, D.G., Wassef, A.A., *et al.* (2003). Effect of divalproex combined with olanzapine or risperidone in patients with an acute exacerbation of schizophrenia. *Neuropsychopharmacology*, **28**(1), 182–92.

19. Wassef, A.A., Dott, S.G., Harris, A., *et al.* (2000). Randomized, placebo-controlled pilot study of divalproex sodium in the treatment of acute exacerbations of chronic schizophrenia. *Journal of Clinical Psychopharmacology*, **20**(3), 357–61.

20. Citrome, L., Casey, D.E., Daniel, D.G., *et al.* (2004). Adjunctive divalproex and hostility among patients with schizophrenia receiving olanzapine or risperidone. *Psychiatric Services*, **55**(3), 290–4.

21. Hollander, E., Allen, A., Lopez, R.P., *et al.* (2001). A preliminary double-blind, placebo-controlled trial of divalproex sodium in borderline personality disorder. *The Journal of Clinical Psychiatry*, **62**(3), 199–203.

22. Frankenburg, F.R. and Zanarini, M.C. (2002). Divalproex sodium in the treatment of women with borderline personality disorder and bipolar II disorder: a double-blind placebo-controlled pilot study. *The Journal of Clinical Psychiatry*, **63**(5), 442–6.

23. Hollander, E., Swann, A.C., Coccaro, E.F., *et al.* (2005). Impact of trait impulsivity and state aggression on divalproex versus placebo response in borderline personality disorder. *The American Journal of Psychiatry*, **162**(3), 621–4.

24. Bernus, I., Dickinson, R.G., Hooper, W.D., *et al.* (1997). The mechanism of the carbamazepine-valproate interaction in humans. *British Journal of Clinical Pharmacology*, **44**, 21–7.

25. Keck, P.E. Jr., McElroy, S.L., Tugrul, K.C., *et al.* (1993). Valproate oral loading in the treatment of acute mania. *The Journal of Clinical Psychiatry*, **54**, 305–8.

26. McElroy, S.L. and Keck, P.E. (1995). Antiepileptic drugs. In *The American psychiatric press textbook of psychopharmacology* (eds. A.F. Schwartzberg and C.B. Nemeroff), pp. 351–75. American Psychiatric Press, Inc., Washington, DC.

27. Post, R.M. (1995). Carbamazepine. In *Comprehensive textbook of psychiatry/VI* (6th edn) (eds. H. Kaplan and B. Sadock), pp. 1964–72. Williams & Wilkins, Baltimore.

28. Maxmen, J.S. and Ward, N.G. (1995). *Psychotropic drugs: fast facts* (2nd edn). W.W. Norton and Company, Inc., New York.

29. Levy, R.H. and Kerr, B.M. (1988). Clinical pharmacokinetics of carbamazepine. *The Journal of Clinical Psychiatry*, **49**(Suppl. 4), 58–61.

30. Van Amelsvoort, T., Bakshi, R., Devaux, C., *et al.* (1994). Hyponatremia associated with carbamazepine and oxcarbazepine therapy: a review. *Epilepsia*, **35**, 181–8.

31. Spiller, H.A., Krenzelok, E.P., and Cookson, E. (1990). Carbamazepine overdose: a prospective study of serum levels and toxicity. *Journal of Toxicology. Clinical Toxicology*, **28**, 445–58.

32. Hansen, D.K., Dial, S.L., Terry, K.K., *et al.* (1996). In vitro embryotoxicity of carbamazepine and carbamazepine-10,11-epoxide. *Teratology*, **54**, 45–51.

33. Weisler, R.H., Kalali, A.H., Ketter, T.A., and SPD417 Study Group. (2004). A multicenter, randomized, double-blind, placebo-controlled trial of extended-release carbamazepine capsules as monotherapy for bipolar disorder patients with manic or mixed episodes. *The Journal of Clinical Psychiatry*, **65**(4), 478–84.

34. Weisler, R.H., Keck, P.E. Jr, Swann, A.C., *et al.* (2005). Extended-release carbamazepine capsules as monotherapy for acute mania in bipolar disorder: a multicenter, randomized, double-blind, placebo-controlled trial. *The Journal of Clinical Psychiatry*, **66**(3), 323–30.

35. Ketter, T.A., Post, R.M., and Worthington, K. (1991). Principles of clinically important drug interactions with carbamazepine. I. *Journal of Clinical Psychopharmacology*, **11**, 198–203.

36. Ketter, T.A., Post, R.M., and Worthington, K. (1991). Principles of clinically important drug interactions with carbamazepine. II. *Journal of Clinical Psychopharmacology*, **11**, 306–13.

37. Spina, E., Pisani, F., and Perucca, E. (1996). Clinically significant pharmacokinetic drug interactions with carbamazepine. An update. *Clinical Pharmacokinetics*, **31**, 198–214.

38. Fitton, A. and Goa, K. (1995). Lamotrigine: an update of its pharmacology and therapeutic use in epilepsy. *Drugs*, **50**, 691–713.

39. Goodwin, G.M., Bowden, C.L., Calabrese, J.R., *et al.* (2004). A pooled analysis of 2 placebo-controlled 18-month trials of lamotrigine and lithium maintenance in bipolar I disorder. *The Journal of Clinical Psychiatry*, **65**(3), 432–41.

40. Calabrese, J.R., Bowden, C.L., Sachs, G.S., *et al.* (1999). A double-blind placebo-controlled study of lamotrigine monotherapy in outpatients with bipolar I depression. Lamictal 602 Study Group. *The Journal of Clinical Psychiatry*, **60**(2), 79–88.

41. Bowden, C.L., Calabrese. J.R., Sachs, G., *et al.* (2003). A placebo-controlled 18-month trial of lamotrigine and lithium maintenance treatment in recently manic or hypomanic patients with bipolar I disorder. *Archives of General Psychiatry*, **60**(4), 392–400.

42. Calabrese, J.R., Bowden, C.L., Sachs, G., *et al.* (2003). A placebo-controlled 18-month trial of lamotrigine and lithium maintenance treatment in recently depressed patients with bipolar I disorder. *The Journal of Clinical Psychiatry*, **64**(9), 1013–24.

43. McElroy, S.L., Zarate, C.A., Cookson, J., *et al.* (2004). A 52-week, open-label continuation study of lamotrigine in the treatment of bipolar depression. *The Journal of Clinical Psychiatry*, **65**(2), 204–10.

44. Goodwin, G.M., Bowden, C.L., Calabrese, J.R., *et al.* (2004). A pooled analysis of 2 placebo-controlled 18-month trials of lamotrigine and lithium maintenance in bipolar I disorder. *The Journal of Clinical Psychiatry*, **65**(3), 432–41.

45. Chattergoon, D.S., McGuigan, M.A., Koren, G., *et al.* (1997). Multiorgan dysfunction and disseminated intravascular coagulation in children receiving lamotrigine and valproic acid. *Neurology*, **19**, 1442–4.

46. Calabrese, J.R., Suppes, T., Bowden, C.L., *et al.* (2000). A double-blind, placebo-controlled, prophylaxis study of lamotrigine in rapid-cycling bipolar disorder. Lamictal 614 Study Group. *The Journal of Clinical Psychiatry*, **61**(11), 841–50.

47. Normann, C., Hummel, B., Scharer, L.O., *et al.* (2002). Lamotrigine as adjunct to paroxetine in acute depression: a placebo-controlled, double-blind study. *Journal of Clinical Psychiatry*, **63**(4), 337–44.

48. Barbosa, L., Berk, M., and Vorster, M. (2003). A double-blind, randomized, placebo-controlled trial of augmentation with lamotrigine or placebo in patients concomitantly treated with fluoxetine for resistant major depressive episodes. *The Journal of Clinical Psychiatry*, **64**(4), 403–7.

49. Tiihonen, J., Hallikainen, T., Ryynanen, O.P., *et al.* (2003). Lamotrigine in treatment-resistant schizophrenia: a randomized placebo-controlled trial. *Biological Psychiatry*, **54**(11), 1241–8.

50. Kremer, I., Vass, A., Gorelik, I., *et al.* (2004). Placebo-controlled trial of lamotrigine added to conventional and atypical antipsychotics in schizophrenia. *Biological Psychiatry*, **56**(6), 441–6.

51. van Passel, L., Arif, H., and Hirsch, L.J. (2006). Topiramate for the treatment of epilepsy and other nervous system disorders. *Expert Review of Neurotherapeutics*, **6**(1), 19–31.

52. McElroy, S.L., Arnold, L.M., Shapira, N.A., *et al.* (2003). Topiramate in the treatment of binge eating disorder associated with obesity: a randomized, placebo-controlled trial. *The American Journal of Psychiatry*, **160**(2), 255–61.

53. Diener, H.C., Tfelt-Hansen, T., Dahlof, C., *et al.* MIGR-003 study group. (2004). Topiramate in migraine prophylaxis-results from a placebo-controlled trial with propranolol as an active control. *Journal of Neurology*, **251**(8), 943–50.

54. McIntyre, R.S., Mancini, D.A., McCann, S., *et al.* (2002). Topiramate versus bupropion SR when added to mood stabilizer therapy for the depressive phase of bipolar disorder: a preliminary single-blind study. *Bipolar Disorder*, **4**, 207–13.

55. Chengappa, K.N., Rathore, D., Levine, J., *et al.* (1999). Topiramate as add-on treatment for patients with bipolar mania. *Bipolar Disorder*, **1**, 42–53.

56. Bahk, W.M., Shin, Y.C., Woo, J.M., *et al.* (2005). Topiramate and divalproex in combination with risperidone for acute mania: a

57. McElroy, S.L., Arnold, L.M., Shapira, N.A., *et al.* (2003). Topiramate in the treatment of binge eating disorder associated with obesity: a randomized, placebo-controlled trial. *The American Journal of Psychiatry*, **160**(2), 255–61.

58. Silberstein, S.D., Schmitt, J., Neto, W., *et al.* (2004). Topiramate in migraine prevention: results of a large controlled trial. *Archives of Neurology*, **61**(4), 490–5.

59. Hoopes, S.P., Reimherr, F.W., Hedges, D.W., *et al.* (2003). Treatment of bulimia nervosa with topiramate in a randomized, double-blind, placebo-controlled trial, 1. Improvement in binge and purge measures. *The Journal of Clinical Psychiatry*, **64**(11), 1335–41.

60. Johnson, B.A., Ait-Daoud, N., Akhtar, F.Z., *et al.* (2004). Oral topiramate reduces the consequences of drinking and improves the quality of life of alcohol-dependent individuals: a randomized controlled trial. *Archives of General Psychiatry*, **61**(9), 905–12.

61. Dannon, P.N., Lowengrub, K., Gonopolski, Y., *et al.* (2005). Topiramate versus fluvoxamine in the treatment of pathological gambling: a randomized, blind-rater comparison study. *Clinical Neuropharmacology*, **28**(1), 6–10.

62. Nickel, M.K., Nickel, C., Mitterlehner, F.O., *et al.* (2004). Topiramate treatment of aggression in female borderline personality disorder patients: a double-blind, placebo -controlled study. *The Journal of Clinical Psychiatry*, **65**(11), 1515–19.

63. Goa, K.L. and Sorkin, E.M. (1993). Gabapentin. *Drugs*, **46**, 409–27.

64. Serpell, M.G. and Neuropathic Pain Study Group. (2003). Gabapentin in neuropathic pain syndromes: a randomized, double-blind, placebo-controlled trial. *Pain*, **99**, 557–66.

65. Morello, C.M., Leckband, S.G., Stoner, C.P., *et al.* (1999). Randomized, double-blind study comparing the efficacy of gabapentin with amitriptyline on diabetic peripheral neuropathy pain. *Archives of Internal Medicine*, **159**, 1931–7.

66. Pande, A.C., Crockatt, J.G., Janney, C.A., *et al.* (2000). Gabapentin in bipolar disorder: a placebo-controlled trial of adjunctive therapy. *Bipolar Disorders*, **2**, 249–55.

67. Vieta, E., Manuel-Goikolea, J., Martinez-Aran, A., *et al.* (2006). A double-blind, randomized, placebo-controlled, prophylaxis study of adjunctive gabapentin for bipolar disorder. *The Journal of Clinical Psychiatry*, **67**, 473–7.

68. Pande, A.C., Pollack, M.H., Crockatt, J., *et al.* (2000). Placebo-controlled study of gabapentin treatment of panic disorder. *Journal of Clinical Psychopharmacology*, **20**(4), 467–71.

69. Pande, A.C., Davidson, J.R., Jefferson, J.W., *et al.* (1999). Treatment of social phobia with gabapentin: a placebo-controlled study. *Journal of Clinical Psychopharmacology*, **19**(4), 341–8.

70. Wagner, K.D., Kowatch, R.A., Emslie, G.J., *et al.* (2006). A double-blind, randomized, placebo-controlled trial of oxcarbazepine in the treatment of bipolar disorder in children and adolescents. *The American Journal of Psychiatry*, **163**(7), 1179–86.

71. Croissant, B., Diehl, A., Klein, O., *et al.* (2006). A pilot study of oxcarbazepine versus acamprosate in alcohol-dependent patients. *Alcoholism, Clinical and Experimental Research*, **30**(4), 630–5.

72. McElroy, S.L., Kotwal, R., Guerdjikova, A.I., *et al.* (2006). Zonisamide in the treatment of binge eating disorder with obesity: a randomized controlled trial. *The Journal of Clinical Psychiatry*, **67**(12), 1897–906.

73. McElroy, S.L., Suppes, T., Keck, P.E. Jr., *et al.* (2005). Open-label adjunctive zonisamide in the treatment of bipolar disorders: a prospective trial. *The Journal of Clinical Psychiatry*, **66**(5), 617–24.

74. Ghaemi, S.N., Zablotsky, B., Filkowski, M.M., *et al.* (2006). An open prospective study of zonisamide in acute bipolar depression. *Journal of Clinical Psychopharmacology*, **26**(4), 385–8.

75. Pollack, M.H., Roy-Byrne, P.P., Van Amerigen, M., *et al.* (2005). The selective GABA reuptake inhibitor tiagibine for the treatment of

randomized, open-label study. *Progress in Neuro-Psychopharmacology & Biological Psychiatry*, **29**, 115–21.

generalized anxiety disorder: results of a placebo-controlled study. *The Journal of Clinical Psychiatry*, **66**(11), 1401–8.

76. Connor, K.M., Davidson, J.R., Weisler, R.H., *et al.* (2006). Tiagabine for posttraumatic stress disorder: effects of open-label and double-blind discontinuation treatment. *Psychopharmacology*, **184**(1), 21–5.

77. Carpenter, L.L., Schecter, J.M., Tyrka, A.R., *et al.* (2006). Open-label tiagabine monotherapy for major depressive disorder with anxiety. *The Journal of Clinical Psychiatry*, **67**(1), 66–71.

78. Schwartz, T.L., Azhar, N., Husain, J., *et al.* (2005). An open-label study of tiagabine as augmentation therapy for anxiety. *Annals of Clinical Psychiatry*, **17**(3), 167–72.

79. Suppes, T., Chisholm, K.A., Dhavale, D., *et al.* (2002). Tiagabine in treatment refractory bipolar disorder: a clinical case series. *Bipolar Disorders*, **4**(5), 283–9.

80. Zhang, W., Connor, K.M., and Davidson, J.R. (2005). Levetiracetam in social phobia: a placebo controlled pilot study. *Journal of clinical Psychopharmacology*, **19**(5), 551–3.

81. Feitner, D.E., Crockatt, J.G., Dubovsky, S.J., *et al.* (2003). A randomized, double-blind, placebo-controlled, fixed-dose, multicenter study of pregabalin in patients with generalized anxiety disorder. *Journal of Clinical Psychopharmacology*, **23**(3), 240–9.

82. Rickels, K., Pollack, M.H., Feitner, D.E., *et al.* (2005). Pregabalin for treatment of generalized anxiety disorder: a 4-week, multicenter, double-blind, placebo-controlled trial of pregabalin and alprazolam. *Archives of General Psychiatry*, **62**(9), 1022–30.

83. Montgomery, S.A., Tobias, K., Zornberg, *et al.* (2006). Efficacy and safety of pregabalin in the treatment of generalized anxiety disorder: a 6-week, multicenter, randomized, double-blind, placebo-controlled comparison of pregabalin and venlafaxine. *The Journal of Clinical Psychiatry*, **67**(5), 771–82.

84. Pande, A.C., Feitner, D.E., Jefferson, J.W., *et al.* (2004). Efficacy of the novel anxiolytic pregabalin in social anxiety disorder: a placebo-controlled, multicenter study. *Journal of Clinical Psychopharmacoly*, **24**(2), 1419.

85. United States Food and Drug Administration (January 31, 2008). *Information for Healthcare Professionals - Suicidality and Antiepileptic Drugs.*

## 6.2.7 Drugs for cognitive disorders

Leslie Iversen

### Introduction

Cognitive disorders are among the most difficult of all nervous system illnesses to treat as they affect the most complex and least clearly understood aspects of brain function. Animal studies cannot accurately mirror the complexities of human cognition, and there are few, if any, animal models of human cognitive illnesses. As so few drugs have been found to exert clinically significant effects, animal models for testing novel cognition-enhancing agents have unknown predictive value. However, progress has been made in recent years with improved international agreement on the criteria used to approve new cognition-enhancing drugs, and the introduction of new drugs for the treatment of dementia.

### Alzheimer's disease

It is important to define the objective of drug treatment in this, the most common of all forms of senile dementia. Alzheimer's disease

(**AD**) is a progressive illness; drug treatment could treat the symptoms without influencing the course of the disease, or it might seek to delay or arrest the progressive cognitive deterioration which such patients suffer. Although the latter aim is the subject of intensive research in academic and industrial laboratories,[1] there are no drugs that target the underlying pathology, and only palliative treatments are, as yet, available.

The approval of new medicines for the symptomatic treatment of AD in recent years has led regulatory agencies to define more clearly what criteria should be used in assessing the clinical benefits derived from drug treatment. AD is a disease characterized by disturbances in higher cortical function, including disorders of recent memory, language function, praxis, visual perception, abstract thinking, and decision making. A variety of composite dementia assessments designed to provide an overall summary of cognitive status, for example the Mini Mental State Examination (**MMSE**), Alzheimer's Disease Assessment Scale-Cognition (**ADAS-Cog**), and the Brief Cognitive Rating Scale are used.[2] Most studies with cholinesterase inhibitors in AD have used ADAS-Cog (a 70-point scale), and a two to three-point improvement for the drug-treated group versus placebo at 6 months has generally been accepted. However, statistically significant, but small, drug-induced improvements in cognitive assessment scores do not necessarily represent a clinically significant improvement to the patient or to their doctor; they must be supplemented by evidence of clinical improvement, using some form of Clinical Global Impression of Change as an outcome measure, usually rated by a clinician on a seven-point scale.

The development of agreed scientific and clinical standards for the approval of new drugs has largely eclipsed most of the older drugs that had been used in the treatment of AD and other dementias, since none of them can meet these standards. The older drugs include a range of cerebral vasodilators (e.g. dihydroergotoxin, papaverine, isoxsuprine, cinnarizine) and the so-called 'nootropics' (e.g. piracetam, oxiracetam, aniracetam), which were widely used in some European countries, as well as the so-called 'metabolic enhancers' (e.g. idebenone and indeloxazine) which were popular for a while in Japan.

### Cholinergic agents

Attention has focused instead on the cholinergic agents. The 'cholinergic hypothesis' of dementia. was boosted by the discovery in the 1970s that cholinergic neurones are particularly damaged or absent from the brains of patients dying with AD, and that the extent of damage to the cholinergic system correlates with the severity of dementia in life.[3] In AD the damage appears to be particularly severe in the system of cholinergic neurones located deep in the forebrain in the nucleus basalis of Meynert, whose fibres branch extensively and innervate most areas of the cerebral cortex. This neuronal system forms part of the ascending reticular activating system, which plays a key role in the process of selective attention—essential for the laying down of new memories. Consequently, there has been considerable interest in the possibility that 'cholinergic replacement therapy' might relieve the symptoms of AD, in the same way that dopamine replacement therapy has successfully been employed in the treatment of Parkinson's disease. The most successful approach so far has been the use of inhibitors of the enzyme acetylcholinesterase.

**Inhibitors of acetylcholinesterase** have been known since the nineteenth century with the discovery of physostigmine, a plant product used as an arrow-tip poison. Irreversible organophosphate inhibitors of acetylcholinesterase were later developed as chemical warfare agents ('nerve gases'), and for more peaceful uses as insecticides. Despite their colourful past, low doses of this class of compounds have proved effective as cognitive enhancers in a wide range of animal tests, including those in which cholinergic function is deliberately impaired.[4] The first clinical trials in patients with AD were performed with physostigmine, and confirmed that the drug had significant beneficial effects on cognitive performance in AD patients.[5] However, it has limited usefulness because, although it is absorbed rapidly, it has only a very short half-life in plasma. This means that to obtain any sustained cognitive benefit it has to be given in doses that are sufficiently high to elicit a number of adverse side-effects; thus, the therapeutic window was very narrow.

Subsequently four other cholinesterase inhibitors with improved profiles have gained approval for use in AD: **tacrine, donepezil, rivastigmine, and galantamine**, but tacrine is no longer actively marketed owing to liver toxicity. Clinical data from several thousand patients with AD involved in trials with these cholinesterase inhibitors are now available.[6–8] The first of these to gain approval in 1997 was donepezil. Results of large-scale clinical trials with donezepil and the other cholinesterase inhibitors over periods of 15 and 24 weeks have yielded similar results for the three compounds in patients with mild to moderately severe AD. The drugs caused small but significant improvements in the ADAS-Cog, CIBIC, and MMSE scores. The most common side-effects were transient mild nausea, insomnia, and diarrhoea. Not all patients with AD will benefit from treatment with cholinesterase inhibitors; the proportion ranges from 30 to 50 per cent; although the clinical benefits of drug treatment in patients showing a response can persist for up to 24 months.

The approval of cholinesterase inhibitors for the treatment of Alzheimer's disease was an important landmark. They are reasonably well tolerated and produce significant, if modest, beneficial effects in patients with mild to moderately severe AD. However, they have not gained immediate and universal acceptance. In some countries (e.g. the United Kingdom) it has been argued that the drugs are too costly and provide at best only a modest improvement.

Some studies have also found the cholinesterase inhibitors to be effective in treating the cognitive deficits in vascular dementias, but the effects are small and less consistent. Rivastigmine has also been shown to have beneficial effects in treating the cognitive deficits in Parkinson's disease with dementia.[9] The cholinesterase inhibitors may thus find other applications as cognitive enhancers in conditions other than AD.

An alternative approach to cholinergic replacement therapy has been to develop **drugs that mimic acetylcholine** and act as agonists at the muscarinic cholinergic receptors in brain, but which, unlike acetylcholine itself, are bioavailable and brain-penetrant. Attention has focused on the discovery and development of muscarinic agonists that show selectivity for the $m_1$-receptor subtype, which is the predominant form present in the cerebral cortex. The most thoroughly studied cholinomimetic to date is xanomeline, a compound that acts as a highly potent and selective $m_1$-receptor agonist. Clinical effects were assessed in a multicentre study of 343 patients with AD.[10] Patients on the highest dose showed significant improvement when assessed using the ADAS-Cog scale and also showed a significant overall global improvement using CIBIC. In addition to cognitive improvements, patients receiving xanomeline also exhibited significant behavioural improvement, with dose-dependent reductions in vocal outbursts, suspiciousness, delusions, agitation, and hallucinations. Xanomeline is unlikely to be used in the treatment of AD because of its relatively short duration of action, but these results suggest that further research on cholinomimetics may still be justified.

An entirely different pharmacological approach is exemplified by the drug **memantine**, the first to be approved for the treatment of moderate to severe AD. Memantine is thought to act by virtue of its ability to block the NMDA sub-type of glutamate receptors in the brain. Clinical trials in AD showed small but significant beneficial effects on cognitive tests and in global clinical outcome, but curiously the effects were most notable in patients with advanced stage disease and less in patients with mild to moderate AD.[11] Although the effects of memantine are small, it remains the only effective treatment for advanced stage AD.

## Attention-deficit hyperactivity disorder

Attention-deficit hyperactivity disorder (**ADHD**) is one of the most thoroughly studied disorders in child psychiatry, and the increasingly common use of stimulant drugs to treat this disorder has become the focus of much public attention and debate in recent years.[12] ADHD is defined in terms of three key features: lack of sustained attention, impulsivity, and hyperactivity. According to the DSM-IV definition the diagnosis of ADHD now includes more than 10 per cent of children.[13]

Because of the interest in the drug treatment of ADHD, a number of assessment tools have been developed. These include the widely used Conners' Teacher Rating Scale, the Conners' Parent Rating Scale, and a variety of tests designed to measure hyperactivity, problem behaviour, attention, and other aspects of cognition, as well as academic performance.[14]

The most commonly used drugs are the psychostimulants **amfetamine** and **methylphenidate**. Methylphenidate (Ritalin®) is by far the most widely prescribed. In more than 100 published trials these drugs have been found to have significant beneficial effects on all three key symptoms of ADHD in approximately 70 per cent of the treated children, and also in an adult form of ADHD.[15] Amfetamine (Adderall®) is approved for treatment of adult ADHD (not licensed in UK).

The mechanism of action of all three agents is similar; they act principally as inhibitors of the dopamine-uptake mechanism in the brain and promote the release of this neurotransmitter, thus stimulating dopaminergic mechanisms. The drugs also act to an important extent on noradrenaline-containing neurones to promote an increased release of this monoamine.[16] This may be relevant;a selective inhibitor of the noradrenaline transporter in brain, **atomoxetine**, has been approved as the first non-scheduled stimulant for the treatment of ADHD in both children and adults.[17]

Another non-amfetamine **modafinil** is also non-scheduled and is widely used in the United States for the treatment of ADHD,[18] although the drug has not yet gained regulatory approval from FDA because of possible serious adverse skin reactions. The mode of action of modafinil is unknown but it is used for the treatment of narcolepsy.

It is paradoxical that stimulant drugs, whose actions include an ability to promote hyperactivity, should have a calming effect on hyperactive children. One explanation is that actions of these amfetamine derivatives show the 'rate dependency' typical of other central nervous system agents, i.e. they tend to stimulate low rates of behaviour and to suppress high rates.[19] An alternative view is that the relatively low doses of amphetamines used in the treatment of ADHD would not have stimulant effects even in normal healthy adults. There are few animal models that can be used in the study of psychostimulant use or ADHD. Mice that are genetically engineered to delete the genes for the dopamine and other monoamine transporters have proved valuable.[20] Animals which lack the dopamine transporter have elevated levels of dopamine in their brains and are behaviourally hyperactive. Paradoxically, d-amfetamine decreases activity in these animals, in keeping with the 'rate-dependency' hypothesis.[20]

The use of amfetamines, particularly methylphenidate, has increased rapidly during the past 30 years, particularly in the United States where in some states more than 10 per cent of school-age boys receive the drug.[12] The use of amfetamines in Europe has been at a much lower level so far, although their use in ADHD has also been increasingly rapidly.[12] In turn, such widespread use of psychostimulants creates problems about diversion and abuse.[12]

## Further information

'Cognition Enhancers' in Drugs Futures 2025—[www.foresight.gov.uk/Brain_Science_Addiction].

'Drug Treatment of Alzheimer's Disease', Royal College of Psychiatry—[www.rcpsych.ac.uk/mentalhealthinformation/olderpeople/drugtreatmentofalzheimers.aspk].

'Methylphenidate, atomoxetine and dexamfetamine for attention deficit hyperactivity disorder (ADHD) in children and adolescents—guidelines.' National Institute for Clinical Excellence UK, March 22, 2006. [http://www.nice.org.uk].

## References

1. Moreira, P.I., Zhu, X., Nunomura, A., et al. (2006). Therapeutic options in Alzheimer's disease. Expert Review of Neurotherapeutics, 6, 897–910.
2. Gershon, S., Ferris, S.H., Kennedy, J.S., et al. (1994). Methods for the evaluation of pharmacological agents in the treatment of cognitive and other deficits in dementia. In Clinical evaluation of psychotropic drugs: principles and guidelines (eds. R.F. Prien and D.S. Robinson), pp. 467–99. Raven Press, New York.
3. Bartus, R.T., Dean, R.L., Beer, B., et al. (1982). The cholinergic hypothesis of geriatric memory dysfunction. Science, 217, 408–17.
4. Rupniak, N.M.J., Steventon, M.J., Jennings, C.A., et al. (1989). Comparison of the effects of four cholinomimetic agents on cognition in primates following disruption by scopolamine. Psychopharmacology, 99, 189–95.
5. Giacobini, E. (1998). Cholinesterase inhibitors for Alzheimer's disease therapy: from tacrine to future applications. Neurochemistry International, 32, 413–19.
6. Birks, J. and Harvey, R.J. (2006). Donepezil for dementia due to Alzheimer's disease. Cochrane Database Systematic Reviews, (1), CD001190.
7. Loy, C. and Schneider, L. (2004). Galantamine for Alzheimer's disease. Cochrane Database Systematic Reviews, (4), CD001747.
8. Birks, J., Grimley Evans, J., Lakovidou, V., et al. (2006). Rivastigmine for Alzheimer's disease. Cochrane Database Systematic Reviews, (4), CD001191.
9. Maidment, I., Fox, C., and Boustani, M. (2006). Cholinesterase inhibitors for Parkinson's disease dementia. Cochrane Database Systematic Reviews, (1), CD004747.
10. Bodick, N.C., Offen, W.W., Levey, A.I., et al. (1997). Effects of xanomeline, a selective muscarinic receptor agonist, on cognitive function and behavioral symptom in Alzheimer's disease. Archives of Neurology, 54, 465–73.
11. McShane, R., Areosa Sastre, A., and Minakaran, N. (2006). Memantine for dementia. Cochrane Database Systematic Reviews, (2), CD003154.
12. Iversen, L.L. (2006). Speed, ecstasy, ritalin: the science of amphetamines. Oxford University Press, Oxford.
13. American Psychiatric Association. (2000). Diagnostic and statistical manual of mental disorders (4th edn, Text Revision) (DSM-IV-TR). American Psychiatric Association, Washington, DC.
14. Conners, C.K. (1998). Rating scales in attention deficit hyperactivity disorder: use in assessment and treatment monitoring. The Journal of Clinical Psychiatry, 59(Suppl. 7), 24–30.
15. Wender, P.H. (2001). ADHD: attention-deficit hyperactivity disorder in children, adolescents and adults. Oxford University Press, Oxford.
16. Solanto, M.V. (1998). Neuropsychopharmacological mechanism of stimulant drug action in attention-deficit hyperactivity disorder: a review and integration. Behavioural Brain Research, 94, 127–52.
17. Kratochvil, C.J., Vaughan, B.S., Daughton, J.M., et al. (2004). Atomoxetine in the treatment of attention deficit hyperactivity disorder. Expert Review of Neurotherapeutics, 4, 601–11.
18. White, R.F. and Giorgadze, A. (2006). A randomized, double-blind, placebo-controlled study of modafinil film-coated tablets in children and adolescents with attention-deficit hyperactivity disorder. Journal of the American Academy of Child and Adolescent Psychiatry, 45, 503–11.
19. Robbins, T.W. and Sahakian, B.J. (1979). Paradoxical effects of psychomotor stimulant drugs in hyperactive children from the standpoint of behavioural pharmacology. Neuropharmacology, 18, 931–50.
20. Gainetdinov, R.R., Sotnikova, T.D., and Caron, M.G. (2002). Monoamine transporter pharmacology and mutant mice. Trends in Pharmacological Sciences, 23, 367–73.

# 6.2.8 Drugs used in the treatment of the addictions

Fergus D. Law and David J. Nutt

Medical treatment of the addictions remains controversial, with addiction itself viewed as a lifestyle problem, a hijacking of brain systems by drugs, or as a medical illness. Many of these controversies may be avoided by taking a goal-oriented approach to treatment, in which clinical objectives are defined, and both medications and psychological interventions are used to facilitate progress towards these. The effectiveness of medications is maximized when they are used as one component of a comprehensive treatment plan.

There are no 'magic bullets' in addiction treatment—the same pharmacological principles apply to these drug treatments as to any other. Drugs need to be given in effective doses, at appropriate intervals, allowed time to reach steady state, and also to dissipate when terminated on the basis of their half-life. Some drugs also have an abuse potential of their own (e.g. opiates, sedative-hypnotics) especially those with a rapid onset of action, and such drugs need to be particularly closely monitored and controlled, to minimize their diversion and misuse.

## Medications in perspective

The clinical goal-oriented approach requires clarity about the clinical objectives at each phase of the treatment process. A typical treatment plan involves three primary clinical objectives:

- drug and psychosocial stabilization
- detoxification when appropriate
- prevention of relapse or recurrence.

Stabilization with a substitution treatment (e.g. methadone or buprenorphine in opiate addiction) involves prescribing a pharmacological equivalent to the abused drug to stop illicit use, crime, etc. It allows time for stabilization to occur and to consider later objectives. Stabilization itself may be either short-term with the primary goal of terminating illicit drug use 'on top' of the prescription, or longer-term where it is commonly known as maintenance. The goals of maintenance are either psychosocial stabilization in preparation for detoxification, or harm reduction in patients where abstinence is not practicable or safe. Unless a sufficient degree of stabilization has been achieved prior to detoxification, the chances of success are strictly limited. The harm-reduction goal has generated much controversy, but one of its major benefits is the reduction in the spread of HIV among injecting drug users. In this group stable long-term maintenance treatment is preferable to repeated cycles of premature discontinuation followed by relapse to uncontrolled drug use with its attendant elevated risk of death from overdose as tolerance wanes. Monitoring by using drug screens and clinical assessments is required to ensure that patients do not use 'on top' of their prescription.

## Specific drugs used in addiction treatment

This chapter deals with methadone, levacetylmethadol (LAAM), codeine and dihydrocodeine tartrate, buprenorphine, clonidine, lofexidine, naltrexone, naloxone, acamprosate, disulfiram, and clomethiazole (chlormethiazole), and covers addiction indications only. Many of these drugs are not licensed for use in addiction treatment (e.g. methadone tablets and injection), or are currently licensed in only one or a few countries (e.g. clonidine in Germany, lofexidine in the United Kingdom).

## Methadone[1,2] (Methadose®, Physeptone®, Synastone®)

This is a long-acting opioid analgesic which has been the mainstay of opioid substitution treatment, but is often difficult to stop due to its prolonged withdrawal syndrome.

**Pharmacology**: it is a strong full μ-opioid agonist.

**Types of compounds available**: it is available in liquid, injectable, and tablet formulations.

**Pharmacokinetics**: $t_{max}$ 2 to 4 h after oral dosing; 1 h after intramuscular injection; its half-life is 25 h.

**Side-effects**: as with other μ-opioids, its side-effects include mental blunting, sweating, constipation, nausea, and analgesia.

**Toxic effects**: acute overdose leads to respiratory depression and pulmonary oedema.

**Indications**: opiate maintenance, stabilization, and detoxification; it is also indicated for use during pregnancy.

**Contraindications**: respiratory or severe liver disease, monoamine oxidase inhibitors; caution should be exercised in elderly people.

**Interactions**: respiratory depression especially in combination with other sedative drugs; metabolism affected by hepatic enzyme induction and inhibition; plasma levels are affected by HAART drugs.

**Effects of withdrawal**: these include moderate but prolonged abstinence syndrome, especially poor sleep.

**Dosage and administration**: single daily dose, occasionally twice daily; dose depends on the level of dependence—if unknown, initially 10 to 20 mg daily. The minimum dose that covers withdrawal symptoms for 24 h should be given, and increased by 5 to 10 mg as necessary. Close monitoring is necessary by clinical assessment and drug screen. Some centres use intravenous preparations in those who don't respond to oral preparations.

## LAAM[3] (ORLAAM®)

LAAM is a methadone variant with a much longer half-life, requiring only three visits a week for full supervision of medication. However, take-home medication is not allowed and its use is restricted to specialist clinics and is reserved for patients who have failed other treatments. Its licence in Europe has been withdrawn due to QTc prolongation.

**Pharmacology**: it is a synthetic μ-opioid agonist with active metabolites which are more potent than the parent drug.

**Types of compounds available**: aqueous solution.

**Pharmacokinetics**: $t_{max}$ 2 to 4 h; duration of action is 48 to 72 h; half-lives for LAAM and its metabolites are 2 to 4 days; it takes 2 weeks to reach steady state.

**Side-effects**: too rapid escalation of the dose may result in sedation, orthostatic hypotension, poor concentration, and overdose.

**Toxic effects**: as for methadone; QTc prolongation; overdose occurs with too frequent (daily) dosing, use of multiple drugs, or 'on-top' use due to impatience with its slow onset of action.

**Indications**: opiate maintenance, stabilization, and detoxification.

**Contraindications**: pregnancy (transfer to methadone); QTc prolongation prior to induction of treatment; dose should be reduced in elderly people, and in renal and hepatic impairment.

**Interactions**: as for methadone; other drugs prolonging QTc interval.

**Effects of withdrawal**: as for methadone, but with a milder withdrawal syndrome due to longer $t_{1/2}$.

**Dosage and administration**: pre-treatment ECG to identify prolonged QTc intervals, repeated 12–14 days after initiating treatment and periodically thereafter to rule out alterations to the QTc; give three times a week or on alternate days; increase dose by 20 to 40 per cent when transferring form 48 h to 72 h dosing interval. Transfer methadone to LAAM by giving 1.2 to 1.3 times the daily methadone dose; and LAAM to methadone by waiting at least 48 h and then giving 0.8 times the LAAM dose. If low or unknown tolerance, the initial dose is 20 to 40 mg three times weekly. Adjust dose in 5- to 10-mg steps, but no more frequently than weekly at the most. Strongly warn patients of the risk of supplementation with street drugs especially prior to steady state. LAAM is detected by urine screens for methadone.

## Buprenorphine[4,5] (Subutex®, Suboxone®, Temgesic®, Buprenex®)

Advantages over methadone and other full μ-agonists are its safety in overdose, the attenuation of the drug 'high' during on-top use, and its low levels of psychological reinforcement and withdrawal symptomatology during detoxification.

**Pharmacology**: a partial μ-opioid agonist, which explains the ceiling on respiratory depression; slow onset of action; dissociates slowly from the μ-receptor.

**Types of compounds available**: 0.2-, 0.4-, 2- or 8-mg sublingual tablets, or 0.3-mg ampoules for injection; it is also available in combination with naloxone in a 1:4 ratio (Suboxone®) to reduce misuse if diverted.

**Pharmacokinetics**: sublingual tablets absorbed rapidly into the buccal mucosa and released slowly into the blood stream; $t_{max}$ 2 to 6 h.

**Side-effects**: withdrawal symptoms if either too little or too much is given; nausea and vomiting are rare in addicts.

**Toxic effects**: as for methadone, but less constipation and respiratory depression.

**Indications**: opiate maintenance, stabilization, and detoxification, including in pregnancy; may be especially suitable for opioid antagonist-assisted withdrawal; no dosage adjustment needed in renal failure or elderly people.

**Contraindications**: severe respiratory disease; use with care in severe liver disease.

**Interactions**: rare; sedation with benzodiazepines.

**Effects of withdrawal**: there is a mild but delayed withdrawal syndrome.

**Dosage and administration**: initial dose is 0.8–4 mg increasing by 4 to 8 mg daily until the required dose level is reached; usual daily dose 8 to 32 mg; doses above 12 mg may be given on alternate days; minimize withdrawal symptoms after long-term use by reducing by 1 mg every 3 to 4 days or less often; buprenorphine-assisted heroin detoxification by rapid reduction over 5 to 10 days; the injectable form is not recommended for use in addiction treatment. Monitor clinical state and perform drug screens for compliance and on-top use.

## Codeine phosphate and dihydrocodeine tartrate[6,7] (DF118 Forte®, DHC Continus®)

Advantages over methadone occur in situations where long-acting opioids may be inappropriate. These are often preferred by patients, and by doctors treating the young, low-dose users, and in acute situations (e.g. in police custody). Disadvantages are its ease of misuse, high levels of psychological reinforcement due to its rapid onset of action, and its unfavourable side-effect profile.

**Pharmacology**: it is a weak short-acting μ-opioid agonist.

**Types of compounds available**: Codeine: 15-, 30- and 60-mg oral tablets, linctus, syrup and injection; dihydrocodeine tartrate: 30- or 40-mg oral tablets for use three to six times a day, and a 60-, 90-, or 120-mg slow-release preparation (DHC Continus) for use every 12 h; also parenteral preparation and elixir.

**Pharmacokinetics**: peak plasma levels at 1 to 2 h; half-life 3.5 to 4.5 h.

**Side-effects**: it is more likely to cause sedation, dizziness, stimulation, euphoria, constipation, histamine release, psychomimetic effects, and disturbing dreams than other opioids.

**Toxic effects**: precipitation of life-threatening exacerbations of asthma; in overdose, coma with myotonic twitching, grand mal convulsions, and rarely rhabdomyolysis may occur.

**Indications**: opiate maintenance, stabilization, and detoxification

**Contraindications**: acute exacerbations of asthma, lower respiratory tract infection, respiratory depression, and hepatic failure, increased intracranial pressure; caution should be exercised in renal impairment and elderly people.

**Interactions**: as for methadone; it may enhance the effects of warfarin.

**Effects of withdrawal**: mild withdrawal syndrome.

**Dosage and administration**: dose depends on level of dependence; monitor clinical state and urine screen to confirm compliance and termination of on-top use.

## Naltrexone[8–11] (Nalorex®, Opizone®)

Naltrexone is used to maintain abstinence in detoxified opiate addicts during the period of highest vulnerability to relapse following detoxification. It blocks the 'high' produced by opiates and promotes the extinction of conditioned responses. It also has a role in alcohol misuse and ultra-rapid opioid detoxification. Nalmefene is a related long-acting μ receptor antagonist that has a licence for alcoholism in some countries.

**Pharmacology**: it is a long-acting non-selective opioid antagonist.

**Type of compound available**: 50-mg oral tablet.

**Pharmacokinetics**: $t_{max}$ 1 h; duration of action is dose related, and a single dose can be effective for up to 48 h.

**Side-effects**: opiate withdrawal syndrome may occur on induction; occasionally, gastrointestinal irritation, headaches, arthralgia, flattening of mood, and rash occur.

**Toxic effects**: severe opioid withdrawal in dependent addicts lasting 2 days; reversible liver toxicity at high dose in obese and elderly people; liver function tests should be monitored especially if baseline tests are impaired.

**Indications**: prevention of impulsive relapse following detoxification in opioid users; opioid antagonist-assisted withdrawal; it reduces the reinforcing effects of alcohol.

**Contraindications**: acute hepatitis or liver failure, and active peptic ulcer; caution should be exercised in hepatic or renal impairment.

**Interactions**: competitive opioid blockade, so potentially can be overcome using very high opiate doses.

**Effects of withdrawal**: none, but risk of opioid overdoes following withdrawal (loss of toerance).

**Dosage and administration**: treatment initiated following LFTs and opioid-negative urine screen (or a negative naloxone challenge). Twenty-five mg is given on the first day, and then 50 mg daily for 3 to 6 months. Thrice-weekly dosing (100/100/150 mg) may occasionally improve compliance. Supervision of consumption by a supportive person, urine tests to monitor compliance, and regular reviews are very important in maximizing effectiveness.

## Naloxone[12] (Narcan®)

Naloxone is a short-acting antagonist used in the treatment of opioid overdose, during detoxification, and naltrexone induction. Take home naloxone may be used to treat opiate overdoses in the community by patients trained in its use.

**Pharmacology:** it is a short-acting competitive opioid antagonist.

**Types of compounds available:** it is available in injectable form for intramuscular, intravenous, or subcutaneous use.

**Pharmacokinetics:** half-life 1 to 2 h.

**Side-effects:** withdrawal in opiate-dependent subjects; nausea and vomiting; rarely, high blood pressure and pulmonary oedema can occur.

**Toxic effects:** very occasional deaths due to acute pulmonary oedema, extreme hypertension, and ventricular arrhythmias have occurred in those with known myocardial disease.

**Indications:** naloxone reverses the effects of opioid overdose, and in high doses may help in overdose due to alcohol and benzodiazepines. Naloxone is also occasionally used as the diagnostic test of opioid dependence, and as a challenge test prior to naltrexone initiation. It is also used for opioid antagonist-assisted withdrawal, and in combination with oral opiate agonists to reduce misuse by the injectable route (e.g. Suboxone®). In neonates it is used for the reversal of the effects of opioids given to mothers during labour.

**Contraindications:** none if not opioid dependent (safe in neonates, children, pregnancy, elderly people); caution is advisable in opioid dependence, painful conditions, and cardiovascular disease.

**Interactions:** severe hypertension following reversal of coma due to clonidine overdose.

**Effects of withdrawal:** none.

**Dosage and administration:** in opioid overdose, give 0.4 to 2 mg intravenously (5 to 10 µg/kg in neonates and children) and repeat at 2- to 3-min intervals until desired response; may also be given intramuscularly in overdose; lower doses are used in adults (0.1–0.2 mg) to reverse opioid-induced respiratory depression, but higher doses are needed with buprenorphine and σ-receptor agonists. Continue naloxone by infusion or repeated injection if necessary to maintain recovery. During naltrexone induction, give 0.2 mg parenterally followed by 0.8 mg 30 min later (or 0.6 mg 30 s later if given intravenously). In equivocal cases give 1.6 mg.

## Clonidine hydrochloride[13, 14] (Catapres®, Dixarit®)

Clonidine is an $\alpha_2$-adrenoceptor agonist used to suppress some symptoms of opioid withdrawal, especially methadone-assisted withdrawal. It is ineffective for subjective symptoms, muscle/bone aches, stomach cramps, and insomnia.

**Pharmacology:** clonidine is an antihypertensive agent that decreases central and peripheral (sympathetic) noradrenergic activity by stimulating presynaptic receptors in the locus coeruleus.

**Types of compounds available:** it is available as tablet, liquid, sustained release capsule, and transdermal preparation; the tablet is licensed in Germany.

**Pharmacokinetics:** $t_{max}$ 90 min; half-life of 20 to 25 h

**Side-effects:** it causes hypotension, sedation, dry mucous membranes, bradycardia, depression, impotence, constipation and diarrhoea, sleep disturbance, fluid retention, headache, euphoria, and Raynaud's phenomenon.

**Toxic effects:** a clonidine withdrawal syndrome may occur on abrupt withdrawal or non-compliance; paralytic ileus, psychotic features, or depression can also occur; coma or severe sedation can occur on acute overdose.

**Indications:** rapid opiate withdrawal and opiate antagonist-assisted withdrawal; it is also used as adjunct for alcohol, benzodiazepine, and nicotine withdrawal.

**Contraindications:** low baseline blood pressure, disorders of cardiac pacemaker activity and conduction, cardiovascular and cerebrovascular disease, and porphyria; caution is necessary in renal and hepatic impairment, peripheral vascular disease, and where there is a history of depression or psychosis.

**Interactions:** combinations with sedative drugs; phenothiazines may increase hypotension. Tricyclic antidepressants may block its effects.

**Effects of withdrawal:** an increase in sympathetic activity with symptoms mimicking the opiate withdrawal syndrome may occur 18 to 72 h after the last dose on abrupt termination. Blood pressure rebound is rare when used for less than 1 month. The effects are minimized by gradual withdrawal.

**Dosage and administration:** expertise is needed to monitor cardiovascular signs and adjust dose during a clonidine detoxification over 1 to 3 weeks. Start clonidine after discontinuation of the opioid. Following a test dose, 0.1 mg tablets are given four to six times daily building up to 2 mg daily over a few days in inpatients but half this dose in outpatients. Patches applied once weekly and supplemented by tablets if withdrawal symptoms occur. Frequent monitoring for hypotension and bradycardia is needed.

## Lofexidine[13–15] (BritLofex®)

Lofexidine is an analogue of clonidine, but easier to use because there is less hypotension and sedation.

**Pharmacology:** as for clonidine; differences occur possibly because it is more potent at the A subtype of $\alpha_2$-adrenoceptors.

**Types of compounds available:** 0.2-mg oral tablets; these are licensed in the United Kingdom only.

**Pharmacokinetics:** $t_{max}$ 3 h; half-life of 15 h.

**Side-effects:** these are the same as for clonidine, but with markedly less hypotension and other side-effects.

**Toxic effects:** as for clonidine; it has little rebound effect on blood pressure, and no psychiatric complications or misuse has been reported.

**Indications and contraindications:** as for clonidine.

**Interactions:** as for clonidine.

**Effects of withdrawal:** as for clonidine, but less rebound.

**Dosage and administration:** treat for 1 to 3 weeks; dose may be started before opiate is stopped; on day 1, give 0.8 mg in divided doses, and build up by 0.4 to 0.8 mg daily. Aim for a minimum of 1.6 mg daily in four divided doses, increasing to a maximum daily dose of 2.4 mg. Plan for a peak in the dose when the peak of withdrawal symptoms are expected. Blood pressure should be monitored 2 h after the initial dose, and daily as the dose is increasing. After peak opiate withdrawal lofexidine should be withdrawn gradually over at least 2–4 days. The dose should be reduced by 0.2–0.4 mg daily.

## Acamprosate (calcium acetylhomotaurinate)[16,17] (Campral EC®)

Acamprosate is a non-aversive agent used to maintain abstinence in alcohol-dependent patients during the most vulnerable period following detoxification, which may work as an anticraving agent.

**Pharmacology**: this is not fully understood. It affects the brain's γ-aminobutyric acid (inhibitory) and glutamate (excitatory) systems.

**Types of compounds available**: oral enteric-coated tablets containing 333 mg acamprosate.

**Pharmacokinetics**: $t_{max}$ 5 h; half-life 21 h; steady state after 7 days.

**Side-effects**: there are a range of dose-related side-effects which are mainly mild and transient, including diarrhoea and other gastrointestinal effects, pins and needles in the limbs, skin pruritus, confusion, and sexual effects. Transient reductions in blood pressure occur in those with alcohol-induced hepatic cirrhosis.

**Toxic effects**: hypercalcaemia is a theoretical possibility following overdose.

**Indications**: maintenance of abstinence following alcohol detoxification; it is suitable for use in those with liver dysfunction.

**Contraindications**: renal impairment and severe hepatic failure.

**Interactions**: concomitant food decreases bioavailability.

**Effects of withdrawal**: none.

**Dosage and administration**: begin treatment as soon as possible after detoxification, and continue for 1 year. Four tablets a day (2–1–1) with meals if body weight is less than 60 kg, but six tablets a day (2–2–2) if over 60 kg. The drug should be continued during alcohol relapses.

## Disulfiram[18–20] (Antabuse®)

An unpleasant disulfiram-ethanol reaction occurs when alcohol is consumed, acting as a deterrent or punishment if drinking occurs. Disulfiram is used under specialist supervision during periods of vulnerability to relapse.

**Pharmacology**: disulfiram is an aldehyde dehydrogenase inhibitor leading to the accumulation of acetaldehyde after ethanol consumption.

**Types of compounds available**: 200-mg oral tablets.

**Pharmacokinetics**: inhibition of alcohol dehydrogenase develops slowly over 12 to 24 h and peaks at 48 h.

**Side-effects**: relatively non-toxic on its own, but may cause drowsiness, fatigue, halitosis, nausea, vomiting, and a decrease in libido. With alcohol, disulfiram causes nausea, vertigo, anxiety, blurred vision, hypotension, chest pain, palpitations, tachycardia, facial flushing, and throbbing headache. Symptoms can last 3 to 4 days, but may persist for 1 week. Symptoms may occur even with small amounts of alcohol, but 25 to 50 per cent of patients experience little or no reaction at standard doses.

**Toxic effects**: the disulfiram-ethanol reaction may be very severe with respiratory depression, cardiovascular collapse, cardiac arrhythmias, coma, cerebral oedema, hemiplegia, convulsions, and death. Chronic treatment and overdose may cause high blood pressure, hepatotoxicity, and neuropsychiatric complications.

**Indications**: it is used as a deterrent to the use of alcohol and maintenance of abstinence, especially if there is high motivation and good compliance in the patient.

**Contraindications**: cardiac failure, cardiovascular or cerebrovascular disease, hypertension, peripheral neuropathy, psychosis, severe personality disorder, suicide risk, pregnancy, and breast feeding. It should be used with caution in hypertension, diabetes mellitus, epilepsy, impaired hepatic or renal function, respiratory disorders, cerebral damage, and hypothyroidism, as it may exacerbate these conditions. Caution should be exercised in the elderly.

**Interactions**: caution with phenytoin, diazepam, chlordiazepoxide, theophylline, warfarin, and caffeine metabolism; acute psychosis or confusional state may occur with metronidazole. Concurrent tricyclic antidepressants may exacerbate the disulfiram-ethanol reaction and cause a toxic confusional state.

**Effects of withdrawal**: none but restoration of alcohol dehydrogenase depends on *de novo* enzyme synthesis which occurs over 6 or more days.

**Dosage and administration**: after 24 h without alcohol, give 800 mg as a single dose on day 1, then reduce dose over 5 days from 100 to 200 mg daily. Effectiveness is dose related. Blood pressure should be monitored regularly if the patient is taking over 500 mg/day. Compliance is improved with monitoring (carbon disulphide breath test) and supervision. Patients should be warned not to ingest any alcohol, including alcohol in food, liquid medicines, and even toiletries. An alcohol challenge test may be done in specialist centres. The patient should be reviewed every 6 months at a minimum. Alcohol should be avoided for at least 1 week on terminating disulfiram.

## Clomethiazole (edisylate)[21] (Heminevrin®)

Clomethiazole (previously known as chlormethiazole) is a sedative-hypnotic-anxiolytic which also inhibits the metabolism of alcohol resulting in a more gradual elimination of alcohol from the body.

**Pharmacology**: it is an agonist at the picrotoxin/barbiturate site of the GABA-A receptor, a glutamate antagonist, and an inhibitor of alcohol dehydrogenase.

**Types of compounds available**: oral and parenteral forms.

**Pharmacokinetics**: $t_{max}$ 1 h (oral dosing); plasma half-life is 4 h but is double this in elderly people.

**Side-effects**: conjunctival irritation, nasal congestion, tingling in the nose, headaches, and reversible elevation of liver function tests.

**Toxic effects**: respiratory depression, sudden fall in blood pressure, anaphylactic reactions, and death (often due to combination with alcohol).

**Indications**: acute alcohol withdrawal and delirium tremens in inpatients.

**Contraindications**: alcohol addicts who continue to drink, pulmonary insufficiency, pregnancy, and lactation; caution is advised in renal impairment, severe liver damage, and cardiac and respiratory disease.

**Interactions**: alcohol and diazoxide may cause severe respiratory depression. Plasma levels are increased by cimetidine. It causes severe bradycardia with propranolol.

**Effects of withdrawal**: rebound insomnia and anxiety (as with other sedative drugs).

**Dosage and administration**: titrate using three or four daily doses according to patient response. Initially give 2 to 4 capsules, then 9 to 12 in divided doses over the next 24 h, 6 to 8 capsules on day 2, 4 to 6 on day 3, reducing it to 0 by day 6 to 9 in order to avoid dependency. Only use it by infusion where resuscitation facilities are available; initially give 3 to 7.5 ml/min, then reduce dosage to 0.5 to 1 ml/min (infusion no longer available in UK).

## Further information

British National Formulary (BNF) www.bnf.org.
NIDA (National Institute on Drug Abuse) www.nida.nih.gov.
SAMHSA (Substance Abuse and mental health services administration). www.samhsa.gov

## References

1. Lingford-Hughes, A.R., Welch, S., and Nutt, D.J. (2004). Evidence-based guidelines for the pharmacological management of substance misuse, addiction and comorbidity: recommendations from the British Association for Psychopharmacology. *Journal of Psychopharmacology*, **18**, 293–335.

2. NICE. (2007). *Methadone and buprenorphine for the management of opioid dependence. NICE technology appraisal guidance 114.* National Institute for Health and Clinical Excellence, London.

3. Clark, N., Lintzeris, N., Gijsbers, A., *et al.* (2002). LAAM maintenance vs methadone maintenance for heroin dependence. *The Cochrane Database of Systematic Reviews*, (2): CD002210.

4. Law, F.D., Myles, J.S., Daglish, M.R.C., *et al.* (2004). The clinical use of buprenorphine in opiate addiction: evidence and practice. *Acta Neuropsychiatrica*, **16**, 246–74 (with erratum at 2004, **16**, 326).

5. Nutt, D.J. (1997). Receptor pharmacology of buprenorphine. *Research and Clinical Forums*, **19**, 9–15.

6. Krausz, M., Verthein, U., Degwitz, P., *et al.* (1998). Maintenance treatment of opiate addicts in Germany with medications containing codeine—results of a follow up study. *Addiction*, **93**, 1161–7.

7. Robertson, J.R., Raab, G.M., Bruce, M., *et al.* (2006). Addressing the efficacy of dihydrocodeine versus methadone as an alternative maintenance treatment for opiate dependence: a randomized controlled trial. *Addiction*, **101**, 1752–9.

8. Gonzalez, J.P. and Brogden, R.N. (1988). Naltrexone. A review of its pharmacodynamic and pharmacokinetic properties and therapeutic efficacy in the management of opioid dependence. *Drugs*, **35**, 192–213.

9. NICE. (2007). *Naltrexone for the management of opioid dependence. NICE technology appraisal guidance 115.* National Institute for Health and Clinical Excellence, London.

10. Srisurapanont, M. and Jarusuraisin, N. (2005). Opioid antagonists for alcohol dependence. *The Cochrane Database of Systematic Reviews*, (1): CD001867.

11. Minozzi, S., Amato, L., Vecchi, S., *et al.* (2006). Oral naltrexone maintenance treatment for opioid dependence. *The Cochrane Database of Systematic Reviews*, (1): CD001333.

12. Handal, K.A., Schauben, J.L., and Salamone F.R. (1983). Naloxone. *Annals of Emergency Medicine*, **12**, 438–45.

13. Gowing, L., Farrell, M., Ali, R., *et al.* (2004). Alpha2 adrenergic agonists for the management of opioid withdrawal. *The Cochrane Database of Systematic Reviews*, (4): CD002024.

14. Kahn, A., Mumford, J.P., Rogers, G.A., *et al.* (1997). Double-blind study of lofexidine and clonidine in the detoxification of opiate addicts in hospital. *Drug and Alcohol Dependence*, **44**, 57–61.

15. Strang, J., Bearn, J., and Gossop, M. (1999). Lofexidine for opiate detoxification: a review of recent randomised and open controlled trials. *American Journal on Addictions*, **8**, 337–48.

16. Littleton, J. (1995). Acamprosate in alcohol dependence: how does it work? *Addiction*, **90**, 1179–88.

17. Wilde, M.I. and Wagstaff, A.J. (1997). Acamprosate: a review of its pharmacology and clinical potential in the management of alcohol dependence after detoxification. *Drugs*, **53**, 1038–53.

18. Banys, P. (1988). The clinical use of disulfiram (Antabuse): a review. *Journal of Psychoactive Drugs*, **20**, 243–60.

19. Heather, N. (1993). Disulfiram treatment for alcohol problems: is it effective and, if so, why? In *Treatment options in addiction: medical management of alcohol and opiate abuse* (ed. C. Brewer), pp. 1–18. Gaskell, London.

20. Brewer, C. (1984). How effective is the standard dose of disulfiram? A review of the alcohol-disulfiram reaction in practice. *The British Journal of Psychiatry*, **144**, 200–2.

21. Majumdar, S.K. (1990). Chlormethiazole: current status in the treatment of the acute ethanol withdrawal syndrome. *Drug and Alcohol Dependence*, **27**, 201–7.

# 6.2.9 Complementary medicines

Ursula Werneke

Complementary medicines pose a particular challenge to medical practitioners who may feel that their patients need conventional treatment but often find themselves out of their depth when patients ask about complementary therapies. Pharmacological options include herbal medicines, certain foods, and nutritional supplements such as vitamins and minerals. Physical treatments include acupuncture, massage, and osteopathy to name a few. Treatments, which purport to achieve their effects through changes in internal 'energy flow' include reiki, reflexology, healing, and therapeutic touch, and also homeopathy and traditional Chinese acupuncture. All these treatments are either used alternatively, i.e. instead of, or complementary, i.e. in addition to, conventional medicine. In patients with mental health problems, depending on the definition and inclusion criteria, estimates of the prevalence of complementary medicine use range from 8 per cent to 57 per cent. Depression and anxiety seem to be the most common indications.[1]

## Herbal remedies and supplements

### Principles of treatment

Herbal remedies and supplements may come in many different forms and formulations. Since they are currently not subject to the same regulatory requirements as conventional medicines they can vary substantially in contents and dose even if they purport to contain the same ingredients. The pharmacological properties of an extract or a supplement may depend on many different factors (Table 6.2.9.1).

## Condition-specific remedies

### Cognitive enhancers

Cognitive enhancers are either used in the treatment of dementia to enhance mental performance or prevent cognitive decline in healthy people. One strategy aims at increasing choline availability, e.g. by inhibiting acetylcholine esterase. Alternative non-cholinergic neuroprotective strategies have been postulated. These rely on antioxidants scavenging free radicals thereby reducing neurotoxicity or anti-coagulants and increasing cerebral blood flow.[4] Suggested herbal cognitive enhancers for which some positive trial evidence has been collated include ginkgo (*Ginkgo biloba*), panax

**Table 6.2.9.1** Determinants of pharmacological properties of complementary medicines

| Factor | Problem | Example |
|---|---|---|
| Material production | Quality may depend on plant material used, time of harvesting, geographical location, or other environmental factors | St John's wort extracts prepared from the flowers are more potent than extracts prepared from the leaves |
| Extraction method | Determines remedy composition | Alcoholic valerian extracts may be safer than aqueous extracts such as teas because harmful volatile substances (valepotriates) are eliminated more easily. The resulting extracts may be less potent though, since valepotriates have GABAergic properties.[2] Conversely, aqueous kava extracts may be safer than alcoholic extracts because liver protective substances such as glutathione are retained |
| Standardization | Difficult to achieve if active ingredient is unknown | St John's wort is based on the extract traditionally standardized on hypericin, a photosensitive red pigment. However, current evidence suggests that standardization should be based on hyperforin, which inhibits the reuptake of monoamines[1] |
| Dosing | Depends on standardization | 300 mg of St John's wort extract standardized on 0.5% or 5% hyperforin most likely have different pharmacodynamic effects |
| Contamination | Increased and sometimes unexpected toxicity | Contamination with e.g. fertilizer residuals or heavy metals. Association of eosinophilicmyalgic syndrome and some 5-hydroxy-tryptophan products may be at least in part due to contamination of some batches |
| Adulteration | May lead to serious side effects and drug interactions falsely ascribed to the remedy *per se* | Adulterants include steroids, NSAIDs, anticonvulsants, benzodiazepines, hypoglycemic agents, erectogenic agents, and warfarin[3] |

ginseng (*Panax ginseng*), hydergine (*Claviceps purpurea*), sage (*Salvia officinalis*), and vitamin E. The potential side effects can be derived from the purported mechanisms of action. For example, remedies increasing the cerebral blood flow such as ginkgo may increase the risk of cerebral haemorrhage. *Panax ginseng* has been associated with manic episodes and hydergine can lead to ergot poisoning unless dosed carefully. Some sage species can lower the seizure threshold. Others contain camphor, which can be toxic in high doses.[2] Also, evidence is emerging that taking vitamin E above the recommended level may increase all-cause mortality.[5]

## Anxiolytics and sedatives

Drugs considered to be either anxiolytics or sedatives essentially have the same underlying mechanisms of action. The stronger an agent the more sedating it will be, leading to coma in extreme cases. Four mechanisms of action have been implicated; binding to γ-aminobutyric acid (GABA) receptors leading to hyperpolarization of the cell membrane through increased influx of chlorine anions; inhibition of excitatory amino acids (EAA) thereby also impairing the ability to form new memories; sodium channel blockade, reducing depolarization of the cell membrane; and calcium channel blockade, reducing the release of neurotransmitters into the synaptic cleft.[4] The most commonly used CAMs for anxiolysis and sedation, such as valerian (*Valeriana officinalis*), passion flower (*Passiflora incarnata*), kava (*Piper methysticum*), and German chamomile (*Matricaria recutita*) are GABAergic. Lemon balm (*Melissa officinalis*) has cholinergic and GABAergic properties. For other plant remedies, including hops (*Humulus lupulus*), oats (*Avena sativa*), lavender (*Lavendula angustifolia*), and starflower also known as borage (*Borago officinalis*), the actual mechanism of action remains unknown. Melatonin regulates the circadian rhythm and also has some GABAergic properties although trial evidence remains inconclusive. Some of these remedies can potentially have serious side effects. For instance, kava extracts have been associated with significant and potentially fatal hepatotoxicity. Starflower contains γ-linolenic acid that may lower the seizure threshold. Some passion flower extracts may contain cyanide components. As expected, all remedies in this class can lead to drowsiness when taken in high doses and can potentiate the effect of synthetic sedatives.

## Antidepressants and mood stabilizers

Most complementary antidepressants are thought to work through serotonergic and noradrenergic pathways. The most robust clinical data are available for St John's wort (*Hypericum perforatum*), having been extensively reviewed in meta-analyses.[1] Hyperforin, inhibiting the reuptake of monoamines, is thought to be the most likely active component. Supplements, such as S-adenosylmethionine (SAMe), folic acid, L-tryptophan, and 5-hydroxytryptophan are components or co-factors in the serotonin synthesis. For SAMe, equivalence to tricyclic antidepressants has been demonstrated. However, SAMe is very expensive and a suitable oral formulation may be difficult to obtain. Selenium has also been suggested but the mechanism of action, albeit still unclear, seems to be different. Its antioxidant properties may reduce nerve cell damage. Selenium also facilitates conversion from thyroxin (T4) to thyronine (T3), and T3 substitution is one possible augmentation strategy for antidepressants. As for lithium, the therapeutic index is narrow. Omega-3 fatty acids are known to stabilize membranes and to facilitate monoaminergic, serotonergic, and cholinergic neurotransmission. The currently available evidence supports the use of eicosapentaenoic acid on its own or in combination with docosahexaonic acid as adjunctive treatment.[6] Serotonergic remedies should not be combined with each other or with conventional antidepressants because of the increased risk of serotonin syndrome. Equally, herbal antidepressants may induce mania in vulnerable patients although current evidence relies on case reports only. Finally L-tryptophan and 5-hydroxytryptophan should be avoided until the associated risk of eosinophilic myalgic syndrome is fully explained.

## Remedies for psychosis

Rauwolfia (*Rauvolfia serpentina*) extracts were traditionally used before synthetic antipsychotics became widely available. Several alkaloid derivatives including reserpine were introduced in the 1950s. They block vesicular storage of monoamines so that the presence of monoamines in the cytoplasm is prolonged, enabling them to be more easily degraded by monoamine oxidases. In consequence, the amount of neurotransmitter available on depolarization of the cell membrane is reduced.[4] On the one hand, this may lead to a reduction of dopamine and the resolution of psychotic symptoms. On the other hand, less serotonin and noradrenaline will be available, which explains why drugs such as reserpine may precipitate depression. An alternative strategy is the augmentation of antipsychotic treatment with omega-3-fatty acids, but the results of clinical trials remain inconclusive and larger trials will be needed to clarify effectiveness.[6,7]

## Remedies for movement disorders

Attempts have been made to treat tardive dyskinesia with antioxidants. This approach relies on the assumption that tardive dyskinesia is not only due to dopamine receptor super-sensitivity but is also related to oxidative tissue damage induced by antipsychotics. Clinical trials suggest that vitamin E may prevent the progression of tardive dyskinesia. One trial found actual improvement. However, the benefits have to be offset against taking vitamin E long-term, particularly when higher than recommended daily doses are used.[5] A far more powerful antioxidant than vitamin E is melatonin attenuating dopaminergic activity in the striatum as well as hypothalamic dopamine release.[8]

## Remedies for the treatment of addiction

Only few plants have been identified as having the potential to counter addiction. Such may be ibogaine, derived from the West African shrub *Tabernanthe iboga*. It has hallucinogenic properties, and has been used to counter nicotine, cocaine, and opiate addiction. It causes dose-dependent CNS stimulation ranging from mild excitation and euphoria to visual and auditory hallucinations. The therapeutic value of ibogaine is limited since it is highly neurotoxic and can cause irreversible cerebellar damage. A synthetic derivative with similar reported effects, but without cerebellar toxicity is 18-methoxycoronaridine (18-MC).[4] Between 1990 and 2006, twelve deaths after ibogaine use were reported. More deaths may have occurred but may not have been reported due to the 'underground nature of ibogaine treatment'. Passion flower and valerian, by virtue of their GABAergic properties, may ameliorate withdrawal symptoms. Kudzu, Japanese arrowroot (*Pueraria lobata*), has traditionally been used for the treatment of alcohol hangover. The active ingredient, puerarin, counteracts the anxiogenic effects associated with alcohol withdrawal.[9]

## Examples of remedies commonly used for chronic somatic conditions

Many different remedies are available for somatic conditions. Their use may be problematic in chronic conditions such as cancer or HIV where the therapeutic margin of conventional medicines is narrow.[10] For example, echinacea (*Echinacea purpurea*) is used to boost immune system. This may be detrimental where immunosupression is desired since echinacea may potentially stimulate the growth of malignant or infectious cell lines. Patients with breast cancer may often resort to phytoestrogens such as soy (*Glycine max*), wild yam (*Dioscorea alata*), or liquorice (*Glyccyrhiza glabra*) to reverse the effects of antiestrogenic therapies such as tamoxifen. Phytoestrogens, however, can theoretically stimulate breast cancer cells and thus should be advised against in this patient group. Liquorice is a popular ingredient of many traditional Chinese medicines and may cause hypokalemia if used excessively. Evening primrose (*Oenothera biennis*) oil is a popular remedy for premenstrual syndrome and mastalgia. Like starflower it contains γ-linolenic acid and may lower the seizure threshold or reduce the efficacy of antiepileptic drugs.

# Drug interactions

Determining interactions between complementary and conventional medicines can be extremely difficult. In the first instance, the clinician must be prepared to consider such a possibility and take a corresponding history. As often, association does not prove causality. Drug interactions can be distinguished into pharmacodynamic and pharmacokinetic interactions. Pharmacodynamic interactions occur when remedies act as agonists, antagonists or inverse agonists to conventional medicines. Additive toxicity, e.g. hepatotoxicity due to pyrrolizidine alkaloids, or increase of coagulability due to coumarinic constituents may also be of concern. Pharmacokinetic interactions include interactions with the cytochrome microsomal enzyme system (CYP) or membrane transporter proteins expressed through the ABC cassette genes (Table 6.2.9.2).[1,2,11,12]

## The CYP system

The pharmacokinetics of most anticancer drugs is highly variable and may be genetically determined. For instance, the oxidative metabolism depends on the CYP system. The effects of CYP inducers and inhibitors are essentially differential depending on whether metabolites are more or less active (Table 6.2.9.2). If metabolites are less active than the original agent, CYP inhibitors increase whereas inducers reduce therapeutic effectiveness. Conversely, if metabolites are more active than the original agent, CYP inhibitors reduce whereas as inducers increase therapeutic effectiveness. Often such interactions have only been studied *in vitro* and it remains unclear whether they translate into tangible clinical effects.[11,12] In clinical practice, it is often possible to monitor combination of medicines more closely or to adjust the doses of conventional drugs in the required direction rather than to advise discontinuation of complementary remedies. Interactions with CYP 3A4 are of particular concern, since this enzyme metabolizes up to 60% of all clinically used drugs including HIV protease inhibitors, HIV non-nucleoside reverse transcriptase inhibitors, warfarin, ciclosporin, oral contraceptives, digoxin, theophylline, anticonvulsants, and various psychoactive drugs.[13]

## ABC transporters

The ABC cassette genes represent proteins binding to ATP and use this energy to drive various molecules through cell membranes. The transport is mostly unidirectional. The ABC genes have been mainly explored for their capacity to cause multi-drug resistance in cancer chemotherapy.[12] Thus remedies exerting such effects may be of particular interests to the liaison psychiatrist. The most commonly known transporter is p-glycoprotein involved in the

**Table 6.2.9.2** Examples of potential drug interactions of commonly used psychotropic remedies

| Remedy | Pharmacodynamic | Pharmacokinetic |
|---|---|---|
| Ginkgo | Antithrombolytic agents | 1A1, 1A2, 2B1/2, 2C9, **2C19***, 3A1, **3A4** inhibition |
| Panax ginseng | Insulin and oral hypoglycaemics, antithrombolytic agents, MAOIs (phenelzine), loop diuretics | 1A1, 1A2, 1B1, 2C9, 2C19, **2D6**, 2E1 inhibition3A4 inconclusive; p-glycoprotein inhibition |
| Hydergine | Serotonergic antidepressants, choline-esterase inhibitors | |
| Vitamin E | Anticoagulants and antiplatelet drugs; prevention of nitrate tolerance possible; ↑ effect of sildenafil and related phophodiesterase-5 inhibitors possible; ↓ effect of chemotherapies relying on oxidative stress | CYP 3A11 induction |
| Valerian | ↑ Effect of sedatives | **CYP 3A4** and p-glycoprotein inhibition |
| Passion flower | Anticoagulants, ↑ effect of sedatives | CYP 3A4 inhibition |
| Kava | ↓ Effect of levodopa | Potentiation of liver toxicity of other drugs CYP 1A2, 2C9, 2C19, 2D6, 3A4 and 4A9/11 inhibition |
| Melatonin | Anticoagulants, ↑ effect of sedatives; ↓ effect of chemotherapies relying on oxidative stress | |
| St John's wort | Serotonergic antidepressants | CYP 3A4, 1A2, 2C9, **3A4**and **2E1** induction:, p-glycoprotein induction |
| Omega 3 fatty acids | ↑ Effect of warfarin, aspirin and non- steroidal anti- inflammatory drugs | CYP 3A4 and p-glycoprotein inhibition |
| Rauwolfia | ↑ Effect of anti- psychotics and barbiturates; ↓ effect of levodopa; severe bradycardia with digitalis glycosides; hypertension in combination with sympathomimetics | |
| Iboga | Cholinergic and anticholinergic drugs | |
| Echinacea | ↓ Effect of immunosuppressants | CYP **2A1**, 2C9, and **3A4** inhibition, CYP 3A4 induction also possible depending on extract |
| Evening primrose oil | Other drugs reducing seizure threshold, anticoagulants | 1A2, 2C9, 2C19, 2D6, 3A4 inhibition |

*Bold font: *In vivo* evidence available.

transport of many psychotropic drugs through the blood brain barrier. St John's wort, valerian, and panax ginseng are remedies shown to change p-glycoprotein activity (Table 6.2.9.2).[11,12] However, whether such effects are sufficiently powerful to affect conventional treatments remains unclear.[14]

## Conclusions

At present, the evidence base for the use of psychotropic complementary medicines is extremely limited. Due to the large variability of formulations it can be extremely difficult to conduct clinical trials with replicable results even if a candidate plant has been identified. Pooling results of existing trials in meta-analyses may be unhelpful if the trials are too small or heterogenous or if the analysis is not adjusted for the extract types used. Equally, systematic pharmacovigilance is difficult to implement in the absence of a regulatory framework.

Clinicians need to be aware that patients may use complementary therapies regardless of the evidence available and should inquire about such forms of self-medication. Pattern of use may vary with cultural background and health beliefs. Given the complex pattern of potential interactions, conventional health care professionals should not be afraid to discuss complementary use with their patients. For instance, complementary medicines should be considered a potential cause when the clinical presentation, the

treatment result, adverse effects, or even diagnostic investigations are unusual or unexpected. Equally, patients should be encouraged to disclose information about complementary medicines to health care professionals. On the one hand, discussions need to be conducted sensitively in order to avoid alienating patients who may feel that they have not been taken seriously or have been criticized for using complementary medicines. On the other hand, uncritical encouragement of potentially harmful or inappropriate use of complementary medicines may possibly lead to litigation.(15) In most cases, remedies may not have to be discontinued if conventional treatments are closely monitored and adjusted. A constructive discussion about complementary medicines may potentially be a gateway towards enhancing compliance with conventional treatments.

## Further information

Memorial Sloan-Kettering Cancer Center: Cancer Information: Integrative Medicine: www.mskcc.org. Keyword: herbs.
National Centre for Complementary Alternative Medicines / National Institute of Health: http://nccam.nih.gov.
Royal Botanic Gardens, Kew: Education: Resources: Information Sheets: www.rbgkew.org.uk/ksheets/.
Royal College of Psychiatrists: Mental Health Information: Therapies: Complementary and Alternative Medicines 1 & 2: www.rcpsych. ac.uk/mentalhealthinformation/therapies.aspx.

The Prince of Wales Foundation for Integrated Health: http://www.fih.org.uk/.

## References

1. Werneke, U., Turner, T., and Priebe, S. (2006). Complementary alternative medicine in psychiatry: a review of effectiveness and safety. *The British Journal of Psychiatry*, **188**, 109–21.
2. Natural Medicines Comprehensive Database. (2007). Keyword: product search. www.naturalmedicines.com.
3. Ernst, E. (2002). Adulteration of Chinese herbal medicines with synthetic drugs: a systematic review. *Journal of Internal Medicine*, **252**, 107–13.
4. Spinella, M. (2001). *The psychopharmacology of herbal medicine*. MIT Press, Cambridge.
5. Food Standards Agency. Expert Group on Vitamins and Minerals. (2003). *Safe upper levels for vitamins and minerals*. www.foodstandards.gov.uk.
6. Freeman, M.P., Hibbelen, J.R., Wisner, L.K., et al. (2006). Omega-3 fatty acids: evidence base for treatment and future research in psychiatry. *The Journal of Clinical Psychiatry*, **67**, 1954–67.
7. Joy, C.B., Mumby-Croft, R., and Joy, L.A. (2003). *Polyunsaturated fatty acid supplementation for schizophrenia (Cochrane review)*. In *The Cochrane Library*, Issue 4, John Wiley & Sons, Ltd., Chichester, UK.
8. Lohr, J.B., Kuczenski, R., and Niculescu, A.B. (2003). Oxidative mechanisms and tardive dyskinesia. *CNS Drugs*, **17**, 47–62.
9. Overstreet, D.H., Keung, W.M., Rezvani, A.H., et al. (2003). Herbal remedies for alcoholism: promises and possible pitfalls. *Alcoholism: Clinical and Experimental Research*, **27**, 177–85.
10. Labriola, D. and Livingston, R. (1999). Possible interactions between dietary antioxidants and chemotherapy. *Oncology (Williston Park)*, **13**, 1003–8.
11. Sparreboom, A., Cox, M.C., Acharya, M.R., et al. (2004). Herbal remedies in the United States: potential adverse interactions with anticancer agents. Journal of Clinical Oncology, **22**, 2489–503.
12. Sparreboom, A., Danesi, R., Ando, Y., et al. (2003). Pharmacogenomics of ABC transporters and its role in cancer chemotherapy. *Drug Resistance Updates*, **6**, 71–84.
13. Committee of Safety in Medicine & Medicines Control Agency. (2000). Reminder: St John's wort (*Hypericum perforatum*) interactions. *Current Problems in Pharmacovigilance*, **26**, 6–7.
14. Morris, M.E. and Zhang, S. (2006). Flavonoid-drug interactions: effects of flavonoids on ABC transporters. *Life Sciences*, **78**, 2116–30.
15. Cohen, M.H. and Eisenberg, D.M. (2002). Potential physician malpractice liability associated with complementary and integrative medicinal therapies. *Annals of Internal Medicine*, **136**, 596–603.

# 6.2.10 **Non-pharmacological somatic treatments**

## Contents

6.2.10.1 Electroconvulsive therapy
Max Fink

6.2.10.2 Phototherapy
Philip J. Cowen

6.2.10.3 Transcranial magnetic stimulation
Declan McLoughlin and Andrew Mogg

6.2.10.4 Neurosurgery for psychiatric disorders
Keith Matthews and David Christmas

## 6.2.10.1 **Electroconvulsive therapy**

Max Fink

### Introduction

Convulsive therapy (ECT or electroshock) is an effective treatment for those with severe and persistent emotional disorders. It is safe for patients of all ages, for those with debilitating systemic illnesses and during pregnancy. It relieves symptoms in a briefer time than do psychotropic drugs. To achieve remission, treatments are usually given three times a week for two to seven weeks. To sustain recovery, treatments are continued either weekly or biweekly for several months. The overall duration of the treatment course is similar to that of the psychotropic medications frequently used for the same conditions.

The treatment is severely stigmatized and its use is discouraged, even interdicted, in the belief that the electricity or the seizures irreversibly damage the brain.[1–5] Few physicians are tutored in its use and facilities are limited making ECT unavailable to many who would benefit. The ease in the use of psychotropic medications, and neither greater efficacy nor greater safety, encourages their preferential use as ECT is relegated to the 'last resort.' In countries where psychotropic medications are expensive, ECT is prescribed, but the expense for anesthetics limits its use to its unmodified form.

Despite these hurdles of stigma, expense and lack of training, its use has persisted for more than 70 years. Indeed, its use is increasing. Whole societies where it was interdicted at the end of the 20th century, as in the Netherlands, Germany, Austria, Italy, and Japan, interest and usage has increased, texts have been written or translated, and local psychiatric societies formed to encourage its use.[4–6]

### Origins

At the turn of the century when malarial fevers were used to treat patients with neurosyphilis, it was deemed possible to treat one illness by developing another. Reports that patients with dementia praecox were relieved of their psychosis after suffering convulsions supported a concept of an antagonism between epilepsy and psychosis. An explanation was seen in the reports that the concentrations of brain glial cells in patients with dementia praecox were low and in those with epilepsy were high.[7] Was it possible that the root of schizophrenia lay in the paucity of glia and would their increase relieve the illness?

After testing ways to induce a grand mal seizure in animals, Ladislas Meduna, a Hungarian neuropathologist and psychiatrist, on January 24, 1934, injected camphor-in-oil into a man with the catatonic form of schizophrenia. The patient seized and recovered without incident. Following the model of malarial fever therapy, Meduna repeated the injections every three days, and after the fifth seizure, the patient, for the first time in four years, talked spontaneously and fed and cared for himself. After three additional treatments he was discharged home, returned to work, and was well when Meduna left Hungary in 1939.[7]

Chemically induced seizures, either with camphor or pentylenetetrazol (Metrazol), were rapidly adopted worldwide as the treatment for dementia praecox, but the treatments were painful and frightening, so alternative means were sought. In 1938, the Roman psychiatrists Ugo Cerletti and Luigi Bini demonstrated the ease of administration and the efficiency of electrically induced seizures. Quickly, 'electroconvulsive therapy' (ECT, electroshock) became the commonest method of inducing seizures and is the standard induction today.[4–5,8]

## For whom is ECT effective?

Established DSM diagnoses are usually cited as the indications for ECT. The diagnoses are imprecise, however, offering heterogeneous population samples. A syndromic view offers more homogeneous populations for treatment.[9–11]

*Defined by DSM Classification.* The DSM defined conditions for which ECT is prescribed are cited in established texts[12–15] (Table 6.2.10.1.1). The breadth of its clinical efficacy across major DSM diagnostic classes is striking, reflecting commonalities in the pathophysiology of different disorders. This experience challenges the concept that DSM classified disorders are distinct biological abnormalities, and supports the 19th century concept of a unitary psychosis.[16]

ECT is *not* useful for a patient with neurosis, situational maladjustment, personality disorder (character pathology), or drug dependence. It is of limited benefit for anyone with a lifelong history of mental and emotional dysfunction, unless the onset of the present illness is acute and well defined, or affective, psychotic, or catatonic features dominate the presentation[12–15] (Table 6.2.10.1.2).

*Defined by syndrome.* DSM-III and DSM-IV classify illnesses based on the check-off of symptoms modified by duration criteria. The DSM criteria identify heterogeneous populations that do not support useful treatment algorithms or the search for biological roots of the illnesses. Clinical syndromes describe more homogeneous populations, often substantiated by biological tests and/or a high specificity of interventions. Melancholia, psychotic depression, catatonia, delirious mania, and acute schizophrenia are syndromes that are particularly responsive to ECT (Table 6.2.10.1.3). These syndromes are not readily identified in the established classification systems. Summary descriptions are offered here; the interested reader will find more extensive descriptions in the cited literature.

### (a) Depressive mood disorders

Convulsive therapy is most effective against mood disorders, depression and mania. Depressive mood disorders are dominated by sadness, hopelessness, fears, and thoughts that life is no longer worth-living. Variants are recognized, dominated by vegetative and motor abnormality (melancholia), by delusions (psychotic depression), by severe cognitive deficit (pseudodementia), or by catatonia.[14]

While all variants respond to induced seizures, some also respond to other specific treatments. Melancholic and pseudodementia patients respond to tricyclic antidepressants. Psychotic depressed patients require high doses of both antidepressant and antipsychotic medications.[11] Anticonvulsant sedative drugs, the barbiturates and the benzodiazepines, are useful in catatonic patients.[9]

### (i) Melancholia

Motor signs (retardation or agitation) and vegetative symptoms of inability to sleep, feeding, and weight loss are its features. Work, sex, and family are disregarded. Thoughts of suicide are prominent.[10–11]

**Table 6.2.10.1.1** DSM defined clinical diagnoses in which ECT is effective[11]

| Major depressive disorder | |
|---|---|
| single episode | [296.2x]** |
| recurrent | [296.3x]** |
| **Bipolar disorder** | |
| mania | [296.4x]** |
| depressed | [296.5x]** |
| mixed type | [296.6x]** |
| not otherwise specified | [296.70]** |
| **Atypical psychosis** | **[298.90]** |
| **Schizophrenia** | |
| catatonia | [295.2x] |
| schizophreniform | [295.40] |
| schizo-affective | [295.70] |
| **Catatonia** | |
| Schizophrenia, catatonic type | [295.2x] |
| Catatonic disorder due to a medical condition | [293.89] |
| Malignant catatonia | [293.89] |
| Neuroleptic malignant syndrome | [333.92] |
| **Delirium** | |
| Due to a general medical condition | [293.0] |
| Due to substance intoxication | |

\* from Fink, 1999

\*\* specifier for psychosis

Hypercortisolemia is characteristic of the syndrome.[17] Cortisol metabolism is influenced by hypothalamic, pituitary, and adrenal interactions. Melancholic patients exhibit elevated serum levels of cortisol, obtunded diurnal rhythmicity, and serum levels remain elevated despite an administered dose of dexamethasone. The abnormality is measurable by the dexamethasone suppression test (DST) or its variant, the dexamethasone/corticotrophin releasing factor test (Dex/CRH). Elevated cortisol levels normalize with treatment and become abnormal again with relapse. In the 1980s, the specificity of the DST was considered poor for the major depressions defined by DSM-III and the test was discarded. But the re-assessment of the literature and recent reports find the test as

**Table 6.2.10.1.2** DSM diagnoses in which ECT is ineffective[11]

| Dementia and Amnestic Disorders | [293.0, 290.xx, 294.xx] |
|---|---|
| Substance-related Disorders | [303.xx, 291.x, 304.x, 292.x] |
| Anxiety and Somatiform Disorders | [300.xx] |
| Factitious Disorders | [300.xx] |
| Dissociative Disorders | [300.1x, 300.6] |
| Sexual Dysfunctions | [302.xx, 625.8, 608.89, 607.84, 608.89, 625.8] |
| Sleep Disorders | [307.xx, 780.xx] |
| Impulse disorders | [312.3x] |
| Adjustment disorders | [309.xx] |
| Personality disorders | [301.xx] |

**Table 6.2.10.1.3** ECT responsive syndromes

Mood disorders
  Depression
    Melancholia
    Psychotic (Delusional) depression
  Mania
    Mixed States (mania, depression)
    Rapid cycling mania
    Depressive phase of bipolar disorder
    Delirious mania

Psychosis
  Acute schizophrenia
  Postpartum psychosis

Catatonia
  Hypokinetic catatonia (Kahlbaum Syndrome)
  Excited catatonia (delirious mania, oneiroid state)
  Malignant catatonia (NMS, TSS)

Other
  Delirium
  Suicide risk
  Status epilepticus (SE< NCSE)

\* from Fink, 1999.

both sensitive and specific for melancholic depression, where it has a positive predictive value.[11,18]

After an extensive review of the literature, Taylor and Fink (2006) concluded that classifying mood disorder patients as either melancholic or non-melancholic offered more homogeneous populations with better outcomes with TCAs and ECT than did the DSM classification of major depression and bipolar disorder.[11] In their formulation, melancholia is a syndrome of depressive mood, with motor and vegetative abnormalities and with evidence of cortisol abnormality.

### (ii) Delusional (psychotic) depression

Overwhelmed by feelings of helplessness, hopelessness, and worthlessness, the patient believes others are watching or talking about him, reporting voices when no one is present. He imagines that events depicted on a television or movie screen apply directly to him. This form is labelled psychotic depression and is remarkably responsive to ECT.

In 1975, Glassman and his associates at Columbia University reported that only three of 13 delusional depressed patients (23 per cent) improved when they were treated with high doses of imipramine, while 14 of 21 non-delusional patients (66 per cent) improved under the same treatment.[18] Nine of the 10 unimproved delusional patients responded well to ECT. These findings have been repeatedly verified.[11,12]

In a study of 437 depressed hospitalized patients treated with imipramine in doses of 200 to 350 mg/day for 25 days or longer, 247 (57 per cent) were evaluated as recovered and were discharged.[19] When the 190 unimproved patients were treated with bilateral ECT, 156 (72 per cent) were recovered. Most of the depressed patients who had not improved with imipramine were delusional as well as depressed.

Only a third of delusional depressed patients recover when treated with antidepressant drugs alone and half recover with antipsychotic drugs alone.[11, 19–20] Two-thirds of those treated with ECT or with high doses of both antidepressant and antipsychotic drugs regain their health.

In a two-year study of late-life depression, 47 per cent of the delusional depressed patients treated with medication relapsed earlier and more often than the nondelusional depressed (15 per cent), indicating that delusional depression is particularly resistant to medication.[21] It is, however, so amenable to ECT that it is considered a primary indication for its use.[11–14] But the condition is difficult to diagnose making inadequate treatment common. In a three-hospital research study of ECT and continuation medications, only 2 of 52 delusional depressed patients had adequate courses of medication treatment before they were referred for ECT.[22] The same failure was found in another multi-center study with only 5 of 106 patients failing adequate courses of treatment before referral to ECT.[23]

Many reviews find psychotic depression to have a more severe pathophysiology and just using the same treatments as for non-psychotic depression, even at much higher doses is not adequate.[11,12] Yet, bilateral ECT is remarkably effective. In a multi-site collaborative ECT study, of 253 patients with unipolar major depression, 77 were psychotic depressed. Their remission rate was 95 per cent compared to 83 per cent for the non-psychotic depressed, with the speed of response faster for the psychotic depressed patients.[24, 25]

### (iii) Pseudodementia (reversible dementia)

Because the depressed patient ignores daily events, little of what happens to him is registered and memory is compromised. The condition is hardly distinguishable from Alzheimer's dementia. The onset is usually more rapid and severe compared to the onset of a structural dementia, and patients often report a history of prior depressive episodes.[11,14]

Because the syndrome is not well known, patients are often sent to nursing home care. An example of a 58-year old woman who developed a reversible dementia and was not adequately treated for eight years is reported. Once the diagnosis was considered, antidepressant treatment relieved the syndrome and returned the patient to a more normal family life.[14]

### (iv) Catatonia

When the patient is mute, sitting rigidly in a chair or lying motionless on his bed, and unresponsive to questions and commands, he appears as in a stupor. The state is called *catatonia* or *depressive stupor*. Catatonia is seen among patients with many DSM diagnoses.[9] It is discussed in detail below.

### (b) Manic mood disorders

A mood disorder dominated by grandiosity, expansiveness, feelings of increased power and energy, and excitement, can last for hours, days, weeks, or months. Even after it is relieved, it may recur or alternate or combine with episodes of depression. When the switches occur within one or a few days, the experience is labelled *rapid cycling*, a malignant form of the illness. *Bipolar disorder* is the label applied to both mania and mixed forms of the illness.[11,26]

Disturbances in eating and sleeping, thinking, memory, and movement are features of mania. The patient does not sleep, eats poorly, loses weight, and concentrates thoughts poorly. Memory is impaired, often severely; he may be so disorganized as to appear demented and delirious. Melancholia, psychosis, pseudodementia, and catatonia variations are commonly seen.

Delirious mania is a striking form of mania. A normal person suddenly becomes excited, restless, and sleeps poorly, fears that neighbors are watching him, and is easily frightened. He may hide in the house or leave it abruptly, dressed inappropriately, sometimes naked, and wander about the streets. His hallucinations are vivid, his thoughts disorganized. Confusion alternates with mutism, posturing, rigidity, and stereotyped repetitive movements. Physical exhaustion even to the point of death occurs.[11,27]

Before ECT, patients were sedated with opiates, bromides, or chloral and many died of poor care, inanition, and pneumonia. A 1994 summary of the reports of manic patients treated with ECT finds 371/562 (66 per cent) remitted or showed marked clinical improvement.[28] The introduction of chlorpromazine and other sedative drugs quickly replaced ECT for efficacy and ease of use. But when chlorpromazine and other antipsychotic drugs were used in place of ECT, the doses often carried the risks of sudden death and neuroleptic malignant syndrome, as well as tardive dyskinesia and tardive dystonia.[9]

Anticonvulsant drugs are now preferentially recommended, even though the evidence for their efficacy is poor. Many authors encourage the use of lithium for immediate relief and for prophylaxis. In 438 manic patients treated with ECT or lithium, 78 per cent of the ECT treated group showed marked improvement compared to 62 per cent of those treated with adequate doses of lithium and 56 per cent of those treated with inadequate doses.[29] The group receiving neither ECT nor lithium fared least favourably with only 37 per cent improved.

No matter the array of medications and polypharmacy for mania, ECT is an effective alternative.

## (c) Catatonia

Muscular rigidity, posturing, negativism, mutism, echolalia, echopraxia, and stereotyped mannerisms, the signs of catatonia, appear suddenly and immobilize patients.[9] When the disorder is transient, it may be disregarded, but when it persists, it threatens life. Patients undergo forced feeding and develop bedsores, muscular atrophy and pulmonary embolization. Repeated bladder catheterizations induce infections.

Catatonia is recognized in patients with affective illnesses, both depression and mania, in patients with systemic disorders, and in those with toxic brain states caused by hallucinogenic drugs. For decades, the prevailing belief was that each instance of catatonia represented schizophrenia. The major classification systems in psychiatry—DSM-III and IIIR of the American Psychiatric Association and the International Classification of Diseases (ICD-IX, ICD-X)—assigned patients with catatonia to the diagnosis of schizophrenia, catatonic type. Few patients were treated with anticonvulsant sedatives or ECT, despite their known efficacy, because neither was recommended for schizophrenia. This short-sighted view was somewhat corrected in the 1994 classification system of the American Psychiatric Association (DSM-IV), which recognized catatonia as secondary to systemic illness in the class of "*Catatonic disorder due to . . . . (Indicate the General Medical Condition)* [293.89]".[30] The experience that catatonia is not limited to patients with "schizophrenia" has led to the call for a separate category in DSM-V.[9,31]

Catatonia is defined by the persistence of two or more characteristic motor signs for more than 24 h in a patient with a mental disorder.[9,31] Posturing and staring can be observed, but most signs require elicitation in the examination. The accepted motor signs and a formal examination are cited in catatonia rating scales.[9] An intravenous challenge of lorazepam or amobarbital verifies the diagnosis in more than 2/3 patients with catatonia, and a positive test response augurs well for high dose benzodiazepine therapy. When this treatment fails, ECT is effective, although the treatment schedule may require daily treatments.

Catatonia may be transitory or may persist for months or years. It appears in many guises.[9,32] Prominent examples are *malignant (pernicious) catatonia* (MC) with a high risk of death and the *neuroleptic malignant syndrome* (NMS) that follows on the administration of neuroleptic drugs.

### (i) Malignant catatonia

Descriptions of patients who develop an acute febrile delirium with excitement or stupor dot the literature. They often exhibit signs of catatonia. Vegetative dysregulation is often severe and death was a frequent feature before the introduction of ECT. Descriptions by Bell (1849), Stauder (1934), and Bond (1950) highlight the lethal nature of the syndrome. In 1952, Arnold and Stepan described patients in whom ECT rapidly relieved malignant catatonia, but to avoid mortality it had to be used within the first five days.[9]

### (ii) Neuroleptic malignant syndrome (NMS)

A toxic response to neuroleptic drugs evinced by fever, motor rigidity, negativism, mutism, and cardiovascular and respiratory instability is a toxic response to neuroleptic drugs. It is indistinguishable from malignant catatonia.[9,32] It is an MC variant as the diagnostic criteria and effective treatments are the same as for MC. MC occurs with almost all neuroleptics, most commonly with the high-potency agents like haloperidol, fluphenazine, and thiothixene, but also with atypical neuroleptics.

One hypothesis explains the syndrome as a consequence of an excessive reduction in the amount of brain dopamine. Those who believe this association prescribe the dopamine agonists bromocriptine or levodopa and relieve muscular rigidity by prescribing the muscle relaxant dantrolene. Neither of these treatments has proved effective and dantrolene use is associated with considerable toxicity.[33] These are best not used and patients are best treated with sedative anticonvulsants and ECT.

### (iii) Toxic serotonin syndrome (TSS)

A toxic syndrome is occasionally described in association with the SSRI antidepressant drugs. TSS is similar to MC with prominent gastrointestinal symptoms. The diagnosis and treatment follows the protocol for MC.[9]

## (d) Psychosis

A severe impairment of thought characterized by delusions is a feature of many psychiatric conditions, notably manic delirium, psychotic depression, post partum depression, and toxic psychosis. It is broadly defined as a psychosis and diagnosed within the major class of psychoses as schizophrenia. In this class ECT is hardly considered. But when we consider the efficacy of ECT in the psychotic variants of the mood disorders, we appreciate that ECT is an effective treatment of psychosis.[34]

Convulsive therapy was introduced for the treatment of dementia praecox and was widely and quickly adopted. Comparisons with chlorpromazine found both treatments effective in acute and severe short-term illnesses, but neither was useful in chronic states. Chlorpromazine was favoured since its cost is considerably less and its image better. As more patients failed to respond to medications, however, a cadre of 'medication resistant' psychotic patients developed. Families asked whether anything else could be done to better the patients' lives. Friedel (1986) augmented a failed course of thiothixene therapy with ECT, returning each of nine patients to community life. The finding was replicated in the successful augmentation in 8/9 psychotic patients.[34]

Clozapine was described as a treatment for psychotic patients who had failed to respond to two different antipsychotics. As the experience with this treatment grew, clinicians were again faced with treatment failures and ECT augmentation was tried. A synergy for ECT and clozapine was described and offers an effective treatment for patients who have failed conventional antipsychotics and clozapine.[34]

It is reasonable to consider ECT in the treatment of psychosis, whether in an affective illness or in schizophrenia. For the affective illnesses, ECT is used alone. In schizophrenia, ECT is effective alone or in augmenting neuroleptics.[34]

### (e) Delirium

Acutely ill psychotic patients often exhibit disturbances in consciousness and are confused. Delirium is common in toxic states, either drug induced (alcohol being the most common), or secondary to drug withdrawal, or associated with systemic illnesses. Delirium is a feature of acute manic states (e.g. delirious mania) and the confusional state described as oneirophrenia. With few resources to treat acute psychoses, ECT was applied with favourable results.[14,35] The relief of delirium by ECT is an unrecognized effect that warrants consideration as an alternative to the risks of high potency neuroleptic drugs inducing NMS (MC).

### (f) Neurological syndromes

ECT is well appreciated in catatonia, but it is also useful in status epilepticus (SE), non-convulsive status epilepticus (NCSE), and Parkinsonism.

#### (i) Status epilepticus

SE and NCSE are emergency conditions with high mortality rates. The pathophysiology is the persistence of seizures as biochemical inhibitory mechanisms fail to terminate a seizure.[36] Despite ever larger doses of anticonvulsant medications, proceeding from lorazepam to phenytoin, phenobarbital, and general anesthesia with midazolam, propofol, or barbiturates, patients persist in SE and NCSE.

ECT is another effective intervention. During the course of electroconvulsive therapy, the seizure threshold rises, encouraging seizure termination. The first report of the relief of intractable epilepsy by ECT in 1943 has been sporadically verified.[37]

An explanation for this application is physiologically interesting. The strength of a seizure can be judged by the immediate rise in serum prolactin after a sustained epileptic seizure. Within the hour after a seizure, the level of serum prolactin indicates whether the seizure is a cerebral grand mal event or a pseudoseizure. Serum prolactin levels do not rise in SE but remain normal. This suggests that the SE seizures are partial or incomplete and that they fail to stimulate an inhibitory termination process. But even in patients in SE, ECT elicits maximal seizures, making it a reasonable alternative to general anesthesia as a treatment for intractable seizures.

#### (ii) Parkinsonism

In treating older depressed patients with concurrent Parkinsonism with ECT, motor and facial rigidity were also relieved. In Parkinsonism, brain dopamine levels are reduced, making dopamine agonists effective treatments. In ECT, brain and CSF levels of dopamine increase. Experiments in Parkinsonian patients without mood disorder found motor rigidity to be relieved.[38] For those patients who are not relieved by conventional treatments, periodic ECT has been helpful. Continuation treatments, like continuation pharmacotherapy, are necessary to sustain the benefit.

### (g) Suicide

All psychiatric disorders carry the risk of suicide. ECT reduces this drive. The impact of medications on suicide risk is not well defined but compared to ECT, the efficacy is less favourable.[6,11] Comparisons of ECT and TCAs across different treatment eras find the frequency of suicides decreased in the ECT era. A study of the psychiatric status of 519 patients six months after discharge from hospital treatment for depression found 0.8 per cent of the ECT treated patients had made a subsequent suicide attempt compared to 4.2 per cent for those rated as receiving adequate and 7 per cent of those receiving inadequate courses of antidepressant drugs. At the 6-month follow-up no suicides were reported in 34 women treated with ECT, but two suicides occurred in the 84 patients treated with antidepressants (2.4 per cent).[39]

In a study of the expressed suicide intent (changes in Item 3 of the HAMD rating scale) in 148 patients treated with ECT, the baseline average score was 1.8. It reduced to 0.1 in 72 responders and to 0.9 in 76 non-responders. For the total sample, there was a greater decrease in the suicide item scores than in the overall HAMD scores.[40]

In another study of 444 patients referred for ECT, 131 had high expressed suicide intent scores.[6] The scores dropped to zero in 106 (80.9 per cent) with treatment, occurring in 38.2 per cent (50/131) after 3 ECT (one week), in 61.1 per cent (80/131) after 6 ECT (two weeks); and in 76.3 per cent (100/131) after nine ECT (three weeks).

ECT's effect on the death rate in the mentally ill, particularly those with mood disorders, must be a major consideration in treatment recommendations.

## Principles of treatment

*When to consider ECT?* Psychotropic drugs and psychotherapy are the first treatments of the psychiatrically ill, with referral to ECT when these treatments fail. Since ECT is effective in medication treatment failures, would it not be wise to spare patients a prolonged illness and risks of suicide by offering ECT as the initial treatment? ECT is indeed considered the first treatment when there is a need for a rapid, definitive response, as in suicidal patients who require constant observation and restraint, in hyperactive patients who may be at risk of harm to themselves or others, in those with malignant disorders as malignant catatonia, neuroleptic malignant syndrome, or delirious mania, or in those whose lives are in jeopardy from systemic illness. It is also preferred in those patients who have had a prior illness that responded well to ECT or who have had a poor experience with medications.[11–15]

How many failed trials of medications are reasonable before ECT is considered? For some patients, especially those whose practitioners are not knowledgeable about ECT, medication trials become interminable and ECT is considered only when the patient seeks care elsewhere. A reasonable guideline is derived from the experimental trials with clozapine, an agent with life-threatening risks.[41] To put patients at risk and yet obtain the possible benefits of clozapine, the researchers decided that patients should not be offered clozapine unless they had experienced two unsuccessful courses of neuroleptic treatment. A similar standard seems reasonable for recommending ECT. After patients have failed two different courses of medications at adequate doses and for adequate periods, ECT is to be considered.

Financial considerations affect the decision. If the patient is severely ill and has only a limited ability to pay for extended care, repeated unsuccessful medication trials are unwarranted. All practitioners should balance the cost of medication trials and the effective use of ECT.

*Consideration of age.* ECT is an accepted treatment for adults. For decades, the attitudes of child and adolescent psychiatrists precluded consideration of ECT for their patients except the most devastatingly ill. The acknowledged safety of ECT in adults relaxed prejudices against its use and led to more treatment trials. Once it became clear that the response of adolescents was similar to that of adults, the attitude changed and ECT is now an accepted treatment for adolescents with the same illnesses that are successfully treated in adults.[42]

ECT is probably effective in similar conditions in children, but their expression of mood and psychotic disorders is different than in adults and difficult to interpret. The published experience in the few children treated with ECT finds that conditions that respond in adults and adolescents also respond in children.

ECT is widely used in geriatric patients. Indeed, it is increasingly called on when the side effects of medications become intolerable and when medication trials fail. The safety of modern ECT is such that even the frailest and systemically ill elderly can be safely treated with ECT. We acknowledge no absolute contraindication to ECT other than the lack of skill of the clinicians.[11–15]

## The treatment process

*Consent.* The referral of a patient to an ECT service starts the treatment process. As in surgical treatment, the patient and family members are educated as to the risks and processes of the treatment course, and a signed voluntary consent, witnessed by a family member if possible, is obtained. In response to the turmoil of the 1970s when a draft for an unwelcome war led to widespread questioning of authority, attacks on ECT as a forced involuntary treatment led the profession to suggest procedures for informed voluntary consent. These procedures are well established.[1,2,4,12]

An explanation of why the treatment is recommended, specific anticipated benefits and risks, the names of the responsible physicians, and a statement that the patient may, at any time, discontinue the treatment are elements of a valid consent.[4,13,14] Although voluntary consent is the basis for ECT in almost all Western countries, provisions for involuntary treatment for patients who may not be able to understand the severity of their illness nor the need for treatment is provided in state laws with courts authorizing treatment. In a few venues, surrogate consent by family members is accepted. Educational videotapes and books for laymen support the consent process.[4,12,43]

*Procedures.* Treatments are usually given in an equipped room with access to the in-patient wards. Increasingly, as more than half the treatments are given to out-patients, units are established with ready access to the community.[12,13]

Prior to treatment, systemic medical examinations usually advised for general anaesthesia are completed. These include complete blood count, electrocardiogram, and urinalysis. If systemic illness is present, the treatment is optimized. Often, an anaesthesiologist will examine the patient and the record before treatment, obtaining a separate anaesthesia consent. Although no medical examinations relative to the ECT process are required, some centers unnecessarily insist on pre-treatment brain scans and EEG for all patients.

*Anaesthesia.* When curare and succinylcholine were introduced to modify the convulsion, patients thought they were suffocating as respiratory muscles relaxed. Momentary amnesia was provided by a barbiturate and the combination of barbiturate-induced amnesia and succinylcholine muscle relaxation became standard procedure.[8,12] When psychiatric practice changed from an office to a hospital venue, and anaesthesiologists administered medications, misunderstanding of the role of anaesthesia ensued and the benefits of treatments were reduced by high anaesthetic doses that made effective seizures difficult. Present practice is detailed in anaesthesiology texts.[44]

*Monitoring and electrode placement.* To monitor the physiologic effects of induced seizures, EEG and ECG electrodes are applied. To monitor the motor seizure, a blood pressure cuff is usually applied to the calf of one leg, inflated before the administration of a motor relaxant to observe the motor seizure duration. Two stimulating electrodes are required for ECT. In the early years, the electrodes were applied to both temples, with the maximum energies passing through the intervening brain tissues, especially the centrencephalic structures of the hypothalamus and pituitary. Relocating the electrodes on one side of the head to avoid stimulating the dominant temporal lobe led to seizures with less immediate impact on cognition. 'Right unilateral ECT' (RUL-ECT) became popular until clinicians realized that the efficacy of such treatments was significantly less than through bilateral electrodes (BL-ECT).[8,12]

At one time we believed that any seizure was therapeutic, but we now know that this is not so. A seizure with EEG or motor durations under 20 sec rarely develops a full grand mal convulsion. At first, effective treatments were characterized as those with a motor seizure of at least 25 sec. But not all seizures of such length are effective. Seizures induced through unilateral electrodes at near-threshold energies (experimentally identified as 1.5 and 2.5 times the calibrated seizure threshold) are not as effective as seizures induced through bilateral electrode placements.[45] Energies for seizure inductions in unilateral ECT must be at least 6 to 8 times the calibrated seizure threshold to achieve equal efficacy; at such high energies the advantage in minimizing immediate memory effects is lost.[46] As there is a linear relationship between age and seizure threshold, the energy levels with modern devices that deliver brief pulse electrical currents for BL-ECT is estimated by the half-age formula.[47] In devices that deliver 500 mC of energy at 100 per cent, the energy level for the first induction is set at half the patient's age. The quality and duration of the EEG seizure are a guide to later induction energies. In present clinical practice, electrodes are applied to both temples (BT-ECT) or over the outer canthus of each eye in 'bifrontal' (BF-ECT) placement. While the advantages of BF-ECT and BT-ECT are being assessed in large studies, their efficacy seems equivalent. There is little justification for the use of RUL-ECT in clinical practice.

We now rely on the ictal EEG to define an effective treatment, and modern ECT devices record either one or two channels of brain electrical activity. The typical ictal EEG presents a build-up of energies, then high-voltage spike activity mixed with high-voltage slow waves (3–6 Hz), followed by trains of lesser voltage slow waves, and an abrupt end to the electrical activity with electrical silence. Such EEG patterns, generally of 35–130 sec in duration, are associated with motor seizures that are 10–20 per cent shorter. If seizures do not show these well-defined phases, we repeat the treatment at different energy settings until a robust EEG sequence is elicited.[11–15]

A rise in the post-ictal serum prolactin is another index of seizure adequacy. Grand mal seizures release brain peptides into the CSF and blood. Serum prolactin, easily measured, rises rapidly reaching a peak at about 25–30 min, and falls to a baseline level within 2 h. The absence of a dramatic rise in serum prolactin is a sign of inadequate treatment.[48]

*The ECT course.* Occasionally a single treatment relieves a disorder, but such instances are so rare as to be noteworthy. The basic course is more often between 6 and 20 treatments. These are usually given three times a week at the onset and, after the symptoms show some relief, are reduced to twice or once a week. The resolution of catatonia (MC, NMS) is frequently accomplished in three to five treatments but these are best administered daily. Depressive disorders require 6–12 treatments for resolution. Manic and psychotic disorders require 20 or more treatments.

Discontinuing treatment at the point of immediate resolution of symptoms is associated with high relapse rates. Continuation treatment, often continuation ECT, is as essential a part of ECT management as it is for pharmacotherapy.[49,50]

*Continuation treatments.* High relapse rates are the most common complaint in ECT practice. When patients are given a short course of treatments, early relapse is common. Because ECT is complex, frightening, and expensive, patients seek the shortest course of treatment, and physicians accede by prescribing a limited number of treatments on referral or at the time the patient signs the consent.[4]

Short courses of treatments may relieve symptoms but relapse is quick.[49,50] Continuation treatment is necessary. Two recent studies guide present practice. In a 3-hospital collaborative study of depressed patients referred for ECT, remitted patients were randomly assigned to 6-month courses of medication. Relapse rates were 84 per cent for placebo, 60 per cent for nortriptyline and 39 per cent for the combination of lithium and nortriptyline under serum level control.[50] In the 4-hospital collaborative study, depressed patients treated with bitemporal ECT were randomly assigned to continuation with ECT or the same lithium and nortriptyline combination. The 6-month relapse rates were 32 per cent for continuation medication and 37 per cent for continuation ECT.[49] These rates are statistically indistinguishable in the two studies.

*ECT and psychotropic drugs.*[12, 51] With the exception of antipsychotics, we lack evidence of synergy between psychotropic drugs and ECT.[11,12,14] TCA, MAOI, and SSRI antidepressants are usually discontinued during an ECT course. Anticonvulsants and sedative drugs affect seizure thresholds and may interfere with efficacy. ECT augmentation of antipsychotics is seen as safe and effective.

When ECT is administered to a patient with clinically effective serum lithium levels, generally seen as 0.8–1.2 mEq/l, there is the risk of a post-seizure delirium. If lithium treatment is sustained during ECT, the dosages are reduced so that the serum lithium levels do not rise above 0.6 mEq/l on treatment days.

Systemic drugs, especially those used to treat cardiovascular disorders, may put the patient at risk for hypotension, ataxia, or exaggerated cognitive deficits, but these effects can be easily managed, so they are usually continued during ECT.

Inducing adequate seizures in patients who have been receiving benzodiazepines may be difficult. Intravenous flumazenil, the benzodiazepine antagonist, effectively minimizes the inhibiting effects of benzodiazepines. Such use is encouraged for patients with catatonia or mania who have been treated with benzodiazepines.[9]

## Risks and contraindications

Bone fractures, tardive seizures, and cardiac arrhythmias were common risks of early ECT, but the routine use of muscle relaxation with succinylcholine markedly reduced them.[8,12] Headache, tongue injury, and post-seizure delirium continue to be systemic risks. Headaches respond to analgesics, delirium to benzodiazepines, and tongue injury can be prevented by the proper application of bite-blocs. The principal risks of ECT today are cognitive effects and unacceptable relapse rates.

In a post-seizure delirium, which occurs in about 10 per cent of the treatments, the patient is poorly aware of where he is and may thrash about and be confused. It is more common in the first and second treatments than in later ones. Reassurance, calm talk, and gentle handling of movements that might be harmful can usually allay such states. If the restlessness does pose risks, it can be calmed by intravenous diazepam.

Persistent amnesia is the most dreaded risk of ECT.[12–15] Patients usually forget the personal events that occurred during the illness and treatment. On treatment days, both the anesthesia and the seizure alter cognition, temporarily interfering with the memory of events. In the first decades of ECT use, adequate ventilation was not assured and untoward effects on cognition were profound and frequent. But changes in practice have reduced these effects. Ventilation with pure oxygen, changes in the type of electrical current and the amounts of energy, and selected electrode placement reduced the effects on cognition, so that within a few weeks after the course is over, the patients' performance on memory tests usually surpasses their pre-treatment abilities.

*Contraindications.* There are no systemic illnesses that preclude the administration of ECT when the treatment is clearly warranted. Some conditions — severe hypertension, uncontrolled cardiac arrhythmia, bleeding tendencies, recent myocardial infarction, increased intracranial pressure, and a brain or cerebrovascular lesion — call for special care. The case literature offers suggestions for the appropriate treatment with ECT of patients with these conditions.[12–15]

## Mechanism of action

When convulsive therapy was introduced, its most prominent side effect was amnesia, and much debate centered on whether amnesia was, in fact, the mechanism for improving thought and mood. Experiments with different electrode placements discouraged this explanation.[4,12]

Others focused on the physiologic effects of seizures, especially the changes in the interseizure EEG. Such changes were found to be necessary, but not sufficient, for recovery.[8,52] Interest in this hypothesis is revived by recent studies.[53]

Explanations based on neurohumours and their receptors are important in our present views of the action of drug therapies. These are also cited to explain the benefits of ECT. The experimental data fail to support these explanations.[8,12,54]

Meduna thought that the concentration of glia was a factor in illness and that seizures elicited increased gliosis and recovery.[6] Recent reports cite increased neurogenesis as an active brain response to induced seizures.[55]

My view is that the neuroendocrine system is the most likely agent for the clinical changes brought about by induced seizures.[8,56] Neuroendocrine dysregulation is prominent in patients with the mental disorders for which ECT is effective. Thyroid, adrenal, sex gland, and hypothalamic dysfunction are common in patients with disorders in mood, thought, motor activity, feeding, sleep, sex, growth, and maturation. Indeed, every aspect of body physiology and mental activity is affected by these glands, as exemplified by the action of the adrenal glands in depressive mood disorders.

In the severely depressed patients, the adrenal glands produce too much cortisol.[17, 18, 56] The high blood levels disrupt the normal diurnal rhythms of other glandular discharges, and the glands do not respond to the usual feedback mechanisms. The most prominent features of depression — failure to eat, loss of weight, inability to sleep, loss of interest in sex, inability to concentrate thoughts, and difficulties in memory — are distortions of the functions regulated by the neuroendocrine glands in a self-adjusting feedback.

Each seizure stimulates the hypothalamus to discharge its hormones, which causes the pituitary gland to discharge its products, which then affects the level of cortisol. The first effects of this cascade are transitory, but repeated seizures restore the normal interactions of the hypothalamic-pituitary-adrenal axis. Feeding and sleep become normal, followed by motor activity, mood, memory, and thought.

How does a seizure elicit such profound changes in physiology? In ECT, the currents from the stimulating electrodes on each temple pass through the central parts of the brain, stimulating both the hypothalamus to discharge its hormones and the centrencephalic structures to produce a bilateral grand mal seizure. (One of the flaws in unilateral electrode placement is that the currents have to take indirect routes to affect the pertinent areas of the brain.) The massive amounts of hypothalamic and pituitary hormones that enter the bloodstream during ECT are measurable within a few minutes. They circulate throughout the body, affecting all the body's cells — a compelling and welcome sign of recovery.

After some courses of ECT, the return to normal endocrine function persists. At other times, the glands revert to their abnormal activities and the mental disorder becomes evident again. In these cases, repeated stimulation of the hypothalamus and the pituitary by continuation ECT restore and sustain normal glandular functions and support a normal mental state.

## Suggested replacements for ECT

Although Meduna's experiments and numerous studies of ECT and sham ECT support the seizure as evidence of the brain changes essential to a therapeutic benefit, the introduction of electricity focussed attention away from the seizure and onto electricity as the medium for the treatment's efficacy. This interest is not new. Soon after Galvani and Volta demonstrated that electric currents could stimulate nerves and muscles, medical applications were enthusiastically sought. The first electrical experiments in the mentally ill are ascribed to Gale in New York State in 1802 and Aldini in Italy in 1803.[3,16,54] Electrical experiments were publicly demonstrated by Franklin, Mesmer, and Marat in the first years of the 19th century. Little benefit was recorded and most efforts are best considered quaint explorations.[3] At the time of World War I, faradization was a treatment for hysteria and applied in the military.[57]

During the second half of the 20th century, many techniques have been suggested as replacements for ECT, the latest being transcranial magnetic stimulation (rTMS), vagus nerve stimulation (VNS), and deep brain stimulation (DBS).[58] In rTMS rapidly alternating magnetic fields are delivered to stimulate the brain. At very high intensities, a seizure may be induced and some experiments have been undertaken to compare the seizure induced by magnetic currents with those induced by electric currents. The technique, called magnetic seizure therapy (MST), is reported to have a mild antidepressant effect.[58]

In VNS an electrical stimulator is implanted in the chest wall and electrodes are threaded through the neck to the left vagus nerve. The stimulator is similar to that used to reduce seizures in patients with severe epilepsy. The side effects of hoarseness, nausea, and vomiting are common. In DBS, the stimulating electrodes are placed in the brain, a technique occasionally used in severe Parkinsonism. We lack sufficient evidence for the efficacy of rTMS, VNS and DBS in psychiatric disorders to warrant their routine clinical use.

Device manufacturers who seek a market for their products encourage the technologies. The bad image and the stigma of ECT make its replacement the basis for exploration. At the time of this writing (Spring, 2007), no evidence has been published that any of these techniques have persistent therapeutic effects, and none are replacements for ECT.

## The future in ECT

Induced seizures effectively allay severe psychiatric disorders. The treatment's stigma, however, inhibits its use and research into its mechanism. When neuroscientists recognize the unique nature of the seizure — a phenomenon that is ubiquitous in animal life — and seek to understand its biology, they will then seek ways to replace the gross process of induced seizures by more acceptable interventions. Understanding the mechanism will clarify the aetiology of psychiatric disorders. ECT will be replaced when we understand its mechanism better; for the present, continued usage is assured since no alternative intervention with its efficacy and safety is in our *materia medica*.

## Further information

Abrams, R. (2001). *Electroconvulsive Therapy* (4th edn.). Oxford University Press, New York

Fink, M. (1999). *Electroshock: Restoring the Mind.* Oxford University Press, New York.

Taylor, M.A. Fink, M. (2006). *Melancholia: Diagnosis, Pathophysiology and Treatment of Depressive Illness.* Cambridge University Press, Cambridge UK.

American Psychiatric Association. (2001). *Electroconvulsive Therapy: Recommendations for Treatment, Training and Privileging.* Washington DC.

Scott, A.I.F. (Ed.) (2004). *The ECT Handbook,* (2nd edn.). Royal College of Psychiatrists, London.

Ottosson, J-,O, Fink, M. (2004). *Ethics in Electroconvulsive Therapy. Brunner-Routledge,* New York.

Shorter, E. and Healy, D. (2007). H*istory of the Shock Therapies.* Rutgers University Press, New Brunswick, NJ.

# References

1. Fink, M. (1991). Impact of the antipsychiatry movement on the revival of electroconvulsive therapy in the United States. *Psychiatric Clinics of North America,* **14**(4), 793–801.
2. Fink, M. (1997). Prejudice against ECT: competition with psychological philosophies as a contribution to its stigma. *Convulsive Therapy,* **13**(4), 253–65; discussion 66–8.
3. Kneeland, T.W., and Warren, C.A.B. (2002). *Pushbutton psychiatry: a history of electroshock in America.* Westport, Conn.: Praeger.
4. Ottosson, J.-O., Fink, M. (2004). *Ethics in electroconvulsive therapy.* Brunner–Routledge, New York.
5. Shorter, E., and Healy, D. (2007). *Shock Therapy: The History of Electroconvulsive Treatment in Mental Illness.* Rutgers UP; New Brunswick, in press.
6. Kellner, C.H., Fink, M., Knapp, R., *et al.* (2005). Relief of expressed suicidal intent by ECT: a consortium for research in ECT study. *American Journal of Psychiatry,* **162**(5), 977–82.
7. Meduna, L. (1985). Autobiography. *Convulsive Therapy,* **1**, 43–57; 121–38.
8. Fink, M. (1979). *Convulsive therapy: theory and practice.* Raven Press, New York.
9. Fink, M., and Taylor, M.A. (2003). *Catatonia: a clinician's guide to diagnosis and treatment.* Cambridge University Press, Cambridge, New York.
10. Parker, G., and Hadzi–Pavlovic, D. (1996). *Melancholia: a disorder of movement and mood: a phenomenological and neurobiological review.* Cambridge Unniversity Press, Cambridge, New York, USA.
11. Taylor, M.A., Fink, M. (2006). *Melancholia: the diagnosis, pathophysiology, and treatment of depressive illness.* Cambridge; New York: Cambridge University Press; 2006.
12. Abrams, R. (2002). *Electroconvulsive therapy.* (4th ed.) Oxford Unversity Press, Oxford, New York.
13. American Psychiatric Association. (2001). *Committee on Electroconvulsive Therapy.* Weiner, R.D. The practice of electroconvulsive therapy: recommendations for treatment, training, and privileging: a task force report of the American Psychiatric Association. (2nd edn.) American Psychiatric Association, Washington, DC.
14. Fink, M. (1999). *Electroshock: restoring the mind.* Oxford University Press, New York.
15. Scott, Ae. (2004). *The ECT Handbook.* (2nd edn.) London: Royal College of Psychiatrists.
16. Shorter, E. (1997). *A history of psychiatry: from the era of the asylum to the age of Prozac.* John Wiley & Sons, New York.
17. Carroll, B.J., Curtis, G.C., Mendels, J., *et al.* (1976). Neuroendocrine regulation in depression. II. Discrimination of depressed from nondepressed patients. *Archives of General Psychiatry,* **33**(9), 1051–8.
18. Fink, M. (2005). Should the dexamethasone suppression test be resurrected? *Acta Psychiatrica Scandinavica,* **112**(4), 245–9.
19. Avery, D., and Lubrano, A. (1979). Depression treated with imipramine and ECT: the DeCarolis study reconsidered. *American Journal of Psychiatry,* **136**(4B), 559–62.
20. Kroessler, D. (1985). Relative Efficacy Rates for Therapies of Delusional Depression. *Convulsive Therapy,* **1**(3), 173–82.
21. Flint, A.J., and Rifat, S.L. (1998). Two–year outcome of psychotic depression in late life. *American Journal of Psychiatry,* **155**(2), 178–83.
22. Mulsant, B.H., Haskett, R.F., Prudic, J., *et al.* (1997). Low use of neuroleptic drugs in the treatment of psychotic major depression. *American Journal of Psychiatry,* **154**(4), 559–61.
23. Rasmussen, K.G., Mueller, M., Kellner, C.H., *et al.* (2006). Patterns of psychotropic medication use among patients with severe depression referred for electroconvulsive therapy: data from the Consortium for Research on Electroconvulsive Therapy. *Journal of ECT,* **22**(2), 116–23.
24. Husain, M.M., Rush, A.J., Fink, M., *et al.* (2004). Speed of response and remission in major depressive disorder with acute electroconvulsive therapy (ECT): a Consortium for Research in ECT (CORE) report. *Journal of Clinical Psychiatry,* **65**(4), 485–91.
25. Petrides, G., Fink, M., Husain, M.M., *et al.* (2001). ECT remission rates in psychotic versus nonpsychotic depressed patients: a report from CORE. *Journal of ECT,* **17**(4), 244–53.
26. Goodwin, F.K., and Jamison, K.R. (1990). *Manic–depressive illness.* Oxford University Press, New York.
27. Fink, M. (1999). Delirious mania. *Bipolar Disorders,* **1**(1), 54–60.
28. Mukherjee, S., Sackeim, H.A., Schnur, D.B., *et al.* (1994). Electroconvulsive therapy of acute manic episodes: a review of 50 years'experience. *American Journal of Psychiatry,* **151**(2), 169–76.
29. Black, D.W., Winokur, G., Nasrallah, A., *et al.* (1987). Treatment of mania: a naturalistic study of electroconvulsive therapy versus lithium in 438 patients. *Journal of Clinical Psychiatry,* **48**(4), 132–9.
30. American Psychiatric Association. (1994). *Task Force on DSM–IV. Diagnostic and statistical manual of mental disorders: DSM–IV.* (4th edn.) Washington, DC: American Psychiatric Association.
31. Taylor, M.A., and Fink, M. (2003). Catatonia in psychiatric classification: a home of its own. *American Journal of Psychiatry,* **160**(7), 1233–41.
32. Fink, M., and Taylor, M.A. (2001). The many varieties of catatonia. *European Archives of Psychiatry and Clinical Neuroscience.,* **251** (Suppl 1), I8–13.
33. Caroff, S.N. (2004). *Catatonia: from psychopathology to neurobiology.* (1st ed.) American Psychiatric Pub, Washington, DC.
34. Fink, M., and Sackeim, H.A. (1996). Convulsive therapy in schizophrenia? *Schizophrenia Bulletin,* **22**(1), 27–39.
35. Fink, M. (2000).The interaction of delirium and seizures. *Seminars in Clinical Neuropsychiatry,* **5**(2):93–7.
36. Lowenstein, D.H., and Alldredge, B.K. (1998). Status epilepticus. *New England Journal of Medicine.,* **338**(14), 970–6.
37. Fink, M., Kellner, C.H. and Sackeim, H.A. (1999). Intractable seizures, status epilepticus, and ECT. *Journal of ECT,* **15**(4), 282–4.
38. Fall, P.A., Ekman, R., Granerus, A.K., *et al.* (1995). ECT in Parkinson's disease. Changes in motor symptoms, monoamine metabolites and neuropeptides. *Journal of Neural Transmission. Parkinson's Disease and Dementia Section,* **10**(2–3), 129–40.
39. Avery, D., and Winokur, G. (1978). Suicide, attempted suicide, and relapse rates in depression. *Archives of General Psychiatry,* **35**(6), 749–53.
40. Prudic, J., and Sackeim, H.A. (1999). Electroconvulsive therapy and suicide risk. *Journal of Clinical Psychiatry,* 60 Suppl 2, 104–10; discussion 11–6.
41. Kane, J., Honigfeld, G., Singer, J., *et al.* (1988). Clozapine for the treatment–resistant schizophrenic. A double–blind comparison with chlorpromazine. *Archives of General Psychiatry,* **45**(9), 789–96.
42. Rey, J.M., and Walter, G. (1997). Half a century of ECT use in young people. *American Journal of Psychiatry,* **154**(5), 595–602.

43. Fink, M. (1986). Informed ECT for Patients and Families. Lake Bluff: Somatics, Inc.

44. Folk, J.W., Kellner, C.H., Beale, M.D., *et al.* (2000). Anesthesia for electroconvulsive therapy: a review. *Journal of ECT*, **16**(2), 157–70.

45. Abrams, R. (2002). Stimulus titration and ECT dosing. *Journal of ECT*, **18**(1), 3–9; discussion 14–5.

46. McCall, W.V., Reboussin, D.M., Weiner, R.D., *et al.* (2000). Titrated moderately suprathreshold vs fixed high–dose right unilateral electroconvulsive therapy: acute antidepressant and cognitive effects. *Archives of General Psychiatry*, **57**(5), 438–44.

47. Petrides, G., and Fink, M. (1996). The 'half–age' stimulation strategy for ECT dosing. *Archives of General Psychiatry*, **12**(3), 138–46.

48. Abrams, R., and Swartz, C. (1990). *The Technique of ECT.* Lake Bluff: Somatics, Inc.

49. Kellner, C.H., Knapp, R.G., Petrides, G., *et al.* (2006). Continuational ectroconvulsive therapy vs pharmacotherapy for relapse prevention in major depression: a multisite study from the Consortium for Research in Electroconvulsive Therapy (CORE). *Archives of General Psychiatry*, **63**(12), 1337–44.

50. Sackeim, H.A., Haskett, R.F., Mulsant, B.H., *et al.* (2001). Continuation pharmacotherapy in the prevention of relapse following electroconvulsive therapy: a randomized controlled trial. *Journal of the American Medical Association*, **285**(10), 1299–307.

51. Fink, M., and Kellner, C.H. (1993). ECT and Drugs: Concurrent Administration. *Convulsive Therapy*, **9**(4), 237–40.

52. Fink, M., and Kahn, R.L. (1957). Relation of electroencephalographic delta activity to behavioral response in electroshock; quantitative serial studies. *A. M. A. Archives of Neurology and Psychiatry*, **78**(5), 516–25.

53. Sackeim, H.A., Luber, B., Katzman, G.P., *et al.* (1996). The effects of electroconvulsive therapy on quantitative electroencephalograms. Relationship to clinical outcome. *Archives of General Psychiatry*, **53**(9), 814–24.

54. Shorter, E., and Healy, D. (2007). *History of the Shock Therapies.* Rutgers University Press, New Brunswick.

55. Fink, M. (2004). Induced seizures as psychiatric therapy: Ladislas Meduna's contributions in modern neuroscience. *Archives of General Psychiatry*, **20**(3), 133–6.

56. Fink, M. (2000). Electroschock revisited. *American Scientist*, **88**(2), 162–7.

57. Eissler, K.R. (1986). *Freud as an expert witness: the discussion of war neuroses between Freud and Wagner-Jauregg.* International Universities Press, New York.

58. Lisanby, S.H. (2004). *Brain stimulation in psychiatric treatment.* American Psychiatric Pub, Washington, DC.

## 6.2.10.2 **Phototherapy**

Philip J. Cowen

## Introduction

Phototherapy or artificial bright-light treatment, has been used in the management of a number of medical disorders including psoriasis and hyperbilirubinaemia of the newborn. From the point of view of psychiatric treatment, the notion that light might help people with certain psychological symptoms has an ancient lineage. For example, Wehr and Rosenthal[1] cite Aretaeus who suggested in the second century AD that 'lethargics are to be laid in the light and exposed to the rays of the sun (for the disease is gloom)'. In 1898,

a ship's physician named Frederick Cook recorded that the 'languor' which affected members of an Antarctic expedition during the winter darkness could be relieved with bright artificial light.[1]

The first systematic study of phototherapy as a psychiatric treatment was carried out in 1984 by Rosenthal *et al.*[2] who used bright artificial light to treat patients with the newly identified syndrome of seasonal affective disorder. Seasonal affective disorder is a recurrent mood disorder in which patients experience regular episodes of depression in autumn and winter with remission in spring and summer. Since then phototherapy has become the mainstay of the treatment of seasonal affective disorder, particularly in patients with atypical depressive features such as hyperphagia and hypersomnia. Phototherapy has also been used as an investigational treatment in other psychiatric disorders but the evidence for its efficacy in these conditions less established.

## Mechanism of action

### Light and seasonal and circadian rhythms

Animals and humans show circadian and seasonal rhythms in aspects of their physiology and behaviour that are influenced by environmental cues or *zeitgebers*. The light–dark cycle is believed to be one of the most important *zeitgebers* regulating circadian and seasonal rhythmicity in mammals. Mammalian circadian rhythms are driven by an 'oscillator' in the suprachiasmatic nucleus of the hypothalamus. Environmental light influences the activity of this nucleus via a neuronal pathway which runs from the retina to the hypothalamus. Thus appropriately timed bright light is able to advance or delay endogenous circadian rhythms.[3]

Lewy *et al.*[4] suggested that in patients with seasonal affective disorder the delayed onset of dawn in the autumn causes endogenous circadian rhythms to become phase-delayed with respect to clock time and the sleep–wake cycle. Bright-light treatment is able to correct this abnormality by phase advancing circadian rhythms, thereby re-synchronizing them with the sleep–wake cycle. This proposal is supported by the fact that controlled trials show that in most patients morning phototherapy is more effective than evening phototherapy.[5] While this hypothesis gives a good account of how bright-light treatment might ameliorate the symptoms of seasonal affective disorder, its possible efficacy in other conditions such as non-seasonal depression is difficult to explain by this mechanism.

### Light treatment and monoamines

It is possible that bright-light treatment, through its interaction with the hypothalamus, could alter the circadian activity of the monoamine neurotransmitters involved in mood regulation. For example, some studies have shown that the antidepressant effects of phototherapy can be reversed by treatments that diminish both catecholamine and serotonin neurotransmission.[6] This has been taken as evidence that the antidepressant effects of bright light are mediated via activation of serotonin and catecholamine pathways. An alternative explanation is that in the absence of concomitant drug treatment, recovered depressed patients are vulnerable to depletion of these neurotransmitters in any case. However, effects of bright light on monoamines could account for the therapeutic effects of light in mood disorders other than winter depression.

## Forms of phototherapy

The most common form of phototherapy uses a light box, which contains fluorescent tubes mounted behind a translucent plastic-diffusing screen. Depending on the fluorescent tubes employed, the light emitted is either full spectrum, which contains a little ultraviolet light, or cool white light which has no ultraviolet. The light box usually rests on a table or desk at about the eye level of a seated subject. The output of different light boxes varies but is usually between 2500 and 10 000 lux. Light sources producing 10 000 lux are more expensive but allow a reduced duration of exposure (30 min compared with 120 min) to secure a therapeutic effect.[7]

Phototherapy has also been administered using head-mounted units or light visors. These instruments are attached to the head and project light into the eyes allowing subjects to remain mobile while receiving treatment. While light visors are more convenient to use than light boxes, results from placebo-controlled trials have not been encouraging.[7]

Another form of light therapy involves the use of dawn-simulating alarm clocks. These clocks are programmed to simulate the illumination that would be experienced out of doors during sunrise on a spring day.[8] In practice, the clocks begin a gradual illumination of the bedroom about 2 h before normal wake time, increasing to a maximum of about 250 lux at the point of waking. Overall the effects of dawn-simulation in the treatment of winter depression seem equivalent to those of bright-light treatment[9] and patients often find dawn-simulating clocks more convenient (although a partner sleeping in the same room may not).

### Adverse effects

Generally phototherapy is well tolerated although mild side effects occur in up to 45 per cent of patients early in treatment. These include headache, eye strain, blurred vision, eye irritation, and increased tension. Insomnia can occur particularly with late-evening treatment. Rare adverse events that have been reported include manic mood swings and suicide attempts, the latter putatively through light-inducing alerting and energizing effects prior to mood improvement. Whether these rare events are actually adverse reactions to the light is uncertain. There is no evidence that phototherapy employed in recommended treatment schedules causes ocular or retinal damage.

## Indications and contraindications to light treatment

### Seasonal affective disorder

The best established indication for light treatment is seasonal affective disorder where patients experience autumn and winter depressions. Clinical predictors of a response to light treatment include the following:

♦ Increased sleep

♦ Increased appetite and winter weight gain

♦ Carbohydrate craving

♦ Afternoon slump in energy

♦ Complete remission of symptoms in the summer

Several controlled trials have assessed the efficacy of bright-light treatment in the treatment of winter depression. In a meta-analysis of nine randomized studies, Golden et al.[9] found a significant benefit of bright light over dim light control with an effect size of 0.84 (95 per cent confidence interval, 0.6–1.08). A similar benefit was apparent for six studies of dawn simulation which had a mean effect size of 0.73 (95 per cent confidence interval, 0.37–1.08). While these data are compelling it needs to be remembered that it is often difficult to arrange a placebo treatment that will match the therapeutic expectation of bright light or dawn simulation.

### Other mood disorders

Patients with more typical melancholic symptoms (e.g. weight loss and insomnia) do less well with bright-light treatment, even when the disorder is seasonal in nature. However, bright light has also been used in the treatment of non-seasonal depression both as a sole treatment as an adjunct to more conventional therapy. The evidence for the efficacy of bright light for this indication is less established but a Cochrane review[10] suggested that morning light treatment was significantly better than control treatment when applied as an adjunct to drug treatment or sleep deprivation. Most of these studies were of short-term duration and there are suggestions that the added benefit of light therapy does not persist when treatment stops.[11] In these studies, hypomania was more common in light-treated subjects. Phototherapy may also be of benefit in other conditions characterized by depressed mood and overeating (e.g. premenstrual dysphoria and bulimia nervosa). The literature contains reports of a number of controlled trials in such disorders where light treatment has improved depression ratings. However, the difficulty of distinguishing the specific and placebo effects of bright-light treatment relative to dim light control makes the current data difficult to interpret.

### Circadian rhythm disorders

Because bright light is an effective *zeitgeber* for circadian rhythms it may also have a useful place in the treatment of disorders characterized by circadian rhythm disturbances. Such disorders encompass a range of conditions including phase-delayed or phase-advanced sleep disorder, jet lag, and problems related to shift work. In addition, disturbances of the sleep–wake cycle are common in older people with cognitive impairment. There are several reports of the utility of light treatment in these conditions; however, there is a paucity of randomized trial data.[7]

### Contraindications

There are no absolute contraindications to phototherapy, except the obvious caveat that since the therapeutic effect depends on retinal activation, subjects must have sufficient visual function to allow this to occur. Otherwise it would seem prudent to avoid phototherapy in patients with pronounced and untreated agitation because this symptomatology could be worsened. In addition, evening phototherapy may worsen insomnia.

A substantial minority of patients with seasonal affective disorder meet criteria for bipolar II disorder, raising the concern that phototherapy may trigger hypomania in such individuals. Particular caution might be needed in patients with a bipolar I syndrome. Some regimes of phototherapy might lead to a degree of sleep deprivation which could also destabilize mood in bipolar patients.

## Interactions

One of the advantages of phototherapy in seasonal affective disorders is that the use of antidepressant drugs may be avoided. Despite this, many patients with winter depression use phototherapy concomitantly with antidepressant medication without an obvious potentiation of adverse effects. However, a case report described apparent serotonin toxicity where phototherapy was combined with selective serotonin re-uptake inhibitors.[7]

Like bright light, the pineal hormone, melatonin, also has the ability to shift the timing of circadian rhythms[2] and theoretically melatonin taken at an inappropriate time of day could offset the antidepressant effect of light. It is also possible that bright-light treatment could exacerbate the ability of some drugs (e.g. chlorpromazine, St John's Wort) to cause skin photosensitivity reactions.[7]

## Effects of withdrawal of phototherapy

If a patient with seasonal affective disorder responds to light treatment, withdrawal of treatment during the period of seasonal vulnerability leads to a return of symptomatology within a few days. It may be possible, however, to lessen the daily duration of treatment particularly towards the end of winter without inducing relapse. Otherwise cessation of light treatment does not seem to cause a specific withdrawal syndrome.

## Administration of phototherapy

Since the best established indication for phototherapy in psychiatry is seasonal affective disorder, the following account will describe the use of bright-light treatment in winter depression. One of the major practical difficulties in phototherapy is the time needed to administer treatment. For this reason a 10 000 lux light box may be preferred because the daily duration of treatment can be reduced to 30 min. It seems likely that cool-white light and full-spectrum light have equivalent clinical efficacy, but because cool-white light is free of ultraviolet light it is theoretically safer and should be preferred.

The balance of evidence suggests that bright-light treatment of winter depression is most effective when administered in the early morning.[4] However, treatment given later in the day may be effective for some patients. In an initial trial, therefore, it is best to recommend early morning treatment but to advise the patient that the timing of therapy can eventually represent a balance of therapeutic efficacy and practical convenience. Treatment in the late evening should be avoided because of the possibility of sleep disruption.

Early-morning phototherapy should start a few minutes after waking. Subjects should allow themselves a 30 min duration of treatment with a 10 000 lux light source. They should seat themselves about 30 to 40 cm away from the light box screen. They should not gaze at the screen directly but face it an angle of 45° and glance across it once or twice each minute.

The antidepressant effect of light treatment usually appears in a few days but in controlled trials up to 3 weeks can be needed before the therapeutic effects of bright light exceed those of placebo treatment. If no benefit is noted after the third week of therapy, light treatment should probably be abandoned. As noted above mild side effects are common in the early stages of treatment but usually settle without specific intervention. If they are persistent and troublesome the patient can sit a little further away from the light source or reduce the duration of exposure. Exposure should also be reduced or stopped if elevated mood occurs.

Once a therapeutic response has occurred it is usually necessary to continue phototherapy up to the usual time of natural remission, otherwise relapse will occur. It may be possible, however, to lower the daily duration of treatment. Phototherapy can also be started in advance of the anticipated episode of depression as this may have a preventative effect; however, the evidence for this is limited and doubts have been expressed.[7,12]

## Further information

Centre for Environmental Therapeutics. http://www.cet.org.

Seasonal Affective Disorder Association. http://www.sada.org.uk.

Eagles, J.M. (2003). Reading about seasonal affective disorder. *The British Journal of Psychiatry*, **182**, 174–6.

## References

1. Wehr, T.A. and Rosenthal, N.E. (1989). Seasonality and affective illness. *The American Journal of Psychiatry*, **146**, 829–39.

2. Rosenthal, N.E., Sack, D.A., Gillin, C., *et al.* (1984). Seasonal affective disorder: a description of the syndrome and preliminary findings with light therapy. *Archives of General Psychiatry*, **41**, 72–80.

3. Arendt, J. and Broadway, J. (1987). Light and melatonin as *zeitgebers* in man. *Chronobiology International*, **4**, 273–82.

4. Lewy, A.J., Sack, R.L., Miller, S.L., *et al.* (1987). Antidepressant and phase-shifting effects of light. *Science*, **206**, 710–13.

5. Terman, J.S., Terman, M., Lo, E.S., *et al.* (2001). Circadian time of morning light administration and therapeutic response in winter depression. *Archives of General Psychiatry*, **58**, 69–75.

6. Neumeister, A., Turner, E.H., Matthews, J.R., *et al.* (1998). Effects of tryptophan depletion versus catecholamine depletion in patients with seasonal affective disorder in remission with light therapy. *Archives of General Psychiatry*, **55**, 524–30.

7. Eagles, J.M. (2004). Light therapy and the management of winter depression. *Advances in Psychiatric Treatment*, **10**, 233–40.

8. Terman, M. and Terman, J.S. (2006). Controlled trial of naturalistic dawn simulation and negative air ionization for seasonal affective disorder. *The American Journal of Psychiatry*, **163**, 2126–33.

9. Golden, R.N., Gaynes, B.N., Ekstrom, R.D., *et al.* (2005). The efficacy of light therapy in the treatment of mood disorders: a review and meta-analysis of the evidence. *The American Journal of Psychiatry*, **162**, 656–62.

10. Tuunainen, A., Kripke, D.F., and Endo, T. (2007). Light therapy for non-seasonal depression. http://www.cochrane.org.reviews/en/ab004050.html.

11. Martiny, K., Lunde, M., Unden, M., *et al.* (2006). The lack of sustained effect of bright light in non-seasonal major depression. *Psychological Medicine*, **36**, 1247–52.

12. Partonen, T. and Lonnqvist, J. (1996). Prevention of winter seasonal affective disorder by bright-light treatment. *Psychological Medicine*, **26**, 1075–80.

# 6.2.10.3 **Transcranial magnetic stimulation**

## Declan McLoughlin and Andrew Mogg

## Introduction

Transcranial magnetic stimulation (TMS) is a means of non-invasively stimulating the cerebral cortex using a hand-held coil applied to the scalp. In recent years TMS has been increasingly used to target neuronal circuitry implicated in neuropsychiatric disorders.

A key milestone in the development of TMS occurred in 1831 when Michael Faraday discovered the phenomenon of electromagnetic induction whereby a time-varying magnetic field can induce electrical currents through a conductor lying in proximity to the field. The French biophysicist D'Arsonval in 1896 induced phosphenes, vertigo, and syncope in human subjects by placing an induction coil around their heads. In the late 1950s, Kolin stimulated peripheral nerves (the frog sciatic nerve) with a magnetic field and a few years later the same technique was used in human subjects, inducing muscle twitching by applying a pulsed magnetic field over the ulnar, peroneal, and sciatic nerves.

In the mid-1980s, Barker and colleagues in Sheffield developed a magnetic stimulator to directly stimulate the human motor cortex.[1] They applied a circular coil, through which a large (4000 A), brief (110 μs) current was passed to the scalp. The resulting pulsed magnetic field was used to stimulate the motor cortex, evoking movements in the contralateral limbs and is known as transcranial magnetic stimulation. This ability to non-invasively stimulate the motor cortex with a magnetic field soon replaced high-voltage transcutaneous electrical stimulation for assessing central motor conduction times and mapping corticospinal pathways in a variety of neurological conditions. In the late 1980s machines capable of delivering multiple TMS pulses were developed. Repetitive TMS (rTMS), unlike single pulses of TMS can produce effects that last after the period of stimulation. For example, it has been shown that rapid rTMS (at frequencies of 5 Hz and greater) enhances motor excitability whereas slow rTMS (at 1 Hz or less) transiently depresses excitability.[2] The underlying principle of rTMS treatment is that the normal balance of excitatory and inhibitory processes within certain neuronal pathways may be disrupted in psychiatric conditions such as depression. Stimulating the brain using rTMS provides a means of increasing and decreasing excitation and inhibition in these pathways, having a neuromodulatory effect and allowing a focal targeting of specific neuronal circuitry.

## Mechanism of action

The underlying mechanisms of the effects of rTMS remain poorly understood. This is in part because, as with attempting to understand the mode of action of psychotropic medication, it is difficult to establish links between cellular and physiological changes and alterations in emotion, thinking, and behaviour. Techniques used to try to better understand the molecular and physiological effects of rTMS have included neuroimaging and animal studies.

Neuroimaging has demonstrated that rTMS may exert effects on the brain at a considerable distance from the site of stimulation. For example, serial positron emission tomography scanning has been used to measure regional cerebral blood flow in medication-free patients with major depression before and after courses of fast and slow rTMS administered over the left prefrontal cortex.[3] It has been demonstrated that fast rTMS causes increases in regional cerebral blood flow in bilateral frontal, limbic, and paralimbic areas whereas slow rTMS caused decreases in blood flow in the right prefrontal cortex, left medial temporal cortex, and left basal ganglia and amygdala.

It has been suggested that rTMS of the left prefrontal cortex may modulate brain function by an effect on dopamine release. Elevated extracellular dopamine concentrations in the dorsal hippocampus have been demonstrated in the brains of rats who received rTMS. However, one of the problems with using animal models of rTMS is that currently small rTMS coils are not available and it is therefore impossible to focally stimulate one particular area of the small rodent brain. In humans it has been shown that rTMS to the dorsolateral prefrontal cortex can induce the release of dopamine in the ipsilateral caudate nucleus.[4]

## Side-effects

Being non-invasive and not requiring a general anaesthetic, rTMS is considered to be a relatively safe treatment and few side-effects have been reported. The most significant potential side-effect is the risk of unintended seizure induction. There have been six reports to date of seizure induction in healthy volunteers. In half of these, very high stimulation intensities and frequencies were used. There have only been three reports of seizures in patients receiving rTMS and one of these patients had a pre-existing diagnosis of temporal lobe epilepsy. Researchers generally follow safety guidelines that exclude high-risk patients, (e.g. those with a stroke, brain tumour or pre-existing epilepsy) from receiving rTMS. These guidelines also suggest limits to the intensity, frequency, and stimulus duration of the rTMS used.[5]

The most common side-effect of rTMS is headache or facial discomfort that is the result of direct stimulation of muscle and nerves in proximity to the coil. Approximately 10–30 per cent of subjects experience these symptoms, which are generally short-lived and well-tolerated.

## Technique

rTMS equipment comprises a stimulator unit, booster modules, a laptop computer, and a figure-of-eight coil. The stimulator unit contains the charging circuitry, energy storage capacitors, control electronics and discharge, and safety circuitry. It is connected to booster modules, which charge the high-voltage capacitors, enabling trains of high-intensity magnetic stimulation to be produced. The stimulating coil consists of tightly wound copper wire in a figure-of-eight through which a rapidly alternating electric current passes to produce a pulsed magnetic field. Various stimulation parameters including train duration, frequency of stimulation, stimulus intensity, and length of inter-train interval can be altered using computer software.

rTMS treatment is delivered via the figure-of-eight coil applied to the scalp surface. Typically, prior to treatment, TMS will be used to map the motor area of the right abductor pollicis brevis (APB), and measure its motor threshold. The stimulus intensity delivered during treatment is then calculated in relation to this motor threshold. The main method of localizing the stimulation site has been to use a fixed point in anatomical relation to a specific motor area, for example the dorsolateral prefrontal cortex has generally been defined as the point 5 cm anterior to the APB motor area in the parasaggital plane. More recently some studies have used magnetic resonance imaging to more accurately delineate the area to be stimulated.

## rTMS and depression

Transcranial magnetic stimulation was first postulated to have potential applications in psychiatry by Bickford and colleagues who noted transient elevation in mood in several healthy subjects who had received single pulses of TMS to the motor cortex.[6] Several small open studies followed that suggested that low frequency rTMS over the vertex may have antidepressant effects. Since the mid 1990s most interest has focussed on high-frequency rTMS applied to the left dorsolateral prefrontal cortex (LDLPFC), a region reported to be underactive in depression. To date there have been approximately 30 randomized trials of real and placebo rTMS in depression. In addition there have been several published meta-analyses including a Cochrane review.[7] This reviewed 16 trials, 14 of which were suitable for quantitative analysis. They found that high-frequency rTMS to the LDLPFC and low-frequency rTMS to the right dorsolateral prefrontal cortex (RDLPFC) were both superior to sham treatment but only for one measure (the Hamilton Depression Rating Scale) and at one time point (immediately after 2 weeks of treatment). The difference between real and sham was not large, leading to the conclusion that at this stage there was not strong evidence to support the use of rTMS as an antidepressant therapy.

There has been considerable heterogeneity between studies. Nearly all the trials have comprised patients with major depressive disorder defined using DSM-IV criteria. However there has been considerable variability with respect to pharmacotherapy received, with some trials specifying treatment resistance (variously defined) and some specifying medication-free participants. In two of the studies patients were started on antidepressant treatment either shortly before or simultaneously with the rTMS treatment.

The choice of appropriate sham condition is an important methodological consideration. There are two main approaches. Most studies have relied on tilting the active coil (usually through 45° or 90° with one or both wings of the coil touching the scalp). However intracerebral voltage measurements in a rhesus monkey have shown that, depending on how the coil is tilted, sham conditions obtained by coil tilting can induce voltages in the brain to levels only 24 per cent below active rTMS.[8] The fact that some 'sham' coils produce significant cortical stimulation may account for some of the benefit seen in those receiving sham stimulation and may underestimate the difference between real and placebo treatment. The other approach is to use a specially designed placebo coil. This looks identical to the real coil and makes the same noise but does not cause any cortical stimulation. However, neither does it cause sensation to the scalp, meaning that subject blinding may still be less effective. Indeed the problem of maintaining

blinding in studies with rTMS continues to be a major methodological issue.

Most studies have given high-frequency rTMS to the LDLPFC, probably as a result of the positive early studies when this area was stimulated. Several investigators have used low-frequency rTMS to the RDLPFC. Low-frequency rTMS is much less likely to induce a seizure and is probably better tolerated by patients. Since slow rTMS has an inhibitory effect in contrast to the excitatory effect of fast rTMS and since there is considerable evidence that the left and right hemispheres have contrasting functions in regulating mood, it could be speculated that slow rTMS to the right cortex may have a similar effect to fast rTMS to the left.

Studies of high-frequency rTMS in depression have generally used stimulation frequencies of 5 to 20 Hz. There is a suggestion from animal studies that higher frequency stimulation may have a greater antidepressant effect but so far the numbers of subjects in human studies have been too low to show if a difference in effect of varying stimulation frequency exists. Likewise, the optimal stimulus intensity, length of treatment course, and total number of stimulations is not yet clear from the published data. However, longer trials with an increase number of stimulations appear to make little difference.[9]

Most of the rTMS studies in depression have been small, the largest until recently having 70 patients. However, recently a much larger industry-sponsored (Neuronetics) trial submitted their findings to the US Food and Drug Administration (FDA), seeking licensing approval for an rTMS device. In this study 301 patients were randomized to real or sham rTMS. Participants received 10 Hz rTMS of the left dorsolateral prefrontal cortex, 3000 pulses per day for 20 days. Although there was a marginal difference between the groups in favour of rTMS at the end of treatment, there was no significant group difference on an intention-to-treat analysis of the primary outcome measure (Montgomery-Åsberg Depression Rating Scale). In January 2007 the FDA Neurological Devices panel considered Neuronetic's application to have its rTMS equipment licensed for therapeutic use. The panel felt that there was insufficient evidence to support its efficacy. The final FDA decision is expected in summer 2007 (website: http://www.fda.gov/cdrh/panel/summary/neuro-012607.html, accessed: 5 June 2007).

In the United Kingdom the National Institute for Clinical Excellence (NICE) has issued recommendations stating 'Current evidence suggests there are no major safety concerns associated with transcranial magnetic stimulation for severe depression but there is no evidence that the procedure has clinically useful efficacy' (website: http://www.nice.org.uk/article.aspx?o=ip346consultation, accessed: 5 June 2007).

## Comparisons with ECT

In addition to comparisons with placebo treatment, rTMS has also been directly compared with ECT in several studies. While ECT is the most effective treatment for severe depression in the short-term its use is limited by several issues, including acceptability to patients, the requirement to be anaesthetized, and the occurrence of side-effects, particularly cognitive side-effects. rTMS could be a potential alternative if it proved effective. In total there have been six published randomized controlled trials to date comparing ECT and rTMS. These trials have all had relatively small numbers of patients, particularly when compared with trials of antidepressant medications. They have either shown rTMS to be less effective or not statistically different from ECT. The most recent and largest trial to date included 46 patients and compared 3 weeks of treatment with rTMS to a course of ECT.[10] The mean reduction in the Hamilton Depression Rating Scale achieved at the end of treatment was 14.1 points in the ECT group, compared with 5.4 points for the rTMS group, translating into a mean percentage reductions from baseline of 58 and 22 per cent, respectively. Overall, ECT was shown to be substantially more effective as a short-term treatment of depression than rTMS.

## rTMS and schizophrenia

While most studies of rTMS within psychiatry have focussed on depression, there has been a growing interest in using rTMS as a possible treatment for schizophrenia. It has been used to treat both auditory hallucinations and to alleviate negative symptoms of schizophrenia.

Auditory hallucinations occur in approximately 70 per cent of patients with schizophrenia and in about a quarter of cases respond poorly if at all to antipsychotic medication. Recent advances in neuroimaging have enabled measurement of neural activity while hallucinations are being experienced and it has been demonstrated that auditory hallucinations are associated with activation in a number of brain areas, including the temporal cortex bilaterally. This area has been targeted in several rTMS studies using slow rTMS to reduce excitability.

The first account of using rTMS to treat auditory hallucinations reported improvement in the severity of hallucinations of three patients with schizophrenia who had 40 min/day of 1 Hz rTMS over 4 days.[11] There have now been 15 published treatment studies of rTMS targeting auditory hallucinations in schizophrenia. Ten sham-controlled trials (involving 212 patients) were included in a recent meta-analysis[12] which concluded that overall rTMS was significantly better than sham stimulation in the treatment of auditory hallucinations.

Negative symptoms of schizophrenia include alogia, avolition, anhedonia, and affective flattening and are associated with attentional impairment and executive dysfunction. Negative symptoms are often resistant to neuroleptic medication and are associated with poor clinical outcome. There is increasing evidence that negative symptoms are related to reduced cortical activation, particularly involving the left prefrontal cortex. Therefore one treatment approach has been to attempt to increase activation within this region. There have been four published randomized controlled studies comparing real and sham rTMS of the left dorsolateral prefrontal cortex to target negative symptoms of schizophrenia, of which three found no difference between real and sham treatments and one found 2 weeks of high-frequency rTMS significantly improved negative symptoms. Novak et al.[13] additionally performed a battery of neuropsychological tests and follow-up patients for 6 weeks after treatment but found no significant differences between treatment groups at either time point for primary or secondary outcome measures. The most recent study[14] did not provide evidence that rTMS to the DLPFC improved negative symptoms of schizophrenia in patients with prominent negative symptoms but did suggest that rTMS may improve cognitive functioning in this patient group, at least in the short-term.

However larger studies with longer periods of follow-up will be required to further examine this preliminary finding.

## rTMS and obsessive–compulsive disorder

There have been several studies that have attempted to treat symptoms of obsessive–compulsive disorder (OCD) by modulating activity in prefrontal and motor circuits using rTMS. The earliest blinded trial of rTMS for OCD included 12 patients and found that a single session of right prefrontal high-frequency cortical stimulation significantly decreased compulsive urges for over 8 h.[15] Obsessive thoughts did not change significantly. This study suggested that rTMS may be a useful probe of neuronal circuitry associated with symptoms of OCD. However a number of subsequent studies have failed to replicate these findings. A Cochrane review in 2003 examined three randomized controlled trials and concluded that there were currently insufficient data to draw conclusions about the efficacy of rTMS in the treatment of OCD.[16]

The most recent, and largest trial of TMS in OCD to date randomly allocated 33 patients with OCD to receive 10 sessions of either active or sham low-frequency (1 Hz) rTMS over the LDLPFC.[17] This study did not demonstrate any difference between real and sham treatments.

## rTMS and other neuropsychiatric disorders

rTMS has been postulated as a potential treatment in a variety of other neuropsychiatric disorders. There is emerging evidence that it may improve some of the motor symptoms of Parkinson's disease. In a recent study six daily sessions of high-frequency rTMS were given to 55 unmedicated patients with Parkinson's disease.[18] Patients received either 10 Hz or 25 Hz rTMS bilaterally to the motor cortex arm and leg areas or to the occipital cortex (control group). It was found that stimulation to the motor areas improved all measures, e.g. walking time, key-tapping speed, and self-assessment and that 25 Hz stimulation yielded greater improvement than 10 Hz. The effect was sustained for a month after treatment and restored by further booster sessions. The authors concluded that 25 Hz rTMS can lead to cumulative and long-lasting benefits on motor performance in Parkinson's disease.

A recent study explored the effect of low-frequency rTMS to the left temperoparietal region on chronic tinnitus.[19] Patients received 1200 stimuli per day for 5 days of either real or placebo treatment in a randomized controlled crossover trial. Overall active rTMS induced a transient, but significant improvement in the symptoms of tinnitus.

rTMS has also been used in an attempt to provide relief from chronic neuropathic pain.[20] A recent review summarized that high-frequency rTMS to the motor cortex is able to produce pain relief but that the effect is brief and that research in this area is required.

rTMS has also been used as a probe of neuronal circuits in dementia and in attention deficit hyperactivity disorder although any possible therapeutic role for it in these conditions appears some way off.

## Summary

rTMS has an increasing role as a useful investigational tool for probing neuronal circuitry in a variety of neuropsychiatric disorders. However its therapeutic value is at present less certain.

The antidepressant efficacy of rTMS has now been investigated for over 15 years and despite initial early enthusiasm there is still not clear evidence for its usefulness as a treatment in depression, reflected in the recent FDA and NICE decisions. Further research is required to identify specific brain regions in specific conditions that may be appropriate targets for treatment with rTMS, allowing tailoring of treatments for individual patients. The recent development of neuronavigational techniques using MRI imaging should aid treatment site localization. Other future research should be directed at establishing optimal rTMS parameters, e.g. the intensity, frequency and number of treatments.

## Further information

http://www.ists.unibe.ch/ is the homepage of the International Society for Transcranial Stimulation. It also provides links to other websites of interest.

George, M.S. and Belmaker, R.H. (eds.) (2007). *Transcranial magnetic stimulation in clinical psychiatry*, p. 289. American Psychiatric Publishing. Arlington, VA. Provides a useful summary of the theoretical and practical aspects of TMS research.

Lisanby, S.H. (ed.) (2004). *Brain stimulation in psychiatric treatment*, p. 153. American Psychiatric Publishing, Washington, DC. Reviews transcranial magnetic stimulation and also other brain stimulation techniques including deep brain stimulation, magnetic seizure therapy and vagus nerve stimulation.

## References

1. Barker, A.T., Jalinous, R., and Freeston, I.L. (1985). Non-invasive magnetic stimulation of human motor cortex. *Lancet*, **1**, 1106–7.

2. Hallett, M. (2000). Transcranial magnetic stimulation and the human brain. *Nature*, **406**,147–50.

3. Speer, A.M., Kimbrell, T.A., Wassermann, E.M., *et al.* (2000). Opposite effects of high and low frequency rTMS on regional brain activity in depressed patients. *Biological Psychiatry*, **48**, 1133–41.

4. Strafella, A.P., Paus, T., Barrett, J., *et al.* (2001). Repetitive transcranial magnetic stimulation of the human prefrontal cortex induces dopamine release in the caudate nucleus. *The Journal of Neuroscience*, **21**, RC157.

5. Wassermann, E.M. (1998). Risk and safety of repetitive transcranial magnetic stimulation: report and suggested guidelines from the international workshop on the safety of repetitive transcranial magnetic stimulation, June 5–7, 1996. *Electroencephalography and Clinical Neurophysiology*, **108**, 1–16.

6. Bickford, R.G., Guidi, M., Fortesque, P., *et al.* (1987). Magnetic stimulation of human peripheral nerve and brain: response enhancement by combined magnetoelectrical technique. *Neurosurgery*, **20**, 110–6.

7. Martin, J.L., Barbanoj, M.J., Schlaepfer, T.E., *et al.* (2002). Transcranial magnetic stimulation for treating depression. *Cochrane Database of Systematic Reviews*, **2**, CD003493.

8. Lisanby, S.H., Gutman, D., Luber, B., *et al.* (2001). Sham TMS: intracerebral measurement of the induced electrical field and the induction of motor-evoked potentials. *Biological Psychiatry*, **49**, 460–3.

9. Loo, C.K., Mitchell, P.B., McFarquhar, T.F., *et al.* (2007). A sham-controlled trial of the efficacy and safety of twice-daily rTMS in major depression. *Psychological Medicine*, **37**, 341–9.

10. Eranti, S., Mogg, A., Pluck, G., *et al.* (2007). A randomized, controlled trial with 6-month follow-up of repetitive transcranial magnetic stimulation and electroconvulsive therapy for severe depression. *The American Journal of Psychiatry*, **164**, 73–81.

11. Hoffman, R.E., Boutros, N.N., Berman, R.M., *et al.* (1999). Transcranial magnetic stimulation of left temporoparietal cortex in three patients reporting hallucinated. "voices" *Biological Psychiatry*, **46**, 130–2.

12. Aleman, A., Sommer, I.E., and Kahn, R.S. (2007). Efficacy of slow repetitive transcranial magnetic stimulation in the treatment of resistant auditory hallucinations in schizophrenia: a meta-analysis. *The Journal of Clinical Psychiatry*, **68**, 416–21.

13. Novak, T., Horacek, J., Mohr, P., *et al.* (2006). The double-blind sham-controlled study of high-frequency rTMS (20Hz) for negative symptoms in schizophrenia: negative results. *Neuroendocrinology Letters*, **27**, 209–13.

14. Mogg, A., Purvis, R., Eranti, S., *et al.* (2007). Repetitive transcranial magnetic stimulation for negative symptoms of schizophrenia: a randomized controlled pilot study. *Schizophrenia Research*, **93**, 221–8.

15. Greenberg, B.D., George, M.S., Martin, J.D., *et al.* (1997). Effect of prefrontal repetitive transcranial magnetic stimulation in obsessive-compulsive disorder: a preliminary study. *The American Journal of Psychiatry*, **154**, 867–9.

16. Martin, J.L., Barbanoj, M.J., Perez, V., *et al.* (2003). Transcranial magnetic stimulation for the treatment of obsessive-compulsive disorder. *Cochrane Database of Systematic Reviews*, **3**, CD003387.

17. Prasko, J., Paskova, B., Zalesky, R., *et al.* (2006). The effect of repetitive transcranial magnetic stimulation (rTMS) on symptoms in obsessive-compulsive disorder. A randomized, double blind, sham controlled study. *Neuroendocrinology Letters*, **27**, 327–32.

18. Khedr, E.M., Rothwell, J.C., Shawky, O.A., *et al.* (2006). Effect of daily repetitive transcranial magnetic stimulation on motor performance in Parkinson's disease. *Movement Disorders*, **12**, 2201–5.

19. Rossi, S., De Capua, A., Ulivelli, M., *et al.* (2007). Effects of repetitive transcranial magnetic stimulation on chronic tinnitus. A randomised, cross over, double blind, placebo-controlled study. *Journal of Neurology, Neurosurgery, and Psychiatry*, **78**, 857–63.

20. Leo, R.J and Latif, T. (2007). Repetitive transcranial magnetic stimulation (rTMS) in experimentally induced and chronic neuropathic pain: a review. *The Journal of Pain*, **8**, 453–9.

## 6.2.10.4 **Neurosurgery for psychiatric disorders**

Keith Matthews and David Christmas

## Ablative neurosurgery

### Definition

Historical definitions of Neurosurgery for Mental Disorder (NMD), previously known as 'psychosurgery', have either made distinctions between neurosurgery for psychiatric or 'psychological' illness and disorders assumed to have a clearer 'biological' origin (e.g. epilepsy, Parkinsons' disease); or, have emphasized control of behaviour as a therapeutic objective rather than the control of symptoms. A more recent definition, and the one used throughout this chapter is that provided by the UK Royal College of Psychiatrists:[1]

> *A surgical procedure for the destruction of brain tissue for the purposes of alleviating specific mental disorders carried out by a stereotactic or other method capable of making an accurate placement of the lesion.*

### Historical overview

The first attempt at treating psychiatric illness by surgical methods is commonly attributed to Gottlieb Burckhardt, a Swiss psychiatrist, who in 1888 performed 'temporal topectomy' on six patients who were most probably suffering from schizophrenia. His intention was to sever the connections between the frontal lobes and the rest of the brain. Results were mixed: one patient was reported as improved; two were 'quieter'; and two showed no change. However, one patient died; another developed epilepsy; and a further had motor weakness. His results were met with a mixture of ridicule and hostility and he never again wrote on the subject.

In 1935, James Fulton and Carlyle Jacobsen operated on the frontal lobes of two chimpanzees named Becky and Lucy after first studying their responses to frustration in behavioural experiments. They found their behaviour dramatically changed after the surgery. Becky's previous agitated responses to frustration became more passive whilst Lucy was much more agitated. At a London meeting in 1935, they presented their findings to an audience which included Egas Moniz, a Portuguese neurologist.

Moniz teamed up with Almeida Lima, a neurosurgeon, and in a 30-min operation in November 1935, they performed frontal leucotomy on their first patient. The procedure first involved injecting alcohol into the white matter tracts of the frontal lobes, but they later would change to using an instrument of their own design, the leucotome, to extirpate 'cores' of tissue. In 1936, they published their report on the outcomes of 20 patients who were probably suffering from depression, panic disorder, and schizophrenia. One-third were better, one-third were worse, and one-third were unchanged.

Shortly after their paper was published, Walter Freeman, a US neurologist, wrote an enthusiastic review and quickly secured the collaboration of a neurosurgeon, James Watts. They modified the procedure slightly and began practising what Freeman termed bilateral frontal lobotomy. Over the next decade, Freeman became frustrated with the cumbersome requirements of a neurosurgical theatre and team. Adapting a technique first described in the 1930s, Freeman infamously developed the transorbital lobotomy in 1946. Notorious for the initial use of an ice-pick, the procedure involved forcing a tool (an 'orbitoclast') under the upper eyelid and through the base of the skull into the frontal lobes. Also known as the 'ice-pick lobotomy', the relative ease with which the procedure could be performed resulted in the widespread adoption of the technique throughout the United States and Europe. However, it was the indiscriminate overuse of such 'freehand' procedures and the associated adverse effects that occurred in many patients that led to public and professional antipathy towards neurosurgery for psychiatric illness, which peaked in the late 1950s. The introduction of chlorpromazine in 1954 also meant that for the first time there was a non-surgical treatment for schizophrenia.

Despite a reduction in the use of neurosurgery for mental disorder in the late 1950s and early 1960s, the development of stereotactic techniques (which had been demonstrated in 1908 by Horsley and Clarke and adapted for human use in 1947 by Spiegel and Wycis) meant that greater accuracy and greater consistency in neurosurgery could deliver better outcomes in selected patients. Procedures became more selectively and reliably targeted and lesions became more discrete.

## Procedures

All NMD procedures have targeted one or more of three main regions: (i) fronto-limbic connections within the orbital or cingulate cortices; (ii) subcortical limbic circuitry; and (iii) limbic cortex, including the amygdala and cingulate cortex.

Four 'modern' stereotactic procedures have been described with only two remaining in regular usage in the Western World. Anterior capsulotomy is still performed in Cardiff (UK), Spain, Belgium, and Scandinavia, whilst anterior cingulotomy is the procedure of choice in Dundee (UK), Poland, South Korea, and North America.

### (a) Subcaudate tractotomy (SST)

Developed in the United Kingdom by Geoffrey Knight in 1965, lesions were originally created using radioactive Yttrium$^{90}$ rods. SST targets the white matter tracts of the 'substantia innominata' connecting the orbital cortex to limbic regions, and probably involved lesioning the nucleus accumbens.

### (b) Anterior capsulotomy (ACAPS)

Described by Jean Talairach in 1949 and further developed by Lars Leksell for the treatment of chronic pain, ACAPS places lesions in the anterior limb of the internal capsule—a large white matter bundle connecting the frontal cortex with the thalamus and limbic structures. Lesions are generated using focused gamma radiation (gammacapsulotomy) or thermal damage (thermocapsulotomy). (See figure 6.2.10.4.1 for typical ACAPS lesions.)

### (c) Anterior cingulotomy (ACING)

The cingulate gyrus was first proposed as a target by John Fulton in the late 1940s. Hugh Cairns, an English neurosurgeon and a friend of Fulton's, performed 'cingulectomy' in 1948. The less destructive 'cingulotomy' was first performed by Eldon Foltz and Lowell White in 1962 for the treatment of pain. (See figure 6.2.10.4.2 for typical ACING lesions.)

### (d) Limbic leucotomy

First developed by Desmond Kelly in 1973, it represented a combination of cingulotomy and subcaudate tractotomy lesions.

## Indications

During the 1960s and 1970s, a variety of other operations were explored as treatments for hypersexuality, aggression, and criminality. These included hypothalamotomy and amygdalotomy. Reports of outcomes from such interventions were often favourable, but interpretation has been complicated by issues of diagnosis, patient selection, and assessment. Such clinical presentations are not considered appropriate indications for surgery today.

Three main indications exist for modern NMD: obsessive-compulsive disorder (OCD); anxiety disorders; and major depression. Only individuals who have experienced chronic, disabling symptoms that have failed to respond after the diligent pursuit of available treatments (pharmacological and psychological) should be considered for ablative neurosurgery.

There are few absolute contraindications to NMD. There is no evidence to support the use of NMD as a treatment for eating disorders, schizophrenia, or personality disorders. However, where these exist as significant comorbid conditions alongside depression or OCD, these do not represent absolute contraindications and careful consideration is required.

## Ethical considerations

One of the most persistent concerns for the public and for health professionals is that NMD is used to treat patients in the absence of informed consent. Although the absence of informed consent was likely to be an issue for early procedures, to the best of our knowledge, all contemporary centres performing NMD today insist upon the patient's ability to give informed consent. In Scotland, the Mental Welfare Commission must authorize any proposed NMD as being in the patient's best interests and must confirm that the patient is capable of providing informed consent. In England and Wales, the Mental Health Act Commission has a duty to set-up multi-disciplinary panels to authorize NMD for consenting patients under Section 57 of the Mental Health Act, 1983. Similarly, in most other countries where the procedure is available, the procedure can only go ahead with the approval of an independent review board.

## Criteria for NMD

General criteria for suitability show little variation between centres. Key inclusion and exclusion criteria for NMD in Dundee are shown below in Table 6.2.10.4.1.

## Outcomes from NMD

Whilst placebo-controlled trials are considered the ideal assessment for intervention trials, they have frequently been described as unethical in the case of NMD. Despite this, there have been three isolated double-blind trials, involving a total of 6 patients. Despite suggestions of non-response in all cases, follow-up was brief and there is inadequate detail to make informed judgements of outcome.

### (a) Combined outcomes for different procedures

Comparisons across studies are of limited value due to differences in procedure, patient characteristics, and the use of different rating scales. However, Spangler et al.[2] reviewed outcomes from different procedures and for different indications, defining a positive outcome as being a score of 1 or 2 on the Clinical Global Impression (Improvement) scale.[2] Positive outcome rates were: ACAPS (67 per cent); ACING (61 per cent); SST (37 per cent); and limbic leucotomy (67 per cent). The most effective procedures for affective disorder and OCD (respectively) were limbic leucotomy followed by ACING. The least effective procedure for both disorders (and overall) was SST.

**Table 6.2.10.4.1** Inclusion and exclusion criteria for NMD

| Inclusion criteria | Exclusion criteria |
| --- | --- |
| 1. Age ≥20 years | 1. Age <20 years |
| 2. *Legal status*: both formal and informal patients can be considered | 2. Failure to fulfil ICD-10 criteria for a suitable indication |
| 3. *ICD-10 diagnosis of*: severe depressive episode; recurrent depressive disorder, current episode moderate to severe; bipolar affective disorder, current episode severe depression | 3. *Primary diagnosis of*: substance misuse; organic brain syndrome; adult personality disorder; pervasive developmental disorder |
| 4. *Duration of episode of illness*: minimum of 3 years, with at least 2 years of unremitting symptoms despite active treatment. Only in exceptional circumstances would a duration<5 years be considered | 4. Absence of evidence of an adequate therapeutic trial of psychological treatment |
| 5. *Consent*: the patient must be capable of providing sustained, informed consent | 5. Absence of evidence of extensive trials of adequate pharmacological treatment |

### (b) Anxiety disorders

The crude rate of improvement following NMD (all procedures) for anxiety disorders ($n = 290$) is 77 per cent.[1] More recent reports of ACAPS would support a claim to effectiveness but this may be at the expense of significant adverse effects (apathy and dysexecutive symptoms).

### (c) Obsessive-compulsive disorder

The combined rate of 'Completely Improved' or 'Improved' outcomes following SST is 52 per cent. More recent studies involving ACAPS or ACING report improvements on the Yale-Brown Obsessive-Compulsive scale (Y-BOCS) in the region of 30 per cent. Despite this relatively low figure, approximately 85 per cent of patients ($n = 478$) will have a marked or lesser improvement following NMD for OCD.[1]

### (d) Depression

There is only one report of outcomes from ACAPS for depression. Herner (1961) described outcomes for 19 patients with a 'depressive state'.[3] Outcomes included: 'permanent improvement' (74 per cent); unchanged (5 per cent); and worse (5 per cent). In all 75 per cent experienced permanent side effects.

Spangler et al. (1996) reported that 53 per cent of those with affective disorder ($n = 10$) responded to ACING, with a 60 per cent response rate in unipolar depression.[2] Dougherty et al. (2003) reported a mean reduction in Beck Depression Inventory (BDI) score of 33 per cent in 13 patients following ACING.[4] With regards to limbic leucotomy, there are few studies looking at outcomes solely in depression but Mitchell-Heggs (1976) reported that 7 of 9 patients with depression improved after surgery.[5]

### (e) Bipolar disorder

There are only two reports of NMD for bipolar disorder, both following SST.[6,7] Each involved small numbers ($n = 9$) but described improvements in cycle frequency with a greater effect on manic episodes than depression. Improved drug responsiveness was also alleged.

## Mechanism of action

The mechanism of action of NMD is unknown, but almost all neurosurgical procedures involve lesioning white matter tracts connecting the prefrontal cortex with the thalamus, cingulate gyrus, and areas of the limbic system such as the amygdala and hippocampus. Neuroimaging studies have suggested that this circuitry is dysfunctional in depression and interrupting parts of these circuits may rectify emotional and cognitive processing within these brain areas. In the case of OCD, there is compelling evidence that symptoms arise from functional circuits connecting the frontal cortex, thalamus, and basal ganglia and that lesioning parts of this circuit may serve to eradicate many of the symptoms.

## Adverse effects

### (a) General adverse effects

Transient adverse effects such as headache are relatively common and tend to resolve in the first week after surgery. Post-operative confusion can occur in 3–10 per cent of patients with higher rates following SST. Incontinence is relatively uncommon with modern procedures, but the reported rates are: 1.1 per cent after SST;

5.5 per cent after ACING; and 9.5 per cent with limbic leucotomy. Apathy has been reported to occur in up to 24 per cent of patients following limbic leucotomy, but not all studies report its occurrence and this is likely to be a relatively high estimate. The incidence of weight gain varies greatly: 6.2 per cent after SST; 65.5 per cent after ACAPS; and 5.5–21.4 per cent after ACING. Similarly, there is wide variation in the reported rates of seizures: 1.6–3.3 per cent after SST; 0–7.7 per cent after ACAPS; 1–9 per cent after ACING; and 14.2 per cent after limbic leucotomy. Finally, suicide rates range from 1 per cent after SST to 12 per cent after ACING but these rates may reflect differing severities of illness.

### (b) Effects on personality

It is certainly the case that early procedures such as leucotomy had marked effects on the personality and behaviour of large numbers of patients. However, with the advent of stereotactic procedures and more focused lesions, the effects on personality appear to be mild, sometimes even absent. It is acknowledged, however, that it is difficult to make robust appraisals of personality without assessment tools designed for such a purpose and in the context of symptom reduction in chronic illnesses.

Most published studies have reported normalization of personality traits following modern procedures such as ACING and ACAPS. In addition, there is a trend towards reductions in neuroticism and increases in extraversion. There are some recent reports of adverse effects on executive function following ACAPS for anxiety disorders[8] but many such studies lack preoperative assessments of personality making conclusions difficult to draw.

### (c) Effects on neuropsychological function

As with personality changes, the detrimental effects of earlier procedures upon neuropsychological functioning were probably significant. However, the majority of studies reporting neuropsychological outcomes from ACAPS, ACING, and limbic leucotomy from the early 1970s onwards report either no deterioration on general measures (such as IQ, attention, memory) post-operatively or, more frequently, improvement. It is likely that improvements in performance are mediated through symptom reduction.

## Vagus nerve stimulation (VNS)

### Overview

The vagus nerve is the longest of the 12 cranial nerves and 80 per cent of its fibres are sensory afferents. These fibres terminate in the nucleus tractus solitarius, sending ascending fibres to the forebrain via the locus coeruleus and parabrachial nucleus. The vagus nerve, therefore, provides an access route to modify information which is processed in brain regions involved in mood regulation.

VNS involves the subcutaneous implantation of a programmable pulse generator in a location similar to a cardiac pacemaker. Electrodes connect the generator to the left cervical portion of the vagus nerve. Stimulation is delivered in an intermittent pattern (typically 30 s every 5 min) but parameters are changed using a palmtop computer and a programming wand held over the pulse generator.

VNS was first used to treat epilepsy in 1988 and became available for the treatment of refractory partial seizures in 1994. The first trials in depression began in 1998.

### Outcomes in depression

There are a number of short, open trials of VNS which typically report a 3-month response rate (≥50 per cent reduction in the 24-item Hamilton Rating scale for Depression; $HRSD_{24}$) of 30–40 per cent, and a remission rate ($HRSD_{24} \leq 9$) of approximately 15 per cent.

Larger, 12-month trials have demonstrated 12-month response rates of 27.2–46 per cent and remission rates of 15.8–29 per cent.[9,10] In a 12-month controlled comparison of VNS versus Treatment-As-Usual (TAU), George et al.[11] reported response rates of 27 per cent for VNS + TAU versus 13 per cent for TAU. Such improvements appear to be maintained at 2 years, with response rates of 42 per cent and remission rates of 22 per cent.[12] In the only randomized, controlled trial of VNS, Rush et al.[13] reported 10-week response rates on the $HRSD_{24}$ of 15.2 per cent in the VNS group versus 10.0 per cent in the placebo group, changes which were non-significant.[13] Despite positive results in uncontrolled trials, definitive evidence of efficacy remains elusive.

### Adverse effects

Most adverse effects are related to stimulation, and in most people they are fairly mild and improve over time. Many can be managed by altering the stimulation parameters. In the initial stages, common effects are: hoarse voice (53 per cent); headache (23 per cent); neck pain (17 per cent); cough (13 per cent); and dyspnoea (17 per cent). At 12-months, the only adverse effect to persist at rates higher than 10 per cent is hoarse voice (21 per cent).[9]

## Deep brain stimulation (DBS)

### Overview

As with VNS, DBS has evolved from a treatment for neurological disorders to a putative intervention for psychiatric illness. The most

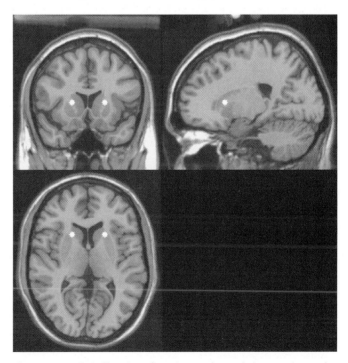

**Fig. 6.2.10.4.1** Typical locations of anterior capsulotomy lesions superimposed upon normalized T1 MRI scan.
Lesions not to scale.

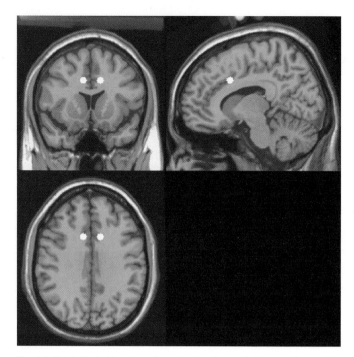

**Fig. 6.2.10.4.2** Typical locations of anterior cingulotomy lesions superimposed upon normalized T1 MRI scan. Lesions not to scale.

effective targets for OCD and depression have yet to be determined but a number of possible locations for stimulation exist. However, DBS should be considered as an experimental treatment for both disorders.

The procedure involves the bilateral implantation of electrodes using stereotactic guidance with post-operative confirmation of location using MR scanning. The electrodes are connected to a generator typically implanted in the abdomen. Following surgery, the stimulation settings are programmed using immediate/short-term changes in symptoms as a guide.

### DBS for obsessive-compulsive disorder

The most common target for DBS for OCD, thus far, has been ventral portion of the anterior limb of the internal capsule, the same site as ablative anterior capsulotomy. In a double-blind cross-over trial of anterior capsular stimulation in four patients Nuttin *et al.* (2003) reported reductions in symptoms of 36.8 per cent which were maintained after 21 months. In a small case series of four patients Abelson *et al.*[14] described marked improvements in one patient, with a lesser improvement in another. Greenberg *et al.* (2006) reported responses (≥35 per cent reduction in Y-BOCS score) in 4 out of 8 patients with DBS in the internal capsule.

Other proposed targets include the nucleus accumbens and the ventral caudate nucleus, but all targets may involve stimulation of a common anatomical area.

### DBS for depression

In the only published report of DBS for depression, Mayberg *et al.*[15] stimulated the white matter tracts of the subgenual cingulate gyrus in six patients. Four patients were responders whilst two showed no change. Randomized on-off-on-off trials confirmed a stimulation-related improvement which was associated with a reduction in local cerebral blood flow in the subgenual cingulate and dorsolateral prefrontal cortex.

### Adverse effects

Adverse effects that have been reported include: throbbing or buzzing sensations; nausea; and jaw tingling. A number of reports have described problems with battery life with the stimulators being replaced every 5 to 12 months. Battery failure has often been associated with a recurrence of symptoms over a few days which has been associated with marked depressive symptomatology and suicidal ideation. One study has reported a suicide, but commented that this was unrelated to stimulation. Numbers of reported cases are too small to determine if this is indeed the case.

## Conclusions

Despite its chequered past, modern NMD bears little similarity to historical freehand procedures. Advances in neuroimaging mean that anatomical substrates for depression and OCD are being elucidated. Ablative procedures such as ACAPS and ACING are unlikely to undergo randomized controlled trials but prospective clinical audit suggests that such procedures may offer improvement to selected patients with treatment-refractory depression and OCD. Interventions such as VNS and DBS offer the possibility of double-blind testing but as yet there is insufficient evidence to suggest that such procedures offer greater effectiveness.

## Further information

Freeman, C., Crossley, D., and Eccleston, D. (2000). *Neurosurgery for mental disorder. Report from the Neurosurgery Working Group of the Royal College of Psychiatrists.* Royal College of Psychiatrists, London.

Binder, D.K. and Iskandar, B.J. (2000). Modern neurosurgery for psychiatric disorders. *Neurosurgery,* **47**, 9–21.

Feldman, R.P., Alterman, R.L., and Goodrich, J.T. (2001). Contemporary psychosurgery and a look to the future. *Journal of Neurosurgery,* **95**, 944–56.

George, M.S., Rush, A.J., Sackeim, H.A., *et al.* (2003). Vagus nerve stimulation (VNS): utility in neuropsychiatric disorders. *International Journal of Neuropsychopharmacology,* **6**, 73–83.

Malone, D.A., Greenberg, B.D., and Rezai, A.R. (2004). The use of deep brain stimulation in psychiatric disorders. *Clinical Neuroscience Research,* **4**, 107–12.

## References

1. Freeman, C., Crossley, D., and Eccleston, D. (2000). *Neurosurgery for mental disorder. Report from the Neurosurgery Working Group of the Royal College of Psychiatrists.* Royal College of Psychiatrists, London.
2. Spangler, W.J., Cosgrove, G.R., Ballantine, H.T. Jr., *et al.* (1996). Magnetic resonance image-guided stereotactic cingulotomy for intractable psychiatric disease. *Neurosurgery,* **38**, 1071–6.
3. Herner, T. (1961). Treatment of mental disorders with frontal stereotaxic thermo-lesions: a follow-up study of 116 cases. *Acta Psychiatrica Scandinavica,* **36**(Suppl. 158), 1–140.
4. Dougherty, D.D., Weiss, A.P., Cosgrove, G.R., *et al.* (2003). Cerebral metabolic correlates as potential predictors of response to anterior cingulotomy for treatment of major depression. *Journal of Neurosurgery,* **99**, 1010–7.
5. Mitchell-Heggs, N., Kelly, D., and Richardson, A. (1976). Stereotactic limbic leucotomy—a follow-up at 16 Months. *The British Journal of Psychiatry,* **128**, 226–40.

6. Lovett, L.M. and Shaw, D.M. (1987). Outcome in bipolar affective disorder after stereotactic tractotomy. *The British Journal of Psychiatry*, **151**, 113–16.

7. Poynton, A., Bridges, P.K., and Bartlett, J.R. (1988). Resistant bipolar affective disorder treated by stereotactic subcaudate tractotomy. *The British Journal of Psychiatry*, **152**, 354–8.

8. Rück, C., Andreewitch, S., Flyckt, K., *et al.* (2003). Capsulotomy for refractory anxiety disorders: long-term follow-up of 26 patients. *The American Journal of Psychiatry*, **160**, 513–21.

9. Marangell, L.B., Rush, A.J., George, M.S., *et al.* (2002). Vagus nerve stimulation (VNS) for major depressive episodes: one year outcomes. *Biological Psychiatry*, **51**, 280–7.

10. Rush, A.J., Sackeim, H.A., Marangell, L.B., *et al.* (2005). Effects of 12 months of vagus nerve stimulation in treatment-resistant depression: a naturalistic study. *Biological Psychiatry*, **58**, 355–63.

11. George, M.S., Rush, A.J., Marangell, L.B., *et al.* (2005). A one-year comparison of vagus nerve stimulation with treatment as usual for treatment-resistant depression. *Biological Psychiatry*, **58**, 364–73.

12. Nahas, Z., Marangell, L.B., Husain, M.M., *et al.* (2005). Two-year outcome of vagus nerve stimulation (VNS) for treatment of major depressive episodes. *The Journal of Clinical Psychiatry*, **66**, 1097–104.

13. Rush, A.J., Marangell, L.B., Sackeim, H.A., *et al.* (2005). Vagus nerve stimulation for treatment-resistant depression: a randomized, controlled acute phase trial. *Biological Psychiatry*, **58**, 347–54.

14. Abelson, J.L., Curtis, G.C., Sagher, O., *et al.* (2005). Deep brain stimulation for refractory obsessive-compulsive disorder. *Biological Psychiatry*, **57**, 510–6.

15. Mayberg, H.S., Lozano, A.M., Voon, V., *et al.* (2005). Deep brain stimulation for treatment-resistant depression. *Neuron*, **45**, 651–60.

# 6.3

---

# Psychological treatments

## Contents

6.3.1 **Counselling**
Diana Sanders

6.3.2 **Cognitive behaviour therapy**

    *6.3.2.1* **Cognitive behaviour therapy for anxiety disorders**
    David M. Clark

    *6.3.2.2* **Cognitive behaviour therapy for eating disorders**
    Zafra Cooper, Rebecca Murphy, and Christopher G. Fairburn

    *6.3.2.3* **Cognitive behaviour therapy for depressive disorders**
    Melanie J. V. Fennell

    *6.3.2.4* **Cognitive behaviour therapy for schizophrenia**
    Max Birchwood and Elizabeth Spencer

6.3.3 **Interpersonal psychotherapy for depression and other disorders**
Carlos Blanco, John C. Markowitz, and Myrna M. Weissman

6.3.4 **Brief individual psychodynamic psychotherapy**
Amy M. Ursano and Robert J. Ursano

6.3.5 **Psychoanalysis and other long-term dynamic psychotherapies**
Peter Fonagy and Horst Kächele

6.3.6 **Group methods in adult psychiatry**
John Schlapobersky and Malcolm Pines

6.3.7 **Psychotherapy with couples**
Michael Crowe

6.3.8 **Family therapy in the adult psychiatric setting**
Sidney Bloch and Edwin Harari

6.3.9 **Therapeutic communities**
David Kennard and Rex Haigh

## 6.3.1 Counselling

Diana Sanders

### Introduction

People seek counselling for many reasons. Sometimes those who have had no previous need for mental health services are literally stopped in their tracks by life events—illness, family breakdown, intolerable stresses. People with long-term difficulties may turn to counselling when they feel the statutory services are not able to meet their needs, or as an adjunct to health care provision. With greater social mobility and the separation of family members, counselling increasingly provides the care and support previously offered within local communities. The provision and acceptability of counselling is on the increase. Counselling is possibly the most commonly delivered form of psychological therapy[1,2] and the British Association for Counsellors and Psychotherapists have over 30 000 members, with equivalent numbers in other countries. Professional training programmes in counselling have mushroomed in response to demand. Counsellors are found in many statutory and voluntary settings—mental health, primary care and medical settings, workplaces, drug and alcohol services, voluntary and charitable organizations, trauma services, and educational settings—as well as in private practice.

But what exactly is counselling? What do counsellors do? Is counselling the same as psychotherapy? And, is it an effective form of treatment? Although counselling is a major growth area within mental health, it can be difficult for consumers and purchasers of counselling services to know what kind of counselling and counsellor to use, with lack of clarity about what works for whom. There are many different models of counselling, types of counsellor and many different training courses. It is difficult to make clear distinctions between counselling and psychotherapy. Much of the work of counsellors has not historically been amenable to standard methods of evaluation, and research is relatively new. Currently there is no statutory regulation for the term 'counsellor', which means that people are able to practise as counsellors without registration or accreditation. By definition, people who seek counselling are likely to be vulnerable, and the issue of public protection is paramount.

The aim of this chapter is to clarify these issues and examine the place of counselling in psychiatry. The chapter begins by looking at the definition of counselling, and how counselling is both similar to, and distinct from, psychotherapy. The chapter goes on to look at the key features of counselling, and different models of counselling. Although counselling can and is used for many psychological difficulties, the chapter selects specific problems where there is evidence that it is an effective intervention: mild to moderate depression, adjustment difficulties, bereavement, trauma, and relationship problems. I then consider counselling in different settings, again selecting a few which illustrate the work of counsellors—primary care, mental health settings, student counselling, and the workplace—looking at the way counselling can be adapted according to the needs of the service. The chapter concludes by looking at issues of training, quality, and standards, commenting on the need for the control of an ever-developing profession without loss of the growing availability of effective counselling services to those in need.

## Defining counselling

No single definition of either counselling or psychotherapy exists in spite of many attempts in Britain, North America, and elsewhere to arrive at one.[3] Currently, neither the British Association of Counselling and Psychotherapy (BACP) nor the American Counseling Association has either proprietary rights of the terms or even official definitions, although, as discussed below, the move towards statutory regulation for counselling and psychotherapy may ensure greater clarity for practitioners and consumers.

At its broadest, counselling is conceptualized as a way of helping or assisting others to make their own adjustment and decisions in the face of life problems. Counselling aims to offer a safe relationship within which the individual can explore personal difficulties and, through developing a deeper understanding of themselves, move towards change. The Department of Health defines counselling as . . . a *form of psychological therapy that gives individuals an opportunity to explore, discover, and clarify ways of living more resourcefully, with a greater sense of well being. Counselling may be concerned with addressing and resolving specific problems, making decisions, coping with crises, working through conflict, or improving relationships with others.*[4]

In contrast with other forms of psychological therapy, where the focus may be on treating specific problems, many counselling models give equal if not more weight to the *process* of change. The journey through which a client goes—to greater understanding, awareness, and resolution—is as important as the outcome. Counsellors practise within all therapeutic approaches, strongly influenced by humanistic, experiential, and psychodynamic principles. They tend not to link their work to diagnostic categories, preferring to see each client as an individual, and using an approach matching the client's needs rather than diagnosis. Counsellors may define themselves by the model they practise—for example, humanistic or psychodynamic—and/or by the type of problems they work with, such as bereavement or relationship counsellors.

Counselling may also be defined in terms of *key elements* and *goals*,[5] as shown in Table 6.3.1.1. Again, the key elements and goals illustrate the variation within counselling. For example, what is meant by counselling ranges from providing a safe arena for people to gain understanding and insight, to offering more direction and guidance leading to decision-making and problem-solving.

**Table 6.3.1.1** The key elements and goals of counselling (Reproduced from Feltham, C. What are counselling and psychotherapy? In The Sage Handbook of Counselling and Psychotherapy, (eds. C. Feltham and I. Horton), pp. 3–10, copyright 2006, Sage Publications.)

| The key elements of counselling | The goals of counselling |
|---|---|
| ◆ Listening and talking methods of addressing psychological and psychosomatic problems and change | ◆ Support, psycho-education and guidance |
| ◆ An unstructured and non-directive form of therapy, using the therapeutic relationship as an active ingredient in promoting change | ◆ Insight and understanding |
| | ◆ Self actualization and personality change |
| | ◆ Adjustment, symptom reduction and 'cure' |
| ◆ Counselling operates largely without medication or other physical interventions | ◆ Problem-solving and decision-making |
| ◆ Counselling may be concerned not only with mental health but with social, spiritual, philosophical and other aspects of living | ◆ Crisis intervention and management |
| ◆ Professional forms of counselling are based on formal training, accreditation and on-going supervision and professional development | ◆ Risk management (e.g. genetic counselling) |

## Counselling and psychotherapy

Much of the above can also be applied to psychotherapy and parts of this chapter do indeed overlap significantly with psychotherapy. There may well be variation between countries in what is defined as counselling or psychotherapy. Counselling and psychotherapy each have distinct features including different historical roots. *Psychotherapy* arose from the seminal works of Freud in the late nineteenth and twentieth centuries, and in the past, psychotherapists tended to offer a long-term psychodynamic approach. Now, however, psychotherapy also includes interpersonal, humanistic, and cognitive models. In the United States, *counselling* was originally linked with vocational guidance, personnel management, and the workplace,[5] and as such was much more advisory and directive than the analytic processes of psychotherapy. Carl Rogers, the founder of non-directive counselling in the 1940s, initiated the movement away from practical guidance and problem-solving towards collaborative and person-centred models, forming the basis of counselling today.

Differences between psychotherapy and counselling tend to relate more to the individual psychotherapist's or counsellor's training and interests and to the setting in which they work, rather than to any intrinsic difference in the two activities. In medical and mental health settings, psychotherapists are more likely to work with patients with severe psychological disorders, offering long-term therapy, whereas counsellors may concentrate on difficulties amenable to short-term work—mild to moderate psychological disorders, relationship difficulties, or bereavement. Counsellors who work for voluntary agencies or in educational settings such as schools and colleges usually concentrate more on the 'everyday' problems and difficulties of life than on severe psychological disorders, although agencies such as MIND, Alcoholics Anonymous, or

Narcotics Anonymous offer counselling to people with serious mental illnesses. In private practice, however, a counsellor's work will overlap with that of a psychotherapist.

In a pragmatic vein, Feltham states that *practitioners and the public stand to gain much more from the assumption of commonality than from spurious or infinitesimal distinctions . . . little is to be gained practically from further controversy about professional titles and distinctions.*[5] In 2000, the British Association for Counselling lent weight to greater rapprochement by becoming the British Association for Counselling and Psychotherapy. On a practical level, it is interesting that many recipients of 'talking therapies' other than counselling, such as psychotherapies, cognitive-behaviour therapy and problem-focused discussions with GPs, psychiatrists, or nurses, say that they have received *counselling*, reinforcing Feltham's plea that the issue of definition and distinction is academic rather than of practical value.

### Counselling skills and counselling practice

*Counselling skills* are integral to the practice of psychiatry and all the 'helping professions', as basic ingredients of effective interviewing, accurate history-taking, diagnosis, and treatment-planning.[6] The skills of listening, summarizing, reflecting, checking, understanding, gaining rapport, and communicating enable other people to feel understood. They are essential for engagement and eliciting information, especially when the person is afraid, in pain, or mistrustful. The health worker's counselling skills may influence the patient's collaboration with an active participation in treatment, and thereby the outcome of a wide range of medical and even surgical treatments. Many helping and health professionals such as social workers, occupational therapists, probation officers, and speech and communication therapists use counselling skills as an integral part of their work but would not be seen as primarily counsellors.

In contrast, counsellors as *professionals*, who use counselling as a specific intervention, work in many areas of mental health practice alongside psychotherapists, clinical and counselling psychologists, psychiatrists, psychiatric nurses, and social workers.[7] For professional counsellors, counselling skills are central to their work.

Counselling as a specific planned intervention in psychiatry can be differentiated into two broad and overlapping categories, defined by aims into *decision-making* and *treatment*:

- *Decision-making* is an important ingredient in many forms of therapeutic counselling but, conversely, some forms of decision-oriented counselling (e.g. genetic counselling) embody no explicit therapeutic intention.

- Counselling as a primary *treatment* for problems is used in the management of a range of conditions as an adjunct to other interventions including medication, as an integral component of a multimodal treatment method (e.g. crisis intervention), or as a specific treatment in its own right (e.g. for postnatal depression).

### Counselling psychology

As well as professional counsellors, counselling psychologists have a particular role to play within counselling provision in mental health. The area of counselling psychology, now developing in the United Kingdom in line with other parts of the world, is a distinctive profession within applied psychology, which aims to foster the psychological development of the individual and help people develop more effective and fulfilled lives. It is based on the fundamental tenets of counselling, but in addition aims to integrate the application of psychological theory and research into its practice.[8] Counselling psychologists use a variety of therapeutic models, including person-centred, psychodynamic, and cognitive. Although the training of counsellors can be varied, as discussed below, counselling psychologists undergo standardized post-graduate doctorate training leading to chartered status within the British Psychological Society, or equivalent in other countries.

## Is counselling an effective method of treatment?

Despite the proliferation of counsellors in many areas of medicine and psychiatry, counselling has tended to lag behind medicine and other health care professions in engaging in and promoting research to establish its effectiveness and efficacy.[9] The nature of counselling can mean that standard methods such as RCTs are not appropriate means of evaluation, whereas qualitative research methodology is better able to assess meaningful changes.[10] However, counselling as a profession is now engaging in better quality research, concentrating on outcomes in routine practice as well as qualitative analysis. New practice-based methods of evaluation, such as CORE (Clinical Outcomes in Routine Evaluation), and the aggregation of data across UK NHS counselling services can lead to national benchmarks. Methods of case-study research, and the development of measures of the client's perspective on psychological distress, PSYCHLOPS,[11] enable more client-focused research. Such emphasis on evidence-based practice will lead to more careful targeting of specific counselling approaches to specific problems,[3] clearer information for the public and will improve counselling's parity with other health care professions.

Currently, counselling has an image that it is more appropriate for people with mild to moderate difficulties. The Department of Health[4] recommends that counselling should not be the main intervention for people with severe and complex mental health problems or personality disorders. Patients who are adjusting to life events, illnesses, disabilities, or losses may benefit from brief therapies such as counselling. However, counsellors such as those in primary care and the voluntary sector are already offering an important and valued service. Although people with more serious and enduring mental health difficulties require primarily psychiatric and pharmacological intervention, offering emotional support, advice, and problem-solving can form an important, although under-researched, part of their care.

## The core conditions of counselling and the therapeutic relationship

Counselling depends primarily on the interaction between the counsellor and client, what goes on in that interaction and the qualities of both client and counsellor. Carl Rogers'[12] definition of the conditions necessary for therapeutic change was a radical departure from traditional psychotherapeutic practice, in emphasizing the *qualities* and *attitudes* of the counsellor rather than specifying what the counsellor must *do*. His work led to the following as *necessary* and *sufficient* conditions for therapeutic change:

- The client is in a state of *incongruence*, being vulnerable or anxious.

- The therapist is *congruent* and *genuine* in the relationship with the client.

◆ The therapist experiences *unconditional positive regard* for the client.

◆ The therapist experiences an *empathic understanding* of the client's frame of reference or way of seeing things.

◆ The therapist feels *non-possessive warmth* towards the client.

◆ The client *perceives* the therapist's unconditional positive regard and empathic understanding.

These core conditions have been used and developed in many models of counselling and therapy; even therapies traditionally seen as more technical have always maintained their importance.[13] *Empathy*, for example, a core condition which is central to all good therapeutic relationships, enables clients to know that they are heard and understood. At its simplest, empathy is a simple restatement of someone else's words. At its richest, it involves ... *a fearless exploration of another's inner world, a sensing of meanings unspoken, a compassionate naming of pain ... the fullest empathy does not censor or discriminate. It sees the world as the other person sees it.*[14]

While Rogers took the view that such core conditions are both necessary and sufficient for therapeutic change to occur, other models of counselling have defined such conditions as necessary but not in themselves sufficient for change. However, the core conditions remain the bedrock upon which counselling is practised.

### The therapeutic relationship

Across very diverse treatments, including cognitive and psycho-pharmacological,[15] measures of the strength of the relationship, or alliance, have been the strongest and most consistent process correlates of treatment outcome.[3,16] Clients who have strong alliances with their therapists tend to have better outcomes.

Although recognized as an essential component of change, different models have different conceptual and practical approaches to the relationship. Three examples illustrate the differences:

◆ Person-centred models take a here-and-now perspective, looking at the immediate interaction between client and counsellor. The client's perception of the therapist's empathy, unconditional positive regard, and congruence enables therapeutic change.

◆ Cognitive models regard the relationship as necessary but not sufficient for therapeutic change. The relationship is primarily collaborative, with an active, working bond formed between client and counsellor to facilitate the tasks of therapy.

◆ Psychodynamic models distinguish the real relationship between client and counsellor, and the transference relationship, consisting of both client transference and therapist counter transference. The working alliance therefore is only partly based in reality, also containing aspects of both parties' histories.

## Counselling methods and techniques

There have always been many approaches to counselling and psychotherapy, and this diversity grew into a veritable 'multiverse' during which some authors estimated that there were over 400 brand therapies in existence. There are also different settings and agencies which offer counselling—clinics, institutes, health centres, or voluntary bodies, each with its own particular features. Within each model and setting, there are different formats of counselling including self-help materials on CD-rom and the Internet, as well as individual, couple, group, family, and organizational.

Such a range can be confusing to potential clients and organizations, and the question of what works, for whom, and in which setting, has to be central in matching client, problem, therapy, and therapist.

Specific models of counselling are usually differentiated by a number of factors:

◆ Basic assumptions or philosophy

◆ Formal theory of human personality and development

◆ Clinical theory defining the goals, principles, and processes of change

◆ Therapeutic skills and techniques[17]

One useful distinction exists between *schools* of counselling and *theoretical approaches*.[18] A theoretical approach presents a single position regarding the theory and practice of counselling, whereas a school is a grouping of different theoretical approaches with common characteristics(see Table 6.3.1.2).

The three main schools are humanist-existential, psychodynamic, and cognitive behavioural. Humanistic-existential models will be described in detail, with briefer mention of psychodynamic and cognitive behavioural models, which are covered in other chapters. The section on methods also looks at the trend towards integration and eclecticism within counselling, whereby counsellors use a variety of methods and approaches adopted from different models. Although not clearly fitting into any one school, information-giving and *problem-solving* are counselling methods widely used in psychiatry, and are therefore described first.

### Information-giving and problem-solving

*Giving information* is an important part of all medical and psychiatric practice, reflecting an open and collaborative approach to treatment, providing patients and their carers with the material necessary for informed decision-making. For example, for people with schizophrenia or those who misuse alcohol, the provision of information about the diagnosis, causes, and potential consequences of their condition is essential for mobilizing motivation and compliance with treatment. Giving information about the actions and potential side-effects of a prescribed medication enables people to

**Table 6.3.1.2** Overview of counselling schools and main approaches (Reproduced from Nelson-Jones, R. *Theory and practice of counselling and therapy* (4th edn.), copyright 2006, Sage Publications.)

| |
|---|
| **Psychodynamic school** |
| Classical psychoanalysis (Sigmund Freud) |
| Analytical therapy (Carl Jung) |
| **Humanistic-existential school** |
| Person-centred therapy (Carl Rogers) |
| Gestalt therapy (Fritz Perls) |
| Transactional analysis (Eric Berne) |
| Existential therapy (Irvin Yalom and Rollo May) |
| **Cognitive behavioural school** |
| Behaviour therapy (Ivan Pavlov, BF Skinner and Joseph Wolpe) |
| Rational emotive behaviour therapy (Albert Ellis) |
| Cognitive therapy (Aaron Beck) |
| Multimodal therapy (Arnold Lazarus) |

play an active role in pharmacological intervention. Information-giving is always crucial when communicating a diagnosis and fundamental to counselling for risk, as in genetic counselling, and to any intervention in which the individual is helped to make decisions.

Psycho-educative methods have a place in most models of counselling and psychotherapy, but have specific importance in problem-solving and cognitive behavioural models. For example, a psychologist or counsellor may describe to the client a psychological model of a specific condition, such as the cognitive model of panic, to help the client understand their particular symptoms.

Information-giving and psycho-education involves more than just giving information to a passive recipient. Wherever possible the individual's curiosity about their condition is promoted, encouraging them to ask questions and, when appropriate, to find their own answers. The Socratic method and guided learning are central to cognitive approaches. Information is not provided in a didactic fashion, but in response to the client's questions, as client and therapist are engaged in collaborative enquiry. Whatever the information given, the practitioner checks whether the client has understood the information and its meaning. Information-giving is rarely the endpoint of an intervention, serving instead as the basis for decision-making or continuing therapeutic work.

***Problem-solving*** has been used and empirically validated as a specific treatment, particularly for depression, and is used by many cognitive behavioural and humanistic counsellors. Problem-solving forms a major part of brief solution-focused therapy.[19] From a problem-solving perspective, depression results from the interaction between negative life events, current problems, and deficient problem-solving abilities, and therefore facilitating solving problems is a means to alleviate depression.[20] Therapist and client work collaboratively to identify and prioritize key problem areas, break them down into specific manageable tasks, solve problems, and develop appropriate coping behaviours. The approach involves several stages:

- Identification and formulation of the client's problem(s)
- Setting clear and achievable goals
- Generation of alternatives for coping
- Selection and operationalization of a preferred solution
- Evaluation of progress, with further problem-solving as necessary

Research in the United Kingdom has shown that problem-solving delivered by general practitioners is as effective as pharmacological treatment for moderate and major depression in primary care.[21,22] The intervention can be extremely useful for clients who do not want or cannot tolerate pharmacological treatment and is recommended in NICE guidelines as a treatment for mild depression. It can be offered by counsellors, general practitioners, and nurses, and may be a means to improve treatment adherence for people with psychotic disorders, as part of a psycho-educational intervention including motivational interviewing.[23]

***Brief solution-focused therapy*** developed from its roots in family therapy to applications in counselling, mental health, group work, education, drug and alcohol work, social work, and business. It is the preferred mode of working for counsellors in the workplace, given its brief and focused approach. The model arose from family

therapists' observations that clients made significant changes when focusing on their preferred futures rather than on current problems. By articulating solutions, and building on existing skills and strengths, clients saw their problems in a different light and could effect change.

The 'miracle question' is a classic method of solution-focused therapy which is integrated into other models. The client is asked to think about and describe waking up one day to find that all problems have vanished. The counsellor explores the impact of the miracle on people and situations. The question enables the client to get into a problem-solving cognitive set, enabling identification of what needs to happen for the problems to change. The method has been studied in a range of client groups and settings, including with repeat offenders in the forensic service, and can produce positive outcomes.[19]

## Humanistic and existential models

Humanistic and existential approaches include person-centred therapy, gestalt therapy, transactional analysis, and existential approaches. Of these, the person-centred model is the most well known, and the one that comes most readily to mind when describing the philosophy of counselling.

***Client-centred***, or ***person-centred*** as it is more often called, counselling originates from the work of Carl Rogers, whose emphasis on the recognition and empowerment of the help-seeker challenged the perceived authoritarianism of both the medical model and psychoanalysis. The model highlights respect for the person, and adopts the optimistic assumption that each person has an inner potential for healthy development and achievement, or 'self-actualization'. Person-centred approaches often use the analogy of a plant to describe the concept of growth and change. No one can make a plant grow, but if the plant is provided with the right conditions—water, light, soil, nutrients—then it will become the best plant it can be. Person-centred therapy assumes that people have an inbuilt motivation to change, and also have the skills necessary with which to effect changes. Rogers' model of counselling is non-directive. The counsellor's task is to create the core relationship conditions of empathy, warmth, unconditional positive regard, and genuineness, described above, in which the client's inner resources and potential will be unlocked, leading to the spontaneous resolution of problems and developmental growth.

The central features of person-centred counselling form the bedrock of other models of counselling, including cognitive approaches. Carl Rogers, in initiating the person-centred approach, has also had a wide influence in the helping professions—the term 'person-centred' is used frequently in policy documents and guidelines within health care organizations, as one of the standards of service and as a philosophy of health care.

While a non-directive and reflective approach has value, and may be useful for initial data-gathering and supportive work, caution must be applied to the use of Rogerian counselling in psychiatry. Resource constraints require practitioners to impose time limits on counselling, which therefore must be more focused and 'active'. Furthermore, very disturbed people may be unable to access an inner potential for spontaneous change and growth, implicit within the client-centred model. There are some for whom a reflective non-directive approach may be harmful, risking an overwhelming upsurge of avoided or forgotten memories of traumatic experiences without providing methods for coping with them.

Victims of childhood sexual abuse or other destructive experiences may be re-traumatized by unstructured reflective counselling.

It is likely that the person-centred approach will continue to form the basis of good counselling and psychotherapeutic practice regardless of the model used, with increased emphasis on more 'skills-based' approaches such as cognitive behavioural and other models that lend themselves more easily to measurement, structured working, and evidence-based practice.

*Gestalt therapy* was originated by Fritz Perls, who described his approach as dealing with the total existence of a person, rather than being primarily occupied with symptoms or character structure.[24] Gestalt therapy argues that the past is past and the future unknowable, therefore the focus of counselling should be the present moment—an approach, interestingly, espoused by the development of mindfulness in psychiatry and psychotherapy.[25] The goal of therapy is to put clients in touch with what they are thinking, feeling, and sensing, in the here and now, and how they restrict or limit themselves by continual focus on the past or future. Gestalt therapists regard the therapeutic relationship as a 'working' relationship, with client and counsellor taking responsibility for themselves. Attaining awareness is an essential aim within the relationship.

Gestalt therapy uses many techniques, including dream-work and psychodrama. The classic 'two chair' method of gestalt therapy enables clients to work with 'unfinished business' which may be influencing current problems. For example, a client with memories of a difficult relationship with a parent is encouraged to have a dialogue with the parent in the empty chair, to see both client and parent's point of view. The client may put themselves, metaphorically, in the empty chair, to enable greater understanding and acceptance of the self.

Research has only recently played a role in the development of gestalt theory and practice. Most of the studies concern the effectiveness of the two-chair method, an approach which is being integrated into other models, for example Greenberg's[26] emotion-focused psychotherapy, and cognitive approaches.[13]

*Transactional analysis (TA)* was founded by Canadian psychiatrist Eric Berne, and provides a theory of personality, child development, and psychopathology as well as a theory of counselling. The method assumes, as for other person-centred approaches, that people are born with a drive for growth and health—the 'I'm OK, you're OK' life position. TA characterizes the personality into three groups of 'ego states'—parent, adult, and child, each with behavioural, social, historical, and phenomenological aspects. Psychopathology arises from the repetition of unhelpful life scripts, or patterns of being, often learned early in life. Counselling enables the individual to identify and modify problematic patterns.

Very little research has been conducted into the effectiveness of TA as a therapy although many theoretical concepts and practical techniques have been assimilated into psychotherapy and counselling.[27] The method has also led to the concept of the 'reflective practitioner', a theme embodied by the BPS Division of Counselling Psychology.

*Existential approaches* originated in applied philosophy, and focus on helping people to come to terms with life in all its confusing complexity. Rather than curing people of pathology, the aim is to help people deal with the contradictions, dilemmas, and paradoxes of everyday existence.[28] Anxiety and depression, rather than to be avoided, are to be embraced and understood in order to live life to the full. The main method is conversational, enabling clients to confront rather than avoid the reality of situations.

Although existential approaches may sound idealized and unrealistic, much of existential therapy aims to help people build confidence and competence in tackling everyday problems. The methods and approaches have very little outcome research, because of the opposition of existential therapists to what is seen as the reductionist tendencies of research—i.e. what is effective in therapy is not open to evaluation using standard methodology. It may be that the approach offers a number of factors which can be usefully integrated into other, more evidence-based models, such as the focus on validating experience, creation of meaning to enable traumatic events to be processed, and authenticity.

## Cognitive behavioural approaches

Cognitive behaviour therapy (CBT) is currently receiving excellent press internationally, and occupies a central place in the move towards evidence-based practice. NICE recommends CBT more often than other therapeutic approaches for many psychological problems. Despite its popularity and evidence-base, cognitive approaches have not been readily embraced by the counselling world.[13] The structured and focused approach, and use of techniques to promote change, rested uncomfortably with counsellors trained in client-centred approaches, and cognitive therapy was felt to pay insufficient attention to the therapeutic relationship and to the influence of past events on current problems. However, the last few years have seen a major change in the way cognitive therapy is being adopted within counselling, and a large proportion of counsellors integrate at least some of the approaches into their work.

The attraction of cognitive therapy to counsellors is increasing, with more overt focus placed on the therapeutic relationship, long-term approaches, and schema-focused work inherent in newer models, which enables counsellors to abandon their prejudices against CBT.[29] There is enormous scope for counsellors to adopt cognitive therapy in a more systematic and rigorous manner, particularly in light of the empirical evidence supporting its effectiveness and increasing demand for briefer interventions.[13] However, counsellors trained in different schools of counselling can be tempted to borrow specific methods from cognitive therapy, such as monitoring negative thoughts, and to use them in an eclectic way. The risk is that the effective components of the approach such as collaboration, structure, focus and homework, may be lost, thus diluting CBT's established effectiveness.

## Psychodynamic counselling

Psychodynamic counselling[30] draws from the theoretical traditions of Alderian therapy, Jung's analytical psychology, Freudian psychoanalysis, and Kleinian psychodynamic therapy. Psychodynamic approaches pay particular attention to past experience, particularly adverse relationship experiences during early life, the continuing influence of which may be mediated by unconscious processes. These are seen to influence attachment patterns, psychosocial development, and later psychological functioning. Unconscious processes derived from early experiences contribute to the generation and maintenance of abnormal psychological states. In psychodynamic counselling and psychotherapy, these unconscious processes may be identified through examining transference and counter-transference in the therapeutic relationship.

The search for the personal meaning of the client's problem or symptoms is central to psychodynamic counselling. The counsellor encourages clients to talk about their difficulties, but also to reflect and gain insight on spontaneous associations and attitudes towards the counsellor as potential sources of information about the presenting problems. Insight alone may be sufficient to enable clients to spontaneously bring about the required changes in their lives. Psychodynamic counselling may also use methods akin to problem-solving and behavioural experiments to facilitate identification and rehearsal of new and more adaptive interpersonal strategies.

### Eclectic-integrative approaches

Many practitioners assimilate conceptual and practical way of working that can be attributed to more than one theoretical perspective, formulating the client's difficulties and choosing a mix of methods using more than one theoretical framework. Formally working with a variety of models and methods may be described eclectic or integrative.[31] Such generic therapies often emphasize non-specific factors such as building the therapeutic alliance and engendering hope. Whether this gives the best of each world, or risks the worst of all, is very much open to question, and by nature, eclectic therapy is difficult to standardize for RCTs. The worst kind of *eclecticism* may be an arbitrary pick-and-mix approach, whereby a generically skilled counsellor trains in a variety of approaches and applies these with clients in a way in which he or she deems best. There is little evidence that such an approach is any more effective than the core conditions of counselling allow. Lazarus[32] describes *technical eclecticism*, the drawing of interventions from different sources without necessarily subscribing to their founding discipline. Wherever possible, technically eclectic therapists use treatments based on empirical evidence and client need.

*Integration*, in contrast, combines identifiable and specific aspects of models in a predetermined way, allowing the evolution of a defined form of therapy such as *cognitive analytic therapy*.[33] *Psychodynamic interpersonal therapy* offers NHS counsellors a point of convergence between predominantly humanistic counselling and more clinically and dynamically orientated approaches often used within psychiatry.[34]

Integration and eclecticism in counselling and therapy will no doubt continue to develop as the nature of clients' problems and the ways of doing therapy evolve. Environmental and technological changes may lead to increasing use of the Internet in counselling and psychotherapy, with face-to-face interactions possible even when client and counsellor are in different locations. It is essential that new counselling approaches are thoroughly supported by empirical evidence so we do not see creeping eclecticism washing out the effectiveness of established methods.

## Applications of counselling to specific conditions

Depending on the settings in which they work, counsellors need to be equipped to work with clients with a range of psychological difficulties. For example, the primary care counsellor's caseload is likely to include client difficulties ranging from mild to moderate anxiety or depression to bereavement and relationship problems. Whether or not counselling is an effective intervention for the range of problems seen in these settings has not yet been clearly established. The following looks at counselling for problems where there is good evidence for effectiveness.

### Common psychological problems

A Cochrane systematic review[35] compared counselling with normal GP care for people suffering from anxiety, depression, or stress disorders. The authors concluded that overall, significant benefits were seen in mental health improvement from counselling compared with usual GP care, or GP care plus antidepressant treatment, in the short-term (up to 4 months). However these benefits were not maintained in the longer term, over 9 to 12 months. Counselling may be more effective for depression than as a treatment for anxiety. Barrowclough et al.[36] compared CBT with supportive counselling (SC) in the treatment of anxiety symptoms in older adults. The CBT group did better than the SC group following treatment, and at follow-up. Overall, cognitively orientated models of counselling and therapy are more effective for depression and anxiety in the long-term than generic counselling. However, counselling may enable people to recover more quickly from depression, and is therefore a valuable and valued intervention.

### Counselling for adjustment disorder

Adjustment disorder is defined as a problematic response to a normal stressor, not caused by another mental health problem or bereavement. Such stressors include normal transitions such as leaving home, migration, adverse interpersonal experiences (e.g. relationship breakdown), and unexpected losses such as redundancy. Individual vulnerability can play a part in a person's reaction to life changes, such as previous losses or other adversity, social or cultural isolation, economic deprivation or physical illness.

Counselling is recommended as the first line of treatment for people having difficulty adjusting to life events, illnesses, disabilities or losses, including childbirth and bereavement.[4] The counselling relationship is an important source of security when much has changed in the person's life. The client is helped to identify the stressors, to explore the personal significance of the changes experienced, and to express the emotions generated. It can be necessary to examine unresolved past experiences which may impact on the current adjustment—for example, an individual may not begin to come to terms with redundancy until he recognizes and addresses his unresolved feelings about being abandoned by a parent in childhood. Problem-solving methods are used to identify adaptive goals and ways they may be achieved. The counsellor may encourage the client not to use unhelpful solutions such as denial, excessive use of alcohol, or emotional suppression. The aim is for the client to resolve the crisis themselves.

### Relationship problems

Government statistics from both the United States and the United Kingdom show that an ever-growing proportion of marriages fail, with around one in two marriages ending in divorce and an even higher rate in other relationships. Many divorces and relationship problems involve children under the age of 16. A number of specialized services have evolved, including pre-marital counselling, counselling for sexual problems, infertility counselling, bereavement and divorce counselling, and counselling for those involved in second and subsequent relationships.[37] Telephone counselling and drop in services are frequently used by individuals and couples aiming to clarify the problems and find appropriate help. The kind of issues couples bring to relationship counselling include:

◆ Communication difficulties

◆ Conflicts in need between different parties

◆ Extra-relationship affairs

◆ Sexual problems

◆ Conflicts as parents

◆ Gender role changes

◆ Violence

◆ Substance abuse

◆ Jealousy or possessiveness

Because of the wide range of difficulties, relationship counsellors tend to offer a variety of interventions rather than working within one therapeutic model, and it is unclear whether any one theoretical approach is generally more effective than another.[38] Brief, dynamic work can start the process of internal change, so that the couple is able to work on their own to practise new patterns of relating. Brief, focused work can offer immediate and early solutions to issues which might otherwise threaten the relationship. Longer interventions may be required for couples dealing with major life events and experiences, and offer the opportunity to look at childhood and other roots of persistent or destructive patterns of relating.

The effectiveness of counselling depends a great deal on the willingness of participants to engage in a process which can be painful, challenging often long-established patterns of relating, and one partner in the relationship may be more enthusiastic than the other to promote change. Research shows that many of those who experience relationship counselling understand themselves better, become less emotionally disturbed and understand their partner and relationships better.[39] In some cases, a good outcome is for the relationship to end, in a way which causes least disruption to all parties including children. In the latter case, referral to other agencies may be essential, such as when child protection issues are involved.

### Grief counselling

Grief is not a pathological state in itself, and most people emerge from the natural grieving process in a healthy way. Counselling has a role both in facilitating grieving for those who experience difficulties in the process, and in helping those with complex grief reactions.[40] Counselling might involve more than one person in a bereaved family or other grouping, for example the college friends of a student killed in an accident.

In health settings grief counselling is undertaken by trained professionals or volunteers, and in the community by self-help voluntary agencies such as Cruse (in the United Kingdom) or groups attached to hospices.[41] Voluntary agencies are often staffed by people who have themselves experienced bereavement, and group counselling in this context provides a valuable opportunity for acceptance, sharing of experience, and the hope borne out of talking with others who have already come to terms with their loss.

The research on grief counselling[42] shows that professional services and professionally supported voluntary and self-help services can reduce the risk of psychiatric and physical problems following bereavement, and reduce the risk level of 'high-risk' widows to that of a 'low-risk' group. Reid et al.[43] found that support by hospice volunteers of high-risk bereaved relatives substantially reduced their levels of anxiety and need for medical care.

### Drug and alcohol problems

Drug and alcohol dependence and related problems generate many controversies about their nature and treatment, such as whether people diagnosed as alcoholics can ever return to harm-free, controlled drinking, and the motivation and ability of those addicted to drugs and alcohol to change. Many volunteer agencies offer drug and alcohol treatments, advocating a multifaceted approach, with a combination of methods drawn from motivational interviewing, person-centred and cognitive behavioural therapy known as 'motivational enhancement therapy'. There are several different models of drug and alcohol use, including that of Narcotics Anonymous, similar to Alcoholics Anonymous, who view substance abuse as a pre-existing, biochemical abnormality, necessitating life-long abstinence. Other views seek to minimize the harm caused by drugs and alcohol, by reducing risks, reducing intake, and possibly changing to another, less harmful substance. A third view sees addiction as a pattern of inappropriate coping: cognitive behavioural principles are used to recognize and deal with situations likely to lead to drug use.

A major trial in the United States randomized 487 patients to one of four, 6-month, treatments. All treatments included group drug counselling following a 12-step model, focusing on achieving abstinence. The group program was offered either alone, or in combination with individual drug counselling, CBT or individual supportive-expressive psychotherapy. Attrition rates in all groups were high, with only 28 per cent completing treatment. All interventions led to a reduction in drug use, but the greatest reduction was for individual plus group counselling.[44]

### Counselling for recent and past trauma

Increased public awareness of global trauma arising from natural disasters, war, and terrorism, has led to the development of psychological interventions designed to prevent the onset of post-traumatic stress disorder (PTSD) in those exposed to traumatizing events. However, after many years of early interventions in the form of active single-session 'debriefing' for individuals and groups, there is no evidence for their effectiveness in preventing PTSD. One of the problems in the field is the tendency to 'medicalize' normal distress in traumatic situations, leading to the construction of 'disaster therapists', perhaps with limited understanding of the culture in which the disaster occurred, ready to offer advice and counselling to survivors who may not see themselves as having a mental health problem.[45]

There is also no evidence that non-directive counselling is effective in treating acute stress disorder, which itself constitutes a risk factor for PTSD.[46] Short individualized preventive interventions in the style of 'psychological first aid' may be most effective.

There is no evidence that non-directive or reflective counselling is effective in the treatment of post-traumatic stress disorder. The advocates of counselling for post-traumatic stress disorder describe active-focused methods such as cognitive behaviour therapy,[47] and using debriefing, to enable people to build a cognitive and emotional account of their experiences. Given that many clients with PTSD are, understandably, mistrustful or avoidant, the methods have to be used within the context of a sound therapeutic relationship, meeting the core counselling conditions.

### Postnatal depression

Postnatal depression is often mild and remits spontaneously for many women. However, effective treatment is important because of the potential adverse effect on the child's emotional and cognitive development. Home-based counselling is as effective as antidepressant medication in the treatment of postnatal depression, and is more acceptable to mothers.[48] Counselling can be delivered by health visitors trained in cognitive behavioural counselling methods.[49] The research suggests that depressed mothers benefit from an opportunity to talk about their concerns, not all of which necessarily focus on their baby, with a receptive and non-judgemental professional person. Counselling and other psychological interventions are highly acceptable to mothers with postnatal depression, and preferred over pharmacological treatment. If counselling and other forms of psychotherapy enable women to recover from postnatal depression more rapidly than usual care, this alone may be a valuable service to offer in addition to routine care.

## Counselling settings

Counselling takes place in a large number of settings relevant to psychiatry. These include primary care, general medical settings, student counselling services, workplace counselling services, and the voluntary sector. These settings will be described below, aiming to discuss the ways in which counselling may be best adapted to the individual settings, with indications of outcome data on effectiveness.

### Counselling in primary care

Primary care is one of the most conspicuous areas of growth in counselling, stimulated by greater demands for alternatives to medication for emotional problems, and by continuing debate about the most effective way of managing mental health problems in primary care. The Layard report on the need for CBT for depression and NICE guidelines stress the importance and effectiveness of psychological interventions including counselling, with a particular focus on CBT. It is likely that the number of counsellors who practice CBT will grow in order to meet demand.

In the United Kingdom, around half of general practices employ a qualified counsellor and the majority meet national criteria for good practice.[50] The development of UK primary care counselling is no doubt part of a wider international trend towards more accessible counselling services at the primary care level.

Counsellors in primary care are a diverse group, in the patients that they see, the counselling models used, and the length of counselling offered. Those identified as primary care counsellors include practice nurses, health visitors, and district nurses trained in counselling skills; clinical and counselling psychologists; community psychiatric nurses, and social workers, and qualified counsellors and psychotherapists. Counselling in primary care is usually provided through one of three main service delivery models[51]:

♦ Counsellors based in GP practices and provided by a local agency or cooperative

♦ Managed counselling services provided by the PCT or mental health trust, with counsellors based in GP practices or a central site

♦ Voluntary agencies (in cases where PCTs have contracts to refer to externally managed services in the voluntary sector)

Counsellors are valued in primary care for a number of reasons,[52] providing time for patients to talk through and reflect on problems, where general practitioners are unable to spend the necessary time on individual patients, as well as a valued alternative or addition to pharmacotherapy. Counselling in primary care also facilitates early identification and intervention for mental health difficulties.

Counsellors in primary care need to be flexible in the way that they work, using different models as appropriate to each client. They also need to be flexible about boundaries and confidentiality, communicating with general practitioners and other health professionals as appropriate. Counselling is generally six to eight 50-min sessions, with a maximum of 20 sessions, and therefore focusing on presenting difficulties rather than long-term issues. The role of the counsellor is varied, and may include offering individual or group counselling, offering advice or training to primary care staff on managing mental health problems, and general consultation.

Despite the growth and popularity of counselling in primary care, it is not clear how effective it is compared to other models such as CBT. Studies have shown mixed findings.[9] Trials comparing counselling for anxiety and depression with usual general practitioner care, CBT, and anti-depressant medication have shown significantly greater clinical effectiveness of counselling compared to usual general practitioner care in the short-term but not in the long-term.[53–55] For people with chronic depression, there were no significant differences between usual care, CBT and short-term psychodynamic counselling,[56] although at 12 months, both psychological therapies were superior to usual care. Counselling in primary care can be cautiously reported as a valuable service, particularly for people with mild to moderate emotional disturbance as well as bereavement and relationship difficulties. Clients improve in the short-term, and the service is appreciated and valued by general practitioners and patients. Primary care services are probably best offered as a range of mental health services, linking closely with community mental health services.

### Counselling in general medical settings

Medical patients are understandably at higher risk of psychological difficulties compared to the general population, and many hospital departments and clinics employ counsellors as part of the multidisciplinary team to meet patients' psychosocial needs.[57] Counselling benefits patients in many hospital settings such as gastroenterology, cardiology, obstetrics, and gynaecology, the families of children with medical problems and disabilities and patients with diabetes, renal failure, disfigurement, cancer, head injuries, and chronic conditions such as multiple sclerosis.[58] Counsellors offer what is becoming increasingly limited in medicine—time. A large amount of psychosocial adjustment is needed in most serious illnesses and conditions, and counsellors in health care settings are assisting people cope with potentially life's most challenging moments.

For some conditions, such as HIV/AIDS and genetically transmitted illnesses, counselling forms an important aspect of treatment. From its outset, HIV/AIDS attracted the attention of psychological therapists, since at first there was little else to offer to help people deal with a strange and potentially fatal illness. A range of professional and voluntary services grew to support those infected. The stages of the illness present different needs, from pre-testing counselling, dealing with the emotional, social, and physical consequences of a positive diagnosis, and managing the adjustment to living with a chronic condition. *Genetic counselling* is specialized branch of counselling practice with increasing applications within psychiatry. In the coming years, the expected identification of susceptibility genes for psychiatric disorders may bring new opportunities and expectations from patients and families for psychiatric genetics.[59]

Counselling is usually offered through referral to a specific hospital department or ward-based counsellor. Many health care workers and hospital chaplains use counselling skills, which are generally regarded as supportive and therapeutic for patients. This does not replace the need for managed counselling services delivered by trained and professional therapists.

## Counselling in educational settings

Counselling services in college and university settings cater for students with a wide range of issues. Because of their age and developmental stage, many students have problems adjusting to the new freedoms and demands of college life and also face the developmental challenges of adolescence and young adulthood—conflicts between dependence and independence, psychosexual development, issues to do with self and body image and eating disorders. Other common difficulties include financial, study, and interpersonal problems. Mature students may also contend with the stress of juggling study with children and home-life, and being minorities within a younger peer group. With increasing admissions of overseas students, issues such as identity and loneliness will also arise.

Student counselling services are often arranged so that practical (e.g. financial guidance or careers counselling) and psychological help are offered separately to provide discreet and confidential access. Most clients refer themselves, but may be referred by staff or the student's doctor. Services need to include or work closely with psychiatrists and other mental health professionals in order to meet the needs of students with mental illness. The majority present with less severe emotional or psychological problems, but these may be highly disruptive to their studies and social integration.

Short-term counselling is usually appropriate for students, partly because of their urgency and the structure of the academic year, but also because their natural developmental potential enables most young people quickly to change. This process may be accelerated even more by the intelligence inherent in students, though emotional development can lag behind intellectual development. The task of counselling has been likened to helping the young person back on to the track of normal psychosexual development. More severe derailments, however, may require longer counselling, specialized psychotherapy, or psychiatric treatment.

## Counselling in the voluntary sector

Counselling within the voluntary sector has vastly increased, with a growing number of support groups and voluntary organizations offering counselling, mainly on self-referral basis. The most well known in the United Kingdom include Alcoholics Anonymous, Cruse Bereavement Care, Relate for relationship difficulties, and the Samaritans, with equivalent organizations in other countries. Many mental health charities offer support, befriending, and counselling at a 'grassroots' level; some, such as MIND in the United Kingdom, are organized nationally, whereas others operate at a local level. These organizations contribute a great deal to mental health provision, offering the opportunity to talk through and reflect on problems, and in offering support to individuals with more severe mental health problems and their families.

The interface between voluntary and statutory services is varied and at times uncomfortable, with the two sharing different models of care, philosophies, and policies on issues such as confidentiality. There is less research on the effectiveness of counselling provision within the voluntary sector, although one study has shown it to be at least as effective as statutory provision and is often carried out by appropriately trained staff.[60]

## Counselling in the workplace

Mental health and employment are known to be significantly related: satisfaction at work is positively correlated with mental health and the unemployed experience higher rates of mental health problems compared to those in employment. The provision of workplace counselling has steadily expanded over the past 20 years, with more than 75 per cent of medium and large organizations in Britain and North America making counselling available to their staff. Counselling may be part of a benefits package, occupational health, human resources or a service brought in to help with specific problems, such as redundancy. Workplace counselling can be viewed as the application of methods of brief psychological interventions that have been shown to be effective in other settings. However, a distinctive strength of seeing a counsellor in the workplace is that the counsellor will be sensitive to the combination of personal and work pressures that the person may present. Workplace counselling is a systemic, as well as individual, intervention in that the organization that pays the counsellor is always present, consciously or unconsciously, influencing the number of sessions and confidentiality boundaries.

Counselling for work-related difficulties is effective in reducing stress-related problems at work and sickness.[61,62] Those who receive counselling are highly satisfied, believing it helps them resolve their problems. Clinically significant improvement in levels of anxiety and depression are reported in 60–75 per cent of clients. Counselling is associated not only with reduction in sickness absence but also improvement in other organizational outcomes such as more positive work attitudes, fewer accidents, and enhanced work performance.

The main provision of counselling at work include employee assistance programmes (EAPs) and specialized staff counselling services.

*Employee assistance programmes* were first introduced in the United States after the Second World War, to rehabilitate oil-industry employees with alcohol problems. EAPs have become widespread in North America and are increasing in the United Kingdom. They are reported to achieve good results in terms of the percentage of employees who are rehabilitated for work, the reduction in alcohol consumption, improvement of work performance, and cost savings to the company.[63]

EAPs provide a comprehensive confidential counselling service to employees and their families, allowing employee's problems to be identified and resolved at an early stage, and are normally incorporated into the company's benefits package as a form of private emotional health care. EAPs include 24-h access, telephone counselling, and helplines as well as individual counselling offered at short notice. One of the advantages of counselling organized through EAPs as opposed to in-house staff counselling is improved confidentiality: staff may be reluctant to use counselling services at work if they are not convinced of full confidentiality, and if they fear their career prospects may be adversely affected.

*Staff counselling services*: many private and public sector organizations now have in-house counselling services.[61] One of the first was set-up by the Post Office in the early 1980s, in recognition of the need to provide emotional and psychological support to employees. Mental health issues, mainly anxiety and depression, formed 46 per cent of the caseload, as well as relationship problems, alcohol problems, bereavement, assault, physical illness or disability, and social problems. Staff counselling schemes are now promoted by many health and education authorities, the Royal College of Nursing, the British Medical Association, and MIND at Work. Problem-solving and cognitive methods of counselling appear to be the most valuable models for workplace settings.[61]

Evaluation of the London Transport Counselling and Trauma Unit showed that the service made huge savings in its first year of operation, in terms of reduced sickness absence and other treatment costs. Research from the United States indicates a return for every dollar invested in Employee Assistance Programmes of between $3 and $7.[61,62] Other benefits may be less quantifiable but nevertheless valuable. For example, a qualitative study[64] of police officers and support staff who had received counselling for work-related difficulties, showed that many described themselves as learning something new and useful about themselves as a result of counselling. For example, an experienced detective stated, *I am 100 per cent better at listening now to a person.*

### Telephone and electronically delivered counselling

*The telephone* is a valuable method of counselling, as shown by organizations such as The Samaritans. Telephone helplines respond to millions of calls each year, and offer a means of talking about feelings and gaining support, information, and advice. The telephone is excellent for crisis intervention and short-term work—one of the key reasons why people phone telephone helplines is because they are in crisis and want to talk anonymously and confidentially.

The telephone and teleconferencing can also be used to conduct some or all of a course of individual or group counselling, or as an adjunct to pharmacological treatment. Telephone advice and structured counselling improved outcome and satisfaction for clients starting antidepressant medication,[65] and also improved adherence to medication.[66]

*Electronically delivered counselling*: since the mid-1990s, new forms of text technology—the Internet, chatrooms, email, and mobile phone texting—are being developed to deliver counselling and psychotherapy. There is an increasing body of evidence that using text to conduct a therapeutic relationship is not only possible but also in many cases more desirable than face-to-face interaction. Electronically delivered counselling has been addressed by counselling organizations in the United Kingdom, United States and internationally, with published guidelines on issues such as confidentiality and data protection, contracting and informed consent, assessment of suitability of clients, boundaries, and practitioner competence.[67] The International Society for Mental Health

Online (http://www.ismho.org/) was formed in 1997 to 'promote the understanding, use and development of online communication, information, and technology for the international mental health community'.

Working electronically has benefits those who cannot access therapy because of, for example, disability or geography. Communicating from a distance can make for a more honest and open relationship, clients diverging information or issues which they would find difficult to discuss face-to-face. Such disinhibition may be empowering—clients having a cathartic experience, so they can then disappear into cyberspace—or potentially hazardous, with traumatic issues remaining unresolved. Although the evaluation of such services is in its infancy, and there are many issues to be addressed, such as practitioner competence and confidentiality, electronic forms of mental health provision are likely to increase. They provide a means of providing help to clients who not only cannot but do not wish to meet with a helper, clients who have been traditionally excluded from mental health provision.

## Counselling accreditation, training, and registration

The number of counsellors and psychotherapists in the United Kingdom and other countries is growing rapidly. Professional status and accountability are key concerns about counselling and counsellors, along with other providers of non-medical health care[68]—in the past, anyone could practise as a counsellor, with no standards of training, supervision, or attachment to a regulatory body. As a result, the vulnerable users of such practitioners are at risk. However, there is a strong move within counselling towards clear standards of training and accreditation, to be able to provide an effective and accountable service to the public.

For full *accreditation*, professional counsellors are required to follow, as a minimum, a 3-year full-time training course in the theory and practice of counselling. The standards required are covered by two main organizations in the United Kingdom, with equivalents in other countries:

◆ The British Association of Counselling and Psychotherapy, which offers accreditation for counsellors from a variety of disciplines, mainly humanistic and psychodynamic.

◆ The British Psychological Society, which offers accredited chartered status for counselling psychologists, trained to meet standards in applied psychology.

The requirements for accreditation or registration vary between organizations. Common requirements are a minimum of 450 taught contact hours and 450 h of supervised practice, evaluated via case studies and process reports; academic knowledge of counselling theory and research; personal counselling or psychotherapy; and, for the British Psychological Society, research skills and experience. The qualification requires that practitioners follow a code of practice and ethics, stipulating ethical practice, the need for supervision, appropriate confidentiality, and other standards for professional practice.

One of the problems in accreditation is ensuring that counsellors have followed a known and recognized training course. Alongside the expansion of interest in counselling, the number of counselling courses rises each year, ranging from short evening classes in active listening and short courses in counselling skills for health professionals, to full-time training leading to professional accreditation or chartering. A recent review of UK training found that many psychotherapy and counselling organizations are small, and a significant number of training providers are linked to no external quality assurance systems, 63 per cent having no professional body recognition.[69] There are a large number of titles for both training courses and individual counsellors and psychotherapists, which can only cause confusion to both potential trainees and the public. The review[69] made a number of recommendations to improve the quality of training courses, to lead to greater standardization.

A further change within counselling is the move towards registration. Currently there is no statutory protection for using the terms 'counsellor' or 'psychotherapist', and therefore no means for the prevention of bad practice or abuse. Without registration through a professional body, clients may have no redress for incompetent practice. The National Service Framework for mental health, which sets clear standards for the delivery of effective services, emphasize the importance of 'talking therapies' but stresses the need to register counsellors, psychotherapists, and psychologists. The registering organizations are now moving towards statutory registration and legal protection for the terms counsellor, psychologist, and psychotherapist; and at the time of writing, definitive legislation is likely to be in place by 2008 or so. In the meantime, it is vital that the public and health professionals are aware of the need to seek help only from qualified practitioners of counselling.

## Conclusions

For psychiatrists and other mental health care professionals, it can be difficult to make sense of the range of counselling models available, and it is therefore not surprising that potential purchasers and consumers are similarly confused about the nature and advisability of seeking counselling. Counselling has only recently been subject to the rigorous evaluation necessary to meet the standards of evidence-based practice. The most central aspects of counselling, the therapeutic relationship, and qualitative nature of the work, can be difficult to evaluate using established research methodology.

However, counselling is an evolving profession, moving away from, but not forgetting, its roots in Rogerian and psychoanalytic practice, and working hard to meet standards of effectiveness, evaluation, registration, and accountability.

Far more attention is being paid to evaluation, with the development of research paradigms suited to counselling. Systematic evaluation will eventually make it possible to identify, on the basis of clear evidence, the indications for specific models of counselling as well as their limitations. Issues of training, standards, ethics, and accountability are being addressed, to enable counselling to become fully consolidated and integrated within mental health services.

Counselling is a vital part of psychiatry for many reasons. There is a significant gap between the demand for psychological therapy and the available supply. One proposal to overcome this problem is to increase efficiency of provision through the adoption of briefer 'minimal interventions' within stepped care models.[70] Counselling is likely to play an increasingly important part of provision of psychological therapies, particularly for those with mild to moderate mental health problems and social and relationship difficulties.

It makes sense for interventions to be offered at an early stage of difficulties: while many problems do resolve on their own, people welcome the support and understanding that counselling can offer, and it is valuable in hastening recovery from emotional distress. Counselling may be appropriate as part of the treatment for people with serious mental illness, offered by psychiatric nurses, social workers, occupational therapists, and workers in the voluntary sector.

Although CBT is being advocated as the treatment of choice for many psychological problems, there is a risk that over-enthusiastic endorsement of the benefits of CBT at the expense of other models may lead to a gap in care: not everyone responds to cognitive approaches, and even when they do, the level of recovery varies. Therefore, the breadth and repertoire of counsellors can add a variety and richness to mental health care provision. *It is this aspect of the human condition, the recognition that we must learn to 'weep for the plague, not just cure it', that is an essential component of meaningful therapy and meaningful relationships. When we experience what seems awful and horrible in our lives, we often take solace in knowing that another person understands, or, at least, is attempting to understand, our pain.*[71]

## Acknowledgements

My thanks to Dr Sietske Boeles and Frank Wills for comments on earlier drafts of the chapter.

## Further information

Bower, P. and Rowland, N. (2006). Effectiveness and cost effectiveness of counselling in primary care. *Cochrane Database Systematic Review* **3**: Art. No. CD001025.

Feltham, C. and Horton, I. (eds.) (2006). *The Sage handbook of counselling and psychotherapy* (2nd edn). Sage, London.

Nelson-Jones, R. (2006). *Theory and practice of counselling and therapy* (4th edn). Sage, London.

Roth, A. and Fonagy, P. (2005). *What works for whom? A critical review of psychotherapy research* (2nd edn). Guildford Press, New York.

Woolfe, R., Dryden, W., and Strawbridge, S. (eds.) (2003). *Handbook of counselling psychology* (2nd edn). Sage, London.

## Resources

The British Association of Counselling and Psychotherapy represents counsellors and psychotherapists in the United Kingdom, with information, training and accreditation: www.bacp.co.uk.
Website for MIND, with information about counselling: www.mind.org.uk.
American Counseling Association: www.counseling.org.
American Mental Health Counselors Association: www.amhca.org.
Canadian Counselling Association: www.ccacc.ca.
Australian Counselling Association: www.theaca.net.au.
European Association for Counselling: www.eacnet.org.

## References

1. Chilvers, C., Dewey, M., Fielding, K., *et al.* (2001). Antidepressant drugs and generic counselling for treatment of major depression in primary care: randomised trial with patient preference arms. *British Medical Journal*, **322**, 772–5.

2. Sibbald, B., Addington-Hall, J., Brenneman, D., *et al.* (1996). *The role of counsellors in general practice.* Royal College of General Practitioners, London.

3. Roth, A. and Fonagy, P. (2005). *What works for whom? A critical review of psychotherapy research* (2nd edn). Guilford Press, New York.

4. DOH. (2001). *Treatment choice in psychological therapies and counselling: evidence based clinical practice guidelines.* Department of Health, London.

5. Feltham, C. (2006). What are counselling and psychotherapy? In *The Sage handbook of counselling and psychotherapy* (eds. C. Feltham and I. Horton), pp. 3–10. Sage, London.

6. Burnard, P. (2006). *Counselling skills for health professionals* (4th edn). Nelson Thornes Ltd., Cheltenham.

7. Dryden, W. (2007). *The handbook of individual therapy* (5th edn). Sage, London.

8. Woolfe, R., Dryden, W., and Strawbridge, S. (eds.) (2003). *Handbook of counselling psychology* (2nd edn). Sage, London.

9. Rowland, N. and Goss, S. (eds.) (2000). *Evidence-based counselling and psychological therapies: research and applications.* Routledge, London.

10. McLeod, J. (2002). *Qualitative research in counselling and psychotherapy.* Sage, Thousand Oaks, CA.

11. Ashworth, M., Shepherd, M., Christey, J., *et al.* (2004). A client-generated psychometric instrument: the development of 'PSYCHLOPS'. *Counselling and Psychotherapy Research*, **4**, 27–31.

12. Rogers, C. (1957). The necessary and sufficient conditions of therapeutic personality change. *Journal of Consulting and Clinical Psychology*, **21**, 95–103.

13. Sanders, D. and Wills, F. (2006). *Cognitive therapy: an introduction.* Sage, London.

14. Tolan, J. (2006). *Skills in person-centred counselling and psychotherapy*, p. 18. Sage, London.

15. Krupnick, J., Stosky, S., Simmens, S., *et al.* (1996). The role of the therapeutic alliance in psychotherapy and pharmacotherapy outcome: findings in the national institute for mental health treatment of depression collaborative research program. *Journal of Consulting and Clinical Psychology*, **64**, 532–9.

16. Hubble, M., Duncan, B., and Miller, S. (eds.) (1999). *The heart and soul of change: what works in therapy.* American Psychological Association, Washington, DC.

17. Horton, I. (2000). Models of counselling and psychotherapy. In *The Sage handbook of counselling and psychotherapy* (eds. C. Feltham and I. Horton), pp. 234–6. Sage, London.

18. Nelson-Jones, R. (2005). *The theory and practice of counselling psychology* (4th edn). Sage, London.

19. O'Connell, B. (2005). *Solution-focused therapy* (2nd edn). Sage, London.

20. D'Zurilla, T. and Nezu, A. (2006). *Problem-solving therapy: a positive approach to clinical intervention* (3rd edn). Springer Publishing Company, Springer.

21. Mynors-Wallis, L., Gath, D., Day, A., *et al.* (2000). Randomised controlled trial of problem solving treatment, antidepressant medication, and combined treatment for major depression in primary care. *British Medical Journal*, **320**, 26–30.

22. Huibers, M., Beurskens, A., Bleijenberg, G., *et al.* (2003). The effectiveness of psychosocial interventions delivered by general practitioners. *Cochrane Database of Systematic Reviews*, **2**, CD003494.

23. Staring, A., Mulder, C., van-der-Gaag, M., *et al.* (2006). Understanding and improving treatment adherence in patients with psychotic disorders: a review and a proposed intervention. *Current Psychiatry Reviews*, **2**, 487–94.

24. Perls, F., Hefferline, R., and Goodman, D. (1994). *Gestalt therapy: excitement and growth in the human personality.* Souvenir Press, London.

25. Segal, Z., Williams, J., and Teasdale, J. (2002). *Mindfulness-based cognitive therapy for depression: a new approach to preventing relapse.* Guilford, New York.

26. Greenberg, L. (2002). *Emotion focused psychotherapy: coaching clients to work through their feelings.* American Psychological Association, Washington, DC.

27. Novey, T. (2002). Measuring the effectiveness of transactional analysis: an international study. *Transactional Analysis Journal*, **32**, 8–24.

28. Spinelli, E. (2007). *Practising existential psychotherapy: the relational world.* Sage, London.

29. Wills, F. (2006). CBT: can counsellors help fill the gap? *Healthcare Counselling and Psychotherapy*, **6**, 6–9.

30. Jacobs, M. (2006). *The presenting past: the core of psychodynamic counselling and therapy* (3rd edn). Open University Press, Milton Keynes.

31. O'Brien, M. and Houston, G. (2007). *Integrative therapy: a practitioner's guide* (2nd edn). Sage, London.

32. Lazarus, A. (2005). Multimodal therapy. In *Current psychotherapies* (eds. R. Corsini and D. Wedding), pp. 337–71. Thomson Brooks/Cole, Belmont, CA.

33. Ryle, A. and Kerr, I. (2002). *Introducing CAT principles and practice.* Wiley, Chichester.

34. Jenkins, P. (2003). Psychodynamic interpersonal therapy: bridging the gap within the medical model. *Healthcare Counselling and Psychotherapy*, **3**, 15–18.

35. Bower, P., Rowland, N., and Hardy, R. (2003). The clinical effectiveness of counselling in primary care: a systematic review and meta-analysis. *Psychological Medicine*, **33**, 203–15.

36. Barrowclough, C., King, P., Colville, J., *et al.* (2001). A randomized trial of the effectiveness of cognitive-behavioural therapy and supportive counselling for anxiety symptoms in older adults. *Journal of Consulting and Clinical Psychology*, **69**, 756–62.

37. Hill, D. (2006). Relationship problems. In *The Sage handbook of counselling and psychotherapy* (eds. C. Feltham and I. Horton), pp. 453–7. Sage, London.

38. Jacobson N. and Gurman, A. (eds.) (2002). *Clinical handbook of couple therapy.* Guildford, New York.

39. McCarthy, P., Walker, J., and Kain, J. (1998). *Telling it as it is: the client experience of Relate counselling.* Newcastle Centre for Family Studies, Newcastle.

40. Worden, J. (2005). *Grief counselling and grief therapy: a handbook for the mental health practitioner* (3rd edn). Bruner-Routledge, Hove.

41. Parkes, C., Relf, M., and Couldrick, A. (2002). *Counselling in terminal care and bereavement.* BPS Blackwell, Oxford.

42. Parkes, C. (2001). *Bereavement: studies of grief in adult life* (3rd edn). Taylor & Francis, Philadelphia.

43. Reid, D., Field, D., Payne, S., *et al.* (2006). Adult bereavement in five English hospices: types of support. *International Journal of Palliative Nursing*, **12**, 430–7.

44. Crits-Christoph, P., Siqueland, L., McCalmont. E., *et al.* (1999). Psychosocial treatments for cocaine dependence: national institute on drug abuse collaborative cocaine treatment study. *Archives of General Psychiatry*, **56**, 493–502.

45. Summerfield, D. (2006). Survivors of the tsunami: dealing with disaster. *Psychiatry*, **5**, 255–6.

46. Wessely, S. and Deahl, M. (2003). Psychological debriefing is a waste of time. *The British Journal of Psychiatry*, **183**, 12–14.

47. Foa, E., Keane, T., and Friedman, M. (eds.) (2004). *Effective treatments of PTSD.* Guildford, New York.

48. Cooper, P., Murray, L., Wilson, A., *et al.* (2003). Controlled trial of the short- and long-term effect of psychological treatment of post-partum depression. *The British Journal of Psychiatry*, **182**, 412–19.

49. Appleby, L., Hirst, E., Marshall, S. *et al.* (2003). The treatment of postnatal depression by health visitors: impact of brief training on skills and clinical practice. *Journal of Affective Disorders*, **77**, 261–6.

50. Mellor-Clark, J., Simms-Ellis, R., and Burton, M. (2001). *National survey of counsellors working in primary care: evidence for growing professionalization?* Royal College of General Practitioners, London.

51. BACP. (2006). *Shaping effective counselling services in health care: case studies of service delivery and outcomes*. British Association of Counselling and Psychotherapy, Rugby.

52. Keithley, J., Bond, T., and Marsh, G. (eds.) (2002). *Counselling in primary care*. Oxford University Press, Oxford.

53. Bower, P. and Rowland, N. (2006). Effectiveness and cost effectiveness of counselling in primary care. *Cochrane Database of Systematic Reviews*, **3**, CD001025.

54. King, M., Sibbald, B., and Ward, E. (2000). Randomised controlled trial of non-directive counselling, cognitive-behaviour therapy and usual general practitioner care in the management of depression as well as mixed anxiety and depression in primary care. *Health Technology Assessment*, **4**, 1–83.

55. Ward, E., King, M., Lloyd, M., et al. (2000). Randomised controlled trial of non-directive counselling, cognitive-behaviour therapy, and usual general practitioner care for patients with depression. I: clinical effectiveness. *British Medical Journal*, **321**, 1383–8.

56. Simpson, S., Corney, R., Fitzgerald, P., et al. (2000). A randomised controlled trial to evaluate the effectiveness and cost-effectiveness of counselling patients with chronic depression. *Health Technology Assessment*, **4**, 1–83.

57. Thomas, P., Davison, S., Rance, C. (eds.) (2001). *Clinical counselling in medical settings*. Brunner-Routledge, London.

58. Davis, H. and Fallowfield, L. (1996). *Counselling and communication in health care*. John Wiley & Sons, Chichester.

59. Finn, C. and Smoller, J. (2006). Genetic counseling in psychiatry. *Harvard Review of Psychiatry*, **14**, 109–21.

60. Moore, S. (2006). Voluntary sector counselling: has inadequate research resulted in a misunderstood and underutilised resource? *Counselling and Psychotherapy Research*, **6**, 221–6.

61. Greenwood, A. (2006). *Counselling for staff in health service settings*. Royal College of Nursing, London.

62. McLeod, J. and Henderson, M. (2003). Does workplace counselling work? *The British Journal of Psychiatry*, **182**, 103–4.

63. Carroll, M. and Walton, M. (eds.) (1999). *Handbook of counselling in organisations*. Sage, London.

64. Millar, A. (2002). Beyond resolution of presenting issues: clients' experiences of an in-house police counselling service. *Counselling and Psychotherapy Research*, **2**, 159–66.

65. Simon, G., Ludman, E., Tutty, S., et al. (2004). Telephone psychotherapy and telephone care management for primary care patients starting antidepressant treatment: a randomized controlled trial. *The Journal of the American Medical Association*, **292**, 935–42.

66. Tutty, S., Simon, G., and Ludman, E. (2000). Telephone counseling as an adjunct to antidepressant treatment in the primary care system. A pilot study. *Effective Clinical Practice*, **3**, 170–8.

67. Goss, S. and Anthony, K. (eds.) (2003). *Technology in counselling and psychotherapy. A practitioner's guide*. Palgrave Macmillan, Basingstoke.

68. DOH. (2006). *The regulation of the non-medical healthcare professions*. Department of Health, London.

69. Aldridge, S. and Pollard, J. (2005). *Interim report to the Department of Health on initial mapping project for psychotherapy and counselling*. British Association for Counselling and Psychotheraphy, Rugby.

70. Bower, P. and Gilbody, S. (2005). Stepped care in psychological therapies: access, effectiveness and efficiency: narrative literature review. *The British Journal of Psychiatry*, **186**, 11–7.

71. Leahy, R. (2001). *Overcoming resistance in cognitive therapy*. Guildford, New York.

# 6.3.2 **Cognitive behaviour therapy**

## Contents

6.3.2.1  Cognitive behaviour therapy for anxiety disorders
David M. Clark

6.3.2.2  Cognitive behaviour therapy for eating disorders
Zafra Cooper, Rebecca Murphy, and Christopher G. Fairburn

6.3.2.3  Cognitive behaviour therapy for depressive disorders
Melanie J. V. Fennell

6.3.2.4  Cognitive behaviour therapy for schizophrenia
Max Birchwood and Elizabeth Spencer

## 6.3.2.1 **Cognitive behaviour therapy for anxiety disorders**

David M. Clark

### Introduction

Cognitive behaviour therapy for anxiety disorders is a brief psychological treatment (1 to 16 sessions), based on the cognitive model of emotional disorders. Within this model, it is assumed that it is not events per se, but rather people's expectations and interpretations of events, which are responsible for the production of negative emotions such as anxiety, anger, guilt, or sadness. In anxiety, the important interpretations, or cognitions, concern perceived physical or psychosocial danger. In everyday life, many situations are objectively dangerous. In such situations, individuals' perceptions are often realistic appraisals of the inherent danger. However, Beck[1] argues that in anxiety disorders, patients systematically overestimate the danger inherent in certain situations, bodily sensations, or mental processes. Overestimates of danger can arise from distorted estimates of the likelihood of a feared event, distorted estimates of the severity of the event, and/or distorted estimates of one's coping resources and the availability of rescue factors. Once a stimulus is interpreted as a source of danger, an 'anxiety programme' is activated. This is a pattern of responses that is probably inherited from our evolutionary past and originally served to protect us from harm in objectively dangerous primitive environments (such as attack from a predator). The programme includes changes in autonomic arousal as preparation for flight/fight/fainting and increased scanning of the environment for possible sources of danger. In modern life, there are also situations in which these responses are adaptive (such as getting out of the path of a speeding car). However, when, as in anxiety disorders, the danger is more imagined than real, these anxiety responses are largely inappropriate. Instead of serving a useful function, they contribute to a series of vicious circles that tend to maintain or exacerbate the anxiety disorder.

Two types of vicious circle are common in anxiety disorders. First, the reflexively elicited somatic and cognitive symptoms of anxiety become further sources of perceived danger. For example, blushing can be taken as an indication that one has made a fool of oneself, and this may lead to further embarrassment and blushing; or a racing heart may be taken as evidence of an impending heart attack and this may produce further anxiety and cardiac symptoms. Second, patients often engage in behavioural and cognitive strategies that are intended to prevent the feared events from occurring. However, because the fears are unrealistic, the main effect of these strategies is to prevent patients from disconfirming their negative beliefs. For example, patients who fear that the unusual and racing thoughts experienced during panic attacks indicate that they are in danger of going mad and often try to control their thoughts and (erroneously) believe that if they had not done so, they would have gone mad.

Within cognitive models of anxiety disorders, at least two different levels of disturbed thinking are distinguished. First, negative automatic thoughts are those thoughts or images that are present in specific situations when an individual is anxious. For example, someone concerned about social evaluation might have the negative thought, 'They think I'm boring', while talking to a group of acquaintances. Second, dysfunctional assumptions are general beliefs, which individuals hold about the world and themselves which are said to make them prone to interpret specific situations in an excessively negative and dysfunctional fashion. For example, a rule involving an extreme equation of self-worth with social approval ('Unless I am liked by everyone, I am worthless') might make an individual particularly likely to interpret silent spells in conversation as an indication that others think one is boring.

Cognitive behaviour therapy attempts to treat anxiety disorders by (a) helping patients identify their negative danger-related thoughts and beliefs, and (b) modifying these cognitions and the behavioural and cognitive processes that normally maintain them. A wide range of procedures are used to achieve these aims, including education, discussion of evidence for and against the beliefs, imagery modification, attentional manipulations, exposure to feared stimuli, and numerous other behavioural assignments. Within sessions there is a strong emphasis on experiential work and on working with high affect. Between sessions, patients follow extensive homework assignments. As in cognitive behaviour therapy for other disorders, the general approach is one of collaborative empiricism in which patient and therapist view the patient's fearful thoughts as hypotheses to be critically examined and tested.

# Background

## Historical development of cognitive behaviour therapy

Modern cognitive behaviour therapy for anxiety owes its development to pioneering work since the 1950s and 1960s in which the principles of classical conditioning were applied to the understanding and treatment of phobias.[2] It was argued that (a) phobic stimuli are conditioned stimuli that acquired their aversive properties by being paired on one or more occasions with a traumatic event, and (b) avoidance is the main reason why phobias fail to extinguish. This suggestion led naturally to the development of various forms of exposure therapy, in which patients were systematically exposed to phobic stimuli. Initially therapists were concerned that elicitation of strong anxiety responses would be counter-therapeutic so exposure was very gradual, often starting with brief, imaginal presentations, followed by relaxation. Subsequent research showed that such a gentle approach was unnecessary and relatively rapid, in vivo exposure became the norm. By the mid-1970s, it was clear that up to 70 per cent of phobics obtained worthwhile

improvements from in vivo exposure.[3] However, many were less than fully recovered and it was not clear how exposure therapy could be applied to non-phobic anxiety states (such as panic disorder and generalized anxiety disorder). In an attempt to enhance treatment effectiveness further, researchers attempted to identify additional factors that might maintain anxiety. Several cognitive processes outlined below received empirical support. As a consequence, more comprehensive cognitive behavioural treatments that attempt to modify a range of maintaining factors were developed. This chapter describes these treatments.

## Cognitive content of anxiety disorders

Although there is no substitute for a careful assessment of each patient's ideation, research shows that most anxiety disorders are characterized by a specific type of fearful ideation and successful therapy generally focuses on such ideation.[4]

### (a) Panic disorder

Panic disorder is characterized by a fear of an immediately impending internal disaster (e.g. heart attack, cessation of breathing, mental derangement) and a sense of loss of control over physical and mental functions. Many of panic patients' negative thoughts can be viewed as misinterpretations of normal bodily sensations (such as palpitations or a slight feeling of breathlessness). Indeed, cognitive theorists[5] argue that panic attacks result from a vicious circle in which catastrophic misinterpretations of body sensations lead to an increase in anxiety and associated sensations, which are in turn interpreted as further evidence of impending, internal disasters (e.g. heart attack, fainting, going mad). Panic disorder with agoraphobia is often also accompanied by fear of the interpersonal consequences of attacks (e.g. 'I'll make a fool of myself').

### (b) Social phobia

Social phobia is characterized by exaggerated fears of being evaluated, of having one's weaknesses exposed, and of being judged adversely by other people. While in feared social situations, the social phobic continually monitors his or her performance, fears that this performance will be viewed as evidence that he or she is inept, boring, or stupid, and expects that such judgements will have dire long-lasting implications (loss of status or worth and failure to achieve key goals such as friendship, marriage, promotion). Often social phobics have excessively high standards for social performance (e.g. 'My speech must be perfectly fluent', 'I must always appear intelligent and witty'). Typically, social anxiety is triggered when individuals have a strong desire to convey a particular, favourable impression of them and have marked insecurity about their ability to do so.

### (c) Generalized anxiety disorder

Generalized anxiety disorder is characterized by excessive worry about a number of life circumstances (e.g. finance, health, work, children, etc.) and the subjective impression that the worry is difficult to control.[6] Beck et al.[7] suggested that generalized anxiety disorder patients are anxious about many topics because their beliefs about themselves and the world make them prone to interpret a wide range of situations and circumstances in a threatening fashion. Although their beliefs are quite varied, Beck suggested that they mainly revolve around issues of acceptance, competence, responsibility, and control, as well as the symptoms of anxiety. Borkovec et al.[8] have shown that, compared with non-patients, the worry of general anxiety disorder patients involves less imagery about specific feared outcomes and more verbal rumination in which problems are cast in a more abstract, more difficult to solve, form. Wells[9] has highlighted the importance of positive and negative beliefs about worry (meta-cognition).

### (d)  Obsessive–compulsive disorder

Obsessive–compulsive disorder is characterized by intrusive and distressing thoughts, impulses, or images about possible harm coming to oneself or others. Thoughts with a similar content to the intrusions of obsessional patients (e.g. a young mother having an intrusive thought about dropping her baby) are common in the general population.[10] For this reason, it has been suggested that the key cognitive abnormality in obsessive–compulsive disorder is not the content of obsessional thoughts, but rather the way the thoughts are interpreted.[11] In particular, it would appear that obsessional patients interpret recurrent obsessional thoughts and impulses as a sign that something terrible will happen, for which they will be responsible. For example, the young mother mentioned above may think that because she had a thought of dropping her baby, she is very likely to do so, despite finding the idea repugnant. In order to prevent the feared consequences of their obsessional thoughts, patients engage in a wide range of 'putting right' acts including (when relevant) washing and checking.

### (e)  Post-traumatic stress disorder

Surveys[12] indicate that unwanted, intrusive, and distressing memories and the other symptoms of post-traumatic stress disorder (avoidance of reminders and hyperarousal/numbing) are common immediately after traumatic events. Over the next few months many people recover but in a subgroup post-traumatic stress disorder becomes chronic. It is the latter group that normally present for treatment. Research indicates that chronic post-traumatic stress disorder is associated with appraising the traumatic event and/or its sequelae in a manner that would produce a sense of serious current threat to one's view of oneself and/or the world.[13] Examples are given in Table 6.3.2.1.1. There is also evidence that chronic post-traumatic stress disorder tends to be associated with a fragmented memory for the traumatic event and that recovery is associated with developing a more coherent narrative.[14,15]

## Why do negative thoughts and beliefs persist?

If the world is not as dangerous as anxiety disorder patients assume, why do they not notice this and correct their thinking? For many patients with chronic anxiety disorders, the persistence of their fears can seem strangely irrational, at least at first glance. Consider, for example, panic disorder patients who think during their panic attacks that they are having a heart attack. Before they come for treatment they may have had several thousand panic attacks, in each one of which they thought they were dying, but they are not dead. Despite what might appear to an outsider as stunning disconfirmation of their belief that a panic attack can kill, their thinking has not changed.

Several factors that appear to prevent patients from changing their negative thinking are outlined below. Such factors are important because reversing them is likely to be a particularly efficient way of treating anxiety disorders.

### (a)  Avoidance, escape, and safety-seeking behaviours

Early conditioning theorists identified avoidance of, and escape from, feared stimuli as important factors in the maintenance of anxiety disorders. It is easy to see how avoidance of a feared situation (e.g. a supermarket for an agoraphobic) or escape from the situation before a feared event (e.g. a panic attack) occurs could prevent phobics from disconfirming their fears. However, situational avoidance/escape is not so obviously relevant to non-phobic anxiety and some phobics regularly endure feared situations without marked improvement in their fears. Salkovskis[16] introduced the concept of in-situation safety behaviours to deal with this problem. In particular, Salkovskis suggested that while in feared situations most patients engage in a variety of (often subtle) behaviours that are intended to prevent, or minimize, a feared outcome. For example, cardiac concerned panic disorder patients may sit down, rest, and slow down their breathing during attacks and believe, erroneously, that performing these safety behaviours is the reason why they did not die. Experimental studies have confirmed that (a) anxious patients engage in safety behaviours while in feared situations, and (b) dropping these behaviours facilitates fear reduction.[4]

Recent work[17] has highlighted several other important features of safety behaviours. First, although termed 'behaviours', many are internal mental processes. For example, patients with social phobia who are worried that what they say may not make sense and will sound stupid, often report memorizing what they have said and comparing it with what they are about to say, whilst speaking. If everything goes well, patients are likely to think 'It only went well because I did all the memorizing and checking; if I had just been myself people would have realized how stupid I was'. In this way their basic fear persists. Second, it is common for patients to engage in a large number of different safety behaviours while in a feared situation. Table 6.3.2.1.2 illustrates this point by summarizing the safety behaviours used by a patient who had a fear of blushing, especially while talking to men whom she thought other people would think were attractive. Third, safety behaviours can create some of the symptoms that patients fear. For example, responding to a feeling of breathlessness in panic attacks by breathing more quickly and deeply (hyperventilating) can enhance the feeling of being short of breath. Similarly, post-traumatic stress disorder patients who are concerned that unwanted intrusive recollections of the trauma mean they are going mad and often try hard to suppress such recollections. Unfortunately, active suppression increases the probability that the intrusion will occur. Fourth, some safety

**Table 6.3.2.1.1** Some examples of idiosyncratic negative appraisals leading to a sense of current threat in post-traumatic stress disorder

| What is appraised? | Negative appraisal |
|---|---|
| Fact that trauma happened | 'Nowhere is safe' |
| One's behaviour/emotions during trauma | 'I cannot cope with stress'; 'It was my fault' |
| *Initial post-traumatic stress disorder symptoms* | |
| Irritability, anger outbursts | 'My personality has changed for the worse' |
| Flashbacks, intrusive recollections, and nightmares | 'I'm going mad'; 'I'll lose control of my emotions' |
| *Other people's reactions after trauma* | |
| Positive responses | 'They think I am too weak to cope on my own |
| Negative responses | 'Nobody is there for me'; 'I can't rely on other people' |

**Table 6.3.2.1.2** Safety behaviours associated with a fear of blushing

| Feared outcome | Safety behaviour intended to prevent feared outcome |
|---|---|
| 'My face (and neck) will go red' | Keep cool (open windows, drink cold water, avoid coffee, wear thin clothes) |
| | Avoid eye contact. If in a meeting, pretend to be writing notes |
| | Keep topic of conversation away from 'difficult' issues |
| | Tell myself the man is not really attractive. He's no more than a 2 (out of 10) |
| 'If I do blush, people will notice' | Wear clothes (scarf, high collar) that would hide part of the blush |
| | Wear make-up to hide the blush |
| | Put hands over face. Hide face with long hair |
| | Stand in a dark part of the room |
| 'If people notice, they will think badly of me' | Provide an alternative explanation for the red face, e.g. 'it's hot in here'. |
| | 'I'm in a terrible rush today', 'I'm recovering from flu', etc. |

behaviours can draw other people's attention to problems that patients wish to hide. For example, a secretary who covered her face with her arms whenever she felt she was blushing discovered that colleagues in her office were much more likely to look at her when she did this than when she simply blushed. Finally, some safety behaviours influence other people in a way that tends to maintain the problem. For example, the tendency of social phobics to monitor continually what they have said, and how they think they come across, often makes them appear distant and preoccupied. Other people can interpret this as a sign that the phobic does not like them and, as a consequence, they respond to the phobic in a less warm and friendly fashion.

### (b) Attentional deployment

Selective attention plays an important role in maintaining some anxiety disorders. Patients with panic disorder or hypochondriasis fear certain bodily sensations and symptoms, believing they indicate the presence of a serious physical disorder (heart attack, cardiac disease, cancer, etc.). Such patients have often had several medical investigations that indicate they do not have the physical illness(es) they fear, but they are not convinced. One reason appears to be that their fears lead them to focus attention on relevant parts of their bodies and, as a consequence of this attentional deployment, they become aware of benign bodily sensations that other people do not notice.[5] The presence of such sensations is then taken by the patient as evidence that a serious physical illness has been missed. (Hypochondriasis is classified as a somatoform disorder in DSM-IV[6] and as a somatization disorder in ICD-10.[18] However, it has many features in common with anxiety disorders and can be conceptualized as such for the purposes of psychological treatment).

Social phobia appears to be associated with two attentional biases. First, when in feared social situations, patients with social phobia report becoming highly self-focused, constantly monitoring how they think and feel they are coming across, and paying less attention to other people.[17] Reduced processing of other people

means that social phobics have less chance to observe other people's responses in detail and, therefore, are unlikely to collect from other people's reactions information that would help them to see that they generally come across more positively than they think. Second, there is some evidence that when social phobics do focus on other people, they are particularly good at detecting negative reactions[19] and are poor at detecting positive reactions.

### (c) Spontaneously occurring images

Spontaneously occurring images are common in anxiety disorders and also appear to play a role in maintenance. Patients with social phobia often report 'observer-perspective' images in which they see themselves as if viewed from outside.[20] Unfortunately, in their images they do not see what a true observer would see, but rather their fears visualized. For example, a teacher who was anxious about talking with colleagues in coffee breaks noticed that before speaking she felt tense around her lips. The tension would trigger an image in which she saw herself with a twisted and contorted mouth, looking like 'the village idiot'. At that moment, she was convinced everyone else thought she was stupid. Negative images are also used as information in other anxiety disorders. For example, obsessional patients who have images of committing a repugnant act (e.g. stabbing one's child) take the occurrence of the image as evidence that they are in danger of performing the act. Similarly, patients with post-traumatic stress disorder report that flashbacks increase the perceived likelihood of a future trauma.

### (d) Emotional reasoning

A further source of misleading information that can enhance patients' perception of danger is anxiety itself.[21] For example, social phobics often think they look as anxious as they feel, but in general this is not the case.[22] Similarly, generalized anxiety disorder patients often take feeling on edge as a sign that something bad is about to happen.

### (e) Memory processes

Some anxiety disorders are associated with a tendency for the selective recall of information that would appear to confirm the patient's worst fears. For example, high socially anxious individuals selectively recall negative information about the way they think they have appeared to others in the past when anticipating a stressful social interaction.[22] Similarly, patients with hypochondriasis selectively recall illness-related information. In post-traumatic stress disorder, a failure to elaborate memories at the time of the trauma and enhanced associative learning appear to play a key role in maintaining the re-experiencing symptoms.[13]

### (f) Rumination

Anxious patients often spend protracted periods of time ruminating about negative things that could happen in the future and about how bad they would be. They may also ruminate about things that they feel have gone wrong in the past. Studies by Davey and Matchett[23] indicate that such rumination can enhance fear. There are several ways in which rumination might operate. First, thinking about an event may directly increase its subjective probability. Second, selectively focusing on past negative events, feelings, and impressions may further enhance the perceived likelihood of future danger. Third, rumination is rarely focused on constructively processing perceived threats, but instead often seems to elaborate the threats or make them more abstract and hence difficult to deal with. For example, patients with post-traumatic stress disorder often ask themselves 'Could I have done something different?' during their traumatic event without thinking through in detail what their alternative options might have been, and how feasible they would have been at the time.

## Treatment

### Assessment interview

Table 6.3.2.1.3 summarizes the main topics covered in the assessment interview. The aims of the interview are as follows: (a) to obtain a detailed description of the patient's fears and behaviour; (b) to identify maintaining factors; (c) to normalize the problem; (d) to develop a model of the problem that can be used to guide treatment.

The interview would start by asking the patient to provide a brief description of the main presenting problem(s). For example, intense anxiety attacks, anxious apprehension, and avoidance of places where the attacks seem particularly likely or would be embarrassing. The interviewer then obtains a detailed description of a recent occasion when the problem occurred or was at its most marked. This would include the situation ('Where were you?', 'What were you doing?'), bodily reactions ('What did you notice in your body?', 'What sensations did you experience?'), thoughts ('At the moment you were feeling particularly anxious, what went through your mind? What was the worst that you thought might happen? Did you have an image/mental picture of that? How do you think you looked?'), behaviour ('What did you do?'), and the behaviour of others ('How did X react?', 'What did X say/do?'). Having obtained a detailed description of a recent occasion, the interviewer should check whether the occasion was typical. If not, further descriptions of other recent occasions should be elicited to provide a complete picture.

**Table 6.3.2.1.3** Summary of topics to be covered in assessment interview

| |
| --- |
| Brief description of presenting problem(s) |
| For each problem |
|   Detailed description of a recent occasion when problem occurred/was at its most marked |
|     Situation |
|     Bodily reaction |
|     Cognitions |
|     Behaviour |
|   List of situations when the problem is most likely to occur/be most severe |
|   Modulators (things making it better or worse) |
|   Possible maintaining factors |
|     Avoidance of situations/activities |
|     Safety behaviours |
|     Attentional deployment |
|     Faulty beliefs |
|     Attitudes and behaviour of others |
|     Medication |
|   Beliefs about cause of the problem |
|   Previous treatment (types, whether successful) |
|   Onset and course |
| Personal strengths and assets |
| Social and financial circumstances |

Next a list of situations in which the problem is most likely to occur or is most severe is elicited ('Are there any situations in which you are particularly likely to have a panic attack?'), together with information about modulators ('Are there any things that you notice make the symptoms stronger/more likely to occur?', 'Are there any things that you've noticed make the symptoms less likely/less severe/more controllable?').

Possible maintaining factors should be identified, including the following:

◆ avoidance of situations or activities ('What situations/activities do you avoid because of your fears?')

◆ safety behaviours ('When you are afraid that X might happen, is there anything you do to try to stop it happening?')

◆ attentional deployment ('What happens to your attention when you are worried about X? Do you focus more on your body? Do you become self-conscious?')

◆ faulty beliefs (e.g. an obsessive–compulsive disorder patient, believing that thinking something can make it happen)

◆ attitudes and behaviour of significant others ('What does Y think about the problem?'; 'What does Y do when you are particularly anxious?')

◆ current medication

There are several ways in which excessive use of both prescribed and non-prescribed medications can maintain anxiety disorders. For example, painkillers and tranquillizers can cause derealization and sleep disturbance respectively, and drinking before social occasions prevents disconfirmation of one's social fears.

It is also important to assess patients' beliefs about the cause of their problems as some beliefs may make it difficult for patients to engage in therapy. For example, patients with post-traumatic stress disorder who think the best way of dealing with a painful memory is to push it out of their mind are unlikely to engage in imaginal reliving of the event until this belief is dealt with.

Finally, a brief description of the onset and subsequent course of the problem should be obtained. This description should particularly focus on factors, which may have been responsible for initial onset and for fluctuations in the course of the symptoms and is primarily used to make the development of the problem seem understandable to the patient.

It is not always possible to obtain all the information needed for a cognitive behavioural formulation in an assessment interview. Sometimes it is necessary to follow-up the interview with homework assignments in which the patient collects more information to clarify the formulation. For example, a hypochondriacal patient who was concerned that palpitations meant that she had cardiac disease was asked to record what she did each hour and how many palpitations she experienced. To her surprise, palpitations were not associated with exercise, as she expected, but rather were most common when she was sitting quietly, reading, watching television, or studying. This realization helped convince her that her problem may be disease preoccupation rather than a faulty heart.

### Developing an idiosyncratic model of the patient's problem

Assessment ends with the development of an idiosyncratic version of the cognitive model. In particular, therapists aim to show patients how the specific triggers for their anxiety produce negative automatic thoughts relating to feared outcomes and how these are maintained by safety behaviours and other maintenance processes. The model is usually drawn on a whiteboard, so that patient and therapist can look at it and discuss it together. Figure 6.3.2.1.1 shows an example for a panic disorder patient. His panic attack started with a twinge in his chest muscles, and he then had the thought, 'There is something wrong with my chest area, maybe I am having a heart attack'. This interpretation made him start to feel anxious, his chest muscles tightened up more, he started to feel dizzy, his heart raced more, and he then thought, 'I'm dying, I'm having a heart attack', and also, interestingly, 'If I don't die, people will notice I'm anxious and think it is odd'. He then engaged in a series of safety behaviours to try to prevent himself from dying. He thought he had read somewhere that paracetamol (aminacetophen) is good for people with heart problems and so he took a paracetamol. This is incorrect information, but the key point is that he believed it. He also sat down and rested, took the strain off his heart, and took deep breaths, trying to slow down his heart rate. He believed that the main reason he had not died was that he had engaged in the safety behaviours. The reader will also notice that some of the safety behaviours (taking deep breaths and monitoring the heart) will also have augmented his feared symptoms.

Figure 6.3.2.1.2 shows a further example with a social phobic patient. The patient's main fear was that other people would think she was stupid and boring. The situation used to develop the model was a recent coffee break at work during which the patient had difficulty joining a conversation with colleagues. When attempting to join the conversation she had the thought, 'I'll sound stupid and everyone will think I am dumb'. In order to prevent herself from sounding stupid, she engaged in an extensive set of safety behaviours which (a) prevented her from discovering that her spontaneous thoughts are interesting to other people, (b) made her appear preoccupied and uninterested in her colleagues, and (c) made her excessively self-conscious. While self-conscious, she became particularly aware of anxiety symptoms (sweaty palms, stiff muscles

around her mouth) that she thought other people might see, and indeed, had an image of herself in which she looked very strange, with a twisted and rigid mouth and appeared stupid.

Normally idiosyncratic models of the form illustrated in Figs 6.3.2.1.1 and 6.3.2.1.2 will be developed at the end of the first interview, and certainly not later than the second session. Such models are used as blueprints to help therapist and patient organize and develop the rest of therapy.

## Monitoring progress

Once treatment has started, it is important to monitor progress continually in order to decide whether a particular treatment procedure is working or whether the case needs reformulating and new treatment procedures need to be implemented. Usually patients are asked to complete a small number of self-report questionnaires before each therapy session. Typically, these include frequency and severity ratings for the main anxiety problems (often using simple 0–8 Likert-type scales), a measure of negative thoughts, and general measures of anxiety and depression (such as the Beck Anxiety Inventory[24] and the Beck Depression Inventory[25]). Table 6.3.2.1.4 summarizes some of the most commonly used weekly measures. In some instances these are supplemented by more individualized diaries and ratings. More global standardized measures of symptom severity are also often administered at the beginning, middle, and end of therapy in order to provide normative data (see Table 6.3.2.1.4).

Notice a twinge in
my chest muscles

'There is something wrong
in my chest area. Maybe
I'm having a heart attack'

Anxious

**Safety behaviours**
Take paracetamol
Rest
Take deep breaths
Monitor my heart

'My heart will stop
and I'll die'. 90% belief
'People will notice I
am anxious' 25%
belief

Muscles tighten up
in chest and back
Dizzy
Unreal
Racing heart
Dry throat

**Fig. 6.3.2.1.1** A cognitive model of a patient's panic attacks. (Reproduced from Clark, D.M., Panic disorder: from theory to therapy.
In *Frontiers of cognitive therapy* (ed. P.M. Salkovskis), pp. 318–344, Copyright 1996, Guildford Press, New York.)

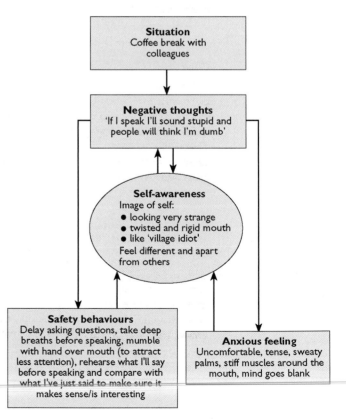

**Fig. 6.3.2.1.2** A cognitive model for a patient with social phobia.

# Plates for Chapter 2.3.1

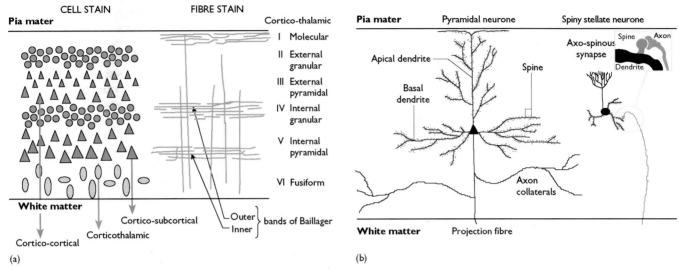

**Plate 1** (a) Laminar structure of the cerebral neocortex; (b) excitatory amino acid using spiny neurones of the neocortex.

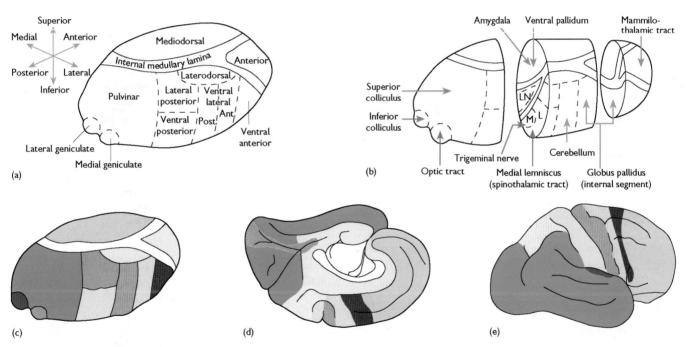

**Plate 2** (a) The thalamus is shown as if removed from the brain at the top, with the individual major nuclei indicated. (b) Schematic diagram showing the isolated thalamus divided approximately at the middle of its anteroposterior extent; the arrows indicate known sources of major subcortical afferents to the individual named nuclei. (c) The diagram of the isolated thalamus shown in (a) with the individual main nuclei colour coded. (d), (e) Schematic diagrams of the cerebral surfaces (medial and lateral) showing the regions of cortex colour coded to correspond to the main thalamic nuclei with which they have major connections.

## Plates for Chapter 2.3.6

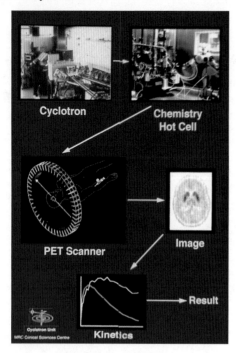

**Plate 3** Steps in the production and use of PET radio-isotopes.

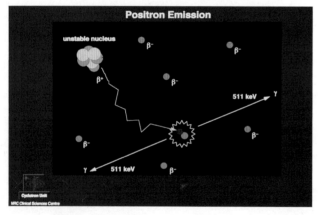

**Plate 4** Principles of positron emission: $\beta^-$ is an electron and $\beta^+$ is a positron. Two high-energy gamma rays ($\gamma$) are produced on annihilation of a positron by an electron

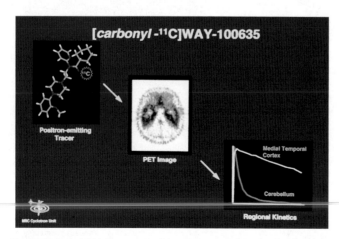

**Plate 5** Use of a PET radiotracer to image 5-HT$_{1A}$ receptors in the human brain.

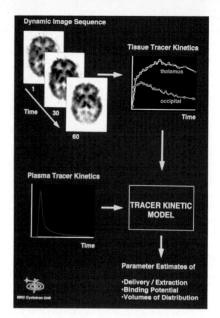

**Plate 6** Steps in the data analysis of a PET radiotracer.

## Plates for Chapter 2.3.7

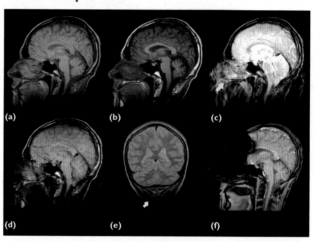

**Plate 7** Spin echo MR images and artefacts. Top row, spin echo images: left, proton density image (TR = 2000 ms, TE = 20 ms); middle, $T_1$-weighted image (TR = 350 ms, TE = 20 ms); right, $T_2$-weighted image (TR = 2000 ms, TE = 90 ms). The arrow on the $T_2$-weighted image indicates blurring caused by movement (swallowing) during acquisition. Bottom row, examples of poor tissue contrast and susceptibility artefact: left, spin echo image showing poor contrast due to injudicious prescription of pulse sequence (TR = 350 ms, TE = 90 ms); middle, bulk susceptibility artefact; right, ferromagnetic susceptibility artefact caused by a metallic hairgrip.

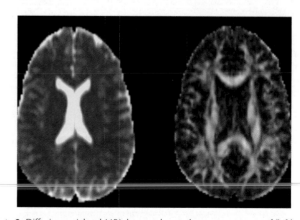

**Plate 8** Diffusion-weighted MRI data can be used to generate maps of (left) the apparent diffusion coefficient (**ADC**) and (right) the anisotropy of diffusion. Diffusion of protons is most rapid and isotropic in cerebrospinal fluid, and least rapid and most anisotropic in white matter. White matter is clearly defined by relative hyperintensity in the anisotropy map.

## Plates for Chapter 2.3.7 *(continued)*

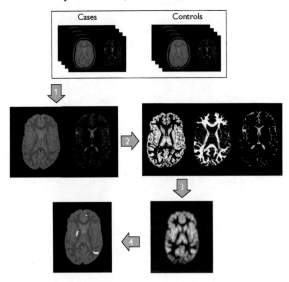

**Plate 9** Steps in computerized image analysis. Dual-echo (fast spin echo) data are acquired from several cases and controls in a cross-sectionally designed study. Extracerebral tissue is removed (1) from each image before segmentation or tissue classification (2). Tissue-calssified images are registered with a template image in standard space (3) before hypothesis testing (4). Voxels or clusters, which demonstrate a significant difference in tissue class volume between groups, are colour coded.

**Plate 11** Activation map. Generically activated voxels are colour coded against a grey-scale background of gradient echoplanar imaging data. The grid respresents the standard Talairach-Tournoux Space;[12] z-coordinates for each slice are shown at the bottom left. Colour codes the timing and power of a periodic response to a covert verbal-fluency experiment. Blue voxels show increased magnetic resonance signal during condition B (repeat a word covertly); light blue represents a greater power of response than dark blue. Red voxels show increased magnetic resonance signal during condition. A (generate a word beginning with a cue letter); yellow and orange represent a greater power of response than dark red. The voxel-wise probability of a false-positive error is $p = 0.0001$. The main areas activated during conditioin A are the dorsolateral prefrontal cortex, inferior frontal gyrus, and supplementary motor area; the main areas activated during condition B are the medial parietal cortex and posterior cingulate gyrus.

## Plates for Chapter 2.3.8

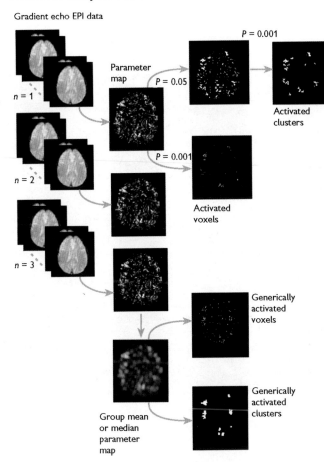

**Plate 10** Steps in computerized data analysis. Gradient echoplanar imaging data have been acquired from three subjects under identical conditions. The time series at each voxel is analysed to estimate a measure or parameter of the experimental effect, which is represented as a parameter map. Significantly activated voxels or clusters can be identified in each individual image. Parameter maps can be averaged over individuals and generically activated voxels or clusters identified over the group of subjects. The power to detect activation is enhanced by cluster-level analysis and by combining data from several subjects.

## Plate for Chapter 4.1.3

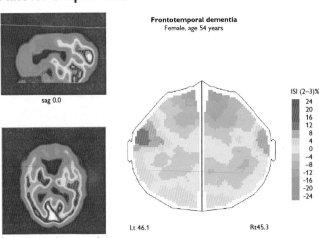

**Plate 12** Regional cerebral blood flow (rCBF) measured using SPECT with exametazine (left) and the Xenon-133 inhalation method (right) in a 54-year-old female with clinical signs of FTD. The variation of regional cerebral blood flow is measured with xenon-133, above (red) or below (green) the average flow level, as indicated by the colour code. The patient showed the first signs of personality change, and stereotypy of speech and behaviour at the age of 48 years. EEG was normal, and CT and MRI showed slight frontal cortical atrophy. The regional cerebral blood flow measurement with xenon-133 showed a normal average flow level and marked bilateral, frontal flow decreases. The SPECT scan showed a severe perfusion deficit in the frontal and anterior cingulate cortex. (Courtesy of Department of Neurophysiology, University Hopital, Lund, Sweden.)

## Plate for Chapter 4.2.1

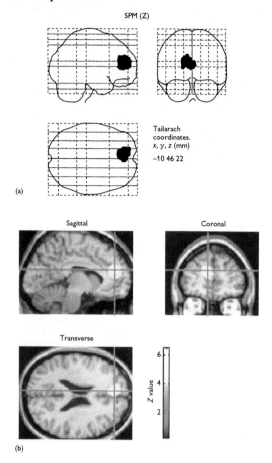

**Plate 13** Area of activation during opiate craving: (a) [$^{15}$O]H$_2$O PET SPM image; (b) area of activation superimposed on magnetic resonance image.

## Plate for Chapter 4.5.6

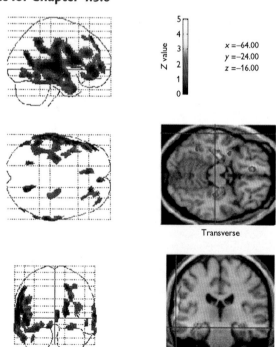

**Plate 14** Statistical parametric maps (p < 0.001) for reductions in grey matter densities in subjects with chronic refractory depression compared with controls. Effects are controlled for age. (Reproduced with permission from P.J. Shah *et al.* (1998). Cortical grey matter reductions associated with treatment-resistant chronic unipolar depression: controlled MRI study. *British Journal of Psychiatry*, **72**, 527–32.)

## Plates for Chapter 6.2.10.4

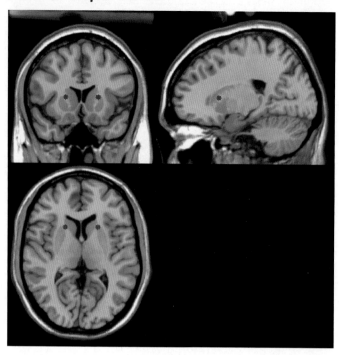

**Plate 15** Typical locations of anterior capsulotomy lesions superimposed upon normalized T1 MRI scan. Lesions not to scale.

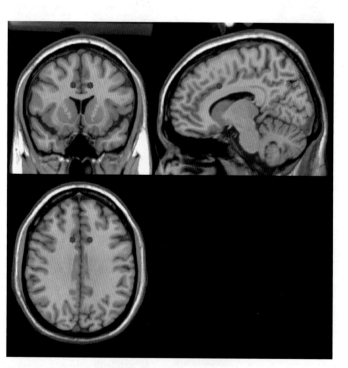

**Plate 16** Typical locations of anterior cingulotomy lesions superimposed upon normalized T1 MRI scan. Lesions not to scale.

## Treatment procedures

A wide range of procedures can be used to modify patients' negative beliefs and linked maintenance processes. For clarity the procedures are described separately. However, in practice the techniques are closely interwoven. Within a given session, therapists will usually use a mixture of discussion and experiential techniques to help patients to challenge convincingly their negative beliefs. As with cognitive behaviour therapy for other disorders, patients are given extensive homework assignments and it is assumed that a sizeable amount of therapeutic change is the result of homework assignments.

### (a) Identifying patients' evidence for their negative beliefs

Anxiety disorder patients usually have reasons for believing that the things they fear are dangerous, however strange their fears may seem. The therapist, therefore, tries to 'get inside the patient's head' and see what the evidence is. Often the evidence is an event or piece of information that the patient has misinterpreted. Identifying and correcting such misinterpretations can be helpful. For example, a panic disorder patient believed that experiencing high anxiety could kill her. When asked by the therapist what her evidence was, she explained that she had seen it happen. Further enquiry revealed she had entered Dresden the day after the fire bombing of that city by the allies during the Second World War and had helped search for survivors. When opening up cellars below demolished houses, she repeatedly observed that the occupants were either dead or behaved in a dazed confused manner, even though the fire had not entered their cellars. She concluded that fear had killed the occupants or sent them mad. However, further questioning from the therapist revealed that the cellar occupants all had bright cherry-red lips. This allowed the therapist to explain that they were suffering from carbon monoxide poisoning, not the effects of intense fear. This correction considerably reduced the patient's fear of anxiety.

### (b) Education

Education about the symptoms of anxiety is often helpful, especially if it directly targets patients' idiosyncratic fears and concerns. For example, post-traumatic stress disorder patients often think their flashbacks and emotional outbursts mean they are going mad or have permanently changed for the worse. In such cases, detailed assessment of the patient's post-traumatic stress disorder symptoms and explanation that each are common reactions to a trauma can greatly help. Similarly, panic disorder patients with cardiac concerns often cite left-sided chest pain as evidence for their belief that they have a cardiac disorder. In such cases discussion of Fig. 6.3.2.1.3 (from a study of chest pain in patients referred to a cardiac clinic[26]) is useful. In particular, the patient discovers that left-sided chest pain is more characteristic of non-cardiac chest pain than of either confirmed angina or myocardial infarction. Further questioning helps patients to see that the association between left-sided pain and attacks is probably a consequence of their fears. That is to say, they can experience pain on either side of the chest but only panic when it is on the left side. Finally, patients with obsessive–compulsive disorder who are perturbed by the apparently repulsive and unusual nature of their intrusive thoughts often benefit from reviewing Rachman and De Silva's classic

**Table 6.3.2.1.4** Commonly used measures for monitoring progress

| Anxiety disorder | Measure | | |
|---|---|---|---|
| | Symptoms | Thoughts | Global severity |
| Panic disorder | Panic Rating Scale[63] Panic Diary[63] BAI[33] BDI[2] | Agoraphobic Cognitions Questionnaire[65] | Fear Questionnaire[64] Mobility Inventory[66] |
| Social phobia | Social Summary Scales (Table 4) BAI[33] BDI[2] | Social Cognitions Questionnaire[53] | Liebowitz Social Anxiety Scale[67] Social Performance Scale[68] Social Interaction Anxiety Scale[68] Social Phobia and Anxiety Inventory[69] |
| Generalized anxiety disorder | BAI[33] BDI[2] | Worry Domains Questionnaire[70] Thought Control Questionnaire[72] | Penn State Worry Questionnaire[71] Spielberger State Trait Inventory[73] |
| Obsessive-compulsive disorder | BAI[33] BDI[2] | Responsibility Interpretations Questionnaire[74] | Padua Inventory[75] Yale–Brown Obsessive Compulsive Scale[76] |
| Post-traumatic stress disorder | Post-traumatic Diagnosis Scale[77,78] BAI[33] BDI[2] | Post-traumatic Cognitions Inventory[79] Personal Beliefs and Reactions Scale[81] | Impact of Events Scale[80] Post-traumatic Diagnosis Scale[78] |

Owing to their length, the Post-traumatic Cognitions Inventory and the Personal Beliefs and Reactions Scale are not suitable for weekly administration.

BAI, Beck Anxiety Inventory; BDI. Beck Depression Inventory.

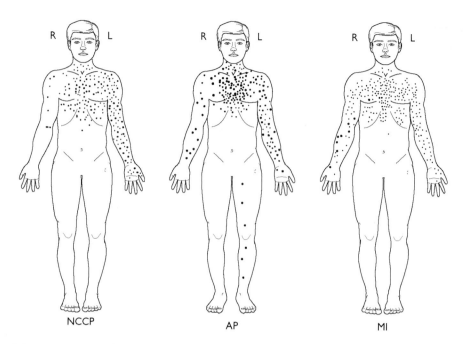

**Fig. 6.3.2.1.3** Distribution of chest pain in patients referred to a cardiac clinic and subsequently diagnosed as non-cardiac chest pain (NCCP), angina pectoris (AP), or myocardial infarction (MI). (Reproduced from Beunderman, R. *et al.* (1998), Differentiation in prodromal and acute symptoms of patients with cardiac and non-cardiac chest pain, In *Advances in theory and practice in behaviour therapy* (ed. P.M.G. Emmelkamp, *et al.*), Copyright 1998, Swets and Seitlinger, Taylor and Francis Group, an informa business.)

paper[10] which demonstrated that thoughts with identical content to obsessional intrusions are common in the general population.

### (c)  Identifying observations that contradict patients' negative beliefs

As anxiety disorder patients' beliefs about the dangerousness of feared stimuli are generally mistaken, patients have often experienced a number of events that contradict their beliefs before they come into therapy. Therapists can make considerable progress, even in an assessment interview, by spotting these events and helping patients understand their significance. For example, panic disorder patients who are worried that their symptoms mean they are about to have a heart attack, often report that in some attacks something unexpected happened to distract them (e.g. a telephone call) and then their symptoms went away. Therapists could then pause and help the patient understand what this means, perhaps asking, 'Would a cardiologist prescribe telephone calls as a treatment for a heart attack?' The patient would probably answer 'No', to which the therapist might reply, 'If telephone calls would not stop a heart attack, how might they work? If the problem was the negative thought, could they help (by distracting one from the thoughts)?'

### (d)  Imagery modification

Images play an important role in many anxiety disorders. Most images represent feared catastrophes and can be treated as predictions to be tested (see behavioural experiments below). However, when the images are stereotyped and repetitive it is often also necessary to work directly with the images and to restructure them explicitly.

The problem with anxiety-related images is that they seem very realistic at the time they occur and, as a consequence, greatly enhance fear. A common restructuring technique involves discussing with the patient whether the image is realistic. Once it is intellectually agreed that the image is an exaggeration, patients are asked to recreate intentionally the negative image and to hold it in mind until they start to feel anxious. They are then asked to transform it into a more realistic image, or an image, which convincingly indicates that the original image was unrealistic. A common observation is that patients' spontaneous images generally stop at the worst moment. For example, agoraphobic patients who fear fainting in a supermarket might see themselves collapsed on the floor, but not see themselves getting up, recovering, and going home. A useful transformation in such cases is to 'finish out' the image by asking patients to run it on until they see the positive resolution. Of course, sometimes simply running on an image does not produce a positive resolution. For example, a patient who feared she would go mad frequently experienced an image of two men in white coats entering her house to take her away to a locked ward. In the image, the men were extremely powerful and she felt powerless. Transformation, following suggestions from her, involved shrinking the men and then turning them into ridiculous looking (and hence non-threatening) white poodles.

An interesting observation about spontaneous imagery is that it often fails to incorporate positive information that would seriously undermine the impact of the image, even when the patient has such information. For example, a mother whose children died in a house fire, repeatedly experienced intrusive flashbacks in which she saw the house going up in flames and smelled burning flesh, despite having seen her children in the mortuary, knowing that they had not been burnt, but instead were rapidly overcome by fumes.

For imagery restructuring to be effective it is important that it is not done as a cold, intellectual exercise, but instead includes eliciting the affect normally associated with the image. Transformation may have to be done in several steps. It is often best to start with the most threatening aspect of the image. Possible alternative images should be generated by patients, rather than simply imposed by the therapist.

### (e) Cognitive restructuring

All the above techniques are examples of cognitive restructuring in which the therapist provides information and asks a series of questions to help the patients challenge their fearful thoughts and images. A list of some of the questions that can be particularly useful for helping anxiety disorder patients challenge their negative thoughts is given in Table 6.3.2.1.5. Further useful questioning techniques can be found in Chapter 6.3.2.3.

It is sometimes helpful to use graphical methods for discussing alternatives to negative thoughts. In situations where there are several non-threatening alternative explanations for a feared event, pie charts are particularly useful. When constructing a pie chart the therapist draws a circle which is meant to represent all the possible causes of a particular event and asks the patient to list all the possible non-catastrophic causes of the event and allocate a section of the circle to each cause. At the end of the exercise, there is often very little of the circle left for the patient's negative explanations. Figure 6.3.2.1.4 illustrates the use of a pie chart to challenge a generalized anxiety disorder patient's belief that he would be 100 per cent responsible for people not enjoying themselves at his dinner parties. The belief was preventing him from making new social contacts after a painful divorce. Pie charts are particularly helpful for dealing with distorted beliefs about responsibility and hypochondriacal concerns (e.g. 'Headaches mean I have a brain tumour').

When considering the worst that could possibly happen in a feared situation patients frequently ignore the fact that there are many intermediate events, each with a probability of less than 1, which have to occur for the catastrophe to be realized. The inverted pyramid can be a good way of representing this. Figure 6.3.2.1.5 shows an example with a patient who was afraid of blushing. His worst fear was that other people would think they were greatly superior to him if he blushed. Whenever he felt his face becoming hot, he was convinced other people were thinking they are superior to him and gloating. However, careful discussion helped him to see that there were many intermediate steps between him feeling hot and the feared outcome. Once the conditional probabilities were taken into account, there was only a minute chance that his worst fear would be correct.

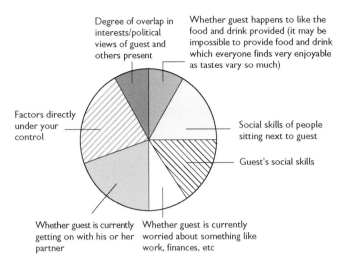

**Fig. 6.3.2.1.4** A pie chart representing factors that might contribute to guests enjoying themselves at a dinner parties to challenge a generalized anxiety disorder patient's belief that he would be 100 per cent responsible for people not enjoying themselves. (Reproduced from Clark, D.M., Anxiety states: panic and generalized anxiety, In *Cognitive therapy for psychiatric problems: a practical guide* (ed. K. Hawton, *et al.*), pp. 52–96. Copyright 1989 with permission from Oxford University Press.)

It is important to remember that anxiety results from overestimating the cost of feared events as well as their probability. Discussions aimed at modifying perceived cost are often helpful. This can be true even in cases where it might seem obvious that the feared event is objectively costly. For example, in hypochondriacal patients who are worried about dying, therapists may be tempted to focus exclusively on whether or not the patients are likely to die from the symptoms they are concerned about. Accepting that dying is a bad thing, the therapist may not be inclined to ask, 'What would be so bad about dying?' However, Wells and Hackmann[27] found that many hypochondriacal patients have distorted beliefs and images about death and the process of dying. For example, they think that when they die they will remain conscious and will continue to experience all the pain they had up to that point. Such people can benefit greatly from discussion of their beliefs about the cost of dying.

**Table 6.3.2.1.5** Useful questions for challenging anxiety-related thoughts

---

What is the evidence for this thought?

Is there any alternative way of looking at the situation?

Is there an alternative explanation?

How would someone else think about the situation?

Are you focusing on how you felt, rather than on what actually happened?

Are you setting yourself an unrealistic or unobtainable standard?

Are you forgetting relevant facts or overfocusing on irrelevant facts?

Are you thinking in all-or-nothing terms?

Are you overestimating how responsible you are for the way things work out?

What if the worst happens? What would be so bad about that? How could you cope?

How will things be x months/years afterwards?

Are you overestimating how likely the event is?

Are you underestimating what you can do to deal with the problem/situation?

---

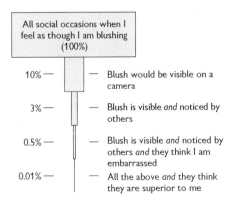

**Fig. 6.3.2.1.5** An inverted pyramid representing conditional probabilities between 'feeling hot' and 'others thinking they are superior to you' constructed for a patient who was afraid of blushing.

### (f) *In vivo* exposure to feared situations, activities, and sensations

Systematic exposure to feared and avoided situations has a long history in cognitive behaviour therapy and is one of the most effective ways of helping patients to discover that the things they are afraid of will not happen or are more manageable than they anticipate. Initially, exposure was often conducted in imagination but it is now known that *in vivo* exposure is a more effective way of dealing with situational fear.[3] During the 1970s and 1980s the dominant framework for exposure was habituation. It was assumed that repeated prolonged exposure was required to achieve fear reduction. More recent cognitive formulations have suggested that exposure is likely to be optimally effective when set-up in a way that maximizes the extent to which patients are able to disconfirm their fears, and considerable attention is now devoted to setting up exposure assignments in a way that will maximize cognitive change. Before entering a feared situation, patients are asked to specify what is the worst they think could happen, how likely they think it is, and what they would normally do to prevent the feared catastrophe (safety behaviours). They are then asked to enter the feared situation while dropping their safety behaviours and to observe carefully whether the feared outcome occurs. Afterwards, discussion focuses on whether the feared catastrophe occurred. If it did not, how does the patient explain its non-occurrence? Was it because the patient now thinks the feared outcome is unrealistic or does the patient think it was because of 'luck' or the continued use of safety behaviours? In the latter two instances, further exposure assignments with further encouragement to drop safety behaviours are required.

In addition to avoiding feared situations, anxiety disorder patients can also avoid feared sensations. Such avoidance is particularly prominent in panic disorder. For example, because of their fears about the meaning of increases in heart rate, dizziness, sweating, and other autonomic cues, panic disorder patients often avoid exercise. Increasing exercise can be an excellent way of helping them to challenge their negative beliefs, as can other ways of inducing bodily sensations such as ingesting caffeine, and hyperventilating. In each instance, the key point is to help patients discover that they can experience intense physical sensations without dying, losing control, or experiencing some other catastrophe.

Table 6.3.2.1.6 shows a record sheet that can be useful for planning and summarizing the results of exposure assignments, with illustrations from patients with social phobia and agoraphobia. Because of the intensity of patients' fears, and their tendency to attribute good outcomes to 'luck', it is often necessary to move up a hierarchy of feared situations and to consolidate successes by repetition.

In obsessive–compulsive disorder, the compulsive rituals act as safety behaviours and it is necessary to ensure that patients refrain from engaging in rituals (which are often also termed 'putting right' acts) during exposure assignments. This procedure is called 'exposure and response prevention'. For example, obsessional washers would be asked to 'contaminate' themselves by touching feared objects and then not put things right by washing. Similarly, obsessional checkers may be asked to expose themselves to activities that would normally provoke their checking (e.g. turning on the gas cooker) and then refrain from checking more than would be normal. In both instances, patients usually find that although exposure initially provokes considerable distress, the distress systematically declines during prolonged response prevention.[28]

Unlike most phobic fears, the fears of obsessive–compulsive disorder patients (e.g. developing a fatal disease from touching an object that is believed to be contaminated) often cannot be disconfirmed during a single or indeed multiple, exposure assignments. Discussing this issue, Salkovskis[11] has suggested that exposure and response prevention may work by providing patients with a different understanding of their problems. In particular, the decline

**Table 6.3.2.1.6** Record sheet for noting behavioural experiments

| | Situation | Prediction | Experiment | Outcome | What I learned |
|---|---|---|---|---|---|
| | | (What exactly did you think would happen? How would you know?) (Rate belief 0–100%) | (What did you do to test the prediction?) | (What actually happened? Was the prediction correct?) | (1) Balanced view (rate belief 0–100%)? (2) How likely is what you predicted to happen in future (Rate belief 0–100%) |
| Social phobic patient | Coffee break; sitting with other teachers; trying to join in the conversation | If I just say things as they come into my mind, they'll think I'm stupid (50%) | Say whatever comes into my mind *and* watch them like a hawk; don't focus on myself; this only gives me misleading information (such as images of myself as the 'village idiot'), and means I can't see them | I did it and I watched the others; one of them showed interest and we talked; she seemed to quite enjoy it | I am probably more acceptable than I think (70%) |
| Agoraphobic patient | Shopping in a supermarket | I will feel dizzy and have a panic attack (90%). Unless I grip the trolley tightly or sit down at that moment, I collapse (80%) | Go into the supermarket. When I start to feel dizzy, remind myself it is just anxiety, my heart rate is up and I can't faint. Then move away from the trolley and stand unsupported | I felt dizzy but didn't faint, even though I didn't sit down or hold on to the trolley | Feeling dizzy in anxiety attacks will not make me faint (60%) |

in distress during exposure and response prevention helps the patient to discover that they are suffering from a worry problem, rather than being in objective danger.

### (g) Imaginal exposure in post-traumatic stress disorder

Although imaginal exposure is rarely used in most anxiety disorders, it plays an important role in the treatment of post-traumatic stress disorder. It is known[29] that avoidance of thinking about the traumatic event is an important predictor of persistent post-traumatic stress disorder. In the light of this finding, clinicians have attempted to treat post-traumatic stress disorder by repeated, imaginal reliving of the traumatic event, and controlled trials[30] have shown that this technique is effective. At this stage it is not known why reliving works. One suggestion is that the intrusive symptoms of post-traumatic stress disorder are the result of a fragmented and disorganized memory for the trauma that is poorly integrated with other autobiographical information. Reliving might, therefore, facilitate the production of a more organized narrative account of the event that can be placed in the broader context of the individual's life.[13,31] Two types of imaginal reliving have been used in controlled trials: writing out details of the event and reliving the event in imagery. In either case, it seems important to focus not only on what happened, but also on patients' feelings and thoughts, both at the time and now, looking back at the event. Problematic idiosyncratic meanings that can be addressed with cognitive restructuring are often identified during reliving exercises.

### (h) Behavioural experiments

Behavioural experiments play a central role in the treatment of anxiety disorders. In a behavioural experiment, therapist and patient plan and implement a behavioural assignment that will provide a test of a key belief. The *in vivo* exposure assignments outlined above are examples of behavioural experiments. Several further examples are given to illustrate the technique.

Patients with post-traumatic stress disorder often think their intrusive recollections mean they are going mad or losing control in some way, and as a consequence, try to push the intrusions out of their mind. If this problem is identified during the first session of therapy, therapists often conduct an experiment to illustrate the undesired consequences of thought suppression. For example, the therapist might say to the patient, 'It doesn't matter what you think about in the next few minutes as long as you don't think about one particular thing. The thing is a fluorescent green rabbit eating my hair!' Most patients find they immediately get an image of the rabbit and have difficulty getting rid of it. Discussion then helps them to see that an increase in the frequency of target thoughts is a normal consequence of thought suppression. This result can then be used to set-up a homework assignment in which the patient is asked to collect data to test the idea that thought suppression may be enhancing intrusions. The experiment involves not trying to push the intrusions out of one's mind, but instead just letting them come and go, watching them as though they were a train passing through a station. Often patients report this simple experiment produces a marked decline in both the frequency of intrusions and the belief that they are a sign of impending insanity or loss of control.

Patients with social phobia often overestimate the significance of their anxiety symptoms for other people. A useful behavioural experiment to illustrate this point involves having either the patient or the therapist conduct a survey in which other people are asked for their views about the feared symptom. For example, in the case of fear of blushing, other people might be asked:

Why do you think people blush?
Do you notice other people blushing?
Do you remember it?
Do you think badly about people who blush?
If you do, what do you think about them?'

A further helpful experiment can involve intentionally displaying a feared symptom (e.g. handshaking or forgetting what one is talking about) and closely observing other people's responses. A particularly effective behaviour experiment for modifying social phobics distorted self-images involves the use of video feedback. Patients are asked to engage in a difficult social task while being videotaped. Afterwards they are asked to describe in detail how they think they appeared. They are then asked to view the video, watching themselves as though they are watching a stranger, ignoring memories of how they felt and simply focusing on how they would look to other people. In this way they often discover that they come across better than they would expect on the basis of their self-imagery. This experiment is often a powerful way of correcting distorted self-images.

Patients with panic disorder or hypochondriasis persistently think that normal bodily signs and/or symptoms are caused by a serious physical disorder. Numerous behavioural experiments can be used to demonstrate the correct, innocuous causes of their symptoms. For example, reading pairs of words which represent patient's illness interpretations (e.g. palpitations-dying, breathlessness-suffocate) has been shown to induce feared sensations.[5] Similarly, reproducing patients' fear-driven behaviours can produce the very symptoms the patients take as evidence for a serious physical illness. For example, patients who feel short of breath in a panic attack often respond by breathing quickly and deeply (hyperventilation), which paradoxically produces more breathlessness. Similarly, patients who are concerned about cancer may palpate body parts and then take the resulting soreness or discomfort as evidence of the presence of cancer.

### (i) Therapy notes

Over a series of sessions therapist and patient will generate a substantial number of arguments against the patient's fearful beliefs. In order to maximize the impact of this accumulation, patients are asked to keep a running record of evidence against their beliefs in a notebook that can easily be consulted at times of doubt. Table 6.3.2.1.7 shows an illustrative example from a panic disorder patient's notebook. At the start of therapy, the patient had been concerned that there was something seriously wrong with his heart.

### (j) Anger management

Although anxiety is the predominant problematic emotion in anxiety disorders, some patients also report significant problems with other emotions such as depression and anger. Techniques for dealing with depression can be found in Chapter 6.3.2.3. Some empirically validated techniques for dealing with anger are described here. Although presented in the context of anger accompanying anxiety disorders, these techniques are also relevant to anger in other disorders and to people without an Axis I disorder.

**Table 6.3.2.1.7** A panic disorder patient's notebook: evidence for the two alternative explanations for chest pains

| 'There is something seriously wrong with my heart' | 'My problem is my belief that there is something wrong with my heart' |
|---|---|
| 1 *I hear my heart thumping sometimes, even in my ear.* But because of my fears I focus on my body and that makes me notice it. When I notice it I get anxious and that makes it louder because my heart beats are bigger | 1 I think I am dying in a panic attack and that thought makes me anxious, producing many more sensations and setting up a vicious circle |
| 2 *I have chest and rib tightness throughout the day.* But cardiac patients don't. They get chest pain (often crushing and more localized) during heart attacks. It is muscle tension due to work stress. It is mild after a good night's sleep and easier at weekends. It is worst after a stressful day at work | 2 Distraction sometimes helps. That makes sense if the problem is my thoughts. It does not make sense if the problem is a heart attack. The same argument applies to leaving the situation. That would not stop a heart attack but it makes me feel more comfortable and undermines the negative thoughts |
| 3 *I occasionally get tingling in my fingertips.* But this is a common symptom of anxiety. Also deep breathing—which I do when I think there is something wrong—causes tingling | 3 I get symptoms most often at the end of the day, when I have come to expect them and have time to dwell on them |
|  | 4 I have proved to myself that there is nothing wrong with my heart with vigorous exercise. All that happens is that my heart beats faster and pumps harder, as it should do in order to supply my muscles with the energy they need |

Reproduced from Clark, D.M. Panic disorder: from theory to therapy. In Frontiers of cognitive therapy (ed. P.M. Salkovskis), pp. 318–44. Copyright 1996, Guilford Press. New York.

### (k) Cognitive content and other assessment issues

Anger is triggered when other people are seen to have broken one's personal rules about what is right and fair.[1] Angry individuals invariably think that they have been badly treated and ascribe their perceived ill treatment to intention or unacceptable neglect on the part of others. A key first step in assessment is to help patients become aware of their automatic thoughts during periods of anger. It is also helpful to keep a record of the situations and behaviours of other people that routinely trigger anger. Review of such triggers often reveals a particular theme and an implicit rule that the patient thinks other people should abide by. A detailed description of how the person behaves when angry and what effect the behaviour has on others is also essential.

### (l) Intervention

As patients' rules about the way that others should behave are often highly idiosyncratic, a useful tactic involves asking patients to consider whether the problem is assuming that others hold the same rule as them when they do not. This can help reduce the conviction that others' actions are actively malicious. Other useful questions include the following.

- Is there any other explanation for what happened?
- Did the other people know that their actions would harm me?
- Am I mind-reading?
- Am I over-applying the 'shoulds'?
- What are the advantages and disadvantages of responding with anger?
- Are there other ways I could behave which will be more likely to put things right/help me to get over it?

Although identifying and changing anger-related thoughts is a useful tactic, it is important to remember that anger is an action-orientated emotion. When angry, patients have a strong compulsion to hit out verbally or physically, and have great difficulty in thinking rationally. For patients with recurrent anger problems, it is often useful to teach them first to pause and relax or remove themselves from the anger-provoking situation before trying to challenge their thoughts and to delay taking action (such as writing angry letters to others) until they have calmed down and had time to consider the appropriateness/usefulness of the action. To enhance further the generalizability of thought-challenging work, it is often useful to summarize the answers to typical anger-related thoughts on a flash card that patients can carry around and consult whenever they become angry.

Anger can sometimes be the result of chronic under-assertiveness, with patients' fears preventing them from making their point of view known until they feel overwhelmed and irritated by the demands placed on them. In such cases, discussion of the fears that prevent earlier and more appropriate assertion and role-playing in which the patients try out and evaluate ways of communicating their views to others in a prompt and constructive fashion can be helpful.

## Indications and contraindications

Cognitive behaviour therapy is suitable for most patients with anxiety disorders and the low dropout rates reported in many controlled trials[4,32] suggest that it is well tolerated. In cases with additional severe comorbid problems (e.g. alcohol dependence, depression) it is sometimes necessary to bring these problems under control before starting cognitive behaviour therapy for anxiety. Concurrent use of prescription anxiolytic medication (benzodiazepines, tricyclics, selective serotonin reuptake inhibitors) is not a contraindication. At one time it was thought that anxiolytics may facilitate treatment by helping patients to confront their fears more quickly. However, there is little evidence that concurrent medication enhances initial response.[32] In addition, combining medication (alprazolam or imipramine) with cognitive behaviour therapy has been shown to produce poorer long-term outcome than cognitive behaviour therapy alone in panic disorder.[33] The latter result suggests that if a patient is not already taking anxiolytic medication, it is probably best to start treatment with cognitive behaviour therapy alone. Medication might then be added at a later stage, if response to cognitive behaviour therapy alone is poor.

## Efficacy

Controlled trials involving comparisons with other psychological interventions and waiting-list control groups indicate that cognitive behaviour therapy is an effective and specific treatment for panic disorder, social phobia, specific phobia, generalized anxiety disorder, hypochondriasis, obsessive–compulsive disorder, and post-traumatic stress disorder.[4,32] Results comparing immediate response to cognitive behaviour therapy alone and pharmacotherapy alone have been mixed, with superiority for cognitive behaviour therapy, equivalence for cognitive behaviour therapy, and superiority for pharmacotherapy all being reported. In contrast to the immediate response data, the follow-up analyses after medication discontinuation that are currently available favour cognitive behaviour therapy.[34] However, the database is modest and further research is required. For anger problems, controlled trials have shown that the cognitive behavioural procedures described here are effective.[35]

## Training and supervision

Most controlled trials have used therapists who have received specialized training in cognitive behaviour therapy and there is some evidence that deviation from therapy protocols and/or poor implementation is associated with less good outcome.[36] For these reasons, clinicians are likely to benefit from specialized training and supervision. Where local training institutes exist, it is wise to take advantage of their expertise. Even when no local institute is available, expert cognitive behaviour therapists from established centres often travel internationally to deliver workshops and supervision. Several professional organizations run regular training workshops and can be contacted through the Internet. The organizations include the British Association of Behavioural and Cognitive Psychotherapies (http://www.babcp.org.uk), the Association of Behaviour and Cognitive Therapies (www.abct.org), the International Association of Cognitive Psychotherapy (http://www.cognitivetherapyassociation.org), the American Psychological Association (http://www.apa.org), and the American Psychiatric Association (www.psych.org). A comprehensive list of the competencies required for the main cognitive behaviour therapies for anxiety disorders can be found at: http://www.ucl.ac.uk/clinical-health-psychology/CORE/CBT_Framework.htm

## Further information

A number of texts describe the theory and practice of cognitive behaviour therapy for specific anxiety disorders[37–39] and for anger problems[40] in considerable detail. Texts are frequently updated. Readers interested in the latest therapy guides are recommended to visit the following websites: www.oup.com, www.oup.com/us/ttw, www.guilford.com, www.wiley.com. Video illustrations of therapy sessions are also available for some anxiety disorders (see ABCT, American Psychological Association, and Guilford Press websites).

## References

1. Beck, A.T. (1976). *Cognitive therapy and the emotional disorders.* International Universities Press, New York.
2. Rachman, S. (1996). The evolution of cognitive behaviour therapy. In *Science and practice of cognitive behaviour therapy* (eds. D.M. Clark and C.G. Fairburn), pp. 3–26. Oxford University Press, Oxford.
3. Marks, I.M. (1975). Behavioural treatment of phobic and obsessive-compulsive disorders. In *Progress in behavior modification* (eds. M. Hersen, R.M. Fisher, and P.M. Miller), **1**, pp. 66–158. Academic Press, New York.
4. Clark, D.M. (2004). Developing new treatments: on the interplay between theories, experimental science and clinical innovation. *Behaviour Research and Therapy*, **42**, 1089.
5. Clark, D.M. (1996). Panic disorder: from theory to therapy. In *Frontiers of cognitive therapy* (ed. P.M. Salkovskis), pp. 318–44. Guilford, New York.
6. APA. (1994). *Diagnostic and statistical manual of mental disorders* (4th edn). American Psychiatric Association, Washington, D.C.
7. Beck, A.T., Emery, G., and Greenberg, R.L. (1985). *Anxiety disorders and phobias: a cognitive perspective.* Basic Books, New York.
8. Borkovec, T.D., Ray, W.J., and Stober, J.W. (1998). A cognitive phenomenon intimately linked to affective, physiological, and interpersonal behavioral processes. *Cognitive Therapy and Research*, **22**, 561–76.
9. Wells, A. (2000). *Emotional disorders and metacognition: innovative cognitive therapy.* Wiley, Chichester.
10. Rachman, S.J. and De Silva, P. (1978). Abnormal and normal obsessions. *Behaviour Research and Therapy*, **16**, 233–48.
11. Salkovskis, P.M. (1985). Obsessional–compulsive problems: a cognitive-behavioural analysis. *Behaviour Research and Therapy*, **23**, 571–83.
12. Kessler, R.C., Sonnega, A., Bromet, E., *et al.* (1995). Posttraumatic stress disorder in the National Comorbidity Survey. *Archives of General Psychiatry*, **52**, 1048–60.
13. Ehlers, A. and Clark, D.M. (2000). A cognitive model of posttraumatic stress disorder. *Behaviour Research and Therapy*, **38**, 319–45.
14. Brewin, C.R. and Holmes, E.A. (2003). Psychological theories of posttraumatic stress disorder. *Clinical Psychology Review*, **23**, 339–76.
15. Foa, E.B., Molnar, C., and Cashman, L. (1995). Change in rape narratives during exposure therapy for posttraumatic stress disorder. *Journal of Traumatic Stress*, **8**, 675–90.
16. Salkovskis, P.M. (1996). The cognitive approach to anxiety: threat beliefs, safety-seeking behaviour, and the special case of health anxiety and obsessions. In *Frontiers of cognitive therapy* (ed. P.M. Salkovskis), pp. 48–74. Guilford Press, New York.
17. Clark, D.M. and Wells, A. (1995). A cognitive model of social phobia. In *Social phobia: diagnosis, assessment and treatment* (eds. R. Heimberg, M. Liebowitz, D.A. Hope, and F.R. Schneier), pp. 69–93. Guilford Press, New York.
18. WHO. (1992). *International statistical classification of diseases and related health problems* (10th edn). WHO, Geneva
19. Veljaca, K.A. and Rapee, R.M. (1998). Detection of negative and positive audience behaviours by socially anxious subjects. *Behaviour Research and Therapy*, **36**, 311–21.
20. Hackmann, A., Surawy, C., and Clark, D.M. (1998). Seeing yourself through others' eyes: a study of spontaneously occurring images in social phobia. *Behavioural and Cognitive Psychotherapy*, **26**, 3–12.
21. Arntz, A., Rauner, M., and Van den Hout, M. (1995). If I feel anxious, there must be danger: ex-consequential reasoning in inferring danger in anxiety disorders. *Behaviour Research and Therapy*, **33**, 917–25.
22. Mansell, W. and Clark, D.M. (1999). How do I appear to others? Social anxiety and processing of the observable self. *Behaviour Research and Therapy*, **37**, 419–34.
23. Davey, G.C.L. and Matchett, G. (1994). Unconditioned stimulus rehearsal and the retention and enhancement of differential 'fear' conditioning: effects of trait and state anxiety. *Journal of Abnormal Psychology*, **103**, 708–18.
24. Beck, A.T. and Steer, R.A. (1993). *Beck anxiety inventory manual.* Psychological Corporation, San Antonio, TX.
25. Beck, A.T. and Steer, R.A. (1993). *Beck depression inventory.* The Psychological Corporation, San Antonio, TX.
26. Beunderman, R., Van Dis, H., Koster, R.W., *et al.* (1988). Differentiation in prodromal and acute symptoms of patients with cardiac and

non-cardiac chest pain. In *Advances in theory and practice in behaviour therapy* (eds. P.M.G. Emmelkamp, W.T.A.M. Everaerd, F. Kraaimaat, and M.J.M. van Son). Swets & Zeitlinger, Amsterdam.

27. Wells, A. and Hackmann, A. (1993). Imagery and core beliefs in health anxiety: content and origins. *Behavioural and Cognitive Psychotherapy*, **21**, 265–73.

28. Rachman, S.J., De Silva, P., and Roger, G. (1976). The spontaneous decay of compulsive urges. *Behaviour Research and Therapy*, **14**, 445–53.

29. Ehlers, A., Mayou, R.A., and Bryant, B. (1998). Psychological predictors of chronic posttraumatic stress disorder after motor vehicle accidents. *Journal of Abnormal Psychology*, **107**, 508–19.

30. NICE. (2005). *Post-traumatic stress disorder (PTSD): the management of PTSD in adults and children in primary and secondary care (Clinical Guideline 26)*. National Institute for Clinical Excellence, London, UK (www.nice.og).

31. Foa, E.B. and Riggs, D.S. (1993). Post-traumatic stress disorder in rape victims. In *Annual review of psychiatry* (eds. J.M. Oldham, M.B. Riba, and A. Tasman), pp. 273–303. American Psychiatric Association, Washington, DC.

32. Nathan, P.E. and Gorman, J.S. (eds.) (2002). *A guide to treatments that work*. Oxford University Press, New York.

33. Barlow, D.H., Gorman, J.M., Shear, M.K., *et al.* (2000). Cognitive-behavioral therapy, imipramine, or their combination for panic disorder. A randomized controlled trial. *Journal of the American Medical Association*, **283**, 2529–36.

34. Clark, D.M. and Wells, A. (1997). Cognitive therapy for anxiety disorders. In *Review of psychiatry* (eds. L.J. Dickstein, M.B. Riba, and J.M. Oldham), pp. 9–44. American Psychiatric Press, Washington, DC.

35. Del Vecchio, L. and O'Leary, K.D. (2004). Effectiveness of anger treatments for specific anger problems: a meta-analytic review. *Clinical Psychology Review*, **24**, 15–34.

36. Schulte, D., Kunzel, R., Pepping, G., *et al.* (1992). Tailor-made versus standardized therapy of phobic patients. *Advances in Behaviour Research and Therapy*, **14**, 67–92.

37. Hawton, K.E., Salkovskis, P.M., Kirk, J., *et al.* (1989). *Cognitive behaviour therapy for psychiatric problems*. Oxford University Press, Oxford.

38. Wells, A. (1997). *Cognitive therapy of anxiety disorders: a practice manual and conceptual guide*. Wiley, Chichester, UK.

39. Barlow, D.H. (ed.). (2007). *Clinical handbook of psychological disorders* (4th edn). Guilford Press, New York.

40. Howells, K. (1998). Cognitive behavioural interventions for anger, aggression and violence. In *Treating complex cases* (eds. N. Tarrier, A. Wells, and G. Haddock), pp. 295–318. Wiley, Chichester.

41. Spielberger, C.D., Gorsuch, R.L., and Lushene, R.E. (1970). *Manual for the state—Trait anxiety inventory*. Consulting Psychologists Press, Palo Alton, CA.

42. Clark, D.M., Salkovskis, P.M., Hackmann, A., *et al.* (1994). A comparison of cognitive therapy, applied relaxation and imipramine in the treatment of panic disorder. *British Journal of Psychiatry*, **164**, 759–69.

43. Marks, I. and Mathews, A.M. (1979). Brief standard self-rating for phobic patients. *Behaviour Research and Therapy*, **17**, 263–7.

44. Chambless, D.L., Caputo, G.C., Bright, P., *et al.* (1984). Assessment for fear of fear in agoraphobics: the Body Sensations Questionnaire and the Agoraphobia Cognitions Questionnaire. *Journal of Consulting and Clinical Psychology*, **52**, 1090–7.

45. Chambless, D.L., Caputo, G.C., Jasin, S.E., *et al.* (1985). The mobility inventory for agoraphobia. *Behaviour Research and Therapy*, **23**, 35–44.

46. Fresco, D.M., Coles, M.E., Heimberg, R.G., *et al.* (2001). The Liebowitz social anxiety scale: a comparison of the psychometric properties of self-report and clinical-administered formats. *Psychological Medicine*, **31**, 1025–35.

47. Mattick, R.P. and Clarke, J.C. (1998). Development and validation of measures of social phobia scrutiny fear and social interaction anxiety. *Behaviour Research and Therapy*, **36**, 455–70.

48. Turner, S.M., Beidel, D.C., Dancu, C.V., *et al.* (1989). An empirically derived inventory to measure social fears and anxiety: the social phobia and anxiety inventory. *Psychological Assessment*, **1**, 35–40.

49. Tallis, F., Davey, G.C.L., and Bond, A. (1994). The Worry Domains Questionnaire. In *Worrying: perspectives on theory, assessment and treatment* (eds. G. Davey and F. Tallis). Wiley, Chichester.

50. Molina, S. and Borkovec, T.D. (1994). The Penn State Worry questionnaire: psychometric properties and associated characteristics. In *Worrying: perspectives on theory, assessment and treatment* (eds. G. Davey and F. Tallis). Wiley, Chichester.

51. Wells, A. and Davies, M. (1994). The Thought Control Questionnaire: a measure of individual differences in the control of unwanted thoughts. *Behaviour Research and Therapy*, **32**, 871–8.

52. Salkovskis, P.M., Wroe, A.L., Gledhill, A., *et al.* (1999). Responsibility attitudes and interpretations are characteristic of obsessive compulsive disorder. *Behaviour Research and Therapy*, **38**, 347–72.

53. Van Oppen, P., Hoekstra, R.J., and Emmelkamp, P.M.G. (1995). The structure of obsessive-compulsive symptoms. *Behaviour Research and Therapy*, **33**, 15–23.

54. Goodman, W.K., Price, L.H., Rasmussen, S.A., *et al.* (1989). The Yale-Brown Obsessive-Compulsive Scale (YBOCS) Part 1: development, use and reliability. *Archives of General Psychiatry*, **46**, 1006–11.

55. Foa, E., Riggs, D.S., Dancu, C.V., *et al.* (1993). Reliability and validity of a brief instrument for assessing post-traumatic stress disorder. *Journal of Traumatic Stress*, **6**, 459–73.

56. Foa, E., Ehlers, A., Clark, D.M., *et al.* (1999). The post-traumatic cognitions inventory (PTCI): development and validation. *Psychological Assessment*, **11**, 303–14.

57. Horowitz, M.J., Wilner, N., and Alvarez, W. (1979). The Impact of Event Scale: a measure of subjective stress. *Psychosomatic Medicine*, **41**, 209–18.

58. Mechanic, M.B. and Resick, P.A. (1993). The personal beliefs and reactions scale: assessing rape-related cognitive schemata. *Paper presented at the 9th annual meeting of the International Society for Traumatic Stress Studies*, San Antonio, TX.

59. Clark, D.M., Ehlers, A., Hackmann, A., *et al.* (2006). Cognitive therapy and exposure plus applied relaxation in social phobia: a randomised controlled trial. *Journal of Consulting and Clinical Psychology*, **74**, 568–78.

## 6.3.2.2 **Cognitive behaviour therapy for eating disorders**

Zafra Cooper, Rebecca Murphy, and Christopher G. Fairburn

### Introduction

The eating disorders provide one of the strongest indications for cognitive behaviour therapy. This bold claim arises from the demonstrated effectiveness of cognitive behaviour therapy in the treatment of bulimia nervosa and the widespread acceptance that cognitive behaviour therapy is the treatment of choice.[1] Cognitive behaviour therapy is also widely used to treat anorexia nervosa although this application has not been adequately evaluated. Recently its use has been extended to 'eating disorder not otherwise specified' (eating disorder NOS),[2] a diagnosis that applies to over 50 per cent of cases,[3] and emerging evidence suggests that it is just as effective with these cases as it is with cases of bulimia nervosa.

In this chapter the cognitive behavioural approach to the understanding and treatment of eating disorders will be described. The data on the efficacy and effectiveness of the treatment are considered in the chapters on anorexia nervosa and bulimia nervosa (see Chapters 4.10.1 and 4.10.2 respectively), as is their general management.

## The cognitive behavioural account of the maintenance of eating disorders

Although both the DSM and ICD schemes for classifying eating disorders encourage the view that anorexia nervosa and bulimia nervosa are distinct clinical states, consideration of their clinical features and course over time does not support this.[4] Patients with anorexia nervosa, bulimia nervosa, and eating disorder NOS have many features in common, most of which are not seen in other psychiatric disorders, and studies of their course indicate that most patients migrate between these diagnoses over time. This temporal movement, together with the fact that the disorders share the same distinctive psychopathology, has led to the suggestion that common 'transdiagnostic' mechanisms are involved in the persistence of eating disorder psychopathology.[5]

Anorexia nervosa, bulimia nervosa, and most cases of eating disorder NOS are united by a distinctive core psychopathology: patients over-evaluate the importance of their shape and weight and their ability to control them. According to the cognitive behavioural view it is this dysfunctional scheme of self-evaluation that is of central importance in maintaining these disorders. Whereas most people evaluate themselves on the basis of their perceived performance in a variety of domains of life, people with eating disorders judge themselves primarily in terms of their shape and weight and their ability to control them. Most of their other clinical features can be understood as stemming directly from this 'core psychopathology', including the extreme weight-control behaviour (i.e. the dieting, self-induced vomiting, laxative misuse, and over-exercising), the various forms of body checking and avoidance, and the preoccupation with thoughts about eating, shape, and weight. Fig. 6.3.2.2.1 provides a 'transdiagnostic' representation (or 'formulation') of the main processes involved in the maintenance of eating disorders.

The only feature that is not obviously a direct expression of the core psychopathology is binge eating, present in all cases of bulimia nervosa, many cases of eating disorder NOS and some cases of anorexia nervosa. The cognitive behavioural theory proposes that binge eating is largely a product of attempts to adhere to multiple extreme, and highly specific, dietary rules. These patients' tendency to react in a negative and extreme fashion to the (almost inevitable) breaking of these rules results in even minor dietary slips being interpreted as evidence of poor self-control. Patients respond to this perceived lack of self-control by temporarily abandoning their efforts to restrict their eating. This produces a highly distinctive pattern of eating in which attempts to restrict eating are repeatedly interrupted by episodes of binge eating. The binge eating maintains the core psychopathology by intensifying patients' concerns about their ability to control their eating, shape, and weight. It also encourages further dietary restraint, thereby increasing the risk of further binge eating.

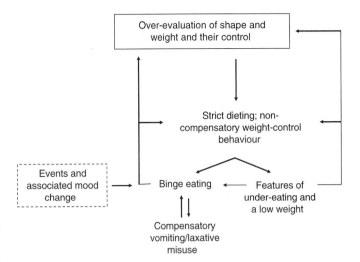

**Fig. 6.3.2.2.1** The transdiagnostic 'template' formulation of the maintenance of eating disorders. (Reproduced from Fairburn, C.G., *Cognitive behavior therapy and eating disorders*, Copyright 2008, Guilford Press, NY).

Three further processes also maintain binge eating. First, difficulties in the patient's life and associated mood changes increase the likelihood that they will break their dietary rules. Second, binge eating temporarily ameliorates such mood states and distracts patients from thinking about their difficulties. Third, if the binge eating is followed by compensatory vomiting or laxative misuse, it is also maintained because patients' mistaken belief in the effectiveness of such 'purging' undermines a major deterrent to their binge eating. They do not realize that purging has little effect on energy absorption.[6]

Patients with anorexia nervosa share the distinctive core psychopathology of those with bulimia nervosa and eating disorder NOS. The major difference between patients with anorexia nervosa and those with other eating disorders lies in the fact that in anorexia nervosa under-eating predominates and therefore patients become extremely underweight. This has certain physiological and psychological consequences (see Chapter 4.10.1) that contribute to the persistence of the eating disorder.[7] For example, delayed gastric emptying results in a sense of fullness even after eating modest amounts of food and secondary social withdrawal magnifies patients' isolation from the influence of others.

The composite 'transdiagnostic' formulation shown in Fig. 6.3.2.2.1 represents the core processes that maintain any eating disorder. The specific maintaining processes operating in any patient depend upon the nature of the eating disorder psychopathology present. In some cases only certain of the processes are active (for example, in most cases of binge-eating disorder), but in others (for example, cases of the binge eating/purging subtype of anorexia nervosa) most are operating. The formulation highlights the maintaining processes that need to be addressed in treatment, thereby allowing the clinician to design a bespoke treatment to fit the individual patient's psychopathology.

### Evidence for the cognitive behavioural account

There is a sizeable body of research that supports the cognitive view of the maintenance of eating disorders.[8] This includes descriptive and experimental studies of the clinical characteristics of these patients and the research on dietary restraint and 'counter-regulation' (a possible analogue for binge eating).[9] There is also strong indirect support from a large body of research indicating that cognitive behaviour therapy based on this model has a major and lasting impact on bulimia nervosa (see Chapter 4.10.2) and emerging evidence that this is also true of eating disorder NOS. Further support comes from the finding that 'dismantling' the cognitive behavioural treatment for bulimia nervosa by removing those procedures designed to produce cognitive change attenuates its effects and results in patients being markedly prone to relapse.[10] Direct support comes from studies that have shown that dietary restraint appears to mediate this treatment's effect on binge eating[11] and that continuing over-evaluation of weight and shape in those who have recovered in behavioural terms is predictive of subsequent relapse.[12,13]

## Transdiagnostic cognitive behavioural treatment of eating disorders

There follows a brief description of cognitive behaviour therapy for eating disorders. Full details are provided elsewhere.[14] The treatment is outpatient-based and, as applied in research settings, involves 20 individual treatment sessions over 20 weeks for the 80 per cent or more of patients who are not significantly underweight (body mass index over 17.5). The remaining patients with a body mass index of 17.5 or below receive 40 sessions over 40 weeks. The indications for the treatment are the presence of an eating disorder of clinical severity. It is not appropriate for those whose psychiatric state, general physical health, or degree of weight loss is such that they cannot safely be treated on an outpatient basis.

The treatment has four stages.

### (a) Stage one

The aims of the first stage are as follows: to educate patients about treatment and the disorder; to engage the patient in treatment and change, and to introduce and establish a pattern of regular eating and weekly weighing. This stage comprises approximately eight sessions which are held twice weekly over 4 weeks.

#### (i) Jointly creating the formulation

This is usually done in the first treatment session. The therapist draws out the relevant sections of Fig. 6.3.2.2.1 incorporating the patient's own experiences and terms. This helps patients to realize both that their behaviour is comprehensible and that it is maintained by a variety of self-perpetuating mechanisms which are open to change. The formulation provides a guide to what needs to be targeted in treatment if patients are to achieve a full and lasting recovery.

#### (ii) Establishing real-time self-monitoring

This is the ongoing 'in-the-moment' recording of eating and other relevant behaviour, thoughts, feelings, and events (see Chapter 4.10.2 for an example monitoring record). Self-monitoring is initiated in the first session and continues throughout treatment. It serves two purposes: it assists in the identification of the patient's problems and progress and, more importantly, it facilitates change by helping patients address problems as they occur.

#### (iii) Establishing 'weekly weighing'

The patient and therapist check the patient's weight once a week and plot it on an individualized weight graph. Patients are strongly encouraged not to weigh themselves at other times. Weekly in-session weighing has several purposes: first, it provides patients with accurate data about their weight at a time when their eating habits are changing; second, it provides an opportunity for the therapist to help patients interpret the numbers on the scale, which otherwise they are prone to misinterpret and, third, it addresses the important maintaining processes of excessive body weight checking or its avoidance.

#### (iv) Providing education

From the second session onwards, an important element of treatment is education about weight and eating since many patients have misconceptions that maintain their eating disorder. The following topics need to be covered:

◆ Body weight and its regulation: the body mass index and its interpretation; natural weight fluctuations; and the effects of treatment on weight.

◆ Physical complications of binge eating, self-induced vomiting, the misuse of laxatives and diuretics, and the effect of the eating disorder on hunger and fullness.

◆ Ineffectiveness of vomiting, laxatives, and diuretics as a means of weight control.

◆ Adverse effects of dieting: the types of dieting that promote binge eating; dietary rules versus dietary guidelines.

To provide reliable information on these topics, patients are asked to read relevant sections from one of the authoritative books on eating disorders[6,15,16] and their reading is discussed in subsequent treatment sessions.

#### (v) Establishing 'regular eating'

The establishment of a pattern of regular eating is fundamental to successful treatment whatever the form of the eating disorder. It addresses an important type of dieting ('delayed eating'); it displaces episodes of binge eating and, for underweight patients, it introduces regular meals and snacks that can be subsequently increased in size. Early in treatment (usually by the third session) patients are asked to eat three planned meals each day, plus two (or if underweight three) planned snacks and they are asked not to eat between them. Patients may choose what they eat at these times with the only conditions being that the meals and snacks are not followed by any compensatory behaviour and that there should rarely be more than a 4-hour interval between these occasions of eating. The new eating pattern should take precedence over other activities but should not be so inflexible as to preclude the possibility of adjusting timings to suit the patients' commitments each day.

Patients should be helped to adhere to their regular eating plan and to resist eating between the planned meals and snacks. Two rather different strategies may be used to achieve this: the first involves helping patients to identify activities that are incompatible with eating or make it less likely, and the second is to help patients to recognize that the urge to eat is a temporary phenomenon. Through using these strategies patients learn to distance themselves from the urge to eat which they find gradually fades with time.

#### (vi) Involving significant others

The treatment is primarily an individual treatment for adults and hence it does not actively involve others. Despite this, it is our practice to see 'significant others' with the patient if this is likely to facilitate treatment and the patient is willing for this to happen. There are two specific indications for involving others: if others could help the patient in making changes or if others are making it difficult for the patient to change by, for example, commenting adversely on eating or appearance.

### (b) Stage two

Stage two is a transitional stage which generally comprises two appointments, a week apart. Whilst continuing with the procedures introduced in stage one the therapist and patient conduct a joint review of progress to date, identify problems still to be addressed, revise the formulation if necessary, and design stage three.

### (c) Stage three

The aim of this stage is to address the key mechanisms that are maintaining the patient's eating disorder. The order in which these mechanisms are addressed depends upon their relative importance in maintaining the particular patient's psychopathology. There are generally 8-weekly appointments.

#### (i) Addressing the over-evaluation of shape and weight

The first step involves explaining the concept of self-evaluation and helping patients identify the life domains which contribute to their judgement of themselves. The relative importance of these domains can be visually represented on a pie chart, which for most patients is dominated by a large slice representing shape and weight and controlling eating.

The patient and therapist then identify the problems inherent in this scheme for self-evaluation. Briefly there are three related problems: first, the over-evaluation of shape and weight tends to marginalize other domains and thus self-evaluation is overly dependent on performance in one area of life; second, the area of controlling shape and weight is one in which success is elusive, thus undermining self-esteem; and third, the over-evaluation leads to behaviour which is unhelpful and which itself maintains the disorder.

The final step in educating about self-evaluation involves identifying its three main expressions which occur to varying degrees in different patients. These are body checking, body avoidance, and feeling fat. The therapist explains how these behaviours and experiences serve to maintain and magnify the patient's concerns about shape and weight and it is agreed therefore that they need to be addressed in treatment.

#### (ii) Addressing body checking and avoidance

Patients are often not aware that they are engaging in body checking and that it is maintaining their body dissatisfaction. The first step in addressing body checking involves obtaining a detailed account of the behaviour by asking patients to record it. An example monitoring record is shown in Fig. 6.3.2.2.2. Patients are then helped to realize that body checking is not a helpful way of assessing their

Day ......Friday............    Date ......6th Sept ............

| Time | Food and drink consumed | Place | * | V/L | Checking (what done, time taken) | Place | Context and comments |
|------|------|------|------|------|------|------|------|
| 7.45 | 1 piece of toast with butter and | Kitchen | | | | | Not hungry but know I should have breakfast |
| 8.15 | marmite. 1 cup of tea | | | | Looking at stomach and thighs in bedroom mirror while getting dressed (2 mins) | Bedroom | Depressing. Can't see any muscles – only fat. |
| 10.30 | 1 apple & diet coke | Office | | | Scrutinisng stomach in mirror standing sideways (1 min) | Office toilet | Ok |
| 11.15 | | | * | | | | How can it be so fat?? Have hardly eaten anything today! |
| 12.30 | Cheese and tomato sandwich & banana and kit kat | Canteen | | | Feeling and pinching stomach while sitting at desk (10mins) | Office | Chocolate was too much. Feel too full. myself sick. |
| 1.30 | | | | | | | Fat disgusting flesh. Feel massive. |
| 3.10 | Cup of coffee and 1 yoghurt | Office | | | Assessing shape of woman on street (10secs) | Office – through window | Had planned to have other 1/2 of chocolate bar. Can't do it, am already too fat! |
| 3.30 | Water | | | | | | Feel unhappy. Wish I was as thin as her. Can't accurately compare myself to others – never really sure what my shape is. Frustrating. |
| 6.45 | Salad with tuna 1 glass of red wine | Living room | | | Looking at reflection in window while doing dishes (5mins) | Kitchen | Still want more food but won't let myself since might lose control. |
| 7.30 | | | | | | Bathroom | |
| 8.10 | | | * | V | Touching and pinching stomach and thighs while having a bath (15mins) | | I'm so huge! Wish I was tall and elegant. How depressing. |
| 9.30 | 1 kit kat and half a crunchie 1 glass of red wine | Living room | | | | | Feel disgusted. Am I ever going to get rid of this fat? |
| | | | | | | | Feel fat! Too much chocolate today. Have to get rid of the food. Go to bed to stop thinking about it. |

**Fig. 6.3.2.2.2** An adapted monitoring record illustrating body checking.

shape or weight as it provides unreliable and biased information. Certain forms of body checking are best stopped altogether. In the case of more normative checking such as mirror use, education should stress that, as with other forms of body checking, what one finds depends to an important extent upon how one looks (e.g. scrutiny of perceived flaws tends to magnify them). For patients who avoid seeing their bodies, the therapist needs to explain that this too maintains dissatisfaction. Patients need to be encouraged to get used to the sight and feel of their body. Participation in activities that involve a degree of body exposure can be helpful, for example, swimming.

### (iii) Addressing 'feeling fat'

'Feeling fat' is an experience reported by many women but the intensity and frequency of this feeling appears to be far greater among people with eating disorders. Feeling fat is a target for treatment since it tends to be equated with being fat (irrespective of actual shape and weight) and hence maintains body dissatisfaction. Although this topic has received little research attention, clinical observation suggests that in many patients feeling fat is a result of mislabelling certain emotions and bodily experiences. It may be addressed by helping patients appreciate that feeling fat tends to be triggered by the occurrence of certain negative mood states (e.g. feeling bored or depressed) or by physical sensations that heighten body awareness (e.g. feeling full, bloated, or sweaty). Patients can then be encouraged to question the feeling when it occurs and correctly label and address the underlying triggering state using a problem-solving approach.

### (iv) Developing marginalized domains for self-evaluation

Tackling the expressions of the over-evaluation of shape and weight will gradually reduce it. At the same time, it is also important to encourage the patient to increase the number and significance of other domains for self-evaluation. Although this is an indirect means of diminishing the over-evaluation of shape and weight, it is nevertheless a powerful one.

### (v) Exploring the origins of the over-evaluation

Towards the end of stage three it is often helpful to explore the origins of the patient's sensitivity to shape, weight, and eating. An historical review can help to make sense of how the problem developed and evolved, highlight how it might have served a useful function in its early stages and help patients distance themselves from the past. If a specific event appears to have played a critical role in the development of the eating problem, the patient should be helped to reappraise this from the vantage point of the present.

### (vi) Addressing dietary restraint

A major goal of treatment is to reduce, if not eliminate altogether, strict dieting. This dieting has two aspects: an attempt to limit eating termed 'dietary restraint' and actual under-eating in physiological terms termed 'dietary restriction'. 'Regular eating' will already have addressed one form of dietary restraint (delayed eating). Patients need to recognize that their multiple extreme and rigid dietary rules lead to preoccupation with food and eating, encourage binge eating and impose practical and social restrictions. It should therefore be agreed that dietary restraint needs to be addressed. To do this, the patient's various dietary rules should be identified together with the beliefs which underlie them. The patient should be helped to break the rules in order to test the beliefs in question and to learn that the feared consequences that maintain the dietary rule (typically sudden weight gain or binge eating) are not an inevitable result of breaking it. With patients who binge eat it is important to pay particular attention to food avoidance and to help them systematically reintroduce such foods into their diet.

### (vii) Addressing event-triggered changes in eating

Among patients with eating disorders, eating habits may change in response to outside events. The change may involve eating less, stop eating altogether, overeating or binge eating. If these changes persist into stage three, they should be addressed by helping patients to tackle the triggering events using a problem-solving approach and by helping patients to accept the occurrence of intense-mood states and identify ways (that are not harmful) of modulating their moods.

### (d) Stage four

The aims in stage four are to ensure that the changes made in treatment are maintained over the following months and that the risk of relapse is minimized in the long term. There are three appointments, each 2 weeks apart. During this stage, as part of their preparation for the future, patients discontinue self-monitoring and transfer from in-session weighing to weighing themselves at home.

To maximize the chances that progress is maintained the therapist and patient jointly devise a specific plan for the patient to follow over the following few months until a post-treatment review appointment. Typically this includes further work on body checking, food avoidance, and perhaps further practice at problem-solving. In addition, the therapist encourages patients to continue their efforts to develop new interests and activities.

There are two elements to 'relapse prevention'. First, patients must have realistic expectations regarding the future. A common problem is that many hope never to experience any eating difficulties again. It needs to be explained that this makes them vulnerable to relapse since it encourages a negative reaction to even minor setbacks. Patients should be told to expect lapses with the eating problem continuing to be their Achilles' heel. The goal is for patients to identify setbacks as early as possible, view them as a 'lapse' rather than a 'relapse', and use a well-developed plan to deal with them. Thus, the second element of relapse prevention is the construction of such a plan. The therapist and patient should review the components of treatment with the aim of identifying the principles and procedures that were most relevant and helpful and devise a plan for the future incorporating this information.

## Underweight patients

When treating patients who are underweight (most are cases of anorexia nervosa but some are cases of eating disorder NOS) three main modifications to the treatment are required: the motivation of these patients needs to be enhanced, their state of starvation needs to be corrected, and significant others are more likely to be involved. As a result treatment needs to be considerably longer.

### (a) Enhancing motivation to change

The poor motivation of these patients needs to be addressed from the outset of treatment. There are various ways of enhancing motivation[17] including focusing on establishing a sound therapeutic relationship, ensuring that the patient feels understood, making it clear that one is working on behalf of the patient and not their relatives or concerned others, accepting the patient's beliefs and values as genuine and comprehensible, and adopting an experimental approach in which the therapist and patient together explore the advantages and disadvantages of making changes. This includes educating the patient about the physiological and psychological effects of starvation; for example, impaired concentration, preoccupation with food and eating, sleep disturbance, sensitivity to cold, ritualistic eating, social withdrawal, and enhanced fullness secondary to delayed gastric emptying.[7] It is best to focus particularly on those features that the patient views as a problem and explain how they tend to perpetuate the eating disorder. In addition, an exploration of the broader impact of the eating problem on the patient's life is important. When exploring the advantages and disadvantages of change, it is important to draw a distinction between the short-term and long-term consequences of change since patients tend to focus on the immediate present rather than the future.

### (b) Restoring a healthy weight

Unless the weight loss is rapid or extreme, or the patient's health is endangered by physical complications, weight restoration can usually be accomplished on an outpatient basis. Before focusing on weight gain, however, it is best to devote several sessions to establishing a collaborative working relationship and to developing a joint formulation and treatment plan. Thereafter, weight gain and the subsequent maintenance of a healthy weight must be an integral part of treatment. A target weight range should be identified in excess of a body mass index of 19.0.

The weight gain should be gradual and steady (at an average rate of about 0.5 kg/week). This requires an energy surplus to be established. This can be achieved by providing patients with energy-rich drinks to supplement their food intake (which should be increased such that it is sufficient to maintain their current weight). The energy-rich drinks may be viewed as weight restorative 'medicine' designed to produce the energy surplus. The drinks should be phased out once the target weight range has been reached. Whilst regaining weight patients should be helped to address their shape and weight concerns and dieting in much the same way as described above. Once a satisfactory weight has been reached patients need time to learn how to maintain their weight in a normal manner.

### (c) Involving the significant others

Weight regain is a protracted process that takes considerable time and effort on the part of the patient. If the patient lives with others it can be helpful to involve them if doing so is consistent with the nature of their relationship. Significant others can help the patient choose what to eat and provide guidance concerning portion sizes. This is likely to be especially important with younger patients (many underweight patients are adolescents) who are still living at home with their parents.

## Acknowledgements

We are grateful to the Wellcome Trust for its support. CGF holds a Principal Research Fellowship (046386). ZC and RM are supported by a programme grant (046386).

## Further information

Fairburn, C.G. (2008). *Cognitive behavior therapy and eating disorders.* Guilford Press, New York.
*The International Journal of Eating Disorders.*

## References

1. National Institute for Clinical Excellence. (2004). *Eating disorders—core interventions in the treatment and management of anorexia nervosa, bulimia nervosa and related eating disorders.* NICE Clinical Guideline No. 9. NICE, London. www.nice.org.uk

2. American Psychiatric Association. (1994). *Diagnostic and statistical manual of mental disorders.* American Psychiatric Association, Washington, DC.

3. Fairburn, C.G. and Bohn, K. (2005). Eating disorder NOS (EDNOS): an example of the troublesome 'not otherwise specified' (NOS) category in DSM-IV. *Behaviour Research and Therapy,* **43,** 691–701.

4. Fairburn, C.G. and Harrison, P.J. (2003). Eating disorders. *Lancet,* **361,** 407–16.

5. Fairburn, C.G., Cooper, Z., and Shafran, R. (2003). Cognitive behaviour therapy for eating disorders: a 'transdiagnostic' theory and treatment. *Behaviour Research and Therapy,* **41,** 509–28.

6. Fairburn, C.G. (1995). *Overcoming binge eating,* pp. 48–54. Guilford Press, New York.

7. Garner, D.M. (1997). Psychoeducational principles in treatment. In *Handbook of treatment for eating disorders* (eds. D.M. Garner and P.E. Garfinkel), pp. 145–77. Guilford Press, New York.

8. Vitousek, K.M. (1996). The current status of cognitive–behavioral models of anorexia nervosa and bulimia nervosa. In *Frontiers of cognitive therapy* (ed. P. Salkovskis), pp. 383–418. Guilford Press, New York.

9. Polivy, J. and Herman, C.P. (1993). Etiology of binge eating: psychological mechanisms. In *Binge eating: nature, assessment and treatment* (eds. C.G. Fairburn and G.T. Wilson), pp. 173–205. Guilford Press, New York.

10. Fairburn, C.G., Jones, R., Peveler, R.C., *et al.* (1993). Psychotherapy and bulimia nervosa: the longer–term effects of interpersonal psychotherapy, behaviour therapy and cognitive behaviour therapy. *Archives of General Psychiatry,* **50,** 419–28.

11. Wilson, G.T., Fairburn, C.G., Agras, W.S., *et al.* (2002). Cognitive-behavioral therapy for bulimia nervosa: time course and mechanisms of change. *Journal of Consulting and Clinical Psychology,* **70,** 267–74.

12. Fairburn, C.G., Peveler, R.C., Jones, R., *et al.* (1993). Predictors of 12–month outcome in bulimia nervosa and the influence of attitudes to shape and weight. *Journal of Consulting and Clinical Psychology,* **61,** 696–8.

13. Fairburn, C.G., Stice, E., Cooper, Z., *et al.* (2003). Understanding persistence in bulimia nervosa: a 5-year naturalistic study. *Journal of Consulting and Clinical Psychology,* **71,** 103–9.

14. Fairburn, C.G. (2008). *Cognitive behavior therapy and eating disorders.* Guilford Press, New York.

15. Cooper, P.J. (1995). *Bulimia nervosa and binge eating: a guide to recovery.* Robinson, London.

16. Schmidt, U. and Treasure, J. (1993). *Getting better bit(e) by bit(e).* Erlbaum, Hove.

17. Vitousek, K., Watson, S., and Wilson, G.T. (1998). Enhancing motivation for change in treatment–resistant eating disorders. *Clinical Psychology Review,* **18,** 391–420.

## 6.3.2.3 **Cognitive behaviour therapy for depressive disorders**

Melanie J. V. Fennell

## Introduction

This chapter describes A.T. Beck's cognitive behaviour therapy (CBT) for depression.[1] Beck's is probably the most fully developed, comprehensively evaluated, and widely disseminated cognitive behavioural approach to depression. Additionally, CBT is an effective treatment for a range of acute psychiatric disorders, shows promise for severe mental illness and personality disorder, and is thus helpful not only with primary depression, but also with a range of comorbid conditions.

### Central characteristics of CBT

The general principles and nature of CBT are described elsewhere. Two specific points relate to depression:

#### (a) Demands of CBT

Given the nature of depression, CBT challenges both therapist and patient. It requires **active engagement** (e.g. willingness to carry out self-help assignments), yet depressed patients often lack motivation and energy. It is based on a **friendly collaboration**, yet depressed people often find it hard to talk and clinicians may find their negativity aversive. It is an **educational approach**, using written materials and record sheets, yet depressed patients often have concentration and memory difficulties. Its stance is **optimistic**, yet depressed patients are often afraid (or convinced) that change is impossible. Therapists should be alert to these difficulties, understand them as aspects of depression rather than blaming the patient ('She must want to be depressed') or themselves ('I'm no good at this'), and maintain a persistent, problem-solving stance.

#### (b) Advantages of CBT

Nonetheless, CBT has real advantages for depressed patients. Its **structure** discourages rumination, and helps patients to focus systematically on their difficulties. Its emphasis on a warm **therapeutic relationship** encourages empathy, while its **goal orientation** implies that change *is* possible. The **coherent model** of human functioning, on which it is based, allows it to address many issues, including depression itself, comorbid conditions, problems in living, long-standing difficulties (such as low self-esteem), patients' responses to therapy and therapist, and therapists' responses to patients. Its **emphasis on collaboration and on transfer of knowledge and skill** empowers patients to become their own therapists and to take control of their lives.

## Background

Beck's interest in the role of cognition grew out of his practice as a psychoanalytical therapist. Dissatisfied with analytical understandings of depression, he became curious about the role of the negative thinking he observed in depressed patients.[2–4] Beck's clinical observation and research consistently showed the thinking of depressed people to be dominated by self-derogation, negative expectations, overwhelming problems and responsibilities, deprivation and loss, and escapist and suicidal wishes, themes fuelled by systematic biases in information processing. He suggested that patients could recover from depression by learning to re-evaluate everyday cognitions, and to understand the long-standing idiosyncratic schemas under lying them.

This early scientist–practitioner stance has remained central CBT, stimulating an integrated flow of experimental investigation, practice development, and research into treatment efficacy, which has continued to the present day. The first successful outcome trial of CBT for depression appeared in 1977.[5] A detailed treatment manual emerged shortly afterwards.[1] Thirty years of randomized controlled trials now support the treatment's effectiveness.[6] Like other short-term focused psychological treatments, it has consistently proved as effective as antidepressant medication post-treatment. It reduces the likelihood of relapse by about 50 per cent, and this effect endures,[7] and can be enhanced by booster sessions in the months following treatment.[8] Thus CBT emerges as surprisingly cost-effective.[9] With adequate training and supervision equivalent results can be achieved even with severe depression and high comorbidity.[10,11]

## Technique

### Cognitive case conceptualization

#### (a) Enduring cognitive vulnerability to depression

The **cognitive model of depression** proposes that enduring cognitive structures and processes shape how everyday experience is interpreted, and are in turn reinforced by these interpretations. This model (Fig. 6.3.2.3.1) forms the basis for an **individualized conceptualization**, developed and shared with the patient, which informs and guides therapy. It suggests that **experience** (loss, events with lasting implications for self-worth)[12,13] leads people to reach **fundamental conclusions** about themselves, others, and the world ('basic' or 'core' beliefs, or schemas). They devise **guidelines for living** ('conditional assumptions'), which allow them to operate in the world, assuming the truth of those conclusions. Using schemas and rules to organize experience and guide behaviour is a normal part of human functioning. However, where schemas are globally negative (e.g. 'I am inferior') and assumptions extreme and resistant to change (e.g. stringent perfectionism), they become counterproductive. Evidence for **cognitive vulnerability** to depression prior to first onset is now emerging,[14] as is evidence that recurrent episodes leave an tendency to re-experience depressogenic processing patterns in the presence of mild, normal depressed mood ('cognitive reactivity').[15,16]

#### (i) *Relationship between thinking and other aspects of depression*

Dysfunctional beliefs and assumptions are **activated by events** that match the person's particular sensitivities. So a person with negative beliefs about the self whose psychological well-being depends on love and approval might become depressed after experiencing rejection. Activation of the system results in an upsurge of '**negative automatic thoughts**'—'negative' in that they are associated with painful emotions, and 'automatic' in that they pop into the person's mind rather than being a product of reasoned reflection. Such thoughts reflect **processing biases** such as overgeneralization. Depression is characterized by biased negative thoughts about the self (e.g. 'I'm useless'), the world (e.g. 'My situation is intolerable'), and the future (e.g. 'Nothing will ever change'). The latter (hopelessness) is central to suicidality.

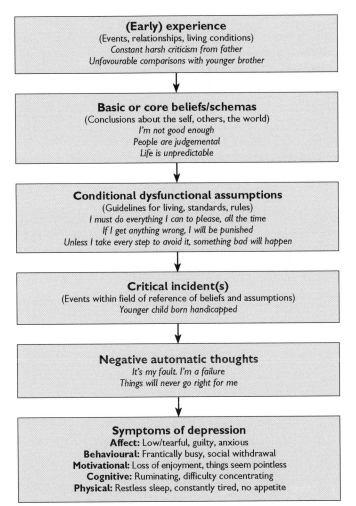

**Fig. 6.3.2.3.1** Cognitive model of depression.

The more depressed people become, the more negative thoughts they think, and the more they believe them. The more negative thoughts they think and the more they believe them, the more depressed they become. Thus depression is maintained by **vicious circles** in which negative thinking and other symptoms reinforce one another. Experimental and clinical research reflects this **reciprocal relationship between affect and cognition**: modifying depressive thinking modifies depressed mood, while modifying depressed mood modifies depressive thinking.

### (ii) Objectives of CBT for depression

The first goal is to **break the vicious circle** described above by teaching patients to work effectively with negative automatic thoughts. Attention then turns to cognitive predisposing factors (beliefs, assumptions) in order to **reduce vulnerability** and decrease the likelihood of future episodes. The aim is not to teach realistic thinking *per se*, but rather to help patients to resolve their problems by teaching them cognitive behavioural skills.

### (iii) Overview of CBT for depression

Treatment usually proceeds through the following **stages**:

◆ diagnosis, assessment, problem identification

◆ cognitive interventions designed to reduce the frequency of negative thoughts

◆ behavioural assignments intended to tackle behavioural and motivational deficits

◆ monitoring, questioning, and testing negative automatic thoughts (the main body of therapy)

◆ relapse prevention.

Patients usually move from one stage to the next as each is mastered. The **starting point varies**: severely depressed patients often begin with simple behavioural interventions, whereas relatively mild depressions may immediately be amenable to cognitive work. At each stage, **cognitive and behavioural interventions are closely integrated**.[17] Thus behavioural interventions such as activity scheduling present opportunities to identify, question, and test negative thoughts, while work on thoughts and assumptions is closely linked to changes in behaviour.

Traditionally, **up to 20 sessions** of therapy are offered, twice weekly for 4 weeks and once weekly thereafter. Most patients respond within about 15 sessions. Some do well with 4–6 sessions, but severe chronic depressions may require more than 20 sessions, as well as shorter, more frequent sessions early on. Post-treatment boosters help to increase confidence and consolidate and extend skill. Sessions start with agenda-setting (prioritizing what to work on), homework review, and feedback on the previous session. After the day's main topics have been discussed, more homework practice is agreed to ensure generalization and reinforce new learning. Key points are summarized, and the therapist asks for reactions to the session, including anything that has been uncomfortable or unclear.

## Indications and contraindications

CBT was developed as a treatment for moderate-to-severe unipolar depression,[1] and has been consistently effective with this population. However, good average results in outcome trials conceal wide variations in responsiveness.[18] Consistent predictors of treatment response remain elusive.

Patients presenting with endogenous symptoms are as likely to respond well as non-endogenous patients. However, results for severe depression[19] and bipolar disorder[20] remain somewhat conflicting.

Some factors may facilitate a positive response; well-developed pre-existing cognitive and behavioural coping skills, acceptance of the cognitive model, willingness to engage in self-help assignments, an early focus on teaching specific cognitive-therapy skills, ease of access to thoughts and feelings, problem specificity, and ability to form a collaborative alliance. Such criteria can be explored at assessment, especially if it is divided into two sessions with a simple intervening homework assignment.

Patients who are unsuitable for short-term CBT[21] may nonetheless respond to a modified approach with:

◆ greater emphasis on socialization and on cultivating a solid working relationship

◆ more extended behavioural work

◆ more work on enduring depressogenic schemas in the later stages of treatment

◆ more emphasis on integration with antidepressant medication

◆ more careful attention to environmental factors (including not only life stresses and family relationships, but also the ward and health-care team)

Finally, given that CBT and antidepressant medication generally produce similar results, the patients' wish for psychological treatment should also be taken into account.

## Selection procedure

### Diagnosis: recognizing and labelling depression

CBT was designed for moderate-to-severe major unipolar depression. The diagnostic criteria for major depressive episode,[22] remarkably consistent for over 30 years, describe a symptom pattern (including cognitive features) that has been recognized throughout history, and appears basically consistent across age, gender, race, and culture. However, the relative emphasis on different symptoms and the manner in which distress is expressed varies, and assessment procedures should be adapted to explore cultural context. Additionally, sociocultural factors necessarily influence belief systems, and therapists should be sensitive to such differences, rather than assuming that their own assumptions are shared by their patients.

### Severity

Severity should be taken into account when deciding whether concurrent (or alternative) physical treatments or hospitalization are necessary, and in determining where to begin within CBT. Severity can be assessed through clinical interview (e.g. intensity, pervasiveness, and reactivity of depressed mood; extent of behavioural and interpersonal deficits). The **Beck Depression Inventory** (BDI-II)[23] a well-established self-report measure of depression, provides a rapid overview of symptoms. Weekly completion allows clinicians to observe overall progress, as well as tracking scores on particular items, e.g. hopelessness. Hopelessness and suicidality should be routinely assessed[24] and any sign of suicide risk investigated in-depth.[25]

### Clinical interview

Interview assessment for CBT includes the following:

#### (a) Symptoms and associated cognitions

Negative automatic thoughts both trigger and enhance symptoms of depression (Table 6.3.2.3.1). Identifying meanings attached to symptoms prepares the ground for more helpful perspectives (e.g. 'These are symptoms of depression, not a reflection of my worth as a person').

#### (b) Impact on functioning

It is important to establish how depression affects relationships, work performance, and leisure time. It may be necessary to take practical steps to improve the patient's situation (e.g. gradual reintroduction to work).

#### (c) Coping strategies

The more depressed the patient, the more likely that she/he has adopted coping strategies which help in the short-term, but are in the longer-term self-defeating (e.g. alcohol or drugs, social withdrawal, bed). Therapist and patient can discuss the pros and cons of these, and how cognitive behavioural strategies might be more beneficial. The aim is for patients to reach the point of trying more adaptive coping strategies for themselves.

**Table 6.3.2.3.1** Negative automatic thoughts and symptoms of depression

| Symptoms | Negative automatic thoughts |
| --- | --- |
| *Behavioural* | |
| Lowered activity level | I can't do it. It won't work. |
| Procrastination | I'll never get it done. It's too much for me. |
| *Motivational* | |
| Loss of energy | It's too much effort. I'll wait till I fell better. |
| Loss of pleasure, interest | I won't enjoy it. What's the point? I can't be bothered. |
| *Affective* | |
| Sadness | I've lost everything important to me. |
| Guilt | I'm letting everybody down. |
| Anger | Why can't people just leave me alone? |
| Shame | What must everyone think? |
| Anxiety | I'm not going to be able to cope. |
| *Cognitive* | |
| Indecisiveness | Whatever I do will go wrong. |
| Poor concentration | I must be going senile. |
| *Physical* | |
| Loss of sleep | If this goes on, I won't be able to function. |
| Loss of appetite | I'm going to make myself ill. |
| Loss of sexual appetite | Our marriage is at an end. |
| *Other* | |
| Suicide | This is unbearable. There is no other way out. |
| Problems in living | There's nothing to be done. |

#### (d) Onset of current episode

Information about the onset of episodes may provide valuable clues about beliefs and assumptions. For example, a young woman became depressed when her husband took a job abroad, and was away for long periods. She believed that he would not have done so if he truly loved her. In fact, he had taken the job because it paid exceptionally well and the savings they could make would allow them to start the family they had been planning. The therapist noted the patient's interpretation of her husband's behaviour, and later in therapy used this clue as a starting point to identify long-standing doubts about her attractiveness, and a linked dysfunctional assumption: 'If someone is not there for me all the time, it means they don't care about me'.

#### (e) Background

#### (i) Previous treatment

Many depressed patients presenting for CBT have already received other treatment (most commonly antidepressant medication and counselling). The therapist should inquire about the **outcome** of such treatment, and **what the patient makes of it**. Depressed patients often conclude that the incomplete success of prior treatment means that they will also be unable to benefit from this new approach. Such thoughts can be worked with using straightforward cognitive behavioural methods (identify, question, test). When the patient has received psychological therapy, it is often helpful to ask **what they learned** from it. If they feel they learned nothing, this may predispose them to approach CBT with pessimism.

Alternatively, if they learned something of value, CBT can build on this positive experience.

### (ii) Expectations of CBT

These may reflect general pessimism about change, especially if patients know nothing about the approach. Those who have heard or read about CBT, and are aware of outcome data, may be more optimistic, although still anxious lest it fail to help *them*. Others may have heard negative reports (e.g. that it is mechanistic and fails to address deep issues). **Non-defensive discussion** of expectations allows doubts and misconceptions to be addressed, as well as encouraging open-mindedness and continued frank feedback from the patient.

### (iii) Early experience and resultant beliefs and assumptions

CBT is **conceptualization driven,**[26] **closely based on the cognitive model of depression**. In order for patients to understand how their problems developed, and that current beliefs are learned opinions rather than reflections of fact, it is helpful to know about relevant formative experiences. This is particularly true when working with severe, chronic problems, and personality disorders. However, **obtaining historical information is often not an immediate priority**. It is more important initially to convey the hopeful message that something can be done to change things for the better. Therefore details about history, beliefs, and assumptions may not be explored until work on behavioural deficits and negative automatic thoughts has produced a reduction in hopelessness and depressed mood. That said, where patients are relatively mildly depressed, psychologically minded, and able to articulate their difficulties with ease, a draft conceptualization incorporating historical information, beliefs, and assumptions sometimes emerges even from the initial assessment.

## Managing treatment

### (a) Starting treatment

The **first treatment interview has four main objectives**:

- to establish a warm, collaborative therapeutic **alliance**

- to list specific **problems and** associated **goals**, and select a first problem to tackle

- to educate the patient about the **cognitive model**, especially the vicious circle that maintains depression

- to give the patient first-hand experience of the focused, workman-like, empirical **style** of CBT.

These convey two important messages: (1) it is possible to make sense of depression; (2) there is something the patient can do about it. These messages directly address hopelessness and helplessness.

### (i) Identifying problems and goals

The **problem list** usually includes symptoms of depression. It may also contain aspects of other disorders (e.g. panic attacks), problems in living (e.g. family conflicts), and, in some cases, long-standing psychological problems (e.g. fear of intimacy). Developing the list provides the therapist with a 'map of the territory', which suggests possible targets for intervention, as well as an opportunity to foster the therapeutic relationship by demonstrating empathy. It suggests that apparently chaotic experience can be broken down into manageable problem areas. **Goal identification** then implies that progress is possible.

### (ii) Introducing the cognitive model of depression

The therapist's next task is to demonstrate **how negative thinking influences emotion and behaviour**, relating this to the patient's experience using material derived from the session. The therapist explains that the patient will learn to notice negative automatic thoughts, to stand back, question them, and develop more realistic and helpful perspectives. Patients are often doubtful about their ability to do this. It is important therefore to present **CBT as a learning opportunity** during which skills can be acquired, step by step, with the therapist's guidance. The therapist is not obliged to convince patients that CBT will work for them, but a willingness to try it in practice is essential.

### (iii) Where to start?

A **first treatment target** is chosen towards the end of the first session, and an appropriate **homework** task agreed upon. Suitable homework tasks include: observing a recording of the session and noting important points (this assignment follows every session), reading assignments,[27] and self-monitoring assignments. The initial target varies. Where patients are only relatively mildly depressed, and remain active and capable of experiencing interest and pleasure, monitoring negative automatic thoughts can begin right away. Where the depression is more severe, with significant behavioural and motivational deficits, it is best to begin with behavioural interventions.

### (b) Behavioural interventions

### (i) Reducing rumination

In severe depression, access to more positive perspectives may be blocked by depressed mood, making modifying negative automatic thoughts difficult or impossible. At the same time, depressed patients spend a great deal of time ruminating about their difficulties and shortcomings.[28] Learning to **direct attention elsewhere** reduces the frequency of negative thoughts and hence improves mood. This palliative measure will not resolve the patient's problems, but its impact reinforces the model, and feeling somewhat better can facilitate more constructive thinking.

### (ii) Monitoring activities

Lowered activity levels and loss of interest and pleasure are often central to depression, and interventions designed to address them are known to be powerful in their own right.[19] Early behavioural interventions serve to **maximize engagement in activities providing a sense of pleasure and mastery**. This has a direct impact on mood, and provides opportunities to test negative thoughts that block engagement and, in a more global sense, prevent recovery (e.g. 'I can't do anything to change how I feel').

Patients record what they do, hour by hour, on a Weekly Activity Schedule (Fig. 6.3.2.3.2). Each activity is rated **0–10 for Pleasure (P)** and **Mastery (M)**. P ratings indicate how enjoyable the activity was, and M ratings how much of an achievement it was. 'P' is usually easily understood, but M can present difficulties. Depressed people often feel that nothing they do is an achievement, perhaps because most of their activities are routine ('What's so special about that?') or do not meet their standards ('I should have done more'). M should therefore be explained as 'an achievement, *given how you felt at the time*'. Thus even simple activities (e.g. making a cup of tea) are real achievements when patients are hampered by low mood and loss of energy. Ratings should be made immediately

Name _____                    Week beginning _____

| | Monday | Tuesday | Wednesday | Thursday | Friday | Saturday | Sunday |
|---|---|---|---|---|---|---|---|
| 9–10 | | | Bed (P5, M0) | Take kids to school (P0, M9) | Bed (P4, M0) | | |
| 10–11 | | | Bed (P4, M0) | Shopping with friends | Bed (P0, M0) | | |
| 11–12 | | | Bed (P2, M0) | ↓ (P6, M7) | Bed (P0, M0) | | |
| 12–1 | | | Bed (P1, M0) | Lunch with friend (P7, M3) | Up, shower, dress (P2, M7) | | |
| 1–2 | | | Bed (P0, M0) | Went for a walk (P7, M5) | Lunch, read paper (P3, M4) | | |
| 2–3 | | | Up, shower, dress (P0, M5) | Gardening (P4, M7) | Therapy Session | | |
| 3–4 | | | Pick up kids from school (P3, M7) | Pick up kids from school (P1, M3) | | | |
| 4–5 | | | Tea with friends (P4, M9) | Tea & TV with kids (P5, M2) | | | |
| 5–6 | | | Tea with friends (P6, M7) | Ironing (P0, M5) | | | |
| 6–7 | | | Get supper (P2, M5) | Get supper (P1, M5) | | | |
| 7–8 | | | Read with kids (P8, M3) | Read with kids (P7, M3) | | | |
| 8–12 | | | TV (P3, M1) Bed (P8, M0) | TV (P4, M0) Bed (P9, M0) | | | |

**Fig. 6.3.2.3.2** Weekly activity schedule. P, pleasure; M, mastery.

after each activity, since retrospective ratings may be distorted by negatively biased recall. In addition, it is helpful for patients to **review each day**, asking questions like: 'What worked for me?' 'What did not work?' 'What do I need more of? Less of? Different?'

### (iii) Planning activities

Once self-monitoring is mastered, **each day is planned in advance on an hour-by-hour basis**. This:

◆ provides a structure and helps with setting priorities

◆ averts the need to keep making decisions about what to do next

◆ reduces what may seem like chaos to a manageable list

◆ increases the chances that activities will be carried out

◆ enhances patients' sense of control.

A pattern of activities is sought in which **mastery and pleasure are balanced and maximized**. The plan is likely to contain a blend of obligations (e.g. the ironing) and pleasures (e.g. listening to music). Avoided tasks can be included, broken down into manageable steps ('graded task assignment'). Again, it is helpful for patients to review each day in detail, identifying unhelpful thoughts to be worked on in the next therapy session (e.g. 'If I can't complete the task, I might as well not bother at all'). Thus the cognitive element is present even when behaviour change is the primary target.

### (c) Working with negative automatic thoughts

Once behavioural methods have been mastered, patients learn to **identify, question, and test negative automatic thoughts**. The main tool here is the Dysfunctional Thoughts Record (Fig. 6.3.2.3.3). The example summarizes a lengthy discussion that took place when a patient experienced a serious setback midway through treatment.

### (i) Identifying negative automatic thoughts

Patients learn to **record upsetting incidents** as soon as possible after they occur (delay makes it difficult to recall thoughts and feelings accurately). They learn:

1 **To identify unpleasant emotions** (e.g. despair, anger, guilt), signs that negative thinking is present. Emotions are rated for intensity on a 0 to 100 scale. These ratings (though the patient may initially find them difficult) help to make small changes in emotional state obvious when the search for alternatives to negative thoughts begins. This is important, since change is rarely all-or-nothing and small improvements may otherwise be missed.

2 **To identify the problem situation**. What was the patient doing or thinking about when the painful emotion occurred (e.g. 'waiting at the supermarket checkout', 'worrying about my husband being late home')?

3 **To identify negative automatic thoughts associated with the unpleasant emotions**. Sessions direct the therapist towards asking: 'And what went through your mind at that moment?' Patients become aware of thoughts, images, or implicit meanings that are present when emotional shifts occur, and record them word-for-word. Belief in each thought is also rated on a 0 to 100 per cent

| Date | Emotion(s) *What did you feel? How bad was it (0–100%)?* | Situation *What were you doing or thinking about?* | Automatic thoughts *What exactly was running through your mind? Write your thoughts down, word for word. How far did you believe each of them (0–100%)?* | Alternative views *What alternatives are there to the automatic thoughts? How far do you believe each of them (0–100%)?* | Outcome *1. How far do you now believe the original thoughts (0–100%)? 2. How do you now feel (0–100)? 3. What can you do now (action plan, experiment)?* |
|------|------|------|------|------|------|
| Thurs | Depressed (95%) Hopeless (90%) | Three terrible days | I'm back to square one—I've lost everything I learned (100%) | Not true — even now, I'm not as bad as when I came into hospital (100%)<br><br>I am doing my housework, looking after the children, doing my job. I am getting some satisfaction out of it — it's not a total failure (75%) | 1. (60%)<br><br>2. Depressed (70%) Hopeless (35%)<br><br>3. Accept setbacks as part of recovery, not the end of the world. |
| | | | There's no point in doing anything. Nothing will work (100%) | I've been feeling very bad, but setbacks are to be expected — disappointment at the contrast with last week makes it worse (100%) | Make a detailed plan to help me deal with these feelings if they come again. |
| | | | I've tried everything now, and nothing has changed (100%) | I've been getting this therapy for 7 weeks — I've been depressed for 3 years. It's not surprising I haven't got over it completely. Already I can manage 75% of my depression, as opposed to 25% (100%) | Keep using what I have learned to deal with my depression |
| | | | I've failed again (100%) | This setback is not my failure —it is part of the problem (80%) | |
| | | | I will always be like this (100%) The only solution is to kill myself (95%) | Suicide is not the answer. Keep working on your thoughts. The past 7 weeks, and today, show it can work (100%) | |

**Fig. 6.3.2.3.3** Dysfunctional thoughts record.

scale (100 per cent represents complete belief, 50 per cent a moderate degree of belief, and so on). Again, this helps to make small changes in conviction evident at the next stage.

The skill of identifying painful emotions and associated thoughts is best learned if therapist and patient **work through examples on the sheet** before the patient self-monitors independently. Therapists can make sure that patients understand what is required, and are prepared for possible difficulties. For example, patients sometimes avoid recording thoughts because doing so is upsetting. Therapists can reassure them that this phase will pass once they learn to answer their thoughts, and suggest that they follow recording by engaging in an absorbing and pleasurable activity. Sometimes thoughts recorded do not seem to 'fit' the emotion experienced; in this case, therapists may need to help patients to **'unpack' the meaning of the thought** (for example, 'That didn't go too well' may turn out to mean 'I'm a total failure'). Time taken to learn accurate self-monitoring varies; many patients acquire the skill within a few days, but others take much time and coaching.

### (ii) Questioning negative automatic thoughts

Once patients can record thoughts and feelings, they learn to **search for alternative views**, writing these in the fifth column of the Dysfunctional Thoughts Record. There is no such thing as a 'right' answer to a negative thought; the 'right' answer is the one that helps the patient to feel better and handle the situation more constructively.

Accordingly, the therapist's task is not to suggest alternatives, but rather to elicit them through **'guided discovery'**, a process of sensitive questioning, which allows patients to reach new interpretations independently. It is helpful for therapists to develop a personal 'library' of questions, through discussion with colleagues, observation of other therapists, attendance at workshops, and reading. Productive areas of inquiry include:

1 **What is the evidence?** Processing biases in depression mean that patients give weight to information consistent with prevailing perspectives at the expense of information, which suggests that they may not be wholly true. The therapist thus needs to examine 'evidence' believed to support the thought, and also to seek information that might contradict it.

2 **What alternative views are there?** Questions such as the following can prompt alternative perspectives: 'How would you have reacted to this before you became depressed?' 'What is your perspective on this when you feel relatively well?' 'What might someone whose views you trusted make of this?' 'If someone you cared about came to you with this problem, what would you say?'

3 **What are the advantages and disadvantages of this way of thinking?** This approach is particularly helpful with self-critical thinking. Patients often believe that self-criticism is an effective way of bringing about change; in fact, it only intensifies depression. Patients who habitually self-criticize can be helped to draw

up an analysis of pros and cons. Apparent advantages (e.g. 'It keeps me on my toes') may in fact be outweighed by disadvantages (e.g. 'It paralyses me').

4 **What are the biases in my thinking?** The tendency to make inferential errors such as overgeneralization has already been mentioned. Learning to recognize these can be helpful, especially when patients regularly make the same mistake.

Alternatives reached by questioning negative automatic thoughts are recorded on the Dysfunctional Thoughts Record. The patient rates them for degree of belief, to ensure that they are *sufficiently* convincing (they do not require belief ratings of 100 per cent). If alternatives are not at all convincing, they will have no impact on the strength of the original automatic thoughts or associated emotions. These are now re-rated in the final column as a check that plausible alternatives have been found.

As with self-monitoring, these skills are **best learned by working through examples in session** before the patient attempts to answer thoughts independently. Even then, patients are sometimes unable to find alternatives, especially if emotion is high. This is quite normal, given that questioning one's thoughts is a complex skill. It may be helpful to leave searching for alternatives until the storm is past. Sometimes alternatives make no difference to the original thoughts or emotions. This may be because the patient has reservations about their validity ('Yes, but . . . '), which can dealt with like other negative thoughts. Alternatively, it may be that non-verbal methods (e.g. imagery work, experiential learning) are necessary to facilitate emotional change, or that the resistant thought is a more or less direct statement of an underlying belief of much longer duration, which will take longer to change.

### (iii)  Testing negative automatic thoughts: what can I do now?

It is important that cognitive changes brought about by questioning are consolidated through **behavioural experiments.**[17] These are often designed to test out the validity of the new perspective by seeking further information or acting differently and observing the results. They may also include practical plans to solve genuine life problems and to deal with the trigger situation differently should it occur again.

### (d)  Ending treatment

Although most episodes of depression are time-limited, **relapse and recurrence are common**—the more so, the more episodes a person has experienced. CBT therefore emphasizes working on cognitive vulnerability factors, summarizing and consolidating learning, and preparing for possible setbacks. A new approach, *Mindfulness-Based Cognitive Therapy*,[29] which integrates elements of CBT with intensive meditation practice, has been developed specifically to tackle this problem. Its effectiveness with patients who have experienced three or more episodes of depression has been demonstrated in two clinical outcome trials.[30,31]

### (i)  Re-evaluating dysfunctional assumptions

Once patients are skilled at answering negative automatic thoughts, attention turns to dysfunctional assumptions that make them vulnerable to depression. Often these emerge from information gathered earlier, for example repeating themes in Dysfunctional Thoughts Records. They may also be identified using a 'downward arrow' technique, which involves identifying situations that typically distress the patient, and associated thoughts. Instead

of responding directly to these, the therapist asks: 'If that was true, what would it mean to you?' This question (or variants) is repeated until a general assumption or rule, relevant to a range of situations, emerges. The validity of the rule is then questioned and tested. This process normally takes several sessions to complete. A helpful sequence of questions is given below (these are not exhaustive:

1 **Where did this rule come from?** Identifying the source of a dysfunctional assumption (e.g. parental criticism) often helps to encourage distance by suggesting that its development is understandable, though it may no longer be relevant or useful.

2 **In what ways is the rule unrealistic?** Dysfunctional assumptions do not fit the way the world works. They operate by extremes, which are reflected in their language (always/never rather than some of the time; must/should/ought rather than want/prefer/would like).

3 **In what ways is the rule helpful?** Dysfunctional assumptions are not usually wholly negative in their effects. For example, perfectionism may lead to genuine high-quality performance. If such advantages are not recognized and taken into account when new assumptions are formulated, the patient may be reluctant to move forward.

4 **In what ways is the rule unhelpful?** The advantages of dysfunctional assumptions are normally outweighed by their costs. Perfectionism leads to rewards, but it also undermines satisfaction with achievements and stops people learning from constructive criticism.

5 **What alternative rule might be more realistic and helpful?** Once the old assumption has been undermined, it is helpful to formulate an explicit alternative (e.g. 'It is good to do things well, but I am only human-sometimes I make mistakes'). This provides a new guideline for living, rather than simply undermining the old system.

6 **What needs to be done to consolidate the new rule?** As with negative automatic thoughts, re-evaluation is best made real through experience: behavioural experiments. These encourage patients to challenge specific examples of old rules, as well as testing out the validity of new ones by acting as if they were true and observing the results This systematic work may need to continue for weeks or indeed months, given that assumptions have often been in place for many years.

### (ii)  Re-evaluating negative core beliefs

Negative thoughts often disappear as patients recover, whether the depression is treated by psychological means or not. Sometimes, however, they reflect enduring beliefs about the self, the world (including other people), or the future, which if left untouched may predispose the patient to become depressed again. Methods for dealing with these have primarily been developed in the context of CBT for personality disorder,[32,33] but can often be used within short-term CBT. This is important, given limited resources.

The cognitive model suggests that negative beliefs contributing to vulnerability to depression are (like dysfunctional assumptions) based on early learning, and maintained by a consistent bias in favour of information, which confirms them, and against information, which contradicts them. Therapists help patients to become aware of this bias, to question the 'evidence' that upholds the negative beliefs (much as the 'evidence' in favour of negative automatic thoughts is questioned), and to search actively for information which contradicts it. Once a relevant belief has been identified (e.g. 'I am no good') and rated for degree of belief (0–100 per cent), the suggestion is introduced that this may be more of an opinion than a fact (work at the level of automatic thoughts should have prepared the ground for this idea). If possible, the patient is asked to suggest a more positive alternative (e.g. 'If you were not 'no good', how would you like to be?'), and belief in the alternative (which is likely to be low) is also rated. The alternative provides a new 'address' at which to store information inconsistent with the old belief. However, it is not always possible to find one at this stage (e.g. when the patient has predicated his or her life on the belief and accumulated a large body of supporting evidence). In this case, an alternative may only become available once the old belief has been systematically weakened.

Supporting 'evidence' may include events from the distant past, which have been interpreted in a self-derogatory way (e.g. childhood abuse), as well as later experiences (e.g. a broken marriage) and everyday events of the kind already recorded on the Dysfunctional Thoughts Record. Each item is questioned, and new and more adaptive interpretations arrived at. In addition, patients are asked to record evidence that would support a more positive alternative to the old belief (e.g. examples of their strengths and skills). The success of these interventions is assessed by repeatedly rating the degree of belief in the old system, as well as in the new alternatives. This work too may take a considerable time, especially if negative beliefs have had a sizeable impact on the person's life. Where treatment time is limited for practical reasons, clinicians may find it helpful to space out later sessions, ensuring that intervening weeks are used to consolidate and extend within-session work.

### (iii) Consolidating learning: 'blueprints'

Preparation for ending treatment begins with the treatment contract. The implication of offering a limited number of sessions is that treatment will end, and that patients will acquire the skills necessary to deal with depression independently. Throughout therapy, they are encouraged to take increasing responsibility for determining session content, making practical suggestions, devising homework assignments, summarizing learning, and applying new skills in fresh areas. Written session summaries and therapy tapes encourage reflection and consolidation.

At the end of treatment, gains are summarized in a personal action plan or 'blueprint for the future'. The blueprint is confined to one or two sheets of paper, guides continued learning, and helps deal with relapse or recurrence. It draws on the case conceptualization, session notes, homework records, reading materials, and the like. The therapist should examine sessions, records, etc. independently, so that the plan is drawn up jointly, nothing important is forgotten, and the patient goes away with as full a summary as possible. The following questions provide a useful framework:

1 **How did my problems develop?** (unhelpful beliefs and assumptions, the experiences that led to their formation, events precipitating onset)

2 **What kept them going?** (maintenance factors)

3 **What did I learn from therapy that helped?** (techniques (e.g. activity scheduling) and ideas (e.g. 'I can do something to influence my mood'). Techniques should be detailed so that patients

know exactly what to do should depression recur. Examples of handouts and record sheets can be included.)

4 **What were my most unhelpful negative thoughts and assumptions? What alternatives did I find to them?** (summarized in two columns)

5 **How can I build on what I have learned?** (a solid, practical, clearly specified action plan)

### (iv) Preparation for setbacks

The blueprint should also be used to plan for relapse. It is helpful right at the beginning of treatment to tell patients that, however well they do, they may well experience a setback at some point, not least because periods of low mood are a normal part of human experience. CBT will not prevent the patient from ever having another moment's distress; it will provide tools for dealing with distress more effectively. This information can help patients to respond with less fear and despair when they do encounter setbacks.

Preparation for setbacks can be framed by the following questions:

1 **What might lead to a setback for me?** For example, future losses (e.g. children leaving home) and stresses (e.g. financial difficulties), i.e. events which impinge on patients' vulnerabilities and are thus liable to be interpreted negatively. For people who have experienced recurrent depression, mild normal low mood (without any major environmental stimulus) can act as a trigger for negative thinking which, if unchecked, can spiral down into clinical depression.

2 **What early warning signs do I need to be alert for?** Feelings, behaviours, and symptoms that might indicate the beginning of another depression are identified and listed, using careful analysis of this and previous episodes and of fluctuations in mood occurring during treatment.

3 **If I notice that I am becoming depressed again, what should I do?** Clear simple instructions, which will make sense despite low mood, are needed here. Specific ideas and techniques summarized earlier in the blueprint should be referred to. General encouragement can also be included (e.g. 'Don't panic'), as well as a specific plan for what to do if cognitive behavioural methods do not lift mood within a specified period (e.g. contact the general practitioner about medication, contact the therapist for telephone discussion or booster sessions, contact emergency services or telephone helplines in the event of serious suicidal thoughts). Recontacting therapists is often difficult, as patients may feel that they have failed or them down. Therapists should make it clear that they consider it a sign of courage to ask for further help, not a sign of weakness.

### (e) Training

Cognitive behaviour therapy for depression is a sophisticated treatment, requiring theoretical knowledge, research familiarity, and clinical expertise. The latter is best developed through practical training and close supervision. Core skills have been operationalized in measures of therapist competency, such as the *Cognitive Therapy Scale*,[34] which allow practitioners to judge for themselves whether they are indeed practising cognitive behaviour therapy and to monitor skills development.

Treating depressed patients with cognitive behaviour therapy is a challenge, especially with severe, chronic, and relapsing depressions and depression comorbid with other conditions. Therapist competency (the ability to carry out the treatment as intended and to an adequate standard) has a direct impact on outcome. Thus the need for experienced therapists, and for adequate training and ongoing supervision, especially with more difficult groups, cannot be overemphasized.[10,11]

Where established training institutes exist, it is wise to take advantage of their expertise. Even where no local institute is available, expert therapists from established centres often travel internationally to deliver conferences, workshops, seminars, and supervision—notably the triennial World Congress of Cognitive and Behaviour Therapies.

However, novice therapists will sometimes have little option but to supervise themselves, using clinical texts as a knowledge base. Therapists at all skill levels will benefit from regularly monitoring audio or video recordings of their treatment sessions, using the *Cognitive Therapy Scale* to identify strengths and areas in need of improvement. Even if no more experienced practitioner is available, peer supervision with interested colleagues is helpful. It provides external feedback on clinical practice, and makes other forms of learning possible (role play, study groups, etc.).

### (f) Self-care

Depression is an infectious disease. It is easy for psychological therapists (especially if relatively inexperienced) to become contaminated by patients' hopelessness. Therefore supervision should include a focus on the therapist's own thoughts and feelings. Therapists with a substantial proportion of depressed clients should also ensure that they leaven their day by planning life-enhancing and pleasurable experiences, and should be prepared to use cognitive behavioural methods to address their own negative thoughts.

## Training and supervision

The Beck Institute for Cognitive Therapy and Research in Philadelphia, Pennsylvania, runs extramural courses and training programmes (www.beckinstitute.org), as does the Oxford Cognitive Therapy Centre (www.octc.co.uk), who also offer a selection of CBT oriented booklets for patients and clinicians. The Academy of Cognitive Therapy offers information about CBT, training in CBT, certification as a cognitive therapist, and (once a member) access to a ListServe on which issues relating to theory, research, and clinical practice can be discussed with experienced cognitive therapists (www.academyofcognitivetherapy.org) The International Association of Cognitive Psychotherapy (www.cognitivetherapyassociation. org) also has a ListServe and hosts regular conferences in member countries. Different countries also have their own national organizations promoting CBT, for example, the American Association for Behavioural and Cognitive Therapies (www.aabt.org), the Australian Association for Cognitive and Behavioural Therapies (www.aabct.org), and the British Association for Behavioural and Cognitive Psychotherapies (www.babcp.com). These will be able to offer information about training opportunities.

## Further information

A number of texts describe the theory and practice of CBT for depression in some detail.[1,17,21] Practical ideas can also be found in self-help texts for patients.

### For the clinician:

Beck, J.S. (1995). *Cognitive therapy: basics and beyond*. Guilford Press, New York.

Fennell, M.J.V. (1989). Depression. In *Cognitive behaviour therapy for psychiatric problems: a practical guide* (eds. K. Hawton, P.M. Salkovskis, J. Kirk, and D.M. Clark). Oxford Medical Publications, Oxford.

Fennell, M. J. V., Westbrook, D., and Benneth-Levy, J. (2004). Depression. In *The Oxford guide to behavioural experiments in cognitive therapy* (eds. J. Benneth-Levy, G. Butler, M.J.V. Fennell, *et al.*). Oxford University Press, Oxford.

### For the patient:

Beck, A.T. and Greenberg, R.L. (1974). *Coping with depression*. Available from The Beck Institute of CBT and Research, GSB Building, City Line and Belmont Avenues, Suite 700, Bala Cynwyd, Philadelphia, PA 19004–1610, USA.

Burns, D.D. (1980). *Feeling good*. New American Library, New York.

Butler, G. and Hope, A. (2007). *Manage your mind* (2nd edn). Oxford University Press, Oxford.

Fennell, M.J.V. (1999). *Overcoming low self-esteem*. Constable Robinson, London.

Gilbert, P. (1996). *Overcoming depression*. Constable Robinson, London.

Greenberger, D. and Padesky, C.A. (1995). *Mind over mood*, Chap. 10. Guilford, New York.

Westbrook, D. (1999). *Coping with depression*. Available from: Oxford Cognitive Therapy Centre, Dept of Clinical Psychology, Warneford Hospital, Oxford OX3 7JX, UK.

### Subjective experience:

Solomon, A. (2002). *The noonday demon*. Simon & Schuster, New York.

Styron, W. (1991). *Darkness visible*. Jonathan Cape, London.

Wolpert, L. (1999). *Malignant sadness*. Faber, London.

Current research and theoretical developments are best followed through professional journals (primarily psychiatry and clinical psychology—see the reference list for examples), available in libraries and through the Internet.

## References

1. Beck, A.T., Rush, A.J., Shaw, B.F., *et al.* (1979). *Cognitive therapy of depression*. Guilford Press, New York.

2. Beck, A.T. (1963). Thinking and depression: 1. Idiosyncratic content and cognitive distortions. *Archives of General Psychiatry*, **9**, 324–33.

3. Beck, A.T. (1964). Thinking and depression: 2. Theory and therapy. *Archives of General Psychiatry*, **10**, 561–71.

4. Beck, A.T. (1967). *Depression: clinical, experimental and theoretical aspects*. Harper and Row, New York.

5. Rush, A.J., Beck, A.T., Kovacs, M., *et al.* (1977). Comparative efficacy of cognitive therapy and pharmacotherapy in the treatment of depressed outpatients. *Cognitive Therapy and Research*, **1**, 17–37.

6. Hollon, S.D., Thase, M.E., and Markowitz, J.C. (2002). Treatment & prevention of depression. *Psychological Science in the Public Interest*, **3**, 39–77.

7. Paykel, E.S., Scott, J., Cornwall, P.L., *et al.* (2005). Duration of relapse prevention after cognitive therapy in residual depression: follow-up of controlled trial. *Psychological Medicine*, **35**, 59–68.

8. Jarrett, R.B., Kraft, D., Doyle, J., *et al.* (2001). Preventing recurrent depression using cognitive therapy with and without a continuation phase. *Archives of General Psychiatry*, **58**, 381–8.

9. Vos, T., Corry, J., Haby, M.M., *et al.* (2005). Cost-effectiveness of cognitive-behavioural therapy and drug interventions for major depression. *The Australian and New Zealand Journal of Psychiatry*, **39**, 683–92.

10. DeRubeis, R.J., Hollon, S.D., Amsterdam, J.D., *et al.* (2005). Cognitive therapy vs. medications in the treatment of moderate to severe depression. *Archives of General Psychiatry*, **62**, 409–16.

11. Hollon, S.D., DeRubeis, R.J., Shelton, R.C., *et al.* (2005). Prevention of relapse following cognitive therapy vs. medications in moderate to severe depression. *Archives of General Psychiatry*, **62**, 417–22.

12. Ingram, R.E. (2003). Origins of cognitive vulnerability to depression. *Cognitive Therapy & Research*, **27**, 77–88.

13. McGinn, L.K., Cukor, D., and Sanderson, W. (2005). The relationship between parenting style, cognitive style and anxiety and depression: does increased early adversity influence symptom severity through the mediating role of cognitive style? *Cognitive Therapy & Research*, **29**, 219–42.

14. Alloy, L.B., Abramson, L.Y., Whitehouse, W.G., *et al.* (2006). Prospective incidence of first onsets and recurrences of depression in individuals at high and low cognitive risk for depression. *Journal of Abnormal Psychology*, 115, 145–56.

15. Segal, Z.V., Gemar, M., and Williams, S. (1999). Differential cognitive response to a mood challenge following successful cognitive therapy or pharmacotherapy for unipolar depression. *Journal of Abnormal Psychology*, **108**, 3–10.

16. Lau, M.A., Segal, Z.V., and Williams, J.M.G. (2004). Teasdale's differential activation hypothesis: implications for mechanisms of depressive relapse and suicidal behaviour. *Behaviour Research and Therapy*, **42**, 1001–17.

17. Fennell, M.J.V., Westbrook, D., and Bennett-Levy, J. (2004). Depression. In *The Oxford guide to behavioural experiments in cognitive therapy* (eds. J. Bennett-Levy, G. Butler, M.J.V. Fennell, *et al.*). Oxford University Press, Oxford.

18. Tang, T.Z., DeRubeis, R.J., Beberman, R., *et al.* (2005). Cognitive changes, critical sessions, and sudden gains in cognitive-behavioural therapy for depression. *Journal of Consulting and Clinical Psychology*, **73**, 168–72.

19. Dimidjian, S., Hollon, S.D., Dobson, K.S., *et al.* (2006). Randomized trial of behavioural activation, cognitive therapy, and antidepressant medication in the acute treatment of adults with major depression. *Journal of Consulting and Clinical Psychology*, **74**, 658–70.

20. Scott, J., Payken, E., Morris, R., *et al.* (2006). Cognitive behavioural therapy for severe and recurrent bipolar disorders. Randomised controlled trial. *The British Journal of Psychiatry*, **188**, 313–20.

21. Moore, R.G. and Garland, A. (2003). *Cognitive therapy for chronic and persistent depression*. Wiley, Chichester, UK.

22. American Psychiatric Association. (1994). *Diagnostic and statistical classification of diseases and related health problems* (4th edn). American Psychiatric Association, Washington, DC.

23. Beck, A.T., Ward, C.H., Mendelson, M., *et al.* (1961). An inventory for measuring depression. *Archives of General Psychiatry*, **4**, 561–71.

24. Beck, A.T., Weissman, A., Lester, D., *et al.* (1974). The measurement of pessimism: the Hopelessness Scale. *Journal of Consulting and Clinical Psychology*, **42**, 861–5.

25. Beck, A.T. (1993). *Beck scale for suicide ideation* (*manual*). Psychological Corporation, San Antonio.

26. Persons, J.B. (1989). *Cognitive therapy in practice: a case formulation approach*. Norton, New York.

27. Beck, A.T. and Greenberg, R.L. (1974). *Coping with depression*. Available from The Beck Institute of Cognitive Therapy and Research, GSB Building, City Line and Belmont Avenues, Suite 700, Bala Cynwyd, Philadelphia, PA 19004–1610, USA.

28. Papageorgiou, C. and Wells, A. (2003). *Depressive rumination: nature, theory and treatment*. Wiley, Chichester.

29. Segal, Z.V., Williams, J.M.G., and Teasdale, J.D. (2002). *Mindfulness-based cognitive therapy for depression: a new approach to preventing relapse*. Guilford, New York.

30. Teasdale, J.D., Segal, Z.V., Williams, J.M.G., *et al.* (2000). Reducing risk of recurrence of major depression using Mindfulness-Based Cognitive Therapy. *Journal of Consulting and Clinical Psychology*, **68**, 615–23.

31. Ma, J. and Teasdale, J.D. (2004). Mindfulness-based cognitive therapy for depression: replication and exploration of differential relapse prevention effects. *Journal of Consulting and Clinical Psychology*, **72**, 31–40.

32. Padesky, C.A. (1994). Schema change processes in cognitive therapy. *Clinical Psychology and Psychotherapy*, **1**, 267–78.

33. Beck, A.T., Freeman, A., Davis, D.D., *et al.* (2004). *Cognitive therapy of personality disorders*. Guilford Press, New York.

34. Young, J.E. and Beck, A.T. (1980). *Development of an instrument for rating cognitive therapy: the cognitive therapy scale*. University of Pennsylvania, Philadelphia, PA.

## 6.3.2.4 Cognitive behaviour therapy for schizophrenia

Max Birchwood and Elizabeth Spencer

### Introduction

Cognitive behaviour therapy (**CBT**) for schizophrenia focuses on the core psychotic symptoms of hallucinations and delusions. Other psychosocial approaches to psychosis (e.g. intervention with families and to promote medication compliance) also frequently use CBT techniques. In this chapter, however, we focus on CBT for delusional beliefs and other psychotic phenomena and review evidence for its efficacy.

### Background: assumptions and common components

The CBT approach to psychotic symptoms comprises two different strands each with their own theoretical basis, although of late these two approaches have become conjoined in practice.

#### Coping strategy enhancement

The first approach is inspired by the stress-vulnerability model of schizophrenia. Vulnerability here is viewed as a 'black box', drawing mainly on the biomedical tradition. It is assumed that stressors capable of triggering or exacerbating symptoms may be generated or modulated by the individual. For example, stressors emanating from the social environment are modulated by the patient's own appraisal of their stressfulness and his or her coping strategies.

Another class of stressors consists of the symptoms themselves. It is assumed that certain strategies used to cope with symptoms are unhelpful and generate stress in the individual, in turn, exacerbating symptoms. These strategies are conventionally divided into affective strategies (e.g. relaxation, sleep, etc.), behavioural strategies (being active, drinking alcohol, etc.), and cognitive strategies (distraction, challenging voices, switching attention away from voices, etc.). This underpins the approach known as Coping Strategy Enhancement[1] whereby patients are offered a range of strategies which are implemented in an empirical fashion to determine their effectiveness in symptom control. For example, Falloon and Talbot[2] documenting the coping strategies used by voice-hearers, concluded that those who had multiple strategies available to them were more able to cope with their voices. Tarrier[3] on the other hand, focusing on a wider range of psychotic symptoms, concluded that those who applied strategies consistently tended to fare the best. This approach views the individual as an active agent who attempts to reduce the threat or distress posed by psychotic symptoms, but does not concern itself with the content or meaning that psychotic symptoms may have to the individual. There is also, in this approach, assumed to be a fundamental discontinuity between normal and abnormal functioning that comes about once the biological vulnerability is 'online'.

## CBT for delusions and hallucinations

The second CBT strand draws its theoretical strength from the cognitive therapy approach.[4] Early work in this area focused on the similarity between normal (but strongly held) beliefs and delusions, in terms of the psychological processes at play in their maintenance. For example, Brett-Jones et al.[5] showed that delusions, like everyday beliefs, lead the individual to recruit evidence to support them and to de-emphasize or dismiss contradictory evidence. Continuing the exploration of the continuity between normal and delusional beliefs, Birchwood and Chadwick[6] argued that certain beliefs about voices' power may be considered as a quasi-rational response to anomalous experience, with the meaning attributed to them in terms of identity, power, and the consequence of disobedience determining distress and behaviour in relation to the voice. Other work has drawn on the cognitive therapy approach in depression, which emphasizes the importance of evaluative beliefs about the self (e.g. self-worth) in the genesis and maintenance of depressed mood.[7] The application of this to psychosis also emphasizes evaluative beliefs about the self. The precise relationship between self-evaluative beliefs and delusional thinking is a much debated issue of the present time. It has been argued, for example, that delusions may serve the function of defending the individual from the full impact of low self-worth through blaming others for negative events rather than the self. This is the so-called 'paranoid defence'.[8] The content of psychotic thinking often reflects such personal issues. For example, for the patient who has been sexually abused, this theme tends to crop up in the content of voice activity or in the supposed identity of the voice.[6]

This early work has been elegantly drawn together in a cognitive model of psychosis by Phillipa Garety and her colleagues. In a seminal paper[9] they propose a model of the cognitive processes leading to the positive symptoms of psychosis. In brief, positive symptoms in psychosis are hypothesized to begin with basic cognitive disturbances with lead to ambiguous sensory input, the intrusion into consciousness of unintended material from memory, or to difficulties with the self-monitoring of intentions and actions, such that they are experienced as alien. This result in anomalous conscious experiences such as actions being experienced as unintended, racing thoughts, thoughts appearing to be broadcast, and thoughts experienced as voices.

However, the authors argue that such anomalous experiences alone do not develop into full-blown psychotic experiences unless an individual appraises them as externally caused and personally significant. Such appraisals are the results of particular reasoning processes (e.g. data gathering bias or externalizing attributional style), dysfunctional personal schemas (e.g. low self-esteem born of adverse social experience), emotional states (e.g. anxiety and depression), and appraisal of the experience of illness.

This model integrates the two strands of cognitive therapy. It suggests, for example, that the reduction in dysfunctional emotional states through, for example, coping strategy enhancement, will contribute to alterations in the attributions, which are important in the formation and maintenance of the positive symptoms. Similarly, it provides a theoretical basis for the basic techniques traditionally used in the second strand of CBT. Such techniques encourage the individual to weigh evidence that contradicts a delusion as a strategy to compensate for the basic information-processing abnormality, challenge negative self-schemata, and combat depression.

## Evaluation

In recent years the volume of trials evaluating CBT for psychosis has greatly expanded, with approximately 20 such studies now reported. Most of these have been conducted in the United Kingdom among patients with chronic schizophrenia. The strength of the data is now sufficient for The UK National Institute for Clinical excellence to state that cognitive behavioural therapy should be available as a treatment option for people with schizophrenia.[10]

An up-to-date review[11] reporting the analysis of 19 studies of CBT for positive symptoms in schizophrenia, found a mean effect size of 0.37. The authors concluded that 74 per cent of these studies achieved small effect sizes, 32 per cent moderate effect sizes, and 16 per cent large effect sizes in improving positive psychotic symptoms, relative to standard psychiatric care. Furthermore, they argued that this is unlikely to be due to publication bias. The effect sizes for CBT versus standard treatment among patients with chronic illness were greater than those among acutely ill patients. This may have been due to a ceiling effect caused by the effectiveness of medication in reducing symptoms in floridly ill inpatients. Similarly, the better the design of the trial, the smaller the treatment effect size, suggesting that CBT is not the panacea for all psychotic ills that it may have originally appeared.

With regard to relapse prevention, CBT appears to be more successful when the intervention is focused on relapse prevention, rather than relapse prevention being one of a series of components.[11] For example, Gumley and his colleagues[12] were able to demonstrate that a group of patients with psychosis receiving targeted CBT for relapse prevention had almost half the rate of relapse over a 12-month period compared with a similar group receiving treatment as usual (18.1 versus 34.7 per cent). In this study, the CBT treatment consisted of an engagement phase, early signs of relapse monitoring with a personalized questionnaire, and targeted CBT at the first sign of impending relapse.

While large, pragmatic trials of CBT treatment packages have yielded the above favourable results, investigating the active elements of the interventions is difficult because CBT for psychosis now refers to a wide range of treatments.

Furthermore, although the conceptual basis of CBT emphasizes the link between emotion, cognition, and behaviour, modifying emotion in psychosis has been relatively neglected in CBT trials, in favour of outcomes based on modification of delusions and hallucinations themselves.

It has been proposed that CBT should be focused into more targeted interventions aimed at emotional dysfunction or distress and/or behavioural anomaly in psychosis that is directly or indirectly linked to psychosis symptoms.[13] This approach recognizes that while changing the psychosis symptoms might not always be possible, it may well be feasible to change the affective consequences of the symptoms or the diagnosis. This affective change may have further benefits in reducing the severity of the psychosis experience *per se*.

For example:

1 CBT can be used to reduce distress, depression, and problem behaviour associated with commanding voices, without changing the frequency or content of the voices themselves.[14]

2 CBT can focus on anxiety, depression, and interpersonal difficulty in individuals at high risk of developing psychosis.[15]

3 CBT can focus on the relapse prodrome to prevent relapse in psychosis.[12]

4 CBT can focus on 'comorbid' depression and social anxiety, including the patient's appraisal of the diagnosis and its stigmatizing consequences.[16]

5 CBT can be used to reduce stress reactivity, thereby increasing resilience to life stress and preventing psychotic relapse.[17]

6 CBT can be used to increase self-esteem and social confidence in people with psychosis.[18]

## Management

### Coping strategy enhancement

Coping strategy enhancement involves developing a coping repertoire and over-rehearsing it to facilitate an automatic coping response.[19] It can either be used to improve an individual's attempts to cope with his or her voices by developing an understanding of factors that trigger or improve the voices, or to test the reality of thoughts about the voices.

For example, therapy with a patient who hears threatening and frightening voices exacerbated of being alone might involve: An explicit congratulation on the strength involved in withstanding the voices' incessant activity; strengthening of coping strategies involving seeking company and social support; and the use of a personal stereo for distraction.

### Cognitive therapy to challenge delusions and dysfunctional assumptions

The application of cognitive therapy in challenging of delusions and dysfunctional beliefs draws upon the approach described by Chadwick *et al.*[20] and builds upon the pioneering work of Chadwick and Lowe.[21]

Engaging patients is perhaps the greatest challenge facing a therapist. It is noticeable that many individuals either never attend or do so for a few sessions and then stop. Once individuals get past the opening strategies of cognitive therapy they usually see therapy through. Careful attention to appropriate therapeutic technique can maximize client engagement. Similarly, Kuipers *et al.*[22] report that a response to CBT in their study was associated with greater cognitive flexibility concerning delusions at baseline. This suggests that the sufferer may need some small degree of insight into the fact that he might be mistaken, to benefit from cognitive therapy for delusions.

The process involves six basic steps as summarized in Table 6.3.2.4.1.

**Table 6.3.2.4.1** A summary of the steps in cognitive therapy for delusions

1 Viewing delusions as beliefs, not facts

2 Developing a rationale for questioning the delusion

3 Weakening delusions

4 Utilizing inconsistency and irrationality

5 Reformulating delusions as reactions to, and attempts to make sense of, specific experience

6 Assessing the delusion and alternative, and empirical testing

#### (a) Viewing delusions as beliefs, not facts

The first technical difficulty to be encountered is the necessary move to aid the client in conceptualizing a delusion as a belief and not a fact. This move is an essential part of CBT for all emotional problems, but is difficult at the best of times. With depression, for example, patients often struggle to appreciate that their sense of worthlessness, which is so concrete to them, is actually a belief they hold and is different from a knowledge of events and facts. With delusions there is the added complication that the therapist might be perceived as being just another person who disbelieves the patient.

There are two central points to bear in mind when seeking to reconceptualize delusions as beliefs, not facts—why it is being done and how it is done.[20]

The purpose of clarifying that delusions are beliefs, not facts, is to empower the patient and offer a way of easing his or her distress. If the patient really is being persecuted by a powerful organization, or has a radio transmitter and receiver in his head, neither he nor the therapist can actually change this. The patient feels that he knows this as a fact, with the consequence that he feels frustrated and helpless as well as distressed. However, if the patient only believes this to be true, then he gains the freedom to examine his beliefs and perhaps change his distressing feelings and behaviour and experiences himself. In this sense it is in his best interest for the delusion to be false.

How this process takes place is critical. The process of Socratic questioning is not one of persuading a patient that he is wrong and that you, the therapist, are right. This mistake is made all too often. Rather, in Socratic dialogue the therapist helps the patient to draw on his own doubt and experience in order to realize that there are other ways in which he is able to make sense of his experience. So, when the therapist pursues the conceptual step of clarifying that a delusion is only a belief, the patient's own doubt, past or present, his own contradictory experience and behaviour, and concern about the possibility that the delusion is wrong are accessed. Many patients have 'double awareness' of delusions—on the one hand they believe them firmly and are distressed and disturbed by them, yet on the other hand they behave in ways that contradict the delusion, and they believe that working with a therapist might ease the problem. Finally, the therapist must accept that it is acceptable if the patient does not alter his belief. The process is 'collaborative empiricism, not indoctrination'.[17]

#### (b) Developing a rationale for questioning the delusion

Patients are usually used to being told by family and carers that their beliefs are wrong, that they are deluded. It is easy for a therapist to prepare the intervention well and embark on it before the patient is clear of the purpose and possible benefit, thus causing early loss of engagement. It is revealing to turn the engagement question on its head and to consider why a patient should ever wish to engage in therapy. With emotional problems patients identify their problems as depression, anger, anxiety, guilt, etc.; with delusions and hallucinations this is not so—patients predominantly present problems which they believe are actual events (persecution, voices, passivity). This means that they have no clear objective and therefore have no particular motivation to engage. The key reason for a patient to reconsider delusional beliefs is that it will help him feel less distress and it will free him to behave differently and to pursue the things he wants more directly. What the therapist does gradually through the unfolding cognitive assessment is to clarify with the patient that he is experiencing emotional and behavioural problems, and that these are tied to his beliefs (delusional and evaluative). The therapist then needs to explore with the patient how the delusion affects his life and how his life would be different (i.e. better or worse) if the delusion were false.[20] In this way, the therapist slowly encourages the patient to view the delusion not as an important discovery but as a belief that results in distress (e.g. fear, anxiety) and causes him to behave in ways which he would rather not (e.g. avoid things he would otherwise like to do).

### (c) Weakening delusions

Disputing comprises four elements:[20]

◆ The evidence for the belief is challenged, in inverse order of its importance to the delusion.

◆ The internal consistency and plausibility of the delusional system is questioned.

◆ Following Maher,[23] the delusion is reformulated as being an understandable response to, and way of making sense of, specific experience, and a personally meaningful alternative is then constructed.

◆ The individual's delusion and the alternative are assessed in the light of the available information.

◆ Challenging the evidence for the belief.

Watts *et al.*[24] argued that a danger when trying to modify delusions, indeed, all strongly held beliefs, was psychological reactance, whereby too direct an approach served only to reinforce the belief. They offered two principles to minimize this possibility: begin with the least important belief, and also work with the evidence for the belief rather than the belief itself.

Accordingly a 'verbal challenge' of delusions begins by questioning the evidence for the belief, and this process begins with the least significant item of evidence and works up to the most significant one. Our preferred approach is that with each item of evidence the therapist questions the patient's delusional interpretation and puts forward a more reasonable and probable one. The customary approach in CBT is for the patient to be asked to generate the alternative interpretation(s), rather than the therapist supply one, but we have found that for certain patients this conventional tactic is a weak intervention.

When the therapist questions the evidence for a delusion there are two distinct but related objectives. One is to encourage the patient to question and perhaps even to reject the evidence for his or her belief, and in this way perhaps to undermine the patient's conviction in the delusion itself. For some individuals challenging the evidence is a very powerful intervention and one that produces a substantial reduction in delusional conviction. However, more commonly this does not happen, but challenging evidence is still valuable in that it does impart insight into the connection between events, beliefs, affect, and behaviour. This is the second objective of challenging evidence, namely to convey the essentials of the ABC approach, i.e. that strongly held beliefs influence affect, behaviour, and cognition (i.e. interpretation) for all people. Core beliefs recruit or bias everyday inferences and automatic thoughts. However, this means that people often impose an interpretation on to events, which is unwarranted, and because we are prone towards selectively processing information that confirms our beliefs, this goes undetected. In other words, it is understandable that a patient should interpret a particular event in line with his delusion because this is merely one occurrence of a general tendency, and confirmation bias, common to all of us. In therapy, it is helpful to convey the ordinariness and normality of this process with everyday examples.

Having considered the alternatives, the patient is then asked to rate his conviction about each; regardless of how convinced he remains that the delusional interpretation is correct, it is usual to move on to the next piece of evidence. The therapist does not have to change what the patient thinks, but only to offer a fresh insight into the way he is thinking.

### (d) Utilizing inconsistency and irrationality

Although delusions contain differing degrees of inconsistency and irrationality, they all seem to contain some. For example, Margaret believed that she could not act or make a decision without reference to her voice; however, she described periods when she was relaxed and the voices quiescent where she would be making decisions. Such inconsistencies can be therapeutically useful.

### (e) Reformulating delusions as reactions to, and attempts to make sense of, specific experience

We always construe a delusion as both a reaction to and an attempt to make sense of certain puzzling and often threatening experience. It is an understandable and reasonable attempt to find meaning at a time when the individual is bewildered, anxious, and frightened. But, the delusion carries a cost in terms of distress and disturbance, which the individual might not otherwise experience. This is how delusions may be explained to patients.[23]

At this stage the therapist has commenced the process of challenging the delusional belief, re-formed the delusion as an attempt to make sense of certain experiences (e.g. primary symptoms, trauma) and raised the idea that the delusion is psychologically functional (i.e. it eases puzzlement) and perhaps linked to evaluative beliefs.

### (f) Assessing the delusion and alternative, and empirical testing

Finally, the patient and therapist need to assess the delusion and alternative in the light of the available evidence and previous discussion. The therapist may spell out the advantages of the alternative interpretative framework, which can also be discussed by relating it to the patient's experiences.

It is an integral part of CBT that the belief or assumption under consideration be tested empirically. Such reality testing involves planning and performing an activity that validates or invalidates a belief, or part of a belief.

When working with delusions, we set up a clear alternative belief in opposition to the delusion, clarifying with the patient in advance precisely what has to happen for each to be supported and refuted. For example,[20] Alison believed that by repeating her voice's command (e.g. 'The price of milk *will* rise a billion times') it would actually happen by transmitting the thought to a member of the government who would act upon it. The empirical test involved repeating the voice and purchasing milk before and after doing so, predicting that within 2 weeks the price of milk would at least double. If it did not, the alternative (that the power to change events was very weak) would be strengthened.

### Cognitive therapy for beliefs about auditory hallucinations

The above techniques can be applied to challenge beliefs about 'voices' using the following three steps:

#### (a) Assessment

Assessing the personal meaning a voice has for a person is the defining feature of the cognitive approach to assessing auditory hallucinations. The delusional beliefs found to be most significant are those relating to a voice's identity, purpose, power, knowledge, and the consequences of compliance and resistance. The semi-structured interview schedule developed by Chadwick and Birchwood[6,25] is recommended.

#### (b) Disputing beliefs about voices

The thrust of the therapist's challenge is that the beliefs are reasonable and understandable reactions to, and attempts to make sense of, the auditory hallucinations. The therapist reviews evidence and inconsistency, and plans tests, with the aim always of evaluating two possible meanings: that the beliefs are true, a discovery, or that they are reasonable and understandable, but mistaken. As ever, it is vital that the therapist really practises Socratic questioning and works collaboratively. This involves drawing out patients' own doubts, puzzlement, double awareness, critical faculty, etc., rather than forcing a contradiction on them.

The major piece of evidence for the delusional beliefs is always the actual voices, especially their content—these are, after all, the activating events that the delusions are invoked to explain. The role of beliefs is critical because individuals usually attribute voices with a power and knowledge that goes well beyond what they have actually said. Several examples of challenging follow.

It is really quite common for beliefs about compliance (e.g. 'If I don't do what my voice says I will be punished') not to fit patients' experiences, and perhaps it is only their emotional impact which prevents patients from abandoning them. Kate, for example, believes 'If I drop my guard the voices will kill me', but in fact she has dropped her guard on many occasions without consequence. This might be pointed out as follows. 'Kate, you say that the voices have the power to kill you and you must be on your guard constantly. I certainly appreciate the fear that this must create. What puzzles me though is that your guard is often down, like when you are asleep. How is it that they have not succeeded in all these years?'

The appearance of being all knowing (omniscience) is a vital aspect of many voices[22] and often features as a key piece of evidence that the identity of the voice is superhuman. It leaves individuals feeling exposed and vulnerable and very prone to guilt and shame. Alice believes that her voice is a prophet endowed with the ability to foretell the future. In particular, the voice anticipates exactly the arrival of her husband home from work each day. To begin the process of questioning she was asked: 'Let's suppose for a moment that the voice cannot foretell the future; can you think of any other possible explanations for last night's prediction?' One such possibility was that the voice was making a very safe guess.

#### (c) Testing beliefs about control

A useful strategy is to use a procedure whereby the patient and therapist learn to engineer situations to start or increase the probability of hearing voices, and then to stop or reduce them. In this way the patient gains a surprising degree of control over the voice. The initial assessment provides information about cues that provoke voices for a particular individual; concurrent verbalization is known to stop or diminish voices temporarily. This information is combined in the following five steps.

- Identify cues that increase and decrease voices.
- Practise the use of 'increasing' and 'decreasing' strategies within a session.
- Propose the notion that 'control' requires the demonstration that voice activity can be turned up/on or down/off.
- In sessions encourage the patient to initiate or increase voice activity for short periods then reduce or stop it.
- Elicit changes in the patient's belief about his control over the voices.

The above process has been applied in a targeted way to the special case of beliefs about command hallucinations. These are high-risk, distressing, and relatively common symptoms of schizophrenia.

For example, Byrne and her colleagues[26] have developed a specific cognitive therapy for command hallucinations, which draws on the above techniques. Using the methods of collaborative empiricism and Socratic dialogue, the therapist seeks to engage the client to question, challenge, and undermine the power beliefs, then to use behavioural tests to help the client gain disconfirming evidence against the beliefs. These strategies are also used to build clients' alternative beliefs in their own power and status, and finally, where appropriate, to explore the origins of the schema so clients have an explanation for why they developed those beliefs about the voice in the first place. They were able to show that this process produce significant reductions in compliance behaviours and favourable changes in beliefs about the power, superiority and need to comply with the voices, despite the frequency, loudness, and content of the voices staying the same.[14]

### Conclusion

CBT for psychosis is a rapidly developing field, and one that has borne considerable fruit in terms of providing effective treatments and a basis upon which a dialogue between the patient and the professional can take place about matters of great concern and a source of much distress.

## Further information

Nelson, H. (2005). *Cognitive behavioural therapy with delusions and hallucinations: a practice manual* (2nd edn). Nelson Thornes, Cheltenham.

Morrison, A.P. (2002). *A casebook of cognitive therapy for psychosis.* Brunner/Routledge, London.

Byrne, S., Meaden, A., Trower, P., et al. (2006). *A casebook of cognitive behaviour therapy for command hallucinations: a social rank theory.* Routledge, London.

## References

1. Tarrier, N., Yusupoff, L., Kinney, C., et al. (1998). Randomised controlled trial of intensive cognitive behavioural therapy for patients with chronic schizophrenia. *British Medical Journal*, **317**, 303–7.

2. Falloon, I.R.H. and Talbot, R. (1981). Persistent auditory hallucinations: coping mechanisms and implications for management. *Psychological Medicine*, **11**, 329–39.

3. Tarrier, N. (1987). An investigation of residual positive symptoms in discharged schizophrenic patients. *British Journal of Clinical Psychology*, **26**, 141–3.

4. Beck, A.T., Rush, A., Shaw, B., et al. (1979). *Cognitive therapy of depression.* Guilford, New York.

5. Brett-Jones, J., Garety, P., and Hemsley, D.R. (1987). Measuring delusional experiences: a method and its application. *British Journal of Clinical Psychology*, **26**, 257–65.

6. Birchwood, M. and Chadwick, P.D. (1997). The omnipotence of voices. II. Testing the validity of the cognitive model. *Psychological Medicine*, **27**, 1345–53.

7. Garety, P.A., Kuipers, L., Fowler, D., et al. (1994). Cognitive behavioural therapy for drug resistant psychosis. *The British Journal of Medical Psychology*, **67**, 259–71.

8. Bentall, R.P. and Kinderman, P. (1998). Psychological processes and delusional beliefs: implications for the treatment of paranoid states. In *Outcome and innovation in psychological treatment of schizophrenia* (eds. T. Wykes, N. Tarrier, and S. Lewis), pp. 119–44. Wiley, Chichester.

9. Garety, P.A., Kuipers, A.E., Fowler, D., et al. (2001). A cognitive model of the positive symptoms of psychosis. *Psychological Medicine*, **31**, 189–95.

10. National Collaborating Centre for Mental Health. (2003). *Schizophrenia: full national clinical guideline on core interventions in primary and secondary care.* Royal College of Psychiatrists and the British Psychological Society, London.

11. Tarrier, N. and Wykes, T. (2004). Is there evidence that cognitive behavioural therapy is an effective treatment for schizophrenia? A cautious or cautionary tale. *Behaviour Research and Therapy*, **42**, 1377–401.

12. Gumley, A., O'Grady, M., McNay, L., et al. (2003). Early intervention for relapse in schizophrenia: results of a 12-month randomized controlled trial of behavioural therapy. *Psychological Medicine*, **33**, 419–31.

13 Birchwood, M. and Trower, P. (2006). The future of cognitive behavioural therapy for psychosis: not a quasi-neuroleptic. *British Journal of Psychiatry*, **188**, 107–8.

14. Trower, P., Birchwood, M., and Meaden, A. (2004). Cognitive therapy for command hallucinations: randomised controlled trial. *British Journal of Psychiatry*, **184**, 312–20.

15. Morrison, A.P., French, P., Walford, L., et al. (2004). Cognitive therapy for the prevention of psychosis in people at ultra-high risk: randomised controlled trial. *British Journal of Psychiatry*, **185**, 291–7.

16. Iqbal, Z., Birchwood, M., and Chadwick, P. (2000). Cognitive approach to depression and suicidal thinking in psychosis. 2. Testing the validity of a social ranking model. *British Journal of Psychiatry*, **177**, 522–8.

17. Myin-Germeys, I., Delespaul, P., and van Os, J. (2005). Behavioural sensitization to daily life stress in psychosis. *Psychological Medicine*, **35**, 733–41.

18. Hall, P.L. and Tarrier, N. (2003). The cognitive behavioural treatment of low self esteem in psychotic patients: a pilot study. *Behaviour Research Therapy*, **41**, 317–32.

19. Tarrier, N. (1992). Management and modification of residual psychotic symptoms. In *Innovations in the psychological management of schizophrenia* (eds. M. Birchwood and N. Tarrier), pp. 38–72. Wiley, Chichester.

20. Chadwick, P.D., Birchwood, M., and Trower, P. (1996). *Cognitive therapy for delusions, voices and paranoia.* Wiley, Chichester.

21. Chadwick, P.D.J. and Lowe, C.F. (1990). Measurement and modification of delusional beliefs. *Journal of Consulting and Clinical Psychology*, **58**, 225–32.

22. Kuipers, E., Garety, P., Fowler, D., et al. (1997). London-East Anglia randomised controlled trial of cognitive behavioural therapy for psychosis. I. Effects of the treatment phase. *The British Journal of Psychiatry*, **171**, 319–27.

23. Maher, B.A. (1988). Anomalous experience and delusional thinking: the logic of explanation. In *Delusional beliefs* (eds. F. Oltmans and B.A. Maher), pp. 5–22. Wiley, New York.

24. Watts, F., Powell, E., and Austin, S.V. (1973). The modification of abnormal beliefs. *The British Journal of Medical Psychology*, **46**, 359–63.

25. Chadwick, D. and Birchwood, M. (1994). The omnipotence of voices. A cognitive approach to auditory hallucinations. *British Journal of Psychiatry*, **164**, 190–201.

26. Byrne, S., Meaden, A., Trower, P., et al. (2005). *A casebook of cognitive behaviour therapy for command hallucinations: a social rank theory approach.* Routledge, London.

## 6.3.3 **Interpersonal psychotherapy for depression and other disorders**

Carlos Blanco, John C. Markowitz, and Myrna M. Weissman

### Introduction

Interpersonal psychotherapy (IPT) is a time-limited, diagnosis-focused therapy. IPT was defined in a manual. Research has established its efficacy as an acute and chronic treatment for patients with major depressive disorder (MDD) of all ages, as an acute treatment for bulimia nervosa, and as adjunct maintenance treatment for bipolar disorder.[1–9] The research findings have led to its inclusion in treatment guidelines and increasing dissemination into clinical practice.

Demonstration of efficacy in research trials for patients with major depressive episodes (MDEs) has led to its adaptation and testing for other mood and non-mood disorders. This has included modification for adolescent and geriatric depressed patients[10,11] patients with bipolar[12] and dysthymic disorders;[13,14] depressed HIV-positive[15] and depressed pregnant and postpartum patients;[16,17] depressed primary care patients;[18] and as a maintenance treatment to prevent relapse of the depression.[5] Most of the modifications have been relatively minor and have retained the general principles and techniques of IPT for major depression.

Non-mood targets have included anorexia, bulimia, substance abuse, borderline personality disorder, and several anxiety disorders. In general, outcome studies of IPT have suggested its promise for most psychiatric diagnoses in which it has been studied, with the exceptions of anorexia, dysthymic disorder, and substance use disorders.[14,19,20]

IPT has two complementary basic premises. First, depression is a medical illness, which is treatable and not the patient's fault. Second, depression does not occur in a vacuum, but rather is influenced by and itself affects the patient's psychosocial environment. Changes in relationships or other life events may precipitate depressive episodes; conversely, depressive episodes strain relationships and may lead to negative life events. The goal of treatment is to help the patient solve a crisis in his or her role functioning or social environment. Achieving this helps the patient to gain a sense of mastery over his or her functioning and relieves depressive symptoms.

Begun as a research intervention, IPT has only lately started to be disseminated among clinicians and in residency training programmes. The publication of efficacy data, the promulgation of practice guidelines that embrace IPT among antidepressant treatments, and economic pressures on length of treatment have led to increasing interest in IPT. This chapter describes the concepts and techniques of IPT and its current status of adaptation, efficacy data, and training. The chapter provides a guide to developments and a reference list, but not a comprehensive review.

## Background

IPT traces its theoretical and clinical origins to the interpersonal psychoanalytic theory of Meyer and Sullivan and builds on work of other relational theory including object relations, particularly with regard to attachment. However, it applies this theory within a conceptual and clinical framework that differs significantly from that of Sullivan and much of relational theory. In contrast with psychoanalytically inspired schools of thought, IPT sees its goals in treating depression and other medical disorders, rather than trying to change overall personality. Pragmatically, IPT opts to narrow its focus to address the area of interpersonal life that seems to require the most immediate attention.

Acknowledging the importance of personality and early experience, IPT emphasizes the role of recent stressful events in triggering depression and other psychiatric disorders in vulnerable individuals, while it also recognizes the protective role social supports play against psychopathology. Nevertheless, IPT is less interested in discerning the *cause* of a depressive episode (since it assumes the aetiology of depression to be multifactorial) than in using the connection between current life events and the onset of depressive symptoms to help the patient understand and combat the episode of illness.

Compared to other psychotherapies, such as psychoanalytic psychotherapy or even cognitive behavioural therapy, IPT is relatively young. It is less concerned about maintaining an established orthodoxy than about adapting itself to the needs of the patient. Although IPT theorists have taken into account theoretical developments in psychiatry and related fields, much of IPT's evolution has been based on the results of clinical trials. As investigations continue into IPT as a treatment for different disorders and populations, further modification of its theoretical aspects as well as techniques are likely.

## Indications

IPT research has demonstrated its efficacy for major depressive disorder across a range of patient ages and contexts, and for bulimia nervosa. One large trial indicates its efficacy (modified as interpersonal social rhythms therapy, or IPSRT) as an adjunctive treatment for bipolar disorder.[6] Lesser evidence suggests the potential benefits of IPT for several anxiety disorders.[21,22] IPT has shown no advantages over control psychotherapies for dysthymic disorder or substance abuse disorders.[14,20] For depressed adolescents, IPT has shown not only efficacy but effectiveness in a school-based programme.[10,11]

Both the physician and patient guides in primary care guidelines for depression list IPT, cognitive behavioural therapy (CBT), behavioural, brief dynamic, and marital therapy as treatments for depression. IPT is spreading from its initial research base in the United States. The IPT manual has been translated into Italian, German, Japanese, Spanish, and French, and is being used ever more widely around the world. Descriptions of IPT have appeared in Spanish, Norwegian, Finnish, and Dutch journals. An International Society for Interpersonal Psychotherapy, established at the American Psychiatric Association Annual meeting in May 2000 in Chicago, has a growing membership and biennial international meetings in 2004 and 2006, and maintains a bibliography of studies.

Because IPT focuses clinically on the social context of the depressive episode, researchers have sometimes adapted IPT when applying it to different treatment populations, developing manuals for different age groups or subpopulations, and occasionally adding focal problem areas. IPT has also been used at different lengths, in different formats, in one pilot couple's adaptation, and as a telephone intervention. Nonetheless, all these adaptations involve the basic principles that constitute IPT: a no-fault definition of the patient's problem as a medical illness, excusing the patient from blame for his or her symptoms; and a continual focus on the relationship between the patient's moods and life situation. The continuing growth of IPT research precludes an exhaustive description of studies. This chapter presents a selection of key research trials of IPT for mood and other disorders (see **Efficacy**) and offers selected references for further reading.

## Contraindications

Although formal contraindications (i.e. situations in which IPT would worsen the patients' situation) are not known, IPT was never intended to function as a monotherapy for patients with psychotic depression or bipolar disorder. In addition, three controlled trials have found no benefit of IPT as a treatment for substance use disorders.

## Conducting IPT

Each of the four IPT interpersonal problem areas has discrete goals for therapist and patient to pursue. The therapist helps the patient relate life events to mood and other symptoms. In this section we outline the phases of IPT, as well as common strategies and techniques used in IPT treatment. We also outline some differences with cognitive behavioural therapy, to which it is often compared.

### Phases of treatment

As an acute treatment, IPT has three phases. The *first phase*, generally covering sessions 1–3, includes diagnostic evaluation, psychiatric history, and setting the treatment framework. The therapist reviews symptoms, diagnoses the patient as depressed according to DSM-IV (or ICD-10) criteria, and gives the patient the sick role. The psychiatric history includes the 'interpersonal inventory', which is not a structured instrument but a careful review of the patient's past and current social functioning and close relationships, their patterns, and mutual expectations. The relationships are examined to see to what extent they are satisfactory, whether there have been recent changes in those relationships, or whether the patient desires to change them. As part of this review, the therapist commonly links the main social and interpersonal situations of the patient's life to the onset of depressive symptoms.

During the opening phase the therapist also sets a time limit for the acute treatment, generally between 12 and 16 sessions. The optimal number of sessions for IPT requires further research. One study suggests that as few as eight sessions may be effective for some patients, but similar to pharmacological treatment, different doses (i.e. number of IPT sessions) might be necessary for different patients. Sessions are generally scheduled weekly. This allows sufficient time to pass that things will happen in the patient's outside life, on which the treatment focuses. Yet it is frequent enough to maintain momentum and thematic continuity. However, in certain cases logistical difficulties (e.g. due to a general medical illness) might require less frequent sessions.

At the end of the first phase, the therapist links the depressive syndrome to the patient's interpersonal situation focusing on one of the four interpersonal problem areas: (1) *grief*; (2) interpersonal *role disputes*; (3) *role transitions*; or (4) *interpersonal deficits*. Once the patient explicitly accepts this formulation as the focus for treatment, IPT enters its middle phase.

It is important to keep treatment focused on a simple theme. Any formulation necessarily simplifies a patient's life narrative. Although some patients may present with multiple interpersonal problems, the goal of the formulation is to isolate one or, at most, two salient problems related to the patient's mood disorder (whether as precipitant or consequence). More than two foci would risk diffusing the treatment and diluting its efficacy. Sometimes a number of interpersonal problems contribute to the depressive episode, making it apparently difficult to choose a focus. However, research has shown that IPT therapists agree in choosing foci, and patients find those foci credible. Moreover, resolution of the interpersonal treatment focus appears to correlate with symptomatic improvement.

An important task of the initial phase requires deciding whether or not to use medication. A growing literature suggests that combined treatment with antidepressants and IPT works at least as well as, but is not always superior to IPT alone. Thus, except for very severe cases or possibly the elderly, the choice between IPT alone or combined with medication relies more on cost, availability of resources, and patients' preference than on existing empirical evidence.

The *middle phase* involves approaches specific to the chosen interpersonal problem area. For **Grief**—complicated bereavement following the death of a loved one—the therapist facilitates mourning and helps the patient find new activities and relationships to compensate for the loss. **Role disputes** are conflicts with significant others: a spouse, a child, other family members, co-workers, or a close friend. The therapist helps the patient explore the relationship, the nature of the dispute, and available options to negotiate its resolution, including ending the relationship. **Role transition** includes change in life status: for example, beginning or ending a relationship or career, moving, promotion, demotion, retirement, graduation, having a baby, or diagnosis of another medical illness. The patient learns to manage the change by mourning the loss of the old role, recognizing positive and negative aspects of the new role, and taking steps to master this new role.

**Interpersonal deficits** are used as a focus for patients who lack any of the first three focal life situations. Such patients are isolated or lack social skills, have problems in initiating or sustaining relationships. The goal is to help the patient to develop new relationships and skills. Some patients who fall into this category may in fact suffer from dysthymic disorder or social anxiety disorder, for which separate strategies have been developed.

The *final phase* of IPT, occupying the last 2–4 sessions of acute treatment, builds the patient's newly acquired sense of independence and competence by recognizing and consolidating therapeutic gains. Compared to psychodynamic psychotherapy, IPT de-emphasizes termination: it is a bitter–sweet graduation from successful treatment. The sadness of separating from the therapist is contrasted with depressive feelings.

If the patient has not improved, the therapist emphasizes that the *treatment* has failed, not the patient, and that alternative effective treatments, such as medication or other psychotherapies exist. If the treatment has succeeded, the therapist underscores the patient's competence to function without further therapy by emphasizing that the depressive episode has improved because of the patient's actions in changing a life situation. The therapist also helps the patient to anticipate triggers for and responses to depressive symptoms that might arise in the future.

Patients with multiple prior MDE's or significant residual symptoms, who successfully complete acute treatment but remain at high risk for relapse or recurrence, may contract for maintenance therapy as acute treatment draws to a close. At the end of the treatment (acute or maintenance, depending on the case) the patient is also explicitly told that, should depression recur, the patient should immediately seek treatment, just as the patient would do if any other medical illness recurred.

## Techniques

Readers new to IPT will find that much of what we describe below sounds familiar and overlaps with other psychotherapies. Thus, on one level, IPT demands few novel skills from therapists and is relatively easy to learn.

The challenges of IPT lie not in the use of any individual technique, but in organizing these approaches to establish and maintain a coherent primary treatment focus and to resist the temptations of digressing into clinical material outside that focus. Additional challenges may arise from 'unlearning' reflexive responses from prior training experiences such as making transference-focused interventions (for psychodynamic therapists) or identifying automatic cognitions and schemas (for cognitive therapists). In our exposition of strategies and techniques, we focus on major depressive disorder, the first and still best tested indication for IPT, although the same principles may apply to other disorders.

### (a) General strategies

IPT is organized around four important concepts.

### (i) Psychoeducation

The therapist helps the patient to recognize that the problem is a common medical illness, a mood disorder, with a predictable set of symptoms, not the personal failure or weakness of the patient. IPT therapists define depression as a treatable condition that is not the patient's fault. This definition displaces guilt from the patient to the illness, decreases the patient sense of isolation by feeling part of a larger group (those with depression), and provides hope for a response to treatment.

Underscoring this approach, IPT therapists give depressed patients the 'sick role'. This role temporarily excuses them from what their illness prevents them from doing while assigning them the task of working as patients in order to recover their previous healthy role. The resolution of the sick role is to regain the healthy, euthymic role by the end of treatment. The time-limited structure of IPT also energizes patients and protects against regression during treatment.

### (ii) Focusing on the positive

IPT therapists take an empathic, supportive, and encouraging stance. They emphasize their patients' successes, although they also commiserate on their difficulties. 'Focusing on the positive' means underscoring positive events; it does *not* mean ignoring negative affect. By doing this, IPT therapists may facilitate the therapeutic alliance that is crucial to good outcome. By solving an interpersonal crisis—a complicated bereavement, a role dispute or transition, or an interpersonal deficit—the IPT patient has the dual opportunity to improve his or her life situation and simultaneously relieve the symptoms of the depressive episode.

This coupled formula, validated by randomized controlled trials in which IPT has been tested, can be offered with confidence and optimism. Symptomatic relief may correlate with the degree to which the patient solves his or her interpersonal crisis. This therapeutic optimism, while not specific to IPT, very likely provides part of its power in remoralizing the patient.

### (iii) Focus on the present, not the past

IPT deals with current rather than past interpersonal relationships, focusing on the patient's immediate social context. The IPT therapist attempts to intervene in depressive symptom formation and social dysfunction rather than addressing enduring aspects of personality, which are difficult to assess accurately during an episode of an Axis I disorder. However, IPT does build new social skills such as self-assertion and increased ability to understand interpersonal exchanges, which may be as valuable as changing personality traits.

### (iv) Link mood to life events

A core strategy of IPT is constant attention to the link between the patient's current mood state and recent interpersonal experiences. Stressful life events and negative interpersonal encounters trigger lower mood and can lead to depressive episodes in vulnerable individuals. Conversely, depressed mood impairs social functioning, which can lead to further negative life events. IPT is postulated to work by helping the patients manage interpersonal relationships more effectively, which leads to improved mood. Improved mood then allows patients to more effectively manage interpersonal experiences in an iterative fashion.

Unlike psychodynamic psychotherapy, IPT *does not* focus on early childhood experiences and long-standing familial dynamics.

Thus, the patient's current mood state is linked to recent experiences rather than those rooted in the distant past. Nor does IPT focus on transferential material, except in the relatively rare instance when problems arise in the therapeutic alliance. Thus the treatment highlights recent experiences outside the office.

### (b) Specific techniques

To achieve the general goals of IPT, the following techniques are frequently used:

1 *An opening question*: 'how have things been since we last met?', which leads the patient to provide an interval history of mood and events. The therapist begins each session after the first one with this tactic. It is common, particularly at the beginning of the treatment that the patient will focus exclusively either on the mood or on a recent event. When that occurs, the therapist gently asks about the other aspect and helps the patient connect mood and recent events.

2 *Communication analysis*, a detailed recreation of recent, affectively charged circumstances. This detailed analysis often helps the patient uncover nuances of the interpersonal exchanges that had been missed prior to the session.

3 An exploration of the patient's wishes and options, to help the patient realize and voice the desired outcomes.

4 *Decision analysis*, to help the patient integrate communication analysis, the wishes and options and the constraints of the situation and decide on a specific course of action.

5 *Role-playing*, to help the patient rehearse that course of action before implementing in real life.

## Similarities and differences with other psychotherapies

Because IPT and CBT are the two best empirically supported psychotherapies, they are often compared. [23] IPT shares with CBT an orientation towards making the patient feel understood, a 'here and now' focus, a general feeling of hope and optimism, psychoeducation, and the use of role-playing to favour the acquisition of new skills. It addresses interpersonal issues in a manner familiar to marital therapists. Although like CBT a time-limited treatment targeting a syndromal constellation (e.g. major depression), IPT is considerably less structured, and focuses on interpersonal problem areas rather than automatic thoughts. IPT overlaps to some degree with psychodynamic psychotherapies, yet IPT also meaningfully differs from them: in its focus on the present, not the past; its focus on practical, real-life change rather than self-understanding; its medical model; and its avoidance of the transference and of genetic and dream interpretations.

## Efficacy

### Research findings: IPT for mood disorders

IPT outcome research is ongoing, with new studies published every year. What follows is a selection of key research trials of IPT for mood and other disorders. For some of these trials, IPT was adapted in a separate treatment manual, but in all cases the general principles of the treatment remained the same.

### (a) Acute treatment of major depression

IPT was first tested as an acute antidepressant treatment in a four-cell, 16-week randomized trial. This compared weekly IPT, amitriptyline (AMI), their combination, and a monthly supportive psychotherapy treatment for 81 outpatients with major depression.[24,25] The outcome of patients receiving amitriptyline and IPT was similar and superior to that of supportive psychotherapy. Patients who received both amitriptyline and IPT had better depression outcomes and better scores on a range of social adjustment measures including overall adjustment, work performance, and communication than those on amitriptyline alone, suggesting an additive effect of IPT on medication treatment. At 1-year follow-up, many patients sustained improvement from the brief IPT intervention, and IPT patients had developed significantly better psychosocial functioning whether or not they received medication. This effect on social function was not found for AMI alone and had not been evident for IPT at the end of the 16-week trial.

Still probably the most important study to date involving IPT is the National Institute of Mental Health Treatment of Depression[24,25] Collaborative Research Program (TDCRP), investigators randomly assigned 250 outpatients with major depression to 16 weeks of IPT, CBT, or either imipramine (IMI) or placebo with clinical management.[2] Most subjects completed at least 15 weeks or 12 treatment sessions. Patients with milder depression (defined as a 17-item Hamilton Depression Rating Scale [HDRS] score <20) improved equally in all four treatments. For more severely depressed patients (HDRS>20), IMI worked fastest and most consistently better than placebo. IPT and IMI were comparable on several outcome measures, including HDRS, and superior to placebo for more severely depressed patients. In some analyses, IPT appeared to be slightly superior to CBT. CBT was not superior to placebo among the more depressed patients.

A follow-up study of TDCRP subjects 18 months later found no significant difference in recovery among remitters (who had minimal or no symptoms after the end of treatment, sustained during follow-up) among the four treatments.[26] Thirty per cent of CBT, 26 per cent of IPT, 19 per cent of imipramine, and 20 per cent of placebo subjects initially randomized to those treatments remitted and remained in remission during that time span. Among acute remitters, relapse over the 18-month follow-up was 36 per cent for CBT, 33 per cent for IPT, 50 per cent for imipramine (medication having been stopped at 16 weeks), and 33 per cent for placebo. The authors concluded that, for many patients, 16 weeks of specific treatments were insufficient to achieve full and lasting recovery.

## Special populations and settings

### (a) Depressed primary care patients

There has been a study comparing IPT and nortriptyline with usual care for depressed patients in a primary care setting. If patients were hospitalized for a general medical condition, IPT was continued in the hospital when possible. Depressive symptom severity declined more rapidly with either nortriptyline or IPT than in usual care. Approximately 70 per cent of treatment completers receiving nortriptyline or IPT, but only 20 per cent in usual care, had recovered after 8 months. Subjects with a lifetime history of comorbid panic disorder had a poorer response across treatments, compared to those with major depression alone.

### (b) Depressed HIV-positive patients (IPT-HIV)

IPT has also been investigated for depressed HIV patients (IPT-HIV), emphasizing common issues among this population including concerns about illness and death, grief and role transitions. A randomized study echoing the TDCRP of 101 HIV-positive patients with depressive symptoms found IPT and imipramine each superior to CBT and supportive therapy. Many patients reported improvement in depressive physical symptoms that they had mistakenly attributed to HIV infection. IPT may have been a better fit than CBT for these patients due to the extreme life events they faced at the height of the HIV epidemic.

### (c) Peripartum depression

Pregnancy and the postpartum also provide natural role transitions as an IPT focus. Exploring these role transitions addresses the depressed pregnant woman's self-evaluation as a parent, physiologic changes of pregnancy and postpartum, and altered relationships with the spouse or significant other and with other children. Timing and duration of sessions are adjusted in response to bedrest, delivery, obstetrical complications, and childcare. Postpartum mothers may bring children to sessions. As with depressed HIV-positive patients, telephone sessions, and hospital visits are sometimes necessary. A controlled clinical trial comparing IPT to a didactic parent education group in depressed pregnant women showed advantages for IPT. A study of depressed postpartum women found superiority of IPT over a wait-list control group. A small randomized trial has also suggested the possibility that group IPT may serve to prevent MDD relapse during the postpartum period.

### (d) Conjoint IPT for depressed patients with marital disputes (IPT-CM)

Marital conflict can precipitate or complicate depressive episodes. Some clinicians believe that individual psychotherapy for patients in marital disputes may lead to premature rupture of marriages. Researchers at Yale University developed a manual for conjoint therapy of depressed patients with marital disputes (IPT-CM). IPT-CM includes the spouse in all sessions and focuses on the current marital dispute. Eighteen patients with major depression linked to the onset or exacerbation of marital disputes were randomly assigned to 16 weeks of either individual IPT or IPT-CM. Patients in both treatments showed similar reductions in depressive symptoms, but patients receiving IPT-CM reported significantly better marital adjustment, marital affection, and sexual relations. These pilot findings require replication with a larger sample and other control groups.

### (e) Depressed adolescents (IPT-A)

IPT has also been modified to incorporate adolescent developmental issues. Three randomized trials, one of them conducted in Puerto Rico, have shown the efficacy of IPT-A. It is important to note that in the Puerto Rico study, the only one that also included CBT in the design, IPT appeared superior to CBT in certain measures (e.g. self-esteem and social adaptation), consistent with the findings of the TDCRP and the study of depressed HIV-positive patients.

### (f) Maintenance treatment

Based on the success of IPT as acute treatment for MDD, the recurrent nature of mood disorders, and the efficacy of medication in preventing relapse and recurrence, IPT was adapted as a once monthly maintenance treatment for MDD (IPT-M). This was a novel development and allowed the first real testing of psychotherapy as a maintenance treatment for patients who had remitted from acute depression. Since IPT-M begins with patients who have remitted, its goal is to maintain the remitted state. Both patient and therapist are vigilant for early signs of interpersonal problems similar to those of which the patient and therapist previously identified as associated with the onset of the patient's most recent depressive episode. At the same time, the therapist works to enhance strengths that appear to have been present prior to the patient's illness or began to emerge as the most recent depressive episode remitted. In contrast with the acute phase application of IPT, which usually focuses on one or at most two interpersonal problem areas, IPT-M may shift problem areas over time. Three studies have compared medication and IPT as maintenance treatment for MDD.

In the first study, 128 outpatients with recurrent depression initially treated with combined high dose (>200 mg/day) imipramine and weekly sessions of IPT. [4,5] Responders remained on high-dosage medication while IPT was tapered to a monthly frequency during a 4-month continuation phase. Patients who remained remitted were then randomly assigned to 3 years of either: (1) imipramine plus clinical management; (2) imipramine plus monthly IPT; (3) monthly IPT alone; (4) monthly IPT plus placebo; or (5) placebo plus clinical management.

Both IPT and imipramine were significantly superior to the placebo group in delaying MDD relapse. Imipramine was superior to IPT-M in the ability to prevent relapse. The group that received IPT with imipramine had a numerically lower rate of recurrence at 1 year (16 per cent) than the group on imipramine alone (40 per cent), but those results were not statistically significant. Two different studies have had very similar findings in comparisons of IPT and nortriptyline for geriatric patients with recurrent major depression. [7,27]

Further study is required to determine the efficacy of IPT relative to newer medications (e.g. selective serotonin-reuptake inhibitors), and the efficacy of dosages other than once monthly maintenance IPT. A study of differing doses of maintenance IPT for depressed patients in Pittsburgh has not found differences in outcome based on frequency of sessions.[28] Perhaps optimal dosing of maintenance IPT depends on individual patients' needs.

The success of IPT in treating MDD has led researchers to investigate its efficacy in bipolar and dysthymic disorder.

### (i) Bipolar disorder

The modification of IPT used as an adjunct to medication in the treatment of bipolar disorder is called interpersonal and social rhythm therapy (IPSRT). Its use rests on the hypothesis that disruptions of social rhythms are destabilizing for bipolar patients and contribute to trigger their relapse. By decreasing the number and intensity of those disruptions, IPSRT should improve the course of bipolar disorder. The behavioural component helps to protect sleep patterns and limit the disruptions that may provoke mania; the IPT approach to depression remains largely the same.

After stabilizing bipolar I patients with appropriate pharmacotherapy and either IPSRT or intensive clinical management, patients were randomized again to either IPSRT or clinical management for preventive treatment.[6] They found that participants assigned to IPSRT acutely had longer survival times to a new affective episode, irrespective of maintenance treatment assignment. Participants in the IPSRT group had higher regularity of social rhythms at the end of the acute treatment, and this increased regularity of social rhythms during the acute treatment mediated the reduced likelihood of recurrence during the maintenance treatment. Further research appears necessary to more firmly establish the optimal timing and treatment duration of IPSRT.

### (ii) Dysthymic disorder

A modification of IPT for dysthymic disorder[29] encourages patients to reconceptualize what they have considered their lifelong character flaws as ego-dystonic, chronic mood-dependent symptoms: as chronic but treatable 'state' rather than immutable 'trait'.

Three randomized trials have examined the efficacy of IPT in dysthymic disorder. In the first study, 35 patients with an ICD-10 diagnosis of dysthymia with or without comorbid MDD were randomized to moclobemide alone ($n = 19$) or moclobemide plus IPT ($n = 16$). Patients were assessed with the 17-item Hamilton Rating Scales for Depression (HAM-D), the Global Assessment Scale (GAS), and the Quality of Life and Satisfaction Questionnaire at baseline, 12, 24, and 48 weeks. Both groups showed statistically significant improvement in all measures across time. There were no differences between the two treatments at week 12. However, patients in the combined group had statistically better scores than the patients in the moclobemide group on all outcome variables at weeks 24 and 48.

In the second study, 707 adults in primary care clinic with DSM-IV dysthymic disorder were randomized, with or without past and/or current MDD (15 per cent of the sample had current MDD), to treatment with sertraline alone (50–200 mg), IPT alone (10 sessions), or sertraline with IPT combined.[30] At the end of treatment, response rates were 60 per cent for sertraline alone, 47 per cent for IPT alone, and 58 per cent for sertraline with IPT. After an additional 18-month naturalistic follow-up phase, there were no statistically significant differences in symptom reduction between sertraline alone and sertraline with IPT. However, both were more effective than IPT alone in reducing depressive symptoms. It is important to note, though, that IPT was given as a brief treatment, while sertraline was generally continued for the full 2 years of the study.

A third study compared IPT adapted for the treatment of dysthymia (IPT-D), brief supportive psychotherapy, sertraline, and combined IPT-D/sertraline for patients with pure dysthymic disorder (i.e. without 'double' depression) in 94 subjects treated over 16 weeks.[14] Patients improved in all conditions, with the cells including sertraline pharmacotherapy showing superiority over psychotherapy alone in response and remission. The results of this study are consistent with an emerging literature suggesting that pharmacotherapy may acutely benefit patients more than psychotherapy. In conjunction with the other studies in patients with dysthymic disorder, it suggests that IPT alone may not be an efficacious treatment for dysthymic disorder.

## IPT for non-mood disorders

The efficacy of IPT as an antidepressant treatment has led to its adaptation as a treatment for other psychiatric disorders, based on the premise that life events are ubiquitous.

### (a) Bulimia

Fairburn *et al.* modified IPT for the treatment of bulimia, eliminating the use of the sick role and of role-playing in order to contrast distinct therapeutic strategies in comparing IPT and CBT. Initial trials showed that although CBT worked faster to relieve bulimic symptoms, IPT had longer-term benefits comparable to CBT and superior to a behavioural control condition.[1] A subsequent multisite trial found CBT superior to IPT.[9]

Following a model closer to the original IPT principles, Wilfley *et al.* modified IPT in a group format (IPT-G) and compared it to group CBT and a wait-list control for 56 women with non-purging bulimia.[8] The initial IPT phase was conducted individually. The interpersonal area for almost of all subjects was formulated as 'interpersonal deficits'. At termination, binge eating decreased in the IPT-G and CBT groups, but not in the control condition. Results persisted at 1-year follow-up. A randomized clinical trial of 162 women, comparing group IPT, and CBT for 20 sessions over 20 weeks, yielded similar results.

A research group in Christchurch, New Zealand studied the application of IPT to anorexia nervosa.[19] In their trial, neither IPT nor CBT showed efficacy as an outpatient treatment, consistent with the general anorexia outcome literature.

#### (b) Anxiety disorders

IPT has not yet been tested in controlled studies for anxiety disorders. Promising results have been found in for social anxiety disorders, PTSD, and panic disorder.[22, 31–33] Several groups are currently conducting controlled trials for these disorders.

#### (c) Substance abuse

IPT has failed to demonstrate efficacy in three clinical trials for patients with substance dependence.[20, 34, 35] These negative studies suggest limits to the range of utility of IPT as a main treatment for substance use disorders, but do not necessarily preclude its use to treat MDD comorbidity in those patients.

#### (d) Other applications

Research groups are testing the applicability of IPT to body dysmorphic disorder, chronic somatization in primary care patients, depressed patients postmyocardial infarction, depressed cancer patients, borderline personality disorder, insomnia, and other disorders. The IPT focus on life events suggests its potential applicability to patients with medical illness.

#### (e) IPT by telephone

Because many patients avoid or have difficulty reaching an office for face-to-face treatment, IPT and IPC are being tested as a treatment delivered over the telephone. Weissman and Miller conducted a successful pilot feasibility trial comparing IPT by telephone to wait-list control in 30 patients with recurrent major depression, and found IPT to be the superior control condition in reducing depressive symptoms and improving psychosocial functioning.[36] Neugebauer and colleagues found telephone IPC a helpful intervention for women with subsyndromal depression following a miscarriage.[37, 38]

#### (f) Interpersonal counselling (IPC)

Many patients presenting for treatment, particularly outside mental health settings, report psychiatric symptoms but do not meet threshold criteria for a psychiatric disorder. Nonetheless, their symptoms can be debilitating, interfering with their daily functioning, and often result in increased use of general medical services. Interpersonal counselling (IPC), based on IPT, was designed to treat distressed primary care patients who do not meet full syndromal criteria for psychiatric disorders. IPC is administered for a maximum of six sessions by health care usually by professionals who lack formal psychiatric training such as nurse practitioners. The first session can last up to 30 min; subsequent sessions are briefer.

IPC therapists assess the patient's current functioning, recent life events, occupational and familial stressors, and changes in interpersonal relationships. They assume that such events provide the context in which emotional and bodily symptoms occur. Klerman and colleagues studied 128 patients in a primary care clinic who scored 6 or higher on the Goldberg General Health Questionnaire (GHQ), randomizing them to IPC or to usual care without psychological treatment.[39] Over an average of 3 months, often receiving only one or two IPC sessions, IPC subjects showed significantly greater symptom relief on the GHQ than controls, especially mood improvement. IPC subjects were more likely to subsequently make use of mental health services, suggesting a new awareness of the psychological aspect of their symptoms.

### Predictors of response to IPT

Five studies have examined predictors of response to IPT. Analyses of the TDCRP data identified general predictors of response to MDD treatment, as well as predictors for specific treatment modalities.[40,41] Seven patient characteristics predicted outcome across treatments: social dysfunction (higher social function predicted better response), cognitive dysfunction (better cognitive function predicted better response, particularly to CBT), expectation of improvement (higher expectation predicted better response), therapeutic alliance (a stronger alliance predicted better response), endogeneity of depression (endogenous depression tended to have better response, a finding supported by another study examining the relationship between EEG patterns and response to IPT in depressed patients[42]), double depression (its presence predicted poorer outcome), personality traits (their presence predicted worse response), and duration of current episode (longer duration was associated to worse response). In addition prior social adjustment, as measured by previous attainment of a marital relationship and higher satisfaction with social relationships in general, differentially predicted good response to IPT. This finding is consistent with reports in the general psychotherapy literature documenting that various indicators higher baseline psychosocial functioning predict good psychotherapy response. Two other studies suggest that comorbidity tends to worsen the prognosis of treatment with IPT alone, but not the prognosis of combined treatment.[43,44]

### Summary of research findings

IPT has demonstrated efficacy as an acute and maintenance monotherapy and as a component of combined treatment for major depressive disorder. It also appears to have utility for other mood and non-mood syndromes, although the evidence for these is sparser. It has not shown benefit for substance use disorders or as a monotherapy for dysthymic disorder. Since monotherapy with either IPT or pharmacotherapy is likely to suffice for most patients with major depressive disorder, combined treatment is probably best reserved for severely or chronically ill patients. How best to combine time-limited psychotherapy with pharmacotherapy—for which patients, in what sequence, etc.—is an exciting area for future research.

## Training

Until recently, IPT therapists were few, and practiced almost exclusively in research studies. Publications supporting its efficacy have led to clinical demand for this empirically supported treatment. IPT training is now increasingly included in professional workshops and conferences, with training courses conducted at University centres in Canada, the United Kingdom, continental Europe, Asia, New Zealand, and Australia. IPT is taught in a small but growing minority of psychiatric residency training programmes in the United States and as well as some family practice and primary care training programmes.

Although the principles and practice of IPT are relatively straightforward, any psychotherapy requires innate therapeutic ability, comfort with the so-called common factors of psychotherapy: tolerating and exploring affect, helping the patient to feel understood, engendering hope, etc. IPT training requires more than reading the manual: psychotherapy is learned by doing. Most IPT training programmes are designed to help experienced therapists refocus their treatment by learning new techniques, not to teach novices psychotherapy. Candidates should have a graduate clinical degree (MD, Ph.D., MSW, RN), several years of experience conducting psychotherapy, and clinical familiarity with the diagnosis of patients they plan to treat.

The IPT training in the TDCRP became the model for subsequent research studies. It included a brief didactic programme, reading the manual, and a practicum in which the therapist treated 2–3 patients under close supervision monitored by videotapes of the sessions. For research certification, we continue to recommend at least two or three successfully treated cases with hour for hour supervision of taped sessions.

Although many clinicians would like a formal certificate or diploma in IPT, there is no gold standard of IPT proficiency and no accrediting board. When IPT practice was limited to research settings, this posed no problem: one research group taught another, in the manner described above. As IPT spreads in clinical practice, the educational and accreditation process for IPT requires further study. The newly created International Society for Interpersonal Psychotherapy (ISIPT) may provide an appropriate forum in which to discuss these increasingly important issues.

## Future directions

The history of IPT has been a succession of outcome trials. These studies have helped to define diagnostic indications for this treatment, but we know far less about the dosage and indications of IPT than about antidepressant medication. Future outcome trials may continue to define the scope of efficacy (response to treatment under ideal conditions) and effectiveness (response to treatment in more general clinical settings) of IPT. These should include both tests for different diagnoses, such as the anxiety disorders, testing of dosage—optimal frequency and duration of IPT sessions—and also studies of the sequencing of IPT with other treatments. Other research may help to determine the cost-effectiveness and potential cost-offset of IPT as a treatment that improves both symptoms and social functioning.

Most of the work on IPT to date has focused on treatment outcome. By contrast, little is known about the process aspects in IPT such as the specific value of many IPT interventions. Although it appears that solving an interpersonal problem area correlates with treatment outcome, it is unclear, for example, whether the choice of a particular treatment focus over other makes a difference for patients, or whether particular sorts of life events are helpful or unhelpful foci. Patient and therapist characteristics may also potentially influence treatment outcome.

Finally, while the initial work on IPT was conducted in the United States, over the last few years, IPT trials have also been conducted in other countries. As those studies continue to be conducted, it will become easier to discern to what extent IPT addresses topics are universal across cultures.

In summary, IPT is a time-limited, forward-looking, pragmatically focused psychotherapy that defines psychiatric disorders as treatable medical illnesses and links them to the patient's current social situation. This strategy has proved efficacious for patients with major depression and bulimia, and shows promise for other mood and non-mood disorders.

## Further information

Elkin, I., Shea, M.T., Watkins, J.T., et al. (1989). National Institute of Mental Health treatment of depression collaborative research program: general effectiveness of treatments. *Archives of General Psychiatry*, **46**, 971–82.

Weissman, M.M., Markowitz, J.C., and Klerman, G.L. (2000). *Comprehensive guide to interpersonal psychotherapy*. Basic Books, New York.

Weissman, M.M., Markowitz, J.C., and Klerman, G.L. (2007). *Clinician's quick guide to interpersonal psychotherapy*. Oxford University Press, New York.

Website of the International Society of Interpersonal Psychotherapy: http://www.interpersonalpsychotherapy.org/

## References

1. Fairburn, C.G., Jones, R., Peveler, R.C., et al. (1993). Psychotherapy and bulimia nervosa. Longer-term effects of interpersonal psychotherapy, behavior therapy, and cognitive behavior therapy. *Archives of General Psychiatry*, **50**(6), 419–28.

2. Elkin, I., Shea, M.T., Watkins, J.T., et al. (1989). National Institute of Mental Health Treatment of Depression Collaborative Research Program. General effectiveness of treatments. *Archives of General Psychiatry*, **46**(11), 971–82; discussion 983.

3. Klerman, G.L. and Weissmann, M.M. (1987). Interpersonal psychotherapy (IPT) and drugs in the treatment of depression. *Pharmacopsychiatry*, **20**(1), 3–7.

4. Frank, E., Kupfer, D.J., Wagner, E.F., et al. (1991). Efficacy of interpersonal psychotherapy as a maintenance treatment for recurrent depression: contributing factors. *Archives of General Psychiatry*, **48**, 1053–9.

5. Frank, E., Kupfer, D.J., Perel, J.M., et al. (1990). Three-year outcomes for maintenance therapies in recurrent depression. *Archives of General Psychiatry*, **47**(12), 1093–9.

6. Frank, E., Kupfer, D.J., Thase, M.E., et al. (2005). Two-year outcomes for interpersonal and social rhythm therapy in individuals with bipolar I disorder. *Archives of General Psychiatry*, **62**(9), 996–1004.

7. Reynolds, C.F. III, Frank, E., Perel, J.M., et al. (1999). Nortriptyline and interpersonal psychotherapy as maintenance therapies for recurrent major depression: a randomized controlled trial in patients older than 59 years. *The Journal of the American Medical Association*, **281**(1), 39–45.

8. Wilfley, D.E., Welch, R.R., Stein, R.L., et al. (2002). A randomized comparison of group cognitive-behavioral therapy and group interpersonal psychotherapy for the treatment of overweight individuals with binge-eating disorder. *Archives of General Psychiatry*, **59**(8), 713–21.

9. Agras, W.S., Walsh, B.T., Fairburn, C.G., et al. (2000). A multicenter comparison of cognitive-behavioral therapy and interpersonal psychotherapy for bulimia nervosa. *Archives of General Psychiatry,* **57**(5), 459–66.

10. Mufson, L., Dorta, K.P., Wickramaratne, P., et al. (2004). A randomized effectiveness trial of interpersonal psychotherapy for depressed adolescents. *Archives of General Psychiatry,* **61**, 577–84.

11. Mufson, L., Weissman, M.M., Moreau, D., et al. (1999). Efficacy of interpersonal psychotherapy for depressed adolescents. *Archives of General Psychiatry,* **56**(6), 573–9.

12. Frank, E., Cyranowski, J.M., Rucci, P., et al. (2002). Clinical significance of lifetime panic spectrum symptoms in the treatment of patients with bipolar I disorder. *Archives of General Psychiatry,* **59**(10), 905–11.

13. Markowitz, J.C. (1994). Psychotherapy of dysthymia. *American Journal of Psychiatry,* **151**, 1114–21.

14. Markowitz, J.C., Kocsis, J.H., Bleiberg, K.L., et al. (2005). A comparative trial of psychotherapy and pharmacotherapy for "pure" dysthymic patients. *Journal of Affective Disorders,* **89**(1–3), 167–75.

15. Markowitz, J.C., Svartberg, M., and Swartz, H.A. (1998). Treatment of HIV-positive patients with depressive symptoms. *Archives of General Psychiatry,* **55**, 452–7.

16. Spinelli, M.G. (1997). Interpersonal psychotherapy for depressed antepartum women: a pilot study. *The American Journal of Psychiatry,* **154**(7), 1028–30.

17. Spinelli, M.G. and Endicott, J. (2003). Controlled clinical trial of interpersonal psychotherapy versus parenting education program for depressed pregnant women. *The American Journal of Psychiatry,* **160**(3), 555–62.

18. Schulberg, H.C., Block, M.R., Madonia, M.J., et al. (1996). Treating major depression in primary care practice. Eight-month clinical outcomes. *Archives of General Psychiatry,* **53**(10), 913–9.

19. McIntosh, V.V., Jordan, J., Carter, F.A., et al. (2005). Three psychotherapies for anorexia nervosa: a randomized, controlled trial. *The American Journal of Psychiatry,* **162**(4), 741–7.

20. Rounsaville, B.J., Glazer, W., Wilber, C.H., et al. (1983). Short-term interpersonal psychotherapy in methadone-maintained opiate addicts. *Archives of General Psychiatry,* **40**(6), 629–36.

21. Lipsitz, J.D., Fyer, A.J., Markowitz, J.C., et al. (1999). Open trial of interpersonal psychotherapy for the treatment of social phobia. *The American Journal of Psychiatry,* **156**(11), 1814–16.

22. Bleiberg, K.L. and Markowitz, J.C. (2005). A pilot study of interpersonal psychotherapy for posttraumatic stress disorder. *The American Journal of Psychiatry,* **162**(1), 181–3.

23. Markowitz, J.C., Svartberg, M., and Swartz, H.A. (1998). Is IPT time-limited psychodynamic psychotherapy? *Journal of Psychother Practice and Research,* **7**(3), 185–95.

24. DiMascio, A., Weissman, M.M., Prusoff, B.A., et al. (1979). Differential symptom reduction by drugs and psychotherapy in acute depression. *Archives of General Psychiatry,* **36**(13), 1450–6.

25. Weissman, M.M. (1979). The psychological treatment of depression. Evidence for the efficacy of psychotherapy alone, in comparison with, and in combination with pharmacotherapy. *Archives of General Psychiatry,* **36**(11), 1261–9.

26. Shea, M.T., Elkin, I., Imber, S.D., et al. (1992). Course of depressive symptoms over follow-up. Findings from the National Institute of Mental Health Treatment of Depression Collaborative Research Program. *Archives of General Psychiatry,* **49**(10), 782–7.

27. Reynolds, C.F. III, Frank, E., Kupfer, D.J., et al. (1996). Treatment outcome in recurrent major depression: a post hoc comparison of elderly ("young old") and midlife patients. *The American Journal of Psychiatry,* **153**(10), 1288–92.

28. Frank, E., Kupfer, D.J., Buysse, D.J., et al. (2007). Randomized trial of weekly, twice-monthly, and monthly interpersonal psychotherapy as maintenance treatment for women with recurrent depression. *The American Journal of Psychiatry,* **164**(5), 761–7.

29. De Mello, M.F., Myczcowisk, L.M., and Menezes, P.R. (2001). A randomized controlled trial comparing moclobemide and moclobemide plus interpersonal psychotherapy in the treatment of dysthymic disorder. *Journal of Psychother Practice Research,* **10**(2), 117–23.

30. Browne, G., Steiner, M., Roberts, J., et al. (2002). Sertraline and/or interpersonal psychotherapy for patients with dysthymic disorder in primary care: 6-month comparison with longitudinal 2-year follow-up of effectiveness and costs. *Journal of Affective Disorders,* **68**(2–3), 317–30.

31. Lipsitz, J.D., Gur, M., Miller, N.L., et al. (2006). An open pilot study of interpersonal psychotherapy for panic disorder (IPT-PD). *The Journal of Nervous and Mental Disease,* **194**(6), 440–5.

32. Lipsitz, J.D., Gur, M., Vermes, D., et al. (2007). A randomized trial of interpersonal therapy versus supportive therapy for social anxiety disorder. *Depression and Anxiety,* **25**(6), 542–53

33. Lipsitz, J.D., Fyer, A.J., Markowitz, J.C, (1999). Open trial of interpersonal psychotherapy for the treatment of social phobia. *The American Journal of Psychiatry,* **156**(11), 1814–6.

34. Carroll, K.M., Fenton, L.R., Ball, S.A., et al. (2004). Efficacy of disulfiram and cognitive behavior therapy in cocaine-dependent outpatients: a randomized placebo-controlled trial. *Archives of General Psychiatry,* **61**(3), 264–72.

35. Carroll, K.M., Rounsaville, B.J., and Gawin, F.H. (1991). A comparative trial of psychotherapies for ambulatory cocaine abusers: relapse prevention and interpersonal psychotherapy. *The American Journal of Drug Alcohol Abuse,* **17**(3), 229–47.

36. Miller, L. and Weissman, M. (2002). Interpersonal psychotherapy delivered over the telephone to recurrent depressives. A pilot study. *Depression and Anxiety,* **16**(3), 114–7.

37. Neugebauer, R., Kilne, J., Bleiberg, K., et al. (2007). Preliminary open trial of interpersonal counseling for subsyndromal depression following miscarriage. *Depression and Anxiety,* **24**(3), 219–22.

38. Neugebauer, R., Kline, J., Markowitz, J.C., et al. (2006). Pilot randomized controlled trial of interpersonal counseling for subsyndromal depression following miscarriage. *The Journal of Clinical Psychiatry,* **67**(8), 1299–304.

39. Klerman, G.L., Budman, S., Berwisk, D., et al. (1987). Efficacy of a brief psychosocial intervention for symptoms of stress and distress among patients in primary care. *Medical Care,* **25**(11), 1078–88.

40. Sotsky, S.M., Glasss, D.J., Shear, M.T., et al. (1991). Patient predictors of response to psychotherapy and pharmacotherapy: findings in the NIMH Treatment of Depression Collaborative Research Program. *The American Journal of Psychiatry,* **148**(8), 997–1008.

41. Barber, J.P. and Muenz, L.R. (1996). The role of avoidance and obsessiveness in matching patients to cognitive and interpersonal psychotherapy: empirical findings from the treatment for depression collaborative research program. *Journal of Consulting & Clinical Psychology,* **64**(5), 951–8.

42. Thase, M.E., Buysse, D.J., Frank, E., et al. (1997). Which depressed patients will respond to interpersonal psychotherapy? The role of abnormal EEG sleep profiles. *The American Journal of Psychiatry,* **154**(4), 502–9.

43. Frank, E., Shear, M.K., Rucci, P., et al. (2000). Influence of panic-agoraphobic spectrum symptoms on treatment response in patients with recurrent major depression. *The American Journal of Psychiatry,* **157**(7), 1101–7.

44. Brown, C., Suhulberg, H.C., Madonia, M.J., et al. (1996). Treatment outcomes for primary care patients with major depression and lifetime anxiety disorders. *The American Journal of Psychiatry,* **153**(10), 1293–300.

# 6.3.4 Brief individual psychodynamic psychotherapy

Amy M. Ursano and Robert J. Ursano

## Introduction

Interest in brief dynamic psychotherapy has flourished in recent years. The psychodynamic psychotherapies, including brief psychodynamic psychotherapy, aim to change behaviour through new understanding and the recognition of maladaptive patterns of behaviour enacted since childhood but not previously observed. Through this process, perceptions, expectations, beliefs, and, therefore, behaviours and feelings are altered.[1]

Historically, 'brief psychotherapy' and 'long-term psychotherapy' were used synonymously with 'supportive' and 'explorative' psychotherapy, respectively. However, brief and long-term describe only the duration rather than the technique, focus, or goal of treatment.[2] The time limits of brief dynamic psychotherapy give it a unique character and distinguish it from long-term psychotherapy and psychoanalysis. Because of its limited goals, the brief dynamic psychotherapist must confront his or her ambitiousness and perfectionism as well as any exaggerated ideal of personality structure and function.

Psychotherapy in general, and brief individual psychodynamic psychotherapy in particular, is perhaps the most elegant form of micro-neurosurgery. Psychotherapy strives to alter behaviour (i.e. cognitions, affects, and actions) with verbal interchange—fundamentally to change neurone A that used to connect to neurone B so it will now connect to neurone C. Although the therapist in the individual psychodynamically derived psychotherapies does not 'require' behavioural change, the end result of the therapist's technical expertise is to achieve behavioural change, including changes in well-being, physical health, social supports, and societal productivity as well as symptomatic relief. As in all of medicine, both non-specific and specific curative factors affect the outcome of this work. The non-specific curative factors—abreaction, the provision of new information, and maximizing success experiences—are present in all forms of medical treatment including brief psychotherapy. Brief individual dynamic psychotherapy also has specific technical interventions and procedures above and beyond the non-specific curative factors. As in other medical therapies, there are contraindications and dangers in the use of this treatment.

## Background

Evolving from psychoanalysis in the mid-twentieth century, brief individual psychodynamic psychotherapy, like other psychodynamic treatments, is based on the principle that meanings and past experience play an important role in behaviour and illness. Although psychoanalysis is now a lengthy procedure usually requiring a number of years to complete, the early psychoanalytic literature, including Freud's first cases, contain histories of successful short analyses. During the first 30 years of psychoanalysis, it was unusual for treatments to extend beyond 1 year.[3] Ferenczi was the first analyst to advocate shortening psychoanalysis. He advocated

'active therapy' a more directive, focused, and briefer treatment. Rank was the first one to explicitly to set a time limit on treatment. Ferenczi and Rank[4] articulated the advantages of brief dynamic psychotherapy.

Following the Second World War, the interest in psychoanalysis resulted in greater demand for psychotherapy and increased pressure to develop briefer treatments. In the mid-1940s, Alexander and French advocated shortening treatment by decreasing the frequency of sessions in order to minimize regression. They proposed to focus treatment on the present rather than the past, using historical conflicts to inform the therapist in providing the best corrective emotional experience for the patient in the present.

The community-based mental health treatment movement, the increasing cost of mental health care, and the rise of managed care in the United States; have stimulated efforts to find briefer forms of psychotherapy. Contemporary brief individual psychodynamic psychotherapy is heavily influenced by the British School's development of brief focal psychotherapy. Balint sponsored a workshop of experienced psychoanalytic psychotherapists, which focused on clinical evaluation and attempted to understand which patients might be suitable for briefer treatment. After Balint's death, Malan carried on the work of the group. At the Tavistock clinic, Malan developed and applied the principles of psychodynamic treatment to brief treatment, delineating methods for evaluating process and outcome variables. He emphasized the importance of therapeutic planning and the identification of a focal conflict.

Concurrently, Sifneos, at the Massachusetts General Hospital, was studying brief psychotherapy.[5,6] Sifneos developed 'short-term anxiety-provoking psychotherapy' as a technique and theory with strict inclusion and exclusion criteria for choosing patients. Davanloo broadened the focus of the brief psychodynamic psychotherapies to include more than one conflict. He also expanded the inclusion criteria to individuals with character pathology and chronic phobic and obsessional neuroses, and advocated actively confronting resistances. Mann's time-limited psychotherapy identified a central issue related to the meaning of time, as the focus of the treatment. Mann related this to the patient's difficulties in confronting loss and separation and the reality of time and death.

In recent years, brief psychotherapy has become increasingly research based. Strupp, Luborsky, and Horowitz have all introduced manualized focused psychodynamic treatments which substantially contribute to our research understanding of this treatment modality.

## Brief dynamic psychotherapy technique

### (a) Evaluation and setting

The evaluation is particularly important in brief individual psychodynamic psychotherapy because of the need for rapid and accurate assessment. In contrast to longer term treatments, brief individual psychodynamic psychotherapy does not offer the luxury of time to re-evaluate and correct mistakes. Although at times we think of psychotherapy as beginning as soon as the doctor sees the patient, this is a hyperbole, used to underscore the importance of interpersonal and transferential elements in the initial meeting with the patient. In fact, it is extremely important, particularly in brief individual psychodynamic psychotherapy, to distinguish the diagnostic interviews from the ongoing treatment.

The interventions and technical procedures performed during the evaluation phase, usually one to four sessions, are substantially different from the technical aspects of brief individual psychodynamic psychotherapy itself. The evaluation phase includes the diagnosis, consideration of the interaction among the patient's ego strength, physical health, and selection variables, and the treatment recommendation, including considering the option that no treatment is indicated.

As in all medical treatments, brief individual psychodynamic psychotherapy is given to patients rather than to diseases. The ability to participate in brief individual psychodynamic psychotherapy process requires the patient to be able to access his or her fantasy life in an active and experiencing manner (i.e. psychologically minded) and, importantly, is able to get up and leave this process behind at the end of a session and not be lost in reverie or uncontrolled fantasies or fears. Note that this does not mean the patient requires a 'high IQ'. In fact, a high IQ, when accompanied with rigidity, intellectualization, and rumination, as is often seen, can be a contraindication to a brief psychodynamic treatment since these defences can be quite formidable. The availability of interpersonal support in the patient's real environment and the patient's ability to experience and simultaneously observe highly charged affective states are necessary to a successful treatment. Individuals who are in an emergent crisis (e.g. imminently suicidal, psychotic, recent major life trauma) and therefore are very concerned and focused on the real events in their life cannot enter into a brief psychodynamic psychotherapy without first having a period of supportive treatment. A true life crisis does not allow the patient the opportunity to explore fantasies.

Negotiation with the patient is an important part of reaching a treatment decision in brief individual psychodynamic psychotherapy. The patient must rapidly feel a part of the treatment and committed to the process. The process of setting a time limit at the beginning of the treatment can be an important element in decreasing the dropout rate from this form of treatment,[7] particularly with the patient who is concerned about dependency, 'becoming addicted' to the therapist, or who needs to maintain a substantial sense of control. What is dealt with in treatment can only be what the patient is able to bring into focus, what the patient can tolerate talking about, and what he or she can tolerate the therapist talking about.[8] Although this is not different than other psychodynamic treatments, the limited time of brief individual psychodynamic psychotherapy means that there is limited ability to interpret multiple defences that might open new areas of exploration.

### (b) Technique

The rapid establishment of the therapeutic alliance is critical to brief individual psychodynamic psychotherapy.[9] Identifying the patient's initial anxieties related to beginning therapy is an important technique in the early sessions of brief individual psychodynamic psychotherapy in order to assure the alliance and to establish the conditions under which the patient can favourably hear and respond to the interpretations that the therapist will later give. As the therapy unfolds, the therapist operates on the hypothesis that each session is related to the previous one. The therapist strives in each session to identify the continuity of meaning related to the treatment focus that is present but hidden.[10] This continuity is driven by the 'experience bias' of the patient, and his or her tendency to experience the world in a certain way due to unique developmental experiences that have moulded his or her perception, interpersonal beliefs, and expectations.[11]

Brief individual psychodynamic psychotherapy is more focused, and more 'here and now' oriented with fewer attempts to reconstruct the developmental origins of conflicts than the extensive reworking of personality undertaken in longer term psychotherapies. Through the exploration of the patient's metaphors and symbols, both defensive patterns and disturbances in present interpersonal relations are identified in the treatment setting as well as in the patient's life. The importance of being able to hear what the patient has to say and to understand its meaning remains central as in other psychoanalytically oriented treatments.

**Free association and inquiry**: Free association is part of the technique of brief individual psychodynamic psychotherapy. But what constitutes free association—as in all dynamic therapies—requires thoughtful consideration. In its most basic form, and particularly highlighted in brief individual psychodynamic psychotherapy, free association means that the patient is free to choose what they wish to talk about. This rather direct definition emphasizes that free association is always relative. In addition, in brief dynamic psychotherapy, the patient is always somewhat more task focused that in open-ended treatments or psychoanalysis and this focus should not be discouraged by the therapist. Rather it is the therapist's task to hear the themes in the patient's concerns. The therapist asks questions, directs the patient's attention, and uses benign neglect, i.e. avoids some areas of conflict that cannot be dealt with at this time or in a short period of time. The therapist identifies those spots at which free association breaks down (the presence of a defence) or at which the narrative is carrying a single emotional story out of the patient's awareness. As in all dynamic treatments, often when the patient is able to talk freely and with a coherent narrative about their conflicts, the work of the treatment is completed.

**Defence and transference**: Brief individual psychodynamic psychotherapy emphasizes understanding (a) the mechanisms of defence used by the patient to decrease anxiety and other uncomfortable feelings associated with areas of conflict which are out of awareness, and (b) the characteristic transference relationships which distort the patients response to their adult world. Typically these two areas, defence and transference, create the world of meaning and expectations in which the patient lives. The techniques of the brief psychodynamic psychotherapy are directed towards clarifying these areas and presenting them to the patient to increase understanding and in this manner change symptoms and behaviour. Often only one defence is concentrated on in a given brief treatment. As the defence is clarified, the transference relationship may become evident. The developmental narrative of how the patient came to see the world in the way he or she does, provides the 'glue' through which the patient can integrate this knowledge into their life experience and behaviours, and recall it for practice and future use.

The brief individual psychodynamic psychotherapy therapist, similar to longer term psychodynamic work, must both enhance the patient's observing capacity in order that the transference can be observed by the patient and therapist, and create the therapeutic situation in which the patient can hear the therapist's interpretations in a useful manner. Dreams, as well as slips of the tongue and symptoms, can provide an avenue to the understanding of unconscious conflict which can be taught and explored with the patient. The therapist strives to interpret both the triangle of anxiety (wish-defence-anxiety) and the triangle of insight (transference figure in the present—the therapist/patient interaction—transference figure from the past).

Frequently, when the transference is most evident, other elements of the past are simultaneously experienced in the patient's life. In brief individual psychodynamic psychotherapy these can be particularly important to the patient's understanding the feeling elements of the transference in a mutative manner since the depth and intensity of the transference is much less and much briefer than in long-term work. In contrast, however, the presence of a recent precipitant to the patient's problems, as is usually the case in brief psychodynamic psychotherapy, can considerably intensify transference responses and be a central element in developing the psychodynamic understanding for the patient. The transference experience—the transference, the life experiences being relived, and particularly the precipitant—provide the web of meaning that is the focus of interpretation and the mutative force in brief individual psychodynamic psychotherapy.

Often the transference in brief individual psychodynamic psychotherapy is paternal or maternal, but it has also been noted that, perhaps due to the time-limited nature of the work, sibling and transference figures from adolescence may more often be recalled in brief individual psychodynamic psychotherapy. The transference is rarely as deep as that seen in long-term treatment. It requires a skilled eye to note and bring the transference to the attention of the patient in a manner that is neither intrusive nor offensive.[12] Interpretations usually occur over several sessions, in the middle or later third of the treatment, during which past, present, and transference experiences are linked together. In the context of the affective arousal associated with this transference experience and the simultaneous understanding of the experience, behavioural change occurs and the patient's ability to perceive previously hidden feelings and relationships as well as his or her view of the future and the past can change.

**Countertransference**: Countertransference is also an important element in brief individual psychodynamic psychotherapy as in other psychodynamic treatments.[13] Analysis of countertransference reactions can allow the therapist to recognize subtle aspects of the transference relationship and to understand the patient's experience better. Because of the more active stance, the brief psychodynamic psychotherapist can be particularly prone to countertransferences that show up as over-involvement or aggression. In addition, the brief time available for treatment can make recovery from countertransference errors quite difficult.

### (c) Medication

Medication is frequently used in conjunction with brief psychodynamic psychotherapy. This can complicate the treatment and its progress as well as aid in symptom recovery. The therapist must explore the meaning of the medication and its role in the patient's view of himself or herself and interpersonal strengths and vulnerabilities. At times, brief individual psychodynamic psychotherapy can also serve as an alternative to medication treatment for less severe symptoms or when medication is contraindicated. Medication may have also begun during the initial brief psychodynamic psychotherapy and then continued after the psychotherapy has formally stopped and the patient is followed with less frequent meetings to monitor medication. This sequence has many advantages including resolving present stressors and precipitants, encouraging medication compliance, and ongoing medical follow-up after therapy either in maintenance or intermittent frequency. Another course of brief dynamic therapy may be indicated at a later date if the response to combined treatment is ineffective or if new problems appear. Greater education of clinicians and research on this combined and sequential treatment is needed.

### Comparison of the brief psychodynamic psychotherapies

The work of Malan, Sifneos, Mann, and Davanloo shows substantial overlap in each author's goals, selection criteria, technique, and duration of treatment.[14] The goals of all of these models of brief psychotherapy include facilitating health-seeking behaviours and mitigating obstacles to normal growth. From this perspective, brief psychotherapy focuses on the patient's continuous development throughout adult life and the context-dependent appearance of conflict, depending on environment, interpersonal relationships, biological health, and developmental stage. This picture of brief psychotherapy supports modest goals that require the therapist to refrain from perfectionism. Malan, Sifneos, Mann, and Davanloo also seem to agree with Stierlin's[15] contrast between brief psychotherapy's use of the 'propitious moment' and long-term treatment's use of 'a shared past' between therapist and patient. Both the propitious moment and the shared past carry psychotherapeutic advantages and disadvantages, emphasizing certain technical possibilities and limiting others.

**Selection criteria**: Many of the selection criteria emphasized by Malan, Sifneos, Mann, and Davanloo are common to all kinds of psychodynamic psychotherapy. However, unique selection criteria are required due to the brief duration of treatment. Patients in brief psychodynamic psychotherapy must be able to engage quickly with the therapist, terminate in a short period of time, and be able to carry on much of the working through and generalizing of the treatment effects on their own.

The necessity for greater independent action by the patient requires that the patient have high levels of ego strength, motivation, and responsiveness to interpretation. Sifneos's rather unique emphasis on intelligence as a criterion may be related to his anxiety-provoking interpretations, which require a broader educational context in order to be understood. The importance of the rapid establishment of the therapeutic alliance underlies a substantial number of the selection and exclusion criteria.

**Focus of brief psychotherapy**: All authors mention the central importance of the focus in brief psychotherapy, and therefore the evaluation sessions to determine this focus. Mann formulates the focus to the patient in terms of the patient's fears and pain. However, he would probably agree with Malan, Davanloo, and Sifneos in the importance of constructing the psychodynamic focus at a deeper level in one's own understanding of the work being done. Maintaining the focus is the primary task of the therapist. This enables the therapist to deal with complicated personality structures in a brief period of time. Resistance is limited through benign neglect of potentially troublesome but non-focal areas of the personality. The elaboration of techniques for establishing and maintaining the focus of treatment is critical to all brief individual psychodynamic psychotherapies.

**Transference**: The manner and rapidity in which transference is dealt with vary considerably among proponents of brief individual psychodynamic psychotherapy. Malan takes a more typical psychoanalytic approach of waiting for transference to become resistance before it is interpreted. Sifneos, in his emphasis on the Oedipal relationship, is more aggressive in handling the deep conflictual areas of transference material. Davanloo is confrontational in developing a transference experience. This confrontational style may at times confuse the patient's experience of the real and the transferential therapist. However, Davanloo often treats severe obsessional disorders. In these cases, the need to increase the patient's affective awareness is high. These may be the patients in which this particular technique is most useful. Aggressive, competitive, and hostile feelings, which might otherwise remain firmly defended, may thus become available to these patients.

**Countertransference**: The role of countertransference in brief psychotherapy is as complicated as it is in long-term treatment. Countertransference issues related to the aggressive techniques used by Sifneos and Davanloo have been observed. Countertransference experiences related to termination and loss can also be prominent.[16] The goal-directed techniques of brief psychotherapy limit the development of regressive countertransference responses.[13]

**Duration of treatment**: There is remarkable agreement on the duration of brief psychotherapy. Although the duration ranges from 5 to 40 sessions, authors generally favour 10 to 20 sessions. The duration of treatment is critically related to maintaining the focus within the brief psychotherapy. Shlien et al.[17] have found in Rogerian therapy, a correlation between the number of sessions and recovery. In general, they report an increasingly successful outcome (measured by the patient's self-concept) up to about 20 sessions. Howard et al.[18] using a meta-analytical technique, found 75 per cent of patients showing some improvement by 26 sessions. However, this study includes a wide range of types of treatment. When treatment extends beyond 20 sessions, the therapist frequently may find himself or herself enmeshed in a broad character analysis without a focal conflict. Change after 20 sessions may be quite slow. Clinical experience generally supports the idea that brief individual psychodynamic psychotherapy should be between 10 and 20 sessions although more complicated cases will require greater length of treatment. Often extending treatment beyond 20 sessions is recognition that treatment will be beyond 40 or 50 sessions.

Brief psychodynamic psychotherapy for depression, narcissistic disturbances, panic disorder, substance abuse, and post-traumatic stress disorder have been described.[14,19] Horowitz et al.[20] have described brief psychotherapy focused on the stress responses evidenced by various personality styles. He emphasizes that this psychotherapy is directed towards dealing with the process of the stress response and not character change. However, his outcomes indicate that selected character changes are possible in some areas. The distinction between recovery from a disruption in homoeostatic balance, reconstitution of self-esteem and self-concept, and changes in character structure require further exploration.

**Critical points**: The identification of critical points during brief psychotherapy, when the 'danger' of becoming a long-term treatment is most acute, clarifies the technical handling of brief psychodynamic psychotherapy. At these points, the therapist often notes an increasing vagueness of the goals of the treatment, decreased activity by the therapist, and the emergence of the transference as the central element. These variables indicate the potential of a short-term psychotherapy becoming a long-term treatment. The fourth to sixth hour of weekly 12-session therapy is often a point at which incipient or potential regression may suddenly appear. The patient at this time is testing the boundaries of the treatment. Action by the therapist is required if a brief psychotherapy is to remain exactly that—brief. The study of technical interventions, which occur at these critical moments, will further elucidate the technical handling of limited regression in brief psychodynamic psychotherapy.

**Malan and the Tavistock group: focal psychotherapy**: Developed from the workshops of Balint and Malan, focal psychotherapy is an example of applied psychoanalysis.[21] Malan has carried on Balint's earlier work.[22,23] Previous attempts to develop brief forms of psychoanalytic psychotherapy primarily involved the use of 'activity' which was frequently equated with manipulation. On the contrary, Malan emphasized the importance of choosing and maintaining a narrow focal area to be dealt with in a brief period of time. He stresses the importance of finding the appropriate focus in the patient's story and consistently interpreting the focal problem area.[23] Through selective attention and neglect, the therapist maintains the focus and completes a brief psychotherapy. The importance of determining the focus underscores the value of the diagnostic process, including the psychodynamic assessment of the patient prior to the initiation of psychotherapy.[24]

Malan identifies the following factors as leading to the lengthening of treatment: resistance, overdetermination, a need for working through the roots of conflict in early childhood, transference, dependence, negative transference connected with termination, and the transference neurosis. In addition, some therapist characteristics may lengthen treatment. These include a tendency towards passivity, a sense of timelessness conveyed to the patient, therapeutic perfectionism, and a preoccupation with deeper earlier experiences. All of these factors must be dealt with in order to maintain a brief therapy. For Malan, identifying a focal conflict acceptable to the patient is critical to a successful outcome (Table 6.3.4.1). In addition, the patient must have the capacity to think in feeling terms, demonstrate a high motivation, and exhibit a good response to trial interpretations made during the evaluation phase. Patients who have had serious suicidal attempts, drug addiction, long-term

**Table 6.3.4.1** Brief psychodynamic psychotherapies

| **Goal of treatment** |
| --- |
| Identify the defence, the anxiety, and the impulse |
| Link the present, the past, and the transference |
| **Focus of treatment** |
| Internal conflict present since childhood |
| **Selection criteria** |
| Patient is able to think in feeling terms |
| Highly motivated |
| Good response to trial interpretation |
| **Duration of treatment** |
| Up to 1 year |
| Mean 20 sessions |
| **Termination** |
| Set definite termination date at beginning of treatment |

hospital stays, more than one course of electroconvulsive therapy, chronic alcoholism, incapacitating severe chronic obsessional symptoms, severe chronic phobic symptoms, or gross destructive or self-destructive acting-out are excluded from treatment. The patient is also excluded from focal psychotherapy if the therapist anticipates any of the items in Table 6.3.4.2.

For Malan, the criteria in Table 6.3.4.2 represent specific dangers. If the therapist cannot make contact with the patient, or low motivation or rigid defences are present, it will be difficult to form an effective therapeutic working alliance within a short time. Complex or deep-seated issues, which must be dealt with to resolve a conflict area, require a longer period of treatment. Difficult transference relationships may also prevent timely termination or lead to premature termination. The occurrence of severe depressive or psychotic episodes during treatment can be a danger to the patient and require adjunctive treatments. Thus, Malan takes seriously the time limitation in brief therapy, which requires the rapid establishment of a therapeutic alliance and the ability to terminate therapy without the development of unexpected serious symptoms.

Malan, in contrast with other practitioners, does not automatically exclude patients with serious psychopathology. He sees the balance between motivation and focality as the primary criteria. A patient with only moderate motivation but a highly focal conflict might be accepted into treatment. Similarly, a patient with high motivation but not as focal a conflict might also be accepted into treatment with the hope that clarification of the focus would occur in a short period of time.

Identifying the precipitating factors, early traumatic experiences, or repetitive patterns can indicate the area of internal conflict present since childhood and the possible focus of treatment. The therapist should assess the congruence between the current conflict and the 'nuclear' or childhood conflict during the evaluation phase. The patient's response to interpretations about aspects of this conflict may lead to acceptance into treatment. According to Malan, the greater the probability that the conflict area will manifest itself in the transference, the more positive the outcome will be.

Malan is less concerned with technique than with the importance of choosing the focus. He employs the usual technical procedures of psychoanalytic psychotherapy and emphasizes the importance of making interpretations of the transference and connecting these to current and past relationships. This 'triangle of insight' (the transference, the current relationship, and the past relationship) leads to the patient's cure. Overall, the goal is to clarify the nature of the defence, the anxiety, and the impulse, which the

**Table 6.3.4.2** Exclusion criteria for Malan's and the Tavistock group's brief focal psychotherapy

---

1. Therapist is unable to make affective contact with the patient during the evaluation
2. Therapist anticipates that extended work will be needed
   To generate motivation
   To decrease rigid defences
   To reach complex or deep-seated issues
   To resolve unfavourable, intense transference, or dependence which may develop
3. Depressive or psychotic disturbance may intensify and place the patient at risk

---

patient is experiencing, and to link these to the present, the past, and the transference. Once the defence and the anxiety are clarified, the link to the past can be made. The interpretation that links to the past may be experienced as reassuring by the patient because of its emphasis on the conflict belonging to the world of fantasy rather than to the world of the present. Malan emphasizes transference interpretations as the most therapeutically effective interpretations because of their 'here and now' character.

In the brief therapy unit at the Tavistock Clinic, a time limit was almost always given at the beginning of treatment. For trainees this was usually 30 sessions. However, in his publications, Malan indicates a mean of 20 sessions for those cases with favourable outcomes. The longer time for trainees gives the opportunity to correct mistakes that might occur. In some published cases, therapy was extended up to 1 year (46 sessions). In general, Malan advocates the importance of a definite date rather than a number of sessions. Practically speaking, this eliminates the need for the patient and therapist to keep count of the number of sessions and eliminates complications related to whether or not to make up sessions that the patient has missed. Such a time limit gives a definite beginning, middle, and end to the therapy. It helps to concentrate the patient's material and the therapist's work, to maintain the focus, and decrease the diffuseness that might lead into long-term work.

**Sifneos: short-term anxiety-provoking psychotherapy:** Sifneos emphasizes the importance of patient selection because of the anxiety-provoking nature of his brief psychotherapy techniques (Table 6.3.4.1). He distinguishes anxiety-provoking therapy from anxiety-suppressing therapy, commonly referred to as supportive psychotherapy. For short-term anxiety-provoking psychotherapy, the patient must be of above average intelligence and have had at least one meaningful relationship with another person during his or her lifetime. The patient who has had such a relationship will be able to withstand the anxiety produced by the therapy and to develop rapidly a mature collaborative relationship with the therapist. This criterion tends to exclude narcissistic disorders. In addition, the patient must be highly motivated for change, not only for symptom relief. Sifneos also identifies several criteria for the patient selection based on the presentation of the patient during the evaluation. The patient must have a specific chief complaint. If the patient has a number of complaints, Sifneos asks the patient which complaint is of top priority. The patient's ability to identify one conflict area and to postpone work on others is taken as an indication of the patient's ability to tolerate anxiety. Sifneos looks for patients with anxiety, depression, phobias, conversion, and mild obsessive-compulsive features or personality disorders involving clear-cut interpersonal difficulties. During the evaluation, the patient must show an ability to interact with the evaluating psychiatrist, to express feelings, and to show some flexibility.

Sifneos is one of the few authors who clarifies his assessment of motivation. He defines motivation as including the patient's ability to recognize symptoms as psychological, a tendency to be introspective and honest about emotional difficulties, and a willingness to participate in the treatment situation. In addition, motivation includes curiosity, willingness to change as well as a willingness to make reasonable sacrifices, and a realistic expectation of the results of psychotherapy.

Sifneos focuses on the Oedipal conflict and does not expect a good outcome in dealing with other than Oedipal conflict areas.

The majority of failures using short-term anxiety-provoking psychotherapy have occurred in patients who complained of reactive depression following the loss of a loved one. He believes that this failure is due to the non-triangular (non-Oedipal) origins of the ambivalent feelings in some patients. In such cases, when the issue of termination arises, the patient regresses and an impasse is reached.

During the initial phase of psychotherapy, the therapist must establish good rapport with the patient in order to create a therapeutic alliance. The therapist uses anxiety-provoking confrontations in order to clarify issues around the patient's early life situation and present-day conflict. The therapist avoids areas such as passivity, dependence, and acting-out, which might lead to extensive regression. The use of anxiety-provoking confrontations in a direct attack on the patient's defences distinguishes short-term anxiety-provoking psychotherapy from other brief psychotherapies. Although it is made clear to patients during their evaluation that the psychotherapy is expected to last only a few months, no specific number of sessions or termination date is given. Interviews are held weekly and last for 45 min. The vast majority of treatments last from 12 to 16 sessions, and none go beyond 20 sessions. The aggressive confrontational style of this treatment underscores the importance of excluding pre-Oedipal problems and the importance of countertransference reactions in the therapist related to being too aggressive.

**Mann: time-limited psychotherapy:** Mann has focused on the specific limitation of time in brief psychotherapy. Mann sees the variable of time as a specific operative factor in psychotherapy as well as an element in its curative effect.[25,26] The experiences of the timelessness of treatment and of the treatment's termination are significant elements in Mann's view of the psychotherapeutic process.

Usually there are two to four evaluation meetings prior to beginning psychotherapy. Mann limits psychotherapy to a total of 12 treatment hours, distributed according to patient need. This may result in weekly 30-min sessions for 24 weeks or twice weekly hour-long sessions for 6 weeks. In practice, however, nearly all patients are seen in once-weekly 45- or 50-min sessions for 12 weeks. Mann admits having chosen the number 12 somewhat arbitrarily; however, his clinical experience indicates that somewhere between 10 and 14 sessions is a sufficient number. Mann emphasizes the importance of a uniform number of sessions for evaluating the psychotherapeutic process among different therapists. In this way, the relationship between the patient's presenting problems and psychotherapeutic technique can be more easily studied. Also, the provision of a specific number of sessions can be more easily accepted by the patient as a typical medical 'prescription'. Finally, the setting of a specific last session in the initial contract with the patient allows the therapy to have a clear beginning, middle, and end (see Table 6.3.4.1).

Mann indicates a number of exclusionary criteria: serious depression, acute psychosis, borderline personality organization, and the inability to identify a central issue. Mann sees Sifneos' criteria as primarily excluding borderline patients. He does not agree with Sifneos' emphasis on superior academic or work performance.

To some extent, Mann initially minimized selection as a central issue for brief psychotherapy. Later, Mann expanded his selection criteria by emphasizing the importance of the patient's ego strength as measured by prior work performance and past relationships.[26]

Patients who may have difficulty engaging and disengaging rapidly from treatment are excluded. This includes schizoid patients, certain obsessional patients, patients with strong dependency needs, some narcissistic patients, some depressive patients who will not be able to form a rapid therapeutic alliance, and some patients with psychosomatic disorders who do not tolerate loss well.

According to Mann, the selection of the central issue for the psychotherapy is the critical event. It is the vehicle through which the patient is engaged in the work of therapy and on which a successful outcome depends. Mann looks for a central issue that is developmentally and adaptively relevant and has been recurrent over time. He describes this issue as the patient's 'present and chronically endured pain' and characterizes it as preconscious. Mann has further described the central issue as including a particular image of the self.[25] The central issue formulated in terms of time, affect, and an image of the self is the 'paradigm of the transference' expected to emerge in treatment. The therapist's statement of the central issue is a clarification, which can be readily recognized, felt, and held onto by the patient. Time-limited psychotherapy is intended to resolve this present and chronically endured pain and the patient's 'negative self-image'. The therapist frames the central issue to the patient in terms of a general statement about feelings.

Mann and Goldman[26] described in detail the phrasing of the central issue to the patient. It is the central issue that specifies the therapeutic contract and the goal of the therapy. In the case of a 41-year-old depressed woman who was preoccupied with her husband and children being even a minute late, Mann suggested the central issue: 'You've encountered extreme life situations and have managed them remarkably well ... yet you fear and have always feared that despite your best efforts you will lose everything'. In a 31-year-old married man attempting to gain a college degree who was consumed with a fear of failing, Mann suggested the central issue: 'Because there have been a number of sudden and very painful events in your life, things always seem uncertain, and you are excessively nervous because you do not expect anything to go along well. Things are always uncertain for you'.[26]

Mann uses the usual psychoanalytic psychotherapy techniques: defence analysis, transference interpretation, and genetic reconstruction. Transference is interpreted from within the central identified conflict area and in terms of the adaptive processes of the patient. However, Mann does not confront the patient. In general, his interventions are very close to the conscious material provided by the patient. Mann identifies specific dynamic events that unfold during the 12 sessions. The opening sessions are understood as filled with the unconscious magical expectation that past pains will now be resolved. During the initial phase, the therapist makes few comments and accepts the positive transference of the patient. Important aspects of the current problem, defence mechanisms, coping styles, and genetic roots of the central issue become clearer during this phase. In the middle four sessions, resistance is likely to appear, as well as the negative transference. The patient experiences the frustration that all of the wished for changes may not occur. In the ending phase of treatment, termination and the patient's resistances to termination in the face of unresolved problems in other areas of life are prominent.

Mann sees the importance of confronting separation and termination issues as critical to the success of brief psychotherapy. Frequently, the patient unconsciously reveals an awareness that the mid-point of treatment has come. The patient experiences separation from the transference-invested therapist as a separation from an ambivalently experienced person from the past, without having achieved the fantasized magical resolution. The goal is to enable the patient to separate from the transference-invested therapist less ambivalently than he had done from this earlier important figure. Consequently, both the resolution of the central issue and the unfolding of an attachment-separation process in the 12-session treatment contract are intimately related through the development and interpretation of the transference.

**Davanloo: broad-focus short-term dynamic psychotherapy:** Davanloo writes about broad-focus short-term dynamic psychotherapy.[27] His selection criteria include patients with an Oedipal focus, those with a loss focus, and those with multiple foci. Davanloo is particularly interested in patients suffering from long-standing obsessional and phobic neuroses. His research data indicate that 30 to 35 per cent of the psychiatric outpatient population can benefit from this mode of therapy. Most information about his technique is derived from the publication of cases, presentations, and brief descriptions of his research that accompany case presentations.

The initial evaluation is a specific focused interview in which the patient's defences against 'true' feelings are gently but consistently confronted. Davanloo says that this is not a universal technique for the initial interview and cautions on its use with patients with severe psychopathology. Selection is based on psychological mindedness, the quality of the patient's interpersonal relations, and, in particular, on the presence of at least one meaningful relationship in the patient's past. The patient's ability to tolerate and experience anxiety, guilt, and depression are important (Table 6.3.4.1). The patient must be motivated to complete the treatment process and to resolve neurotic problems. His or her ability to respond to interpretation is an important selection criterion. In particular, response to transference interpretations, which link the transference with the present and the past, is a critical feature in the assessment for broad-focus short-term dynamic psychotherapy. Davanloo finds no value in criteria based on severity and duration of illness. Finally, the presence of flexibility in the ego's defensive pattern and a lack of use of the primitive defences of projection, splitting, and denial are important factors in selecting patients.

The technique Davanloo uses in therapy is a continuation of that used in the initial interview. The emotional experience of the patient in the transference is emphasized. The patient is 'gently but relentlessly' confronted about his defences against feelings in the transference relationship and in the past. All the usual techniques of psychoanalytic psychotherapy are employed: defence analysis, transference interpretations, and genetic reconstruction. Dreams and fantasy materials are also used. Transference interpretations tend to be made early. Because of the confrontive style, a strong therapeutic alliance is necessary. Patients frequently experience hostile, angry feelings towards the therapist because of being confronted. Davanloo actively pursues the patient's defences against recognizing the anger and its transference elements. Davanloo warns therapists that passive dependent and obsessional characters may develop a symbiotic transference relationship. This may be avoided through active confrontation and selection of patients. The active confrontation of defences and early transference interpretations tend to mobilize powerful affects and memories early on in treatment.

Davanloo recommends from 5 to 40 sessions, depending on the patient's conflict area (Oedipal versus multiple foci) and other selection criteria. In general, his treatments fall between 15 and 25 sessions. He does not recommend setting a specific termination date but rather makes clear to the patient that treatment will be short. Shorter time periods (5–15 sessions) are chosen for patients with a predominantly Oedipal focus, longer durations (20–40 sessions) for the more seriously ill group.

## Comparison of psychodynamic, cognitive, and interpersonal brief psychotherapies

Interpersonal psychotherapy[28,29] and cognitive behavioural psychotherapy[30] derive from the psychodynamic model and therefore share many common elements with brief psychodynamic psychotherapy but with distinct approaches and interventions. All three modalities, interpersonal psychotherapy, cognitive behavioural therapy, and brief individual psychodynamic psychotherapy, are complex methods of treatment that must be custom-tailored to the individual patient. Brief by definition, they all lack the extended working through and application period of psychoanalysis and intensive (long-term) psychodynamic psychotherapy. All demand a high degree of clinical judgement and considerable experience to acquire competency. The relationship between the therapist and patient and the establishment of a therapeutic alliance are essential (Table 6.3.4.3).

**Table 6.3.4.3** Comparison of the brief dynamic psychotherapy with cognitive psychotherapy and interpersonal psychotherapy

| | Brief dynamic psychotherapy | Cognitive psychotherapy | Interpersonal psychotherapy |
|---|---|---|---|
| Free association | ++ | + | + |
| Directiveness | + | +++ | ++ |
| Neutrality | +++ | +++ | +++ |
| Time-limited | +++ | +++ | +++ |
| Defence analysis | +++ | +++ Schema/distortions | + |
| Transference | +++ Interpersonal | + | +++ patterns |
| Behavioural interventions | — | +++ | + |
| Published manuals | + | ++ | ++ |
| Concurrent use of medication | ++ | +++ | +++ |
| Empirical research indicates efficacious treatments | + | +++ | +++ |
| Training in long-term dynamic psychotherapy helpful | +++ | + | +++ |

While sharing many similarities, it is ultimately in the conception of the problem, the goals, and therapeutic interventions that these treatments differ. It is unclear to what extent behavioural changes may be attributed to the similarities or differences between treatments. All psychotherapies, including brief individual psychodynamic psychotherapy, interpersonal psychotherapy, and cognitive behavioural therapy teach new skills-problem-solving skills directed at how to resolve interpersonal and emotional problems when they arise. Differences among these psychotherapies in their interventions are more striking than the differences in their goals or the problem areas they identify for therapeutic work. In psychodynamic psychotherapy the structure of the session is determined by the flow of the patient's thoughts and their interaction with the therapist's interpretive comments. In contrast, cognitive and interpersonal psychotherapies use more directive, structured, and behavioural interventions. Whereas the brief individual psychodynamic psychotherapy like other psychodynamic psychotherapies relies on the patient to activate and practice new behaviours without direction. The therapist remains an empathic interpreter, a sharer of the patient's experience and perspective. While in other therapies, especially cognitive, the therapist may direct, prescribe, enjoin, educate, or role play.

## Practical problems in brief psychodynamic psychotherapy

The choice of focus is perhaps the most important and the most difficult aspect of brief individual psychodynamic psychotherapy. It is helpful to identify several foci during the evaluation process, recognizing that there are inevitably several conflict areas active at any one time in a patient's life. Then the therapist can begin the process of thinking through what the treatment of each focus would entail (Table 6.3.4.4).

The therapist can begin to decide which focal conflict will be more difficult to reach in a brief period of time, which will threaten the therapeutic alliance more and therefore require a deeper working relationship that may take more time, and which focus requires interpreting more primitive defences and therefore may be more complicated.

Choice of a particular focus can also create more family or external disruption or support which can aid or disrupt the treatment.

Use of medication requires carefully explaining to the patient the relationship of the medication to the psychotherapy. Often the medication treatment will continue beyond the psychotherapy.

**Table 6.3.4.4** Identifying and selecting the focal conflict in brief dynamic psychotherapy

| Identifying the focal conflict |
| --- |
| *Explore* |
| Precipitant of symptoms |
| Early life traumas |
| Repetitive patterns of behaviour |
| Listen for inhibitions/avoidance |
| Watch for conflicts about success as well as loss/failure |
| Selection among several foci |
| Choose the focus that is presently active |
| Use trial interpretation to identify active focus |
| Select focus related to only one transference figure |

If repeated complicated medication alterations are needed or if serious side effects of the medication occur, the psychotherapy plan may have to be altered to allow time to understand them from the patient's perspective.

New therapists are often concerned about setting the date of termination at the time of the evaluation, fearing that they may not be able to complete the work by the deadline. Supervision with an experienced colleague can be very helpful to assure confidence and avoid mistakes that may lengthen the treatment. Alternatively, the new therapist may feel too much relief in setting the termination date when treating a very dependent patient and therefore miss the intensity with which the patient is attached and experiencing the therapist as an important, needed, or feared figure from the past.

The management of missed sessions should be made clear at the beginning of treatment. Usually it is best not to 'make up' the sessions, but to keep to the termination date. If the therapist is concerned about this as a potential issue in the treatment, the therapist may wish to plan several additional sessions in the overall treatment to assure this can be discussed and understood therapeutically. Of course if an emergency arises it is always appropriate to schedule appointments as needed for the health and safety of the patient.

The patient who 'divulges' new 'secret' information near the end of the treatment is a challenge to all therapists. Understanding to what extent this represents narcissistic, or sociopathic issues, fear of the therapist or the treatment, or the emergence of hope for the future or a transference enactment will determine how to respond.

Brief individual psychodynamic psychotherapy is best learned in conjunction with the skills of longer term psychodynamic psychotherapy. In the longer work, the therapist will be able to see more easily the possible conflict areas and think about the sequencing of the treatment of these, i.e. which is closer to the patient's awareness or which is more defended. In addition there is more time to correct errors and repair untoward events in the therapeutic relationship. The brief individual psychodynamic psychotherapist will have less time to correct mistakes and must more quickly identify conflict areas and assess their relative importance and potential for resolution through treatment.

## Efficacy: research and evaluation

The brief psychodynamic treatments have a small empirical database. Much further research is needed.[31] In general, studies have supported the efficacy of this treatment approach. However, methodological issues are prominent in most research in this area. The development of handbooks for treatment has gone far in improving research in the psychoanalytically oriented brief treatments.[19,32–34]

The effectiveness of psychotherapy in general, is not argued as in the past.[8,35–37] Brief psychodynamic psychotherapy has been shown to have an effect size similar to many other medical treatments. Short-term psychodynamic psychotherapy has shown modest to moderate, often sustained gains for a variety of patients.[38] However, the question of which psychotherapy is suitable for which patient and by which therapist is still unclear. The cost-effectiveness of psychotherapeutic treatment remains hotly debated and is a focus of substantial research.[9,39,40] Individual psychotherapy has been shown to result in fewer days of hospital stay for patients on medical or surgical services of a general hospital. In health clinics or health maintenance organizations, brief psychotherapy decreases the number of visits to primary health care providers, reduces the number of laboratory and radiographic studies, decreases the number of prescriptions given, and, overall, reduces direct health care costs. Recently summaries of the cost-offset effects of outpatient mental health treatment, the majority of which were short-term are hopeful but not unambiguous. One study found outpatient psychotherapy resulted in a 33 per cent average reduction in medical care utilization. Furthermore, these reductions occurred mostly in the more expensive, inpatient medical services. In another study, 72 patients with significant emotional problems and treated only by internists in a general medical clinic were compared with 62 patients who, in addition to being treated by internists for medical problems, received 10 weekly psychotherapy visits. Both groups had approximately an equal degree of emotional disturbance. At 4-month and 1-year follow-ups, the brief psychotherapy group reported significantly more global improvement than the non-psychotherapy group. Also, more patients in the brief psychotherapy group became employed at 1-year follow-up than in the non-psychotherapy group. This study suggests specific beneficial effects of brief psychotherapy when used in a medical setting by skilled psychotherapists. Combining psychotherapy with antidepressant medication has also been shown to give the best outcome at 1 year when compared to either treatment alone. Whether a therapist keeps to a consistent frame of reference in the treatment may also be a predictor of success if brief individual psychodynamic psychotherapy, regardless of what that perspective is.[41]

Malan's finding of the importance of making the transference-parent link for the successful outcome of treatment is significant and requires further exploration.[2] One reanalysis of Malan's data confirmed his finding and one did not.[42] In addition, one replication of this finding has been published.[43] Importantly, more recently, the overuse of transference interpretations has been shown to lead to poorer outcome. The therapeutic alliance, particularly when measured from the patient's perspective, has a consistent although modest contribution to outcome.[9,44] It has been shown that independent of the type of treatment and early clinical improvement, the therapeutic relationship contributes directly to the positive therapeutic outcome.[45]

The quality of the therapeutic interaction and the handling of the transference and countertransference appears to be critical to success or failure in brief individual psychodynamic psychotherapy.[34] Patients treated by therapists who have not been professionally trained, may, on average, be as improved as patients treated by professional brief dynamic therapists. However, such non-experienced therapists run out of relevant material and are unwilling to continue to treat patients over an extended period of time.[46] One of the important tasks of training in psychotherapy may be the development of the ability to 'endure' with the patient and, over time, with numbers of patients. Technical training and a theoretical framework may allow the therapist to maintain a sense of competence, direction, and interest in the work which the non-professional therapist cannot.

Interpersonal psychotherapy and cognitive-behavioural therapy have been much more extensively studied than dynamic psychotherapy, particularly in combination with medications. Recently, telephone psychotherapy with cognitive behavioural therapy in primary care settings when initiating antidepressant medication has been shown to improve clinical outcome.[47,48] To the extent that these treatments share techniques and outcomes, similar results might be expected with brief dynamic psychotherapy; however, this still needs to be shown. Focal directive psychotherapies generally appear to be more effective than traditional unstructured psychodynamic psychotherapy for a number of types of patients, but a delineation of which psychotherapy for which patient over what time and with which medication remains to be demonstrated. Good clinical sense dictates combined treatments with matching the patient's cognitive and affective style with treatment type and making medication compliance a focus of any psychotherapy. Additionally, further research of brief psychodynamic psychotherapies in specific psychiatric disorders as well as across the life span are needed.[49,50]

## Conclusion

Brief dynamic psychotherapy is an important treatment for numerous disorders, primarily the adjustment, anxiety, and mood disorders. Both alone and in combination with medication brief dynamic psychotherapy is an effective part of the treatment armamentarium. Clinicians should be trained in the brief as well as the longer term treatments and their use as brief, intermittent, and maintenance treatments. Skill in the longer term psychotherapies is important to developing skill in the brief dynamic psychotherapy where the needs for rapid establishment of the therapeutic alliance and the accurate assessment of transference and defence patterns are important.

Empirical studies comparing well-defined brief dynamic psychotherapy with cognitive and interpersonal psychotherapies are limited. Future research must address which form of brief psychotherapy may be most helpful for which patient. An individual's preferred learning path-what he or she may see and observe most easily such as thoughts or feelings or interpersonal relations-may be an important variable in determining which brief psychotherapy for which patient. State, trait, and contextual variables will influence this learning modality. The process of change in brief individual psychodynamic psychotherapy, a process of altering neuronal organization through verbal means, is influenced by the patient's diagnosis, medications, past history, cognitive style, developmental stage, and affective availability, as well as the doctor–patient match.

## Further information

Ursano, R.J., Sonnenberg, S., and Lazar, S. (2004). *Concise guide to psychodynamic psychotherapy: principles and techniques of brief, intermittent and long term psychodynamic psychotherapy*. American Psychiatric Press, Washington, DC.

Levinson, H., Butler, S.F., Powers, T.A., *et al.* (2002). *Concise guide to brief dynamic and interpersonal psychotherapy* (2nd edn). American Psychiatric Publishing Inc., Washington, DC.

Luborsky, L. and Luborsky, E. (2006). *Research and psychotherapy: the vital link*. Jason Aronson, Lanham MD.

Dewan, M.J., Steenbarger, B.N., and Greenberg, R.P. (eds.) (2004). *The art and science of brief psychotherapies: a practitioner's guide*. American Psychiatric Publishing Inc., Arlington, VA.

## References

1. Gabbard, G.O. (1994). *Mind and brain in psychiatric treatment*. Institute of Pennsylvania Hospital Strecker Award Monograph Series 31. Pennsylvania Hospital, Philadelphia, PA.

2. Ursano, R.J. and Silberman, E.K. (1988). Individual psychotherapies. In *Textbook of psychiatry* (eds. J.A. Talbott, R.E. Hales, and S.C. Yudofsky), pp. 855–89. American Psychiatric Press, Washington, DC.

3. Michels, R. (1997). Psychodynamic psychotherapy in modern psychiatry. *Journal of Practical Psychiatry and Behavioral Health*, **3**, 95–8.

4. Ferenczi, S. and Rank, O. (1925). *The development of psychoanalysis.* Nervous and Mental Diseases Publishing Company, New York.

5. Sifneos, P.E. (1972). *Short-term psychotherapy and emotional crisis.* Harvard University Press, Cambridge, MA.

6. Sifneos, P.E. (1984). The current status of individual short-term dynamic psychotherapy and its future: an overview. *American Journal of Psychotherapy*, **37**, 472–83.

7. Sledge, W.H., Moras, K., Hartley, D., *et al.* (1990). Effect of time-limited psychotherapy on patient dropout rates. *The American Journal of Psychiatry*, **147**, 1341–7.

8. Crits–Christoph, P. and Barber, J.P. (eds.) (1991). *Handbook of short-term dynamic psychotherapy.* Spectrum, New York.

9. Ursano, A.M., Sonnenberg, S.M., and Ursano, R.J. (in press). Physician patient relationship in psychiatry (3rd edn) (eds. A. Tasman, J. Kay, and J.A. Lieberman). Wiley & Sons, Ltd., West Sussex, England.

10. Coleman, J.V. (1968). Aims and conduct of psychotherapy. *Archives of General Psychiatry*, **18**, 1–6.

11. McGuire, M. (1965). The process of short-term insight psychotherapy. *The Journal of Nervous and Mental Disease*, **141**, 83–94.

12. Frances, A. and Perry, S. (1983). Transference interpretations in focal therapy. *The American Journal of Psychiatry*, **140**, 405–9.

13. Klan, H. and Frances, A. (1984). Countertransference in focal psychotherapy. *Psychotherapy and Psychosomatics*, **41**, 38–41.

14. Levinson, H., Butler, S.F., Powers, T.A., *et al.* (2002). *Concise guide to brief dynamic and interpersonal psychotherapy* (2nd edn). American Psychiatric Press, Washington, DC.

15. Stierlin, H. (1968). Short-term versus long–term psychotherapy in the light of a general theory of human relationships. *British Journal Medical Psychology*, **41**, 357–67.

16. Hoyt, M. and Farrell, D. (1984). Countertransference difficulties in a time–limited psychotherapy. *International Journal of Psychoanalytic Psychotherapy*, **10**, 191–203.

17. Shlien, J.M., Mosik, H.H., and Dreikurs, R. (1962). Effective time limits: a comparison to psychotherapy. *Journal of Counselling Psychology*, **9**, 31–4.

18. Howard, K., Kopta, S., Krause, M., *et al.* (1986). The dose-effect relationship in psychotherapy. *The American Psychologist*, **41**, 159–64.

19. Milrod, B.L., Busch, F.N., and Cooper, A.M. (eds.) (1996). *Manual of panic-focused psychodynamic psychotherapy.* American Psychiatric Press, Washington, DC.

20. Horowitz, M.J., Marmar, C., Krupnick, J., *et al.* (1984). *Personality styles in brief psychotherapy.* Basic Books, New York.

21. Balint, M., Ornstein, P., and Balint, E. (1972). *Focal psychotherapy.* Lippincott, Philadelphia, PA.

22. Malan, D.H. (1975). *A study of brief psychotherapy.* Plenum Press, New York.

23. Malan, D.H. (1980). *Toward the validation of dynamic psychotherapy.* Plenum Press, New York.

24. Ursano, R.J., Sonnenberg, S., and Lazar, S. (2004). *Concise guide to psychodynamic psychotherapy: principles and techniques of brief, intermittent and long term psychodynamic psychotherapy.* American Psychiatric Press, Washington, DC.

25. Mann, J. (1980). *Time–limited psychotherapy.* Harvard University Press, Cambridge, MA.

26. Mann, J. and Goldman, R. (1995). *A casebook in time-limited psychotherapy.* Jason Aronson, New York.

27. Davanloo, H. (ed.) (1980). *Short-term dynamic psychotherapy.* Jason Aronson, New York.

28. Markowitz, J.C. (ed.) (1998). *Interpersonal psychotherapy.* American Psychiatric Press, Washington, DC.

29. Klerman, G.L., Weissman, M.M., Rounsaville, B.J., *et al.* (1984). *Interpersonal psychotherapy of depression.* Basic Books, New York.

30. Beck, A.T. and Rush, A.J. (1995). Cognitive therapy. In *Comprehensive textbook of psychiatry*, Vol. VI (eds. H.I. Kaplan and B.J. Sadock), pp. 1847–57. Williams and Wilkins, Baltimore, MD.

31. Kay, J. (1997). Brief psychodynamic psychotherapies: past, present and future challenges. *Journal of Psychotherapy Practice and Research*, **6**, 330–7.

32. Luborsky, L. (2000). *Principles of psychoanalytic psychotherapy: a manual for supportive expressive treatment.* Basic Books, New York.

33. Miller, N.E., Luborsky, L., Barber, J.P., *et al.* (eds.) (1993). *Psychodynamic treatment research.* Basic Books, New York.

34. Strupp, H.H. and Binder, J. (1984). *Psychotherapy in a new key: time-limited dynamic psychotherapy.* Basic Books, New York.

35. Gabbard, G.O., Lazar, S.G., Hornberger, J., *et al.* (1997). The economic impact of psychotherapy: a review. *The American Journal of Psychiatry*, **154**, 147–55.

36. Lazar, S.G. (ed.) (1997). *Extended dynamic psychotherapy: making the case in an era of managed care.* Psychoanalytic inquiry supplement. Analytic Press, Hillsdale, NJ.

37. Crits–Christoph, P. (1992). The efficacy of brief dynamic psychotherapy: a meta-analysis. *The American Journal of Psychiatry*, **149**, 151–8.

38. Abass, A.A., Hancock, J.T., Henderson, J., *et al.* (2007). *Short-term psychodynamic psychotherapies for common mental disorders* (*Review*), pp. 1–47. The Cochrane Collaboration, John Wiley & Sons, Ltd, New York.

39. Ursano, R.J. and Silberman, E.K. (1999). Psychoanalysis, psychoanalytic, psychotherapy, and supportive psychotherapy. In *Textbook of psychiatry* (eds. R.E. Hales, S.C. Yudofsky, and J.A. Talbot), pp. 1157–84. American Psychiatric Press, Washington, DC.

40. Wiborg, I.M. and Dahl, A.A. (1996). Does brief dynamic psychotherapy reduce the relapse rate of panic disorder? *Archives of General Psychiatry*, **53**, 689–94.

41. Barbar, J.P., Crits–Christoph, P., and Luborsky, L. (1996). Effects of therapist adherence and competence on patient outcome in brief dynamic therapy. *Journal of Consulting and Clinical Psychology*, **64**, 619–22.

42. Hoglend, P. (1996). Long-term effects of transference interpretations: comparing results from a quasi-experimental and a naturalistic long-term follow-up study of brief psychotherapy. *Acta Psychiatrica Scandinavica*, **93**, 205–11.

43. Marziali, E.A. (1984). Prediction of outcome of brief psychotherapy from therapist interpretive interventions. *Archives of General Psychiatry*, **41**, 301–4.

44. Joyce, A.S., Ogrodniczuk, J.S., Piper, W.E., *et al.* (2003). The alliance as mediator of expectancy effects in short-term individual therapy. *Journal of Consulting and Clinical Psychology*, **71**, 672–9.

45. Zuroff, D.C. and Blatt, S.J. (2006). The therapeutic relationship in the brief treatment of depression: contributions to clinical improvement and enhanced adaptive capacities. *Journal of Clinical Psychology*, **74**, 130–40.

46. Strupp, H.H. (1980). Success and failure in time-limited psychotherapy: with special reference to the performance of lay counselors. *Archives of General Psychiatry*, **37**, 831–41.

47. Simon, G.E., Ludman, E.J., Tutty, S., *et al.* (2004). Telephone psychotherapy and telephone care management for primary care patients starting antidepressant treatment: a randomized controlled trial. *The Journal of the American Medical Association*, **292**, 935–42.

48. Ludman, E.J., Simon, G.E., Tutty, S., *et al.* (2007). A randomized trial of telephone psychotherapy and pharmacotherapy for depression: continuation and durability of effects. *Journal of Consulting and Clinical Psychology*, **75**, 257–66.

49. Leichenring, F, Rabung, S, and Leibing, E. (2004). The efficacy of short-term psychodynamic psychotherapy in specific psychiatric disorders. *Archives of General Psychiatry*, **61**, 1208–16.
50. Shefler, G. (2000). Time-limited psychotherapy with adolescents. *Journal of Psychotherapy Practice and Research*, **9**, 2.

# 6.3.5 Psychoanalysis and other long-term dynamic psychotherapies

Peter Fonagy and Horst Kächele

## Introduction

### Basic assumptions

The term psychodynamic psychotherapy has no specific referent. It denotes a very heterogeneous range of psychological treatment approaches which arguably have in common an intellectual heritage of psychoanalytic theory. Psychoanalytic theory itself is no longer based on a unitary body of ideas[1] but a number of ideas appear to be core to most psychodynamic approaches. These notions are:

(a) A shared notion of psychological causation, that mental disorders can be meaningfully conceived of as specific organizations of an individual's conscious or unconscious beliefs, thoughts, and feelings.

(b) Psychological causation extends to the non-conscious part of the mind, and to understand conscious experiences, we need to refer to other mental states of which the individual is unaware.

(c) The mind is organized to avoid unpleasure arising out of conflict[2] in order to maximize a subjective sense of safety.[3]

(d) Defensive strategies are a class of mental operations that seem to distort mental states to reduce their capacity to generate anxiety, distress, or displeasure. Individual differences in the predisposition to specific strategies have often been used as a method for categorizing individuals or mental disorders.[4,5]

(e) Varying assumptions are made concerning normal and abnormal child and adolescent development but therapists are invariably oriented to the developmental aspects of their patients' presenting problems.[6]

(f) Relationship representations linked with childhood experience are assumed to influence interpersonal social expectations including the transference relationship with the therapist[7] and to shape the representations of the self.[8–11]

(g) These relationship representations inevitably re-emerge in the course of psychodynamic treatments.[12]

### Brief overview of theories

Psychoanalytic theory has evolved from the work of Freud following two broadly separate paths which converged over the past 25 years only to separate again. In the United States followers of the Vienna school in the 1950s and 1960s evolved a systematic psychology of the ego, a conflict-oriented complex psychological model of the mind and its disturbances.[13] In Europe, only Anna Freud and her followers in London pursued this tradition of psychoanalytic thought.[14] Based on the Berlin school of Karl Abraham, Melanie Klein and her followers established a distinct approach focusing on the understanding of disturbance rooted in infantile destructiveness and sadism.[15] Some psychoanalysts, influenced by Klein and the idea of the pathogenic nature of the experiences of infancy, gradually discarded the mechanistic psychology of drives and psychology of internal structures in favour of theories of intrapsychic interpersonal relationships (object-relations theory).[16]

As these schools developed in the United Kingdom, their influence travelled across the Atlantic. First, Kohut, strongly influenced by Winnicott (albeit without explicit acknowledgement), evolved a psychoanalytic psychology of the self.[17] Shortly after, Kernberg arrived at an imaginative integration of ego-psychological and Kleinian ideas.[18] In the meantime, in the United Kingdom, the Kleinian movement rapidly progressed in their understanding of psychoanalytic clinical experience, moving beyond Klein's original work and integrating some of the key features of the Anna Freudian and the British object-relations traditions.[19] In the United States, disillusionment with the false certainty provided by ego-psychology became intense throughout the late 1970s and early 1980s and a radical change in psychoanalytic thinking took place with the emergence of the interpersonal relational perspective, which is in part rooted in the work of Harry Stack Sullivan.[20,21] The relational psychoanalysis of the 1980s and 1990s consolidated several lines of thought initiated by justified critiques of traditional analytic theory[22]; including feminism, the hermeneutic-constructivist critique of the analyst's authority, infancy research, and, closely related to this, the intersubjectivist-phenomenological philosophy of mind—as well as a general political movement to improve and democratize access to analytic ideas and training.[23]

There are many other new psychoanalytic theoretical approaches, bringing the field increasingly close to total fragmentation.[24] This is because the emergence of new approaches in no way signals the demise of any previous orientations, most of which continue to enjoy considerable popularity among specific groups of psychoanalysts.

### Psychoanalytic therapy as treatment

The history of psychoanalysis as a therapeutic approach is rather different. Broadly speaking, it may be argued that psychoanalysis and other long-term psychodynamic therapies are predominantly verbal, interpretive, insight-oriented approaches which aim to modify or re-structure maladaptive relationship representations. It is implicitly assumed that genetic and early environmental factors give rise to partial, unintegrated, and generally troublesome relationship representations (e.g. a helpless 'infant' requiring total care from an adult, a self with exaggerated sense of power, and entitlement requiring constant confirmation from outside) that lie at the root of psychological disturbance. It is believed that the integration of these partial representations into more complex schemata, primarily but not exclusively through the use of insight, leads to improved internal and social adjustment.

Psychoanalysis is the most intensive form of these long-term therapies. The analysand attends treatment three or more times a week over a period of years. The use of the couch and the instruction to the analysand to free associate have been considered hallmarks. The distinction between psychoanalysis and other forms of psychotherapy is normally made in terms of the frequency of sessions rather than in terms of the therapeutic stance of the analyst. It is difficult to avoid the conclusion that in the absence of plausible, theoretically based criteria for what is or is not psychoanalytic, against the background of an overwhelming diversity of theoretical frameworks, psychoanalysts have attempted to find common ground in readily identifiable treatment parameters. This problem arises as a consequence of an extremely loose relationship between psychoanalytic theory and clinical practice.[24] It is an indisputable fact that, whereas theory has evolved extremely rapidly in the last half of the twentieth century and continues to change, psychoanalytic practice has, until recently, changed surprisingly little and continues to provide the core of the psychoanalytic identity. On the other hand, the follow-along study by Sandell *et al.*[25] found that psychoanalysis and psychoanalytic psychotherapy were 'separate things'. When psychotherapy was performed using mainly psychoanalytic techniques, it was less effective than psychotherapy performed with modified and adjusted techniques (that is, not performed as an 'as-if analysis'). The findings from the Stockholm study suggest that psychoanalysis and psychoanalytic psychotherapy may be separate endeavours, although how exactly they differ is far from clear.

In this chapter we will not consider the theoretical richness of this field but instead will focus on the clinical constructs which run across the diverse intellectual approaches. The intersection of the two is perhaps clearest in one area which we shall consider in some detail—namely, the therapeutic action of long-term psychoanalytically oriented psychotherapeutic treatment.

## Background

### Historical development of the psychoanalytic approach to treatment

As is well known, Freud's discovery of the talking cure[26] was really that of an intelligent patient (Anna O) and her physician (Breuer). The patient reported that certain symptoms disappeared when she succeeded in linking up fragments of what she said and did in an altered state of consciousness (which we might now call dissociative) with forgotten impressions from her waking life. Breuer's remarkable contribution was that he had faith in the reality of the memories which emerged and did not dismiss the patient's associations as products of a deranged mind. The patient's response to treatment was probably less complete than Breuer and the young Freud had hoped[27] but the 'treatment' defined the basic elements of the 'cathartic' method-linking memory of trauma (the circumstances of her experience of her father's death) to her many symptoms.

At first Freud rigorously pursued the traumatogenic origins of neuroses. Later, when confronted by evidently incorrect statements, he modified his theory, assuming consistency between recollection and childhood psychic reality rather than physical reality.[28] The issue of accuracy of memories of childhood sexual trauma remains controversial, although its relevance to psychoanalytic technique is at best tangential.[29] Freud's technique, however, was dramatically modified by his discoveries. The intense emotional relationship between patient and physician, which had its roots in catharsis following hypnotic suggestion, had gradually subsided into what was principally an intellectual exercise to reconstruct the repressed causes of psychiatric disturbance from the fragments of material

derived from the patient's associations. It was a highly mechanistic approach reminiscent of a complex crossword puzzle. In the light of therapeutic failures, however, Freud once more restored the emotional charge into the patient–physician relationship.[30] However, in place of hypnosis and suggestion, he used the patient's emotion, signs of transference of affect and affective resistance which were manifest in the analytic relationship. Instead of seeing the patient's intense emotional reaction to the therapist as an interference, Freud came to recognize the importance of transference as a representation of earlier relationship experiences which could make the reconstruction of those experiences in analysis highly meaningful to that individual.[31]

Freud's early clinical work evidently lacked some of the rigour which came to characterize classical psychoanalysis.[32] His occasional encouragement to his patients to join him on holiday might now be considered a boundary violation.[33] What is perhaps less well known is that Freud remained somewhat sceptical about the effectiveness of psychoanalysis as a method of treatment.[34] Indeed, autobiographies of some of his patients testify to his great flexibility as a clinician and use of non-psychoanalytic techniques, including behavioural methods.[35] Nor was Freud the only clinician to use psychoanalytic ideas flexibly. The Hungarian analyst Sandór Ferenczi should be credited with the discovery of the treatment of phobic disorders by relaxation and exposure[36] although many of his well-intentioned actions were criticized by contemporaries and more recently on arguable ethical grounds.[37]

The technique of psychoanalysis after Freud's death came to be codified. Those (such as Alexander and French and Freda Fromm-Reichmann) who attempted to revive or retain Freud's original clinical flexibility were subjected to powerful intellectual rebuttals.[38] In reality, psychoanalysts probably continued to vary in the extent to which they observed the ideals of therapeutic neutrality, abstinence, and a primarily interpretive stance, but these deviations could no longer be exposed to public scrutiny for fear of colleagues' forceful condemnation. Personal accounts of analyses with leading figures yield fascinating insights into variations in technique, principally in terms of the extent to which the analyst made use of a personal relationship.[39] There has been an ongoing dialectic throughout the history of psychodynamic approaches between those who emphasize interpretation and insight and those who stress the unique emotional relationship between patient and therapist as the primary vehicle of change. The controversy dates back to disputes concerning the work of Ferenczi and Rank[40] but re-emerged with the first papers of Balint and Winnicott in London opposing a Freudian and Kleinian tradition, and somewhat later in the United States with Kohut and more subtly Loewald opposing classical ego psychology.

In the last two decades, the pluralistic approach of modern psychoanalysis has brought out into the open many important dimensions along which psychoanalysts' techniques may vary. In particular, the recent trend to consider analyst and patient as equal partners engaged in a mutual exploration of meaning[41] directly challenged many of the classical constructs. The emphasis on the mutual influence of infant and caregiver shaped the emerging relational model of therapy as a two-person process in which there was little room for a detached analyst with pretensions of 'objectivity'. Drawing on the assumption that humans are predisposed towards two-person co-constructed systems that provide a context for psychic change, the quality of engagement between therapist and patient became the core of therapeutic action. What changes the mind is not the insights gained but learning from the interactional experience of being with another person. Neither the analyst nor the patient can be considered as forging meaning; rather, meaning is co-constructed.

## Technique—principal features

### Neutrality and abstinence

Based in the classical framework of libidinal theory, Freud made an explicit injunction against the analyst giving in to the temptation of gratifying the patient's sexual desire.[42] Obviously, this is primarily an ethical issue. However, within the psychoanalytic context it also justifies the analyst's stance of resisting the patient's curiosity or using the therapeutic relationship in any way that consciously or unconsciously could be seen as motivated by the need to gratify their own hidden desires. Within this classical frame of reference, the patient must also agree to forgo significant life changes where these could be seen as relevant to current psychotherapeutic work. In practice, such abstinence on the part of the patient is rare. Yet long-term psychodynamic treatment may founder if the emotional experiences of the therapy are obscured by the upheavals of significant life events.

The primary function of abstinence is to ensure the neutrality of the therapist. The analyst assumes an attitude of open curiosity, empathy, and concern in relation to the patient. The therapist resists the temptation to direct the patient's associations and remains neutral irrespective of the subject matter of the patient's experiences or fantasies. While it is easy to take this issue too lightly, (and it is perhaps this aspect of the psychoanalyst's therapeutic stance which makes them most vulnerable to ridicule), it is probably genuinely critical for the therapist to retain emotional distance from the patient to a degree which enables the latter to bring fantasies and fears of which they feel uncertain. Nevertheless, neutrality at its worst denies the possibility of sensitivity; recent literature on the process and outcome of psychotherapy makes it clear that the therapist's genuine concern for the patient must become manifest if significant therapeutic change is to be achieved.[43] The quality of the alliance is one of the better predictors of outcome[44] and alliance is impacted by the patient's attachment style and quality of object-relations.[45]

### Mechanisms of defence

The term 'psychic defences' may risk reification and anthropomorphism (precisely who is defending whom against what?) yet the existence of self-serving distortions of mental states relative to an external or internal reality is generally accepted, and frequently demonstrated experimentally.[46–48] Within classical psychoanalytical theory and its modern equivalent (ego psychology), intra-psychic conflict is seen as the core of mental functioning.[49] Here defences are seen as adaptations to reduce conflict. Within many object-relations theories, defences are seen as helpful to the individual to maintain an authentic or 'true' self-representation or a nuclear self.[17] Models of representations of relationships are of course often defensive. Traumatic experiences may give rise to omnipotent internal working models to address a feeling of helplessness. Within attachment theory, defences are construed as assisting in the maintenance of desirable relationships.[50] The Klein–Bion model makes limited use of the notion of defence

mechanisms but uses the term in the context of more complex hypothetical structures called defensive organizations.[19] The term underscores the relative inflexibility of some defensive structures, which are thus best conceived of as personality types. For example, narcissistic personality disorder combines idealization and destructiveness; genuine love and truth are devalued. Such a personality type may have been protective to the individual at an earlier developmental stage, and has now acquired a stability or autonomy which must be rooted in the emotional gratification which such a self-limiting form of adaptation provides.[51]

Irrespective of the theoretical frame of reference, from a therapeutic viewpoint clinicians tend to differentiate between so-called primitive and mature defences based on the cognitive complexity entailed in their functioning.[52] In clinical work, primitive defences are often noted together in the same individual. For example, individuals loosely considered 'borderline' tend to idealize and then derogate the therapist. Thus they maintain their self-esteem by using splitting (clear separation of good from bad self-perception) and then projection. Projective identification[53] is an elaboration of the process of projection. An individual may ascribe an undesirable mental state to the other through projection but when the other can be unconsciously forced to accept the projection and experience its impact, the defence becomes far more powerful and stable. The analyst's experiencing of a fragment of the patient's self-state, has in recent years been considered an essential part of therapeutic understanding.[54]

Whether in fantasy or in actualized form, through projective identification the patient can experience a primitive mode of control over the therapist. Bion argued that when the self is experienced as being within another person (the therapist) the patient frequently attempts to exert total control over the recipient of the projection as part of an attempt to control split-off aspects of the self. Bion[55] also argued that not all such externalizations were of 'bad' parts of the self. Desirable aspects of the self may also be projected, and thus projective identification can be seen as a primitive mode of communication in infancy. There are other aspects of projective identification which we commonly encounter clinically. These include the acquisition of the object's attributes in fantasy, the protection of a valued aspect of the self from internal persecution through its evacuation into the object, and the avoidance or denial of separateness. It is thus a fundamental aspect of interpersonal relationship focused on unconscious fantasy and its appreciation is critical for the adequate practice of long-term psychotherapy.[56]

Classifications of defences have been frequently attempted[52,57–61] and often as a method for categorizing individuals or mental disorders.[4,5] An attachment theory-based classification rooted in the notion of habitual deactivation or hyperactivation of the attachment system ('attachment style') has achieved general acceptance.[62,63] Deactivating ('avoidant' or 'dismissing') strategies include suppression of ideas related to painful attachment experiences, repressing painful memories, minimizing stress and distress, segregated mental systems that result in the defensive exclusion of distressing material from the stream of consciousness.[64,65] Ingenious experimental studies have shown that individuals who habitually use avoidant defences are more efficient, when instructed, at suppressing conscious thoughts and associated feelings about a romantic partner leaving them for someone else[66] and are more likely to attribute their own unwanted traits to others (projection) which serves to both increase self-other differentiation and enhance self-worth.[67] In a further, remarkable study the same group of researchers demonstrated that the above advantages of the suppression strategy of those using avoidant defence fall away in the laboratory situation if a cognitive load is placed on the participant which then leaves them literally defenceless so that they experience a heightened rebound of previously suppressed thought about painful separation.[68] The cognitive and socio-cognitive strategies associated with reducing anxiety or displeasure and enhancing safety, which both the attachment theory and psychoanalytic literatures tend to refer to as defences, are perhaps better thought of not as independent classes of mental activity or psychological entities but as a pervasive dynamic aspect of complex cognition interfacing with attachment relationships and emotional experience. Some mechanisms of defence are thought to be more characteristic of the less severe psychological disorders (e.g. depression, anxiety, obsessive–compulsive disorders, etc.). It is beyond the scope of this chapter to consider the various defence mechanisms in detail.

## Modes of therapeutic action

The primary mode of the therapeutic action of psychoanalytic psychotherapy is generally considered to be insight.[69] Insight may be defined as the conscious recognition of the role of unconscious factors on current experience and behaviour. Unconscious factors encompass unconscious feelings, experiences, and fantasies. The psychodynamic model has been seen as a model of the mind that emphasizes repudiated wishes and ideas which have been warded off, defensively excluded from conscious experience. In our view this is a narrow and somewhat misleading way to define the therapeutic mechanism for approaches that are considered as psychodynamic. The psychodynamic approach is better seen as a stance taken to human subjectivity that is comprehensive, and aimed at understanding all aspects of the individual's relationship with her or his environment, external, and internal. Freud's great discovery ('where id was, there ego shall be', Freud[70] p. 80), often misinterpreted, points to the power of the conscious mind radically to alter its position with respect to aspects of its own functions, including the capacity to end its own existence through killing the body. Psychodynamic, in our view, refers to this extraordinary potential for dynamic self-alteration and self-correction—seemingly totally outside the reach of non-human species. Engaging with this potential to bring change through understanding, is the science and the art of the psychodynamic clinician.

Conscious insight is more than mere intellectual knowledge[71,72] or descriptive insights. Prototypically, psychodynamic therapy achieves demonstrated or ostensive insights which represent a more direct form of knowing, implying emotional contact with an event one has experienced previously. Working with what is non-conscious is at the heart of the dynamic approach to bringing about psychological change because of the force that awareness of unconscious expectations can bring to the interpretation of behaviour. Although specific formulations of the effect of insight depend on the theoretical framework in which explanations are couched, there is general agreement that insight has its therapeutic effect by in some way integrating mental structures.[72] Kleinian analysts[73] tend to see the healing of defensively created splits in the patient's representation of self and others as crucial. Split or part-objects may also be understood as isolated representations of intentional beings whose motivation is insufficiently well understood for these to be seen as coherent beings.[74] In this case insight could be seen as a development of the capacity to understand internal and external objects in mental state terms, thus lending them coherence and consistency.[75] The same phenomenon may be described as an increasing willingness on the part of the patient to see the interpersonal world from a third person's perspective.[76]

A simple demonstration to the patient of such an integrated picture of self or others is not thought to be sufficient.[31] The patient needs to 'work through' a newly arrived integration. Working through is a process of both unlearning and learning: actively discarding prior misconceptions and assimilating learning to work with new constructions. The technique of working through is not well described in the literature, yet it represents the critical advantage of long-term over short-term therapy.[77] Working through should be systematic and much of the advantage of long-term treatment may be lost if the therapist does not follow through insights in a relatively consistent and coherent manner.

In contrast to the emphasis on insight and working through are those clinicians who, as we have seen, emphasize the 'relationship aspect' of psychoanalytic therapy (Balint, Winnicott, Loewald, Mitchell, and many others). This aspect of psychoanalytic therapy was perhaps most eloquently described by Loewald when he wrote about the process of change as: 'set in motion, not simply by the technical skill of the analyst but by the fact that the analyst makes himself available for the development of a new 'object-relationship' between the patient and the analyst . . .'(Loewald, 1960, pp. 224–5).[78] Sandler and Dreher[79] have recently observed 'while insight is aimed for it is no longer regarded as an absolutely necessary requirement without which the analysis cannot proceed'. There is general agreement that the past polarization of interpretation and insight on the one hand, and bringing about change by presenting the patient with a new relationship on the other, was unhelpful. It seems that patients require both, and both may be required for either to be effective.[80]

Controversy remains even if all accept that neutrality is an impossible and undesirable fiction and that patient and therapist affect each other in myriad mutually influencing ways. Projective identification is seen as occurring in a bidirectional interpersonal field between analyst and patient—a model clearly adapted from Kleinian approaches to infant-caregiver interaction.[23] If we take this perspective seriously, we have to concede that all analytic interventions change the situations into which they are introduced, and their content and style always reflect the analyst's countertransference/response to the treatment situation.[81] Relational psychoanalysis advocates making the interactional influence of analyst upon patient explicit. As Levenson[82](p. 9) put it, the key therapeutic question is not 'what does this mean?' but rather 'what is going on around here?' The therapist will 'act' on the patient; this is not a therapeutic disaster but rather a potentially progressive and certainly inevitable part of the process.

It has been suggested that change in analysis will always be individualized according to the characteristics of the patient or the analyst.[83] For example, Blatt[84] suggested that patients who were 'introjective' (preoccupied with establishing and maintaining a viable self-concept rather than establishing intimacy) were more responsive to interpretation and insight. By contrast, anaclitic patients (more concerned with issues of relatedness than of self-development) were more likely to benefit from the quality of the therapeutic relationship than from interpretation. Taking a second look at large-scale outcome investigations Blatt found strong evidence for the oft made but rarely demonstrated claim of patient personality—therapeutic technique fit.[85]

# Indications and contraindications and selection procedures

Medical treatments normally have indications and contraindications. In psychodynamic treatment the term 'suitability' indicates a looser notion of the appropriateness of the approach.[86] Nevertheless, based primarily on clinical experience, some writers have arrived at specific criteria for long-term psychodynamic therapy.[87] Some authors have also suggested relatively systematic methods of assessment yielding both diagnostic and prognostic information.[88] The majority of psychodynamic clinicians, however, rely on clinical judgements based on interpersonal aspects of their first meeting with the patient.[71] The three areas of assessment are personal history, the content of the interview, and the style of the presentation.

A history of one good relationship has been traditionally regarded as a good indicator.[89] By contrast, a history of psychotic breakdown, severe obsessional states, somatization, and lack of frustration tolerance are generally considered contraindications. For example, a challenging set of re-analyses of the Treatment of Depression Collaborative Research Program found that the trait of perfectionism was associated with poor outcome, and could undermine the therapeutic alliance and the patient's satisfaction with social relations, limiting their improvement in the course of brief treatment for depression.[90]

Empirical literature, to the meagre extent that this is available, suggests that many of the presuppositions about suitability are unfounded. It was, for example, assumed that patients who manifested more serious mental illness, especially disturbances in reality testing, were unsuitable for psychoanalysis; however, a recent study showed that some patients with serious disturbances in reality testing were able to benefit from psychoanalysis when their analysts were able to tolerate and analyse this level of psychopathology.[91] What does seem to be consistent is that severity of symptoms, as well as functional levels in work and relationships, are correlated with the outcome of psychotherapy[92]—although no single patient variable is a strong predictor of outcome. This is why the effects of psychotherapy, good and bad, can sometimes be surprising.

Prediction based on the content of assessment interviews is hard. In general, the presence of some kind of 'mutuality' between therapist and patient is a positive indicator. Some clinicians offer 'trial interpretations' which summarize their initial impressions, and a positive thoughtful response to these is regarded a good indication. The capacity to respond emotionally within the assessment session is a further indicator.[93] Motivation for treatment is harder to ascertain. Most patients express enthusiasm for the treatment, which falls away once they are asked to confront unpleasant or unflattering parts of themselves.

More recently, psychodynamic therapists have given increasing consideration to the style of the patient's discourse during assessment rather than its content. Holmes,[94] for example, attempts to identify whether patients' narrative styles are avoidant (sparse and dismissing of interpersonal issues) or enmeshed and entangled (excessive current anger about past hurts and insults). The findings of one study indicate that, in a severely personality disordered population at least, the avoidant type of patient has a better prognosis in psychodynamic therapy.[95] A further relevant capacity is reflective function or mentalization, often reflected in narrative; this has been variously described as seeing oneself from the outside,[96] reflecting on one's inner world[87] or having fluidity of thought.[97]

# Managing treatment

## Starting treatment

### (a) Establishing parameters

Most psychodynamic therapists, explicitly or implicitly, convey objectives and expectations to their patients. The details of this agreement normally include arrangements for a time and a place as well as the length and frequency of sessions. Usually a tentative idea is offered as to the likely duration of therapy: 'It is likely to take years rather than months.' Most therapists also describe the expected behaviour of the patient and the therapist: 'I would like you to be as open and honest with me as possible and say absolutely everything that comes into your mind. This is the fundamental rule.' In fact it is very likely, in view of the variety of such agreements that tend to be made, that its emotional context is more relevant than the specific items agreed upon. Such a 'contract' implies recognition by both patient and therapist that the process of therapy needs protecting and that it is important enough to require a sacrifice from both parties.

In the treatment of severe personality disorders, contracts may have an additional important function—that of protecting the therapy from incessant enactments, self-harming, parasuicidal gestures, and so on. In Kernberg's approach to the treatment of borderline patients, the patient formally undertakes not to seek the therapist's help outside of office hours, not to engage in acts of violence and to deal with self-destructive acts through normal medical channels.[98] Whilst such agreements are commonly made in long-term therapy, it is by no means clear that they are either essential or useful. For example, in an alternative form of psychodynamic therapy, Mentalization-Based Treatment (MBT), contracts are not recommended.[99]

### (b) Formulation of patients' problems

An important part of initiating any psychosocial treatment is arriving at least at a preliminary formulation of the patient's problems. In the case of psychodynamic therapies this represents a special challenge because of the diversity of the possible theories to draw on. In principle, psychodynamic formulations would identify key unconscious conflicts, central maladaptive defences, unhelpful unconscious fantasies and expectations, deficits in personal development, and so on. The complexity of such formulations is such that agreements are hard to arrive at even when clinicians follow similar orientations. In the absence of a generally accepted format for formulating the patient's problems, a list of key parameters for the level of maturity of personality organization may be offered:

(a) the maturity of relationship representations (three or more persons versus just a self-other dimension)

(b) the maturity of psychic defences (primarily based on projective versus internalizing processes)

(c) the extent of whole as opposed to part object-relations (e.g. whether a person is represented as performing more than a single function for the patient)

(d) the general mutuality of the relationship patterns described; the quality of attachment to others.

It should be noted that psychodynamic formulations tend to change as treatment progresses. Indeed, Winnicott described psychoanalysis as 'an extended form of history taking'.[100] Within certain psychodynamic approaches formulation is communicated formally to patients (e.g. by letter in cognitive analytic therapy Ryle[101]).

## The middle phase

### (a) Supportive and directive interventions in psychodynamic therapy

Supportive techniques are used both explicitly and implicitly in psychodynamic treatment. They include offering explicit support and affirmation; offering reassurances concerning, for example, irrational anxieties about the therapeutic arrangements; expressing concern and sympathy to a patient who has suffered a recent loss; and general empathy for the patient's anxieties and struggles with the treatment.[102]

From a psychodynamic point of view, such supportive interventions are by no means straightforward. For example, Feldman[103] illustrated how patients may sometimes experience the therapist's submission to a demand for reassurance as a source of anxiety rather than comfort. They may be unconsciously aware that the therapist's true stance is not compatible with reassurance and therefore face anxieties about the therapist's weakness in allowing themselves to be manipulated. By contrast, Kohut's[17] emphasis on interpersonal empathy was probably a welcome antidote to the somewhat rigid interpretive stance of American ego psychologists, particularly for those whose history of psychosocial deprivation meant that they had experienced little by way of genuine warmth or concern in the past.

The most common use of supportive and directive techniques in psychodynamic psychotherapy are in the service of the therapy itself. Elaborative techniques (e.g. the simple question: 'Could you tell me more?') are undoubtedly directive in specifying a topic of interest, but at the same time may be crucial antecedents to interpretive work. Clarification stands in between supportive and interpretive interventions. It is a restatement in the therapist's words of the patient's communication. It may also be crucial in offering a verbal (symbolic) label for a confused set of internal experiences which the patient is poorly equipped to represent coherently. Confrontation is also in between a directive and an interpretive approach. At its gentlest, confrontation may involve the therapist simply identifying an inconsistency in the patient's communication and bringing this to the patient's attention. For example: 'You seem to express no sadness about this loss, yet in the past you claimed to have cared a great deal for him'.

### (b) Regression

An important facet of psychoanalysis and long-term psychodynamic therapy is the activation and exploration of parts of the patient's personality which may be normally hidden behind an over-riding demand to adapt to the demands of every day life. Access to these aspects of personality is achieved through the process of regression.

It has been suggested that rather than encouraging regression, the process is best conceived of as inhibiting 'an anti-regressive function' in much the same way that certain intimate interpersonal experiences, large group situations, and alcohol appear to bring out the more infantile aspects of our character.[104] Some psychoanalysts consider regression to be crucial to successful psychoanalytic treatment, but others consider the concept and its clinical application outmoded and counterproductive.[105] The extent to which a particular treatment involves significant regression appears to be a function of the patient's personality as well as the therapist's particular approach. Fear of regression is an important source of resistance to long-term psychotherapy, particularly amongst those with previous experience of psychotic episodes.[104]

### (c) Resistance

Resistance is inevitably encountered in any long-term psychodynamic treatment. In fact, the presence of resistance is implied by the term dynamic, which suggests psychic forces both pulling against and pushing towards change. Like regression, resistance fluctuates in the middle stage of treatment. In borderline and narcissistic disorders, the patient's intense resistance signals the patient's desperation to protect extremely fragile self-esteem. In less severe cases, what appears to be at issue is preventing a painful integration of experience, such as the integration of love and hate directed towards the same object.[106]

In clinical practice resistance takes a variety of forms. In repression resistance, the patient may experience a temporary difficulty in gaining access to particular ideas and feelings; for example, failing to remember dreams. In transference resistance the patient may appear to wish to keep their relationship with their therapist at an extremely superficial level. In a negative therapeutic reaction the increase of symptomatology occurs alongside therapeutic progress. In Freud's formulation this may be attributed to unconscious guilt. It is quite likely that in at least some patients this form of resistance against psychotherapy is part of a pervasive so-called 'envious' predisposition to eradicate any aspect of their life that they experience as 'good' but beyond their immediate control.[107]

### (d) The experience of the transference

Patients may experience a whole range of feelings about an analyst including love, admiration, excitement or anger, disappointment, and suspicion. The feelings appear to have little to do with the therapist's actual personality as different patients are likely to bring quite disparate feelings about the same analyst at the same time. While clearly not realistic, the actual nature of transference experience and its use in therapy is quite controversial.[108] Object-relations theorists consider the analyst a vehicle onto which an internal object (a person, an aspect of a person, the self, or an aspect of the self) is projected.[109] Clearly internal objects are representations which are heavily distorted by both fantasy and defensive processes.

For John Bowlby[64] transference feelings are based on expectations gathered through past relationship experience with an attachment figure. Patients resist understanding of the past relationship by insisting on repeating it. Bowlby's[110] suggestion that therapists function as secure bases implies that psychodynamic therapists are, in part, conducting attachment therapy as inevitably they serve as attachment figures for their patients. There is accumulating evidence for this claim[111–114] with a number of studies linking specific transference schemas and attachment.[115–117] Many analysts do not accept such an isomorphism between past and present. Rather, they see it as something which gives coherence to the patient's experience of the analytic relationship—an aspect of narrative rather than a representation of the historical realities of the patient's experience.[118] In contrast, analysts who work in the Klein–Bion frame of reference see transference as providing an inevitably accurate picture of the patient's current internal world.[119] For example, a transference where the analyst is idealized may reflect psychotic anxieties in the patient linked to an intensification of the death instinct. The idealization serves to protect both the patient and the analyst from fantasized destruction which threatens to engulf them both. Marcia Cavell[120] demonstrated that these alternative models of transference have their philosophical roots in the debate between correspondence and coherence models of truth.

There is significant debate regarding from what point and how much psychoanalytic therapists should work 'in the transference'. Some analysts are inclined to see transference as pertinent to every aspect of the psychoanalytic situation. For example, Joseph[119] considers the therapeutic situation in toto as mirroring the internal state of the patient. Thus the therapeutic alliance or the 'real relationship'[121] are regarded as subsumed under the transference relationship. In this context it makes little sense to interpret anything other than the transference from the very beginning of the analysis. By contrast, Strachey[122] understood transference as an attempted externalization of the patient's superego. Unlike other people in the patient's life, the analyst does not accept this externalization, whether it is idealized, denigratory, or judgemental. The analyst conveys his or her understanding of the externalization by a so-called 'mutative interpretation'. While Strachey implied that only interpretation of the transference is therapeutic, his view clearly admits other aspects of the therapeutic relationship. Other therapists, particularly Freudian psychoanalysts, regard transference interpretations as an important but not uniquely therapeutic way of providing the patient with insight and consider the almost exclusive reliance on understanding the patient through their thoughts and feelings about their therapists as unhelpful and even dangerous.[123] The only systematic investigation of this technical controversy, where patients were randomly assigned to a transference and a non-transference-oriented psychological therapy, could not show a significant difference between the overall effectiveness of these two treatments, although there was a tendency for those with more dysfunctional object-relationship representations to do better in therapy which used transference interpretations.[124,125]

The nature of the transference appears to systematically relate to specific clinical groups and hence may have an aetiological significance. For example, specific transference patterns appear to characterize particular groups of narcissistic patients.[17] The 'mirroring' transference is one where patients crave the approbation and admiration of the therapist. This may be a consequence of the failure of the original self-objects (parents) in their mirroring function. If this transference is undermined by premature interpretations, an opportunity for restoring self-esteem is lost. The 'idealizing' transference also enables the patient to address a deficiency in self-esteem by secretly identifying with the object of admiration (the analyst). If the analyst destroys this idealized image, within Kohut's framework, this is equivalent to a direct attack on the patient's self-regard. Other analysts would suspect that behind such an exaggeratedly positive image lies the patient's

true image of the analyst as frustrating or inadequate, an image which is simply placed out of harm's way by the idealization. An interesting empirical study of clinicians' experience of the transference with personality disordered patients was reported from Drew Westen's laboratory.[115] The study identified five transference dimensions: angry/entitled, anxious/preoccupied, avoidant/counterdependent, secure/engaged, and sexualized which were associated in predictable ways with Axis II pathology and confirmed that the way patients interact with their therapists can provide important data about their personality, attachment patterns, and interpersonal functioning.

Commonly, transference includes an erotic component, regardless of the age or even the gender of the analyst.[126] Admitting to such feelings may border on the unacceptable for some patients. Attachment theorists may suggest that sexual fantasies are used in the service of obtaining the attention of an unresponsive attachment figure.[127] Eroticized transference, relatively common in severely traumatized patients, represents an expression of a need for sexual gratification which, in the context of the therapy, is not considered by the patient as unrealistic.[71] Some view this phenomenon as an indication of an immature mode of representing internal reality, where only the physically observable outcome is believed to be real.[128]

### (e) Experience of the countertransference

Countertransference is a somewhat controversial concept in psychoanalytic clinical work. The therapist during the course of an intensive long-term treatment is likely to have a range of feelings which are related to the patient's current experience but which may serve to either illuminate or obscure this. Some countertransference experiences may be instances of projective identification and thus can be appropriately attributed to the patient,[129] whereas others are likely to be the analyst's neurotic emotional reactions to the patient's behaviour or the material he or she brings. For Freud,[130] countertransference was always of this latter type, a neurotic reaction which was likely to obstruct psychoanalytic treatment. It was not until Paula Heimann[131] pointed out that the analyst's feelings and thoughts could contain important clues about the patient's unconscious mental state that countertransference started to be seriously considered as part of the analyst's therapeutic armamentarium. Those following an interpersonalist tradition saw the recognition of the complementarity of the therapeutic relationship as highly appropriate. From this point of view, the assumption of perfect neutrality on the part of the analyst who is a participant as well as an observer is both an anathema and an anachronism.[132] The psychotherapeutic process is more accurately viewed as a complex mixture of complementary interpersonal processes which establish themselves in 'custom designed' configurations in each treatment.[133]

The therapist's feelings may be either complementary to or concordant with those of the patient.[134] Concordant countertransferences are the product of primitive, empathic processes within the therapist who 'feels' for the patient, who may unconsciously react to experiences implied but not yet verbalized by the patient; for example, inexplicable overwhelming sadness. Complementary countertransferences tend to occur when the patient treats the analyst in a manner consistent with interpersonal interactions within a past relationship. Most commonly this occurs when the patient treats the therapist as he or she experienced being treated as a child. This is known as the 'reverse transference'.[135]

The mechanisms of countertransference are poorly understood. To assert that countertransference functions via projective identification merely brings one poorly understood phenomenon to account for a second even less well understood one. Sandler[136] suggested that an instantaneous process of automatic mirroring of one's partner in an act of communication accounted for concordant countertransference. The process, which he termed primary identification, was non-conscious and could be brought into awareness only upon reflection. Recent work on the mirror neurone system[137,138] suggests that the fundamental mechanism that allows us to understand the actions and emotions of others involves the activation of the mirror neurone system for actions and the activation of visceromotor centres for the understanding of affect. An alternative account suggests that a secondary mode of encoding is available within language whereby the use of a language of pretend gestures at the phonemic, syntactic, or even semantic level enables the communicator to address directly the unconscious of the recipient of the communication.[139] In other words, anything that can be said in gestures may be communicated unconsciously through language, through phonemic distortion, intonation, and other paralinguistic features and picked up impressionistically by the therapist.

When either concordant or complementary countertransferences mobilize defensive processes within the analyst, countertransference is in danger of becoming disruptive to therapeutic understanding. The analyst may react by unconsciously withdrawing from the therapeutic relationship. For example, in the case of a concordant countertransference where the patient's feelings of inadequacy create a similar feeling in the analyst, the analyst's vulnerability in this area may lead him or her to become defensively angry or excessively motivated to demonstrate his or her efficacy. There may be no simple way of regulating such reactions and the only reasonable strategy might be to carefully monitor one's style of relating, noting anything that is unusual. A number of analysts have pointed to the importance of reflectiveness in this context.

Some feelings in relation to the patient are not provoked either by the patient's projections or the neurotic feelings these give rise to in the therapist. It required someone of the stature of Donald Winnicott[140] to make the self-evident observation that the provocative behaviour of certain patients (particularly those in the borderline spectrum) can lead to a normal reaction of 'objective hate'. These reactions are merely indications of the therapist's humanity. Analytic understanding of these sometimes intense reactions to patients helps, but models of countertransference ill-fit such experiences. The objective study of countertransference has had to wait for a recent ingenious methodological development from Westen's laboratory.[141] The Countertransference Questionnaire yielded eight clinically and conceptually coherent factors that were independent of clinicians' theoretical orientation: (i) overwhelmed/disorganized, (ii) helpless/inadequate, (iii) positive, (iv) special/overinvolved, (v) sexualized, (vi) disengaged, (vii) parental/protective, and (viii) criticized/mistreated. Countertransference patterns were systematically related to patients' personality pathology across therapeutic approaches, suggesting that clinicians, regardless of therapeutic orientation, can make diagnostic and therapeutic use of their own responses to the patient.

## (f) Interpretation

Interpretive interventions are at the core of psychoanalytic and psychodynamic treatment. However, the importance of interpretation is often exaggerated in relation to other aspects of the therapy. It is a sobering reminder that follow-up studies of long-term psychodynamic therapies invariably demonstrate that patients remember their analyst not for their interpretive interventions, rarely remembering individual interpretations, but rather for their 'emotional presence', regardless of the analyst's therapeutic perspective.[142]

Interpretations may be classified according to the aspect of a conflict they aim to address: the defence, the anxiety, or the underlying wish or feeling. Similarly, the content of the interpretation may be used in classifying interpretations: whether it relates to external reality, the transference relationship, or childhood relationships. In principle, in the earliest phases of treatment interpretations relating to current events are most common and, as the treatment progresses, transference issues and the patient's past may increasingly take over as foci of analytic work. Interpretations should start with the patient's anxiety, by identifying the defence used by the patient to protect himself from repudiated wishes and affects. In reality, these are guidelines that are rarely followed in practice. For example, very long-term treatments tend to end up being principally supportive explorations of the patient's current experience.[143] Furthermore, interpretations of the distant past tend to be least helpful to individuals with severe personality disorders.[144] Working in the so-called 'here and now' is more effective with those patients whose representation of the past is unreliable and distorted.[145]

Steiner[146] distinguished analyst-centred from patient-centred interpretations. The former refers to comments on the patient's reactions in terms of what the patient thinks may be going on in the analyst's mind, while the latter directly addresses the analyst's perception of the patient's non-conscious mental state. In either case the patient is directly learning about how minds interact in the context of social relationships. The distinction is important since when patient-centred interpretations are used exclusively the therapist may appear to be persecutory and not to be cognizant of the patient's genuine difficulties in being in an intimate relationship with another person. Others have argued, that at least in the case of severe personality disorder, interpretations, if they were to have therapeutic value, should focus on the patient's understanding of thoughts and feelings in themselves or in others at the level of what was conscious rather than unconscious, what patients could discover for themselves rather what they received as a communication from a 'mind expert'.[147] This implies that interpretation of the transference is about helping the patient represent their own and their therapist's mental states in the treatment room in all their complexity but with a stance conveying enquiry and playful curiosity about something that is not readily knowable (the mental state of the other is always opaque) with the aim of making thinking about thoughts and feelings safe again rather than communicating powerful insights.

The idealization of the transference has led some therapists to neglect interpretation of the patient's behaviour outside of the therapy. Most clinicians now agree that a balance needs to be struck between these two approaches. Treatment which is over-focused on the transference becomes a claustrophobic enclave.[148] In certain instances, the direct communication of the therapist's experience of frustration (objective hate in Winnicott's terms) may help to break a rigid repetitive pattern in the therapy.[149] Disclosing the therapist's experience is one of the cutting edges of the relational approach to psychodynamic therapy.[150] In cases where the therapeutic alliance falters, perhaps following an empathic failure on the part of the therapist, it turns out that the recovery of the alliance may have particular therapeutic value both in showing the possibility of repair[151] but also as an opportunity to understand misunderstanding, an ideal opportunity for the recovery of mentalization.[152]

### Ending treatment

The ending of psychoanalytic therapy is often idealized in clinical descriptions. As there is little agreement on the goals of psychoanalytic therapy,[79] it is hardly surprising that there is little general agreement about when ending is appropriate. Desirable final outcomes are mostly stated in terms of the process of treatment and are thus mostly specified in theoretical terms (e.g. increased awareness of impulses and fantasies, a reintegration of aspects of the self lost through projective identification, the capacity to engage in self-analysis, etc.). All these, even if observable in the course of treatment, are only loosely related to the aims the patient might have in concluding a lengthy treatment process.

The patient's own goals tend to be outcome rather than process goals and are more easily defined: the decline of symptoms, improved relationships, greater well-being, increased capacity for work, higher self-esteem, a capacity for assertiveness. As such changes are clearly achievable without psychodynamic treatment, many psychodynamic clinicians erroneously regard such criteria for ending as superficial. Independent evidence will be required to show that the achievement of process aims results in a more permanent or general achievement of outcome aims, in order to validate process aims as an appropriate criterion for ending.

Ending itself, of course, is a process. There is significant disagreement between authors, however, as to its nature; it has been labelled among other things as a mourning,[153] a detachment,[71] and a maturation.[154] It is inevitable that there is disappointment and disillusionment at the ending of long-term therapy as what is achieved is never quite the same as what has been hoped for.[155] Also, the patient loses the object who has been available as a receptacle for projections.[146] It is not surprising then, that symptoms sometimes return, even if only briefly, as part of the process of termination and the full benefit is not seen until some months after termination.[25] There is general agreement, however, that with these unconscious issues worked through the ending of therapy requires no special form of intervention on the part of the therapist.

## Efficacy

It is often said that there are no studies on the effectiveness of psychoanalysis and long-term psychodynamic psychotherapy. In fact, this is not true. There are a number of comprehensive reviews[156–160] and they tend to come to similar conclusions. There is considerable evidence for the effectiveness of psychoanalytic approaches but definitive randomized controlled trials of its efficacy are still lacking.

The Boston Psychotherapy study[161] compared long-term psychoanalytic therapy (two or more times a week) with supportive therapy for clients with schizophrenia in a randomized controlled design. On the whole clients who received psychoanalytic therapy fared no better than those who received supportive treatment. In a partial-hospital RCT[162,163] the psychoanalytic arm of the treatment included therapy groups three times a week as well as individual therapy once or twice a week over an 18 month period.

The Stockholm Outcome of Psychotherapy and Psychoanalysis Project[164–166] followed 756 persons who received national insurance funded treatment for up to 3 years in psychoanalysis or psychoanalytic psychotherapy. The groups were matched on many clinical variables. Four or five times weekly analysis had similar outcomes at termination when compared with one to two sessions per week psychotherapy. During the follow-up period, psychotherapy patients did not change but those who had had psychoanalysis continued to improve, almost to a point where their scores were indistinguishable from those obtained from a non-clinical Swedish sample.

The German Psychoanalytic Association undertook a major follow-up study ($n = 401$) of psychoanalytic treatments undertaken in that country between 1990 and 1993.[159,167] Between 70 per cent and 80 per cent of the patients achieved (average 6.5 years after the end of treatment) good and stable psychic changes according to the evaluations of the patients, their analysts, independent psychoanalytic and non-psychoanalytic experts, and questionnaires commonly applied in psychotherapy research. The evaluation of mental health costs showed a cost reduction through fewer days of sick leave during the 7 years following the end of long-term psychoanalytic treatments. In the absence of pre-treatment measures it is impossible to estimate the size of the treatment effect.

The Research Committee of the International Psychoanalytic Association recently prepared a comprehensive review of North American and European outcome studies of psychoanalytic treatment.[157] Four case record studies, 13 naturalistic pre-post or quasi-experimental studies, nine follow-up studies, and nine experimental studies were identified. In addition, six process-outcome studies were also reviewed. The committee concluded that existing studies failed to demonstrate unequivocally the efficacy of psychoanalysis relative to either alternative treatment or active placebo. Studies showed a range of methodological and design problems including absence of intent to treat controls, heterogeneous patient groups, lack of random assignments, failure to use independently administered standardized measures of outcome, etc.

Another overview[168] suggested that psychoanalytic treatments may be necessary when other treatments proved to be ineffective. The authors concluded that psychoanalysis appears to be consistently helpful to patients with milder disorders and somewhat helpful to those with more severe disturbances. More controlled studies are necessary to confirm these impressions. A number of studies testing psychoanalysis with 'state of the art' methodology are ongoing and are likely to produce more compelling evidence over the next years. Despite the limitations of the completed studies, evidence across a significant number of pre-post investigations suggests that psychoanalysis appears to be consistently helpful to patients with milder (neurotic) disorders and somewhat less consistently so for other, more severe groups. Across a range of uncontrolled or poorly controlled cohort studies, mostly carried out in Europe, longer intensive treatments tended to have better outcomes than shorter, non-intensive treatments (demonstration of a dose-effect relationship). The impact of psychoanalysis was apparent beyond symptomatology, in measures of work functioning and reductions in health care costs. Studies report results which other psychotherapies have not been able to achieve; some studies show very long-term benefits from psychoanalytic treatment; the results tend to be highly consistent across studies; some of the populations studied have been larger than most better controlled treatment trials. So whereas it is true to say that little that is definite can be stated about the outcome of psychoanalysis, a number of suggestive conclusions may be drawn and these are listed below.

Across a number of studies and measures psychoanalysis has been shown to benefit the majority of those who are offered this treatment[169] and can bring the functioning of a clinical group to the level of the normal population.[167] Completed treatments tend to be associated with greater benefits.[170] On the whole longer treatments have better outcomes[171] and intensive psychoanalytic treatment is generally more effective than psychoanalytic psychotherapy,[25] but its superiority sometimes only becomes apparent on long-term follow-up.[172] Psychoanalysis can lead to a reduction in health care related use and expenditure[173] and this is maintained for a number of years after therapy ends[174] but it does not invariably achieve this.[166] Psychoanalytic treatment can lead to a reduction in the use of psychotropic medication amongst inpatients.[175] Long-term psychoanalytic therapy can reduce symptomatology in severe personality disorders such as BPD[162,176,177] and these improvements are maintained.[163]

## Training

Training in psychoanalytic psychotherapy and psychoanalysis has three components: a personal psychoanalytic psychotherapy, theoretical training, and supervised clinical practice. A variety of trainings are available, although in most countries there is only one training organization that is recognized by the International Psychoanalytic Association. Training is long, chiefly because of the length of supervised treatments. Training standards are carefully monitored by national and international bodies.

## Conclusion

Psychoanalysis is hardly a practical treatment alternative for the twenty-first century. The principles derived from this treatment, however, have powerfully influenced other psychotherapeutic approaches, whether long-term or short-term therapy or psychiatric care more generally, particularly in the United States. At the time of its invention, it was the unique effective psychosocial treatment method for psychiatric disorder which offered a genuine alternative to the sometimes barbaric and generally ineffective treatment methods available. Not surprisingly, its proponents adopted an almost religious zeal in defending its value against alternative approaches. While understandable, such an attitude has no place in the sophisticated evidence base underpinning multi-agency service planning. Psychoanalytic clinicians face a challenge in identifying their niche in the complex mental health care delivery systems of the twenty-first century.

## Further information

Budd, S. and Rusbridger, R. (eds.) (2005). *Introducing psychoanalysis: essential themes and topics*. Routledge, London.

Fonagy, P. and Target, M. (2003). *Psychoanalytic theories: perspectives from developmental psychopathology*. Whurr, London.

Yeomans, F.E., Clarkin, J.F., and Kernberg, O.F. (eds.) (2002). *A primer of transference-focused psychotherapy for the borderline patient*. Jason Aronson, Northvale, NJ.

## References

1. Fonagy, P. and Target, M. (2003). *Psychoanalytic theories: perspectives from developmental psychopathology*. Whurr, London.

2. Smith, H.F. (2003b). Conceptions of conflict in psychoanalytic theory and practice. *The Psychoanalytic Quarterly*, **72**, 49–96.

3. Sandler, J. (2003). On attachment to internal objects. *Psychoanalytic Inquiry*, **23**, 12–26.

4. Bond, M. (2004). Empirical studies of defense style: relationships with psychopathology and change. *Harvard Review of Psychiatry*, **12**(5), 263–78.

5. Lenzenweger, M.F., Clarkin, J.F., Kernberg, O.F., *et al.* (2001). The inventory of personality organization: psychometric properties, factorial composition, and criterion relations with affect, aggressive dyscontrol, psychosis proneness, and self-domains in a nonclinical sample. *Psychological Assessment*, **13**(4), 577–91.

6. Fonagy, P., Target, M., and Gergely, G. (2006). Psychoanalytic perspectives on developmental psychopathology. In *Developmental psychopathology: theory and methods*, Vol. 1 (2nd edn) (eds. D. Cicchetti and D.J. Cohen), pp. 701–49. John Wiley & Sons, Inc., New York.

7. Brumbaugh, C.C. and Fraley, R.C. (2006). Transference and attachment: how do attachment patterns get carried forward from one relationship to the next? *Personality and Social Psychology Bulletin*, **32**(4), 552–60.

8. Adler, G. and Buie, D. (1979). Aloneness and borderline psychopathology: the possible relevance of some child developmental issues. *The International Journal of Psycho-analysis*, **60**, 83–96.

9. Eagle, M. (2003). Clinical implications of attachment theory. *Psychoanalytic Inquiry*, **23**(1), 27–53.

10. Mikulincer, M. and Shaver, P.R. (2004). Security-based self representations in adulthood: contents and processes. In *Adult attachment: theory, research and clinical implications* (eds. W.S. Rholes and J.A. Simpson), pp. 159–95. Guilford, New York.

11. Winnicott, D.W. (1958). The capacity to be alone. In *The maturational processes and the facilitating environment*, pp. 29–36. International Universities Press, New York, 1965.

12. Westen, D. and Gabbard, G.O. (2002). Developments in cognitive neuroscience. II. Implications for theories of transference. *Journal of the American Psychoanalytic Association*, **50**(1), 99–134.

13. Hartmann, H. (1939). *Ego psychology and the problem of adaptation*. International Universities Press, New York, 1958.

14. Freud, A. (1965). *Normality and pathology in childhood: assessments of development*. International Universities Press, Madison, CT.

15. Klein, M. (1948). On the theory of anxiety and guilt. In *Envy and gratitude and other works, 1946–1963*. (eds. M. Masud and R. Khan) Delacorte Press, New York, 1975.

16. Fairbairn, W.R.D. (1952). *An object-relations theory of the personality*. Basic Books, New York, 1954.

17. Kohut, H. (1984). *How does analysis cure?* University of Chicago Press, Chicago.

18. Kernberg, O.F. (1976). *Object relations theory and clinical psychoanalysis*. Aronson, New York.

19. Rosenfeld, H. (1987). *Impasse and interpretation*. Tavistock Publications, London.

20. Aron, L. and Harris, A. (eds.) (2005). *Relational psychoanalysis: innovation and expansion*, Vol. II. Analytic Press, Hillsdale, NJ.

21. Sullivan, H.S. (1953). *The interpersonal theory of psychiatry*. Norton, New York.

22. Mitchell, S.A. and Aron, L. (eds.) (1999). *Relational psychoanalysis: the emergence of a tradition*. Analytic Press, Hillsdale, NJ.

23. Seligman, S. (2003). The developmental perspective in relational psychoanalysis. *Contemporary Psychoanalysis*, **39**, 477–508.

24. Fonagy, P. (2003). Some complexities in the relationship of psychoanalytic theory to technique. *The Psychoanalytic Quarterly*, **72**, 13–48.

25. Sandell, R., Blomberg, J., and Lazar, A. (2002). Time matters. On temporal interactions in psychoanalysis and long-term psychotherapy. *Psychotherapy Research*, **12**, 39–58.

26. Freud, S. and Breuer, J. (1895). Studies on hysteria. In *The standard edition of the complete psychological works of Sigmund Freud*, Vol. 2 (ed. J. Strachey), pp. 1–305. Hogarth Press, London.

27. Castelnuovo-Tedesco, P. (1994). On rereading the case of Anna O: more about questions that are unanswerable. *Journal of the American Academy of Psychoanalysis*, **22**, 57–71.

28. Freud, S. (1899). Screen memories. In *The standard edition of the complete psychological works of Sigmund Freud*, Vol. 3 (ed. J. Strachey), pp. 301–22. Hogarth Press, London.

29. Fonagy, P. and Target, M. (1997). Perspectives on the recovered memories debate. In *Recovered memories of abuse: true or false?* (eds. J. Sandler and P. Fonagy), pp. 183–216. Karnac Books, London.

30. Freud, S. (1912a). The dynamics of transference. In *Standard edition of the complete psychological works of Sigmund Freud*, Vol. 12, (ed. J. Strachey) pp. 97–109. Hogarth Press and the Institute of Psycho-Analysis, London.

31. Freud, S. (1914). Remembering, repeating, and working through. In *The standard edition of the complete psychological works of Sigmund Freud*, Vol. 12 (ed. J. Strachey), pp. 145–56. Hogarth Press, London.

32. Jones, E. (1953). *The life and work of Sigmund Freud*, Vol. I. Basic Books, New York.

33. Celenza, A. and Gabbard, G.O. (2003). Analysts who commit sexual boundary violations: a lost cause? *Journal of the American Psychoanalytic Association*, **51**(2), 617–36.

34. Freud, S. (1937). Analysis terminable and interminable. In *The standard edition of the complete psychological works of Sigmund Freud*, Vol. 23 (ed. J. Strachey), pp. 209–53. Hogarth Press, London.

35. Walter, B. (1946). *Theme and variations*. Knopf, New York.

36. Ferenczi, S. (1930). The principle of relaxation and neocatharsis. *The International Journal of Psycho-analysis*, **11**, 428–43.

37. Szecsödi, I. (2007). Sándor Ferenczi–the first intersubjectivist. *Scandinavian Psychoanalytic Review*, **30**(1), 31–41.

38. Eissler, K.R. (1953). The effect of the structure of the ego on psychoanalytic technique. *Journal of the American Psychoanalytic Association*, **1**, 104–43.

39. Guntrip, H. (1975). My experience of analysis with Fairbairn and Winnicott. *International Review of Psychoanalysis*, **2**, 145–56.

40. Ferenczi, S. and Rank, O. (1925). *The development of psychoanalysis*. International Universities Press, Madison, CT, 1986.

41. Altman, N., Briggs, R., Frankel, J., *et al.* (2002). *Relational child psychotherapy*. The Other Press, New York.

42. Freud, S. (1915). Observations on transference love. In *The standard edition of the complete psychological works of Sigmund Freud*, Vol. 12 (ed. J. Strachey), pp. 157–71. Hogarth Press, London.

43. Lambert, M. (ed.) (2004). *Bergin and Garfield's handbook of psychotherapy and behavior change*. Wiley, New York.

44. Orlinksy, D.E., Ronnestad, M.H., and Willutski, U. (2004). Fifty years of psychotherapy process-outcome research: continuity and change. In *Bergin and Garfield's handbook of psychotherapy and behavior change* (ed. M. Lambert), pp. 307–90. Wiley, New York.

45. Pinsker-Aspen, J., Stein, M., and Hilsenroth, M. (2007). Clinical utility of early memories as a predictor of early therapeutic alliance. *Psychotherapy: Theory, Research, Practice, Training*, **44**, 96–109.

46. Blagov, P.S. and Singer, J.A. (2004). Four dimensions of self-defining memories (specificity, meaning, content, and affect) and their relationships to self-restraint, distress, and repressive defensiveness. *Journal of Personality*, **72**(3), 481–511.

47. Lyons-Ruth, K. (2003). Dissociation and the parent-infant dialogue: a longitudinal perspective from attachment research. *Journal of the American Psychoanalytic Association*, **51**(3), 883–911.

48. Shamir-Essakow, G., Ungerer, J.A., Rapee, R.M., *et al.* (2004). Caregiving representations of mothers of behaviorally inhibited and uninhibited preschool children. *Developmental Psychology*, **40**(6), 899–910.

49. Brenner, C. (1982). *The mind in conflict*. International Universities Press, New York.

50. Walins, D.J. (2007). *Attachment and psychotherapy*. Guilford Press, New York.

51. Steiner, J. (2000). Containment, enactment and communication. *The International Journal of Psycho-analysis*, **81**(2), 245–55.

52. Vaillant, G.E. (1992). *Ego mechanisms of defense: a guide for clinicians and researchers*. American Psychiatric Association Press, Washington, DC.

53. Klein, M. (1946). Notes on some schizoid mechanisms. In *Developments in psychoanalysis* (eds. M. Klein, P. Heimann, S. Isaacs, and J. Riviere), pp. 292–320. Hogarth Press, London.

54. Heimann, P. (1956). Dynamics of transference interpretation. *International Journal Psycho-analysis*, **37**, 303–10.

55. Bion, W.R. (1962). *Learning from experience*. Heinemann, London.

56. Greatrex, T. S. (2002). Projective identification: how does it work? *Neuro-Psychoanalysis*, **4**, 187–97.

57. Fraiberg, S. (1982). Pathological defenses in infancy. *The Psychoanalytic Quarterly*, **51**, 612–35.

58. Freud, A. (1936). *The ego and the mechanisms of defence*. International Universities Press, New York, 1946.

59. Horowitz, M.J. (1995). Defensive control states and person schemas. In *Research in psychoanalysis: process, development, outcome* (eds. T. Shapiro and R.N. Emde), pp. 67–89. International Universities Press, Madison, CT.

60. Kaye, A.L. and Shea, M.T. (2000). Personality disorders, personality traits, and defense mechanisms. In *Handbook of psychiatric measures* (ed. Task Force for the Handbook of Psychiatric Measures), pp. 713–49. American Psychiatric Association, Washington, DC.

61. Spitz, R. (1961). Some early prototypes of ego defenses. *Journal of the American Psychoanalytic Association*, **9**, 626–51.

62. Cassidy, J. and Kobak, R.R. (1988). Avoidance and its relation to other defensive processes. In *Clinical implications of attachment* (eds. J. Belsky and T. Nezworski), pp. 300–23. Erlbaum, Hillsdale, NJ.

63. Mikulincer, M. and Shaver, P.R. (2003). The attachment behavior system in adulthood: contents and processes. In *Advances in experimental social psychology*, Vol. 35 (ed. M.P. Zanna), pp. 53–152. Academic Press, San Diego, CA.

64. Bowlby, J. (1980). *Attachment and loss, Vol. 3: loss: sadness and depression*. Hogarth Press and Institute of Psycho-Analysis, London.

65. George, C. and West, M. (2001). The development and preliminary validation of a new measure of adult attachment: the adult attachment projective. *Attachment & Human Development*, **3**(1), 30–61.

66. Fraley, R.C. and Shaver, P.R. (1997). Adult attachment and the suppression of unwanted thoughts. *Journal of Personality and Social Psychology*, **73**(5), 1080–91.

67. Mikulincer, M. and Horesh, N. (1999). Adult attachment style and the perception of others: the role of projective mechanisms. *Journal of Personality and Social Psychology*, **76**(6), 1022–34.

68. Mikulincer, M., Dolev, T., and Shaver, P.R. (2004). Attachment-related strategies during thought suppression: ironic rebounds and vulnerable self-representations. *Journal of Personality and Social Psychology*, **87**(6), 940–56.

69. PDM Task Force. (2006). *Psychodynamic diagnostic manual*. Alliance of Psychoanalytic Organizations, Silver Spring, MD.

70. Freud, S. (1933). New introductory lectures on psychoanalysis. In *The standard edition of the complete psychological works of Sigmund Freud*, Vol. 22 (ed. J. Strachey), pp. 1–182. Hogarth Press, London.

71. Etchegoyen, H. (1991). *The fundamentals of psychoanalytic technique*. Karnac, London.

72. Thomä, H. and Kächele, H. (1987). *Psychoanalytic practice. I. Principles*. Springer-Verlag, New York.

73. Spillius, E.B. (2001). Freud and Klein on the concept of phantasy. *The International Journal of Psycho-analysis*, **82**(2), 361–73.

74. Gergely, G. (2000). Reapproaching Mahler: new perspectives on normal autism, normal symbiosis, splitting and libidinal object constancy from cognitive developmental theory. *Journal of the American Psychoanalytic Association*, **48**(4), 1197–228.

75. Allen, J.G. (2006). Mentalizing in practice. In *Handbook of mentalization based treatments* (eds. J.G. Allen and P. Fonagy), pp. 3–30. Wiley, Chichester.

76. Britton, R. (1998). *Belief and imagination*. Routledge, London.

77. Lipsius, S.H. (2001). Working through in psychoanalytic psychotherapy: an alternative and complementary path. *Journal of the American Academy of Psychoanalysis*, **29**, 585–600.

78. Loewald, H.W. (1960). On the therapeutic action of psycho-analysis. *The International Journal of Psycho-analysis*, **41**, 16–33.

79. Sandler, J. and Dreher, A.U. (1996). *What do psychoanalysts want? The problem of aims in psychoanalysis*, Vol. 24. Routledge, London and New York.

80. Chodorow, N.J. (2003). The psychoanalytic vision of Hans Loewald. *The International Journal of Psycho-analysis*, **84**, 897–913.

81. Hoffman, I.Z. (2006). The myths of free association and the potentials of the analytic relationship. *The International Journal of Psycho-analysis*, **87**(Pt 1), 43–61.

82. Levenson, E. (1983). *The ambiguity of change*. Basic Books, New York.

83. Pine, F. (1998). *Diversity and direction in psychoanalytic technique*. Yale University Press, New Haven, CT.

84. Blatt, S.J. (2004). *Experiences of depression: theoretical, clinical and research perspectives*. American Psychological Association, Washington, DC.

85. Blatt, S.J., Auerbach, J.S., Zuroff, D.C., *et al.* (2006). Evaluating efficacy, effectiveness, and mutative factors in psychodynamic psychotherapies. In *Psychodynamic diagnostic manual* (ed. PDM Task Force). Alliance of Psychoanalytic Organizations, Silver Spring, MD.

86. Varvin, S. (2003). Which patients should avoid psychoanalysis, and which professionals should avoid psychoanalytic training? A critical evaluation. *Scandinavian Psychoanalytic Review*, **26**, 109–22.

87. Coltart, N. (1988). Diagnosis and assessment for suitability for psycho-analytic psychotherapy. *British Journal of Psychotherapy*, **4**, 127–134.

88. Kernberg, O.F. (1981). Structural interviewing. *The Psychiatric Clinics of North America*, **4**, 169–95.

89. Piper, W.E., Ogrodniczuk, J.S., McCallum, M., *et al.* (2003). Expression of affect as a mediator of the relationship between quality of object relations and group therapy outcome for patients with complicated grief. *Journal of Consulting and Clinical Psychology*, **71**(4), 664–71.

90. Shahar, G., Blatt, S.J., Zuroff, D.C., *et al.* (2003). Role of perfectionism and personality disorder features in response to brief treatment for depression. *Journal of Consulting and Clinical Psychology*, **71**(3), 629–33.

91. Leuzinger-Bohleber, M. (2002). A follow-up study critical inspiration for our clinical practice? In *Outcomes of psychoanalytic treatment. Perspectives for therapists and researchers* (eds. M. Leuzinger-Bohleber and M. Target). Whurr Publishers, London and Philadelphia.

92. Clarkin, J.F. and Levy, K.N. (2004). The influence of client variables on psychotherapy. In *Bergin & Garfield's handbook of psychotherapy and behavior change* (ed. M.J. Lambert), pp. 194–226. Wiley, New York.

93. Piper, W.E., Joyce, A.S., Azim, H.F.A., *et al.* (1994). Patient characteristics and success in day treatment. *Journal of Nervous and Mental Diseases*, **179**, 432–8.

94. Holmes, J. (2003). Borderline personality disorder and the search for meaning: an attachment perspective. *The Australian and New Zealand Journal of Psychiatry*, **37**(5), 524–31.

95. Fonagy, P., Leigh, T., Steele, M., *et al.* (1996). The relation of attachment status, psychiatric classification, and response to psychotherapy. *Journal of Consulting and Clinical Psychology*, **64**, 22–31.

96. Sandler, J., Dare, C. and Holder, A. (1992). *The patient and the analyst* (2nd edn). Karnac, London.

97. Limentani, A. (1972). The assessment of analysability: a major hazard in selection for psychoanalysis. *The International Journal of Psycho-analysis*, **53**, 351–61.

98. Kernberg, O., Clarkin, J.F., and Yeomans, F.E. (2002). *A primer of transference focused psychotherapy for the borderline patient*. Jason Aronson, New York.

99. Bateman, A.W. and Fonagy, P. (2004b). *Psychotherapy for borderline personality disorder: mentalization based treatment*. Oxford University Press, Oxford.

100. Winnicott, D.W. (1965). *The maturational process and the facilitating environment*. Hogarth Press, London.

101. Ryle, A. (2004). The contribution of cognitive analytic therapy to the treatment of borderline personality disorder. *Journal of Personality Disorders*, **18**(1), 3–35.

102. Gorman, H.E. (2002). Growing psychoanalysis. *Canadian Journal of Psychoanalysis*, **10**(1), 45–69.

103. Feldman, M. (1993). The dynamics of reassurance. *The International Journal of Psycho-analysis*, **74**, 275–85.

104. Sandler, J. and Sandler, A.M. (1994). Theoretical and technical comments on regression and anti-regression. *The International Journal of Psycho-analysis*, **75**, 431–9.

105. Inderbitzin, L.B. and Levy, S.T. (2000). Regression and psychoanalytic technique. *The Psychoanalytic Quarterly*, **69**(2), 195–223.

106. Smith, H.F. (1997). Resistance, enactment, and interpretation: a self-analytic study. *Psychoanalytic Inquiry*, **17**(1), 13–30.

107. Cairo-Chiarandini, I. (2001). To have and have not: clinical uses of envy. *Journal of the American Psychoanalytic Association*, **49**, 1391–404.

108. Smith, H.F. (2003a). Analysis of transference: a north American perspective. *The International Journal of Psycho-analysis*, **84**, 1017–41.

109. Kernberg, O.F. (1984). *Severe personality disorders: psychotherapeutic strategies*. Yale University Press, New Haven, CT.

110. Bowlby, J. (1988). *A secure base: clinical applications of attachment theory*. Routledge, London.

111. Diamond, D., Stovall-McClough, C., Clarkin, J.F., *et al.* (2003). Patient-therapist attachment in the treatment of borderline personality disorder. *Bulletin of the Menninger Clinic*, **67**(3), 227–59.

112. Farber, B.A., Lippert, R., and Nevas, D. (1995). The therapist as attachment figure. *Psychotherapy*, **32**, 204–12.

113. Mallincrodt, B., Porter, M., and Kivlighan, M. (2005). Client attachment to therapist, depth of in-session exploration and object relations in brief psychotherapy. *Psychotherapy: Theory, Research, Practice, Training*, **42**, 85–100.

114. Parish, M. and Eagle, M.N. (2003). Attachment to the therapist. *Psychoanalytic Psychology*, **20**(2), 271–86.

115. Bradley, R., Heim, A.K., and Westen, D. (2005). Transference patterns in the psychotherapy of personality disorders: empirical investigation. *The British Journal of Psychiatry*, **186**, 342–9.

116. Eames, V. and Roth, A. (2000). Patient attachment orientation and the early working alliance: a study of patient and therapist reports of alliance quality and ruptures. *Journal of Psycho-Therapy Research*, **10**, 421–34.

117. Waldinger, R.J., Seidman, E.L., Gerber, A.J., *et al.* (2003). Attachment and core relationship themes: wishes for autonomy and closeness in the narratives of securely and insecurely attached adults. *Psychotherapy Research*, **13**(1), 77–98.

118. Spence, D.P. (1982). *Narrative truth and historical truth. Meaning and interpretation in psychoanalysis*. Norton, New York/London.

119. Joseph, B. (1985). Transference: the total situation. *The International Journal of Psycho-analysis*, **66**, 447–54.

120. Cavell, M. (1994). *The psychoanalytic mind*. Harvard University Press, Cambridge, MA.

121. Hausner, R.S. (2000). The therapeutic and working alliances. *Journal of American Psychoanalytic Association*, **48**(1), 155–87.

122. Strachey, J. (1934). The nature of the therapeutic action of psychoanalysis. *The International Journal of Psycho-analysis*, **15**, 275–92.

123. Couch, A.S. (2002). Extra-transference interpretation. *Psychoanalytic Study of the Child*, **57**, 63–92.

124. Hoglend, P., Amlo, S., Marble, A., *et al.* (2006). Analysis of the patient-therapist relationship in dynamic psychotherapy: an experimental study of transference interpretations. *The American Journal of Psychiatry*, **163**(10), 1739–46.

125. Hoglend, P., Johansson, P., Marble, A., *et al.* (2007). Moderators of the effect of transference interpretation in brief dynamic psychotherapy. *Psychotherapy Research*, **17**(2), 162–74.

126. Bollas, C. (1994). Aspects of the erotic transference. *Psychoanalytic Inquiry*, **14**(4), 572–90.

127. Bowlby, J. (1977). The making and breaking of affectional bonds. II. Some principles of psychotherapy. *The British Journal of Psychiatry*, **130**, 421–31.

128. Fonagy, P., Gergely, G., Jurist, E., *et al.* (2002). *Affect regulation, mentalization and the development of the self*. The Other Press, New York.

129. Spillius, E.B. (1992). Clinical experiences of projective identification. In *Clinical lectures on Klein and Bion* (ed. R. Anderson), pp. 59–73. Routledge, London.

130. Freud, S. (1912b). Recommendations to physicians practising psychoanalysis. In *The standard edition of the complete psychological works of Sigmund Freud*, Vol. 12 (ed. J. Strachey), pp. 109–120. Hogarth Press, London.

131. Heimann, P. (1950). On countertransference. *The International Journal of Psycho-analysis*, **31**, 81–4.

132. Renik, O. (1998). The analyst's subjectivity and the analyst's objectivity. *The International Journal of Psycho-analysis*, **79**, 487–97.

133. Mitchell, S.A. (1997). *Influence and autonomy in psychoanalysis*. Analytic Press, Hillsdale, N.J.

134. Racker, H. (1968). *Transference and countertransference*. Hogarth Press, London.

135. King, P. (1978). Affective response of the analyst to the patient's communications. *The International Journal of Psycho-analysis*, **59**, 329–34.

136. Sandler, J. (1993). Communication from patient to analyst: not everything is projective identification. *British Psycho-Analytical Society Bulletin*, **29**, 8–16.

137. Gallese, V., Keysers, C., and Rizzolatti, G. (2004). A unifying view of the basis of social cognition. *Trends in Cognitive Sciences*, **8**(9), 396–403.

138. Rizzolatti, G. and Craighero, L. (2004). The mirror-neuron system. *Annual Review of Neuroscience*, **27**, 169–92.

139. Fonagy, P. and Target, M. (2007). The rooting of the mind in the body: new links between attachment theory and psychoanalytic thought. *Journal of the American Psychoanalytic Association*, **55**(2), 411–56.

140. Winnicott, D.W. (1949). Hate in the countertransference. *The International Journal of Psycho-analysis*, **30**, 69–75.

141. Betan, E., Heim, A.K., Zittel Conklin, C., *et al.* (2005). Countertransference phenomena and personality pathology in clinical practice: an empirical investigation. *The American Journal of Psychiatry*, **162**(5), 890–8.

142. Leuzinger-Bohleber, M., Stuhr, U., Ruger, B., *et al.* (2003a). How to study the 'quality of psychoanalytic treatments' and their long-term effects on patients' well-being: a representative, multi-perspective follow-up study. *The International Journal of Psycho-analysis*, **84**(Pt 2), 263–90.

143. Blum, H.P. (1989). The concept of termination and the evolution of psychoanalytic thought. Annual meeting of the American Psychoanalytic Association (1987, Montreal, Canada). *Journal of the American Psychoanalytic Association*, **37**, 275–95.

144. Bateman, A.W. and Fonagy, P. (2006). *Mentalization based treatment for borderline personality disorder: a practical guide*. Oxford University Press, Oxford.

145. Fonagy, P. (1999). Memory and therapeutic action (guest editorial). *The International Journal of Psycho-analysis*, **80**, 215–23.

146. Steiner, J. (1993). *Psychic retreats: pathological organisations in psychotic, neurotic and borderline patients*. Routledge, London.

147. Fonagy, P. and Bateman, A. (2006). Progress in the treatment of borderline personality disorder. *The British Journal of Psychiatry*, **188**, 1–3.

148. O'Shaughnessy, E. (1992). Enclaves and excursions. *The International Journal of Psycho-analysis*, **73**, 603–11.

149. Symington, N. (1983). The analyst's act of freedom as agent of therapeutic change. *International Review of Psycho-analysis*, **10**, 783–92.

150. Ehrenberg, D. (1993). *The intimate edge*. Norton, New York.

151. Safran, J.D. (2003). The relational turn, the therapeutic alliance, and psychotherapy research: strange bedfellows or postmodern marriage? *Contemporary Psychoanalysis*, **39**, 449–75.

152. Bateman, A.W. and Fonagy, P. (2004a). Mentalization-based treatment of BPD. *Journal of Personality Disorders*, **18**(1), 36–51.

153. Klein, M. (1950). On the criteria for the termination of a psychoanalysis. *The International Journal of Psycho-analysis*, **31**, 78–80.

154. Payne, S. (1950). Short communication on criteria for terminating analysis. *The International Journal of Psycho-analysis*, **31**, 205.

155. Pedder, J. (1988). Termination reconsidered. *The International Journal of Psycho-analysis*, **69**, 495–505.

156. Bachrach, H.M., Galatzer-Levy, R., Skolnikoff, A., *et al.* (1991). On the efficacy of psychoanalysis. *Journal of the American Psychoanalytic Association*, **39**, 871–916.

157. Fonagy, P., Kachele, H., Krause, R., *et al.* (2002). *An open door review of outcome studies in psychoanalysis* (2nd edn). International Psychoanalytical Association, London.

158. Lazar, S.G. (ed.) (1997). *Extended dynamic psychotherapy: making the case in an era of managed care*. Analytic Press, Hillsdale, NJ.

159. Leuzinger-Bohleber, M. and Target, M. (eds.) (2002). *The outcomes of psychoanalytic treatment*. Whurr, London.

160. Richardson, P., Kachele, H., and Renlund, C. (eds.) (2004). *Research on psychoanalytic psychotherapy with adults*. Karnac, London.

161. Stanton, A.H., Gunderson, J.G., Knapp, P.H., *et al.* (1984). Effects of psychotherapy in schizophrenia. I. Design and implementation of a controlled study. *Schizophrenia Bulletin*, **10**, 520–63.

162. Bateman, A.W. and Fonagy, P. (1999). The effectiveness of partial hospitalization in the treatment of borderline personality disorder-a randomised controlled trial. *The American Journal of Psychiatry*, **156**, 1563–9.

163. Bateman, A.W. and Fonagy, P. (2001). Treatment of borderline personality disorder with psychoanalytically oriented partial hospitalization: an 18-month follow-up. *The American Journal of Psychiatry*, **158**(1), 36–42.

164. Blomberg, J., Lazar, A., and Sandell, R. (2001). Outcome of patients in long-term psychoanalytical treatments. First findings of the Stockholm outcome of psychotherapy and psychoanalysis (STOPP) study. *Psychotherapy Research*, **11**, 361–82.

165. Grant, J. and Sandell, R. (2004). Close family or mere neighbours? Some empirical data on the differences between psychoanalysis and psychotherapy. In *Research on psychoanalytic psychotherapy with adults* (eds. P. Richardson, H. Kächele, and C. Renlund), pp. 81–108. Karnac, London.

166. Sandell, R., Blomberg, J., Lazar, A., *et al.* (2000). Varieties of long-term outcome among patients in psychoanalysis and long-term psychotherapy: a review of findings in the Stockholm outcome of

psychoanalysis and psychotherapy project (STOPP). *The International Journal of Psycho-analysis*, 81(5), 921–43.

167. Leuzinger-Bohleber, M., Stuhr, U., Ruger, B., *et al.* (2003b). How to study the quality of psychoanalytic treatments and their long-term effects on patients' well-being: a representative, multi-perspective follow-up study. *The International Journal of Psycho-analysis*, 84, 263–90.

168. Gabbard, G.O., Gunderson, J.G., and Fonagy, P. (2002). The place of psychoanalytic treatments within psychiatry. *Archives of General Psychiatry*, 59(6), 505–10.

169. Fonagy, P. (2006). Evidence-based psychodynamic psychotherapies. In *Psychodynamic diagnostic manual* (ed. PDM Task Force). Alliance of Psychoanalytic Organizations, Silver Spring, MD.

170. Bachrach, H.M., Weber, J.J., and Murray, S. (1985). Factors associated with the outcome of psychoanalysis. Report of the Columbia psychoanalytic research center (IV). *International Review of Psychoanalysis*, 12, 379–89.

171. Erle, J. and Goldberg, D. (1984). Observations on assessment of analyzability by experienced analysts. *Journal of the American Psychoanalytical Association*, 32, 715–37.

172. Sandell, R., Blomberg, J., Lazar, A., *et al.* (1997). *Findings of the Stockholm outcome of psychotherapy and psychoanalysis project (STOPPP)*. Paper presented at the Annual Meeting of the Society for Psychotherapy Research, Geilo, Norway.

173. Dührssen, A. (1962). Katamnestische Ergebnisse bei 1004 Patienten nach analytischer Psychotherapie. *Psychosomatic Medicine*, 8, 94–113.

174. Breyer, F., Heinzel, R., and Klein, T. (1997). Kosten und Nutzen ambulanter Psychoanalyse in Deutschland (Cost and benefits of outpatient psychoanalytic therapy in Germany). *Gesundheitsökonomie und Qualitätsmanagement*, 2, 59–73.

175. Bateman, A.W. and Fonagy, P. (2003). Health service utilization costs for borderline personality disorder patients treated with psychoanalytically oriented partial hospitalization versus general psychiatric care. *The American Journal of Psychiatry*, 160(1), 169–71.

176. Clarkin, J., Levy, K.N., Lenzenweger, M.F., *et al.* (2007). Evaluating three treatments for borderline personality disorder: a multiwave study. *The American Journal of Psychiatry*, 164, 922–8.

177. Giesen-Bloo, J., van Dyck, R., Spinhoven, P., *et al.* (2006). Outpatient psychotherapy for borderline personality disorder: randomized trial of schema-focused therapy vs transference-focused psychotherapy. *Archives of General Psychiatry*, 63(6), 649–58.

# 6.3.6 **Group methods in adult psychiatry**

John Schlapobersky and Malcolm Pines

## Introduction

After a century of development, group therapy is today one of the most widely practised treatment methods in psychiatry with an extensive literature. There are three principles common to its wide range of applications. First, the therapist calls the 'community' into the consulting room where, together with the therapist, it becomes the therapeutic agent. Second, the therapist assembles a group of people who can contribute to a commonly held resource from which its members can each derive benefits. And third, the therapist does nothing for them in the context of the group, that they can do for themselves, and one another.

This chapter starts by providing a conceptual framework that differentiates methods, models, and applications for the practice of group therapy in adult psychiatry. After classification of the different methods and applications we discuss the main theoretical models; explore the dynamic life of therapy groups; consider some of the key clinical issues facing practitioners; their applications to a range of patient populations and settings; their evaluation and justification and their historical evolution this century. In the conclusion we consider the planning of group services and the training of their practitioners. This revision of the chapter has brought it up-to-date with the contemporary literature in a field that has seen a great deal of innovation since the original 2000 edition.

The developing evidence base for group psychotherapy is 'Guardedly optimistic. The literature has become stronger and deeper and is capable of supporting evidence-based treatment recommendations for some patient populations.' The evidence base for the effectiveness of group psychotherapy has been growing with the field. Some 700 studies, spanning the past three decades, have shown that the group format consistently produced positive effects with diverse disorders and treatment models.[1] These show that both individual and group psychotherapy will effect much the same set of results. For group therapy to be effective it has to utilize those therapeutic factors originally laid out by Foulkes[2] and later by Yalom[3]—the group has to be the primary focus of therapy; patients need to be well selected; and therapists need to be adequately trained. The chapter will address these questions of focus, selection, and training.

Although the two authors of this chapter are both group analysts, we have set out to provide a full account of the wide range of group work practice. The United Kingdom is our own working location which lends emphasis to the chapter but it is compiled with sources and references that address the international field and it gives attention to current literature in many countries including North and South America and Continental Europe.

## Basic methods

In Fig. 6.3.6.1 we have used two simple factors—therapeutic goals and group leadership—to provide a simple classification of the many different methods.

### Therapeutic goals

Groups will be more or less specific in their therapeutic goals. For example, those catering for a homogeneous population with a commonly defined problem whose solution provides the basis for entry to the group—such as overcoming drink or drug dependence—are classified here with specific goals. Groups that provide psychoanalytic psychotherapy, whether run according to Interpersonal, Tavistock, or Group-Analytic models, are classified here with nonspecific goals. There is a wide range of variation between these extremes and within each of these main psychodynamic models.

### Leadership

The more the leader directs the group, the more prominent he becomes as the group's 'model object'. The less the leader directs the group, the more scope there is for the emergence of unconscious dynamics and for attention to transference and counter-transference. In this case, therapy progresses through the development of relationships. The greater the leadership activity, the more likely it

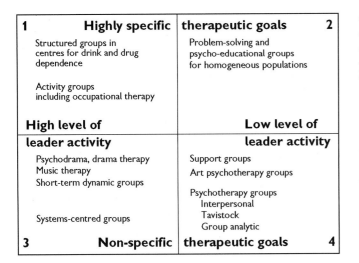

| 1 | **Highly specific** | **therapeutic goals** | 2 |
|---|---|---|---|
| Structured groups in centres for drink and drug dependence | | Problem-solving and psycho-educational groups for homogeneous populations | |
| Activity groups including occupational therapy | | | |
| **High level of** | | **Low level of** | |
| **leader activity** | | **leader activity** | |
| Psychodrama, drama therapy Music therapy Short-term dynamic groups | | Support groups Art psychotherapy groups | |
| Systems-centred groups | | Psychotherapy groups Interpersonal Tavistock Group analytic | |
| 3 | **Non-specific** | **therapeutic goals** | 4 |

**Fig. 6.3.6.1** A simple classification of group methods.

is that group members are being offered a technique or skill in the setting of a group. The lower this activity, the stronger will be the relational content of the therapy and the therapist's skills of fostering relationships will equip the group to work developmentally and in depth on both the obvious and hidden issues that its members bring. The three principal psychodynamic methods discussed in The principal model of psychodynamic group therapy below share a non-directive philosophy with subtle but significant differences between their models of practice.

Using these two basic indicators—specificity of goals and levels of leadership activity—the four quadrants in the diagram provide us with a simple way of 'placing' the different group therapies.

### Goal-specific therapy with high level of leader activity: quadrant 1

In many drug and alcohol dependency regimes, participants are required to fulfil obligations tied to each stage of a structured programme. They move forward when stage-specific obligations are fulfilled. As the novice moves up, he/she becomes a trainer to the newcomers with the therapist(s) directing the process in active terms. Cognitive therapy given in a group setting uses the group as an assembly who learn from and discuss with the expert. Dependency on a shared and valued leader, and attention to group dynamics amplify the learning and some group cohesion develops, but this is not the primary focus of the therapy.

### Goal-directed with lower level of leader activity: quadrant 2

Problem-solving or psycho-educational groups for homogeneous populations, such as those set up for eating disorders or offenders, which are run along analytic lines, can be placed in this category. Although there are clear and directed goals, the leader's level of activity is confined to a facilitating, linking, or enabling one, followed by analysis and interpretation. Group discussion and cohesion amplify the affective experience and enhance the learning.

### Non-specific goals with high level of leader activity: quadrant 3

In **psychodrama groups**, leadership is explicitly vested in the psychodrama director. The needs and goals of group members are

diffuse and often diverse and, in psychiatric practice, will have to do with relief from mental suffering. The psychodrama director can draw on many techniques. Affective arousal can be high so the power of sharing through discussion and the sympathy; and empathy of group members towards one another become powerful therapeutic tools. Strong conflict arousal and its subsequent resolution is similarly therapeutic.

**Systems-centred therapy** (as developed by Agazarian)[4] similarly provides a high level of leadership activity for groups that have non-specific goals. Short-term dynamic groups are frequently constituted with non-specific goals but are run over 10 or 20 sessions by leaders who maintain a high level of involvement and direction, often demarcated according to the different stages of the group's progress.

### Non-specific goals with low level of leader activity: quadrant 4

The goals of group-analytic or psychoanalytic group therapy are most frequently diffuse and non-specific involving relief from symptoms and other forms of suffering; personal growth; and psychological change. There are three main schools considered in this chapter—the Interpersonal (Yalom), Tavistock (Bion or group-as-a-whole), and the Group-Analytic. They share non-specific goals and have low levels of leader activity but differ from one another in how the leadership role and function is understood and discharged. They share assumptions about the importance of unconscious individual and group dynamics and look to the group for its transformational potential. Their differences affect the way in which transference and counter-transference is understood and worked with. There is a comparative appraisal of these models below.

## The application of basic methods

We now provide a more detailed overview of the current field and offer a brief set of training requirements for practitioners in each of the methods discussed.

The field can be divided into **five basic methods**—activity, supportive, problem-solving, psycho-educational, and psychodynamic. The first three methods are goal-specific as indicated by their descriptions, the fourth is less specific and the fifth is a non-directive analytic psychotherapy. In supportive and problem-solving groups, therapeutic leadership can be highly directed or not, depending on the approach. Activity and psycho-educational groups will inevitably have a high level of directed group leadership, whilst psychodynamic groups have a much lower level of directed group leadership. All five methods rely on the same basic procedures—the selection and grouping of a number of people seeking help who have regular meetings together with one or more well-trained therapist(s).

### Activity groups

The most vulnerable and disturbed patients can be placed in therapy groups defined by an activity that provides a convening function such as exercise or cooking. They can then be used to create conditions for a wide range of secondary functions that foster affiliations, develop social skills, address unspoken anxieties, and express troubling emotions. Occupational therapists and nurses using art media or other socially syntonic activity like gardening or hair-dressing have been developing a wide range of group services in both acute and rehabilitation psychiatry for many years.[5] The approach has been used in a wide range of other settings including medical rehabilitation, rehabilitation with refugees, social work and fostering, and adoption programmes. Groups that keep the original activity as their primary focus, working with art media for example, need to be differentiated from those which use such media to develop an analytic focus on psychological work. The arts psychotherapies belong to this latter group. They have non-specific therapeutic goals and might, as in the case of music therapy, have a high level of leadership activity or, in the case of art therapy, have a low level of leadership activity.

Whilst therapists do not engage in the uncovering and exploration of unconscious dynamics, they will need leadership abilities, capabilities in organizing group activities, and should have a basic understanding of psychopathology and group dynamics.

## Supportive groups

These groups function as a form of social support providing containment, the improvement of social skills, and the enhancement of participants' capacities for social adaptation. They aim to reduce the deleterious effects of social isolation, bring people out of withdrawal into a social context, and provide opportunities for problem sharing. They cater to patient populations with longstanding personality disorders not open to uncovering exploration; those with chronic mental and physical illness,[6] physical handicap, mental retardation, and carers for those with any of these problems. They will often allow a certain amount of psychoeducation with the group leader influencing members' attitudes as in the case, for example, of a group for young sexually active adults with learning disability who might receive guidance on contraception.

Whilst therapists do not engage in the uncovering and exploration of unconscious dynamics, they will need leadership abilities, capabilities in organizing group activities, and should have a basic understanding of psychopathology and group dynamics.

## Problem-solving groups

Group therapy is provided for a set of referral criteria to resolve a defined and sometimes circumscribed problem. Alcoholics Anonymous, Alanon, Gamblers Anonymous, and groups for people with poor impulse control, eating disorders, or other habitual problems such as smoking, are a few of the examples. These groups can take on many of the features of long-term support groups, in that they offer ego-supportive and adaptive resources, providing an extended service for monitoring by the patient or by professionals, without necessarily committing members to the deeper and more radical analytic work entailed by a psychodynamic group. In many cases, the problem-solving focus provides a convening frame by which to engage a population who are soon drawn into psychodynamic work that sees them through profound changes. Many of the groups run by clinicians in primary hospital care—occupational therapists, nurses, doctors, and psychologists—take this form. The Group Work Programme at the Medical Foundation For Victims Of Torture in London is another example (see also section on trauma in special population, below).

Where they cater for the more severely disturbed, staff will need to be well-trained in one of the core professions. They will

need leadership abilities, capabilities in organizing group activities, should have a basic understanding of psychopathology, and be sufficiently well-trained to explore the dynamic group issues that lead from the problem back to the personality structure of their membership. If therapeutic goals involve major changes in personality and social functioning, this will involve the uncovering and exploration of unconscious dynamics.

## Psycho-educational groups

The original groups for servicemen with war neurosis at Northfield took this form in which people were given the role of students of their disorders rather than 'sick' people. Patients become open to new information and are better able to unlearn maladaptive attitudes about the nature of their disorder. This more cognitive approach can be applied in homogeneous problem-solving groups. Information can be provided through lectures, discussions, and suitable reading material. There are different ways of lowering anxiety and uncovering maladaptive and inappropriate attitudes towards such problems as anxiety states, phobias and obsessions, and psychosomatic disorders. Many of the groups run for those with serious physical illness (see also section on the medically ill in special populations, below) take this form. And there is often a major psycho-educational component in support groups—for example, those with chronic mental illness who can be helped to understand and cope with delusions, hallucinations, and the stigma of illness.[7] (see also section on the mentally ill in special populations, below)

Staff need leadership abilities; capabilities in organizing group activities, a basic understanding of psychopathology, and need to be sufficiently well-trained in their chosen problem area to be able to relate its educational focus to thematic group issues. If therapeutic goals involve major changes in personality and social functioning, this will involve the uncovering and exploration of unconscious dynamics.

## Psychodynamic groups

There are supportive, problem-solving, and psycho-educational components in all psychodynamic groups, but the description 'psychodynamic' is reserved for those in which the declared goal is lasting personal change through a non-directive, free-associative therapy. The range of different group contexts is so varied that—at first sight—they might appear to have little in common. But there will be common principles offering therapy to a group of people on an in-patient unit recovering from psychosis and meeting thrice weekly; those in a secure unit for violent offenders meeting once weekly; and those—including mental health trainees—attending a group in private practice once or twice weekly. These principles can be summarized in the table, Table 6.3.6.1 below.

Within these parameters therapy is part of the cultural domain of all shared, conversational experience in which people struggle with meaning—in congregational life, in the confessional, in theatre, narrative or poetry.[8,9]

Staff need to be trained to the level already described. They need good leadership ability, capabilities in organizing group activities, and a good understanding of psychopathology. Beyond these requirements, therapeutic goals will involve major changes in personality and social functioning involving the uncovering and exploration of unconscious dynamics. So staff will need access to a

**Table 6.3.6.1** Organizing principles for group therapy

1  Members will have been chosen by the therapist.

2  They will have chosen to join and participate.

3  They will be expected to justify their place by reliable attendance and participation.

4  The work will be governed by a psychotherapeutic contract.

5  The contract will include definitions of confidentiality and other boundaries.

6  A therapeutic alliance with individual members will be established either prior to their joining the group or during the early stages of their attendance in the group.

7  Agreed parameters will include the duration and time-boundaries of the group as well as its membership and composition.

8  Groups can be homogeneous or heterogeneous.

9  Groups may have a fixed time limit or continue on a slow–open basis for many years.

10  Groups may have a stable and fixed, or a rotating membership with empty places taken by new members.

range of specialized training opportunities which should provide psychodynamic theory, clinical supervision and, ideally, some opportunity for the practitioners' own personal development.

# The contemporary field and its history

The paradigm shift that led to a vision of the group as a whole began over a period of time and in a number of locations. Trigant Burrow coined the term group analysis in the USA in the 1920s.[10,11] Further development in the years after World War II period enabled workers to recognize the dynamics of groups and institutions and led to group and family therapy, milieu therapy, and therapeutic community concept and practice.

## Second World War

In Britain and the US, during the Second World War, an appreciation of group psychology led to a wide range of innovations, the most important of which included:

- The use of group methods for selection and allocation of work responsibilities
- Studies of group morale
- The integration of psychiatric knowledge to the management of large groups through the role of the command psychiatrist
- The treatment of acute and prolonged battle stress and the rehabilitation of returned prisoners of war.

Clinicians used the opportunities created within army psychiatry to apply methods developed in the pre-war years.[12] Brigadier J.R. Rees, Director of the Tavistock Clinic in the 1930s, largely created this opportunity in the British Army. His Tavistock colleagues formed an 'invisible college' and were responsible for signal achievements in the advances in selection and treatment.[13]

Foremost amongst these were Northfield, the military hospital near Birmingham where S.H. Foulkes was a senior medical officer.[14] A refugee from Nazi Germany, Foulkes brought with him from the Frankfurt Institute the revised understanding of Freudian theory that was also to prove influential in the US. In the New School for Social Research, New York, and in the work of Neo-Freudians like

Erich Fromm, Frieda Fromm-Reichman, and social theorists like Adorno, Marcuse, and Norbert Elias, psychoanalysis and Marxist theory were brought into a new, creative relationship.[15] In the United Kingdom Foulkes first developed his approach to group therapy in Exeter before the war and was able to apply it successfully on a large scale to the treatment of war neuroses at Northfield.

## Post-war period

Group psychotherapy moved from inspirational and didactic models to psychodynamic and analytic ones in the post-war period.

### (a) United Kingdom

The Group-Analytic Tradition: Foulkes gathered around him a small group of clinicians and others who developed his ideas and practises. Drawing on the ideas of Trigant Burrow, they called it group analysis and later established the Group-Analytic Society, and trained generations of clinicians. His first book written in the heat of the Northfield experience outlined the basics of his approach.[16] Other publications followed and, with Malcolm Pines, training courses were established which lead to the founding of the Institutes of Group Analysis and Family Therapy, the Association of Family Therapists, and Association of Therapeutic Communities. There are now training courses in group analysis in many centres in the United Kingdom and continental Europe. The Journal, *Group Analysis*, established by Foulkes, continues to be the major publication in European group psychotherapy. Group-analytic psychotherapy has undergone clinical evaluation by a number of clinicians.[17–19]

The 'Tavistock' Approach: The approach originates in the work of Bion, Ezriel, Sutherland, and their colleagues. It shares with group analysis an interest in the underlying pattern of object relations in groups but, under the influence of Bion—its major exponent—his 'basic assumption theory' is applied to the exclusion of almost everything else. (Bion's monograph was his only publication on groups and marked the end of his interest in the subject.[20]) The approach has been especially influential in staff training and consultancy which, given the slender theoretical foundations on which it rests, suggests a wide responsiveness in the field of basic assumption theory. The approach has undergone further development in the United States where it is often referred to as group-as-a-whole. When employed as a therapy, it can overlook the individuality of a group's members, disturbing some patients whose experience of the group situation can repeat early developmental traumas of neglect and misunderstanding by caretakers. Malan's study of effectiveness[21] raised serious questions about the model's efficacy in its clinical applications but its training applications continue to influence the field.

### (b) United States
#### (i) Early pioneers

**Jacob Moreno** was the innovator of group psychodrama, a pioneer form of group psychotherapy.[22] He also introduced sociometry, a scientific method for the study of group affiliations and conflicts, widely accepted and used by social psychologists. **Slavson** was an educationalist of psychoanalytic persuasion who became the central figure in the early development of group psychotherapy. His clinical influence, particularly with groups for the parents of children in difficulty, and his focus on the dynamics of projection in groups has been of lasting importance.[23] His organizational efforts lead to the formation of the American Group Psychotherapy

Association. **Emanuel Schwartz** began to apply psychoanalytic ideas to group psychotherapy in the late 1930s and was later joined by **Alexander Wolf**.[24, 25] In their approach, people underwent an individual psychotherapy in the setting of a group, a kind of parallel process alongside their fellow patients, with attention focused on the transferential relationship between each individual and their therapist. The approach has been of lasting importance in creating a clinical framework for combining individual and group therapy. Foulkes' criticism at the time was that the approach overlooked any systematic use of group-specific process. In contrast to their 'psychotherapy in the group' he offered group analysis as a clinical alternative, describing it as 'psychotherapy by the group'.

### (ii) Irving Yalom

Yalom's interpersonal approach is influenced by the interpersonal psychotherapy of Sullivan and Frank. His *Theory And Practice of Group Psychotherapy*, now in its fifth edition and written jointly with Leszcz, is the first systematic account of groups informed by research and remains one of the most influential books in the field.[3] Yalom's later text on inpatient group psychotherapy systematized group work in that setting.[26]

### (iii) The contemporary field

There are many centres of excellence, a wide range of methods and models and an empirical base grounded in research. The most useful single text is by Rutan and Stone, now in its fourth edition.[27] Collections by Kaplan and Sadock[28] and by Alonso and Swiller[29] cover the field. Psychoanalytic models have a rich diversity of theory with contributions from object relations, self psychology, and social systems theory.[30] The Modern Group movement is amongst the most innovative, beginning with a classic text by Spotnitz[31] and developing through an active training programme, a journal, *The Modern Group,* and publications by Ormont[32] and others.

### (iv) South America

There is a vigorous field of development throughout South America that draws on both the Tavistock and Group Analytic traditions but is informed by independent sources based largely on the work of Pichon-Riviere. Tubert-Oklander and Hernandez de Tubert have introduced this approach, referred to as Operative Groups, to the English-speaking world.[33]

### (v) Continental Europe

Group methods have played an active part in the reconstruction of mental health services throughout Europe in the post-war period. Distinctive approaches are emerging. Those in Germany include psychosomatic practice[34] and the Gottingen model.[35] The journal of the Heidelberg Institute of Group Analysis gives access to a vigorous field. A major research study is in process, based in Germany, in which therapists throughout Europe are taking part and which aims to provide a detailed evaluation of group therapy, its patients, and its therapists.[36] Other distinctive developments include those in Italy[43] and original training models, for example, those in Greece[37] and Norway.[38]

## Principal models of psychodynamic group therapy

### The therapist

The therapist is responsible to the group— and to the institution in which it is set—for achieving and maintaining professional competence and should have a level of training appropriate to the task. A formal qualification in psychotherapy is the ideal training. This will have included theory, personal therapy for the therapist, and clinical supervision. Mental health professionals from all disciplines make an active contribution to a rich and diverse service with the training requirements of theory and supervision arranged at their workplace. The opportunity to run a group is provided in most psychiatric and psychology training programmes. Many centres and training institutions offer training in group methods and several are wholly committed to the training of group therapists who have their own professional associations in the UK and internationally. Private once- or twice-weekly analytic groups are now regarded by many mental health professionals as the therapy of choice for their personal development. Other requirements for a good therapist are listed in table 6.3.6.2.

### (a) Making a beginning

The establishment of a group begins as a management task in the definition of its goals, recruitment of its members, protection of its setting, venue and timetable, and in the maintenance of its ongoing life. It evolves as a therapeutic task in which the therapist is responsible for maintaining a therapeutic attitude to the individual members and to the group as a whole. Powerful affects and attitudes will be directed towards her which she will monitor and transform into verbal and non-verbal therapeutic responses.

The therapeutic rationale will allow the therapist to be discriminating and consistent about interventions of various kinds during the life of the group and what follows below provides an orientation—based on the dynamic elements of structure, process and content—to the three main models used in the UK.

## Structure, process, and content: the dynamic elements of a group

Regardless of the therapist's method, people usually start in groups with a form of serial monologue. Out of this arise the capacities to talk and listen that are often undeveloped or even non-existent at the outset of therapy but which are its core constituents. From talking and listening comes self-disclosure and out of this social exchange identification emerges, which in due course leads to dialogue and differentiation. So the conductor must give a place to monologue whilst, at the same time, cultivating dialogue—the exchange between members or sub-groups—and, ultimately,

**Table 6.3.6.2** Requirements for therapeutic competence

**Requirements for therapeutic competence include:**

1 The ability to follow complex interactions and processes.

2 The ability to discriminate between appropriate activity and a containing form of silence.

3 A reflective attitude and the capacity to consider and reflect upon the processes concerning both the individual members and the group as a whole.

4 An eye for both the visible and invisible group and a curiosity about the unconscious or otherwise hidden aspects of a group's life. This will require the therapist's access to their own internal process and a capacity to make use of it.

5 A therapeutic rationale for action related to the group tasks and leadership requirements including the psychopathology of the individuals, their psychodynamics, and group dynamics.

promoting discourse, defined here as the free interaction of participants in the flexible and complex exchange that distinguishes the communication of a group.

Structure describes the more enduring aspects of any group's makeup, the 'architecture' of its interpersonal relations conceptualized first in terms of the setting and its boundaries and then conceptualized in the bond between each individual, the therapist(s), and the group as a whole. Process describes the fluid and dynamic fluctuations of emotion and experience, the business of relating and communicating, the changes of association and inter-member responses. The content of a group's exchange is in its visible and audible events, in the narrative line and dramatic content of peoples' encounters, the topics raised, their thematic development, and the extent to which they are explored or avoided.

As Fig. 6.3.6.2 illustrates, each of these three dynamic elements has a determining influence on each of the others. For example, a group in which there was a problem caused by the institution's failure to honour its commitment to reliable space for regular meetings, would have a serious structural problem. Intrusion, relocation, or a conflict over space might then emerge in the content of the members' associations as they talked about shared past experience. The therapist would need to decide whether to direct the process towards the connection between past and present anxieties, or reassurance that the therapist would—from now on—be able to protect their space.

### (a) Overview of the Interpersonal, Tavistock, and Group-Analytic Models

In the Interpersonal school, intra-group interactions, including those between its members and the leader, are taken in their totality, but differentiating the leader as a different 'sort' of person from the others. In the Tavistock model, a two-body psychology is used to analyse the interchange between the leader and the group taken as a whole. The therapist's principal role is in the analysis and interpretation of defences against primitive anxieties (or basic assumptions). The Group-Analytic Model calls on elements of both foregoing models. Like the Tavistock model it considers the leader as structurally different to other group members but like the Interpersonal model, it encourages the leader to work in the group with individuals. A three-body psychology is used to understand the role of the leader who is referred to here as the conductor.

Therapy proceeds through the dynamic interaction between each individual, the conductor, and the group as a whole.

### (b) The model of interpersonal group therapy

The focus is on interpersonal learning as a primary mechanism of change. The group provides the antidote to maladaptive interpersonal beliefs and behaviours through feedback from others and encouragement to experiment with healthier behaviours first within the group and then outside. The joint examination of intra-group transference reactions allows members to replace processes that have a historical origin in the 'there and then', the dynamic past, with those more appropriate to the 'here and now', the dynamic present. The approach emphasizes the educational opportunities of working in the 'here and now' of the group. The therapist takes the responsibility for leading the group towards awareness of these interpersonal dynamics and their expressions. There is also greater therapist transparency than in other psychodynamic approaches with the therapist modelling desired behaviours, sharing the reactions to events in the group directly, and being open to feedback from other group members.

As the diagram indicates, interpersonal dynamics are kept at the forefront of members' attention by the therapist. This sets a pattern in which the content of members' discussions and the process of their interactions gives the group its agenda. The interpersonal approach places the therapist amongst other members of the group without giving him a distinctive structural identity and omits any formal demarcation for the boundaries of the group as a whole.

The model provided the early descriptive research on the phases of small groups, on the basis of which Yalom tabulated the **curative factors** in a group's life (see Table 6.3.6.3).

This construction has been very influential. Yalom's use of the term 'curative' poses many problems for those clinicians who see the goals of therapy involving personal growth and change. He did much to address this difficulty by singling out the last of his 'curative' factors—existential issues—for special treatment in a subsequent text.[49]

### (c) The Tavistock model

Bion's ideas have an explanatory power and simplicity of application that continues to prove illuminating.[40] In a group at any

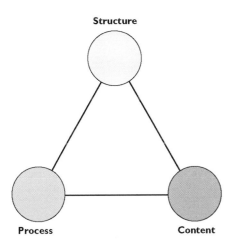

**Fig. 6.3.6.2** The dynamic elements of a group.

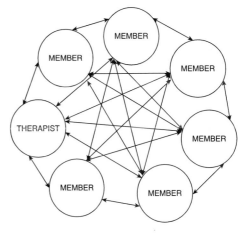

**Fig. 6.3.6.3** The elements of an interpersonal group.

**Table 6.3.6.3** Yalom's curative factors

1   Instillation of hope
2   Universality
3   Imparting information
4   Altruism
5   Corrective recapitulation of primary family group
6   Development of socializing techniques
7   Imitative behaviour
8   Interpersonal learning
9   Group cohesiveness
10  Catharsis
11  Existential factors

point in time, its culture and climate are governed by primitive, unconscious anxieties that impede its capacities for rational work in which the person or representation of the leader plays a crucial part. The anxieties, organized into one of three categories, referred to as **basic assumptions**, are dependency, fight or flight, and pairing. They affect the group as a whole in which only one basic assumption is believed to be operative at any point in time. Bion saw basic assumptions as interfering with the 'work group', the more rational, higher-level functioning of the group and its members. The therapist's key task lies in understanding and interpreting the operative basic assumption to the whole group. The meaning of individuals' experience is subsumed by this understanding of the whole. This therapist-centred approach sees transference only as directed towards the therapist who represents authority. In **dependency**, the group tries to elicit protection through passive or dependent behaviour. In **fight/flight** they will attack the therapist or some other issue; or retreat and withdraw. And in **pairing** they may create a group illusion that some magical form of rescue may arise from the dilemmas of group life through charged partnerships. Hopper has introduced a fourth basic assumption that he calls **massification/aggregation** in which the defensive structures of groups or societies in crisis is thought to entail either a rigid fusion of identities excluding individuality, or extensive withdrawal preventing mutuality.

The two-body psychology used here enforces a series of clinical constraints that reduce the complexity of group interaction to a bi-personal exchange between therapist and group taken as a whole. As Fig. 6.3.6.4 illustrates, intra-group dynamics are considered only in their entirety for what they reveal about the unconscious state of the group as a whole, and for what they indicate about the nature of the group's relationship with the therapist. Figure 6.3.6.4 illustrates how the therapist stands outside the group in a stance that is not only neutral and dispassionate but also opaque and withholding of self.

Ezriel, basing his work on Bion, developed his theory of **common group tension**.[41] He believed that the group would be caught up at any given time in a commonly shared conflict centred on the unconscious fear of catastrophe, what he called **the dreaded state**. People would avoid a state in the group—say one in which they talked about sad feelings—because of the unconscious fear that talking about sadness would lead to a dreaded state, in this case a depressive collapse. A group would be driven into unconscious, defensive organization—what he called **the required state**—to keep sadness at bay. For example, an extended period of manic humour, the required state, would help prevent **the avoided state**, sadness, and this would in turn protect against the dreaded state. Interpretations would allow members to become increasingly aware of the underlying catastrophic fears and reduce their need for defensive organization.

Horwitz calls Ezriel's approach 'deductive', in that it relates individual's contributions only to the common group tension. He realized that this deductive approach was clinically unproductive and developed, what he called an 'inductive' method which is group-centred.[42] Interventions are first addressed to individual members in the group. Only after working with patients individually does the therapist introduce a common theme that binds them together. Thus the therapist, as in the Group-Analytic model, works on a figure/ground basis in which individual contributions are valued and explored in their own right before they are contextualized in the life of the group as a whole.

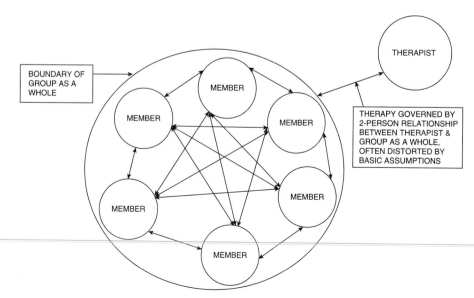

**Fig. 6.3.6.4** The elements of a Tavistock group.

Another approach, **focal conflict theory**, as developed by Whitaker and Lieberman[43] is similar to Ezriel's in focussing the therapist on a conflict that becomes his point of emphasis, but it answers Horwitz's criticisms. On their account, underlying **disturbing motives** in group behaviour are acted against by unconscious, **restrictive solutions**. On their account the therapist—by focusing on such key conflicts—helps give members access to the unconscious anxieties and once these have been relieved they can construct more **enabling solutions** to the shared dilemmas of the group. The idea of focal conflicts, conceived of in these broader terms, has become an integral part of the Group-Analytic model.

#### (d) The Group-Analytic model

This approach integrates important aspects of the two preceding models but introduces a number of new elements. As Fig. 6.3.6.5 suggests, the therapist is encouraged to address the individual as well as the whole group and considers the more conscious and individual dynamics as well as the unconscious and potentially destructive whole-group dynamics. The approach is guided by an integrated set of concepts relating structure, process, and content to one another in which the group conductor works both as therapist and as group member to foster and cultivate the ordinary language of shared conversational experience. He will at times take up the position of the group's manager, and at other times he will speak personally as one of its members. Groups may begin with a relatively high level of leadership activity, referred to as **dynamic administration**, which is flexibly reduced with a decrescendo of responsibility as the group becomes the therapist and the leadership function is devolved upon its membership who becomes active co-therapists in each other's treatment[44]. Figure 6.3.6.6 indicates how, in this approach, at one key moment in the group its theme can focus on structural dynamics that link one member to both the therapist and to the group as a whole. The web of interconnecting dynamics between any one member and all the others, is summarized by 'the group as a whole', and this is called on to represent the inter-connecting latticework of relationships that includes all the members and the therapist.

#### (c) The Matrix

As Fig. 6.3.6.6 indicates, the conductor is inside and a part of the group, the structural elements of which provide a way of understanding the crucial links between each member, the conductor and the group as a whole. The triangle by which the group's psychological objects are linked to each other illustrates one of the 6 corresponding patterns of connection. When replicated for each of the 6 members, the diagram will produce a **matrix** of relational patterns, a complex relational field that will undergo change in terms of alliances, sub-groups, and polarizations. This concept of the matrix is crucial in group analytic theory. It allows us to accept that all events in a group will become part of an unconscious network that is intrapsychic, interpersonal, and transpersonal. The developing matrix creates the capacity to receive, contain, and eventually transform individuals' contributions, fostering integration at the individual level as it does so in the group as a whole.

Free-floating discussion: Free floating discussion is the group-analytic equivalent of free-association. The term originates in Foulkes' own writing and describes a set of key clinical concepts in therapeutic practice that distinguish the group-analytic approach. The language of the group is discussed in the dynamic life of groups, below.

Group-specific process: These processes, also mapped out originally by Foulkes, have been studied further by Pines[45] and by Agazarian and Peters.[46] The key concept of **resonance** describes the unconscious communication of emotion. The group provides its members with a wide field of meaning which is explored as they **mirror** one another's experience, find their emotions **amplified** by association with one another, and find **condensed**, sometimes highly aroused, cathartic experience, moments charged with significance.

Content analysis: Foulkes described four levels at which the content of the group's discussion can be analysed in the search for meaning.[47] In the Tavistock model this is the therapist's exclusive task, whereas here interpretation is only one amongst a number of others. The therapist's overall stance is to foster communication and educate the group's members about the dynamic links between the group's structure, the content of the discussion, and the form

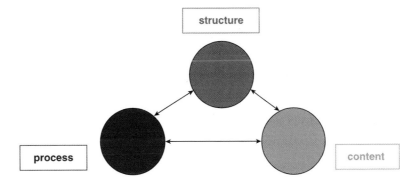

**1: Group activity**      * Psychotherapy in the group, by the group, including the conductor

**2: Group conductor**      * As therapist
      * As group member

**3: Group matrix**      * The ordinary language of shared conversational experience in which people struggle with meaning

**4: The dynamic elements of a group:**

structure

process

content

**Fig. 6.3.6.5** Group Analytic psychotherapy.

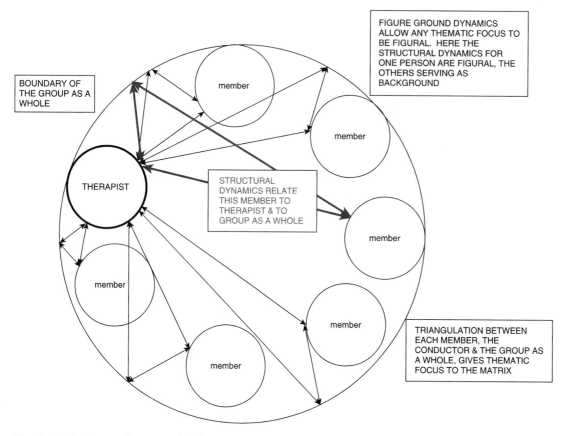

**Fig. 6.3.6.6** The elements of a group-analytic theory.

in which it takes place. Figure 6.3.6.7 illustrates the conductor's therapeutic role in relation to each of these dynamic elements of the discussion.

### (f) Recent developments in group-analytic psychotherapy

The role of dreams in group psychotherapy has been reconsidered.[48] Friedman described two of the unconscious functions they serve in group therapy—requests for containment and influence on relations with the dream audience.[49] Lipgar and Pines[50] work towards an integration of the ideas and methods of Bion and Foulkes with discussion from an international panel. Nitsun[51] considers sexuality in group psychotherapy: sexual identity, boundary transgression, erotic connection, dissociation of desire, the group as witness, erotic transference and counter-transference, and the effectiveness of psychotherapy.

### (g) The conductor as therapist and group member

At times of coherence, when the members are close in the shared experience of a moment, or when there is an issue charged with meaning, the group-analytic approach comes into its own. The symbolic content of the discourse might evolve in the language content, the flux of interactions, or the attention given to an individual's problems. The conductor needs to be able to model this use of imaginative play—with images, associations, or exchanges—and then stand back to allow members to take the enquiry forward. Cox[52] shows how images can safely hold experience too painful or brittle to tolerate much analysis. People discover that images can touch the depths before they stir the surface, giving access to

profoundly felt and deeply hidden concerns. When used and played with in this way, **the mutative use of metaphor** provides the whole group with a vehicle for change. Other aspects of the therapist's activity are summarized in Table 6.3.6.4.

## The dynamic life of groups

In the sections that follow we draw on our own Group-Analytic model to examine a range of clinical considerations and make them as relevant as possible to the widest range of practitioners, regardless of their own models.

### Group development theory

Many schemata have been proposed, usually derived from time-limited experiential and study groups but some of these can provide a useful orientation. Bennis and Shepard,[53] followed by Yalom, write about the initial stages of **orientation**, involving a search for structure and goals, dependence on the leader, and concern with boundaries. Their second stage is characterized by **conflict**, particularly over **norms**, authority, and control. Their third stage is achieved with a high level of group **coherence** that allows for inter- and intra-personal exploration. They acknowledge that the boundaries between phases are not clear and that a group never graduates permanently from any one phase.

In slow open groups, especially, this idea of discrete phases has its limits. The group-analytic approach provides a cyclic model in which focal issues such as affection, intimacy, personal history, and change, are understood and struggled with repeatedly. A group

| DYNAMIC ELEMENTS | CONDUCTOR'S THERAPEUTIC ROLE |
|---|---|
| **A: Structure** | **A: Dynamic administration** |

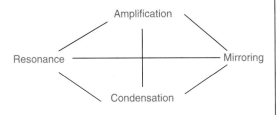

Individual
Conductor ——————— Group-as-a-whole

**A: Dynamic administration**

1  Group selection and composition
2  Managing the setting
3  Managing boundaries, membership and time issues

**B: Process**

Amplification
Resonance ——————— Mirroring
Condensation

**B: Facilitate members' participation and reflective analysis**

1  Allow and cultivate free-floating discussion
2  Location of group preoccupations and focal conflicts
3  Translation from language of unconscious symptoms to conscious behaviour – "ego training in action"

**C: Content**

The shared experience of the group analysed at 4 levels:

1  Current level
2  Transference level
3  Projective level
4  Primordial or archaic level

**C: Analysis and interpretation**

The conductor working as both therapist and group member:

1  Therapist provides holding, containment and reflection
2  Analysis of transference issues
3  Interpretation and therapist's use Of counter-transference
4  Mutative use of metaphor and allegory

**Fig. 6.3.6.7** Structure, process, and content—the conductor's therapeutic map.

**Table 6.3.6.4** The therapist's activity

**A: Leadership and analysis**

1  Model a capacity for open, direct communication
2  Maintain therapeutic neutrality
3  Attend to boundary events
4  Provide holding and containment
5  Withhold personal material
6  Drawn on counter-transference for
7  Reflection on group events
8  Bring events from background to foreground, or vice versa
9  Provide linking communications
10  Clarification and confrontation with individuals
11  Attention to omissions, avoidance, denial
12  Maintain silence

**B: Interpretation**

1  Locate group preoccupations
2  Translate from the language of unconscious (individual and group) behaviour
3  Interpret or provide metaphorical constructions for
   I  Defences and resistances
   II  Transference and projective process
   III  Archaic and primordial experience

understands in these terms struggles with **developmental tasks** rather than phases, in the course of which it is the individuals who enjoy growth, differentiation, and progressive change.

**(a) Developmental stages and thematic focus**

Figure 6.3.6.8 provides a map of these developmental tasks conceived of in logical rather than sequential terms. The way in which one person comes into the group will be different to the arrival of another. The terms on which one person joins will have a determining influence on each of the stages they pass through. For example, preoccupations about how someone came into the group—the terms of their engagement—might be resolved only when the person leaves perhaps one, three, or five years later, when they have to assess the outlook for their future as they look back over the years spent in therapy. So the diagram can be used as a thematic map for one person's journey through therapy, or as a way of appraising the stage reached by the group as a whole.

Early stages are dominated by the anxiety of being involved in a new situation and by questions about other group members. Preoccupations are likely about boundary issues, confidentiality and security. In the second stage, those familiar with psychotherapy—or otherwise accustomed to talking about themselves—will be at an advantage. There will be a range of tensions about group norms and disclosures, reasons for joining and discrepant levels of confidence about using the group. In the third stage, members will defend against intimacy with one another and struggle with questions of trust, attachment, and affiliations. In the fourth stage, as members become increasingly able to trust the group with self-disclosure, observed changes might become manifest as self-exploration yields the beneficial experience of individuation and differentiation. In the concluding stage, people prepare for departure and find themselves comparing points of difference between changes achieved in the group and the state of their lives outside—generalising from the arena of therapy to that of real life. Has therapy made a lasting difference? Will it be maintained outside?

### The language of the group

Foulkes suggested that 'symptoms, in themselves unsuitable for sharing, exert, for this very reason, an increasing pressure upon the individual to express them'.[54] The group equips the person to transform the mute and inchoate language of symptoms into a socially understandable form of discourse. Following publication of Schlapobersky's paper, The Language of the Group, there is increasing interest in characterizing group phases in terms of the language that predominates, using theory from discourse analysis and the Foulksian concept of free-floating discussion.[16]

It is possible to differentiate between three primary forms of speech that arise in the matrix of any group. At the most basic level **monologue**—speaking alone (with or without an audience)—is a form of individual self-expression. At the next level **dialogue**—a conversation between two people—is the form of communication that distinguishes a bipersonal exchange. And at the third level **discourse**—the speech pattern of three or more people—allows the free interaction of all its participants in a flexible and complex exchange that distinguishes the communication of a group. These patterns of speech are universal cultural forms arising in all communication and are present in the life of every group, although in no set order. Monologue can be understood as a soliloquy, dialogue as the resolution of opposites or the search for intimacy, and discourse as the work of a chorus. The use of free-floating discussion allows a pattern of exchange to move freely between these different speech forms, each of which constitutes a distinctive type of communication. It is through this movement—from monologue through dialogue to discourse and back again—that the group-analytic method comes into its own, creating an arena in which the dialectic between the psyche and the social world helps to refashion both.[13,14]

### Leadership

The group analyst works as both group member and therapist, beginning with dynamic administration, assuming an active role in a new group and allowing a **decrescendo** of his own role as the group gains authority. He is responsible for helping the group with the **location** of disturbance in its process and for providing a balance between analytic and integrative forces whilst manifest content is translated into language that describes the unconscious. Transference is prominent but the work is undertaken in the dynamic present. Foulkes' account in the following passage,[55] of the conductor at work in a group, stands in dramatic contrast to Freud's account of the psychoanalyst at work behind the couch:

> He treats the group as adults on an equal level to his own and exerts an important influence by his own example . . . representing and promoting reality, reason, tolerance, understanding, insight, catharsis, independence, frankness, and an open mind for new experiences. This happens by way of a living, corrective emotional experience.

Disturbed, narcissistic, or borderline patients bring to the group more primitive psychic structures and processes that put strain on the resources of other group members. Such patients can create turmoil in which the leader's task is to maintain the group at a more mature level of psychic organization. By responding to part-object relationships and processes on the level of whole-object relations, containing responses can be established. Progressively, these help to build for the disturbed patient a more benign world of inner object relationships and processes. More disturbed patients desperately seek attention in ways that are inappropriate and disruptive. This search for **attention** arises because the patient cannot establish a sense of **connection** between herself and the processes of the group. Mirroring and resonance can steadily come to replace these isolated and fragmentary responses allowing the patient to attain—for the first time—a coherent sense of self and a capacity to recognize the identity of others.

#### (a) The dynamics of change

As noted above, Yalom cited 11 'curative' factors responsible for change in groups. Foulkes believed there were four key group-specific factors: mirroring, exchange, social integration, and activation of the collective unconscious. Tschuschke and Dies[56] have identified five key factors that they could study empirically (Table 6.3.6.5).

#### (b) Binding forces: alliance, cohesion, and coherence

*Group alliance* has as its major focus the quality of the relationship that develops between each individual member and the therapist(s). These alliances grow as each individual develops a transference relationship to the therapist and can feel that their own particular individual dynamics are recognized. Group cohesion used to be compared to the concept of therapeutic alliance in individual psychotherapy but current research shows that alliance (defined as the affective bond that develops between each group member and the therapist) can be differentiated from group cohesion.

*Group cohesion* describes the bonds between group members, their attitudes, and their commitment to therapeutic work, in particular

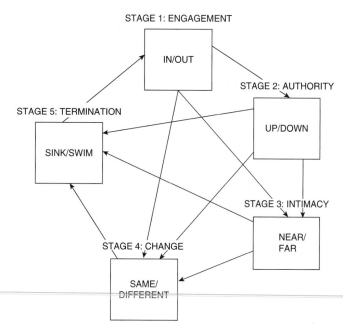

**Fig. 6.3.6.8** Developmental stages and thematic focus.

**Table 6.3.6.5** Five factors in the dynamics of change open to empirical evaluation[56]

| 1 Cohesiveness | Closely related to 2 & 3 as determining factors that influence outcome in 4 and 5 |
|---|---|
| 2 Self-disclosure | Closely related to 1 & 3 as determining factors that influence outcome in 4 and 5 |
| 3 Feedback | Closely related to 1 & 2 as determining factors that influence outcome in 4 and 5 |
| 4 Interpersonal learning output | Evidence of working through process seen in 4 |
| 5 Family re-enactment | Findings of change in these patterns provides evidence of enduring psychic change |

their feelings of attraction and dependency. These processes are interdependent and in combination they provide optimal conditions for positive group process and outcome.[57]

*Group coherence* is a more evolved group state requiring but going beyond cohesion. It evolves as a semantic matrix, built on the earlier, relational matrix. When a group moves through support and understanding to be able to recognize and work through conflict, it can achieve a sense of containment.[58] At this stage the group becomes a more complex, self-evolving, and self-defining entity capable of reaching deeper levels of exploration, acceptance, and understanding.

#### (c) Corrective emotional experience
The concept was introduced by Alexander to describe the patient's recognition of discrepancies between present and past experience. Grotjahn, a colleague of his, applied this to the group, describing it as 'the corrective family experience'.

> There is a built-in correction of the transference phenomena through the peer relationship in groups. An analyst is trained to let the transference neurosis to grow to full bloom. Members of a group are neither trained nor willing to accept such projections . . . and will correct them. This is the basis of a corrective therapeutic family experience.[59]

Oedipal, sibling, and pre-oedipal constellations are activated in group therapy and can be worked through as the members play parts in each other's family scenarios.[60] The task of the therapist interprets transference and helps the group as a whole to develop coherent norms of understanding and responsiveness that equip its members to go beyond the private preoccupations that might have brought them into therapy. Garland calls this **taking the non-problem seriously**.[61]

#### (d) Resonance, mirroring, and other dynamic processes
Foulkes described the group as 'a hall of mirrors'. Each person, he thought, could see aspects of themselves reflected in the personality and behaviour of others and could often more easily recognize these aspects of the self than by direct introspection. We cannot know ourselves in the absence of reflective mirroring, the feedback and information we obtain from others according to our presence and behaviour in the group brings us to a greater awareness of who we are. Resonance in the group is the unconscious communication of emotion by which the other process dynamics—like mirroring, amplification and condensation—are effected.

### Insight and outsight, regressive and progressive forces in groups
The dictum, 'where id was, ego shall be', coined originally by Freud to ground the psychoanalytic enterprise in an easily comprehensible principle, has been superseded for group workers by the idea of **ego training in action**, coined by Foulkes. It emphasizes two related issues. The first is that **insight**—the understanding of the self— is related to **outsight** defined as the understanding of the other(s). And the second is that people find growth and change as much in what they do for others—**progressive behaviour**—as in what others can do for them—**regressive behaviour**. So the group is designed to create an arena in which there is continuous flux between these different elements.

#### (e) Imitation, identification, internalization, and differentiation
*(i) Imitation*
From early in infancy, we observe and copy what others do. A therapeutic group is designed to create conditions in which imitative behaviour, or modelling, can be experienced, monitored, and understood. It brings the group members closer together and, as it develops into identification and internalization, it increases the cohesiveness of the group.

*(ii) Identification*
Peoples' predominant modes of relatedness to one another— such as compliance, avoidance, dominance, receptivity, exploitation, and need—become apparent in the group. The group exposes these patterns of relatedness to reveal how the internal objects with which members have identified can be externalized and encountered in the group through projection and introjection. Members compel each other to play and re-play the dramas of their interior lives and past injuries in the 'here and now' of group experience.

*(iii) Internalization*
Intimacy with others is developed through the exchange of understanding. As it is given and received, it allows for new forms of intimacy within the self. **Constructive** experience in the group is taken in and becomes part of the self. This can allow the recognition and reappraisal or **deconstruction** of repetitive patterns and fixed, maladaptive characteristics. And this can lead to the **reconstruction** of the self in the concluding phases.

*(iv) Differentiation*
Over time people become aware of significant differences in their reactions, emotions, and psychological structures. Examples are increased tolerance of affect, understanding and modification of self-inflicted pain, diminution of guilt and shame, retrieval of lost aspects of the self, increased openness with others, increased spontaneity and creativity, and, most critically, feelings of tolerance for or forgiveness of the self, for the constraints into which it has been driven by past injury and present defence.[62]

#### (f) Personal and group resistances
Some resistances are manifestations in the group of the characteristic defences of the members, evident in their interpersonal behaviour. Others are resistances of the group as a whole, shown in blockage of free-floating discussion, opposition to group interaction, sub-grouping, and opposition to the deepening and broadening of the group's exploration. A constructive function of resistances should be kept in mind when monitoring the pace at which both individuals and the group can progress without experiencing

overwhelming anxiety. Resistances can protect people from fears of loss of self and identity; and from fears of engulfment through excessive intimacy. Resistances then become opportunities for understanding fear of change, for the re-working early developmental patterns, and for discovering the freedom that can follow release from excessive internal control.

### (g) The anti-group

Nitsun developed an understanding of the anti-group, bringing together the work of Bion and Foulkes.[63] He introduced the concept to help understand the negative experiences therapists face in periods of stagnation, hostile silence, severe conflict in or premature departure from the group, or negative feelings about the work of the group. These situations can arise when the group recapitulates early experiences of loss, deprivation, anger and envy or in an effort to avoid these emotions. Negative emotions can then be projected towards the group and the conductor who represent early care-givers. These feelings can be worked on when the therapist uses counter-transference to recognize and verbalize projected feelings. The idea of **negative elaboration** (see below) is a useful guide in this process.

## Basic clinical issues

### Dynamic administration

#### (a) Selection and composition

Group composition is the therapist's first and most enduring contribution to the group for its membership will determine the outcome of therapy. Preparing patients for treatment with several individual sessions or, if necessary, an extended programme of preparatory work will provide the therapist and patient with a basis for judgement about therapeutic prospects. Preparatory work has been found likely to enhance participation and reduce drop-out rates, although findings are not conclusive.[64]

The criteria for selection are exclusive rather than inclusive since most patients seeking psychotherapy can be accommodated in a group, provided a suitable one is available. The selection process should take into account both the patient needs and the composition of the group. A service should, ideally, provide a selection of groups into which people can be placed both according to their needs and characteristics, and those of the particular group. Selection criteria aim to optimize the 'fit' between the needs and resources of the individual and those of the group.

Table 6.3.6.6 lists inclusion criteria, while Table 6.3.6.7 gives a shortlist of excluding criteria. Lists of this kind should be used with caution. In general, at least four inclusive criteria should be found amongst those to be included in outpatient, dynamic psychotherapy groups with a mixed population. If there are four exclusion criteria, one should be very wary about including the person in a group. However, there are many exceptions.

The criteria in Tables 6.3.6.6 and 6.3.6.7 hold good for mixed groups and outpatient services generally. With homogeneous groups for special populations, the range of potential candidates is much wider, for example, Hearst describes a population of severely deprived mothers drawn entirely from those on the exclusion list.[65]

#### (b) Homogeneous and heterogeneous groups

Homogeneous groups: Are for people with similar symptomatic or diagnostic pictures, such as phobias, anxiety, or depression. Such

**Table 6.3.6.6** Inclusion criteria for psychodynamic groups (at least four of these criteria should be present, for someone to join a group)

1  Motivation to address personal issues, to resolve problems
2  Willingness to try and participate
3  Some experience of successful relationships in childhood or present
4  Some interest in exploring and understanding the self
5  Some capacity to talk, listen, and relate
7  Some interest in others
8  Some sense that being amongst others could be helpful
9  Some ability to sympathize or empathize with others' needs and problems
10  Some indication of future reliability in attendance

**Table 6.3.6.7** Exclusion criteria for psychodynamic groups[66] (if four or more of these criteria are present, then questions should be raised about inclusion)

1  Those in acute crisis
2  Prior history of broken attendance in therapy
3  Major problems of self-disclosure
4  Major problems with reality testing, i.e. paranoid projections or psychosis
5  Pathological narcissism
6  Difficulties with intimacy generalized into personal distrust
7  Defences that rely excessively on denial and disassociation
8  Emotional unavailability
9  Tendency to be verbally subdued or withdrawn
10  Tendency to be hostile and aggressive, verbally or otherwise

groups offer more immediate support to members, are better attended, and provide faster symptomatic relief. However they may remain at a more superficial level with less interpersonal learning.[67]

Homogeneous groups are also used for those with similar personality structure or life-history, particularly those in socially extreme categories. For example, men with histories of sexual violence or women who have suffered rape or torture may be treated.

Heterogeneous groups: Melnick and Woods[67] suggest that group composition should be guided by an optimal balance between conditions ensuring group maintenance or homogeneity, and those maximizing interpersonal learning or heterogeneity. A group which shares one strong characteristic—a diagnosis such as an eating disorder, or a personal attribute like intelligence—can accommodate a diversity of presenting problems or social backgrounds. If, on the other hand, the members are similar in social background, diversity can be incorporated on another basis, such as diagnosis. Thygesen[68] found that diversity enabled group members to recognize and work with differences in mental and emotional attitudes, life histories, and developmental problems. Recognizing and working with difference develops emotional resources, promotes flexibility, and the tolerance of emotional tension. And it encourages the group to move from **cohesion**, in which security is based on identification, to **coherence** in which relationships are based on differentiation.

It is useful also to identify members likely to be isolated from the rest of the group by age, ethnicity, gender, personality, or problems or a history that noone else shares, for they are likely to find the group experience threatening. We do not put a patient into a position of being isolated.

## Managing the structure, setting, and time boundaries

### (a) Optimal and sub-optimal size

The optimal number for small group psychotherapy, ranging from five to nine, is determined by practical considerations. A smaller number than this minimum is likely to have an active attendance of only two or three and will not necessarily generate the corporate energy to produce movement. A group larger than this will exceed the number that can be taken into one person's confidence in a face-to-face exchange.

**Sub-optimal groups** can provide valuable therapy under good conditions.[69] Low and irregular attendance is often associated with a problematic composition, particularly if there is a high proportion of members with character disorders and borderline features. Their inner sense of deprivation and loss can make the group seem unreliable and threatening which can be reinforced if the therapist is seen to be in difficulty. Therapists who can maintain an understanding attitude and positive commitment to the group's future will usually find the situation settles into a working nucleus of members that can then be built upon.

### (b) Setting and time-boundaries

The therapist supplies, creates, and maintains the setting throughout the group's life. This requires attention to such matters as meeting times, punctual beginnings and endings, confidentiality, the predictable frequency of its meetings and breaks, and the general guarantee of a stable background.

Every aspect of the group's life, including absences, departures, late attendance, and extra-group communication in terms of letters, phone calls, and messages, referred to generically as **boundary events**, are open for discussion. Boundary events are interpreted for the meaning they might hold for the life of the group as a whole. This is a task initiated by but not confined to the therapist. Also, the setting itself—to which each member is seen to contribute—comes to acquire a capacity to **hold** the individual members and **contain** their anxieties and insecurities. The issue of containment is of great importance, as is the discovery—by people who may have no belief in themselves as responsible members—that they can take responsibility for themselves and expect responsibility from others. The group is thus responsible not only for the nurture, acceptance, and security of its members, but also for their containment, the setting of limits and the maintenance of consistent authority. The therapist will often have to lead the way in modelling both roles for the group's members.

## Fostering therapeutic norms and a culture of enquiry

The therapist encourages the sharing of experience and helps to balance participation, recognition, and translation. The thrust of a group's life is towards greater shared involvement and the expression of emotions. The expression of feeling may arise in the recounting of members' life-situations and their reasons for therapy—**narrative emotion**—or it may arise in the interpersonal encounters engendered by the telling—in the **drama** of 'here and now'. Therapy becomes effective when the problems that brought the patient into treatment become recognizable in their interpersonal encounters. At this point the affect lodged in the narrative will interact with the drama of the group's current emotions,

creating opportunities for corrective emotional experience. As the group progresses from **constructive** to **deconstructive**, and ultimately to **reconstructive**, experience, it will encompass gesture, behaviour, body-language, and other non-verbal communication, and actions that convey feelings when emotions have no words.

## Guidelines for intervention

There are four modalities of time and place in any therapy group. The content of the exchange might be located in the past outside the group, the past inside the group, the present outside the group, and the present in the group.

Free-floating discussion will carry the focus of the exchange between these different modalities. The therapist's task is to follow the interaction, to use interventions sparingly and strategically, to cultivate a reflective curiosity for which Table 6.3.6.8 offers some pointers, and to work towards a progressive shift in the focus of attention, from no. 1, in Fig. 6.3.6.9 towards 4, via 2 and 3. A group governed by narrative in its free-floating discussion is likely to be dominated either by the the group's own past or by the past of its members outside the group or by their current lives outside. A group governed by members' intense experience of one another in the present, is likely to be governed by the drama of immediate encounter and understanding. The corrective recapitulation of early family life is likely to arise when the issues that predominate in no's 1, 2, and 3, are translated into issues that prevail in 4, where they can be addressed in the present which allows new resolutions to be forged.

## Groups for special populations

Nine distinctive clinical populations or approaches merit special mention. Some pose distinctive problems for group workers and, as we indicate in the section on borderline patients, they sometimes need co-therapists working together in the group.

**Table 6.3.6.8** Interventions in time and place

| | |
|---|---|
| 1 | Address process rather than content |
| 2 | Help members recognize aspects of themselves in others and accept the viewpoints of others on themselves |
| 3 | Monitor the intensity of participation to allow an enabling pace so members can develop resources to deal with the intimacies of each others' lives |
| 4 | Establish a sense of enquiry about the fluctuations of mood and outlook, and a sense of curiosity about thematic movement between the different modalities of time and place |
| 5 | Help the group recognize role configurations taken up by individuals (therapist's assistant or rival, joker, complainer) |
| 6 | Hold in mind the gestalt of figure and ground. If someone stands out, what is the background against which they do so? If the ground changes the underlying pattern of the group, how might the figural person be affected? |
| 7 | Help the group recognize sequences and patterns |
| 8 | Help the group decode and find meaning in the constructive, deconstructive, and reconstructive elements of its exchange |
| 9 | Work towards the coherency of the group |
| 10 | Foster the integration and integrity of its members |

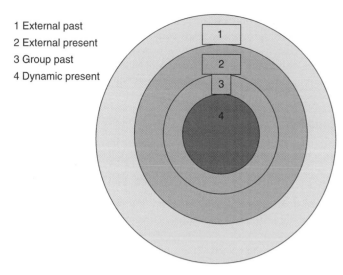

1 External past
2 External present
3 Group past
4 Dynamic present

**Fig. 6.3.6.9** Location of group discourse in time and place.

## Intensive outpatient psychotherapy heterogeneous groups for mixed populations

Group analytic psychotherapy has come into its own as a treatment modality in out-patient settings in the context of clinical agencies in public and private Health Services. Table 6.3.6.9 gives a picture of patients' clinical needs in the private practice of John Schlapobersky over a twenty-year period. Some attempt has been made to indicate how these categories are mapped against those in ICD 10 and DSM IV.

### The medically ill

Groups have been used successfully for people with diseases of the cardiovascular, endocrine, gastro-intestinal, pulmonary, neurological, and renal systems. Amongst the applications are groups for those with renal dialysis and organ transplantation; chronic conditions such as diabetes, irritable-bowel syndrome, and rheumatic disease; and life-threatening conditions such as metastatic cancers.

Groups usually have members with a single disorder, last for 20 sessions or fewer, and are psycho-educational in purpose. They emphasize compliance with treatment regimes and opportunities to share and explore the affective consequences of the conditions. The focus is on helping patients come to terms with the complaint; make changes in lifestyle, including diet, exercise, work, and recreation; deal with the inevitable anxieties about death, stigma, demoralisation, feared dependency, and loss of control; and resolve issues in relationships with loved ones and care staff. Clinicians write of how, despite their brevity, these groups provide a forum for sometimes profound exchange about major existential issues including pain, fear, and impending death.[70]

Evaluation indicates such groups are effective in improving quality of life and, to some extent, in prolonging its duration even with metastatic cancer.[71] Improved survival correlates significantly with enhanced, active coping. Spiegel reported a significant, near-doubling of survival effects in 86 women with metastatic breast cancer treated for one year with weekly, supportive-expressive group therapy.[72,73]

### The chronic mentally ill

In North American literature there are consistent findings that schizophrenic patients do best in support groups that help them manage their symptoms and devise coping strategies for day-to-day problems.[74] Group discussion is used to help overcome problems of social isolation, develop social skills and coping resources, and learn about maladaptive interactions evident in the 'here and now' of the group. The leader creates a sense of safety and security with supportive feedback. Areas that people find helpful include the management of symptoms, expression of emotion, and relationships with others. Groups are less valued for acquiring insight or receiving guidance about the illness, medication, or economic problems. Interpretations that reveal or explore unconscious conflicts, particularly transferential issues between members or with the therapist, are more likely to be harmful than helpful.[75] Patients respond positively to an interactive, open, and safe group environment, with gradually increased cohesion, decreased avoidance, and decreased conflict.[10]

Recently, Resnik[76] has described the use of insight-orientated psychotherapy with delusional problems using psychoanalytic principles in long-term group psychotherapy for psychotics.

## Borderline personality disorders

Working with these patients can pose difficult clinical problems based on their 'stable instability', including their inability to form a stable therapeutic alliance, mood oscillations, poor impulse control, limited reflective ability, painful states of psychic emptiness, followed by self destructive acting-out including self-destructive gestures and self-mutilation, violence; substance abuse, sexual acting out, and eating disorders. Some attempts at short-term group therapy combining cognitive behavioural approaches with the psychodynamic have shown promise. Longer therapies in out-patient groups have been encouraging but have not been evaluated. Good results are reported with in-patient applications at, for example, The Cassel and Henderson Hospitals, and in other forensic settings where day hospital group treatments are followed by outpatient group therapy in a carefully monitored programme.[77]

Homogeneous outpatient groups do not do well because the members use similar 'primitive' defences of splitting, projection and denial, and have not acquired a stable sense of identity. They are suspicious of close interpersonal contact and have little capacity to care for or be cared for by others. Such groups lack cohesion, are pervaded by a sense of pessimism, hostility, rivalry, and easily fragment. Self-destructiveness is turned onto the group and its therapists who may experience intense counter-transference feelings of frustration, despair, and anger.

These problems can be managed in the containing setting of closed or specialized institutions. However, it is generally better to place one or two borderline patients in an otherwise well-functioning group where other members will not always respond to borderline pathology at the same primitive level. They may—like the adult carers of children—respond with understanding, find ways of setting limits, and expect co-operation with the task at hand. After sometime, lengthy periods in which borderline patients maintain a frustrating presence on the margins of the group, or make themselves felt in aggravating terms at its very centre, they can acquire resources to take part in the group's work in more mature terms. This combination of borderline and neurotic members in a carefully composed group can benefit both parties. Borderline members will often have an unerring accuracy of perception about others, they can shake the group into more active interactions, and may not collude with others' neurotic defences.

**Table 6.3.6.9** Categories of clinical need catered for by intensive, outpatient group therapy with mixed populations (many of those who join groups are found in more than one of these categories of need)

| 1. High dependency need including: | 2. Problematic reactions to traumatic life events including: | 3. Character problems including: | 4. Serious relational problems including: | 5. Selected people with borderline personality disorders including | 6. Training of mental health professionals including: | 7. Those seeking personal growth or understanding including: |
|---|---|---|---|---|---|---|
| a Recovery from serious or enduring mental and physical illness<br>b Help with the resolution of moderate psychiatric symptoms<br>c Resolving addiction and substance abuse | a Loss, injury, illness, disorder, infertility<br>b Massive psychic and physical trauma<br>c Adult sequelae of child sexual abuse | a Immaturity and developmental problems<br>b Chaotic life situations<br>c Problems of identity and meaning<br>d Problems of gender, sexuality, and orientation<br>e Occupational problems | a Intimacy avoidance<br>b Recurrent broken relationships<br>c Intractable conflicts | Those with insight who both need and can tolerate containment | Psychotherapists, psychiatrists, psychologists, social workers, clergy | People who would have previously sought this through individual psychoanalysis |

(John Schlapobersky: Group-Analytic Practice & Southwood Practice: 1987–2007)

Category 1: Corresponds to Axis I in DSM IV and Groups F1–4 in ICD 10.

Category 2: Corresponds to Axes III, IV, & V in DSM IV and Group F5 in ICD 10.

Category 3: Corresponds to Axes IV and V in DSM IV and Group F8 in ICD 10.

Category 4: Corresponds to Axis V in DSM IV and Group F8 in ICD 10.

Category 5: Corresponds to Axis II in DSM IV and Group F6 in ICD 10.

The containing resources of the other members that set the norms and values of the group can slowly be internalized by the borderlines. As with many of these specialist areas, therapists working with these populations will need to acquaint themselves with the literature, have ongoing supervision and may—to begin with—work more fruitfully in co-therapy.

For a review of group psychotherapy for personality disorders see [78, 79].

## Forensic groups

Group therapy has been used for forensic populations, previously thought untreatable. Pioneering work has been done in the UK in special hospitals,[80,81] in prisons such as Grendon,[82] and great strides have been made in outpatient services at the Portman Clinic in London.[83] Therapeutic community treatment for mentally disordered offenders in North America and Western Europe has been reviewed by Lees, Manning, and Rawlings.[84]

The aim of forensic group therapy is to help patients find words, rather than actions, to express impulses and compulsions. A major part of the group's work is to provide psychic space for perspective, negotiation, recognition, acceptance, and verbalization of hurt. Sharing the past and present can make it accessible as internalized, persecutory, and vengeful monologues are brought into dialogue.

In Britain, the Probation Service is the agency most actively involved in the groupwork with offenders.[85] A report for the NHS Centre for Reviews and Dissemination (CRD Report 17) reviews studies of therapeutic communities and small groups and indicates that these show the most promising results of any form of treatment for anti-social personality disorders.[86]

## Trauma

Group work with trauma victims is a comparatively new field but one in which there is a vigorous range of applications. The most comprehensive overview is Van der Kolk's text.[87] There are groups for survivors of sexual abuse,[88] war trauma,[89] and torture and other forms of organized violence. Group work applications to traumatized children and adolescents is discussed in reference 90 and more generally in reference 91.

At the Medical Foundation for The Care of Victims of Torture in London, a group work programme caters for refugees and asylum-seekers. The groups provide psychotherapy for massive psychic and physical trauma, for problems of displacement and exile, and for trans-cultural problems.[92] The diversity of different kinds of groups, including a range of activity, problem-solving, and psychodynamic groups, ensures that people can be provided with an environment in which they can each realize their own potential for self-healing. The programme is grounded in commitment to human rights, to team-work that addresses counter-transference issues, and to principles of positive intervention to counter emotions of hopelessness, and despair.[93,94]

## Couples groups

These groups cater for people in stable but troubled relationships in which there is some form of pernicious collusion. The approach can provide symptom relief and personality change in even severe difficulties with relationships that last but do not work. Family therapy is concerned with the systemic function served by symptoms. Psychoanalysis is concerned with the origins of the symptoms in object relationships. Group analysis provides a bridge between these paradigms, helping therapists find a point of intervention between marital and object relationships.

In a group, the process moves between the psychology of the individuals and the dynamics of their marriages. This interplay between the pair and the person—the interactive and historical dynamics—is part of the group's free-floating discussion. The therapist uses this interplay, following the patterns of the group's progress and making interpretations. Work is at times transferential, other times, systemic techniques are used to address immediate issues.[95] Themes to which the group resonates are amplified and members are helped to condense from this discourse, the kind of personal knowledge that promotes growth and change. There is insufficient evaluation of the method's efficacy, but experience in hospital and private practice is very encouraging.[96]

### The elderly

This is an area of relatively new therapeutic exploration. A range of groups has been found useful in helping the aged to face their problems, improve their functioning, and feel happier about themselves. The groups include those offering support, activity, psycho-education, problem-solving, and insight, and takes place in many settings. Common themes include the ubiquity of loss, the acceptance of death, and the value of humour in lightening mood.[97]

### Brief therapy in groups

Spurred by economic and managerial pressures a distinctive modality has evolved. Sessions are held weekly and number between 6 and 30. Characteristics that differentiate brief from long-term therapy include: clearly defined therapeutic goals agreed at the outset, the early establishment of a therapeutic alliance, active and flexible therapeutic style, a focus on 'here and now' group process, the maintenance of time awareness, monitored in stage-specific terms, and the vigorous, directed exploration of thematic content.

Short-term groups may be homo- or heterogeneous. Homogenous groups have proved effective in helping patients deal with loss and grief, the consequences of trauma and abuse, and common problems coping with physical illness and disability. Heterogenous groups require more psychodynamic commonalities such as shared problems in inter-personal relationships, the ability to recognize and work on psychological issues, and the ability to cope with the speed and intensity of the process. Those who lack psychological sophistication or are not motivated for self-exploration, are not suited.

### Research and evaluation

The general trends in literature show ample empirical confirmation that group treatments represent a powerful therapeutic intervention. A comprehensive overview of literature described positive outcomes with alcoholism, anxiety disorders, bereavement, bulimia, depression, schizophrenia, and sexual abuse.[98] There is also evidence of the adverse outcomes in group psychotherapy which can guide the clinicians training for the work.[99]

#### (a) Outcome research

A meta-analysis of 58 controlled studies of psychotherapy for the treatment of depression showed that in comparison to a waiting list control the average treated patient was better off than 80 per cent of the controls.[100] The efficacy of group and individual therapy was almost identical. Tyllitski[101] also reported no appreciable difference between individual and group therapy effectiveness, both doing better than the control condition. Budman et al. found significant improvement in time-limited individual and group therapies. It seems that most patients who are suitable for psychotherapy will benefit in either modality.

#### (b) Process research
##### (i) Preparation of patients for group therapy
In a review of 20 controlled or comparative studies, Piper and Perrault[102] found that preparation has a positive effect upon attendance but that it could not be shown to have a direct effect on outcome.

##### (ii) Therapist activity
Development of constructive group norms will depend on factors such as careful group composition and leadership style. Foulkes' idea that the conductor has, at first, a relatively high rate of activity which decreases as the group develops its own resources for psychological work has been supported by later research findings.[103]

##### (iii) Group process variables
Research on therapeutic factors (e.g. self-disclosure and feedback) and leadership technique indicate that members in well-established groups are engaged in many different types of psychological work. They are less group-centred and more likely to be confronting the personal distress and maladaptive interpersonal styles that brought them to treatment in the first place.[104]

##### (iv) Therapeutic factors
In a study of long-term in-patient groups, Tschuschke and Dies[105] investigated five therapeutic factors: cohesiveness, self-disclosure, feedback, interpersonal learning-output, and family re-enactment. All five therapeutic factors were associated with clinical improvement with group cohesiveness, an important ingredient. They suggested that **affective integration** into the group, that is the high and positive emotional relatedness to co-members, promotes the capacity to disclose and leads to more frequent and intense feedback from fellow patients. It appeared that feedback given earlier in the group had a stronger relationship to treatment outcome. This may suggest that **interpersonal feedback** needs time to be assimilated and worked through before it can be utilized effectively. There are significant differences between successful and unsuccessful patients in terms of level of group cohesion and amount of self-disclosure. Patients who disclose little and do not feel drawn to the group receive relatively little meaningful interpersonal feedback and become neglected. They concluded that **cohesiveness, self-disclosure**, and **feedback** and together promote **interpersonal learning** within the group.

These findings were confirmed by the author's later studies, the most recent of which was published in 2007[106] and by recent independent studies using different parameters; see, for example, references [107–109].

## Conclusion: planning a service

For group psychotherapy to be effective the group has to be the primary focus of therapy; patients need to be well selected; and therapists need to be adequately trained. Therapeutic competence is not a function of mastering the literature so much as it is the outcome of experience in the group situation itself. Courses introducing different group methods are now widely available throughout the UK, Continental Europe, and the USA. Group training is also provided in many general training programmes and, along with clinical supervision, is offered in many health and other service agencies.

Long-term **outpatient** group therapy of 100 sessions or more is effective and economic in producing lasting benefits for patients with a wide range of medical and psychiatric symptoms, interpersonal problems, traumatic life experiences, character and personality disorders. **In-patient** group therapy is an effective resource in the context of acute units working with crisis, and in secure units working with long-term problems. **Short-term** group therapy for selected conditions requires careful composition of the group and an active, flexible therapeutic approach.

We have not tried to cover the range of group services and approaches for children. Chapters by Schamess[110] and by Kymissis[111] cover group work with children and adolescents, respectively. Further reading is available in Evan's text[112] and Melzack.[113]

There are economic arguments for group therapy. In one study, the quality of improvement between individual and group therapy of psychiatric patients was not significantly different but the cost of the service was different. Cost savings were calculated as the reduction in medical consultations and hospital attendance, and lost workdays. For those treated with psychotherapy of any kind, the cost of treatment was 25 per cent per patient less than it was for those who did not receive psychotherapy. The cost of group psychotherapy per patient was about a third less than for individual psychotherapy.[114]

## Further information

A. Bateman, D. Brown and J. Pedder's (2000) *Introduction To Psychotherapy* (Routledge) sets group therapy in the context of other psychotherapies. D. Stock Whittaker's (1995) introduction, *Using Groups To Help People* (Routledge) and M. Aveline and W. Dryden's (1988) *Group Psychotherapy In Britain Today* (Open University Press) give a general overview of UK practice in the past. There are three good texts that introduce the group-analytic approach. The most recent by H, Behr and L. Hearst (2005) is *Group Analysis: A Meeting of Minds* (John Wiley). W. Barnes, S. Ernst and K. Hyde have written a recent overview, (1999) *An introduction to groupwork: a group-analytic perspective* (Palgrave Macmillan). And an earlier text by D. Kennard (1993) *The Workbook of Group Analysis* (Routledge) provides a clinically grounded study of practitioners at work. The range of other books in the International Library of Group Analysis and the journals, *Group Analysis, Group, and The International Journal of Group Psychotherapy* give access to the many specialist applications discussed here.

## References

1. Burlingame, G.M., Mackenzie, K.R., Strauss, B. (2005). Small-group treatment. Evidence for effectiveness and mechanisms of change. Ch.14. In *Bergin and Garfield's Handbook of psychotherapy and behaviour change.* (ed. M.J.Lambert), New York. Wiley.
2. Foulkes, S.H. and Anthony, J. (1957). *Group psychotherapy: the psychoanalytic approach.* Penguin, Harmondsworth. (Maresfield Reprint, Karnac Books London 1989.
3. Yalom, I. and Leszcz, M. (2005). *The theory and practice of group psychotherapy.* Basic Books, New York.
4. Agazarian, Y. (1997). *Systems-centred therapy for groups.* Guilford Press, New York.
5. Creek, J. (ed.) (1997). *Occupational therapy and mental health.* Churchill Livingstone, Edinburgh.
6. Stone, W. (1996). *Group psychotherapy for people with chronic mental illness.* Guilford, New York.
7. Kanas, N. (1999). Group therapy with schizophrenic and bipolar patients. In G*roup psychotherapy of the psychoses* (eds. V. Schermer and M. Pines), pp. 129–47. Jessica Kingsley, London.
8. Schlapobersky, J. (1993). The language of the group: monologue, dialogue and discourse in group analysis. In *The psyche and the social world: developments in group- analytic theory (*eds. D. Brown and L. Zinkin), pp. 211–31. Routledge, London.
9. Schlapobersky, J. (1996). A group-analytic approach to forensic psychotherapy: from the speech of hands to the language of words. In *Forensic psychotherapy: crime, psychodynamics and the offender patient. Vol. 1: Mainly theory* (ed. C. Cordess and M. Cox), pp. 227–43. Jessica Kingsley, London.
10. Abse, W. (1979). Trigant Burrow and the inauguration of group analysis in the USA. *Group Analysis,* **3**, 218–29.
11. Lewin, K. (1951). *Field theory and the social sciences.* Harper and Rowe, New York.
12. Trist, E., Murray, H. (1990). T*he social engagement of social science Vol. 1, section 1.* University of Pennsylvania Press, Philadelphia, PA.
13. Pines, M. (1991). A history of psychodynamic psychiatry in Britain. In *Textbook of psychotherapy in clinical practice* (ed. J. Holmes), pp. 75–86. Churchill Livingstone, Edinburgh,
14. Harrison, T. (2000). *Bion, Rickman, Foulkes and the Northfield Experiment: Advancing on a different front.* Jessica Kingsley, London.
15. Elliott, A. (1999). *Social theory and psychoanalysis in transition. Chapter 2, Free Association Books,* London. pp. 46–76.
16. Foulkes, S.H. (1948). *Introduction to group analytic psychotherapy.* Heinemann, London. (Maresfield Reprint, Karnac Books, London 1991.)
17. Dick, B. M. (1975). A ten year study of out-patients analytic group therapy. *British Journal of Psychia*try **127**, 365–75. Lorentzen, S. (2000) An assessment of change after long-term psychoanalytic group treatment. *Group Analysis* (in press).
18. Sigrell, B. (1992). The long-term effects of group psychotherapy. A thirteen year follow up study. *Group Analysis,* **25**, 333–52.
19. Lorentzen, S. (2000). An assessment of change after long-term psychoanalytic group treatment. *Group Analysis,* **33**.
20. Bion, W.R. (1961). *Experiences in groups.* London: Tavistock.
21. Malan, D. (1976). A follow up study of group psychotherapy. *Archives of General Psychiatry 33*, 1303–15.
22. Moreno, J. L. (1953). *Who shall survive? Foundations of sociometry, group psychotherapy and psychodrama.* Beacon House, New York.
23. Slavson, S. (1940). Group psychotherapy. *Mental Hygiene,* **24**, 36–49.
24. Wolf, A. (1949). The psychoanalysis of groups—1. *American Journal.of Psychotherapy,* **3**, 525–58.
25. Wolf, A. (1950). The psychoanalysis of groups—2. *American Journal of Psychotherapy,* **3**, 16–50.
26. Yalom, I. (1983). *In-patient group psychotherapy.* Basic Books, New York.
27. Rutan, J.S. and Stone, W. (2007). P*sychodynamic group therapy* (Fourth Edition). Guilford Press, New York.
28. Kaplan, H.I. and Sadock, B.J. (eds) (1993). *Comprehensive group psychotherapy.* Williams and Wilkins, Baltimore, MD.
29. Alonso, A. and Swiller, H.I. (eds) (1993). *Group therapy in clinical practice.* American Psychiatric Press, Washington, DC.
30. Ashbach, C. and Schermer, V. (1987). *Object relations, the self and the group.* Routledge, London.
31. Spotnitz, H. (1961). *The couch and the circle.* Knopf, New York.
32. Ormont, L.R. (1992). *The group therapy experience: from theory to practice.* St. Martin's Press, New York.

33. Tubert-Olander, J. and de Tubert, R.H. (2004). *Operative Groups*. Routledge, London.

34. Janunsen, P. (1994). *Psychoanalytic therapy in the hospital setting*. Routledge, London.

35. Koenig, K. and Lindner, W.V. (1994). *Psycho-analytic group therapy*. Jason Aaronson, New York.

36. Tschuschke, V. (2000). The P.A.G.E. study: early treatment effected of long-term outpatient group therapies-first preliminary results. *Group Analysis*, 33, 3, 397–411.

37. Tsegos, I.K. (1995). Further thoughts on group-analytic training. *Group Analysis*, 28, 313–26.

38. S. Lorentzen (1990). Block training in Oslo: the experience of being both organiser and participant in the Norwegian Psychiatric Association group psychotherapy training programme. *Group Analysis*, 23, 361–82.

39. May, R. and Yalom, I.D. (1989). Existential Psychotherapy. In *current psychotherapies* (eds. R. Corsini and D. Wedding.) pp. 363–402. F.E. Peacock, Itasca, Ill.

40. Bion, W. (2000). *Experiences in Groups*. Routledge, London (First published by Tavistock, 1961).

41. Ezriel, H. (1950). A psycho-analytic approach to group treatment. *British Journal of Medical Psychology*, 23, 56–74.

42. Horwitz, L. (1977). A group-centred approach to group psychotherapy. *International Journal Group Psychothererapy*, 27, 423–39.

43. Whitaker, D.S. and Lieberman, M.A. (1964). *Psychotherapy through the group process*. Tavistock, London.

44. Pines, M., Hearst, L. and Behr, H. (1982). Group analysis (group analytic psychotherapy). In *basic approaches to group psychotherapy and group counselling*. (ed. G. Gazda), pp. 132–178. Charles C. Thomas, Springfield Ill.

45. Pines, M. (1982). Reflections On Mirroring: 5th. Foulkes Lecture. *Group Analysis*, 15 (Supplement). Reprinted in Pines, M. (1998) *Circular reflections: selected papers on group analysis and psychoanalysis*. Jessica Kingsley, London, pp. 17–39.

46. Agazarian, Y., Peters, R. (1981). *The visible and invisible group: two perspectives on group psychotherapy*. Routledge, London.

47. Foulkes, S.H. (1964). *Therapeutic group analysis*. Allen and Unwin, London. (Maresfield Reprint, Karnac, London1984).

48. Pines, M. and Hearst, L. (1993). Group Analysis in *Comprehensive Group Psychotherapy*. (eds Kaplan I. and Sadock, J.) Williams & Wilkins, Baltimore.

49. Friedman, R. (2008). Dreamtelling as a request for containment: three uses of dreams in groups. *International Journal of Group Psychotherapy*, 58, 3, 327–44.

50. Lipgar, R. and Pines, M. (2003). *Building On Bion: Vol. 1: Roots; Vol. 2: Branches*. Jessica Kingsley, London.

51. Nitsun, M. (2006). *The group as an object of desire: exploring sexuality in group therapy*. Routledge, London.

52. Cox, M. and Theilgaard, A. (1987). *Mutative metaphors in psychotherapy: the Aeolian mode*. Tavistock Press, London.

53. Bennis, W.G. and Shepard, H.A. (1956). A theory of group development. *Human Relations*, 9, 415–37. Reprinted in *Sensitivity training and the laboratory approach* (eds. R. Golembiewski and A. Blumberg) pp. 91–115. F.E. Peacock, Itasca, Ill.1970.

54. Foulkes, S.H. (1964). *Therapeutic group analysis*. George Allen and Unwin, London. pp. 51–2, 176–77.

55. Foulkes, S.H. (1964). *Therapeutic group analysis*. George Allen and Unwin, London. p. 57.

56. Tschuschke, V. and Dies, R.R. (1994). Intensive analysis of therapeutic factors and outcome in long-term inpatient groups. *International Journal of Group Psychotherapy*, 44, 185–208.

57. Marziali, C. et al. (1997). The contributions of group cohesion and group alliance to the outcome of group psychotherapy. *International Journal Group Psychotherapy*, 47, 4, 475–97.

58. Pines, M. (1986). Coherence and its disruption in the development of self. *British Journal of Psychotherapy*, 2, 3, 180–85. Reprinted in Pines, M. (1998) *Circular Reflections: selected papers on group analysis and psychoanalysis*, Chapter 12. Jessica Kingsley, London. pp. 211–23.

59. Grotjahn, M. (1977). *The art and technique of analytic group therapy*. Jason Aaronson, New York. p. 14.

60. Pines, M. (1990). Group analysis and the corrective emotional experience: is it relevant? *Psychoanalytic Inquiry*, 10, 3, 389–408.

61. Garland, C. (1982). Group analysis: taking the non-problem seriously. *Group Analysis*, 15, 4–14.

62. Pines, M. (1995). The universality of shame: a psychoanalytic approach. *British Journal of Psychotherapy*, 11, 346–57.

63. Nitsun, M. (1996). *The anti-group: destructive forces in the group and their creative potential*. Routledge, London.

64. Salvendy, J.T. (1993). Selection and preparation of patients and organisation of the group. In *Comprehensive group psychotherapy* (ed. H.I. Kaplan and B.J. Sadock). Williams and Wilkins, Baltimore, MD.

65. Hearst, L. (1998). The restoration of the impaired self in psychoanalytic treatment. In *Borderline and narcissistic patients in treatment* (ed. N. Slovinska-Holy) International University Press, New York. Chapter 7.

66. Roback, H.B. and Smith, M (1987). Patient attrition in dynamically oriented treatments in groups. *American Journal of Psychotherapy*, 144, 426–31.

67. Melnick, J. and Woods, M. (1976). Analysis of group composition: research and theory for psychotherapeutic and growth-oriented groups. *Journal of Applied Behavioural Science*, 12, 493–512.

68. Thygesen, B. (1992). *Diversity as a group-specific factor. Group Analysis* 25, 175–86.

69. Zelakowski, P. (1998). The sub-optimal group. *Group Analysis*, 31, 491–504.

70. Stern, M.J. (1993). Group therapy with medically ill patients. In *Group therapy in clinical practice* (ed. A. Alonso and H.I. Swiller), pp. 185–200. American Psychiatric Press, Washington, DC.

71. Leszcz, M. and Goodwin, P. (1998). The rationale and foundation of group psychotherapy with metastatic breast cancer. *International Journal of Group Psychotherapy*, 48, 245–73.

72. Spiegel, D., Bloom, J.R. and Yalom, I.D. (1981). Group support for patients with metastatic cancer. *Archives of General Psychiatry*, 38, 527–33.

73. Spiegel, D. (1999). *Supportive group therapy with cancer patients*. Basic Books, New York.

74. Kanas, N. (1999). Group therapy with schizophrenic and bipolar patients. In *Group psychotherapy of the psychoses* (eds. V. Schermer and M. Pines) Jessica Kingsley, London.

75. Kapur, R. (1993). The effects of group interpretations with the severely mentally ill. *Group Analysis*, 26, 411–32.

76. Resnik, S. (1987). *The theatre of the dream*. The New Library of Psychoanalysis, London; and (1995) *Mental Space*. Karnac. London.

77. Chiesa, M. and Fonagy, P. (2000). The Cassel Hospital personality disorder study. *British Journal of Psychiatry (forthcoming)*.

78. Wilborg,T. and Karterud, S. (2001). The place of group psychotherapy in the treatment of personality disorders. *In Current Opinion in Psychiatry*, 14/2, 125–30.

79. Karterud, K., Oyvind, U. (2004). Short-term day programmes for patients with personality disorders. What is the optimal composition? *Nordic Journal Psychiatry*, 58(3) 243–49.

80. Cox, M. (1986). The 'holding function' of dynamic psychotherapy in a custodial setting: a review. *Journal of the Royal Society of Medicine*, 79, 162–64.

81. Kennard, D. (1993). Group therapy at Rampton. Group Work Co-ordinating Committee, Rampton Hospital.

82. Genders, E. and Player, E. (1995). *Grendon: A study of a therapeutic prison*. Clarendon, Oxford University Press.

83. Welldon, E. (1994). Forensic Psychotherapy. In *Handbook of psychotherapy*, (eds. P. Clarkson and M. Pokorny), pp. 470–93. Routledge, London.

84. Lees, J., Manning, N. and Rawlings, B. (2000). Therapeutic community effectiveness: A systematic international review of therapeutic community treatment for people with personality disorders and mentally disordered offenders. *CRD Report 17: University of York NHS Centre for Reviews and Dissemination.*

85. Brown, A., Caddick, B. (eds) (1993). *Groupwork with offenders.* Whiting and Birch, London. p. 2.

86. Welldon, E. and Wilson, P. (2006). Special edition of Group Analysis, Forensic Psychotherapy. *Group Analysis*, 39.1.

87. Van der Kolk, B. (1993). Groups for patients with histories of catastrophic trauma. In *Group therapy in clinical practice* (ed. A. Alonso and H.I. Swiller). American Psychiatric Press, Washington, DC. pp. 289–305.

88. Hall, Z., Mullee, M. and Thompson, R. (1995). A clinical and service evaluation of group therapy for women survivors of childhood sexual abuse. In *Research Foundations for Psychotherapy Practice* (eds. M. Aveline and D.A. Shapiro). Wiley, Chichester.

89. Lifton, R. (1983). *The broken connection.* Basic Books, New York.

90. Greene, L.R. (ed.) (2005). Special Edition of the International Journal of Group Psychotherapy: Children & Adolescents in the Aftermath of 9/11: Group Approaches Towards Healing, Trauma and Building Resilience, July 2005.

91. Weinberg, H. and Nuttman-Shwartz, O. (eds) (2005). Special Edition of Group Analysis on Trauma, Vol. 38 No 2, June 2005.

92. Schlapobersky, J. and Bamber, H. (1988). Rehabilitation with victims of torture. In *Refugees—The trauma of exile.* pp. 206–22. Nijhoff, The Hague.

93. Woodcock, J. (1997). Groupwork with refugees and asylum seekers. In *Race and groupwork*, (eds. T. Mistry and A. Brown), pp. 254–77. Whiting and Birch, London.

94. Callaghan, K. (1996). Torture—the body in conflict: The role of movement psychotherapy. In *Arts Approaches to Conflict*, (ed. M. Liebmann). Jessica Kingsley, London.

95. Benun, I. (1986). Group Marital Therapy: A Review. *Sexual and Marital Therapy*, **1**, 61–74.

96. Skynner, A.C.R. (1986). Recent developments in marital therapy. In *Explorations with families: group analysis and family therapy: selected clinical papers of Robin Skynner.* Routledge, London.

97. Lesecz, M. (1997). Integrated group psychotherapy for the treatment of depression in the elderly. *Group* **21**, 89–113.

98. Dies, R.R. (1993). Research on group psychotherapy: overview and clinical applications. In *Group therapy in clinical practice*, (eds. A. Alonso and H.I. Swiller), pp. 475–6. American Psychiatric Press, Washington DC.

99. Roback, H. (2000). Adverse outcomes in group therapy. *Journal of Psychotherapy Practice and Research*, **9**, 113–22.

100. Robinson, L.A., Berman, J.S. and Niemeyer, R. (1990). Psychotherapy for the treatment of depression: a comprehensive review of controlled outcome research. *Psychological Bulletin*, **108**, 30.

101. Tyllitski, C.J. (1990). A meta-analysis of estimated effect sizes for group versus control treatments. *International Journal of Group Psychotherapy*, **40**, 215–24.

102. Piper., W.E., Perrault, E.L. (1989). Pre-therapy preparation for group members. *International Journal of Group Psychotherapy* **39**, 17–34.

103. Lorentzen, S. and Heglund, P. (2004). Predicting change in long-term group psychotherapy. *Psychotherapy and Psychosomatic Medicine*, **73**, 1. 125–135; and Lorentzen, S. (2006) Contemporary Challenges For Research. In *Group Analysis*, 3, 321–340; and Mace, C., (2006) Setting the world on wheels: some clinical challenges of evidence-based practice. In *Group Analysis*, 39, 3, 304–20.

104. Dies, R. R. (1993). Research on group psychotherapy: overview and clinical applications. In *Group therapy in clinical practice*,

(eds. A. Alonso and H.I. Swiller), p. 502. American Psychiatric Press, Washington DC.

105. Tschuschke, V. and Dies, R.R. (1994). Intensive analysis of therapeutic factors and outcome in long-term inpatient groups. *International Journal of Group Psychotherapy*, **44**, 183–214.

106. Tschuschke, V., Anbeh, T., Kiencke, P. (2007). Evaluation of long-term analytic outpatient group therapies. In *Group Analysis*, **40**, 1, 140–59.

107. Lorentzen, S., Bogwald, K. and Hogland, P. (2002). Change during and after long-term analytic psychotherapy. *International Journal of Group Psychotherapy*, **52**(3) 419–29.

108. Terlidou, C., Moschonas, D., Kakitsis, P., Manthouli, M., Moschona, T., Tsegos, I. (2004). Personality changes after the completion of long-term group psychotherapy. *Group Analysis*, **37**, 3, 401–18.

109. Conway, S., Audin, K., Barkham, M., Mellor-Clark, J. and Russell, S. (2003). Practice based evidence for a brief time-intensive multi-modal therapy guided by group-analytic principles and methods. *Group Analysis* **36**, 3, 413–35.

110. Schamess, G. (1994). Group psychotherapy with children. In *Comprehensive group psychotherapy* (ed. H.I. Kaplan and B.J. Sadock). Williams and Wilkins, Baltimore, MD. pp. 560–77.

111. Kymissis, P. Group psychotherapy with adolescents. In *Comprehensive group psychotherapy* (ed. H.I. Kaplan and B.J. Sadock), pp. 577–84. Williams and Wilkins, Baltimore, MD.

112. Evans, J. (1998). *Active analytic group therapy for adolescents.* Jessica Kingsley, London.

113. Melzak, S. (ed.) (2000). *Children in exile: therapeutic and psychotherapeutic work in the clinic and the community.* Jessica Kingsley, London.

114. Heinzel, R. (2000). Outpatient psychoanalytic individual and group psychotherapy in a nationwide follow-up study in Germany. *Group Analysis*, **33**, 353–72.

# 6.3.7 **Psychotherapy with couples**

Michael Crowe

## Introduction and background

There is an ongoing crisis in the institution of marriage, at least in Western cultures. There has for some time been a tendency to idealize marriage, and at the same time social forces are operating which tend to undermine it.[1] These influences have probably made a contribution to the increasing divorce rate, as well as the tendency for fewer couples to marry, and have probably also led to an increase in the number of couples seeking help with their relationships.

In the United Kingdom, for example, the number of marriages taking place each year has fallen for the first time in living memory, and the number of divorces is still steadily increasing, reaching 40 per cent of marriages in 1996.[2] There are also a large number of 'common-law' marriages, often with children, as well as more transient cohabiting or non-cohabiting sexual relationships, both heterosexual and homosexual. The stability of these relationships is, of course, not recorded in the marriage or divorce statistics, and the rate of breakup can only be guessed at; however, it is very probable from clinical experience that in these non-marital relationships there is a higher than 40 per cent incidence of breakup. In the wake of these changes, there are a large number of single-parent families and 'reconstituted' or blended families, as reviewed by Robinson,[3] and there is a decreasing proportion of children who are being brought up in the traditional nuclear family with two biological parents.

In addition to these new factors affecting marriage in the early 21st century we should also be aware of the fact that many countries, especially those in the developed world, have a multicultural society, and that immigrant cultures have different attitudes to marriage and family life. For example, families from the Indian subcontinent often prefer to arrange marriages for their children, and in some cases insist that the couple live in the husband's parents' house. On the other hand, West African couples often leave their children in Africa to be looked after by family members for long periods of time, while the parents work or study in the West.

In the last few years, Gay marriage or Civil Partnership has been recognized in many western countries. Couples in Gay relationships have many of the same problems and satisfactions as heterosexual couples, and in addition, must live with fairly widespread negative attitudes and homophobia from neighbours, family and society generally. Their relationships have to be, if anything, stronger than heterosexual ones to survive these pressures, and may be more in need of therapy.

Couple therapy must be able to take account of these factors, and whilst much of what is contained in this chapter will relate to heterosexual married British couples living with their biological children, it should be understood that there are many other types of relationship which can be helped using a similar approach, with appropriate changes of emphasis. In a later section, there will be some additional discussion of the specific problems relating to couples from other cultures, and ways of managing these.

## Couple counselling and couple therapy

The concept of couple counselling dates from the 1920s when in the United States the American Association for Marital Counselling was formed; in the United Kingdom the Marriage Guidance Council (now called Relate) was founded in 1938. Counselling mainly took the form of giving advice on practical issues, but in more recent years, Relate counselling has been orientated more towards psychodynamic approaches, and favours a longer-term involvement with the couple. Couple counselling continues in both countries, and the great majority of couples seeking help with their relationships are seen by couple counsellors, rather than any other types of therapist.

The distinction between couple counselling and couple therapy is not an easy one, because many of the interventions are similar. In a simplistic sense therapy attempts to make a more radical difference to the couple's functioning than counselling, which has the general aim of improving adjustment to the situation as it is. However, many forms of both couple therapy and couple counselling are based on a theoretical formulation which is derived from a related school of individual psychotherapy (for example, cognitive behavioural or psychodynamic). Thus, theoretical formulations in the resultant couple work are so different between therapies (e.g. psychodynamic as against behavioural) that a particular form of counselling may have more in common with a related form of couple therapy than that therapy itself has with another type of couple therapy.

## Psychoanalytic/psychodynamic couple therapy

Couple therapy using a psychodynamic model began in the United Kingdom in 1948, when Dicks and his colleagues founded the Institute of Marital Studies. The theories and techniques involved have been ably reviewed by Daniell[4] and Clulow.[5] The central concept used is that the inner (unconscious) world of the two partners determines their interaction and their response to changing circumstances. It is as though each partner has an internal blueprint, both of themselves and each other, formed partly by observation but also partly by the influence of earlier intimate attachment experiences with parents, siblings, or friends. These influences may actually determine the choice of partner, and the nature of each partner's patterns of attachment (secure or insecure) will affect the ways in which they cope with the stresses of the new relationship. There may then be projections which lead one partner to attribute motives such as hostility or sadism to the other, whereas in fact this is a split-off and denied characteristic of the first partner. Other consequences of this unconscious process may include the system of shared fantasies and defences which builds up as the relationship continues.

In therapy, four premises are used, which inform a relatively long-term and open-ended series of sessions. The first is that a person's emotional health is related to his or her capacity to manage both internal conflict and external stress: it is important to be able to experience fear as well as trust, pain as well as pleasure, doubt as well as certainty, frustration as well as satisfaction. Secondly, significant relationships can be used to resurrect, but also change, inflexible patterns of behaviour established in the past. Thirdly, unconscious processes need to be taken into account when attempting to understand problems in relationships. Fourthly, change takes time because it requires a reordering of perceptions of self and others, perhaps with the help of transference interpretations by the therapist involving both partners.

Therapy in this mode may be carried out by one therapist seeing both partners, but is more often done by two therapists either seeing the couple together or in parallel individual sessions, using one partner with one therapist, with joint supervision of the two therapists. An intriguing aspect of this therapeutic format is that sometimes the two cotherapists find themselves interacting in unfamiliar ways, in sessions and between sessions, which are thought to represent the projection of fantasies and feelings by the couple on to the therapists; the therapists' understanding of these projections in their joint supervision may play a role in advancing the therapy itself. If these insights are used to inform the therapists' interaction with the couple, the individual partners may then be made aware of their own conflicts, fantasies, and projections, and thus be able to give up some of their repetitive patterns of behaviour and withdraw damaging projections.

The psychoanalytic approach has been an important source of theoretical ideas in couple therapy, especially the concepts of attachment and loss developed by Bowlby.[6] It has also the distinction of being the first theory to be adapted to this area of work. There are, however, some drawbacks to working in this way, as enumerated by Wile.[7] He sees the emphasis on negative impulses and emotions (e.g. dependence, narcissism, sadism, manipulation, and exploitation) as painting a rather unflattering and negative picture of the couple in therapy, and perhaps therefore reducing their motivation to continue. A more serious problem with the approach is that the psychodynamic concepts, whether of defence mechanisms, projections, or shared fantasies, are treated as if they were as real as observed behaviour, whereas in fact they must remain assumptions based on hypothetical constructs, and are really only valuable in so far as the therapy based on them is effective.[1]

The question of efficacy is raised later in the chapter, but it must be stated here that the psychodynamic therapies for couple problems have only seldom been submitted to controlled trial, and then usually in a relatively short-term form. The therapy may be quite long term, and the improvements seen are usually not dramatic, so that in the last analysis the approach has to remain of uncertain value.

## Behavioural couple therapy

The behavioural approach, in contrast, makes no assumptions about internal conflicts or underlying mechanisms in the individuals. The approach was initiated in 1969 by Stuart[8] and Liberman[9] as behavioural marital therapy. They worked from the principles of operant conditioning and made the assumption that couples who were having difficulties were either giving each other very low levels of positive reinforcement or were using punishment or negative reinforcement to coerce each other into behaving differently. The remedy that they proposed for this situation was to help the partners to learn how to persuade each other to conform to the desired pattern of behaviour by the use of prompting and positive reinforcement. Thus, complaints would be transformed into requests and requests into tasks agreed by both partners.

Behavioural marital therapy relies on the therapist's observation of the couple's behaviour in the session and on the problems they report from the previous week or equivalent timespan. There are two types of therapeutic activity in behavioural marital therapy. The first is reciprocity negotiation, in which the partners request changes in behaviour on each side and negotiate how this can be achieved through mutually agreed tasks. The second is communication training, in which the partners are encouraged to speak directly and unambiguously to each other about feelings, plans, or perceptions, and to feed back what they have heard and understood. In both these approaches, the deeper meanings behind a particular piece of behaviour are ignored, the emphasis being on change in the interaction both in the here and now and in the immediate future. The approach has been the subject of many controlled trials (see below), and is of proven efficacy.

## Cognitive behavioural and rational–emotive couple therapy

Aaron Beck,[10] in his cognitive behavioural approach to couple therapy, identifies in the communication of disturbed couples many of the problems found in the thinking of depressed patients, and attempts to correct these. Thus, he tackles misunderstandings, generalizations, untested assumptions, and automatic negative thoughts by challenging assumptions, reducing unrealistic expectations, relaxing absolute rules, improving the clarity of the communication and focusing on the positive rather than the negative.

Similarly, Albert Ellis (reviewed by Dryden[11]) uses a rational-emotive approach to couple problems. Here, the main focus is on the use of words; terms such as 'intolerable' are replaced by (for example) 'difficult to accept', and the couple are encouraged to express desires rather than demands. There is an analysis of the repetitive cycles of cognitive and behavioural disturbance, in which each partner may attribute the other's behaviour to a negative motive and assume that nothing can be done about it. The general thrust of this therapy is similar to that of Beck, but with a more lively and less formalized approach in the session.

## Systems therapy for couple problems

The systems approach to couple therapy derives partly from concepts developed by Minuchin[12] and Haley,[13] and partly from the work of Selvini Palazzoli *et al.*[14] All these pioneers worked predominantly with families rather than couples, but many of their ideas and techniques are relevant to the treatment of couples. Although the systems approach to therapy has broadened and deepened since the 1980s, many of the early concepts are still very useful.

A central concept in thinking about couple relationships is 'enmeshment', by which is meant an excessive involvement in what is essentially the private business of another person. It is quite common to find an enmeshed relationship between parents and their teenage children, in which both sides find it very hard to 'let go'. It can also be found in couple relationships where one partner wants to be closer than the other, and a conflict arises as to what is the best distance to maintain. Systems therapy aims to help them to find a compromise 'distance' which suits them both, and thereby to reinforce the necessary 'boundaries' which people need in maintaining their individuality within a relationship.

The concept of circular causality is also central to systems work. This enables the couple to get away from the idea that one person is necessarily to blame for a particular situation by considering the continuous cycle of cause and effect in which A's actions may be caused by B's actions and also B's may equally be caused by A's. Thus, systems therapists, when approaching a couple problem, do not focus on one partner's behaviour, but rather on the pattern of interaction obtaining in the relationship. They will then try to effect a change in which both partners contribute actively to the solution of the problem.

Systems therapists have many techniques at their disposal, including those which increase the couple's understanding of the system they are participating in. These include family genograms (a form of family tree construction which leads to discussion of transgenerational influences or 'systems over time'), family 'sculpting' (in which the members position themselves and each other wordlessly to represent their current relationships), and the discussion of 'family myths' and stories. More active techniques, designed to play a part in changing the family interaction, include creating conflict in the session, giving homework tasks, and the use of 'paradoxical injunctions' in which the therapist tells the family to continue with the current interaction because, even though it is problematic, it seems to be protecting them from worse consequences. These more active techniques will be dealt with in more detail in the main part of this chapter on behavioural–systems therapy.

## Mixed or eclectic approaches

Most couple therapists use a mixture of techniques, and it seems that this is probably an inevitable consequence of the difficulties involved in applying one therapeutic method rigorously in a clinical setting. A number of specific combinations have been advocated, and will be briefly mentioned here.

The first is the psychodynamic-behavioural approach of Segraves.[15] In this, the basic underlying cause of marital disturbance is assumed to be the partners' conflicting internal and unconscious projections, and their interactions. The therapy, however, is not only directed at helping them to understand these (as in psychodynamic therapy) but also to increase their negotiating and communicating skills (as in behavioural marital therapy).

The second is a more comprehensive mixture of theory and technique, known as the intersystem model, and advocated by Weeks.[16] This tries to take account of the individual, interactional, and intergenerational aspects of couple relationships, and combines them in what is probably closest to a systems model, but with more emphasis on the psyche of the individual. Interventions are on both a conjoint and individual basis, and the techniques of decentring (see below) and paradoxical injunctions are often used.

The third eclectic approach is that of Spinks and Birchler.[17] This is called behavioural–systems marital therapy, and makes use of behavioural marital therapy as the main form of intervention, moving into the systems mode when 'resistance' emerges. There are many similarities between this form of treatment and the one described in the main part of this chapter, but our 'behavioural–systems approach' is more integrated as between the two components of the method.

The fourth eclectic approach which should be mentioned is that of Berg-Cross.[18] She uses rational-emotive, sociocognitive, systemic, psychodynamic, humanistic, and theological concepts to understand and modify couple relationships. Like that of Weeks, her approach gives the therapist a very wide canvas to work on, but may lose some of the focus by being very general and all-embracing.

## The behavioural–systems approach to couple therapy

Behavioural–systems couple therapy is the approach that will be described in detail in the present chapter, and although it is only one of several approaches to couple problems, it has the advantage of spanning two of them, and issues such as indications for therapy and assessment are shared with both the pure behavioural and systemic approaches. It is the method developed at the Maudsley Hospital Couple Therapy Clinic in the 1980s. It has been expounded at greater length by Crowe and Ridley,[1] and like some of the other eclectic models mentioned above it combines two different approaches, behavioural marital therapy and systems family therapy. The behavioural dimension, similarly to that described by Stuart (8) and Jacobson and Margolin,[19] consists of the relatively straightforward methods of reciprocity negotiation and communication training. The systems dimension is more complicated, and involves systems thinking, structural moves during the session, tasks and timetables for the couple between sessions, and the use of paradox. The method was developed in a predominantly psychiatric setting, and has been found to be particularly suitable for those couples where one or both partners has psychiatric problems in addition to their relationship difficulties. It is also useful as an adjunct to psychosexual therapy where a sexual dysfunction or a sexual motivation problem seems to be connected with relationship issues.

The method should be thought of as a series of menus from which the practitioner can choose techniques rather than as a set course of therapy beginning at one point and ending at another. Thus, the various components of behavioural–systems couple therapy can be incorporated at any time in the therapy session, although in practice, negotiation, communication training, and structural moves are usually employed in the earlier part of the session, while tasks, timetables, and paradox are usually reserved for the 'message' at the end, and are linked to homework assignments to be carried out between sessions.

The different techniques of behavioural–systems couple therapy can be thought of as belonging to a kind of hierarchy. The so-called 'hierarchy of alternative levels of intervention (ALI)'[1] links each type of intervention with a particular set of clinical problems and makes recommendations as to the type of intervention that is appropriate. The ALI hierarchy is shown in diagrammatic form in Fig. 6.3.7.1. As may be seen, where the couple appear to have greater rigidity in their behaviour, where they show more symptoms, and where they show more reluctance to accept the relationship as the focus of work, the therapist needs to move to the systems end of the hierarchy, and use more ingenuity in the development of interventions. If, however, the couple accept the interactional focus and show willingness to recognize the part that the relationship is playing in maintaining the problems, the therapist may be quite comfortable and effective working behaviourally. By and large, the preference is to work behaviourally, since this implies collaborating with the couple and accepting their stated goals, whereas the systems approach puts the therapist into a more managing role, deciding what is best for the couple and suggesting tasks that may not be what they would expect. It should be emphasized that the therapist may at any stage move up or down the hierarchy, according to the couple's response: an increase in flexibility shown by the couple could be the trigger for the therapist to begin working in a more behavioural way, whereas an increase in rigidity or a failure to respond to behavioural work could be met by a more systemic approach.

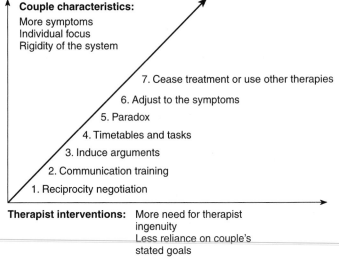

**Fig. 6.3.7.1** The alternative levels of intervention hierarchy.

## Indications and contraindications

If there is a relationship problem identified by either the couple or their advisers, even if there are also individual psychiatric or behavioural problems, and if the couple are willing to attend together, then in most cases they are suitable for behavioural–systems couple therapy. The breadth of the therapeutic approach, the fact that the behavioural techniques are of proven efficacy (see below), and the fact that the systemic interventions are suitable for those with more psychiatric symptoms or similar problem behaviours, all give the therapy a wide range of positive indications.

### (a) The nature of the problem

Clearly those with relationship problems such as arguments and tensions are highly suitable for couple therapy. Another related indication is those relationships in which one partner (who might be attending a counsellor or psychiatrist alone) spends much time complaining about the absent partner's behaviour. A third indication is where the health of one partner suffers following the other partner's individual therapy.

Many problems with sexual function would be suitable for couple therapy, including those couples where there is a disparity in sexual desire, or those where one partner has a specific phobia for sex. In some such cases there is also a need for individual therapy, especially where one partner is the survivor of earlier childhood sexual abuse.

Many people with depression or anxiety, especially those where there is also poor self-esteem, may be suitable for couple therapy. There are often aspects of the illness that are exacerbated by problems in the relationship. Indeed, in a study by Leff *et al.* in 2000[20] it was shown that couple therapy was an effective and acceptable form of treatment for couples in whom one partner was depressed.

Where jealousy is present the problem usually affects the non-jealous partner to a greater or lesser extent, and here it would almost always be useful to have at least a few conjoint sessions with the couple, as suggested by De Silva.[21]

Some problems are perhaps less amenable to couple work, and among these are, for example, phobias which seem unconnected with home life in any way, and post-traumatic stress reactions where the event happened away from the partner. Some alcoholic and drug-addicted patients have so much of their existence involved with the addiction that they are not available emotionally to do couple work, and the work would at that stage be wasted on them. Similarly, those with an acute psychosis would, at the time they are acutely ill, be unavailable to this kind of therapy, and should not be offered it. However, in both cases, when the acute crisis is over and the addiction or psychosis is under control, it would be very appropriate to offer them some kind of couple therapy, even if this had limited aims and expectations. Some of the most useful psychological interventions in schizophrenia, after the acute illness has resolved, involve the nearest relative, as shown by McFarlane.[22]

### (b) Degree of connection with the relationship

Some problems in individuals have been in existence long before they entered the present relationship. If this is the case, the therapist should consider whether it is best to embark on couple therapy or whether individual therapy would be better. However, even when there seems no causal connection with the relationship, the effect of the problem on the partner may be such as to warrant at least one or two couple sessions.[23]

### (c) Availability and willingness for joint therapy

If the partner of a patient is unavailable or unwilling to attend for therapy, it may be appropriate to let the situation be, and not offer treatment. In some immigrant couples, for example those from the Indian subcontinent, there are cultural reasons given for a wife not attending therapy, and we usually have to respect these. However, in both situations it is sometimes right to put some pressure on the absent partner to attend, because the reasons for non-attendance may be relevant to the couple problems we are trying to treat.

### (d) Is the relationship continuing?

If the person who is asking for therapy is going through a divorce or equivalent breakup of a relationship, it may not be appropriate or possible to treat both partners. However, in some cases there is good work to be done in arranging a more satisfactory breakup, in terms of domicile and care of any children. This 'mediation' work is increasingly being done, and many of the processes are similar to those of couple therapy.

## Assessment and selection

This is not an easy process, because there is a dearth of research on the types of couple problem presenting for treatment and on the outcome of treatment itself. However, on the basis of the referral letter (usually from a GP or psychiatrist) the therapist will usually arrange a preliminary session with the couple. The only reason not to see the couple in the first instance is that they are not willing to attend as a couple, or the problem is seen clearly as an individual one (see above).

Another, more subtle, form of selection occurs during the first therapy session, when the couple are in contact with the process of therapy. In this session, the therapist considers the ability of the partners to empathize with each other, their pattern of communication, their stage in the 'family life cycle' (see below) with its associated stresses, and their flexibility in response to simple therapeutic interventions. He or she will attempt to use reciprocity negotiation or other straightforward techniques of therapy, partly as a treatment trial, and partly to see whether the couple is ready for this kind of intervention. If not, the therapist can move to a more systemic approach, or decide after a few visits that there is no future at this point in further therapy of this kind, and that something else (e.g. individual therapy) is needed (Fig. 6.3.7.1).

## The process of therapy: beginning and continuing

Behavioural–systems couple therapy is essentially a short-term therapy involving perhaps 5 to 10 sessions of 60 minutes each, over a period of 3 to 6 months. Although the therapy was developed in a room with a one-way screen and live supervision, it is quite possible to use behavioural–systems couple therapy in any conventional consulting room without a team or live supervision. If the one-way screen is used, the therapist and the team (which may include students as well as experienced colleagues) begin by reading the referral letter and the biographical questionnaires which the couple will have completed, and discuss the case with a view to formulating the problem from an interactional point of view. This may involve, for example, thinking about the couple's stage in the 'family life cycle' (e.g. birth of the first child or the 'empty nest'), any recent event such as a bereavement or a new relationship, or the diagnosis of a serious illness. Hypotheses about the possible causation of the recent problems are not necessarily thought of as 'true' explanations, but have the function of informing the therapist's thinking and suggesting what level of the ALI hierarchy to choose at the initial meeting and what strategy to employ in the session.

There are several important issues to address in the first session, which functions both as a kind of assessment and as the beginning of the therapeutic work. It is necessary:

- to remain in control;
- to develop rapport with both partners, without favouring either;
- to maintain the momentum of the session and the interactional focus;
- to maximize the opportunities for the couple to experience a change in the nature of their interaction.

A particularly useful move at some stage in the first session, and one which we almost always use, is to ask the partners to talk directly to each other rather than the therapist; this is the so-called 'decentring' technique originated by Minuchin.[12] Keeping this configuration for as much as possible of the session enables the therapist to observe the couple's typical pattern of interaction, to intervene as a 'theatrical producer' rather than a diplomatic negotiator, to avoid as far as possible taking sides, and to encourage the kind of negotiation which hopefully the couple will be able to carry on at home without the presence of a third party. It is not necessary to remain decentred for the whole session, but if it does not happen at all in the first session, an opportunity for effective work will have been lost.

It may be difficult to remain decentred in the face of pressures from one or both partners to talk to the therapist directly. One way to participate while still remaining decentred is to request the partners to ask each other questions to which the therapist would like to know the answer. For example, one might say: 'Could you ask your partner what she thinks about your coolness on this matter?' or 'Perhaps your partner disagrees with you; could you check with him?'. In this way the couple can continue to talk to each other in the decentred position without undue 'triangling in' of the therapist.

One situation which causes particular problems for the behavioural–systems therapist is where one partner persists with monologues, either about his or her own symptoms and problems or about the partner's unreasonable behaviour. This is a perfectly acceptable way to present a problem in one-to-one therapy, but in couple therapy it slows down the interaction and prevents the therapist focusing on the relationship. One way to overcome this is by decentring, but in some couples this is too difficult, and another possibility is to ask the non-verbal partner to comment on the spokesperson's problems. This can provoke a minor crisis in the couple, and lead to the spokesperson realizing that the problems are not all one-sided. It is a technique related to circular questioning, and is used fairly extensively in family therapy see Chapter 6.3.8

Another obstacle to progress is the situation in which the partners have intractable arguments, perhaps about other family members. If such battles continue to dominate the sessions the therapist may have to devise a method for putting them 'on ice for the time being' and concentrating instead on negotiating everyday problems to do with the house or the children.

Momentum may also be slowed by the therapist's own style of working. Students of the behavioural systems approach may need to 'unlearn' some of their otherwise good therapeutic habits such as being a good and empathetic listener. They may be able to achieve this by decentring or by asking circular questions in order to refocus on the interaction and increase momentum.

On the other hand, it is still important for the therapist to be able to feel and show empathy to the two individuals in therapy. The difficulty may be that to show empathy to one partner may be interpreted by the other as side-taking. A possible remedy lies in a particular skill, which, however, is not easy to acquire, of saying something to show that one has understood one partner without antagonizing the other. One way to develop this skill is for the therapist not to become emotionally involved in the issues, but to concentrate on the process of interaction, thinking all the time in terms of balance and communication rather than worrying about the rights and wrongs of what is being discussed. This must be done while still showing respect to both the partners, taking their problems seriously, and at the same time conveying hope that they can be solved.

It is also very helpful for the partners themselves to be in touch with each other emotionally and take each other seriously. Some individuals are very good at communicating, but only at an intellectual level, and cannot express empathy with each other. Their interaction is like that of fellow committee members, and they tend to suppress any expression of feelings such as sadness or anger which are 'not on the agenda'. In other couples, there is an imbalance, with one partner expressing feelings openly and the other being exclusively logical and self-controlled. In both situations it is necessary to help them to communicate both intellectually and emotionally, encouraging the self-controlled individual to be more open and the person who is emotionally open to try to be more restrained at times.

### Ending the session

Every session must have an ending, and the purpose in the behavioural–systems approach is to send the couple away with something to work at in the weeks before the next session. About two-thirds of the way through a supervized session the therapist will usually go behind the one-way screen, turning off the camera and closing the shutters (although when working alone this luxury is not available and the therapist must work independently to end the session on a positive note). The team and the therapist then spend about 15 minutes in discussion, planning the 'message' to be given to the couple at the end. Part of this discussion will centre round the team's thinking about the significance of the problems from a systems point of view, but part will also be concerned with how the therapist can help the couple to change their interaction.

The introduction to the message will give the date of the next appointment, and usually also contains some positive and sympathetic comments for both partners. It is important as far as possible to keep them both 'on side' at this stage, so that it would be unwise to say something which could be seen by either partner as favouring the other one. A good example of an introductory comment would be: 'The team and I are aware of the great difficulties you are experiencing, but we think you have what is basically a good relationship, and you are both working hard to improve things'.

The message itself will vary according to the level of the hierarchy at which the therapy is being pitched. If it is mainly a session of reciprocity negotiation the main theme may be simply to reiterate the negotiated plans for both partners which have emerged from the earlier discussion. If, however, the therapist is working more systemically, the message may contain a task, a timetable, or a paradoxical injunction which is designed to alter both the behaviour of the couple and the way they conceptualize their relationship. In some cases, it is appropriate to use a 'split-team' message , in which one part of the team is said to favour a more behavioural task while the other part believes that that will be impossible to achieve and therefore prefers to 'prescribe the symptom'.

The final part of the message is again likely to reiterate the positive sentiments of the introduction. There are good therapeutic reasons for this, in that people tend to remember the positive things that they hear about themselves, and may then link these to the more specific tasks or injunctions that are given with them. In many cases we also send a written copy of the message to the couple, so that they can think it over between sessions and not forget what has been discussed.

Where therapists are working alone, they will be unable to have the 15 minute break in the session, but it is always useful to spend a little time thinking about the message to be given at the end of the session, and to think what other team members might have said or suggested for a final message.

## Specific techniques in behavioural–systems couple therapy

### (a) Reciprocity negotiation

Within the alternative levels of intervention hierarchy, reciprocity negotiation is at the lowest level, relating closely to the goals that the couple themselves has set, and depending on a fairly co-operative attitude on both sides. The partners state their complaints in everyday terms, and the task of the therapist is then to help them to achieve a compromise by each doing what the other partner wants in a reciprocal way.

Reciprocity negotiation is partly based on operant conditioning and partly on the social exchange theory of Thibault and Kelley.[24] The assumption is that satisfaction in marriage and other intimate relationships is based on a relatively equal and high level of input by each partner of positive (i.e. rewarding) behaviour and a relatively low input of negative or unacceptable behaviour. Problematic marriages have a low level of these mutually rewarding behaviours on both sides, or may have a gross imbalance in the input from the two different partners. Instead of exchanging positive behaviour, the partners may use coercive methods to try and force the other to stop doing those things of which they disapprove.

The remedy proposed by behavioural marital therapy is that each partner should state their **complaints**, but that these complaints should then be translated into **wishes** for an alternative way of behaving which is more acceptable, and, as a second stage, into **tasks**. It is very useful to concentrate on practical, domestic issues for these tasks, as these are easily grasped, frequently repeated, and more likely to be remembered than more abstract tasks. In principle the tasks for each partner should be linked and reciprocal, but if this is not possible a 'bank account' approach can be used in which each partner builds up a fund of good behaviour

and they work out at the end of a period of time whether it has been mutually acceptable. In moving from complaints to tasks one also moves from past to future, and this is one of the most characteristic features of reciprocity negotiation. The therapist is thus more interested in what will happen next week than in what happened last week or last year.

The way that reciprocity negotiation is used in behavioural–systems couple therapy is a little different from its use in behavioural marital therapy. We will usually have the couple in a decentred position while negotiating, and feel that this helps the process both to be effective, and to translate more successfully to their home setting. We also use it quite briefly at different stages of therapy, rather than as the mainstay of therapy throughout.

The tasks developed for each partner in reciprocity negotiation should be:

1 specific,

2 positive,

3 repeatable,

4 practicable, and

5 acceptable to both partners.

They should also be concerned with everyday activities, rather than once-only events such as arranging an overseas holiday. Sometimes sexual problems can be brought in to the negotiation.

Reciprocity negotiation is a well-tried and effective method of couple therapy in those who accept that they have marital problems. It is also an advantage that the therapist here works in a way which is straightforward and takes an adult-to-adult approach. But it is also, in our setting, a way of assessing whether the couple are ready for this sort of intervention; if not, they can be offered a more systemic input until they are more ready to negotiate.

### (b) Communication training

The second strategy in the alternative levels of intervention hierarchy is training in communication. This too is part of the behavioural marital therapy spectrum, but not so exclusively, because work on communication is part of most types of couple therapy. The characteristic feature of the form of communication training used in our setting, however, is that it aims for efficient and clear communication, with positive and constructive requests rather than complaints. Other forms of communication training[25] emphasize other skills such as empathy, reflective listening, and supportive comments. In the present form of communication training these are also issues to be considered, but the main emphasis is on issues such as reducing misunderstandings, ensuring that both partners have an equal say, and helping them both to speak from the 'I' position.

Problems encountered in couple therapy amenable to communication training include:

- lack of empathy
- inability to express emotion
- failing to listen
- monologues with no break for feedback
- one partner the spokesperson and the other silent
- mind-reading (i.e. A knowing better than B what is in B's mind)

- sting in the tail (a positive comment followed by a criticism)

- wandering off the topic

- continual criticism.

In carrying out communication training, the therapist first decentres him- or herself, and asks the couple to converse about a relevant topic. When a problem of communication arises the therapist acts as a 'director' and asks them to discuss the topic in another way. If the problem observed is one of lack of empathy, this may include asking one partner to attend to the emotional state of the other, and perhaps to feed back his or her understanding. If it is of inability to express emotion, the therapist may try to intensify the interaction, pointing out the way in which they are holding back their emotions, and encouraging more expressiveness.

The next three problems are connected: failing to listen, talking in monologues, and the 'spokesperson' problem. Remedies can be decentring, encouraging each partner to speak for him- or herself, stopping the talkative partner (perhaps by asking them to listen to what the other partner has to say), and cutting any monologues short by asking for feedback from the other partner. In dealing with mind-reading one may have to be quite diplomatic, because the process is rather similar to psychotherapeutic interpretation, and some partners may feel that this is a legitimate way of giving insight; however, it should be tactfully blocked, usually by asking the partner whose mind is being 'read' to say whether that is what he or she really thinks.

The 'sting in the tail' is dealt with usually by simply pointing it out, but in some cases it can be neutralized by asking the speaker to restate the idea the opposite way round with the 'sting' first. An example of this is given by a man who said 'I realize you were hurt by what I did, but I had no intention to harm you (i.e. you are being oversensitive)'. He was asked to rephrase it as 'I had no intention to harm you, but I realize that you must have been hurt', and his wife found this much more acceptable, because she could respond to the more positive part of the comment.

The problems of wandering off the topic and continuous criticism are often rather intractable. One way, however, of keeping them to task is to bring them back frequently to the problem first presented, and ask whether they can concentrate on solving it. In the case of mutual criticism, one way of coping is to slow down the interaction so that each partner speaks only after the therapist has intervened to reframe what has just been said.

As with reciprocity negotiation, communication training is used not as a self-contained therapy in itself, but rather as part of a menu of techniques to be chosen according to the problem presented or observed at the time.

### (c) Structural moves in session

The main interventions under this heading are raising arguments (or heated discussions) in the session, reversed role play, and 'sculpting'.

There are many couples in which there is a reluctance to enter any sort of conflict. They avoid differences of opinion, and pretend that there is agreement on almost every issue. The more dominant partner, usually more at ease verbally, effortlessly takes the spokesperson role. The other partner is either silent much of the time or spends much effort placating the other in order to reduce conflict.

One strategy with such couples is to ask them to argue (or, to put it more acceptably, to have a **heated discussion**) about a fairly trivial topic. An example of this might be whether the toilet seat should be left up or down after it has been used. It must be a genuine difference of opinion, and not simply one manufactured for the purpose, but it is important that it should be of a trivial nature, as otherwise the couple may feel inhibited about discussing it.

They are then asked to discuss the issue with the therapist observing, and the therapist particularly encourages the more submissive partner to participate with enthusiasm. It may be necessary to ask him or her to speak louder, or to ask the other partner to listen more carefully to what the quiet partner has said, but the therapist should not take sides as such. What is being dealt with is not the issue itself, but the process of arguing. The outcome does not matter, except that the submissive partner should not be allowed to 'get away with' their usual tactic of giving in for the sake of peace. The couple may 'agree to differ' or the submissive partner may have a better than usual hearing, and even win the argument.

This intervention is particularly useful for those couples where there is a degree of depression in the quieter partner, or where the quieter partner is very reluctant to be involved sexually, and is blaming him- or herself.

Another intervention in session which can have an impact on the interaction is the '**reversed role play**'. Here the couple is asked to discuss a particular issue, but they are asked to act as if they were the other partner, even perhaps changing chairs for the purpose. The exercise is useful for some couples who have difficulty understanding each other's point of view, and may promote better mutual understanding.

A third intervention in session is the use of '**sculpting**', in which the partners position themselves and each other wordlessly in a kind of tableau to express some aspects of the relationship. For example, a wife who feels herself excluded from her husband's life may place him looking away from her, while her husband might place the two arm-in-arm and facing the same way. Neither position would represent the objective truth, but each would gain some understanding of the views of the other. The different views could also be the subject for discussion in session or during 'homework'. As with reversed role play, sculpting, with the accompanying 'experiential' insight, can be useful in those couples where there is little understanding of the other's point of view.

### (d) Timetables and tasks

These are perhaps the most frequently used of our interventions. They are always given as part of the 'homework' at the end of the session, and may be of a behavioural nature or more systemic. Systems tasks are usually used for behaviour which is thought of as being out of control. Thus, they may be used in a couple where there is a jealous partner: this partner would be asked to raise his or her doubts about the other's fidelity, but only at a specified time each day and for a limited period (e.g. half an hour). If the topic comes up at any other time, they are asked to postpone any discussion till the appointed time. This can be frustrating for the jealous partner, although he or she will perhaps be reassured that the other will give the topic his or her full attention at the set time: but for the other partner it can come as a great relief that the issue of jealousy is at last under some sort of control, even in this simple form.

A timetabled task may be used in other situations, for example, when one partner has a series of complaints which the other is rejecting. The couple can again be asked to discuss the issue only at certain times and for a limited duration. The advantage of a timetable under these circumstances is that the therapist does not have to adjudicate as to who is right or wrong in the content of the argument, but simply deals with the process of arguing by asking the couple to raise their legitimate complaints at home at an appropriate but limited time.

Another frequently used timetable is the 'talk' timetable, in which a couple who do not communicate very often are asked to set a time each day or evening when they can get together for a discussion about the day's events. In cases where there are difficulties with empathy, it may be useful in addition to ask each partner at the daily talk session to repeat back what the other one has said to reassure the other that they have understood what is meant.

One situation which responds particularly well to timetabling is where the male partner is very keen on sex and the female (while not having a sexual dysfunction as such) is much less enthusiastic. Here the partners are encouraged to reach a compromise on the agreed frequency at which sexual relations might occur, and then they agree on a suitable timetable. The day of the week has to be fixed in advance, since if this is not done the usual arguments will ensue as to whether sex should take place that night, and they are also asked to make the chosen night something special, with perhaps a dinner and the telephone disconnected. If, however, the enthusiastic partner suggests sex on another night, the other can simply remind him that it has been arranged and that they should stick to the arrangement. This remedy may seem somewhat crude, and it is often simply a temporary measure. However, it can be said to have virtually saved some relationships, because it takes the heat out of the sexual conflict which could otherwise lead to divorce, and its use can open up the discussions in subsequent sessions to include non-sexual topics which would otherwise be pushed out by the sexual issue.

It should be mentioned here that many relationship problems have a sexual and a general dimension. When the sexual difficulty is motivational rather than dysfunctional, it is often most productive to deal with it in couple relationship therapy either alone or in combination with psychosexual therapy. In such a case it is quite appropriate to suggest techniques such as the Masters and Johnson 'sensate focusing'[26] in addition to the couple therapy approaches already mentioned.

### (e) Paradoxical interventions

Paradox is a relatively infrequently used option in couple therapy (Fig. 6.3.7.1), and is brought in when other methods are ineffective or where the couple relationship seems so rigid that no other intervention can be used. The rationale for paradox depends on a systemic hypothesis which states that the homeostatic forces in the system may be so strong that no straightforward intervention will alter it. All systems tend towards a resistance to change, but in some the resistance is maintained by powerful forces which themselves seem to be informed by extreme anxiety.[14] In these couples or families the only intervention likely to succeed in changing the system is one which prohibits change, but for unacceptable reasons. Although the above explanation is somewhat unsatisfactory, paradox remains in practice a technique which can unlock an otherwise stuck relationship and get the couple back on course for continued therapy.

Paradox is always applied with care and in a sympathetic manner. A common form is to 'prescribe the symptom', that is to advise the couple that it is best 'for the time being' to persist with both the behaviour complained of and the reciprocal behaviour in the other partner. The reason given for this conclusion is a plausible, but challenging and perhaps unacceptable, explanation based on systemic understanding of the relationship.

In using paradox the therapist should think in four stages. First, there should be a positive connotation of the 'symptom' and the reciprocal behaviour. Secondly, there should be a rehearsal of why they are at present helpful for the couple. Thirdly, a statement should be made of the hypothesized feared consequences if the behaviours were to stop. Fourthly, the symptom and the reciprocal behaviour should be prescribed. A case example may make this process a little clearer.

---

**Case Study:** A couple who presented with depression in the wife (Edna) and a rather overprotective attitude on the husband, George's, side were in therapy for some weeks without much progress. Following a session in which the therapist asked many questions of both of them about the circumstances and consequences of the depressive episodes, the paradox was presented as follows. 'This depression seems in some ways to be quite good for you as a couple, because it enables Edna to help George by giving him a role in life as her protector. If the depression were to disappear it might be difficult for you both to continue your peaceful relationship, because the differences between your views and ideals would become very clear and you might argue all the time. So for the time being it is better for Edna to remain depressed and for George to be her spokesman and protector'.

This intervention led to quite an outburst from the wife, who up to that time had always been very quiet, and she began to talk of some of the differences of opinion that they had actually had. The husband looked rather disconcerted, and questioned the therapist's reasoning. In the next two sessions the couple reversed their imbalance to some extent, the wife became more assertive than the husband, and her depression became less severe.

---

The paradox can thus be a powerful mechanism for change, but it must be used with some caution, since an instruction given paradoxically may be taken literally. So it would be inappropriate to include in a paradox any instructions to break the law, to harm oneself or others, or to act irresponsibly. If given as recommended, however, the paradox can unlock a 'stuck' system and put the couple on the road to change and improvement.

In a team setting it is probably best to use a **'split team'** message rather than a paradox as such. This presents the paradox as above, but in the form of an alternative, for example in the form of a disagreement between the therapist and the supervising team. 'I feel that you can carry on with the tasks that I have been giving you, but my team think I am being naïve, and that you really need the depressive symptoms and the overprotection to keep your marriage from falling apart'. The effect is similar, but the impact is softened somewhat by this technique.

## Couple therapy with couples from other cultures

As mentioned above, most western countries are now multicultural, and a significant minority of those seeking therapy, especially in urban centres, are from immigrant backgrounds. Probably the most frequently seen in Britain are those of South Asian origin, but Eastern European, African and African- Caribbean couples are also seen quite often. In the USA there are many people of Latin American and Oriental backgrounds, and here again these will be more commonly encountered in urban settings. The author's experience is mainly with South Asians, and the examples will be mainly from this group.

Cultural factors in counselling have been highlighted by d'Ardenne and Mahtani,[27] and include the need for awareness in the counsellor that he or she also comes from a specific culture which may be just as difficult for the client to comprehend as the client's is to the counsellor. They emphasize the need for humility in the face of difference, and the responsibility of the counsellor to check with the clients before making assumptions about their lifestyles and beliefs. Their advice on the use of interpreters is that unofficial interpreters, including members of the clients' own families, should be discouraged because they are inclined to act as therapists themselves, may translate inaccurately, may ignore cultural differences and may even exploit the clients. It is better to use official interpreters, though this may become expensive to the treatment unit, and the interpreters themselves may translate inaccurately in accord with what they think the therapist wants to hear. Ideally a unit would have multilingual counsellors, but this is not always practicable. In practice, it is often possible with a modicum of understanding of the language for a couple relationship therapist to carry out therapy in English without an interpreter, but with a little bit of necessary translation by the partner whose English is better.

Little has been written specifically on cultural factors in relationship therapy, but Ahmed and Bhugra[28] have reviewed the role of culture in sexual dysfunctions, and their observations are also relevant to couple therapy. They emphasize the need to adapt the techniques of 'western' sex therapy to accommodate the cultural backgrounds of the patients, in particular the gender roles in the culture, and they highlight the risks of ignoring these in therapy.

Couple therapists need to be flexible in regard to the aims of therapy in these couples, which may be rather different from the typical white British couple, and there may also be limits to the kind of therapeutic change possible. For example, a couple from South Asia may be orientated towards a male dominated marital pattern, and both partners may be reluctant to accept the kind of equal relationship that typical couple therapy would expect. In other cases, the more traditional male partner may be concerned to retain the traditional dominance, while the (more westernized) woman may be demanding equality. Similar problems may arise in couples who come from different cultures, and there are clearly more interracial relationships developing as the cultures become more integrated.

Religious considerations may bring difficulties to therapy. Strict Muslim couples may be reluctant to attend therapy together, particularly with a male therapist, because of the difficulty of the wife talking to a male stranger. Masters and Johnson[26] found that one of the most reliable prognostic factors in their therapy was the negative effect of any strong religious belief on the outcome. It has also been observed that in a sexual dysfunction clinic Asian couples were more likely than white couples to default from therapy, a finding put down to their pursuit of organic explanations for the problems and educational and language barriers.[29]

Similarly African-Caribbean couples will have different aims and limitations from white British couples. The father in these families may traditionally be more of an absentee, and leave the upbringing of the children to his partner, who becomes the main authority figure in the family. Again, the therapist must remain aware of possible differences from his/her own culture, and remember that the key consideration is the wishes and wellbeing of the couple rather than any imposed set of rules derived from theory. In particular it is usually impossible to persuade the man to take a more active role in child care, even when the woman wants this, and their relationship will usually remain 'semi-detached'.

One particular 'problem constellation' which the author has seen many times is that of an Englishman married to a North American woman. This should theoretically present no problems, as the language and cultures of both are similar. However, they are divided by the tendency for the British man to be reserved and sometimes resentful and the American woman to be outspoken and critical. Such difficulties have also been found with couples from other disparate backgrounds, such as North American and Latin American partners, and Southern European and British couples. These differences in outlook can lead to repetitive quarrels, in which neither partner can understand where the other is coming from, and often there is also a lack of sexual contact between them. In therapy it is usually necessary to explain each partner to the other, using positive terms and helping them to appreciate the cultural differences without condemning the partner. Then they can usually cooperate with reciprocity negotiation and communication training.

Although the examples given are mainly of South Asian and Western couples, the principles for dealing with cross-cultural relationships of all sorts are basically similar. The therapist needs to respect the differences between their culture and his/her own, trying not to impose solutions which are alien to the couple's own culture. In those cases where they each come from a different background, the general approach is to try to build bridges between them, and use the techniques of behavioural systems therapy to solve their difficulties.

## Efficacy of couple therapy

The efficacy of couple therapy is not an easy topic to discuss. Problems arise as to how one should assess efficacy, and while most authors would agree that a measurable improvement in marital adjustment is a valid measure of improvement, some authors dismiss that as being too subjective or too superficial. On the other hand, to use an objective criterion such as divorce as an outcome variable might be seen as being too strict on the therapy, since divorce happens for many reasons, and it might not actually be a bad outcome in some relationships.

A review of efficacy in couple therapy has been carried out by Baucom et al.[30] They did a very thorough search of the literature, and made some far-reaching and challenging observations. They comment that the untreated improvement rate is very low in couple problems, and that many of the non-behavioural approaches are of unproven efficacy. They conclude however that behavioural marital therapy (comparing mean effect size over a series of 17 independent controlled outcome studies) is an efficacious and specific intervention for marital distress. The improvement is likely to last for up to a year after treatment but there is less certainty over longer follow-up periods. The addition of cognitive restructuring to behavioural couple therapy did not add anything to the efficacy, but the numbers were rather small.

Snyder and Wills[31] evaluated the outcomes of behavioural versus insight-orientated marital therapy, and found that there was equal improvement in the two conditions, with both being superior to waiting list controls. There was, however, a difference at follow-up, with more of those who had had behavioural therapy divorcing than those who had had insight-orientated therapy.

In a controlled study of behavioural versus interpretative couple therapy, Crowe[32] found that both approaches were effective, but that the behavioural approach produced results more quickly. The follow-up at 18 months showed both methods to be of lasting efficacy, with no differences between them at that point.

Another treatment approach, emotion-focused therapy,[33] has produced good results with couples in therapy. As with behavioural couple therapy the couples improved significantly more than those on a waiting list, but this therapy seems less effective in couples with higher levels of distress.

In one of the relatively few studies on the efficacy of systems-orientated couple therapy. Emmelkamp *et al.*[34] evaluated the effects of behavioural versus systems couple therapy, and concluded that the two approaches had very similar results, but both did better than waiting-list controls.

The London Depression Study[20] (see above) found that systemic couple therapy produced good improvement not only in terms of the couple satisfaction but also on the depression in the depressed partner. The therapy was also associated with a lower drop-out rate than the antidepressant condition, and was thus more acceptable to the patients and their partners.

Thus, the two components of behavioural–systems couple therapy have both been validated by outcome research, although at a much higher level for the behavioural than the systemic. It would be desirable to carry out research on the combined therapy, but this has not yet been done, and the best that can be said is that it is a combination of two probably effective treatment approaches, and therefore likely to be effective.

## Training

Training for work with couples using a behavioural–systems approach has been thoroughly reviewed by Crowe and Ridley.[1] It requires an ability in the therapist to understand and use different approaches, and an ability to adapt ones activity to the needs of the couple. Before beginning to work as a couple therapist the trainee should have a basic understanding of the dynamics of couple and family interaction, the phases of human development, the impact on the individual of life events, sexual function and interaction and the impact of physical illness on couple and family relationships. These can be dealt with in the traditional seminar format, in which the trainee can also learn about theoretical and technical aspects of the approach to couple therapy itself. It is also important in selecting candidates for training to ensure that they have some experience of counselling individuals or of being in a therapeutic role, for example as a nurse or doctor.

In addition to the seminars there are also more active training sessions in which the trainee is given the technical skills to carry out therapy. The latter take three main forms: role play, observation, and supervized practice. In role play the trainees are encouraged to use either an existing couple or a fictional one and role play a couple therapy session. Ideally they should each, in different exercises, have the opportunity to play the husband, wife, therapist, and observer in therapy.[35] This helps both in the development of technical skills and in learning to be empathetic to clients through having experienced the client role. In role play the trainee can practise any of the techniques required in therapy, but it is perhaps especially useful in the area of communication training, in which the therapist needs to be alert to the problems shown by the partners and able to apply the appropriate technique smoothly and effectively.

In observation and supervision other aspects of the therapy can be taught, especially the more systemic methods such as arguments, reversed role play, and the framing of messages. The trainees move quite quickly from live observation of therapy in the clinic to being firstly a co-therapist and then the sole therapist in the session, supported and supervised by the trainer and the observation team on the other side of the screen. It is in this activity that trainees begin to display their skills or deficits as therapists, and the trainer must be able to assess progress at this stage and take remedial action if a trainee does not seem to be working as well as expected.

## Conclusions

The field of couple therapy is a wide and varied one, and there are almost as many different approaches to treatment as in individual psychotherapy. The relatively brief therapeutic method presented here, behavioural systems couple therapy, is an eclectic one, taking techniques from two approaches of proven efficacy and combining them into a flexible and versatile therapy capable of being used in a wide variety of presenting problems. These include simple relationship problems, psychosexual problems, and such psychiatric conditions as anxiety, depression, and morbid jealousy. It is relatively easy to teach, and although it has not yet been subjected to controlled trials it can be assumed to be no less effective than its component therapies which are both effective. It has recently also been recommended in a package for self-help[36] with homework exercises and theoretical explanations to be used without the intervention of a therapist. There are few contraindications for the therapy, and it can be used both as a therapy in its own right or as an adjunctive therapy in, for example, the treatment of depression, psychosis or sexual dysfunctions. It can thus be a useful addition to the various methods available for the reduction of distress, whether in couples or individuals.

## Further information

Crowe, M. and Ridley, J. (2000). *Therapy with Couples: a behaviouralsystems approach to marital and sexual problems* (2nd edn.). Blackwells Science, Oxford.

Clulow, C. (ed.) (2001). *Adult Attachment and Couple Therapy*. Brunner Routledge, London.

### Organizations which provide information about how to obtain couple therapy

British Association for Sexual and Relationship Therapy www.basrt.org.uk
British Association for Counselling and Psychotherapy www.bacp.co.uk
United Kingdom Council for Psychotherapy www.psychotherapy.org.uk
Institute of Family Therapy www.instituteoffamilytherapy.org.uk
American Association for Marriage and Family Therapy www.aamft.org

### Organizations which provide information on training in Sexual and Relationship Therapy

British Association for Sexual and Relationship Therapy www.basrt.org.uk

Porterbrook Clinic, Sheffield (Sheffield Hallam University) www.
porterbrookclinic.org.uk

London South Bank University ww.lsbu.ac.uk/psychology

University of Central Lancashire: Lancashire School of Health and
Postgraduate Medicine www.uclan.ac.uk

Relate Institute, Doncaster www.relate.org.uk

American Association for Marriage and Family Therapy www.aamft.org

## References

1. Crowe, M. and Ridley, J. (2000). *Therapy with couples: a behavioural–systems approach to marital and sexual problems* (2nd edn). Blackwell Science, Oxford.

2. National Statistics Office (1998). *Population trends*. HMSO, London.

3. Robinson, M. (1991). *Family transformation through divorce and remarriage*. Tavistock Press, London.

4. Daniell, D. (1985). Marital therapy: the psychodynamic approach. In Marital therapy in Britain, Vol. 1 (ed. W. Dryden), pp. 169–94. Harper and Row, London.

5. Clulow, C. (ed.) (2001). *Adult Attachment and Couple Psychotherapy*. Brunner Routledge, London.

6. Bowlby, J. (1969). Attachment and loss, Vols 1 and 2. Hogarth Press, London.

7. Wile, D.B. (1993). *Couples therapy, a nontraditional approach* (2nd edn). Wiley, Chichester.

8. Stuart, R.B. (1980). *Helping couples change*. Guilford Press, New York.

9. Liberman, R.P. (1970). Behavioural approaches in family and couple therapy. *American Journal of Orthopsychiatry*, **40**, 106–18.

10. Beck, A. (1988). *Love is never enough*. Harper and Row, New York.

11. Dryden, W. (1985). Marital therapy, a rational emotive approach. In Marital therapy in Britain, Vol. 1 (ed. W. Dryden), pp. 195–221. Harper and Row, London.

12. Minuchin, S. (1974). *Families and family therapy*. Tavistock Press, London.

13. Haley, J. (1980). *Leaving home*. McGraw Hill, New York.

14. Selvini Palazzoli, M., Boscolo, L., Cecchin, G., et al. (1978). *Paradox and counter–paradox*. Aronson, New York.

15. Segraves, R.T. (1982). *Marital therapy: a combined psychodynamic–behavioural approach*. Plenum Medical, New York.

16. Weeks, G.R. (1989). *Treating couples, the intersystem model of the Marriage Council of Philadelphia*. Brunner–Mazel, New York.

17. Spinks, S.H. and Birchler, G.R. (1982). Behavioural–systems marital therapy: dealing with resistance. *Family Process*, **21**, 169–85.

18. Berg–Cross, L. (1997). *Couples therapy*. Sage, Thousand Oaks, CA.

19. Jacobson, N.S. and Margolin, G. (1979). *Marital therapy: strategies based on social learning and behavioral exchange principles*. Brunner–Mazel, New York.

20. Leff, J., Vearnalls, S., Brewin, C.R., et al. (2000) The London depression intervention trial. Randomized controlled trial of antidepressants v. couple therapy in the treatment and maintenance of people with depression living with a partner: clinical outcome and costs. *British Journal of Psychiatry*, **177**, 95–100.

21. De Silva, P. (1997) Jealousy in couple relationships: nature, assessment and therapy. *Behaviour Research and Therapy*, **35**, 937–85.

22. McFarlane, W. (2000) Psychoeducational multi-family groups. Adaptations and outcomes. In *Psychosis: Psychological Approaches and their Effectiveness*. (ed. B. Martindale, A. Bateman, M. Crowe and F. Margison) Gaskell, London.

23. Crowe, M. (2005) Couples and mental illness. *Sexual and Relationship Therapy*, **19**, 309–10.

24. Thibault, J.W. and Kelley, H.H. (1959). *The social psychology of groups*. Wiley, New York.

25. Olson, D.H., McCubbin, H.I., Barnes, H., et al. (1983). *Families: what makes them work*. Sage, Los Angeles, CA.

26. Masters, W.M. and Johnson, V.E. (1970). *Human sexual inadequacy*. Little, Brown, Boston, MA.

27. d'Ardenne, P. and Mahtani, A. (1989). *Transcultural Counselling in Action*. Sage, London.

28. Ahmed, K. and Bhugra, D. (2007). The role of culture in sexual dysfunction. In *Psychiatry: Sexual Disorders and Psychosexual Therapy*. (ed M.Crowe). Medicine Publishing (Elsevier), London.

29. Bhui, K. (1998). Psychosexual care in a multi-ethnic society. *Journal of Social Medicine*, **91**, 141–3.

30. Baucom, D.H., Shoham, V., Mueser, K.T., et al. (1998). Empirically supported couple and family interventions for marital distress and adult mental health problems. *Journal of Consulting and Clinical Psychology*, **66**, 53–88.

31. Snyder, D.K. and Wills, R.M. (1989). Behavioural versus insight orientated marital therapy: effects on individual and interpersonal functioning. *Journal of Consulting and Clinical Psychology*, **57**, 39–46.

32. Crowe, M.J. (1978). Conjoint marital therapy: a controlled outcome study. *Psychological Medicine*, **8**, 623–36.

33. Johnson, S.M. and Greenberg, L.S. (1985). Differential effects of experiential and problem–solving interventions in resolving marital conflict. *Journal of Consulting and Clinical Psychology*, **53**, 175–84.

34. Emmelkamp, P.M.G., van der Helm, M., MacGillavry, D., et al. (1984). Marital therapy with clinically distressed couples: a comparative evaluation of system–theoretic, contingency contracting and communication skill approaches. In *Marital interaction: analysis and modification* (ed. K. Hahlweg and N. Jacobson), pp. 36–52.Guilford Press, New York.

35. van Ments, M. (1983). *The effective use of role–play. A handbook for teachers and trainers*. Kogan Page, London.

36. Crowe, M. (2005) *Overcoming Relationship Problems*. Constable Robinson, London.

# 6.3.8 Family therapy in the adult psychiatric setting

Sidney Bloch and Edwin Harari

The term 'family therapy' covers a range of approaches. At one extreme, it is a method which seeks to help an individual patient. At the other extreme, the focus is on the relationships between people; according to this view psychopathology reflects recurring, problematic interactive patterns among family members. Midway between the two positions is one that views the family as acting potentially either as a resource or a liability for an identified patient. In this chapter, we cover the spectrum but confine ourselves to the adult psychiatric setting.

## A historical and theoretical context

The family has long been recognized as a core aspect of social organization. The folklore of all cultures emphasize the family's role to mould the character of its members. In the past 150 years academic disciplines, such as anthropology and sociology, have studied the various forms of family structure found in different cultures, and at different times. Since the 1960s, psychiatry has also developed a clinical and research interest in the family beyond that of genetics.

Scattered through Freud's writings are interesting comments about marital and family relationships and their possible roles in both individual normal and abnormal development.[1] His description of unconscious processes like introjection, projection, and identification illuminate how individual experiences may be transmitted across generations. In 1921, J.C. Flugel published the first comprehensive psychoanalytic account of family relationships.[2] Influenced by Anna Freud, Melanie Klein, and Donald Winnicott, the child guidance movement in Britain, mainly consisting of social workers, devised a model of one therapist working with the disturbed child and another with the mother. The two clinicians then collaborated in order to appreciate how the mother's anxieties distorted her perception and handling of her child, leading to developmental difficulties.

## Proliferation of theoretical schools

### Psychoanalytic and related approaches

Things took a different turn in the United States where Nathan Ackerman[3] began in the 1950s to treat families with a disturbed child, using psychodynamic principles. An interest in working with two or more generations arose concurrently with 'transgenerational'-oriented family analysts using object–relations concepts. Thus, Murray Bowen[4] noted that the capacity of psychotic children to differentiate from their families, while still retaining a sense of age-appropriate belonging, was impaired by the effects of unresolved losses and other trauma in parental and grandparental generations. He also devised the genogram, a schematic depiction of family structure, with a notation for notable events; this remains a standard part of family assessment (see below).

Boszormenyi-Nagy and Spark[5] similarly addressed the transgenerational theme, describing how relationships were organized around a ledger of entitlements and obligations, which conferred on each family member a sense of justice or injustice about their situation. This, in turn, reflected childhood experiences of neglect or sacrifices made on another relative's behalf for which redress was sought in adult life.

### Systems-oriented (see later)

Bowen[4] also introduced the principles of 'systems theory' into family therapy. A system is defined as a set of interrelated elements that function as a unity within a particular environment and where the whole is larger than the sum of the parts. 'General systems theory', propounded in the 1940s by a German biologist,[6] contains among its key concepts the place of hierarchy and the emergence of new features in the system as it transforms itself, necessarily, from one level of organization to another. A family is an example of a partially open system that interacts with both its biological and socio-cultural environments and changes over time to accommodate developments such as the advent of a first child or the death of a grandparent.

Working with delinquent youth, Salvador Minuchin recognized the relevance of systems thinking. The youngsters often came from poor, emotionally deprived families, headed by a demoralized single parent (usually the mother) who alternated between excessive discipline and helpless delegation of responsibilities to a child or to her own critical mother. Since these families were beyond the reach of conventional 'talking' therapies, Minuchin applied action-oriented techniques which enabled him to 'join' the family and to re-establish an adaptive hierarchy and effective boundaries between subsystems (marital, parent–child, siblings).

Later, treating 'psychosomatic families' where the problem was a child or adolescent suffering from anorexia nervosa, unstable diabetes or asthma, Minuchin and his colleagues noted that these families, while intact and articulate, were often enmeshed. Members avoided challenging the apparent sense of family unity. Typically, marital conflict was detoured through the symptomatic child, resulting in maladaptive coalitions between parent and child (sometimes between grandparent and child) and the involvement of third parties (e.g. helping agencies) in family life; loss of hierarchy and boundaries ensued. Because words were used to avoid change in these well-educated families, non-verbal strategies were devised to face unspoken fears of conflict and change.[7]

Jay Haley's 'strategic therapy'[8] combined features of Minuchin's model with ideas of Milton Erickson whose techniques had skilfully exploited the notion that a covert message lurks behind explicit communication, which defines the power relationship between family members. Related theoretical developments took place in Palo Alto, California in the 1950s, where a group of clinicians, together with the anthropologist Gregory Bateson,[9] observed that implicit in communication were tacit, non-verbal 'meta-communications' which defined the ties between participants. A contradictory quality between these two levels of communication—in which messages carried persuasive, moral, or coercive force for the recipient—formed part of what they called a 'double-bind'; this form of entrapment was proposed, albeit erroneously, as a possible basis for the formal thought disorder found in schizophrenia.[10,11]

#### (a) Systems-oriented models: further developments

All the above system-oriented views assume that family functioning can be objectively studied. However, therapists are not value-free and may actively orchestrate changes in accordance with their preferred theoretical model; neglected in these circumstances are therapists' biases and their influence.

This tendency probably reflected the determination of family therapists to distance themselves from psychoanalytical theory; but it also led them to neglect the family's past history and changes through the lifecycle, including the relevance of traumatic events.

In response to this criticism there was a shift away from a problem-focused approach, which had typified most communication-based views of psychopathology. The so-called Milan school[12] (see course of therapy below), whose founders were psychoanalysts, launched profound conceptual changes in how to approach the family, particularly in interviewing them. Another innovation was the participation of observers behind a one-way screen whose task was to offer hypotheses about the family-plus-therapist system to the protagonists.

A Norwegian group[13] took the idea one step further by developing the 'reflecting team dialogue'. Here, following a session, the family could observe the therapeutic team discussing their problems and possible causes, and what factors might have prompted them to seek certain remedies—especially those they had persevered with despite the clear lack of effectiveness.

#### (b) Post-modern developments

Family therapists also began to ask whether families might be hampered from trying out new ways to solve their difficulties because of the ways they themselves had interpreted their past experiences or unwittingly absorbed the explanatory narratives of external 'experts' or society at large.

This led to a shift from considering the family as a system defined by its organizational structure to a linguistic-based one. According to this view the narrative a family relates about themselves is a means to integrate in specific ways their past experience and its significance. Other 'stories' are excluded from consideration. For instance, when a family with an ill member talk to health professionals, the conversations inevitably revolve around problems (a problem-saturated description). The family ignore times when problems were absent or minimal, or when they were confined to manageable proportions. A different story might be told if they were to examine the factors that could have led, or still lead, to better outcomes than those currently deemed pathological.

Several narrative-based approaches apply these concepts.[14–16] Philosophically, they align themselves with post-modernism, a movement which challenges the idea that there is a fundamental truth or grand theory known only by the expert.

### (c) Criticism of systems approaches

Many criticisms have been levelled at systems-based approaches, these include:

- disregard of the subjective experiences of family members

- neglect of the family's history

- inattention to unconscious motives in interpersonal behaviour

- not addressing the issue of unequal power in a family, particularly violence against women and child abuse, and

- ignoring various forms of injustice based on societal attitudes regarding gender, ethnicity, and class.

This critique has led to integrating systems-oriented and psychoanalytic concepts, particularly those derived from object–relations theory.[17–20] Specific disorders such as schizophrenia[21] and anorexia nervosa[22] have been targeted. Another noteworthy variant of integration is Byng-Hall's[23] synthesis of attachment theory, systems-thinking, and a narrative approach.

Another criticism of systems-oriented approaches is minimizing the impact of material reality, such as physical handicap, or biological factors, in the causation of mental illness, as well as sociopolitical phenomena like unemployment, racism, and poverty. These are obviously not merely the result of social constructions or linguistic games and the distress they may inflict on people are potentially considerable.

The 'psycho-educational' approach and 'family crisis intervention' have arisen in the context of the burden that severe mental illness, particularly schizophrenia, places on the family and the potential for members to influence dramatically the course of the condition. This has led to a series of family interventions:

- educating the family about the nature, cause, course, and treatment of schizophrenia

- providing the family with opportunities to discuss their difficulties in caring for the patient, and to devise pertinent strategies

- clarifying the role of conflict, not only about the illness but also about other relational issues

- regularly evaluating the impact of the illness on the family, both individually and collectively

- helping to resolve other conflicts possibly aggravated by the demands of caring for a enduringly ill person.

This type of work may be done with a single family or with several families meeting together, known as Multiple-Family Group Treatment (MFGT). The latter has emerged as a powerful adjunct to conventional individual-based treatment of schizophrenia, bipolar disorder, major depression, obsessive-compulsive disorder, somatization disorder, and an array of chronic medical conditions. Good results have been achieved in reducing the relapse rate, duration, and frequency of hospitalization and in boosting compliance with medication.[24] Family crisis intervention, initially devised for families with a schizophrenic relative but since applied to other clinical states, operates on the premise that deterioration or a request by the family to hospitalize a member may reflect change in a previously stable pattern of family functioning. Convening an emergency meeting with the patient, spouse, and other key family members may help to avoid admission. Social and institutional forces outside the family often contribute to a crisis, and may precipitate a psychotic episode in a vulnerable member. The 'open dialogue' model of family crisis interviewing, developed in Finland, fosters discussion about such forces, using concepts and techniques derived from, *inter alia*, the Milan school, narrative approaches, and psychodynamic thinking; this integrated perspective has much potential.[25]

## Indications

A measure of controversy has dogged the issue of what constitutes the indications for family therapy. Pioneering practitioners claimed, somewhat overzealously, that their methods were suited to most conditions. A more balanced view since the mid-1990s encompasses a consensus that considering the systemic context is advantageous in assessing and treating any psychiatric problem. However, it does not follow that family therapy is the treatment of choice (or even indicated).

Family therapy, it should be stressed, does not constitute a unitary approach, with one principal purpose. The diversity of theoretical models we have alluded to above, with their corresponding techniques, should make this obvious. Regrettably, attempts to link indications to specific models have contributed little to the field.

It has also become clear that DSM or ICD diagnoses do not serve well as a basis for determining indications for family interventions. DSM has a minuscule section, the V diagnoses, covering 'relational problems'; these are limited in scope and not elaborated upon.[26] We are only informed that the problem in relating can involve a couple, a parent, and child, siblings, or 'not otherwise specified'. ICD neglects this relational area entirely.

In mapping out indications, we need to avoid blurring family assessment and family therapy. A patient's family may be recruited in order to gain more knowledge about diagnosis and treatment. This does not necessarily lead to family therapy. Indeed, it may point to marital therapy or to long-term supportive therapy. Thus, we need to distinguish carefully between an assessment family interview and family therapy *per se*.

A typology of family psychopathology, which might allow us to differentiate one pattern of dysfunction from another and so map out corresponding interventions, remains elusive. Empirical evidence is inconclusive and clinical consensus lacking. An inherent difficulty is in selecting dimensions of family functioning central to creating a typology.[27] Communication, cohesiveness, adaptability, boundaries between family members and subgroups, and level of conflict are a few of the contenders offered (see our own classification below).

There are no clear correlates between conventional diagnoses and family type. Efforts to establish links, such as an anorexia nervosa family[28] or a psychosomatic family[29] have not been fruitful. Similarly, investigations into the family and schizophrenia have yielded no durable results.[4,10] Clinicians and researchers have reluctantly accepted that models of effective family-based treatment for mental illness may not necessarily follow an understanding of the apparent causes of a condition in terms of observed disturbances in family relating. This complex matter is helpfully reviewed by Eisler regarding studies of the treatment of anorexia nervosa, but has implications for the entire field.[30]

What follows is our attempt to distil clinical and theoretical contributions.[31] Given the considerable overlap in clinical practice, categories are not mutually exclusive; and a family may require family therapy based on more than one indication. We should stress that family dysfunction is obvious in certain clinical situations and covert in others, often being concealed by a specific member's clinical presentation. Six categories emerge:

1 The problem manifests in explicit family terms and the therapist readily notes the family's dysfunction. For example, a marital conflict dominates, with repercussions for the children; or tension between parents and an adolescent child dislocates family life with everyone ensnared in conflict. In these situations the family is the target of intervention by dint of its clear dysfunctional pattern, and family therapy undoubtedly is the treatment of choice.

2 The family has experienced a disruptive life event which has led to its dysfunction. These events are either predictable or accidental and include, for instance, suicidal death, financial embarrassment, diagnosis of a serious physical illness, and the unexpected departure of a child from home. Any family stability that prevailed previously has been disturbed; the ensuing disequilibrium becomes associated with family dysfunction and/or the development of symptoms in one or more members. Family efforts to rectify the situation may inadvertently aggravate it.

3 Continuing, demanding circumstances in a family are of such a magnitude as to lead to ineffective adjustment. The family's resources may be stretched to the hilt; external sources of support may be scanty or unavailable. Typical situations are chronic physical illness, persistent or recurrent psychiatric illness, and the presence of a frail elderly member.

4 An identified patient may have become symptomatic in the context of a dysfunctional family; symptoms are in fact an expression of that dysfunction. Depression in a mother, an eating problem in a daughter, alcohol misuse in a father, through family assessment, are adjudged to reflect underlying family difficulties.

5 A family member is diagnosed with a conventional condition such as schizophrenia, agoraphobia, obsessive-compulsive disorder, or depression; the complications are the adverse reverberations within the family stemming from that diagnosis. For example, the son with schizophrenia taxes his parents in ways that exceed their 'problem-solving' capacity; an agoraphobic woman insists on the constant company of her husband in activities of daily living; a recurrently depressed mother comes to rely on the support of her eldest daughter. In these circumstances, members begin to respond maladaptively to the diagnosed relative, which paves the way for a deterioration of her condition, manifest as an enduring or relapsing course.

6 Thoroughly disorganized families, buffeted by many problems, are viewed as the principal target of help. This is apposite, even though, for instance, one member abuses drugs, another is prone to violence, and a third manifests antisocial behaviour. Regarding the family as the core dysfunctional unit is the rationale rather than a focus on each member's individual problems.

To reiterate, family therapy may not be the only treatment indicated. Thus, in helping a disturbed family struggling to deal with a schizophrenic member, supportive therapy and medication for the patient are usually as pertinent as any family treatment. Similarly, an indication for family therapy does not negate the possible use of another psychological approach for one or more family members. For instance, an adolescent striving to separate and individuate may benefit from individual therapy following family treatment (or in parallel with it), while his parents may require a separate programme to focus on their sexual relationship.

## Contraindications

These are self-evident and therefore mentioned only briefly.

1 The family is unavailable because of geographical dispersal or death.

2 Shared motivation for change is lacking. One or more members may wish to participate, but their chances of benefiting from a family approach are likely to be less than if committing themselves to individual therapy. We need to distinguish here between poor motivation and ambivalence; in the latter, the assessor teases out factors that underlie it and may encourage the family to engage.

3 The level of family disturbance is so severe or long-standing, or both, that a family approach seems futile, according to the best possible clinical judgement. For example, a family that has fought bitterly and incessantly for years is unlikely to engage in the constructive purpose of exploring their patterns of functioning.

4 Family equilibrium is so precarious that the inevitable turbulence[32] arising from family therapy is likely to lead to decompensation of one or more members; for example, a sexually abused adult may do better in individual therapy than by confronting the abusing relative.

5 The patient is too incapacitated to withstand the demands of family therapy. Someone in the midst of a psychotic episode or buffeted by severe melancholia is too affected by the illness to engage in family work.

6 An identified patient acknowledges family factors in the evolution of his problem, but seeks the privacy of individual therapy to explore it, at least initially. For example, a university student struggling to achieve a coherent sense of identity may benefit more from her individual pursuit of self-understanding. Such an approach does not negate an attempt to understand the contribution of family factors to the problem.

## Assessment

Family assessment, an extension of individual psychiatric assessment, adds a broader context to the formulation. The range and pace of the enquiry depends on the specifics of the case. Its phases are history from the patient, a provisional formulation concerning the relevance of the family, an interview with one or more members, and a revised formulation. In some cases, it is clear from the outset that the problem resides in the family group, thus rendering the phases below superfluous.

### History from the patient

The most effective way to obtain a family history is by constructing a family tree. Apart from showing the structure, it allows relevant information about noteworthy life events and a range of family features to be added. Scrutiny of the tree also provides a source of issues warranting exploration and, eventually, the potential for formulating hypotheses.

Personal details such as age, date of birth and death, occupation, education, and illness are recorded for each member, as well as critical family events (for example, migration, crucial relationship changes, notable losses, and achievements), and the quality of relationships. For an excellent discussion of the family tree—its construction, interpretation, and clinical uses—see McGoldrick and Gerson.[33] (See Fig 6.3.8.1 for genogram conventions.)

Useful principles are to work from the presenting clinical problem to the broader context, from the current situation to its historical origins and evolution, from 'facts' to inferences, and from non-threatening to more sensitive themes.

Questions are best preceded by a statement such as: 'In order to understand your problems better I need to know something of your background and your current situation'. This can be enriched by questions that allude to interactive patterns: 'Who knows about the problem? How does each of them see it? Has anyone else in the family faced similar problems? Who have you found most helpful and least helpful so far? What do they think needs to be done'. Attitudes of family members can be thus explored and light shed on the clinical picture.

### The presenting problem and changes in the family

Questions to understand the current context include: 'What has been happening recently in the family? Have there been any changes (e.g. births, deaths, illness, losses). Has your relationship with family members changed? Have relationships in the family altered?'

### The wider family context

A broader enquiry flows logically in terms of other family members to be considered, and in the time span of the family's history. Other significant figures, which may include caregivers and professionals, should not be forgotten.

Apart from information about the extended family's structure, questions about their response to major events can be posed: for example, 'How did the family react when your grandmother died? Who took it the hardest? How did migration affect your parents?'

Relationships are explored at all levels, covering those between the patient and other members and between these other members. Conflicted ties are particularly illuminating. Understanding who takes what 'roles' is also useful: 'Who tends to take care of others? Who needs most care? Who tends to be the most sensitive to what is going on in the family?' Asking direct questions about members is informative, but a better strategy is to seek the patient's views about their beliefs and feelings and to look for differences between members: 'What worries your mother most about your problem? What worries your father most?' Several lines of enquiry may reveal differences.

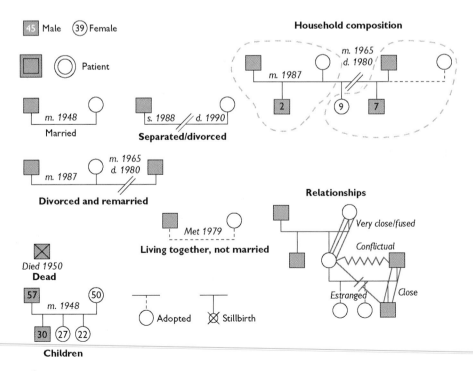

**Fig. 6.3.8.1** Genogram conventions.

◆ Pursuing sequential interactions: 'What does your father do when you say your depressions are dreadful? How does your mother respond when your father advises you to pull up your socks? How do you react when she contradicts him?'

◆ 'Ranking' responses: 'Everyone is worried that you may harm yourself. Who worries most? Who is most likely to do something when you talk about suicide?'

◆ Looking for relational changes since the problem: 'Does your husband spend more or less time with you since your difficulties began? Has he become closer or more distant from your daughter?'

◆ Hypothetical questions dealing with imagined situations: 'How do you think your relationship with your wife will change if you don't improve? Who would be most likely to notice that you were getting better?'

Triadic questions help to gain information about relationships which go beyond pairs; for example: 'How do you see your relationship with your mother? How does your father see that relationship? How would your mother react to what you have told me if she were here today?'

## Making a provisional formulation

Two questions arise from the above interview—how does the family typically function and are there any family features relevant to the patient's problems?

### (a) How does the family typically function?

A schema to organize ideas about family functioning builds from simple to complex observations: structure, changes, relationships, interaction, and the way in which the family works as a whole.

◆ The family tree will reveal the many family structures possible—single-parented, divorced, remarried, siblings with large age gaps, adoptees. Unusual configurations invite conjecture about inherent difficulties.

◆ Data will be obtained about notable family changes and events; the timing of predictable transitions is pertinent. Have external events coincided with these transitions (times at which the family may be more vulnerable)? How has the family met such changes?

◆ Relationships refer to how members interact with one another. What is the degree of closeness and emotional quality (e.g. warm, tense, rivalrous, hostile)? Major conflicts may be noted, as may be overly intense relationships.

◆ Particular interactive patterns may become apparent which go beyond pairs. Triadic relationships are more revealing about how a family functions overall. A third person is often integral to defining the relationship between another pair. A conflict, for instance, may be re-routed through the third person, preventing direct resolution. A child may act in coalition with one parent against the other or with a grandparent against a parent.

◆ At a higher level of abstraction, the clinician notes how the family works as a whole. Particular patterns (possibly a series of triads) may emerge that may have recurred across generations. For example, mothers and eldest sons have fused relationships, with fathers excluded, while daughters and mothers-in-law are in conflict.

Idiosyncratic shared beliefs may be discerned, explaining much of the way the family does things. 'Rules' governing members' behaviour towards one another or to the outside world may flow from these beliefs. For example, a family may hold that 'You can only trust your own family; the outside world is always dangerous'; they may therefore avoid conflict at any cost, and prohibit seeking external support.

Evidence of family difficulties may be found at each of these five levels. If they are, the question arises whether these do or do not relate to the patient's problems.

### (b) Are family factors involved in the patient's problems?

Links between family functioning and the patient's problems take various forms, but the following categories cover most situations:

◆ the family as reactive

◆ the family as a resource, and

◆ the family in problem maintenance

Often, more than one will apply.

## The family as reactive

The patient's illness, or its exacerbation, may have occurred at a time of family upheaval. While the precipitant for the upheaval may have been inherent in the illness itself, an escalating combination of the two may pertain. The illness may have occurred in the face of family stress; it pressurizes the family all the more, and this in turn exacerbates the illness.

## The family as a resource

The family may be well placed to assist in treatment. This may be as straightforward as supervising medication, ensuring clinic attendance, and detecting early signs of relapse, or providing a home environment that promotes and maintains recovery. The family may also call on friends and agencies, professional or voluntary, to offer support.

## The family in problem maintenance

Interactions revolving around the patient's illness may act to maintain it.

1 First, the illness becomes a way of 'solving' a family problem, the best that can be achieved. For example, anorexia nervosa in a teenager due to attend a distant university may lead to her abandoning this plan since she feels unable to care for herself. Were she to leave, parental conflict would become more exposed and her mother, with whom the patient is in coalition against her father, would find herself unsupported. The illness therefore keeps the patient at home and enmeshed in the parental relationship, and also provides a focus for shared concerns and an ostensible sense of unity.

2 Maintenance of the illness does not solve a family problem but may have done so in the past. An interactive pattern persists even though it lacks utility. In the previous example, the father's mother died 9 months later. His wife subsequently expressed feelings of closeness which he had not experienced for years; their relationship gradually improved. Both parents, however, continued to treat their daughter as incapable of achieving

autonomy, reinforcing her own uncertainty about coping independently if she were to recover.

3 Persistence of illness reflects a perception by the family of themselves and their problems, to which they are bound by the persuasive power of the narrative they have shaped for themselves. This often stems from the health care professional's explanatory schema.

### Interview with key informants

The clinician will by now have made an initial assessment of the patient's problems and of the family context. The next step is an interview with one or more informants, usually family members, to corroborate the story, to fill in gaps, to determine influences impinging on the patient, and to recruit others to help. A family meeting is most effective to accomplish these goals.

Implementing the session may prove difficult since the patient may oppose it for all sorts of reasons: symptoms have been kept secret, he regards it as unfair to burden others, he is ashamed of seeing a psychiatrist, he is fearful the family will be blamed, he is suspicious of them, and so forth. These concerns need ventilating, particularly if the family context is pivotal and it is likely that treatment will be enhanced by their involvement. The patient will agree in most cases. Where the safety of the patient or others is threatened, refusal may be overridden on ethical grounds. Otherwise, refusal must be respected. A family session can be suggested again after a more trusting relationship has been established.

Who should be seen depends on the purpose of the interview; generally, all those living in the household are likely to be affected by the patient's illness. The more family factors pertain, the more desirable the attendance by all. The patient's views are sought since he will provide insight into the members he deems crucial to his 'story'.

### The family interview

Much information will have been garnered by the time the family is seen. The clinician should consider any biases that may have infiltrated her thinking about the family, and how best to avoid being drawn into alliances. A non-judgemental stance is paramount.

Introductions are made in the initial phase. Names and preferred modes of address are clarified. The clinician then explains the meeting's purpose, details of which may well influence future participation. She invites everyone to share views about the nature and effects of problems they face.

The clinician has an idea about how the patient's problems relate to family function, and can test it out by asking probing questions and observing interactions. This is kept to herself since it is unhelpful for a hypothesis to be offered prematurely. Instead, details about everyday events are sought and inferences drawn later. For example, rather than focusing on 'closeness', questions can be asked about time spent together, whether intimate experiences are shared, who helps with family tasks, and so on.

Triadic relationships can be scrutinized both through questioning (what does A do when B says this to C?) and observation (what does A do when B and C reveal tensions?). The scope for such 'circular' questioning (a method ushered in by the Milan school) is enhanced if several members participate. A third person may be asked to comment on what two others convey to each other when a particular event occurs. This strategy of not posing questions to

which the family may have stereotypical responses challenges them to think about their relationships in a fresh way.

Information is elicited that elaborates the family tree. Observations may be made concerning family structure and functioning; for example, who makes decisions, who controls others and in what areas, the quality of specific dyadic relationships, conflict, alliances, how clearly people communicate and how they solve problems. The discussion then extends to all spheres of family life: beliefs, traditions, rules, and values.

Throughout the interview the clinician affirms the experiences of all family members. Concerns are attended to and the members' strengths and efforts acknowledged.

The interview concludes with a summary of what has emerged. The clinician may wish to continue the assessment or recommend family therapy. If the latter, an explanation of its aim and rationale is then given.

Arrangements are made for a follow-up session, purportedly the launch of family therapy *per se*, but in essence a continuation of 'work' in progress.

### Revised formulation

Since new information becomes available at each point, the initial formulation is revised as necessary.

Five observational levels —of structure, transitions, relationships, patterns of interaction, and global functioning—are re-examined in terms of the family as reactive, resourceful, or problem-maintaining. We now turn to the course of family therapy.

## The course of therapy

With a family approach agreed upon, therapy begins. However, when a family is referred as a group on the premise that the problem is inherently a family one, it is made explicit that the initial stage incorporates assessment.

Given the plethora of 'schools' of family therapy it would be laborious to chart the course of treatment based on each. We shall focus on the Milan approach,[12] but stress that it has undergone refinements. Our account highlights core features but first we comment briefly on the different roles the therapist may assume.

## Role of the family therapist

Beels and Ferber,[34] early observers of possible roles for family therapists, divide them into 'conductors' and 'reactors'; this differentiation remains useful since it transcends schools. Virginia Satir[35] is a good illustration of the conductor given that she espoused the notion of family therapist as a teacher who shares her expertise in how to communicate well by setting goals and the direction of treatment. She guided the family to adopt a new form of language to resolve communication problems, which she saw as the root of their troubles. Additionally, the therapist instils confidence, promotes hope for change, and makes them feel comfortable. Conductor-type therapists are explicit authorities, who intervene actively.

The therapist as reactor resonates with, and responds to, what the family exhibits to her. Psychoanalytically oriented and 'pure' systems therapists are representative since they typically share observations about patterns of relating that emerge. We will illustrate this in our account of the Milan school.[12]

## The Milan approach

With assessment complete, the therapist (sometimes a pair) meets the family for about an hour. With her preparatory knowledge, she develops a hypothesis about the nature of the family's dysfunction. She has the opportunity on observing patterns *in vivo* to confirm her notions. Patterns usually emerge from the start, making the therapist's job correspondingly easier. Apart from hypothesis-testing, another key task is to engage the family so they will be motivated to reattend. We could interpolate a dictum here: a primary aim of the first session is to facilitate a second session. A vital element in encouraging engagement is for the therapist to promote a sense of curiosity in family members so that they raise questions about themselves and the family as a group.[36]

The chief strategy is circular questioning.[37] Its main purpose is to address the family's issues indirectly; this avoids applying pressure on members and possibly inviting their resistance. For example, the therapist questions an adolescent about how his parents get on with each other, a mother about how her husband relates to the eldest son, a grandmother about which grandchild is closest to the parents, and so forth. This generates illuminating data about individual members and about the family as a group. In this phase, it helps to clarify the hypothesis and to engage participants. It also affords the therapist a greater facility to remain neutral. Because the system and not a patient is the target of change, the therapist is wary of showing any bias.

Various options are then available. If the therapist works as part of a team, her colleagues have busily observed the proceedings through a one-way screen. The family's consent for this will of course have been obtained. During a break, the team—observers and therapist(s)—pool impressions.[38] This is always enlightening since team members note something that others have missed. A consensus evolves, conclusions are drawn and converted into 'messages'. The therapist returns to the family to convey them. The actual messages and their oracular quality comprise a potent intervention, but not necessarily more cogent than circular questions made during the working session. We should mention here that the narrative school has brought with it a de-emphasis on the 'message' on the grounds that 'truth' is a shared construction.

One to three messages are usually given, with maximal clarity. These have a range of purposes including promotion of inter-sessional 'work'. Homework may be assigned and another session planned (unless termination was set for this point). Meetings commonly occur 3 to 4 weeks apart, and for good reason. During this time, the family, armed with new ideas, tackle them in their day-to-day lives. It is not critical how they go about it but that they do so. As Cecchin has posited,[36] the family's interest in their functioning should have been so aroused that they will be motivated to continue looking at themselves between sessions.

The varied nature of the message makes them classifiable.[39] Messages are supportive, hypothesis-related, or prescriptive. First, the message has a reassuring and encouraging quality and is not related to the hypothesis. A *complimentary message* might be that 'The team were impressed by how open you all were in the session', and a *reassuring message* that 'This is tantamount to a new start for the family and uncertainties are likely'.

*Hypothesis-related messages* refer to the hypothesis worked out by the team, and may assume diverse forms. It may be stated directly; for example, 'Susan has assumed the role of therapist for her parents

and sister to save the family from breaking up'. There may be reference to change such as, 'The team sees John taking responsibility; John and his father's improved relationship has enabled this to occur'. The family may be offered choices related to the hypothesis; for instance, 'The family could risk openness or remain self-preoccupied'. *Paradoxical messages* are a means to communicate a hypothesis which invites the family to revisit a feature of their functioning so that the family's difficulties are positively promoted and explicitly encouraged; for example, 'The team sense that your problem is working for the good of your marriage; sticking with your illness can save the marriage'. More creatively, the paradox may be split, in that the family are told about a divergence of opinion in the team[40]; for instance, some members believe it is too risky for them to communicate openly, others suggest the family can begin to do so. Through a *prescriptive message* the family is given a task. This may or may not be related to the hypothesis. For example, the family is urged to meet on their own before the next session to explore what inhibits a member from relating closely to the others.

Whatever the form of message, the therapist de-emphasizes the pathological status of the patient and applies what the Milan school calls *positive connotation*. This brilliant innovation rests on the premise that all behaviour is purposeful, and that the purpose can be construed positively. An adolescent's 'open grieving' is reframed as sparing the family the anguish of grief. This quality of message calls for creative thinking and flies in the face of the customary view of symptoms as evidence of psychopathology. Again, curiosity enters the picture as the family hears a positive communication concerning an issue they hitherto regarded as abnormal.

The process described continues in succeeding meetings, with attention also paid to family life between sessions. Duration of therapy depends on how entrenched the family dysfunction is rather than on the status of the patient's problems. Thus, systemic change is aimed for, with the family invited to consider a substitute mode of functioning that is feasible and safe. In practice, the number of sessions ranges from 1 to 12. If progress has not been made by about the seventh session, it is likely that alternate ways of helping family and/or patient are needed.

## Ending therapy

Termination issues are less profound than in individual or group therapy. The reason is obvious. The family has come as a living unit and will continue as such. Even when the therapist is a pure conductor, the family's intrinsic resources are highlighted so that they can be drawn on after the therapist's departure. Determining the end-point is not usually problematic. There is a shared sense that the work has been accomplished.

A hypothesis (or set of hypotheses) has been introduced, tested, and confirmed. The family system has been examined so that impediments are recognized and understood and better modes of functioning devised and implemented. The family is not required to leave functioning optimally. Instead, termination occurs when there is agreement that the family feels confident to try out newly discovered options.

As alluded to earlier, this may be determined alongside a judgement that the identified patient (or another family member) requires another form of therapy in their own right. An adolescent who has felt unable to separate and individuate is a good example. While family work has explored the system that hindered his 'graduation', the sense prevails that he could benefit further from individual or group therapy. In another example, the parents may conclude, with the therapist's support that they have an agenda which is not pertinent to their children and is therefore best undertaken in couple therapy.

## Problems encountered in therapy

Where assessment has been carried out diligently and motivation for change sustained, treatment proceeds smoothly. A crisis may still buffet the group but, rather than being derailed, the family regard it as a challenge with which to grapple.

Family treatment does not always succeed. Indeed, deterioration may occur, albeit in a small percentage of cases. What common difficulties are encountered? The non-engaging family is problematic in that while evidence points to the need for family intervention, members cannot participate in the task, usually because they resist letting go of 'the devil they know'. In another variation, engagement of some members may fail. This is particularly so in the case of fathers who, in the wake of their denial, tend to see the target of therapy as the identified patient rather than the family as a group. This belief may apply to any member.

Missed appointments may punctuate therapy, often linked to turbulent experiences between sessions or apprehension about what a forthcoming session may engender. Like any psychotherapy, drop-out is possible. On occasion, this is appropriate in that the indication for family therapy was misconstrued. In other circumstances, drop-out is tantamount to failure and may stem from such factors as therapist ineptitude, unearthing of family conflict which they cannot tolerate, and inappropriate selection of a family based on faulty assessment.

Given that the family continues as a living group during treatment, they are exposed to all manners of vicissitudes, and these may disrupt the therapeutic work. For example, an overdose by the patient, abrupt marital separation, or admission to a psychiatric hospital may take its toll and undermine treatment.

In discussing termination, we commented on outcome. Not all families will benefit. The family's dysfunction may be so intractable that it proves impervious to change, hypotheses may be 'off the mark', the family may lack sufficient psychological-mindedness, members may retreat in the face of change because of insecurity, and so forth.

Occasionally, dependency becomes a problem as the family discards any vestige of autonomy and only feels secure in the authoritative hands of the therapist. The latter may inadvertently foster such dependency by assuming undue authority, so precluding any sense of a growing partnership. The family's inherent resources are then not permitted expression.

Finally, part of the family may harbour a secret that threatens the principle of open communication. The therapist may be inveigled into a subgroup, although knowing that secrets are not conducive to the therapeutic process. For example, a wife calling the therapist to say she has been having an affair but cannot divulge this to her husband or children lest she hurt them imposes a burden on the therapist and the process (see Bloch et al.[27] for an overview of confidentiality in family therapy).

Sound clinical judgement is required in all these situations. Since no ready-made prescriptions are available, the therapist must be aware that difficulties may occur even in a highly motivated, well-selected family. The general principle, however, is to prevent their evolution if at all possible or to recognize them early and 'nip them in the bud'.

## Research in family therapy

Selective reviews of the vast research literature in family therapy have been provided by Carr.[41,42] Larner[43] has examined political and conceptual issues raised by family therapists' attempts to conform to the criteria of evidence-based practice while Stratton and his colleagues[44] have looked at the impact of such research on clinicians. An argument for the continuing relevance of single-case studies has been mounted by Datillio[45] and the possibilities of conducting qualitative research in a systems model by Burck.[46]

The long-standing debate between the role of 'common basic factors' versus 'model-specific factors', which has bedevilled research in individual therapy, also pertains to family therapy. Simon[47] has proposed a testable hypothesis, rich in its implications, that the most effective model is one whose concepts and values most closely resemble the world view of the therapist. He offers this as a conceptual bridge between the two approaches to therapeutic research, although he curiously says nothing about the family's world view.

Modifying the psychoeducational model of family-based treatment to incorporate clinically relevant socio-cultural factors has been proposed for the treatment of adolescents and young adults suffering from schizophrenia[48] and depression.[49]

In appraising the contemporary state of family therapy research in adult clinical psychiatry, we may be cautiously optimistic. Immense strides have been made in developing theoretical concepts. As can be seen in the first section of the chapter, we have a rich array of therapeutic approaches.[50] On the other hand, the growth occurred at a dizzy pace, with the inevitable consequence of overload. How can we make sense of so many offerings? Is integration needed to forestall fragmentation? Have we reached the point to pause and reflect? Are we in a position to evaluate the effectiveness of diverse approaches, and for various types of clinical problems?

Observers of the research[51,52] have pointed to a complicating factor in contemplating future work, namely the therapist assembling a natural group, of varying composition, in which the principal goal is to improve its functioning. We face the conundrum of what constitutes optimal outcome and how it is best measured. We can best illustrate this by citing Asen and his colleagues.[53] In their trial of family therapy they had agreed to apply multidimensional measures to assess outcome—at individual, dyadic, and family system levels. At follow-up they noticed changes at the first two levels, but not in the family as a whole. The latter involved ratings of such aspects as communication, boundaries, adaptability, and competence. The researchers were candid in sharing their doubts about how to deal with the divergent findings. Several interpretations were offered: for example, no change was achieved in family functioning, the instrument of family functioning was non-reactive to treatment since it was a trait measure, and an inappropriate model of therapy was applied in the first place. The group concluded that the 'assumptive worlds' of therapists and researchers were under scrutiny rather than the families themselves.

A group in Oxford[54] encountered similar difficulties in their study of consecutive families treated in an adult family therapy clinic. Whereas two-thirds of the identified patients were judged improved at termination, only half the families were rated as functioning at a better level. Again, the investigators were left with questions of how to determine what had actually been achieved.

A methodologically simpler method is to focus only on the identified patient. The work of Hafner *et al.*[55] exemplifies this choice— a case-controlled evaluation of family therapy in an inpatient setting with subsequent hospital admission data as the chief outcome criterion. Satisfactory as this study is in design, the omission of a family-system outcome measure leaves us ignorant about the level of family functioning following the intervention.

With these tricky matters in mind, what does research need to sort out? The diffuse question of whether family therapy works is of little utility, and is reminiscent of the sterile debate that typified individual psychotherapy outcome research for decades.[56] While subsequent meta-analyses demonstrated that psychological interventions overall exerted useful effects across a range of conditions, the field was still open to the criticism that efficacy of a specific approach for a particular clinical state remained unanswered. Family therapy should not repeat the same mistake; instead of posing the futile question of whether family therapy is effective in adult psychiatry, we should ascertain whether a specific family therapeutic approach, whose character is well identified and measurable, is useful for both the identified patient, with a specific clinical presentation, and his family's functioning, again well defined.

We have good examples of such research. Many intervention studies of families with a schizophrenic member have carefully described the principles of treatment, its rationale, process aspects, and outcome measures in the patient and (in some cases) the family.[57–60]

As mentioned earlier, multiple family group therapy (MFGT) is emerging as the preferred psychosocial intervention for adolescents and young adults with schizophrenia. A comparison with the 'open dialogue' model we mentioned earlier has not been conducted, and may not be feasible, since the latter is part of a comprehensive treatment paradigm.[61] A Danish study[62] which combined MFGT with assertive community-based treatment of young people with schizophrenia reported improvement not only of psychotic features (both positive and negative), but also a decline in use of alcohol and illicit drugs. Given the major problem of co-morbidity, this is a welcome development.

MFGT has also been directed to helping the caregivers of patients with schizophrenia. In a randomized controlled trial, Hazel *et al.*[63] found that those in the treatment programme for over a 2-year period experienced greater relief from distress compared to controls, but they were not able to determine the mechanism for this effect.

Work in the area of affective disorders and family therapy has been innovative, with MFGT, again, gaining popularity.[64] As in schizophrenia, the family treatment aims to reduce members' hostility and criticism expressed toward the depressed patient.

An excellently designed and executed study on anorexia and bulimia nervosa illustrates how outcome research can contribute to the clinical sphere.[65] In a well-controlled study, patients were randomized to either family therapy or 'routine individual supportive therapy', following their discharge from a weight-restoration programme. The family intervention focused on providing the members with information about the eating disorder and the effects of starvation. Parental anxiety was acknowledged and efforts made to help them take control of their daughter's diet. In parallel

with improved physical status, therapy turned progressively to typical adolescent issues of autonomy and how these might be achieved. Overall, a structural approach was applied, with systemic and strategic methods added as necessary. Applying these principles to groups of families with adolescents with anorexia nervosa appears to be useful.[66]

While the above studies concerning particular diagnoses, and involving an identified patient, is necessary for progress,[67] this does not preclude outcome studies where the family system is the main target of change. We illustrate this with a particular form of family grief therapy.[68] The model was derived from earlier empirical research on the outcome of family grieving in an oncology setting. A 13-month follow-up yielded five family clusters, two of which were distinctly dysfunctional, two functional, and an intermediate group vulnerable to maladaptive grieving. Three dimensions of family relational functioning were critical: cohesiveness, conflict, and expressiveness. The researchers then developed a treatment model highlighting the goals of promoting cohesiveness, expressiveness, and optimal management of conflict. A screening instrument was found which could readily identify dysfunctional families. A randomized controlled trial was then carried out which showed certain family types benefiting but others remaining unchanged, and a small group even being made worse.[69]

This necessarily schematic account of research on family therapy in adult psychiatry points to action needed in future. We can best summarize what investigators should strive for as: 'Specificity is of the essence'.

## Training

From charismatic figures devising innovative methods of family therapy, the field has developed into a worldwide enterprise, with dozens of books, scores of training courses, several journals, and a busy programme of national and international conferences and workshops on offer.[70] Formal training may be given as follows[71]:

1 University-based programmes that regard family therapy as a distinct professional pursuit, with a corresponding corpus of knowledge, and offer degree courses at various academic levels.

2 Free-standing institutes that also see family therapy as a distinct discipline and provide training, generally part-time and of briefer duration than university-based programmes.

3 Within university-affiliated hospitals and clinics that arrange professional training in psychiatry, psychiatric nursing, psychology, social work, and occupational therapy. Although there is a tremendous diversity in the above programmes, most include:

- ◆ Supervision of clinical work with the experienced practitioner (and perhaps other students) observing the trainee and family from behind a one-way screen. Some clinicians however consider the one-way screen as dehumanizing. They advocate instead a model of co-therapy between trainee and supervisor, often with other students sitting in the same room as the family.

- ◆ Video recording the trainee's work, which she then reviews with the supervisor and fellow students, is widely used. Tapes conducted by eminent therapists are also popular.

Whether training requires familiarity with concepts and techniques of diverse schools or whether it is preferable to develop expertise in only one school remains an open question. The free-standing institutes tend to be run by practitioners of a particular school so that, after a mostly cursory overview of the field, training concentrates on a specific model. Wendel and his colleagues[72] have proposed a model of training for multidisciplinary mental health settings which places most emphasis on integrating empirically derived knowledge; flexibility is a crucial feature for facilitating its optimal application.

## Conclusion

Family therapy has the potential to play a major role in the adult psychiatric setting. As we have commented above, research reveals several promising developments. Clinicians should seriously consider applying this mode of treatment; they will be much rewarded in doing so.

## Further information

Luepnitz, D.A. (1988). *The family interpreted: feminist theory in clinical practice*. Basic Books, New York.

Byng-Hall, J. (1995). *Rewriting family scripts. Improvisation and systems change*. Guilford, London.

Kissane, D. and Bloch, S. (2002). *Family focused grief therapy*. Open University Press, Buckingham, UK.

## References

1. Sander, F. (1978). Marriage and family in Freud's writings. *Journal of the American Academy of Psychoanalysis*, **6**, 157–74.
2. Flugel, J.C. (1921). *The psychoanalytic study of the family*. Hogarth, London.
3. Ackerman, N.W. (1958). *The psychodynamics of family life*. Basic Books, New York.
4. Bowen, M. (1971, 1981). *Family therapy in clinical practice*. Aronson, New York. (For an incisive critique of Bowen's theoretical contributions, see Miller, R., Anderson, S., and Keala, D. (2004). Is Bowen theory valid? A review of basic research. *Journal of Marital and Family Therapy*, **30**, 453–66.)
5. Boszormenyi-Nagy, I. and Spark, G.M. (1984). *Invisible loyalties: reciprocity in intergenerational family therapy*. Brunner-Mazel, New York.
6. von Bertalanffy, L. (1968). *General systems theory: foundation, development, applications*. Braziller, New York.
7. Minuchin, S. and Fishman, H.C. (1981). *Family therapy techniques*. Harvard University Press, Cambridge, MA.
8. Haley, J. (1976). *Problem-solving therapy*. Jossey-Bass, San Francisco, CA.
9. Bateson, G. (1972). *Steps to an ecology of mind*. Ballantine, New York.
10. Bateson, G., Jackson, D.D., Haley, J., *et al.* (1956). Toward a theory of schizophrenia. *Behavioural Science*, **1**, 251–64.
11. Bateson, G., Jackson, D.D., Haley, J., *et al.* (1962). A note on the double-bind. *Family Process*, **2**, 154–61.
12. Selvini-Palazzoli, M., Boscolo, L., Cecchin, G., *et al.* (1980). Hypothesising-circularity-neutrality: three guidelines for the conductor of the session. *Family Process*, **19**, 3–12.
13. Andersen, T. (1991). *The reflecting team: dialogues and dialogues about dialogues*. Norton, New York.
14. Anderson, H. and Goolishian, H.A. (1988). Human systems as linguistic systems: preliminary and evolving ideas about the implications for clinical theory. *Family Process*, **27**, 371–93.
15. De Shazer, S. (1985). *Keys to solution in brief therapy*. Norton, New York.
16. White, M. and Epston, D. (1990). *Narrative means to therapeutic ends*. Norton, New York.
17. Flaskas, C. and Perlesz, A. (eds.) (1996). *The therapeutic relationship in systemic therapy*. Karnac Books, London.
18. Braverman, S. (1995). The integration of individual and family therapy. *Contemporary Family Therapy*, **17**, 291–305.
19. Cooklin, A. (1979). A psychoanalytic framework for a systemic approach to family therapy. *Journal of Family Therapy*, **1**, 153–65.
20. Luepnitz, D.A. (1988). *The family interpreted: feminist theory in clinical practice*. Basic Books, New York.
21. Ciompi, L. (1988). *The psyche and schizophrenia. The bond between affect and logic*. Harvard University Press, Cambridge, MA.
22. Dare, C. (1997). Chronic eating disorders in therapy: clinical stories using family systems and psychoanalytic approaches. *Journal of Family Therapy*, **19**, 319–51.
23. Byng-Hall, J. (1995). *Rewriting family scripts. Improvisation and systems change*. Guilford, London.
24. McFarlane, W.R. (ed.) (2002). *Multiple family groups in the treatment of severe psychiatric disorders*. Guilford, New York.
25. Seikkula, J. and Olsen, M. (2003). The open dialogue approach to acute psychosis: its poetics and micropolitics. *Family Process*, **42**, 403–18.
26. American Psychiatric Association. (1994). *Diagnostic and statistical classification of diseases and related health problems* (4th edn). American Psychiatric Association, Washington, DC.
27. Bloch, S., Hafner, J., Harari, E., *et al.* (1994). *The family in clinical psychiatry*. Oxford University Press, Oxford.
28. Minuchin, S., Rosman, A., and Baker, L. (1978). *Psychosomatic families: anorexia nervosa in context*. Harvard University Press, Cambridge, MA.
29. Stierlin, H. (1989). The psychosomatic dimension: relational aspects. *Family Systems Medicine*, **7**, 254–63.
30. Eisler, I. (2005). The empirical and theoretical base of family therapy and multiple family day therapy for adolescent anorexia nervosa. *Journal of Family Therapy*, **27**, 104–31.
31. Clarkin, J., Frances, A., and Moodie, J. (1979). Selection criteria for family therapy. *Family Process*, **18**, 391–403.
32. Jenkins, H. (1989). Precipitating crises in families: patterns which connect. *Journal of Family Therapy*, **11**, 99–109.
33. McGoldrick, M. and Gerson, R. (1985). *Genograms in family assessment*. Norton, New York.
34. Beels, C. and Ferber, A. (1969). Family therapy: a view. *Family Process*, **8**, 280–332.
35. Satir, V. (1967). *Conjoint family therapy*. Science and Behaviour Books, Palo Alto, CA.
36. Cecchin, G. (1987). Hypothesizing, circularity, and neutrality revisited: an invitation to curiosity. *Family Process*, **26**, 405–13.
37. Tomm, K. (1987). Interventive questioning: part II. Reflexive questioning as a means to enable self-healing. *Family Process*, **26**, 167–83.
38. Selvini, M. and Selvini Palazzoli, M. (1991). Team consultation: an indispensable tool for the progress of knowledge. Ways of fostering and promoting its creative potential. *Journal of Family Therapy*, **13**, 31–52.
39. Allman, P., Bloch, S., and Sharpe, M. (1992). The end-of-session message in systemic family therapy: a descriptive study. *Journal of Family Therapy*, **14**, 69–85.
40. Papp, P. (1980). The Greek chorus and other techniques of paradoxical therapy. *Family Process*, **19**, 45–58.
41. Carr, A. (2005). Thematic review of family therapy journals in 2004. *Journal of Family Therapy*, **27**, 399–421.
42. Carr, A. (2006). Thematic review of family therapy journals in 2005. *Journal of Family Therapy*, **28**, 420–39.
43. Larner, E. (2004). Family therapy and the politics of evidence. *Journal of Family Therapy*, **26**, 17–39.
44. Stratton, P., McGovern, M., Wetherall, A., *et al.* (2006). Family therapy practitioners researching the reactions of practitioners to an outcome measure. *Australian and New Zealand Journal of Family Therapy*, **27**, 199–207.
45. Datillio, F. (2006). Case-based research in family therapy. *Australian and New Zealand Journal of Family Therapy*, **27**, 208–13.

46. Burck, C. (2005). Comparing qualitative research methodologies for systemic research: the use of grounded theory, discourse analysis and narrative analysis. *Journal of Family Therapy*, **27**, 237–62.

47. Simon, G. (2006). The heart of the matter: a proposal for placing the self of the therapist at the centre of family therapy, research and training. *Family Process*, **45**, 331–44.

48. Weisman, A., Duarte, E., Koneru, V., *et al.* (2006). The development of a culturally-informed, family-focused treatment for schizophrenia. *Family Process*, **45**, 171–86.

49. Breland-Noble, A.M., Bell, C., and Nicolas, G. (2006). Family first: the development of an evidence-based family intervention for increasing participation in psychiatric clinical care and research in depressed African-American adolescents. *Family Process*, **45**, 153–69.

50. Gurman, A. and Kniskern, D. (eds.) (1991). *Handbook of family therapy*, Vol. II (2nd edn). Brunner-Mazel, New York.

51. Gurman, A., Kniskern, D., and Pinsof, W. (1986). Research on marital and family therapy. In *Handbook of psychotherapy and behaviour change* (3rd edn) (eds. S. Garfield and A. Bergin), pp. 565–624. Wiley, New York.

52. Bednar, R., Burlingame, G., and Masters, K. (1988). Systems of family treatment: substance or semantics? *Annual Review of Psychology*, **39**, 401–34.

53. Asen, K., Berkowitz, R., Cooklin, A., *et al.* (1991). Family therapy outcome research: a trial for families, therapists, and researchers. *Family Process*, **30**, 3–20.

54. Bloch, S., Sharpe, M., and Allman, P. (1991). Systemic family therapy in adult psychiatry: a review of 50 families. *The British Journal of Psychiatry*, **159**, 357–64.

55. Hafner, J., MacKenzie, L., and Costain, W. (1990). Family therapy in a psychiatric hospital: a case-controlled evaluation. *Australian and New Zealand Journal of Family Therapy*, **11**, 21–5.

56. Alexander, J., Holtzworth-Munroe, A., and Jameson, P. (1994). The process and outcome of marital and family therapy: research review and evaluation. In *Handbook of psychotherapy and behaviour change* (4th edn) (eds. A. Bergin and S. Garfield), pp. 595–630. Wiley, New York.

57. Falloon, I., Boyd, J., and McGill, C. (1986). *Family care of schizophrenia: a problem-solving approach to the treatment of mental illness*. Guilford, New York.

58. Dixon, L. and Lehman, A. (1995). Family interventions for schizophrenia. *Schizophrenia Bulletin*, **21**, 631–43.

59. Mueser, K. and Bellack, A. (1995). Psychotherapy and schizophrenia. In *Schizophrenia* (eds. S. Hirsch and D. Weinberger), pp. 626–48. Blackwell Science, Oxford.

60. McFarlane, W., Dixon, L., Lukens, E., *et al.* (2003). Family psychoeducation and schizophrenia. A review of the literature. *Journal of Marital and Family Therapy*, **29**, 223–45.

61. Alanen, Y., Lehtinen, V., Lehtinen, K., *et al.* (2000). The Finnish integrated model for early treatment of schizophrenia and related psychosis. In *Psychosis: psychological approaches and their effectiveness* (eds. B. Martindale, A. Bateman, M. Crowe, and F. Margison), pp. 235–65. Gaskell, London.

62. Peterson, L., Jeppesen, P., Thorup, A., *et al.* (2005). A randomised multicentre trial of integrated versus standard treatment for patients with first-episode psychotic illness. *British Medical Journal*, **331**, 1065–69.

63. Hazel, N., McDonell, M., Short, R., *et al.* (2004). Impact of multiple-family groups for outpatients with schizophrenia on caregivers' distress and resources. *Psychiatric Services*, **55**, 35–41.

64. Keitner, G.I., Drury, L.M., Ryan, C.E., *et al.* (2003). Multiple family group therapy for major depressive disorder. In *Multiple family groups in the treatment of severe psychiatric disorders* (ed. W. Mcfarlane), pp. 244–67. Guilford, New York.

65. Russell, G.F., Szmukler, G., Dare, C., *et al.* (1987). An evaluation of family therapy in anorexia nervosa and bulimia nervosa. *Archives of General Psychiatry*, **44**, 1047–56.

66. Sholz, M., Rix, M., Sholz, K., *et al.* (2005). Multiple family therapy for anorexia nervosa: concepts, experiences and results. *Journal of Family Therapy*, **27**, 132–46.

67. Rowe, C. and Liddle, H. (2003). Substance abuse. *Journal of Marital and Family Therapy*, **29**, 97–120.

68. Kissane, D. and Bloch, S. (2002). *Family focused grief therapy*. Open University Press, Buckingham.

69. Kissane, D., McKenzie, M., Bloch, S., *et al.* (2006). Family focused grief therapy: a randomized controlled trial in palliative care and bereavement. *The American Journal of Psychiatry*, **163**, 1208–18.

70. Liddle, H. (1991). Training and supervision in family therapy: a comprehensive and critical analysis. In *Handbook of family therapy*, Vol. II (2nd edn) (eds. A. Gurman and D. Kniskern), pp. 638–97. Brunner-Mazel, New York.

71. Goldenberg, I. and Goldenberg, H. (1996). *Family therapy: An overview*. Brooks-Cole, Pacific Grove, CA.

72. Wendel, R., Gouze, K., and Lake, M. (2005). Integrative module-based family therapy: a model for training and treatment in a multidisciplinary mental health setting. *Journal of Marital and Family Therapy*, **31**, 357–70.

# 6.3.9 Therapeutic communities

## David Kennard and Rex Haigh

### Introduction

Two of the best-known pioneers of therapeutic communities, Tom Main and Maxwell Jones, defined them as follows:

> An attempt to use a hospital not as an organization run by doctors in the interests of their own greater technical efficiency, but as a community with the immediate aim of full participation of all its members in its daily life and the eventual aim of the resocialization of the neurotic individual for life in ordinary society.[1]

> What distinguishes a therapeutic community from other comparable treatment centres is the way in which the institution's total resources, staff, patients, and their relatives, are self-consciously pooled in furthering treatment. That implies, above all, a change in the usual status of patients.[2]

Today therapeutic communities can be defined by a number of common features, but a word of warning. For reasons of historical coincidence, the term is used in the fields of mental health and addictions to refer to two somewhat different treatment models. In the addiction field they are also known as hierarchical, drug-free or concept-based therapeutic communities, or simply addiction therapeutic communities,[3] in contrast to the more democratized programmes in mental health. The two models have similar goals but their methods differ, although there are signs of increasing rapprochement between them. This chapter deals mainly with therapeutic communities in mental health, but reference will also be made to addiction therapeutic communities and those in long-term care settings. It is worth noting that those admitted to a therapeutic community for treatment are usually referred to as residents, clients, or members, rather than as patients.

## Defining beliefs

Certain beliefs about human relationships and the nature of therapy are central to therapeutic communities.

1 Staff are not completely 'well' and residents are not completely 'sick'. There is a basic equality as human beings between staff and residents, who share many of the same psychological processes and experiences.

2 Whatever the symptoms or behaviour problems, the individual's difficulties are primarily in his or her relationships with other people.

3 Therapy is essentially a learning process, both in the sense of learning new skills—how to relate to others or deal more appropriately with distress—and learning to understand oneself and others.

## Defining principles

A study of one of the best-known therapeutic communities, Henderson Hospital,[4] identified four principles or 'themes' that have come to be widely associated with therapeutic community treatment.

Four principles of therapeutic community treatment

♦ **Democratization** Every member of the community should share equally in the exercise of power in decision-making about community affairs.

♦ **Permissiveness** All members should tolerate from one another a wide degree of behaviour that might be distressing or seem deviant by ordinary standards.

♦ **Communalism** There should be tight-knit intimate sets of relationships, with sharing of amenities (dining room etc.), use of first names, and free communication.

♦ **Reality confrontation** Residents should be continuously presented with interpretations of their behaviour as it is seen by others in order to counteract their tendency to distort, deny, or withdraw from their difficulties in getting on with others.

## Defining aspects of current practice

The generalizability of these principles to newer therapeutic communities is now being questioned and others are developing theoretical frameworks for different therapeutic communities.[5] In 2002, a quality network including most British therapeutic communities started, the 'Community of Communities', with the explicit aim of defining good practice and improving it. In 2006 the first version of 'Core Standards' was published.[6] This comprised 16 standards which were derived from consensus and consultation exercises to determine what practitioners and service users thought reflected the underlying values of therapeutic communities.

Box 6.3.9.1 illustrates a sample of eight of the standards. Note that 'all community members' should be taken to include both resident or client members, and staff.

# Background

## Evolution of different types of therapeutic community

Communities providing sanctuary for mentally ill people have been known as far back as the fourteenth century at Geel in Belgium.

In 1796 the Retreat was opened by the Quakers in York, England, where personal relationships and social expectations in a family-like atmosphere enabled previously dangerous and unpredictable individuals to control and modify their behaviour.[7] This model, known as 'moral treatment', strongly influenced the creation of asylums in Britain and the United States in the first half of the nineteenth century. In the early twentieth century, pioneers in therapeutic education, inspired by a Christian belief in the therapeutic power of love and by Freud's new method of psychoanalysis (see Chapter 3.1), created residential schools for maladjusted children that demonstrated most of the practices and attitudes outlined above.[8] The modern equivalent of communities such as Geel can be found in the intentional communities run by third sector (voluntary) organizations such as l'Arche and the Camphill communities for people with learning disabilities. (The term 'intentional community' avoids language that implies clinical responsibility or a focus on therapy or change, and has been defined as 'a relatively small group of people who have created a whole way of life for the attainment of a certain set of goals'.) A number of therapeutic communities for children and young people now exist as voluntary organizations in the educational sector, as progressive schools, and as long-term treatment units for very disturbed children.

The history of mental health therapeutic communities for adults began during the Second World War, when the psychoanalyst Wilfred Bion was put in charge of the training wing at Northfield Military Hospital in Birmingham, England. His brief attempt in 1943 to establish a therapeutic community failed, but was soon followed by others who were more successful: Tom Main, S. H. Foulkes, and Harold Bridger at Northfield, and Maxwell Jones at Mill Hill Hospital, London. In dealing with psychiatric casualties among soldiers they developed a radical new approach, which was first described in a series of papers in 1946. One of these coined the term 'therapeutic community'.[1] Main and Jones continued to develop different versions of this new method after the war, Main as director of the Cassel Hospital and Jones at Belmont Hospital Industrial Neurosis Unit, which was renamed the Henderson

---

**Box 6.3.9.1** Core standards for therapeutic communities

1 The whole community meets regularly

2 All community members work alongside each other on day-to-day tasks

3 All community members share meals together

4 All community members can discuss any aspects of life within the community

5 All community members create an emotionally safe environment for the work of the community

6 All community members participate in the process of a new client member joining the community

7 There is an understanding and tolerance of disturbed behaviour and emotional expression

8 Positive risk taking is seen as an essential part of the process of change

Hospital in 1958. The Cassel Hospital continues as an inpatient psychotherapy hospital, and Henderson Hospital replicated itself in 2000 to serve national needs for 'severe personality disorder' provision by founding Main House in Birmingham and Webb House in Crewe.

The creation of the National Health Service in 1948 provided the stimulus to address the major problems of institutionalization revealed in a number of studies of large mental hospitals in the United Kingdom and United States.[9,10] In the 1950s and 1960s social psychiatry was in the ascendancy and a number of these hospitals developed what Clark called the 'therapeutic community approach'.[11] In the 1970s and 1980s concepts of collective responsibility fell from favour and individualism prevailed, with a decline in the fortunes of therapeutic communities. The 1990s and 2000s have seen a revival of interest in therapeutic communities within more specific mental health contexts, including prisons, personality disorder services, and for the management of people with enduring mental illness in the community. The problem of degraded and poorly functioning inpatient units is now being addressed by attention to establishing and maintaining 'therapeutic environments' in acute settings, in a direct parallel to the 'therapeutic community approach' 40 years earlier.[12,13]

Alongside these developments two other types of therapeutic community have emerged. In 1958 a self-help organization in the United States called Synanon became the prototype for concept-based therapeutic communities for ex-addicts. Phoenix House and Daytop were two major programmes that grew from this, and today therapeutic communities modelled on them can be found in more than 50 countries worldwide.[3] A development that grew out of the antipsychiatry movement in the 1960s is known at Soteria. These are small low-stress family-like environments where psychosis is responded to with intensive therapeutic support rather than medication. These communities are mainly found in Europe.[14]

### Scientific background

Therapeutic communities have drawn on the concepts of psycho-analysis, group analysis (see Chapter 6.3.6), humanistic and integrative psychotherapies, and on sociological studies of mental hospitals which identified phenomena such as the total institution[10] and patterns of behaviour associated with psychiatric treatment in institutions.[15] They are also underpinned by studies of the impact of unconscious processes in organizations,[16,17] and by anthropological studies such as that of Rapoport[4] which found a typical pattern of oscillation in the therapeutic community.

A developmental model based on the 'required emotional experiences' of attachment, containment, communication, inclusion, and agency has been proposed by Haigh.[18] This identifies ways in which a range of psychological theories and approaches are relevant to therapeutic community practice, and illustrates how they are replicated in the structures and culture of a therapeutic community. It also proposes that disturbance of 'primary emotional development' (which all humans undergo early in life) can to some extent be made good by a satisfactory experience of 'secondary emotional development' in a therapeutic community.

### Technique—how change is brought about

Since the therapeutic community *is* the treatment, managing treatment involves attention to two parallel processes: the progress of each resident through the community, and the effective functioning of the therapeutic community as a whole. Responsibility for managing these two processes ultimately belongs to the staff, though it is shared with the residents when the community is functioning well.

Most if not all the treatment in a therapeutic community takes place in groups and in the everyday life of the community, although some also use individual psychotherapy. The essence of the therapeutic community technique has been encapsulated in two phrases.

1 A *living–learning* situation: this refers to the fact that everything that happens between members of a therapeutic community in the course of living together, and in particular when a crisis occurs, is used as a learning opportunity.[19]

2 *Culture of enquiry*: this refers to the creation not just of certain structures but of a basic culture among the staff of 'honest enquiry into difficulty'. There is a conscious effort to identify and challenge dogmatic assertions or accepted wisdoms.[20]

The basic mechanism of change is not difficult to explain. The therapeutic community provides a wide range of lifelike situations in which the difficulties a member has experienced in their relationships with others outside are re-experienced, with regular opportunities in small group and community meetings to examine and learn from these difficulties. If the therapeutic community is to work as a therapeutic method, all its constituent parts described in this chapter must be in good-working order. This requires a process by which new members adopt the values of the community, emphasizing openness, responsibility, and active participation, and in turn pass these on when the next new members arrive. To operate this mechanism requires both staff and residents to fulfil a number of roles (Box 6.3.9.2).

### Staff training

The need for specialized training for leading or working as a staff member in a therapeutic community has been a matter of some debate.[21] There is an argument that the emphasis on egalitarianism and democratization means that this form of treatment is best delivered by people without special training who can just 'be themselves'. Unqualified social therapists often form a key part of the staff complement. However, the other argument is now increasingly accepted, that while being oneself is an important part of the staff role (see above), therapeutic community work requires a high level of skill and knowledge in a number of areas, together with a well-developed capacity for open honest discussion and reflection.

Training courses exist in the United Kingdom, Finland, Norway, the Netherlands, and Greece, but there is no set standard or curriculum. Some relevant theoretical training is obtainable as part of group therapy and systemic therapy courses, and the case has also been made for a placement in a therapeutic community to be part of professional training in psychiatry and psychotherapy. The benefits include learning at first hand about the treatment of personality disorders, experience of group-based treatment, and working as a member of a multi-disciplinary team, thus gaining first-hand experience of institutional dynamics and the way individuals react to their wider social networks. One of the most popular short courses in the United Kingdom and the Netherlands

**Box 6.3.9.2** Staff and client/resident roles in a therapeutic community

| Role | Role activity of client/resident members | Role activity of staff members |
|---|---|---|
| Participation and involvement in the daily life of the community ('Living–learning') | To explain how the community works to those referred, to visitors, and new members | To spend informal time with client/residents (those who appear aloof may be challenged about this) |
| | To take responsibility for various tasks which contribute to the running of the community | To work alongside clients/residents in day-to-day tasks |
| | To contribute to various 'extras' such as being involved in teaching and research | To monitor other staff members' emotional involvement and consider in supervision |
| | To notice and include those who isolate themselves | |
| Contributing to and managing therapeutic processes ('Culture of enquiry') | To use identification to challenge or support peers | To use therapeutic interventions in groups of various modalities (e.g. group analytic, psychodrama, art therapy, CBT) |
| | To be open to the challenge and support of one's peers | To encourage client/resident members to take a therapeutic role, in some cases delegating responsibility for out-of-hours support to them |
| | To support those in crisis, often including out-of-hours | |
| | To maintain community structures such as rules and timekeeping | |
| Responsibility for decision-making and 'Democratization' | To make decisions about day-to-day and domestic matters, including rotas and elections | To decide the level of decision-making which would be optimal for the therapeutic benefit of the client group, according to their capabilities and needs |
| | To participate in decisions about therapeutic matters (e.g. deciding consequences of breaking rules) | To monitor the functioning of the therapeutic environment and titrate the level of staff input and leadership required |
| | To be involved in planning local events and service developments (e.g. open days, starting new groups) | To ensure good communication with managers, commissioners, referrers, clinical colleagues, and other relevant organizations |
| | Senior and ex-members can offer invaluable support in maintaining effective external relations (e.g. with organizational executives) | |

is a brief residential simulated therapeutic community.[22] Here, 20 to 30 health professionals live together for a few days in the roles of residents with a 'staff' group working with them. This provides a valuable opportunity to experience at first hand the workings and impact of this form of treatment.

## Indications and contraindications

Universal indications for therapeutic community treatment are difficult to give. Modified therapeutic communities have been developed for people with different types and levels of psychiatric disorder, and even the same therapeutic community may fluctuate in its capacity to absorb difficult members. An individual's suitability will need to be judged in relation to a particular therapeutic community at a particular time. Having made this caveat, the general indications and contraindications will usually apply (Box 6.3.9.3).

## Pathways and process: phases in the therapeutic journey

There are usually four distinct but overlapping phases in a member's journey to and through a therapeutic community:

*Engagement phase*: Referral, preparation, and selection procedures are an integral part of therapeutic community practice, involving both the prospective member and existing residents as active participants in the process, which start with referral or self-referral. Many prospective members of therapeutic communities are wary or fearful of the forthcoming therapy, and need support and encouragement to persist. This is often effectively delivered by current or ex-members, arranged in partnership with voluntary agencies, or with internet support groups. During this time, any regular support from mental health teams or other agencies should continue.

*Assessment and preparation phase*: When a decision to proceed towards formal treatment has been made, several arrangements may need to be made. These include formal assessment processes, practical planning, and agreeing a treatment contract. This work is frequently arranged through the use of an 'assessment and preparation group', which is also designed to be a time-limited foretaste of what the treatment phase entails. The assessment process can be undertaken in this group itself, in smaller groups, or with individual appointments. The practical planning involves matters such as arranging childcare, securing stable accommodation, and agreeing plans for medication and risk management. It also includes an

**Box 6.3.9.3** Indications and contraindications for therapeutic community treatment

| Indications | Indications for specialized TC | Contraindications |
| --- | --- | --- |
| **Diagnosis of:** | | |
| ◆ Personality disorder | First episode psychosis | Physically dependent addictions |
| ◆ Self-harm | Serious and enduring mental illness | Current mania |
| ◆ Adjustment disorders | Less than 18 years old | Depression with severe retardation |
| ◆ Recurrent depressive disorders | Learning disabilities | Dementia |
| ◆ Bipolar disorder | Perpetrators of sexual abuse | Dangerously low weight |
| ◆ Intractable anxiety disorders | | Antisocial PD with history of intimidation and deception |
| ◆ Eating disorder | | No capacity for social involvement |
| ◆ Addictions | | Inability to see problems in terms of relationships |
| | | Unwillingness to engage in informal, intimate, and open style of relating with professionals |
| **Age:** | | |
| No age limits: young children to elderly members can show benefit | | Belief that only experts can help |

explicit treatment contract, which may be a verbal agreement about understanding the community rules, or a formal written and signed agreement.

*Treatment phase*: This usually begins with a formal 'case conference' or 'selection panel' including current community members with a decision made by voting. Subsequent therapy programmes vary considerably: from 1 day per week to whole-time residential; from predominantly sociotherapy to a range of psychoanalytic, cognitive behavioural, humanistic and interpersonal and systemic groups; from a few weeks duration to several years, either time-limited or open-ended; and from group size of less than 6 to more than 50. Some communities include individual therapy, but others consider this inimical to the group dynamic process. A modal or typical programme would be for between 3 and 5 days per week, with all interventions in groups comprising a mixture of community meetings, small therapy groups, shared lunch, and informal time together. A typical community would have between 12 and 24 members divided into three small groups, who would stay for 12 to 18 months. Suitable arrangements would be in place for crisis meetings to be called at short notice, as would a system for members to support each other out-of-hours.

During the first few weeks of treatment the new member will be feeling his or her way, forming attachments to one or two others, but still wary of the groups. After the first month or two he or she will begin participating more actively in the groups, taking part in the full life of the community with certain role responsibilities, helping and supporting other members. This will probably include experience of situations similar to those triggering referral, such as having to deal with authority, fear of failure, feeling rejected or abandoned, situations evoking rivalry and competition, or many others. As before, these may trigger destructive or violent impulses towards the self or another person, or the experience of other symptoms of distress. Through the group meetings the member is confronted with the effects of their behaviour on fellow members and the meaning of the behaviour or symptoms is explored, making full use of the insights and understanding of fellow members. Through this repeated process the member gradually comes to experience himself and others differently. As one member wrote: *Bit by bit, almost grudgingly, the fact dawned on me that I wasn't surrounded by forty sticks of furniture but by Jim, Gary, Jane . . .* [23]

*Re-entry phase*: Until recently, many therapeutic communities had a 'cliff-edge' ending, where one day members are able to have the community's full emotional and practical support, and the next are not allowed to contact any other members. Although this has some theoretical justification in terms of 'coming to term with endings', and has strong advocates amongst ex-members of therapeutic communities, it is now generally considered better practice to support members over the leaving process, and then into re-establishing mainstream social networks. This can be done with a specific 'leavers group', that members join while in the full treatment phase and continue afterwards, for either a fixed or indefinite period. These groups normally include a practical focus, and are social and supportive rather than exploratory and therapeutic. For those who are ready and able, they can have objectives of securing employment or education for members. In the case of prison-based therapeutic communities for ex-addicts the provision of drug-free housing and vocational training have been found to improve success rates. [24]

As well as planned endings there are various other types of ending. Some members may leave prematurely, unable to cope with therapy; some may be 'voted out' by the community for a serious or repeated transgression of community rules. Such endings do not necessarily indicate a treatment failure, although the longer members remain the more likely they are to benefit.

## Research evidence

The effectiveness of therapeutic communities has been investigated in relation to different clinical problems, which are discussed separately.

### Personality disorders

Until recently there has been little systematic evidence of the efficacy of therapeutic communities for treating personality disorders, and disagreement over whether those who did benefit were really suffering from psychopathic or personality disorder. While efficacy in this area is still questioned (see Chapter 4.12.7), the picture has recently become clearer with the publication of the first systematic review of therapeutic community treatment for people with personality disorders.[25] The authors carried out a full search of therapeutic community publications and grey literature, collecting over 8000 references from 38 countries. These were reduced to 29 research studies that met the criteria of randomized controlled trial design (eight studies) or comparative or controlled studies that reported raw data and used conservative outcome criteria (e.g. reconviction rates rather than psychological improvement). A meta-analysis found that 19 studies showed a positive effect within the 95 per cent level of confidence while the remaining 10 straddled the neutral score. The overall summary log odds ratio was −0.567, with a 95 per cent confidence interval, −0.524 to −0.614. The authors concluded that there is strong evidence for the effectiveness of therapeutic communities. A more recent systematic review assessed evidence for interventions for people with PD in general and for dangerous and severe personality disordered offenders and made clear recommendations about the most promising treatment interventions for PD in use or currently in development. The reviewers covered therapeutic community programmes; cognitive, behavioural, cognitive behavioural, and psychodynamic psychotherapies; pharmacological and physical treatments. They concluded that 'the TC model currently has the most promising evidence base in this poor field'.[26]

### Offending behaviour

Therapeutic communities have been established in prisons to deal with disruptive, violent inmates, and also with the underlying problems of antisocial personality disorder. Results at Barlinnie Special Unit in Scotland demonstrated substantial reductions in violent incidents within prison. Reconviction studies carried out at Grendon, a prison run entirely on therapeutic community lines, found that prisoners had lower rates of reconviction, fewer custodial sentences, and fewer reconvictions for violent offences than prisoners on the Grendon waiting list who never went there. Those who stayed at Grendon longer than 18 months showed the greatest reductions in reconviction rates. Re-offending rates have also been found to be lower in the former Federal Republic of Germany for prisoners in Social Therapeutic Institutions than those receiving standard prison sentences.[27] In 2004, the 'Democratic Therapeutic Community Core Model' was accredited as a treatment programme for use in prisons in England and Wales. Such programmes must show evidence of their capacity to impact on dynamic risk factors known to be associated with re-offending. Risk factors that therapeutic communities have been found to have a positive influence on include negative attitudes towards authority, identification with antisocial role models, and acceptance of responsibility for offending behaviour.

### Drug dependence

Therapeutic communities for drug dependence use the hierarchical or concept-based model. These form one part of the range of treatments for drug abuse, which includes other residential models such as Christian communities and the Minnesota model, as well as methadone maintenance programmes and psychotherapy. Therapeutic communities for drug dependence, often modified to suit different local cultures, can now be found in many European and international countries as well as in the United States where they originated. Although the model began, and continues, as a residential peer-support programme in the community, it has adapted well to secure environments, and concept-based therapeutic communities for drug dependence have been established in American prisons since the mid-1980s, accompanied by a growing number of aftercare programmes providing employment and drug-free accommodation. Several national studies have evaluated the outcome of these programmes. Randomized controlled trials show that no-treatment groups have a higher level of recidivism than those who complete treatment in a prison therapeutic community, and that recidivism is further reduced by participation in a community aftercare therapeutic community.[24] Since 1995 a number of these therapeutic communities have also been established in English prisons. The general conclusion, for both secure and non-secure therapeutic communities, is that residents who stay in programmes for longer periods have lower rates of drug use and criminal behaviour and higher rates of employment than those who stay for shorter times. However, there are no direct comparisons between therapeutic communities and other treatment models, and it is likely that therapeutic communities are successful for those who are well motivated. Although this may be only a relatively small proportion of all drug abusers, studies, and admission policies, suggest those who enter these high intervention therapeutic communities tend to be severely addicted and damaged, often dually diagnosed with personality disorder, and less likely to respond to low intervention treatments.[28]

### First episode psychosis

A small number of therapeutic communities have been developed in the United Kingdom, United States, Switzerland, and Germany on the principle that first episodes of psychosis can be effectively treated in low-stress family-like settings providing round the clock personal support, with no or minimal use of neuroleptics. This has become known as the Soteria model. Two Soteria houses, in California and Berne, have been subjected to randomized or matched control trials comparing them with usual hospital treatment. One study found that completing subjects with schizophrenia exhibited a large effect size benefit with Soteria treatment, especially in the areas of psychopathology, work, and social functioning. Length of stay in Soteria Berne was initially longer but this was subsequently reduced to less than the admission ward. In both studies the 2-year outcomes were at least as good in the Soteria group and less antipsychotics were prescribed for the Soteria group.[14] A 20-year study of an acute psychiatric ward in Finland found that people with acute psychotic episodes and borderline conditions seemed to benefit from the therapeutic community model with a high level of support, negotiation, order, and organization.

### Severe and enduring mental illness

The therapeutic community approach[11] has been widely used in large mental hospitals to counter the effects of institutionalization and to mobilize the residual capacity of those suffering from chronic mental illness for social relationships, purposeful employment, and personal responsibility. The method was as much about improving the sense of purpose and morale of the staff and the general quality of life in the institutions as it was about clinical improvement, and its success was demonstrated in the way some large old mental hospitals were turned into centres of excellence.

With the re-provision of services for people with enduring mental illness in the community, therapeutic community principles have been found to be an effective way of structuring staffed hostels and homes. In one version of this, the 'ward in a house', the model is close to the original practice of the York Retreat, an antecedent of therapeutic communities (see above).[29] The challenges presented by the severely mentally ill chemical user have also been addressed using a modified therapeutic community with some evidence of success. Three main modifications required to the TC structure were increased flexibility, decreased intensity, and greater individualization.[30]

### Children and adolescents

Therapeutic communities for children and adolescents were first developed in the field of therapeutic education almost a century ago, and now exist for a variety of needs: learning disability, delinquency, and emotional disturbance. Little systematic evaluation has been carried out. A survey of 186 children in nine therapeutic communities for emotionally disturbed children found evidence of increased stability and hopeful outcomes for those who stayed. A 20-year follow-up of 28 children in one community reported evidence of long-term improvement.[31]

Wright and Richardson, reviewing the current state of research for therapeutic communities for children and young people, conclude that, 'when rigorous quality controls are introduced there are as yet too few studies to draw any aggregated conclusions. Perhaps the clearest qualified statement would be that there is low-level evidence that some residential therapeutic placements produce changes in the mental and social functioning of some young people who have been unable to cope with family life'.[32]

### Learning disabilities

Long-term residential communities for adults with learning disabilities exist in the charitable sector in many countries around the world. These are value based rather than evidence based. There is some evidence that many families express a strong preference for village-style communities such as the Camphill for their mentally handicapped relatives.[33]

## Further information

Campling, P. and Haigh, R. (eds.) (1999). *Therapeutic communities: past, present and future.* Jessica Kingsley, London.

Campling, P., Davies, S., and Farquharson, G. (2004). *From toxic institutions to therapeutic environments.* Gaskell, London.

Community of Communities. (2006). *Service standards for therapeutic communities.* Royal College of Psychiatrists, London.

Kennard, D. (1998). *An introduction to therapeutic communities* (2nd edn). Jessica Kingsley, London. www.therapeuticcommunities.org—website of the Association of Therapeutic Communities.

## References

1. Main, T. (1946). The hospital as a therapeutic institution. *Bulletin of the Menninger Clinic,* **10**, 66–70.
2. Jones, M. (1968). *Social psychiatry in practice,* pp. 85–6, Penguin, Harmondsworth.
3. Rawlings, B. and Yates, R. (2001). *Therapeutic communities for the treatment of drug users.* Jessica Kingsley, London.
4. Rapoport, R.N. (1960). *Community as doctor.* Tavistock, London.
5. Campling, P. and Haigh, R. (eds.) (1999). *Therapeutic communities: past, present and future.* Jessica Kingsley, London.
6. Community of Communities. (2006). *Service standards for therapeutic communities.* Royal College of Psychiatrists, London.
7. Tuke, S. (1813). *Description of the retreat.* Reprinted by Process Press, London, 1996.
8. Bridgeland, M. (1971). *Pioneer work with maladjusted children.* Staples Press, London.
9. Barton, R. (1959). *Institutional neurosis.* John Wright, Bristol.
10. Goffman, I. (1961). *Asylums.* Doubleday, New York; Penguin, Harmondsworth, 1968.
11. Clark, D.H. (1965). The therapeutic community—concept, practice and future. *The British Journal of Psychiatry,* **131**, 553–64.
12. Campling, P., Davies, S., and Farquharson, G. (2004). *From toxic institutions to therapeutic environments.* Gaskell, London.
13. Hardcastle, M., Kennard, D., Grandison, S., *et al.* (2007). *Experiences of mental health in-patient care: narratives from service users, carers and professionals.* Routledge, London.
14. Ciompi, L. and Hoffman, H. (2004). Soteria Berne: an innovative milieu therapeutic approach to acute schizophrenia based on the concept of affect-logic. *World Psychiatry,* **3**, 140–6.
15. Stanton, A. and Schwartz, H. (1954). *The mental hospital.* Basic Books, New York.
16. Menzies, I. (1960). A case-study in the functioning of social systems as a defence against anxiety. *Human Relations,* **13**, 95–121.
17. Main, T. (1957). The ailment. *British Journal of Medical Psychology,* **30**, 129–45.
18. Haigh, R. (1999). The quintessence of a therapeutic environment. In *Therapeutic communities: past, present and future* (eds. P. Campling and R. Haigh), Chap. 20. Jessica Kingsley, London.
19. Jones, M. (1968). *Social psychiatry in practice,* pp. 105–12. Penguin, Harmondsworth.
20. Main, T. (1983). The concept of the therapeutic community: variations and vicissitudes. In *The evolution of group analysis* (ed. M. Pines), pp. 197–217. Routledge and Kegan Paul, London.
21. Roberts, J. (1998). Questions of training. In *An introduction to therapeutic communities* (ed. D. Kennard). Jessica Kingsley, London.
22. Rawlings, B. (2005). The temporary therapeutic community—a qualitative evaluation of an ATC training weekend. *Therapeutic Communities,* **26**, 6–18.
23. Mahoney, N. (1979). My stay at the Henderson Therapeutic Community. In *Therapeutic communities: reflections and progress* (eds. R.D. Hinshelwood and N. Manning), pp. 76–87. Routledge and Kegan Paul, London.
24. Wexler, H. (1997). Therapeutic communities in American prisons. In *Therapeutic communities for offenders* (eds. E. Cullen, L. Jones, and R. Woodward), pp. 161–79. Wiley, Chichester.
25. Lees, J., Manning, N., and Rawling, B. (1999). *Therapeutic community effectiveness. A systematic international review of therapeutic community treatment for people with personality disorders and mentally disordered offenders.* CRD Report 17, NHS Centre for Reviews and Dissemination, University of York, York.
26. Warren, F., Preedy-Fayers, K., McGauley, G., *et al.* (2003). *Review of treatments for severe personality disorder.* Home Office Online Report 30/03, Home Office, London.
27. Rawlings, B. (1999). Therapeutic communities in prisons: a research review. *Therapeutic Communities,* **20**, 177–93.
28. Yates, R. and Wilson, J. (2001). The modern therapeutic community: dual diagnosis and the problem of change. In *Therapeutic communities for the treatment of drug users* (eds. B. Rawlings and R. Yates). Jessica Kingsley Publishers, London and Philadelphia.
29. Leff, J. and Trieman, N. (1997). Providing a comprehensive community psychiatric service. In *Care in the community: illusion or reality* (ed. J. Leff), pp. 189–201. Wiley, Chichester.

30. Sacks, S. (2000). Co-occurring mental and substance use disorders: promising approaches and research issues. *Substance Use and Misuse*, **35**, 2061–93.

31. Rose, M. (1997). *Transforming hate to love: an outcome study of the Peper Harow treatment process for adolescents*. Routledge, London.

32. Wright, J.C. and Richardson, P. (2003). The challenge of research. In *Therapeutic communities for children and young people* (eds. A. Ward, K. Kasinski, J. Pooley, and A. Worthington), pp.244–53. Jessica Kingsley, London.

33. Cox, C. (1995). The case for village communities for people with learning disabilities. *British Journal of Nursing*, **4**, 1130–4.

**6.4**

# Treatment by other professions

**Contents**

6.4.1 Rehabilitation techniques
W. Rössler

6.4.2 Psychiatric nursing techniques
Kevin Gournay

6.4.3 Social work approaches to mental
health work: international trends
Shulamit Ramon

6.4.4 Art therapy
Diane Waller

## 6.4.1 Rehabilitation techniques

W. Rössler

The goal of psychiatric rehabilitation is to help disabled individuals to establish the emotional, social, and intellectual skills needed **to live, learn, and work in the community** with the least amount of professional support.[1]

Rehabilitation practice has changed the perception of mental illness. Enabling disabled people to live a normal life in the community causes a shift away from a focus on an illness model towards **a model of functional disability**. As such, other outcome measures aside from clinical conditions become relevant. Social role functioning including social relationship, work, and leisure as well as quality of life and family burden are of major interest for the people affected living in the community.[25]

The relevance of psychosocial and environmental problems is reflected in the DSM-IV and ICD-10. Axis IV of DSM-IV and codes Z55–Z65 and Z73 of ICD-10 are assigned for reporting psychosocial and environmental problems that may affect the diagnosis, treatment, and prognosis of mental disorders.

### The International Classification of Functioning, Disability and Health

Long-term consequences of major mental disorders might be described using different dimensions. A useful tool was provided by the International Classification of Impairment, Disability and Handicaps (ICIDH), first published by the World Health Organization in 1980. The ICIDH has been recently revised. The revised '**International Classification of Functioning, Disability and Health**' (ICF) includes a change from negative descriptions of impairments, disabilities and handicaps to neutral descriptions of body structure and function, activities and participation. A further change has been the inclusion of a section on environmental factors as part of the classification. This is in recognition of the importance of the role of environmental factors in either facilitating functioning or creating barriers for people with disabilities. Environmental factors interact with a given health condition to create a disability or restore functioning, depending on whether the environmental factor is a facilitator or a barrier.

ICF is a useful tool to comprehend chronically mentally ill in all their dimensions including impairments at the structural or functional level of the body, at the person level concerning activity limitations and at the societal level with respect to restrictions of participation. Each level encompasses a theoretical foundation on which a respective rehabilitative intervention can be formulated.

### Target population

During the course of psychiatric reforms the predominant objective of psychiatric rehabilitation was to resettle patients from large custodial institutions to community settings. Today all patients suffering from severe mental illness require rehabilitation. The core group is drawn from patients with the following:

◆ persistent psychopathology

◆ marked instability characterized by frequent relapse

◆ social maladaptation.[28]

There are other definitions currently used to characterize the chronically mentally ill. But they all share some common elements, that is a diagnosis of mental illness, prolonged duration, and **role incapacity**.

Although the majority of the chronically mentally ill have the diagnosis of schizophrenic disorders, other patient groups with psychotic and non-psychotic disorders are targeted by psychiatric rehabilitation. Up to 50 per cent of people with severe mental illness carry **dual diagnoses** especially in combination with substance abuse.

## The role of the psychiatrist in rehabilitation

Psychiatric rehabilitation is by its very nature, **multidisciplinary;** because of the many different competencies required. Monitoring medication is a key task of the psychiatrist.

Pharmacotherapy in psychiatric rehabilitation needs some special consideration. Symptom control does not necessarily have the highest priority as some side effects of pharmacological treatment can weaken a person's ability to perform his social roles, and impair vocational rehabilitation. Many patients living in the community **want to take responsibility for their medication** themselves. This also includes the varying of medication without consultation within certain limits.

The starting point for an adequate understanding of rehabilitation is that it is concerned with the individual person in the context of his or her specific environment. Psychiatric rehabilitation is regularly **carried out under real life conditions**. Thus, rehabilitation practitioners have to take into consideration the realistic life circumstances that the affected persons are likely to encounter in their day-to-day living.

A necessary second step is helping disabled persons to **identify their personal goals**. Motivational interviews provide a sophisticated approach to identify the individuals' personal costs and benefits associated with the needs listed.[8] This makes it also necessary to assess the individuals' readiness for change.[15] Functional assessment and individual goal setting are prerequisites of a differentiated rehabilitation intervention plan and should be repeated in different stages of the rehabilitation process.

The rehabilitative planning process **focuses on the patient's strengths**. Irrespective of the degree of psychopathology of a given patient, the rehabilitation practitioner must **work with the 'well part of the ego'** as 'there is always an intact portion of the ego to which treatment and rehabilitation efforts can be directed' (Lamb 1984[2]). This leads to a closely related concept: the aim of restoring hope to people who suffered major setbacks in self-esteem because of their illness. As Bachrach[2] states 'it is the kind of hope that comes with learning to accept the fact of one's illness and one's limitations and, proceeding from there'.

Psychiatric rehabilitation **concentrates on peoples' rights as a respected partner** and **endorses their involvement and self-determination** concerning all aspects of the treatment and rehabilitation process. These rehabilitation values are also incorporated in the **concept of recovery**.[9] Within the concept of recovery, the **therapeutic alliance** plays a crucial role in engaging the patient in his or her own care planning. It is essential that the patient can rely on his or her therapist's understanding and trust as most of the chronically mentally ill and disabled persons lose close, intimate, and stable relationships in the course of the disease. Recent research has suggested that social support is associated with recovery from chronic diseases, greater life satisfaction, and enhanced ability to cope with life stressors.[24] Therefore, psychiatric rehabilitation is also an exercise in network building.

## Current approaches

Psychiatric rehabilitation aims at **changing the natural course** of the disease. Yet, there is no consensus among rehabilitation researchers on what rehabilitation actually does accomplish. Some understand rehabilitation as an approach to help disabled people to compensate for impairments and to function optimally with the deficiencies they have. Other researchers assume that rehabilitation helps the patient to recover from the disorder itself, while the contributing factors to the healing process are not clear.

The overall philosophy of psychiatric rehabilitation comprises two intervention strategies. The first strategy is individual-centered and aims at **developing the patient's skill** to interact with a stressful environment. The second strategy is ecological and is directed towards **developing environmental** resources to reduce potential stressors. Most disabled people need a combination of both approaches.

As a general rule people with psychiatric disabilities tend to have the **same life aspirations** as people without disabilities in their society or culture. They want to be respected as autonomous individuals and lead a life as normal as possible. As such they mostly desire (1) their own housing, (2) an adequate education and a meaningful work career, (3) satisfying social and intimate relationships, and (4) participation in community life with full rights.

### Housing

The objective of psychiatric reforms since the mid-50s of the 20th century has been to resettle chronically mentally ill persons from large custodial institutions to community settings. Providing sheltered housing in the community for the long-term patients of the old asylums was one of the first steps in the process of deinstitutionalization. Most long-stay patients can successfully **leave psychiatric hospitals and live in community settings**.

Ideally, a **residential continuum** (RC) with different housing options should be provided. RC ranges from round-the-clock staffed sheltered homes to more independent and less staffed sheltered apartments, which eventually allow individuals moving to independent housing in the community. Critics of RC contended that (1) up to date RC is rarely available in communities, (2) that RC does not meet the varying and fluctuating needs of persons with serious mental illnesses, and (3) that RC does not account for individuals' preferences and choices. **Supported housing**, i.e. independent housing coupled with the provision of support services emerged in the 1980s as an alternative to RC. Supported housing offers flexible and individualized services depending on the individual's demands. In the meantime, rehabilitation research could demonstrate that supported housing is a realistic goal for the majority of people with psychiatric disabilities.[23] Once in supported housing, the majority stay in housing and are less likely to become hospitalized. Other outcomes do not yield consistent results.

### Work

The beneficial effects of work on mental health have been known for centuries.[11] Therefore, **vocational rehabilitation** has been a core element of psychiatric rehabilitation since its beginning. Vocational rehabilitation is based on the assumption that work not only improves activity, social contacts, etc., but may also promote gains in related areas such as self-esteem and quality of life, as work and employment are a step away from dependency and a step closer to integration into society. **Enhanced self-esteem** in turn improves adherence to rehabilitation of individuals with impaired insight.

Vocational rehabilitation originated in psychiatric institutions where the lack of activity and stimulation led to apathy and withdrawal of their inpatients. Long before the introduction of medication, occupational and work therapy contributed to sustainable improvements in long-stay inpatients. Today occupational and work therapy are not any longer hospital-based but represent the starting point for a wide variety of rehabilitative techniques teaching vocational skills.

Vocational rehabilitation programs in the community provide a series of **graded steps to promote job entry or re-entry**. For less disabled persons, brief and focused techniques are used to teach how they can find a job, fill out applications, and conduct employment interviews. In transitional employment, a temporary work environment is provided to teach vocational skills, which should enable the affected person to move on to competitive employment. But all too often, the gap between transitional and competitive employment is so wide that the mentally disabled individuals remain in a temporary work environment. Sheltered workshops providing pre-vocational training also quite often prove a dead end for the disabled persons.

One consequence of the difficulties in integrating mentally disabled individuals into the common labour market has been the steady growth of cooperatives, which operate commercially with disabled and non-disabled staff working together on equal terms and sharing in management. The mental health professionals work in the background providing support and expertise.

Today, the most promising vocational rehabilitation model is **supported employment** (SE). In SE, disabled persons are placed in competitive employment according to their choices as soon as possible, and receive all support needed to maintain their position.[4] The support provided is continued indefinitely. Participation in SE programs is followed by an increase in the ability to find and keep employment.[7] Links were also found between job tenure and non-vocational outcomes, such as improved self-esteem, social integration, relationships, and control of substance abuse.[4,29] It was also demonstrated that those who had found long-term employment through SE had improved cognition, quality of life, and better symptom control.[17]

Although findings regarding SE are encouraging, some critical issues remain to be answered. Many individuals in SE obtain unskilled part-time jobs. Since most studies only evaluated short (12–18 months) follow-up periods, the long-term impact remains unclear. Currently, we do not know which individuals benefit from supported SE and which do not.[20] After all, we have to realise that the integration into the labour market does by no means only depend on the ability of the persons affected to fulfil a work role and on the provision of sophisticated vocational training and support techniques but also on the **willingness of society to integrate** its most disabled members.

## Building relationships

In recent years, social skills training packaged in the form of modules with different topics has become very popular and has been widely promulgated. The modules focus on medication management, symptom management, substance abuse management, basic conversational skills, interpersonal problem solving, friendship and intimacy, recreation and leisure, workplace fundamentals, community (re-)entry, and family involvement. Each module is composed of skill areas. The skills areas are taught in exercises with demonstration videos, role-play and problem solving exercises, and *in-vivo* and homework assignments.[14]

The results of several control studies suggest that disabled individuals **can be taught a wide range of social skills**. Social and community functioning improve when the trained skills are relevant for the patient's daily life, and the environment perceives and reinforces the changed behaviour. Unlike medication effects, benefits from skills training occur more slowly. Furthermore, long-term training has to be provided for positive effects.[3] Overall, social skills training have been shown to be effective in the acquisition and maintenance of skills and their transfer to community life.[13]

## Keeping relationships

As a consequence of deinstitutionalization the **burden of care** has increasingly fallen on the relatives of the mentally ill. Informal caregiving significantly contributes to health care and rehabilitation.[31] Fifty to ninety per cent of disabled persons live with their relatives following acute psychiatric treatment. This is a task many families do not choose voluntarily. Caregiving imposes a significant burden on families. Those providing informal care face considerable adverse health effects, including higher levels of stress and depression, and lower levels of subjective well being, physical health and self-efficacy. Additionally, not all families are equally capable of giving full support to their disabled member and are not willing to replace an insufficient health care system. Caregivers regularly experience higher levels of burden when they have poor coping resources and reduced social support. But **families also represent support systems**, which provide natural settings for context-dependent learning important for recovery of functioning. As such, there has been a growing interest in helping affected families since the beginning of care reforms.

One area of interest deals with the expectations of relatives concerning the provision of care. Relatives quite **often feel ignored**, not taken seriously, and also feel insufficiently informed by health professionals. They also may feel that their contribution to care is not appreciated or that they will be blamed for any patient problems. It certainly is no surprise that there is a lot of frustration and resentment among relatives considering the physical, financial and emotional family burden.

**Family intervention programs** have produced promising results. Family intervention is effective in lowering relapse rate, and also in improving outcome e.g., psychosocial functioning. Possibly, family intervention can reduce family burden. Furthermore, the treatment gains are fairly stable.[21] But we also have to appreciate, that it is not clear what the effective components of the different models are. Additionally, family interventions differ in frequency and length of treatment. There are also no criteria for the minimum amount of treatment necessary.

Finally, we have to be aware that most family interventions were developed in the context of western societies during deinstitutionalization. Family caregiving might be quite different in a **different cultural context**. This refers to other cultures in total as well as to minority groups in western societies.[31]

## Participation in community life with full rights

Practitioners often are confronted with the **deleterious effects of stigma and discrimination** in the lives of people with serious mental illnesses. Numerous studies have examined stigmatizing attitudes toward people with mental illness.[12] In recent years, the scientific interest in the perspective of the labelled individual has increased too. There is extensive empirical evidence of the negative consequences of labelling and perceived stigmatization. These include demoralization, low quality of life, unemployment, and reduced social networks.[10,19] Once assigned the label 'mental illness' and having become aware of the related negative stereotypes, the affected individuals expect to be rejected, devalued or discriminated against. This vicious cycle decreases the chance of recovery and normal life.

On the other hand, well-integrated people with mental illness exhibit better outcomes regarding psychopathology and quality of life. The importance of social integration is underlined even more when considering the subjective availability of support: perceived social support predicts outcome in terms of recovery from acute episodes of mental illness, community integration, and quality of life.[27,30]

On the basis of comprehensive research in this area during the last decade, several strategies have been developed to fight the stigma and discrimination suffered by those who have mental illnesses.[30] Different research centres developed interventions directed to specific target groups relevant for de-stigmatization, e.g., students[18] or police officers.[22] Persons in contact with mentally ill individuals quite often have a more positive attitude. Contact with the mentally ill persons also reduces social distance,[12] which is a strong argument in favour of community psychiatry. Other initiatives have targeted stigma by means of more comprehensive programs. The World Psychiatric Association launched one of the internationally best-known programs in 1996 (www.openthedoors.com). All these initiatives make clear that efforts in re-integrating persons with serious mental illness into community life must be accompanied by measures on the societal level.

The core elements of modern psychiatric rehabilitation are summarized in Box 6.4.1.1

## Developing environmental resources

Effective psychiatric rehabilitation requires **individualized and specialized treatment**, which has to be embedded in a comprehensive and coordinated system of rehabilitative services. But even

when a variety of services are available, they are poorly linked in many cases, and costly duplication may occur.

While developing community support systems it became obvious that there is a **need to coordinate and integrate the services** provided as each involved professional concentrates on different aspects of the same patient. Therefore, as a key coordinating and integrating mechanism, the concept of **case management** (CM) originated. CM focuses on all aspects of the physical and social environment. The core elements of CM are the assessment of patients' needs, the development of comprehensive service plans for the patients, and arrangement of service delivery.[26]

Over the past two decades, a variety of different models of CM have been developed which exceed the original idea that CM mainly intends to link the patient to needed services and to coordinate those services. Today most clinical case managers also provide direct services in the patient's natural environment. This model is called **Intensive Case Management** (ICM). ICM on its part is difficult to distinguish from **Assertive Community Treatment** (ACT).

Stein and Test have developed the basic compounds of ACT in the 1970's.[33] The original program was designed as a community based alternative to hospital treatment for persons with severe mental illnesses. A comprehensive range of treatment, rehabilitation, and support services in the community is provided through a multidisciplinary team. ACT is characterized by an assertive outreach approach i.e., interventions are mainly provided in the natural environment of the disabled individuals.[32]

Research on CM and ACT yielded 'mixed' results.[6] While the traditional office-based CM approach obviously is less successful, the ACT model was found to be more beneficial when compared with standard care.[16] ACT can reduce time in hospital,[20] but has moderate or only little effects on improving symptomatology and social functioning. The differing features of the respective services might explain the international variation. Six regularly occurring features of successful services were identified: smaller case loads, regularly visits at home, a high percentage of contacts at home, responsibility for health and social care, multidisciplinary teams, and a psychiatrist integrated in the team.[5]

## References

1. Anthony, W. (1979). *The principles of psychiatric rehabilitation.* University Park Press, Baltimore, MD.
2. Bachrach, L.L. (2000). Psychosocial rehabilitation and psychiatry in the treatment of schizophrenia – what are the boundaries? *Acta Psychiatr Scand Suppl* **407**, 6–10.
3. Bellack, A.S. (2004). Skills training for people with severe mental illness. *Psychiatr Rehabil J*, **27**(4): 375–91.
4. Bond, G.R. (2004). Supported employment: evidence for an evidence-based practice. *Psychiatr Rehabil J*, **27**(4): 345–59.
5. Burns, T, Catty, J, Wright, C. (2006). De-constructing home-based care for mental illness: can one identify the effective ingredients? *Acta Psychiatr Scand Suppl*, **429**, 33–5.
6. Burns, T, Fioritti, A, Holloway, F. *et al.* (2001). Case management and assertive community treatment in Europe. *Psychiatr Serv*, **52**(5), 631–6.
7. Cook, J.A., Leff, H.S., Blyler, C.R. *et al.* (2005). Results of a multisite randomized trial of supported employment interventions for individuals with severe mental illness. *Arch Gen Psychiatry*, **62**(5), 505–12.
8. Corrigan, P.W., McCracken, S.G., Holmes, E.P. (2001). Motivational interviews as goal assessment for persons with psychiatric disability. *Community Ment Health J*, **37**(2), 113–22.

---

**Box 6.4.1.1** Core elements of psychiatric rehabilitation

- multidisciplinary
- carried out under real life conditions
- identify patient's personal goals
- focus on the patient's strengths
- work with the 'well part of the ego,
- concentrate on people's rights as a respected partner
- endorse their involvement and self-determination
- build a therapeutic alliance

9. Farkas, M., Gagne, C., Anthony, W. *et al.* (2005). Implementing recovery oriented evidence based programs: identifying the critical dimensions. *Community Ment Health J*, **41**(2), 141–58.

10. Graf, J., Lauber, C., Nordt, C. *et al.* (2004). Perceived stigmatization of mentally ill people and its consequences for the quality of life in a Swiss population. *J Nerv Ment Dis*, **192**(8), 542–7.

11. Harding, C., Strauss, J., Hafez, H. *et al.* (1987). Work and mental illness. I. Toward an integration of the rehabilitation process. *Journal of Nervous and Mental Disease*, **175**, 317–26.

12. Lauber, C., Nordt, C., Falcato, L. *et al.* (2004). Factors influencing social distance toward people with mental illness. *Community Ment Health J*, **40**(3), 265–74.

13. Liberman, R.P., Glynn, S., Blair, K.E. *et al.* (2002). In vivo amplified skills training: promoting generalization of independent living skills for clients with schizophrenia. *Psychiatry*, **65**(2), 137–55.

14. Liberman, R.P., Kopelowicz, A. (2002). Teaching persons with severe mental disabilities to be their own case managers. *Psychiatr Serv* **53**(11), 1377–9.

15. Liberman, R.P., Wallace, C.J., Hassell, J. (2004). Rehab rounds: Predicting readiness and responsiveness to skills training: the Micro-Module Learning Test. *Psychiatr Serv*, **55**(7), 764–6.

16. Marshall, M. (1996). Case management: a dubious practice. BMJ, **312**(7030), 523–4.

17. McGurk, SR., Mueser, K.T. (2003). Cognitive functioning and employment in severe mental illness. *J Nerv Ment Dis*, **191**(12), 789–98.

18. Meise, U., Sulzenbacher, H., Kemmler, G. *et al.* (2000). ["…not dangerous, but nevertheless frightening". A program against stigmatization of schizophrenia in schools]. *Psychiatr Prax*, **27**(7), 340–6.

19. Mueller, B., Nordt, C., Lauber, C. *et al.* (2006). Social support modifies perceived stigmatization in the first years of mental illness: a longitudinal approach. *Soc Sci Med* 2006, **62**(1), 39–49.

20. Mueser, K.T., Bond, G.R., Drake, R.E. *et al.* (1998). Models of community care for severe mental illness: a review of research on case management. *Schizophrenia Bulletin*, **24**, 37–74.

21. Pilling, S., Bebbington, P., Kuipers, E. *et al.* (2002). Psychological treatments in schizophrenia: I. Meta-analysis of family intervention and cognitive behaviour therapy. *Psychol Med*, **32**(5), 763–82.

22. Pinfold, V., Huxley, P., Thornicroft, G. *et al.* (2003). Reducing psychiatric stigma and discrimination–evaluating an educational intervention with the police force in England. *Soc Psychiatry Psychiatr Epidemiol*, **38**(6), 337–44.

23. Rog, DJ. (2004). The evidence on supported housing. *Psychiatr Rehabil J*, **27**(4), 334–44.

24. Rogers, E.S., Anthony, W., Lyass, A. (2004). The nature and dimensions of social support among individuals with severe mental illnesses. *Community Ment Health J*, **40**(5), 437–50.

25. Rössler, W. (2006). Psychiatric rehabilitation today: an overview. World Psychiatry **5**(3), 151–7.

26. Rössler, W., Fätkenheuer, B., Löffler, W. *et al.* (1992). Does case management reduce the rehospitalization rate? *Acta Psychiatrica Scandinavica*, **86**, 445–9.

27. Rössler, W., Salize, H.J., Cucchiaro, G. *et al.* (1999). Does the place of treatment influence the quality of life of schizophrenics? *Acta Psychiatr Scand*, **100**(2), 142–8.

28. Royal College of Psychiatrists (1996). *Psychiatric rehabilitation* (revised edition). Gaskell, London.

29. Ruesch, P., Graf, J., Meyer, P.C. *et al.* 2004). Occupation, social support and quality of life in persons with schizophrenic or affective disorders. *Soc Psychiatry Psychiatr Epidemiol*, **39**(9), 686–94.

30. Rusch, N., Angermeyer, M.C., Corrigan, P.W. (2005). Mental illness stigma: concepts, consequences, and initiatives to reduce stigma. *Eur Psychiatry*, **20**(8), 529–39.

31. Schulze, B., Rössler, W. (2005). Caregiver burden in mental illness: review of measurement, findings and interventions in 2004–2005. *Current Opinion in Psychiatry*, **18**, 684–91.

32. Scott, J.E. and Dixon, L.B. (1995). Assertive community treatment and case management for schizophrenia. *Schizophrenia Bulletin*, **21**, 657–68.

33. Stein, L.I. and Test, M.A. (1980). Alternative to mental hospital treatment. I. Conceptual model, treatment program, and clinical evaluation. *Archives of General Psychiatry*, **37**, 392–7.

# 6.4.2 **Psychiatric nursing techniques**

Kevin Gournay

## Background

Psychiatric nursing as an entity has really only evolved since the Second World War. Psychiatric nurses (now often referred to as mental health nurses in the United Kingdom and Australasia) can now be found in most countries of the developed world, although in the developing world, psychiatric nursing is still not defined as a specific discipline. In many countries, psychiatric hospitals are still staffed by untrained 'Attendants' who may have some supervision from general trained nurses. Nevertheless, a number of initiatives, notably those of the Geneva Initiative in Psychiatry[1] in Eastern Europe and the former Soviet Union and the World Health Organization in African countries, have provided specific training in psychiatric nursing techniques.

The development of psychiatric nursing across the world needs to be seen in the context of changing and evolving patterns of mental health care. De-institutionalization, with the attendant setting up of community mental health teams, has prompted a range of innovations in psychiatric nursing and the psychiatric nurse of today, who in the United States and Europe is likely to be a university graduate, is a very different person to that of the nurse working in the post-Second World War asylums of 40 years ago.

In this chapter, we examine the development of psychiatric nursing in some detail and particularly emphasize the role of psychiatric nurses working in the community. Community psychiatric nursing first developed in the United Kingdom nearly 50 years ago and this model has been followed in countries such as Australia and New Zealand. However, this community role has not developed to any great extent in the United States, where the main presence of psychiatric nursing remains in hospital-based care. Furthermore, in the United Kingdom and Australasia, the development of community initiatives has seen the role of the psychiatric nurse blurring with that of other mental health professionals. Chapters such as this cannot really do justice to the whole range of techniques used by psychiatric nurses; neither can it examine in any detail the differences between psychiatric nursing practices across the world. However, a description of psychiatric nursing in six important areas will provide the reader with an appreciation of the range and diversity of psychiatric nursing skills:

- Inpatient care
- Psychosocial interventions in the community
- Prescribing and medication management

- Cognitive behaviour therapy
- Primary care
- Psychiatric nursing in the developing world.

## Psychiatric nursing in inpatient settings

In the past three decades the population in psychiatric hospitals across the developed world has fallen dramatically in England from 160 000 to 30 000 beds over a period of 25 years and the duration of inpatient care in the United Kingdom in 2007 is approximately 36 days. However, today's inpatients are a population with much greater levels of illness than was previously the case; they tend to be more treatment-resistant, have complex problems, and display high levels of substance abuse and violence.[2] As a corollary of this, a greater proportion of patients are now detained under mental health legislation. Inpatient facilities consist of acute psychiatric units, local secure units, and high secure psychiatric hospitals for those patients who pose high levels of danger to themselves and others. In the United Kingdom, four high secure hospitals contain approximately 1600 patients. It should also be noted that, due to the large numbers of people with psychiatric problems in prisons, there are now several hundred psychiatric nurses employed in prison settings to carry out a range of assessment and treatment procedures. In addition, the NHS also has a number of 'in reach' schemes, which include sending NHS staff into prisons on a sessional basis.

Given that community care in the western World is now the norm, inpatient care is now seen as a short-term measure with the dual purposes of stabilizing the patient's condition and keeping the patient safe. Psychiatric nurses have a role to play in the overall assessment of the patient and, given that the nurse is—literally—with the patient 24 h a day, the observation of the patient's mental state and behaviour is of considerable importance. Unfortunately, this is an area where, outside the United States, a number of problems exist and suicide rates by inpatients are unacceptably high.[3] In the United States, inpatient wards tend to be much more secure than wards in countries such as the United Kingdom and Australia and, therefore, the incidence of inpatient suicide is much lower. The *UK National Confidential Inquiry into suicides and homicides*[3] demonstrates that nearly 200 suicides by inpatients occur every year, with hanging on the ward itself being still prevalent at unacceptably high levels. Recently the National Institute for Health and Clinical Excellence (NICE)[4] has published guidelines, which include the observation of patients at risk. This guidance sets out very careful protocols for the observation of patients at risk and includes recommendations regarding the prevention of absconding. In the United Kingdom and Australia, open-door policies still operate in acute psychiatric units and it is being increasingly recognized that balancing the rights of the patients against safety is a difficult issue. Nurses also have a major role to play in providing patients and their families with information about condition and treatment. We also know that there are interventions that can be applied by nurses, which would lead to improved outcomes. For example, Drury et al.[5] showed that a cognitive behavioural therapy package improved longer-term outcomes. Similarly, Kemp et al.[6] showed that motivational interviewing and psychoeducation methods produced clear, clinical, and economic benefits in patients who have compliance problems with medication.

With regard to the containment of violent behaviour, which is now so common in inpatient settings, nurses in the United Kingdom have been assisted by very comprehensive evidence-based guidance from the National Institute for Health and Clinical Excellence (NICE),[4] which sets out clear guidance on the use of de-escalation techniques and control and restraint, as well as providing a comprehensive algorithm for the use of rapid tranquillization. In respect of rapid tranquillization, nurses are now provided with the necessary skills to observe and monitor patients following rapid tranquillization, including the use of pulse oximetry and blood pressure. Whilst nurses in Australasia use the same methods of managing violent behaviour as nurses in the United Kingdom, psychiatric nurses in most European countries and in the United States use various forms of mechanical restraint and a very wide range of devices, including belts, straps, nets, and jackets. Whilst it needs to be recognized that there are a range of social and cultural influences that determine how violence in mentally ill people is managed, it is important to note that the evidence base for all forms of violence management, including rapid tranquillization, is very poor and a Cochrane review found that there is no evidence base for the use of seclusion and restraint.[7]

## Psychosocial interventions in the community

In order to appreciate the current practice of psychiatric nurses working in the community, it is important to say something about the historical context. Until the early 1980s, community psychiatric nurses (CPNs) in the United Kingdom were generally based in large, Victorian psychiatric hospitals and worked mostly within a consultant psychiatrist team responsible for the follow-up of patients after discharge from hospital. Their main responsibilities were the administration of medication and the provision of general, supportive care, mostly to people with schizophrenia, the elderly with functional and organic illnesses, and to people with other serious and enduring mental illnesses. Initial research on the effectiveness of community psychiatric nurses produced very positive results. In a randomized trial conducted by Paykel et al.[8] CPNs were compared with psychiatric registrars in the provision of aftercare for patients who had suffered an acute episode requiring hospitalization. In general terms, this study showed that there was an equivalent outcome on clinical, social, and economic measures. Some 20 years ago, CPNs in the United Kingdom began to diversify their practice and separated themselves from consultant psychiatrists, attaching themselves to primary care settings and taking referrals directly from GPs. By 1990, a national survey showed that 40 per cent of CPNs worked in primary care.[9] The vast majority of this work involved treating people with depression, anxiety, and adjustment disorder, using counselling-based approaches. Whilst this work by CPNs became very popular with GPs and mental health professionals in general, research into the effectiveness of their work demonstrated that they were largely ineffective. Gournay and Brooking[10] carried out a randomized controlled trial involving 11 CPNs, working in six primary care settings in North London. In this study, 177 patients were randomized to either routine continuing care from their GP or to CPN intervention. The majority of patients had adjustment disorders and various states of general depression and anxiety. Patients, in both the CPN and continuing GP care groups, showed significant improvement on a range of measures, clinical status, and social functioning but, at post-treatment and follow-up, there was no difference in outcomes demonstrated. Patients allocated to CPNs showed high levels of dropout (50 per cent) and patient satisfaction rating did not correlate with outcome measures. An economic analysis[11] showed that, per unit of health gain, CPN intervention was very expensive compared with interventions for people with schizophrenia. The Paykel and Gournay and Brooking studies still represent the only research evidence regarding the efficacy of CPNs working with common mental disorders.

During the early 1990s a National Review of Psychiatric Nursing in the United Kingdom led to CPNs refocusing their efforts on the seriously mentally ill and this trend has been followed in Australasia. In the last decade there has been a wide range of psychiatric nursing developments in respect of psychosocial interventions. The initial impetus for this development came from the Thorn Programme, this initiative taking its name from the Sir Jules Thorn Trust, a charitable foundation that provided the funds to inaugurate the first 3 years of the training programme for nurses, commencing in 1992. The initiative was originally led by Dr Jim Birley who, with a group of colleagues from other professions, became impressed by the work of nurses working in cancer care. Birley's initial aim was to train a substantial number of nurses specifically dedicated to the care of people with schizophrenia and their relatives. Indeed, Birley, who was one of the pioneers of Social Psychiatry in the United Kingdom, noted that the families of people with schizophrenia were often in great need of intervention. Previous work in Manchester[12] had confirmed that nurses could be trained in family intervention skills which in turn led to positive outcomes for the patient and family. This training in family work formed the basis of what has now become a more general initiative to train nurses in various evidence-based psychosocial interventions for schizophrenia. The Thorn Initiative has now become the national model of training in psychosocial interventions in the United Kingdom and similar programmes to Thorn have been set-up in Australasia and some European countries. The psychosocial interventions used by nurses are as follows:

- Assertive community treatment
- Family interventions for schizophrenia
- Cognitive behavioural techniques for managing hallucinations and delusions
- Approaches with dual diagnosis
- Medication management.

In addition to psychosocial interventions, training programmes for psychiatric nurses working in the community, now also include approaches to improve the physical health of people with serious mental health problems and nurses are now taking a more active lead in ensuring that this very vulnerable population obtains appropriate medical services including physical screening and health promotion activities. At the time of writing, there are also, in several parts of the United Kingdom, specific training programmes for nurses aimed at helping patients with chronic mental illness to deal with obesity, lack of exercise, and smoking.

On a cautionary note, there are now several studies[13] which demonstrate that more intensive case management may not be effective,

the possible reason being that one needs to provide nurses with suitable levels of training in community approaches. In the UK700 study[13] mentioned above the nurses involved only received a few hours training in case management approaches, whist nurses undertaking basic psychosocial interventions training such as a Thorn diploma will receive 250 h of classroom instruction in addition to supervised practice. Whilst there have been considerable numbers of nurses trained in the above-mentioned evidence-based psychosocial interventions, unfortunately there are still many nurses working in the community without such training. Whilst their general psychiatric nursing skills will be reasonably sound, their impact on patient care will be somewhat limited.

In the early part of the twenty-first century, psychiatric nurses working in the United Kingdom, Europe, and Australasia are increasingly working in specialist community teams, for example, assertive outreach services, early intervention teams and crisis intervention, and home treatment teams. Whilst these approaches are commonly used across the United States, such teams are likely to be staffed by case managers who have backgrounds in social work and social care and psychiatric nurses are unlikely to be employed in large numbers. In the United States, psychiatric nurses are often specifically employed to run medication clinics, probably for reasons of cost, whilst in the United Kingdom, approximately 50 per cent of community mental health teams carrying out a very wide range of psychosocial functions are likely to be CPNs.

## Prescribing and medication management

The work of Kemp et al.[6] who showed that motivational interviewing and psychoeducation methods produced good outcomes for patients who were non-compliant with their medication, led to the development of medication management training for nurses in the United Kingdom. Gray et al.[14] using a cluster randomized controlled trial, where 60 CPNs were randomly assigned to medication management training or carrying on with their usual treatment as usual, demonstrated that the nurses who had received medication management training produced very clear benefits in patients with schizophrenia. The study demonstrated a significantly greater reduction in patients' overall psychopathology for the trained group, compared with treatment as usual. At the end of the 6-month study period, the improvement in positive and negative symptoms for the trained nurses over the control was statistically and clinically significant. This training is now used by, literally, thousands of nurses in the United Kingdom, Australasia, and some non-English speaking countries in Europe. Whilst this training, which comprised a number of components, including improving the pharmacological knowledge of the nurses, the use of side effect monitoring and motivational interviewing for non-compliant patients, a European multi-centre trial, which tested adherence therapy as a treatment package over and above routine clinical care and delivered mostly by psychologists and psychiatrists, showed that the treatment package was no more effective than health education in improving quality of care.[15] Both studies raised a number of questions concerning the very complex issue of treatment compliance with medication and the specific difficulties associated with measurement of compliance itself and of patient insight.

Arguably, the most important recent development in psychiatric nursing has been the advent of nurse prescribing. This began more than a decade ago in the United States, where nurses have prescriptive authority in virtually all states. The situation in the United States is, however, complex with a considerable variation in the level of prescriptive authority across the United States from complete independence to being able to prescribe under a physician protocol. In turn, the educational requirement for nurse prescribers also varies considerably. However, most states have fairly comprehensive regulations concerning not only course content, but also hours of instruction and supervision. The Website of the American Psychiatric Nurses,[16] provided at the end of this chapter, provides very detailed state-by-state information. In 2006, United Kingdom legislation was passed that means nurses may prescribe almost independently,[17] although—as in the United States—there is a variation across the country in terms of training and practice. Across nursing more generally, the law in the United Kingdom means that provided it is within their area of specialist work, nurses may independently prescribe any drug (including controlled substances such as opiates). By contrast to the different legislative frameworks that exist in the United States, the legislative framework for the United Kingdom is unitary. However, interpretation of that framework in the United Kingdom seems to vary between NHS services. There are now similar nurse prescribing initiatives in Australasia, where because of the nature of rural and remote populations, the development of nurse prescribing seems very logical.

At present, there are no randomized controlled trial data to compare nurse prescribing with more conventional doctor prescribing, neither is there any substantial data on patient efficacy. The advantages of nurse prescribing have been clearly set out in a *Maudsley discussion paper* by Gournay and Gray[18] and these include the delegation of routine prescribing tasks to nurses, so that psychiatrists may concentrate their prescribing efforts on difficult-to-manage patients who may be treatment-resistant and/or non-compliant and those patients who have substantial physical health co-morbidity. Another advantage might be that CPNs, who are case managers, may be able to spend more time than their psychiatrist colleagues in the detailed evaluation of effectiveness and side effect monitoring and management.

## Cognitive behaviour therapy

For more than 35 years, nurses in the United Kingdom have been trained to provide psychological treatment to patients with various mental health problems. These developments began in 1972, when Isaac Marks, a psychiatrist working at the Maudsley hospital, began a 3-year experiment to determine whether nurses could be trained to deliver behavioural interventions for neurotic disorder. Isaac Marks was one of the first to recognize that the workforce of psychologists would be insufficient to deliver evidence-based treatment. Subsequently, Marks[19] published data which demonstrated both the clinical and economic effectiveness of nurses working with neurotic disorders in primary care. Over the years, training programmes for nurses have developed and now nurses are trained in a variety of university and clinical settings alongside their psychology colleagues in the practice of evidence-based psychological treatments, i.e. cognitive behaviour therapy for a very wide range of disorders. Whilst the original efforts to train nurses were centred on techniques for the treatment of phobias and obsessive–compulsive disorder, nurses are now trained more comprehensively in cognitive behavioural methods, which encompass treatment techniques

used in the treatment of depression, schizophrenia, and personality disorders. In recent years there has been a small, but significant, growth in the United Kingdom of psychiatric nurses employed as psychological therapists. However, this trend has not been replicated in Australasia or Europe, where legislative frameworks prevent nurses from obtaining full accreditation as psychological therapists. In the United States, the situation is variable. Nevertheless, the American Psychiatric Nurses' Association membership comprises a significant number of nurses who have full accreditation as therapists in their respective states. Such nurses are now often prepared at a post-doctoral level and their expertise is arguably equivalent to that of their clinical psychologist colleagues.

## Primary care

Following the refocus of CPNs efforts on people with schizophrenia and other serious and enduring illnesses, there have recently been a number of United Kingdom policy developments that will lead to more psychiatric nurses being employed in primary care settings. This trend follows the recognition that many people with common mental health problems do not receive evidence-based treatment or, if they do, they are subject to long periods on waiting lists. Psychiatric nurses are now being trained to provide brief evidence-based interventions in primary care and also to provide important assessment and screening functions, so as to ensure that patients who need the services of the community mental health teams are suitably referred and those who can be managed at primary care level are provided with appropriate treatments. Nurses are now also increasingly involved in the delivery of computerized cognitive behaviour therapy, which, as a recent NICE review demonstrated,[20] is effective in the treatment of a wide range of mental health problems. This method of treatment is particularly important given the scarcity of skilled therapist resources. Psychiatric nurses are therefore increasingly involved in the running of 'Computer clinics', which now use a very wide variety of treatment packages for a whole range of disorders. Whilst most of these packages come at a cost, there are now free to access programmes on the Internet. These include 'Moodgym',[21] a programme for the self-help treatment of depression, which is based on a cognitive behavioural approach and developed in Australia at the Australian National University in Canberra. Moodgym has been evaluated and its use is supported by positive randomized trial data.[22]

## Psychiatric nursing in the developing world

As noted above, there have been a number of training initiatives in the former communist countries of Eastern Europe and the former Soviet Union.[1] Nevertheless, the numbers of trained psychiatric nurses across this region still remains fairly small. It is also clear that the skills of psychiatric nurses, in these countries, are compromised by the relatively poor general standards of mental health care.

With the exception of South Africa, psychiatric nursing is very poorly developed in the African continent. However, the World Health Organization has a number of projects that aim to integrate mental health into primary care provision. For example, the Ministry of Health in Kenya, the Kenyan Psychiatric Association, and the Kenyan Nursing Council are working with the UK Department for International Development on a 5-year programme that began in 2005, which has the ambitious aim of training 3000 primary care workers with some skills in very basic mental health care.

In Asia, psychiatric nursing is becoming increasingly recognized and there are now substantial training initiatives in the Indian subcontinent and China. Nevertheless, the numbers of psychiatric nurses who are needed in those vast countries are very great and, at present, the best way of describing the psychiatric nursing presence would be to say that it is sparse and patchy, with most nurses working in the large cities. An additional problem is that, where reasonable standards of education and training exist (and this applies particularly to India and China) there is a considerable loss to immigration to the developed world—to countries such as the United Kingdom and the United States, where the recruitment and retention of psychiatric nurses is an ongoing problem, and is financially very attractive.

There is obviously enormous potential for the development of psychiatric nursing across the developing world and, although current initiatives have focused on providing nurses with basic skills, there is obviously enormous potential for the provision of evidence-based psychosocial interventions and, given the tremendous shortage of psychiatrists in many countries, nurse prescribing (providing that the nurses have received adequate education and training) could obviously potentially provide widespread benefits for a substantial proportion of the literally millions of people whose illnesses are currently untreated.

## Conclusion

Psychiatric nursing is a relatively new profession, which has evolved over the past 50 years, from a branch of general nursing, where the main role focused on the custodial care of people with chronic serious and enduring mental illnesses—such as schizophrenia—to the present day situation, where nurses are, in the developing world at least, more likely to be university graduates who may be employed in a number of very diverse roles. The setting for these roles could be in inpatient settings, where custodial care is challenging, to say the least, to the community with roles involving psychosocial interventions within primary health care teams, to inpatient and community settings where nurses are increasingly autonomous prescribers of medication or psychological therapists. It is pleasing to note that the education and training of psychiatric nurses is gradually becoming more evidence based and policy makers are apparently much more aware of the need to provide focused skill sets on populations of need.

## Further information

From values to action: The Chief Nursing Officer's review of mental health nursing (2006)—England—http://www. dh.gov.uk/en/Publicationsandstatistics/Publications/ PublicationsPolicyAndGuidance/DH_4133839

American Psychiatric Nurses Association—http://www.apna.org/i4a/pages/ index.cfm?pageid=1

Newell, R. and Gournay, K. (2008). *Mental health nursing: an evidence based approach* (2nd edn). Elsevier, London.

Australian and New Zealand College of Mental Health Nursing—http:// www.acmhn.org/index.html

## References

1. Geneva Initiative Training. http://www.geneva-initiative.org/pages/ projects/projects.asp
2. Healthcare Commission. (2005). The National Audit of Violence 2003–2005. www.healthcarecommission.org.uk
3. National Confidential Inquiry. (2006). *Avoidable deaths: five year report of the National Confidential Inquiry into suicide and homicide by people with a mental illness*. University of Manchester. www.medicine.manchester.ac.uk/suicideprevention/nci/useful/ avoidable_deaths.pdf
4. National Institute for Health and Clinical Excellence (NICE) (2005). Violence. The short-term management of disturbed/violent behaviour in psychiatric inpatient settings and emergency departments. *Clinical Guidelines 25*. www.nice.org.uk
5. Drury, V., Birchwood, M., Cochrane, R., *et al.* (1996). Cognitive therapy in recovery from acute psychosis, a controlled trial. *The British Journal of Psychiatry*, **169**, 593–607.
6. Kemp, R., David, A., Hayward, P., *et al.* (1998). Compliance therapy, an 18 month follow up. *The British Journal of Psychiatry*, **5**, 228–35.
7. Sailas, E. and Fenton, M. (2002). Seclusion and restraint for people with serious mental illnesses. *The Cochrane Library*, (1). Update Software, Oxford.
8. Paykel, E., Mangen, S., Griffith, J., *et al.* (1982). Community psychiatric nursing for neurotic patients: a controlled trial. *The British Journal of Psychiatry*, **140**, 573–81.
9. White, E. (1990). *The third quinnenial survey of CPNs*. Department of Nursing Studies, University of Manchester.
10. Gournay, K. and Brooking, J. (1994). The CPN in primary care: an outcome study. *The British Journal of Psychiatry*, **165**, 231–8.
11. Gournay, K. and Brooking, J. (1995). The CPN in primary care: an economic analysis. *Journal of Advanced Nursing*, **22**, 769–78.
12. Brooker, C., Fallon, I., Butterworth, A., *et al.* (1994). The outcome of training community psychiatric nurses to deliver psychosocial intervention. *The British Journal of Psychiatry*, **165**, 222–30.
13. Burns, T., Fiander, M., Kent, A., *et al.* (2000). Effects of caseload size on the process of care of patients with severe psychotic illness: report from the UK700 trial. *The British Journal of Psychiatry*, **177**, 427–33.
14. Gray, R., Wykes, T., Edmonds, M., *et al.* (2004). Effect of a medication management training package for users on clinical outcomes for patients with schizophrenia: cluster randomised controlled trial. *The British Journal of Psychiatry*, **185**, 157–82.
15. Gray, R., Leese, M., Bindman, J., *et al.* (2006). Adherence therapy for people with schizophrenia. *The British Journal of Psychiatry*, **189**, 508–14.
16. American Psychiatric Nurses' Association. www.apna.org
17. Extended Nurse Prescribing. http://www.dh.gov.uk/en/Publicationsandstatistics/Publications/ PublicationsPolicyAndGuidance/DH 4006775
18. Gournay, K. and Gray, R. (2001). *Should mental health nurses prescribe? Maudsley discussion paper*. Institute of Psychiatry, London.
19. Marks, I. (1985). *Nurse therapists in primary care*. RCN Publications, London.
20. National Institute for Health and Clinical Excellence (NICE) (2006). The clinical and cost effectiveness of computerised cognitive behaviour therapy for depression and anxiety. *Technology Appraisal 51*. NICE, London. http//www.nice.org.uk/
21. Moodgym website: http://moodgym.anu.edu.au/
22. Christensen, H., Griffiths, K.M., and Jorm, K. (2004). Delivering interventions for depression by using the internet: randomised controlled trial. *British Medical Journal*, **328**, 265.

## 6.4.3 **Social work approaches to mental health work: international trends**

Shulamit Ramon

### The historical development of mental health social work

Social work was formally established in most European countries and North America at the end of the nineteenth century, before it took off gradually in other countries. It usually developed out of charitable work, which focused on financial support for poor families. The second main strand in social work was represented by the Settlement Movement, which concentrated on improving the communal life of poor people by living with them, using community work methods to support and empower.

The major impetus to developing mental health social work at the beginning of the twentieth century was related to the work of leading psychiatrists and psychologists with shell-shocked (PTSD) soldiers during the First World War.[1] This approach lead to the establishment of the psychodynamically oriented Tavistock Clinic in London, where the first British psychiatric social worker was appointed in 1920.[2] Stuart[3] argues that American mental health social work in the pre-1920 period concentrated more on care in the community in its social, rather than its administrative or psychological meaning, than after 1920, when it shifted further to the psychological dimension.

Social workers in both the children and the adults outpatient services provided comprehensive psychosocial history of the child/adult and their family, enabled parents, teachers, and partners of adult clients to understand the underlying psychological reasons for the index client's mental ill health, and guided them as to how they could actively support that family members.[2] It was only in the 1950s that qualified psychiatric social workers began to work in hospitals.

Since the 1970s all English-speaking countries have also opted for deinstitutionalization as their core mental health policy, leading to the closure of many of their psychiatric hospitals, replacing them by community-based services and by small psychiatric wards in general hospitals.[4,5] With the notable exception of Italy,[6,7] most continental European countries have opted for bed reduction coupled with less extensive community services.

The trend towards deinstitutionalization is formally adhered to also in Latin America, but thus far is only practised in some small-scale projects.[8,9] This applies also to Asia. MHSWs (mental health social workers) there focus mainly on sorting out benefits, though some are based in rehabilitation focused facilities where they work on connecting users to educational and employment opportunities.[10]

This fundamental change has led to the relocation of MHSWs away from institutions into community services,[5] to a renewed interest in rehabilitation, and more recently also in the newly defined recovery.[11]

The paralleled development of private, for-profit mental health services especially—but not exclusively—in the United States, has led to a further shift in the location of MHSWs and their work focus. Most United States MHSWs are to be found today working as psychotherapists in private practice or in managed care residential units.[12] In the latter they work with users who have long-term mental illness to a per capita budget.

Although the not-for-profit sector has grown considerably with the focus on care in the community, MHSWs work there only in certain countries in which the public sector has either been reduced or never played the major part it does in the United Kingdom (e.g. the Netherlands, Hong Kong).

### Underpinning values

Social work, including its mental health branch, is ethically governed by a set of values, which are expected to be universal and adhered to in everyday practice,[13] even though its implementation may prove at times to be problematic in terms of balancing care and control.

The values are derived from the liberal collectivist, humanistic, tradition of the twentieth century in which social work has developed.

The core values are social justice, respect for people who social workers meet at their most vulnerable state, readiness to help in a way which will enable the client to retain dignity, self-determination, and enhance their problem-solving abilities. Social workers are expected to take an active stance against any type of discrimination. Furthermore, social workers are committed to pursing a psychosocial approach in any type of their practice, and believe that most clients have the potential to grow and positively change.

Several elements stand out as central to MHSW:

1 The right to fail—this comes as part of the right to self-determination, in that social workers are aware that risk needs to be taken at times to enable people to grow and develop, or as a basic human right of making a mistake. When social workers take this right seriously, they are able to have a genuine discussion with clients as to the pros and cons of risk-taking, of learning from success as much as of learning from failure.[14,15]

2 The wish to take an active stance against discrimination applies to working well with clients who come from ethnic minorities, from sexual orientation minorities, and to combating stigma against mental illness in one's practice.

3 The adherence to a psychosocial approach entails ensuring that both the psychological and the social aspects of users' lives are attended to, an issue of importance in mental health where often biological aspects are attended to, but the psychosocial ones are not getting the same priority.[16]

### Conceptual developments
#### Psychodynamic approaches

As outlined above, mental health social work originated within the psychodynamic fold, though social workers did not practice psychoanalysis as a work method.

Social workers have tended to select from the range of psychodynamic perspectives those theories, which were more focused on the ego, rather than on the id or the unconscious. The impact of ego psychology was/is in evidence in terms of understanding how people come to develop and maintain mental distress and mental illness, the importance of family dynamics, and of attachment to significant others.[17, 18, 19, 20]

American social workers developed the crisis approach in its application to all areas of social work.[21] Based on Erickson's notion of the normal crisis every person goes through when moving from one stage of life to another, major life events may lead initially to adverse reactions. However, with professional support people can reorganize their reactions more constructively, reduce the duration of these reactions, be more ready for change at the point of crisis, and learn how to improve their coping strategies and emotional responses. The problem-solving approach also originated from the United States, developed by Perlman.[22] Although the psychodynamic understanding of relationships is in evidence in her work, she focused on the process of social work with individuals and families (casework) and the client–worker relationships, beginning with the presenting problem.

The identification of child abuse, especially child sexual abuse, and its implications for the mental health of children and adults in the 1970s and the 1980s led to refocusing on the psychodynamic approach among social workers in this area[23] at a time in which all other approaches have paid less attention to the impact of such abuse on mental health.

## Learning theory applications in social work

### Behavioural social work

Behavioural social work developed in the United States in the 1950s, and is a leading approach in relation to people with milder forms of mental illness and problems of living.[24] Its application within social work does not differ in any significant way from its application within psychiatry or psychology. In this sense it is not a social work approach. A number of influential texts appeared in the United Kingdom which demonstrated the research evidence pertaining to the effectiveness of the approach in a number of social work areas.[25]

### Task-centred social work

This orientation takes further the crisis perspective and the lessons from learning theories and behaviour modification.

Reid and Epstein[26, 27], as well as Marsh and Doel,[28] proposed that people work better on their problems if focused on specific targets and if the problem-solving effort leads to success, however small. Research evidence demonstrated the usefulness of this approach to different aspects of social work, such as direct work with children and their parents, as well as with people suffering from mild mental distress symptoms.

### The social dimension in mental health social work

Social workers and theorists interested in the social dimension began usually from the assumption that inequality in opportunities and in civic participation due to poverty may increase the rate of mental illness among poor people. This assumption follows Merton's classical matrix of the reactions to the gap between social goals and means, in which mental illness is a reaction of people who accept socially desirable goals, but withdraw from obtaining them after being frustrated in doing so, whilst at the same time not adopting antisocial means (as in criminal behaviour) or developing an alternative model of society (social rebels).

This strand of thinking was reinforced in the 1960s and 1970s by the application of Marxist thinking and the combined impact of the deviancy and anti-psychiatry orientations.[29] Discrimination on the basis of age, ethnicity, gender, or sexual orientation was added in the 1980s to the likely social factors which foster inequality.

Social workers accepted the logic presented by sociologists such as Goffman and Scheff[30, 31, 32] that the stigma attached to mental illness is largely irreversible, as it is accepted both by others and by the individual concerned who in turn internalizes his or her poor social status.

Interestingly, although accepting the enormity of the labelling process, social workers did not count themselves among the labellers.

The appeal of the anti-psychiatry approach for social workers related to acknowledging the price of labelling for the individual concerned, and the considerable shortcomings of a system focused on the psychiatric hospital and medication in which psychological and social factors were largely ignored.

Today the social perspective implies a greater focus on social inclusion, supporting users and carers-led initiatives, ensuring financial support side-by-side with the critique of the medicalized approach to mental health and illness, of modernity and post-modernity.[16]

A more recent strand of this approach is outlined in the critical social work, which applies a post-modern perspective to the analysis of where social work is, as well as the issues and dilemmas related to mental health social work. Bainbridge[33] highlights the need to focus on the social dimension and sociological understanding of mental ill health in social work, as well as on issues of power and empowerment.

#### (a) The social role valourization (SRV) and the strength approach

This approach was initially developed by psychologists in the field of learning difficulties.[34–37]

SRV accepts the deviancy approach up to the point at which the impact of labelling and segregation is said to be irreversible. Conversely, SRV is focused on reversing the devaluation of the disabled person and the group, while accepting that a disability exists. The devalued existence can be reversed by the combined impact of the following:

♦ enabling those who have been segregated to live in the community by providing them with the opportunities to do so and the support they require for this purpose

♦ enhancing the competencies of the disabled person

♦ changing their public image, in part by their positive presence in ordinary settings in the community

♦ upgrading the state of the physical settings in which a disabled group is treated, lives, and works

♦ changing the derogatory language used in both professional and lay circles in describing people with disabilities.

Its protagonists are critical of professional attitudes, knowledge, and skills, including those of social workers (see Wolfensberger).[35] Yet as a group social workers have within their repertoire more of the attitudes, knowledge, and skills required by this approach than any other mental health profession. Furthermore, SRV offers an interesting and comprehensive combination of psychological and social dimensions; for an application to how it can work with the Nearest Relative in mental health.[38]

In the United States and Canada, but much less so in the United Kingdom, SRV came into prominence within social work through the **strengths** model of social work.[39] The model is unique in concentrating on the strengths the person and his or her environment possess, and how these could be harnessed to solve the specific problem and lead to an improvement in the person's quality of life. Coming together with a focus on following people's ambitions (as long as these are within socially acceptable norms), this orientation has led to useful and positive outcomes in care management.[40] A further development of the strengths model is the growing interest in focusing on enhancing resilience in mental health social work.[41]

Interestingly, the approach has been adopted by other mental health professionals in the field of employment without acknowledging the debt to social work.

## Legally anchored MHSW

The social mandate of social work is anchored within legal and policy frameworks; this applies to MHSW too.

### Securing benefits

In all countries social workers are gatekeepers to and advocates for securing benefits either in cash (e.g. disability allowance, Direct Payment agreement) or in kind (e.g. housing, clothing). They often have to make the claim in addition to the client, verify the claim as against eligibility criteria, secure supporting documents from other professionals, at times negotiate with other agencies (e.g. social security, health, education), and in a number of countries they are indeed located in social security services (e.g. Portugal, Israel).

While this work is considered to be routine, its importance in the life of poor people cannot be underestimated. The evidence highlights that most people with enduring mental illness are poor,[42] and that remaining poor is a strong counter-indication to becoming mentally healthy. Furthermore, the evidence related to Direct Payment in mental health,[43] which enables users to take the driving seat as to how they spend their budget in agreement with the local authority and mental health trust, illustrates the social inclusion and recovery value of such a scheme which clearly comes out of the strengths model.

Knowledge of the available resources and eligibility is needed for this type of work, as well as the ability to inform users and enable them to participate as deserving partners.

In a large number of countries this is the main social work task in mental health (e.g. Brazil, Greece, Italy, Ireland, Portugal, and Poland).

### The approved social worker

This role illustrates an enhanced legal position for MHSWs; its fullest form is practised in the United Kingdom.

The approved social worker was developed in Britain to provide a complementary measure to the psychiatric perspective within the 1982 amendments to the 1959 Mental Health Act.

Social workers were seen as suitable professional figures who would represent the psychosocial angle in parallel to the psychiatric view in the following instances:

- assessing people when an application has been made for a compulsory admission to a psychiatric unit
- the follow-up to such an admission
- mental health review tribunals (established within the 1959 Mental Health Act)
- work with the Nearest Relative[38]
- coordinate the multi-disciplinary assessment, which needs to be carried out by a psychiatrist and a GP in addition to the social worker. This assessment has to be carried out within a specified limited period of time.

Each of these tasks calls for somewhat different knowledge and skills, as well as emphasis and use of a range of more generic skills.[44] In each task social workers are asked not to replicate the psychiatric assessment but to compliment it. For example, they have to look for the least restrictive alternative to the hospitalization before they can recommend a hospital admission, rather than diagnose mental illness. Social workers have an autonomous position as they can disagree with the views of the other professions. The role requires exercising more social control than care, a contested issue within social work.

Training to become an approved social worker requires 60 days of academic input and supervised practice initially, followed by 5 days refresher training annually. Individual social workers can take it up after 2 years of post-qualification work experience. This compares with 2 days training for general practitioners and 1 day for psychiatrists.

Most of the activities undertaken by MHSWs with adults since 1983 are related to meeting the requirements of this role. Existing evidence[45] highlights that in most cases ASWs are working to a good standard. The role also offered MHSW a higher status and pay, but came with the price tag of giving up most of their previous activities, such as family work, group and community work, and work with users who have minor mental illness. However, the proposed new English Mental Health Act[46] includes the introduction of AMHPs (Approved Mental Health Practitioners) who can come from any mental health discipline, but likely to be nursing because of the numerical dominance of nurses in the English mental health service. ASWs are unhappy at being dethroned of their unique legal role, arguing that nurses do not have the same background training for psychosocial understanding and intervention.

Workforce research into ASWs[47] has highlighted a recent steady decrease in the number of ASWs, a high number of workers approaching retirement age and low morale, factors likely to have played a part in the government's wish to introduce other professions to this role. There are currently 4500 ASWs, a minority in the total workforce of social workers in England which stands at 46 000.

While current ASWs and MHSWs will be able to be part of the AMHP workforce, this change may also enable them to reclaim some of their previous roles and activities.

### Care management

In all English-speaking countries and a number of European countries (e.g. the Netherlands, Slovenia), MHSWs are also often engaged in one form or another of care management, which follow the specific laws and regulations of each country (e.g. the Care in the Community 1990 Act in England).

Care management (not be confused with managed care) is a form of coordinating the assessment, planning, and interventions with people who require long-term care, including in mental health. It is aimed at preventing fragmentation and duplication of professional input and services, as well as ensuring that services follow the user's needs, and not vice versa as was—and still is—the case all too often. While in the United Kingdom, psychiatrists are formally the nominated care manager since 1995, and CPNs are the professionals in more frequent contact with the users, in other countries such as Australia, New Zealand, and Canada, social workers are often the nominated care coordinator.

Care management can be practised in a variety of ways, ranging from a purely administrative orientation, through clinical care management, to one anchored within the strengths and recovery orientations.[40, 48, 49] The choice is often dictated by the managers of a local authority or a mental health trust.

### Community treatment orders (CTOs)

CTOs constitute a third legally defined area in which MHSWs are engaged. They originated in the United States, and exist in a variety of formats in Canada, Australia, and the United Kingdom.[50–52] They represent a response to the escalation of concerns about risk avoidance in the field of mental health, closely related to the growing fears of risk raised by modernity and post-modernity,[54, 55] and reinforced more recently by fears of terrorism as a particularly threatening type of risk. It is indicative that this preoccupation is not shared between North and South Europe; it is much more prominent in the North.

Following a legal process, CTOs enable the nominated mental health professional to require a service user to adhere to specific restrictions, such as to live in a certain facility or to present themselves for interventions at specific locations. This measure has been introduced to ensure that users with long-term mental illness who lead a disorganized life (e.g. often do not comply with medication, live rough, misuse substances, mishandle money, misagreed appointments, and get into trouble with the law) will have a safety net, which structures their lives. There is some evidence of the effectiveness of CTOs,[48, 49] but it seems restricted to specific subgroups within the broader category of people with severe and enduring mental illness.

Social workers are often the nominated professionals responsible for the agreed plan and enforcement of the CTO. This puts them in a somewhat conflictual position regarding the desired focus on care in social work, as it is tilted more towards the control element.[56]

### Non-legally anchored MHSW

The constraints on this type of work come not only from the primacy of legally sanctioned work, but also from working within welfare bureaucracies, for a private employer interested primarily in profit, or for an impoverished not-for-profit service.

Despite these constraints, we have examples of good and innovative MHSW practice in most countries, which include:

◆ Successful attachment to primary care was established as early as 1965 in London, with the social workers, their clients, and the general practitioners expressing satisfaction with this way of working. Nevertheless, this form was largely abandoned owing to the focus on statutory responsibilities.

◆ Social workers pioneered collective user involvement approach during the early 1980s[57] some years before it became fashionable in wider circles.

◆ Applying self-directed group and community work approach to working with mothers of abused children, empowering them to take control over their lives.[58]

◆ Initiating de-institutionalization in social care institutions in Slovenia.[59]

◆ Creating family support teams[60] where most staff members are social workers providing brief assessment and consultation to families of children with minor mental distress, and are often successful in preventing the need for referral to more expensive services.

◆ Establishing the Building Bridges project in which parents with mental health difficulties and their children are supported together as well as separately.[61]

◆ Creating The Faith Links project, a multi-faith project within an inpatient service in which users, volunteers, and social workers plan joint activities which follow users' spiritual wishes.[62]

◆ Supported education and employment schemes in mental health initiated by social workers.[63]

## Conclusion

Mental health social work is a broad, rather than a rigorous, church. Since the 1980s social workers have gained in professional status by the introduction of the roles of the approved social worker (or licensed to carry out civil commitment in the American context), care co-ordinators, managers of managed care facilities, or psychotherapists. These gains have come at a price outlined in the text above.

Often the cost of closer collaboration within the multi-disciplinary framework has led to the risk of giving up the attempt to hold on to, and further develop, an alternative and complimentary perspective from that of psychiatrists, nurses, or psychologists, as well as raising doubts as to the uniqueness of MHSW.

The increased narrowness of the role is not simply the byproduct of the legal framework. It is also due to increased specialization within mental health on the one hand, and the effects of neo-liberal policies globally on public sector funding on the other hand.

The move to privately contracted work, either in managed care or in psychotherapy so apparent in the United States, is yet another outcome of neo-liberal policies which fragments MHSW. As a trend we are likely to see growing beyond the United States, the increased concentration of mental health social workers within the private sector does not bode well for a profession whose value base focuses on the need to protect the more vulnerable and stigmatized populations, and to provide the dual perspectives of psychosocial input.

Mainly due to governmental pressure related to fear of risk and its potential political fallout, the focus on working exclusively with people experiencing long-term severe mental illness has contributed to the increasing narrowness of the role of social workers in most First World countries. The paralleled withdrawal of social work involvement with people who have milder forms of mental distress within public sector and not-for-profit services, and its increased availability only to those who can afford it, is a reflection of this situation.

The core qualities of belief, optimism, and caring of MHSWs identified in a cross-national research[64] coupled with the ability of MHSW to innovate as highlighted in this chapter, illustrate the optimistic scenario for positive change within this branch of social work. However, unless theory building and research aspects are given the importance they deserve within MHSW globally, including an inevitable critical dimension of the existing system, mental health social work is likely to be no more than a reflection of the developments in other professions. This will not only mean curtailing its autonomous potential, but also the impoverishment of the multi-disciplinary framework as a whole of a crucial dimension necessary for its comprehensive work, as exemplified in some recent work on the social aspects of MHSW.[16]

In addition, mental health social work will have to develop a much stronger policy making function, if it is to provide a more responsive, effective, and comprehensive service to users, relatives, and the communities in which these people live.

## Further information

Norman, E. (ed.) (2000). *Resiliency enhancement: putting the strength perspective into social work practice*. Columbia University Press, New York.

Ramon, S. and Williams, J.E. (eds.) (2005). *Mental health at the crossroads: the promise of the psychosocial approach*. Ashgate Publishing, Aldershot.

Tew, J. (ed.) (2005). *Social perspectives of mental health*. Jessica Kingsley, London.

## References

1. Dicks, H. (1970). *Fifty years of the Tavistock*. Tavistock Publications, London.
2. Timms, N. (1964). *Social casework*. Routledge and Kegan Paul, London.
3. Stuart, P.H. (1997). Community care and the origins of psychiatric social work. In *Social work in mental health: trends and issues* (ed. U. Aviram), pp. 25–37. Haworth Press, New York.
4. Goodwin, S. (1997). *Comparative mental health policy: from institutional to community care*. Sage, London.
5. Shera, W., Aviram, U., Healy, B., *et al.* (2002). Mental health systems reform: a multi country comparison. *Social Work in Health Care*, **35**, 547–75.
6. De Leonardis, O., Mauri, D., and Rotelli, F. (1986). *Deinstitutionalisation: a different path: the Italian mental health reform*, health promotion, Vol. 2, pp. 151–65. WHO Cambridge University Press.
7. Ramon, S. (ed.) (1990). *Psychiatry in transition: British and Italian experiences*. Pluto Press, London.
8. Vasconcelos, E.M. (2005). Structural issues underpinning mental health care and psychosocial approaches in developing countries: the Brazilian case. In *Mental health at the crossroads: the promise of the psychosocial approach* (eds. S. Ramon and J.E. Williams), pp. 95–108. Ashgate Publishing, Aldershot.
9. Ramon, S. and Williams, J.E. (2005). *Mental health at the crossroads: the promise of the psychosocial approach*. Ashgate Publishing, Aldershot.
10. Fung Sheung Chee, B., Law Ka Sin, J., and Lee Yuk Yee, K. (2006). *Clubhouse model in an Asian culture*, 5th International Conference on health and mental health social work, December, Hong Kong.
11. Ramon, S., Healy, B., and Renouf, N., (2007). Recovery from mental illness as an emergent concept and practice in Australia and the UK. *International Journal of Social Psychiatry*, **53**, 108–22.
12. Cohen, G.A. (2003). Managed care and the evolving role of the clinical social worker in mental health. *Social Work*, **48**, 34–43.
13. Beckett, C. and Maynard, A. (2005). *Values and ethics in social work*. Sage, London.
14. McDermott, R. (ed.) (1975). *Self determination in social work*. Routledge and Kegan Paul, London.
15. Ramon, S. (2006). Risk avoidance and risk taking in mental health social work. In *Knowledge in mental health: reclaiming the social* (eds. L. Sapouna and P. Hermann), pp. 39–56. Nova Publications, New York.
16. Tew, J. (ed.) (2005). *Social perspectives of mental health*. Jessica Kingsley, London.
17. Parad, H.J. (ed.) (1958). *Ego psychology and dynamic casework*. American Family Services Association, New York.
18. Hutton, J.M. (ed.) (1977). *Short-term contracts in social work*. Routledge and Kegan Paul, London.
19. Yellowly, M. (1980). *Psychoanalysis and social work*. Van Nostrand, New York.
20. Howe, D. (1995). *Attachment theory for social work practice*. Macmillan, London.
21. Golan, N. (1978). *Treatment in crisis situations*. Free Press, New York.
22. Perlman, H. (1957). *Social casework—a problem-solving process*. Chigaco University Press, Chigaco, IL.
23. Perlberg, R. and Miller, A. (eds.) (1992). *Gender and power in families*. Routledge, London.
24. Gambrill, E.D. (1977). *Behaviour modification*. Jossey-Bass, San Francisco, CA.
25. Hudson, B. and Macdonald, E. (1986). *Behavioural social work: an introduction*. Macmillan, London.
26. Reid, W.J. and Epstein, L. (1972). *Task centered casework*. Columbia University Press, New York.
27. Jackson, V.H. (1996). Behavioral managed care: a social work perspective. *Behavioral Health Management*, 22–3.
28. Marsh, P. and Doel, M. (1993). *Task-centred social work*. Ashgate, Aldershot.
29. Leonard, P. and Corrigan, P. (1978). *The Marxist approach to social work*. Macmillan, London.
30. Goffman, I. (1961). *Asylums*. Penguin, Harmondsworth.
31. Laing, R.D. (1965). *The divided self: an existential study in sanity and madness*. Penguin, Harmondsworth.
32. Scheff, T. (ed.) (1975). *Labelling madness*. Prentice-Hall, Englewood Cliffs, NJ.
33. Bainbridge, L. (1999). Competing paradigms in mental health practice and education. In *Transforming social work practice: postmodern critical perspective* (eds. B. Pease and J. Fook), pp. 179–94. Routledge, London.
34. Nirje, B. (1969). The normalisation principle and its human management implications. In *Changing patterns in residential services for the mentally retarded* (eds. R. Kugel and W. Wolfensberger), pp. 255–87. President's Committee on Mental Retardation, Washington, DC.
35. Wolfensberger, W. (1983). Social role valorisation: a proposed new term for the principle of normalisation. *Journal of Mental Retardation*, **21**, 234–9.
36. Ramon, S. (ed.) (1991). *Beyond community care: normalisation and integration work*. Mind/Macmillan, Basingstoke.
37. Brandon, D. (1991). Implications of normalisation work for professional skills. In *Beyond community care: normalisation and integration work* (ed. S. Ramon), pp. 35–55. Mind/Macmillan, London.
38. Rapaport, J. (2005). The informal caring experience: issues and dilemmas. In *Mental health at the crossroads: the promise of the psychosocial approach* (eds. S. Ramon and J. Williams), pp. 155–70. Ashgate Publishing, Aldershot.
39. Saleebey, D. (ed.) (1992). *The strengths perspective in social work practice*. Longman, New York.

40. Rapp, C. (1998). *The strengths perspective of case management with persons suffering from severe mental illness.* Oxford University Press, Oxford.

41. Norman, E. (ed.) (2000). *Resiliency enhancement: putting the strengths approach into social work practice.* Columbia University Press, New York.

42. Pilgrim, D. and Rogers, A. (2003). *Mental health and inequality.* Palgrave, Macmillan, Basingstoke.

43. Glasby, J. and Lester, H. (2002). *Social work and direct payment.* Policy Press, Bristol.

44. Barnes, M., Bowl, R., and Fisher, M. (1990). *Sectioned: social services and the 1983 Mental Health Act.* Routledge, London.

45. Hatfield, B. and Robinshaw, P. (1994). The use of compulsory powers by approved social workers in five local authorities: some trends over two years. *Journal of Mental Health*, **3**, 339–50.

46. Rapaport, J. (2006). New roles in mental health: the creation of the approved mental health practitioner. *Journal of Integrated Care*, **14**, 37–46.

47. Huxley, P., Evans, S., Webber, M., *et al.* (2005). Staff shortages in the mental health workforce: the case of the disappearing social worker. *Health and Social Care in the Community*, **13**, 504–13.

48. Kanter, J. (1989). Clinical case management: definition, principles, components. *Hospital and Community Psychiatry*, **40**, 361–8.

49. Brandon, D., Atherton, K., and Brandon, A. (1996). *Handbook of care planning.* Positive Publications, London and ref. 26.

50. Hiday, V.A. and Scheid-cook, T.L. (1991). Outpatient commitment for "revolving door" patients compliance and treatment. *Journal of Nervous and Mental Disease*, **179**, 83–8.

51. Campbell, J., Brohpy, L., Healy, B., *et al.* (2006). International perspectives on the use of community treatment orders: implications of mental health social workers. *British Journal of Social Work*, **36**, 1101–18.

52. Canvin, K., Bartlett, A., and Pinfold, V. (2002). A "bittersweet pill to swallow": learning from mental health service users' responses to compulsory community care in England. *Health and Social Care in the Community*, **10**, 361–9.

53. Stanley, N. and Manthorpe, J. (2004). *The age of the inquiry.* Routledge, London.

54. Beck, A. (1992). *The risk society.* Sage, London.

55. Rose, N. (2002). *Powers of freedom: reframing political thought.* Cambridge University Press, Cambridge.

56. Thompson, P. (2003). Devils and deep blue seas: the social worker in-between. *Journal of Social Work Practice*, **17**, 35–47.

57. Hennelly, R. (1990). Mental health resource centres. In *Psychiatry in transition: British and Italian experiences* (ed. S. Ramon), pp. 208–18. Pluto Press, London.

58. Mullender, A. and Ward, D. (1991). *Self-directed groupwork.* Whiting and Birch, London.

59. Flaker, V., Cizely, M., Ferle, Z., *et al.* (2004). Special care homes: the vision: a project of the community of social institutions in Slovenia. *Journal of Social Work, Faculty of Social work*, University of Ljubljana, Ljubljana, Slovenia.

60. Debell, D. and Walker, S. (2003). *Norfolk family support teams: an evaluation of the first two years.* Anglia Ruskin University, Cambridge.

61. Diggins, M. (2000). Innovation as a professional way of life—the building bridges project for parents-users of mental health services and their children. In *A stakeholder approach to innovation in mental health services* (ed. S. Ramon), pp. 77–93. Pavilion, Brighton.

62. Jones, J. (2006). *The faith links project—equality and diversity in Brent, central and north west London.* Mental Health NHS Trust, London.

63. Mowbray, C.T., Collins, M.E., and Bellamy, C.D. (2005). Supported education for adults with psychiatric disabilities: an innovation for social work and psychosocial rehabilitation practice. *Social Work*, **50**, 7–20.

64. Ryan, M., Merighi, J.R., Healy, B., *et al.* (2004). Belief, optimism and caring: findings from across-national study of expertise in mental health social work. *Qualitative Social Work*, **3**, 411–29.

## 6.4.4 Art therapy

Diane Waller

### The fundamental principles of art therapy/art psychotherapy

#### Definitions

Descriptions of art therapy from two of the oldest and largest professional associations, the British Association of Art Therapists and the American Art Therapy Association refer to: the use of art materials for self-expression and reflection in the presence of a trained art therapist. Art therapy uses the flexible, creative problem-solving potential of art-making to improve and enhance the physical, mental, and emotional well-being of individuals of all ages. The relationship between the therapist, client, and their artwork is of central importance. Art therapy can be used on a one-to-one and group basis.

Art therapy (or art psychotherapy, both titles are protected by law) in the United Kingdom is firmly rooted in psychodynamic and humanistic concepts and practices appropriate to public sector settings, and adapted to the social and mental health of the client. It is a broad-based discipline, involving substantial knowledge of the visual arts, individual and group psychotherapy, social and communication sciences, and the impact of culture on health.[1]

#### Main premises

- That visual image-making is an important aspect of the human learning process;

- That art made in the presence of an art therapist may enable a person to get in touch with feelings that cannot easily be expressed in words;

- That the creative process helps people to resolve conflicts and problems;

- That art can act as a 'container' for powerful emotions and be a means of communication between client(s) and therapist;

- That the image can serve to illuminate the transference in the case of a psychodynamic approach.

Engagement in image-making is of central importance although clients do not need any prior experience of or skill in art, as the aim is not to produce a 'good' piece of art that can be exhibited. The images made in art therapy may embody thoughts and feelings, be a bridge between the 'inner world' and outer reality, be a mediator between unconscious and conscious, hold and symbolize past, present, and future aspects of a client's life. Ambivalence and conflict can be stated and contained within an image. In art therapy the client tries to give form to what seem to be inexpressible or unspeakable feelings, which they can then share with the art therapist.

The focus of the transference (bringing feelings from the past into the present), can be onto the art object rather than to the therapist directly, adding a 'third dimension' to the therapeutic process.[2-4]

An important aim, as with all psychotherapy, is to bring about change. Positive change may occur when a client can direct their strong feelings into making art and when the therapist helps the client to tell their story through the art. How, when, and if change occurs obviously depends on their capacity to engage with this process and needs much time and patience while the client builds confidence. For verbally inarticulate clients, or those who use words defensively, engagement with the art materials gives the opportunity to understand self and environment, communicate emotions to the therapist, receive feedback, and encouragement.

## The historical development of art therapy in the United Kingdom, United States, and Europe

There are parallels in the development of art therapy in the United Kingdom and United States, early history being shared with that of group analytic psychotherapy as a phenomenon of the Second World War rehabilitation movement.[5-7] In the 1940s and 1950s art therapists were simply artists working in hospitals who emphasized the healing role of art. In 1963, the British Association of Art Therapists was formed from this small group of artists and art educators, who set themselves the task of defining and extending the activity, preparing standards for training in the higher education sector, informing the public and other professionals of the potential of art therapy, and working towards a career and salary structure in the National Health Service (NHS). The first *postgraduate trainings* began in the late 1960s. The positive response of the NHS and other organizations to art therapy's beneficial impact led to a petition being made for statutory regulation under the old Council for Professions Supplementary to Medicine in 1991, approved in 1997, after which art therapists, along with music and dramatherapists had their own federal Board at the Council. They were transferred to the Health Professions Council in 2001. Training in the United Kingdom is now at Master's level, in four universities in England, one in Scotland, one in Northern Ireland, and usually follows a degree in art and design. Study of psychotherapeutic principles, visual art, and practical placement are important elements in the training. Elsewhere in Europe the picture is very different with some countries sharing the UK standards, others having no training or a great variety of trainings in both the public and private sector. The United States, Australia, and New Zealand have the same requirements of a Master's level qualification in order to practice. (See website references for more information.)

## The development of art therapy with specific client groups

One of art therapy's main advantages as a treatment is its flexibility. It can be used with many different client groups and some of these are discussed as follows:

### Children

Many founder art therapists in the United Kingdom and United States were art teachers and were influenced by the 'child-centred'

approach to art education that developed in the 1930s. American pioneer Kramer considered that it was art activity itself that had inherent healing properties; and that within a secure relationship with the therapist, a child could sublimate their destructive and aggressive feelings by producing an object, which would symbolize those feelings, prevent them being acted out and lead to more insight and control. This often led to change in behaviour.[8]

Others pioneers from the United States gave examples of how group work could enable angry and shameful feelings to be shared among the group members as well as the therapist, to the relief of the child as well as his peers.[9] Many art therapists specializing in work with children attest to the importance of play and to the role of art materials in allowing regression in the form of mess-making. This seems to be particularly beneficial for children who have suffered sexual abuse[10-12] due to the loosening of control that happens when a child becomes deeply immersed in the physical process of painting and is able to lower defences as a result. Materials may be smeared, spilled, and wasted and it is important that the therapist maintains control of the boundaries and is able to tolerate a high level of anxiety as the child attacks the therapeutic space.[13]

Art therapy is helpful for children suffering from chronic constipation, faecal overflow soiling, and also 'antisocial behaviour' and Aldridge[14] pointed out the relationship she observed between food, painting, and faeces while working with neglected and abused children in the context of a social services Unit and how mess-making was important in their creative development. Ambridge[15] discussed how images may be used to reflect mother–child relationships with children who have been sexually abused and are often so traumatized that they cannot speak about their experiences.

The physical involvement in the art materials in enabling regression and essentially in receiving containment and acceptance from the therapist is very important to all the children mentioned above.

Dubowski[16,17] used a Developmental Art Therapy approach in research with children with learning difficulties, aiming to help the child to achieve his or her maximum potential. Understanding creativity and mark-making in early childhood is as important in this model as understanding psychodynamics. Studies made by Kellog[18] of over 100 000 children's scribbles inform our understanding of the developmental process leading to production of meaningful marks. Visual problem-solving through picture-making is developed between the age of about 18 months (when hand-eye co-ordination has developed to the extent that they can grasp an implement and direct it to a picture surface while attending to the activity) and 4 years, by which time most have developed the capacity to make recognizable pictures endowed with symbolic meaning.[19] This model draws on insights from art educationists, most recently Matthews.[20,21] Art therapists have also contributed to the emotional and educational development of children with Autism.[22,23]

Art therapists also occasionally work with families and this is an emerging area of interest.

### People with learning difficulties

Stott and Males[24] were among the first British art therapists to write about their work in a large hospital with people who had lived in institutions most of their lives. They suggested that art therapy offered a means of communication and of self-expression through which difficulties of life in an institution, such as loss of identity, could be eased. Their goals were: to find the art medium of most use to each resident, bearing in mind any physical handicaps; to set-up the art therapy sessions at regular times and in the same place; record and report the results of sessions; to enable maximum communication to take place. For some long-term residents, the art therapy studio became an 'oasis' in the desert of the hospital and they gained an identity as 'artist'.

Their work was continued by a generation of art therapists concerned about the effects of institutionalization on long-stay residents. Drawing on Gardner's work concerning the categories of personal and spatial intelligence[25] Rees set-up a qualitative research project using a detailed observational schedule with a group of women with severe learning difficulties in a single-sex locked ward, conducted over 3 years to investigate clients' use of physical space and its potential symbolic significance. Rees found that by relating to physical and spatial aspects of their environment, some clients discovered an effective way of maintaining some level of psychological and emotional integration. They were helped to manage their often overwhelming feelings and to develop a stronger identity in their, albeit, very restricted environment.[26] Strand used a group interactive art therapy model with a group of learning disabled clients whom she observed to be suffering from loss and despair as a result of their emotional needs being neglected.[27]

Now that people with learning difficulties mainly live in the community, art therapists are now able to assist clients in developing resources to manage their day-to-day activities, and to improve their quality of living—particularly social interaction—through engagement in creative activity, often in groups. Insights from earlier work on institutionalization and exclusion now inform art therapy with older residents in care homes.

## Offenders

Liebmann used art therapy within probation services to address 'offending behaviour' directly[28] summarizing the benefits to offenders as follows: as a means of non-verbal communication, important for the high percentage of offenders who have poor verbal skills, conversely with those who use words defensively; to release angry and aggressive as well as shameful and embarrassed feelings and provide an acceptable way of looking at and dealing with difficult emotions; client and therapist together could look back at the images over a series of sessions, see patterns and note developments; active participation is required, helping to mobilize those who may not be voluntary clients and bring about favourable behavioural changes that outlast the session itself. Liebmann devised strategies to help offenders gain insight into their behaviour, for example, the comic strip where the client is asked to draw an important life event within frames, the sequences of which can then be discussed and alternative options suggested.[29] This approach combines some elements of cognitive behavioural therapy with a psychodynamic approach, providing a structure, which is empathetic but on the other hand does not collude with offending behaviour, nor accept it as inevitable.

Teasdale produced a set of Guidelines while working in the prison service. These focus on inmates and on the prison environment, reinforce many of the points above, such as using art therapy to support prisoners in coping with their imprisonment, address feelings of separation, isolation, loss, low self-esteem. Specific advice is offered for conducting art therapy within a prison context.[30]

### People with psychotic illness

From the 1940s art therapists have worked with long-stay clients in psychiatric hospitals modifying the effects of institutionalization through detailed attention to communication when even the most psychotic patients could communicate through images and have this acknowledged. Now that people with psychosis increasingly live in the community and cope with the challenges of everyday life the focus is on issues of independence, isolation, building relationships, managing the illness, and its impact on self and family.[31]

Work with acutely psychotic clients, on the other hand, takes place on wards, is normally brief and aimed at helping the client to interact positively with others usually in 'open' studio groups with a rapidly changing population, or for those in a serious acute state, on a one-to-one basis. Drawing on process-oriented psychology McClelland[32] has devised a new model using art therapy to work directly on the acute state itself, requiring an active and assertive therapist style and meeting the client in their own 'language' however bizarre this may seem.

### Older people

With older people's mental health and well-being coming under increased government scrutiny, this is an area where art therapy has much potential to be beneficial. Art therapists in this field have noted that attention to loss, fear of illness and dying, feelings of helplessness and dependency is necessary in alleviating depression. Recent art therapy research with older people with dementia showed some improvements in mental acuity, calmness, sociability, and physical competence following 40 weekly sessions of group work, compared to no change in the control.[33]

As with other client groups, engaging in creative activity can also provide an outlet for frustrations to do with ageing, as well as possibly leading to a challenging and rewarding hobby.

### Physical illness

Art therapy is used with people suffering from cancer, including terminal cancer[34,35] as well as with other long-term and progressive illnesses or conditions such as multiple sclerosis, ME, kidney disease, effects of stroke, Parkinson's disease, and in palliative care to manage anxiety and fear about death and dying. The aims are to assist clients in coping with the emotional impact of their illness, enabling expression of feeling, relieving depression and stress, and improving their quality of living.

**Other areas** where promising work is going on: with eating disorders, drug and alcohol addiction, and with refugees and asylum seekers, many of whom have been the victims of war, of torture and are suffering extreme stress; also with the moderately to severely depressed and those who have work and relationship difficulties.

## Contextual issues

In the United Kingdom, over 50 per cent of art therapists work within the NHS where they may form part of the psychological therapies or occupational therapy department, or be autonomous. Others practise in Social Services, Education, Home Office, non-Statutory services, and a fairly small percentage work privately or are self-employed.

All are capable of assessing the suitability of the client for art therapy. Exclusion criteria are minimal. Initial interviews usually explain that the client does not have to be 'good at art' and that art therapy is not a 'painting class' but that it may arouse strong and sometimes difficult feelings. All therapists are trained to work with individuals and groups, to function as members of multi-disciplinary teams, to manage health and safety issues concerning preparation and maintenance of the art therapy space, liaising regularly with medical, nursing, teaching, or other appropriate staff in the interests of the client. Ethical standards are laid down by the Health Professions Council as for the other arts therapists (drama and music and also dance) with whom there is regular contact.

## Research

There is a substantial body of qualitative research in art therapy, however much of this would not meet the criteria for evidence-based practice required by today's public sector. Currently there is very little about art therapy within National Institute of Clinical Excellence guidelines, which have tended to emphasize quantitative studies. This is unfortunate as it gives the impression of a profession without a strong evidence base, which is not so as the flourishing Art Therapy Practice Research Network and a growing body of literature demonstrates.[36,37]

A few books and papers emerging from control group studies feature evaluations of art therapy groups with older people with moderate to severe dementia[38] and with schizophrenia. In 2006, the UK Health Technology Assessment supported a consortium headed by Crawford, Killaspy, and Waller (University of London) for a multi-centre random control group study of art therapy and schizophrenia. The Master's level training in art therapy requires a substantial dissertation, and a significant percentage of art therapists continue to doctorate research designed to use and test the hypotheses emerging from over 60 years of detailed casework.

## Further information

British Association of Art Therapists: www.baat.org.

Health Professions Council: www.hpc-uk.org (Art, Drama and Music Therapy).

International Society for the Study of the Psychopathology of Expression and Art Therapy: http//www.online-art-therapy.com/

American Association of Art Therapists: www.arttherapy.org.

## References

1. Quality Assurance Agency. (2004). *Benchmark statements for arts therapies*, www.qaa.ac.uk.
2. Dalley, T. (ed.) (1987). *Art as therapy*, pp. 6–19. Tavistock, London.
3. Schaverien, J. (1987). The scapegoat and the talisman: transference in art therapy. In *Images of art therapy* (eds. T. Dalley, *et al.*), pp. 74–108. Tavistock, London.
4. Schaverien, J. (1992). *The revealing image: analytical art therapy in theory and practice*. Routledge, London.
5. Waller, D. (1991). *Becoming a profession: the history of art therapy in Britain*. Routledge, London.
6. Waller, D. (2004). *Art therapists: pragmatic rebels*. Goldsmiths College, London (Inaugural Lecture May 2001).
7. Hogan, S. (2001). *The healing arts: the history of art therapy*. Jessica Kingsley, London.
8. Kramer, E. (1971). *Art therapy with children*. Schocken Books, New York.
9. Rubin, J. (1978). *Child art therapy*. Van Nostrand Reinhold, New York.
10. Lee Drucker, K. (2001). Why can't she control herself? Case study. In *Art therapy with young survivors of sexual abuse* (ed. J. Murphy), pp. 101–25. Brunner-Routledge, Hove and New York.
11. Lillitos, A. (1990). Control, uncontrol, order and chaos: working with children with intestinal motility problems. In *Working with children in art therapy* (ed. C. Case), pp. 72–88. Routledge, London.
12. Sagar, C. (1990). Working with cases of child sexual abuse. In *Working with children in art therapy* (ed. C. Case), pp. 89–114. Routledge, London.
13. Waller, D. (2006). Art therapy and Children: how it leads to change. *Clinical Child Psychology and Psychiatry*, **11**, 271–82.
14. Aldridge, F. (1998). Chocolate or shit: aesthetics and cultural poverty in art therapy with children. *Inscape*, **3**, 2–9.
15. Ambridge, M. (2001). Using the reflective image within the mother-child relationship. In *Art therapy with young survivors of sexual abuse* (ed. J. Murphy), pp. 69–85. Brunner-Routledge, Hove.
16. Dubowski, J. (1984). Alternative models for describing the development from scribble to representation in children's graphic work. In *Art as therapy* (ed. T. Dalley), pp. 45–61. Tavistock, London.
17. Dubowski, J. (1989). Art versus language (separate development during childhood). In *Working with children in art therapy* (ed. C. Case), pp. 7–22. Tavistock/Routledge, London.
18. Kellog, R. (1970). *Analysing children's art*. National Press Books, California.
19. Dubowski, J. and James, J. (1998). Arts therapies with children with learning difficulties. In *Development and diversity: new applications in art therapy* (ed. D. Sandle), pp. 41–56. Free Association Books, London and New York.
20. Matthews, J. (1999). *The art of childhood and adolescence: the construction of meaning*. Falmer Press, London.
21. Matthews, J. (2003). *Drawing and painting: children and visual representation*. Paul Chapman, London.
22. Evans, K. and Rutten-Saris, M. (1998). Shaping vitality affects: enriching communication: art therapy for children with autism. In *Development and diversity: new applications in art therapy* (ed. D. Sandle), pp. 57–77. Free Association Books, London and New York.
23. Tipple, R. (2003). The interpretation of children's art work in a paediatric disability setting. *Inscape*, **8**, 48–59.
24. Stott, J. and Males, B. (1984). Art therapy for people who are mentally handicapped. In *Art as therapy* (ed. T. Dalley), pp. 111–26. Tavistock, London.
25. Gardner, H. (1984). *Frames of mind: the theory of multiple intelligences*. Paladin, London.
26. Rees, M. (1995). Making sense of marking space: researching art therapy with people who have severe learning difficulties. In *Art and music therapy and research* (eds. A. Gilroy and C. Lee), pp. 117–37. Routledge, London and New York.
27. Strand, S. (1990). Counteracting isolation: group art therapy for people with learning difficulties. *Group Analysis*, **23**, 255–63.
28. Liebmann, M. (ed.) (1994). *Art therapy with offenders*. Jessica Kingsley, London.
29. Liebmann, M. (1998). Art therapy with offenders on probation. In *Development and diversity: new applications in art therapy* (ed. D. Sandle), pp. 104–20. Free Association Book, London.
30. Teasdale, C. (2002). *Guidelines for arts therapists working in prisons*. Department for Education and Skills/HM Prison Service, Prisoners' Learning and Skills Unit.
31. Killick, K. and Schaverien, J. (1997). *Art psychotherapy and psychosis*. Routledge, London and New York.

32. McClelland, S. (1992). Brief art therapy in acute stages: a process-oriented approach. In *Art therapy: a handbook* (eds. D. Waller and A. Gilroy), pp. 189–208. Open University Press, Buckingham.

33. Rusted, J., Sheppard, L., and Waller, D. (2006). A multi-centre randomized control group trial on the use of art therapy for older people with dementia. *Group Analysis*, **39**, 517–36.

34. Pratt, M. and Wood, M. (eds.) (1998). *Art therapy in palliative care.* Routledge, London and New York.

35. Waller, D. and Sibbett, C. (eds.) (2005). *Art therapy and cancer care.* McGraw-Hill, Maidenhead.

36. Karkou, V. and Sanderson, P. (2006). *Arts therapies: a research based map of the field.* Elsever, London.

37. Gilroy, A. (2006). *Art therapy, research and evidence based practice.* Sage, London.

38. Waller, D. (ed.) (2002). *Arts therapies and progressive illness.* Brunner-Routledge, Hove and New York.

# Indigenous, folk healing practices

## Wen-Shing Tseng

## What are indigenous, folk healing practices?

Indigenous, folk healing practices are nonorthodox therapeutic practices based on indigenous cultural traditions, operating outside of official (modern) healthcare systems.[1] These practices are often validated by experience, but are not founded on scientific principles. Indigenous healing practices are observed in 'primitive' or 'pre-industrialized' societies as well as in modern or developed societies. All healing practices or psychotherapies are more or less culturally influenced, including modern and orthodox psychotherapies, but indigenous healing practices are described as 'culturally embedded' because they are often intensely embedded in the cultural systems in which they were invented and in which they are practised. They are, therefore, usually very difficult to transplant to entirely different cultural settings, where they do not have the same meaning or legitimacy.[2]

While indigenous healing practices function in general as healing methods for problems, they are not usually considered by either the healer or the clients to be psychological therapy for the clients' emotional or psychological problems. Rather, they are recognized as religious ceremonies or healing exercises related to supernatural or natural powers. However, from a mental health point of view, the indigenous healing practices often provide psychotherapeutic effects for the clients, and can be considered as folk psychotherapy.

Anthropologists have studied folk healing practices as a part of cultural behaviour. Recently, cultural psychiatrists have become interested in examining indigenous healing practices from clinical perspectives to explore the similarities and differences that exist between folk healing practices and modern psychotherapy, and to disclose the therapeutic mechanisms that are operating in and being utilized by indigenous healing practices. Many people in developed societies utilize folk healing practices as adjunctive to their primary (modern) therapy or as their main way to get help. Therefore, it is relevant for the modern psychiatrists to know what they are and the possible therapeutic mechanism they offer, or the possible negative effects they may receive by utilizing such indigenous healing practices.

Various practices are covered by the loosely defined terms, indigenous or folk healing. Religious healing practices and ceremonies are closely related to a specific religion. Shamanism involves a spirit medium. Divination, or various kinds of fortune-telling, including astrology or physiognomy, may be used by people to solve their psychological problems or to seek answers for life problems, and, therefore, can be viewed as folk counselling practices as well. Furthermore, the practice of meditation, a self-training exercise used to obtain tranquility, growth of mind, and prevention of emotional problems, can be considered a folk healing practice if one defines psychotherapy very broadly, as not only treating a suffering person but also providing a means for preventing problems and improving the quality of a person's mental life.[3]

No matter what terms are used, indigenous healing practices share some common features. They are invented and utilized by local people for the purpose of solving problems or treating suffering—therefore, they are called indigenous in contrast to universal. They are distinctly different from the modern (Western or orthodox) professional medical approaches—thus, they are called folk practices. Most of them are supernaturally oriented and remote from any scientific orientation. Such indigenous practices are usually rooted in traditional beliefs and folk interpretations of problems, and, thus, are closely related to cultural beliefs.

## Subdivision of various healing practices

Based on their core nature and their basic therapeutic orientation, healing practices observed in different societies can be subdivided into different categories namely, supernatural orientation (such as spirit mediumship, religious healing ceremony, and divination); nature orientation (such as fortune-telling, astrology, and meditation); medical-physiological orientation (such as mesmerism, acupuncture, and herb medicine); and socio-psychological orientation (such as Zen training, Alcoholics Anonymous, est, and most modern psychotherapy).[4,5] It is recognized that such subdivisions are arbitrary, and often overlap. Yet these subcategories will help us to understand various healing practices that exist on a spectrum which includes the supernatural, natural, physiological, and psychological.

### Spirit mediumship (trance-based healing system)

Spirit mediumship broadly refers to a situation in which the healer or the client, or both, experiences alternate states of consciousness in the form of dissociation or a possessed state at the time of the healing ritual. From a psychotherapeutic point of view, it is important to distinguish which person is in an alternative state of consciousness, as the mechanism of therapy differs depending on whether it is the healer or the client who is dissociating.

## (a) Shamanism

It is speculated that the geographic heartland of shamanism is Central and North Eurasia, with widespread diffusion to Southeast Asia and the Americas.[3] Through a religious ceremony, a shaman can work himself into a trance state in which he is possessed by a god. The rhythmic singing, dancing, or praying (quiet meditation) seems to assist the self-induction of the trance state. Among native healers in North and South America, a psychedelic substance (such as may be found in cactus) is frequently used to induce an altered state of consciousness and a special psychic experience for the healing performance. Whether the altered state of consciousness is substance- or self-induced, the healer is considered to be possessed by a supernatural power. The client can then consult the supernatural through the shaman for instructions on dealing with his or her problems.

The causes of problems are usually interpreted according to the folk concepts held by the culture—involving such things as loss of the soul, sorcery, spirit intrusion, or violation of taboos. Disharmony with nature may also be interpreted as the cause of problems. Coping methods are usually magical in nature, such as: prayer, the use of charms, or the performance of a ritual ceremony for extraction or exorcism. Utilizing supernatural powers, acting as an authority figure, making suggestions, and providing hope are some of the main mechanisms for healing provided by the shaman. The goal of the healing practice is to resolve the problems that a client is encountering.

## (b) Zar ceremonies

The term *zar* refers to a ceremony as well as a class of spirits. *Zar* ritual is observed primarily in Muslim societies in the Mideast, including Ethiopia, Egypt, Iraq, Kuwait, Sudan, and Somaliland. *Zar* ritual is different from shamanism in that, in addition to the healer, the client also experiences the dissociated or possessed state.

The *zar* ceremony is primarily a female activity. All of those attending the ceremony wear new or clean clothing to please the spirits. The main patient usually wears a white gown, as much gold jewelry as possible, and is heavily perfumed. The ceremony master begins the ceremony with a song and drumming. When a spirit associated with some person in the audience is called, that person begins to shake in her seat, dancing, and trembling until she falls, exhausted, to the floor. Before the spirit consents to leave, it usually demands special favours, such as jewellery, new clothing, or expensive foods. It is the duty of the relatives and friends to gather around the prostrate woman and pacify the spirit. The whole tone of the ceremony is one of propitiation and persuasion, rather than coercion. The ceremony ends with an animal sacrifice and a feast.

The *zar* ceremony is primarily an adult female activity reflecting social conditions of sex-separation, low female status, restriction of women from religious participation, an unbalanced sex ratio, marital insecurity, and relative isolation. The *zar* ceremony provides women an ideal situation for relief of persistent and regular anxieties and tensions arising from their life conditions. The goods demanded during the ceremony are all things that their husbands should provide. This fulfills a woman's wish for attention and care.

Emotional catharsis, fulfillment of unsatisfied desire, and compensation for the suppressed female role are some of the therapeutic mechanisms working in this kind of therapeutic ritual. Restoring balance in real life is the implicit goal of this culture-embedded healing practice.[6]

## Religious healing ceremonies

A distinction needs to be made between religion and a religious healing ceremony. Religion refers to a system of belief in a divine or superhuman power or spiritual practice. As a part of a religion, some people may perform special ceremonies for the purpose of healing certain problems or disorders. There are various kinds of religious healing ceremonies observed in different societies that are considered by mental health workers to serve a therapeutic function for their participants.

## (a) Sprit dancing ceremony

As observed among Salish-speaking Indians of the Pacific Coast of North America, healing ceremonies utilize psychological mechanisms and processes similar to those in brainwashing. The initiate has to go through three major therapeutic approaches: depatterning through shock treatment (such as physical restraint, blindfolding, hitting, kinetic stimulation, or intensive acoustic stimulation, followed by lying still, being forbidden to talk, and starvation); physical training (such as daily running, jumping into ice-cold waters, or frequent rounds of dancing); and, finally, indoctrination.[7]

## (b) Sacrificial ritual

An example is found in Yoruba, Africa. A person's problems were identified by palm nuts tossed by the diviner. It was usually interpreted that the person or a member of his family had offended the family *orisa* (the lineage deity) or some other spirit. Then, the sacrifice of a certain animal was prescribed for resolution. In the sacrifice, the supplicant passed his bad luck or illness to the animal, and the animal was killed in the supplicant's stead. The healing power of the ritual lies in its reassurance and generation of conviction. The ritual demonstrates that proper curative steps are being taken.[8]

## (c) The religious ceremony of mourning

This is practised among members of the Spiritual Baptist Church in the West Indies. In a desire for spiritual strength and other benefits, church members volunteer to participate in the practice. After ceremonial washing and anointing, the mourners are isolated in a small chamber at the back of the church, where they remain for a period of 7 days. During that time, each individual prays, fasts, and experiences dreams and visions. The mourners claim they obtained beneficial psychological relief on their moods; attainment of the ability to foresee and avoid danger; improvement in their decision-making abilities; cures for physical illnesses; and heightened facility to communicate with God.[9]

## (d) Snake-handling cult

An extremely different form of religious ritual was a snake-handling cult in the southern United States. As part of cult activities, members, in trance states, handled poisonous snakes as a sign of being blessed by God. Occasionally, some of the members died when they were bitten by the snakes. Although forbidden by the government to perform such cult rituals, these activities still exists. The gratification of emotional excitement was interpreted as one of the effects sought by cult members—even at the risk of their lives.[10]

### (e) Christian religious healing

It is important to know that religious healing ceremonies are not only observed in primitive societies or among uncivilized populations, but are quite common in many industrialized societies, as well. In Christian religious healing, there is a broad spectrum of beliefs and activities, ranging from Christian Science to the fundamentalism of healers such as Oral Roberts to the Roman Catholic rite of anointing of the sick. The participating client is provided with the hope for supernatural resources against disease, thus increasing his or her security and sense of well-being.[11]

Thus, in various forms of religious healing ceremonies, the therapeutic operation is carried out through the ritual of prayer, testimony, sacrifice, reliving experience, or even spirit possession. Assurance, suggestions, and generation of conviction are some of the healing mechanisms utilized in the practices. The aims of therapy are to heal the problems and give a certain perspective to the client's life.

## Divination

Divination refers to the act or practice of trying to foretell the future or the unknown by occult means. It relies on mysterious, magic, or religious methods. Since the interpretation of divine instruction is usually provided by the diviner himself, or an interpreter, the interaction between the diviner/interpreter and the client becomes an important variable.

There is a range of methods of divination. Some methods are very simple, while others are more complicated. For example, in Nigeria, Africa, the divination practised by the Nsukka Ibo (called *Afa*) is carried out by casting four strings containing half-shells of the seeds of the bush mango;[12] and by the people in Yoruba (known as *Ifa*) by tossing palm nuts.[8] In the divination practised in some parts of Africa, the diviner simply offers a certain sign himself. For example, divination may occur while his hand is shaking, with the belief that he is guided by a supernatural power to give instructions.

In ancient China, turtle shells or the bones of big animals were burned during divination ceremonies and divine instruction was interpreted through the cracks made from the heat. An elaborate divination system called *chien* has been developed in China, and a modified version is used in Japan. To obtain answers to questions about their lives, some Chinese or Japanese will visit temples for divination. After a sincere prayer to the god of the temple, the person will ask for divine instruction, which is provided through a fortune stick that the person selects. Corresponding to the number on the stick, there is a fortune paper with an answer written on it. This practice is called *chien* drawing in Chinese,[13] or *kujibiki* in Japanese.

No matter what method of divination is practised, the basic therapeutic operation is performed to provide a clear-cut answer for the problems presented. Thus, it is helpful psychologically for a client to find a definite way to address his problems. Naming effects are among the healing mechanisms operating in divination. It is assumed that human life is under the influence of supernatural regulation. It is the basic goal of the person seeking help to find the proper way to comply with the universe through divine instruction.

### (a) Fortune-telling

The system of reference shifts from the supernatural to the natural in the practice of fortune-telling. Based on the concepts of microcosm and macrocosm, fortune-telling is oriented to the basic belief that human life and behaviour are parts of the universe. The nature of the problems is usually explained in terms of an imbalance of vital forces or disharmony with the natural principles that rule the universe. The objective of the practice is to help the client find out how to live compatibly with nature and adjust to the environment more harmoniously.

Based on the sources of information used, fortune-telling can be divided into several groups. In astrology, there is a basic belief that a person's life is correlated to and influenced by the movement of the stars, thus, their movement becomes the essential source of information for predicting one's life course. For the Chinese, an ancient record of universal change, the Oracle of Change (*Yi-Jing*), is used for fortune-telling. A person's date and time of birth, and the number of strokes in the Chinese character for his or her name, is the information needed to calculate an individual's fortune.

Physiognomy is based on the assumption that there is a close correlation between the mind and the body and that one's character, life, and fortune can be read by examining one's physical features. It is assumed that a person is born with a certain predisposition, which is shown in his physical appearance and will lead him to manifest certain behaviour patterns. A physiognomist tries to help a client understand his own character and behaviour patterns, learning how to make good use of his talents and, at the same time, make up for his shortcomings.

Although the basic assumption underlying fortune-telling is that every person has a predetermined course of life, such fate is not absolutely unchangeable—it may be subject to modification. Thus, it is not a completely passive acceptance of fate, but allows room for adjustment. Finding a way to adjust your own fortune is the purpose of fortune-telling.

Even though the basic orientation shifts from a supernatural to a natural one, and the sources of practice rely on the rules of nature, the therapeutic operation, like divination, is still characterized by offering folk-natured interpretation and providing concrete guidance for a client in making choices. Based on the concepts of microcosm and macrocosm, complying with the fundamental rules of nature is the basic goal of the practice.

## Common therapeutic factors

Reviewing various forms of folk therapy, it has been pointed out that the core of the effectiveness of different methods of religious and magical healing seems to lie in their ability to arouse hope by capitalizing on the patient's dependency on others.[14] Comparing the healing practices carried out by witch doctors and psychiatrists, it has been pointed out that they share a common root. Both kinds of therapists are able to decrease the client's anxiety by identifying what is wrong with him—that is, to name the cause of the problems, providing the effect of the Rumpelstiltskin principle; the therapist presents certain personal qualities that are admired by the culture and contribute to the therapy; the client's expectations of therapy, and the emotional arousal that is usually enhanced by the therapeutic setting, the therapist's belief in himself, and his reputation; the emerging sense of learning and mastery that the client obtains through therapy; and finally, the techniques of therapy that enhance the basic components of psychotherapy. It is clear that folk healing practices and modern psychotherapy share a number of nonspecific therapeutic mechanisms.[15] It has been indicated that traditional healing practices have several advantages over cosmopolitan modern medicine, namely: cultural congeniality, maximal use of the personality of the healer, a holistic approach, accessibility and availability (particularly for developing areas), effective use of affect and altered states of consciousness, collective therapy management, and cost-effectiveness.[1] It is important to recognize that both folk healing and modern therapy utilize symbols and metaphors for interpretation and suggestions.[16] In contrast to modern psychotherapists, some folk healers make use of symbolic interpretations and suggestions to enhance the effects of healing.

## Attitudes towards indigenous healing practices

Different points of view exist among scholars, clinicians, and public health workers regarding whether or not to encourage or discourage indigenous folk healing practices in various societies. Some people (particularly modern clinicians) see folk healing as merely superstitious and primitive, insisting that such out-of-date practices should be discouraged or prohibited. Others (such as cultural anthropologists and cultural psychiatrists) consider these folk practices to be interesting subjects for academic study—examining the therapeutic elements that are utilized in these primitive healing practices, and why such supernaturally oriented therapeutic exercises are still popular among some groups. Still other people (such as some community health workers) believe that, due to the shortage of professional personnel available in the community, the existence of folk therapies should be supported. The position was taken that any folk healing practice that is proven (or at least considered) to be helpful to the client and useful to the community deserves the support and encouragement of clinicians as well as administrators.

## Final comments: clinical implications

The comparative study of indigenous healing practices and modern psychotherapy has revealed the existence of certain universal elements of the healing process that operate as important factors for therapy, whether the therapy is carried out in a primitive or modern form. The universal and nonspecific healing factors identified are: the cultivation of hope, the activation of surrounding support, and the enhancement of culturally sanctioned coping. The study of indigenous healing practices has also pointed out the existence of supernatural dimensions of healing power, which are less intentionally utilized in modern therapy.

Despite the general usefulness of folk therapies, the ill effects of some have not been widely studied and reported. Yet, clinical observation has disclosed that some folk therapists cause harm to the clients who seek their services. Under the guise of treatment, tricking a client out of his money by deceit or fraud, or sexual involvement with a client, are examples of disreputable behaviour that are occasionally reported. Harming a client by prescribing dangerous substances, and physically injuring or even killing a client by accident during the performance of an exorcism, are other examples of serious complications that have occurred.

No matter what position is taken, there is one simple fact that deserves attention, namely, that there exists a wide range of professional quality among so-called folk healers, and different motivations for practice. Some are benign healers motivated by a desire to serve, while others are not. Some are well-trained in their particular professions and know how to practice within its limitations, while others are not—and are liable for malpractice. The major problem is that, from a public health point of view, in most societies, there still are no formal guidelines for regulating folk therapy, as there are for modern therapy. Folk therapy, whether it is shamanistic practice or faith healing, should be subject to periodic surveys and reevaluation by the public health administration, as is modern clinical work, so that its benefits to clients can be protected and any potential malpractice can be prevented. If any folk therapist refuses to be examined and regulated, he or she should be discouraged or prevented from practicing.

## Further information

Tseng, W.S. (1999). Culture and psychotherapy: review and practical guidance. *Transcultural Psychiatry*, **36**(2), 131–79.

Tseng, W.S. (2003). 7: Culturally competent psychotherapy. In *Clinician's guide to cultural psychiatry* (ed. W.S. Tseng), pp. 291–342. Academic Press, San Diego.

## References

1. Jilek, W.G. (1994). Traditional healing in the prevention and treatment of alcohol and drug abuse. *Transcultural Psychiatric Research Review*, **31**(3), 219–58.

2. Tseng, W.S. (2001). *Handbook of cultural psychiatry*, pp. 515–37. Academic Press, San Diego.

3. Prince, R. (1980). Variations in psychotherapy procedures. In *Handbook of cross-cultural psychology: psychopathology*, Vol. 6 (eds. H.C. Triandis and J.G. Draguns). Allyn and Bacon, Boston.

4. Tseng, W.S. and Hsu, J. (1979). Culture and psychotherapy. In *Perspectives on cross-cultural psychology* (eds. A.J. Marsella, R.G. Tharp, and T.J. Ciborowski). Academic Press, New York.

5. Tseng, W.S. (1999). Culture and psychotherapy: review and practical guidance. *Transcultural Psychiatry*, **36**(2), 131–79.

6. Kennedy, J.G. (1967). Nubian *zar* ceremonies as psychotherapy. *Human Organization*, **26**(4), 185–94.

7. Jilek, W.G. (1976). Brainwashing as therapeutic technique in contemporary Canadian Indian sprit dancing: a case in theory building. In *Anthropology and mental health: setting a new course* (ed. J. Westermeyer). Mounton Publishers, Paris.

8. Prince, R. (1975). Symbols and psychotherapy: the examples of Yoruba sacrificial ritual. *Journal of American Academy of Psychoanalysis*, **3**(3), 321–38.

9. Griffith, E.E.H. and Mahy, G.E. (1984). Psychological benefits of spiritual Baptist mourning. *The American Journal of Psychiatry*, **141**(6), 769–73.

10. La Barre, E.H. (1962). *They shall take up serpents: psychology of the southern snake-handling cult*. University of Minnesota Press, Minneapolis.

11. Hufford, D. (1977). Christian religious healing. *Journal of Operational Psychiatry*, **8**(2), 22–7.

12. Shelton, A.J. (1965). The meaning and method of *Afa* divination among the northern Nsukka Ibo. *American Anthropologist*, **67**, 1441–5.

13. Hsu, J. (1976). Counseling in the Chinese temple: a psychological study of divination by Chien drawing. In *Culture-bound syndromes, ethnopsychiatry, and alternate therapies* (ed. W.P. Lebra). University Press of Hawaii, Honolulu.

14. Frank, J.D. (1961). *Persuasion and healing: a comparative study of psychotherapy*. Schocken Books, New York.

15. Torrey, E.F. (1986). *Witchdoctors and psychiatrists: the common roots of psychotherapy and its future*. Harper & Row Publishers, New York.

16. Kirmayer, L.J. (1993). Healing and the invention of metaphor: the effectiveness of symbols revisited. *Culture, Medicine and Psychiatry*, **17**(2), 161–95.

# SECTION 7

# Social Psychiatry and Service Provision

**7.1 Public policy and mental health** *1425*
Matt Muijen and Andrew McCulloch

**7.2 Service needs of individuals and populations** *1432*
Mike Slade, Michele Tansella, and Graham Thornicroft

**7.3 Cultural differences care pathways, service use, and outcome** *1438*
Jim van Os and Kwame McKenzie

**7.4 Primary prevention of mental disorders** *1446*
J. M. Bertolote

**7.5 Planning and providing mental health services for a community** *1452*
Tom Burns

**7.6 Evaluation of mental health services** *1463*
Michele Tansella and Graham Thornicroft

**7.7 Economic analysis of mental health services** *1473*
Martin Knapp and Dan Chisholm

**7.8 Psychiatry in primary care** *1480*
David Goldberg, André Tylee, and Paul Walters

**7.9 The role of the voluntary sector** *1490*
Vanessa Pinfold and Mary Teasdale

**7.10 Special problems** *1493*

7.10.1 The special psychiatric problems of refugees *1493*
Richard F. Mollica, Melissa A. Culhane, and Daniel H. Hovelson

7.10.2 Mental health services for homeless mentally ill people *1500*
Tom K. J. Craig

7.10.3 Mental health services for ethnic minorities *1502*
Tom K. J. Craig and Dinesh Bhugra

# Public policy and mental health

## Matt Muijen and Andrew McCulloch

## Introduction

Public policy, and specifically national public policy, is one of the key factors that affects the practice of psychiatry, the shape of mental health services, and the environment within which mental health services work. The specific content of public policy varies greatly across the world and often even across neighbouring countries. It is therefore impossible within the space of this chapter to undertake systematic international comparisons. This chapter gives an overview of:

(a) what policy is and why it might be important;

(b) types of policy and policy development internationally;

(c) international structures and organizations that are relevant to the scope and content of policy, especially in the field of human rights which is often the starting point for policy;

(d) the breadth of policy activity that is relevant to mental health—stretching beyond the health ministry and health policy—and the partnerships that are necessary to tackle the mental health of individuals and populations.

## What is public policy?

Koontz and Weihrich[1] define policy or policies as 'General statements or understandings which guide thinking on decision making.' This definition implies that:

1 policy may be stated in writing (statute, guidance, or statement) or may be unwritten and disseminated through management or political chains of command only;

2 policies may exist at various organizational levels albeit here we are mainly concerned with national policies;

3 policy is only one factor in any final management or clinical decision. Other factors will often be more important, and clinical behaviour is notoriously resistant to policy influence except where certain behaviour is directly prohibited.[2]

Therefore, the policy needs to be understood as just one of the factors which determine the nature and state of mental health services and mental health promotion or public mental health within a society.

In many developed countries, the management of the public sector has seen major changes over the last two decades, shifting from a hierarchical and bureaucratic administration to a model of 'managerialism'.[3] In the old model policy making and administration was separated, and governments were responsible for the provision of services often via related public sector agencies. The new model, inspired by business,[4] is characterized by governments introducing competition and market principles and involving the private sector in providing services, setting measurable objectives, and introducing performance management with the aim of delivering higher efficiency. This has affected professionals such as psychiatrists by shifting accountability for good medical practice as judged by peers to reporting on outputs to managers as specified by contracts and practice guidelines. Nevertheless, in most cases strong professional accountability remains, creating a dual accountability that may be appropriate but is always challenging and sometimes conflicting.

## Mental health public policy

Public policy in mental health is driven by a range of influences and interests which policy makers will attempt to balance. Positive drivers, that is factors that encourage the development of progressive mental health policies, include:

◆ epidemiological evidence of the prevalence and the contribution of mental disorders to the burden of disease;

◆ evidence for effective and efficient interventions;

◆ public interest as expressed by politicians and the media;

◆ campaigns by NGOs and professional groups;

◆ human rights considerations;

◆ pressure from patient and family organizations;

◆ growing public expenditure.[5]

The strong interface between mental health issues and human rights explains the importance of human rights conventions and declarations in the shaping of policies and legislation, especially in countries where mental health policy and practice are less developed historically. Negative drivers, that is, factors that limit the commitment of policy makers, include budget limitations, competition from other priority areas, discrimination, and the perception that mental health is not a fruitful area for investment.

## The function of mental health policy

Mental health policy may serve a variety of functions ranging from the purely political and presentational through to delivering on a moral or social imperative. Often policy is mixed in function, enabling politicians to make a statement on an important human rights or social issue whilst also achieving real improvements for people with mental illness and delivering on economic targets. Mental health policy will also affect delivery of other aspects of policy in relation to crime, housing, education, and health. Thus, a coherent set of social policies cannot be developed without addressing mental health in some way. Mental health has been called a 'wicked' social policy issue (see Bogdanor for a discussion of such issues)[6] because it is hard to define, to address, and to deliver on tangibles, but unless we do, many of our social aspirations will not be fully realizable. Finally, the stated mission or desired outcome of policy may vary—for example some countries may have goals in terms of reduced prevalence of an outcome such as suicide, others may wish to achieve de-institutionalization.[7]

# Broader public policy and mental health

Whilst policy on mental health services *per se* is likely to be the concern of the health ministry, the impact of other public policy on both mentally ill people, and the practical application of psychiatry may be even bigger. People with severe or persistent common mental health problems often face social exclusion and face difficulties with issues including housing/shelter, employment, education, and welfare or welfare benefits. All mental health professionals in all countries of the world will be aware of how much these issues can affect the lives of people with mental illness and indeed clinical outcomes. Box 7.1.1 summarizes some of the main relevant policy areas which will impact on mental health services.

It should be clear from only brief examination of this table that achieving a totally coherent mental health policy presents huge challenges:

- The views of different parties and the priorities of many different government departments must be reconciled;

- Policy must integrate horizontally—for example, across health, education, and local government, and vertically from small organizations up to government;

- The non-measurable side of what is offered is very important to the stakeholders—services must be responsive, caring, joined up and visible to users, carers, and the general public—yet these features of services are hard to influence from central government;

- The needs and demands are so large and diverse it is difficult to construct and resource a coherent system for delivery even in the richest countries;

- Achieving equity and balancing resource allocation across groups of people suffering from a range of mental disorders with different prevalence and causing a different burden to self, families, and communities. Different groups of disorders require different investment producing different potential benefits yet such decisions must often be made on the basis of ambiguous information whilst subject to conflicting pressures from advocacy groups, communities, media, colleagues, government ministries, and parliament.

**Box 7.1.1** Policy links for mental health across government

| Government department or ministry (generic description may not accord with structures in all countries) | Mental health relevant policy responsibility (Examples) |
| --- | --- |
| Department of health/health and social services | Primary mental health care. Human resources for health and social care services. Finance for health and social care. Specialist mental health care policy. Public mental health or mental health promotion |
| Department of employment/ social welfare | Welfare benefits for people with mental health problems. Employment rights and protection. Occupational health |
| Department of education | Education on mental health issues as part of wider curricula in schools and higher education. Healthy schools. Higher education for relevant vocational qualifications |
| Department of criminal justice/internal security | Diversion of mentally ill offenders from the criminal justice system. Public security |
| Department of housing/ communities and local government/regions | Housing for mentally ill people. Community development. Urban policy |
| Department for constitutional affairs/human rights | Protection of those who lack capacity |
| Treasury or finance ministry | Financing of the above at a macro level. Strategic value for money |

(The authors after Jenkins *et al.* (2002))

## Comparative policy

It can be argued that mental health policies in most countries fall within four broad groupings:

1 Provision for the basic protection of human rights of people with mental illness or those lacking mental capacity;

2 As one together with a simple health care policy to provide for the health care needs of people with serious mental illnesses;

3 The above but with a more comprehensive health and social care policy which addresses primary and specialist care needs for various groups of disorders;

4 A comprehensive cross-sectoral mental health policy that addresses care, public mental health, and broader issues such as housing.

No country in the world has a fully comprehensive policy although developed countries such as New Zealand, Australia, several

European countries, and states of Canada and the United States have advanced policies. This reflects the nature and resources of these societies, and does not necessarily result in differences in prevalence or outcomes.[8]

## Human right conventions and legislation

Human rights have historically been a fundamental driver for the development of mental health policy in most countries of the world. The current Human Rights conventions derive from the United Nations, and are binding once they are ratified by member states following adoption by the United Nations General Assembly. The Universal Declaration of Human Rights was adopted in 1948. This was followed in 1966 by the International Covenant on Political and Civil Rights (ICCPR) and the International Covenant on Economic, Social and Cultural Rights (ICESCR), in combination known as the International Bill of Rights. None of the conventions directly addresses issues related to mental health care, although the right to the highest attainable standard of physical and mental health is included in Article 12 of the ICESCR. In non-binding general comments, the committee on Economic, Social and Cultural Rights specified that right to health covers availability, accessibility with a strong emphasis on equality and non-discrimination, and acceptability including cultural sensitivity and quality. The obligation of signatories to provide information on detentions and measures taken to prevent abuse for people admitted to mental hospitals is important.[9]

In 1991, the United Nations General Assembly adopted 'the principles for the protection of persons with mental illness and the improvement of mental healthcare', better known as the MI principles, which remains a key reference document for national mental health legislation. The document outlines 25 principles, stressing the importance of non-discriminatory practice within the health care system. The rights to which patients with mental health problems are entitled, according to the MI principles, include the right to live and work as far as possible in the community, and the right to the best available treatment and care in the least restrictive settings in conditions suited to the cultural background of the patient. The principles also set out expectations for confidentiality, the protection of autonomy, and the conditions for involuntary detention. In combination the principles offer a good foundation for modern mental health policies and legislation. Although the document is not legally binding, it is clearly stated that member states are expected to implement these principles fully.

An essential principle, confirmed by the World Conference on Human Rights in 1993, is that all human rights are universal, equally applying to people with disabilities and mental disorders. This is a strong driver for national governments to deliver anti-discrimination legislation, guidance, and practice.

## International agencies

There are several relevant regional agencies that represent countries, including political organizations such as the European Union, the Council of Europe and the European Court of Human Rights, the African Commission on Human and People's Rights, and the Inter-American Court of Human Rights. All have produced conventions and declarations pertinent to people with mental health problems, some legally binding.[10]

The World Health Organization (WHO), the specialist health agency of the United Nations, is mandated by its constitution to support member states in all health areas, including mental health. Its core functions include to:

◆ propose conventions, agreements and regulations, and make recommendations with respect to international health matters;

◆ assist governments, upon request, in strengthening health services;

◆ promote improved standards of teaching and training in the health, medical, and related professions;

◆ study and report on, in cooperation with other specialized agencies where necessary, administrative and social techniques affecting public health and medical care from preventive and curative points of view, including hospital services and social welfare.

In 2001, WHO dedicated the World Health Report to mental health. The report entitled 'New Understanding, New Hope' urges member states 'to seek solutions for mental health that are already available and affordable'.[11] The report formulates a set of 10 recommendations for member states to address the challenges faced in various areas of mental health. By adopting the report (World Health Assembly Resolution WHA 55.10), governments have committed themselves to implement its recommendations to strengthen primary care and develop accessible and affordable community-based mental health services.

At WHO regional level there have been several declarations and action plans that elaborated the principles of the World Health Report 2001, and reinforced the commitment by governments to delivery. Examples include the Caracas Declaration for the Americas, anticipating the World Health Report, and the European Declaration for Mental Health signed in Helsinki 2005.

## Why public mental health policy?

Although the governments of most countries accept a role for public policy in the regulation, commissioning, funding, resourcing, and provision of mental health care, particularly for persons with severe and enduring mental health problems, a case still should be made why mental health care cannot be left to a combination of the private market and civil society to deliver without central intervention. As we have argued, when national systems are compared, considerable variation emerges, even within developed countries. In some, the role of government is limited to regulation of independent health insurance groups that purchase from independent providers, and the public funding of a safety net for expensive acute care or long-term conditions. In other countries all parts of the health system are state owned and tax funded.

The World Bank produced a report on this question,[12] scrutinizing the arguments for public financing of mental disorders as compared to other conditions that compete for public money. In their opinion, disease burden, cost-effectiveness of interventions, and externalities are not sufficient arguments since these are not unique to mental health. However, the potential of catastrophic cost, the risk of insurance market failure, and the place of involuntary treatment and consequent issues of human rights are all disproportionately present in mental health care and plead in favour of a public role. One could add to this that stigma and discrimination may negatively affect the availability and access to mental health services if left to market forces together with the argument advanced above that comprehensive social policies cannot logically leave out mental health.

## Economic impact of disease burden

An important argument for the view that mental health should be central to health care and public policy in general is the burden of disease evidence, addressed elsewhere in this book (cross ref). The realization that mental disorders contribute so much to the overall burden of disease puts mental health care at least on an equal footing with other groups of disorders that have long been recognized as posing a major public health challenge such as infectious disease, cancer, and heart disease. Even more startling is the very high proportion of years lived with disability attributable to mental health problems and the days lost to employment due to mental health conditions. The majority of mental health problems contributing to disability are anxiety and depression and the burden of substance misuse and organic disorders in developed countries is also very high, and rising.

From a public policy perspective, this means that the consequences of mental health problems are no longer only an issue of health care, but are central to macro-economic national interests, particularly at times of skills shortages. This has become connected with the interest in the mental well-being of the population, based on the observation that level and growth in Gross National Product (GNP) is only very marginally associated with status of mental well-being of the population, and in some cases even inversely correlated.[13] This has resulted in the conclusion by economists that government's macro-economic policies should not simply be driven by the aim to maximize the Gross National Product and the income of its citizens. Rather, the 'happiness' of the population should become the prime driver of policy making.[14] Governments have consequently seen a need to stimulate the employment of people with mental disorders, both as part of the social inclusion agenda and to reverse the very high and increasing cost of mental disability. This could be considered as a somewhat symptomatic approach ignoring the more systemic problem of job stress and insecurity in very competitive market economies. However, there is also no doubt that loss of employment is a disastrous event for individuals and families in its own right, whether considered from an emotional, social, or financial perspective. The strong association of unemployment with divorce, mental illness, suicide, all factors associated with social exclusion[15] in their own right, supports the case for increasing employment rates, if not exclusively so. A challenge mental health services are facing is to identify the most appropriate and effective response to such broader societal needs as many of the levers for change lie outside the health care sector.

## The scope of mental health public policy development

The scope of mental health policy making has broadened, as reflected in the content of international declarations. During the second half of the twentieth century mental health policy and expenditure was focused on people with severe and enduring conditions cared for in institutional settings. Increasingly the focus is broadening to incorporate mental health promotion and prevention and treatment of common mental disorders, including a key role for primary care. The reasons for this include:

- an increased demand for the treatment of stress and depression;
- the development of community-based services, lowering the threshold to access for, and acceptability of care;
- the growing evidence base for a range of interventions such as cognitive behavioural therapy (CBT);
- increased media interest in common mental disorders and their treatment;
- the reduction of stigma of common mental disorders;
- growing affluence in many countries making privately purchased therapies more affordable;
- an awareness that mental health problems are associated with many social determinants of health, including inequality, and macro-economic conditions;
- the co-morbidity between mental health problems and many physical diseases including diabetes and CHD, affecting mortality, and recovery rates;
- an awareness of the cost of mental illness to society, and the evidence of cost-effective promotion and prevention activities.

All these have major consequences for public policy. The complex interface between public mental health activities and mental illness services demands a multi-agency approach, crossing the responsibilities of government departments and local services and requires 'joined up government'. This requires clear policies with explicit objectives and targets, specifying responsibilities for delivery and funding. It requires the active ownership of mental health issues beyond the health care sector and its advocacy by leading practitioners across a range of sectors and disciplines.

## Policy implementation

The growing range and complexity of mental health-related activities requires explicit strategies outlining the vision and values of reform, the planned service organization, capital and human resource implications, financing, quality monitoring, and human rights protection. The number of countries in the world with such detailed mental health policies as defined above is still low but growing. There are also many examples of good strategies, whether at national, state, regional, or local level, that have produced impressive change, and guidance for the drafting of policy and legislation is available.[16]

The common factors in countries with a successful track record of change include:

- full commitment by government;
- national consultation exercises, gaining the views and support of key stakeholders;
- clear and consistent communication of objectives;
- realistic and sustained resource allocation;
- workforce strategies including education and training.

However, there are also examples of countries that have drafted comprehensive strategies that have not been implemented.

Failure of implementation will create cynicism that may obviate future attempts. Main factors that lead to failure include:

1 Poor connection between the strategy and reality, and lack of focus. In some instances strategies are written by foreign experts ignorant of local circumstances. Other examples are of strategies that are based on ideology and are overambitious, repeating the content of declarations without taking into account local needs and resources.

2 Lack of financial commitment or poor grasp of the financial costs of a new model of care, causing rejection by the finance ministry or inability to deliver locally.

3 Neglect of the human resource implications. New models tend to require more staff with new skills, and implementation can create high levels of anxiety that need to be confronted.

4 Lack of consultation with professional groups, users, carers, and communities, who therefore reject or resist the strategy.

5 Insufficient joint planning either across government or with partner organizations that will carry responsibilities for the funding and delivery of essential components such as social care, housing, and employment. Incentives will need to be created for various groups such as professionals and the private sector to support the strategy. Added to this is the need to align incentives across different areas, and to prevent the development of perverse incentives, leading to conflicts of interest.[17]

6 Lack of a long-term perspective. It is often possible to develop local model services, but generalization to national and sustainable programmes requires different approaches.

7 Lack of all party political support. It is unlikely reform will be initiated and embedded within the lifetime of a single parliament/administration or under the governance of the same minister of health. Unless political support is strong across the political spectrum, the risk of reversal due to weak commitment or even hostility to previously agreed plans is high.

## Human resources

Any strategy must include plans for sufficient staff with the right attitudes, skills, and competencies. The growing demand for mental health care has increased the need for staff. Many countries around the world are looking for ways to remedy staff shortages, particularly of doctors and nurses. Three approaches can be distinguished:

◆ increase of national recruitment;

◆ creation of different roles and responsibilities for staff;

◆ international recruitment.

Although the increase of training places is on the face of it an obvious approach, it does not solve the problem immediately since the lag time between the creation, for example, of a medical training place and the production of a psychiatrist will be at least 10 years. The availability of training places assumes that places will be filled with able candidates, which is also not always the case. In some poorer countries students reject the option to become mental health workers due to stigma, poor working conditions, and poor pay.

An important alternative strategy is to take a more comprehensive competency-based approach, and analyse the roles and responsibilities

of staff groups that are available and could be equally effective, sometimes even at lower cost. A potential example of this is nurse prescribing.[18] A step further is the creation of new workforce roles, compatible with the direction of reform. Community-based services may require a multi-disciplinary team involving a larger proportion of social workers and psychologists instead of only doctors and nurses. One could also consider new types of community workers focusing on prevention or early intervention, or support workers for patients with severe and enduring disorders. A primary care-based approach may suggest the development of mental health expertise for primary care workers. In practice, however, such models tend to create additional demands for staff and change roles of existing staff, rather than reducing the need for the specialists who remain in short supply.[19]

A short cut to solving staff shortages is international recruitment, setting up a three-way dilemma between ethical recruiting practice, the interest of both receiving and sending countries, and the benefit of individuals. In some trade zones the free migration of employees, including health care staff, is a basic right. It is also hard to argue that health care staff living in poverty and insecurity should be deprived of the opportunity to improve their lives by working in rich and secure countries. Developed countries argue that it is their responsibility to ensure access to health care for their population, although some consideration for the consequences of the country of origin should be shown. Ethical recruitment guidelines have been developed, distinguishing between active recruitment, that is deliberately setting out to attract staff, and passive recruitment, offering open opportunities, for example, by advertising in an international journal. The presence of a bilateral memorandum of agreement is also a indication of good practice.[20] It has to be recognized that international recruitment is not a phenomenon limited to western host countries. It is a global process, with a stream of staff following the trail of higher salaries.

## Funding

If it is accepted that the public sector is responsible for the funding of mental health care, the total amount and by implication the proportion of the health budget to be allocated to mental health has to be determined, whether at a national, regional, or local level. In theory this could be calculated on the basis of a population needs assessment, matching the level of need with the cost of interventions. Many countries have performed epidemiological surveys with a sufficient degree of precision to allow an estimate of the prevalence of diagnostic groups.[21] It is more challenging to take account of the cost of treatment. Attempts to determine the costs of specific interventions are possible in research settings. However, in psychiatry, the cost variation even within homogeneous diagnostic groups attributable to factors such as severity, age, co-morbidity, ethnicity, geography, and social context, as well as supply factors such as the range of treatments and delivery options, make any prediction imprecise, as demonstrated by the challenge of developing Diagnosis Related Groups (DRGs) for mental health care.[22]

The variation of spending on mental health across countries is striking. About 20 per cent of countries in the world dedicate less than 1 per cent of the total health budget on mental health, and a few more than 10 per cent as reported in the WHO Atlas project (2005),[23] with a strong positive correlation between the mental health budget and GDP. Thus, the poorest countries have a very low public spending on mental health, although this ignores the importance of out of pocket payments in many of these countries, sometimes with catastrophic impact on families.

Variations over time of the proportion of health budget allocated to mental health tend to be minor. This suggests that proportion of budget allocated to mental health can be attributed to static factors such as historical spending, often based on running costs of hospitals, adjusted by political priorities and influenced by factors such as advocacy and level of stigma. We do not know of any example of a national formula of rational health budget allocation at treasury/finance ministry level, although a number of countries use a psychiatric needs index to inform sub-national spending decisions.

## Equitable resource allocation

A decision on basis of equity needs to balance the burden of disease for patients, families, and the community (see Chapter 7.5), intensity of human suffering, and the cost-effectiveness of treatment relative to other health conditions. In developed countries budgets can be expected to cover basic needs and simple evidence-based practices across all disease groups. It would be hard to accept in Western Europe or North America that patients have no access to treatments for conditions such as tuberculosis or schizophrenia. Some rationing in a variety of implicit or explicit forms is usually in place for expensive new technologies or costly treatments for common and mild conditions. Whilst mental health has few hi-tech interventions, interventions like CBT would be highly expensive if applied to more than defined subgroups of patients.

In poor countries with very low mental health budgets, many lives will depend on the decision how best to invest the scarce resources in order to gain the greatest cost-effectiveness as measured by DALYs averted. Cost-effectiveness studies have found that episodic treatment with older antidepressant drugs is the most cost-effective treatment in poor countries, whereas the treatment of schizophrenia is relatively more expensive.[24] Even more challenging is to decide on the merit of allocation across disease groups, for example, tuberculosis versus mental health.[25] However, one has to take into account that figures are based on averages, and ignore the very great personal and community benefits that some individual interventions can offer. In mental health, it also has to be considered that interventions are not only about treatment of diseases, but also involve in many instances action against major human rights abuses and the consequences of neglect, such as patients with schizophrenia locked up for years or children ignored in institutions. It is hard to put monetary values on such decisions, and this yet again places mental health activities beyond a narrow health treatment perspective, but shows it as one component of broad public policy making. The challenge is to keep mental health high on the agenda of all public policy makers, rather than it being allowed to slip down every government department's list of priorities.

## Further information

Moniz, C. and Gorin, S.H. (2006). *Health and mental health care policy: a biopsychosocial perspective*. Allyn and Bacon, Boston.

Knapp, M., McDaid, D., Mossialos, E., *et al.* (2006). *Mental health policy and practice across Europe*. Open University Press, Maidenhead.

Brody, E. and Kemp, D.R. (eds.) (1993). *International handbook of mental health policy*. Greenwood Press, Westport.

Jenkins, R., McCulloch, A., Friedli, L., *et al.* (2002). *Developing a national mental health policy*. Maudsley Monograph. The Psychology Press, Hove.

## References

1. Koontz, H. and Weihrich, H. (1988). *Management*. McGraw Hill, New York.
2. McCulloch, A. and Cohen, A. (2007). *Mental health policy and primary mental health care: present and future*. Chapter in Mental health care policy and primary mental health care: present and future. Royal College of General Practitioners, London.
3. Hughes, O.E. (1994). *Public management and administration*. St. Martin's Press, New York.
4. Peters, T. and Waterman, R. (1982). *In search of excellence: lessons from America's best Run Companies*. Harper and Row, New York.
5. Friedman, B. (2005). *The moral consequences of economic growth*. Oxford University Press, Oxford.
6. Bogdanor, V. (2005). *Joined up government*. Oxford University Press, Oxford.
7. Jenkins, R., McCulloch, A., Friedli, L., *et al.* (2002). *Developing a national mental health policy*. Maudsley Monograph 43. The Psychology Press, Hove.
8. Jablensky, A., Sartorius, N., Ensberg, G., *et al.* (1992). Schizophrenia: manifestations, incidence and cause in different cultures—a World Health Organization ten country study. *Psychological Medicine Monograph*, (Suppl. 20), 1–97.
9. WHO. (2005). *WHO resource book on mental health, human rights and legislation*. World Health Organization, Geneva.
10. WHO. (2005). *WHO resource book on mental health, human rights and legislation*. World Health Organization, Geneva.
11. WHO. (2001). *World Health Report 2001: mental health: new understanding, new hope*. World Health Organization, Geneva.
12. Beeharry, G., Whiteford, H., Chambers, D., *et al.* (2002). *Outlining the scope for public health sector involvement in mental health*. The World Bank, Washington, DC.
13. Offer, A. (2006). *The challenge of affluence*. Oxford University Press, Oxford.
14. Layard, R. (2006). *Happiness. Lessons from a new science*. Penguin Books, London.
15. Warr, P. (1987). *Work, unemployment and mental health*. Oxford University Press, Oxford.
16. WHO. (2003). *WHO mental health policy and service guidance package: organization of services for mental health*. World Health Organization, Geneva.
17. Muijen, M. and Ford, R. (1996). The market and mental health: intentional and unintentional incentives. *Journal of Interprofessional Care*, **10**, 13–22.
18. Department of Health. (2006). *From values to action: the chief officer's review of mental health nursing*. Department of Health, London.
19. Muijen, M. (2006). Challenges for psychiatry: delivering the mental health declaration for Europe. *World Psychiatry*, **5**, 113–17.
20. McIntosh, T., Torgerson, R., and Klassen, N. (2007). The ethical recruitment of internationally educated heath professionals: lessons from abroad and options for Canada. Canadian Policy Research Networks, Ottawa, Ontario.
21. WHO World Mental Health Survey Consortium. (2004). Prevalence, severity and unmet need for treatment of mental disorders in the

World Health Organization World Mental Health surveys. *The Journal of the American Medical Association*, **291**, 2581–9.

22. Burgess, P., Pirkis, J., Buckingham, W., *et al.* (1999). Developing a casemix classification for specialist mental health services. *Casemix*, **4**.

23. WHO. (2005). *Atlas: mental health resources in the world 2005*. World Health Organization, Geneva.

24. WHO. (2006). *Dollars, DALYs and decisions: economic aspects of the mental health system*. World Health Organization, Geneva.

25. Jamison, D.T., Breman, J.G., Measham, A.R., *et al.* (2006). *Disease control priorities in developing countries* (2nd edn). World Bank/Oxford University Press, New York.

# Service needs of individuals and populations

Mike Slade, Michele Tansella, and Graham Thornicroft

## Introduction

The importance of needs assessment has been one of the most consistent themes to emerge from the evolution of community mental health services. However, the concept of 'need' is used in different, and sometimes contradictory, ways. The aim of this chapter is to

- define needs assessment
- consider different approaches to assessing needs, both at the individual and at the population levels
- discuss how needs assessments can be applied in real-world settings in planning and delivering clinical care.

## Defining needs

At its simplest, a need involves a lack of something. But of what? In operational terms the concept of need is usually applied to a difficulty (in this case in relation to a person with mental illness) for which a possibly effective intervention exists. By implication an experienced difficulty for which there is no known effective intervention is therefore not defined as a need.[1] The clearest categorization of such needs was identified by Brewin, who grouped definitions of need within mental health care into three categories: lack of health, lack of access to services or institutions, and lack of action by mental health workers.[2] Approaches to need within each of these three categories will be reviewed.

### (a) Needs for improved health

The psychologist Maslow established probably the best-known hierarchy of need, when he formulated a theory of human motivation.[3] In his model, fundamental physiological needs (such as the need for food) underpin the higher needs of safety, love, self-esteem, and self-actualization. He proposed that people are motivated by the requirement to meet these needs, and that higher level needs could only be met once the lower and more fundamental needs were met. The clinical relevance of this theory is that it implies a hierarchy of clinical priorities—interventions to meet basic physiological need (e.g. to ensure adequate food supply) should take priority over interventions to foster, for example, self-esteem.

In practice health-related needs are often considered in a widely defined way. In England, for example, the requirement to base the provision of services on level of need was first made explicit in the National Health Service and Community Care Act,[4] which defined need as *the requirements of individuals to enable them to achieve, maintain, or restore an acceptable level of social independence or quality of life*. This requirement was retained when national standards for mental health services were set.[5] This involves **needs-led** care planning—basing care for an individual patient on an assessment of their health and social needs. The needs-led approach offers many benefits:

1 The overall level of need gives guidance about which part of the mental health system should treat the patient, for example that people with less disabling mental disorders should be seen in primary care settings.[6]

2 Needs assessment can improve the comprehensiveness of case formulations and care plans by incorporating a broad range of health determinants, such as poor housing or lack of social support.

3 Explicit identification of need can support clinician–patient discussions about care priorities, which is associated with improved treatment satisfaction[7,8] and compliance.[9,10]

4 Identification of needs helps to identify the contribution of services outside the psychiatric sector.

5 Needs-led care can facilitate more individualized treatment planning than diagnosis-driven approaches, by more closely matching the help offered to patient's needs and by explicitly identifying problems which require the involvement of both health and other agencies.

Needs-led care planning focussing on health can be differentiated from the assessment of care needs. Assessing care needs involves identifying whether the patient will benefit from a predefined menu of interventions, and by definition will not identify all unmet needs for individual patients. Assessment of need at the patient level should therefore be a separate process from decisions about what care or treatment to provide. There are, however, other reasons to assess needs for services, which we now review.

### (b) Needs for services

The second category of need is a requirement for a particular type of service. At the population level, it is possible to use epidemiological methods to develop prevalence for different disorders, which can be translated into estimates of the need for services. A recent epidemiological survey in the United States, for example, found very considerable unmet need of the population level nationwide.[11] This study identified that between 1990–92 and 2001–03 the overall annual period prevalence of mental illnesses remained constant at between 29.4 and 30.5 per cent. Among these cases, however, there was an increase in the proportion who received any treatment at all, rising from 20.3 to 32.9 per cent between the two time periods. The inverse is however very revealing, namely that the most recent data show that 67 per cent of people with mental disorders in the United States receive no treatment. The situation is worse in other countries. A recent comparative international study of depression found that 0 per cent of patients in St Petersburg received evidence-based treatment in primary care, and only 3 per cent were referred on to specialist mental health care.[12] The inability of patients to afford out-of-pocket costs was the primary barrier to care for 75 per cent of the depressed Russian patients studied.

International comparisons of population-level needs have been conducted in recent years. The ESEMed Study, for example, carried out cross-sectional surveys in Belgium, France, Germany, Italy, the Netherlands, and Spain among 8796 representative members of the general population. Individuals with a 12-month mental disorder that was disabling or that had led to use of services in the previous 12 months were considered in need of care. The study found that about 6 per cent of the sample was defined as being in need of mental health care. Nearly half (48 per cent) of these people reported no formal health care use, so that 3.1 per cent of the adult population had an unmet need for mental health care. In contrast, only 8 per cent of the people with diabetes had reported no use of services for their physical condition.[13]

### (c) Needs for action

In health care, the concept of need has been taken to mean the ability to benefit in some way from health care, and thus distinguished from demand (what the person asks for) and supply (services given).[14] For example, the MRC Needs for Care Assessment Schedule is premised on the assumption that need is 'a normative concept which is to be defined by experts'.[15]

Using this approach, an Australian study compared current and optimal treatment for 10 high-burden mental disorders in Australia.[16] This found that current levels of treatment at current coverage avert 13 per cent of the overall burden attributable to these disorders. Providing optimal treatment at current coverage would avert 20 per cent of the burden, and optimal treatment at optimal coverage would avert 28 per cent. The development of a more robust treatment evidence base makes this innovative approach to informing public policy more possible, and the approach can be recommended for evidence-based policy initiatives.

### Patient and staff perceptions of need

There has been a long-standing recognition that differences in perceptions of need can exist, in particular between staff and patient. In the 1990s the emphasis was put on acknowledging these differences, but then prioritizing the staff perspective. For example,

UK policy stated that *all users ... should be encouraged to participate to the limit of their capacity. ...Where it is impossible to reconcile different perceptions, these differences should be acknowledged and recorded.*[17] Several societal and scientific developments challenge this prioritization of staff over patient perspectives.

First, general societal changes towards consumerism and an emphasis on rights have produced more assertive mental health service users. Easier access by patients to internet-based information reduces the knowledge disparity. Reduced societal trust in the authoritative expert has eroded the position power of mental health staff. The emphasis put on choice and empowerment raise patient expectations of being more than passive recipients of care.[18,19]

Second, the prioritization of staff perspectives has been actively challenged by an increasingly vociferous and organized user movement. This opposition has found its voice in the 'recovery' movement, which emphasizes the meaning and values of the patient, and the need for services to foster self-management rather than dependency. There has been widespread international policy support for recovery-focussed services[20] although there can be tensions between what professionals construe as their duty of care and being led by the patient perspective on need, which can create ethical dilemmas. Care planning which emphasizes agreement between staff and patients may have additional advantages. A recent study in Verona showed staff–patient agreement on needs was significantly associated with better treatment outcomes both rated by the patient and by staff (psychopathology, social disability, global functioning, subjective quality of life, and satisfaction with care).[21] Similarly, there is emerging evidence that crisis plans (advanced statements) which are jointly agreed between staff and patient can be cost-effective in reducing compulsory admission to hospital.[22,23] Such emerging findings indicate that needs assessment and care planning, which are based on negotiation and jointly agreed analyses of problems and interventions, are likely to become increasingly important in future.

Finally, emerging empirical evidence strongly supports the positioning of the patient perspective at the heart of needs assessment and care planning. Evidence from several studies consistently shows differences between staff and patient perspectives on need,[24,25] so the two perspectives are not interchangeable. Empirical research suggests two reasons for basing care on the patient rather than staff assessment of need. First the patient rating is more stable than the staff rating.[26] Second, longitudinal studies indicate a causal relationship between patient-rated (but not staff-rated) unmet need and quality of life.[27–29] If the goal of mental health services is to improve quality of life, then best available evidence indicates that the patient's perspective on their unmet needs should drive care planning.

### Assessing needs

In this section we identify specific approaches to assessing needs.

### (a) Individual-level needs assessment measures

Several standardized approaches to the assessment of patient-level need have been developed, primarily in the United Kingdom. These have shown a transition along a continuum, from an initial focus on assessment of need as an objective state to be defined by experts following careful assessment, towards those which emphasize the subjective nature of needs assessment.

The earliest standardized needs assessment measure was the **Medical Research Council Needs for Care Assessment (NFCAS)**.[30]

The NFCAS assesses the need for further action by health care professionals, and links identification of a need with a predefined list of actions. This raises two problems. First, the emphasis on identifying available interventions which would be at least partly effective is problematic, given the complexities of deciding that a treatment has not worked. Second, updating the list of actions has proved problematic. However, as Bebbington notes, 'the inevitable value judgements inherent in the procedure have the virtue of being public and consequently accessible to argument'.[31] An important variation of the NFCAS is the **Cardinal Needs Schedule (CNS)**,[32] which also considers patient willingness to accept help and level of carer concern. Training is needed for using both the NFCAS and the CNS, and they are primarily used for research purposes.

At the other end of this continuum are needs assessment measures which emphasize individual difference and the subjective nature of need. The **AVON Mental Health Measure** was developed by service users, and assesses physical, social, behaviour, access, and mental health domains.[33] It can take up to 20 min for completion by the patient and 5 min by the staff, and its development has emphasized external validity over other psychometric properties. The **Carers and Users Experience of Services (CUES)** was developed by service users and staff, and assesses 16 domains: the place you live, money situation, the help you get, the way you spend time, your relationships, social life, information/advice, access to services, choice of mental health services, relationship with mental health workers, consultation and contact, advocacy, stigma, any treatment, access to physical health services, and relationship with physical health workers.[34] Completion can take up to 30 min. Neither AVON nor CUES have become widely used in mental health services.

The **Camberwell Assessment of Need (CAN)**[35] spans both ends of the continuum. It assesses 22 domains of health and social need, and a key development is that it records staff and patient views separately, without giving primacy to either perspective. Research (CAN-R), clinical (CAN-C), and brief versions (CANSAS) of the CAN have been developed for adults of working age with severe mental health problems,[36] and it has been translated in 22 languages. Variants have been developed for people with learning disabilities and mental health problems (CANDID),[37] mentally disordered offenders (CANFOR),[38] older adults (CANE),[39] and mothers with mental health problems (CAN-M).[40] An updated web resource for the CAN is available at www.iop.kcl.ac.uk/prism/can.

The CAN has become the most widely used needs assessment measure internationally,[41] and is the standardized needs assessment measure which is most relevant to routine clinical practice. The short version, CANSAS, can be recommended for routine use in community services. Two specific approaches have been empirically shown to produce patient-level benefit. First, the patient-rated two-way communication (2-COM) measure is an amended version of the CAN which gives the patient the opportunity to identify unmet needs and also prioritize those which they wish to discuss with their clinician.[42] Asking patients to complete 2-COM before an outpatient appointment and then using that information in the appointment was associated with greater patient satisfaction and more likelihood of treatment change.[7] Second, a structured approach to collating and feeding back staff and patient ratings for CANSAS and other assessments led to a reduction in psychiatric

admissions, probably because of earlier intervention during relapse,[43] and improvements in patient-rated unmet need and quality of life for higher premorbid IQ patients.[44] Routine use of CANSAS brings patient-level benefits, and empirical evidence indicates the clinical focus should be on assessment and interventions for patient-rated, rather than staff-rated, unmet needs.

### (b) Population-level needs assessment measure

Measures to assess population-based needs can be classified by the data and by the analytic approaches they use. Three types of data are commonly used. The most readily accessible documents the use of current mental health services. While this can be criticized as reflecting only current service provision, its ready availability and nationwide coverage means that is extensively used.

Simple population-based samples are very inefficient in estimating the prevalence of relatively rare conditions such as schizophrenia. Studies thus tend to use two-stage procedures, with a relatively brief initial screening process applied to a large number of people followed in-depth interviews for a selected few. 'Booster' samples, perhaps including all the known psychiatric patients for the areas surveyed, may be sought through mental health services.[45] Population surveys depend on the identification of randomly sampled individuals. Some types of mental health problems, notably substance misuse, are commonly associated with socially marginal lifestyles, making it likely that sufferers will be systematically under-represented by traditional population sampling approaches. More sophisticated sampling approaches, such as capture–recapture methods, have been used for these situations.[46]

The third type of data relates to the views of local people. Local needs assessment studies entail a structured approach to eliciting the views of service users, their carers, interested voluntary sector organizations, and all statutory agencies with responsibilities in the area. Smith[47] has described how this type of study can be integrated into the overall planning process.

Government initiatives in England have tried to base the allocation of money between areas on the morbidity as well as the size of their populations. This has led to studies modelling this variation. The first widely used index[48] was developed on the basis of consensus between GPs about patient characteristics associated with high use of primary care services. While developed for wider purposes, this was shown to relate reasonably closely to variations in psychiatric admission. Later indices have been established by statistical modelling exercises seeking to quantify the relationship between social variables measured in censuses and either service use,[49] or population-based epidemiological findings. The variation between places in the prevalence of the less severe types of mental illness commonly dealt with in primary care is less than that for problems usually managed by specialist mental health services, which again is much less than that observed for forensic services. Thus models developed for one level of care should not be used to estimate patterns of need for other levels.

In practice, no single approach to assessing the needs of a population will suffice. Needs assessment at this level requires the integration of many perspectives. The Kings Fund review of London's mental health Services[50] illustrates how a detailed perspective can be assembled from many fragments of evidence, each of which would be inadequate in isolation. Recent examples of population-level needs assessment from the United States, Canada, and

New Zealand also reveal that epidemiological studies may not produce data that corresponds directly to needs, and that some sub-populations, for example particular ethnic groups, may be less well represented in such approaches, unless considerable methodological care is taken.[51–53]

If a mental health practitioner is asked to join a committee to plan services, for example, for a local catchment area, what approach is helpful to identify and use population-level needs? Table 7.2.1 indicates a series of steps to find the best available information on population prevalence rates.[54]

As Table 7.2.1 shows, we consider that the best possible information would be local epidemiological data on the occurrence of mental disorders, using a standard system of classification, alongside a measure of the needs for treatment among the prevalent cases identified.[55] Since these assessments are expensive and time-consuming, most sites will not have access to such recent local data. If the data in step (1) are not available then we suggest that country/regional epidemiological data (2) are used instead, and are then weighed for local socio-demographic characteristics. But if such larger scale prevalence data are not available, then a third option is to use international rates from 'comparison' countries or regions, again weighted for local socio-demographic characteristics (3). The results in this case will be less accurate because they are based on the additional assumption that the data can be transferred between countries. A newer set of techniques that offer considerable promise are rapid appraisal/rapid assessment techniques. These are methods to undertake brief assessments of population needs which are focussed upon key focussed questions, for example on how primary care services should be augmented to treat people with depression, and example of these approaches have been used to positive effect in South Africa.[56–58]

In some cases, none of the data described in steps 1–3 will be available, and then the next option (4) is to use a number of experts, some of whom may be from the local area, to produce a consensus statement on the local rates and characteristics of people with mental illness. Such a data synthesis can be based on the best available views, taking into account local factors (e.g. levels of non-health service provision, family support, traditions, degree of affluence, or migration). This pragmatic approach will yield data which are accurate enough to use for local service planning purposes.

This raises the important topics of coverage and focussing. *Coverage* means the proportion of people who receive treatment who could benefit from it.[59] *Focussing* refers to how far those people who actually receive treatment in fact need it: do they have any form of mental illness?[60] Even in the most well-resourced countries one can find both low coverage and poor focussing.[61,62] From the public health perspective, therefore, the key issue is the appropriate use of resources, whatever the level of resources actually available, namely to increase both coverage and focus.

### (c) The relationship between individual and population-level needs

We have argued in this chapter that the provision of care for individual patients should be based on assessment of their health and social needs. Can these individual assessments be aggregated to inform service? For population-level service planning, the key question is what types of interventions to provide, and with what capacity. Therefore data from individual needs assessments cannot simply be aggregated to inform service development decisions. While it is theoretically feasible to undertake routine standardized needs assessments on all patients within a service, this approach alone has three drawbacks. Firstly, despite the developing evidence reviewed earlier about the benefits of routine use of standardized outcome assessments, this remains the exception rather than the norm.[63,64] Secondly, there is not yet a sufficiently developed information infrastructure to support the national collection, management, and analysis of such data, despite this being a priority identified two decades ago.[65] Thirdly, even if individual needs assessments were nationally aggregated, the diversity of views (patient, staff, carer, taxpayer) would make a shared interpretation of the data problematic.

## Conclusion

In this chapter we have emphasized that it is of central importance when planning mental health service for populations, to do so on the basis of (i) the occurrence of mental disorders in that particular population, (ii) the impairments caused by these disorders that require interventions, (iii) the nature and level of needs among these people, (iv) identifying from among these needs those which are unmet, and then (v) prioritizing new service development on the basis of these unmet needs, including a range of social supports and services (such as housing or employment opportunities, outside the mental health system), the requirements for enhanced physical/general health care, as well as improvements in the provision of specific mental health services. For all of these sectors there is an increasingly clear call from service user/consumer groups for involvement in these priority-setting planning exercises.[18,19]

At the level of individuals with mental illness, there is a similar trend to increasingly involve service users/consumers in assessing needs, with emerging evidence that this produces a more comprehensive basis for care planning. Indeed in the last decade there has been an important conceptual shift away from the view that professionals defined 'needs' while consumers stated 'demands', to a better appreciation of the many advantages to be gained from identifying, as far as possible, unmet needs in a joint and consensual way as a basis for action.

**Table 7.2.1** Ways to measure or estimate local population mental health prevalence

---

(1) Actual local epidemiological data on psychiatric morbidity and disability for the particular area by age, sex, ethnicity, social status, and degree of urbanicity

(if not available)
↓

(2) Country/regional epidemiological data weighed for local socio-demographic characteristics

(if not available)
↓

(3) International data from 'comparable' countries or regions, adjusted for local socio-demographic characteristics

(If 1, 2, 3 not sufficient)
↓

(4) Best estimates and expert synthesis and interpretation based on other sources of local information and opinions (e.g. extent of non-health service provision, family support, local traditions, or migration)

---

# Further information

Andrews, G. and Henderson, S. (eds.) (2000). *Unmet need in psychiatry*. Cambridge University Press, Cambridge.

Lasalvia, A. and Ruggeri, M. (2007). Multidimensional outcomes in 'real world' mental health services: follow-up findings from the South Verona Project. *Acta Psychiatrica Scandinavica Supplementum*, **437**(S116), 3–77.

Thornicroft, G. (2001). *Measuring mental health needs* (2nd edn). Gaskell, Royal College of Psychiatrist, London.

Thornicroft, G., Becker, T., Knapp, M., et al. (2006). *International outcome measures in mental health. Quality of life, needs, service satisfaction, costs and impact on carers*. Gaskell, Royal College of Psychiatrists, London.

Thornicroft, G. and Tansella, M. (2008). *Better mental health care*. Cambridge University Press, Cambridge.

Regularly updated web site for the Camberwell Assessment of Need is available at: http://www.iop.kcl.ac.uk/prism/can

# References

1. Brewin, C.R. (2001). Measuring individual needs for care and services. In *Measuring mental health needs* (2nd edn) (ed. G. Thornicroft), pp. 273–90. Gaskell, London.

2. Brewin, C. (1992). Measuring individual needs for care and services. In *Measuring mental health needs* (eds. G. Thornicroft, C. Brewin, and J. Wing). Gaskell, Royal College of Psychiatrists, London.

3. Maslow, A. (1954). *Motivation and personality*. Harper & Row, New York.

4. House of Commons (1990). *National health service and community care act*. HMSO, London.

5. Department of Health. (1999). *Mental health national service framework*. HMSO, London.

6. Tansella, M. and Thornicroft, G. (1999). *Common mental disorders in primary care*. Routledge, London.

7. van Os, J., Altamura, A.C., Bobes, J., et al. (2004). Evaluation of the two-way communication checklist as a clinical intervention. *The British Journal of Psychiatry*, **184**, 79–83.

8. Lasalvia, A., Bonetto, C., Malchiodi, F., et al. (2005). Listening to patients' needs to improve their subjective quality of life. *Psychological Medicine*, **35**, 1655–65.

9. Haynes, R.B., McDonald, H.P., and Garg, A.X. (2002). *Interventions for helping patients to follow prescriptions for medications*. Cochrane Library Update Software, Oxford.

10. Gray, R., Leese, M., Bindman, J., et al. (2006). Adherence therapy for people with schizophrenia. European multicentre randomised controlled trial. *The British Journal of Psychiatry*, **189**, 508–14.

11. Kessler, R.C., Demler, O., Frank, R.G., et al. (2005). Prevalence and treatment of mental disorders, 1990 to 2003. *The New England Journal of Medicine*, **352**, 2515–23.

12. Simon, G.E., Fleck, M., Lucas, R., et al. (2004). Prevalence and predictors of depression treatment in an international primary care study. *The American Journal of Psychiatry*, **161**, 1626–34.

13. Alonso, J., Codony, M., Kovess, V., et al. (2007). Population level of unmet need for mental healthcare in Europe. *The British Journal of Psychiatry*, **190**, 299–306.

14. Stevens, A. and Gabbay, J. (1991). Needs assessment needs assessment. *Health Trends*, **23**, 20–3.

15. Bebbington, P. and Rees, S. (2001). Assessing the need for psychiatric services at the district level: using the results of community surveys. In *Measuring mental health needs* (2nd edn) (ed. G. Thornicroft). Gaskell, Royal College of Psychiatrist, London.

16. Andrews, G., Issakidis, C., Sanderson, et al. (2004). Utilising survey data to inform public policy: comparison of the cost-effectiveness of treatment of ten mental disorders. *The British Journal of Psychiatry*, **184**, 526–33.

17. Department of Health Social Services Inspectorate. (1991). *Care management and assessment: practitioners' guide*. HMSO, London.

18. Chamberlin, J. (2005). User/consumer involvement in mental health service delivery. *Epidemiologia e Psichiatria Sociale*, **14**, 10–4.

19. Rose, D., Thornicroft, G., and Slade, M. (2006). Who decides what evidence is? Developing a multiple perspectives paradigm in mental health. *Acta Psychiatrica Scandinavica Supplementum*, **429**(S113) 109–14.

20. New Freedom Commission on Mental Health. (2005). *Achieving the promise: transforming mental health care in America*. Department of Health and Human Services, Rockville, MD.

21. Lasalvia, A., Bonetto, C., Tansella, M., et al. (2007). Does staff-patient agreement on needs for care predict a better mental health outcome? A 4 year follow-up in a community service. *Psychological Medicine*, doi 10.1017/S0033291707000785.

22. Henderson, C., Flood, C., Leese, M., et al. (2004). Effect of joint crisis plans on use of compulsory treatment in psychiatry: single blind randomised controlled trial. *British Medical Journal*, **329**, 136.

23. Flood, C., Byford, S., Henderson, C., et al. (2006). Joint crisis plans for people with psychosis: economic evaluation of a randomised controlled trial. *British Medical Journal*, **333**, 729.

24. Lasalvia, A., Ruggeri, M., Mazzi, M.A., et al. (2000). The perception of needs for care in staff and patients in community-based mental health services. The South-Verona Outcome Project 3. *Acta Psychiatrica Scandinavica*, **102**, 366–75.

25. Hansson, L., Vinding, H.R., Mackeprang, T., et al. (2001). Comparison of key worker and patient assessment of needs in schizophrenic patients living in the community: a Nordic multicentre study. *Acta Psychiatrica Scandinavica*, **103**, 45–51.

26. Slade, M., Leese, M., Taylor, R., et al. (1999). The association between needs and quality of life in an epidemiologically representative sample of people with psychosis. *Acta Psychiatrica Scandinavica*, **100**, 149–57.

27. Slade, M., Leese, M., Ruggeri, M., et al. (2004). Does meeting needs improve quality of life? *Psychotherapy and Psychosomatics*, **73**, 183–9.

28. Lasalvia, A., Bonetto, C., Malchiodi, F., et al. (2005). Listening to patients' needs to improve their subjective quality of life. *Psychological Medicine*, **35**, 1655–65.

29. Slade, M., Leese, M., Cahill, S., et al. (2005). Patient-rated mental health needs and quality of life improvement, *The British Journal of Psychiatry*, **187**, 256–61.

30. Brewin, C., Wing, J., Mangen, S., et al. (1987). Principles and practice of measuring needs in the long-term mentally ill: the MRC needs for care assessment. *Psychological Medicine*, **17**, 971–81.

31. Bebbington, P. (1992). Assessing the need for psychiatric treatment at the district level: the role of surveys. In *Measuring mental health needs* (eds. G. Thornicroft, C. Brewin, and J. Wing). Gaskell, Royal College of Psychiatrists, London.

32. Marshall, M. (1994). How should we measure need? *Philosophy, Psychiatry and Psychology*, **1**, 27–36.

33. Lelliott, P. (2000). What do people want from specialist mental health services and can this be routinely measured in routine service settings? *Behavioural and Cognitive Psychotherapy*, **28**, 361–8.

34. Lelliott, P., Beevor, A., Hogman, J., et al. (2001). Carers' and users' expectations of services—user version (CUES-U): a new instrument to measure the experience of users of mental health services. *The British Journal of Psychiatry*, **179**, 67–72.

35. Phelan, M., Slade, M., Thornicroft, G., et al. (1995). The Camberwell assessment of need: the validity and reliability of an instrument to assess the needs of people with severe mental illness. *The British Journal of Psychiatry*, **167**, 589–95.

36. Slade, M., Loftus, L., Phelan, M., et al. (1999). *The Camberwell assessment of need*. Gaskell, London.

37. Xenitidis, K., Slade, M., Bouras, N., *et al.* (2003). *CANDID: Camberwell assessment of need for adults with developmental and intellectual disabilities.* Gaskell, London.

38. Thomas, S., Harty, M., Parott, J., *et al.* (2003). *The forensic CAN: Camberwell assessment of need forensic version (CANFOR).* Gaskell, London.

39. Reynolds, T., Thornicroft, G., Abas, M., *et al.* (2000). Camberwell assessment of need for the elderly (CANE). Development, validity and reliability. *The British Journal of Psychiatry*, **176**, 444–52.

40. Howard, L., Slade, M., O'Keane, V., *et al.* (eds.) (2008). *The Camberwell assessment of need for pregnant women and mothers with severe mental illness.* Gaskell, London.

41. Evans, S., Greenhalgh, J., and Connelly, J. (2000). Selecting a mental health needs assessment scale: guidance on the critical appraisal of standardized measures. *Journal of Evaluation in Clinical Practice*, **6**, 379–93.

42. van Os, J., Altamura, A.C., Bobes, J., *et al.* (2002). 2-COM: an instrument to facilitate patient-professional communication in routine clinical practice, *Acta Psychiatrica Scandinavica*, **106**, 446–52.

43. Slade, M., McCrone, P., Kuipers, E., *et al.* (2006). Use of standardised outcome measures in adult mental health services: randomised controlled trial. *The British Journal of Psychiatry*, **189**, 330–6.

44. Slade, M., Leese, M., Gillard, M., *et al.* (2006). Premorbid IQ and response to routine outcome assessment. *Psychological Medicine*, **36**, 1183–92.

45. Jenkins, R., Bebbington, P., Brugha, T., *et al.* (1997). The National Psychiatric Morbidity surveys of Great Britain-strategy and methods. *Psychological Medicine*, **27**, 765–74.

46. Hay, G. and McKeganey, N. (1996). Estimating the prevalence of drug misuse in Dundee, Scotland: an application of capture-recapture methods. *Journal of Epidemiology and Community Health*, **50**, 469–72.

47. Smith, H. (1998). Needs assessment in mental health services: the DISC framework. *Journal of Public Health Medicine*, **20**, 154–60.

48. Jarman, B. (1983). Identification of underprivileged areas. *British Medical Journal (Clinical research ed.)*, **286**, 1705–9.

49. McCrone, P., Thornicroft, G., Boyle, S., *et al.* (2006). The development of a local index of need (LIN) and its use to explain variations in social services expenditure on mental health care in England. *Health & Social Care in the Community*, **14**, 254–63.

50. Johnson, S., Ramsay, R., Thornicroft, G., *et al.* (1997). *London's mental health. The report of the Kings Fund Commission.* Kings Fund Publishing, London.

51. Messias, E., Eaton, W., Nestadt, G., *et al.* (2007). Psychiatrists' ascertained treatment needs for mental disorders in a population-based sample. *Psychiatric Services*, **58**, 373–7.

52. Kumar, S., Tse, S., Fernando, A., *et al.* (2006). Epidemiological studies on mental health needs of Asian population in New Zealand. *The International Journal of Social Psychiatry*, **52**, 408–12.

53. Hanson, L., Houde, D., McDowell, M., *et al.* (2006). A population-based needs assessment for mental health services. *Administration and Policy in Mental Health*, **34**, 233–42.

54. Thornicroft, G. and Tansella, M. (1999). *The mental health matrix: a manual to improve services.* Cambridge University Press, Cambridge.

55. Thornicroft, G. (2001). *Measuring mental health needs* (2nd edn). Gaskell, Royal College of Psychiatrists, London.

56. Flisher, A.J., Lund, C., Funk, M., *et al.* (2007). Mental health policy development and implementation in four African countries. *Journal of Health Psychology*, **12**, 505–16.

57. Lund, C. and Flisher, A.J. (2006). Norms for mental health services in South Africa. *Social Psychiatry and Psychiatric Epidemiology*, **41**, 587–94.

58. Lund, C. (2002). *Mental health service norms in South Africa.* PhD thesis. University of Cape Town, Cape Town.

59. Habicht, J.P., Mason, J.P., and Tabatabai, H. (1984). Basic concepts for the design of evaluations during programme implementation. In *Methods for the evaluation of the impact of food and nutrition programmes. Food and nutrition bulletin* (eds. D.R. Sahn, R. Lockwood, and N.S. Scrimshaw), pp. 1–25. The United Nations University, New York.

60. Tansella, M. (2006). Recent advances in depression. Where are we going? *Epidemiologia e Psichiatria Sociale*, **15**, 1–3.

61. World Health Organisation (2005). *Mental health action plan for Europe.* World Health Organisation, Copenhagen.

62. World Health Organisation (2005). *Mental health declaration for Europe.* World Health Organisation, Copenhagen.

63. Gilbody, S.M., House, A.O., and Sheldon, T.A. (2002). Psychiatrists in the UK do not use outcome measures. *The British Journal of Psychiatry*, **180**, 101–3.

64. Valenstein, M., Mitchinson, A., Ronis, D.L., *et al.* (2004). Quality indicators and monitoring of mental health services: what do frontline providers think? *The American Journal of Psychiatry*, **161**, 146–53.

65. Ellwood, P. (1988). Outcomes management–a technology of patient experience. *The New England Journal of Medicine*, **318**, 1549–56.

# Cultural differences care pathways, service use, and outcome

Jim van Os and Kwame McKenzie

This chapter discusses the influence of culture on the route an individual takes to access treatment for psychological distress and the treatment received. Culture is difficult to measure. All categories of cultural variables have different meanings and measure different things. Research into them leads to different hypotheses. Given this reality, there is no need to join the cul-de-sac argument of whether one or the other is the most important. In the discussion below, the roles of ethnicity and of socio-economic, political, community, national, and other factors that help to define the culture of an individual or a group are acknowledged. Associations with pathways to care, service use, and outcome will be presented.

## Care pathways

### Cultural variation in pathways through care

At the beginning of the pathway to care, the individual displays cognitive, physical, or behavioural changes. They or their family, friends, or wider community interpret these as in need of some remedy. The individual's personal resources and then informal resources of family and friends are often triggered to help deal with the problem. These may lead to resolution but if they do not they may lead to presentation through an ever more distant and 'professional' array of caregivers, help agencies, and formal medical services. Most help for psychological problems is not given by mental health services. Interventions and their perceived success or failure move an individual along a pathway.

Pathways through care have differing directions and durations. These depend on where the pathway starts, the presenting symptoms, and psychosocial and cultural factors in the individual, their community, and the services used. Pathways are not random, they are structured and set by a dialogue between the individual, the community, and the code of the statutory services and the law set within that country.[1]

At each level the aim of care is to help the individual move down to less professional interventions until they are either back in the community or at the lowest intensity of care that meets their needs. Traditionally, care pathways have considered routes to getting treatment but with de-institutionalization, social inclusion and the recovery model, pathways out of care need to be considered more widely.

### International comparisons

Cultural variation in pathways to care for a mental health problem is readily, though crudely, demonstrated through international comparisons. For example, in an international study of the pathways to care of 1554 patients newly referred to the mental health services in 11 centres in different countries, the majority of patients (63–80 per cent) were referred by their general practitioner in United Kingdom, Spain, Portugal, Czechoslovakia, Cuba, Mexico, and Aden Democratic Republic of Yemen. Only between 0–15 per cent of patients in these centres had referred themselves, with the exception of Mexico (24 per cent). In Kenya, only 7 per cent were referred by general practitioners but 72 per cent were referred by a hospital doctor. In Pakistan and India, a quarter of patients were referred by general practitioners, a quarter by hospital doctors, a third were self-referred, and 11–17 per cent were referred by religious healers. In Indonesia, both primary care and native healer referrals constituted each around a third of all referrals. The differences between these 11 centres largely reflected the people's choice of first port of call for a psychiatric problem.[2]

International differences in pathways are also reflected in primary health care studies. In a 14 country World Health Organization (WHO) investigation, the proportion of attendees with anxiety and depression as defined by the Composite International Diagnostic Interview (CIDI) varied five-fold across centers. Asian sites reported the lowest rates and European and South American sites the highest. The differences in prevalence may reflect a combination of demographic differences between attendees, true differences in population prevalence, the differential availability of other culture-specific pathways to care for the psychologically distressed, and differential sensitivity of the CIDI in picking up psychiatric disorder in different cultures.[3]

Geographically less dispersed countries also demonstrate significant differences in care pathways. In a recent study of 6 Eastern European countries, the percentage of new patients with schizophrenia who first sought care from psychiatric services ranged from 69 per cent in Bucharest (Romania) to 47 per cent in Zagreb (Croatia). Thirteen percent of patients first sought care from general practitioners in Strumica, Macedonia but 47 per cent in Zagreb. The police were the first port of call in 8 per cent of cases in Bucharest but for none in Zagreb.[4]

This study used the 'encounter form' developed for the WHO which can be used to map and quantify pathways to care (Fig. 7.3.1).

Marked differences in pathways to care also exist within countries and groups. The increase in the use of involuntary admission of African-Caribbeans in the UK and African-Americans in the US is well documented. The reasons for this are unclear but some argue that it reflects service configuration.[5] More recently, increased involuntary admission rates have been reported in the Maori population of Auckland, New Zealand.[6]

Geographic and ecological factors may also contribute to variation in pathways to care within a country. In a Canadian province, involuntary admissions were shown to be related to the size of a community and its proximity to the hospital. Thus, involuntary admission rates were increased if a community was close to the hospital. Rates were also higher in both densely populated inner city areas as well as in cities of less than 500 people. The higher rates of involuntary admission in small towns may be related to a decreased likelihood of being tolerated or remaining anonymous.[7] Despite a similar mental health act, involuntary admissions in Greenland were found to be twice as high as they were in Denmark or the Faroe Islands. The excess risk was associated with the higher homicide rate, lower psychiatric bed availability, lower access to psychiatric care, small settlements, and increased alcohol consumption and violence in Greenland.[8]

## Factors associated with cultural variation in pathways

How interpersonal or cultural factors are translated into differences in pathways has rarely been assessed. However, a number of factors have been identified that contribute to cross-national and cross-ethnic differences.

The family may play an important role. An American study reported that Chinese patients were kept for extended periods of time within their families at the beginning of pathways, while Anglo-Saxons and Central Europeans were referred by their relatives or themselves to a range of mental health and social agencies. Native Americans tended to be referred by people other than relatives or themselves.[9] In another study, both Asians and African-Americans showed more extended family involvement, and the involvement of key family members tended to be persistent and intensive in Asians. Ethnicity was also associated with the length of delay, Asians showing the longest delay and white people, the shortest.[10]

The history of and the way that institutions promote themselves can affect the attitude minority patients have to them and so their likelihood of using them. For example, the view of American hospital services by ethnic minority patients has been tarnished by the American Medical Association's support for segregated wards until the 1960s.[11]

The experience of illness is a culturally shaped phenomenon. The monitoring of change, the understanding of symptoms, the language used to present symptoms, and the fears that accompany symptoms are all suffused with cultural interpretations.[12] Cultural differences in displaying distress are most obviously seen in culture-bound syndromes but are present in the content of delusions and somatic presentation of distress. Somatic symptoms are located in multiple systems of meaning that serve diverse psychological and social functions. In one study, the experience of neurotic patients in India was labeled depressive by clinicians using DSM-IIIR, whereas the patients emphasized their somatic experience.[13] Such discrepancies between professional theory and patients' experience may have an impact on the recognition and treatment of psychiatric disorder. For example, ethnic difference between the doctor and the patient or linguistic/communication problems had previously been offered as reasons for British general practitioners missing depression in South Asian women. However, South Asian doctors are also more likely to miss

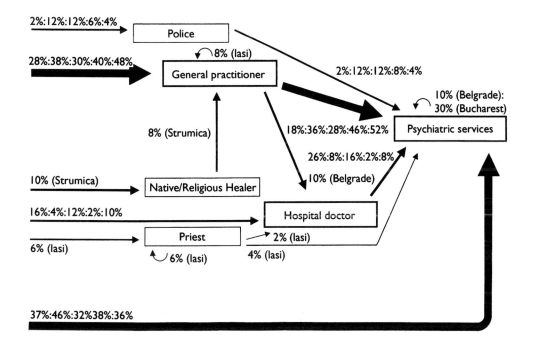

**Fig. 7.3.1** Pathways to psychiatric care in Belgrade, Bucharest, Iasi, Strumica and Zagreb. Percentage of those taking each step for each centre respectively, for carers involved in more than 5 per cent of pathways. Steps occurring in only one or two centres are indicated as a single figure followed by the centre name in brackets. (Curved arrows above carer boxes indicate recursive pathways, where patients have gone from one to another of the same type of carer). Reproduced from Gater, R., Jordanova, V., Maric, N. et al. (2003). Pathways to psychiatric care in Eastern Europe. *British Journal of Psychiatry*, **186**, 529–35, copyright 2003, The Royal College of Psychiatrists.

depression in South Asian women.[14] Thus, rather than 'ethnic match', the culture of medicine may be the important determinant of recognition of depression in this group and its treatment. Longer delays in first contact with a mental health professional,[10] reduce likelihood of successful drug treatment,[15] and poorer outcomes[16] have been reported in groups of Asian patients. The mismatch between patient experience and culture of medicine appears ubiquitous. In Turkey, psychiatric patients with somatic presentations were shown to have longer delays because they went to see hospital doctors first before being referred to a psychiatrist.[17] A study in Nigeria found that a large proportion of depressed patients initially received another diagnosis because of somatic presentation.[18] However, emphasis on somatic experience on the part of the patient does not preclude the patient's recognition of psychological factors, and addressing culturally shaped experience of illness can help clinicians determine underlying aetiology and understand patients with challenging somatic symptoms.[19]

Beliefs about why the problem has arisen, shape the pathway into care. How important this is depends on how different a culture's models of illness and treatment are from that of the service providers. For example, in a study of help-seeking behaviour of families of patients with schizophrenia in India, most of those who believed in supernatural causation consulted indigenous healers first and those who identified schizophrenia as a medical problem consulted practitioners of modern medicine.[20] Similarly, a study in Ghana found that a perceived supernatural cause of mental health problems was associated with a marked reduction in the likelihood of consulting a mental hospital facility.[21] Surveys among Chinese Americans and Mexican Americans show that[22,23] the association between help-seeking, service and acculturation is mediated, amongst others, by beliefs and explanatory models of psychiatric symptoms. Patient satisfaction is highest if the explanatory model of the patient is matched with that of the service provider.[24] Mental health-care professionals are also prone to differences in explanatory models. For example, a comparison between mental health-care professionals in Saudi Arabia and the UK revealed that the staff in the UK believed in a greater range of possible causes and diagnoses for auditory hallucinations than staff in Saudi Arabia. Differences in belief were associated with different expectations regarding efficacy of possible treatments.[25]

Pathways to care are shaped by public opinion and stigma. Such factors can also contribute to the resources that a society will give, and where and by whom treatment is given. A population survey in Germany showed that the lay public generally held psychotherapy in high esteem and the vast majority of respondents rejected pharmacotherapy for psychological problems. Psychoanalysis was the most popular approach in the western part of Germany but in eastern Germany the preference was for group therapy.[26]

Similarly, because psychiatric practice remains to a large degree opinion-based within Europe, differences exist between national samples of psychiatrists with regard to the diagnosis, aetiology, treatment, and outcome of psychiatric disorders such as schizophrenia. Cultural divergence is especially evident with regard to differential emphasis on psychodynamic and biological approaches,[27] and the level of availability of psychotherapy within the health service in European countries appears to be associated with the dominant therapeutic culture of psychiatrists.[28]

The quality of mental health legislation, and, perhaps more importantly, the degree to which correct implementation is enforced have an effect on care pathways. Increased stigma of psychotic illness and fear of public safety have led to compulsory treatment in the community becoming law in the UK. This could change pathways to and through care.[29] In the Netherlands, a weak and impractical act has been criticized for denying patients with severe mental illness the treatment they need. In Spain, to date no specific mental health act exists. In countries like the United Kingdom and France, involuntary admission is in practice, a largely clinical decision, and therefore more easily to put into effect compared with, for example, The Netherlands and most of Germany where the decision is ultimately made by the judiciary. In the United Kingdom and France, the police may bypass medical referral and take people behaving strangely in a public place directly to a psychiatric hospital. This has been shown to be an important pathway for certain ethnic minority groups, such as African-Caribbeans in the United Kingdom.[30]

## Filters on the pathway to care and service use

### Filter permeability and service use

The majority of people in psychological distress never present to formal health services. If formal help is sought, the likelihood of receiving such help is influenced by the permeability of a number of filters (see Chapter 7.8). For example, once the decision to seek formal help is taken, actual receipt of help depends on the ability of the professional at the first port of call (usually primary care services) to recognize the presence of mental disorder. The permeability of subsequent filters determines the rate with which patients move from primary care service to specialist mental health outpatient services, and from specialist outpatient to hospital-based psychiatric services and back down the hierarchy.

### (a) Cross-ethnic differences

There are important cross-ethnic and cross-national differences in the permeability of filters along the pathway to care. Recognition of symptoms by mental health professionals is an important factor. Recognition of distress is dependent on the way symptoms are elicited. For instance, the recognition by primary care doctors of psychiatric disorder in African-Caribbeans and South Asians in the United Kingdom has been shown to be poor.[31] There are a number of reasons for this including differences between the symptoms expected by doctors and those presented.[12] Despite the fact that they visit their general practitioner more often, women of South Asian origin with depression are less likely to be diagnosed and treated than white British women. Detection of depression depends on the doctor's skill but also whether the patient tells the general practitioner about her worries. Those who believed that a doctor was the right person to deal with depression were found to be more likely to disclose information and more likely to be diagnosed and treated.[12] South Asian women are less likely than white British women to think that a doctor was the right person to deal with depression.[32] A one-year follow-up of the sample of the Epidemiologic Catchment Area Program revealed that African-Americans, Hispanics, and other minorities were much less likely to have consulted with a professional in the specialized mental health care sector than white people. The odds of consultation in African-Americans was less than one-quarter of that in white people even after adjustment for confounders.[33] Similarly,

African-American children and adolescents may also remain under-treated although they may have higher levels of symptomatology.[34] Differences between American ethnic groups are also apparent in populations with identical insurance coverage.[35] Hence, these findings[36] suggest low permeability of filters on the pathway to mental health care. Reasons for this may include that African-Americans are less inclined to seek professional help because of increased tolerance to depressive symptoms, but also because of fear of hospital admission.[37] In comparison to all other ethnic groups, African-Americans make more use of emergency rooms for routine psychiatric care.[38]

Despite the low permeability of the filters on the pathway to care there is an over-representation of African-Caribbeans and African-Americans at the level of hospital-based psychiatric services. Possible mechanisms for this include failure of community services to engage mentally ill African-Caribbean men[39] and bypass of the usual filters by, for example, compulsory admission to hospital with or without police involvement.[40] It has been shown that police involvement and compulsory admission to hospital is strongly associated with the absence of general practitioner involvement.[41] Levels of perceived violence and rates of involuntary admission may be due to stereotyped attitudes of the police and mental health professionals or may be in part due to a higher rate of presentation of psychosis that is superimposed on intact premorbid personalities. It has been suggested that reactive forms of psychotic illness in African-Caribbeans are wrongly labelled as schizophrenia.[42] Higher functioning, less withdrawn patients may be perceived as constituting a higher risk by police and mental health professionals. Another factor is that, despite low rates of recognition by general practitioners, African-Caribbeans are most likely to be referred on to a specialist, followed by white people and then people from south Asia even when socioeconomic class and diagnosis are taken into account.[31]

## (b) Cross-national differences

Cross-national differences in filter permeability and service use are difficult to examine. Service organization plays an important role. For example, compared with south Manchester, in the United Kingdom, closer integration between community and inpatient psychiatric services in south Verona, Italy, resulted in a greater permeability of the filter between inpatient and community care, as evidenced by higher hospital admission rates and shorter lengths of stay. Conversely, greater permeability of the general practitioner referral filter in south Manchester resulted in more referrals, and therefore higher treated incidence and prevalence rates of psychiatric disorder.[43] Similarly, compared with the more institution-based system in Groningen, in The Netherlands, the south Verona community-based system provided for a higher degree of continuity of care across services for patients with schizophrenia.[44]

Because of convergence in methodology, fascinating material on cross-national differences in the dynamic balance between psychological distress, need for care, and actual treatment received is now available from large prevalence surveys of representative samples in different countries. Comparative data are available on three large population studies in three countries. In the United States and Ontario (Canada), samples representative of all non-institutionalized individuals aged 18 to 54 years were examined using the Composite International Diagnostic Interview (CIDI) in 1990 and samples of people aged 18 to 64 years in The Netherlands were examined in 1996 (Nemesis Study).[45–47]

The three studies show that help-seeking rates among individuals with a diagnosable disorder vary widely. The contact rate with any type of formal or informal service was lowest in the United States (33.9 per cent) and not far from twice as high in The Netherlands (56.7 per cent) (Table 7.3.1). Among individuals with a diagnosable disorder, ambulatory service use in the general medical sector was much higher in Ontario and The Netherlands than in the United States, especially among those with more severe comorbid

**Table 7.3.1** Prevalence of CIDI disorder and service use in three countries

| | 12-month prevalence | Service use | | | |
| | | General medical[a] | Ambulatory mental health[b] | Any service | Perceived need for care in non-users of professional services |
| --- | --- | --- | --- | --- | --- |
| *National Comorbidity Survey* | | | | | |
| No disorder[c] | 54.0 | 2.6 | 2.6 | 7.6 | |
| One disorder | 15.7 | 5.6 | 8.3 | 18.8 | 8.4 |
| Two disorders | 12.0 | 10.2 | 18.6 | 33.9 | |
| *Ontario* | | | | | |
| No disorder' | 65.6 | 1.5 | 1.2 | 3.3 | |
| One disorder | 127 | 9.7 | 6.3 | 17.8 | 5.4 |
| Two disorders | 5.9 | 24.3 | 23.5 | 39.4 | |
| *Nemesis* | | | | | |
| No disorder[c] | 58.8 | 3.8 | 1.8 | 6.1 | |
| One disorder | 15.3 | 15.5 | 7.8 | 22.5 | 3.8 |
| Two disorders | 8.1 | 42.8 | 30.3 | 56.7 | |

[a] Non-psychiatrist physician in any setting or allied health professional in a general medical setting.

[b] Psychiatrist or psychologist in any setting or allied health professional (e.g. nurse, social worker) in a psychiatric or addiction treatment setting.

[c] No lifetime history of any disorder at all.

Weighted data from Kessler *et al.*[45] and Bijl *et al.*[47]

disorders. Individuals in the United States with more severe disorders were less likely to use services in the health-care sector as a whole, but if treatment from self-help and other sources is included, the difference between Ontario and Nemesis on the one hand, and the United States on the other, is attenuated. This suggests that low permeability of the primary care access and primary care referral filters in the United States may lead to increased use of non-professional services to fill the gap.

Table 7.3.1 shows that the higher the contact rates with professional services of individuals with a CIDI diagnosis, the lower the number of individuals who were not using professional services but felt they were in need of such help (level of unmet need) (Table 7.3.1). Such differences in the population level of unmet need are important from the point of view of public health. For example, if 90 per cent in a population of 200 million are non-users of professional services for mental health problems, then the difference between 8.4 per cent (United States) and 3.8 per cent (The Netherlands) in perceived need is a difference of 9.2 million individuals.

The substantial differences in mental health care provided by the general practitioner are likely to have an equally substantive impact on the likelihood of receiving appropriate management. Thus, the proportion of patients with major depression (as defined in DSM-IIIR) in the previous 12 months who received appropriate medication management, defined as a combination of antidepressant medication use and four or more visits to any health-care provider within the previous 12 months, was much higher in Ontario (14.9 per cent) than in the United States (7.3 per cent). This difference was especially marked for the lowest income groups in the two countries. Individuals in the lowest income groups in the United States were found to be 7.5 times less likely to make contact with either general or specialty health-care providers than their peers in Ontario. For the highest income groups, however, contact rates differed only by a factor 2.1.[48] These data suggest that economic barriers play an important role in determining the permeability of the filters on the pathway to care. In a United Kingdom national survey, 16 per cent of patients with a depressive episode in the past week according to the Revised Clinical Interview Schedule were current users of antidepressant medication.[49]

Because the majority of the population does not have a mental disorder, even a small degree of service use by this large segment of the population will take up a considerable part of the total capacity of mental health services. Thus, Katz *et al.*[50] noted that because of the relatively high rates of perceived need for care and help-seeking among individuals without a CIDI diagnosis in the United States, total mental health outpatient service use was higher in that country than in Ontario. Although diagnosis is only an imperfect indicator of need for care, the results nevertheless suggest that the mismatch between need and care in the population is greater in the United States than in Ontario.

A long-standing debate exists whether and how financing of mental health care can be used to maximize the fit between need and care in the population. A frequently expressed concern is that universal coverage will lead to an increase of people with little need using services of unproven value. The opposite argument, however, is that limitations in coverage will result in service use that is poorly matched to need. Although it is thought that differences in type of insurance system have an impact on demand and utilization of mental health services,[51] systematic comparisons between

countries have been lacking. The systems of coverage in the United States, Canada, and The Netherlands are different in many respects. In Ontario, universal and relatively comprehensive coverage for mental health services exists, with no or minimal limits on inpatient stays or outpatient visits for mental health services, and minimal patient cost sharing. In The Netherlands, almost all mental health care is covered under the Exceptional Medical Expenses Act, and is available to the entire population. A comprehensive range of public services exists, with few supply-side controls. In the United States, at least 16 per cent of the population is uninsured, and even for the insured mental health coverage is increasingly limited. Although the public health system provides mental health care at little or no cost to the poor and the uninsured, supply-side controls severely and increasingly limit access. Therefore, the results of the comparisons between the three countries do not support the frequently expressed reservation that expansion of insurance coverage for mental health disorders results in an increase in unnecessary use of services. Of the three countries considered, those with broad mental health coverage actually treated a similar number or more people with severe mental illness, but less people who never had a history of mental illness.

## Treatment and response

Culture has an important influence on the type of service received. There are reports that African-Caribbean and African-American patients receive antipsychotic medications in a higher prescribed dose, and more frequent use of injectable preparations is made.[30,52–57] Asian patients have been reported to receive lower doses.[58,59] Some ethnic minority groups may receive less information about side-effects,[60] which may result in less vigilance with regard to onset of problems such as tardive dyskinesia. In the United States and the United Kingdom, ethnic minority patients are less likely to receive psychological treatment.[61,62] In the United States, African-American children have substantially lower rates of receiving methylphenidate.[63,64] Such differences may be related to differences in explanatory models of African-American parents, and differences in the rate with which African-American parents receive appropriate information about attention deficit–hyperactivity disorder from the doctor.[65]

There are several important considerations with regard to outcome in relation to cultural variables.[66] The first is that services offered may not be equally efficacious for different groups of people. For example, Chinese, Japanese, Filipino, Korean, and Southeast Asian Americans who were treated in the same setting in Los Angeles County showed different outcomes. Filipinos were under-represented in the system, whereas Southeast Asians were over-represented and had higher rates of service utilization. Despite this, Southeast Asians showed less improvement than the other groups, even after controlling for diagnosis and initial level of functioning.[67] The second is that treatment uptake may differ between groups.[33] In the United Kingdom and the United States, uptake of treatment with antipsychotic medication may be higher in white patients, though the overall influence of ethnicity remains small.[68] The third consideration is that the expectations about the desired endpoint of treatment may not be the same for different groups of people. For example, the expectations of British Asian and white people relating to the process and outcome of a psychological intervention were shown to be different in one study.[69]

Outcome may improve if therapists receive information about their clients' cultural background and expectations before treatment.[70] Perhaps the most important consideration is that outcome is a multidimensional concept defying summary statements. For example, clinical outcome in terms of usual symptom severity and risk of self-harm may be better in African-Caribbean patients with psychosis as compared with white people, yet risk of imprisonment and compulsory admission may be greater,[71] as may be the frequency of relapse[72] and the rate of dissatisfaction with services.[73]

However, it is interesting to note that a recent pan-European study has concluded that despite the fact that differences in health-care systems may affect service provision and cost, the impact of such differences on outcome may be less marked. More work needs to be undertaken on cultural differences in care pathways and treatment to see if they change outcomes.[74] Moreover, at an individual level, recent work has failed to show differences in the duration of untreated psychosis between African Caribbeans and whites in the UK,[75] even though they have different pathways to care at first admission indicating that the impact of cultural or ethnic differences in pathways can be difficult to predict.

### Pathways out of care

Pathways out of care are complex and have multiple influences. An important influence is the pathway into care because the relationship set up with services at first contact determines, in part, the trajectory of the clinical career of a patient. Moreover, in specific circumstances, such as where the criminal justice system is involved, certain responsibilities may be placed on services which constrain the ability to discharge patients. There has been little research which aims to understand ethnic differences in pathways out of care.[76] This reflects the fact that the focus of studies to date has been to document any inequalities in access to care.

Pathways out of statutory sector care are influenced by the effectiveness of treatment strategies, the illness models and treatment preferences of patients, the structure and funding of clinical services, the availability of and access to nonstatutory sector support and also the socio-cultural context in which people live.

Effectiveness is a combination of the efficacy of a treatment and the real world context which influences outcomes. Though there may be differences in the efficacy of drugs by racial group, differences in compliance are more likely to be important,[77] and there are well documented differences in adherence to treatment programs which may lead to differences in rates of patients leaving care.[78]

Adherence has been linked to differences in illness models but in psychosis the level of discord between patient and treatment service illness models are not consistently associated with differences in outcome.[79] This may reflect the fact that preferred alternative treatment outside statutory mental health services are not available or that services are more coercive with patients who do not fully subscribe to their model.

The structure and funding of clinical services is important. Filters out of care can be porous—an example of this is Ontario, where rehabilitation is mainly offered by local community based organizations which may have better links with the community and so make transition out of care easier. They also have limited responsibility for their clients compared to the UK and may be less risk averse. Risk averse service cultures can lead to delay in discharge

from care.[80] Moreover, putting the onus on risk can mean that ethnic groups who are considered more risky have particular difficulty in getting out of care.

Prevailing law also shapes pathways out of care. Such laws may be applied differently to some ethnic groups. For instance, in New Zealand, the Maori population is more likely to be detained on community treatment orders thus delaying movement out of statutory service care.[81]

The availability of nonprofessional support and the structure of some cultural groups may affect pathways. Those of South Asian origin with severe mental illness spend less time in hospital and outpatient care. Family support is cited as the reason for this. Socio-cultural mores are important but also geographic concentration; dispersed refugee and asylum groups with limited access to community support may stay longer in services than would be expected from their symptoms. But socially cohesive groups can be a double-edged sword. One study has demonstrated higher rates of re-admission in areas with high social capital which arguably could be a result of high levels of health norm policing and low levels of tolerance for deviance.[82]

Socio-economic factors also need to be kept in mind when considering the capacity of communities to offer care. The decreased resources available to low income groups will be important in determining the level of burden they will be able to accept.

## Further information

World Health Organization: up to date information on the health with a good archive, research tools and data as well as a section which summarizes health systems organization and funding for each of the countries in the world. http://www.who.int/en/

World Association of Cultural Psychiatry: free newsletter and journal on cross cultural psychiatry issues at: http://www.waculturalpsychiatry.org/

National Institute for Clinical Excellence in the UK has developed a pathways approach to improving mental health services for people with schizophrenia backed by algorithms and research evidence: http://www.schizophreniaguidelines.co.uk/nice_implementation/pathways_to_care.php.

## References

1. Rogler, L.H. and Cortes, D.E. (1993). Help-seeking pathways: a unifying concept in mental health care. *American Journal of Psychiatry*, **150**, 554–61.
2. Gater, R., de Almeida e Sousa, B., Barrientos, G., *et al.* (1991). The pathways to psychiatric care: a cross-cultural study. *Psychological Medicine*, **21**, 761–74.
3. Üstün, T.B. and Sartorius, N. (eds.) (1995). *Mental illness in genera health care*. Wiley, New York.
4. Gater, R., Jordanova, V., Maric, N., *et al.* (2003). Pathways to psychiatric care in eastern Europe. *British Journal of Psychiatry*, **186**, 529–35.
5. Bhui, K., Stansfeld, S., Hull, S., *et al.*(2003). Ethnic variations in pathways to and use of specialist mental health services in the UK. Systematic review. *British Journal of Psychiatry*, **182**, 105–16.
6. Wheeler, A., Robinson, E., Robinson, G., *et al.* (2005). Admissions to acute psychiatric inpatient services in Auckland, New Zealand: a demographic and diagnostic review. *NZ med J*, **118** (1226): u1752.
7. Malla, A. and Norman, R.M.G. (1988). Involuntary admissions in a Canadian province: the influence of geographic and population factors. *Social Psychiatry and Psychiatric Epidemiology*, **23**, 247–51.
8. Engberg, M. (1991). Involuntary commitment in Greenland, the Faroe Islands and Denmark. *Acta Psychiatrica Scandinavica*, **84**, 353–6.

9. Lin, T.Y., Tardiff, K., Donetz, G., et al. (1978). Ethnicity and patterns of help-seeking. Culture in Medicine and Psychiatry, 2, 3–13.

10. Lin, K.M., Inui, T.S., Kleinman, A.M., et al. (1982). Sociocultural determinants of the help-seeking behavior of patients with mental illness. Journal of Nervous and Mental Disorders, 170, 78–85.

11. King, G. (1996). Institutional racism and the medical health complex: a conceptual analysis. Ethnicity and Disease, 6, 30–46.

12. Kleinman, A. (1991). Rethinking psychiatry. Free Press, New York.

13. Weiss, M.G., Raguram, R., and Channabasavanna, S.M., et al. (1995). Cultural dimensions of psychiatric diagnosis. A comparison of DSM-IIIR and illness explanatory models in south India. British Journal of Psychiatry, 166, 353–9. Erratum: British Journal of Psychiatry, 167, 119 (1995).

14. Jacob, K.S., Bhugra, D., Lloyd, K.R., et al. (1998). Common mental disorders, explanatory models and consultation behaviour among Indian women living in the UK. Journal of the Royal Society of Medicine, 91, 66–71.

15. Cornwell, J. (1998). Do general practitioners prescribe antidepressants differently for South Asian patients? Family Practice, 15, S16–18.

16. Ying, Y.-W. and Hu, L.-T. (1994). Public outpatient mental health services: use and outcome among Asian Americans. American Journal of Orthopsychiatry, 64, 448–55.

17. Kilic, C., Rezaki, M., Üstün, T.B., et al. (1994). Pathways to psychiatric care in Ankara. Social Psychiatry and Psychiatric Epidemiology, 29, 131–6.

18. Makanjuola, J.D. and Olaifa, E.A. (1987). Masked depression in Nigerians treated at the Neuro–Psychiatric Hospital Aro, Abeokuta. Acta Psychiatrica Scandinavica, 76, 480–5.

19. Handelman, L. and Yeo, G. (1996). Using explanatory models to understand chronic symptoms of Cambodian refugees. Family Medicine, 28, 271–6.

20. Banerjee, G. and Roy, S. (1998). Determinants of help-seeking behaviour of families of schizophrenic patients attending a teaching hospital in India: an indigenous explanatory model. International Journal of Social Psychiatry, 44, 199–214.

21. Fosu, G.B. (1995). Women's orientation toward help-seeking for mental disorders. Social Science and Medicine, 40, 1029–40.

22. Wells, K.B., Hough, R.L., Golding, J.M., et al. (1987). Which Mexican-Americans underutilize health services? American Journal of Psychiatry, 144, 918–22.

23. Ying, Y.-W. and Miller, L.S. (1992). Help-seeking behavior and attitude of Chinese Americans regarding psychological problems. American Journal of Community Psychology, 20, 549–56.

24. Callan, A. and Littlewood, R. (1998). Patient satisfaction: ethnic origin or explanatory model? International Journal of Social Psychiatry, 44, 1–11.

25. Wahass, S. and Kent, G. (1997). A cross-cultural study of the attitudes of mental health professionals towards auditory hallucinations. International Journal of Social Psychiatry, 43, 184–92.

26. Angermeyer, M.C. and Matschinger, H. (1996). Public attitude towards psychiatric treatment. Acta Psychiatrica Scandinavica, 94, 326–36.

27. van Os, J., Galdos, P., Lewis, G., et al. (1993). Schizophrenia sans frontieres: concepts of schizophrenia among French and British psychiatrists. British Medical Journal, 307, 489–92.

28. van Os, J. and Neeleman, J. (1994). Caring for mentally ill people. British Medical Journal, 309, 1218–21.

29. Department of Health (2007) regulatory impact assessment of mental health bill available at dh.gov.uk/prod_consum_dh

30. Dunn, J. and Fahy, T.A. (1990). Police admissions to a psychiatric hospital. Demographic and clinical differences between ethnic groups. British Journal of Psychiatry, 156, 373–8.

31. Rawaf, S. and Bahl, V. (1998). Assessing health needs of people from minority ethnic groups. Royal College of Physicians of London.

32. Lloyd, K.R., Jacob, K.S., Patel, V., et al. (1998). The development of the Short Explanatory Model Interview (SEMI) and its use among primary-care attenders with common mental disorders. Psychological Medicine, 28, 1231–7.

33. Gallo, J.J., Marino, S., Ford, D., et al. (1995). Filters on the pathway to mental health care. II. Sociodemographic factors. Psychological Medicine, 25, 1149–60.

34. Cuffe, S.P., Waller, J.L., Cuccaro, M.L., et al. (1995). Race and gender differences in the treatment of psychiatric disorders in young adolescents. Journal of the American Academy of Child and Adolescent Psychiatry, 34, 1536–43.

35. Scheffler, R.M. and Miller, A.B. (1989). Demand analysis of mental health service use among ethnic subpopulations. Inquiry, 26, 202–15.

36. Brown, D.R., Ahmed, F., Gary, L.E., et al. (1995). Major depression in a community sample of African Americans. American Journal of Psychiatry, 152, 373–8.

37. Sussman, L.K., Robins, L.N., Earls, F., et al. (1987). Treatment-seeking for depression by black and white Americans. Social Science and Medicine, 24, 187–96.

38. Neighbors, H.W. (1986). Ambulatory medical care among adult black Americans: the hospital emergency room. Journal of the National Medical Association, 78, 275–82.

39. Bhui, K., Brown, P., Hardie, T., et al. (1998). African-Caribbean men remanded to Brixton Prison—psychiatric and forensic characteristics and outcome of final court appearance. British Journal of Psychiatry, 172, 337–44.

40. Morgan, C., Mallett, R., Hutchinson, G., et al. (2005). On behalf of the ÆSOP Study Group Pathways to care and ethnicity II; Source of referral and help seeking. A Report From the ÆSOP (Aetiology and Ethnicity in Schizophrenia and Other Psychoses) Study. British Journal of Psychiatry, 186, 290–6.

41. Cole, E., Leavey, G., King, M., et al. (1995). Pathways to care for patients with a first episode of psychosis. A comparison of ethnic groups. British Journal of Psychiatry, 167, 770–6.

42. Littlewood, R. and Lipsedge, M. (1978). Migration, ethnicity and diagnosis. Psychiatric Clinics of Basel, 11, 15–22.

43. Amaddeo, F., Gater, R., Goldberg, D., et al. (1995). Affective and neurotic disorders in community-based services: a comparative study in south Verona and south Manchester. Acta Psychiatrica Scandinavica, 91, 386–95.

44. Sytema, S., Micciolo, R., Tansella, M., et al. (1997). Continuity of care for patients with schizophrenia and related disorders: a comparative south Verona and Groningen case-register study. Psychological Medicine, 27, 1355–62.

45. Kessler, R.C., Frank, R.G., Edlund, M., et al. (1997). Differences in the use of psychiatric outpatient services between the United States and Ontario. New England Journal of Medicine, 336, 551–7.

46. Katz, S.J., Kessler, R.C., Frank, R.G., et al. (1997). The use of outpatient mental health services in the United States and Ontario: the impact of mental morbidity and perceived need for care. American Journal of Public Health, 87, 1136–43.

47. Bijl, R.V., Ravelli, A., Van Zessen, G., et al. (1998). Prevalence of psychiatric disorder in the general population: results from The Netherlands mental health survey and incidence study. Social Psychiatry and Psychiatric Epidemiology, 33, 587–95.

48. Katz, S.J., Kessler, R.C., Lin, E., et al. (1998). Medication management of depression in the United States and Ontario. Journal of General Internal Medicine, 13, 77–85.

49. Meltzer, H., Gill, B., Petticrew, M., et al. (1995). OPCS surveys of psychiatric morbidity. Report 1: the prevalence of psychiatric morbidity among adults aged 16–64 living in private households in Great Britain. HMSO, London.

50. Katz, S.J., Kessler, R.C., Frank, R.G., et al. (1997). The use of outpatient mental health services in the United States and Ontario: the impact of mental morbidity and perceived need for care. American Journal of Public Health, 87, 1136–43.

51. Frank, R.G. and McGuire, T.G. (1986). A review of studies of the impact of insurance on the demand and utilization of specialty mental health services. *Health Services Research*, **21**, 241–65.

52. Citrome, L., Levine, J., Allingham, B., *et al.* (1996). Utilization of depot neuroleptic medication in psychiatric inpatients. *Psychopharmacology Bulletin*, **32**, 321–6.

53. Segal, S.P., Bola, J.R., Watson, M.A., *et al.* (1996). Race, quality of care, and antipsychotic prescribing practices in psychiatric emergency services. *Psychiatric Services*, **47**, 282–6.

54. Lawson, W.B. (1996). Clinical issues in the pharmacotherapy of African-Americans. *Psychopharmacology Bulletin*, **32**, 275–81.

55. Price, N., Glazer, W., Morgenstern, H., *et al.* (1985). Demographic predictors of the use of injectable versus oral antipsychotic medications in outpatients. *American Journal of Psychiatry*, **142**, 1491–2.

56. Shubsachs, A.P., Huws, R.W., Close, A.A., *et al.* (1995). Male Afro-Caribbean patients admitted to Rampton Hospital between 1977 and 1986—a control study. *Medicine, Science and Law*, **35**, 336–46.

57. Strakowski, S.M., Shelton, R.C., Kolbrener, M.L., *et al.* (1993). The effects of race and comorbidity on clinical diagnosis in patients with psychosis. *Journal of Clinical Psychiatry*, **54**, 96–102.

58. Rosenblat, R. and Tang, S.W. (1987). Do oriental psychiatric patients receive different dosages of psychotropic medication when compared with occidentals. *Canadian Journal of Psychiatry*, **32**, 270–4.

59. Bond, W.S. (1991). Ethnicity and psychotropic drugs. *Clinical Pharmacology*, **10**, 467–70.

60. Benson, P.R. (1984). Drug information disclosed to patients prescribed antipsychotic medication. *Journal of Nervous and Mental Disease*, **172**, 642–53.

61. Olfson, M. and Pincus, H.A. (1994). Outpatient psychotherapy in the United States. II. Patterns of utilization. *American Journal of Psychiatry*, **151**, 1289–94.

62. Littlewood, R. and Lipsedge, M. (1997). *Aliens and alienists*. Routledge, New York.

63. Zito, J. M., Safer, D. J., dos Reis, S., *et al.* (1997). Methylphenidate patterns among Medicaid youths. *Psychopharmacology Bulletin*, **33**, 143–7.

64. Zito, J. M., Safer, D. J., dos Reis, S., *et al.* (1998). Racial disparity in psychotropic medications prescribed for youths with Medicaid insurance in Maryland. *Journal of the American Academy of Child and Adolescent Psychiatry*, **37**, 179–84.

65. Bussing, R., Schoenberg, N.E., Perwien, A.R., *et al.* (1998). Knowledge and information about ADHD: evidence of cultural differences among African-American and white parents. *Social Science and Medicine*, **46**, 919–28.

66. McKenzie, K. and Murray, R.M. (1998). *Risk factors for mental illness in African-Caribbeans*. Department of Health Conference on Culture, Ethnicity and Mental Health. Department of Health, London.

67. Ying, Y.W. and Hu, L.T. (1994). Public outpatient mental health services, use and outcome among Asian Americans. *American Journal of Orthopsychiatry*, **64**, 448–55.

68. Bebbington, P.E. (1995). The content and context of compliance. *International Clinics in Psychopharmacology*, **5**, 41–50.

69. Balabil, S. and Dolan, B. (1992). A cross-cultural evaluation of expectations about psychological counselling. *British Journal of Medical Psychology*, **65**, 305–8.

70. Yamamoto, J., Acosta, F. X., Evans, L.A., *et al.* (1984). Orienting therapists about patients' needs to increase patient satisfaction. *American Journal of Psychiatry*, **141**, 274–7.

71. McKenzie, K., van Os, J., Fahy, T., *et al.* (1995). Psychosis with good prognosis in Afro-Caribbean people now living in the United Kingdom. *British Medical Journal*, **311**, 1325–8.

72. Birchwood, M., Cochrane, R., Macmillan, F., *et al.* (1992). The influence of ethnicity and family structure on relapse in first-episode schizophrenia. A comparison of Asian, Afro-Caribbean, and white patients. *British Journal of Psychiatry*, **161**, 783–90.

73. Parkman, S., Davies, S., Leese, M., *et al.* (1997). Ethnic differences in satisfaction with mental health services among representative people with psychosis in south London: PRiSM Study 4. *British Journal of Psychiatry*, **171**, 260–4.

74. Becker, T., Kilian, R. (2006). Psychiatric services for people with severe mental illness across western Europe: what can be generalized from current knowledge about differences in provision, cost and outcomes of mental health care *Acta Psychiatr Scan*, Suppl 429, 9–16

75. Morgan, C., Fearon, P., Hutchinson, G., AESOP Study Group., *et al.* (2006) Duration of untreated psychosis and ethnicity in the AESOP first-onset psychosis study. *Psychological Medicine,* **36**(2), 239–47

76. EPIC group (2007). ww.wolfson.qmul.ac.uk/psychiatry/epic/docs/SRper cent20Keyper cent20Summary.pdf accessed

77. Lin, K.M., Anderson, D., Poland, R.E., *et al.* (1995). Ethnicity and psychopharmacology. Bridging the gap. *Psychiatr Clin North Am.* **18**(3), 635–47.

78. Sue, S., Fujino, D. C., Hu, L. T., *et al.* (1991). Community mental health services for ethnic minority groups: a test of the cultural responsiveness hypothesis. *J Consult Clin Psychol*, **59**(4), 533–40.

79. Rosemarie McCabe, PhD and Stefan Priebe, MD. (2004). Explanatory models of illness in schizophrenia: comparison of four ethnic groups *The British Journal of Psychiatry,* **185**, 25–30

80. Lelliott, P. and Audini, B. (2003). Trends in the use of Part II of the Mental Health Act 1983 in seven English local authority areas. Br J Psychiatry, **182**, 68–70.

81. Gibbs, A., Dawson, J., Forsyth, H., (2004). Maori experience of community treatment orders in Otago, New Zealand. *Aust N Z J Psychiatry*, **38**(10), 830–5s

82. McKenzie, K. (2000). Neighborhood, safety and mental health outcomes. Postingnumber 28, 2000. Social Capital Lets Talk. Socialcapital@tome. worldbank.org

# 7.4

# Primary prevention of mental disorders

## J. M. Bertolote

Despite the demonstration of the possibility of preventing some forms of mental disorders, many mental health professionals continue to underestimate the possibilities of primary prevention in their field. This is due to:

1 a lack of clear concepts when referring to this issue;

2 the fact that the effective prevention of mental and neurological disorders often falls outside the usual remit of mental health professionals (in many cases it falls outside the health sector altogether).

These two factors are discussed below, in addition to an indication of actions which effectively prevent some forms of mental disorders.

## Prevention

In the late 1950s, Leavell and Clark[1] proposed a three-level concept of prevention (primary, secondary, and tertiary), covering almost all medical actions. Their innovative approach must be understood in relation to what they also called the horizon of the natural history of the disease process: under natural circumstances, a disease will proceed from a prepathological period through its early stages, evolving either to partial or full recovery (or cure), or to death; in the case of partial recovery, there may be chronification or sequelae. Prevention, in this sense, refers not only to the appearance of the disease but also to any further worsening or complication of it once it has appeared.

### Primary prevention

The primary prevention level covers what is otherwise referred to as both health promotion and specific protection, and is best exemplified by, for example, adequate nutrition and immunization against specific diseases by vaccines. Whereas, in this example, adequate nutrition is totally non-specific (it contributes to enhancing the overall resistance to several diseases without conferring any specific protection against any), vaccination is highly specific in relation to a single condition. Rational-specific protection is fully dependent on a reasonable knowledge of the aetiology of the disease (or, at least, its mode of transmission) in order to be effective.

### Secondary prevention

The secondary prevention level refers to early detection and treatment of diseases. Usually the bulk of the medical activity, its main preventive goal is to avoid chronicity and the establishment of irreversible sequelae. It is dealt with more specifically in Part 6 of this book.

### Tertiary prevention

The tertiary prevention level largely corresponds to rehabilitation. It enters into operation once the disease process has been established and aims at reducing as much as possible damages caused by the disease process, preserving intact functions, and restoring and/or compensating impaired functions, disabilities, and handicaps.

On one hand, this conceptual model was highly instrumental in providing an impetus towards preventive activities in the medical field as a whole but, on the other hand, it so popularized the term prevention that it almost lost its powerful message. Therefore, it is important to retain the idea of primary prevention as a synonym of specific protection, referring to methods designed to avoid the occurrence of a specific disorder or groups of disorders. It comprises those measures applicable to a particular disease or group of diseases in order to intercept their causes before they affect people, and should be differentiated not only from treatment and rehabilitation, but also from mental health promotion.

The main obstacle for the prevention of many mental disorders is the limited knowledge about their aetiology. Admittedly, there are very promising and exciting hypotheses concerning the causes of three mental disorders which represent the greatest burden, namely, depression, schizophrenia, and dementia. They are, nevertheless, nothing more than hypotheses. The most successful examples of prevention of diseases refer to those whose aetiology (cause and/or mode of transmission) is relatively well-known. There are historical examples of the prevention of some conditions based on false assumptions about or without a good knowledge of their aetiology (for example, the eradication of malaria in ancient Rome, and the control of the London cholera epidemics by John Snow in the nineteenth century). However, it does not seem appropriate for health professionals and scientists to base their actions on chance or false assumptions, even though the result might be opportune to the population.

As implied by the need to intercept causes of a particular disease or groups of diseases (with a common cause), the concept of prevention calls for a high degree of specificity concerning the target condition or conditions. In the medical field, it led to successful programmes for the prevention of, for example, diarrhoeal diseases (such as typhoid), hypertension, coronary heart disease, breast cancer, and unwanted pregnancies, rather than of infectious diseases, cardiovascular diseases, cancer, or obstetrical problems. Unfortunately, in the mental health field there has not been a great concern with the specification of the target condition, and the prevention of 'mental disorders' (as a whole) became a label soon associated with failure and disinterest.

## Mental disorders

What is understood as 'mental disorders' comprises a variety of quite diverse clinical conditions in terms of aetiology, symptomatology, clinical course, prognosis, and response to treatment. Therefore, whenever the prevention of mental disorders is referred to, an effort must be made to obtain some precision.

From a nosological point of view, most of the mental disorders are conceptually at a syndromal level; depression, schizophrenia, and dementia are appropriate examples. In this respect, dementia is one step ahead of the other two, in so far as vascular dementia is now clearly differentiated from Alzheimer's disease, with important implications for prevention.

Therefore a strategic shift is necessary in order to obtain greater efficiency in the successful prevention of some mental disorders. The first step is for an effort to be as specific as possible in relation to the target condition: for instance Down syndrome or phenylketonuria instead of intellectual disorder, foetal alcohol syndrome, delirium tremens instead of alcoholism, and vascular dementia and dementia following brain injury instead of dementia in general.

The second step applies to those conditions which cannot be meaningfully broken down into more specific conditions, such as schizophrenia or depression. In these cases, the target is displaced from the appearance of the conditions towards future relapses, once a first episode has occurred; this conveniently applies to schizophrenia, depression, and dependence on alcohol and other drugs.

Finally, there are some violent behaviours, such as suicide, parasuicide, and violence against others, the control (and prevention) of which are largely expected by society to come from the field of mental health. They do not characterize a mental disorder in particular, but are frequently associated with one or more of them. Their prevention, therefore, requires specifically dedicated interventions.

With this wide range of issues considered as mental disorders, it becomes clear that the coverage of their prevention goes well beyond the limits of this chapter. A detailed conceptual approach to the prevention of mental and psychosocial disorders can be found in a recent publication of the World Health Organization (**WHO**).[2]

## Prevention of mental disorders

From a practical point of view there are three groups of conditions for which efficient preventive action has been documented.

1 Mental disorders with known aetiology: this mostly includes those disorders demonstrated to have an organic basis, ranging from the 'historical' general paresis and dementing disorders (e.g. vascular dementia, pellagra, and dementias associated with infectious and parasitic diseases such as malaria and HIV infection) to several forms of intellectual disorder (Down syndrome, foetal alcohol syndrome, phenylketonuria, and intellectual disorder due to iodine deficiency).

2 Mental disorders without a well-established aetiology but with a relatively predictable course: these are chronic disorders with a recurrent relapsing fluctuating pattern, such as schizophrenia, mood disorders (unipolar and bipolar), and alcohol dependence syndrome.

3 Psychosocial problems strongly associated with mental disorders: these range from violence (domestic and other) to suicide and staff burnout.

### Mental disorders with known aetiology

#### (a) Infectious diseases

Prevention of this group of disorders has by far yielded the greatest success. The demonstration in 1911 by Noguchi and Moore of the brain infection by *Treponema pallidum* as the cause of general paresis[3] opened the way in 1917 to its treatment by malaria therapy, and later to its prevention with penicillin; this is now a landmark in the history of medicine. The discovery of the aetiology of pellagra also led to its prevention and control, leading to the prevention of one type of dementia associated with alcoholism and avitaminosis.

These two once very frequent diseases have almost completely disappeared and there are many experienced psychiatrists who never come across a single case of either; with them also disappeared the history of their successful control. Although the same success has not yet been achieved in relation to vascular dementia, the control of hypertension and atherosclerosis (e.g. through the reduction of salt and fat intake) can significantly reduce brain damage and ensuing dementia (vascular or multi-infarct dementia).

In some developing countries, meningitis and malaria (and, to a lesser extent, inadequately treated epilepsy) are important causes of permanent brain damage which can also lead to dementing disorders. The environmental control of malaria and other brain infections, of which bacterial meningitis is the most important, and their early and prompt treatment can reduce the impact of the infection on the brain and prevent these forms of dementia (or intellectual disorder, depending on the age of onset).

More recently, it has been demonstrated that in some people infected with HIV, the initial manifestations of AIDS are accompanied by some forms of mental disorder, such as mood disorders or dementia.[4] The prevention of these forms of mental disorders follow the same measures as for the prevention of AIDS in general. However, it is not yet certain if the newer combined treatments (bi- and tritherapy) can alter the course of AIDS when brain damage due to HIV has been confirmed.

#### (b) Intellectual disorder (mental retardation)

Up to 15 per cent of cases of intellectual disorder could be prevented by dealing with the causes that lead to it. A recent WHO publication[2] has set detailed guidelines for the prevention of some forms of this condition, namely, Down syndrome, foetal alcohol syndrome, phenylketonuria, and iodine deficiency syndrome.

These preventive actions are both efficient and affordable even in very poor regions of the world.

- *Down syndrome*—The primary prevention of Down syndrome can be successfully achieved through the control of the age at which women become pregnant: ideally, the age range during which the risk is minimal is between 16 and 35 years, after which the risk increases almost exponentially, as shown in Fig. 7.4.1. Amniocentesis is a procedure that can be very useful for the *in utero* diagnosis of Down syndrome (as well as of other problems and malformations). Where it is culturally and morally acceptable, and legally permitted, a therapeutic abortion is viewed by some as another primary prevention measure.

- *Iodine deficiency*—The world population at risk of intellectual disability due to iodine deficiency is approximately 1 billion and it still occurs in large numbers in some regions of the globe.[6] However, it can be very efficiently and cheaply prevented through the addition of iodine to salt, milk, flour, or water, or, in special situations, through injections of an oily solution containing iodine.[7]

- *Phenylketonuria*—Intellectual disorder due to phenylketonuria can also be successfully prevented through the early identification of children at risk who then receive a phenylalanine-free diet throughout their lives.[8]

- *Foetal alcohol syndrome* (FAS)—Intellectual disorder and malformations seen in FAS syndrome can be prevented if women stay away from alcohol during pregnancy, more particularly during the first trimester, or at least keep their alcohol intake below the dangerous limit of 15 g of ethanol per day.[9]

Table 7.4.1 summarizes actions which can effectively prevent some forms of intellectual disorder. Prevention of intellectual disorder is discussed further in Chapter 10.3.

## Mental disorders without a well-established aetiology but with a relatively predictable course

In this group of disorders, the target for prevention is not the disorder itself, whose aetiology is not clearly established, but the

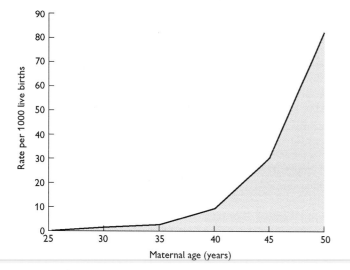

**Fig. 7.4.1** Estimated risk of Down syndrome by related age. (Data from Gottesman.[5] Taken from the contribution of genetic factors to the common psychopathologies © World Health Organization, www.who.int )

**Table 7.4.1** Action to prevent mental retardation

| Condition | Preventive action |
| --- | --- |
| Iodine deficiency disorders | Iodize salt or water supply<br>Treat individuals at risk with iodized oil or Lugol's solution |
| Down syndrome | Discourage pregnancies in women over the age of 35 years<br>If appropriate, provide amniocentesis to women over the age of 35 years |
| Foetal alcohol syndrome | Use simple screening test to identify women at risk<br>Discourage women from drinking alcohol during pregnancy<br>Alert women that drinking around the time of conception increases the risk to the child |
| Phenylketonuria | Screen all newborn babies for phenylketonuria<br>Treat with a special low-phenylalanine diet<br>Discourage pregnancies in women with phenylketonuria |

occurrence of further episodes of the disorder, since these are chronic recurrent disorders. Three good examples of this are mood disorders, schizophrenia, and alcohol dependence syndrome.

### (a) Mood disorders

In addition to the use of antidepressants and neuroleptics to treat episodes of depression and mania, respectively, it has been demonstrated that the appropriate use of lithium salts can prevent the reappearance of new episodes of disease, or at least increase the disease-free periods and reduce both their duration and severity. The use of lithium salts, also called psychoprophylactics, is now a standard procedure for the treatment and management of mood disorders and this use can be considered as a form of prevention of mood disorders (see Chapter 4.5.8).

### (b) Schizophrenia

Although no evidence of a definite cause of schizophrenia is yet available, it can be reasonably controlled through the use of psychopharmacotherapy and psychosocial interventions. Relapse rates (measured by number of hospital readmissions or days in hospital) decrease significantly when persons with schizophrenia adhere to some specific pharmacological regimens and are exposed, together with their relatives, to psychoeducational programmes.[10] These usually include some social skills training for the patient and information about the disease and the management of expressed emotions for the relatives. Unfortunately, schizophrenia is a very long-lasting condition, even lifelong, and most studies on the combination of those two approaches have not yet gone beyond a follow-up of 48 months, thus limiting the full appreciation of its long-term efficiency.

### (c) Alcoholism

This term refers to both the alcohol dependence syndrome and other forms of problematic use of alcohol. For people in either category, whenever total abstinence is an unachievable or undesirable goal, the intake reduction, particularly when in connection with risk or dangerous situations, may become the target for prevention. There are several therapeutic techniques usually revolving around brief interventions that are useful to help people significantly to reduce their alcohol and their exposure to problems associated with it (harm reduction). One should neither forget nor minimize the positive impact of self-help groups (such as Alcoholics Anonymous) in helping some people to achieve sobriety.

## Psychosocial problems strongly associated with mental disorders

### (a)  Violent behaviour

In this category, the immediate target condition is not strictly a mental disorder. However, its close connections with some forms of mental disorder or symptoms make their prevention of immediate concern in the mental health field. Domestic violence (spouse and child beating) is strongly associated with substance abuse;[11] some types of mental disorders are potent risk factors for suicide (see below), and stress and anxiety are at the roots of the burnout syndrome seen in health workers (see below).

Extremely violent behaviour (and crime) is not associated with severe mental disorders (such as schizophrenia) as usually portrayed by the media.[12,13] On the contrary, it is more frequently associated with some types of personality disorders (e.g. antisocial, poor impulse control, aggressive) and with substance use, of which the most prevalent is alcohol. Hence, the control of substance use disorders (in itself a case of secondary prevention) can be seen as an example of primary prevention of domestic violence. The focus of prevention should be broadened from the individual perspective (the substance user) to the social group (the family) which is not exposed to the direct organic effects of alcohol, but nonetheless suffers from its indirect effects.

### (b)  Suicide

Despite the long-standing sociological tradition of considering suicide as a phenomenon associated with the social condition known as anomia,[14] the medical profession tends to see it primarily as a medical problem. Probably both are right. Among the demonstrated risk factors for suicide there are both social factors (anomy, old age, masculine gender, social isolation) and medical problems (chronic, painful, and incurable diseases and, most of all, psychiatric disorders and psychological problems). Several European studies have indicated that approximately 80 per cent of all cases of suicide are associated with alcohol use and depression combined.[2] This indicates the appropriateness of targeting the treatment of these two conditions (another secondary prevention intervention) regarding the prevention of suicide. However, given the broad social implications of suicide, treatment of mental disorders alone has not yet produced a significant reduction of suicide rates.

Hence the importance of a paradigmatic change which views suicide on a ecological perspective that considers the suicidal act as the immediate target for prevention and not just suicidal intention or ideation as subsumed by the traditional medical (and psychiatric) model.[2] It is now firmly established that the control of the availability of means to commit suicide can greatly contribute to the reduction of mortality rates from suicide. According to WHO,[2] steps to prevent suicide can be taken in the following areas:

- psychiatric treatment
- gun control
- gas detoxification
- control of toxic substances

- responsible media reporting.

  Corresponding actions to prevent suicide include:
- identification and treatment of people suffering from depression
- restriction of access to guns
- detoxification of domestic gas and car emissions
- controlling the availability of toxic substances and medicines
- downtoning reports of suicide in the media
- erection of physical barriers to deter jumping from high places.

A more detailed discussion about the prevention of suicide can be found in Chapter 4.15.4.

### (c)  Staff burnout

Freudenberger[15] first used the term 'staff burnout' to describe a 'syndrome of exhaustion, disillusionment and withdrawal in voluntary mental health workers'. The concept has aroused considerable interest in the caring professions, and the publication of a large number of articles and books on the subject suggests that burnout is a major problem in health services.[2]

Indeed, with the general trend towards community-based care in many parts of the world, burnout is now a problem faced by all caregivers, including the relatives of people suffering from chronic disorders.

There is no single accepted definition of burnout; however, there is general agreement that the syndrome has three major characteristics, which are observed in various caregivers, particularly health workers and family members:

- emotional exhaustion
- depersonalization
- a reduced feeling of personal accomplishment.

The two approaches most frequently employed to prevent staff burnout are:

- Stress management (at the individual level);[16] and
- Supervisor training (at the organizational level).[17]

Table 7.4.2 summarizes actions which contribute to the prevention of burnout among health care staff, at different levels of intervention.

## Who is responsible for primary prevention?

As indicated in the introduction of this section, one of the obstacles to a greater involvement of mental health professionals in preventive action stems from the fact that the effective actions for the

**Table 7.4.2**  Action to prevent staff burnout

| |
|---|
| Avoid making unrealistically high demands of caregivers |
| Ensure that all workers have some rewarding tasks |
| Train caregivers in time-management and relaxation techniques |
| Modify jobs that are proving too stressful |
| Encourage the formation of support groups |
| Consider the possibility of part-time employment |
| Encourage workers to participate in decisions which affect them |

prevention of several mental disorders often falls outside their usual remit and in many cases falls outside the health sector altogether, as indicated in Table 7.4.3. Although this is true, it does not mean that mental health professionals do not have a major role to play in three areas: advocacy, information generation, and supervision.

Perhaps mental health professionals need to reconsider their potential role in primary prevention; for instance, they could develop their potential to act as advocates and advisers to professionals in other sectors. As Eisenberg[18] has argued:

> what matters is not the mode of action of the agent, the venue in which it is applied, or the academic discipline of the practitioner, but the effectiveness of the measure in preventing diseases manifested by disturbances in mental function.

At any rate, prevention is unquestionably a public health priority. Accordingly, WHO has recently published a book on this aspect of prevention, whose reading is strongly recommended.

**Table 7.4.3** Agents for prevention

| Condition | Effective agents for prevention |
| --- | --- |
| Mental retardation | |
| Down syndrome | Family planning professionals |
| | Obstetricians/midwives |
| | Women's associations |
| Foetal alcohol syndrome | General health-care personnel |
| | Substance abuse professionals |
| | Family planning professionals |
| | Obstetricans/midwives . |
| | Educators |
| | Women's associations |
| Phenylketonuria | Obstetricians/midwives |
| | Paediatricians |
| | Nutritionists |
| Iodine deficiency | General health-care personnel |
| | Nutritionists |
| | Groups involved in salt production/trade |
| | Water supply personnel |
| | Educators |
| Depression | Mental health workers |
| | Rehabilitation officers |
| Schizophrenia | Mental health workers |
| | Rehabilitation officers |
| Alcohol dependence syndrome | General health workers |
| | Mental health workers |
| | Self-help groups |
| Violence | General health workers |
| | Mental health workers |
| | Paediatricians |
| | Justice officers |
| | Police officers |
| Suicide | Mental health workers |
| | General health workers |
| | Agricultural and environment authorities |
| | Journalists |
| | Pharmaceutical industry |
| | Car industry |
| | Traffic authorities |
| | Authorities in charge of provision of domestic gas |
| | Gun control authorities (including legislators) |
| Burnout | Occupational health workers |
| | General health workers |
| | Staff counsellors |
| | Trade unions |
| | Staff associations |
| | Personnel officers |
| | Job supervisors |
| | Self-help groups |

## Further information

Bertolote, J.M. (ed.) (1965). *Primary prevention of mental, neurological and psychosocial disorders.* World Health Organization, Geneva.

Leavell, H.R. and Clark, E.G. (1965). *Preventive medicine for the doctor in his community: an epidemiological approach* (3rd edn). McGraw-Hill, New York.

World Health Organization. (2004). *Prevention of mental disorders: effective interventions and policy options.* World Health Organization, Geneva.

## References

1. Leavell, H.R. and Clark, E.G. (1965). *Preventive medicine for the doctor in his community: an epidemiological approach* (3rd edn). McGraw Hill, New York.

2. Bertolote, J.M. (ed.) (1998). *Primary prevention of mental, neurological and psychosocial disorders.* World Health Organization, Geneva.

3. Schneck, J.M. (1960). *A history of psychiatry.* C.C. Thomas, Springfield, IL.

4. Maj, M. (1990). Psychiatric aspects of HIV-1 infection and AIDS. *Psychological Medicine*, **20**, 547–63.

5. Gottesman, I. (1982). *The contribution of genetic factors to the common psychopathologies.* World Health Organization, Geneva.

6. Hetzel, B.S. (1986). Mental defect due to iodine deficiency: a major international public health problem that can be eradicated. In *Science and service in mental retardation* (ed. J.M. Berg), pp. 297–306. Methuen, London.

7. Dunn, J.T. and van der Haar, F. (1990). *A practical guide to the correction of iodine deficiency.* International Council for Control of Iodine Deficiency Disorders, Adelaide.

8. World Health Organization. (1985). *Community approaches to the control of hereditary diseases: report of a WHO advisory group.* World Health Organization, Geneva.

9. Smith, I.E., Lancaster, J.S., Moss-Wells, S., *et al.* (1987). Identifying high-risk pregnant drinkers: biological and behavioural correlates of continuous heavy drinking during pregnancy. *Journal of Studies on Alcohol*, **48**, 304–9.

10. Leff, J. and Waughn, R. (1981). The role of maintenance therapy and relative expressed emotion in relapse of schizophrenia: a 2-year follow up. *The British Journal of Psychiatry*, **139**, 102–4.

11. Regier, D.A., Farmer, M.E., Rae, D.S., *et al.* (1990). Comorbidity of mental disorders with alcohol and other drug abuse: results from the Epidemiological Catchment Area (ECA) study. *The Journal of the American Medical Association*, **264**, 2511–18.

12. Barbato, A. (1998). Psychiatry in transition: outcomes of mental health policy shift in Italy. *The Australian and New Zealand Journal of Psychiatry*, **32**, 673–9.

13. Aldige, H.V. (1992). Civil commitment and arrests: an investigation of the criminalization thesis. *The Journal of Nervous and Mental Disease*, **180**, 184–91.

14. Durkheim, E. (1990). *Le suicide*. Presse Universitaire de France, Paris.

15. Freudenberger, H.J. (1974). Staff burn out. *Journal of Social Sciences*, **30**, 159–65.

16. Meichenbaum, D. and Jaremko, M.E. (1983). *Stress reduction and prevention*. Plenum Press, New York.

17. Kilburg, R.C., Nathan, P.E., and Thoreson, R.W. (eds.) (1986). *Professionals in distress: issues, syndrome and solutions in psychology*. American Psychological Association, Washington, DC.

# Planning and providing mental health services for a community

Tom Burns

## Introduction

The aim of this chapter is to assist clinicians and managers review and plan services effectively for their local population. Severe psychiatric disorders manifest themselves in social relations and often disrupt social structures; they have wide-ranging consequences and services need to be comprehensive. Health and social care have been intertwined in psychiatry from its origins—it is neither feasible nor sensible to ignore the wider context of their management.

## Mental health services research

The last 30 years have seen an explosion of Mental Health Services Research alongside the shrinking and closure of mental hospitals (see Chapter 7.6). Policy considerations, particularly cost containment and public safety, have influenced the research agenda which is disproportionately Anglophone (from the United States, United Kingdom, and Australasia) and focused on new services developed as alternatives to institutional care with staffing and motivation that are not easily generalizable. More routine practices, crucial for safe and effective care, have been relatively neglected by researchers.

## Scope of chapter

This chapter is mainly devoted to describing the essential components of a mental health service—its 'building blocks'. It will then consider how they relate to one another, how they can be prioritized, and how integrated into an effective local service linking into other essential services. Lastly it will stress how their inevitable evolution should be monitored.

Services for adults (increasingly referred to as 'adults of working age' indicating 18–65 years) will be used as the template. In many settings these may be the only services, stretching to accommodate all comers. In better resourced health care systems a range of specialized services have evolved from this basic model and are described elsewhere in this section (refugees 7.10.1, homeless 7.10.2, and ethnic minorities 7.10.3).

## Building blocks of mental health services: care and treatment

Most mental health treatments (whether psychological, pharmacological, or social) are based on face-to-face interviews and do not require sophisticated equipment or buildings. Institutions (the asylums) evolved for social care of disabled individuals, to protect them while they recovered and, sometimes, to protect society from them. Patients needing long-term institutional care are now relatively few but psychiatry is judged on how they are managed and service planners must pay them due attention.

## Inpatient beds

No comprehensive service can survive without access to 24 h nursing supervision for acute episodes of severe illness. These include patients at risk from neglect or suicide or those lacking insight. Wards usually accommodate 10–20 patients. It is rarely possible to effectively staff and run stand-alone units of less than 3–4 such wards (30–60 beds). Ward size is a trade-off between privacy and domesticity against effective supervision. Single rooms are preferable, affording maximal privacy and, while initially expensive, improve flexibility and reduce conflict.

Smaller, more flexible, units such as 'crisis houses' offering 24 h care are a useful complement to inpatient wards, but not a replacement. Ward design and management are increasingly crucial as improved community care concentrates involuntary and disturbed inpatients in them.

## How many acute beds?

'How many beds do we need for our local population?' is often the first question asked by planners or managers. Unfortunately there is no reliable or precise answer to this. We know that supply will drive use (perceived as need)—beds are rarely left unfilled despite enormous variation in their availability. It is also surprisingly difficult to collect useable figures on bed usage nationally or internationally because of differences in methods of reporting and also the profusion of overlapping and rarely defined local terms (e.g. night hospitals, crisis homes, step-down wards). The levels of external accommodation provision (e.g. hostels, day care) clearly also impact the need for acute beds. Similarly need for beds will reduce as community services become more comprehensive and robust.

European provision of general acute beds in 2000 in the public sector ranged from 128 per 100 000 in the Netherlands to 6 per 100 000 in Northern Italy. However, unless we know the pattern of care (in particular the level of private and social services care) these figures tell us relatively little. The United Kingdom has little parallel private care and here acute beds needed for a population of 250 000 have been estimated to range from 50 to 150 plus 5 to 20 secure or intensive care beds[1] dependent on morbidity (generally much higher in large urban settings). London figures for the mid-1990s were very close to this range, averaging 73 for outer and 110 for inner London, but with increased secure provision, particularly in the deprived inner city. The authors predicted a similar range of 24 h supervised hostel need (40–150 per 250 000 population) and London use was somewhat higher (99 and 162 per 250 000, respectively) but with a markedly wider range.

Current bed usage in the United Kingdom is closer to the 50 per 250 000 and well below this in stable communities. This reflects both the establishment of specialized home-treatment and assertive outreach teams and the expansion of forensic care but also a shift in expectations and practice. The average duration for admissions has been steadily reducing over the last three decades. Figures can be misleading as they are heavily skewed by short (1–2 day) admissions but the current admission for an uncomplicated psychotic relapse is likely to be between 3 and 6 weeks.

### Longer inpatient care

Acute inpatient wards admit patients for weeks or a couple of months. Rapid discharge is anticipated and regimes emphasize openness and independence. Even within a local service some patients will require longer or more secure care because of illness severity or for legal reasons. Modern rehabilitation practice restricts long-stay wards to patients whose behaviour is persistently unacceptable to local communities. Forensic and secure services are usually a regional or national rather than local responsibility.

### Diagnosis-specific wards

Alcohol and substance abuse wards have been long established (especially in Scandinavia and Central Europe) and diagnosis- or disorder-specific wards are increasingly common. Wards for specialized patient groups such as anorexia nervosa or resistant schizophrenia provide highly specific regimes. These are generally an adjunct to acute admission wards rather than an alternative. Some services are organized in disorder-specific wards (e.g. a psychosis unit, a psychosomatic ward) *instead* of general wards. Such specialization is not possible in comprehensive services for populations of less than about 1 000 000. For smaller populations this increased specialization must be balanced against reduced flexibility and energy wasted in 'boundary disputes'.

### Day care

Day care is provided either in day-hospitals or day-centres, with little consistency in the terms or practices. Patients attend usually from 1 to 5 days a week for a half or whole day before returning to their homes in the evening. It is particularly valuable when families are out at work but can offer support at evenings and weekends or for very isolated patients.

Generally day-hospitals are provided by health services, include medical and nursing staff and can offer treatments (e.g. the prescription and monitoring of medication, psychotherapies). Day-hospitals were a significant feature in the move of mental health services from mental hospitals to District General Hospital sites. However their role has been more uncertain since community teams have expanded and taken on much of their therapeutic role. Many services have scaled down or even closed their day-hospitals relying more on social services for day care. Day-hospitals have had a problem of isolating themselves from service needs, locked in time with a static patient group. Comprehensive services can, undoubtedly, survive well without them, so if they are to be established it is essential that there are strong links into local teams who can exercise some control over their clientele and their activity.

Day-centres, provided by social care organizations, can rarely provide treatments or employ clinical staff. However overlap is wide with services highly specific to local context (e.g. a drop-in day-centre may be the main provider of psychiatric assessment and treatment in areas of high social mobility and homelessness). Generally day-centres provide long-term social support and day-hospitals focused interventions and treatments.[2] The 'Club House' is a specialized rehabilitation day centre, popularized in the United States, which emphasizes useful normal work and where members take responsibility for running the centre with minimal supervision. Many day units now function in the evening and at weekends.

Acute day-hospitals in Europe and partial hospitalization in the United States have been energetically proposed as alternatives to inpatient care[3] but have had little impact. While day-hospitals never achieved their anticipated prominence they serve specific groups well (e.g. mothers with small children or protracted treatment of eating disorders or personality problems). Day care is problematic in rural settings but adaptations such as travelling day-centres (i.e. a team that moves from setting to setting on specific days) or a weekly open day run by the community team are worth considering.

## Supported accommodation and residential care

Many patients remain well outside hospital only with adequate support. At its most basic this implies stable, affordable accommodation. For many, however, supervision is needed to ensure self care, continued medication, and to anticipate and defuse crises. This can be provided by voluntary agencies, social services, or health services. Voluntary agencies tend to be more efficient at providing long-term residential care[4] but they may be reluctant to accept risky patients (e.g. with a history of violence or substance abuse). A mixed economy works best and the need for health services supported accommodation depends on the vigour of local voluntary and social services. While some purpose built units exist, the accommodation is usually shared adapted houses to promote integration and reduce stigma.

Supported or sheltered accommodation is subject to a bewildering terminology but can be considered at four basic levels of increasing need:

1 *Group homes*. These have no regular staff and are reserved for relatively independent patients visited by staff from their own community teams.

2 *Day-staffed hostels*. One or two staff are present each day to support and monitor patients (encouraging cooking and cleaning, etc). They would usually not provide specific treatment but liaise with the community team about it.

3 *Night-staffed hostels*. Non-clinical staff sleep over in the hostel to provide greater safety and availability.

4 *24h staffed/nursed hostels*. On-site clinical staff are available overnight either sleeping in or, sometimes, awake. These are expensive hostels and generally restricted to patients with long-term severe illnesses (including sometimes those compulsorily detained). Night-staffed hostels tend to be larger usually with 10–20 residents as opposed to 4–8 in day staffed ones.

Most comprehensive local services provide levels 1 and 2 and most social services undertake to provide level 3. Level 4 is relatively rare and would usually serve a population of 500 000–1 000 000.

## Office-based care and outpatient clinics

In insurance-based systems many psychiatrists run individual office practices and manage patients on their own. In state-funded systems this is rare; most work in outpatient clinics or mental health teams. Both approaches should be considered when planning and providing public mental health services, paying particular attention to financial regulations that can inhibit integration and development (comprehensive planning may pose a significant threat to their livelihood and be resisted). Office-based practice remains widespread but neglected in academic and policy publications. It tends to be narrow in remit (usually either psychotherapy or pharmacotherapy) and is poorly equipped for managing severe disorders.

Outpatient clinics ('polyclinics' or 'dispensaries') are an essential part of modern services increasingly replacing office practice. Psychiatrists and psychologists may still operate independently within them but with access to enhanced resources and second opinions. In the public sector outpatient clinics may operate either alongside community mental health teams (CMHTs) or as part of them (which works better for severe illness).[5] They provide an efficient, predicable format for assessments, treatment, and monitoring.

## Community mental health centres (CMHCs)

Mental hospitals, for all their faults, had no problems coordinating care; what little was available was all in the same place. Outpatient clinics expanded to Community Mental Health Centres (CMHCs) providing a wide range of services located in shared buildings (e.g. depot clinics, a day-hospital, psychotherapy services). The failure of the early US CMHCs demonstrated that relying entirely on patients to attend fails to engage the more ill and also that down-playing the 'medical model' made it impossible to recruit psychiatrists, further distancing practice from the severely ill.

Most CMHTs are based in CMHCs sharing accommodation with other CMHTs and services (e.g. day care). They provide an important safeguard in sustaining clinical standards and reducing the professional isolation in dispersed community services. This is a particularly important safeguard for community teams which can otherwise easily become idiosyncratic and rigid in their practice if not forced into regular contact with others.

## Multidisciplinary Community mental health teams (CMHTs)

Most community mental health services consist of varied forms of multidisciplinary CMHT consisting of psychiatrists, nurses, social workers and often psychologists, and occupational therapists. The staffing of these teams will vary but their strength is that regular meetings to assess and review the management of patients incorporates their varied professional perspectives and allocates tasks based on skills and needs. Developed initially in France and the United Kingdom and championed latterly in Italy they have seen further specialization from North America and Australia.

## The generic sector CMHT ('The CMHT')

### Who it is for

The CMHT is *the* fundamental building block of modern community mental health services. It originated as mental hospital catchment areas (often covering a whole city or county) were divided into sectors of 50–100 000 inhabitants to permit ongoing care. The aim was that it should be possible for most of the team to have some familiarity with most of its complex and long-term patients and to have some *personal* knowledge of its referrers and community resources. Current sector size in Western Europe ranges from 20–50 000 population, determined both by resources (shrinking as investment increases) and by the local configuration. As more specialized teams are established the CMHTs remit may be reduced and sector size consequently increased keeping its caseload fairly constant. 200–250 is considered the maximum for most teams to exploit multidisciplinary working. The number is less in services for highly complex and difficult patients.

CMHTs offer assessment and care for patients discharged from psychiatric units and those who cannot be adequately treated in primary care or in the private sector. They should prioritize severe mental illnesses (SMI—e.g. psychoses and severe affective disorders). However diagnosis is not all—complications from social adversity, personality difficulties, or substance abuse can make secondary mental health care necessary even for apparently 'minor' disorders. Tools to clarify this threshold[6] have been of limited use and most teams rely on clinical assessments. In countries with limited private care CMHTs also treat mild and transient disorders. CMHTs can be remarkably inefficient if little thought is given to their structure and thresholds. To work well, there needs to be agreement on their purpose, clientele and systems of management and they have often suffered from lack of clarity and leadership.

### Staffing and management

CMHT staffing varies enormously and there is no uniform model. Teams of less than 6 can rarely provide comprehensive care or cross-cover while teams of more than about 12–15 start to become unwieldy, overwhelmed with management and information transfer. CMHTs emphasize skill-sharing and a degree of generic working and have evolved an informal, democratic style[7] which often means confusion over clinical leadership (originally provided informally by senior medical staff). With increased staff numbers and treatment complexity 'team managers' now coordinate workload with a role which varies from the purely administrative to setting clinical priorities and supervising staff. Establishing a clear understanding of clinical leadership in CMHTs (without inhibiting initiative and creativity) is essential for effective functioning. If leadership and management are separated (common with a strong medical presence) the roles need to be well defined and relationships good.

## Assessments

The key to good care is accurate assessment (see Chapter 1.8.1). Most commonly psychiatrists conduct initial assessments (usually in an outpatient clinic) and involve the team members in treatment. Increasingly other team members have taken a role in assessments, either individually or jointly with the psychiatrist. Although this issue generates strong feelings there is surprisingly little research into it. With highly developed primary care non-medical assessments may be effective but otherwise medical time should prioritize assessments. With severely ill patients home-based assessments pay considerable dividends.[8,9]

## Case management

Most CMHT staff act as clinical case managers[10,11] with responsibility for coordination, delivery, and review of care for their patients. The caseloads of staff members should be explicitly limited (usually 15 to 30) and reviews recorded and systematic. In the United Kingdom this has been formalized as the Care Programme Approach.[12] Fig. 7.5.1 shows a care plan indicating a patient's needs or problems, the interventions proposed to meet them, who is responsible and who is informed, plus an agreed date for review. Such concise structured paperwork (as with the risk assessment and contingency plan (Fig. 7.5.2)) can be adapted to any service, coordinates complex care and serves as a natural focus for clinical reviews. The level of detail needs to be clinically (not managerially) determined.

## Team meetings

CMHTs need 1–2 regular meetings (each usually 1.5–2 h) per week for both clinical and administrative business. The degree of structure depends on team style and remit.

### (a) Allocation of referrals

Referrals can be allocated by who is first available or by matching the clinical problem against available skill and training. Time discussing allocations before assessment is generally unprofitable and most well-established teams delegate the task to the manager or a senior clinician.

### (b) Patient reviews

Reviews should be held for (i) *new patients*, (ii) *routine monitoring*, and (iii) *discharge*. Reviews can range from simply reporting the problem and proposed treatment in uncomplicated cases through to detailed, structured, multidisciplinary case-conferences including other services (e.g. GP, housing, child protection). *New patient* reviews are an excellent opportunity for providing a broad, experienced overview, and ensuring rational and fair allocation to

caseloads. *Routine monitoring* is often overlooked yet probably the most important for team efficiency. It should be systematic and not only responsive to crises and problems. It shapes and redirects treatment and identifies patients ready for discharge. The burden on individual staff members is regularly monitored. Routine monitoring is a legal requirement of the Care Programme Approach and good practice in all case management. *Discharge reviews* are an excellent opportunity for audit and learning within the team.

### (c) Managing waiting lists and caseloads

Effective CMHTs need to guarantee prompt access. *Routine assessments* should be within 2–4 weeks. Sooner is rarely productive and delays above 3 weeks result in a rapidly rising rate of failed appointments.[13] *Urgent assessments* (most psychotic episodes) need to be seen within a week, usually within a couple of days. *Emergency assessments* are for those associated with immediate risk (e.g. hostile behaviour or suicidal intent) and need to be seen the same day.

A practical approach to waiting lists is to count the assessments in the preceding year and allocate routine appointments for 20 per cent more. Thus a team with 400 assessments the preceding year allocating nine slots a week will have one available weekly for emergencies. Rapid routine assessment reduces pressure for urgent and emergency referrals more efficiently than emergency rotas.

## Communication and liaison

Team meetings ensure internal communication but CMHTs need good links with a wide network of professional colleagues. Structured liaison is advisable with primary care and general hospitals in addition to routine letters. Hospital links may be between specific CMHTs and wards or CMHTs may provide input to patients from their sectors in the absence of dedicated liaison psychiatry services.

### (a) General practice liaison

Much of mental health care is delivered in primary care (see Chapter 7.8) and effective coordination is essential. GP liaison systems range from informal contact through to shared care and co-location of CMHTs in GP Health Centres.[14] An effective system comprises regular, timetabled meetings between the two teams or a 'link' CMHT member attending the GP health centre. Monthly meetings where shared and complex patients are discussed are highly time-efficient because of prompt problem solving and crisis anticipation. However it is important to be clear about responsibilities, fudging boundaries is risky.

### (b) Liaison with other agencies

The same principles apply to liaison with other agencies (social services, housing, charitable, and voluntary sector providers). Whether regular meetings are cost-effective will depend on the volume of shared work but showing up and meeting people (even just once) pays enormous dividends in improved relationships and understanding. Professional confidentiality and information sharing is more sensitive.

## Assertive Outreach (AO) Teams

The most replicated and researched specialist CMHT is the AO Team. The original US model[9] improved clinical and social outcomes with substantially reduced hospitalization at slightly lower cost.

## CPA REVIEW

Patient's name: Jenny T

Address: 56 Acacia Avenue

Phone:

Date of birth: 09.06.61

GP: Dr Findlay

Phone:

CMHT: West Central

Phone:

New patient: ~~YES~~/NO

If NO, date of review: 20.10.07

Diagnosis:

1...Major depressive disorder..... F 32 .0

2.............................................. F __ __.__

**You must consider the following:** 1) Mental health, including indicators of relapse; 2) Physical health; 3) Medication; 4) Daytime activity; 5) Personal care / living skills; 6) Carers, family, children and social network; 7) Forensic history; 8) Alcohol or substance misuse 9) Cultural factors; 10) Housing/finances/legal issues.

Complete a **risk assessment** and include: **i) a crisis plan; ii) a contingency plan**

| Assessed needs or problem | Intervention | Resp.of |
|---|---|---|
| 1. Depressed mood, apathetic and self critical | • Regular home visits, assess mental state<br>• Encourage compliance with antidepressants<br>• Encourage activity – take to shops etc | BJ |
| 2. Suicidal thoughts | • Explore severity (+/- plans) at each visit<br>• Support mother and husband who are scared of suicidal thoughts | BJ/ Cons |
| 3. Daughter's school problems | • Maintain links with class teacher<br>• Keep family informed of her progress | BJ |
| 4. Plan for recovery | • Link with support group when mood lightens<br>• Help reapply for part-time cleaning job | BJ |

Professionals involved in care:  ✔ Dr     Psychologist   ✔ CPN    OT    ✔ SW    Ward Nurse    ACT    Other

Present at planning meeting:  ✔ Dr    ✔ Psychologist   ✔ CPN    OT    ✔ SW    Ward Nurse    ACT    Other

Copy given to patient?    YES/~~NO~~        Copy sent to GP?    YES/~~NO~~

Care co-ordinator(print): **Billie Jarvis (BJ)**          **Phone**

Care co-ordinator (signature): .................................................          **Date of next review: 20.04.08.**

Job title: **CPN**                **Patient's signature:**...................................

| On Supervision Register? | **~~YES~~/NO** | Care management? YES/~~NO~~ | Risk history completed? YES/~~NO~~ |
|---|---|---|---|
| On Supervised Discharge? | **~~YES~~/NO** | Relapse + risk plan required? YES/~~NO~~ | |

**Fig. 7.5.1** Care programme review document.

| CONFIDENTIAL: RELAPSE AND RISK MANAGEMENT PLAN | | | |
| --- | --- | --- | --- |
| **Name:** Alastair W | | | |

**Categories of Risk Identified:**

| | | | |
| --- | --- | --- | --- |
| Aggression and violence | ~~YES~~/NO | Severe self-neglect | YES/~~NO~~ |
| Exploitation (self or others) | YES/~~NO~~ | Risk to children & young adults | YES/~~NO~~ |
| Suicide and self-harm | YES/~~NO~~ | | |
| Other (please specify} ........................... | | | |

**Current factors which suggest there is significant apparent risk:**
(For example: alcohol or substance misuse; specific threats; suicidal ideation; violent fantasies; anger; suspiciousness; persecutory beliefs; paranoid feelings or ideas about particular people)

Continued excessive drinking—especially when depressed. Makes him more suspicious and hostile.

**Clear statement of anticipated risk(s):**
(Who is at risk; how immediate is that risk; how severe; how ongoing)

Clear risk to strangers (not family or staff), usually in bars. Often when poor medication compliance.

**Action Plan:**
(Including names of people responsible for each action and steps to be taken if plan breaks down)

Relapse plan discussed and agreed—to increase antipsychotics and contact when concerned with people plotting ('to help you cope with them').
If he feels seriously threatened to seek admission through the emergency room

**Date Completed:**    xx/xx/xx         **Review date:**    xx/xx/xx

**Fig. 7.5.2** Risk assessment and contingency plan.

AO teams (Box 7.5.1) are costly and consequently reserved for the most difficult ('hard to engage' or 'revolving-door') psychotic patients with frequent, often dangerous, relapses and poor medication compliance plus alcohol or drug abuse, significant personality difficulties, and offending behaviour.

AO emphasizes proactive outreach—visiting patients at home even when they are reluctant. It exploits enhanced team working with daily meetings and several members actively involved with most patients both for safety considerations and also reflecting patients' extensive needs. The culture is of very practical working (taking patients shopping, sorting out accommodation, delivering medicines daily if need be) well beyond traditional professional boundaries.

Despite strongly expressed convictions there is little evidence that AO teams need to slavishly follow the original model[15,16] and local clinical adjustments are both sensible and justified. If embedded in a comprehensive system there is little need for a 24 h service, most staff establish strong individual relationships with patients and caseloads are usually more than the recommended 1:10. Where CMHTs function well AO teams take only patients who cannot be stabilized despite their support.

If CMHTs provide outreach and a comprehensive treatment then the extra AO resources may add little. Improved outcomes follow only from additional effective treatments (e.g. daily Clozapine visits in resistant schizophrenia); it is not outreach itself that is therapeutic. Whether AO will improve care (and, if so, how many teams are needed for how many patients) will depend on current services.

### Ethics in community mental health care

Balancing patients' welfare with their autonomy and their rights with those of their families and the wider community are sharply revealed in AO teams. These teams regularly visit patients who vigorously and clearly reject them. When does intensive support become intrusion? When does professional persistence tip over into coercion or disrespect?

Compulsion was traditionally identified with the buildings of the old asylums or left to the family (as it still is in many parts of the world). With expanded community care, compulsion, and coercion (either explicitly in the form of legal requirements or informally through professional or social pressure[17]) are now a pervasive feature of practice. Improved legal and professional scrutiny makes compulsory treatment possible in the community. Most developed countries have enacted forms of community treatment order ('mandated community treatment', 'outpatient committal') mainly for the care of young psychotic individuals

---

**Box 7.5.1  ACT core components**

- Assertive follow-up.
- Small caseloads (1:10–1:15).
- Regular (daily) team meetings.
- Frequent contact (weekly to daily).
- *In vivo practice* (treatment in home and neighbourhood).
- Emphasis on engagement and medication.
- Support for family and carers.
- Provision of services using all team members.
- Crisis stabilization 24 h a day, 7 days a week.

without insight into their need for ongoing treatment. The introduction of these provisions has generally been controversial but their operation not so.

Community treatment orders have the advantage of legal scrutiny unlike most of the ethical dilemmas facing CMHT and AO staff in their day-to-day work. These require discussion case-by-case. How proper is it to inform neighbours if a patient may pose a risk to them but will not give consent? Is it right for a patient, heavily dependent on his parents, to deny them information on his treatment? What does a case manager do when they know their client is doing something illegal? Most professionals share the goal of maximizing their patient's autonomy while minimizing significant risks. Guidelines exist only for extreme circumstances. Teams should be encouraged in regular discussion of these issues.

## Crisis teams

Crisis teams play a crucial role where local services are poorly developed (they may be the *only* community services) or in city centres with many transient and homeless patients. They must prioritize rapid response and accessibility. Most teams will see patients immediately, certainly the same day. Their clinical aims and staffing are essentially similar to the acute functioning in CMHTs. They are best located alongside CMHTs or in the emergency rooms of general hospitals with 24 h availability. Liaison services (see Chapter 5.7) can often incorporate and manage hospital-based crisis teams.

### Crisis Resolution/Home Treatment (CR/HT) Teams

The CR/HT team model, developed in Australia[18] and currently implemented in the United Kingdom and Europe, reflects increased consumer demand for access in crises and a desire to reduce inpatient care costs. It draws heavily on AO practice with limited, shared caseloads, flexible working, extended access, and an emphasis on outreach. Reduction in hospitalization offsets much of their cost[19] but this needs to be considerable as with two daily shifts and on call overnight needs a staff of about 15 for a caseload of 30 proposed for a population of 150 000.[20] They target patients who would otherwise be in hospital and focus on the severely mentally ill with intensive visiting (usually daily for a limited period) and considerable practical support and work with patients' social networks; most aim for a maximum of 6 weeks involvement. Such intensive team working requires highly effective communication and the teams meet daily (often twice at shift handovers). Information transfer is burdensome and liaison with CMHTs complex requiring absolute clarity on local arrangements for clinical responsibility.

### Variations in practice and sustainability

The CR/HT teams may reduce the need for hospital care[18,21] but how much will vary. The UK model is precisely specified (including who it should and should not care for, Box 7.5.2) but practice varies considerably. A full 24 h service is rarely needed, an on-call facility to the emergency room and police station at night usually suffices. Contact frequencies are generally lower, patients stay with the service longer than anticipated and they are inevitably referred individuals recurrently in crisis (often with alcohol and relationship problems) who cannot easily be refused care but would not be 'otherwise in hospital'. Good medical staffing is needed and CMHT

responsibilities need to be carefully negotiated, mutually agreed and crystal clear if to be avoided. These realities need to be carefully considered before deciding to establish such teams.

Crisis services may have a relatively limited lifespan[22] but can be a very successful way to improve local access, gain familiarity with at-risk populations, and then consolidate as a more comprehensive service. Sometimes, however, they become overwhelmed with inappropriate referrals or patients who cannot be referred on and close.

### Crisis houses and respite care

Crisis houses allow admission with a minimum of formality and often with reduced supervision compared to hospitals. They are usually small (4–8 beds) in a domestic setting and take people for days, occasionally a week or two. They are favoured for vulnerable women and early intervention services. Most have one staff member sleeping in overnight and a couple on during the day with support from patients' case managers. They are very welcome for a minority of patients but do not replace inpatient care and need careful supervision to avoid becoming chaotic or blocked.

### Adjunct or replacement for CMHTs?

The three teams outlined above comprise the fundamental building blocks of most community services. AO and CR/HT teams have been proposed as substitutes for CMHTs, particularly when there are problems with local CMHTs. However both experience and research evidence[23] suggests that they are rarely durable without effective CMHTs to relate to. They should be considered to improve the quality of care in otherwise well-functioning services rather than cost-saving shortcuts.

## Highly specialized and diagnosis-specific teams

There are various specialized teams, generally organized on a regional level. These are not essential local services but impact on them—both in terms of removing some of the clinical obligations and the need to ensure clear and negotiable thresholds.

### Early Intervention Teams (EIS)

Concern that a long duration of untreated psychosis (DUP) confers poorer prognosis[24] has led to the development of EIS teams which many would now argue should be standard provision. Developed mainly from Australian and UK models[25,26] they vary remarkably even despite a detailed prescription for UK teams. Some down-play diagnosis in favour of easy access, others restrict to schizophrenia, some emphasize a 'youth service' while others take all first episode patients irrespective of age.[7] Even more confusing there are three quite different activities which may, or may not, be part of the service (Box 7.5.3).

The core of EIS is a specialized CMHT which case-manages first episode psychosis patients protecting social networks and functioning (keeping patients at college or work, an emphasis on family interventions, etc.) assuming a return to premorbid functioning. Crisis and respite houses are preferred to hospital. Some EIS teams conduct public awareness campaigns, lecturing in schools and colleges.[27] A minority of research teams attempt to identify and treat 'ultra-high risk' patients to prevent progression to psychosis.[28]

### Forensic and rehabilitation teams

Community-focused services face particular difficulties in treatment-resistant patients, particularly those with socially unacceptable or offending behaviour. Such patients fit poorly into open wards and specialized forensic teams provide care where offending behaviour and danger to others predominates. Some provide community services (intensive case management of dangerous patients) with an emphasis on risk assessment and management. Integrating them with general services can be problematical.

### Rehabilitation

A significant number of patients remain disabled despite best treatments and require long-term management of disability rather than episode-based care. Rehabilitation teams generally serve patients who cannot survive without supervised accommodation even when at their best. They include the diminishing cohort of old long-stay patients and increasingly a very disturbed 'new long-stay' population with comorbid substance abuse and behavioural disturbances.

## Diagnostic-specific teams

Highly specialized teams for individual disorders (e.g. eating disorders, personality disorders, bipolar patients) concentrate specific skills and provide specialized treatments and are usually provided at regional level. They usually have stronger advocates than CMHTs, both from professionals and families of sufferers, and the opportunity costs (see below) of establishing them need careful thought.

## Planning services

### Step-wise planning and adaptation

Planning mental health services for a given community rarely starts with a clean sheet. In such circumstances there are excellent texts, both general and specific to mental health. Tansella and Thornicroft's 'matrix' model[29] is particularly thorough and structured (see Chapter 7.2). It covers the process from establishing service principles and needs assessment (at national, regional, and local levels) through to monitoring and reviewing the cycle of planning and provision. They propose a hierarchical approach depending on the level of mental health spend.[30] Case identification and outpatient treatments in primary care are the priority for low income countries and only with increased resources the establishment of a secondary care mental health service (usually a form of generic CMHT). Not until these are well-established are specialist and inpatient services indicated. This process must, however, take account of what is already in place.

### Local population needs assessment

Psychiatric morbidity varies considerably with social deprivation and is much higher in cities than in stable rural or suburban settings (see Chapter 2.7). At the regional and national level comparative need can be predicted fairly well from established indexes incorporating levels of migrants, overcrowding, poverty, etc. Catchment areas should broadly reflect these differences. At the more local level these figures are of limited value. How does one factor in travelling time or known differences in the quality of primary care? A process of negotiation is best to agree local allocation following these general guidelines. However a concentration of hostels for the mentally ill or homeless or the presence of a railway station or international airport may swamp these differences. These should be provisionally estimated in planning but then regularly monitored and reviewed.

### Opportunity costs and unintended consequences

Planning mental health services has become based on international evidence, often including cost-effectiveness analyses, i.e. is there more overall patient health gain for the same input (see Chapter 7.7)? However these rarely address the opportunity costs across a whole system. For example one form of day hospital may be more cost-effective for its patients than another day hospital, but is diverting nurses from an inpatient unit to staff that day hospital a net gain? Rigorous intervention studies of large systems are formidably difficult to conduct and even more so to interpret.

The impact of enthusiasm and the migration of the best staff to such research services can be especially misleading.[31] Successful new services are always reported but there is less consistency in reporting when a service may have lost its efficacy or was abandoned.[5,22] It is best to visit examples of services that are proposed and not to always assume that what works for them will necessarily work for you.[15]

---

**Box 7.5.3 Components of early intervention teams**

- **Case management**—ongoing care of identified patients
- **Early Identification**—awareness-raising campaigns for psychoses
- **High risk and prodromal** patient identification and treatment

Manpower is often as significant a resource limitation as funding, hence the need for a system-wide appraisal. Also, though expressed as costs, these decisions include wider judgements of values and expectations rather than simply outcomes.[30] Local and national objectives also matter, not just clinical ones (e.g. public safety now dominates much mental health planning).

### Cultures and funding

Health care cultures, their structures and their funding systems vary enormously. Services must be congruent with them otherwise they will not survive. Occasionally service planners can influence the system but more often have to adapt to it. Obtaining relatively small changes in funding arrangements (or external governance) can deliver quite major improvements. However caution is needed as unintended consequences and perverse incentives may arise. Enthusiastic clinicians are often blind to the risks of over-prescription which can lock in outmoded practices (e.g. a highly specific form of day hospital or crisis facility) that after opening is found not to have the level of need predicted but may be so rigidly prescribed that it cannot be adapted.

How 'integrated' mental health care should be is a highly local decision. Well-established systems often strive for integration with general medicine or, increasingly, with social services to reduce both discrimination and administrative barriers to integrated care. For less confident services the value of a distinct, separate, identity can be considerable—not least the ability to protect its resources. The 19th century British mental health reformer Lord Shaftsbury wrestled with the same dilemma.

The task of integration is easily underestimated, particularly the energies required to accommodate contrasting health and social care cultures. Social care, for example, tends to rely on very detailed paperwork and a highly structured system of intensive supervision (reflecting political accountability and previously only minimally trained workforce) as opposed to the high levels of professional autonomy in health care. Agreed compromises need to be reached before integration and the negotiations can be exhausting, but preferable to misunderstandings. The costs and benefits will depend very much on the local situation, relationships and history and should be very carefully weighed up.

### Relationships with the voluntary sector and patients movement

Relations with local non-health statutory services (housing, education, police) and with the voluntary sector will determine much of the success of MH services. Voluntary and private sectors may fill specialist niches left by a monolithic public health care system (as with the NHS in the United Kingdom) or conversely the public system may act as a safety net, for charitable and private provision. Service planners need to exploit the strengths of local providers. Non-statutory services are often more efficient but less comprehensive and may also be less reliable over the long-term. Both may be equally reliant on public funding, differing only in contracts and degrees of independence. Patient and carer advocacy and support organizations are now a major force; effective working with them significantly will enhance both the design and delivery of services (see Chapter 7.9).

## Monitoring and review

Careful monitoring and review are as important as careful planning for several reasons. The long-term, fluctuating nature of disorders, the subjective nature of diagnoses (increasingly self-ascribed) complicate outcome measures and the targeting of services; services can easily drift to those who demand them from those who most need them; treatments (particularly psychological and psychotherapeutic treatments) may evolve over time losing their effective characteristics; needy patients are rarely demanding or well-informed; engaging and motivating them to collaborate in long-term, treatments is difficult.

A consistent effort to deliver even the most basic, proven interventions will make a substantial difference to patient welfare. The PORT study in the United States demonstrated how schizophrenia care was strikingly inconsistent and fell below accepted essentials.[32] Regular audit ensures that services remain targeted on those for whom they were developed and that their application and quality remains good. Monitoring can vary in sophistication—from a simple head count of who is getting what through to careful evaluation of care pathways. The audit review process feeds back into the development process, adjusting and refining it. Even in the most hard-pressed services audit more than rewards its investment.

### Routine outcome measures (ROM)

Audit brings rigour and reflection (often lost in the immediacy of the therapeutic relationship) into the care process. Measurement also serves a training purpose by benchmarking interdisciplinary understandings of symptoms and outcomes. Systematic, periodic recording of patients' clinical or social status is increasingly used in both planning and research. Structured outcomes can be generic (e.g. HoNOS[33]) or for specific disorders (e.g. the Brief Psychiatric Rating Scale[34]) or even locally developed. Their value lies in their consistency of use.

## Conclusions

Planning and providing mental health services requires flexibility and compromise. Epidemiological and service statistics translate poorly to local planning; this remains primarily a practical and political, rather than academic, activity. The scientific evidence is dominated by Anglophone alternatives to hospital care studies but local history, culture, mental health law, and political imperatives cannot be ignored. Mediterranean societies, for example, with strong family supports and fewer isolated psychotic individuals have less interest in AO teams. A high-profile patient homicide, or a strong public endorsement of services by politician or celebrity, can derail years of careful planning.

This chapter has attempted to draw out some principles (Box 7.5.4) for the process but these can only be guidelines. Inevitably the decision will be based on what is *possible* locally. Despite this most solutions draw on a limited number of tried and tested structures described here in some detail. Their balance and configuration depend on what is available for them and around them. Above all the mentally ill and their families deserve reliable and predictable services. Not all change is innovation and research findings should be judged in terms of their sustainability and demonstrated translation from research efficacy to clinical effectiveness.

**Box 7.5.4** Developing local community mental health services

◆ Make a careful inventory of what services exist, and any special local needs.

◆ Consult locally and invest heavily in building coalitions with policy makers, statutory services, and voluntary groups.

◆ Test research evidence for durability and relevance. If possible visit established services and ask 'around the service'.

◆ Monitor and review regularly. Improved consistency of current practice often delivers more than introducing new treatments.

◆ Consider carefully opportunity costs. Include both the impact of a specific improvement across the whole service and the costs of system change itself.

◆ Avoid excessive reorganization—not all change is innovation.

## Further information

Burns, T. (2004). *Community mental health teams*. Oxford University Press, Oxford.

The Mental Health Policy Implementation Guide. (2001). Department of Health, London.

Thornicroft, G. and Tansella, M. (2004). Components of a modern mental health service: a pragmatic balance of community and hospital care: overview of systematic evidence. *The British Journal of Psychiatry*, **185**, 283–90.

Thornicroft, G. and Tansella, M. (1999). *The mental health matrix: a manual to improve services*. Cambridge University Press, Cambridge.

## References

1. Strathdee, G. and Thornicroft, G. (1992). Community sectors of need-lead mental health services. In *Measuring mental health needs* (eds. G. Thornicroft, C.R. Brewin, and J. Wing). Gaskell, London.

2. Catty, J., Goddard, K., and Burns, T. (2005). Social services day care and health services day care in mental health: do they differ? *International Journal of Psychoanalysis*, **51**(2), 151–61.

3. Marshall, M. (2003). Acute psychiatric day hospitals. *British Medical Journal*, **327**, 116–7.

4. Knapp, M., Hallam, A., Beecham, J., *et al.* (1999). Private, voluntary or public? Comparative cost-effectiveness in community mental health care. *Policy and Politics*, **27**(1), 25–41.

5. Wright, C., Catty, J., Watt, H., *et al.* (2004). A systematic review of home treatment services. Classification and sustainability. *Social Psychiatry and Psychiatric Epidemiology*, **39**, 789–96.

6. Slade, M., Powell, R., Rosen, A., *et al.* (2000). Threshold assessment grid (TAG): the development of a valid and brief scale to assess the severity of mental illness. *Social Psychiatry and Psychiatric Epidemiology*, **35**(2), 78–85.

7. Burns, T. (2004). *Community mental health teams*. Oxford University Press, Oxford.

8. Burns, T., Beadsmoore, A., Bhat, A.V., *et al.* (1993). A controlled trial of home-based acute psychiatric services. I: clinical and social outcome. *The British Journal of Psychiatry*, **163**, 49–54.

9. Stein, L.I. and Test, M.A. (1980). Alternative to mental hospital treatment. I: conceptual model, treatment program, and clinical evaluation. *Archives of General Psychiatry*, **37**(4), 392–7.

10. Intagliata, J. (1982). Improving the quality of community care for the chronically mentally disabled: the role of case management. *Schizophrenia Bulletin*, **8**(4), 655–74.

11. Holloway, F., Oliver, N., Collins, E., *et al.*(1995). Case management: a critical review of the outcome literature. *European Psychiatry*, **10**, 113–28.

12. Department of Health. (1990). The care programme approach for people with a mental illness referred to the special psychiatric services. Department of Health, London. Report No.: Joint Health/Social Services Circular HC (90) 23/LASS (90) 11.

13. Burns, T., Raftery, J., Beadsmoore, A., *et al.* (1993). A controlled trial of home-based acute psychiatric services. II: treatment patterns and costs. *The British Journal of Psychiatry*, **163**, 55–61.

14. Burns, T. and Bale, R. (1997). Establishing a mental health liaison attachment with primary care. *Advances in Psychiatric Treatment*, **3**, 219–24.

15. Fiander, M., Burns, T., McHugo, G.J., *et al.* (2003). Assertive community treatment across the Atlantic: comparison of model fidelity in the UK and USA. *The British Journal of Psychiatry*, **182**, 248–54.

16. Burns, T., Marshall, M., Catty, J., *et al.* (2005). *Variable outcomes in case management trials—an exploration of current theories using meta-regression and meta-analysis*: Final Report. Department of Health, London.

17. Monahan, J., Redlich, A.D., Swanson, J., *et al.* (2005). Use of leverage to improve adherence to psychiatric treatment in the community. *Psychiatric Services*, **56**(1), 37–44.

18. Hoult, J. (1986). Community care of the acutely mentally ill. *The British Journal of Psychiatry*, **149**, 137–44.

19. Smyth, M.G. and Hoult, J. (2000). The home treatment enigma. *British Medical Journal*, **320**(7230), 305–9.

20. Department of Health. (2001). The mental health policy implementation guide. Department of Health, London.

21. Johnson, S., Nolan, F., Pilling, S., *et al.* (2005). Randomised controlled trial of acute mental health care by a crisis resolution team: the north Islington crisis study. *British Medical Journal*, **331**(7517), 599.

22. Cooper, J.E. (1979). Crisis admission units and emergency psychiatric services. Public Health in Europe, No. 2. Copenhagen: World Health Organisation.

23. Burns, T., Catty, J., Watt, H., *et al.* (2002). International differences in home treatment for mental health problems. Results of a systematic review. *The British Journal of Psychiatry*, **181**, 375–82.

24. Marshall, M., Lewis, S., Lockwood, A., *et al.* (2005). Association between duration of untreated psychosis and outcome in cohorts of first-episode patients: a systematic review. *Archives of General Psychiatry*, **62**(9), 975–83.

25. Edwards, J., McGorry, P.D., and Pennell, K. (2000). Models of early intervention in psychosis: an analysis of service approaches. In *Early intervention in psychosis: a guide to concepts, evidence and interventions* (eds. M. Birchwood, D. Fowler, and C. Jackson). John Wiley & Sons, New York.

26. Birchwood, M., Todd, P., and Jackson, C. (1998). Early intervention in psychosis. The critical period hypothesis. *The British Journal of Psychiatry—Supplement*, **172**(33), 53–9.

27. McGorry, P. and Jackson, H. (1999). Recognition and management of early psychosis. A preventative approach. Cambridge University Press, Cambridge.

28. McGorry, P.D., Yung, A.R., Phillips, L.J., *et al.* (2002). Randomized controlled trial of interventions designed to reduce the risk of progression to first-episode psychosis in a clinical sample with subthreshold symptoms. *Archives of General Psychiatry*, **59**(10), 921–8.

29. Tansella, M. and Thornicroft, G. (1998). A conceptual framework for mental health services: the matrix model. *Psychological Medicine*, **28**(3), 503–8.

30. Thornicroft, G. and Tansella, M. (2004). Components of a modern mental health service: a pragmatic balance of community and hospital care: overview of systematic evidence. *The British Journal of Psychiatry*, **185**, 283–90.

31. Coid, J. (1994). Failure in community care: psychiatry's dilemma. *British Medical Journal*, **308**(6932), 805–6.

32. Lehman, A.F. and Steinwachs, D.M. (1998). Translating research into practice: the Schizophrenia Patient Outcomes Research Team (PORT) treatment recommendations. *Schizophrenia Bulletin*, **24**(1), 1–10.

33. Orrell, M., Yard, P., Handysides, J., *et al.* (1999). Validity and reliability of the health of the nation outcome scales in psychiatric patients in the community. *The British Journal of Psychiatry*, **174**, 409–12.

34. Overall, J.E. and Gorham, D.L. (1962). The brief psychiatric rating scale. *Psychological Reports*, **10**, 799–812.

# Evaluation of mental health services

## Michele Tansella and Graham Thornicroft

## Introduction

Evaluation is the basis for improving care to people with mental illness. It is vital to know whether interventions are beneficial or harmful, and whether they offer value for money. Mental health interventions need to be understood both in terms of their active ingredients and how they fit within their context.[1] Such combined interventions, often including pharmacological, psychological, and social elements, are the epitome of 'complex interventions'[2] and their evaluation poses considerable challenges. In this chapter we shall discuss *definitions* of evaluation, and go on to discuss *why* evaluate, *what* to evaluate, and *how* to evaluate mental health services. In our conclusion we shall offer an indication of the most important trends in this field in the coming years. The overall approach that we take is centred upon the idea that ongoing evaluative research is of fundamental importance in discovering which interventions are effective, neutral, or harmful, and that such information is essential to deliver better mental health care.

## Evaluation: definitions and conceptual framework

The *Concise Oxford English Dictionary*[3] gives the following definitions of 'evaluation':
**evaluate** (*verb transitive*) **1**. assess, appraise; **2a**. find or state the number or amount of; **2b**. find a numerical expression for.
**evaluation** (*noun*) **1**. appraisal, valuation, assessment; **2**. estimate, estimation, approximation, rating, opinion, ranking, judgement, reckoning, figuring, calculation, computation, determination.

The etymological root of the word therefore refers directly to 'value', although in common usage 'evaluation' now has a more technical connotation. In our view evaluation necessarily requires both the precise measurement of the effects of treatments or services, alongside a contextual understand of the meaning, and value of such results.

A conceptual model that can be used to clarify key issues related to the evaluation of mental health services is the Matrix Model.[4,5] The two *dimensions* of this model are place and time (see Table 7.6.1). Place refers to three geographical levels: (1) country/regional, (2) local, and (3) individual. Time refers to three phases: (A) inputs, (B) processes, and (C) outcomes. In this framework *inputs* relates to all those resources which are necessary before health care can

take place (such as financial and human resources, policies, and treatment guidelines), *processes* refers to all those activities which constitute the delivery of health care (such as outpatient consultations, or hospital admissions), while *outcomes* refers to the consequences of health care (such as changes in symptoms, disability, and quality of life). In relation to the evaluation of mental health services, we shall illustrate in this chapter how inputs and processes need to be measured and understood in their contribution to the outcomes of care.

Historically, the first attempts to evaluate psychiatric practice originated in the mid-nineteenth century as the tabulation of admissions, discharges, and deaths in mental hospitals, simply describing the inputs and processes of care. In recent decades, as more sophisticated research methodologies and more valid and reliable research measures have been developed, so the evaluation of mental health services has increasingly focussed upon the analysis of the outcomes of care. As Sartorius has put it, 'In its most classical form, evaluation denotes a comparison between results and goals of activity',[6] indicating that evaluation has now become a purposeful exercise in which measurements are used as tools to answer specific questions, usually defined a priori at the beginning of a scientific study.

## Why evaluate mental health services?

In our view, the main purposes of mental health service evaluation are to assess the effectiveness and cost-effectiveness of care, either at the organizational (local) or at the patient (individual) level. In the long-term such evidence can be used to provide better services for people with mental illness. For example, evaluation can be applied to comparing differing models of care, such as studies in England showing that home-treatment teams can provide a realistic alternative to emergency hospital admission.[7–9] Evaluation therefore measures the impact of care (outcomes) and also aims to increase understanding of the active ingredients (inputs and processes) which contribute to better outcomes.[1] In fact, a wider range of purposes can be served by the evaluation of mental health services, as shown in Table 7.6.2.

## What to evaluate in mental health services?

In our view the most important focus of evaluation is upon the *outcomes* of care.[10,11] The outcome chosen for any particular

**Table 7.6.1** Overview of the Matrix Model, with examples of inputs, processes, and outcomes

| Place dimension | Time dimension | | |
| --- | --- | --- | --- |
| | (A) Input phase | (B) Process phase | (C) Outcome phase |
| (1) Country/regional level | **1A**<br><br>Mental health budget allocation<br>Mental health laws<br>Government directives and policies<br>Training plans for mental health staff<br>Treatment protocols and guidelines | **1B**<br><br>Performance/activity indicators (e.g. admission rates, compulsory treatment rates) | **1C**<br><br>Overall suicide rates<br>Homelessness rates<br>Imprisonment rates<br>Years lived with disability |
| (2) Local level | **2A**<br><br>Local service budgets and balance for hospital and community services<br>Local population needs assessment<br>Staff numbers and mix<br>Clinical and non-clinical services<br>Working relationships between teams | **2B**<br><br>Service contacts and patterns of service use<br>Pathways to care and continuity<br>Targeting of services to special groups | **2C**<br><br>Suicide rates among people with mental illness<br>Employment rates<br>Physical morbidity rates |
| (3) Individual level | **3A**<br><br>Assessments of individual needs made by staff, service users, and by families<br>Therapeutic expertise of staff<br>Information for service users<br>Information for family members | **3B**<br><br>Content of therapeutic interventions (both psychological, social, and pharmacological)<br>Continuity of clinical staff<br>Frequency of appointments | **3C**<br><br>Symptom severity<br>Impact on caregivers<br>Satisfaction with services<br>Quality of life<br>Disability<br>Met and unmet needs |

evaluation will depend upon the central question addressed and the level at which outcomes are assessed, as shown in Table 7.6.3.

Directly in relation to the population level, a frequently used outcome measure is suicide rate (see cell 1C in Table 7.6.1). Rates of homelessness among mentally ill people (or rates of mental illness among the homeless) can also be used as an outcome indicator of the effectiveness of mental illness policies at the national (or regional) level.

At the local level, outcome indicators useful for evaluation can be made in three ways: (i) by interpolating from regional/national data; (ii) by measuring directly at the local level; and (iii) by aggregating individual-level information up to the local level. For example, rates of suicide and unemployment can be estimated using the first method, or directly measured using the second approach if the appropriate data and resources exist, which will provide more accurate and up-to-date information. The third approach is to aggregate up to the local level information gathered from individual

patients, if institutions providing care to those local patients are willing to cooperate in integrating their datasets.

At the individual level mental health service evaluation increasingly acknowledges the importance of outcomes other than symptom severity.[10,11] Traditionally, **symptom severity measures** have been used most often to assess the effectiveness of the early, mental health treatments. Psychiatrists and psychologists have contributed to the early development of such assessment scales to allow this

**Table 7.6.3** Outcome measures suitable for use in routine clinical practice

| Outcome measure | Place dimension | | |
| --- | --- | --- | --- |
| | Country level | Local level | Individual level |
| Employment status | √ | √ | √√ |
| Physical morbidity | √ | √ | √ |
| Suicide and self-harm | √√ | √ | √√ |
| Homelessness | | √ | √√ |
| Standardized mortality ratios | √ | √ | |
| Symptom severity | | √ | √√ |
| Impact on caregivers | | √ | √ |
| Satisfaction with services | | √ | √√ |
| Quality of life | | √ | √ |
| Disability | | √ | √√ |
| Met and unmet needs for care | | √ | √ |

Key: √ = suitable for use as an outcome, √√ = commonly used as an outcome.

**Table 7.6.2** Main purposes of mental health service evaluation

◆ To assess the outcomes of services in experimental conditions (*efficacy*)

◆ To investigate whether interventions which have demonstrated *efficacy* under experimental conditions are also *effective* in ordinary, routine clinical conditions

◆ To understand the mechanism of action (i.e. active ingredients) of interventions

◆ To inform mental health service investment decisions, for example using health economic data on cost-effectiveness

◆ To raise awareness among planners, policy makers, and politicians of service gaps

◆ To test a priori or to check *post hoc* the value of planning decisions (for example, the closure of mental hospitals)

research to take place.[10,11] While the primary symptoms are clearly important, for most of the more severe mental disorders there is symptom persistence, and, at present, it is unrealistic to see symptom eradication as the sole aim of treatment. Therefore, very often, after the point of maximum symptom relief, when the extent of the ongoing impairments is clear, then the clinical task becomes one of attempting to minimize the consequent disability and handicap.

The importance of the **impact of caring** for people with mental illnesses upon family members and others who provide informal care has long been recognized, but has only been subjected to concerted research relatively recently.[11–13] Such research has shown that it is common for carers themselves to suffer from mental illnesses, most commonly depression and anxiety, and to worry about the future when they may no longer be able to cope. Moreover, many family members are most distressed by the patient's underactivity, and are often poorly informed about the clinical condition, its treatment, and the likely prognosis, as well as being inadequately provided with a practical action plan of what to do in the future should a crisis occur. Indeed, some services continue to convey to families the outmoded idea that carers, especially parents, are in some way to blame for the disorder or for relapses of the condition. The regular provision of information sessions for family members is now a hallmark of a good practice.[14,15]

Patients' **satisfaction with services** is a further domain that has recently become established as a legitimate, important, and feasible area of outcome assessment.[16] This is a recognition of the contribution that service users and their carers can make to outcome assessment. Psychometrically adequate scales in this field are those that adopt a multidimensional approach, assess the full range of service characteristics, are independently administered (so that patient ratings have no consequences upon their future clinical care), and have established validity and reliability.[17]

**Quality of life** ratings have also become prominent during the last decade, and several scales have been constructed that reflect different basic approaches to the topic.[18] The first distinction is between scales that address subjective well-being, compared with those that also measure objective elements of quality of life. The second main point of differentiation is between scales constructed for the general population and those designed for patients suffering from specific disorders, including the more severe mental illnesses.[19] One advantage of quality of life data is that they tend to be popular with politicians, for whom the concept often has powerful face validity.

Among people with longer-term or more complex mental illnesses, the measurement of **disability** is often an important consideration.[20] Increasing importance is also being attached to the **needs** of people with mental illness, where met needs are difficulties faced by people with mental illness in the presence of appropriate interventions.[21] Needs (both met and unmet) may be defined by professionals/experts, or by service users, and in fact there is emerging evidence that service user ratings may be more informative, for example in predicting quality of life.[22–24]

## Psychometric properties of outcome measures

Establishing the psychometric qualities of scales used for service evaluation is a central issue.[4] Among the most important characteristics of outcome scales are validity and reliability. Validity refers to whether a scale actually measures what it is intended to measure. It is conventionally assessed in terms of face validity, content validity, consensual validity, criterion-related validity, and construct validity.

In addition, a rating scale must give repeatable results for the same subject when used under different conditions, i.e. it must be reliable. There are four widely used methods to gauge reliability: inter-rater reliability, test–retest reliability, parallel-form reliability, and split-half reliability. The main issue for the evaluation of mental health services is to use wherever possible scales with known and adequate psychometric properties.

## How to evaluate mental health services

In this section we consider research designs that may be applicable to the range of contexts used in mental health service evaluation.[1] Different types of evidence produced using these designs cannot be considered as equivalent. A hierarchical order has been proposed by Geddes and Harrison[25] as shown in Table 7.6.4.

In terms of research methods or designs which can be used to produce such evidence, they can be considered as: (i) randomized controlled trial (RCT), (ii) quasi-experimental studies, (iii) case-control studies, (iv) cohort studies (prospective or retrospective), (v) cross sectional studies, and (vi) case series and single case studies. Since evaluations of mental health services are usually concerned with complex interventions, it is helpful to have an overall scheme linking different stages of research to test treatment interventions. The Medical Research Council (MRC) framework for the evaluation of complex interventions sets out one such sequence, as shown in relation to anti-stigma interventions in Table 7.6.5. The elements in this scheme can be considered as sequential, or stages 0, 1, and 2 can be seen as one larger iterative activity.[1] Nevertheless, although this gives salience to randomized controlled trial designs, it is important to appreciate that research study designs need to be matched to the purpose of each type of evaluation, as shown in Table 7.6.6.

### Evidence from a meta-analysis of randomized controlled trials

Meta-analysis can be defined as 'the quantitative synthesis of the results of systematic overviews of previous studies', while systematic overviews, in turn, are methods of collating and synthesizing all the available evidence on a particular scientific question.[26] Since randomized controlled trials are often considered to produce the most sophisticated evidence on the efficacy of medical treatments,

**Table 7.6.4** Hierarchy of evidence

| | |
|---|---|
| 1a | Evidence from a meta-analysis of RCTs |
| 1b | Evidence from at least one RCT |
| 2a | Evidence from at least one controlled study without randomization |
| 2b | Evidence from at least one other type of quasi-experimental study |
| 3 | Evidence from non-experimental descriptive studies, such as comparative studies, correlation studies, and case-control studies |
| 4 | Evidence from expert committee reports or opinions and/or clinical experience of respected authorities |

(Reproduced from J.R. Geddes, and P.J. Harrison, Closing the gap between research and practice, *The British Journal of Psychiatry*, **171**, 220–5, copyright 1997, The Royal College of Psychiatrists.)

**Table 7.6.5** Phases of the Medical Research Council framework for the evaluation of complex interventions[1, 2]

| 0 Preclinical | 1 Modelling/manualization | 2 Exploratory | 3 Definitive trial | 4 Long-term implementation |
|---|---|---|---|---|
| Explore relevant theory to ensure best choice of intervention and hypothesis and to predict major confounders and strategic design issues | Identify the components of the intervention and the underlying mechanisms by which they will influence outcomes to provide evidence that you can predict how they relate to and interact with each other | Describe the constant and variable components of a replicable intervention and a feasible protocol for comparing the intervention with an appropriate alternative | Compare a fully defined intervention with an appropriate alternative using a protocol that is theoretically defensible, reproducible, and adequately controlled in a study with appropriate statistical power | Determine whether others can reliably replicate your intervention and the results in uncontrolled settings over the long-term |
| Example: anti-stigma intervention in schools study | | | | |
| Social contact theory[69] | Yes | Completed[70] | Planned | Potential if preceding phases successful |

a meta-analysis conducted on well selected and relevant randomized controlled trials can be seen as the highest order of knowledge. It follows that the quality of systematic overviews is limited by the quality and quantity of the contributory trials (see Table 7.6.7).[27]

Cochrane was the first to emphasize the need to bring together, within specific categories, the results of randomized controlled trials.[28] This approach is now central to evidence-based medicine. Within psychiatric evaluation the first meta-analyses were conducted in the late 1970s, and more information is given on systematic reviews in Chapter 1.10 and 6.1.

An illustration of such an exercise is the systematic overview and meta-analysis is that which reviewed RCTs comparing the outcomes of community mental health teams with those of standard care for patients with severe mental illness and disordered personalities.[29, 30] They found 1200 citations using the search strategy: 70 appeared relevant to the review, but only four studies satisfied the inclusion criteria. The main results of this systematic review are that community mental health team management is associated with fewer deaths by suicide, with fewer people being dissatisfied with services or leaving the studies early. No clear difference was found in admission rates, overall clinical outcomes, or in the duration of inpatient hospital treatment. The authors concluded that community mental health team management is not inferior to non-team standard care in any important respects, and is superior in promoting greater acceptance of treatment. It may also be superior in reducing hospital admissions and avoiding deaths by suicide.

### The randomized controlled trials

The importance of randomized controlled trials within medical research has been expressed by Korn and Baumrind:[31]

**Table 7.6.6** Research aims and appropriate study designs

| Research aim | Appropriate study designs |
|---|---|
| Service description | Cross sectional survey |
| Assess intervention | Quasi-experimental study (e.g. controlled before–after comparison) Randomized controlled trial |
| Identify prognosis for a condition | Cohort study |
| Establish aetiology of a condition | Cohort study Case-control study |

'Randomized clinical trials are the sine qua non for evaluating treatment in man'. According to Barker and Rose: 'the essence of the randomized controlled trial is that the outcome of the treatment given to one group of patients is compared with one or more other groups who are given different treatments or none at all. Allocation of individuals to the treatment and comparison groups is by random selection'.[32]

The advantages of the research design of these studies have been extensively described[33] and are shown in Table 7.6.8 (see also Chapter 1.10 in this book). However, the design limitations of such trials also need to be appreciated, particularly in relation to health service research, as shown in Table 7.6.9.[34]

In addition to the technical limitations of the trial design, there are also situations where randomized controlled trials are not applicable to specific research questions. These can be summarized as conditions in which randomized controlled trials are inadequate, impossible, inappropriate, or unnecessary, as shown in Table 7.6.10. Nevertheless, where they are appropriate, it will be necessary to use explicit criteria to assess the quality of such trials, such as those shown in Table 7.6.11.[35, 36]

It is now common to distinguish between *efficacy trials* (which tend to be explanatory) and *effectiveness trials* (sometimes otherwise called large simple, pragmatic, practical, or management trials).[33, 37–39] This categorical distinction has its uses, although

**Table 7.6.7** Characteristics of systematic overviews

**Questions to ask about papers for potential inclusion in a systematic overview**

- Were the questions and methods clearly stated?
- Were comprehensive search methods used to locate the relevant articles?
- Were explicit methods used to determine which articles were included in the review?
- Was the methodological quality of the primary studies assessed?
- Were the selection and assessment of the primary studies reproducible and free from bias?
- Were the differences in individual study results adequately explained?
- Were the results of the primary studies combined appropriately?
- Were the reviewer's conclusions supported by the data cited?

(Reproduced from S.I. Sackett and J.E. Wennberg, Choosing the best research design for each question, *British Medical Journal*, **315** (7123), 1636, copyright 1997, BMJ Publishing Group Ltd.)

**Table 7.6.8** Advantages of RCTs

- Controls for many confounding variables which may exist
- Eliminates the effects of spontaneous remission
- Eliminates regression to mean
- Eliminates placebo effect
- Independent of rater bias if blindness maintained
- Basis for systematic reviews

for some purposes we may rather see efficacy and effectiveness trials as falling along a continuum. Efficacy trials, which usually precede effectiveness studies, refer to those conducted under more ideal, experimental conditions, while effectiveness trials are RCTs carried out in more routine clinical conditions.[28,40–42] Nevertheless, some important questions, for example the impact of clinical guidelines, may only be researchable in real world settings, and will therefore bypass the efficacy study stage.[43]

Cochrane has defined effectiveness, at the patient level, as assessing whether an intervention does more good than harm when provided under usual circumstances of health care practice.[28] At the level of service provision, Wells has defined effectiveness trials as those which 'duplicate as closely as possible the conditions in the target practice venues to which study results will be applied'.[44] The key differences between efficacy and effectiveness trials are shown in Table 7.6.12, although in practice the differences between these types of trial may not necessarily be as great as the differences between pharmacological, psychological, and service interventions

**Table 7.6.9** Limitations and disadvantages of RCTs designs

1. Difficulties in choosing the unit or level of random allocation
- Should allocation be made at the patient level, the clinician level, the clinical team/practice level, or the locality level?

2. Difficulties in achieving random allocation
- Randomization not possible
- Particular patient groups excluded
- Self-exclusion because of non-consent

3. Difficulties in obtaining consent and in maintaining motivation
- Consent may be inversely proportional to severity of condition
- Consent may be refused because of patient treatment preferences
- Retention with the trial may be affected by patient motivation

4. Difficulties in establishing and maintaining blindness
- Degree of blinding of subjects
- Degree of blinding of staff
- Degree of blinding of raters
- Deactive Hawthorne effect (the effect of being studied upon those being studied)

5. Difficulties related to the experimental conditions
- Concurrent multiple interventions in health service research trials (without a single potentially active ingredient)
- Interactions between treatment components
- Consistency of control ('usual treatment') conditions
- High attrition rates or loss to follow-up
  Large differences between conditions in which trials can take place and those of routine practice

**Table 7.6.10** Situations when RCT designs are not applicable

1. Situations in which experimentation is inadequate
- Poor generalizability—low external validity
- Unrepresentative staff included
- Atypical patients included
- Treatments not standardized

2. Situations in which experimentation is impossible
- Refusal of clinicians to take part
- Ethical objections to the study
- Political barriers
- Legal objections
- Contamination between experimental and control conditions
- Scale of task—trials are required for too many treatments

3. Situations in which experimentation is inappropriate
- Studies conducted to reduce the occurrence of events of very low frequency
- Studies to prevent unwanted outcomes in the distant future

4. Experimentation unnecessary
- When benefit/risk ratio is dramatic
- When there is a small likelihood of confounders

(Reproduced from N. Black (1996), Why we need observational studies to evaluate the effectiveness of health care, *British Medical Journal*, **312** (7040), 1215–18, copyright 1997, BMJ Publishing Group Ltd.)

(such as the dissemination, and related barriers, of proven interventions).[45–47]

In planning effectiveness RCTs, seven sets of issues need to be carefully considered: (i) study question (e.g. is the study question expressed in an answerable way?), (ii) reference population (e.g. what is the reference group or subgroup to which the trial results should be generalized?), (iii) patient sample (e.g. how far does the sample reflect the target population?), (iv) study settings (e.g. how representative are the study settings of routine clinical sites?), (v) study interventions (e.g. is the study intervention manualized, acceptable to patients, and suitable for widespread use?), (vi) control condition (e.g. are the key characteristics of the control condition well described, and do they vary within and between sites?), and (vii) bias (e.g. attrition, blinding, concealment, consent, and

**Table 7.6.11** Criteria to evaluate the quality of an RCT

| Criteria |
| --- |
| 1. Is the hypothesis clearly defined? |
| 2. Is the study population representative? |
| 3. Was patient assignment randomized? |
| 4. Were patients, practitioners, and assessors blind to the experimental intervention? |
| 5. Were the groups similar at the start of the trial? |
| 6. Were the groups treated equally apart from the experimental intervention? |
| 7. Were all those who entered the trial accounted for at its conclusion? |
| 8. Was this in the groups to which they were originally allocated? |
| 9. Are all clinically important outcomes considered? |
| 10. Whose perspective do they reflect? |
| 11. Is the data analysis appropriate? |
| 12. What is the size and precision of the treatment effect? |
| 13. Do the likely benefits outweigh the harms and risks? |
| 14. Is the conclusion supported by the results? |

**Table 7.6.12** Key differences between efficacy and effectiveness trials

|  | **Efficacy trials** | **Effectiveness trials** |
|---|---|---|
| Goal | To estimate efficacy and safety (if relevant) usually of a specific clinical intervention | To estimate relative benefits and risks of approved treatments, clinical interventions, programmes, or policies |
| When | Usually before an intervention is introduced | Post-implementation |
| Diagnosis | Diagnosis by structured interview | Clinical diagnosis or structured interview |
| Inclusion and exclusion criteria | Strict and multiple inclusion and exclusion criteria, typically excluding patients with comorbid physical and psychiatric disorders | Relatively few inclusion and exclusion criteria to optimize external validity of sample |
| Patient sample | Typically enrol highly motivated patients | Attempt to include more representative patients, including those who are ambivalent and who may not adhere to the allocated treatment regime |
| Sample size | At most a few hundred, more often less than 100 | Often larger to enable smaller effect sizes to be identified in heterogeneous populations (e.g. in large simple trials with dichotomous outcomes) |
| Comparator | Placebo and/or single active comparator (for drug trials) Treatment as usual or active control (for psycho-social interventions) | One or more active comparators (for drug trials) Treatment as usual or active control (for psycho-social interventions) |
| Dosing | Fixed or flexible | Flexible dosing in clinically used range |
| Blinding | Triple-blind (i.e. patients, staff, and researchers blind), or double-blind | Double-blind (where possible), or single-blind |
| Duration | 1–4 months | 6 months or more |
| Research sites | Small number of experienced research sites | Dozens of routine treatment sites |
| Delivery of intervention | According to manual or protocol, not a focus of research | Fidelity to manual a key variable, and study may consider barriers to delivery of intervention in routine practice[47] |
| Research protocol | Strictly defined | Deliberately similar to usual practice |
| Adjunctive treatments | Not allowed or strictly limited | Allowed as in usual practice |
| Outcomes | Symptom rating scales and other clinical parameters | A single well-defined, clinically important outcome (for large simple trials) and multiple secondary outcomes, including safety and costs (for practical trials) |

(Reproduced from S. Stroup, Practical clinical trials for schizophrenia, *Epidemiologia e Psichiatria Sociale*, **14**, 132–6, copyright 2005 Il Pensiero Scientifico Editore.)

contamination). These issues are shown in more detail in Tables 7.6.13 and 7.6.14.[48]

## Quasi-experimental studies

The term 'quasi-experiment' was first used to refer to a situation in which the decision about whether an individual does or does not receive the intervention to be evaluated is not under the investigator's control.[49] Random allocation of patients is therefore not made, so selection bias may occur. In other respects, a quasi-experiment aims to apply the logic of randomized controlled trials to the study design, and the researcher tries to reduce this bias by making the study units, in the groups being compared, as alike as possible in terms of the most important characteristics. This approach is known as ***matching***. Characteristics chosen for matching are those expected to influence the outcome (i.e. confounding factor). Therefore, the overriding aim of matching is to reduce the contribution made by the matched variables to the selection bias, although this method is inferior to randomization in that it cannot reduce the selection bias from all other variables.

There are two main approaches to matching. ***Paired matching*** consists of selecting individuals for the comparison group (or groups) who have closely similar characteristics to those included in the experimental group, for example in terms of age, gender, and occupation. This form of prestratification will need to be taken into account at the data analysis stage. A less rigorous variant is *group matching*, which only ensures that there are similar overall proportions of people, for both the experimental and comparison groups, in the various age bands, occupational groups, or other predefined strata used for the variables chosen for matching.

## Non-experimental descriptive studies

The next type of research design included in the hierarchy of evidence is non-experimental descriptive studies. For the sake of clarity and brevity we shall distinguish two types of descriptive study: structured clinical practice and everyday unstructured clinical practice. An example of a descriptive evaluation design is the South Verona Outcome Study.[50,51] This is a prospective study, which aims to

**Table 7.6.13** Criteria to plan effectiveness randomized controlled trials[48]

1. Study question
   - Who defines the aim of the study?
   - What process is used to identify the question addressed?
   - Is the study question expressed in an answerable way? (as a clear hypothesis)
   - Prior evidence of intervention effect size
   - Is the answer to this question really unknown?
   - Why is this question important now?
   - Is there initial evidence from efficacy trials or effectiveness studies? (observational or trials)
   - What is the public health importance of the policy or practice question addressed?
   - What is the clinical necessity of the question?
   - Sample size and statistical power for primary/secondary aims and related hypotheses

2. Reference population
   - What is the reference group (or subgroup) to which the trial results should be generalized?
   - What are their socio-demographic and clinical characteristics?
   - What are the ethnic and cultural characteristics of the target group?
   - What is resource level in this population?
   - What is the nature and standard and coverage of health and social care?
   - At what time point is population identified?

3. Patient sample
   - What are their socio-demographic, and clinical characteristics?
   - What are the inclusion criteria?
   - Not invited to participate rate
   - Non-participation rate
   - Patient preferences
   - What are the exclusion criteria?
   - How far does the sample reflect the target population?
   - What level of heterogeneity is there?
   - Selection of incident or prevalent cases (true incidence/prevalence or treated incidence/prevalence)
   - What are the rates of adherence and non-adherence to treatment as recommended?

4. Study settings
   - Characteristics and representativeness of professional staff
   - Levels of resources available
   - Research oriented culture
   - Staff morale and sustainability of intervention
   - Incentives for research collaboration
   - Opportunities for data linkage
   - Centre/professional non-participation

5. Study intervention
   - Is intervention acceptable?
   - Total time needed to deliver intervention
   - Frequency of interventions
   - Simplicity/complexity of the intervention
   - Single/multi-component intervention
   - Is intervention manualized?
   - Do usual professional staff deliver the intervention during the study?
   - Can treatment process be measured? (fidelity)
   - Degree of fit/feasibility for current practice
   - Exit strategy, who pays after the end of study

6. Control condition
   - Treatment as usual or specific control
   - Acceptability to patients of control condition
   - Cost and feasibility of control condition
   - Variation between control condition within and between sites (fidelity)
   - Are the key characteristics of the control condition well described?

7. Bias
   - Does contamination take place?
   - Degree of blinding
   - Choice of primary and secondary outcomes
   - Perspectives prioritized in outcome choice
   - Time(s) at which outcomes measured
   - Total length of follow-up and late effects
   - Sources of outcome data
   - Respondent burden
   - Consent rate
   - Recruitment rate
   - Attrition/drop-out and follow-up rates

(Reproduced from Tansella, M. Thornicroft, G., Barbui, C. *et al.* Seven criteria for improving effectiveness trials in psychiatry. *Psychological Medicine*, **36**(5) 711–200, copyright 2006, Cambridge University Press.)

assess the outcome of mental health care. Data from this study have been analysed using a multidimensional perspective. Among 354 patients followed up after 6 years of treatment in routine clinical settings the study revealed a complex pattern of emerging and disappearing clinical and patterns of exacerbation and remissions, with both changing frequently over time, but changes in both clinical and social domains were not associated with diagnosis.[52]

## Conclusions

Over the course of the next decade we expect that the following key trends will be of paramount importance. In relation to the focus of research, in many countries a degree of contestability may well develop, in which those who have traditionally identified questions to be addressed by research (investigators) will be challenged by research funders (such as governments and charities) and by the intended beneficiaries of the research (people with mental illness and their family members) to set the research agenda.[53] We can expect governments to direct their research investment towards policy challenges, such as barriers to the implementation of evidence-based practice.[54–56] This may well include the commissioning of research not just on new treatments and services, but also to evaluate already or even long-established models of care. For example, there is relatively little mental health service evaluation about: outpatient services (clinics), inpatient services, or forensic service provision.[57,58] In future, it will be important to evaluate *post hoc* current but unproven service configurations, particularly those that are widespread and expensive, as well as innovative interventions. This will necessitate providing sufficient long-term funding for health service research.

In terms of study design, we anticipate that there will be a relative growth of effectiveness studies, especially RCTs, which attempt to balance internal and external validity.[48] These will more often than in the past specify the precise nature of the control condition, use representative patient samples, and standardized outcomes measures. Less common study designs, such as cluster and preference RCTs will be necessary to tackle complex interventions.[59,60] The recent trend to more often include qualitative assessments within RCTs we expect to accelerate, for example to identity the acceptability of interventions to patients, and to identify the active ingredients (and barriers) to treatment effectiveness.[61–65]

How will the conduct of evaluations of mental health services evolve in the coming years? We can identify a trend for study interventions to be increasingly often manualized. At the same time the patient populations treated will be more often similar to those treated in routine clinical practice. As a consequence, more attention will need to be paid to ways to incentivize clinical staff to participate in research.

Although traditionally research scientists have seen the dissemination of research findings largely in terms of publications in scientific journals,[66] it is likely that research funders will increasingly encourage or even insist upon using effective and target-specific communication methods to reach key audiences with the results of research and their implications, including non-traditional methods such as social marketing.[67] This will be intended to alter the behaviour of service planners, commissioners, practitioners, and service users, so that the results of research do influence the behaviour of these key groups in terms of service decisions, so that they increasingly reflect the evidence both of effective interventions and where the evidence shows lack of effect then to stop ineffective practices and services. Such behaviour change (and an established evidence base for this) may include methods as social marketing, as well as carefully combined interventions such as those used in case management in the treatment of depression.[68]

**Table 7.6.14** Key challenges to the evaluation of mental health services

Focus of research
- Clarifying who is defining research questions
- Including service users and family members in setting research questions
- Asking clear research questions to answer important clinical challenges
- Evaluating already established as well new services
- Providing sufficient funding for long-term health service research

Study design
- Balancing internal and external validity of mental health service evaluation
- Moving from efficacy to effectiveness trials
- Specifying the precise nature of the control condition
- Using representative patient samples
- Using standardized outcome measures
- Combining qualitative and quantitative information

Conduct of research studies
- Manualizing the interventions to be evaluated
- Specifying the key characteristics of the patient groups to be treated
- Incentivizing clinical staff to participate in research

Data analysis and interpretation of findings
- Identifying the active ingredients of effective interventions

Dissemination of research findings
- Using effective and target-specific communication methods to reach key audiences with the results of research and their implications

Implementation of effective interventions
- Implementing the results of evaluation when the evidence is strong enough and decommissioning ineffective practice

## Further information

Thornicroft, G. and Tansella, M. (1999). *The mental health matrix: a manual to improve services.* Cambridge University Press, Cambridge.

Thornicroft, G. and Szmukler, G. (2001). *Textbook of community psychiatry.* Oxford University Press, Oxford.

Tansella, M. and Thornicroft, G. (2001). *Mental health outcome measures* (2nd edn). Gaskell, Royal College of Psychiatrists, London.

Thornicroft, G. (2001). *Measuring mental health needs* (2nd edn). Gaskell, Royal College of Psychiatrist, London.

Fulop, N. and Allen, P. (2002). *Studying the organization and the delivery of the health services: research methods.* Routledge, London.

Thornicroft, G. and Tansella, G. (2004). The components of a modern mental health service: a pragmatic balance of community and hospital care. *The British Journal of Psychiatry*, **185**, 283–90.

Thornicroft, G., Becker, T., Knapp, M., *et al.* (2006). International outcome measures in mental health. Quality of life, needs, service satisfaction, costs and impact on carers. Gaskell, Royal College of Psychiatrists, London.

Slade, M. and Priebe, S. (2006). *Choosing methods in mental health research.* Routledge, London.

Knapp, M.J., McDaid, D., Mossialos, E., *et al.* (2007). *Mental health policy and practice across Europe.* Open University Press, Buckingham.

## References

1. Campbell, N.C., Murray, E., Darbyshire, J., *et al.* (2007). Designing and evaluating complex interventions to improve health care. *British Medical Journal*, **334**(7591), 455–9.
2. Campbell, M., Fitzpatrick, R., Haines, A., *et al.* (2000). Framework for design and evaluation of complex interventions to improve health. *British Medical Journal*, **321**, 694–6.
3. Soanes, C. and Stevenson, A. (2003). *Concise Oxford English dictionary* (11th edn). Oxford University Press, Oxford.
4. Thornicroft, G. and Tansella, M. (1999). *The mental health matrix: a manual to improve services.* Cambridge University Press, Cambridge.
5. Thornicroft, G. and Tansella, M. (2007). *Better mental health care.* Cambridge University Press, Cambridge.
6. Sartorius, N. (1997). Evaluating mental health services. A world perspective. *Epidemiologia e Psichiatria Sociale*, **6**(Suppl. 1), 239–45.
7. Johnson, S., Nolan, F., Hoult, J., *et al.* (2005). Outcomes of crises before and after introduction of a crisis resolution team. *The British Journal of Psychiatry*, **187**, 68–75.
8. Killaspy, H., Bebbington, P., Blizard, R., *et al.* (2006). The REACT study: randomised evaluation of assertive community treatment in north London. *British Medical Journal*, **332**(7545), 815–20.
9. Glover, G., Arts, G., and Babu, K.S. (2006). Crisis resolution/home treatment teams and psychiatric admission rates in England. *The British Journal of Psychiatry*, **189**(5), 441–5.
10. Tansella, M. and Thornicroft, G. (eds.) (2001). *Mental health outcome measures.* Royal College of Psychiatrists, Gaskell, London.
11. Thornicroft, G., Becker, T., Knapp, M., *et al.* (2006). International outcome measures in mental health. Quality of life, needs, service satisfaction, costs and impact on carers. Gaskell, Royal College of Psychiatrists, London.
12. Schene, A., Tessler, R.C., Gamache, G.M., *et al.* (2001). Measuring family or care giver burden in severe mental illness: the instruments. In *Mental health outcome measures* (2nd edn) (eds. M. Tansella and G. Thornicroft), pp. 48–71. Royal College of Psychiatrists, Gaskell, London.
13. Joyce, J., Leese, M., and Szmukler, G. (2000). The experience of caregiving inventory: further evidence. *Social Psychiatry and Psychiatric Epidemiology*, **35**(4), 185–9.
14. Thornicroft, G. and Tansella, M. (2004). The components of a modern mental health service: a pragmatic balance of community and hospital care. *The British Journal of Psychiatry*, **185**, 283–90.

15. Szmukler, G., Kuipers, E., Joyce, J., *et al.* (2003). An exploratory randomised controlled trial of a support programme for carers of patients with a psychosis. *Social Psychiatry and Psychiatric Epidemiology*, **38**(8), 411–8.

16. Ruggeri, M. (2001). Measuring satisfaction with psychiatric services: towards a multi-dimensional, multi-axial assessment of outcome. In *Mental health outcome measures* (2nd edn) (eds. M. Tansella and G. Thornicroft), pp. 34–47. Royal College of Psychiatrists, Gaskell, London.

17. Ruggeri, M., Dall'Agnola, R., Agostini, C., *et al.* (1994). Acceptability, sensitivity and content validity of the VECS and VSSS in measuring expectations and satisfaction in psychiatric patients and their relatives. *Social Psychiatry and Psychiatric Epidemiology*, **29**(6), 265–76.

18. Lehman, A. (2001). Measures of quality of life for people with severe mental disorders. In *Mental health outcome measures* (2nd edn) (eds. M. Tansella and G. Thornicroft), pp. 72–92. Royal College of Psychiatrists, Gaskell, London.

19. Ware, J. and Sherbourn, C. (1992). The MOS, 36 item short-form health survey (SF-36). I. Conceptual framework and item selection. *Medical Care*, **30**, 473–83.

20. Wiersma, D. (2001). Measuring social disabilities in mental health. In *Mental health outcomes measures* (2nd edn) (eds. M. Tansella and G. Thornicroft), pp. 118–32. Royal College of Psychiatrists, Gaskell, London.

21. Thornicroft, G. (2001). *Measuring mental health needs* (2nd edn). Royal College of Psychiatrists, Gaskell, London.

22. Slade, M., Thornicroft, G., Loftus, L., *et al.* (1999). *CAN: the Camberwell Assessment of Need*. Gaskell, Royal College of Psychiatrists, London.

23. Lasalvia, A., Bonetto, C., Malchiodi, F., *et al.* (2005). Listening to patients' needs to improve their subjective quality of life. *Psychological Medicine*, **35**(11), 1655–65.

24. Slade, M., Leese, M., Ruggeri, M., *et al.* (2004). Does meeting needs improve quality of life? *Psychotherapy and Psychosomatics*, **73**(3), 183–9.

25. Geddes, J.R. and Harrison, P.J. (1997). Closing the gap between research and practice. *The British Journal of Psychiatry*, **171**, 220–5.

26. L'Abbe, K.A., Detsky, A.S., and O'Rourke, K. (1987). Meta-analysis in clinical research. *Annals of Internal Medicine*, **107**(2), 224–33.

27. Sackett, D.L., Rosenberg, W.M., Gray, J.A., *et al.* (1996). Evidence based medicine: what it is and what it isn't. *British Medical Journal*, **312**(7023), 71–2.

28. Cochrane, A. (1972). *Effectiveness and efficiency: random reflections on health services*. Nuffield Provincial Hospitals Trust.

29. Tyrer, P., Coid, J., Simmonds, S., *et al.* (2000). Community mental health teams (CMHTs) for people with severe mental illnesses and disordered personality. *Cochrane Database of Systematic Reviews*, (2), CD000270.

30. Simmonds, S., Coid, J., Joseph, P., *et al.* (2001). Community mental health team management in severe mental illness: a systematic review. *The British Journal of Psychiatry*, **178**, 497–502.

31. Korn, E.L. and Baumrind, S. (1991). Randomised clinical trials with clinician-preferred treatment. *Lancet*, **337**(8734), 149–52.

32. Barker, D. and Rose, G. (1979). *Epidemiology in medical practice* (2nd edn). Churchill Livingstone, London.

33. Everitt, B. and Wessely, S. (2004). *Clinical trials in psychiatry*. Oxford University Press, Oxford.

34. Black, N. (1996). Why we need observational studies to evaluate the effectiveness of health care. *British Medical Journal*, **312**(7040), 1215–18.

35. Marriott, S. and Palmer, C. (1996). Clinical practice guidelines: on what evidence is our clinical practice based? *Psychiatric Bulletin*, **20**, 363–6.

36. Macfarlane, W., Dushay, R., Stastny, P., *et al.* (1996). Comparison of two levels of family-aided assertive community treatment. *Psychiatric Services*, **47**, 744–50.

37. Schwartz, D. and Lellouch, J. (1967). Explanatory and pragmatic attitudes in therapeutic trials. *Journal of Chronic Diseases*, **20**(20), 637–48.

38. Peto, R., Collins, R., and Gray, R. (1993). Large scale randomised evidence. *Annals of the New York Academy of Science*, **703**, 314–40.

39. Oliver, S. (1997). Exploring lay perspectives on questions of effectiveness. In *Non random reflections on health services research* (eds. A. Maynard and I. Chalmers), pp. 272–91. British Medical Journal Publications, London.

40. Haynes, B. (1999). Can it work? Does it work? Is it worth it? The testing of healthcare interventions is evolving. *British Medical Journal*, **319**(7211), 652–3.

41. Lilienfeld, A. (1982). The Fielding H. Garrison lecture: ceteris paribus: the evolution of the clinical trial. *Bulletin of the History of Medicine*, **56**, 1–18.

42. Pocock, S. (1983). *Clinical trials: a practical approach*. Wiley, London.

43. Andrews, G. (1999). Randomised controlled trials in psychiatry: important but poorly accepted. *British Medical Journal*, **319**(7209), 562–4.

44. Wells, K.B. (1999). Treatment research at the crossroads: the scientific interface of clinical trials and effectiveness research. *The American Journal of Psychiatry*, **156**(1), 5–10.

45. Proudfoot, J., Goldberg, D., Mann, A., *et al.* (2003). Computerized, interactive, multimedia cognitive-behavioural program for anxiety and depression in general practice. *Psychological Medicine*, **33**(2), 217–27.

46. Wells, K.B., Sherbourne, C., Schoenbaum, M., *et al.* (2000). Impact of disseminating quality improvement programs for depression in managed primary care: a randomized controlled trial. *The Journal of the American Medical Association*, **283**(2), 212–20.

47. Campbell, M., Fitzpatrick, R., Haines, A., *et al.* (2000). Framework for design and evaluation of complex interventions to improve health. *British Medical Journal*, **321**(7262), 694–6.

48. Tansella, M., Thornicroft, G., Barbui, C., *et al.* (2006). Seven criteria for improving effectiveness trials in psychiatry. *Psychological Medicine*, **36**(5), 711–20.

49. Campbell, D.T. and Stanley, J.C. (1996). *Experimental and quasi-experimental designs for research*. Rand-McNally, Chicago, IL.

50. Ruggeri, M., Biggeri, A., Rucci, P., *et al.* (1998). Multivariate analysis of outcome of mental health care using graphical chain models. The south-Verona outcome project 1. *Psychological Medicine*, **28**(6), 1421–31.

51. Lasalvia, A. and Ruggeri, M. (2007). Multidimensional outcomes in 'real world' mental health services: follow-up findings from the south Verona project. *Acta Psychiatrica Scandinavica*, (Suppl.).

52. Lasalvia, A., Bonetto, C., Cristofalo, D., *et al.* (2007). Predicting clinical and social outcome of patients attending 'real world' mental health services: a 6 year multi-wave follow-up. *Acta Psychiatrica Scandinavica*, **116**, (s437), 16–30.

53. Chamberlin, J. (2005). User/consumer involvement in mental health service delivery. *Epidemiologia e Psichiatria Sociale*, **14**(1), 10–4.

54. Magnabosco, J.L. (2006). Innovations in mental health services implementation: a report on state-level data from the U.S. Evidence-based practices project. *Implemention Science*, **1**, 13.

55. Drake, R.E., Becker, D.R., Goldman, H.H., *et al.* (2006). Best practices: the Johnson & Johnson—Dartmouth community mental health program: disseminating evidence-based practice. *Psychiatric Services*, **57**(3), 302–4.

56. Aarons, G.A. and Sawitzky, A.C. (2006). Organizational culture and climate and mental health provider attitudes toward evidence-based practice. *Psychological Services*, **3**(1), 61–72.

57. Szmukler, G. and Holloway, F. (2001). In-patient treatment. In *Textbook of community psychiatry* (eds. G. Thornicroft and G. Szmukler), pp. 321–37. Oxford University Press, Oxford.

58. Becker, T. (2001). Out-patient psychiatric services. In *Textbook of community psychiatry* (eds. G. Thornicroft and G. Szmukler), pp. 277–82. Oxford University Press, Oxford.

59. Medical Research Council. (2002). *Cluster randomised trials: methodological and ethical considerations*. Medical Research Council, London.

60. Howard, L. and Thornicroft, G. (2006). Patient preference randomised controlled trials in mental health research. *The British Journal of Psychiatry*, **188**, 303–4.

61. Lester, H., Tritter, J.Q., and Sorohan, H. (2005). Patients' and health professionals' views on primary care for people with serious mental illness: focus group study. *British Medical Journal*, **330**(7500), 1122.

62. Pope, C., Mays, N., and Popay, J. (2006). How can we synthesize qualitative and quantitative evidence for healthcare policy-makers and managers? *Healthcare Management Forum*, **19**(1), 27–31.

63. Mays, N., Pope, C., and Popay, J. (2005). Systematically reviewing qualitative and quantitative evidence to inform management and policy-making in the health field. *Journal of Health Services Research & Policy*, **10**(Suppl. 1), 6–20.

64. Pope, C., Ziebland, S., and Mays, N. (2000). Qualitative research in health care. Analysing qualitative data. *British Medical Journal*, **320**(7227), 114–16.

65. Mays, N. and Pope, C. (2000). Qualitative research in health care. Assessing quality in qualitative research. *British Medical Journal*, **320**(7226), 50–2.

66. Lewison, G., Thornicroft, G., Szmukler, G., *et al.* (2007). The fair assessment of the merits of psychiatric research. *The British Journal of Psychiatry*, **190**, 314–18.

67. Kotler, P., Roberto, E.L., and Lee, N. (2002). *Social marketing: improving the quality of life*. Sage, New York.

68. Wells, K., Miranda, J., Bruce, M.L., *et al.* (2004). Bridging community intervention and mental health services research. *The American Journal of Psychiatry*, **161**(6), 955–63.

69. Thornicroft, G. (2006). *Shunned: discrimination against people with mental illness*. Oxford University Press, Oxford.

70. Pinfold, V., Toulmin, H., Thornicroft, G., *et al.* (2003). Reducing psychiatric stigma and discrimination: evaluation of educational interventions in UK secondary schools. *The British Journal of Psychiatry*, **182**, 342–6.

71. Sackett, D.L. and Wennberg, J.E. (1997). Choosing the best research design for each question. *British Medical Journal*, **315**(7123), 1636.

72. Stroup, S. (2005). Practical clinical trials for schizophrenia. *Epidemiologia e Psichiatria Sociale*, **14**, 132–6.

# Economic analysis of mental health services

## Martin Knapp and Dan Chisholm

## Introduction

Economics is concerned with the use and distribution of resources within a society, and how different ways of allocating resources impact on the well-being of individuals. Economics enters the health sphere because resources available to meet societal needs or demands are finite, meaning that choices have to be made regarding how best to allocate them (typically to generate the greatest possible level of population health). Economics provides an explicit framework for thinking through ways of allocating resources.

Resource allocation decisions in mental health are complicated by the fact that disorders are common, debilitating, and often long-lasting. Epidemiological research has demonstrated the considerable burden that mental disorders impose because of their prevalence, chronicity, and severity: globally, more than 10 per cent of lost years of healthy life and over 30 per cent of all years lived with disability are attributable to mental disorders.[1] Low rates of recognition and effective treatment compound the problem, particularly in poor countries.

However, disease burden is not in itself sufficient as a justification or mechanism for resource allocation or priority-setting. A disorder can place considerable burden on a population but if appropriate strategies to reduce this burden are absent or extremely expensive in relation to the health gains achieved, large-scale investment would be considered misplaced. The reason is that scarce resources could be more efficiently channelled to other burdensome conditions for which cost-effective responses *were* available. For priority-setting and resource allocation, it is necessary to ask what amount of burden from a disorder can be avoided by using evidence-based interventions, and at what relative cost of implementation in the target population.

Cost and cost-effectiveness considerations enter into health care reform processes, priority-setting exercises within and across health programmes, and regulatory decisions concerning drug approval or pricing. Two broad levels of economic analysis can be distinguished: macro and micro.

## Economic analyses at macro level: the mental health system

Macro-level economic analyses are concerned with how health systems function and what they achieve. What, for example, are the motivations and behaviour of key 'stakeholders', with what implications for access, quality, and costs? What roles do economic forces play and can they be shaped to improve health outcomes and cost-effectiveness? Do different organizational or financial arrangements produce different resource configurations? For example, do markets achieve fairer or more efficient allocations than state bureaucracies? Through their macro analyses, economists can contribute to a better understanding of how health systems can improve utilization of resources (for example, see Box 7.7.1).

While improved psychological well-being in the population is likely to represent the primary goal of the mental health system, there are other (social) goals that could also feature prominently, including quality improvements in service provision, and financial (as well as human rights) protection for people with mental health problems.[2] Meeting these goals is achieved via a number of key health system functions, including resource generation, their allocation via appropriate modes of financing, actual provision of services, and overall stewardship and evaluation of these various functions.[3] Economic analysis contributes to policy formation relating to each of these functions.[4–6]

There are barriers to implementation of evidence-based mental health care in even generously resourced health systems. An insidious barrier is resource insufficiency: mental health services are often grossly under-funded in comparison to both needs and the

---

**Box 7.7.1** The relevance of a health systems perspective

The need for a systems approach to mental health policy and planning is made apparent from a simple illustration: cheap, effective drugs exist for key neuropsychiatric disorders, including tricyclic antidepressants, conventional neuroleptics, and anti-epileptic drugs, which are affordable even to resource-poor countries. The availability and prescription of these drugs to those in need, however, are determined by the extent to which such drugs have been distributed and by the ability of health care providers to detect and appropriately treat the underlying condition. Access to and use of such medications may further be hampered by the private cost of seeking and receiving health care, particularly if it is out-of pocket. User fees, provider incentives, and clinical practice are in turn influenced by the availability of national legislation, regulation, and treatment guidelines.

cost-effectiveness of interventions to meet them. This is a major issue for countries where the proportion of national income devoted to health care is low, or where the proportion of the health budget allocated to mental health is minimal. With limited funds it is difficult to build any kind of service system, because it is difficult to recruit, train, and retain skilled staff.

Even when resources are committed, available services might be poorly distributed, available at the wrong place or time relative to the distribution of needs. They may only be delivered by specialist clinics or concentrated in big cities, or affordable only by wealthier individuals. Improvements to practice take time to work through to improved health outcomes, cost-effectiveness gains or fairer access, even when suitable professionals can be recruited or new facilities opened. Decision makers must think long-term, for the immediate consequences of many interventions could be modest but longer-term benefits immense.[7]

A more general difficulty is that available services do not match what is needed or preferred. Indeed, there may be scant information on population or individual needs, and patients may have few opportunities to participate in treatment decisions. Another problem could be poor coordination of services because of professional rivalry, stultifying bureaucracy or 'silo budgeting' (resources held in one agency's 'silo' cannot be allocated to other uses).

## Economic analyses at micro level: cost-effectiveness

The most frequently posed micro questions relate to the cost-effectiveness of interventions, such as an emphasis on community-based care, the use of new drugs, or the development of secure accommodation. For example, consider what happens following development of a new treatment (say a new medication for schizophrenia). Decision makers want answers to two questions when considering whether to use or recommend this drug. The first is the clinical question: is it effective in alleviating psychotic symptoms and generally improving health-related quality of life? If the answer to the clinical question is 'yes', then there is a second question: is it cost-effective? That is, does the drug achieve the improved outcomes at a cost that is worth paying? The meaning of 'worth' is far from straightforward to establish and laden with controversy.

These two questions sit at the heart of economic evaluation: outcomes must be assessed (and compared between different treatments) and the (relative) costs of achieving them must be examined. Looking only at costs is *not* an economic evaluation.

There are different variants of economic evaluation. They share a common approach to the conceptualization, definition, and measurement of costs, but adopt different approaches when considering and measuring outcomes, primarily because they seek to answer slightly different questions. We set out these differences by discussing the questions a study might address, measuring costs and outcomes, making trade-offs between them, and utility and benefit measurement.

### Question and perspective

The choice of evaluative approach depends on the question to be addressed. If the question is essentially clinical—what is the most appropriate treatment for someone with particular needs in particular circumstances—information is needed on the comparative costs of alternative treatments and comparative outcomes measured in

terms of symptom alleviation, improved functioning, and so on. A cost-effectiveness analysis would be appropriate (see 'Effectiveness measurement' below).

If, to take a broader stance, the question is whether to treat depression rather than spending the funds elsewhere in the health system, then decision makers need to know the costs, but now need an outcome measure that uses a common metric across different health domains. The most common such metric is 'utility' and a cost-utility analysis would be undertaken (see 'Utility measurement' below).

To widen the perspective further, if the question is whether to increase expenditure in the health system or in (say) improving transport or launching a new environmental policy, then an evaluation needs to ask about the comparative costs and impacts of the different options, where 'impact' will need to be measured in a common unit across all public policy areas. The usual choice of broad measure is monetary, leading to cost–benefit analysis (see 'Benefit measurement' below).

The question to be addressed thus influences the type of evaluation needed, but the choices are not mutually exclusive: a single study can support more than one approach if the right measures are used. The broader the question, the lower the likelihood that the outcome measure will be sensitive to the particular circumstances of a specific disorder such as depression, but the greater the usefulness in terms of resource allocation decisions.

Linked to specification of the question to be addressed is the *perspective* of a study. Is the evaluation needed to help resource allocation within a particular agency (such as primary care clinic), or a particular system (such as the health care system), or the whole society? The perspective will determine the breadth of both cost and outcome measurement.

### Cost measurement

Some costs are directly associated with a disorder or its treatment, such as the money spent on medications and services used by patients, and some are more indirect, measuring lost productivity because ill-health can disrupt someone's employment pattern or the social cost of unpaid care provided by families. How broadly the costs are measured will depend upon the purpose of the study.

In carrying out evaluations in practice, economists need data on service use patterns by patients. This information might come from organizational 'billing' systems (recording amounts transferred between purchasers and providers for services used), or from routine information systems that record service contacts, or from research instruments that specifically collect data on service use patterns through interviews with patients, caregivers, or service professionals. One widely used instrument is the Client Service Receipt Inventory.[8]

The next task is to attach unit cost estimates to these service use data. In England, there is an excellent annual compendium of health and social care unit costs, which provides just such figures.[9] In other countries, it might be necessary to estimate unit costs anew. A range of data sources could be used, including government statistics, health system expenditure figures, and specific facility or organization accounts. The main cost categories to be quantified would be:

- salaries of staff employed in patient treatment and care
- facility operating costs (e.g. cleaning, catering)

♦ overhead costs (e.g. personnel, finance)

♦ capital costs for buildings and durable equipment

## Effectiveness measurement

The most intuitive mode of economic evaluation is cost-effectiveness analysis (CEA): it measures costs as set out above, and outcomes along the dimensions that would be recognized by clinicians and used in clinical studies (changes in symptoms, behaviour, functioning, and so on). A CEA can help decision makers choose between interventions aimed at specific health needs. A cost-effectiveness analysis looks at a single outcome dimension—such as change in symptoms—and computes and compares the difference in costs between two treatments and the difference in this (primary) outcome. If one treatment is both more effective and less costly than another, then it would clearly be the more cost-effective of the two. But if it is more effective and *more* costly then a trade-off is needed (see below).

Often the economist will compute cost differences and a range of effectiveness differences (one for each outcome dimension)—an approach sometimes called cost-consequences analysis—which has the advantage of breadth but poses a challenge if one outcome is better and another worse for a particular treatment. It is then not always obvious which treatment is to be preferred, and the decision maker must weigh up the strength of evidence.

## Making trade-offs

If an evaluation finds a new intervention to be both more effective but simultaneously more expensive than an older intervention, which is the more cost-effective of the two? A trade-off must be made between the better outcomes and the higher costs necessary to achieve them.

The classical way of determining this trade-off has been via the derivation of a incremental cost-effectiveness ratio (CER), which divides the extra cost associated with a new intervention by its additional effect (see Box 7.7.2).

More recently, health economists have developed the 'net benefit approach' to explicate the nature of the trade-off (see Box 7.7.3 for an example). It is commonly seen today in the construction of *cost-effectiveness acceptability curves* (CEACs). These curves show the probability that an intervention will be cost-effective for each of a number of pre-specified or implicit valuations of an outcome improvement by the decision maker.

## Utility measurement

One way to overcome the potential problem of different outcome dimensions pointing in different directions is to employ a single,

---

### Box 7.7.3 Example of the net benefit approach in mental health services research

An example of the use of cost-effectiveness acceptability curves comes from a study of computer-delivered cognitive behavioural therapy (CCBT) for anxiety and depression.[10] CCBT was more expensive in health service terms than standard primary care services, but more effective in reducing symptoms. The fitted CEACs showed that, even if the value placed by society on a unit reduction in the Beck Depression Inventory (the primary clinical measure used in the trial) was as little as £40, there was an 81 per cent probability that CCBT would be viewed as cost-effective. Similarly, assigning a societal value of just £5 to each additional depression-free day would result in an 80 per cent probability that CCBT would be cost-effective. The CEAC makes transparent the trade-offs faced by decision makers.

---

over-arching measure. A preference-weighted, health-related quality of life measure could be used. The value of the quality of life improvement is gauged in units of 'utility', usually expressed by a combined index of the mortality and quality of life effects of an intervention. The best known such index is the Quality Adjusted Life Year (QALY).

A cost-utility analysis (CUA) measures the outcome difference between two interventions in terms of QALY gain, and compares this with the difference in costs. CUAs have a number of attractions, including a unidimensional, generic outcome measure that allows comparisons across diagnostic groups, based on an explicit methodology for weighting preferences and valuing health states. But the utility measure may be too reductionist and insufficiently sensitive to changes expected in a particular clinical area such as depression treatment.[11] Nevertheless, cost-utility analyses produce estimates of cost-per-QALY gain from one therapy over another, which can then inform health care resource allocation decisions, such as by the National Institute for Health and Clinical Excellence (NICE) in England and Wales.

## Benefit measurement

Cost–benefit analysis asks whether the benefits of a treatment or policy exceed the costs, helping decision makers to allocate resources across a wide area, for example comparing health care with housing, education, or defence. All costs and outcomes (benefits) are valued in the same (monetary) units. If benefits exceed costs, the evaluation would provide support for the intervention or programme, and vice versa. With two or more alternatives, the intervention with the greatest net benefit would be deemed the most efficient. Cost–benefit analyses are thus intrinsically attractive, but conducting them is especially problematic because of the difficulties associated with attaching monetary values to health outcomes, and especially mental health outcomes. Methodological advances in health economics offer ways to obtain direct valuations of health outcomes by patients, families, or others,[12] but they will not be easy to apply in mental health contexts.

## Design issues

As in clinical evaluation, an important consideration for the review, assessment, and interpretation of economic evidence is research

---

### Box 7.7.2 Calculation of the incremental cost-effectiveness ratio

For example, evaluation of a new antidepressant may show that the cost per treated case of major depression is an extra £500 per year but also results in a lower average symptom score over this period (such as a ten point reduction on the Beck Depression Inventory); the resulting incremental CER would therefore be £50 [£500/10], meaning that each additional unit improvement on the BDI cost £50.

design. Generally speaking, the ideal type of study upon which to base decisions on cost-effectiveness and resource allocation is the one conducted prospectively with two (or more) appropriately sized randomly allocated groups of patients, for whom all conceivable costs and outcomes are measured appropriately, including a comparable measure of outcome (monetized benefits or, more realistically, a utility metric).

Looking across the mental health field, the accumulation of new cost-effectiveness evidence has been uneven, tending to be greater in diagnostic areas where new classes of medication have been launched: the pharmaceutical industry looks to economic evidence to support its marketing. At the same time, health care funding and delivery bodies also want their own independent evidence on new therapies. Consequently, a lot of economic studies of depression followed the licensing of the early selective serotonin-reuptake inhibitors (SSRIs) and later antidepressants with other mechanisms of action. Similarly, the arrival of the atypical antipsychotics and the cholinesterase inhibitors for Alzheimer's disease stimulated a lot of economics research.

We cannot cover all mental health areas here. Instead, in the next three sections, we look at areas where there has been some interesting activity:

- cost-utility analysis of depression treatment in primary care
- cost-effectiveness of interventions for child and adolescent mental health problems
- sectoral cost-effectiveness analysis of mental health interventions in developing countries.

## Cost-utility analysis of depression treatment in primary care

Ten years ago, examples of the application of the cost-utility approach to mental health were hard to find.[11] Since then, there has been an increasing use of the so-called cost-per-QALY approach in mental health evaluations, following recommendations for such analyses by regulatory bodies in Australia, Canada, the United Kingdom, and the United States. In the field of depression, for example, cost-utility analyses have now been carried out for: screening in primary care[13] (annual and periodic screening cost more than $50 000 per QALY, one-off screening below this threshold); newer versus older antidepressant drugs[14]; maintenance treatment for recurrent depression[15,16]; guideline-concordant primary care treatment for women[17]; primary care practice-initiated quality improvement programmes[18]; computerized cognitive behavioural therapy[10]; and ECT versus transcranial magnetic stimulation for 'treatment-resistant' depression.[19] Many of the cost-utility analyses carried out to date employ secondary data and modelling techniques to estimate costs and effects, others have constructed cost-per-QALY estimates alongside clinical trials.

An example of a cost-utility analysis using modelling is that by Revicki et al.[14] who compared treatment for major depression with (a) newer antidepressants (nefazodone and fluoxetine) (b) tricyclics (imipramine) and, for treatment failures, (c) a step approach involving initial treatment with imipramine followed by nefazodone. A decision analysis model was developed to simulate the clinical management pathways and pattern of recurrences of major depression for these alternative treatment strategies to estimate lifetime medical costs and health outcomes (expressed as QALYs).

There were only minor differences in costs and QALYs between nefazodone and fluoxetine, and both these newer antidepressants were estimated to be cost-effective compared to imipramine treatment and the imipramine step approach. The ratios of cost to QALYs gained for these newer antidepressants were deemed to be sufficiently low (below $20 000 per QALY gained) to merit adoption of these treatments in the health system. For example, the extra lifetime cost of nefazodone over imipramine ($1321) resulted in 0.32 added QALYs, giving a ratio of $4065 per QALY gained. Since decision models and their findings are only as good as their underlying assumptions and the quality of the data used to estimate key model parameters, extensive sensitivity analyses were conducted, but these did not alter the conclusions. However, the results did not include indirect costs such as changes in work productivity—important for a societal perspective—and are not readily generalizable to groups other than the targeted population (in this study, 30-year old women with one previous depressive episode).

An example of the empirically based generation of cost-per-QALY information is the randomized controlled trial of practice-initiated quality improvement (QI) for depression,[18] which involved group-level randomization of 46 clinics in six community-based US managed care organizations, either to medication or psychotherapy quality improvement programme (in addition to training and enhanced educational resources). Two QALY measures were derived, one from the Short-From, 12-Item Health Survey (SF-12) plus a standard gamble utility weighting exercise among a local convenience sample, the other with reference to estimated time spent depressed plus values from the literature for lost utility due to depression. Relative to usual care, average health care costs increased by $400–500 per treated patient, while QALY gains were less than 0.025, resulting in an estimated cost per QALY of $15 000–36 000 (QI-medication) and $9500–21 500 (QI-therapy). In addition to these health gains, patients exposed to the quality improvement programmes were employed more days than those receiving usual care.

The envisaged benefit of expressing the results of economic evaluation in these terms lies in the ability to line-up cost-per-QALY estimates for a range of different interventions and disorders, with a view to determining acceptable efficiency against a pre-defined threshold (of, say, $50 000 in the US context), or even constructing 'league tables' summarizing best and worst buys in the health sector. In practice, there remain significant problems in relying on league tables for allocating resources (due to the heterogeneous and context-specific nature of cost-utility studies), while there may be criteria unrelated to efficiency that determine whether a particular intervention is deemed acceptable for reimbursement or inclusion in a defined package of basic health care.

## Cost-effectiveness of interventions for child and adolescent mental health problems

There are hundreds of completed economic evaluations in the depression field, almost all confined to adults of 'working age'. But there is surprisingly little economic evidence on child and adolescent mental health interventions. A systematic review a few years ago found only 14 published economic evaluations, some of rather poor quality.[20] Common problems included small sample sizes, narrow cost measures, short follow-ups, and limited outcome measures. (Guidelines and quality checklists are available for health economist researchers and readers of their outputs.)[21]

Another drawback is that most of the completed economic studies have been undertaken in North America, the United Kingdom, and Australia. But the results of economic evaluations generally do not transfer easily from one health system to another because of differences in system structure and financing, leading to differences in relative costs. It is infeasible and certainly unnecessary to carry-out an evaluation every time a policy decision needs to be taken, but it is also difficult to assess the relevance of economic evidence from another country, especially if its mental health system is markedly different.

An example of a well-conducted cost-effectiveness analysis is the evaluation of a home-based social work intervention for children and adolescents who have deliberately poisoned themselves.[22] The researchers measured suicidal ideation, hopelessness, and family functioning as the main outcomes, and costs were based on patterns of utilization of health, education, social care, and voluntary sector services. Within a randomized controlled trial, involving 162 children aged 16 years or under, they found no significant difference in the main outcomes or costs, although parental satisfaction with treatment was significantly greater in the group that received a new social work intervention compared to those who received routine care.

In another pragmatic randomized trial, a parenting intervention for parents of children at risk of developing conduct disorder (the Incredible Years programme) was compared to wait-list controls. The perspective for cost measurement was the public sector (health, social care, special education); effectiveness was measured by reductions in intensity of behaviour problems.[23] The Incredible Years programme was more effective but also more costly. The researchers found that it would cost £1344 to bring the average child in the intervention group (in terms of behaviour intensity score) to below the clinical cut-off point. A cost-effectiveness acceptability curve was plotted to show the trade-offs between cost and effectiveness.

## Sectoral cost-effectiveness analysis of mental health interventions in developing countries

Cost-effectiveness analysis can also be used to evaluate mental health programmes for whole populations (countries or even world regions). While the burden of neuropsychiatric disease is very high, the resources available to address that burden are extremely low. Given the consequent tension between the need for and the availability of mental health care, plus the fact that effective interventions do exist, the job of cost-effectiveness analysis is to show how much of the burden can be reduced or averted, by doing what, and at what cost.

Through its CHOICE project (choosing interventions that are cost-effective), WHO embarked on an initiative to assemble databases on cost-effectiveness of key health interventions in 14 epidemiological sub-regions of the world.[24] A comparative cost-effectiveness analysis of interventions for reducing the burden of major neuropsychiatric disorders formed part of this programme.[6,25,26] WHO-CHOICE advocates a 'generalized' form of cost-effectiveness analysis, in which costs and effects of current and new interventions are compared to the starting point of 'doing nothing'. Accordingly, the costs and effectiveness of pharmacological and psychosocial interventions in primary care or outpatient

settings for psychiatric disorders were compared in a population model to an epidemiological situation representing the untreated natural history of these disorders. Effects are measured as disability adjusted life years (DALYs) averted (i.e. reduced burden), and costs in international dollars (I\$; one international dollar should buy the same quantity of health care resources in China as in the United States).

Compared to no treatment (natural history), the most cost-effective strategy for averting the burden of psychosis and severe affective disorders in developing regions of the world is a combined intervention of first-generation antipsychotic or mood-stabilizing drugs with adjuvant psychosocial treatment delivered by community-based outpatient services, with cost-effectiveness ratio of I\$4200–5500 in Sub-Saharan Africa and South Asia, rising to more than I\$10 000 in middle-income regions[25] (see Fig. 7.7.1). Currently, the high acquisition price of second-generation antipsychotic drugs makes their use in developing regions questionable on efficiency grounds alone, although this situation stands to change as these drugs come off patent. By contrast, evidence indicates that the relatively modest additional cost of adjuvant psychosocial treatment reaps significant health gains, thereby making such a combined strategy for schizophrenia and bipolar disorder treatment more cost-effective than pharmacotherapy alone.

For more common mental disorders treated in primary care settings (depressive and anxiety disorders), the single most cost-effective strategy is the scaled-up use of older antidepressants (due to their lower cost but broadly similar efficacy to newer antidepressants). However, as the price margin between older and generic newer antidepressants continues to narrow, generic SSRIs should be at least as cost-effective and may therefore represent the treatment of choice in the future. Since depression is commonly recurring, there are also grounds for thinking that proactive care management, including long-term maintenance treatment with antidepressant drugs, represents a cost-effective (if more resource-intensive) way of significantly reducing the enormous burden of depression in developing regions.[27]

The purpose of such an exercise is to locate the relative position of effective and applicable interventions within a wider cost-effectiveness and priority-setting framework. Using the affordability criteria of the WHO Commission for Macroeconomics and Health,[28] this analysis indicates that (a) the most efficient interventions for common mental disorders can be considered very cost-effective (each DALY averted costs less than 1 year of average per capita income), and (b) community-based interventions for severe mental disorders using older antipsychotic and mood-stabilizer drugs meet the criterion for being cost-effective (each DALY averted costs less than three times GDP per capita). These findings therefore provide relevant information regarding the relative value of investing in neuropsychiatric treatment and prevention, and so may help to remove one of many remaining barriers to a more appropriate public health response to mental health needs.

## Conclusion

Economic evaluation provides a means of comparing the costs and outcomes of mental health interventions or programmes, enabling decision makers to assess whether they offer good use of (scarce) resources. An analysis of costs alone, or indeed of outcomes alone,

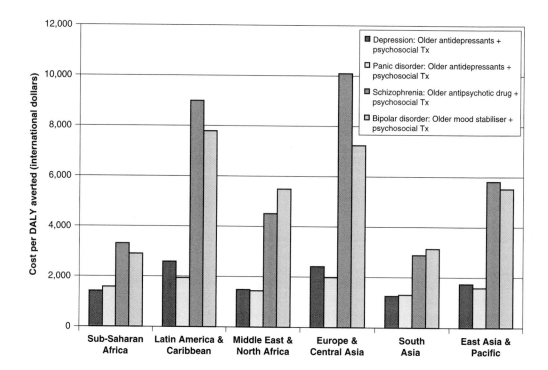

**Fig. 7.7.1** Cost-effectiveness ratios for a basic mental health package in low and middle-income regions of the world.

does not provide such information. The results of well-conducted economic evaluations can be channelled into decision-making processes at a succession of levels.

## Patients, users, and caregivers

Economic evidence can complement clinical decision-making at the patient, user, and caregiver level by comparing costs and consequences of particular treatments. One very pertinent question about any treatment is whether the additional acquisition costs associated with (say) newer antidepressants or second-generation antipsychotics are compensated by better symptomatic response or fewer side effects. Our earlier examples of economic evaluations of treatments for depression and for child and adolescent mental health problems provide this kind of evidence.

## Purchasers and providers

At another decision-making level, those who commission or purchase mental health services need economic data. A core element of local needs assessment and strategic service development by (say) a state health care system or a health maintenance organization concerns the resource implications of changes to, for instance, the hospital/community balance or investment in a new clinic or training of therapists.

## Government and society

Economic evaluations should influence national-level policy and resource allocation decisions. Such evaluations have influenced policy with respect to the substitution of community-based for long-term hospital care, the development of 'assertive outreach' models, the expansion of early intervention initiatives for psychosis, and the overall level of funding. The CHOICE programme aims to provide this kind of evidence.

While adding economic analysis to mental health evaluations introduces an extra dimension that offers a wider assessment of the implications of new or existing courses of action, there can also be limitations. Many economic evaluations fall short of the ideal, whether in terms of sample size, comprehensiveness of cost measurement, outcome assessment, or evidence interpretation. Conclusions based on small-sample randomized trials can often only be tentative, while failure to measure the wider (non-health and non-service) costs associated with two or more treatments may produce misleading and partial results.

Even when it overcomes these limitations, an economic evaluation can never resolve difficult allocative and policy issues; rather, it is one additional tool that, together with evidence on the clinical and social dimensions, can facilitate explicit evidence-based decision-making.

## Further information

Knapp, M.R.J., Funk, M., Curran, C., *et al.* (2006). Economic barriers to better mental health practice and policy. *Health Policy and Planning*, **21**, 157–70. http://heapol.oxfordjournals.org/cgi/content/full/21/3/157

WHO. (2006). *Dollars, DALYs and decisions: economic aspects of the mental health system.* WHO, Geneva, Switzerland. http://www.who.int/mental_health/evidence/dollars_dalys_and_decisions.pdf

Website of WHO's cost-effectiveness work programme (CHOICE): http://www.who.int/choice

## References

1. WHO. (2001). *The World health report 2001; mental health: new understanding, new hope.* WHO, Geneva.
2. WHO. (2004). *Mental health policy, plans and programmes. Mental health policy and service guidance package.* WHO, Geneva.
3. WHO. (2000). *The world health report 2000; health systems; improving performance.* World Health Organization, Geneva.
4. Dixon, A., McDaid, D., Knapp, M., *et al.* (2006). Financing mental health services in low- and middle-income countries. *Health Policy and Planning*, **21**, 171–82.

5. Knapp, M.R.J., Funk, M., Curran, C., *et al.* (2006). Economic barriers to better mental health practice and policy. *Health Policy and Planning*, **21**, 157–70.

6. WHO. (2006). *Dollars, DALYs and decisions: economic aspects of the mental health system*. WHO, Geneva.

7. Scott, S., Knapp, M., Henderson, J., *et al.* (2001). Financial cost of social exclusion: follow-up study of antisocial children into adulthood. *British Medical Journal*, **323**, 191–4.

8. Beecham, J.K.J. and Knapp, M.R.J. (2000). Costing psychiatric interventions. In *Measuring mental health needs* (2nd edn) (eds. G. Thornicroft, C. Brewin, and J.K. Wing), pp. 200–24. Gaskell, London.

9. Curtis, J. and Netten, A. (2005). *Unit costs of health and social care*. Personal Social Services Research Unit, University of Kent, Canterbury.

10. McCrone, P., Knapp, M., Proudfoot, J., *et al.* (2004). Cost-effectiveness of computerised cognitive-behavioural therapy for anxiety and depression in primary care: randomised controlled trial. *The British Journal of Psychiatry*, **185**, 55–62.

11. Chisholm, D., Healey, A., and Knapp, M.R.J. (1997). QALYs and mental health care. *Social Psychiatry and Psychiatric Epidemiology*, **32**, 68–75.

12. Olsen, J.A. and Smith, R.D. (2001). Theory versus practice: a review of 'willingness-to-pay in health and health care. *Health Economics*, **10**, 39–52.

13. Valenstein, M., Vijan, S., Zeber, J.E., *et al.* (2001). The cost-utility of screening for depression in primary care. *Annals of Internal Medicine*, **134**, 345–60.

14. Revicki, D., Brown, R., Keller, M., *et al.* (1997). Cost-effectiveness of newer antidepressants compared with tricyclic antidepressants in managed care settings. *The Journal of Clinical Psychiatry*, **58**, 47–58.

15. Kamlet, M.S., Wade, M., Kupfer, D.J., *et al.* (1992). Cost-utility analysis of maintenance treatment for recurrent depression: a theoretical framework and numerical illustration. In *Economics and mental health* (eds. R.G. Frank and W.G. Manning), pp. 267–91. Johns Hopkins University Press, Baltimore, MD.

16. Hatziandreu, E.J., Brown, R.E., Revicki, D.A., *et al.* (1994). Cost-utility of maintenance treatment of recurrent depression with sertraline versus episodic treatment with dothiepin. *Pharmacoeconomics*, **5**, 246–64.

17. Pyne, J.M., Smith, J., Fortney, J., *et al.* (2003). Cost-effectiveness of a primary care intervention for depressed females. *Journal of Affective Disorders*, **74**, 23–32.

18. Schoenbaum, M., Unutzer, J., Sherbourne, C., *et al.* (2001). Cost-effectiveness of practice-initiated quality improvement for depression; results of a randomized clinical trial. *The Journal of the American Medical Association*, **286**, 1325–30.

19. Knapp, M., Romeo, R., Mogg, A., *et al.* (in press). Cost-effectiveness of transcranial magnetic stimulation vs. electroconvulsive therapy for severe depression: a multi-centre randomised controlled trial. *Journal of Affective Disorders*.

20. Romeo, R., Byford, S., and Knapp, M. (2005). Annotation: economic evaluations of child and adolescent mental health interventions: a systematic review. *Journal of Child Psychology and Psychiatry*, **46**, 919–30.

21. Drummond, M.F. and Jefferson, T.O. (1996). Guidelines for authors and peer reviewers of economic submissions to the BMJ. The BMJ economic evaluation working party. *British Medical Journal*, **313**, 275–83.

22. Byford, S., Harrington, R., Torgerson, D., *et al.* (1999). Cost-effectiveness analysis of a home-based social work intervention for children and adolescents who have deliberately poisoned themselves. Results of a randomised controlled trial. *The British Journal of Psychiatry*, **174**, 56–62.

23. Edwards, R., Ceilleachair, A., Bywater, T., *et al.* (2007). Parenting programme for parents of children at risk of developing conduct disorder: cost effectiveness analysis. *British Medical Journal*, **334**, 682–7.

24. Tan Torres, T., Baltussen, R.M., Adam, T., *et al.* (2003). *Making choices in health: WHO guide to cost-effectiveness analysis*. WHO, Geneva.

25. Chisholm, D. (2005). Choosing cost-effective interventions in psychiatry. *World Psychiatry*, **4**, 37–44.

26. Hyman, S., Chisholm, D., Kessler, R., *et al.* (2006). Mental disorders. In *Disease control priorities in developing countries* (2nd edn) (eds. D. Jamison, J. Breman, A. Measham, *et al.*). Oxford University Press, New York.

27. Chisholm, D., Sanderson, K., Ayuso-Mateos, J.L., *et al.* (2004). Reducing the global burden of depression: a population-level analysis of intervention cost-effectiveness in 14 epidemiologically-defined sub-regions (WHO-CHOICE). *The British Journal of Psychiatry*, **184**, 393–403.

28. Commission on Macroeconomics and Health. (2001). *Macroeconomics and health: investing in health for economic development*. WHO, Geneva.

# Psychiatry in primary care

David Goldberg, André Tylee,
and Paul Walters

## Epidemiology

In recent years, major epidemiological surveys have been carried out in the community in many different countries, in the United Kingdom most recently by the Office of National Statistics (to find this and other surveys go to http://www.statistics.gov.uk/STATBASE/Product.asp?vlnk=8258). The findings in such community surveys can be compared with findings in primary care surveys, when it will be found that the list of common mental disorders is not quite the same, although conditions characterized by symptoms of depression and anxiety are the most common. Rather than considering the detailed diagnoses, it can be helpful to distinguish between 'internalizing disorders', which besides anxiety states and depression, also include the fear disorders like phobias and panic disorder, obsessive-compulsive disorder and many cases of somatization disorder; and 'externalizing disorders' consisting of conduct disorder in childhood, and antisocial behaviour, as well as drug and alcohol disorders in adult life. The former group of disorders are characterized by subjective distress, and typically high levels of anxious and depressive symptoms; while in the latter group abnormalities are in externally observed behaviour.[1]

In community surveys it can be seen that rates of internalizing disorders rise sharply after puberty, are highest between the ages of 35 and 55 and fall thereafter, and that females rates are higher than males at all ages., while rates of externalizing disorders reach their maximum between the ages of 15 and 34, and fall sharply after that, with males rates much higher than female rates at all ages. This is shown in Table 7.8.1 (which does not include antisocial behaviour as reliable data are not available in the community).

## The Goldberg-Huxley Model[2]

This was devised as a framework for comparing the characteristics of patients seen in the community with those in other medical settings, and describing the pathway which people usually follow to mental health care in places where GPs act as 'gatekeepers'. It consists of five levels, separated by four filters. The figures for psychiatric morbidity over 1 year necessitate using estimates of incidence rates, and are therefore much higher than the point prevalence rates reported in community surveys. The essence of the model is the demonstration that most distressed patients will see a doctor over the course of 1 year (filter 1), but only about half of them will have their distress detected (filter 2). Most common mental disorders are treated in primary care, so filter 3 is relatively impermeable, only allowing one in five to pass. Psychiatrists only have any part in the process with the fourth filter, which also holds back most patients. Psychiatrists therefore form their ideas about mental disorders from a highly skewed section of all those with disorders.

## Prevalence of psychiatric disorder in primary care

In the United Kingdom, about 80 per cent of the population consult their doctor in the course of a year, and prevalences among attenders are higher than among the general population.[2] In contrast, specialist mental health services see between 1 and 2 per cent of the population in the course of a year, and admit only about 0.5 per cent to inpatient care, so that primary care deals with the major part of the burden of common mental disorders.

The World Health Organization (WHO) carried out the largest primary care survey in 14 countries[3] but for purposes of comparison only the UK data will be shown here. Table 7.8.2 compares the frequencies and types of mental disorders seen in the community, in primary care, and in psychiatric practice. Mental disorders

**Table 7.8.1** Annual prevalence of mental disorders in the community by type and age, rates per 100 at risk

| Disorder | Gender | 5 to 16 | to 34 | to 54 | to 74 | All (16–75) |
|----------|--------|---------|-------|-------|-------|-------------|
| Internalizing | Male | 3.1 | 11.70 | 16.75 | 9.87 | 13.5 |
| | Female | 4.3 | 20.55 | 21.35 | 14.80 | 19.4 |
| Externalizing | Male | 10.05 | 11.6; 18.9 | 2.25; 10.4 | 0.4; 3.8 | 6.0; 11.9 |
| | Female | 4.35 | 5.3; 5.7 | 0.75; 2.1 | 0.4; 0.5 | 2.3; 2.9 |
| Other | Male | 1.9 | 0.33 | 0.78 | 0.23 | 0.5 |
| | Female | 0.75 | 0.42 | 0.73 | 0.52 | 0.6 |

*Internalizing* = any neurotic disorder. *Externalizing* = conduct disorder for age 5–16; for the remaining age groups the rate for drug dependence is shown first, followed, after the semicolon, by the rate for alcohol dependence. *Other* = psychotic disorders in adults. Source: National Statistics website: www.statistics.gov.uk Crown copyright material is reproduced with the permission of the Controller Office of Public Sector Information (OPSI).

**Table 7.8.2** Prevalence of mental disorder by gender for the community, for primary care attenders, and for admissions to psychiatric beds

| | The community annual prevalence (%) | | Primary care cases consecutive attenders (%) | | Mental hospital inpatients (%) | |
|---|---|---|---|---|---|---|
| | Males | Females | Males | Females | Males | Females |
| Mixed anxiety depression | 6.8 | 10.8 | 2.1 | 4.5 | 9.8 | 17.6 |
| GAD | 4.3 | 4.6 | 4.9 | 14.9 | | |
| Panic | 0.7 | 0.7 | 3.4 | 3.6 | | |
| Phobias | 1.3 | 2.2 | 2.1 | 4.6 | | |
| Neurasthenia | – | – | 6.1 | 21.7 | | |
| Somatoform disorder | – | – | – | 0.5 | | |
| OCD | 0.9 | 1.3 | – | – | | |
| Depression | 2.3 | 2.3 | 13.9 | 18.3 | 17.9 | 27.3 |
| Alcohol dependence | 11.9 | 2.9 | 5.3 | 0.8 | | |
| Drugs dependence | 5.4 | 2.1 | – | – | 30.1 | 14.3 |
| Schizophrenia | 0.6 | 0.5 | – | – | 20.4 | 13.7 |
| Organic, dementia | – | – | – | – | 10.3 | 15.9 |
| Subnormality | – | – | – | – | 7.1 | 5.4 |
| Developmental disorders | – | – | – | – | 5.1 | 5.4 |
| Any Dx | 14.1% | 19.9% | 23.5% | 27.5% | 100% | 100% |

Sources: National Statistics website: www.statistics.gov.uk Crown copyright material is reproduced with the permission of the Controller Office of Public Sector Information (OPSI).

seen in primary care settings are more severe on average than those seen in community surveys, and different disorders predominate. The figures shown are for practices in Manchester with a fairly high prevalence of mental disorders, but the spread of diagnoses is fairly similar in other countries. The ICD-10 criteria only counted somatoform disorders if they were severe and long-standing, and do not count the many patients presenting with unexplained somatic symptoms, which are often accompanied by symptoms typical of anxiety or depression. A more recent study from Denmark[4] has estimated that almost a half of their patients were diagnosed cases of mental disorders, with somatoform disorders being found in about one-third. Patients with established physical illnesses are also at greater risk of mental disorders, and this is especially so if they are disabled by their illness. It can be seen from Table 7.8.3 that disorders admitted to psychiatric hospitals in the United Kingdom are different again from those typically seen in primary care, with organic states, drug and alcohol dependence, schizophrenia and severe depressive states accounting for the majority of cases (Source: http://www.hesonline.nhs.uk/Ease/servlet/ContentServer?siteID=1937&categoryID=202).

A study in 10 European countries shows 28 per cent of consecutive attenders in the United Kingdom to be distressed on a screening interview, but only 6 per cent presented psychological symptoms to their GP. Most of these (5.5 per cent) received a psychiatric diagnosis, but the GPs also diagnosed others as 'psychiatric'—so that their total rate was 15 per cent.[5] These figures are fairly similar to those in Switzerland and the Netherlands, but in stark contrast to those in Eastern Europe. In the Russian Federation, for example, 27 per cent were distressed, but none reported psychological distress to their GPs, and none were diagnosed: however, the GPs identified 3 per cent of their patients as 'psychiatric'. Fairly similar

figures were reported in Estonia, Poland, and Belgium; while figures in Germany, Spain, and Sweden are intermediate (*ibid* 2007; see Fig. 7.8.1). This study also showed that GPs who discuss psychosocial matters with their patients, and look at them are better at diagnosing them—a finding that echoes previous research in the United Kingdom.[2]

It can be seen from Fig. 7.8.1 that most distressed patients—who may well be found to have a mental disorder if interviewed with a research interview—do not mention their distress to their doctor, and that this accounts for failure to diagnose the disorder. Many patients who have not endorsed feelings of distress are nonetheless assessed as mental unwell, either because they are presenting with

**Table 7.8.3** The Goldberg-Huxley Model: Data for Manchester, UK

| | |
|---|---|
| **Level 1**: Community samples<br>*First Filter: The decision to consult* | **250–315/1000/year** |
| **Level 2**: All those seeing GPs found to have a mental disorder<br>*Second filter: GPs ability to detect* | **210–230/1000/year** |
| **Level 3**: Cases recognized by the GP<br>As 'mental disorders'<br>*Third filter: GPs decision to refer* | **101/1000/year** |
| **Level 4**: All those seeing mental health professionals<br>*Fourth filter: Psychiatrist's decision to admit to hospital* | **20.6/1000/year** |
| **Level 5**: Those admitted as inpatients | **3.4/1000/year** |

(Note that these estimates are annual period prevalences, and depend on estimates of annual incidence rates in addition to point prevalence rates. Source: Reproduced from D.P. Goldberg and P.J. Huxley, *Common mental disorders—a bio-social model*, copyright 1992, The Tavistock Institute, London.)

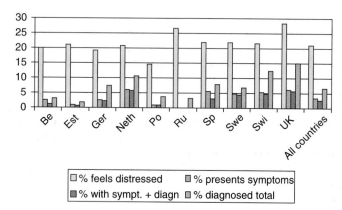

**Fig. 7.8.1** Proportions of population that feel distressed, present symptoms of distress, are diagnosed if they do so, and total number of patients diagnosed, in 10 European countries (Reproduced from P. Verhaak, J. Bensing, and A. Brink-Nuinen, Primary mental health care in 10 European countries: patients' demands and GPs' responses. *European Journal of Psychiatry*, **21**, (1), Zaragoza Jan–Mar 2007, copyright 2007, INO REPRODUCCIONES, S.A.).

unexplained somatic symptoms or because they are under treatment for a mental disorder that has responded to treatment.

## Clinical presentations

### Somatization

Somatization is broadly defined as the expression of psychological distress through physical symptoms. In primary care, most patients present physical symptoms at the onset of an episode of anxiety and depression. This is actually the usual way that new episodes of common mental disorders present in general medical settings, as only about 15 per cent of new episodes present purely in psychological terms.[2]

Primary care somatizers can be subdivided into 'facultative somatizers', who admit to their psychological symptoms and accept a mental disorder diagnosis if appropriately interviewed, and 'pure somatizers' who, despite such an enquiry, still deny the presence of psychiatric symptoms. People have many reasons for preferring to present somatic symptoms to their doctors—they are understandably worried that they may have a new physical disease, they give priority to pains over other symptoms because it is pain that hurts, and they often wish to avoid the stigma of being thought psychologically distressed.

Somatizers may be compared with 'psychologisers', who directly present their psychological problems to their doctors. The former are more likely to report adverse childhood events and periods of childhood illnesses, while the latter have more abnormal attachment behaviours.

### Hidden versus conspicuous morbidity

The ability of GPs to detect psychological disorders among their patients forms the second filter that patients must pass through in order to receive a diagnostic label. This ability varies a good deal between places as well as between disorders. In the WHO study[3] the overall average detection rate was 48.9 per cent, but rates varied from 75 per cent for Verona to 15.9 per cent for Shanghai (62.9 per cent for Manchester). Recognition rates for individual

diagnoses followed these overall rates, with somatization disorder being best recognized, followed by depression. However, these detection rates do not reveal whether the GP is identifying the same patients as the research assessment. In fact, the exact agreement between the two (measured by κ) is rather poor, at only +0.18 for all centres (+0.38 for Manchester).

The second filter is passed when the GP recognizes a mental health problem in the patient, although this will often be without a precise ICD-10 diagnosis. Those recognized by the GP make up the 'conspicuous' morbidity—in fact, just under half of that estimated to be present in the waiting room population by a two-stage case-finding procedure: so that the patients who are not identified can be thought of as the 'hidden morbidity'. These undetected patients continue to consult, but an outsider's inspection of notes and prescriptions, or even discussion with the relevant doctor, will not identify them as patients with psychiatric morbidity. In practice, the 'conspicuous' morbidity may be greater than 50 per cent, as the longitudinal nature of primary care means that patients may be diagnosed in subsequent visits, and this is missed in cross-sectional waiting room studies.[6,7] Kessler *et al.* followed up a cohort of primary care patients over 3 years and found only 14 per cent of patients with depression remained unrecognized at the end of this period.[8] Rost *et al.* followed up 98 depressed patients who had made at least one visit to their GP and found 32 per cent were undetected at 1 year.[9] Despite this, GPs are good at recognizing severe depression, and unrecognized depression tends to be mild.[10–12] The severity of depression in primary care, rather than being defined categorically, may therefore be better conceptualized as running along a continuum from mild to severe. Using a dimensional approach Thompson *et al.* calculated GPs only miss one 'probable' case of depression every 29 consultations.[13]

Doctors better able to detect disorder have the following characteristics:[2]

- Make eye contact with the patient
- Make empathic comments
- Pick up verbal cues
- Pick up non-verbal cues
- Ask directive questions, with a psychological content
- Do not read notes, or look at their computer, while the patient is speaking
- Deal with over-talkativeness
- Deal with today's problem

Data from the WHO study indicate that these 'undetected illnesses' are on an average less severe than those detected by GPs and have a somewhat better outlook. However, the data does not support the view that failure to detect these less severe disorders has serious long-term consequences for the patient[14] although this does not mean that there are not individuals would be better served if their distress was acknowledged.

### The elderly

Mental illness in the elderly is common in primary care. Between 5 and 10 per cent of older adults attending primary care will suffer from depression, though this may be higher in areas of socio-economic deprivation.[15] Older people are less likely to admit to psychiatric problems and more likely to emphasize somatic concerns and present behavioural changes. One study found that only 38 per cent of those identified as depressed through screening in the community had discussed feelings of depression with their GP.[16] This may lead to under-recognition in primary care. Crawford *et al.* found that only 52 per cent of 62 patients identified with clinical depression from a community survey were correctly diagnosed by their GP.[17] The elderly may attribute their symptoms to 'normal ageing', grief, or physical illness, or may fear sigmatization more than younger patients making recognition more difficult. Elderly depressed men may be particularly likely to go unrecognized.[17]

A systematic approach using a collaborative care model may improve depression management for the elderly in primary care. The Improving Mood-Promoting Access to Collaborative Treatment (IMPACT) trial in the United States demonstrated that a primary care collaborative model for late-life depression was more effective than usual care in improving depressive symptoms. It also decreased pain due to osteoarthritis, increased functional abilities, and improved quality of life.[18] The collaborative care model was highly cost-effective[19] and continued to show benefits over a 2-year follow-up period.[20]

The other major condition with which the GP will be involved is dementia. In the United Kingdom, the prevalence rate is approximately 5 per cent for all those over 65, but there is an age-related rise within this band to 25 per cent for those aged over 85. Consultations for organic psychoses reflect this: 370 consultations per 10 000 years at risk for those aged over 75, and 888 per 10 000 years at risk for those aged over 85. However, the management of people with dementia in primary care has been criticized.[21] Up to 75 per cent of patients with moderate to severe dementia and up to 97 per cent of patients with mild cognitive impairment go unrecognized by their GP.[22] Again there may be a number of reasons for this. Dementias have an insidious onset, and sometimes the doctor's familiarity with the patient can militate against spotting change. If a relative also accepts that the changes associated with dementia reflect normal ageing, the diagnosis may be delayed or never made. Only 40 per cent of GPs in the United Kingdom use a specific test to detect dementia, and in a survey of 8051 GPs in England 40 per cent thought an early diagnosis of dementia was not important.[23] Turner *et al.* surveyed GPs knowledge, confidence, and attitudes about dementia and found that despite GPs overall knowledge about diagnosis and management being good, a third lacked confidence in their diagnostic skills and two-thirds lacked confidence in their management of behavioural problems and other associated problems in dementia.[24]

Downs and others conducted a trial of an educational package to improve detection and management of dementia in primary care.[25] In the United States, a trial of collaborative care versus care as usual for patients with dementia in primary care has produced encouraging results.[26] Compared with care as usual, collaborative care (consisting of case management though a senior practice nurse working with the patient's family and integrated in the primary care team, and the use of standard protocols to guide and monitor treatment) resulted in significant improvements in the quality of care and in the symptoms of dementia, without an increase in psychotropic medication use.

# Classification of mental disorders in primary care

## Difficulties with conventional psychiatric taxonomies

The main problem with the International Classification of Diseases, 10th Edition (ICD-10)[27] or Diagnostic and Statistical Manual, 4th Edition (DSM-IV)[28] classifications used by psychiatrists is that they were devised to describe a very different consulting population, they are needlessly complicated, and they do not lead directly to management. Patients usually present a mixture of physical, psychological, and social symptoms expressed in any order, although somatic symptoms are usually first. Some symptoms are repeatedly mentioned and some are mentioned only in passing. Symptoms left to the end may be the most important of all. Symptoms may not fit a psychiatrist's taxonomy. In primary care, patients often have several concurrent problems of a medical, psychological, and social nature.

Most psychologically distressed patients show symptoms of both anxiety and depression. The ICD-10 classification has a mild disorder called 'mixed anxiety depression', since some patients have symptoms of each which together seem sufficient for a diagnosis, although not satisfying the criterion for either disorder on its own. However, this does not solve the problem of the many patients who are above the threshold for both disorders, who are declared 'co-morbid' for two different disorders by conventional psychiatric taxonomy.

An alternative view points out that the two groups of symptoms are strongly correlated with one another (about +0.7) in the consulting population,[2] and thus views them as two related dimensions of symptomatology which tend to co-vary over time. GPs themselves rarely emphasize the distinction between the two groups of symptoms, and there appears to be no evidence that any adverse consequences follow this neglect. For the GP, the diagnostic task can be one of separating the symptoms of depression and anxiety from those of an accompanying physical illness, or of probing for psychiatric morbidity in patients where apparent physical symptoms do not have an organic cause. In primary care settings, 'co-morbidity' refers to patients who have both physical disorders and mental disorders.

## Solutions to the classification problem

Both the major psychiatric classifications—ICD-10 and DSM-IV—offer special versions produced in collaboration with primary care physicians which are deemed suitable for this setting, and roughly correspond to the parent classification. The WHO offers '**ICD10-PHC**'[29] which consists of 26 common conditions, with advice on how they present, the diagnostic features, the differential diagnosis of similar symptoms, essential information for the patient and the carer, advice and support for the patient and the carer, the role of medication, and indications for referral to the mental health services. Information is given about national organizations, and self-help materials, to assist people with particular diagnoses, and advice is given to GPs in particular areas about customizing the system by including information about self-help and support groups for local people.

The '**DSM-IVPC**'[30] on the other hand is organized by symptoms that branch out into diagnostic algorithms. The GP assesses the patient's symptoms and, in workbook fashion, determines the relevant psychiatric diagnoses. The manual is formatted to be concise and practical, with limited use of psychiatric jargon. As a key feature, the chapter devoted to 'Algorithms for Common Primary Care Presentations' presents nine algorithms, headed by the presenting symptoms, for the most common psychiatric concerns encountered in primary care. No advice is given on management or on information to be given to carers.

Given the quantity of printed material that floods into GPs offices, it is doubtful whether many GPs keep such systems on their desks—although they may be incorporated in their computer programs. It is more realistic to use such systems in training new doctors, so that ways of approaching patients and their carers become incorporated in their usual routines, with the system only consulted when an unusual problem presents itself. It can be seen that whereas the DSM-IV system is aimed at formal diagnosis, the ICD10-PHC system is aimed at management once an assessment has been completed.

## The International Classification for Primary Care, (ICPC-2-R)[31]

The classification most widely used by GPs is of course their own, devised under the auspices of the World Organization of National Colleges & Academies ('WONCA'), called the International Classification for Primary Care, '**ICPC-2-R**'. This is a system which classifies all patient data and clinical activity in primary care, taking into account the frequency distribution of problems commonly encountered.

It allows classification of

- the patient's reason for encounter (RFE),
- the problems/diagnosis managed,
- interventions,
- test results, and the
- ordering of these data in an episode of care structure

It has a biaxial structure and consists of 17 chapters, each divided into seven components dealing with

- symptoms and complaints
- diagnostic, screening, and preventive procedures
- medication, treatment, and procedures
- test results
- administrative
- referrals and other reasons for encounter, and
- diseases

It is not clear to what extent all GPs work their way through this complex system, but should they reach the seventh component, there is a rough correspondence with the ICD. Note that multiple disorders can be coded in the same episode, but the extent to which this is done is not clear. Nor does the system provide advice on the management of the various conditions—it is assumed that the clinician knows how to do this.

## The Read codes[32]

The most widely used system in the United Kingdom since the advent of computerization, are the Read codes. This meets the needs of the generalist by including diagnoses, symptoms, and problems. Some very broad reasons for consultation—such as 'anxiousness', 'depressed', and 'headache' are provided. A letter of the alphabet is followed by up to four numerical codes, and there are also about 50 codes for diagnoses such as E204. 'Depression' or E2003 'anxiety with depression', which correspond very roughly to ICD diagnoses. However, no criteria are given, nor any advice on management for these various diagnoses.

None of the above four systems take into account functional impairment and disability, yet clinicians need to consider this in conjunction with the set of symptoms presented by an individual patient. Both diagnosis and current impairment are essential, and may help to explain why up to a quarter of patients with schizophrenia are managed solely in primary care settings[33] whilst some patients with adjustment disorder need referral to the community mental health team.

## Improving the identification of some common disorders

### (a) Aids to accurate detection of depression

Rather than using routine screening questionnaires to all patients, it is more practical to ask the following questions in six groups of patients:

- all those who look or sound depressed, or mention depressive symptoms
- all those with a past history of depression
- all those with significant physical illness causing disability
- all those with diabetes and coronary heart disease, where the risk is higher
- all those with other mental health problems, such as dementia or heavy drinking
- mothers of infants who are either single or are unsupported by a partner or family

Both these questions should be asked:

- During the past month, have you been feeling down, depressed or hopeless?
- During the last month, have you often been bothered by having little interest or pleasure in doing things?

### (b) Aids to accurate assessment of severity of depression

If positive replies are obtained to either of these, assess severity of using the Patient Health Questionnaire-9 (PHQ-9) a questionnaire with nine questions validated for use in primary care,[34] which may assist in ensuring that antidepressant medication is better targeted on those with moderate and severe degrees of depression.

### (c) Aids to the accurate detection of alcohol problems

Other, more recent tools, such as the Drug Abuse Problem Assessment for Primary Care (DAPA-PC),[35] were designed specifically to be administered via computer. While currently popular in the areas of depression and substance abuse, the audience for assessment tools is expanding for a number of reasons, including: convenience, privacy, high-patient satisfaction,[36] decreased provider time, improved validity, and reliability,[37] and decreased expense.

## The management of mental disorders within primary care

### (a) Stepped care

With the introduction of mental health guidelines there has been a shift towards stepped care for mental health problems.[38] Stepped care 'provides a framework in which to organize the provision of services supporting both patients and carers, and healthcare professionals in identifying and accessing the most effective interventions' (see Fig. 7.8.2). Stepped care allows treatment to be provided in steps according to the severity of problems and/or response to treatment, aiming to provide the greatest benefit to most of the people from the resources available. Patients who fail to respond are given the next step on the treatment plan. Stepped care can be delivered by starting at the least invasive step and gradually 'climbing' the steps according to response, thus targeting more intensive treatments to those that that need them, or by 'stratifying' care so that the first treatment step is determined by severity of disorder and thereafter by response.[39] Stepped care was developed in the United States, initially for the management of depression.[40] In the United Kingdom, this model of care has now been recommended for depression,[38] anxiety disorders,[41] obsessive-compulsive disorder,[42] and self-harm.[43]

### (b) Mental health workers based in primary care

Several new possibilities have emerged recently with the advent of the new *graduate mental health workers* in primary care. The NHS plan (DH 2000) was to have 1000 such workers in England and indications are that there are 600–700 in post. Mostly, the posts are similar to assistant psychologists and they generally are trained on a one-day release scheme at local university level in primary care mental health. Many are conducting initial assessment, providing brief psychological interventions such as brief cognitive behaviour therapy (CBT) or problem-solving for common mental health problems and medication management. Many are overseeing the use of self-help written materials and computerized help such as 'Beating the Blues', a computerized CBT programme for depression, which has been shown to be cost-effective.[44] Graduate primary care mental health workers (PCMHWs) also act as advisors on the range of other local services (for example, local library bibliotherapy schemes, and support groups). They have been proved to be effective at increasing patient satisfaction with episodes of care but were found not to improve mental health symptoms or to use the voluntary sector more than usual care.[45] Many PCMHWs are psychology graduates, and they tend to move on after a year or two into much wanted clinical psychology posts, so corporate memory can be diminished. Many other interventions described in level two of the National Institute for Clinical Excellence (NICE) Depression guideline[38] are increasingly applied in primary care—such as exercise schemes, befriending schemes, brief problem-solving, brief CBT, self-help materials, and sleep restoration.

Practice primary care counsellors may in reality be psychologists, psychotherapists, or counsellors depending on their training, expertise, and accreditation. They mostly see adults with common mental health disorders which may include adjustment disorders and losses. They often integrate different models of brief psychotherapeutic treatment depending on their training and the particular patient, and they receive regular supervision. These services may be provided in-house or in a neighbouring practice depending on

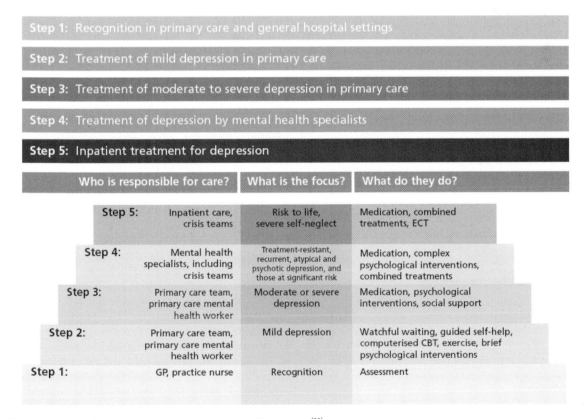

**Fig. 7.8.2** The stepped care model applied to depression. Reproduced with permission.[38]

available space. Some counsellors specialize in providing services for non-English speaking groups and certain patient subgroups such as eating disorders, domestic violence, etc.). Whilst resources are usually limited on occasions they may see patients for longer courses of treatment.

### (c) The role of the primary care nurse

Practice nurses are increasingly involved in chronic disease management within practices and this includes managing mental health conditions whether severe or common. From April 2006, practices have been rewarded in England under the Quality and Outcomes Framework of the General Services Medical Contract[46] for screening their patients with coronary heart disease (CHD) and diabetes for depression and with any newly depressed patients for using a recommended patient self-report instrument to assess baseline severity of depression. The recommended instruments are the Patient Health Questionnaire-9 item (PHQ9),[34] the Hospital Anxiety and Depression Scale (HADS),[47] or the Beck Depression Inventory (BDI).[48] Practice nurses are expected to undertake much of this work as they see the patients with CHD or diabetes for review and therefore they need proper training and supervision. Also rewarded in the GP contract is an annual physical review of all patients on the Severe and Enduring Mental Illness registers (SEMI or SMI)—again usually conducted by practice nurses. Such nurses have traditionally administered depot medication for such patients without much training on the procedure or the accompanying health checks. This training has been improving lately. Expecting an untrained practice nurse to administer depot without support and training is unacceptable, and training is needed in how to give the injection, how to review the suitability of this form of medication, how to monitor for side-effects, how to assess mental state for signs of deterioration, when to involve colleagues or refer to the community mental health team, and crisis management.

Practice nurses have been successfully trained in the assessment and management of depression[49,50] and the use of problem-solving in major depression.[51] Practice nurses have been successfully trained in chronic disease management of the severely mentally ill,[51] whereby they constructed a disease register, a care plan, and 3-monthly structured reviews encompassing psychological, physical, and social well-being. Whilst the practice nurses were diligent and detected problems, there was little evidence that they communicated these to the GPs. There was also a failure to increase health promotion in this group, despite their recognized increased standardized mortality.

Health visitors trained in counselling have been shown to benefit women with postnatal depression,[52] and Appleby et al.[53] have targeted the same group of patients with a nurse-led intervention.

### Primary care mental health services

The primary care team provides the majority of care to people suffering from mental health problems. Though many services remain GP-led, many are becoming increasingly sophisticated with a growing number of professionals involved in the care of people with mental health problems. In England, the Department of Health has produced a guide for improving primary care mental health services.[39]

A number of models for primary care mental health services are described reflecting the need for services to provide care to populations with different needs, resource availability, and relationships with secondary care. Examples include the 'opt-in' or self-referral model, proactive models such as a collaborative care model, 'one-stop shop' models, and focused service models (i.e. services are developed for a specific remit such as common mental disorder or psychosis). The 'opt-in' model is one in which the patient initiates care and follow-up and is the traditional primary care model. In a collaborative care model there is active follow-up and collaboration between patient, primary care health professionals, and when required secondary care professional with the health professional coordinating care. A 'one-stop shop' model provides a single point of access to all mental health services with a triage system determining resource allocation. There is no perfect model, and all have advantages and disadvantages depending on the population needs and availability of resources.

As services develop so the range of primary care mental health professionals is expanding. As well as the traditional primary care professionals—the GP and practice nurse—many practices now have others, including primary care graduate mental health workers and health visitors. Their roles include making assessments, facilitating referrals and movement through the health care system, and delivering treatments. In the United Kingdom, the availability of counselling services is now commonplace in primary care and up to 50 per cent of general practices have on-site counselors.[54] They are referred people with a wide range of common mental disorders and other psychosocial problems such as adjustment disorders. Bower and Roland reviewed the evidence for the effectiveness of counselling in primary care and found it was associated with a modest improvement in short-term outcomes compared to usual care, but was no better than usual care over the longer-term. It did not appear to be any more cost-effective than usual care but patients appeared satisfied with it.[55]

## The primary–secondary care interface

### What GPs expect of psychiatrists

GPs expect psychiatrists to possess and exhibit specialized skills of assessment and management not possessed within the primary health care team. The primary care team may include primary care mental health workers ranging from graduate workers to counsellors, psychotherapists, or psychologists, although if present these are usually extremely thinly spread (i.e. 1–2 sessions per practice per week). GPs do expect their psychiatrists or a named person from the mental health team to be available when they are needed, and they should also make themselves available for incoming telephone calls from the key contact. Because of sheer numbers (in England and Wales there are 12 times as many GPs as psychiatrists) the GP must protect this valuable resource by not overloading it with inappropriate referrals and by obtaining and maintaining certain assessment and management skills that can be used in primary care as well as sharing the care of certain patients under the leadership of secondary care. Referrals will vary widely from practices depending on their own 'in-house' expertise and the presence or absence of any primary care mental health workers or local counselling services. Larger practices often have more in-house expertise and are more likely to have at least one of their GPs who possess more specialized mental health skills. Small practices with one or two partners are less likely to have such skills and may need more support. GPs expect the psychiatrist to provide inpatient care when needed (e.g. serious self-neglect, suicide intent, etc.) and day-patient facilities to provide a place of care, respite, and safety. They can also expect the psychiatrist to use diagnostic facilities and investigations (e.g. scans) as necessary and to provide highly specialized treatments when indicated (e.g. electroconvulsive therapy). Less frequently, the GP may need respite from particular doctor–patient relationships for the longer-term good of both. Referral is also sometimes a result of pressure by the relatives or patient. Where good communication exists between primary and secondary care, these often 'covert' reasons for referral can be openly discussed.

Access to specialist assessment when appropriate is paramount for a primary care service. GPs are not usually trained in specialist assessment and therefore, to match need to services, a psychiatrist, community psychiatric nurse, or psychologist from the community mental health team can perform this function, often in a primary care setting or the patient's home. Other community mental health teams operate an outpatient clinic (which may be moved into the surgery). Often 'true consultancy' is being sought by the GP, whereby he or she may receive advice only. Other practices operate a joint consultation system whereby the specialist and generalist see the patient together and formulate a plan. With recent changes in the configuration of mental health teams in the United Kingdom to provide acute care, early intervention and assertive outreach, in some places the more traditional community mental health teams are being reduced which is often confusing and can be unsettling for practices which have developed relationships with individual psychiatrists and colleagues. Also, if crisis teams work 9 to 5 p.m., yet the GP surgeries are open until 6 or 7 p.m., this can create difficulties for making urgent referrals.

### Ways of organizing the interface

The interface between primary and secondary care is of key importance in the delivery of mental health care. Bower and Gilbody[56] have described a continuum of specialist involvement in primary care mental health with least involvement of secondary care professionals in the education/training model, and increasing involvement through the consultation-liaison model, the collaborative care and the replacement/referral model. In practice, these models are not mutually exclusive. They can complement one another and be adapted to take into account local workforce issues and staff availability.

There are at least four models of working across the interface between primary and secondary care:

1 A **replacement/referral model** is the traditional way in which primary care interfaces with secondary care. In this model, the patient's care is handed over to specialist services by way of a referral, the specialist service only relinquishing care when the patient had been treated. However, over the last 25 years other models have developed.[57] These include:

2 The **consultation-liaison model** allows secondary care professionals to develop ongoing relationships with primary care professionals, not only providing expert advice but also actively liaising with the primary care team, and often attending team meetings or seeing patients jointly with the GP.

3 The **collaborative care model**, as described above has primary care mental health professionals working between primary and secondary care to improve the overall care of patients. These

link-workers can provide active follow-up and access to specialist advice and care as needed.[59]

4 In the **training/education model**, secondary care provides education and training to the primary care team which otherwise functions autonomously utilizing secondary care services when needed via a referral system.

How health services negotiate the interface between primary and secondary mental health services is likely to get increasingly complex as secondary care moves away from centralized care through the community mental health teams, to specialist teams such as assessment and brief treatment teams, early intervention teams, and continuing care teams. It is likely that each of these teams will develop its own model of interfacing with primary care. This may allow for a more fluid interface and closer working relationships between primary care and secondary care teams.[59] However, it needs to be managed appropriately or could lead to confusion of roles and responsibilities.

### Shared care registers and shared care plans

A **shared care register** is usually a computerized record of all patients jointly cared for by the two services. It might consist of all those who have been discharged from hospital in the past 2 years, all those who have been on a psychotropic drugs for longer than a year, and all psychotic patients known to the GP who have not had an admission to the hospital. The record gives information about the key worker, outpatient clinics are held in the surgeries, and 'good practice protocols' can be developed, so that the case register can be audited against what other teams agree is good clinical practice.

**Shared care plans** follow on from this development. Such a plan gives the primary care staff information about symptoms which they may expect while the patient is well, likely symptoms in relapse, the name of the key worker, and full details of whom to contact in an emergency both during the day and at night. The plan makes clear who is responsible for medication, and gives an acceptable alternative should the GP find it necessary to vary the medication. It is essential that these plans are mutually agreed between the two teams, rather than being imposed by one team on the other. GPs in England are now being remunerated for keeping registers of patients with psychotic illnesses, dementia, and learning disabilities.

## Improving the mental health skills of GPs

About half of GP trainees have a 6-month psychiatry hospital attachment, many of which are considered to be unhelpful for a future generalist career.[59] Many GPs have had no higher professional training in mental health and are not required to do so. There are several GPs who may have previously trained in psychiatry or psychotherapy (e.g. cognitive analytic psychotherapy, CBT, family therapy, etc.) before entering general practice and there is a growing national network of GPs with a special interest in psychiatry (GPsis) with the development of a national course for GPsis to Diploma/Masters level organized by PRIMHE, the National Primary Care Mental Health charity for professionals (www.primhe.org). The GPs network covers most regions and greatly overlaps with the National Trailblazer network (www.iop.kcl.ac.uk). Trailblazers was developed 10 years ago by one of the authors (AT) to bring together professionals from primary and secondary care to work together in pairs to build bridges and enhance local services by working on a local service development project together with supervision. Trailblazer courses bring pairs together for tutor and peer supervision of projects for up to a year. To date nearly 1000 GPs, psychiatrists, CPNs, PNs, etc., have participated in this way and trailblazer training centres now run in every region in England, supported by the Regional Care Services Improvement Partnership Development Centres (www.csip.org.uk/regions) of the UK Department of Health. International trailblazers is now part of the International Initiative for Mental Health Leaders (www.IIMHL.org) and runs in New Zealand, United States, and England where there is the added interest of comparing service systems by participants who have exchange visits as modules rotate in the three countries. Trailblazers has been positively evaluated for the adult-centred learning approach.[60] Another well-recognized Quality Improvement Programme with a long history of working in primary care has recently focused its methods on common mental health disorders. The Improvement Foundation (www.improvementfoundation.org.uk) formerly known as the National Primary Care Development Team (www.npdt.org.uk) have been working with 20 PCTs in England using a Plan Do Study Act cycle (PDSA) to help practices improve their depression care.

As there are few opportunities for primary care workers to obtain mental health skills training, one successful distance learning method involves the use of training DVDs. 'Micro-skills' of assessment or treatment of mental health disorders can be demonstrated by real-life general practitioners with actor–patients in 10 min consultations. The learner is then encouraged to practice these skills using role-plays supplied with the DVDs. A series of existing training materials have been put together for the World Psychiatric Association (WPA) which involves two of the authors (DG and AT) and colleagues from the Institute of Psychiatry, and Prof. Linda Gask and her colleagues at Manchester University. The materials in this WPA package cover depression, somatization, chronic fatigue, schizophrenia, anxiety, and dementia (see www.iop.kcl.ac.uk or www.man.ac.uk for further details).

## Summary

At one time, it was asserted that the 'worried well' were treated in primary care, while true mental illnesses were seen by the mental illness services. This was not true when it was asserted, and is even less true now. The great majority of patients with common mental disorders are cared for within primary care, and many of those with severe mental illnesses are only seen in primary care. 'Stepped care' is a model for distributing clinical problems between the services, and 'shared care' refers to the care of patients seen by both primary care and specialist mental health services. Many other workers in primary care now assist GPs with the treatment of mental disorders, and special administrative arrangements within primary care are necessary to ensure that clinical services are available to those with special needs.

In summary, mental disorders in primary care:

- Are an important public health problem
- Frequently present with somatic symptoms
- Are more likely to be detected if the doctor has better communication skills
- Those with disabling physical illnesses are also at greater risk
- Are on average less severe than those seen in specialist care

## Further information

Care Services Improvement Partnership (CSIP). Improving Primary care Mental Health Services. National Institute for Mental Health England, Department of Health. 2006. (www.csip.org.uk/resources/publications/primary-care.html) Accessed 22/3/07. A practical guide to developing and improving mental health services in primary care.

http://guidance.nice.org.uk/topic/behavioural. National Institute for Health and Clinical Excellence's website for guidance on mental and behavioural disorders.

Jenkins, R. (ed.) (2004). *WHO guide to mental and neurological health in primary care. A practical guide to the assessment and treatment of mental disorders in primary care* (2nd edn). Royal Society of Medicine Press, London.

## References

1. Krueger, R.F. (1999). The structure of common mental disorders. *Archives of General Psychiatry*, **56**, 921–6.
2. Goldberg, D.P. and Huxley, P.J. (1992). *Common mental disorders—a bio-social model*. Tavistock, London.
3. Ustun, B. and Sartorius, N. (1995). *Mental disorders in general health care: an international study*. John Wiley, Chichester.
4. Toft, T., Fink, P., Oernboek, E., *et al.* (2005). Mental disorder in primary care: prevalence and co-morbidity among disorders. *Psychological Medicine*, **35**, 1173–84.
5. Verhaak, P., Bensing, J., and Brink-Muinen, A. (in press). Primary mental health care in 10 European countries: patients' demands and GPs' responses. *European Journal of Psychiatry*.
6. Ormel, J. and Tiemens, B. (1995). Recognition and treatment of mental illness in primary care. Towards a better understanding of a multifaceted problem. *General Hospital Psychiatry*, **17**, 160–4.
7. Freeling, P. and Tylee, A. (1992). Depression in general practice. In *Handbook of affective disorders* (ed. E.S. Paykel), pp. 651–6. Churchill Livingstone, Edinburgh.
8. Kessler, D., Bennewith, O., Lewis, G., *et al.* (2002). Detection of depression and anxiety in primary care: follow up study. *British Medical Journal*, **325**, 1016–7.
9. Rost, K., Zhang, M., Fortney, J., *et al.* (1998). Persistently poor outcomes of undetected major depression in primary care. *General Hospital Psychiatry*, **20**, 12–20.
10. Simon, G.E., Goldberg, D., Tiemens, B.G., *et al.* (1999). Outcomes of recognized and unrecognized depression in an international primary care study. *General Hospital Psychiatry*, **21**, 97–105.
11. Dowrick, C.F. (1995). Case or continuum? Analysing GPs ability to detect depression in primary care. *Primary Care Psychiatry*, **1**, 255–7.
12. Wittchen, H.U., Hofler, M., and Meister, W. (2001). Prevalence and recognition of depressive syndromes in German primary care settings: poorly recognized and treated? *International Clinical Psychopharmacology*, **16**, 121–35.
13. Thompson, C., Ostler, K., Peveler, R.C., *et al.* (2001). Dimensional perspective on the recognition of depressive symptoms in primary care: the Hampshire Depression Project 3. *The British Journal of Psychiatry*, **179**, 317–23.
14. Goldberg, D.P., Privett, M., Üstün, B., *et al.* (1998). The effects of detection and treatment on the outcome of major depression in primary care: a naturalistic study in 15 cities. *The British Journal of General Practice*, **48**, 1840–4.
15. Unutzer, J. (2002). Diagnosis and treatment of older adults with depression in primary care. *Biological Psychiatry*, **52**, 285–92.
16. Blanchard, M., Waterreus, A., and Mann, A. (1994). The nature of depression among older people in inner London and the contact with primary care. *The British Journal of Psychiatry*, **164**, 396–402.
17. Crawford, M.J., Prince, M., Menezes, P., *et al.* (1998). The recognition and treatment of depression in older people in primary care. *International Journal of Geriatric Psychiatry*, **13**, 172–6.

18. Unutzer, J., Katon, W., Callahan, C.M., *et al.* (2002). Collaborative care management of late-life depression in the primary care setting: a randomized controlled trial. *The Journal of the American Medical Association*, **288**, 2836–45.

19. Katon, W.J., Schoenbaum, M., Fan, M.Y., *et al.* (2005). Cost-effectiveness of improving primary care treatment of late-life depression. *Archives of General Psychiatry*, **62**, 1313–20.

20. Hunkeler, E.M., Katon, W., Tang, L., *et al.* (2006). Long term outcomes from the IMPACT randomised trial for depressed elderly patients in primary care. *British Medical Journal*, **332**, 259–63.

21. Audit Commission. (2002). *Forget me not: developing mental health services for older people in England*. Audit Commission, London.

22. Gifford, D.R. and Cummings, J.L. (1999). Evaluating dementia screening tests: methodologic standards to rate their performance. *Neurology*, **52**, 224–7.

23. Woods, R.T., Moniz-Cook, E., Iliffe, S., *et al.* (2003). Dementia: issues in early recognition and intervention in primary care. *Journal of the Royal Society of Medicine*, **96**, 320–4.

24. Turner, S., Iliffe, S., Downs, M., *et al.* (2004). General practitioners' knowledge, confidence and attitudes in the diagnosis and management of dementia. *Age and Ageing*, **33**, 461–7.

25. Downs, M., Turner, S., Bryans, M., *et al.* (2006). Effectiveness of educational interventions in improving detection and management of dementia in primary care. *British Medical Journal*, **332**, 692.

26. Callahan, C.M., Boustani, M.A., Unverzagt, F.W., *et al.* (2006). Effectiveness of collaborative care for older adults with Alzheimer disease in primary care: a randomized controlled trial. *The Journal of the American Medical Association*, **295**, 2148–57.

27. ICD-10. (1993). *The ICD-10 classification of mental & behavioural disorders*. WHO, Geneva.

28. American Psychiatric Association. (1994). *Diagnostic & statistical manual of mental disorders* (4th edn). American Psychiatric Association, Washington.

29. WHO. (2001). *Guide to mental health in primary care*. Royal Society of Medicine Press, London.

30. Pingitore, D. and Sansone, R.A. (1998). *Using DSM-IV primary care version: a guide to psychiatric diagnosis in primary care. American Family Physician* **58**, 1347–52. Online at: http://www.aafp.org/afp/981015ap/pingitor.html.

31. WONCA. (2005). *International classification committee ICPC--R: International Classification of Primary Care*. OUP, Oxford.

32. The Clinical Terms Version 3 (The Read Codes) NHS Information authority. (2000). Available at http:\\www.coding.nhsia.nhs.uk.

33. Melzer, D., Hale, A., Malik, S., *et al.* (1991). Community care for patients with schizophrenia one year after hospital discharge. *British Medical Journal*, **303**, 1023–6.

34. Kroenke, K., Spitzer, R.L., and Williams, J.B. (2001). The PHQ-9: validity of a brief depression severity measure. *Journal of General Internal Medicine*, **16**, 606–13.

35. Holtz, K., Landis, R.D., Nemes, S., *et al.* (2001). DAPA-PC: development of a computerized screening system to identify substance abuse in primary care. *Journal of Health Quality*, **23**, 34–7.

36. Kobak, K.A., Taylor, L.H., Dottl, S.L., *et al.* (1997). A computer-administered telephone interview to identify mental disorders. *The Journal of the American Medical Association*, **278**, 905–10.

37. Greist, J.H. (1998). Clinical computing: the computer as clinician assistant: assessment made simple. *Psychiatric Services*, **49**, 467–72.

38. National Institute for Health and Clinical Excellence (NICE) (2007) CG23 Depression (amended). *Management of depression in primary and secondary care*. NICE, London. Available from www.nice.org.uk/CG23.

39. Raistrick, H. and Richard, D. (2006). *Designing primary care mental health services: guidebook*. Care Services Improvement Partnership, Department of Health, Leeds.

40. Katon, W., Von Korff, M., Lin, E., *et al.* (1999). Stepped collaborative care for primary care patients with persistent symptoms of depression: a randomized trial. *Archives of General Psychiatry*, **56**, 1109–15.

41. National Institute for Clinical Excellence. (2004). *Anxiety: management of anxiety (panic disorder, with or without agoraphobia, and generalised anxiety disorder) in adults in primary, secondary and community care*. Clinical Guideline 22. National Institute for Clinical Excellence, London.

42. National Institute for Clinical Excellence. (2006). *Obsessive-compulsive disorder: core interventions in the treatment of obsessive-compulsive disorder and body dysmorphic disorder*. National Clinical Practice Guideline Number 31. National Institute for Clinical Excellence, London.

43. National Institute for Clinical Excellence. (2004). *Self harm: short-term treatment and management*. National Clinical Practice Guideline Number 16. National Institute for Clinical Excellence, London.

44. McCrone, P., Knapp, M., Proudfoot, J., *et al.* (2004). Cost-effectiveness of computerized cognitive behaviour therapy for anxiety and depression in primary care randomised controlled trial. *The British Journal of Psychiatry*, **185**, 55–62.

45. Lester, H., Freemantle, N., Wilson, S., *et al.* (2007). Cluster randomised controlled trial of the effectiveness of primary care mental health Workers. *The British Journal of General Practice*, **57**, 196–203.

46. Quality and Outcomes Framework Information available at http://www.ic.nhs.uk/services/qof.

47. Zigmond, A.S. and Snaith, R.P. (1983). The hospital anxiety and depression scale. *Acta Psychiatrica Scandinavica*, **67**, 361–70.

48. Beck, A.T., Mendelson, M., and Mock, J. (1961). Inventory for measuring depression. *Archives of General Psychiatry*, **4**, 561–71.

49. Wilkinson, G. (1992). The role of the practice nurse in the management of depression. *International Review of Psychiatry*, **4**, 311–6.

50. Mann, A.H., Blizard, R., Murray, J., *et al.* (1998). An evaluation of practice nurses working with general practitioners to treat people with depression. *The British Journal of General Practice*, **48**, 875–9.

51. Mynors-Wallis, L.M., Gath, D.H., Lloyd-Thomas, A.R., *et al.* (1995). Randomised controlled trial comparing problem-solving treatment with amitriptyline and placebo for major depression in primary care. *British Medical Journal*, **310**, 441–5.

52. Holden, J.M., Sagovsky, R., and Cox, J.L. (1989). Counselling in a general practice setting: controlled study of health visitor intervention in treatment of postnatal depression. *British Medical Journal*, **298**, 223–6.

53. Appleby, L., Warner, R., Whitton, A., *et al.* (1997). A controlled study of fluoxetine and cognitive-behavioural counselling in the treatment of postnatal depression. *British Medical Journal*, **134**, 932–6.

54. Mellor-Clark, J., Simms-Ellis, R., and Burton, M. (2001). *National survey of counsellors in primary care: evidence for growing professionalisation*. Royal College of General Practitioners, London.

55. Bower, P. and Rowland, N. (2006). Effectiveness and cost effectiveness of counselling in primary care.[update of Cochrane Database of Systematic Reviews, 2002; (1): CD001025; PMID: 11869583]. *Cochrane Database of Systematic Reviews*, **3**, CD001025.

56. Bower, P. and Gilbody, S. (2005). Managing common mental health disorders in primary care: conceptual models and evidence base. *British Medical Journal*, **330**, 839–42.

57. Gask, L., Sibbald, B., and Creed, F. (1997). Evaluating models of working at the interface between mental health services and primary care. *The British Journal of Psychiatry*, **170**, 6–11.

58. Von Korff, M. and Goldberg D. (2001). Improving outcomes in depression: the whole process of care needs to be enhanced. *British Medical Journal*, **323**, 948–9.

59. Turton, P., Tylee, A., and Kerry, S. (1995). Mental health training needs in general practice. *Primary Care Psychiatry*, **1**, 197–9.

60. Brown, C., Wakefield, S., Bullock, A., *et al.* (2003). A qualitative evaluation of the Trailblazers teaching the teachers programme in mental health. *Learning in Health and Social care*, **2**, 74–82.

# The role of the voluntary sector

Vanessa Pinfold and Mary Teasdale

## What is the mental health voluntary sector?

The voluntary sector plays an important role in the mental health field across the world. Originally set up and run by volunteers, the prime motivation and purpose for this sector is improving the lives of people affected by mental health problems by doing things differently, tirelessly pushing for change, never giving up hope and working alongside service users (also known as patients and consumers) and their families every step of the way. In some countries it has been labelled the 'third sector' to distinguish it from other organizational sectors namely industry (private sector) and government (public or statutory sector).

The voluntary sector is not, however, a cohesive group of organizations and across the mental health community each one operates with its own specific remit. Some of these organizations have become large businesses providing a wide range of services under contract with statutory agencies. Others choose to avoid employing staff and are still run entirely by committed volunteers. Many rely on voluntary donations in order to remain fiercely independent of government. Each has its own aims and mission, core stakeholder group, trustee and membership structures, management systems, governance procedures, and a unique portfolio of activities.

Some mental health organizations focus activities on mental health or emotional well-being specifically (e.g. Finnish Association for Mental Health). Others target a social problem and support all those affected such as charities working with the homeless, refugees, victims of domestic violence, or young offenders, including people with mental health problems. There are organizations that primarily campaign, educate, advocate, lobby, and promote self-help resources such as EUFAMI—an association for families across Europe and SANE Australia. In parts of the world, including Eastern Europe, there are particular challenges in mental health resulting from poverty, dislocation of the population, and insufficient resources for health. Some states, like Armenia, have no mental health services. Here, the Catholic Agency for Overseas Development (CAFOD) is working with Armenia's Association of Child Psychiatrists and Psychologists to provide therapy and mental health care and to increase awareness and understanding in order to overcome prejudice.

Wherever they work, key characteristics of voluntary sector organizations include an independent position, a strong values base, empowerment principles, non-profit distributing of resources, passionate commitment to the work focus, rooted to service user, and carer experiences and they are always striving for changes to provide people with mental health problems better provision and opportunities. Most started as local support groups but some have grown into large national organizations with considerable political leverage. The National Schizophrenia Fellowship (known today as Rethink) was founded in 1972 by a group of families concerned that relatives of people with schizophrenia had no support for themselves. In this chapter we draw on the Rethink experience to illustrate how the voluntary sector contributes to, and shapes, modern psychiatry. Although the English experience does not directly map onto those in other countries across the world, there are similarities and we seek to highlight these through the use of international examples where possible.

## Rethink severe mental illness

Rethink is a membership charity with 7500 members (service users, carers, mental health professionals, the general public) whose mission is 'to support everyone affected by severe mental illness recover a better quality of life'. It adopts a recovery-orientated approach to supporting the individual and their family through periods of ill health and their journey of recovery. This perspective is significantly different from that of clinicians and statutory providers, who have not been through the experiences common to people who suddenly have to cope with severe mental illness. Rethink staff descriptions of their role include:

> *Bridging: linking a person with non-judgemental delivery of services connected with service user and carer experience*

> *Ensuring service users are heard and needs met more holistically*

Initially providing mutual support, the organization later offered information resources which address the problems commonly encountered by service users and carers, like difficulty in gaining access to services or funding for appropriate care. The emphasis is on finding successful strategies which achieve solutions. Advocacy is provided for individuals and families whose needs are not being met. The experiences of service users struggling to cope provide detailed evidence which is used to develop Rethink's policy on the mental health issues which reach the political arena and also as the basis of campaigns on stigma and discrimination. Research and surveys of service user and carer views form the basis of reports on vital issues, like how information can be provided to carers with due respect for the service user's privacy and autonomy. Guidance on good practice may be developed and sometimes training for professionals. Media activity has publicized Rethink's campaigns and using the internet has made dissemination of information cheaper and easier than it used to be.

Rethink's activities also include the provision of front-line services in partnership with the National Health Service and Social Services (statutory sector) for example supported housing schemes, advocacy projects, community resource centres, carer support services, employment and training programmes, school education projects, and mentoring programmes for young people. In 2007, Rethink ran 350 front-line mental health services and employed approximately 1300 staff.

## Does the voluntary sector make a difference?

The voluntary sector makes a substantial contribution to both the image of psychiatry and its practices. For example in New Zealand, the Mental Health Foundation has worked in partnership with the Ministry of Health and other agencies to run a successful anti-discrimination campaign—like minds, like mine (whakaitia te whakawhiu i te tangata) for the past 10 years. This is an internally renowned mental health awareness programme that is transforming how the New Zealand public engages with mental health issues. Non-Governmental Organizations (NGOs) can also bring influence to bear at a national level and bring people together to plan new service models. The World Fellowship for Schizophrenia and Applied Disorders (WFSAD) supported a workshop in East Africa in 2003 where service users and families could meet with government ministers and medical professionals to discuss plans for achieving effective health care delivery. In England, the voluntary sector has collectively ensured that the published clinical guidelines describing best practice for the treatment of schizophrenia in 2002 took note of service user and carer treatment preferences. In India, Action for Mental Illness (ACMI), an advocacy initiative has achieved tax concessions for those with mental illness and their carers and also maintenance allowances equivalent to those provided to people with physical disabilities.

Standards of mental health care delivery vary dramatically—with cases of human rights abuses in psychiatry being documented in some countries and innovative services emerging in others in response to local demands. The voluntary sector can, and does, bring the spotlight on both ends of the service delivery spectrum (good and bad) and demand better for everyone. It also leads the way by developing innovative solutions both in terms of service delivery, public education, and self-management techniques. In the United States, NAMIs Peer-to-Peer Education Course is a 9-week experiential education course on the topic of recovery for anyone with serious mental illness who is interested in establishing and maintaining wellness. In Canada, a family to family network was established for first episode psychosis families by the Canadian Mental Health Association. The recovery model is being pioneered and embraced by the voluntary sector across the world. However, this relatively new approach requires a change of attitude by both service users and professionals as shown by the Scottish recovery network programme.

Common themes tend to emerge through the campaigns of voluntary organizations across the world, in spite of differences in wealth and varying stages of development. In most places the demands are for earlier intervention, better crisis response, more support for families, and less use of physical restraint on the ward when coping with challenging behaviour. The transition to care in the community presented a new set of problems, not least the need for different professional skills and adequate resources. And in the later part of the last century, the controversy over community treatment orders was raging in many countries. Changes in government policy and concerns over access to newer treatments resulted in new alliances in many countries, and the voluntary sector, clinicians and other professionals often learned to work together, recognizing how in alliance they could lobby more effectively for better law and more resources.

An excellent example of successful partnership working in England and Wales has been the formation of a coalition known as the Mental Health Alliance involving 80 organizations. Professional bodies have joined, including the Royal College of Psychiatrists as prominent and active members. The Mental Health Alliance has opposed the government's proposals for reforming the Mental Health Act 1983 for the past 8 years and has managed to achieve some change in the content of the legislation as well as delaying the whole process.

## The role of critical friends

The independence of organizations is an essential characteristic of the voluntary sector. These bodies do occupy the territory of 'critical friends' to both the statutory and private sectors of the mental health community, monitoring activity and speaking out in praise of positive developments but also highlighting when things are wrong.

For example at Rethink experience shows that misdiagnosis can result in inappropriate care and treatment with tragic consequences like imprisonment, suicide, or even homicide. Therefore Rethink supports service users in obtaining expert second opinions. Providing families or individual service users with accurate but understandable information enables them to challenge the opinion of a psychiatrist or medical team if this seems appropriate.

Rethink also advocates for families by using the complaints procedures or by providing legal representation at inquest hearings in order to draw attention to deficiencies in support, care, and treatment. They focus efforts on cases where systemic problems played a part, like a poor approach to risk assessment or refusal to accept information from families. The aim is to persuade the Ombudsmen or coroners to recommend improvements in the local policies and procedures in order to improve the quality of services.

In recent times there has been a spotlight on mental health services' engagement with people from Black and Minority Ethnic groups (BME) in England. The BME voluntary mental health organizations have formed a network which aims to reduce inequalities and promote good practice in mental health for racialized groups. The Network has been very critical of the Government's proposals to amend mental health legislation and has criticized the statutory health sector for failing to meet legal requirements on race equality. Similar issues arise in the United States where the National Council of La Raza (NCLR)—the largest national Hispanic civil rights and advocacy organization in the United States—works to improve opportunities for Hispanic Americans. They report that Latinos are at a disproportionately high risk for depression and other conditions associated with mental illness, and are also much less likely to seek treatment or receive quality culturally and linguistically competent care.

## Conclusion

The voluntary sector is a dynamic and vital part of any mental health system. Rooted in the experiences of mental health service users and carers, voluntary sector organizations across the world ensure that the voices of 'experts by experience' directly influence campaigns, policy debates, service redesign, and project planning and treatment guidelines. The sector is, however, fragile and in some countries organizations are increasingly dependent on state funding which could undermine their autonomy and independence. Psychiatrists can support their local voluntary organizations by joining them—as members, as campaigners, and as educators. The sector can also support psychiatrists, helping to transform the public image of psychiatry and encouraging young people to take

an interest in mental health as a career option. The alliances forged with psychiatrists and their representative bodies are crucial for improving the quality of mental health services and to effectively tackle stigma and discrimination. We do need each other in order to deliver better outcomes for mental health service users and their families.

## Further information

The websites for some of the voluntary organizations referenced in the chapter are:

Rethink: www.rethink.org

Canadian Association for Mental Health: www.camh.ca

EUFAMI—European Federation of Associations of Families of People with Mental Illness: www.eufami.org

Mental Health Foundation in New Zealand: www.mentalhealth.org.nz

National Alliance on Mental Illness: www.nami.org

SANE Australia: www.sane.org

Scottish recovery network: www.scottishrecovery.net

The World Fellowship for Schizophrenia and Allied Disorders (WFSAD): www.world-schizophrenia.org

# 7.10

# Special problems

## Contents

7.10.1 The special psychiatric problems of refugees
Richard F. Mollica, Melissa A. Culhane, and Daniel H. Hovelson

7.10.2 Mental health services for homeless mentally ill people
Tom K. J. Craig

7.10.3 Mental health services for ethnic minorities
Tom K. J. Craig and Dinesh Bhugra

---

## 7.10.1 The special psychiatric problems of refugees

Richard F. Mollica, Melissa A. Culhane, and Daniel H. Hovelson

While the forced displacement of people from their homes has been described since ancient times, the past half-century has witnessed an expansion in the size of refugee populations of extraordinary numbers.[1,2] In 1970, for example, there were only 2.5 million refugees receiving international protection, primarily through the United Nations High Commission for Refugees (**UNHCR**). By 2006, UNHCR was legally responsible for 8.4 million refugees. In addition, it is conservatively estimated that an additional 23.7 million people are displaced within the borders of their own countries. Although similar in characteristics to refugees who have crossed international borders, internally displaced persons do not receive the same protection of international law. Adding all refugee-type persons together, the world is forced to acknowledge the reality that over the past decade more than 10 000 people per day became refugees or internally displaced persons.

The sheer magnitude of the global refugee crisis, the resettlement of large numbers of refugees in modern industrial nations such as Canada, the United States, Europe, and Australia, and the increased media attention to civil and ethnic conflict throughout the world has contributed to the medical and mental health issues of refugees becoming an issue of global concern. This chapter will focus on a comprehensive overview of the psychiatric evaluation and treatment of refugees and refugee communities. Although this mental health specialty is in its infancy, many scientific advances have been made that can facilitate the successful psychiatric care of refugee patients.

## Definition

The definition of a refugee as outlined in the 1951 Convention and 1967 Protocol relating to the Status of Refugees is presented in Box 7.10.1.1.[3] A person or persons who has passed over from one country into another seeking protection from violence and who cannot return to his country of origin because of fear of persecution or injury is considered a refugee according to international law.

The 1951 Convention Relating to the Status of Refugees was drawn up by the United Nations parallel to the creation of UNHCR. This Convention and the subsequent 1967 Protocol establishes

---

**Box 7.10.1.1** Definations according to the 1951 convention and 1967 protocol relating to the status of refugees

**Article 1—Definition of the term 'refugee' A(2)** [Any person who] . . . owing to well-founded fear of being persecuted for reasons of race, religion, nationality, membership of particular social group or political opinion, is outside the country of his nationality and is unable or, owing to such fear, is unwilling to avail himself of the protection of that country; or who, not having nationality and being outside the country of his former habitual residence . . . , is unable or, owing to such fear, is unwilling to return to it. (As amended by Article 1(2) of the 1967 Protocol.)

**Article 33—Prohibition of expulsion or return (refoulement)** (1) No contracting state shall expel or return (refouler) a refugee in any manner whatsoever to the frontiers of territories where his life or freedom would be threatened on account of his race, religion, nationality, membership of a particular social group or political opinion.

international law for the definition of refugees as well as the protection accorded to them. It also articulates the important principle of *non-refoulement* (Box 7.10.1.1), which states that no refugee can be returned to his or her country of origin or any other location where there is any probability that he or she will be harmed. These legal definitions indicate that a refugee is not an economic migrant or a traditional immigrant. Sadruddin Aga Khan, in a seminal report, was one of the first High Commissioners to acknowledge the human rights violations that are primarily responsible for the generation of refugee populations.[4] Corresponding to these international covenants, the international community has focused on the protection of refugees. There are two components to protection that are classically viewed by UNHCR as an essential aspect of its mandate. These two elements include protection against:

1 ongoing violence and potential injury to the refugee including being denied proper asylum and involuntary repatriation;

2 lack of adequate food, water, clothing, and other forms of material assistance.

The UN Declaration of Human Rights adopted by the United Nations in December 1948 and the United Nations Convention against Torture and Other Cruel Inhuman or Degrading Treatment or Punishment adopted in December 1984 extends the basic principles of refugee protection and asylum, and reaffirms the principle of *non-refoulement*. In most refugee crises, not withstanding the political and military barriers to protection, UNHCR and the international community strive to offer refugees a safe asylum and basic humanitarian aid.

## Trauma and torture

By definition, most refugees have experienced traumatic life events of extraordinary brutality. Since the Second World War, empirical studies have investigated the relationship between mass violence, the refugee experience, and psychiatric morbidity. The earliest research focused on survivors of the Nazi concentration camps.[5-8] Shortly after the Second World War, Eitinger and his colleagues gave a detailed account of their medical and psychiatric examinations of concentration camp survivors. They postulated that the traumatizing process had a dual nature. They described the somatic traumas of captivity, such as head injury, hunger, and infections, as leading to a 'psycho-organic syndrome', and the predominately psychological traumas as leading to other psychiatric disorders such as depression. Thygesan's studies of concentration camp survivors in Denmark revealed similar results.[9,10] These early pioneering investigations of the psychosocial sequelae of the Nazi concentration camps established a preliminary baseline of traumatic outcomes for future generations of refugees, many of whom had experienced the trauma of similar experiences in Cambodia, Bosnia-Herzegovina, and elsewhere.

Increasingly, civilian populations carry the burden of ethnic conflict and mass violence. It is now estimated that more than 80 per cent of casualties caused by the recent violence in Africa, Asia, and Europe have primarily affected non-combatants.[11] Extensive research has revealed the major trauma events experienced by refugee populations fall into the eight groups below:

1 material deprivation

2 war-like conditions

3 bodily injury

4 forced confinement and coercion

5 forced to harm others

6 disappearance, death, or injury of loved ones

7 witnessing violence to others

8 brain injury

Every refugee situation will have a range of traumatic events that will fall into each of these categories that are unique or characteristic of a specific conflict. It is essential that the specific types of violence experienced by a given refugee population are well known to the psychiatric clinician who can use this knowledge to assess potential traumatic outcomes.[12] In addition to many unique forms of violence occurring in different refugee settings, the meaning of violent events also differs across cultures. Anecdotal, clinical, and epidemiological evidence suggests that certain categories of refugee trauma are more potent than others in producing psychiatric morbidity and other traumatic outcomes. Brain injury, sexual violence, torture and other forms of bodily injury, coercion, and forced confinement have great potential of causing psychiatric harm in refugees exposed to these events. Consistent with indicators of the 'potency' of specific trauma events, there evidence of a dose–effect relationship between cumulative trauma and psychiatric symptoms.[13] The personal aspects of human suffering associated with specific types of trauma, such as the murder of a child or the disappearance of a family member are still relatively undefined but obviously very difficult.

Many refugees have actually experienced torture. Recent research states that the most significant finding in the last 7 years may be that either torture has become more prevalent worldwide or the total number of events reported has increased, likely as a result of advocacy and elevated media attention.[14] After 25 years of research on treatment work with torture survivors, still no consensus exists for effective interventions within the field.

## Conceptual model of traumatic outcomes

Research on refugees has revealed the persistence of negative health and social outcomes decades after their initial experience of violence and dislocation. Emergence of standardized criteria for psychiatric diagnoses and disability and the demonstrated ability to elicit trauma events through simple screening instruments in culturally diverse populations have allowed evidence to accumulate suggesting a model of traumatic outcomes associated with the refugee experience. This model is primarily based upon the classic epidemiological triad which describes the interaction between host (i.e. the refugee), agent (i.e. traumatic life experiences), and environment (e.g. refugee camp) in the pathogenesis of psychiatric disorders.[15,16] This model, illustrated in Fig. 7.10.1.1, allows equal attention to be given to all aspects of the refugee experience.

The model in Fig. 7.10.1.1 has three major elements. First, it suggests that the major medical outcomes associated with the refugee experience are medical illness, psychiatric disorders, and disability. Second, trauma and the personal and environmental characteristics of the refugee describe the major risk factors associated with violent outcomes. Third, the direction of the causal arrows in the model do not imply a lack of reciprocal relationships where none is indicated; instead they indicate what most investigations consider

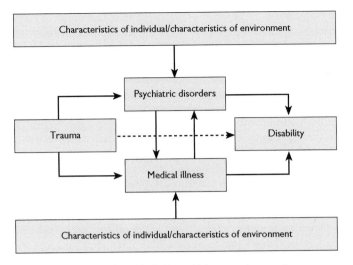

**Fig. 7.10.1.1** Conceptual model of refugee risk factors and traumatic outcomes.

to be the most dominant causal relationship. Despite its limitations, this simple conceptual model can provide the psychiatric professional with a scheme for approaching the refugee patient from either a clinical or public health perspective. The importance of the socio-cultural and political context unique to each refugee situation and its impact on each of the model's pathways cannot be overstated, since refugees come from diverse cultural groups and political experiences.

## Health status and medical illness

Refugees experience many diseases and chronic debilitating conditions, such as starvation and landmine injuries that have both immediate and long-term effects on their physical health. Every refugee situation involves many unique but common acts of violence leading to major medical sequelae. For example, gender-based violence and rape, which were instruments of ethnic cleansing in the Balkans, resulted in pregnancy, medically complicated self-administered abortions, and sexually transmitted diseases.[17] Extensive documentation of refugee survivors of torture describes the medical sequelae of torture and the causal link between refugee trauma and medical mortality and morbidity over time.

Throughout the process of migration, refugees are frequently exposed to infectious diseases and physical or psychological trauma that can have a profound impact on their overall health and well-being. Refugees are at increased risk for diseases such as obesity, diabetes, and heart disease, and often encounter significant barriers to employment and health care when attempting resettle. For these reasons, programmes implemented in the refugees' country of resettlement designed to improve health-seeking behaviours and overall self-care can have a positive, lasting impact on refugees' physical and mental health.[18]

## Psychiatric symptoms and illness

Observations since Kinzie *et al.*[19] and Mollica *et al.*[20] first diagnosed PTSD in Cambodian refugees, have made the cultural validity of PTSD seem almost certain. However, this reality does not negate the importance of culture-specific symptoms related to trauma that are independent of PTSD criteria. Recent large-scale epidemiological studies of refugee populations have confirmed

the high prevalence of major depression and PTSD in Western (e.g. Bosnian[21]) and non-Western (e.g. Cambodian[22] and Bhutanese[23]) refugee communities. The mental health impact of major depression, which presents both as a comorbid disorder with PTSD and alone, is chronic, severely disabling and demands the attention of the clinician working with refugees. Longitudinal data indicates that 45 per cent of Bosnian refugees who met criteria for PTSD, depression or both continued to meet criteria for these disorders 3 years later.[24] Similar results were found in a longitudinal study of Cambodian refugees 20 years after resettling in the United States.[25] As with Western populations, depression in refugees tends to be under-diagnosed and can be expressed as somatic complaints. A study of Vietnamese refugees showed high prevalence based on self-report, but high rate of physician under-diagnosis. Most patients with depression (95 per cent) presented with physical complaints.[26] These finding underscore the importance of depression screening especially in the primary care setting.

New research indicates that there may be memory problems in refugees with PTSD. When asked to recall traumatic events refugees with PTSD reported an increased number of traumatic or torture events over their baseline report, as compared to those with other psychiatric disorders who showed no change or decreases in number of events reported.[27] Substance use disorders are often overlooked in refugee populations but are often comorbid with PTSD.[28] Early in the 1980s reports of Hmong refugees using opium emerged.[29] Substance use disorders have been shown to have a delayed presentation of 5 to 10 years after the initial settlement of the refugee.[30] However, substance use disorders may vary by population. One recent study of Cambodian refugees in the United States reports low rates of alcohol use in the past 30 days.[31] Screening for substance use disorders especially in primary care is important. Complex grief reaction and chronic insomnia are also prevalent in this population.

### (a) Head injury

Clinical evidence is also emerging identifying head injury as a cause of significant psychopathology in refugee survivors. Head trauma is one of the most common forms of torture, so much so that reports of torture almost always imply that some kind of head trauma occurred. Many head injury survivors experience seizures and headaches, as well as behavioural disturbances such as aggressiveness, irritability, and sleep disturbances. Recent research on Vietnamese ex-political detainees who experienced head trauma while in captivity indicates that the number of head injuries is related to a decrease in executive functioning, those with head injury have increased risk of developing PTSD, and had decreased cortical thickness in several brain regions (Mollica *et al.* 2007, unpublished). The long-lasting effects of head trauma are serious and pervasive, affecting both the injured individual and their family. The presence of head trauma in torture victims has been overlooked in past research, but awareness is growing.

### (b) Functional status and disability

Although the functional status of refugees at the emergency and long-term ends of the continuum of the refugee experience has received little attention, the significance of this traumatic outcome is beginning to emerge. Until recently, the standard operating model of refugee protection has not been asked to determine the long-term socio-economic damage caused by the refugee experience. The answer to this question is extremely important to the recovery of societies in which the majority of the population has been displaced. In many societies, the refugee experience is the majority experience, which has strong implications for future socio-economic development. While the prevalence of functional impairment and disability is unknown in refugee populations, a recent epidemiological study of Bosnian refugees in Croatia reveals that functional disability may, in fact, be extremely high, especially in elderly refugees.[21] Furthermore, disability may be exacerbated in refugee survivors who have both chronic medical and psychiatric disorders.

## Psychiatric assessment

This section reviews key factors unique to the psychiatric evaluation and diagnosis of the refugee patient.

### Primary care: the proper setting for a refugee clinic

The psychiatric literature has generally stressed the importance of evaluating and treating refugee patients in a primary health care setting, whether in a refugee camp or in a country of resettlement. Four factors seem to support this viewpoint:

1 refugee patients seldom self-refer to psychiatry;

2 in many societies considerable stigma is associated with psychiatry but not with primary care medicine;

3 the majority of refugees seek out the care of their local medical doctors and indigenous traditional healers for the relief of their emotional suffering;

4 most refugees have associated medical and psychiatric disorders.

Considerable field experience has shown that establishing a mental health programme within a health facility where refugees already seek medical care can result in the highly successful utilization of psychiatric professionals and treatment.

### Cross-cultural psychiatric assessment and diagnosis

Early research describing the psychiatric status of refugee survivors, especially those who had been tortured, refrained from the use of psychiatric diagnoses because of a prevailing perception that the observed symptoms were a normal response to horrific life experiences.[12] Similarly, many medical anthropologists believed that Western psychiatric diagnostic classifications were not relevant to the assessment of suffering in non-Western populations.[32] Despite these reservations, the emergence of standardized diagnostic criteria for major depression and post-traumatic stress disorder (PTSD) have allowed for the cultural validity of these diagnoses to be tested in a number of refugee settings. Cross-cultural research suggests that assessments of psychiatric illness should begin with phenomenological descriptions of folk diagnoses or culture-specific syndromes.[33] Important methods of exploring the validity of DSM-IV diagnoses in cross-cultural settings have included using culturally valid definitions of functioning and mental health problems based on local views of maladaptive thoughts and behaviour in response to distress, not preconceived Western diagnostic categories[34]; however, to date, not a single culture-specific illness associated with the mass violence and torture experienced by refugees has been defined.[35] On the contrary, the criteria for the two major diagnoses associated with violence in Western society, i.e. major depression and PTSD, have been successfully applied

to refugees from many parts of the world. While high rates of PTSD can be measured in refugee patients and traumatized civilians, it is not known if other culture-specific symptoms not part of the DSM-IV criteria that may have greater clinical relevance and meaning to a specific refugee group. A general principle demonstrated by the World Health Organization cross-cultural study of depression,[36] i.e. that while some depressive symptoms may be present across cultures, they may not be the symptoms most strongly endorsed by the patient; this principle may also apply to PTSD. Figure 7.10.1.2 provides an illustration, which can help to address the problem of psychiatric diagnoses in refugee patients. This figure suggests that, until further research is forthcoming, the psychiatric provider needs to determine clinically whether the refugee patient is presenting with scenario A, B, or C.

The high prevalence of psychiatric symptoms associated with trauma in refugee populations neither affirms nor negates the 'normalization' of these symptoms. A narrow medical viewpoint could create a psychiatric redefinition of refugee mental health problems that would place the majority of refugees in a 'mentally ill' box without any access to individual psychiatric care; on the other hand, the hostility of many humanitarian aid workers toward psychiatry has denied the seriously mentally ill refugee legitimate access to psychiatric treatment. There will probably be a compromise at the intersection of public health objectives and the protection goals of humanitarian aid workers. In future, the presence of chronic and severe disability in refugee survivors will be the gold standard which drives the psychiatric and humanitarian rehabilitation of refugee survivors.[37,38]

### Psychiatric screening

If mental health practitioners are to treat refugee patients, they must be able to assess the refugee's major risk factors and traumatic outcomes. Simple screening instruments culturally adapted to the language, trauma, and symptoms of refugee patients have been found to be extremely effective as well as being well received by refugees themselves.[39–41] For example, a simple well-known

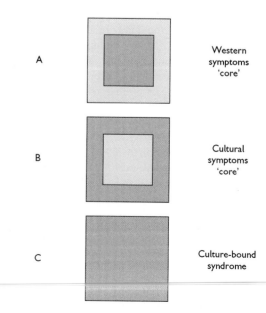

**Fig. 7.10.1.2** Comparison of diagnostic classifications.

screening instrument adapted from the Hopkins Symptom Checklist allowed Indochinese patients for the first time to provide their symptoms with little distress. The development of the Harvard Trauma Questionnaire further revealed that these same patients could provide answers to lists of possible trauma events and symptoms without becoming retraumatized. Overall, two major lessons have been learned from the use of simple checklists with refugee survivors.

1 The checklist acknowledges the traumatic life experiences of the refugee survivors and *de facto* gives them permission to elaborate on the details of their trauma.

2 The checklist, as a simple medical test, helps refugees to 'put words around' events and symptoms that would be too emotionally overwhelming for them in an open-ended interview.

Extensive research regarding appropriate methods of development, translation, and validation of the clinical screening instruments such as the Hopkins Symptom Checklist and Harvard Trauma Questionnaire has been widely disseminated.[29,42]

### Understanding somatic complaints

For years it was considered standard psychiatric wisdom that emotional distress, especially in non-Western patients, was primarily somatic in character; and that, because of their dominant expression of suffering through somatization, these patients were not psychologically minded, making them incapable of participating in psychotherapy or counselling. Extensive clinical experience and scientific studies with refugee patients throughout the world have led to a revision of these previously dominant professional attitudes. While it may be valid that some refugees primarily present their emotional suffering through somatic complaints, it has also been found that it is fairly easy for the medical practitioner to obtain from refugee patients deeper insights into their feelings and their beliefs as to the causes of their emotional distress. Often because of severe victimization, refugees as a group will not readily share their experiences of trauma and related medical and psychiatric injuries unless they are in a highly confidential environment where it is clear that the medical team can be trusted. In fact, the ability of refugee patients to extend themselves beyond their initial somatic complaints, as well as participating in clinical dialogue with the psychiatric practitioner as to the nature of their mental distress, is more the rule than the exception and is a major goal of assessment.[43]

## Psychiatric treatment

### The trauma story

The trauma story emerges as the centrepiece of any treatment approach. Every refugee patient has at least one traumatic experience that figures prominently in his or her life history. The trauma story is a living reality and is present for every patient. The trauma story is also present for the clinician. Yet, the story can be elusive and difficult for both patient and doctor to share. Often times when the patient is ready to tell the trauma story, the clinician is not ready to hear it. More frequently, when the clinician is ready for the patient to tell his or her story, the patient is unwilling. Therefore, one of the major goals of psychotherapy with refugees is to allow the trauma story to emerge gently and become a familiar and acceptable theme, which the refugee is not shamefully hiding

from his or her therapist and ultimately his or her family and community.[44]

#### (a) Debriefing

Although commonly conducted within populations who have experienced trauma, typically by relief workers or crisis counsellors, debriefing has been shown to have negative effects on psychiatric outcomes and should be avoided at all costs.[45] As described above, the trauma story should be allowed to emerge naturally and at the patient's own pace.

#### (b) Treatment

Psychiatric treatment of refugee patients should primarily be based upon standard psychiatric practices for mentally ill patients, including the appropriate use of psychotropic medicines. However, a number of novel therapeutic approaches have been used with refugees. Recent research in refugee populations has indicated that cognitive behavioural therapy (CBT) is efficacious for treatment-resistant PTSD and panic attacks[46,47] and in refugees who have experienced torture.[48] Interpersonal psychotherapy for depression has been found to be useful in rural Uganda.[49] This approach may also be effective with resettled refugees in Western countries. In female veterans of war, prolonged exposure therapy was more effective over time than other interventions for reducing symptoms of PTSD in female veterans of war. It may be possible and beneficial to use prolonged exposure therapy for others with PTSD.[50] Similarly, although no research has specifically examined the effects of therapies such as eye movement desensitization and reprocessing (EMDR) for refugees, positive results have been seen in a variety of different studies done with traumatized populations, including individuals with PTSD. Traditional medicine, which includes diverse health practices, knowledge, and beliefs is widely accepted and practiced worldwide. Traditional medicine typically relies upon local classifications of emotional distress and its treatment can incorporate plant-, animal- or mineral-based medicines, as well as spiritual therapies or massage.[45] Traditional healing approaches were widely used for the Cambodian refugee crisis of the 1990s.[51–53] Although widely used, no conclusive research has yet been done using complementary treatments such as massage, acupuncture or herbal medicine in the treatment of torture survivors.[14] Recent research with Cambodian refugees it was shown that interventions supporting work, altruism, and spirituality for refugees might serve as protective factor for the onset of psychiatric disability.[54]

### Special considerations

A number of special considerations have emerged from the many therapeutic approaches that have been tried with refugees.

### Family focus

Treatment should be directed at the entire family of the identified refugee patient. The refugee crisis tends to initiate a process in which surviving family members become each other's major social support system. The disruption and disintegration of stable communities and traditional social supports place the entire burden of survival upon family members. Sometimes in extreme situations that affect the family unit such as when a refugee is experiencing symptoms of depression, psychosis, or social withdrawal, the psychiatrist must reach out to the patient and establish a one-to-one therapeutic relationship until family members can be of assistance.

## Cultural sensitivity

The cultural sensitivity of refugee mental health practitioners is essential to the proper therapeutic relationship to the refugee patient. This means that the refugee mental health practitioner must be informed as to the type of trauma experienced by the refugee and its socio-cultural meaning, the cultural idioms by which human suffering is expressed in a given community, and the social stigma associated with mental illness. Despite the refugees' own adversity, long-standing social prejudices against mental illness will persist throughout the refugee crisis.

Little cross-cultural literature exists on the relationship between refugee patient, Western professional, and bilingual interpreter. The use of refugees as interpreters can be problematic. Ideally, health professionals from the refugee communities should be recruited to participate in psychiatric intervention. These individuals have had professional medical training as to the importance of confidentiality and can also provide insight into the cultural nuances of the doctor–patient relationship. The use of untrained interpreters from the refugee community should be avoided if at all possible. This is especially true of family members or members of a community or government institution that has previously threatened the security of the refugees. In addition, medical practitioners must respect patient dignity by not allowing young people to interview community elders or males from the community to ask refugee women explicit sexual questions and/or witness or be exposed to an undressed refugee woman during a medical examination. The more the bicultural interpreter can function in the role of a trained mental health paraprofessional, the more successful will be the therapeutic experience of all involved.

## Caring for the seriously mentally ill

Despite numerous biases against psychiatric intervention in refugee populations, psychiatrists are well positioned to treat the seriously mentally ill refugee. In most refugee camps, those in immediate danger are the psychotic and depressed refugees with suicidal ideation. These individuals have difficulty coping with their ongoing crisis and have high mortality rates. Once resettled, these refugees with serious mental health issues need appropriate medical and mental health services.[55]

## Special treatment needs of gender-based violence

Many colleagues in the field of refugee mental health have sought to break the 'conspiracy of silence related to sexual violence'.[32] While this issue has been well documented in refugee communities, it was not until the Bosnian conflict that rape was finally accepted by the international community not as a criminal act but as a crime against humanity. This recognition of gender-based violence as the most common type of torture of women, as well as a major terrorist instrument of war, has contributed to the protection and psychiatric care of sexually abused refugee survivors. While the political will now exists to condemn rape, and to protect refugees from it, the cultural stigma and corresponding social punishments of women considered 'tainted' by sexual violence, sometimes including their murder ('honour killing') by relatives, continues to make the psychiatric care of these survivors extremely difficult. In most cultures, rape remains a secret issue caused by the refugee's extreme resistance to reveal any details to the physician. Psychiatric practitioners must approach this issue with extreme caution in a strictly confidential manner. They must also be aware of the severe consequences to the patient if the rape experience becomes public knowledge, even to the patient's family members.

## Risk and resiliency factors

The pre- and post-conflict personality characteristics of refugees that increase resiliency and reduce psychiatric distress and disability are not known. While certain demographic characteristics have been associated with negative traumatic outcomes, these characteristics may be confounded by other risk factors. Women, especially widows, seem especially vulnerable to negative refugee effects. UNICEF has extensively reviewed those risk factors associated with the vulnerability of refugee children and adolescents.[56] Data from Bosnian refugees correspondingly reveal the high rates of disability associated with trauma and psychiatric comorbidity in the elderly.

Lessons learned from studies of political prisoners in Turkey reveal the importance of a well-established political world view as a major protection against the long-term human suffering associated with torture.[57] Studies of Bhutanese refugees in Nepal confirm the possible protective function of Buddhism in devout refugee practitioners of this religion.[23] Anecdotal reports by refugees themselves consistently confirm the emotional safety that they have found in their spiritual and religious beliefs and practices. Finally, recent research findings concur with the earlier research in concentration camp survivors and prisoners of war that prior psychiatric history and premorbid personality factors may have little effect on the psychiatric sequelae of traumatic refugee experiences. In resettlement countries, opportunities related to family unification, learning to speak the new country's language, and employment have clearly been shown to be associated with decreased psychiatric morbidity over time. Those who provide psychiatric care for refugees must keep in mind the environmental opportunities that can increase their overall resiliency.

## Reducing risk and maximizing resiliency

Figure 7.10.1.1 provides a readily accessible model for psychiatric practitioners to determine how they can reduce the risk factors associated with psychiatric disorders as well as promote the resiliency of the refugee patient. The section on risk factors provides many useful insights into the importance of enhancing the refugee's active role in work, spiritual participation, involvement in altruistic behaviour, and the many other personality and environmental factors that can directly reduce depression and other forms of psychiatric distress.

## Further information

www.hprt-cambridge.org <http://www.hprt-cambridge.org> (Harvard Programme in Refugee Trauma)

http://mentalhealth.samhsa.gov/cmhs/SpecialPopulations/refugmhnew. asp (U.S. Substance Abuse and Mental Health Services Administration, Refugee Mental Health Division)

www.unhcr.org (United Nations High Commission on Refugees)

## References

1. Office of the United Nations High Commissioner for Refugees. (1993). *The state of the world's refugees, 1993: the challenge of protection*, Vol. 9, p. 191. Penguin Books, New York.
2. Office of the United Nations High Commissioner for Refugees. (1997). *The state of the world's refugees, 1997–1998: a humanitarian agenda*, Vol. 12, p. 298. Oxford, England; Oxford University Press, New York.

3. Office of the United Nations High Commissioner for Refugees. (1992). *Handbook on procedures and criteria for determining refugee status: under the 1951 convention and the 1967 protocol relating to the status of refugees*, p. 93. Office of the United Nations High Commissioner for Refugees, Geneva.

4. Independent Commission on International Humanitarian Issues. (1986). *Refugees: the dynamics of displacement: a report for the independent commission on international humanitarian issues*, Vol. 18, p. 152. Zed Books, Atlantic Highlands, NJ, London.

5. Eitinger, L. (1961). Pathology of the concentration camp syndrome. Preliminary report. *Archives of General Psychiatry*, **5**, 371–9.

6. Eitinger, L. (1972). *Concentration camp survivors in Norway and Israel*, p. 199. Martinus Nijhoff, The Hague.

7. Eitinger, L. and Strom, A. (1973). *Mortality and morbidity after excessive stress*. Oslo University Press, Oslo, Norway.

8. Strøm, A.C.S. (1968). *Norwegian concentration camp survivors*. Universitetsforlaget; Humanities Press, Oslo, New York.

9. Thygesen, P. (1980). The concentration camp syndrome. *Danish Medical Bulletin*, **27**(5), 224–8.

10. Thygesen, P., Hermann, K., and Willanger, R. (1970). Concentration camp survivors in Denmark: persecution, disease, disability, compensation. A 23-year follow-up. A survey of the long-term effects of severe environmental stress. *Danish Medical Bulletin*, **17**(3), 65–108.

11. Levy, B.S. and Sidel, V.W. (1997). *War and public health*, Vol. 19, p. 412. Oxford University Press, New York.

12. Mollica, R.F. and Caspi-Yavin, Y. (1992). Overview: the assessment and diagnosis of torture events and symptoms. In *Torture and its consequences* (ed. M. Basoglu), pp. 253–74. Cambridge University Press, Cambridge.

13. Mollica, R.F., *et al.* (1998). The dose-effect relationships between torture and psychiatric symptoms in Vietnamese ex-political detainees and a comparison group. *The Journal of Nervous and Mental Disease*, **186**(9), 543–53.

14. Quiroga, J. and Jaranson, J. (2006). Politically-motivated torture and its survivors: a desk study review of the literature. *Torture*, **15**(2–3), 1–111.

15. Dohrenwend, B.P. (1998). *Adversity, stress, and psychopathology*, Vol. 15, p. 567. Oxford University Press, New York.

16. Susser, M. (1981). The epidemiology of life stress. *Psychological Medicine*, **11**(1), 1–8.

17. Swiss, S. and Giller, J.E. (1993). Rape as a crime of war. A medical perspective. *The Journal of the American Medical Association*, **270**(5), 612–15.

18. Research Triangle Institute. (2005). *Refugee health promotion and disease prevention toolkit*. SAMHSA Center for Mental Health Services, Editor. Rockville, MD.

19. Kinzie, J.D., *et al.* (1990). The prevalence of posttraumatic stress disorder and its clinical significance among Southeast Asian refugees. *The American Journal of Psychiatry*, **147**(7), 913–17.

20. Mollica, R.F., Wyshak, G., and Lavelle, J. (1987). The psychosocial impact of war trauma and torture on Southeast Asian refugees. *The American Journal of Psychiatry*, **144**(12), 1567–72.

21. HPRT. (1998). *Trauma and disability: long-term recovery of Bosnian refugees*. Harvard Program in Refugee Trauma, Cambridge, MA.

22. Mollica, R.F., *et al.* (1993). The effect of trauma and confinement on functional health and mental health status of Cambodians living in Thailand-Cambodia border camps. *The Journal of the American Medical Association*, **270**(5), 581–6.

23. Shrestha, N.M., *et al.* (1998). Impact of torture on refugees displaced within the developing world: symptomatology among Bhutanese refugees in Nepal. *The Journal of the American Medical Association*, **280**(5), 443–8.

24. Mollica, R., Sarajlic, N., Chernoff, M., *et al.* (2001). Longitudinal study of psychiatric symptoms, disability, mortality, and emigration among Bosnian refugees. *The Journal of the American Medical Association*, **286**(5), 546–4.

25. Marshall, G., Schell, T.L., Elliott, M.N., *et al.* (2005). Mental health of Cambodian refugees 2 decades after resettlement in the United States. *The Journal of the American Medical Association*, **294**(5), 571–9.

26. Lin, E., Ihle, L.J., and Tazuma, L. (1985). Depression among Vietnamese refugees in a primary care clinic. *The American Journal of Medicine*, **78**(1), 41–4.

27. Mollica, R., Caridad, K., and Massagli, M. (in press). Longitudinal study of posttraumatic stress disorder, depression, and changes in traumatic memories over time in Bosnian refugees. *The Journal of Nervous and Mental Disease*.

28. Brune, M., *et al.* (2003). Treatment of drug addiction in traumatised refugees. A case report. *European Addiction Research*, **9**(3), 144–6.

29. Westermeyer, J., Lyfoung, T., and Neider, J. (1989). An epidemic of opium dependence among Asian refugees in Minnesota: characteristics and causes. *British Journal of Addiction*, **84**(7), 785–9.

30. Westermeyer, J. (1995). Cultural aspects of substance abuse and alcoholism. Assessment and management. *The Psychiatric Clinics North America*, **18**(3), 589–605.

31. D'Amico, E., Schnell, T.L., Marshall, G.N., *et al.* (2007). Problem drinking among Cambodian refugees in the United States: how big of a problem is it? *Journal of Studies on Alcohol*, **68**(1), 11–17.

32. Goldfeld, A.E., *et al.* (1988). The physical and psychological sequelae of torture. Symptomatology and diagnosis. *The Journal of the American Medical Association*, **259**(18), 2725–9.

33. Westermeyer, J. (1981). Lao folk diagnosis for mental disorders: comparison with psychiatric diagnosis and assessment with psychiatric rating scales. *Medical Anthropology*, **5**, 425–43.

34. Bolton, P. (2001). Local perceptions of the mental health effects of the Rwandan genocide. *The Journal of Nervous and Mental Disease*, **189**(4), 243–8.

35. Simons, R.C. and Hughes, C.C. (1985). *The Culture-bound syndromes: folk illnesses of psychiatric and anthropological interest*. Culture, illness, and healing, Vol. 15, p. 516. D. Reidel; Sold and distributed in the U.S.A. and Canada by Kluwer Academic Publishers, Boston, Hingham, MA.

36. Jablensky, A., *et al.* (1981). Characteristics of depressive patients contacting psychiatric services in four cultures. A report from the WHO collaborative study on the assessment of depressive disorders. *Acta Psychiatrica Scandinavica*, **63**(4), 367–83.

37. Ingstad, B. and Whyte, S.R. (1995). *Disability and culture*, Vol. 10, p. 307. University of California Press, Berkeley.

38. Ormel, J., *et al.* (1994). Common mental disorders and disability across cultures. Results from the WHO collaborative study on psychological problems in general health care. *The Journal of the American Medical Association*, **272**(22), 1741–8.

39. Mollica, R., Caspi-Yavin, Y., and Lavelle, J. (1996). The Harvard Trauma Questionnaire (HTQ) manual: Cambodian, Laotian, and Vietnamese versions. *Torture—Quarterly Journal on Rehabilitation of Torture Victims and Prevention of Torture*, (Suppl. 1), 19–42.

40. Mollica, R.F., *et al.* (1992). The Harvard Trauma Questionnaire. Validating a cross-cultural instrument for measuring torture, trauma, and posttraumatic stress disorder in Indochinese refugees. *The Journal of Nervous and Mental Disease*, **180**(2), 111–6.

41. Willis, G.B. and Gonzalez, A. (1998). Methodological issues in the use of survey questionnaires to assess the health effects of torture. *The Journal of Nervous and Mental Disease*, **186**(5), 283–9.

42. Mollica, R.F., McDonald, L.S., Massagli, M.P., and Silove, D.M. (eds.) (2004). *Measuring trauma, measuring torture*. Harvard Program in Refugee Trauma, Cambridge, MA.

43. Mollica, R.F. and Lavelle, J. (1988). Southeast Asian refugees. In *Clinical guidelines in cross-cultural mental health* (eds. L. Comas-Diaz and E. Griffith), pp. 262–304. Wiley, New York.

44. Mollica, R.F. (2006). *Healing invisible wounds: paths to hope and recovery in a violent world*. Harcourt Press, New York.

45. Mollica, R.F., *et al.* (2004). Mental health in complex emergencies. *Lancet*, **364**(9450), 2058–67.

46. Hinton, D.E., *et al.* (2005). A randomized controlled trial of cognitive-behavior therapy for Cambodian refugees with treatment-resistant PTSD and panic attacks: a cross-over design. *Journal of Traumatic Stress*, **18**(6), 617–29.

47. Hinton, D.E., *et al.* (2004). CBT for Vietnamese refugees with treatment-resistant PTSD and panic attacks: a pilot study. *Journal of Traumatic Stress*, **17**(5), 429–33.

48. Basoglu, M., *et al.* (2004). Cognitive-behavioral treatment of tortured asylum seekers: a case study. *Journal of Anxiety Disorders*, **18**(3), 357–69.

49. Bolton, P., *et al.* (2003). Group interpersonal psychotherapy for depression in rural Uganda: a randomized controlled trial. *The Journal of the American Medical Association*, **289**(23), 3117–24.

50. Schnurr, P.P., *et al.* (2007). Cognitive behavioral therapy for posttraumatic stress disorder in women: a randomized controlled trial. *The Journal of the American Medical Association*, **297**(8), 820–30.

51. Lavelle, J., Tor, S., Mollica, R.F., *et al.* (eds.) (1996). *Harvard guide to Khmer mental health*. Harvard Program in Refugee Trauma, Cambridge.

52. Mollica, R.F., Tor, S. and Lavelle, J. (1998). *Pathway to healing*. Harvard Program in Refugee Trauma, Cambridge.

53. Heigel, J. (1994). Use of indigenous concepts and healers in the care of refugees: some experiences from the Thai border camps. In *Amidst peril and pain: the mental health and well-being of the world's refugees* (ed. A. Marcella). American Psychological Association, Washington, DC.

54. Mollica, R.F., *et al.* (2002). Science-based policy for psychosocial interventions in refugee camps: a Cambodian example. *The Journal of Nervous and Mental Disease*, **190**(3), 158–66.

55. Silove, D., Ekblad, S., and Mollica, R. (2000). The rights of the severely mentally ill in post-conflict societies. *Lancet*, **355**(9214), 1548–9.

56. UNICEF. (1990). *Children and development in the 1990s: a UNICEF source book on the occasion of the World Summit for Children*. UNICEF, New York.

57. Basoglu, M. (1992). *Torture and its consequences: current treatment approaches*, Vol. 13, p. 527. Cambridge University Press, Cambridge, New York.

## 7.10.2 Mental health services for homeless mentally ill people

Tom K. J. Craig

### Definition and demography of homelessness and its link to mental illness

The term 'homeless' has been used to describe populations as diverse as those sleeping in the shelter of a cardboard box, to those sleeping on a friend's floor. Given such wide definition, it is not surprising that estimates of the numbers involved vary greatly from survey to survey and from one country to another. But regardless of the definition, there is consensus that the numbers of homeless people in most Western urban areas increased during the past two decades, reflecting a scarcity of low-cost housing, the erosion of traditional family networks, and downsizing in the organization and delivery of supportive services. Of all these factors, the shortage of affordable accommodation is the most important. For example, in England there has been a 40 per cent increase since 2002 in the number of households on waiting lists for social housing with estimates that a minimum of 20 000 housing units above current government targets are required to simply meet newly arising urgent need.[1]

Compared with a domiciled population, homeless people are less likely to have completed basic education, less likely to have ever held employment, and more likely to have experienced parental neglect and abuse in their childhood.[2]

Given the evidence linking homelessness to poverty and social disadvantage, it is hardly surprising that homeless people report higher rates of psychiatric disorder relative to the general population. While rates vary depending on the particular measure of mental illness adopted by each study and by the homeless population being investigated, most report major psychiatric disorder in 30 to 60 per cent of those using emergency shelters and sleeping rough. The prevalence of schizophrenia and other psychoses is particularly high amongst the middle-aged residents of long-stay hostels, while depression, generalized anxiety, and impulsive self-harm are more typically encountered in younger runaways and adolescent populations. Alcoholism and drug dependency are present in as many as two-thirds of men and a third of homeless women. Co-morbidity of mental illness and substance use disorder is the rule rather than the exception as are the co-occurrence of respiratory disease, infections, trauma, and the physical consequences of poor diet, poor hygiene, and the complications of substance abuse. Of growing concern is the accumulation of older multiply disabled populations in some North American cities.[3]

The typical pattern of service utilization of the severely mentally ill among the homeless population is one of extremes—bursts of involuntary hospital admissions and compulsory treatment interspersed with long periods of neglect and isolation. Many of those who are found sleeping rough or resident in temporary shelters have found their way to these locations as a conscious effort to avoid contact with health and social care professionals and remain unwilling to be part of any structured rehabilitation programme.

### Barriers to care

#### Poverty and isolation

Very few homeless mentally ill people have satisfactory links to family or other supportive social groups. Unemployment is the norm and many have histories of contact with the criminal justice system. The lack of supportive kinship networks mean that there is seldom anyone who has an interest in their welfare and no one on whom services can rely for informal care giving. Affordable housing is likely to be of poor quality and unsupervised. Landlords are reluctant to rent property to someone with a history of destructive behaviour, a criminal record, or manifest mental illness.

#### Barriers arising from the illness

Severe mental illness contributes to incompetence in many aspects of daily life, with impaired social function and problems initiating and executing daily living tasks that require a degree of forward planning. Co-morbid cognitive impairment or substance abuse compound these problems. Many homeless patients will have lost their accommodation as a direct result of their illness, being evicted for failing to keep up with rent payments, neglecting or damaging the property, or following complaints from neighbours.

### Barriers put up by services

The lack of common purpose and co-ordination of social welfare, health, and criminal justice agencies lies at the heart of many difficulties faced by homeless mentally ill people. A young homeless person, for example, may be too chaotic to undertake the retraining programme that is his only route to welfare support, may be unable to register with a local family health centre because of his lack of a permanent address, and may be summarily rehoused without reference to health services involved in his care. Finally, the prejudices of professionals can make services unacceptable and the emphasis on treatment is seldom attractive to a homeless person whose immediate needs are for food, shelter, and security.

## Principles of service organization and delivery

To state the obvious, the solution to problems of homelessness lies in the provision of suitable accommodation, targeted efforts to re-house the most vulnerable, and sufficient longer-term tenancy support to prevent a return to the streets. While many countries have social welfare legislation to assist homeless people, only a minority provide a legally enforceable right to suitable accommodation for vulnerable populations. The Rough Sleepers Initiative in England, provides emergency accommodation for the roofless population and follows this emergency re-housing with a Tenancy Sustainment Programme of flexible practical and emotional support to prevent future accommodation breakdown.[4] This has been very successful in reducing the numbers of rough sleepers though gaps remain, particularly for people suffering from severe mental illness and substance dependency. For these populations, a further tier of service involving specialized mental health provision is needed either as part of an intensive initial stabilization[5] or in the longer-term. While the detail of specialized services varies according to local circumstances, they are all based on a small number of ideological and organizational principles (Table 7.10.2.1).

### Improved inter-agency co-operation

As a first step, most involve a steering group comprising senior representatives of the key stakeholders in health, housing, social

**Table 7.10.2.1** Services for homeless mentally ill people

| Essential components for rehousing |
| --- |
|    Availability of temporary accommodation with a pathway to permanent housing |
|    Capacity to deliver basic needs (shelter, food, income support) |
|    Ongoing practical support to maintain tenancy |
| Specialized mental health service |
|    Steered by a partnership of key stakeholders (housing, health, welfare, etc.) |
|    Multidisciplinary front-line team |
|    Assertive outreach model |
|    Capable of managing mental illness and substance-use disorder |
| Wider context |
|    Community-orientated mainstream psychiatric services |
|    Influence of central and local government policies on health, welfare, and criminal justice |

services, police, and voluntary sectors. These groups oversee the development of services across a wide geographical area—a large sector of a city or state. The members carry sufficient political and managerial authority to be effective in dealing with bureaucratic obstacles that are bound to arise from time to time.

### Providing local multidisciplinary specialist teams

This co-ordination is replicated at the local level through multidisciplinary clinical teams, joint working, and case management. Such partnership ventures have been established in several cities in North America, Europe, and Australia using a variety of organizational approaches ranging from a single multidisciplinary team through 'one-stop shops' where professionals from a variety of backgrounds come together to provide services at a common location.

### Essential components of the specialist service

The management of a homeless mentally ill person involves stages of engagement, stabilization, resettlement, and the eventual transfer of care to mainstream providers. Engagement can take a long time, staff must be prepared to leave the clinic and go to where homeless people congregate. Help with welfare and practical problems may be all that can be done at first but the duty to maintain a therapeutic focus must always be maintained. Stabilization requires the specialist assessment and treatments provided to any mentally ill person, including hospital admission if necessary. The task of resettlement typically involves a compromise between personal preferences, available resources, and the level of support needed to promote rehabilitation. For example, independent accommodation may be a person's first choice but may only be a viable prospect if it can be backed up by weekly visits from the mental health team. Core and cluster arrangements, in which residents have their own flat but receive supervision from an on-site warden within the complex is a particularly effective model for those who have failed in independent accommodation but who reject shared facilities.

The eventual transfer of care to mainstream services can be quite difficult to manage and most follow-up studies suggest that fewer than half of those transferred remain in treatment.

## Conclusion

Specialist multidisciplinary teams for homeless mentally ill people provide an essential safety net for those who have fallen out of the wider mental health care system. They offer distinct advantages in terms of their capacity to work across traditional geographical and bureaucratic barriers, to take the longer-term view of the task of engagement, and to bring together the multiple strands of care across different provider agencies. Introduced as a temporary measure over a decade ago, they are still with us and likely to remain a permanent fixture of urban mental health care.

## Further information

Access to mental health services for people who are homeless or living in temporary or insecure accommodation. A good practice guide: http://www.communities.gov.uk/index.asp?id=1162512

Essential statistics on homelessness in Britain: http:// www.homeless. uk/policyandinfo/facts/statistics

## References

1. National Housing Federation. (2006). *England's housing time-bomb: affordability and supply 2006–11*. National Housing Federation, London. Website: http://www.housing.org.uk/uploads/file/campaigns/tb_england.pdf

2. Bhugra, D. (ed.) (1996). *Homelessness and mental health*. Cambridge University Press, Cambridge.

3. Hahn, J.A., Kushel, M.B., Bangsberg, D.R., *et al.* (2006). The aging of the homeless population: fourteen-year trends in San Francisco. *Journal of General Internal Medicine*, **21**, 775–8.

4. Lomax, D. and Netto, G. (2007). Evaluation of tenancy sustainment teams. Department of communities and local government. http://www.odpm.gov.uk/index.asp?d=1505917

5. Susser, E., Valencia, E., Conover, S., *et al.* (1997). Preventing recurrent homelessness among mentally ill men: a 'critical time' intervention after discharge from a shelter. *American Journal of Public Health*, **87**, 256–62.

# 7.10.3 Mental health services for ethnic minorities

Tom K. J. Craig and Dinesh Bhugra

## Ethnicity, culture, and health care need

Services aimed at minority ethnic populations are all too often developed on the basis of conspicuous morbidity than on any real understanding of the diversity of ethnic minority communities and their wider health needs. For example, in England, while much has been written about ethnicity and psychiatric morbidity, the literature remains largely focused on African-Caribbeans and Asians, while the needs of the Irish, who comprise the largest ethnic community by migration in many parts of the UK are seldom explicitly addressed despite evidence of high rates of suicide and unexplained death many times in excess of the indigenous population.[1] In addition, the large numbers of asylum seekers and refugees who move around the world, brings an increased need for culturally sensitive services. But very few models exist for developing these. The principles of good practice indicate that the start has to be a clear knowledge of the population that will be accessing services and an appreciation of the complicating factors of social disadvantage, material deprivation, and poverty.

There is no doubt that social disadvantage and racial prejudice whether real or perceived are pivotal in determining not only the mental health of minority populations but also the pathways individuals and their families use in seeking help for ill health. Delays in help-seeking can also be due to the stigma of mental illness and to sufferers' fears that they will be misunderstood and mistreated because of differences in culture, language, and racist attitudes within the services. These factors may be more apparent in older individuals and those who were born outside the country who may not be aware of various options available to them. Studies over the past 30 years or more in Britain, the Netherlands, the United States, Canada, and Australia have shown that minority groups have lower access to mental health services, are less likely to receive care, and when they do this is more likely to be of a lower quality. Black people in the UK and the United States are more likely than white people to be compulsorily detained in hospital, to be screened for drug abuse, to receive higher doses of medication and physical rather than psychological therapies. They are over-represented compared with their numbers in the general population, whether in general wards, locked wards, secure units, court diversion schemes, special hospitals, or prisons.[2]

Some of these problems can be attributed to a lack of understanding on the part of mental health practitioners of the cultural beliefs, values, and practices of minority groups with consequent shortcomings in assessment, diagnosis, and the provision of care. While language can be a major obstacle, for many people from minority ethnic groups who speak English the problem is of communication rather than language. The power dynamic that is always present in any clinical consultation is magnified and both patient and doctor will have predetermined expectations of how their interaction will turn out depending upon their experience of previous consultations. Problems in the interaction are likely to be interpreted as arrogance and racism on the one hand and indifference, wariness, or docility on the other. Thus, both missed diagnoses and misdiagnosis may result. A lack of recognition of the personal, social, and cultural problems which influence the presenting patterns of symptoms in different ethnic groups can contribute to the tendency of clinicians to make assumptions and listen out for stereotypical triggers which then prompt a particular therapeutic response. Such triggers include religious euphoria, use of Cannabis in African-Caribbeans, and the 'fatalistic attitude' attributed to Asian patients.

## Culturally competent services

The past decade has seen an emerging consensus that the way forward lies in the development of fully integrated multicultural services with good working links with the local minority community rather than separate services. Such services would provide staff who can understand their client's cultural background and the ways in which this influences the presentation of distress and disorder. There would be closer working links with religious leaders and healers of local ethnic minority communities, female-only areas on wards, and a greater involvement and support of the family in understanding the problems and developing solutions.

In North America,[3,4] Britain,[5] and Australia[6] there has been a significant 'top–down' pressure to shift health care organizations in this direction and several large-scale programmes such as the European 9-country 'Migrant-Friendly Hospitals' initiative[7] have been reported. Although differing in detail, all these programmes share common elements. These principles are outlined in Table 7.10.3.1 setting out the main conclusions in a 'bottom–up' approach in order to emphasize the importance of changes in the attitudes, knowledge, and skills of front-line managerial and clinical staff.

Commonly referred to as 'cultural competence' these attributes include attention to obvious language differences but go further to include history, traditions, beliefs, and values even if the latter differ from those held by the professional. A culturally competent clinician is sensitive to a patient's cultural influences, expressions of distress and help-seeking, and is also aware of their own attitudes and prejudices and how these are in turn shaped by their own cultural background. This objective is achieved through

**Table 7.10.3.1** Organizational steps towards a culturally competent mental health service

---

**1 Workforce level**

Training in 'cultural competence' should be mandatory for all mental health professionals

    (a) Undergraduate programmes

    (b) Post-graduate as continuing professional development

---

**2 Health care provider level**

Provide accommodation, washing, and living space facilities that take into account different cultural and gender definitions of ordinary social behaviour, dignity, and respect.

Senior management responsibility and accountability for:

    (a) Active race equality policies

    (b) Recruitment policy—to increase presence of minority staff and provision of training and support as needed

    (c) Ensure staff have received relevant cultural competency training

Ensure adequate data collection includes a robust estimate of the numbers of ethnic minorities using services with a focus on key areas such as disparities by ethnicity in the use of coercive treatments, dropout from follow-up; differences in the uptake of psychological and pharmacological treatments.

Specialized outreach services targeting mentally ill people in the criminal justice system, homeless, and refugee populations.

Partnership arrangements with NGOs including the provision of volunteer advisors and of translation services that do not rely on relatives or other informal carers.

---

**3 Wider health service level**

At the appropriate Regional or National HMO or Statutory Organization:

    (a) Policy and practice commitment to removing barriers to access, e.g. extend health insurance to the uninsured and closer integration of primary and secondary mental health care

    (b) Collection of good quality demographic information and ethnic monitoring for planning and overseeing services

    (c) Minority representation at all levels of health service planning and delivery

Continue to expand the science base to determine what works best for whom

---

training and a plethora of different cultural competency/diversity courses have sprung up in recent years. A search of the Internet identifies courses in undergraduate nursing, medical, and pharmacy programmes, in post-graduate continuing professional development and as part of wider organizational change and development. While the moral argument for improved cultural competence is hardly contestable, whether or not these training courses are sufficient to effect lasting change in behaviour and the delivery of health care is less certain. The very limited empirical evidence base is predominantly from the United States and shows efficacy in terms of short-term changes in attitudes and knowledge. Evidence is still lacking on which elements of this training are essential and on the downstream effects on service quality that is the real target.

Table 7.10.3.1 also shows the other key steps that have been taken towards developing more culturally sensitive services. Most health service providers have gone some way to providing female-only inpatient wards, more community-orientated service settings and addressing the need for expanding the numbers of people from minority backgrounds in their workforce though it is still all too easy to think that problems with cultural sensitivity can be solved with this alone. Simply hiring people on the basis of nationality, ethnicity, or skin colour will not necessarily ameliorate problems in the service. Typically these staff are the lowest in the hierarchy of power and have the least capacity for influencing either the care of the patient or wider attitudes within the institution. Even when employed in a position of power there is a danger of their appointment being seen as tokenistic.

Another important step involves the elaboration of performance indicators to assess the impact of training and service changes and ethnic monitoring with a focus on key areas such as the use of coercive treatments, treatment discontinuation, and ethnic differences in the uptake of psychological and pharmacological treatments. In the most sophisticated systems this includes both quantitative epidemiological and economic data as well as qualitative inputs from consultation with users, carers, and the general public including community and religious leaders.[8]

Finally, at the wider community level, NGOs have often become the champion of good practice, seen by their users as an antidote to inadequate mainstream care. These small organizations are generally based on consultation with users, carers, and local mental health professionals and are more in tune with the expressed needs of the community. The best have good working relations with mainstream services, and are generally seen as making an important contribution to wider community care. They provide a range of supportive services and are ideal vehicles for health promotion and dissemination of health-related information. Given the need to develop ways of working which promote inclusion of patients, their families, and the community in general, it is impossible to overstate the importance of effective liaison between the voluntary sector and mainstream psychiatric services. People often come into contact with the emergency services because there is a lack of knowledge of the availability of community alternatives and of where to go when distressed. Working with voluntary services will not only contribute to their longevity but also ensure that the complementary treatment modalities they offer are part of the service provided.

Even where these system-wide initiatives are absent or not yet fully implemented, individual clinicians can do a lot to improve the care of minorities within their own service. Finding out the scale of the problem is a good place to start. Are population estimates available from a recent census, is information available from a recent census or from local government sources? More importantly, are there known problems of access for these populations in general or particularly within local mental health services? Are significant numbers not treated because they are held in 'inappropriate' settings in the criminal justice system or because they are mobile populations? In terms of delivering the service, outreach is likely to be the key and this will almost always involve partnership arrangements, developing understanding of key cultural influences including the importance of alternative health perspectives, spirituality and traditional healing. Several innovative services have been developed alongside organizations that 'hold' significant numbers of the minority population such as the Church or the local Mosque or NGOs dealing with specific communities, which can provide a wider social or housing service to minority populations. It is the near universal experience of these services that initial progress is slow with many barriers of mutual misunderstanding and suspicion to overcome. Developing a relationship or even employing someone from the minority culture as a go-between, advisor, or 'cultural consultant' can be helpful though it needs careful preparation to avoid selecting a consultant from the wrong tribal background or at the wrong level of seniority, gender, or language group. Culture broker models have been used in the United States, whereas cultural consultation services happen in parts of the UK and cultural liaison officers are used in parts of Australia. Whatever the choice, it is likely to take time and patience to develop a high level of 'visibility' in the target community as well as a sound understanding of its culture, taboos, and historical context. Where available, cultural supervision from a more experienced practitioner is also helpful. The underlying principle has to be a two-way process, which deals with information from the patient's community and the service provider to ensure that communications are clear.

A few further points can usefully be taken into account in planning the service. First an understanding of local models of illness that determine when and how and of whom help will be sought, second use of local epidemiological data to assess the impact of age and gender on service demand and finally the involvement of the local community to promote a sense of ownership and involvement in the delivery of services.

In conclusion, the diagnosis and treatment of mental ill health among multiethnic populations is probably one of the most complex and contentious challenges in psychiatric service provision. At the heart of this complexity are problems of ignorance, attitude, and failures of communication on all sides. It is also potentially one of the most rewarding endeavours if got right. No one service model is likely to apply to every community, even if people belong to the same ethnic group. The development of specialist psychiatric services may not always be possible or even essential. Instead, the requirements are for approaches that are flexible, sensitive, accessible, and accountable to the people they serve.

## Further information

American Psychological Association guidelines for providers of services to ethnic linguistic and culturally diverse populations: http://www.apa.org/pi/guide.html

Sainsbury Centre for Mental Health. (2002). Breaking the circles of fear http://www.scmh.org.uk

## References

1. Bhugra, D. (2004). *Culture and self-harm*. Psychology Press, Hove.
2. Lipsedge, M. (1993). Mental health: access to care for black and ethnic minority people. In *Access to health care for people from black and ethnic minorities* (eds. A. Hopkins and V. Bahl), pp. 169–83. Royal College of Physicians, London.
3. Office of Minority Health (USA). Assuring cultural competence in health care: recommendations for national standards and an outcome-focused research agenda. www.omhrc.gov/Assets/pdf/checked/Assuring_Cultural_Competence_in_Health_Care-1999.pdf
4. Mental Health: Culture Race and Ethnicity. A supplement to Mental Health: A Report of the Surgeon General. www.surgeongeneral.gov/library/mentalhealth/cre/
5. Department of Health. (2005). *Delivering race equality in mental health care: an action plan for reform inside and outside services and the government's response to the independent inquiry into the death of David Bennett*. HMSO, London. http://www.dh.gov.uk/en/Publicationsandstatistics/Publications/PublicationsPolicyAndGuidance/DH_4100773
6. Royal Australasian College of Physicians. (2005). Policy statement: aboriginal and Torres Strait Islander Health. Available at: http://www.racp.edu.au/index.cfm?objectId=49F4E2A9-2A57-5487-D0597D1ED8218B61
7. Migrant-Friendly Hospitals Initiative. (2004). Available at: http://www.mfh-eu.net/public/home.htm
8. Jordan, J., Dowswell, T., Harrison, S., *et al.* (1998). Health needs assessment. Whose priorities? Listening to users and the public. *British Medical Journal*, **316**, 1668–70.

# SECTION 8

# The Psychiatry of Old Age

**8.1 The biology of ageing** *1507*
Alan H. Bittles

**8.2 Sociology of normal ageing** *1512*
Sarah Harper

**8.3 The ageing population and the epidemiology of mental disorders among the elderly** *1517*
Scott Henderson and Laura Fratiglioni

**8.4 Assessment of mental disorder in older patients** *1524*
Robin Jacoby

**8.5 Special features of clinical syndromes in the elderly** *1530*

  8.5.1 Delirium in the elderly *1530*
    James Lindesay

    8.5.1.1 Mild cognitive impairment *1534*
      Claudia Jacova and Howard H. Feldman

  8.5.2 Substance use disorders in older people *1540*
    Henry O'Connell and Brian Lawlor

  8.5.3 Schizophrenia and paranoid disorders in late life *1546*
    Barton W. Palmer, Gauri N. Savla, and Thomas W. Meeks

  8.5.4 Mood disorders in the elderly *1550*
    Robert Baldwin

  8.5.5 Stress-related, anxiety, and obsessional disorders in elderly people *1558*
    James Lindesay

  8.5.6 Personality disorders in the elderly *1561*
    Suzanne Holroyd

  8.5.7 Suicide and deliberate self-harm in elderly people *1564*
    Robin Jacoby

  8.5.8 Sex in old age *1567*
    John Kellett and Catherine Oppenheimer

**8.6 Special features of psychiatric treatment for the elderly** *1571*
Catherine Oppenheimer

**8.7 The planning and organization of services for older adults** *1579*
Pamela S. Melding

# 8.1

# The biology of ageing

## Alan H. Bittles

## Introduction

Although old age is readily recognizable, methods to define and measure the underlying biological processes are much less amenable to study. For this reason, **life expectancy** has been widely used as a surrogate measure of ageing, as well as to monitor economic progress at national and regional levels. It is generally acknowledged that lifespan is a constitutional feature of the human phenotype, and twin studies have indicated that 25–33 per cent of the variance in human **longevity** is genetic in origin.[1,2] External factors including lifestyle can also exert a major influence, as illustrated by the current mean life expectancies of 79 and 86 years for males and females in Japan, whereas the comparable figures for Botswana are 35 and 33 years, respectively.

The importance of genetic inheritance as a determinant of extended survival has been illustrated by population level studies in Okinawa, an island prefecture of southern Japan with a very high prevalence of long-lived individuals. On the island, the mortality rates of the male and female siblings of centenarians were approximately half those of birth cohort-matched, non-centenarian siblings.[3] These findings parallel an earlier study of the family of Jeanne Calment, who died in France in 1997 aged 122 years. Of her 55 relatives, 24 per cent had lived to >80 years compared to just 2 per cent of a matched control group.[4] However, it remains unclear whether the enhanced lifespan of individuals who exhibit above average longevity is due to a slowing of the overall ageing process or is primarily associated with resistance to major life-threatening pathologies.

The concept of an 'allostatic load', potentially involving the neuroendocrine, sympathetic nervous, immune and cardiovascular systems, and metabolic pathways, has been advanced to describe the lifetime costs of adapting to physical and psychological stresses. According to this hypothesis, while the actions of biological mediators of **stress** can be initially beneficial to health, chronic stimulation results in regulatory imbalance and subsequent pathophysiological changes.[5] Empirical studies have indicated increased physiological dysregulation and functional decline at >70 years of age, which would imply that predicted global increases in the numbers of older persons will be accompanied by disproportionately larger groups of individuals with major age-related pathologies.

## Theories of ageing

While initially popular, it became apparent that single, 'magic bullet' causes of ageing were inappropriate to complex biological species, and with this recognition earlier organ- and system-based theories have gradually been discounted. Conversely, the observation that ageing appears to be initiated at different ages and can proceed at different rates in individual members of a species provides presumptive evidence for the interaction of multiple genetic and non-genetic influences. Two main groups of theories have been formulated, genomic and stochastic, each subdivided into a number of discrete topic headings.

### Genomic theories of ageing

**Genomic theories** premise that ageing is primarily associated with changes in the genetic constitution of the organism. Support for genomic theories stems largely from the characteristic life expectancies of mammalian and non-mammalian species, and theories proposing a primarily genetic basis for ageing were greatly strengthened by the demonstration that human diploid cells exhibited a highly reproducible lifespan when cultured in the laboratory. Although strong evolutionary advantages can be envisaged for genetic control of developmental changes up to and including reproductive adulthood, the existence of genes uniquely encoding ageing seems improbable since few free-living animals or humans have ever succeeded in attaining the maximum lifespan of their species.

### (a) Information transfer

The ability to synthesize functional proteins is dependent on the fidelity of genetic information encoded in the DNA, its unimpaired transcription from DNA to RNA, and translation into peptides and proteins. As each of these processes is subject to inaccuracy, and during the life course of an organism the sequence of information transfer steps is continuously operational, the error potential is large. With increasing chronological age the probability of errors increases, resulting in the accumulation of deleterious mutations late in life.[6] Since a number of the proteins synthesized may be involved as surveillance enzymes to maintain the accuracy of the entire system, feedback mechanisms could lead to its collapse, resulting in a phenomenon initially termed **error catastrophe**.

### (b) Somatic mutation

With the demonstration of an inverse correlation between the lifespan of mammalian species and the incidence of chromosome abnormalities, age-related physiological changes were originally ascribed to accumulated mutations in the nuclear DNA (**nDNA**) of somatic cells. Findings of this nature could, however, be explicable in terms of the ability of an organism to tolerate DNA damage via the repair of damaged molecules, with more than 130 human **DNA repair genes** identified.[7] The capacity of nDNA to resist attack by endogenous reactive species and environmental agents is therefore considerable, which casts doubt on the general applicability of the theory.

### (c) Epigenetic mechanisms

Epigenetic errors, i.e. errors in the control of gene expression rather than mutations in DNA or protein, have been proposed as major primary causal factors in senescence.[8] In promoter regions of genes, hypermethylation silences a gene whereas the hypomethylation of previously methylated sequences permits their expression. The pattern of **DNA methylation** is established during development and is cell type-specific, and changes in methylation can occur both during ageing and in cancer cells. The advantage of epigenetic models of ageing is their lack of requirement for the evolutionary preservation of genes encoding ageing, which in former generations would seldom have been expressed.

### (d) Mitochondrial decline

Mitochondria are subcellular organelles responsible for aerobic energy production in humans and many other species. The mitochondrial genome of ~16.5 kb is characterized by its extremely compact organization, with no protective histones, a lack of excision or recombinational repair mechanisms, and a virtual absence of introns, all of which make it highly susceptible to mutation. Mitochondrial DNA (**mtDNA**) plays a central role in mitochondrial propagation and the maintenance of cellular respiration, but a majority of proteins involved in the regulation of mtDNA transcription, translation and replication, and the mitochondrial respiratory chain, are encoded in the nuclear genome. This design requires the operation of a highly coordinated mechanism for the expression of the nuclear and mitochondrial genomes. The central role of mitochondria in energy production means that defects may be of major metabolic significance, and the demonstration of increased levels of mtDNA deletions and base-substitutions in aged human neurones, heart, and skeletal muscle suggest a causative role for mtDNA mutations in ageing.[9]

### (e) Telomere loss

Telomeres are specialized structures located at the terminus of the DNA helix and critical to the maintenance of DNA stability and replication. The enzyme telomerase which is responsible for telomere synthesis is active during early embryonic and foetal development but its activity is down-regulated in all human somatic cells before birth. As human diploid fibroblasts in culture were shown to progressively lose telomeres, it was hypothesized that telomere length could act as a predictor of the potential *in vitro* lifespan achievable by a cell strain.[10] Humans have a common telomere profile found on lymphocytes, amniocytes, and fibroblasts which appears to be preserved throughout life. However, the rate of telomere loss with ageing varies between chromosomes and there is evidence that, in addition to the common human telomere profile, each person exhibits an individual profile.[11]

Besides ageing, telomere loss has been implicated in a wide range of disease states, including heart disease, stroke, infection, long-term chronic stress, and obesity. Given the apparent relationship between telomere loss and both ageing and age-related pathologies, pharmacological activation of telomerase has been proposed as a potential treatment for chronic or degenerative diseases.[12] As tumour tissue and transformed cells constitutively produce telomerase, any therapeutic intervention of this nature would require careful monitoring.

## Stochastic theories of ageing

**Stochastic theories** of ageing propose that cumulative adverse random changes at the cellular level ultimately overwhelm the capacity of an organism to survive, with ageing representing the preceding period of functional decline.

### (a) Rate of living

An optimum lifespan was achieved by a variety of non-mammalian species when the organisms were maintained at suboptimal temperatures. The further demonstration of an inverse relationship between basal metabolic rate and longevity in mammals was interpreted as evidence that a species lifespan was governed by its **rate of living**, which in turn was correlated with its level of energy expenditure. Theories of this type tend to be imprecise in defining the nature of the factor(s) controlling ageing and lifespan, although it was subsequently proposed that the rate of living theory could be reformulated as a **stress** theory of ageing, with stress resistance and longevity positively correlated.

### (b) Waste product accumulation

Ageing has been ascribed to interference by accumulated waste products in normal cellular metabolism and function, ultimately resulting in dysfunction and death at cellular and organ levels. Lipofuscin, a highly insoluble, pigmented compound derived by auto-oxidation from incompletely degraded cellular materials and detected with advancing age in neurones, cardiac muscle fibres, and the adrenal cortex, has been particularly implicated. Alternatively, the build-up of lipofuscin in older organisms may be secondary to an age-related decline in the function of cellular catabolic processes.

### (c) Macromolecule cross-linkage

Many macromolecules of biological importance develop cross-links with increasing chronological age. The establishment of cross-linkage, whether covalent in nature or due to hydrogen bonding, alters the chemical and physical properties of molecules. Thus cross-linkage of the extracellular protein collagen is believed to be responsible for the loss of elasticity in mammalian blood vessels and skin with advancing age, even though collagen is subject to turnover throughout the lifespan. DNA and RNA also are believed to be potential intracellular targets for cross-linking agents, and changes in their structure could have serious functional implications for cellular information flow.

### (d) Post-synthetic modification

In addition to cross-linkage, molecular aggregation and immobilization that compromises cellular metabolism and function could be caused by post-synthetic modification of proteins, with non-enzymic glycosylation (glycation) particularly associated with ageing. Glycation is initiated by the reaction of glucose with the amino group of lysine residues, which then proceed to form a Schiff base, and progressively more complex compounds collectively termed advanced glycosylation end (AGE) products. As little variation was found in the glycation levels of lens crystallin proteins in subjects aged between 10 and 80 years, post-synthetic mechanisms may be as much an effect as a cause of ageing.

### (e) Free radical damage

The role of **free radicals** in ageing was first proposed over 50 years ago.[13] A wide range of highly reactive free radicals are derived from molecular oxygen, including the superoxide and hydroperoxyl radicals, hydrogen peroxide, hydroxyl radical, and singlet oxygen. The polyunsaturated fatty acid side chains of cell and organelle membranes form highly susceptible targets for the action of **reactive oxygen species (ROS)**, and the resulting lipid peroxidation can result in severe membrane damage and eventual death of the cell. DNA may also be a critical target molecule for free radical damage, with mtDNA especially susceptible because of its proximity to the site of free radical production in the inner mitochondrial membrane.[9] Although a wide variety of antioxidants have been identified in humans, including ascorbate, $\alpha$-tocopherol, $\beta$-carotene, glutathione, and the enzymes superoxide dismutase, peroxidase, and catalase, there has been little experimental evidence that these antioxidants can produce a significant extension in maximum lifespan. However, transgenic mice expressing the free radical scavenger enzyme catalase targeted to mitochondria showed an approximately 20 per cent extension in their mean and maximum lifespans, and concomitant delays in cardiac pathology and cataract development.[14]

## Ageing as an energy crisis

From an evolutionary perspective, it was suggested that senescence was the end-result of an energy conservation strategy operating in somatic cells. During the course of a lifespan, total available energy has to be allocated to a variety of functions, including macromolecular synthesis and degradation, cell and organ maintenance, and reproduction of the species. Since the energy supply is finite, and to ensure propagation of the species by the successful transmission of genes to future generations, a compromise has to be reached between the energy made available for each of these functions. According to the **disposable soma theory**, this accommodation in energy saving is achieved by maintenance of absolute or near absolute accuracy in germ cell replication but less rigorous error correction in somatic cells.[15]

As an organism ages, the demands placed on the free energy pool alter and increase from a primarily anabolic role to meeting the requirements of ever-increasing repair and catabolic functions, including those imposed by specific disease-related insults. If the mitochondrial inner membrane and/or mtDNA is damaged, an organism must increasingly rely on alternative, less efficient pathways for its energy needs, ultimately resulting in a critical shortfall in the energy supply needed to sustain life. In such an **energy crisis**, the somatic cells primarily affected would be post-mitotic cells with high energetic demands, typified by the heart, skeletal muscle, and the brain.

## Dietary modification of ageing

Inherited factors clearly play a major role in ageing, and in determining the human lifespan. But if ageing also is stochastic in nature then it should be possible to modify development of the ageing phenotype by altering the relative influence of contributory environmental variables, including diet.

Dietary (or calorie) restriction, based on a diet reduced in total amount but otherwise nutritionally adequate, is the only method so far proven to increase maximum lifespan in mammals. The original dietary restriction experiments conducted in the 1930s resulted in animals that remained prepubertal as a result of their retarded growth and development.[16,17] In more recent food restriction experiments, rodents have typically been fed a diet corresponding to approximately 60 per cent of the food ingested by *ad libitum* fed controls, commencing either soon after weaning or in young adulthood. Under these circumstances, besides a increase in maximum lifespan the development of tumours and other chronic diseases of late adulthood was slowed.

**DNA microarray** studies into the effects of **calorie restriction (CR)** in mice have indicated a shift in transcriptional patterns towards increased protein turnover and decreased macromolecular damage. Rats maintained on a restricted diet (representing 60 per cent of the control diet) for 36 weeks showed increased transcription of muscle genes involved in ROS scavenging, tissue development, and energy metabolism, with decreased expression of genes involved in signal transduction, stress response, and structural and contractile proteins.[18] CR also was able to maintain ATP production but at the same time reduce age-dependent endogenous oxidative damage.[19]

Preliminary studies conducted on rhesus macaque monkeys aged approximately 20 years and maintained on a reduced caloric intake for 9–10 years have suggested that long-term CR produced beneficial alterations in glycogen metabolism and mitigated the development of insulin resistance in older animals. Although restricted numbers of primates have been studied and few have attained extreme old ages, a wide range of potentially beneficial outcomes have been reported, in particular an improvement in glucose tolerance, a lower core body temperature, an attenuated decline in dehydroepiandrosterone (DHEA) sulphate levels, decreased triglycerides and increased HDL2b, in combination with lower weight, lean body mass and fat, and lower energy expenditure (reviewed in Bittles 2008).

A number of small-scale human studies have been reported, including a 6-day investigation on eight adults and eight pubertal children involving a 50 per cent caloric reduction that resulted in a significant reduction in the nitrogen balance of both adults and children and a decrease in their insulin-like growth factor-1 (IGF-1) levels. Individuals who had voluntarily adopted a restricted food intake for 6 years displayed a wide variety of physiological, metabolic, and biochemical changes, all of which would be consistent with protection against atherosclerosis,[20] and CR alone or with accompanying exercise regimes significantly increased the numbers of mitochondria in skeletal muscle cells while decreasing both energy expenditure and the frequency of mtDNA damage in overweight healthy adults.[21]

## Ageing and the concept of healthy life expectancy

Active Life Expectancy (ALE) is defined as the period of life free of disabilities which interfere with basic Activities of Daily Living (ADL), e.g. eating, getting in and out of bed, bathing and toiletry needs, dressing, and indoor mobility. The concept of healthy life expectancy has been extended by weighting specific physical and cognitive dysfunctions to measure Disability-Adjusted Life Years (DALY) and Quality-Adjusted Life Years (QALY). **Disability Adjusted Life Expectancy (DALE)** is now widely used in epidemiological studies to estimate the number of years that might be expected to be spent in 'full health'. A common finding in developed countries was that although females enjoyed higher DALE scores they also could expect more years of disability at advanced ages. Although measures such as DALE, DALY, and QALY have been criticized on methodological grounds, given global increases in the numbers of elderly individuals, the concept of healthy life expectancy may be increasingly useful in identifying the health and support needs of the aged.

## Discussion

As in other areas of medical science, the Human Genome Project has impacted strongly on research into biological aspects of ageing, and DNA analysis now offers major insights into the development of the ageing phenotype. During the last decade, DNA microarray studies have been adopted to investigate changes in gene expression that accompany ageing.

Initial studies on rodent tissue showed differential gene expression patterns with advancing age, indicative of a marked stress response and lower expression of metabolic and biosynthetic genes. An 'ageing transcriptome' conserved across mammalian species has been identified, comprising deregulation of mitosis, cell adhesion, transport, signal transduction, mitochondrial function, and inflammatory response, and accompanied by a reduction in processes dependent on energy metabolism and mitochondrial function.[22] Subsequent analysis of human tissue based on large-scale DNA microarrays has revealed diverse patterns of both increased and decreased gene expression. However, a study of ~32 000 muscle tissue genes obtained from volunteers aged 16 to 89 years confirmed the existence of a common ageing signature, with altered levels of expression in 250 age-regulated genes and three genetic pathways that correlated both with chronological and physiological age.[23]

Research on adult stem cells may provide key future insights into ageing. Adult stem cells mainly undergo chronological ageing, as in skeletal muscle, or exhibit a combination of chronological and replicative ageing, typified by haematopoietic stem cells.[24] What remains to be determined is whether the overall decline in tissue regenerative capacity with advancing age is caused by intrinsic ageing of stem cells, or is due to increasing impairment of stem cell function in an aged tissue environment. Until this basic question is resolved, the prospect of stem cell therapy as a potential 'treatment' to correct the functional declines and degenerative diseases typical of human ageing will remain a theoretical possibility.

## Further information

Agren, G. and Berennson, K. (eds.) (2007). *Healthy ageing—a challenge for Europe*. Swedish National Institute of Public Health, Stockholm; ISBN 91 7257 481 X.

http://www.healthyageing.nu.

Bittles, A.H. (2008). The biology of human ageing. In *Psychiatry in the elderly* (4th edn) (eds. R. Jacoby, C. Oppenheimer, T. Dening, and A. Thomas). Oxford University Press, Oxford, in press.

Johnson, M., Coleman, P.G., and Bengtson, V.L. (eds.) (2007). *Cambridge handbook of age and ageing*. Cambridge University Press, Cambridge; ISBN 052 182 6322.

National Institute of Aging (NIA); http://www.grc.nia.nih.gov/ *Baltimore Longitudinal Study of Aging*.
*NIA Intramural Research Program 2006 Factbook*.

## References

1. Herskind, A.M., McGue, M., Holm, N.V., *et al.* (1996). The heritability of human longevity: a population-based study of 2872 Danish twin pairs born 1870–1900. *Human Genetics*, **97**, 319–23.
2. Ljungquist, B., Berg, S., Lanke, J., *et al.* (1998). The effect of genetic factors for longevity: a comparison of identical and fraternal twins in the Swedish twin registry. *The Journals of Gerontology. Series A, Biological Sciences and Medical Sciences*, **53**, M441–6.
3. Willcox, B.J., Willcox, D.C., He, Q., *et al.* (2006). Siblings of Okinawan centenarians share lifelong mortality advantages. *The Journals of Gerontology. Series A, Biological Sciences and Medical Sciences*, **61**, 345–54.
4. Robine, J.M. and Allard, M. (1998). The oldest old. *Science*, **279**, 1834–5.
5. Seeman, T.E., McEwen, B.S., Rowe, J.W., *et al.* (2001). Allostatic load as marker of cumulative biological risk: MacArthur studies of successful aging. *Proceedings of the National Academy of Sciences of the United States of America*, **98**, 4770–5.
6. Hughes, K.A., Alipaz, J.A., Drnevich, J.M., *et al.* (2002). A test of evolutionary theories of aging. *Proceedings of the National Academy of Sciences of the United States of America*, **99**, 14286–91.
7. Wood, R.D., Mitchell, M., Sgouros, J., *et al.* (2001). Human DNA repair genes. *Science*, **291**, 1284–9.
8. Holliday, R. (1987). The inheritance of epigenetic defects. *Science*, **238**, 163–70.
9. Kujoth, G.C., Bradshaw, P.C., Haroon, S., *et al.* (2007). The role of mitochondrial DNA mutations in mammalian aging. *PLoS Genetics*, **3**, 0161–73.
10. Harley, C.B., Futcher, A.B., and Greider, C.W. (1990). Telomeres shorten during ageing of human fibroblasts. *Nature (London)*, **345**, 458–60.
11. Graakjaer, J., Londono-Vallejo, J.A., Christensen, K., *et al.* (2006). The pattern of chromosome-specific variations in telomere length in humans shows signs of heritability and is maintained through life. *Annals of the New York Academy of Sciences*, **1067**, 311–16.
12. Harley, C.B. (2005). Telomerase therapeutics for degenerative diseases. *Current Molecular Medicine*, **5**, 205–11.
13. Harman, D. (1992). Free radical theory of aging. *Mutation Research*, **275**, 257–66.
14. Schriner, S.E., Linford, N.J., Martin, G.M., *et al.* (2005). Extension of murine life span by overexpression of catalyse targeted to mitochondria. *Science*, **308**, 1909–11.
15. Kirkwood, T.B.L. (1977). Evolution of ageing. *Nature*, **270**, 301–4.
16. McCay, C.M., Crowell, M.F., and Maynard, L.A. (1935). The effect of retarded growth upon the length of lifespan and upon the ultimate body size. *The Journal of Nutrition*, **10**, 63–79.
17. McCay, C.M., Ellis, G.H., Barnes, L.L., *et al.* (1939). Clinical and pathological changes in aging and after retarded growth. *The Journal of Nutrition*, **18**, 15–25.
18. Sreekumar, R., Unnikrishnan, J., Fu, A., *et al.* (2002). Effects of caloric restriction on mitochondrial function and gene transcripts in rat muscle. *American Journal of Physiology. Endocrinology and Metabolism*, **283**, E38–43.
19. Lopez-Lluch, G., Hunt, N., Jones, B., *et al.* (2006). Calorie restriction induces mitochondrial biogenesis and bioenergetic efficiency. *Proceedings of the National Academy of Sciences of the United States of America*, **103**, 1768–73.
20. Fontana, L., Meyer, T.E., Klein, S., *et al.* (2004). Long-term calorie restriction is highly effective in reducing the risk for atherosclerosis in

humans. *Proceedings of the National Academy of Sciences of the United States of America*, **101**, 6659–63.

21. Civitarese, A.E., Carling, S., Heilbronn, L.K., *et al.* (2007). Calorie restriction increases muscle mitochondrial biogenesis in healthy humans. *PLoS Medicine*, **4**, 0485–94.

22. Wennmalm, K., Wahlestedt, C., and Larsson, O. (2005). The expression signature of *in vitro* senescence resembles mouse but not human aging. *Genome Biology*, **6**, R109.

23. Zahn, J.M., Sonu, R., Vogel, H., *et al.* (2006). Transcriptional profiling of aging in human muscle reveals a common aging signature. *PLoS Genetics*, **2**, e115.

24. Rando, T.A. (2006). Stem cells, ageing and the quest for immortality. *Nature Genetics*, **441**, 1080–6.

## 8.2

# Sociology of normal ageing

## Sarah Harper

## Introduction

Research on the sociology of normal ageing has focused on understanding the paradigms of *successful ageing*. In an apparent reaction to *'disengagement theory'*[1] which proposed that to withdraw from roles and relationships in old age was normal, a new conceptual framework was developed in the late 1960s and 1970s which attempted to explain how individuals adapted to the constraints of ageing and old age. This has been variously measured in terms of good health, high levels of physical and mental functioning, and active engagement with one's social and physical environment. While post-modernism and critical gerontology have attempted to refocus the debate, the emphasis of most research and writing has remained within the framework of understanding, explaining, and even facilitating, 'success' in old age.

There is also a body of research which recognizes the importance of the *life course perspective*, and that throughout an individual's life, he or she is faced with *continuities* and *discontinuities* which have to be negotiated and resolved. Old age is but part of this lifelong process. Changes which occur in later life, such as retirement and widowhood, will lead to discontinuities in roles and relationships, other aspects of our lives will undergo little change allowing continuity. Alongside this, perspectives from anthropology, history and the social constructionist school of thought have also been recently influential.

This chapter will discuss concepts of age, generation, and cohort. It will consider the contribution of the life course approach to understanding ageing, and the manner in which other perspectives, such as social constructionism, narrative psychology and anthropology, have contributed to the sociology of normal ageing.

## Structuring the life course through age

According to Hazelrigg,[2] the concept of age introduces signposts which link memory and anticipation, an iteratively remembered past and an iteratively expected future. Age classification is thus integral to normal organization of consciousness. As Mead's extensive work on life history, reminiscence and autobiography informs us,

*one interacts retrospectively with one's younger selves, recalling earlier states of selfhood in the productive functioning of memory, and interacts prospectively with ones' older selves, anticipating conditions, actions, goal realizations and the like of late states of selfhood.*[1]

For both the individual and society, age conveniently dissects the life course into more manageable components. As a capitalist, industrial system emerged, and individuals moved from domestic units to bureaucratically organized corporations, so age was used to define adulthood and thus labour force participation. Age became the basis for regulating a large population. It defined the responsibilities of citizenship, and for each age related transition there is a stage of preparation, a stage of participation, and a stage of retirement.

Various anthropological studies[2] have highlighted alternative ways in which the life course might be structured. One of the most influential anthropological studies on the sociology of ageing was Cowgill and Holmes[3] work on ageing and modernization, which argued that the marginalization of older people was directly linked to modernization. While extensively debated ever since, this work highlighted the importance and complexity of cultural diversity. The burgeoning of anthropological studies around the concept of age and ageing since the Cwgill and Holmes study have contributed significantly to our understanding of this diversity.

Neither the !Kung nor Herero, hunter-gather and Bantu pastoralist peoples respectively of Botswana, have a concept of chronological age, marking age by physical transitions. Alternatively, the Tuareg, a semi-nomadic peoples in northern Niger, noted age by social transitions—courtship, marriage, childbirth, and grandchildren. Here, life transitions defining the ageing process are predominantly social rather than biological. A girl becomes a women not at menstruation, but at marriage; a women becomes an older women not at menopause but on having a child marry. For the Sukama of north-west Tanzania, ageing is defined through life course events. This emphasizes the social status of elderhood, measured by the wealth of alliances, offspring and livestock, which could not be diminished through ill health or loss of mental capacity. The Gussui of south-western Kenya have a similar notion of elderhood. However, they have adapted this traditional seniority gradation based on networks and affiliations to modern demands,

---

1  G.H. Mead, quoted in Hazelrigg p. 105[2]
2  See Harper for a full reference list to these studies[5]

incorporating such aspects as the role of entrepreneur to the criteria for achieving successful seniority status.

Modern Japanese society still applies a wide variety of terms to different points of the life course indicating complex relationships between chronological age and life transitions and physical appearance. For example, mid-life men and women with children whether or not they are married, will commonly be referred to as uncle and aunt, (*oji-san* and *oba-san*). Similarly, old men and women are frequently given the name of grandfather or grandmother, (*ojii-san* and *obaa san*) regardless of the presence of grandchildren, a characteristic also found in some European countries such as Greece. It is therefore clear that the domination of chronological age, has less salience in some other cultures.

## Generation and cohort

Two further important concepts are generation and cohort. Individuals born within the same time period may be perceived as having a shared history and a common biography. The concept of *generation* is thus the link between an individual life course and the social changes that occur during the historical time of that life course. A generation may thus be thought of as *embodied history*.

Many of these draw on ideas from Mannheim who explored the creation of society through the continuous emergence of new age groups or generations. He argued that if social processes were always carried on and developed by the same individuals then once established, any fundamental social pattern, attitude or intellectual trend would probably be perpetuated. Culture was thus developed by individuals who come into contact anew with the accumulated heritage, that is the role of generations and while the continuous emergence of new individuals results in some loss of accumulated possessions it facilitates re-evaluation of our inventory and teaches us both to forget that which is no longer useful and to covet that which has yet to be won.

The problem for quantitative social scientists is how to disentangle those factors pertaining to the individual life course from those emerging from the historical context. It is here that the concept of cohorts, and cohort analysis has been refined by some to form a more analytical tool in the understanding of age and generational change.

A cohort begins with a particular demography at birth, that is its sex, race and economic composition. Differential mortality may lead to a higher proportion of some sub-groups surviving to old age; social mobility may lead to changes in cohort social status composition; and different historical periods will allow or enhance differential migration in and out of specific cohorts. A more sophisticated analysis places cohorts within specific historical contexts.[4] The *life-stage principle* suggests that disruptive social changes have enduring consequences on the subsequent lives, a particularly marked effect on those vulnerable at the time of occurrence.

## Life course perspective

The life course perspective views old age as part of a life-long process of continuity and change. These can be addressed within four main frameworks: *context, transitions, roles,* and *relationships.*

## Context

A starting point for life course analysis is the acknowledgement of the historical *context* within which different cohorts experience different aspects of the life course to life course perspective. As Harper[5] explores, while, most older men experienced a long period of economic activity followed by abrupt retirement, many older Western women experienced their younger lives within a framework of primary domestic duties, supplemented by intermittent economic activity. As a result, most older women replaced low earning capacity or economic dependence in younger life, with low incomes in old age. Cohorts in mid life, however, have had very different social and economic frameworks within which to live out their lives. Half the labour force in many countries is now female and full-time economic employment, with or without domestic, in particular childcare responsibilities, is becoming a widespread experience for many women. Despite this, there are still considerable income disparities in earning capacity of mid-life men and women. However, it is likely that future cohorts of older women will have higher incomes relative to older cohorts, and a lower gender income disparity.

### Transitions

The processes which occur within these contexts can be understood as a series of life transitions.[6] Key transitions associated with later life are the end of active parenting, grandparenthood, widowhood and retirement. Each of these phases of life which may overlap, may be understood in relation to prior phases, and are mediated by other variables such as gender, class, and race. The transition to grandparenthood, for example, is experienced very differently by men and women, while the end of active parenting and transition to parent of a non-dependent child, the so-called *empty nest syndrome*, is mediated both by gender and by the experience of active parenting itself.

The transition to *widowhood* is one of the most stressful events of later life, with a high prevalence of depression both immediately before (presumably due to anticipation of the event and/or associated care giving) and in the first year following bereavement. Widowhood is likely to lead to lower income but higher social contacts for women, while men maintain their income, but are more likely to lose social contacts, unless they remarry. Over half women over 65 are widowed, rising to four-fifths at 85. Only 17 per cent of men are widowed over 65, rising to 43 per cent by their late 80s. Nearly three-quarters of older men in the UK are married, compared with less than a half of older women. This is explained both by differential life expectancy and the tendency of men to remarry following divorce or widowhood.[7]

The transition to *Grandparenthood* is the current normal experience of old age. US data suggests that more than half the population aged over 55 are in four-generation families and three-quarters of this population are or can expect to be as grandparents, with a prediction that one-third of current grandparents will live to be great grandparents, and one-fifth of all women who reach 80 will spend some time in a five-generation family as great-great-grandmothers. A similar picture may be found in the UK with estimates that three-quarters of adults over 66 years of age are grandparents. The transition from parenthood to grandparenthood, and even great-grandparenthood, determines both an individual's self-identity and subsequent roles and functions as grandparenthood. In addition, the experience of the relationship that the grandchild has with his or her grandparent earlier will partially determine the way they take on the role and relate to their own grandchildren later on in life. Other sociological theories have been applied to the study of grandparenthood. *Role theory* suggests that a successful transition to grandparenthood requires both some socialization to the role, and appropriate life course timing. *Social stress theory* is used to argue that stress associated with transition to grandparenthood is related to the number, type, and context of the transitions and moderated by gender, education, income, and race.[9]

For many individuals, especially men, the transition to *retirement* is abrupt. Although early retirement has increased in Europe over the past twenty five years, most men still retire from full time work in their early-to mid-60s. A successful transition to retirement requires securing both financial security and personal adjustment. Atchley[10] identifies several phases of retirement. Pre-retirement, which may include a combination of both negative and positive feelings towards the impending event; a honeymoon period immediately following the event, which may extend for several years depending on the adjustment and resources, social, financial, and personal, available to the individual; disenchantment and reorientation; and eventually (if successful) stability. This latter stage occurs with the development of a well established set of criteria for making choices and dealing with the challenges and opportunities of this new life phase.

## Roles and relationships

The above transitions—retirement, widowhood, grandparenthood - are also, of course, phases of life with specific roles and relationships. Thus, the transition of retirement also has an associated phase of being retired; that of grandparenthood of being a grandparent; that of widowhood of being a widow or widower.

We can examine two of these—late-life parenting and grandparenting—in the context of negotiating transitions and continuities in family roles and relationships as individuals age.[11] Intergenerational solidarity—shared values, normative obligations and enduring ties—and intergenerational conflict—whereby issues are resolved and relationships move on have been long seen as important components of this. More recently the concept of intergenerational ambivalence has been introduced. This, it is argued, reflects the contradictions which occur with ageing within family relationships These arise both through the desire of parents and children for both help and freedom, and conflicting norms regarding family relationships especially around the issue of care giving.

### (a) Late-life parenting

Increasing longevity also means that most parent-child relationships will be lived out as predominantly non-dependent adult dyads, this is despite the delaying of child birth. The common experience for many parents and children is around 60 years of joint life, of which under one-third is spent in the traditional parent/dependent-child relationship. Around one-quarter of UK women and nearly 40 per cent of US women aged 55–63 still have a surviving parent. These women have thus spent around 60 years a child, some 40 of them in an adult relationship with a living parent. This relies on *re-bonding* in adulthood sometimes also referred to as 'reverse bonding'.[12] Under such experiences we see a loosening of the association between marital and parental roles. As the common

experience of parenthood moves to more than 50 years of shared life, parents and children are adjusting to spending most of their relationship as independent adults. Similarly, husbands and wives are spending fewer of their joint lives as parents of young children. Relationships which have been historically based on a hierarchy which existed in part to support successful reproduction must move to greater equality, both child-parent, and husband-wife, as traditional roles based on parenthood give way to companionate relationships.[12]

### (b) Grandparenting roles[3]

Currently, women can expect to become grandmothers in their 50s and 60s due to the early first age of births in the 1960s and 1970s. In addition, grandparental roles are lasting far longer due to increased longevity, the grandparent is thus more likely to be able to build a relationship with their grandchild into their adulthood. As a result many grandmothers, in particular, now face simultaneous demands as children of frail and dependent parents, mothers and grandmothers, as well as still being in full or part time economic employment.[13]

Grandmothers, in particular maternal grandmothers, are repeatedly attributed with having more influence in almost every value domain over their grandchildren than grandfathers. Research into the role of grandfathers has been limited.[14] However, it has been proposed that men become more nurturing as they get older and it could be hypothesized that these qualities might be expressed in relationships with their grandchildren. Similarly, the need to consider grandfathers as important resources for teenage mothers who are rearing their children, has been stressed. Harper also found that grandfathers could act as replacement partners and replacement fathers in female single parent households.[13]

Various roles of grandparenthood have been identified.[15] Bengtson (1985) for example, identifies five separate symbolic functions of grandparents: being there; grandparents as national guard; family watchdog; arbiters who perform negotiations between (family) members; and participants in the social construction of family history. Harper's study of grandmothers identifies grandmother as carer, replacement partner (confidante, guide and facilitator), replacement parent (listener, teacher and disciplinarian), and as family anchor (transferring values, attitudes and history).[13]

## Complementary perspectives

Our understanding of ageing from a life course perspective has drawn on valuable insights from narrative gerontology and the social constructionist perspective.

### Narrative gerontology

Narrative gerontology's main contribution to the field of ageing has been to the role of the life story in the development of theoretical and empirical approaches to ageing. It presumes that individuals think and act on the basis of stories, which have an external structure and an internal reality. Individuals retell their stories as they progress through their lives to make sense of their lives, and from a sociological perspective this retelling when carried out publicly provides considerable insights into various aspects of an individual's experience of ageing across the life course. There are

---

3  A full reference list on grandparenthood may be found in Harper.[5]

four dimensions to this: the structural story, which reflects the wider societal context inhabited across the life course; the socio-cultural story, which reflects other identities such as ethnicity and gender; the situational story which reflects an individual's roles and relationships; and the interpersonal story, the meanings which the individuals place themselves on their life story.

Writers in this genre of theory have further suggested that individuals experience two types of time. Achenbaum[16] describes this as a *physical outer time* and *a psychological inner time*, or as Kenyon and Randall[17] state *clock time* and *story time*. There may be a tension between the two types of time described as *on time* and *off time*.[18] Hazelrigg[19] suggests that the tension between the two times has been become more extreme within modern society, so dominated by rigid timekeeping. He argues that modern life is lived in two separate registers. On the one hand, most of a life experience is formed directly and indirectly in a highly standardized sequence of institutionalized events—schooling, work, parenting, retirement. These events are regulated by procedural rules and recognized routines, with predictable durations and regulated transitions between events. On the other hand, those aspects of life experiences that are not institutionalized and structurally stabilized in recognized life course sequences tend to have little or no connection to status dimensions or specific locations in the life course. These would include self-image, personal satisfaction, existential aesthetics etc.

Tensions arise when the two registers fail to coincide—*off time*.[18] Examples include middle-aged couples falling in love and publicly exhibiting displays of physical affection and romance, or older people adopting student style lives. Off time may also include the experience of being externally forced, through illness for example, to fall outside the normal behaviour range as defined for one's age. This also includes examples where society takes an individual and places them within a situation which is unusual for their chronological age–for example, a very young person being rapidly promoted within an institution which is very highly age regulated, such as a university, and taking on a professorial mantle.

### Social constructionist approaches

The sociology of ageing has also recently enveloped social constructionist approaches, including phenomenology, symbolic interactionism, and ethnomethodology. These approaches share a subjective orientation to social reality, focusing on describing how individuals negotiate their worlds, rather than trying to explain why. A key area of interest here is the management of identity across the life course and in particular as we age. Examples include, Matthew's[20] seminal work using symbolic interactionist approaches to explore how old women negotiate their own identities when they are continually deluged with negative public stereotypes of infirmity and worthlessness. This is a theme taken up later by Featherstone and Hepworth[21] in their work on the Masks of Ageing. Similarly, Karp[22] uses symbolic interactionist approaches to explore the impact of social messages on the emerging consciousness of men and women in their 50s of their own ageing.

## Conclusion

The sociology of, so-called, normal ageing thus combines perspectives from diverse traditions of thought. This actual measurement of ageing, in terms of health, physical and mental functioning, and active engagement with one's social and physical environment, has combined quantitative social science, epidemiology and political economy. The understanding of these interactions, draws on perspectives from sociology, psychology, and anthropology. In both cases, however, there is now recognition of the importance of context and process, and that, in reality, there is perhaps no single construct of 'normal' ageing. Given this perspective, it is essential that care for older adults is person-centred rather than imposed by professionals.

## Further information

Johnson, M., Bengtson, V., Coleman, P. *et al.* (eds) (2005) *The Cambridge Handbook of Age and Ageing.* Cambridge University Press, New York.

Ageing Horizons: http://www.ageing.ox.ac.uk/ageinghorizons/index.htm

Binstock, R. and George, L. (2005). *Handbook of Ageing and the Social Sciences*. Elsevier, London.

## References

1. Cumming, C., and Henry, W. (1961). *Growing Old*, New York Basic Books.
2. Hazelrigg, L. (1997). On the importance of Age. In *Studying aging and social change: conceptual and methodological issues* (ed. M. A. Hardy). pp. 93–128. Sage Publications, Thousand Oaks.
3. Cowgill, D. and Holmes, L. (eds.) (1972). *Ageing and Modernization*, New York, Apple Century Crofts.
4. Elder, G. H., and O'rand, A. M. (1995). Adult lives in a changing society. In *Sociological perspectives on social psychology* (eds. K. S.Cook, G. A. Fine, & J. S.House), pp. 452–475. Allyn and Bacon, Boston.
5. Harper, S. (2006). *Ageing Societies*. Hodder Arnold, London.
6. Elder, G. H. (1985). Perspectives on the life course. In *Life course dynamics: trajectories and transitions* (ed. G. H. Elder) *1968–1980*. pp.23–49. Cornell University Press, Ithaca.
7. Arber, S. Davidson, K. and Ginn, J. (eds.) (2003). *Gender and Ageing: changing Roles and Relationships*, Maidenhead, Open University Press.
8. Kornhaber, A. (1996). *Contemporary Grandparenting*, New York, Sage.
9. Szinovacz, M. (1997). Grandparents today: a demographic profile. *The Gerontologist*, **38**, 37–52.
10. Atchley, R. (1989). A continuity theory of normal aging, *The Gerontologist*, **29**, 183–90.
11. Giarrusso, R., Silverstein, M., Gans, D., *et al.* (2005). Ageing parents and adult children: new perspectives on intergenerational relationships. In *The Cambridge handbook of age and ageing* (eds. M.L. Johnson, and V. L. Bengston). Cambridge University Press, New York.
12. Harper, S. (2006). *Ageing Societies*. Hodder Arnold, London.
13. Harper, S. (2005). Understanding Grandparenthood. In *The Cambridge handbook of age and ageing* (eds. M.L. Johnson, and V. L. Bengston), Cambridge University Press, New York.
14. Mann, R. (2007). 'Out of the shadows?': Grandfatherhood, age and masculinities', *Journal of Aging Studies*, **21**(4), 271–81.
15. Bengtson, V. (1985) Diversity and symbolism in grandparental roles. In *Grandparenthood* (eds. V. Bengtson, and J. Robertson) Beverly Hills, Sage.
16. Achenbaum, W. A. (1991) Time is the messenger of the Gods: a gerontological metaphor. In *Metaphors of Aging in Science and Humanities* (eds. G. Kenyon, J. Birren, and J. Schroots), pp. 83–101. New York, Springer.

17. Keynon, G., and Randall, W., (1997). *Restorying our Lives: personal growth through autobiographical reflection*. Westport, CT, Praeger.

18. Hagestad, G. O. (1986). Dimension of time and the family. *American Behavioral Scientist*, **29**, 679–94.

19. Hazelrigg, L. (1997). On the importance of Age. In *Studying aging and social change: conceptual and methodological issues* (ed. M. A. Hardy), pp. 93–128. Sage Publications, Thousand Oaks.

20. Matthews, S. (1979). *The Social World of Older Women*. Newbury park, Sage.

21. Featherstone, M., and Hepworth, M., (eds.) (1995). *Images of Ageing*. Sage, London.

22. Karp, D. (1988). A decade of reminders: changing age consciousness between fifty and sixty years old, *The Gerontologist*, 727–38.

# The ageing population and the epidemiology of mental disorders among the elderly

## Scott Henderson and Laura Fratiglioni

In the last decades the ageing of the populations has become a worldwide phenomenon.[1] In 1990, 26 nations had more than 2 million elderly citizens aged 65 years and older, and the projections indicate that an additional 34 countries will join the list by 2030. In 2000, the number of old persons (65+ years) in the world was estimated to be 420 million and it was projected to be nearly 1 billion by 2030, with the proportion of old persons increasing from 7 to 12 per cent.[2] The largest increase in absolute numbers of old persons will occur in developing countries; it almost triples from 249 million in 2000 to an estimated 690 million in 2030. The developing regions' share of the worldwide ageing population will increase from 59 to 71 per cent. Developed countries, which have already seen a dramatic increase in people over 65 years of age, will experience a progressive ageing of the elderly population itself (see Fig. 8.3.1). The global trend in the phenomenon of population ageing has dramatic consequences for public health, health care financing, and delivery systems in the whole world. The absolute number of chronic diseases as well as psychiatric disorders is expected to increase. In this chapter, the epidemiological aspects of the most common psychiatric disorders of the elderly are summarized and discussed.

## Depressive disorders

The epidemiology of depression in the elderly can be approached at three levels: its occurrence in the elderly living in the community, in those reaching primary care, and in the residents of hostels and nursing homes.

### The community

It might be expected that, overall, the prevalence of depressive symptoms and disorders might increase in old age due to the loss of partners, friends, social status, retirement, income, and, above all, declining health. It is surprising, therefore, that surveys of the elderly in the general population have recurrently found rates that are significantly lower than in younger adults. Many of the large national surveys have not included persons aged over 65 years, but two exceptions are Australia, which found a 12-month prevalence of 1.7 per cent for the 65 years and over group compared with 5.8 per cent for all adults; and the New Zealand survey with rates of 2.0 and 8.0 per cent, respectively. It must be emphasized that these data refer to depressive symptoms in the elderly living in the community.

What is so far unproven is that such findings are indeed valid, and if they are, what might explain them.[3] They could be due to sample bias, in which elderly respondents with depressive symptoms may be more likely to decline to be interviewed than younger depressed people. Selective mortality has also been proposed, but cannot account for the size of the difference. It could be due to an error in case ascertainment, by which the interview instrument is not equally valid across age groups. For example, questions about depressive symptoms may be responded to differently by persons aged 20 and 80 years. Another possibility is a cohort effect in much of the Western world, where people born in the second half of the twentieth century have higher rates for depression.[4,5] This seems increasingly likely and may be due to a combination of social and environmental factors.

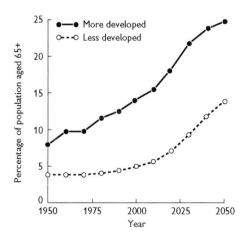

**Fig. 8.3.1** Percentage of the population aged 65+ for more developed and less developed countries. (Reproduced from Kinsella, K. and Velkroff, V.A. The demographics of aging. *Aging Clinical and Experimental Research*, **4**, 59–69, copyright 2002 with permission from Editrice Kurtis S.r.l.)

## Primary care

Unsurprisingly, the prevalence of depressive symptoms is considerably higher in elderly persons consulting their doctor than in the general community. One study in London found a point prevalence of about 30 per cent. Where it has been possible to compare the rates for those cases recognized by their doctor with cases independently ascertained by a research measure, such as a screening instrument or standardized interview, a typical finding is that the general practitioner recognizes about two thirds of the mild cases, rising to some 90 per cent of the moderate to severe ones. Some cases are considered to be depressed when they are not. Another finding is that elderly persons with depressive symptoms may not mention them to their doctor, attributing them to their age and circumstances. These findings have led to programmes offering additional training for GPs and to recommending the use of brief screening tests in primary care. Because diagnosis would lead to appropriate treatment being given earlier in an episode of depressive disorder, its duration would be shortened. Since prevalence is the product of incidence and duration, the prevalence of depression would therefore be expected to fall. This is an example of the application of epidemiology to prevention, which is its ultimate service.

## Depression in hostels and nursing homes

Prevalence rates are also higher in hostels and nursing homes. In the United States, levels as high as 30 to 50 per cent have been reported. It might be thought that the context of living in a nursing home would account for having depressive symptoms. But one study found that the excess over the general population rates was largely accounted for by medical disorders, environmental factors contributing little to the variance. This needs to be studied further because it seems counterintuitive that the social and physical environment, both of which can be modified, could be of little relevance.

What is important is that only about one quarter of cases are recognized. To compound the situation, those cases that are recognized tend to be treated with too low doses of antidepressants. Depressive symptoms are well known to occur comorbidly with cognitive decline and the dementias. These findings from clinical epidemiology have pointed to the need for better case recognition through education of medical and nursing staff, and to the use of routine screening of residents in such settings.

## Suicide

For many decades across the world, the traditional pattern has been for the highest rates of suicide to be in elderly men. This has now changed. In over a third of countries, both developed and less developed, it is younger people who have come to carry the highest rates. The World Health Organization provides a valuable resource for such data, showing rates by age and gender for nearly all countries from 1950 onwards.[6] The pattern varies considerably between countries. For example, in the United Kingdom in 2002, men aged 75 and over had a rate of 10 per 100 000, whereas the highest rate was 18 per 100 000, in men aged 35–44 years. In the United States and in the Russian Federation, the rates for men aged 75 and over were 41 and 89 per 100 000, respectively.

The main risk factors for suicide in the elderly are a past history of an attempt, depressive disorder, physical illness or disability,

chronic pain, recent losses, social isolation, and access to lethal means. While universal interventions are more powerful than selected factors in prevention,[7] these attributes can be used in selective intervention to identify groups at increased risk. Furthermore, being multiplicative, these markers are of great value in individual cases by alerting the clinician to a person needing particular attention. Here is another example of the use of epidemiology for prevention. A systematic review of suicide prevention strategies for all age groups concluded that two interventions did reduce rates: physician education in recognizing and treating depression; and restricting access to lethal means.[8] Both of these interventions have close relevance to the elderly.

## Personality disorders

The subject matter here refers to older people who have enduring attitudes and behaviour that bring difficulties for themselves or for others.[9] There is only sparse information on the prevalence of personality disorders in the general population, let alone specifically in the elderly. One exception, based on a national survey of mental health, found a lifetime prevalence of 6.5 per cent across all age groups with a trend towards lower rates with increasing age.

In clinical practice, it has long been suggested that traits such as impulsivity and externalizing behaviours tend to become less frequent in later life, whereas anxiety-prone, dependent, schizoid, paranoid, or obsessional persons are likely to change little as they age, or to become more so. Bergmann's pioneering enquiries among the elderly of Newcastle upon Tyne found that it was the anxiety-prone and insecure types that had late-onset neurotic disorders. A more recent study of late-life depression found an overall prevalence of comorbid personality disorder of 10–30 per cent. The group formerly known as neurotic and more recently as Cluster C in the DSM classification, had the higher prevalence. The Cluster B group, those with borderline, narcissistic, histrionic, and antisocial traits, were rare. What is not yet established, however, is if this lower prevalence also exists in the general population of the elderly, not just among cases with depressive disorder who have reached treatment in specialist services.

The epidemiology of personality disorders in later life is therefore significant for two reasons. First, some types are associated with increased risk of anxiety, depression, or paranoid states (*vide infra*). Second, there remains much yet to understand about the natural history of the personality disorders across the lifespan.

## Psychosis of late onset

For the functional psychoses of late life, epidemiological information comes from two sources: studies of persons who have reached psychiatric services; and surveys of elderly persons living in the general community.[10] Psychotic symptoms probably exist as a continuum of severity, with only the more developed cases meeting diagnostic criteria. These often, but not always, reach psychiatric services, not uncommonly through being brought to the attention of the police. States phenomenologically similar to those found in clinics do occur in the community in non-trivial numbers. For cases that reach the threshold for a diagnosis by virtue of the range and severity of symptoms and behaviour, it has been proposed that cases with onset after the age of 60 years be called 'very-late-onset schizophrenia-like psychosis'. The syndrome has a 1-year prevalence of 0.1 to 0.5 per cent. For advancing knowledge about the aetiology of schizophrenia, any information on it might be useful in explaining why people with this syndrome have reached the seventh decade or later in life without becoming psychotic, and only then develop it. It is more common in women. This is unlikely to be due to different social visibility or access to services. It is associated with a better premorbid level of social and occupational functioning. Premorbid paranoid or schizoid traits have been implicated and both clinical and community-based studies have found an association with sensory impairment such as deafness or poor eyesight. Personal and environmental factors associated with ageing have been considered, such as physical ill health, bereavement, loss of friends, and loss of income, but these have not been shown to contribute significantly. Genetic factors appear to be less important than in earlier onset schizophrenia.

## Alcohol and drug dependence

It is generally believed that the prevalence of alcohol abuse and dependence declines during adult life and that the elderly have low rates in most communities. This may well be the case, but some other factors have to be considered. Whatever the prevalence, the absolute numbers will rise in the future because of the unprecedented growth in the elderly population. Next, the assumption may be false. In community surveys, errors in the ascertainment of alcohol abuse may lead to an underestimate for older persons. Most screening instruments were developed for use on younger adults, so their validity in the elderly is largely undetermined. Measures of the quantity drunk may mislead because smaller amounts may have an intoxicating effect in persons whose body fat, lean tissue, cerebral reserve, and metabolic function have declined. So the usual cut-off for problem drinking may be set too high for the elderly. One review of screening instruments concluded that the CAGE and MAST-G scales were appropriate, whereas other widely used instruments were not.[11] Next, all the studies have been cross-sectional. The elderly may have lower rates because of a cohort effect, whereby people born in the first half of the twentieth century may have been more moderate drinkers for all their life, compared to the high levels of consumption that are now found in the young of both sexes.

The actual values for prevalence are dependent on the instrument used and the definition used to define problem drinking, alcohol abuse, or dependence.[12] One review of community studies gives a figure of 5.1 per cent using various definitions. Invariably, men have higher rates than women. There is also considerable variation between countries and across different cultures. In identifying cases, a distinction of clinical significance needs to be made between late-onset and long-standing alcohol abuse. In primary care, accident and emergency departments, hospital in-patients, and nursing homes, the prevalence is much higher, yet cases are consistently under-recognized. The use of screening instruments in all of these settings has been advocated to improve this.

Alcohol abuse carries important comorbidity. In addition to all the established medical complications, it is associated with falls, subclinical delirium, cognitive decline, and depression. One study demonstrated a five-fold increase in the risk of developing a psychiatric disorder, especially depression and dementia. Simultaneous use of benzodiazepines, itself common in older persons, is clearly an additional and important factor. Against all this, it should be recalled that moderate alcohol use has been found in population studies to be associated with better mental and cardiovascular health, as well as being subjectively enjoyable.

## Alzheimer's disease and other dementias

In the last two decades the dementia field has registered a tremendous scientific progression in many research areas including aetiology, pathogenesis, clinical aspects, treatment, and prevention. These advances have opened new perspectives, especially concerning definitions and diagnostic criteria, which have a relevant impact on epidemiological research.

Dementia is still defined as a syndrome which includes memory deficits and disturbance of other higher cortical functions; these major symptoms are commonly accompanied, and occasionally preceded, by deterioration in emotional control, social behaviour or motivation. However, it has become apparent that memory impairment may not necessarily be the major or first symptom for dementia subtypes such as frontotemporal dementia (FTD) and vascular dementia (VaD). Furthermore, as the current definition requires impairment severe enough to interfere with daily functioning, in several cases a delay of the diagnosis occurs. For that reason, a new research line has emerged with the aim to detect early Alzheimer's disease (AD) and other dementias, and the terms mild cognitive impairment (MCI) and cognitive impairment no-dementia (CIND) have been proposed to identify those subjects that show a clear cognitive deficit but do not fulfil diagnostic criteria for dementia. Finally, it is well known that dementia syndrome can be induced by many different underlying diseases, and that a differential diagnosis may be difficult for several reasons. AD as well as other dementia subtypes shows heterogeneity with distinct clinical and pathological characteristics; many different dementing disorders overlap in clinical and pathologic features; and different dementing disorders may make a common contribution or interact in causing dementia symptoms. Thus, rather than viewing, for example, AD and VaD as dichotomous entities, it may be more relevant to consider the role of their additive or synergistic interactions in producing a dementia syndrome.[13,14]

Following these new perspectives, in this chapter we will summarize the major findings from the most recent epidemiological research according to three major topics: early detection of AD and other dementias, incidence and risk factors for AD and dementia, and prevalence and impact of the dementing disorders at the individual and societal levels.

### Early detection

As diagnostic criteria for AD require gradual onset of cognitive deficits, it is expected that cognitive disturbances are present already before the diagnosis can be rendered. Cognitive deficits are observable up to 10 years before dementia diagnosis with a sharp decline more evident in the final 3 years,[15] and occurring in episodic memory as well as in other cognitive domains such as executive functioning, verbal ability, visuospatial skills, attention, and perceptual speed.[16] However, our capability to use such early disturbances as a predictive tool of incipient dementia is strongly limited by several concomitant facts: (1) cognitive decline is also present as a function of the normal ageing process; (2) several conditions other than AD may lead to cognitive disturbances in the elderly; and (3) dementia-free patients with cognitive impairment observed in specialized clinical settings are different from cognitively impaired persons detected in the general population.[17]

To overcome these difficulties, different definitions have been proposed, with MCI and CIND being the most commonly used. MCI definition was originally derived in a clinical setting to identify subjects with isolated memory loss (now referred to as the 'amnestic' type) who may be in a preclinical phase of AD. Since then, the view has widened to cover a broader range of cognitive disturbances, and other MCI subtypes have been proposed.[18,19] CIND is derived essentially from population-based studies, and operationalized in slightly different items. Unfortunately, not one of the proposed definitions has shown a sufficiently good predictivity at the community level. Even a highly selected algorithm including subjective memory complaints, and global, and specific (memory/language) cognitive deficits could identify only 18 per cent of the incipient AD cases.[20,21] Although elderly persons with cognitive impairment have a high risk of developing dementia with a rate of about 11 to 50 per cent over 1 to 5 years, not all persons with CIND or MCI develop dementia. A substantial proportion of these persons (24–42 per cent) even improve in their cognitive performances over time.[22] This diverse prognosis supports the notion that AD is not the only causal mechanism underlying cognitive impairment in the non-demented elderly population. Cognitive psychologists have detected lower cognitive performances in elderly persons with deficiency in vitamin $B_{12}$ and folate, elevated homocysteine, thyroid stimulating hormone deficiency, and cardiovascular disease. Physicians found an association between CIND and a number of factors including frailty-related factors such as history of hip fracture and high consumption of multiple drugs, history of psychoses, and depressed mood occurring 3 years before CIND development.[23] Other studies have identified older age, low education, depression, APOE ε4 allele, medicated hypertension, mid-life elevated serum cholesterol, and high diastolic blood pressure, as well as diabetes and anticholinergic medication use as risk factors for MCI.[17]

The prevalence of cognitive impairment—no dementia varies depending on diagnostic criteria with a maximum of 30 per cent.[24] In the younger elderly (e.g. 65–75 years old) cognitive impairment is actually more frequent than dementia disorders.[25] Annual incidence rates vary from 15 per 1000 among persons aged 75–79 years to 98 per 1000 among nonagenarians, when the estimates are corrected for dropouts due to death (Fig. 8.3.2; Ref.[26]). Regardless of the aetiology underlying the cognitive deficits, the high prevalence and incidence highlight the importance of this syndrome in the ageing population. Given that the criteria for cognitive impairment in non-demented persons are still under construction, and that there is no efficacious treatment to stop the possible progression to AD, at the moment we must be cautious with diagnosing MCI, which may cause an unnecessary burden on patients and relatives due to the unclear prognosis. However, it is clinically relevant to identify all persons with cognitive deficits due to treatable conditions such as depression, low-level vitamin $B_{12}$, and use of drugs.

### Incidence and risk factors

Dementia incidence is similar in all continents and from different regions of the world (Table 8.3.1). Slightly lower rates detected in US in comparison with those in Europe and Asia are likely to be due to differences in study designs and case ascertainment.[27] AD accounts for 60–70 per cent and VaD accounts for 15–20 per cent of all dementia cases. The incidence of both AD and dementia increases almost exponentially with age. However, there are inconsistent findings regarding whether the rates continue to increase even in more advanced ages. The apparent decline found in some studies may be an artifact of the poor response rates, survival effects, and nature of populations previously sampled in these very old age groups.[28]

Age is the strongest risk factor for dementia and AD, suggesting that ageing-related biological processes could be implicated in the etiopathogenesis of AD. Further, the strong association with increasing age can be, at least partially, explained by a lifetime cumulative risk to different risk factors. Using this approach, the risk of dementia in late life is considered as a result of complex

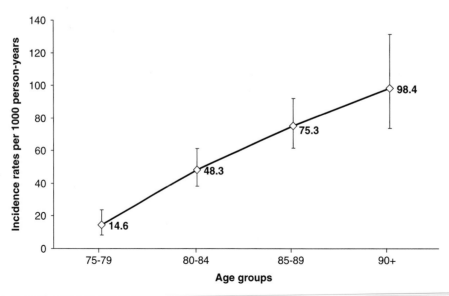

**Fig. 8.3.2** Corrected age-specific incidence rates with 95 per cent confidence intervals of non-dementia cognitive impairment, including the two mutually exclusive definitions of amnestic MCI and CIND. (Reprinted from Alzheimer's and Dementia, 2, L. Fratiglioni, C. Qui, and K. Palmer, vascular cognitive impairment: time for prevention?, 202–4, copyright 2006, with permission from Elsevier.)

**Table 8.3.1** Age-specific prevalence and incidence rates for dementia in the world and different regions: estimated from meta-analyses

| Age groups | Incidence rate (per 1000 person-years) | | | | Prevalence (per 100 population) | | | |
|---|---|---|---|---|---|---|---|---|
| | Worldwide (Gao et al. 1998) | Europe (Fratiglioni et al. 2000) | USA (Jorm and Jolley, 1998) | East Asia (Jorm and Jolley, 1998) | Worldwide (Jorm et al. 1987) | Worldwide (Fratiglioni et al. 1999) | Europe (Lobo et al. 2000) | China (Liu et al. 2003)* |
| 60–64 | 1.1 | — | — | — | 0.7 | 0.9 | — | 0.3 |
| 65–69 | 3.3 | 2.4 | 2.4 | 3.5 | 1.4 | 1.6 | 0.8 | 0.7 |
| 70–74 | 8.4 | 5.5 | 5.0 | 7.1 | 2.8 | 3.5 | 3.0 | 1.3 |
| 75–79 | 18.2 | 16.0 | 10.5 | 14.7 | 5.6 | 6.9 | 5.8 | 2.8 |
| 80–84 | 33.6 | 30.5 | 17.7 | 32.6 | 11.1 | 13.0 | 12.0 | 5.6 |
| 85–89 | 53.3 | 48.6 | 27.5 | 72.1 | 23.6 | 25.2 | 17.4 | 11.8 |
| 90–95 | 72.9 | 70.2 | — | — | — | 35.8 | 28.5 | 23.7 |
| 95+ | 86.8 | — | — | — | — | 48.1 | — | — |

* The dementia cases in this meta-analysis include only Alzheimer's disease and vascular dementia.

(Reproduced from Backman, L., Small, B.J. and Fratiglioni, L. Cognitive deficits in preclinical Alzheimer's disease: current knowledge and future directions. In *New frontiers in cognitive aging* (eds. R.D. Dixon, L. Backman and L.G. Nilsson), pp. 161–77, copyright 2004, with permission from Oxford University Press.)

interactions of genetic susceptibility, biological factors, and environmental exposures experienced over the lifespan. A summary of all these factors is reported in Table 8.3.2, according to different biological mechanisms and grade of scientific evidence. As a part of an initiative of the Swedish Council on Technology Assessment in Health Care, specific criteria to summarize the scientific evidence concerning risk and protective factors for dementia have been proposed. Similar to criteria adopted for other diseases, these criteria first integrate the internal validity with basic causal criteria to weight the study quality, and then they take into account also number and proportion of the included studies reporting a specific association.[29] Moderate or strong evidence supports several genetic, vascular, and psychosocial factors as significantly related to both AD and dementia risk. Whereas implementing preventive strategies targeting the genetic susceptibility is limited, the other two hypotheses can easily lead to prevention programmes.

### (a) Genetic hypothesis

First-degree relatives of AD patients have a higher lifetime risk of developing AD than the general population or relatives of non-demented subjects. Both genetic and environmental factors contribute to the phenomenon of familial aggregation. Twin studies have shown that heritability of AD is about 58 per cent, whereas other variance may be attributable to non-genetic factors.[30] The APOE ε4 allele is the only established susceptibility gene factor for both early- and late-onset AD. The risk effect of APOE ε4 allele decreases with increasing age, and after age 75 years, 15–20 per cent of AD cases are attributable to APOE genotype.[31] Familial aggregation of dementia and AD can be only partially explained by APOE polymorphism, implying that other genetic factors may be active and need to be detected.[32] Several other genes have been examined as possible candidates, but the reports are sporadic or the results are inconsistent.[33]

### (b) Vascular hypothesis

Whereas the reported association between vascular risk factors and dementia risk is expected, due to vascular dementia, several

explanations have been proposed for the association between vascular risk factors and Alzheimer-type dementia: (1) coexistence of vascular factors and AD pathology in the elderly; (2) precipitating effect of cerebrovascular disease or interactive effect between Alzheimer-type and vascular lesions in the brain; and (3) misclassification of mixed dementia as AD. Even if the mechanisms are still not fully understood, prevention may be possible as most vascular risk factors and diseases are modifiable or amenable to prevention and treatment. Controlling high blood pressure in middle age, avoiding mid-life obesity, and appropriately treating diabetes are the major intervention actions. Some studies also show that people who maintain tight control over their blood glucose levels tend to score better on tests of cognitive function than those with poorly controlled diabetes. Indeed, borderline diabetes or impaired glucose tolerance is also linked to an increased risk of dementia and AD in very old people.[34] Finally, to postpone clinical expression of the dementia syndrome in old people, preventing recurrent cerebrovascular disease as well as maintaining sufficient cerebral perfusion by adequately managing heart failure and avoiding very low blood pressure seems to be critical.

### (c) Psychosocial hypothesis

Evidence from both epidemiological and biological studies indicates that factors acting at different periods across life course and having an intellectually stimulating nature may contribute in increasing the neural reserve and therefore promote functionally more efficient cognitive networks to cope with brain pathology and delay the onset of clinical manifestations of dementia. These factors include education, adult-life occupational work complexity as well as late-life social network and intellectually stimulating activities.[29,35] Although physical exercise may reduce the risk of brain damage due to atherosclerosis, the relevance of physical activity itself remains in debate, as most physical activities include also social and mental components. Complex leisure activities with physical, mental, and social components seem to have the most beneficial effect.[36] In addition to the reserve hypothesis, other mechanisms such as premorbid cognitive ability, vascular damage,

**Table 8.3.2** Scientific evidence supporting risk and protective (in italic) factors of dementia and AD by different aetiological hypotheses.

| | Risk and *protective* factors | | | |
|---|---|---|---|---|
| | Vascular | Psychosocial | Genetic | Others |
| **Insufficient or limited scientific evidence** | High cholesterol<br>Cigarette smoking<br>Obesity<br>Late life high BP<br>Late life low BP<br>Heart failure<br>Silent stroke<br>*Moderate alcohol intake*<br>*Dietary factors (e.g. fish and vegetables)* | Depression<br>Low SES<br>*Midlife physical activity*<br>*Late life social network* | Several susceptibility genes | Head trauma<br>Inflammatory markers<br>*NSAIDs*<br>*HRT*<br>Folate and vitamins B12, A, E, and C deficiency<br>Occupational exposure to toxics<br><br>*Antioxidants* |
| **Moderate or strong scientific evidence** | Midlife high BP<br>Diabetes mellitus<br>Clinical stroke<br>Atherosclerosis<br>*Antihypertensive drugs* | Low education<br>*Late life mentally stimulating activities*<br>*Physical activity* | APOE ε4 allele*<br>Familial aggregation | |

Abbreviations: AD = Alzheimer's disease; APOE = apolipoprotein E gene; BP = blood pressure; HRT = hormone replacement therapy; NSAIDs = non-steroidal anti-inflammatory drugs; SES = socioeconomic status.

(Reproduced from Backman, L., Small, B.J. and Fratiglioni, L. Cognitive deficits in preclinical Alzheimer's disease: current knowledge and future directions. In *New frontiers in cognitive aging* (eds. R.D. Dixion, L. Backman and L.G. Nilsson), pp. 161–77, copyright 2004, with permission from Oxford University Press, New York)

neuroprotection, or detection bias may be possible explanations. The most likely effect of a mentally, physically, and socially active life is to postpone the onset of clinical dementia: even delaying dementia onset by 5 years would halve dementia prevalence and substantially decrease the number of dementia cases in the community.

### Prevalence and impact

Despite different inclusion criteria, several meta-analyses of prevalence studies have resulted in strikingly similar results (Ref.[27]; Table 8.3.1). Currently, more than 24 million people in the world have dementia and this number will double in 20 years.[37]

The prognosis of dementia is dramatic. In 3 years, more than 50 per cent of the dementia cases progress to the severe stage. In the Kungsholmen Project, the proportion of severe dementia among prevalent cases increased from 19 per cent at baseline to 48 per cent after 3 years, and to 78 per cent after 7 years. This progression is due to both cognitive and functional decline. The mean annual rate of cognitive decline as measured with the MMSE varies from –4.0 to –2.0 points. Many predictors of a more rapid cognitive decline have been reported such as initial higher cognitive function, functional disability, and brain lesions. The APOE ε4 allele seems not to act as relevant prognostic factor.[38]

Dementia is strongly associated with disability being the major determinant of developing dependence and functional decline over 3 years. Approximately half of the persons who developed functional dependence in a 3-year period can be attributable to dementia.[39] In industrialized countries, mental disease and cognitive impairment are the most prevalent disorders among older adults living in nursing homes or other institutions. However, institutionalization of dementia patients varies depending on age structure, urban or rural residence, and other cultural aspects. In the 75+-year-old population, 70 per cent of incident dementia cases die during the 5 years following the diagnosis, accounting for a mortality rate specific for dementia of 2.4 per 100 person-years. Dementia triplicates the risk of death.[40]

## Conclusion

Mental disorders are common chronic conditions among the elderly people, and the absolute number of subjects with psychiatric disorders will increase dramatically worldwide in the near future due to the ageing of the populations. In addition, the mental disorders have a high impact both at the individual and societal level. Prevention may represent one answer to these challenging conditions. The scientific advances of the last few years have provided sufficiently strong evidence supporting two possible preventative strategies: an active and stimulating lifestyle in late life as well as optimal control of other chronic disease both at middle and late age may decrease the risk of relevant psychiatric disorders such as AD and other dementias.

## Further information

Hybels, C.F. and Blazer, D.G. (2003). Epidemiology of late-life mental disorders. *Clinics in Geriatric Medicine*, **19**, 663–96.

Blazer, D.G. and Hybels, C.F. (2005). Origins of depression in later life. *Psychological Medicine*, **35**, 1241–52.

Jorm, A.F. (2001). History of depression as a risk factor for dementia: an updated review. *The Australian and New Zealand Journal of Psychiatry*, **35**, 776–81.

Ferri, C.P., Prince, M., Brayne, C., *et al.* (2005). Global prevalence of dementia: a Delphi consensus study. *Lancet*, **366**, 2112–17.

Qiu, C., De Ronchi, D., and Fratiglioni, L. (2007). The epidemiology of the dementias: an update. *Current Opinion in Psychiatry*, **20**, 380–5.

Fratiglioni, L. and Wang, H.X. (2007). Brain reserve hypothesis in dementia. *Journal of Alzheimer's Disease*, **12**(1): 11–22.

Fratiglioni, L., von Strauss, E. and Qiu, C., (2007). Epidemiology of the dementias of old age. In *Oxford textbook of old age psychiatry* (eds. R. Jacoby, T. Dening, A. Thomas, and C. Oppenheimer), pp. 391–406. Oxford University Press, Oxford.

## References

1. Kinsella, K. and Velkoff, V.A. (2002). The demographics of aging. *Aging Clinical and Experimental Research*, **4**, 59–69.

2. The US Centers for Disease Control and Prevention. (2003). Public health and aging: trends in aging—United States and worldwide. *The Journal of the American Medical Association*, **289**, 1371–3.

3. Henderson, A.S. (1994). Does ageing protect against depression? *Social Psychiatry and Psychiatric Epidemiology*, **29**, 107–9.

4. Klerman, G.L. and Weissman, M.M. (1989). Increasing rates of depression. *The Journal of the American Medical Association*, **261**, 2229–35.

5. Frombone, E. (1995). Depressive disorders: time trends and possible explanatory mechanisms. In *Psychosocial disorders in young people* (eds. M. Rutter and D.J. Smith). John Wiley & Sons, Chichester.

6. World Health Organization. (2007). Suicide prevention and special programmes. http://www.who.int/mental_health/prevention/suicide/country_reports/en/index.html.

7. Rose, G. (1993). Mental disorder and the strategies of prevention. *Psychological Medicine*, **23**, 553–5.

8. Mann, J.J., Apter, A., Bertolote, J., *et al.* (2004). Suicide prevention strategies: a systematic review. *The Journal of the American Medical Association*, **294**, 2064–74.

9. Burns, A., Bergmann, K., and Lindesay, J. (1998). Key papers in geriatric psychiatry. *International Journal of Geriatric Psychiatry*, **13**, 199–202.

10. Howard, R., Rabins, P.V., Seeman, M.V., *et al.* (2000). Late-onset schizophrenia and very-late-onset schizophrenia-like psychosis: an international consensus. The International Late-Onset Schizophrenia Group. *The American Journal of Psychiatry*, **157**, 172–8.

11. Beullens, J. and Aertgeerts, B. (2004). Screening for alcohol abuse and dependence in older people using DSM criteria: a review. *Aging and Mental Health*, **8**, 76–82.

12. Johnson, I. (2000). Alcohol problems in old age: a review of recent epidemiological research. *International Journal of Geriatric Psychiatry*, **15**, 575–81.

13. Agüero-Torres, H., Kivipelto, M., and von Strauss, E. (2006). Rethinking the dementia diagnoses in a population-based study: what is Alzheimer's disease and what is vascular dementia? A study from the Kungsholmen project. *Dementia and Geriatric Cognitive Disorders*, **22**, 244–9.

14. Fratiglioni, L., Qiu, C., and Palmer, K. (2006). Vascular cognitive impairment: time for prevention? *Alzheimer's & Dementia*, **2**, 202–4.

15. Bäckman, L., Small, B.J., and Fratiglioni, L. (2004). Cognitive deficits in preclinical Alzheimer's disease: current knowledge and future directions. In *New frontiers in cognitive aging* (eds. R.D. Dixon, L. Bäckman, and L.-G. Nilsson), pp. 161–77. Oxford University Press, Oxford.

16. Bäckman, L., Jones, S., Berger, A.K., *et al.* (2005). Cognitive impairment in preclinical Alzheimer's disease: a meta-analysis. *Neuropsychology*, **19**, 520–31.

17. Palmer, K. and Fratiglioni, L. (2006). Is mild cognitive impairment a distinct clinical entity? *Aging Health*, **2**, 763–9.

18. Gauthier, S., Reisberg, B., Zaudig, M., *et al.* (2006). Mild cognitive impairment. *Lancet*, **367**, 1262–70.

19. Portet, F., Ousset, P.J., Visser, P.J., *et al.* (2006). For the MCI working group of the European Consortium on Alzheimer's Disease (EADC). Mild cognitive impairment (MCI) in medical practice: a critical review of the concept and new diagnostic procedure. *Journal of Neurology, Neurosurgery, and Psychiatry*, **77**, 714–18.

20. Palmer, K., Bäckman, L., Winblad, B., *et al.* (2003). Detection of Alzheimer's disease and dementia in the preclinical phase: population-based cohort study. *British Medical Journal*, **326**, 245.

21. Sacuiu, S., Sjogren, M., Johansson, B., *et al.* (2005). Prodromal cognitive signs of dementia in 85-year-olds using four sources of information. *Neurology*, **65**, 1894–900.

22. Palmer, K., Wang, H.X., Bäckman, L., *et al.* (2002). Differential evolution of cognitive impairment in nondemented older persons: results from the Kungsholmen project. *The American Journal of Psychiatry*, **159**, 436–42.

23. Monastero, R., Palmer, K., Qiu, C., *et al.* (2007). Heterogeneity in risk factors for CIND. A population-based longitudinal study from the Kungsholmen project. *The American Journal of Geriatric Psychiatry*, **15**, 60–9.

24. Panza, F., D'Introno, A., Colacicco, A.M., *et al.* (2005). Current epidemiology of mild cognitive impairment and other predementia syndromes. *The American Journal of Geriatric Psychiatry*, **13**, 633–44.

25. De Ronchi, D., Berardi, D., Menchetti, M., *et al.* (2005). Occurrence of cognitive impairment and dementia after the age of 60: a population-based study from Northern Italy. *Dementia and Geriatric Cognitive Disorders*, **19**, 97–105.

26. Caracciolo, B., Palmer, K., Monastero, R., *et al.* (2008). Occurrence of cognitive impairment and dementia in the community: a 9-year long prospective study. *Neurology*, **70**, 1778–85.

27. Fratiglioni, L., von Strauss, E., and Qiu, C. (2007). Epidemiology of the dementias of old age. In *The Oxford textbook of old age psychiatry* (eds. R. Jacoby, T. Dening, A. Thomas, and C. Oppenheimer), pp. 391–406. Oxford University Press, Oxford.

28. Matthews, F. and Brayne, C. (2005). Medical Research Council Cognitive Function and Ageing Study Investigators. The incidence of dementia in England and Wales: findings from the five identical sites of the MRC CFA study. *PLoS Medicine*, **2**, e193.

29. Fratiglioni, L. and Wang, H.-X. (2007). Brain reserve hypothesis in dementia. *Journal of Alzheimer's Disease*, **12**(1), 11–22.

30. Gatz, M., Reynolds, C.A., Fratiglioni, L., *et al.* (2006). Role of genes and environments for explaining Alzheimer disease. *Archives of General Psychiatry*, **63**, 168–74.

31. Qiu, C.X., Kivipelto, M., Agüero-Torres, H., *et al.* (2004). Risk and protective effects of APOE gene towards Alzheimer's disease in the Kungsholmen project: variation by age and sex. *Journal of Neurology, Neurosurgery, and Psychiatry*, **75**, 828–33.

32. Huang, W.Y., Qiu, C.X., von Strauss, E., *et al.* (2004). APOE genotype, family history of dementia, and Alzheimer disease risk: a 6-year follow-up study. *Archives of Neurology*, **61**, 1930–4.

33. D'Introno, A., Solfrizzi, V., Colacicco, A.M., *et al.* (2006). Current knowledge of chromosome 12 susceptibility genes for late-onset Alzheimer's disease. *Neurobiology of Aging*, **27**, 1537–53.

34. Xu, W., Qiu, C., Winblad, B., *et al.* (2007). The effect of borderline diabetes on the risk of dementia and Alzheimer's disease. *Diabetes*, **56**, 211–16.

35. Fratiglioni, L., Paillard-Borg, S., *et al.* (2004). An active and socially integrated life in late life might protect against dementia. *Lancet Neurology*, **4**, 3343–53.

36. Karp, A., Paillard-Borg, S., Wang, H.X., *et al.* (2006). Mental, physical and social components in leisure activities equally contribute to decrease dementia risk. *Dementia and Geriatric Cognitive Disorders*, **21**, 65–73.

37. Ferri, C.P., Prince, M., Brayne, C., *et al.* (2005). Global prevalence of dementia: a Delphi consensus study. *Lancet*, **366**, 2112–17.

38. Agüero-Torres, H., Qiu, C., Winblad, B., *et al.* (2002). Dementing disorders in the elderly: evolution of disease severity over 7 years. *Alzheimer Disease and Associated Disorders*, **16**, 221–7.

39. Agüero-Torres, H., Fratiglioni, L., Guo, Z., *et al.* (1998). Dementia is the major cause of functional dependence in the elderly: 3-year follow-up data from a population-based study. *American Journal of Public Health*, **88**, 1452–6.

40. Agüero-Torres, H., Fratiglioni, L., Guo, Z., *et al.* (1999). Mortality from dementia in advanced age: a 5-year follow-up study of incident dementia cases. *Journal of Clinical Epidemiology*, **52**, 737–43.

## 8.4

# Assessment of mental disorder in older patients

Robin Jacoby

The assessment of older people is not fundamentally different from that of younger patients. The principles of taking history and mental-state examination are the same at any age. But if the goals are common, the routes taken to reach them are not necessarily so. For example, an assessment adequate enough to begin treatment of a 30-year-old woman presenting to an outpatient clinic with a depressive illness might take about an hour and involve speaking only to the patient and perhaps briefly to her partner, whereas the equivalent assessment of an 81-year-old woman in whom uncertainty exists as to whether the diagnosis is that of a depressive or a dementing illness may require more than one interview and necessitate enquiry from several informants. This section will not repeat what can be found in Chapter 1.8.1, but cover only those points which are specific to or need to be emphasized for older patients.

## The referral process

### Who refers?

Whilst the referral process might be the same as for younger patients, it is more often different. In many cases the patient has no idea why, or indeed does not even know or has forgotten that she has been referred. (The feminine gender is used in this chapter because older women are more likely to develop a mental illness and to survive longer than men. However, what is written applies also to men.)

The process has most often been initiated by family members who might not have discussed it with the patient. Many old people live alone with no relatives nearby or even in the same country or state, so that referrals are frequently initiated by friends, neighbours, or other acquaintances, such as local shopkeepers, social services care workers, and people who run luncheon clubs.

### Reasons for referral

In the case of a woman of 30 with a depressive illness, she is referred to a psychiatrist for treatment to effect a remission. However, an older woman of 80 with a similar condition may be referred for a variety of reasons including the following: the primary care doctor might be uncertain of the diagnosis, that is whether it could be dementia; the grown-up children might have removal from home to residential or nursing care as the first item on their agenda; the patient's condition may not be the primary issue—there may be greater concern for her husband who is failing to cope, perhaps to the extent of physically abusing her.

## The informants

A large number of older people seen by psychiatrists are unable to give complete or reliable information about themselves. Frequently, but not invariably, there is a spouse or adult offspring living with the patient. In other cases, however, it is necessary to track down someone less obvious. Neighbours are often helpful at relating recent history, but may know little of past personal or family history. Effort spent in telephoning relatives, even those on the other side of the world, can be invaluable in giving an account of such items as family history or premorbid personality. If an informant is not readily available, for example, because it is night-time in Australia, the psychiatrist should not shelve the task of phoning, but only defer it to the next available opportunity.

Where conflicting information is given by a variety of informants it might be necessary to weigh up the particular 'hidden agenda' of each one. For example, the husband of a demented woman may minimize his wife's behaviour disturbance for fear that she would be 'put away'; whereas the daughter may overstate it in order to support a case for her mother's transfer to a nursing home because her father repeatedly phones her for assistance at all hours of the day and night. Each one of the two informants has cogent reasons for weighting the information, but the psychiatrist and his or her team cannot help to resolve the situation until they understand those reasons.

## Professional informants

Psychogeriatrics is as dependent on multi-disciplinary working as any other branch of psychiatry. Many patients seen for the first time will already be well known to their primary care doctor who will be able to provide invaluable information. The same frequently applies to community psychiatric nurses who now take referrals directly from general practitioners and may themselves be making referrals to the old-age psychiatry service. The psychogeriatrician can save a great deal of time and effort by consulting community psychiatric nurses and general practitioners before seeing the patient or relatives.

## Where to assess the patient

The patient needs to be placed at her maximum advantage to provide clinical information in whatever setting the assessment takes place. This has to be stated explicitly because the doctor is often required to take active steps to ensure it. Account has to be taken of special sensory impairment. Poor vision may need lights to be switched on so that the patient can see who is asking her questions. Distracting noises will make it even more difficult for someone with hearing impairment to grasp what is said. Surprisingly often, this may require a request that the television be switched off. Most importantly, examiners need to sit facing the patient with the lips visible, to speak slowly, and to enunciate words carefully. The patient should then be asked if she can hear properly. Simply shouting at her is not a substitute for these simple steps.

Social customs vary within and between societies. For instance, in the United Kingdom and the United States the use of first names is much more acceptable with younger adults than it was 40 years ago. With the current generation of older patients it is not. For them to be called by their first names unbidden is disrespectful and infantilizing. Even if nurses and other non-medical staff do so, doctors should not use first names, unless specifically invited. Instead, the surname plus appropriate title (Mr, Mrs, etc.) is correct.

## At home

The preferred place to assess older patients is in their own homes, although circumstances sometimes dictate that it will be elsewhere. At home patients feel less intimidated and can be seen within an environment which tells the psychiatrist a great deal that he cannot know in the clinic. If a house is filthy and cold and the patient in a similar state, and if there is reliable information that this is only a recent phenomenon, then it is a powerful descriptor of the patient's inability to cope. However, the converse is not always true; a clean and tidy home may only reflect someone else's willingness to support and care for the patient who could not otherwise do it herself (e.g. a daughter or neighbour). Another advantage of a home assessment is that cognitive disabilities, such as dyspraxia and agnosia, can be tested in an ecologically valid way (making tea, recognition of family members from photographs) that is more acceptable to a patient than being formally tested with the Mini-Mental State Examination.[1]

Assessments at home require more preparation for the doctor than is necessary at outpatient clinics where equipment for physical examination and blood tests are available, for example. It is an obvious courtesy to the patient to let her know of the visit beforehand, but it is also wise to arrange for a suitable informant to be present. Furthermore, some older patients are incapable of letting visitors into their houses and the informant might well first have to facilitate the doctor's access. Elderly patients are much more likely to be suffering from comorbid physical illness which may be the fundamental cause of the mental disorder, for example, pneumonia or a urinary tract infection manifesting delirium. The old-age psychiatrist does not therefore need to adhere rigidly to lines of specialty demarcation but rather be aware of the possibility of and prepared to search for physical illness. The basic equipment for a medical examination, such as a stethoscope, sphygmomanometer, and patellar hammer are items to be taken on home visits. Urine testing strips and a thermometer, especially a low-reading thermometer, are also sometimes useful.

## In a psychiatric hospital

Patients who are assessed after admission to psychiatric beds lack the advantages of being in their own environment, although the opportunity for physical examination is much easier. Another advantage for hospital inpatients is that the assessment can be carried out over a longer period of time, since older people tire more easily and cooperation varies from day-to-day. For example, some demented patients will object to undergoing full cognitive assessment in one go, especially because they are often aware that they are failing. If a few questions are asked in the course of several short sessions, a more accurate and complete picture of the patient's abilities eventually emerges. If the Mini-Mental State Examination is administered in this way, a higher total can be achieved than if an attempt to administer it all at once meets with sullen refusal after the first few questions, with all subsequent ones having to be scored zero.

Information from other informants is as crucial for hospital inpatients as it is for those seen at home. It is usually the responsibility of the house officer or resident to collect the history, and they may be required to telephone several informants in distant and local parts to obtain a full picture which the patient is incapable of providing.

## Liaison visits in general hospitals

Liaison visits to patients in general hospitals make up a considerable part of the old-age psychiatrist's work because comorbid mental and physical illnesses are very common. In spite of the fact that the host nurse's instinct is to lead the visiting psychiatrist straightaway to the patient's bedside, the latter should insist on first reading the case notes (charts) and speaking to the nursing staff who know her best. From the case notes and the prescription cards (medication orders) invaluable information on current and past drug therapy as well as details of the patient's medical history are obtained. Clues as to the patient's mental state are often best gleaned from the records written by the nurses. Nevertheless, non-psychiatrist doctors, surgeons, and nurses are not accustomed to assessment of the mental state and statements such as 'confused' should not be taken at face value, since they stand for anything from slight difficulty in answering complex questions due to anxiety at being in a strange environment to major mental disturbance. As in most other settings, time spent telephoning informants from the general hospital ward is well invested and may permit the visiting old-age psychiatrist to express an opinion on the patient's condition more firmly than would otherwise have been possible.

A useful final step before going to talk to the patient is, if possible, to observe her from a suitable distance. In this way signs of delirium, disruptive behaviour, social interaction, and other phenomena such as dyskinesias may be seen.

When seeing the patient herself, wherever possible she should be taken to a separate room and not examined in an open ward where there are other patients. If it is impossible for the patient to leave her bed, then it is usually feasible to move the bed to a more private place.

## Nursing and residential homes

Much of that which is required for liaison visits to general hospitals applies to assessment in residential or nursing homes, most notably trying to see the patient in a private room away from other residents. Since abuse of elderly people is sometimes an issue in these settings, it is preferable to have at least some time completely alone with the patient first, and if indicated, to check for bruises or other injuries, and secondly to allow the patient to tell the doctor things which she might be frightened to do in front of the staff of the home. Another problem in some nursing and residential homes is that the psychiatrist finds that an untrained or unqualified member of staff accompanies him, the quality of whose information may not be at the level of trained nurses. Careful questioning of several members of staff, attention to written records, and telephone calls to appropriate informants should all improve the quality of the assessment.

## The history

### Family and personal history

As has already been made clear, for many older patients a complete history may have to be obtained from a variety of informants. With the patients themselves a more flexible approach than is taken with younger ones is often needed. Whether intellectual failure is obvious and global or there is only relatively mild cognitive impairment (MCI), for some to give a history that is fully chronologically correct can be too great an effort. The examiner must accept these limitations and try to keep the atmosphere as relaxed as possible. Much more than the young, elderly psychiatric patients perceive the psychiatric interview as an ordeal or a form of trial in which it is easy for them to acquire a sense of failure. This in turn induces anxiety and a vicious spiral of ever worsening performance. One way in which the patient can be put at ease is to reassure her that you will come to her main problem in due course but that it would be good to hear something of her background first. For most older patients the family and personal histories are easier to recall than the confusing events which have led up to the referral. This is not simply good for the patient but for the examiner as well. Amongst the most profitable of pleasures in old-age psychiatry are the life stories of people who have lived during some momentous periods of world history. Furthermore, these stories put patients into a context which makes it much easier to understand why and how they have reacted to the mental illness with which they have presented.

As regards the family history specifically, the examiner needs to be alert to mistakes which could indicate cognitive impairment. A patient may confuse family relationships or misidentify family members quite early in the course of a dementing illness. In other words, inaccurate information from the patient can be as clinically informative as that which is correct. Older patients are not necessarily as sophisticated in medical vocabulary as their children and grandchildren. Therefore, to obtain facts about a possible family history of dementia (an important issue), it may be necessary to ask if any blood relative had 'memory problems' in late life or 'had to go into a home'.

In eliciting the personal history the examiner might need to be aware of the historical context at the time in question. Some older patients, however affluent they may be now, grew up in poverty or other adverse circumstances (e.g. a parent died of tuberculosis during their childhood) which could still be affecting their psychological lives. Similarly, education may have been disrupted in a way that is more unusual nowadays. Some patients, notably women, relate how they missed education because they had to look after their younger siblings after mother died or father was killed, because the remaining parent had to go out to work for the family to survive. A precise enquiry should be made as to educational attainment, and especially the level of literacy and numeracy which may be the only 'baseline' appraisal obtainable for a patient with current dyslexia or dyscalculia.

Whilst it is often very obvious to the examining doctor that a patient has cognitive impairment because of her errors and inconsistencies in giving her personal history, it is very unwise to foreclose on a diagnosis at this stage. Patients with severe depressive illnesses can be even more hesitant than those with, for example, Alzheimer's disease, or show such retardation and lack of concentration on what is being asked that they can portray a clinical picture that is not easily distinguishable from a state of advanced dementia.

### Medical and psychiatric history

The nature of the information required is no different from that in younger patients. However, of particular importance in the older population is past and present medication. Drugs taken at the prescribed dose, at a wrong dose (due to dementia), or drugs no longer intended to be taken and prescribed sometimes quite a long time ago but of which a residual supply remains, are all potent causes of confusion and even frank delirium in old people. It is therefore good practice to ask to see where all medication is kept and to examine each pack or bottle to check that the amount left is approximately proportionate to that which one might expect given the date the drugs were dispensed. Since elderly people are frequently the victims of clinically injudicious polypharmacy, it is common to find a large quantity of current and prescription-expired drugs which the patient is taking on a random basis. To counter this problem proprietary boxes which dispense drugs in daily amounts, such as the Dosette or Nomad systems, are used and can more easily be checked for compliance or overdosing.

### Premorbid personality

Personality is one of the prime determinants of outcome in mental illness at any age, but where older people are concerned too little effort is made, partly for lack of reliable informants, to give a valid assessment of personality. False assumptions are made that someone has always been awkward or cantankerous, whereas it is shown later that they have become so because of frontal-lobe impairment. Similarly, it is sometimes assumed that a woman has always exhibited attention-seeking or manipulative behaviour, when to the surprise of doctors and nurses alike such behaviour disappears following effective treatment for a depressive illness. Every effort should be made to find a reliable informant before reaching such conclusions.

## The mental state examination

### Appearance, behaviour, and the environment

A great deal can be learnt from the appearance of the patient and her home environment. Signs of neglect in both are commonly found. A brief tour of the home may reveal rotten food, little or no food, empty bottles of liquor, evidence of poor hygiene or incontinence, and inadequate heating. The patient may be dirty and unkempt, and clothes may have been put on in the wrong order (dressing dyspraxia). Particular attention should be paid to relatively mild impairment of attention and concentration, since it might betray a delirium which can be treated to achieve a remarkable improvement in the patient's condition. Agitation is another sign to be carefully sought. Sometimes agitation is obvious with behaviour such as pacing and sighing which make it almost impossible to communicate with the patient, but at other times it can be allied to psychomotor retardation and perceptible only in tireless movements of the fingers.

### Talk

Dysphasia in any of its guises is a frequent manifestation of dementia. Sometimes it is obvious, but not always. For example, it may be difficult at first to differentiate between an expressive dysphasia (Broca's dysphasia) and retardation. It is relatively mild or moderate receptive dysphasia (Wernicke's dysphasia), however, which traps the unwary clinician. In such cases the patient may appear to be obtuse, unintelligent, or hard of hearing until it is appreciated that she simply does not understand a considerable proportion of what is said to her.

Even if the patient is not dysphasic, she may be evasive and given to circumlocution. Again, this should not be taken automatically as evidence of a premorbid lack of intelligence or pomposity, since it is frequently used as a camouflage for cognitive impairment. A patient with dementia might say 'Oh of course I know that' or 'I never paid any attention to that sort of thing' when asked to give an item of current affairs.

In manic or hypomanic illness in old-age slow flight of ideas is sometimes missed by inexperienced clinicians or mistaken for evidence of cognitive impairment. Here the normal coherence of thought is disrupted because the patient is distracted from one idea to another, just as in characteristic flight of ideas, but they are delivered at a normal or even slower pace. The latter can occur if a mixed affective state is present.

### Thought content

Much of that which applies to younger patients applies also to older ones and does not need to be mentioned here. However, subtle changes in thought content amounting to a restriction in breadth and a repetitiveness of themes may be noticed. Formal thought disorder which is found in young patients with schizophrenia is extremely rare in the old.

### Mood

Depressive illness is commonly missed in older patients. This is partly because the clinical picture can mimic a dementing illness, so that a history from a reliable informant, as has already been stressed, is mandatory. Another reason is so-called *masked depression* in which the patient denies depressed mood but presents with other symptoms, such as those of apparent physical illness. In this sort of case a reliable account of sleep and appetite disturbance, weight loss, and anhedonia give clues as to the presence of an affective disorder. It should also be remembered that dementia and depressive illness are common disorders and not infrequently occur together, so that the diagnosis of one does not rule out the other.

Older men are still the group most at risk of suicide in most countries of the world where statistics are recorded (see Chapter 4.15.1). The psychiatrist does not shrink from specific enquiry about suicidal thinking in patients of any age, but it can sometimes be difficult to differentiate between a rational desire to die when the time comes and active suicidal ideation. In-depth probing is therefore mandatory and the examiner should not be put off by the patient's attempts to leave the topic, if he or she thinks that there is likely to be risk of self-harm.

### Cognitive examination

In assessing elderly patients more emphasis is usually placed on the cognitive examination than in younger patients. In theory it can be as exhaustive and thorough as assessment by a neuropsychologist, but in the routine practice of old-age psychiatry it usually has to be feasible within the constraints of a consultation which lasts about an hour.

It is in this part of the assessment that the examiner is most likely to lose the patient's cooperation, principally because of the humiliation experienced by some at their own failures. Some patients become angry, indignant, or defensive. Others become anxious and their performance deteriorates. One way to pre-empt this is to preface testing by stressing that this is not a competitive examination and that most people have difficulty answering some of the questions. Correct answers are praised without excessive emphasis and incorrect ones are either treated in a neutral way or given a positive spin by saying, for example, 'Well it's…, but you weren't far off'.

Many old-age psychiatrists and other members of their multi-disciplinary team prefer to use standardized questionnaires, such as the Mini-Mental State Examination,[1] the questionnaire in widest use. It has the advantage that results between and within patients can be compared and progress can be monitored. However, no off-the-shelf test is exhaustive and none produces an adequate cognitive assessment by itself. The clinician therefore needs to have some sort of schema for covering the main areas of cognitive function which would include: memory (in its various aspects) and general information, and naming; the understanding and production of language; praxis (ideomotor and constructional); sensory recognition (gnosis); abstract reasoning; verbal fluency; calculation; left/right orientation; and executive function (the ability to integrate mental processes for goal-directed activity). The list is not exhaustive and some areas may need to be covered in greater detail as the clinical situation demands. Table 8.4.1 gives a guide to cognitive examination based on an extended Mini-Mental State Examination. Clinicians vary in the order and way in which they test individual cognitive functions, and the list in Table 8.4.1 is not intended to be prescriptive.

### Other aspects of the mental state examination

These do not differ in essence from that in younger adults and are not covered in this section.

## Physical assessment

Since physical comorbidity is extremely common, the old-age psychiatrist needs to be able and willing to conduct a basic physical examination. In the patient's home this may not always be easy. For instance, it may not be kind to ask a frail person who takes an hour or more to dress and come downstairs in the morning to return to her bed and undress, but it is usually possible to make a reasonable examination of the arterial pulse, blood pressure, and jugular venous pulse, and to auscultate the heart and lungs when

**Table 8.4.1** Schema for testing cognitive functions based on an extended mini-mental state examination

| Function | Subfunction | Examples |
| --- | --- | --- |
| Orientation | Time | Year, month, date, day, season |
| | Place | Own address or that of hospital, city, county/state, country |
| | Person | Own name (married women sometimes cannot give married name); recognize others by name or function (e.g. you are a doctor) |
| Memory | Immediate recall | Immediate repetition of three objects or a name and (local) address |
| | Delayed recall | Repetition as above but after a distractor task |
| | Long-term recall | Give historical or personal events (that can be verified) |
| | General information | Names of politicians or other VIPs |
| Concentration | | Months of the year in reverse order, counting from 20 back to 1; spelling WORLD forwards then backwards |
| Praxis | Construction | Copy diagram of interlocking pentagons |
| | Ideomotor | Draw a clock and set the hands at a specified time (also a test of executive function) |
| | Dressing | Put on a jacket; undo, and refasten buttons |
| Sensory recognition (gnosis) | Visual including prosopagnosia | Recognize photographs taken from unusual angles and of familiar faces |
| | Auditory | Recognize the doorbell |
| | Tactile | Recognize objects placed in the palm, e.g. coins |
| | Reading | Any sample *but* use large print, e.g. newspaper headlines |
| | Olfactory | Recognize something from the kitchen, e.g. coffee |
| Language | Expressive | Repeat 'no ifs ands or buts' |
| | Understanding | Carry out a three-stage command |
| | Naming | Naming objects of increasing complexity |
| Verbal fluency | | List as many items from a category as possible in 1 min, such as boys' and girls' forenames, or as many words beginning with a specified letter |
| Writing | | Write an ordinary English sentence |
| Calculation | | Not too complex—subtraction of serial sevens from 100 is too difficult for many. A simple sum involving money is better |
| Left–right orientation | | Face–hand test (e.g. left hand to left ear, right hand to left ear); finger recognition on own and examiner's hand |
| Abstract reasoning | | 'In what way are an apple and a banana alike?' 'In what way are a boat and a car similar?' Interpretation of simple proverbs |

Testing one function usually depends on one or more others; for example, most tests depend on understanding of language. Examples are neither prescriptive nor exhaustive.

the patient is seated. Similarly, a partial neurological examination for signs of focal deficits is also possible. However, if something alerts the doctor to the need to examine an undressed and supine patient, the duty should not be shirked, lest a hitherto unsuspected abdominal mass, or a strangulated hernia are missed.

Patients admitted to psychiatric hospital or nursing home beds should all undergo a physical examination. Focal neurological signs may indicate the cause of dementia. Carcinoma of the breast which either dementia or fear has prevented the patient from declaring may be much more treatable than she has believed. All the physical disorders which may be revealed are too numerous to mention, but their detection and treatment nearly always contribute to an improvement in mental function.

### Laboratory investigations

Owing to tight budgetary constraints it is sometimes argued that routine laboratory investigations, such as full blood count and chest radiography, are unnecessary for younger adults. Whether or not this is true, with older patients such tests are strongly advised because the treatment of comorbid physical illness improves mental disorder. Furthermore, a treatable or arrestable cause of

dementia may be found. For patients with dementia the following are recommended: full blood count; serum electrolytes, and creatinine; liver and thyroid function tests; syphilis serology; vitamin $B_{12}$ and red cell folate; chest radiography. Medical and nursing staff should also have a low threshold for sending urine for microbiological examination (see superimposed delirium below). The vexed question of neuroimaging, an expensive procedure, is much discussed and the debate is not easily summarized or resolved. Most space-occupying lesions can be detected, as can many vascular changes. However, there is nothing pathognomonic for Alzheimer's disease on CT, magnetic resonance imaging, or single-photon emission tomography. In Alzheimer's disease, scans may support the diagnosis but not establish it.

## General considerations in the assessment of older psychiatric patients

### Falls

The causes of falls in older people are many and the reader is referred to textbooks of geriatric medicine for a full discussion. However, the old-age psychiatrist needs to be aware that many psychotropic drugs precipitate falls through postural hypotension, with tricyclic antidepressants and neuroleptics being particular offenders. Neuroleptics induce parkinsonism, putting the patient at risk of tripping against rugs or items of furniture. The clinical implications of falls, especially in older women, are serious because patients are at risk of a fractured neck of femur or (less commonly) a subdural haematoma, both of which carry a high mortality.

### Nutrition

Poor nutrition is commonly found in patients presenting to old-age psychiatry services. Even in affluent societies many older people are amongst the most impoverished or feel that they cannot afford good food. Some are too frail to get out to the shops. Others lack motivation to shop and eat because of depressive illness. Patients suffering from dementia may be incapable of shopping and preparing food. Widowers might never have learned to cook. A vitamin $B_{12}$ or folate level at the lower end of the reference range, or even below it, is as often a reflection of poor nutrition as an indication of pernicious anaemia.

### Superimposed delirium

Here it is mentioned only that subacute delirium superimposed on another condition is at risk of not being recognized because it is taken to be a manifestation of the underlying illness, usually dementia. This is particularly the case when a subclinical urinary tract infection occurs in a demented patient. It is of clinical relevance because treatment of the urinary tract infection results in a great improvement in the patient's mental state. On routine assessment particular attention should therefore be paid in the history to evidence of sudden worsening of a stable or only slowly deteriorating condition, and to nocturnal disturbance especially with (usually visual) hallucinations. On examination of the patient herself the level of consciousness, awareness of the environment, attention, and concentration should be noted.

Delirium is described in Chapter 4.1.1, and special features in older people are considered in Chapter 8.5.1.

## Reassessment after treatment

Because so much of psychiatry is practised in the community, it is impossible for all patients to be reassessed by a psychiatrist after treatment. In hospital or outpatient clinics it is feasible, but not for the majority of older patients who live at home. Furthermore, in areas where the population is geographically widespread, it is very difficult if not impossible for many older people, who may be frail and infirm, to travel long distances to attend clinics. Much of the follow-up assessment in old-age psychiatric services is therefore carried out by other members of the multi-disciplinary team, such as psychologists or occupational therapists, but mostly by community psychiatric nurses. It is essential for the psychiatrist to meet regularly with members of the team seeing patients in the community to discuss the progress of individual patients following treatment.

## Further information

Goldberg, D. and Murray, R. (eds.) (2006). *The Maudsley handbook of practical psychiatry* (5th edn). Oxford University Press, Oxford.

Hodges, J.R. (2007). *Cognitive assessment for clinicians* (2nd edn). Oxford University Press, Oxford.

Jacoby, R., Oppenheimer, C., Dening, T. *et al.* (eds.) (2008). *The Oxford textbook of old age psychiatry*. Chap. 10–12. Oxford University Press, Oxford.

## References

1. Folstein, M.F., Folstein, S.E., and McHugh, P.R. (1975). 'Mini-mental state'. A practical method for grading the cognitive state of patients for the clinician. *Journal of Psychiatric Research*, **12**, 189–98.

# 8.5

# Special features of clinical syndromes in the elderly

## Contents

8.5.1 Delirium in the elderly
James Lindesay

    8.5.1.1 Mild cognitive impairment
        Claudia Jacova and Howard H. Feldman

8.5.2 Substance use disorders in older people
Henry O'Connell and Brian Lawlor

8.5.3 Schizophrenia and paranoid disorders in late life
Barton W. Palmer, Gauri N. Savla, and Thomas W. Meeks

8.5.4 Mood disorders in the elderly
Robert Baldwin

8.5.5 Stress-related, anxiety, and obsessional disorders in elderly people
James Lindesay

8.5.6 Personality disorders in the elderly
Suzanne Holroyd

8.5.7 Suicide and deliberate self-harm in elderly people
Robin Jacoby

8.5.8 Sex in old age
John Kellett and Catherine Oppenheimer

## 8.5.1 Delirium in the elderly

James Lindesay

**Note** Dementia in people of all ages is considered in Part 4, Section 4.1, where the following topics are considered: Chapter 4.1.2 Dementia: Alzheimer's disease; Chapter 4.1.3 Frontotemporal dementias; Chapter 4.1.4 Prion disease; Chapter 4.1.5 Dementia with Lewy bodies; Chapter 4.1.6 Dementia in Parkinson's disease; Chapter 4.1.7 Dementia due to Huntington's disease; Chapter 4.1.8 Vascular dementia; Chapter 4.1.9 Dementia due to HIV disease; Chapter 4.1.10 The neuropsychiatry of head injury; Chapter 4.1.11 Alcohol-related dementia (alcohol-induced dementia; alcohol-related brain damage); Chapter 4.1.13 The management of dementia.

### Introduction

Although delirium occurs at all ages, it is most frequently encountered in late life. This is because delirium is the result of an interaction between individual vulnerability factors (e.g. brain disease, sensory impairment) and external insults (e.g. physical illness, medication), the rates of which both increase with age. Our current concept of delirium derives principally from the florid clinical stereotype that has evolved from centuries of clinical observations on younger patients, and it may not be applicable to our historically unique ageing population. In younger adults, a major physical insult is usually necessary to precipitate delirium, which is often a dramatic disturbance. This is not the case in vulnerable elderly patients when relatively mild physical, psychological, or environmental upsets may be sufficient to bring about acute disturbances of mental functioning. These disturbances may be less obvious than in younger patients, particularly if they occur in the context of pre-existing cognitive impairment. Consequently, despite being common and problematic, delirium in elderly patients is frequently missed or misdiagnosed as dementia or depression by medical and nursing staff.[1] This is unfortunate, because delirium is an important non-specific sign of physical illness or intoxication, and if left untreated there may be costly consequences, both for the patient and for health services.

### Clinical features

The clinical features of delirium are described in Chapter 4.1.1. Most delirium in elderly patients is of the quiet hypoactive variety, lacking the more florid disturbances in mood, perception, and behaviour that bring the disorder to clinical notice. Reversible cognitive impairment in elderly patients is associated with reduced conscious level, poor attention, poor contact with the patient, incoherent speech, reduced psychomotor activity, lack of awareness of surroundings, poor orientation, and poor memory.[2] Hyperactive delirium does occur in elderly patients, but it is less pronounced, with the overactivity usually confined to purposeless behaviour such as pulling at the bedclothes. Violent behaviour is uncommon; elderly patients are more likely to injure themselves than others.

## Classification

The ICD-10 and DSM-IV diagnostic criteria for delirium are described in Chapter 4.1.1. They are not entirely concordant; ICD-10 is more restrictive, resulting in the diagnosis of fewer cases.[3] However, the two systems agree on four essential features: disturbance of consciousness, disturbance of cognition, rapid onset/fluctuating course, and evidence of an external cause. Unfortunately, none of these features is specific for delirium as opposed to dementia, and the current diagnostic criteria are poor predictors of outcome, defined in terms of improvement in cognitive function. Reversibility of cognitive impairment may be the most discriminating feature of delirium,[2] but is problematic as a diagnostic criterion since outcome is unknown at the outset.

Another shortcoming of the current classifications of delirium is that they do not recognize the partial and transitory disturbances that are commonly observed in elderly patients. Subsyndromal delirium is common, and is part of a continuum between normality and the full syndrome. Subsyndromal cases are clinically significant, since they have the same risk factors and the same increased mortality as syndromal cases.[4]

## Diagnosis and differential diagnosis

The diagnosis of delirium is a two-stage process: first, diagnose the delirium, and second, identify the underlying cause or causes. The diagnosis of delirium in elderly patients can be problematic, given the predominantly hypoactive clinical picture and the unreliability of 'positive' symptoms. However, it is important to consider the possibility if cognitive decline is rapid, and if any of the recognized signs and symptoms are present. A good informant history from relatives or ward staff is essential to establish the onset and course of the disorder. Routine screening procedures may be useful in identifying patients who develop delirium while in hospital. Brief instruments such as the Mini-Mental State Examination[5] are not diagnostic, but will alert the clinician to any sudden decline in cognitive function. More extended diagnostic instruments are also available, such as the Delirium Rating Scale,[6] the Confusion Assessment Method,[7] and the Delirium Symptom Interview.[8] Another approach to screening for delirium is to identify those at particular risk of developing the disorder. Predictive factors related to the patient include: visual impairment, severity of illness, cognitive impairment, and a blood urea nitrogen/creatinine ratio of 18 or more.[9] Hospital- and treatment-related factors include: use of restraints, malnutrition, use of more than three medications, bladder catheterization, and the number of iatrogenic events.[10] These factors are multiplicative in their effect.

The differential diagnosis of delirium includes most other psychiatric disorders in this age group. These disorders are themselves risk factors for delirium, so the possibility of co-morbidity must always be considered. When in doubt, investigate and manage as delirium until the situation is clear.

### Dementia

Dementia is a major risk factor for delirium, and in practice co-morbidity commonly occurs. However, differential diagnosis is important, as episodes of delirium need to be identified in order for them to be managed effectively. Recent onset and rapid decline of cognitive functioning, from whatever baseline, indicate an episode of delirium until proved otherwise. Delirium in elderly patients can be prolonged, and failure to recover quickly following treatment of the cause does not necessarily indicate an underlying dementia. It is important to have a good history of pre-morbid functioning.

### Depression

Delirium can be difficult to distinguish from severe depression in elderly patients, cognitive impairment associated with severe depression is usually relatively mild in comparison with the affective disturbance, whereas the reverse is true of delirium. The pattern of diurnal variation also varies in the two disorders, with depressed patients tending to be worse in the mornings, and delirious patients in the evenings. Elderly depressed patients are at increased risk of delirium, either through self-neglect or because of the antidepressant treatment they are receiving. Anticholinergic tricyclic drugs are particularly troublesome in this respect. Adverse life events, such as bereavement, may precipitate both depression and delirium in vulnerable individuals.

### Mania

Mania is much less common than delirium in old age, and is often mistaken for it. There may be a previous history of manic-depressive illness, but a proportion of cases of mania in late life are first presentations, usually in association with underlying organic brain disease. Elderly manic patients are often exhausted and dehydrated, and so 'manic delirium' is a common presentation.

### Other disorders

Anxiety states in elderly patients are unlikely to be mistaken for delirium, unless they are particularly severe. Similarly, paranoid states and schizophrenia rarely lead to diagnostic difficulty, although it should be noted that patients with these disorders are at an increased risk of developing delirium, either through self-neglect, or the effects of neuroleptic and anticholinergic medications. A number of other rare conditions in which cognitive, perceptual, affective, and behavioural disturbances occur, such as amnesic syndromes, epilepsia partialis continua, twilight states, the Charles Bonnet syndrome, neuroleptic malignant syndrome, and catatonia, may also resemble delirium. If the history and clinical examination are inconclusive, EEG may be helpful in making the diagnosis.

## Epidemiology

The community prevalence of delirium increases with age, rising to 14 per cent in those aged 85 years and older. In medical and surgical inpatients, the rates of delirium vary considerably (prevalence, 10–30 per cent; incidence, 4–53 per cent), because of methodological and population differences. Similar rates are also found in studies of acute psychogeriatric admissions.[11] Some patient groups, such as those with hip fractures, have consistently higher rates. Other at-risk populations, such as nursing home residents, have received less systematic investigation, but the available evidence suggests that they also have rates of delirium comparable to those found in elderly inpatients.

## Aetiology

Almost any physical illness can give rise to delirium in elderly patients. The most common physical causes are listed in Table 8.5.1.1. In many cases the underlying cause is not obvious, and the delirium may be the most prominent presenting feature. The aetiology is commonly multi-factorial, and all contributory factors need to be identified and treated. As a rule, hyperactive

**Table 8.5.1.1** Common causes of delirium in elderly patients

| Drugs |
| --- |
| Psychotropics |
| Hypnotics |
| Anticonvulsants |
| Anticholinergic drugs |
| Dopamine agonists |
| Analgesics |
| Anaesthetics |
| Alcohol withdrawal |
| **Infection** |
| Urinary tract infections |
| Pneumonia |
| Septicaemia |
| Ulcers, pressure sores, gangrene |
| Endocarditis |
| Postsurgical wound infection |
| **Metabolic and endocrine** |
| Electrolyte abnormalities |
| Uncontrolled diabetes |
| Hyper/hypothyroidism |
| Renal failure |
| Hepatic failure |
| Hypothermia |
| Malnutrition |
| **Cardiovascular** |
| Cardiac failure |
| Myocardial infarction |
| Vascular disease |
| Anaemia/polycythaemia |
| **Respiratory** |
| Pulmonary embolism |
| Pneumothorax |
| Pleural effusion |
| **Intracranial** |
| Trauma |
| Subdural haematoma |
| Stroke |
| Tumour |
| Epilepsy |
| **Gastrointestinal** |
| Perforation |
| Pancreatitis |
| Cholecystitis/cholangitis |
| Haemorrhage |
| Constipation |

delirium is more commonly due to infection and toxic/withdrawal states, whereas hypoactive delirium is more commonly due to metabolic abnormalities.

Drugs are an important cause of delirium in elderly patients, due to age-associated changes in their distribution, metabolism, and excretion. These pharmacokinetic changes are very variable, with the result that toxicity at apparently therapeutic doses is unpredictable. Certain drugs are particularly prone to cause delirium in elderly patients, for example those with anticholinergic activity. Tricyclic antidepressants, thioridazine, and benzhexol are particularly toxic in this respect, but many of the drugs commonly prescribed to elderly patients have some degree of anticholinergic activity, for example, digoxin, prednisolone, cimetidine, ampicillin, and warfarin. Individually, this activity may be small, but the cumulative effect can be significant if patients are on multiple medications.[12] Patients with Alzheimer's disease are particularly prone to develop delirium when given anticholinergic drugs, perhaps because their central cholinergic function is already impaired. In a minority of particularly vulnerable elderly patients, purely environmental and psychological insults are sufficient to cause delirium. The mechanisms of action in these cases are not known, but may involve factors such as sensory deprivation and stress responses via the hypothalamic-pituitary-adrenal axis.

## Course and prognosis

Traditionally, delirium has been regarded as a transient condition that proceeds to either recovery or death. In the majority of cases, the delirium is brief, but about one-third of patients have prolonged or recurrent episodes.[13] Delirium is associated with increased short-term mortality in elderly patients, mainly because of the severity of the underlying illness. Delirium interferes with the processes of diagnosis, treatment, and rehabilitation, and as a result patients have longer hospital stays and higher rates of functional decline and discharge to nursing homes.[14] Increased length of stay and mortality are particularly associated with hypoactive delirium. In general, patients with hyperactive delirium appear to be less severely ill than those with hypoactive delirium; this may be due to differences in the cause of the delirium, or to the fact that hyperactive delirium is more likely to be identified and the causes treated.

Prospective studies have shown that the prognosis, in terms of persistent or recurrent symptoms, is relatively poor in elderly patients.[15] This is probably because those who experience delirium are a vulnerable group who are likely to develop the condition provided there is sufficient external insult. A proportion will also be suffering from a form of dementia, which will increase the vulnerability to delirium as it progresses. There is evidence that delirium is followed by persistent cognitive decline,[16] which raises the possibility that it (or the underlying cause) is a risk factor for the development or exacerbation of dementia.

## Evaluation of treatment

Evidence regarding the efficacy of treatments for delirium is sparse (Chapter 4.1.1). The cholinergic hypothesis of delirium raises the possibility that cholinergic agonists, such as the cholinesterase inhibitors licensed for the treatment of Alzheimer's disease, may be of value in the prevention and treatment of delirium.

# Management

There are four important steps in the management of delirium[17]:

## Address the underlying causes (see above)

## Behavioural control

This aspect of delirium management can be divided into pharmacological and non-pharmacological strategies. Non-pharmacological interventions in delirium are aimed at reducing the confusing, frightening, and disorienting aspects of the hospital environment in which most patients find themselves. They have received little formal evaluation, but features such as good lighting, low noise levels, a visible clock, and the reassuring presence of personal possessions and familiar individuals, such as relatives, are thought to be helpful. Any invasive intervention, including personal care tasks, should be introduced and explained simply, slowly, clearly, and repeatedly before it is carried out. Holding the patient's hand while talking helps to focus attention and provides reassurance.

The drug treatment of the symptoms and behaviours of delirium in the elderly is similar to that of younger patients, although it is necessary to start with lower doses, such as haloperidol 0.5 to 2 mg orally, or intramuscularly if necessary, repeated until the disturbance is controlled. Prescriptions should be for short periods only (up to 24 h) to encourage review of the effects and the necessary dosage. Once the delirium has resolved, the medication should be reduced/discontinued over a period of 3 to 5 days. If the patient cannot tolerate typical or atypical neuroleptic drugs, then a benzodiazepine (for instance, diazepam, lorazepam, or alprazolam) should be used instead.

## Prevent/treat complications

The complications that befall patients with delirium probably contribute to the adverse outcomes associated with this condition. For example, hyperactive delirium is associated with falls during the hospital admission, whereas hypoactive delirium is associated with the development of pressure sores. Other complications of delirium include urinary incontinence, sleep disturbance, malnutrition, and immobilization; all of these problems should be anticipated and prevented where possible.

## Rehabilitation and family support

Given the risk of functional decline following delirium, every effort should be made to return the patient to their pre-morbid level of functioning. ADL capacity should be assessed regularly, and independence encouraged where possible. The patient's family need to be involved in the rehabilitation process, as they will be largely responsible for aftercare following discharge. They should know that delirium is often recurrent, and be advised about the early signs of this. Indeed, delirium is a useful marker of vulnerability, and of the need for more intensive community aftercare.

# Prevention

The modern hospital environment contributes significantly to the development of delirium in elderly patients, and multi-component interventions to improve poor clinical practice have been shown to reduce cost-effectively the incidence of delirium in elderly inpatients.[18] The following areas are important:

- ◆ *Prescribing*
Avoid where possible any drugs with known deliriogenic potential, particularly in at-risk individuals such as those with Alzheimer's disease. There should be regular review of the drug chart, with the aim of keeping the number of drugs to the minimum necessary. Non-pharmacological sleep-promotion strategies should be used in preference to hypnotic drugs.

- ◆ *Ward environment and routines*
These should aim to minimize disorientation, sensory impairment, and sleep deprivation. Patient mobility should be encouraged, as should adequate food and fluid intake. Medical and nursing staff should be trained to recognize and manage delirium.

- ◆ *Surgical routines*
Good preoperative, perioperative, and postoperative care (especially with regard to infection control, blood pressure, and oxygenation) will reduce the risk of postoperative delirium.

# Further information

American Psychiatric Association. (1999). *Practice guideline for the treatment of patients with delirium*. American Psychiatric Association, Washington, DC.

British Geriatrics Society. (2006). *Guidelines for the prevention, diagnosis and management of delirium in older people in hospital*. British Geriatrics Society, London.

Byrne, E.J. (1994). *Confusional states in older people*. Edward Arnold, London.

Lindesay, J., Rockwood, K., and Macdonald, A. (2002). *Delirium in old age*. Oxford University Press, Oxford.

Lipowski, Z.J. (1990). *Delirium: acute confusional states*. Oxford University Press, New York.

# References

1. Bowler, C., Boyle, A., Branford, M., *et al.* (1994). Detection of psychiatric disorders in elderly medical in-patients. *Age and Ageing*, **23**, 307–11.

2. Treloar, A.J. and Macdonald, A.J.D. (1997). Outcome of delirium: Parts 1 and 2. *International Journal of Geriatric Psychiatry*, **12**, 609–18.

3. Liptzin, B., Levkoff, S.E., Cleary, P.D., *et al.* (1991). An empirical study of diagnostic criteria for delirium. *The American Journal of Psychiatry*, **148**, 451–7.

4. Levkoff, S.E., Liptzin, B., Cleary, P.D., *et al.* (1996). Subsyndromal delirium. *The American Journal of Geriatric Psychiatry*, **4**, 320–9.

5. Folstein, M.F., Folstein, S.E., and McHugh, P.R. (1975). Mini-mental state-a practical method for grading the cognitive state of patients for the clinician. *Journal of Psychiatric Research*, **2**, 1891–8.

6. Trzepacz, P.T., Baker, R.W., and Greenhouse, J. (1988). A symptom rating scale for delirium. *Psychiatry Research*, **23**, 89–97.

7. Inouye, S.K., van Dycke, C.H., Alessi, C.A., *et al.* (1990). Clarifying confusion: the confusion assessment method. *Annals of Internal Medicine*, **113**, 941–8.

8. Albert, M.S., Levkoff, S.E., Reilly, C., *et al.* (1992). The delirium symptom interview: an interview for the detection of delirium symptoms in hospitalized patients. *Journal of Geriatric Psychiatry and Neurology*, **5**, 14–21.

9. Inouye, S.K., Viscoli, C.M., Horowitz, R.I., *et al.* (1993). A predictive model for delirium in hospitalised elderly medical patients based on admission characteristics. *Annals of Internal Medicine*, **119**, 474–81.

10. Inouye, S.K. and Charpentier, P.A. (1996). Precipitating factors for delirium in hospitalized elderly persons. Predictive model and interrelationship with baseline vulnerability. *The Journal of the American Medical Association*, **275**, 852–7.

11. Lindesay, J., Rockwood, K., and Rolfson, D. (2002). The epidemiology of delirium. In *Delirium in old age* (eds. J. Lindesay, K. Rockwood, and A. Macdonald), pp. 27–50. Oxford University Press, Oxford.

12. Tune, L., Carr, S., Hoag, E., *et al.* (1992). Anticholinergic effects of drugs commonly prescribed for the elderly: potential means of assessing risk of delirium. *The American Journal of Psychiatry*, **149**, 1393–4.

13. Rudberg, M.A., Pompei, P., Foreman, M.D., *et al.*(1997). The natural history of delirium in older hospitalized patients: a syndrome of heterogeneity. *Age and Ageing*, **26**, 169–74.

14. Inouye, S.K., Rushing, J.T., Foreman, M.D., *et al.* (1998). Does delirium contribute to poor hospital outcome? A three-site epidemiologic study. *Journal of General Internal Medicine*, **13**, 234–42.

15. Levkoff, S., Evans, D., Liptzin, B., *et al.* (1992). Delirium, the occurrence and persistence of symptoms among elderly hospitalised patients. *Archives of Internal Medicine*, **152**, 334–40.

16. Jackson, J.C., Gordon, S.M., Hart, R.P., *et al.* (2004). The association between delirium and cognitive decline: a review of the empirical literature. *Neuropsychological Review*, **14**, 87–98.

17. Marcantonio, E. (2002). The management of delirium. In *Delirium in old age* (eds. J. Lindesay, K. Rockwood, and A. Macdonald), pp. 123–51. Oxford University Press, Oxford.

18. Inouye, S.K., Bogardus, S.T., Charpentier, P.A., *et al.* (1999). A multicomponent intervention to prevent delirium in hospitalized older patients. *The New England Journal of Medicine*, **340**, 669–76.

## 8.5.1.1 Mild cognitive impairment

Claudia Jacova and Howard H. Feldman

### Introduction

Within the cognitive functioning continuum from normal ageing to dementia three broad states can be distinguished: normal functioning for age, clear-cut impairment meeting diagnostic criteria for dementia, and mild cognitive impairment (MCI), which falls below normal but short of dementia in severity (Fig. 8.5.1.1.1). There is active debate over what MCI is, how to define and classify this state, and where to set its borders on the described continuum.[1] Some definitions depict MCI as the tail-end of normal cognitive ageing whereas in other definitions MCI embodies the early clinical manifestation of Alzheimer Disease (AD) and other dementias. In 2003, the key elements of different MCI definitions were integrated into a consensus diagnostic and classification framework,[2] thus establishing some common ground in a field that is still evolving. MCI has also been positioned as a potentially important target for early treatment interventions to delay progression to dementia.

Nosologically, MCI is not currently included as a diagnostic entity in the *Diagnostic and Statistical Manual of Mental Disorders* (DSM-IV-TR)[3] and the *International Classification of Diseases*, 10th revision.[4] The diagnostic categories of *Mild Neurocognitive Disorder* (DSM-IV-TR) and *Mild Cognitive Disorder* (ICD-10) are similar to MCI because they require the presence of cognitive impairment but these categories can only be assigned if a specific neurological or general medical condition can be identified to account for the cognitive symptoms. Much of the current condition

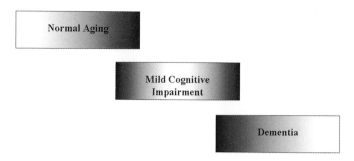

**Fig. 8.5.1.1.1** Theoretical continuum from normal ageing to dementia: darker shading indicates areas of overlap between adjacent states and increased diagnostic challenge. (Reproduced from R. Petersen *et al.* Apolipoprotein E status as a predictor of the development of Alzheimer's disease in memory-impaired individuals, *The Journal of the American Medical Association*, **273**, 1274–78, copyright 1995, The American Medical Association.)

of MCI does not fit as it has no aetiologic specification. Nevertheless, MCI is increasingly a presenting condition in primary and specialized settings of care. Medical practice guidelines have recognized MCI as a risk state for dementia and recommend careful clinical evaluation and monitoring of individuals with this diagnosis.[5,6]

### Nosology

The current nosological entities within the general MCI framework include a variety of definitions and capture overlapping but not identical conditions in the ageing population (Fig. 8.5.1.1.2).

### Age-associated memory impairment (AAMI)

AAMI describes healthy individuals over the age of 50 that experience memory decline. Formal diagnostic criteria require complaints of memory loss, performance on objective memory tests falling at least 1 SD below norms for young individuals, and intellectual functioning normal. AAMI cannot be diagnosed if there is a

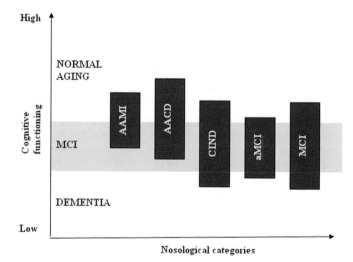

**Fig. 8.5.1.1.2** MCI nosological entities on the continuum from normal ageing to dementia. (Reproduced from H.H. Feldman and C. Jacova, Mild cognitive impairment, *The American Journal of Geriatric Psychiatry*, **13**(8), 645–55, copyright 2005, American Association of Geriatric Psychiatry, Lippincott Williams & Wilkins.)

neurological, psychiatric, or medical condition that can account for the impairment.[7]

### Age-associated cognitive decline (AACD)

The AACD category covers impairments in any domain affected by ageing, including learning, memory, attention, thinking, language, and visuospatial function. There must be self- or informant-reported cognitive decline over at least 6 months and performance on objective cognitive tests at least 1 SD below age- and education-appropriate norms. The cognitive impairment cannot fulfil dementia criteria and is not accounted for by systemic, neurological, or psychiatric disorders.

### Cognitive impairment not dementia (CIND)

CIND includes all individuals that cannot be classified as cognitively normal or as demented. CIND has been applied both in population- and clinic-based studies.[8,9] This diagnostic label is assigned by clinical judgement when there is memory and/or cognitive impairment insufficient to meet DSM criteria for dementia, without exclusions related to underlying aetiologies. There are to date no operational criteria for this category. Because of its inclusiveness CIND encompasses a range of aetiologies that must be disentangled to be clinically meaningful.[8,9]

### Amnestic mild cognitive impairment (aMCI)

This amnestic condition is defined as a clinical disorder that describes a transitional state between normal ageing and AD. It is characterized by memory impairment in the context of otherwise preserved abilities. The diagnostic criteria for aMCI require memory complaint preferably corroborated by an informant, objective memory impairment for age and education, largely normal general cognition, essentially intact activities of daily living (ADLs), and the absence of dementia. Objective memory impairment, though not anchored to a specific cut point, is generally ≥1.5 SD below appropriate norms.[10]

### Mild cognitive impairment (MCI): international working group criteria

The MCI concept has recently been broadened to encompass multiple patterns of cognitive impairment including amnestic, non-amnestic, single- or multiple-domain deficits.[2] In this framework the classification of MCI requires multiple steps. First, individuals should be judged as neither normal nor demented. Second, there should be evidence of cognitive decline, supported by self and/or informant reports, impairment on objective cognitive tests, or evidence of decline over time on these tests. Third, activities of daily living should be mainly preserved, with the provision that complex ADLs can be minimally impaired.[2] Like CIND, this MCI category recognizes multiple aetiologies underlying impairment, and requires their identification.

### Clinical staging scales

Studies of MCI frequently utilize clinical staging scales both to define the inclusion criteria as well as to track outcomes. The Clinical Dementia Rating (CDR) scale[11] distinguishes five stages of dementia severity, with a stage of questionable dementia (CDR 0.5), between the stages of healthy (CDR 0) and mild dementia (CDR 1). CDR 0.5 is most often applied to MCI; however, this stage also can

include those with functional impairment who meet dementia criteria. Similarly, the Global Deterioration Scale (GDS),[12] which distinguishes seven stages of impairment, overlaps with MCI at stage 2 (normal with a subjective complaint) or stage 3 (subtle deficits in cognition and occupational/social activities), whereas individuals with mild dementia may receive a GDS stage 3 or 4. The mapping of MCI onto these staging scales has not yet been fully reconciled.

## Epidemiology

### Prevalence

Prevalence estimates for MCI will naturally vary according to the definition, to age and to the setting. In population-based studies, AAMI has been estimated to affect up to 38.4 per cent, and AACD between 21 and 35.2 per cent, of individuals aged 60 or older.[13] CIND has been reported to affect between 16.8 and 23.4 per cent of individuals aged 65 or older. The prevalence of aMCI has been much lower, at 3 to 6 per cent in similar age groups.[13] Within the broad MCI classification, the multiple domains and single non-memory domain subtypes have been described as roughly twice as frequent as the amnestic subtype, with multiple domain impairment estimated to affect 16 per cent of individuals.[14,15] The prevalence of AACD, aMCI, MCI, and CIND varies with age, with a two- to threefold increase from age 65–74 to >85 in CIND (Fig. 8.5.1.1.3).[8,16] The prevalence of MCI and related conditions within the referral clinic setting is much higher than population estimates.[17]

### Natural history

#### (a) Progression rates to dementia

While the rate of progression to dementia is 1 to 2 per cent per year for cognitively normal individuals aged 65 or older, the rates for all MCI entities are systematically higher and quite variable (Fig. 8.5.1.1.4). Whereas AAMI has low progression rates (1 to 3 per cent per year) and is closest to a normal population, for all other categories most studies report rates between 10 and 15 per cent per

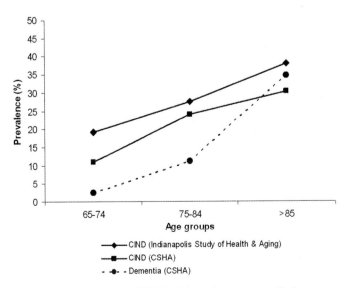

**Fig. 8.5.1.1.3** The prevalence of CIND with increasing age reported in the Canadian study of health and ageing (CSHA)[8] and the Indianapolis study of health and ageing.[16]

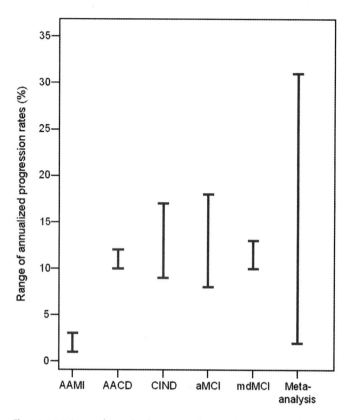

**Fig. 8.5.1.1.4** Range of annualized estimates of progression to dementia in various MCI groups, reported in Refs.[13,14,18]

annum, generally over 5-year periods. A meta-analytic study indicated a mean annual conversion rate of 10.24 per cent, with a range of 2 to 31 per cent. The single most important factor accounting for this heterogeneity was the source of the participants, with subjects referred to specialist services, either geriatric or memory/dementia clinics, progressing to dementia at roughly twice the rate found for community volunteers.[18] In studies of CIND annual rates have been 17 per cent for a dementia clinic-referred cohort, 9 per cent for a population-based cohort.[1,9]

An unresolved question is whether all subjects with MCI eventually develop dementia. In a highly selected aMCI sample with CDR 0.5 followed over 10 years, all subjects eventually progressed to meet dementia criteria.[19] This evidence has been proposed to support the belief that aMCI represents early-stage AD.[19] Other studies with similar length of follow-up have not found as high rates of progression and neuropathologic evidence also suggests more heterogeneity, with up to 50 per cent of subjects with aMCI meeting criteria for AD, and the remainder having varied non-AD abnormalities including vascular lesions, argyrophilic grain disease, or other conditions.[20]

**(b) Reversion rates to normal**

There are consistently proportions of individuals with MCI that will revert back to normal cognitive functioning during follow-up. In population-based studies, this backcrossing has sometimes been particularly high (range 4 to >40 per cent after 1.5 to 5 years).[1] In clinic-referred samples, reversion rates for CIND appear to be lower (14 per cent after 2 years).[9] Reversion may in part be a reflection of an inherent instability in the MCI condition, particularly when it is defined exclusively by psychometric cut points.[1] Reversion appears to be more common when there is no clearly identified aetiology for MCI.[9]

**(c) Mortality risk**

The mortality risk of MCI is near twice the risk of cognitively normal individuals. The estimated relative risk has been 1.5 for AACD, 1.5–1.9 for CIND, and 1.3–1.7 for aMCI while there has been no increased risk reported for AAMI. There is no clear explanation for this increased mortality risk. It is independent of health conditions such as cardiac disease, cerebrovascular disease, diabetes, and malignancies, and it may be related to incipient and eventually full-blown dementia.[21]

## Diagnosis: clinical approach

### Overview

Figure 8.5.1.1.5 depicts a flow chart for the clinical diagnosis of MCI.[2] The diagnostic process begins with an expressed concern about cognitive functioning from the patient and/or informant. The assessment then requires a careful history from the patient and informant, as well as the mandatory administration of objective cognitive testing. An evaluation of social function and ADLs, both instrumental and basic, is performed to determine whether there is impairment sufficient for a dementia diagnosis. A clinical judgement must be made of whether the impairment falls outside of the normal range for age and whether it falls within MCI or dementia. The cognitive profile can further be classified into single amnestic, multiple domains, or single non-memory domain. The final step in the diagnostic process is the determination of the aetiology of MCI.

### Cognitive assessment

The identification of MCI requires evidence of impairment on objective cognitive testing. Generally, a cognitive screening test is needed as a first step. It should be recognized that the most widely used Mini Mental State Examination (MMSE) lacks sensitivity for MCI diagnosis. In turn, two novel instruments (the Montreal Cognitive Assessment, MoCA, and the DemTect) have been shown to reliably discriminate MCI from normal ageing.[22] The effects of age and educational achievement on test performance and the consequent risk of misclassifications must be kept in mind in the clinical assessment. Irrespective of the instrument that is chosen, there should be coverage of episodic memory, executive functioning and language, which are the most frequent presenting problems in MCI.

Neuropsychological testing (NPT) can be helpful where a clear-cut determination of MCI is difficult following the initial assessment. NPT provides information on the pattern of impairment, with identification of the domains affected and reference to standardized scores. Serial NPT may be particularly useful in defining the progression from MCI to mild dementia. The rate of decline on tests of memory, executive functioning and language accelerates during the 3- to 5-year time window before diagnosis of full-blown dementia.[22] NPT also has some predictive utility in addressing the risk of progression from MCI to dementia. Deficits on tests of episodic memory and executive functioning have consistently been found to characterize those with MCI that will develop dementia.[22]

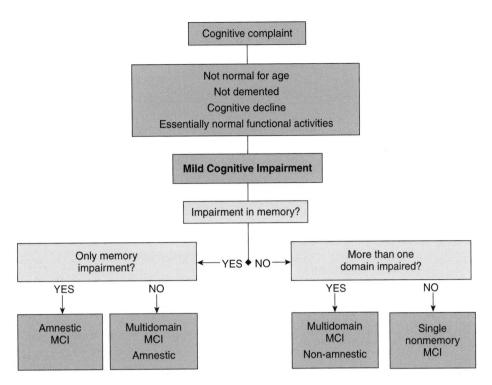

**Fig. 8.5.1.1.5** Diagnostic flow chart proposed by the International Working Group on MCI. (Reproduced from B. Winblad *et al.* (2004), Mild cognitive impairment—beyond controversies, towards a consensus: report of the International Working Group on mild cognitive impairment, *Journal of Internal Medicine*, **256**, 240–6, copyright 2004, John Wiley & Sons, Inc.)

### Neuropsychiatric symptoms (NPS)

NPS may provide a very useful additional domain for evaluation. An estimated 50 to 70 per cent of subjects with MCI have informant-reported NPS. Symptoms of depression, agitation/aggression, anxiety, apathy, and irritability, while at a low level of intensity, nevertheless each have a frequency of >30 per cent. NPS are associated with greater MCI severity and may be predictive of progression to dementia.[23] The evaluation of NPS is recommended within an MCI assessment.

### Aetiology

The determination of aetiology is a final key step in the assessment of MCI. It requires additional laboratory studies as well as consideration of neuroimaging results. Within a cohort of individuals with CIND, the most prevalent aetiologic subtypes were pre-AD, vascular cognitive impairment, cognitive impairment with psychiatric illness, and not otherwise specified (NOS) (Table 8.5.1.1.1). These CIND aetiologic subtypes differed in their functional and psychobehavioural profiles, and in their 2-year prognosis. Pre-AD and vascular CIND had the highest rates of progression to dementia (~40 per cent), with pre-AD subjects developing exclusively probable AD. Psychiatric CIND and CIND NOS had the highest rates of reversion to normal (20 to 30 per cent). Progression to dementia occurred in all aetiologic subtypes (Table 8.5.1.1.1).[9]

## Biomarkers

There are no widely accepted MCI biomarkers at the present time. Research has focused on neuroimaging with MRI and FDG-PET as well as on tau and β-amyloid (Aβ) protein levels in cerebrospinal fluid (CSF).

### Neuroimaging

On structural MRI, individuals with MCI may show volume loss in the medial temporal lobe (MTL) that may presage AD. The key structures of the MTL include the hippocampus and the entorhinal cortex. MTL structures can be rated on visual scales that may

**Table 8.5.1.1.1** Aetiologic subtypes of CIND and their 2-year progression to AD/dementia

| Subtype | Prevalence (% within cohort) | Dementia at 2-years (% within subtype) | AD at 2-years (% within dementia) |
|---|---|---|---|
| Pre-AD | 24.6 | 40.9 | 100 |
| Vascular | 18.1 | 40.0 | 33.3 |
| Psychiatric | 17.3 | 25.0 | 75 |
| Non-AD degenerative | 2.3 | 33.3 | 0 |
| Neurological | 7.3 | 25.0 | 25 |
| Medical | 3.5 | 60.0 | 100 |
| Mixed | 7.6 | 33.3 | 100 |
| Not otherwise specified | 19.3 | 24.2 | 62.5 |

(Reproduced from G.Y. Hsiung et al. (2006), Outcomes of cognitively impaired not demented at 2 years in the Canadian cohort study of cognitive impairment and related dementias. *Dementia and Geriatric Cognitive Disorders*, **22**(5–6), 413–20, with permission from S. Karger A.G, Basel.)

reasonably predict AD.[24] MRI-based predictive algorithms may be better when MTL measures are combined with measures of lateral temporal lobe or anterior cingulate structures, or with performance scores on episodic memory.[24] Both whole brain and MTL atrophy rates are greater in MCI subjects that progress to AD than in those who do not.[25]

The characteristic pattern of AD is to have metabolic reductions in temporoparietal and posterior cingulate regions on [$^{18}$F-]-fluorodeoxyglucose (FDG) PET. This pattern may be seen in individuals with MCI ahead of full-blown disease. Serial PET may show further metabolic deterioration in these areas as well as abnormalities in the ventrolateral prefrontal cortex in subjects who progress to AD.[1] Recently, PET radioligands that bind to cerebral amyloid and potentially to tau proteins have been developed. These include Pittsburgh compound B (PiB) (N-methyl-[$^{11}$C]2-(4'-methylaminophenyl)-6-hydroxybenzothiazole) for amyloid and FDDNP (2-(1-[6-[(2-[$^{18}$F]fluoroethyl)(methyl)amino]-2-naphthyl]ethylidene)malononitrile) for amyloid and tau. Studies with these ligands have revealed higher than normal retention in subjects with MCI, with a pattern that follows the anatomical distribution of AD pathology.[26,27] If longitudinal follow-up confirms that these MCI cases develop AD, PET with PiB or FDDNP could become a diagnostic test for the early identification of AD.[24]

### Cerebrospinal fluid markers

CSF markers can reflect the AD pathogenic process including a reduction in Aβ42 as it aggregates into senile neuritic plaques, as well as an increase in total tau (t-tau) and phospho-tau (p-tau), which signals the hyperphosphorylated state of tau. In MCI, the combination of abnormal Aβ42, t-tau, and p-tau 181 is associated with a 17–20 increased risk of developing AD over 4–6 years. Currently, the utility of these markers is limited by the lack of a standardized assay and the variability in measurements obtained at different laboratories.[28]

## Management and treatment

There are no standard therapies for MCI. A clinical management plan is formulated on an individual basis in consideration of the cognitive pattern of MCI and its aetiology. There are two goals for treatment: first, to alleviate the cognitive symptoms of MCI, and second, to attempt to delay the onset of dementia in those at risk.

### Symptomatic treatment

#### (a) Pharmacotherapy

A 24-week trial of the cholinesterase inhibitor (ChEI) donepezil did not benefit subjects with aMCI on its primary endpoints of delayed recall and global impression of change. There were benefits on secondary measures including the ADAS-cog, neuropsychological tests of attention, and patient-rated global function (Patient Global Assessment, PGA).[29] A longer term trial of donepezil with subjects with aMCI (the Alzheimer's Disease Cooperative Study-Memory Impairment Study, ADCS-MIS) demonstrated benefits on the ADAS-cog, memory and language scores, and global measures including the CDR sum of boxes but these were confined to the first 18 months of treatment.[30]

#### (b) Non-pharmacologic therapies

Cognitive and lifestyle interventions may help the cognitive and behavioural difficulties in MCI. An 8-week cognitive intervention programme to improve memory strategies produced benefits on tests of delayed recall and face-name association, and on self-assessed everyday memory function in subjects with aMCI.[31] A 14-day healthy lifestyle programme with memory training, physical conditioning, relaxation techniques, and a diet plan, showed benefits in subjects with mild self-reported memory complaints. These benefits included improved word fluency and metabolic changes on FDG-PET in dorsolateral prefrontal cortex.[32] Therapeutic approaches of this type require considerable resources, and confirmation in randomized controlled trials (RCTs) is needed before large-scale implementation in MCI can be recommended. Nevertheless these approaches hold some promise.

### Delaying the onset of AD

#### (a) Pharmacotherapy

A considerable number of long and large trials of ChEIs and non-steroidal anti-inflammatory drugs (NSAIDs) have been directed at delaying the time to diagnosis of AD in those with aMCI. In the 3-year ADCS-MIS trial, treatment with donepezil did not have an effect on the primary outcome measure of progression to AD after 36 months. An interesting observation in the study was that carriers of the apolipoprotein E ε4 allele treated with donepezil had a reduced risk of progression to AD at all time points.[30] Similarly, rivastigmine was unsuccessful in delaying the time to diagnosis of AD.[33] A 4-year trial of the COX-2 inhibitor rofecoxib did not show treatment benefits on the primary endpoint of percentage of subjects that were diagnosed with AD nor on secondary measures of cognition and global function.[1] Based on the available data, the long-term use of ChEIs or NSAIDs in MCI, with the goal of delaying AD onset, cannot be recommended.

#### (b) Non-pharmacologic therapies

An expanding literature supports the hypothesis that a cognitively, socially, and physically active lifestyle in late life may reduce the risk for AD.[34] Evidence from RCTs to support this hypothesis is not currently available and it is premature to recommend organized interventions. There would be little perceived harm in promoting an engaged lifestyle as part of the management of MCI.

## The future of MCI

MCI has been a useful construct to focus attention on the cognitive impairment that is going to increase exponentially within our greying societies. It is recognized that MCI is a risk state for developing AD and other dementias. A natural next step will be to develop criteria to diagnose AD earlier. A proposal of research criteria for the early diagnosis of AD has recently been published.[24] The diagnosis builds on a clinical core of early and significant episodic memory impairment and requires in addition the presence of at least one biological footprint of the disease: medial temporal lobe atrophy on structural MRI, abnormal CSF, or reduced temporoparietal glucose metabolism on FDG-PET.[24] Similar frameworks are already in place or will be developed for non-AD dementias. As these frameworks will advance, the concept of MCI will likely be significantly refined and could look quite different by the next edition of this textbook.

## Further information

Petersen, R. (ed.) (2003). *Mild cognitive impairment*. Oxford University Press, New York.

Chertkow, H., Nasreddine, Z., Joanette, Y., *et al.* (2007). Mild cognitive impairment and cognitive impairment, no dementia: part A, concept and diagnosis. *Alzheimer's & Dementia*, 3, 266–82.

Massoud, F., Belleville, S., Bergman, H., *et al.* (2007). Mild cognitive impairment and cognitive impairment, no dementia: part B, therapy. *Alzheimer's & Dementia*, 3, 283–91.

Dubois, B., Feldman, H.H., Jacova, C., *et al.* (2007). Research criteria for the diagnosis of Alzheimer's disease: revising the NINCDS-ADRDA criteria. *Lancet Neurology*, 6(8), 734–46.

# References

1. Feldman, H.H. and Jacova, C. (2005). Mild cognitive impairment. *The American Journal of Geriatric Psychiatry*, 13(8), 645–55.

2. Winblad, B., Palmer, K., Kivipelto, M., *et al.* (2004). Mild cognitive impairment—beyond controversies, towards a consensus: report of the International Working Group on mild cognitive impairment. *Journal of Internal Medicine*, 256, 240–6.

3. American Psychiatric Association. (2000). *Diagnostic and statistical manual of mental disorders* (DSM-IV-TR) (4th text revised edn). APA, Washington, DC.

4. World Health Organization. (1992). ICD-10: international statistical classification of diseases and related health problems (10th revision edn): based on recommendations of the Tenth Revision Conference, 1989 and adopted by the Forty-third World Health Assembly.

5. Petersen, R.C., Stevens, J.C., Ganguli, M., *et al.* (2001). Practice parameter: early detection of dementia: mild cognitive impairment (an evidence-based review). Report of the quality standards subcommittee of the American academy of neurology. *Neurology*, 56, 1133–42.

6. Chertkow, H., Nasreddine, Z., Joanette, Y., *et al.* (2007). Mild cognitive impairment and cognitive impairment, no dementia: part A, concept and diagnosis. *Alzheimer's & Dementia*, 3, 266–82.

7. Crook, T., Bartus, R., Ferris, S.H., *et al.* (1986). Age-associated memory impairment: proposed diagnostic criteria and measures of clinical change—report of a National Institute of Mental Health Work Group. *Developmental Neuropsychology*, 2, 261–76.

8. Graham, J.E., Rockwood, K., Beattie, B.L., *et al.* (1997). Prevalence and severity of cognitive impairment with and without dementia in an elderly population. *Lancet*, 349, 1793–6.

9. Hsiung, G.Y., Donald, A., Grand, J., *et al.* (2006). Outcomes of cognitively impaired not demented at 2 years in the Canadian cohort study of cognitive impairment and related dementias. *Dementia and Geriatric Cognitive Disorders*, 22(5–6), 413–20.

10. Petersen, R.C. (2004). Mild cognitive impairment as a diagnostic entity. *Journal of Internal Medicine*, 256(3), 183–94.

11. Morris, J.C. (1997). Clinical dementia rating: a reliable and valid diagnostic and staging measure for dementia of the Alzheimer type. *International Psychogeriatrics*, 9(Suppl. 1), 173–6.

12. Reisberg, B., Sclan, S.G., Franssen, E. *et al.* (1997). Clinical stages of normal aging and alzheimer's disease: the GDS staging system. *Neuroscience Research Communications*, 13(Suppl. 1), 51–4.

13. Panza, F., D'Introno, A., Colacicco, A.M., *et al.* (2005). Current epidemiology of mild cognitive impairment and other predementia syndromes. *The American Journal of Geriatric Psychiatry*, 13(8), 633–44.

14. Busse, A., Bischkopf, J., Riedel-Heller, S.G., *et al.* (2003). Subclassifications for mild cognitive impairment: prevalence and predictive validity. *Psychological Medicine*, 33(6), 1029–38.

15. Lopez, O.L., Jagust, W.J., DeKosky, S.T., *et al.* (2003). Prevalence and classification of mild cognitive impairment in the cardiovascular health study cognition study: part 1. *Archives of Neurology*, 60(10), 1385–9.

16. Unverzagt, F., Gao, S., Baiuewu, O., *et al.* (2001). Prevalence of cognitive impairment: data from the Indianapolis study of health and aging. *Neurology*, 57(9), 1655–62.

17. Feldman, H., Levy, A.R., Hsiung, G.Y., *et al.* (2003). A Canadian cohort study of cognitive impairment and related dementias (ACCORD): study methods and baseline results. *Neuroepidemiology*, 22, 265–74.

18. Bruscoli, M. and Lovestone, S. (2004). Is MCI really just early dementia? A systematic review of conversion studies. *International Psychogeriatrics*, 16, 129–40.

19. Morris, J.C., Storandt, M., Miller, J.P., *et al.* (2001). Mild cognitive impairment represents early-stage Alzheimer disease. *Archives of Neurology*, 58(3), 397–405.

20. Petersen, R.C., Parisi, J.E., Dickson, D.W., *et al.* (2006). Neuropathologic features of amnestic mild cognitive impairment. *Archives of Neurology*, 63(5), 665–72.

21. Guehne, U., Angermeyer, M.C., and Riedel-Heller, S. (2006). Is mortality increased in mildly cognitively impaired individuals? A systematic literature review. *Dementia and Geriatric Cognitive Disorders*, 21(5–6), 403–10.

22. Jacova, C., Kertesz, A., Blair, M., *et al.* (2007). Neuropsychological testing and assessment for dementia. *Alzheimer's & Dementia*, 3, 299–317.

23. Feldman, H., Scheltens, P., Scarpini, E., *et al.* (2004). Behavioral symptoms in mild cognitive impairment. *Neurology*, 62, 1199–201.

24. Dubois, B., Feldman, H.H., Jacova, C., *et al.* (2007). Research criteria for the diagnosis of Alzheimer's disease: revising the NINCDS-ADRDA criteria. *Lancet Neurology*, 6(8), 734–46.

25. Jack, C.R. Jr, Shiung, M.M., Gunter, J.L., *et al.* (2004). Comparison of different MRI brain atrophy rate measures with clinical disease progression in AD. *Neurology*, 62(4), 591–600.

26. Klunk, W.E., Engler, H., Nordberg, A., *et al.* (2004). Imaging brain amyloid in Alzheimer's disease with Pittsburgh compound-B. *Annals of Neurology*, 55, 306–19.

27. Small, G.W., Kepe, V., Ercoli, L.M., *et al.* (2006). PET of brain amyloid and tau in mild cognitive impairment. *The New England Journal of Medicine*, 355(25), 2652–63.

28. Hansson, O., Zetterberg, H., Buchhave, P., *et al.* (2006). Association between CSF biomarkers and incipient Alzheimer's disease in patients with mild cognitive impairment: a follow-up study. *Lancet Neurology*, 5(3), 228–34.

29. Salloway, S., Ferris, S., Kluger, A., *et al.* (2004). Efficacy of donepezil in mild cognitive impairment: a randomized placebo-controlled trial. *Neurology*, 63, 651–7.

30. Petersen, R.C., Thomas, R.G., Grundman, M., *et al.* (2005). Vitamin E and donepezil for the treatment of mild cognitive impairment. *The New England Journal of Medicine*, 352(23), 2379–88.

31. Belleville, S., Gilbert, B., Fontaine, F., *et al.* (2006). Improvement of episodic memory in persons with mild cognitive impairment and healthy older adults: evidence from a cognitive intervention program. *Dementia and Geriatric Cognitive Disorders*, 22(5–6), 486–99.

32. Small, G.W., Silverman, D.H., Siddarth, P., *et al.* (2006). Effects of a 14-day healthy longevity lifestyle program on cognition and brain function. *The American Journal of Geriatric Psychiatry*, 14(6), 538–45.

33. Feldman, H.H., Ferris, S., Winblad, B., *et al.* (2007). Effect of rivastigmine on delay to diagnosis of Alzheimer's disease from mild cognitive impairment: the InDDEx study. *Lancet Neurology*, 6(6), 501–12.

34. Fratiglioni, L., Paillard-Borg, S., and Winblad, B. (2004). An active and socially integrated lifestyle in late life might protect against dementia. *Lancet Neurology*, 3, 343–53.

# 8.5.2 Substance use disorders in older people

Henry O'Connell and Brian Lawlor

## Introduction

This chapter is divided into three main sections, focussing respectively on alcohol use disorders (AUDs), medication use disorders (MUDs), and use of illegal substances and nicotine, in older people. In each section we focus in detail on definitions and diagnosis, epidemiology, aetiology, clinical features, investigations, screening, management, and prognosis. More is known about AUDs in older people, hence this section is the longest, but MUDs in older people is also a significant problem and abuse of illegal drugs may become increasingly important in future years.

## Alcohol use disorders (AUDs) in older people

### Introduction

The ageing of populations worldwide means that the already significant problem of alcohol use disorders (AUDs) in older people is likely to become even more important in future years. However, AUDs in older people are neglected and underdiagnosed, for the reasons outlined in Table 8.5.2.1, and unless these factors are tackled proactively there exists a real danger of AUDs in older people becoming a silent epidemic, with negative impacts on all aspects of health and well-being[1] (see Table 8.5.2.2).

### Definitions and diagnosis

AUD is a general and broad term, used to include a wide range of alcohol-related problems, as outlined in Table 8.5.2.3. Alcohol status may also change throughout life, with one-third of older people with AUDs developing such problems for the first time in later life (late-onset AUDs). A more severe course of AUD, higher levels of antisocial personality and stronger family histories of AUDs are seen in those with early-onset AUDs.

Because of the effects of physical and cognitive ageing, pharmacokinetic changes, the increased prevalence of comorbid illness, and interactions with prescribed medication, older people are likely to encounter AUDs at levels of intake lower than the general population. Therefore, the recommended levels of intake for the general population (i.e. up to 21 and 14 units per week for men and women, respectively[2]) may be inappropriately high for older people. However, apart from the NIAAA recommendations of no more than one drink per day for older people,[3] there is a lack of guidance on safe levels of alcohol intake, and the pursuit of obvious and 'down and out' drinkers may lead to a significant amount of more subtle and clinically 'silent' AUDs being missed.

Furthermore, the diagnostic criteria used by ICD-10 and DSM-IV used to describe harmful use and alcohol dependence syndrome may not be applicable to older people, as evidence of diagnostic criteria such as craving, compulsion, tolerance, and withdrawal features may be less clear-cut and masked by other medical conditions, and older people may be less likely to encounter the financial, occupational, family and legal consequences of AUDs (see also Table 8.5.2.1 and section on screening).

**Table 8.5.2.1** Reasons for the neglect and underdiagnosis of AUDs in older people

*Patient factors*

Older people may be less likely to volunteer information on alcohol intake/AUDs

Recall of alcohol intake may be inaccurate due to cognitive impairment

Features of AUDs may be atypical or masked (e.g. presenting as falls, confusion)

Pharmacokinetic changes, comorbid illness, and drug-interactions mean alcohol-related problems may arise even at relatively low levels of intake

*Health service factors*

Health care professionals less likely to ask older people about alcohol intake and AUDs

Health care professionals less likely to refer older people for treatment, even when AUD detected

Inappropriate screening and diagnostic tools used

Therapeutic pessimism in treating older people

Inappropriately high levels for 'recommended' or 'healthy' levels of intake

*Family and societal factors*

Family members may be less likely to perceive AUD as a problem in older relatives

Ageist attitudes lead to risk of AUDs in older people being perceived as 'understandable'

AUDs in older people less 'noisy', with less impact on absenteeism, antisocial behaviour, crime

## Epidemiology

The prevalence of AUDs in older people varies depending on the screening and diagnostic criteria used, clinical and socio-demographic characteristics (men having levels 4–6 times higher than women) and the level of severity of AUD being defined. In community-based studies, for example, 2–4 per cent of older people have been estimated to have alcohol misuse or dependence,[4] with higher rates of 16 per cent (men) and 2 per cent (women) when looser criteria such as excessive alcohol consumption are used.[5] Clinical populations of older people have higher levels of AUDs, with emergency department, nursing home and psychiatric inpatients being described as having levels of 14, 18, and 23 per cent, respectively.[6–8]

The true prevalence of AUDs in older people is often underestimated, for the reasons outlined in Table 8.5.2.1. It is likely, however, that the actual levels of alcohol consumption and AUDs do decline with age.[9,10] This decline may be due to factors such as premature death of those with AUDs, reduced physiological reserve and comorbid medical illness leading to reduced alcohol intake, age-cohort effects and age-related changes in social networks, occupational, and financial status.

## Aetiology, risk factors, and associations

These factors can be broadly described as being biological/medical, social, and psychological in nature. Genetic factors are likely to be important in relation to both early-onset[11] and late-onset AUDs.[12] The genetic risk for AUDs may also overlap with risk for other mental disorders such as antisocial personality disorder, other drug use problems, anxiety disorders, and mood disorders.[13] AUDs may have a cause and effect relationship with medical illness.

Important social aetiological factors are likely to include male gender, bereavement, age-cohort effects, culture and ethnicity, religion, and marital status (higher levels of AUDs in divorced and single). Some social factors, such as marital problems, may have a two-way relationship with AUDs.

**Table 8.5.2.2** Physical, neuropsychiatric, and socio-demographic aspects of AUDs in older people

1. Physical factors
*Gastrointestinal*
Hepatic problems: elevated liver enzymes; fatty liver; alcoholic hepatitis; cirrhosis; malignancy
Gastritis, peptic ulcer disease, and bleeding
Oesophageal varices
Acute and chronic pancreatitis

*Malignancies*
Mouth, pharynx, larynx, oesophagus, hepatic, colorectal, pancreatic

*Cardiovascular*
Ischaemic heart disease
Hypertension
Alcohol-induced arrhythmias
Congestive heart failure
Alcoholic cardiomyopathy

*Haematological*
Macrocytosis (acute effect of alcohol intake and due to vitamin B12 and folate deficiency in chronic AUD)
Anaemia (due to gastrointestinal problems)

*Musculoskeletal*
Falls and fractures
Reduced bone density
Myopathy

*Metabolic*
Hypoglycaemia
Hyperuricaemia
Elevated lipids
Diabetes more difficult to control

2. Neuropsychiatric factors
Cognitive impairment and dementia
Frontal lobe impairment
Wernicke–Korsakoff syndrome
Cerebellar cortical degeneration
Central pontine myelinosis
Marchiafava–Bignami disease
Depression
Psychosis
Intoxication
Withdrawal syndrome (may be more difficult to treat in older people)
Suicide

3. Socio-demographic
Male gender
Divorced, widowed, and single status
Social isolation
Upper and lower ends of socio-economic spectrum

4. Other
Alcohol–drug interactions
Aspiration pneumonia
Road traffic and other accidents

Relevant personality factors include the stronger association between antisocial personality, hyperactivity, and impulsivity in 'early-onset' compared to late-onset AUDs, who may have higher levels of 'neuroticism' and depression.[14]

AUDs in older people, as in all populations, may also have a two-way relationship with psychiatric disorders such as depression and anxiety disorders. For example, an older person may begin drinking

**Table 8.5.2.3** Types/levels of severity of AUDs

◆ Excessive alcohol consumption (i.e. drinking above recommended levels)
◆ Binge drinking (i.e. episodic bouts of excessive alcohol intake)
◆ Problem drinkers/harmful use/abuse
◆ Alcohol dependence syndrome
◆ 'Early-onset' versus 'late-onset'

in an effort to self-medicate depressive symptoms, or they may become depressed because of their drinking.[15]

## Clinical features and comorbidity

AUDs in older people are linked to significant morbidity and mortality, affecting practically all aspects of physical, neuropsychiatric and social health and well-being,[1,16] as summarized in Table 8.5.2.2.

Pharmacokinetic changes (reduced physiological reserve, reduced metabolic efficiency, and increased volume of distribution due to a higher fat to lean muscle ratio, leading in turn to relatively higher blood alcohol concentrations in older people) along with the general effects of physical and cognitive ageing, increasing frailty, reduced functional ability, and higher levels of concomitant prescription drug use means that alcohol is relatively more toxic to older people than younger people. Furthermore, as outlined earlier, such toxic effects may be subtle and may be missed or mistaken for other conditions.

AUDs in older people are associated with a wide range of mental disorders, such as depression, psychosis, withdrawal syndromes, cognitive impairment, and dementia[17] (see Table 8.5.2.2) and are also associated with an increased risk of suicide.[18] The relationship between alcohol use and brain damage and dementia is complex,[19] in that AUDs may increase the risk for different types of dementia[20] and there also exist diagnostic entities known as 'amnesic syndrome associated with alcohol use' (ICD-10) or 'alcohol-induced persisting dementia' (DSM-IV). In contrast, light to moderate alcohol use may protect against dementia.[21]

### (a) Clinical assessment

The assessment of AUDs in older people begins with a thorough clinical interview and history of alcohol use (quantity and frequency of drinking, beverage type, drinking context), mental state examination, physical examination and collateral history if available, and with the patient's consent. If indicated by the initial history, additional questions should be asked about features of alcohol dependence syndrome, as they relate to the patient's physical and psychosocial health. Questions should be framed in a sensitive and non-judgemental way, as patients may disengage and be lost to treatment and follow-up if they feel threatened by the assessment procedure.

### (b) Further investigations in AUDs

Following a detailed history and examination, other investigations may be indicated and should be directed by the patient's clinical status. These may include: blood tests to check the following: urea and electrolytes; full blood count; liver function tests; vitamin B12 and folate levels; neuroimaging (CT or MRI brain); gastrointestinal investigations such as ultrasound, CT, or MRI examinations of the abdomen, upper gastrointestinal endoscopy, and liver biopsy; basic cardiovascular investigations such as electrocardiogram and other more detailed investigations if indicated, e.g. echocardiogram and 24 h blood pressure monitoring.

### (c)  Screening for AUDs in older people

Screening programmes should aim to detect both clear-cut and subtle cases of AUDs in older people. It must be remembered that screening tests are not diagnostic in themselves, but positive results should lead on to further investigations. Screening methods may be based on self-report alcohol screening instruments such as the CAGE,[22] the AUDIT,[23] and biophysical measures such as blood tests checking mean corpuscular volume and liver function tests.

A systematic review of self-report alcohol screening instruments in older people[24] revealed that the CAGE was the most widely studied, but that sensitivity and specificity varied depending on the clinical characteristics of the population in question. However, the CAGE is the most well recognized alcohol screening instrument and is quickly and easily administered, so the authors would recommend use of at least this instrument, along with further investigations and assessment scales if problems are detected.

The utility of biophysical screening measures such as carbohydrate-deficient transferrin, liver function tests or the mean corpuscular volume may be less reliable in older people,[25] because of higher levels of comorbid physical illnesses leading in themselves to false-positive and abnormal results. However, they may prove useful when combined with other clinical information, both in the detection of AUDs and monitoring of progress through treatment.

## Management and prevention

*Primary prevention* strategies should focus on individual older people (especially considering that one-third of older people have late-onset AUDs) and can also be directed at the entire population, targeting factors such as ease of access to alcohol, restrictions on alcohol advertising, and education about the adverse effects of drinking. Such primary prevention and public health initiatives tend to be directed towards younger individuals, but they should also take into account the more clinically 'silent' AUDs that may develop in older people.[26]

*Secondary prevention* strategies should focus on older people who already have 'at-risk' drinking, either currently or in the past, and who are at risk of developing worsening problems in the context of diverse factors such as bereavement, social isolation, adjustment to retirement, and physical or psychiatric health problems.

*Tertiary prevention* involves treatment of existing AUDs. Treatment modalities can be divided into biological/medical, social, and psychological. Biological/medical treatments are most important in the acute setting, where detoxification may be required.

Care should be taken with benzodiazepine-assisted withdrawal in older people, in view of the elevated risk of oversedation, confusion, and falls. There are no elderly-specific guidelines on benzodiazepine-assisted alcohol withdrawal in older people. Lorazepam has been identified in one review[27] as the safest choice of benzodiazepine for treatment of alcohol withdrawal in older people, in view of the fact that advancing age and liver disease have little impact on its metabolism, and absorption by the intramuscular route is predictable. In practice, however, it is likely that there is more clinical experience with use of long-acting benzodiazepines

such as chlordiazepoxide. The choice of benzodiazepine used should be based on individual patient characteristics such as previous treatments, current medical status (e.g. degree of hepatic impairment) and an objective measure of withdrawal may help guide the dosing regimen (see Table 8.5.2.4).

Parenteral or oral thiamine should be given to prevent development of the Wernicke–Korsakoff syndrome. A recent review has concluded that, in the emergency department setting, oral thiamine administration is as effective as parenteral administration.[28] Again, however, there are no elderly-specific guidelines, and individual patient characteristics must be taken into account, such as general health, ability to take oral medication, and compliance.

The three medications that are approved by the US Food and Drug Administration to promote abstinence and reduce relapse are Disulfiram, Acamprosate, and Naltrexone.[29] However, the limited efficacy of Disulfiram, combined with the potential for a more severe side-effect profile means it is best avoided in this age group. In contrast, Naltrexone and Acamprosate have been suggested as suitable agents for use in older people.[30]

Psychosocial aspects of treatment should also be explored. This may include addressing social circumstances that may be contributing to the AUD (e.g. personal finances and housing). There is a dearth of evidence on psychotherapeutic approaches to AUDs in older people, but there is some evidence that older people may respond better to psychotherapy in same-age settings,[31,32] and consideration should also be given to support groups such as Alcoholics Anonymous.

## Prognosis

The available literature on the topic suggests that older people are at least as likely, if not more likely, to benefit from treatment of AUDs as younger people.[33,34] However, prognosis in older people is likely to vary widely depending on a number of factors relating to the individual themselves and the nature of their AUD, the presence of family and other support systems and the availability of treatment services, particularly services that are tailored to older people.

**Table 8.5.2.4** The Clinical Institute Withdrawal Assessment for Alcohol-Revised Version (CIWA-Ar) (Reproduced from The South London and Maudsley NHS Trust Prescribing Guidelines, 2005–2006, copyright South London and Mandsley NHS Foundation Trust)

1. Nausea and vomiting
2. Tremor
3. Paroxysmal sweats
4. Anxiety
5. Agitation
6. Tactile disturbances
7. Auditory disturbances
8. Visual disturbances
9. Headaches and fullness in head
10. Orientation and clouding of sensorium

**Severity of alcohol withdrawal**

| | |
|---|---|
| Mild: | <10 |
| Moderate: | 10–20 |
| Severe: | 20+ |

(Items 1–9 are scored from 0–7 and item 10 from 0–4. Maximum possible score is 67)

# Medication use disorders (MUDs) in older people

## Introduction

High levels of prescribing of all types of medications for older people, which may at times be inappropriate, along with factors such as variable compliance, altered pharmacokinetics, reduced functional ability, and increased levels of physical, psychiatric, and cognitive morbidity mean that older people are at higher risk of developing MUDs than any other age group.[35] As with AUDs, clinical features of MUDs may be atypical and masked by other conditions and thus go undetected and untreated.[36]

## Definitions

As with AUDs, older people are affected by a wide range of types and severity of MUD.

The ICD-10 uses the same general principles of intoxication, harmful use, dependence, and withdrawal state that apply to alcohol for use of sedative and hypnotic medications. As with AUDs, elderly-specific criteria are not cited, but the same general principles apply: older people are likely to experience harm at lower levels of use and clinical features guiding diagnosis are more likely to be atypical and masked by other health problems.

Iatrogenic factors are also important, as drugs may be inadequately or underused for treating or preventing conditions, or drugs may be overused, leading to unnecessary exposure of the older individual to adverse effects.[36]

## Epidemiology

Older people comprise 13 per cent of the US population, but they have been estimated to use more than 30 per cent of prescription[37,38] and 35 per cent of OTC drugs:[37] it has been estimated that older people use prescription and OTC medications approximately three times as much as the general population. Furthermore, we know that the risk of MUDs increases with polypharmacy, which is common in older people.[39,40]

Benzodiazepines are the most commonly prescribed psychotropic drugs in older people, with one study of community-dwelling older people in Ireland demonstrating that 17 per cent of participants were prescribed benzodiazepines, with use in females being twice that in males, and 18 per cent of benzodiazepine users taking at least one other psychotropic drug. Furthermore, 52 per cent of benzodiazepine users were prescribed a long-acting benzodiazepine.[41] It has also been reported that depression in older community-dwelling people is more likely to be detected if accompanied by anxiety symptoms, and such individuals are at risk of inappropriate treatment with benzodiazepines.[42]

Use of opiate analgesia is common in older people and is liable to give rise to MUDs. Therefore, use of these medications should be carefully monitored, with due consideration of dose and careful tapering.[43]

## Aetiology, risk factors, and associations

The general principles for aetiology, risk factors, and associations for substance misuse outlined above (see Table 8.5.2.5) also apply to MUDs. Further MUD-specific factors are outlined below in Table 8.5.2.6.

**Table 8.5.2.5** Risk factors for substance abuse in the elderly (Reproduced from R.M. Atkinson (2002), Substance abuse in the elderly, In *Psychiatry in the elderly* (3rd edn.) (eds. R. Jacoby and C. Oppenheimer), copyright 2002, with permission from Oxford University Press).

*Predisposing factors*
Family history (alcohol)
Previous substance abuse
Previous pattern of substance consumption (individual and cohort effects)
Personality traits (sedative–hypnotics, anxiolytics)

*Factors that may increase substance exposure and consumption level*
Gender (men-alcohol, illicit drugs; women-sedative–hypnotics, anxiolytics)
Chronic illness associated with pain (opioid analgesics), insomnia (hypnotic drugs), or anxiety (anxiolytic)
Long-term prescribing (sedative–hypnotics, anxiolytics)
Caregiver overuse of 'as needed', medication (institutionalized elderly)
Life stress, loss, social isolation
Negative affects (depression, grief, demoralization, anger) (alcohol)
Family collusion and drinking partners (alcohol)
Discretionary time, money (alcohol)

*Factors that may increase the effects and abuse potential of substances*
Age-associated drug sensitivity (pharmacokinetic, pharmacodynamic factors)
Chronic medical illnesses
Other medications (alcohol–drug, drug–drug interactions)

## Clinical features and comorbidity

Clinical features and comorbidities associated with MUDs in older people will vary widely depending on the drug being used and patient characteristics such as age, gender, and presence of other physical and neuropsychiatric problems. An outline of clinical features and comorbidities are listed in Table 8.5.2.7.

### (a) Clinical assessment

As with AUDs, a standard clinical assessment involving a history, mental state, and physical examinations and collateral history will form the basis of an MUD assessment. A list of all prescribed and over the counter medications being used, along with their indications for use, should be recorded. Ideally, the patient should be asked to bring with them all medications in their containers, as this will also give an indication as to levels of adherence or compliance. Any reported adverse effects should be recorded, along with

**Table 8.5.2.6** Aetiology, risk factors, and associations of MUDs in older people

*Biological/medical factors*
Genetic predisposition
Chronic medical conditions (e.g. pain)
Age-related pharmacokinetic changes
Interactions: other medications and alcohol
Type of medication (e.g. benodiazepines, analgesics)

*Psychosocial factors*
Depression
Anxiety disorders
Personality disorder
Older age
Female gender
Lower educational level
Separated or divorced status

**Table 8.5.2.7** Clinical features and comorbidity associated with MUDs in older people

| |
| --- |
| *Neuropsychiatric (all psychotropic drugs; benzodiazepines may be particularly problematic)* |
| Delirium |
| Daytime drowsiness |
| Sleep disturbance |
| Depression |
| Anxiety |
| *Physical* |
| Falls |
| Fractures |
| Drug–drug and drug–alcohol interactions |
| Problems related to drug metabolism (e.g. renal and hepatic impairment) |

symptoms and signs indicating underuse, overuse, or intermittent use of medication.

#### (b) Investigations in MUDs

Blood levels of the patient on some prescribed medications may be checked in order to assess levels of compliance and to establish if the blood level is within the therapeutic window for the drug in question (e.g. lithium, carbamazepine). Other biophysical measures may also be indicated that provide proxy measures of medication compliance, such as random or fasting glucose levels and levels of glycosylated haemoglobin, to assess for level of diabetes control and compliance with hypoglycaemic agents or insulin.

#### (c) Screening

There are no routinely used screening measures for MUDs in older people. However, use of a measure such as Beers' criteria[44,45] may be a useful addition to the overall assessment of an older person if an MUD is suspected.

### Management and prevention

#### (a) Primary and secondary prevention

Along with patients themselves, health care workers, family members, and carers all have important roles in the primary and secondary prevention of MUDs in older people. Prescriptions should be reviewed regularly with a view to simplification and rationalization if possible, and the practice of giving 'repeat prescriptions' without clinical assessment should be discouraged.

Community pharmacists have an important role in providing education and advice on the use of both prescription and over the counter medications.

As older people may have physical and cognitive disabilities that interfere with appropriate use of medication,[46] devices such as dosette boxes and combination packs may be helpful.[47,48] Secondary prevention of MUDs in older people should focus on those with a past history of MUD.

#### (b) Tertiary prevention

Tertiary prevention of MUDs in older people will depend on the medication in question and the clinical and socio-demographic profile of the patient. Admission to a medical or psychiatric ward may be required to facilitate reduction or stopping of certain medications, e.g. benzodiazepine detoxification, as outpatient detoxification in older people may be hazardous.

### Prognosis in MUDs

Similar prognostic indicators that apply to AUDs are likely to be relevant to MUDs, and centre on the individual's clinical and socio-demographic characteristics, levels of support, and available services. The duration of abuse and the medication or medications being abused is also of relevance.

## Illicit drug use and nicotine use in older people

Illicit drug use in older people is far less of a problem in comparison to AUDs and MUDs. Lifetime prevalence rates for illicit drug dependence have been estimated as 17 per cent for 18–29 year olds, 4 per cent for 30–59 year olds, and less than 1 per cent for those over the age of 60.[49] Epidemiological Catchment Area data suggest a lifetime prevalence rate for illegal drug use of only 1.6 per cent for older people.[50]

Several other sources of data suggest similarly low rates of illegal drug use among older people. However, the ageing of the 'Baby-boomer' generation is likely to result in a cohort of older people who are healthier and have higher life expectancies than previous generations of older people, but who also carry with them higher rates of illegal drug use.[51]

Principles similar to those seen with AUDs and MUDs apply, in that lower levels of drug intake are required to cause harm and presentation may be atypical and thus go undetected. There is a dearth of evidence in the literature on detoxification and opiate replacement therapies in older populations.

Nicotine use (primarily through cigarette smoking) in older people arguably causes more significant morbidity and mortality than AUDs and MUDs, but the problem tends not to be addressed by psychiatrists, because of a lack of significant neuropsychiatric effects of nicotine use, and a more obvious impact on many aspects of physical health. As with AUDs and MUDs, smoking in older people is treatable, and any comprehensive approach to improving the health of older people, at the individual clinical level or public health level, should involve education about the adverse effects of smoking and efforts at active treatment through the use of nicotine replacement therapies[52] or antidepressants such as nortriptyline or buproprion.[53] However, an important and circular relationship has been described between depression, smoking, and medical illness that complicates smoking cessation in those who have a history of depression.[54]

## Conclusions

In this chapter we have highlighted the importance of AUDs and MUDs in older people, in terms of their prevalence and their important but often underrecognized contribution to morbidity and mortality. AUDs are underdetected, misdiagnosed, and often completely missed in older populations. However, despite ageist and therapeutically pessimistic assumptions, AUDs in older people are as amenable to treatment as in younger people, and treating an AUD in an individual of any age can lead to significant benefits in their quality of life.

Likewise, the wide variety of MUDs in older people may be associated with addiction to medication and the undertreatment and inappropriate treatment of medical and psychiatric conditions. Considering that older people are the highest consumers of prescription medications, screening and treatment programmes for MUDs should also lead to considerable improvements in quality of life, along with financial and other savings.

Misuse of illicit drugs by older people is not generally a major problem at present, but it is virtually certain that consumption of illegal substances by people over 65 will increase in the future.

Greater awareness amongst physicians and other health care providers of the possibility of AUDs and MUDs in their older patients should lead to the development of more comprehensive and age-appropriate prevention and treatment strategies. At the levels of everyday clinical practice and public health policy, greater emphasis should be placed on AUDs and MUDs in older people and further evaluation of dedicated 'same-age' treatment services and settings should be performed.

## Further information

Website of National Institute on Alcohol Abuse and Alcoholism (NIAAA): www.niaaa.nih.gov

Website of Royal College of Psychiatrists: www.rcpsych.ac.uk

O'Connell, H., Chin, A.V., Cunningham, C., et al. (2003a) Alcohol use disorders in elderly people—redefining an age old problem in old age. British Medical Journal, 327, 664–7; www.bmj.com.

Gurnack, A.M., Roland, R., Atkinson, M.D., et al. (eds.) (2001). Treating alcohol and drug abuse in the elderly. Springer, New York.

Barry, K.L., Oslin, D.W., and Blow, F.C. (eds.) (2001). Alcohol problems in older adults: prevention and management. Springer, New York.

## References

1. O'Connell, H., Chin, A.V., Cunningham, C., et al. (2003a). Alcohol use disorders in elderly people—redefining an age old problem in old age. British Medical Journal, 327, 664–7.

2. The Royal Colleges Report. (1995). Alcohol and the heart in perspective: sensible limits reaffirmed. A working group of the Royal Colleges of Physicians, Psychiatrists and General Practitioners. Journal of the Royal College of Physicians of London, 29, 266–71.

3. National Institute on Alcohol Abuse and Alcoholism. (1998). Alcohol alert No. 40. NIAAA, Bethesda, MD. www.niaaa.nih.gov/publications/aa40.htm

4. Adams, W.L. and Cox, N.S. (1995). Epidemiology of problem drinking among elderly people. International Journal of the Addictions, 30, 1693–716.

5. Greene, E., Bruce, I., Cunningham, C., et al. (2003). Self-reported alcohol consumption in the Irish community dwelling elderly. Irish Journal of Psychological Medicine, 20, 77–9.

6. Adams, W.L., Magruder-Habib, K., Trued, S., et al. (1992). Alcohol abuse in elderly emergency department patients. Journal of the American Geriatrics Society, 40, 1236–40.

7. Joseph, C.L., Ganzini, L., and Atkinson, R.M. (1995). Screening for alcohol use disorders in the nursing home. Journal of the American Geriatrics Society, 43, 368–73.

8. Speer, D.C. and Bates, K. (1992). Comorbid mental and substance disorders among older psychiatric patients. Journal of the American Geriatrics Society, 40, 886–90.

9. Adams, W.L., Garry, P.J., Rhyne, R., et al. (1990). Alcohol intake in the healthy elderly. Journal of the American Geriatrics Society, 38, 211–6.

10. Temple, M.T. and Leino, E.V. (1989). Long-term outcomes of drinking: a twenty year longitudinal study of man. British Journal of Addiction, 84, 889–93.

11. Dahmen, N., Volp, M., Singer, P., et al. (2005). Tyrosine hydroxylase Val-81-Met polymorphism associated with early-onset alcoholism. Psychiatric Genetics, 15, 13–6.

12. Tiihonen, J., Hammikainen, T., Lachman, H., et al. (1999). Association between the functional variant of the catechol-O-methyltransferase (COMT) gene and type 1 alcoholism. Molecular Psychiatry, 4, 286–9.

13. Nurnberger, J.I., Wiegand, R., Bucholz, K., et al. (2004). A family study of alcohol dependence: coaggregation of multiple disorders in relatives of alcohol-dependent probands. Archives of General Psychiatry, 61, 1246–56.

14. Mulder, R.T. (2002). Alcoholism and personality. The Australian and New Zealand Journal of Psychiatry, 36, 44–52.

15. Davidson, K.M. and Ritson, E.B. (1993). The relationship between alcohol dependence and depression. Alcohol and Alcoholism, 28, 147–55.

16. Reid, M.C. and Anderson, P.A. (1997). Geriatric substance use disorders. The Medical Clinics of North America, 81, 999–1016.

17. Saunders, P.A., Copeland, J.R., Dewey, M.E., et al. (1991). Heavy drinking as a risk factor for depression and dementia in elderly men. Findings from the Liverpool longitudinal community study. The British Journal of Psychiatry, 159, 213–6.

18. Waern, M. (2003). Alcohol dependence and misuse in elderly suicides. Alcohol and Alcoholism, 38, 249–54.

19. Neiman, J. (1998). Alcohol as a risk factor for brain damage: neurologic aspects. Alcoholism, Clinical and Experimental Research, 22(Suppl. 7), 346S–51S.

20. Letenneur, L. (2004). Risk of dementia and alcohol and wine consumption: a review of recent results. Biological Research, 37, 189–93.

21. Ruitenberg, A., van Sweiten, J.C., Witteman, J.C.M., et al. (2002). Alcohol consumption and risk of dementia: the Rotterdam study. Lancet, 359, 281–6.

22. Ewing, J.A. (1984). Detecting alcoholism: the CAGE questionnaire. The Journal of the American Medical Association, 252, 1905–7.

23. Saunders, J.B. (1993). Development of the alcohol use disorders identification test (AUDIT). Addiction, 88, 791–804.

24. O'Connell, H., Chin, A.V., Hamilton, F., et al. (2004). A systematic review of the utility of self-report alcohol screening instruments in the elderly. International Journal of Geriatric Psychiatry, 19, 1074–86.

25. Luttrell, S., Watkin, V., Livingston, G., et al. (1997). Screening for alcohol misuse in older people. International Journal of Geriatric Psychiatry, 12, 1151–4.

26. O'Connell, H., Chin, A.V., and Lawlor, B.A. (2003b). Alcohol use in Ireland—can we hold our drink? Irish Journal of Psychological Medicine, 20, 109–10.

27. Peppers, M.P. (1996). Benzodiazepines for alcohol withdrawal in the elderly and in patients with liver disease. Pharmacotherapy, 16, 49–57.

28. Jackson, R. and Teece, S. (2004). Oral or intravenous thiamine in the emergency department. Emergency Medicine Journal, 21, 501–2.

29. Williams, S.H. (2005). Medications for treating alcohol dependence. American Family Physician, 72, 1775–80.

30. Barrick, C. and Connors, G.J. (2002). Relapse prevention and maintaining abstinence in older adults with alcohol use disorders. Drugs & Aging, 19, 583–94.

31. Schonfeld, L. and Dupree, L.W. (1995). Treatment approaches for older problem drinkers. International Journal of the Addictions, 30, 1819–42.

32. Kofoed, L.L., Tolson, R.L., Atkinson, R.M., et al. (1987). Treatment compliance of older alcoholics: an elder-specific approach is superior to "mainstreaming". Journal of Studies on Alcohol, 48, 47.

33. Curtis, J.R., Geller, G., Stokes, E.J., et al. (1989). Characteristics, diagnosis and treatment of alcoholism in elderly patients. Journal of the American Geriatrics Society, 37, 310–6.

34. Oslin, D.W., Pettinati, H., and Volpicelli, J.R. (2002). Alcoholism treatment adherence: older age predicts better adherence and drinking outcomes. The American Journal of Geriatric Psychiatry, 10, 740–7.

35. Chutka, D.S., Takahashi, P.Y., and Hoel, R.W. (2004). Inappropriate medications for elderly patients. *Mayo Clinic Proceedings. Mayo Clinic*, **79**, 122–39.

36. Beers, M.H., Baran, R.W., and Frenia, K. (2000). Drugs and the elderly. Part 1: the problems facing managed care. *The American Journal of Managed Care*, **6**, 1313–20.

37. Williams, L. and Lowenthal, D.T. (1992). Drug therapy in the elderly. *The Southern Medical Journal*, **85**, 127–31.

38. Avorn, J. (1995). Medication use and the elderly: current status and opportunities. *Health Affairs*, **14**, 276–86.

39. Chrischilles, E.A., Segar, E.T., and Wallace, R.B. (1992). Self-reported adverse drug reactions and related resource use. A study of community-dwelling persons 65 years of age and older. *Annals of Internal Medicine*, **117**, 634–40.

40. Cadieux, R.J. (1989). Drug interactions in the elderly: how multiple drug use increases risk exponentially. *Postgraduate Medicine*, **86**, 179–86.

41. Kirby, M., Denihan, A., Bruce, I., *et al.* (1999a). Benzodiazepine use among the elderly in the community. *International Journal of Geriatric Psychiatry*, **14**, 280–4.

42. Kirby, M., Denihan, A., Bruce, I., *et al.* (1999b). Influence of anxiety on treatment of depression in later life in primary care: questionnaire survey. *British Medical Journal*, **318**, 579–80.

43. Schneider, J.P. (2005). Chronic pain management in older adults: with coxibs under fire, what now? *Geriatrics*, **60**, 26–8, 30–1.

44. Beers, M.H. (1997). Explicit criteria for determining potentially inappropriate medication use by the elderly. An update. *Archives of Internal Medicine*, **157**, 1531–6.

45. Fick, D.M., Cooper, J.W., Wade, W.E., *et al.* (2003). Updating the Beers criteria for potentially inappropriate medication sue in older adults: results of a US consensus panel of experts. *Archives of Internal Medicine*, **163**, 2716–24.

46. Beckman, A., Bernsten, C., Parker, M.G., *et al.* (2005). The difficulty of opening medicine containers in old age: a population-based study. *Pharmacy World & Science*, **27**, 393–8.

47. Levings, B., Szep, S., and Helps, S.C. (1999). Towards the safer use of dosettes. *Journal of Quality in Clinical Practice*, **19**, 69–72.

48. Ringe, J.D., van der Geest, S.A., and Moller, G. (2006). Importance of calcium co-medication in bisphosphonate therapy of osteoporosis: an approach to improving correct intake and drug adherence. *Drugs & Aging*, **23**, 569–78.

49. Hinkin, C.H., Castellon, S.A., Dickson-Fuhrman, E., *et al.* (2002). Screening for drug and alcohol abuse among older adults using modified version of CAGE. *The American Journal on Addictions*, **10**, 319–26.

50. Anthony, J.C. and Helzer, J.E. (1991). Syndromes of drug abuse and dependence, in psychiatric disorders in America: In *The epidemiologic catchment area study* (eds. L.N. Robins and D.A. Regier). Free Press, New York.

51. Patterson, T.L. and Jeste, D.V. (1999). The potential impact of the baby-boom generation on substance use among elderly persons. *Psychiatric Services*, **50**, 1184–8.

52. Silagy, C., Lancaster, T., Stead, L., *et al.* (2002). Nicotine replacement therapy for smoking cessation. *Cochrane Database of Systematic Reviews*, (4), CD000146.

53. Hughes, J., Stead, L., and Lancaster, T. (2004). Antidepressants for smoking cessation. *Cochrane Database of Systematic Reviews*, (4), CD000031.

54. Wilhelm, K., Arnold, K., Niven, H., *et al.* (2004). Grey lungs and blue moods: smoking cessation in the context of lifetime depression history. *The Australian and New Zealand Journal of Psychiatry*, **38**, 896–905.

## 8.5.3 Schizophrenia and paranoid disorders in late life

Barton W. Palmer, Gauri N. Savla, and Thomas W. Meeks

### Introduction

Estimates of the point-prevalence of paranoia and other psychotic symptoms among persons age ≥ 65 years have ranged from approximately 4 per cent to 6 per cent,[1–3] and may be as high as 10 per cent among those age ≥ 85 years.[4] Although the majority of these symptoms occur as secondary psychoses in the context of Alzheimer's disease or related dementias,[5] the population of people with schizophrenia is ageing along with the general 'greying' of the industrialized world, and mental health care for older adults with schizophrenia is expected to be an increasingly important public health concern.[6]

### Clinical features

Schizophrenia is typified by the presence of two or more of the following categories of core symptoms: delusions, hallucinations, disorganized or catatonic behaviour, disorganized speech (or formal thought disorder), and negative symptoms (such as affective flattening, avolition, or social withdrawal).[7] Older patients tend to have less severe positive symptoms (hallucinations, delusions, disorganized behaviour) than their younger counterparts, but there are few age-related differences in presence or severity of negative symptoms.[8,9]

Most patients with schizophrenia and related primary psychotic disorders also have mild to moderate neurocognitive deficits.[10] There is considerable interpatient heterogeneity in terms of the severity of neuropsychological deficits, but the level of these deficits is a consistent and strong determinant of impairments in everyday functioning[11] and competence or decisional capacity.[12]

In terms of late-life schizophrenia, one common division is between those with earlier onset in adolescence or early adulthood (prior to age 40 or 45 years) versus later-onset (onset ≥ age 40 or 45 years). The latter group may comprise as many as 24 per cent of people with late-life schizophrenia.[13] Relative to similarly aged patients who had earlier onset, those with later-onset schizophrenia tend to have a higher prevalence of paranoid subtype and persecutory delusions, but better premorbid social-occupational functioning, fewer current disorganized symptoms, less severe (although not an absence of) negative symptoms, and less severe neuropsychological impairment. They are also more likely to be women, and tend to respond to lower doses of antipsychotic medication.[3,14,15] The two groups are similar in terms of severity of thought disorder,[16] although patients with very late onset schizophrenia-like psychosis (age of onset ≥ 60 years) tend to have less severe formal thought disorder.[17]

### Classification systems

The term 'schizophrenia' was coined by Eugen Bleuler in the early 20th century, but he wrote of 'the schizophrenias' (plural)[18] as an explicit acknowledgement of the substantial heterogeneity that characterizes this condition. Efforts to group 'the schizophrenias' into meaningful subtypes have been a key part of efforts to define the syndrome itself.[19] Most of the terms describing different subtypes of schizophrenia in the current *Diagnostic and Statistical Manual* (DSM-IV-TR)[7] and in the International Classification of Diseases (ICD-10)[20] [such as paranoid, catatonic, hebephrenic (disorganized), and undifferentiated (simple) subtypes] overlap with the subtypes identified by Kraepelin and or E. Bleuler a century ago. Other subtyping efforts have focused on a variety of dimensions such as positive and negative symptoms, cognitive functioning and/or course, but as true of the clinical subtypes in the DSM-IV-TR and ICD-10, there is invariably substantial intrasubtype heterogeneity.[21]

In regard to late-life schizophrenia, one of the key nosological controversies over the past century has been whether or not the late onset form is actually schizophrenia. Kraepelin's conception of *dementia praecox* in 1896 was that the disorder was defined by onset in adolescence or early adulthood. By 1913, Kraepelin came to acknowledge that early onset was not a universal feature, but the emphasis on early onset remained a potent belief in the field throughout most of the 20th century.[22] On the other hand, interest in late-onset schizophrenia has a long history, including seminal work by Manfred Bleuler, begun in the early 1940s with patients whose symptoms emerged at or after age 40 years.[23]

The term 'late-onset schizophrenia' has occasionally been used interchangeably with the term *late paraphrenia*, although the latter was originally conceptualized as a more circumscribed psychosis with onset at age 60 or 65.[24,25] Unfortunately, the terms 'late-onset schizophrenia,' and *paraphrenia* (with or without the epithet 'late'), and a variety of age cut-offs have been used interchangeably and inconsistently over the years, resulting in considerable confusion in the literature.[22,25] In a 1998 international consensus meeting on this topic, the group consensus suggestion was that the term 'late onset schizophrenia' be reserved for those with onset between ages 40 and 59 years, whereas the term 'very late onset schizophrenia-like psychosis' be used with those whose symptoms first manifest at age 60 or later.[3]

None of the above schizophrenia onset-related categories is represented in the contemporary formal diagnostic systems. The 1980 version of the American Psychiatric Association's *Diagnostic and Statistical Manual* (DSM-III)[26] arbitrarily excluded the diagnosis of schizophrenia if symptoms did not emerge prior to age 45. This exclusion was dropped from the subsequent revision (DSM-III-R),[27] although the DSM-III-R required the specification of 'late onset' if the prodromal phase of illness developed after 45. The latter is the only instance of 'late-onset schizophrenia' appearing as a named condition in one of the major nosological systems. Based on mounting empirical evidence that 'real' schizophrenia could manifest after age 45,[13] the age of onset restrictions as well as the 'late onset' specifier were dropped in the DSM-IV [28] and DSM-IV-TR.[7] Similarly, there is no age-of-onset related restriction or specification under the ICD-10.[20]

## Diagnosis and differential diagnosis

The diagnostic criteria for schizophrenia in the DSM-IV-TR and ICD-10 mention neither current age nor age of onset.[7,20] A key differential diagnosis with older adults is to rule out presence of a secondary psychosis.[29] For instance, among elderly patients, psychotic symptoms most commonly present in the context of dementia, such as Alzheimer's disease, Parkinson's disease, or dementia with Lewy Bodies.[5] The pattern in any one patient may of course vary from normative trends, but in general among those with dementia-related psychotic symptoms, there is a greater propensity for visual over auditory hallucinations, and bizarre content is less common in the delusions than in those of patients with primary psychotic disorders such as schizophrenia.[30]

Delirium may also present as acute psychosis;[31] as with dementia, visual hallucinations and delusions tend to be more common than auditory hallucinations, but the psychotic symptoms associated with delirium can be of any form.[32] Given the high rates of polypharmacy among the elderly as well as age-related changes in pharmacokinetics, it is also important to consider potential acute mental effects of the medications in isolation and in combination.[33] Other differential diagnoses to consider among elderly patients are non-psychotic hallucinations related to bereavement or sensory deprivation.[34,35]

Among the primary psychotic conditions, the standard differential diagnoses and considerations apply in terms of differentiating among schizophrenia, schizoaffective disorder, delusional disorder, brief psychotic disorder, substance-induced psychotic disorder, bipolar disorder with psychotic features, and major depressive disorder with psychotic features.[7]

## Epidemiology

As was noted above, prevalence estimates of paranoia and other psychotic symptoms among persons age $\geq 65$ years have ranged from approximately 4 per cent to 6 per cent,[1–3] but these symptoms are most commonly in the context of a dementia or other medical condition. Estimating the lifetime prevalence of schizophrenia is a methodologically complex endeavour needing additional research attention; recent estimates have ranged from approximately, 0.4 per cent to 1.0 per cent although estimates as high as 1.6 per cent have also been reported.[36,37] The lifetime prevalence of schizophrenia is similar among men and women, and the majority of patients of either gender experience onset in adolescence or early adulthood.[37] However, a consistent finding noted a century ago by E. Bleuler,[18] is that women tend to show later onset than men.[38]

Estimates of the lifetime prevalence of schizophrenia for persons over age 65 have also varied, although the 95 per cent confidence interval estimate from one recent comprehensive study was 0.58 to 1.45 per cent.[37] There have been some epidemiological studies suggesting that the prevalence (current and lifetime) of schizophrenia among elderly persons is lower than that for the younger population. People with schizophrenia have higher mortality due to suicide and physical disorders,[39,40] so there are probably proportionally fewer people with schizophrenia who survive to older age. However, the prevalence of schizophrenia in elderly patients may also have been underestimated in some of the earlier major epidemiological studies.[41] For instance, the Epidemiologic Catchment Area study used the DSM-III criteria, but as was noted above, the DSM-III criteria for schizophrenia arbitrarily required onset of prodromal symptoms prior to age 45, so any cases of later-onset schizophrenia would have been excluded.[41]

## Aetiology

The cause(s) of schizophrenia remains unknown. Both Kraepelin and E. Bleuler correctly suspected that there is a heritable vulnerability to schizophrenia, confirmed by the substantially higher concordance rates among monozygotic twins (estimated at 40 to 50 per cent) relative to dizygotic twins (estimated at 5 per cent to 25 per cent).[42,43] The elevated risk of schizophrenia among first-degree relatives is present among those with schizophrenia onset in middle-age as well as those wither earlier onset relatives.[3] Although some candidate genes have been identified,[44] these efforts remain in an early stage of development. Also, given that even the monozygotic twin concordance rate is substantially below 100 per cent, non-genetic factors clearly have a role in the ultimate expression of the schizophrenia phenotype.

At present, the prevailing model of schizophrenia is that of neurodevelopmentally based aberrations in connectivity of key brain regions and systems.[45,46] Evidence for the neurodevelopment component includes an elevated risk of schizophrenia associated with certain pre- or peri-natal insults or stresses, an increased prevalence of minor facial anomalies among patients with schizophrenia, and an increased prevalence of subtle childhood abnormalities in motor, cognitive, and/or psychosocial development among those who later develop schizophrenia.[45] At the level of neuropathology, Kraepelin expressed some suspicion of involvement of the prefrontal and temporal lobes;[47] these remain areas of interest in schizophrenia research although the current focus is on functional (rather than gross structural) impairments related to the connections among such brain regions or systems.[46]

## Course and prognosis

Schizophrenia is generally a chronic condition, but not necessarily a constantly sustained one in that many patients experience one or more periods of several years of sustained recovery over their lifespan, but periods of relapse are also common.[48] As with other dimensions of this disorder, the long-term course of schizophrenia is also characterized by heterogeneity among patients, as well as methodological challenges in interpreting varied findings in the empirical literature.[49] Some of the factors that have been cited as associated with worse prognosis include poor premorbid functioning, very early and gradual/insidious onset of symptoms, male gender, and a relative prominence of negative symptoms.[49,50] In a recent review of ten long-term longitudinal outcome studies, Jobe and Harrow[48] found that the estimates of 'good outcome' ranged from 21 to 57 per cent. Since most of the long-term research on the course of schizophrenia has been of younger patients as they age, there remains a clear need for longitudinal research to document changes among patients as they age from their 60s, 70s, and 80s. Nonetheless, empirical data do not seem to support Kraepelin's initial suggestion that *dementia praecox* is characterized by a course of progressive decline.[49] In fact, there may be some modest age-related improvements in positive symptoms and perhaps other aspects of psychopathology.[8] Although there is a small subset of 'poor outcome'/ chronically institutionalized patients who seem to be at added risk for cognitive and functional decline in older age,[51] for most patients there is generally no increased (beyond age normal) decline in cognitive functioning among those with early or middle-age onset.[52,53]

## Treatment

Contemporary treatment guidelines for schizophrenia in older adults parallel those for younger adults in that a combination of pharmacological and psychosocial interventions is recommended.[54] Although treatment with antipsychotic medications is a mainstay of effective treatment and management of late-life schizophrenia, selection of the appropriate type and dose of antipsychotic medication in the elderly may be complicated by age-related factors. One of the primary concerns with conventional neuroleptic medications is that they can cause iatrogenic motor abnormalities; older adults are at even greater risk than younger patients to develop tardive dyskinesia and extrapyramidal symptoms, or EPS, (especially parkinsonism) from conventional neuroleptics.[55] The newer ('atypical' or 'second generation') antipsychotic medications have lower (although not absent) associated risk of tardive dyskinesia and EPS, though risks for these motor side effects also vary from one atypical antipsychotic to another.

The current APA treatment guidelines for schizophrenia indicate '*Second-generation antipsychotics are generally recommended over first-generation agents because of their significantly lower risk of inducing extrapyramidal symptoms and tardive dyskinesia in older persons . . . However, the second-generation agents have other clinically significant and common side effects* (pp. 33–34).' In addition to concerns about potential sedation, orthostatic hypotension, and other potential physical or medical side-effects from the newer medications, there has been recent concern about the potentially serious metabolic and cardiovascular side effects.[56] Overall, atypical agents (with the exception of clozapine) have not shown superior efficacy for schizophrenia in direct comparisons with typical antipsychotics.[57] This fact, combined with the lower cost of typical agents, has prompted some experts to question the use of atypical antipsychotics as first-line pharmacotherapy for schizophrenia. In the absence of more definitive evidence, clinicians should discuss these various advantages and disadvantages of specific drugs with patients when choosing drug therapy.

For most antipsychotics (typical or atypical), older adults with schizophrenia generally respond to 50–75 per cent of the doses needed in younger patients and often cannot tolerate the full young adult dose.[58] Side effects that are especially problematic in older adults include anticholinergic effects (e.g. constipation, confusion, urinary retention), orthostatic blood pressure changes (which may lead to falls), and reported increases in stroke and death among persons with dementia receiving antipsychotics (as dementia, of course, becomes more prevalent with increasing age).

Antipsychotic medications are helpful in managing the psychopathologic symptoms of schizophrenia, especially the so-called 'positive symptoms' such as delusions and hallucinations, but they are not a cure. Medications also tend to have little benefit for the 'negative' (e.g. apathy, anhedonia) and cognitive symptoms of the illness. Furthermore, many patients continue to have residual functional disability despite resolution of positive symptoms of psychosis. Thus, the importance of adjunctive treatment with evidenced-based psychosocial interventions in schizophrenia is being increasingly recognized.[59] For instance, investigators at our Research Center have developed or adapted, and validated a number of effective adjunctive psychosocial interventions for older patients with schizophrenia or related psychoses; these include Cognitive Behavioral Social Skills Training,[60]

Functional Adaptation Skills Training,[61] diabetes management/lifestyle modification,[62] and vocational rehabilitation/supported employment.[63] These efforts address a number of dimensions of schizophrenia that are unaffected by pharmacologic treatment alone.

## Management

As noted above, schizophrenia is a chronic condition. In addition, to specific therapies previously described, managing this complex and devastating illness requires careful attention to clinician-patient rapport. This is especially true in persons with severe paranoia and in those who lack insight into their illness. Providing care for someone who does not trust anyone or who sees no reason for treatment can be challenging, but these obstacles can often be overcome by involving family, listening empathically, avoiding premature confrontation about delusions, respecting the increased interpersonal distance many patients require, and identifying the patient's goals and priorities. Management of schizophrenia may often be optimized by multi- and interdisciplinary care to address the many ways in which the illness affects patients' lives. Because there tends to be a high degree of medical comorbidity in persons with schizophrenia (especially older adults), integration of primary care and psychiatric care is often needed. Due to normal age-related physical changes, polypharmacy, and the higher risk of medication side-effects, the long-term management of schizophrenia in older adults demands frequent monitoring of symptoms, overall health, and side-effects. Cross-discipline collaborative care and continuity with the same clinicians can help ensure older persons with schizophrenia achieve the best possible outcomes.

## Further information

Cohen, C. I. (ed.). (2003). *Schizophrenia into later life: Treatment, research, and policy*. American Psychiatric Publishing, Washington, DC.

Lehman, A.F., Lieberman, J.A., Dixon, L.B., *et al.* (2004). Practice guidelines for the treatment of patients with schizophrenia, second edition. *American Journal of Psychiatry*, **161** (2 Suppl), 1–56.

Sharma, T, and Harvey, P. (eds.). (2006). *The early course of schizophrenia*. New York: Oxford University Press.

## References

1. Henderson, A.S., Korten, A.E., Levings, C., *et al.* (1998). Psychotic symptoms in the elderly: a prospective study in a population sample. *International Journal of Geriatric Psychiatry* , 13(7), 484–92.

2. Forsell, Y. and Henderson, A.S. (1998). Epidemiology of paranoid symptoms in an elderly population. *British Journal of Psychiatry*, **172**, 429–32.

3. Howard, R., Rabins, P.V., Seeman, M.V., *et al.*(2000). Late-onset schizophrenia and very-late-onset schizophrenia-like psychosis: an international consensus. The International Late-Onset Schizophrenia Group. *American Journal of Psychiatry*, **157**(2), 172–8.

4. Ostling, S. and Skoog, I. (2002). Psychotic symptoms and paranoid ideation in a nondemented population-based sample of the very old. *Archives of General Psychiatry*, **59**(1), 53–9.

5. Mintzer, J. and Targum, S.D. (2003). Psychosis in elderly patients: classification and pharmacotherapy. *Journal of geriatric psychiatry and neurology*, 16(4), 199–206.

6. Palmer, B.W., Heaton, S.C., Jeste, D.V., *et al.* (1999). Older patients with schizophrenia: challenges in the coming decades. *Psychiatric services*, **50**(9), 1178–83.

7. American Psychiatric Association. (2000). *Diagnostic and Statistical Manual of Mental Disorders - Text Revision*. (4th edn). American Psychiatric Association, Washington, DC.

8. Jeste, D.V., Twamley, E.W., Eyler Zorrilla, L.T., *et al.* (2003). Aging and outcome in schizophrenia. *Acta Psychiatrica Scandinavica*, **107**(5), 336–43.

9. Ciompi, L. (1985). Aging and schizophrenic psychosis. *Acta psychiatrica Scandinavica. Supplementum*, **319**, 93–105.

10. Heinrichs, R.W. and Zakzanis, K.K. (1998). Neurocognitive deficit in schizophrenia: a quantitative review of the evidence. *Neuropsychology*, **12**(3), 426–45.

11. Green, M.F., Kern, R.S., Braff, D.L., *et al.* (2000). Neurocognitive deficits and functional outcome in schizophrenia: are we measuring the 'right stuff'? *Schizophrenia bulletin*, **26**(1), 119–36.

12. Palmer, B.W., Savla, G.N. (in press). The association of specific neuropsychological deficits on capacity to consent to research or treatment. *Journal of the International Neuropsychological Society*, in press.

13. Harris, M.J., Jeste, D.V. (1998). Late-onset schizophrenia: an overview. *Schizophrenia bulletin*, **14**(1), 39–55.

14. Jeste, D.V., Symonds, L.L., Harris, M.J., *et al.* (1997 Fall). Nondementia nonpraecox dementia praecox? Late-onset schizophrenia. *The American journal of geriatric psychiatry* , **5**(4), 302–17.

15. Sato, T., Bottlender, R., Schroter, A., *et al.* (2004). Psychopathology of early-onset versus late-onset schizophrenia revisited: an observation of 473 neuroleptic-naive patients before and after first-admission treatments. *Schizophrenia research*, **67**(2-3), 175–83.

16. Palmer, B.W., McClure, F.S., Jeste, D.V., *et al.* (2001). Schizophrenia in late life: findings challenge traditional concepts. *Harvard Review of Psychiatry* , **9**(2),51–8.

17. Castle, D.J., Wessely, S., Howard, R., et al. (1997). Schizophrenia with onset at the extremes of adult life. *International Journal of Geriatric Psychiatry*, 12(7), 712–7.

18. Bleuler, E. (1950/1911). *Dementia praecox; or, The group of schizophrenias*. International Universities Press, New York.

19. Berrios, G. E., Luque, R., & Villagrán, J. M. (2003). Schizophrenia: A conceptual history. *International Journal of Psychology & Psychological Therapy*, **3**(2), 111–40.

20. World Health Organization. International Statistical Classification of Diseases and Related Health Problems, 10th Revision, Version for 2007. Available via internet at: http://www.who.int/classifications/icd/en/[Accessed June 15, 2007].

21. Palmer, B.W., Nayak, G.V., Jeste, D.V., *et al.* (2003). A comparison of early- and late-onset schizophrenia. In *Schizophrenia into later life* (ed. C., Cohen), pp. 43–75. American Psychiatric Publishing, Washington, DC.

22. Adityanjee, Aderibigbe, Y.A., Theodoridis, D., *et al.* (1999). Dementia praecox to schizophrenia: the first 100 years. *Psychiatry and Clinical Neurosciences*, **53**(4),437–48.

23. Bleuler, M. (1978). *The schizophrenic disorders: Long-term patient and family studies*. Yale University Press, New Haven, CT.

24. Roth, M. (1995). The natural history of mental disorder in old age. *The Journal of Mental Science* , **101**(423), 281–301.

25. Berrios, G.E. (2003). The insanities of the third age: a conceptual history of paraphrenia. *The Journal of Nutrition, Health & Aging*, **7**(6), 394–9.

26. American Psychiatric Association. (1980). *Diagnostic and Statistical Manual* (3rd edn.). Author, Washington, DC.

27. American Psychiatric Association. (1987). *Diagnostic and Statistical Manual* (3rd edn.). Author, Washington, DC.

28. American Psychiatric Association. (1994). *Diagnostic and Statistical Manual of Mental Disorders* (4th edn.). American Psychiatric Association, Washington, DC.

29. Jeste, D.V. and Palmer, B.W. (1998) Secondary Psychoses: An overview. *Seminars in Clinical Neuropsychiatry*, **3**, 2–3.

30. Jeste, D.V., Finkel, SI. (2000 Winter) Psychosis of Alzheimer's disease and related dementias. Diagnostic criteria for a distinct syndrome. The American journal of geriatric psychiatry , 8(1),29–34.

31. Cole, M.G. Delirium in elderly patients. *The American journal of geriatric psychiatry.*

32. Webster, R. and Holroyd, S. (2000). Prevalence of psychotic symptoms in delirium. *Psychosomatics,*41(6),519–22.

33. Marsh, C.M. (1997). Psychiatric presentations of medical illness. *The Psychiatric Clinics of North America*, 20(1), 181–204.

34. Grimby, A. (1993). Bereavement among elderly people: grief reactions, post-bereavement hallucinations and quality of life. *Acta psychiatrica Scandinavica*, 87(1), 72–80.

35. Menon, G.J., Rahman, I., Menon, S.J., et al. (2003). Complex visual hallucinations in the visually impaired: the Charles Bonnet Syndrome. *Survey of Ophthalmology*, 48(1), 58–72.

36. Saha, S., Chant, D., Welham, J., et al. (2005).A systematic review of the prevalence of schizophrenia. *PLoS Medicine*, 2(5), e141.

37. Perala, J., Suvisaari, J., Saarni, S.I., et al. (2007). Lifetime prevalence of psychotic and bipolar I disorders in a general population. *Archives of General Psychiatry*, 64(1), 19–28.

38. Lindamer, L.A., Lohr, J.B., Harris, M.J., et al. (1999). Gender-related clinical differences in older patients with schizophrenia. *The Journal of Clinical Psychiatry*, 60(1), 61–7; quiz 8–9.

39. Black, D.W. and Fisher, R. (1992). Mortality in DSM-IIIR schizophrenia. *Schizophrenia research* , 7(2), 109–16.

40. Joukamaa, M., Heliovaara, M., Knekt, P., et al. (2006). Schizophrenia, neuroleptic medication and mortality. *British Journal of Psychiatry*, 188, 122–7.

41. Hybels, C.F. and Blazer, D.G. (2003). Epidemiology of late-life mental disorders. *Clinics in Geriatric Medicine*, 19(4), 663–96, v.

42. Cardno, A.G. and Gottesman, II. (2000 Spring) Twin studies of schizophrenia: from bow-and-arrow concordances to star wars Mx and functional genomics. *American Journal of Medical Genetics*, 97(1), 12–17.

43. Walker, E., Kestler, L., Bollini, A., et al. (2004).Schizophrenia: etiology and course. *Annual review of psychology*, 55, 401–30.

44. Ross, C.A., Margolis, R.L., Reading, S.A., et al. (2006) Neurobiology of schizophrenia. *Neuron*, 52(1), 139–53.

45. Rapoport, J.L., Addington, A.M., Frangou, S., et al. (2005). The neurodevelopmental model of schizophrenia: update 2005. *Molecular Psychiatry*, 10(5), 434–49.

46. Friston, K.J. and Frith, C.D. (1995). Schizophrenia: a disconnection syndrome? *Clinical neuroscience* , 3(2), 89–97.

47. Kraepelin E. (1971/1919). *Dementia praecox and paraphrenia*. New York: Krieger.

48. Jobe, T.H. and Harrow, M. (2005). Long-term outcome of patients with schizophrenia: a review. *Canadian Journal of Psychiatry*, 50(14), 892–900.

49. Riecher-Rossler, A. and Rossler, W. (1998). The course of schizophrenic psychoses: what do we really know? A selective review from an epidemiological perspective. *European Archives of Psychiatry and Clinical Neuroscience* , 248(4), 189–202.

50. Ram, R., Bromet, E.J., Eaton, W.W., et al. (1992)The natural course of schizophrenia: a review of first-admission studies. *Schizophrenia bulletin* , 18(2), 185–207.

51. White, L., Friedman, J.I., Bowie, C.R., et al. (2006). Long-term outcomes in chronically hospitalized geriatric patients with schizophrenia: retrospective comparison of first generation and second generation antipsychotics. *Schizophr Res*, 88(1–3), 127-34.

52. Heaton, R.K., Gladsjo, J.A., Palmer, B.W., et al. (2001). The stability and course of neuropsychological deficits in schizophrenia. *Archives of General Psychiatry* , 58(1), 24–32.

53. Palmer, B.W., Bondi, M.W., Twamley, E.W., et al. (2003 Winter) Are late-onset schizophrenia spectrum disorders neurodegenerative

conditions? Annual rates of change on two dementia measures. *The Journal of Neuropsychiatry and Clinical Neurosciences*; 15(1), 45–52.

54. Lehman, A.F., Lieberman, J.A., Dixon, L.B., et al. (2004)Practice guideline for the treatment of patients with schizophrenia, second edition. *American Journal of Medical Genetics* , 161(2. Suppl.), 1–56.

55. Jeste, D.V. (2000). Tardive dyskinesia in older patients. *The Journal of clinical psychiatry.* 61 (Suppl 4), 27–32.

56. Newcomer, J.W. and Lieberman, J.A.(2007). Comparing safety and tolerability of antipsychotic treatment. *The Journal of clinical psychiatry* , 68(3), e07.

57. Lieberman, J.A., Stroup, T.S., McEvoy, J.P., et al. (2005). Effectiveness of antipsychotic drugs in patients with chronic schizophrenia. *The New England Journal of Medicine* , 22;353(12), 1209–23.

58. Jeste, D.V., Dolder, C.R., Nayak, G.V., et al. (2005). Atypical antipsychotics in elderly patients with dementia or schizophrenia: review of recent literature. *Harvard Review of Psychiatry* , 13(6), 340–51.

59. Dickerson, F.B., Lehman, A.F. (2006). Evidence-based psychotherapy for schizophrenia. *The Journal of Nervous and Mental Disease* , 194(1), 3–9.

60. Granholm, E., McQuaid, J.R., McClure, F.S., et al. (2005). A randomized, controlled trial of cognitive behavioral social skills training for middle-aged and older outpatients with chronic schizophrenia. *American Journal of Psychiatry* , 162(3), 520–29.

61. Patterson, T.L., Mausbach, B.T., McKibbin, C., et al. (2006). Functional adaptation skills training (FAST): a randomized trial of a psychosocial intervention for middle-aged and older patients with chronic psychotic disorders. *Schizophrenia research* , 86(1–3), 291–9.

62. McKibbin, C.L., Patterson, T.L., Norman, G., et al. (2006).A lifestyle intervention for older schizophrenia patients with diabetes mellitus: a randomized controlled trial. *Schizophrenia research* , 86(1–3), 36–44.

63. Twamley, E.W., Padin, D.S., Bayne, K.S., et al. (2005).Work rehabilitation for middle-aged and older people with schizophrenia: a comparison of three approaches. *The Journal of Nervous and Mental Disease*, 193(9), 596–601.

## 8.5.4 **Mood disorders in the elderly**

Robert Baldwin

### Introduction

This chapter considers some of the commonly asked questions about mood disorders in later life. Is depression in later life a distinct clinical syndrome? How common is it? Is there an organic link, for example to cerebral changes, and if so, is there an increased risk of later dementia? Is it more difficult to diagnose and treat late-life depression, and once treated, is the outcome good, bad, or indifferent? The emphasis will be on depression but bipolar disorder and mania will also be considered.

### Classification

The main mood disorders which older people suffer are classified as: depressive episode, dysthymia, bipolar disorder, and organic mood disorder. Depressive illness and major depression are terms often used synonymously with depressive episode. Current classificatory systems, notably The World Health Organization ICD10 and the DSM Version IV of the American Psychiatric Association, are described in Chapter 4.5.3.

# Depressive episode

## Clinical features

Other than more frequent somatic and hypochondriacal complaints, patients with depression in later life are little different, symptomatically, to younger adults.[1] An exception may be the recently described 'vascular depression' (depression linked to small vessel disease of the brain), in which depressive ideation is less but cognitive impairment and apathy greater. In most cases then the pathoplastic effects of ageing and ill-health are what mainly influence the presentation of depression in later life (Table 8.5.4.1).

An overlap of symptoms due to *associated physical ill-health* may lead to diagnostic difficulty, and determining whether a symptom has arisen predominantly because of affective disorder or a medical condition can be difficult for those without the necessary experience.

Older depressed patients may *minimize feelings of sadness* and instead become *hypochondriacal* (morbidly preoccupied with a fear of illness).[1] Late-onset *neurotic symptoms* (*severe anxiety, phobias, obsessional compulsive phenomena or hysteria*) are usually secondary to depressive illness. Any act of *deliberate self-harm* suggests depression, as elderly people rarely take 'manipulative' overdoses. An overdose in an older person should never be dismissed because its effects, in purely medical terms, were trivial. *All* require psychiatric assessment. Severe depression may mimic dementia. Table 8.5.4.2 highlights the main differences between progressive dementia and the pseudodementia of depression. Pseudodementia is a term which is perhaps waning in use as it has become clear that depressive disorder is commonly associated with cognitive impairment, which may not be reversible, even with adequate treatment of depression. Pseudodementia is often applied to an older depressed patient who, on presentation, appears very confused, with frequent 'don't know' responses. However, the onset of confusion is acute, easily dated, the patients convey their despair non-verbally, and, unlike the person with degenerative dementia, complain vociferously about their memory. Cortical signs (aphasia, apraxia, etc.) suggest a primary dementia with a super-added depression rather than depressive pseudodementia. Wandering off and getting lost suggests dementia but occasional cases are seen of fugue states caused by severe depression mimicking disorganized behaviour in dementia. The key is a good history.

An unusual *behavioural disturbance* may occasionally be a leading symptom of depression. Examples include the onset of incontinence in an older person who feels trapped in a situation of resented dependency in a residential or nursing home, late-onset alcohol abuse or, rarely, shoplifting.

**Table 8.5.4.1** Factors influencing the presentation of depression in older people

| |
|---|
| Overlap of symptoms of physical disorder with those of the somatic symptoms of depression |
| Tendency of older people to minimize a complaint of sadness and instead become hypochondriacal |
| Late-onset neurotic symptoms (severe anxiety, obsessional compulsive symptoms, hysteria) which mask depression |
| Deliberate self-harm which seems medically trivial |
| Pseudodementia |
| Behavioural disturbance such as alcohol abuse or shoplifting |

**Table 8.5.4.2** Characteristics distinguishing depression ('pseudodementia') from dementia

| Dementia | Depression |
|---|---|
| Insidious | Rapid onset |
| Symptoms usually of long duration | Symptoms usually of short duration |
| Mood and behaviour fluctuate | Mood is consistently depressed |
| 'Near miss' answers typical | 'Don't know' answers typical |
| Patient conceals forgetfulness | Patient highlights forgetfulness |
| Cognitive impairment relatively stable | Cognitive impairment fluctuates greatly |
| Higher cortical dysfunction evident | Higher cortical dysfunction absent |

### (a) Vascular depression

In vascular depression, vascular disease is judged to predispose, precipitate, or perpetuate depressive symptoms. Evidence (summarized by Baldwin[2]) includes the following. There is a high rate of structural brain abnormalities in both white matter and basal ganglia grey matter on imaging and on post-mortem examination of older patients with depressive disorder, notably with a late age of onset. Psychomotor change, apathy, and executive dysfunction (leading to slowed responses, failure of initiation, impersistence in tasks, and inefficient memory) occur characteristically in such patients. Strategic lesion location, sufficient to disrupt subcortical-frontal circuitry, is associated with poorer depression outcomes, and progression of such lesions is associated with later incident cases of depression in those not already depressed. The concept of vascular depression is discussed critically under aetiololgy.

## Diagnosis and differential diagnosis

### (a) Assessment

The psychiatric history should include a collateral history as well as drug evaluation (prescribed, 'borrowed', and over-the-counter) and alcohol intake. A cognitive screening test should always be undertaken. A physical evaluation should focus on possible disorders causing an organic mood disorder (Table 8.5.4.3), including medication. Non-selective β-blockers, calcium antagonists, benzodiazepines, and systemic corticosteroids were the main culprits in one study.[3]

Screening questionnaires can be used to help diagnose depression, especially in settings such as medical wards where the prevalence is high, but their results must be informed by clinical judgement. The Geriatric Depression Scale (GDS) (Geriatric Depression Scale website http://stanford.edu/~yesavage/GDS.html) is widely used. It focuses on the cognitive aspects of depressive illness rather than physical depressive symptomatology, and has a simple 'yes/no' format (Table 8.5.4.4). It loses specificity in severe dementia but performs reasonably well in mild to moderate dementia. For rapid screening four questions (1, 3, 8 and 9) can be used.

### (b) Investigations

Table 8.5.4.5 summarizes investigations appropriate for a first episode of depression and a recurrence. A guiding principle is that elderly people are in a more precarious state of homeostasis with their environment because they have less physiological reserve.

**Table 8.5.4.3** Common medical illnesses and drugs that may cause organic mood syndromes

| Medical conditions | Central-acting drugs |
|---|---|
| Endocrine/metabolic | Anti-hypertensive drugs |
| Hypo/hyperthyroidism | β-blockers (especially non-selective) |
| Cushing's disease | Methyldopa |
| Hypercalcaemia | Reserpine |
| Sub-nutrition | Clonidine |
| Pernicious anaemia | Nifedipine, calcium channel agents |
| Organic brain disease | Digoxin |
| Cerebrovascular disease/stroke | Steroids |
| CNS tumours | Analgesic drugs |
| Parkinson's disease | Opioids |
| Alzheimer's disease and vascular dementia | Indomethacin |
| Multiple sclerosis | Anti-parkinson |
| Systemic lupus erythematosus | L-Dopa |
| Occult carcinoma | Amantadine |
| Pancreas | Tetrabenazine |
| Lung | Psychiatric drugs |
| Chronic infections | Neuroleptics |
| Neurosyphilis | Benzodiazepines |
| Brucellosis | Miscellaneous |
| Neurocysticercosis | Sulphonamides |
| Myalgic encephalomyelitis | Alcohol |
| AIDS | Interferon |

Severe depression in a 75-year-old may lead to quite serious metabolic derangement which would be unlikely in a fit 35-year-old.

An electroencephalogram (EEG) can help in differentiating depression from an organic brain syndrome such as delirium or an early dementia. A brain scan is only performed if clinically indicated, for example a rapid-onset depression with neurological symptoms or signs. The Dexamethasone Suppression Test (DST) is less specific for depressive illness than was first thought. It cannot reliably differentiate dementia from depression.

### (c) Differential diagnosis

**Organic mood disorder** is diagnosed when a direct aetiological link can be established between the onset of the mood disorder and an underlying systemic or cerebral disorder (including dementia), or an ingested substance such as medication or alcohol.

**Bipolar disorder** is covered later. **Psychotic illness** (schizophrenia or delusional disorder) may present with marked depressed affect but other symptoms are present. A common depressive delusion in old age is hypochondriasis and sometimes it is difficult to decide whether the patient has a psychotic or an affective disorder. Interpretation depends on which symptoms predominate; if they occur together, it may be appropriate to use the term schizoaffective disorder.

**Table 8.5.4.4** Geriatric Depression Scale

*Instructions:* Choose the best answer for how you have felt over the past *week*.

1. **Are you basically satisfied with your life?** No
2. **Have you dropped many of your activities and interests?** Yes
3. **Do you feel your life is empty?** Yes
4. **Do you often get bored?** Yes
5. Are you hopeful about the future? No
6. Are you bothered by thoughts you can't get out of your head? Yes
7. **Are you in good spirits most of the time?** No
8. **Are you afraid something bad is going to happen to you?** Yes
9. **Do you feel happy most of the time?** No
10. **Do you often feel helpless?** Yes
11. Do you often get restless and fidgety? Yes
12. **Do you prefer to stay at home, rather than going out and doing new things? Yes**
13. Do you frequently worry about the future? Yes
14. **Do you feel you have more problems with your memory than most?** Yes
15. **Do you think it is wonderful to be alive now?** No
16. Do you often feel downhearted and blue (sad)? Yes
17. **Do you feel pretty worthless the way you are?** Yes
18. Do you worry a lot about the past? Yes
19. Do you find life very exciting? No
20. Is it hard for you to start on new projects (plans)? Yes
21. **Do you feel full of energy?** No
22. **Do you feel that your situation is hopeless?** Yes
23. **Do you think most people are better off (in their lives) than you are?** Yes
24. Do you frequently get upset over little things? Yes
25. Do you frequently feel like crying? Yes
26. Do you have trouble concentrating? Yes
27. Do you enjoy getting up in the morning? No
28. Do you prefer to avoid social gatherings (get-togethers)? Yes
29. Is it easy for you to make decisions? No
30. Is your mind as clear as it used to be? No

*Notes:* (1) Answers refer to responses which score '1'; (2) bracketed phrases refer to alternative ways of expressing the questions; (3) questions in bold are for the 15-item version. Threshold for possible depression: >/=11 (GDS30); >/=5 (GDS15); >=2 (GDS4).

**Dysthymia** chiefly occurs in younger adults but may occur in later life in association with chronic ill-health. Where there is a clear onset of depressive symptoms within 1 month of a stressful life event without the criteria for a depressive episode being met, then an *adjustment disorder* may be diagnosed.

## Epidemiology

In the United Kingdom, pervasive depression (a term denoting a depressive syndrome that a psychiatrist would regard as warranting intervention) is found between 8.6 and 14.1 per cent of elderly people living at home. The prevalence of a depressive episode is between 1 and 4 per cent of elderly people living at home.[4] The finding of a high rate of depressive symptoms but a much lower rate of depressive episodes is an epidemiological dilemma which is discussed in Chapter 4.5.4. It is likely that current classification

**Table 8.5.4.5** Investigations for depression in later life

| Investigation | First episode | Recurrence |
|---|---|---|
| Full blood count | Yes | Yes |
| Urea and electrolytes | Yes | Yes |
| Calcium | Yes | Yes |
| Thyroid function | Yes | If clinically indicated, or more than 12 months elapsed |
| B$_{12}$ | Yes | If clinically indicated, or more than 12 months elapsed |
| Folate | Yes | If clinically indicated (for example recent poor diet) |
| Liver function | Yes | If indicated (for example suspected or known alcohol misuse) |
| Syphilitic serology | If clinically indicated (for example relevant neurological symptoms) | Only if clinically indicated |
| CT (brain) | If clinically indicated | If clinically indicated |
| EEG | If clinically indicated | If clinically indicated |

systems overlook many of the late-life depressions found in community studies.

Depression in later life, whether major or 'minor', is associated with worsened medical morbidity, disability, and increased health utilization.[1] Co-morbidity from physical disorder or cognitive impairment is the main determinant of prevalence. Handicap, the disadvantage imposed by a physical impairment and attendant disability, is a further strong predictor of depression.[5] This matters because handicap is amenable to social intervention.

In residential care, nursing homes and medical wards the rates are between 20 and 40 per cent.

## Aetiology

The risk factors for depression in later life are discussed in Chapter 4.5.5. A depressive episode usually arises from a combination of vulnerability factors along with a triggering (precipitating) adverse life event. Avoidant and dependent personality types are associated with late-life depression, and a lifelong lack of a capacity for intimacy is another risk factor.[6] Precipitating life events occur at a similar frequency to other age groups, although health-related events are more common among older people.[6]

The concept of vascular depression suggests new aetiological insights.[2] However, criticisms against vascular depression as a distinct subtype include the difficulty in establishing a temporal link between depression onset and vascular disease and that, if causal, vascular disease is likely to have been present well before old age. Furthermore, in studies of vascular depression the direction of causality is unclear since patients with vascular disease have a high rate of depression, and depression appears to worsen vascular disease, perhaps by direct effects on blood vessel endothelial function and indirectly through poor self-monitoring of health and poor adherence to medical drugs.

If confirmed, the vascular depression hypothesis could lead to antidepressant strategies aimed at improving the underlying vascular impairment as well as mood. In the meantime, a patient presenting late-onset depression should be thoroughly investigated for vascular disease as a potential aetiological contributory factor which should be optimally treated along with the depression.

## Course and prognosis

Across all age groups depressive disorder is prone to persistence. Beekman et al.[7] followed 277 community-dwelling subjects, aged over 55 (most over 75), from a Dutch epidemiological survey. Using multiple assessments of mood over a 6-year period, they found almost half the sample was depressed for more than 60 per cent of the time. Twenty three per cent had true remissions, 12 per cent remissions with recurrence, a third a chronic-intermittent course; another third had chronic depression. Outcomes reported from the community and medical ward patients are worse than those of depressed patients under psychiatric care,[8] possibly linked to undertreatment in the non-specialist settings.

### (a) Comparative outcome

Mitchell and Subramaniam[9] reviewed the literature between 1966 and July 2004, finding 24 publications which could be used to assess outcomes between different age groups. Overall the authors concluded that episodes of depression remitted in later life as well as in other times but with a greater risk of relapse. Two factors seemed to explain this: age of onset (recurrent depression from earlier life conferring a poorer prognosis) and medical comorbidity (with a worse prognosis linked to a later onset). Although these mechanisms differ, the high risk of relapse in late-life depression highlights the need for effective continuation and maintenance phases of treatment, regardless of age of onset.

## Mortality

A number of studies show that depression is an independent risk factor for increased mortality,[1] not accounted for by suicide. Following a cohort of 652 depressed and non-depressed subjects over 3.5 years, Geerlings[10] found that duration, chronicity, and increasing symptoms from baseline were all linked to a higher risk of death, leading them to suggest that adequate treatment may reduce this effect. Physical illness, occult disease (e.g. a carcinoma), poor self-monitoring of health, inactivity, poor adherence to treatments, and effects on the hypothalamic-pituitary-adrenal axis or other endocrine systems are possible factors.

## Factors predictive of outcome

Clinical features that have been shown to be associated with a poorer outcome, include a slower initial recovery, more severe initial depression, duration of illness for more than 2 years, three or more previous episodes, a previous history of dysthymia, psychotic symptoms, and cerebrovascular disease (including vascular depression). Other factors that may affect outcome adversely are chronic stress associated with a poor environment, crime, and poverty as well as a new physical illness, becoming a victim of crime, and poor perceived social support.

The practical message is that to improve the prognosis of depression one must treat episodes early and vigorously and attend to the patient's social supports, and milieu.

### (a) Does depressive disorder predispose to later dementia?

There is growing evidence from epidemiological studies that depression is a risk factor for later cognitive impairment or dementia.[11] Why this might be so is not clear but it is known that chronic depression is associated with hippocampal atrophy in older patients,[12] and that depressed patients may adopt unhealthy lifestyles, which can aggravate the risk factors for vascular disease and later dementia.

## Treatment

Multi-modal management (pharmacological, psychological, and social) within a multidisciplinary framework is as important in late-life as it is at other times of life. Attending to an elderly depressed person's physical health needs, physical environment, and social needs is essential. The goal is remission of all symptoms and not merely improvement, as residual symptoms increase the chance of chronicity. Ageing and frailty result in increased dependency and less ability to adapt in a flexible way to the kinds of adversity that maintain depression. To give a simple example, good chiropody aimed at optimizing mobility can have a major positive impact alongside medical intervention, but no one aspect of treatment should be prioritized over another. Another important principle is patient-centredness. This should include giving the patients as much choice as possible regarding their treatment. Many older depressed patients, if asked, would prefer a psychological approach to medical management and there is good evidence that psychological treatments work well in older adults.[13] Resource limitations are understood, but age alone should not determine the likelihood of receiving a psychological intervention, if preferred.

Collaborative care, whereby, a depression care manager (usually a nurse, psychologist, or social worker) coordinates the care and works closely with both primary care physician and psychiatrist, is an important model for improving outcomes. In the largest study to date, 'IMPACT' from the United States, involving 1801 depressed primary care patients (major depression, 17 per cent; dysthymia, 30 per cent; or both, 53 per cent), at 12 months the Number-Needed-to-Treat (NNT) was highly significant at four in those receiving the intervention.[14]

General principles of pharmacological management include: building a therapeutic partnership with the patient; explanation of how and when antidepressants work; addressing adherence through building therapeutic concordance; tailoring antidepressants drug to the patient; arranging appropriate follow-up.

## Evidence of efficacy

### (a) Antidepressants

Altered pharmacokinetics, different pharmacodynamics, a greater chance of polypharmacy and hence drug interactions and reduced compensatory mechanisms are all important factors which bear upon treatment response in late-life depression.[15] An important practical consequence is to be mindful of greater inter-individual variation in drug-handling in older patients. Patients worry about antidepressants being addictive, which they are not, and that depression means 'senility', which it does not. Psychoeducation is important and can improve adherence to medication recommendations. Recommended starting and therapeutic dosages are listed in Table 8.5.4.6. These are average doses. For some drugs, notably the tricyclics, there is a very wide therapeutic range and higher levels may be required, provided they are tolerated.

A Cochrane systematic review of Randomized Controlled Trials (RCT)[16] found efficacy for antidepressants over placebo in late-life

major depression. However, the analysis could only find 17 suitable studies (two of SSRIs). The NNT averaged four, but was higher for SSRIs. In a further Cochrane systematic review of studies including patients aged over 55 (29 trials), there was no difference in efficacy between tricyclics and SSRIs, but tricyclics were associated with higher withdrawal rates due to side-effects. Patients receiving tricyclic-related antidepressants (Mianserin or Trazodone) had a similar withdrawal rate to SSRIs, leading the authors to conclude that tricyclic-related antidepressants may offer a viable alternative to SSRIs in older depressed patients. The analysis also investigated 'atypical' antidepressants but it was not possible to make recommendations because of low statistical power. Atypicals included the important antidepressants reboxetine, venlafaxine, and mirtazapine.[17]

More recent RCTs have suggested less positive results.[18] Trials involving older adults and with venlafaxine, fluoxetine, citalopram, and escitalopram showed these drugs to be no more effective than placebo. Sertraline and duloxetine were superior to placebo but remission rates, as opposed to response rates, were relatively low in all these studies. Trials which are of insufficient duration and the use of antidepressants for milder depressions, for which they are ineffective, are possible factors.

### (b) Depression in special patient groups

A Cochrane systematic review of antidepressants for depression in dementia found 'weak' evidence for their effectiveness,[19] but there were few admissible trials. This does not mean

**Table 8.5.4.6** Suggested starting and therapeutic doses for antidepressants in the United Kingdom

| Drug | Average therapeutic doses[a] | Average starting doses |
|---|---|---|
| *Tricyclics* | | |
| Amitriptyline | 75–100 | 25 |
| Clomipramine | 75–100 | 10 |
| Dosulepin (dothiepin) | 75–150 | 25–50 |
| Imipramine | 75–100 | 10–25 |
| Nortriptyline | 75–100 | 10–30 |
| Lofepramine | 140–210 | 70–140 |
| *SNRIs* | | |
| Venlafaxine | 150 | 37.5 bd |
| Duloxetine | 60 | 30–60 |
| *SSRIs* | | |
| Fluoxetine | 20 | 20 |
| Fluvoxamine | 100–200 | 50–100 |
| Paroxetine | 20 | 20 |
| Sertraline | 50–150 | 50 |
| Citalopram | 20–40 | 20 |
| Escitalopram | 10 | 5 |
| *Reversible monoamine oxidase inhibitor (RIMA)* | | |
| Moclobemide | 150–600 | 150 bd |
| *5-HT2 receptor blocker* | | |
| Trazodone | 100–300 | 100 |
| *NASSA* | | |
| Mirtazapine | 15–30 | 30 |
| *Others* | | |
| Mianserin | 30–90 | 30 |

[a] See text.

antidepressants are ineffective in depression-related dementia but there is a high rate of spontaneous recovery of depression complicating dementia so that 'watchful waiting' is reasonable for mild-to-moderate cases.

There is little trial data for individual antidepressants in patients with common medical disorders, but in the previously mentioned IMPACT research, both physical function and pain were improved in participants who received active case management compared to usual care.[20,21]

Depression post-stroke is common. A high rate of spontaneous recovery occurs, especially in the first 6 weeks. Studies are underway to assess whether repetitive Transcranial Magnetic Stimulation (rTMS) may be helpful in post-stroke depression. TCAs and SSRIs in standard dosages are effective in post-stroke emotionalism.

### (c) Choice of antidepressant

*Tricyclics* often cause postural hypotension, which may lead to unpleasant dizziness or dangerous falls. Secondary amine tricyclics are generally safer in this respect than tertiary drugs. Poor left ventricular function is a risk, and so are diuretics or antihypertensive medication. Delirium is more likely in medically ill patients.

Behavioural toxicity (affecting vigilance, reaction times, etc.) has been largely ignored in the elderly. Now that so many older people drive and pursue other activities demanding high levels of vigilance, this must be addressed. The *SSRIs* are safer in this respect than tricyclics, except for lofepramine which causes less impairment than the older tricyclics. *Mirtazepine* enhances noradrenergic and serotonergic function via antagonism at the pre-synaptic $\alpha_2$ receptor. Differences in pharmacodynamics and pharmacokinetics are minimal with age. The side effect profile is similar to tricyclics; weight gain and sedation can be troublesome. *Duloxetine*, like venlafaxine is a dual-acting drug. The latter has been subject to cautions, regarding heart disease, at present in the United Kingdom, although recent restrictions have been lifted. Duloxetine has some RCT evidence in older depressed adults.[22] Although a special diet with *moclobemide* is not required, patients should be aware of drug interactions with painkillers and other antidepressants. Co-prescriptions of tricyclic and SSRIs should be avoided. A wash-out period of around 4–5 half-lives of the drug and any active metabolite is advised when transferring from a tricyclic or SSRI to moclobemide (but not from moclobemide to a tricyclic or SSRI).

### (d) Failure to respond to initial treatment

If a patient has made minimal or no recovery after 4 weeks of treatment at optimal dose, then the chances of recovery are slim.[23] The antidepressant may be changed to one of another class but if the patient shows at least 25 per cent improvement and is on an improving trajectory, then augmentation with lithium or a psychological intervention should be considered (see below). Electroconvulsive Treatment (ECT) is safe and effective in older patients. It is recommended when drug treatment has failed, when the patient is in danger of inanition or is acutely suicidal and is probably the treatment of choice for psychotic depression.

### (e) Continuation treatment

Most relapses occur in the first 12 months,[24] so that this is a reasonable time for continuation therapy. Patients must be educated about why they should continue to take medication even when feeling better. In psychotic depression anti-psychotic medication should be continued for 6 months and gradually withdrawn if the patient is well. Following ECT, medication should be continued to avoid relapse. Limited evidence suggests either continuing antidepressants at the acute treatment dose or using lithium.

Older people have been shown to benefit substantially from maintenance therapy,[25] even after a first episode.[24] Maintenance treatment is considered later.

### (f) Resistant depression

Data in the elderly are sparse but the most important consideration is a rational stepped care approach. Before moving up the steps of treatment, the following should be addressed: is the diagnosis correct (for example has a psychotic depression been overlooked)? Is poor tolerance a reason for non-recovery? Does the patient take the tablets? Have psychosocial reinforcing factors (for example, family conflict) been addressed? The steps themselves include optimizing the dose of antidepressant (relevant mainly for older tricyclic antidepressants), changing from one class of antidepressant to another, augmentation with lithium or a psychological intervention and combining antidepressants (for example, a SSRI plus mirtazepine). Finally ECT should be considered as it remains the most effective antidepressant treatment. Using such an approach 80 per cent of patients in one study responded.[26]

### (g) Psychological therapies

Cognitive behavioural therapy (CBT), Interpersonal Psychotherapy (IPT), and psychodynamic psychotherapy have been shown to work in older people,[13] including in group format. CBT and IPT along with family interventions are discussed elsewhere. Problem-solving Treatment (PST) addresses the here and now, focusing on current difficulties and setting future goals.

Psychological interventions may also be important in relapse prevention. Reynolds *et al.*[27] showed in a study of older patients that monthly IPT given in the continuation phase of treatment was more effective than routine care, with combined IPT and antidepressant therapy being the most effective strategy. However, the same group were unable to replicate this in a later study with a group of patients who were somewhat older.[25]

Anxiety management can be an effective adjunctive treatment for depressed patients, especially those recovering from depression but left with residual anxiety, low confidence, or phobic avoidance, any of which can undermine functional improvement. Techniques include progressive relaxation, either alone with a commercial tape, or in groups. Exercise and activity are important both to avoid depression and counter it. Behavioural activation is a technique which can overcome the withdrawal and apathy that so often exists in late-life depression. It works by helping the patient develop a schedule of activities, agreed with the patient, with or without a written diary to support implementation.

Work to support the family and main caregivers is also important.

## Prevention

### (a) Primary prevention

Many prevalent diseases of later life are associated both with depression as well as lifestyle factors: diet, exercise, and obesity. Cole and Dendukuri[28] carried out a meta-analysis of risk factors for late-life depression, finding five which were robustly linked to it. These were bereavement, sleep problems, disability, prior depression, and female gender. Some of these are amenable to a public health preventative approach.

Those most vulnerable to depression will often be in touch with a home care services. This is one area where education about detection could be usefully targeted. Another example is the staff of nursing homes where depression is highly prevalent. Postgraduate training of general practitioners is another way of improving detection via the 'filter' of primary care.

### (b) Secondary prevention

Maintenance treatment with a tricyclic,[24] the SSRIs citalopram[29] and paroxetine[25] or a combining medication with a psychological treatment[27] are effective prevention strategies.

Expert guidelines[30] recommend a minimum of 12 months continuation treatment for a first episode, 24 months for a second, and at least 3 years for three or more episodes. Some clinicians recommend lifelong treatment with antidepressants following even a single episode of major depression on the grounds that a substantial later period morbidity might be reduced. This must be balanced against an increased risk of side effects as patients age.

### (c) Tertiary prevention

Often the emphasis is on basic explanations and on simple instructions about how to manage problems such as frequent hypochondriacal complaints or apathy. Although respite care is usually associated with dementia, there is occasionally a case for it in those with chronic treatment-resistant depression, in order to allow the relative(s) a break.

## Bipolar disorder

Practice guidelines for bipolar disorder are available from the internet. Two are: *British Association of Psychopharmacology* (2003)[31]—http://www.bap.org.uk/consensus/bipolar_disorder.html and the *National Institute for Clinical Excellence (NICE) (2006)*.[32] http://www.nice.org.uk/page.aspx?o=CG38.

## Mania

### Clinical features

Clinical descriptions of mania in late life often portray it as atypical. However, Broadhead and Jacoby[33] found few clinical differences between 35 manic patients over the age of 60 compared to 35 younger manic patients, aged below 40. The younger manic patients were more severely ill but there was no support for the often-held view that there is a greater depressive admixture in older patients.

### Diagnosis and differential diagnosis

The main differential diagnosis of mania in late life lies between a late-onset manic episode and bipolar disorder. In later presentations of bipolar disorder the time between depression and first manic episode can be us much as 15 to 40 years or more. Given this long latency it is easy to overlook bipolar disorder unless a thorough history is taken.

### Epidemiology

Although only about 10 per cent of new onset cases of bipolar disorder occurs after the age of 50 they account for proportionally greater morbidity. Changing demography makes it likely that there will be more cases of bipolar disorder in later life. Episodes can be misdiagnosed; for example a depressive mood swing presenting with withdrawal or a manic one with irritability.

### Aetiology

The phenomenon of conversion to bipolarity after many years of unipolar depression has led to speculation that cerebral organic factors may play a part in the aetiology of late-onset mania. In support of this, cognitive function is significantly impaired in between a fifth and a third of elderly manics.[33,34] Furthermore studies[35] have shown a high rate of neurological disturbance, cerebral deep white matter lesions, and reduced heritability in late-life mania.

The term 'secondary mania' denotes manic illness which starts without a prior history of affective disorder in close temporal relationship to a physical illness or drug treatment and often in the absence of a family history of affective illness. A large number of conditions have been associated with secondary mania, including stroke, head injury, tumours, and non-specific lesions to the right side of the brain.

### Course and prognosis

The prognosis for mania is similar to that for late-life depression; that is, there is an 80 to 90 per cent recovery in the acute phase but relapses and/or recurrences occur over time in about 50 per cent of cases.[35]

### Treatment

As with younger patients, the mainstays of acute treatment are neuroleptics and mood stabilizers which include lithium and anticonvulsants, with ECT reserved for refractory cases. Increasingly atypical antipsychotics are used. These include olanzapine, risperidone, and quetiapine with aripiprazole as a possible new contender. Valproate preparations are the most widely used anticonvulsant in bipolar disorder.

Some general points to consider are: (1) a greater inter-individual variability in drug metabolism, which makes predicting the therapeutic dose difficult. Emergency rapid tranquillization with haloperidol 5 to 10 mg (often with 1 to 2 mg of lorazepam) can be used, but haloperidol has a long half-life and may lead to sudden immobility after a few days; (2) balancing risks caused by overactivity and exhaustion against an increased risk of falls in the elderly when using sedative tranquillizers; (3) an increased risk of confusion and delirium if anticholinergic drugs are given to counteract side effects; and (4) the higher risk of side effects and toxicity from lithium in older patients (including a risk even at what are considered therapeutic doses in younger patient).[35] The optimal treatment dose of lithium is not known. NICE recommends levels of 0.6 to 0.8 mmol/L for adults requiring maintenance lithium. Some old age psychiatrists use lower dosages but the evidence for low dose treatment in older patients is mixed.

The NICE Bipolar Guidance also covers the treatment of bipolar depression. The main message is that antidepressants, if used, should be combined with a mood stabilizer or an antipsychotic because of the risk of a manic switch.

### Prevention

Given the high rate of relapse or recurrence, prophylaxis should be considered in all patients. There has been a steady shift away from lithium to valproate over recent years, although some argue this has occurred ahead of evidence.[36] Also, there is some evidence that lithium may reduce the risk of suicide in bipolar disorder as well as being neuroprotective, possibly reducing the risk of dementia which some population studies have been shown to be raised in affective disorder.[31]

## Further information

CRUSE Bereavement Centre (helpline@crusebereavementcare.org.uk, 0870 167 1677).

Bipolar Organisation (formerly the Manic Depressive Fellowship, http://www.mdf.org.uk/; telephone 08456 340 540 [UK Only]; 0044 207 793 2600 [Rest of world]).

MIND National Association for Mental Health, http://www.mind.org.uk.

Depression Alliance (http://www.depressionalliance.org).

## References

1. Blazer, D.G. (2003). Depression in late life: review and commentary. *Journal of Gerontology: Medical Sciences*, **56A**, 249–65.

2. Baldwin, R.C. (2005). Is vascular depression a distinct sub-type of depressive disorder? A review of causal evidence. *International Journal of Geriatric Psychiatry*, **20**, 1–11.

3. Dhondt, T.D.F., Beekman, A.T.F., Deeg, D.J.H., et al. (2002). Iatrogenic depression in the elderly results from a community-based study in the Netherlands. *Social Psychiatry and Psychiatric Epidemiology*, **37**, 393–8.

4. Copeland, J.R.M., Beekman, A.T.F., Dewey, M.E., et al. (1999). Depression in Europe: geographical distribution among older people. *The British Journal of Psychiatry*, **174**, 312–21.

5. Prince, M.J., Harwood, R.H., Thomas, A., et al. (1998). A prospective population-based cohort study of the effects of disablement and social milieu on the onset and maintenance of late-life depression. The Gospel Oak Project VII. *Psychological Medicine*, **28**, 337–50.

6. Murphy, E. (1982). Social origins of depression in old age. *The British Journal of Psychiatry*, **141**, 135–42.

7. Beekman, A.T., Geerlings, S.W., Deeg, D.J., et al. (2002). The natural history of late-life depression. A 6-year prospective study in the community. *Archives of General Psychiatry*, **59**, 605–11.

8. Cole, M.G. and Bellavance, F. (1997). The prognosis of depression in old age. *The American Journal of Geriatric Psychiatry*, **5**, 4–14.

9. Mitchell, A.J. and Subramaniam, H. (2005). Prognosis of depression in old age compared to middle age: a systematic review of comparative studies. *The American Journal of Geriatric Psychiatry*, **162**, 1588–601.

10. Geerlings, S.W., Beekman, A.T.F., Deeg, D.J.H., et al. (2002). Duration and severity of depression predict mortality in older adults in the community. *Psychological Medicine*, **32**, 609–18.

11. Green, R.C., Cupples, L.A., Kurz, A., et al. (2003). Depression as a risk factor for Alzheimer disease: the MIRAGE study. *Archives of Neurology*, **60**, 753–9.

12. Bell-McGinty, S., Butters, M.A., Meltzer, C.C., et al. (2002). Brain morphometric abnormalities in geriatric depression: long term neurobiological effects of illness duration. *The American Journal of Psychiatry*, **159**, 1424–7.

13. Gatz, M., Fiske, A., Fox, L.S., et al. (1998). Empirically validated psychological treatments for older adults. *Journal of Mental Health and Aging*, **4**, 9–46.

14. Unützer, J., Katon, W., Callahan, C., et al. (2002). Collaborative care management of late-life depression in the primary care setting. *The Journal of the American Medical Association*, **288**, 2836–45.

15. Lotrich, F.E. and Pollock, B.G. (2005). Aging and clinical pharmacology: implications for antidepressants. *Journal of Clinical Pharmacology*, **45**, 1106–22.

16. Wilson, K., Mottram, P., Sivanranthan, A., et al. (2001). Antidepressant versus placebo for depressed elderly (Cochrane Review). In *The cochrane library*. Update Software, Oxford.

17. Mottram, P., Wilson, K., and Strobl, J. (2006). Antidepressants for depressed elderly. *Cochrane Database of Systematic Reviews*, (1): CD003491.

18. Roose, S.P. and Schatzberg, A.F. (2005). The efficacy of antidepressants in the treatment of late-life depression. *Journal of Clinical Psychopharmacology*, **25**, S1–7.

19. Bains, J., Birks, J.S., and Dening, T.D. (2002). Antidepressants for treating depression in dementia. *Cochrane Database of Systematic Reviews*, (4): CD003944.

20. Callahan, C.M., Kroenke, K., Counsell, S.R., et al. For the IMPACT investigators. (2005). Treatment of depression improves physical functioning in older adults. *Journal of the American Geriatrics Society*, **53**, 367–73.

21. Lin, E.H., Katon, W., Von Korff, M., et al. (2003). IMPACT investigators. Effect of improving depression care on pain and functional outcomes among older adults with arthritis: a randomized controlled trial. *The Journal of the American Medical Association*, **290**, 2428–9.

22. Nelson, J.C., Wohlreich, M.M., and Mallinckrodt, C.H. (2005). Duloxetine for the treatment of major depressive disorder in older patients. *The American Journal of Geriatric Psychiatry*, **13**, 227–35.

23. Sackeim, H.A., Roose, S.P., and Burt, T. (2005). Optimal length of antidepressant trials in late-life depression. *Journal of Clinical Psychopharmacology*, **25**, S34–7.

24. Old Age Depression Interest Group. (1993). How long should the elderly take antidepressants? A double blind placebo-controlled study of continuation/prophylaxis therapy with dothiepin. *The British Journal of Psychiatry*, **162**, 175–82.

25. Reynolds, C.F. III, Dew, M.A., Pollock, B.G., et al. (2006). Maintenance treatment of major depression in old age. *The New England Journal of Medicine*, **354**, 1130–8.

26. Flint, A.J. and Rifat, S.L. (1996). The effect of sequential antidepressant treatment on geriatric depression. *Journal of Affective Disorders*, **36**, 95–105.

27. Reynolds, C.F. III, Frank, E., Perel, J.M., et al. (1999). Nortriptyline and interpersonal psychotherapy as maintenance therapies for recurrent major depression: a randomized controlled trial in patients older than 59 year. *The Journal of the American Medical Association*, **281**, 39–45.

28. Cole, M.G. and Dendukuri, N. (2003). Risk factors for elderly community subjects: a systematic review and meta-analysis. *The American Journal of Psychiatry*, **160**, 1147–56.

29. Klysner, R., Bent-Hansen, J., Hansen, H.L., et al. (2002). Efficacy of citalopram in the prevention of recurrent depression in elderly patients: placebo-controlled study of maintenance therapy. *The British Journal of Psychiatry*, **181**, 29–35.

30. Alexopoulos, G.S., Katz, I.R., Reynolds, C.F., et al. (2001). The expert consensus guideline series: pharmacotherapy of depressive disorders in older patients *Postgrad Med Special Report*; (October):1–86, Expert Knowledge Systems, L.L.C, McGraw-Hill Healthcare Information Programs, Minneapolis, US.

31. Goodwin, G.M. (2003). For the consensus group of the British association for psychopharmacology. Evidence-based guidelines for treating bipolar disorder: recommendations from the British association for psychopharmacology. *Journal of Psychopharmacology*, **17**, 149–73.

32. National Institute for Health and Clinical Excellence. (2006). *NICE clinical guideline 38 bipolar disorder: the management of bipolar disorder in adults, children and adolescents, in primary and secondary care*. National Institute for Health and Clinical Excellence, London, UK.

33. Broadhead, J. and Jacoby, R. (1990). Mania in old age: a first prospective study. *International Journal of Geriatric Psychiatry*, **5**, 215–22.

34. Stone, K. (1989). Mania in the elderly. *The British Journal of Psychiatry*, **155**, 220–4.

35. Shulman, K. (1996). Recent developments in the epidemiology, co-morbidity and outcome of mania old age. *Reviews in Clinical Gerontology*, **6**, 249–54.

36. Shulman, K.L., Rochon, P., and Sykora, K. (2003) Changing prescription patterns for lithium and valproic acid in old age: shifting practice without evidence. s, **326**, 960–1.

# 8.5.5 Stress-related, anxiety, and obsessional disorders in elderly people

James Lindesay

Stress-related, anxiety, and obsessional disorders in elderly people are common, distressing, costly to services, and potentially treatable. However, despite their clinical importance, many patients still go untreated, or are treated inappropriately. The specific conditions covered here are described in detail elsewhere; this chapter focuses on the differences and difficulties that are encountered when they occur in old age.

## Classification

The ICD-10 and DSM-IV diagnostic classifications are described in Chapter 1.11. Although the term 'neurotic disorder' is not used in DSM-IV, it is retained in ICD-10 as a collective term for the disorders considered in this chapter. The extensive comorbidity between these conditions and their diagnostic instability over time are also apparent in elderly people, which supports the idea that they are better considered as aspects of a general neurotic syndrome than as discrete diagnostic categories.[1] This model is particularly applicable to elderly patients, whose illnesses are often the result of a long interaction between individual vulnerability, circumstances, and maladaptive responses to distress. Obsessive–compulsive disorder (OCD) is probably not part of a general neurotic syndrome. Although classified with the anxiety disorders in ICD-10 and DSM-IV, it has a number of features that suggest it is a distinct and stable condition with a different aetiology (see Chapter 4.8).

## Clinical features

These disorders have psychological, somatic, and behavioural features. In elderly people, these symptoms and behaviours are similar to those seen in younger patients, but there are some important differences in how they manifest themselves or are perceived by others. Although most neurotic disorders in elderly patients are long standing, an important minority of cases have their onset in old age, and it is these that usually cause the greatest diagnostic difficulties.

### Psychological symptoms

Symptoms of anxiety and depression occur to some extent in all of these disorders in late life. Depressive symptomatology in old age is described elsewhere (see Chapter 8.5.4). Regarding anxiety, the focus of the worries and fears of elderly people is on those issues that are of general concern in this age group (health, finances, crime). The phobias described by elderly people are similar to those seen in younger adults,[2] although some, such as the fear of falling, are more commonly seen in old age. Clinically significant anxieties and fears in elderly people are often dismissed as reasonable purely on grounds of age. In fact, it is physical frailty and the availability of social support that determine elderly people's perceptions of vulnerability and risk, and these rather than age should be considered when deciding whether or not concerns are reasonable.

The clinical features of OCD in old age are similar to those seen in younger patients. Obsessional symptoms rarely appear for the first time after the age of 50 years, and in such cases the possibility of an organic cause such as dementia or a space-occupying lesion should be investigated. They may also form part of a primary affective disorder.

### Somatic symptoms

The somatic symptoms of anxiety are similar at all ages, but in elderly patients there is a greater likelihood of misdiagnosis and inappropriate investigation and treatment. This is particularly true of elderly patients experiencing panic attacks, who tend to be misdirected to cardiologists, neurologists, and gastroenterologists.

### Behavioural disturbance

The psychological and somatic symptoms of anxiety have several adverse behavioural consequences, for example, phobic avoidance, the abuse of sedative drugs and alcohol, and the development of troublesome abnormal illness behaviours such as somatization and hypochondriasis. In elderly patients these behaviours are usually of long standing, but they can develop following the onset of anxiety or depression in old age. In cognitively impaired patients, disturbed behaviour may be the main presenting feature.

## Diagnosis and differential diagnosis

In old age, these disorders usually present in primary care and the general hospital, and clinicians working in these settings need to be able to identify them, and to distinguish them from the other mental and physical disorders that they may accompany or mimic.

### Depression

There is extensive comorbidity between neurotic disorders and depression, and depressive symptoms are an integral component of many neurotic disorders, particularly in old age. It is therefore important to assess to what extent depression forms part of the clinical picture, as this may require treatment in its own right. Depressive disorder that is comorbid with anxiety responds less well to antidepressant treatment, and there is a greater likelihood of relapse and recurrence.

### Dementia

In the early stages, dementia may present with symptoms such as anxiety, and obsessionality. More commonly, anxiety and depression cause subjective cognitive impairment, which may be the presenting symptom. Dementia is associated with higher rates of anxiety, unrelated to severity of cognitive impairment. Patients with vascular dementia may be more vulnerable in this respect.

This anxiety may be associated with the implications of the diagnosis in those patients who retain insight, or a response to psychotic symptoms or misinterpretations of the external environment in those who are more severely affected. The caregivers of people with dementia are also vulnerable to developing depressive and anxiety disorders, particularly if they have a previous psychiatric history.

### Delirium

Although delirium is a relatively quiet disorder in elderly patients (see Chapter 8.5.1), it may be associated with significant affective disturbances, often in response to frightening visual hallucinations and imagined assaults. Conversely, in vulnerable individuals, severe anxiety may be sufficient to precipitate delirium.

### Paranoid states and schizophrenia

Patients suffering from these disorders may experience significant fear and anxiety in response to their psychotic experiences, but this rarely causes diagnostic difficulty. Unusual hypochondriacal ideas may sometimes be difficult to distinguish from monosymptomatic delusional disorders.

### Physical illness

There is an important association between physical illness and neurotic disorders in old age. As a life event, an episode of physical illness may be the cause of neurotic disorder, particularly if it is severe or has sinister implications. For example, mild anxiety symptoms are common following myocardial infarction in old age, and vulnerable individuals may develop a disabling 'cardiac neurosis' focused on their somatic anxiety symptoms. Most cases of agoraphobia that develop after the age of 65 years are not induced by panic but arise following an alarming experience of physical ill health.[1] Follow-up studies of stroke survivors show that conditions such as agoraphobia and generalized anxiety are common, tend to become chronic in a significant proportion of cases, and are associated with poor functional recovery.[3] Chronic disabilities that limit mobility and independence, such as arthritis, balance disorders, and sensory impairments, increase the patient's sense of personal vulnerability and are also associated with elevated rates of anxiety and secondary avoidance.

Neurotic disorders can also cause physical illness by direct or indirect effects on the body. In elderly people, this may come about as the result of many years of harmful anxiety-driven behaviours such as smoking and alcohol abuse.

In terms of differential diagnosis, there is also the problem that a wide range of physical disorders may present with neurotic symptoms, and vice versa. In particular, a number of important cardiovascular, respiratory, and endocrine disorders may present with anxiety or depression and little else in old age.[4] Anxiety symptoms may also be caused by prescribed drugs such as oral hypoglycaemics and corticosteroids, or by excessive intake of caffeine and preparations containing sympathomimetics. In view of this, the clinical assessment should always include a drug history and a physical examination. A physical cause for neurotic symptoms should be considered if there is no past psychiatric history and no life event or other circumstances to account for their onset.

## Epidemiology

While neurotic disorders are relatively uncommon in clinical populations, there are significant prevalence rates in community samples, indicating that they do not pass easily through the filters on the pathway to care. Surveys using different diagnostic criteria produce different rates of disorder, which makes comparisons difficult. However, some general findings include a female preponderance for most disorders, and a fall in prevalence and incidence rates with age. Most elderly people with neurotic disorders developed them before their fifties, but elderly cases of phobic disorder, panic, and OCD tend to be of later onset.[5,6]

## Aetiology

The acquisition and subsequent loss or elaboration of the symptoms of anxiety and depression are determined by the patient's premorbid vulnerability, the particular factors that precipitate the episode of illness (destabilization), and the measures taken by the patient or the doctor to control it (restitution).[7]

### Biological factors

Most of the evidence that biological factors play a role in the development of neurotic disorders derives from studies in younger subjects (see Chapters 4.7.1–4.7.3). These studies indicate that genetic factors contribute significantly to premorbid vulnerability, but the role that they play in old age is not known. Neuroimaging studies of elderly depressed patients provide only limited information about neurotic disorders, suggesting that patients with milder forms of depression and higher anxiety scores are more likely than severely depressed patients to have normal CT scans. It has been suggested that some anxiety disorders following stroke may be related to lesion location.[8]

### Psychosocial factors

#### (a) Social adversity

This may have its effect through higher rates of physical illness and exposure to adverse life events, or by inculcating a sense of poor self-esteem. However, the impact of adversity on self-esteem in old age is not clear, since a hard life may in fact equip one to cope better with the difficulties of old age.

#### (b) Life events

Adverse life events have an important role in determining the onset of depressive and anxiety disorders (see Chapters 4.5.5.1 and 4.7.1–4.7.3). It is the meaning of the event to the individual that is important; loss events lead to depression and threatening events to anxiety. Some types of life events (physical illness, bereavement, retirement, institutionalization) are more common in old age, and are associated with psychiatric morbidity in vulnerable individuals.

Extreme trauma and catastrophe are well known to have adverse psychological consequences, and post-traumatic stress disorder (PTSD) is a recognized diagnosis in ICD-10 and DSM-IV (see Chapter 4.6.2). It is clear from studies of elderly survivors of traumatic experiences such as war and the holocaust that PTSD is often a persistent disorder, and that its onset or recurrence may be precipitated by events many years after the original traumatic experience. PTSD may also develop following trauma in late life, and as in younger subjects it tends to persist.

### (c) Early experience

Early parental loss and childhood physical and sexual abuse are associated with the development of mental disorder in adult life, an effect that persists into old age.[1]

### (d) Relationships

There is evidence that both the quantity and quality of social relationships are important determinants of psychological well-being in old age, and that factors such as smaller social networks are associated with anxiety disorders.[9]

## Course and prognosis

The limited evidence suggests that neurotic disorders in elderly people tend to become chronic and that older age of onset is a predictor of poor outcome, particularly in men.[10] The pattern of symptoms may change over time.[11] Elderly patients with anxiety disorders have an excess mortality.

## Treatment

### Evidence

There is little high-quality evidence available about the effects of treatments for these disorders in elderly patients. Cognitive behaviour therapy (CBT) is of proven benefit in younger adults (see Chapter 6.3.2.1), and there is some evidence that it is also effective in later life.[12] There have been surprisingly few trials of anxiolytic drugs in elderly patients, but there is evidence that antidepressant drugs such as SSRIs and venlafaxine are effective in the treatment of generalized anxiety. In the absence of good evidence for a particular treatment, patient preference, and choice are important considerations.

### Management

Since most patients are seen in primary care and general medical settings, this is where the focus of management should be. The role of specialist old age psychiatry services should be to provide any advice and support that is necessary, which may include assuming responsibility for the most complex cases. Wherever the patient is seen and treated, the following should need consideration from the outset (see also Chapter 8.6):

- a thorough assessment and accurate diagnosis as the basis for the management plan

- the full range of physical and psychological treatment options, including patient education, lifestyle advice, bibliotherapy, and supportive counselling

- clear goals for the treatment plan, agreed if possible with the patient

- an adequate trial of treatment

- the likely duration of treatment

- frequency of review

- any possible adverse consequences, such as dependency, adverse side effects, risk of self-harm.

### (a) Psychological treatments

For the most part, the goals and techniques of CBT are the same for elderly patients as they are for younger adults (see Chapter 6.3.2.1). However, these may require some adaptation to accommodate sensory impairments, physical illness and disability, and cognitive dysfunction.[13] The need to tailor treatment to the individual may limit the value of CBT in a group setting, although this has to be set against the benefits of shared experience and peer support. Group treatment is probably more straightforward with task-centred activities such as anxiety management.

The use of formal psychodynamic approaches to management is currently limited by economic constraints, and the lack of evidence regarding their effectiveness. However, health professionals should have some knowledge of the psychodynamics that underlie the concerns of elderly patients, and the mental defences that they use. They also need to be aware of their own preconceptions and cognitive distortions regarding the experience of old age, the psychological sophistication of elderly people, and their capacity for growth and change.

### (b) Physical treatments

Chapter 8.6 describes the general principles of drug treatment in old age. None of the drugs used to treat anxiety in elderly people is entirely without problems, so they should be prescribed with care.[14] Benzodiazepines are the most commonly used drugs, but they are often prescribed inappropriately. Elderly patients are particularly sensitive to their adverse effects, and drug accumulation may lead to delirium, incontinence, and falls. Compounds with short half-lives and no active metabolites, such as oxazepam, are least problematic, although patients may develop withdrawal symptoms if they are discontinued, or taken erratically. Long-term benzodiazepine use should be avoided where possible, although it may be necessary in a few patients unresponsive to other forms of treatment.

Antidepressant drugs are now the first choice in generalized anxiety and panic, particularly if depressive symptoms are prominent. The use of antidepressants in elderly patients is discussed in Chapter 8.5.4. SSRIs also have a specific effect in OCD. Neuroleptics have only a limited role in the management of anxiety, given their potentially disabling extrapyramidal side effects. However, a short course of low-dose treatment with a drug such as haloperidol or zuclopenthixol may be considered in those unable to tolerate benzodiazepines. Alternatively, sedative antihistamine drugs such as hydroxyzine may be useful. β-blockers are used in younger adults to control the sympathetic somatic anxiety symptoms, but contra-indications such as chronic obstructive airways disease, sinus bradycardia, and heart failure limit their use in elderly patients. Buspirone is an azapirone anxiolytic that is well tolerated by elderly patients, but it takes about 2 weeks to become effective, so is not useful for the management of acute episodes. It is indicated for severe chronic generalized anxiety and in patients where there is risk of dependence or abuse.

## Prevention

The possibilities for primary prevention are limited at present. However, in view of the association with physical illness, there may be an opportunity to intervene and prevent the development of chronic neurotic disability following strokes, heart attacks, and falls. It remains to be seen if the improved management of these disorders earlier in life will result in lower rates of chronicity and recurrence as cohorts age.

## Further information

Lindesay, J. (ed.) (1995). *Neurotic disorders in the elderly*. Oxford University Press, Oxford.

Lindesay, J. (2008). Neurotic disorders. In *The Oxford textbook of old age psychiatry* (eds. R. Jacoby, T. Dening, A. Thomas, and C. Oppenheimer). Oxford University Press, Oxford.

National Institute for Clinical Excellence. (2004). *Anxiety: management of anxiety (panic disorder with or without agoraphobia and generalised anxiety disorder) in adults in primary, secondary and community care*. Clinical Guideline 22. NICE, London (www.nice.org.uk/CG022NICEguideline).

Ruskin, P.E. and Talbot, J.A. (eds.) (1996). *Aging and posttraumatic stress disorder*. American Psychiatric Press, Washington, DC.

Salzman, C. and Lebowitz, B. (eds.) (1991). *Anxiety in the elderly*. Springer, New York.

## References

1. Tyrer, P. (1989). *Classification of neurosis*. Wiley, Chichester.
2. Lindesay, J. (1991). Phobic disorders in the elderly. *The British Journal of Psychiatry*, **159**, 531–41.
3. Astrom, M. (1996). Generalized anxiety disorder in stroke patients. A 3-year longitudinal study. *Stroke*, **27**, 270–5.
4. Pitt, B. (1995). Neurotic disorders and physical illness. In *Neurotic disorders in the elderly* (ed. J. Lindesay), pp. 46–55. Oxford University Press, Oxford.
5. Robins, L. and Regier, D. (eds.) (1991). *Psychiatric disorders in America*. Free Press, New York.
6. Krasucki, C., Howard, R., and Mann, A. (1998). The relationship between anxiety disorders and age. *International Journal of Geriatric Psychiatry*, **13**, 79–99.
7. Goldberg, D. and Huxley, P. (1992). *Common mental disorders: a bio-social model*. Tavistock/Routledge, London.
8. Robinson, R.G. (1998). *The clinical neuropsychiatry of stroke*. Cambridge University Press, Cambridge.
9. Beekman, A.T.F., Bremmer, M.A., Deeg, D.J.H., *et al.* (1998). Anxiety disorders in later life: a report from the longitudinal aging study Amsterdam. *International Journal of Geriatric Psychiatry*, **13**, 717–26.
10. Noyes, R. and Clancy, J. (1976). Anxiety neurosis: a 5-year follow-up. *The Journal of Nervous and Mental Disease*, **162**, 200–5.
11. Larkin, A.B., Copeland, J.R.M., Dewey, M.E., *et al.* (1992). The natural history of neurotic disorder in an elderly urban population. Findings from the Liverpool longitudinal study of continuing health in the community. *The British Journal of Psychiatry*, **160**, 681–6.
12. Mohlman, J. (2004). Psychosocial treatment of late-life generalized anxiety disorder: current status and future directions. *Clinical Psychology Review*, **24**, 149–69.
13. Koder, D.A. (1998). Treatment of anxiety in the cognitively impaired elderly: can cognitive-behavior therapy help? *International Psychogeriatrics*, **10**, 173–82.
14. Suribhatla, S. and Lindesay, J. (2005). Treatment of anxiety disorders. In *Practical old age psychopharmacology*, Chap. 10 (eds. S. Curran and R. Bullock). Radcliffe, Abingdon.

# 8.5.6 Personality disorders in the elderly

Suzanne Holroyd

## Introduction

The study of personality disorder (PD) in late life presents conceptual, diagnostic, and methodological difficulties. By definition, PD is considered a group of personality traits that relatively persistent through adulthood. However, the concept of PD persisting throughout the lifespan contradicts widespread clinical belief that they become less severe with ageing. For example, DSM-IV[1] notes that 'some types of personality disorders . . . tend to become less evident or remit with age'.

There are difficulties in studying PD in the elderly. One is the instability of the definition of PD over time, making it difficult to relate earlier studies to those using current definitions of PD. In addition, diagnostic criteria are subject to criticism when applied to the elderly, in that they may be 'age-biased'.[2,3] Finally, the methodology used to diagnose PD has been highly variable and difficult to interpret between studies.

A major issue is whether personality is fully developed by early adulthood and then remains unchanged, or whether personality continues to develop and change throughout life. The work of McCrae and Costa[4] demonstrated that personality characteristics are relatively stable within individuals over a 30-year period with correlations ranging from 0.7 to 0.8. However, this also demonstrates that complete stability is not there and suggests certain aspects of the personality may still develop and change with ageing. This suggests that PD may also change over the lifespan.

Another issue is whether underlying traits that persist throughout the lifespan can rise to the level of a PD depending on the environment. For example, traits that may be personality disordered in young adult life, such as extreme dependency, may be an appropriate and adaptive trait for an older individual with multiple physical disabilities.[5] Conversely, an individual may have a trait of extreme independence that may be adaptive in earlier life but which leads to distress and maladaptive functioning in a setting requiring dependence, such as a nursing home. Thus it is possible to have a PD diagnosed for the first time in late life, which goes against the very definition of lifelong PD.

## Clinical features

Clinical features of PD and details of their classification are reviewed in Chapters 4.12.2 and 4.12.3. However, there is difficulty in simply relating these criteria, which were developed for younger individuals, to the elderly. Typical diagnostic behaviours that clinicians associate with PD in younger adults may present as different behaviours in the elderly. This may lead clinicians to overlook personality traits and disorders in older individuals. For example, a criterion of antisocial personality disorder is the repeated failure to sustain consistent work, behaviour not applicable to the older retired individual. Yet it is possible that the personality trait of irresponsibility, which led to the loss of jobs earlier in life continues, now appearing as a behaviour such as medicine non-compliance. Some authors have thus argued that the clinical features for some PD are age-biased since certain behaviours are less likely to occur in elderly persons despite the persistence of personality traits.[2,3]

## Diagnosis of personality disorders

Diagnostic criteria for PD are discussed in Chapter 4.12.3. Because features of PD may change with ageing, diagnosis can be difficult. Overlap with Axis I diagnoses such as depression or dementia make the diagnosis even more challenging. For example, depressed elderly people have symptoms normally associated with PD as they may be more dependent, avoidant, resistant, negative, and somatic.[6] In addition, depressed elderly people may view their lives negatively and overestimate personality psychopathology.[7,8]

Clinicians may be reticent to give a personality diagnosis to an individual with multiple medical problems to which maladaptive behaviours may be attributed even if a lifelong history of personality pathology is established.[8] They may also be concerned about the validity of historical information needed to make a PD diagnosis. Therefore, in making a diagnosis of PD, a clinician should take a thorough history from as many reliable outside informants as possible. If the patient is in a state of acute distress with a current Axis I diagnosis such as depression, it is best to defer diagnosis of the PD until the illness is in remission. Otherwise, it is especially important to ask outside informants to think back to when the individual was a younger person, as current symptoms can colour the perception of lifelong personality traits. Asking for specific examples of history such as, details of relationships and job history, legal history, and the like, will be more helpful than just general descriptions of personality.

If behavioural difficulties and personality problems are found to be recent, the clinician needs to search carefully for a superimposed medical condition, or a psychiatric condition such as depression. Clinicians should carefully screen for illnesses such as dementia, stroke, or other neurological disease, or a systemic medical illness. Those with frontal lobe dementia, Alzheimer's disease, or vascular dementia may have personality changes early in their life course.[9–11]

## Epidemiology and aetiology

The prevalence of PD in the elderly varies as to the methodology used and the population studied. It should be noted that no assessment instrument for PD in the elderly has been validated.

### Community studies

Community studies have been the most useful to date. A community study,[12] using the Epidemiologic Catchment Area (**ECA**) data, had 841 subjects examined by psychiatrists using the semi-structured Standardized Psychiatric Examination with DSM-III criteria. Comparing those over the age of 55 with those under 55, older individuals were found significantly less likely to have a PD (6.6 to 10.5 per cent) as compared with younger individuals. This finding was almost entirely due to a three-fold higher prevalence of cluster B PD in those under the age of 55, especially antisocial and histrionic PD. Interestingly, in this study none of the older individuals were found to have cluster A PD. Table 8.5.6.1 summarizes the findings of this large community study. The strengths of this study were that it was a community rather than a clinical sample,

**Table 8.5.6.1** Weighted prevalence (%) of DSM-III personality disorders in a large community study

|  | Age < 55 years | Age > 55 years |
|---|---|---|
| *Cluster A* | 0.1 | 0.0 |
| Paranoid | 0.0 | 0.0 |
| Schizoid | 0.1 | 0.0 |
| Schizotypal | 0.1 | 0.0 |
| *Cluster B* | 6.8 | 2.2* |
| Antisocial | 2.7 | 0.1* |
| Borderline | 0.8 | 0.0 |
| Histrionic | 4.3 | 2.2* |
| Narcissistic | 0.0 | 0.0 |
| *Cluster C* | 3.8 | 4.3 |
| Avoidant | 0.0 | 0.0 |
| Dependent | 0.2 | 0.1 |
| Obsessive–compulsive | 3.6 | 3.3 |
| Passive-aggressive | 0.0 | 1.0 |
| *Any personality disorder* | 10.5 | 6.6* |

* $p < 0.05$

Reproduced from B.J. Cohen *et al.* (1994). Personality disorders in later life. A community study. *British Journal of Psychiatry*, **165**, 493–9, copyright 1994, The Royal College of Psychiatrists.

and subjects were evaluated by psychiatrists using a structured questionnaire. Limitations of this study were those inherent to the study of PD in late life, in that older subjects may have been inaccurate in recalling maladaptive behaviours, outside informants were not used, and lack of non-validated instruments for diagnosing PD in the elderly.

A community study of 43 093 persons, examining alcohol and related conditions across the life span, confirmed that those over 65 years had significantly lower rates of all studied PD including avoidant, obsessive–compulsive, paranoid, schizoid, histrionic, and antisocial, using DSM-IV criteria.[13]

A community survey study of DSM-III PD traits using the Personality Diagnostic Questionnaire revealed that 'dramatic' and 'anxious' personality traits declined up to 60 years of age with a slight increase thereafter, but that 'odd' or 'eccentric' traits showed no change with age.[14]

### Psychiatric populations

In addition to community samples, specific clinical samples have been examined. Limitations of these studies are the possibility of over diagnosis of PD due to symptoms of Axis I diagnoses.

A retrospective study of 2322 psychiatric inpatients with major depression found the prevalence of PD to be 11.2 per cent in those over the age of 65 as compared with 17.2 per cent for those under 65.[15]

Psychiatric inpatient studies suffer from the limitation of diagnosing PD in the face of an acute psychiatric illness requiring hospitalization, making them likely to overdiagnose. Such studies are of very limited value.[16,17]

Unfortunately, outpatient studies have similar limitations when examining those with concurrent Axis I diagnoses. A study of 36 psychiatric outpatients, including those with bipolar disorder, delusional disorder, and schizophrenia, revealed that 58 per cent had a diagnosis of personality disorder.[18] Arguably, diagnosing personality disorder in the face of these disorders is likely to be difficult and result in an overestimation.

### Prevalence summary

A meta-analysis of 11 articles published from 1980 to 1994 of personality disorders based on DSM-III or DSM-IIIR criteria revealed an approximately 10 per cent prevalence of personality disorders in those aged 50 and over.[19] In comparing these studies it was noted that the method of diagnosis affected the prevalence of personality disorder. In conclusion, the authors felt that there was a definite need for well-designed studies using statistically robust samples to assess the true prevalence of personality disorders in late life.

Taking the best studies together—the ECA community study and the meta-analysis—the prevalence of personality disorder in the elderly, as currently defined, ranges from 7 to 10 per cent, with a decrease in prevalence of cluster B diagnoses.

## Course and prognosis

Longitudinal community studies of PD have not been performed. With longitudinal data lacking, only cross-sectional studies are available. However, cross-sectional studies have a variety of limitations, including the possibility of a cohort effect explaining changes in prevalence in late life.

Antisocial personality disorder has been the best studied. The ECA study revealed that antisocial personality disorder declined from a 1-month prevalence of 0.9 per cent for individuals between 25 and 44 years of age to 0 per cent for those over the age of 65. When considering men only, the rate fell from 1.5 per cent in those aged 22 to 44 to 0.1 per cent in those over 65.[20] Supporting this is a study revealing the decline in lifetime prevalence in antisocial personality disorder from between 2.1 and 3.3 per cent to between 0.2 and 0.8 per cent in those aged 65 and older.[21] In addition, antisocial traits, as measured by the Minnesota Multiphasic Personality Index, reveal a decline with ageing.[22] However, a forensic centre study revealed while antisocial PD declined after the age of 27, one-third remained criminally active throughout their lives.[23]

Several hypotheses exist to explain this apparent decline in antisocial personality disorder with ageing. Personality may continue to mature and develop. Early death due to high-risk behaviour or a change in antisocial behaviours to other symptoms including hyperchondriasis, depression, or alcoholism may occur.[23] Also, behaviours such as criminality may decrease in older individuals, but antisocial personality traits remain and are simply more difficult to measure using current diagnostic criteria. Also, decrease in impulsive and aggressive behaviours may correlate with full myelination of frontal, temporal, and parietal cortices that does not occur until 30 or 40 years of age.[24] Changes in brain neurochemistry with ageing, including serotonin and dopamine, may also result in decreased impulsiveness or aggressiveness.[12] Decreased testosterone levels in men with ageing may contribute to a decline in these traits.[25]

Other Cluster B disorders may decline with ageing. The ECA study previously reviewed found a decline in antisocial and histrionic disorder.[23] Another community study supported a decline in histrionic PD with ageing.[26] Interestingly, the pattern of decline varied with gender, with rates remaining constant in women but declining in men. Similarly, a diagnosis of borderline PD is rare in elderly individuals, with only two case reports in the literature.[5] There is conflicting data regarding a decline in cluster A or C diagnoses. A large community study revealed lower rates of both Cluster A and C diagnoses in the elderly.[13] However, a study of schizotypal PD revealed all cases began before 40 years of age and continued lifelong.[27]

Some work has been done on the interaction of PD with Axis I diagnoses. Studies of depressed elderly patients suggest PD is associated with earlier age of depression onset, chronicity, and severity of dysthymia[28,29] however depression may exacerbate or conceal personality traits, thus making firm conclusions of PD in such individuals difficult. In the ECA study, certain Axis I diagnoses were found to be more common with a PD diagnosis. For example, all cases of obsessive–compulsive disorder in older individuals occurred concurrent with a PD.[12] Both generalized anxiety disorder and substance use disorders were more common in the presence of a PD. There were no differences in the prevalence of schizophrenia and major depression in those with or without a PD. The findings need to be confirmed since the group of elderly with PD was small.

A recent interesting study has revealed any PD (DSM-IV criteria) is associated with increased risk of stroke and ischemic heart disease, adding to the possible morbidity of these disorders.[30] However, such results should be viewed with caution as no screening was done to rule out depression or other associated factors that are prevalent in this population and may have led to over diagnosis of PD.

## Treatment and management

Given the relative lack of data regarding PD in the elderly, it is not surprising there is a corresponding lack of information regarding treatment and management. In general, clinicians should have a low threshold for suspecting concurrent psychiatric diagnosis, as major depression, anxiety, substance use disorders or dementia may mimic or exacerbate a personality disorder.[5] Physical and medical problems should be thoroughly evaluated and treated to minimize any associated complaints.

Social and family supports should be explored and maximized. Firm and consistent limits must be set by the clinician for both patients and their families in regard to inappropriate behaviour.[5] Clinicians should also try to determine why the disordered behaviour is occurring at a particular time. For example, placement in a nursing home may be stressful to an individual who has had difficulty forming relationships and is now dependent on a group of caregivers. Psychotherapy with the goal of focusing on current life stresses, the individual's vulnerabilities, and adaptive strategies can help the patient adjust to the current circumstance.[5]

Psychotherapeutic treatments used for personality disorders in younger individuals may be tried although little data exists on their effectiveness for elderly. A study of Dialectical Behavior Therapy (DBT) used in combination with medication to treat elderly depressives with personality disorders revealed better results than just medication. The study is limited in that such results are common in other studies using any psychotherapy with medication versus medication alone and does not support a specific usefulness of DBT in elderly personality disorder. However, the study is the first to use DBT in an older population and shows it is tolerable in this age group.

If possible, psychiatric medication should be avoided unless there is a specific diagnosed condition. This will minimize the possibility of side effects in elderly individuals and avoid dependency and control issues.[5] This is important as elderly individuals with abnormal personality traits have been found to be at higher risk of receiving psychotropic medication.[31]

## Possibilities for prevention

There are no data available for preventing the development of a PD in late life. Clearly, more information is needed on the longitudinal course of diagnosed PD in late life so that information regarding treatment and prevention may be realized.

## Further information

At the time of writing, there are no books or reports that give an overview of personality disorder in the elderly. Further information about specific aspects of the subject can be obtained from the relevant references in the text.

## References

1. American Psychiatric Association. (1994). *Diagnostic and statistical manual of mental disorder* (4th edn). American Psychiatric Association, Washington, DC.

2. Agronin, M.E. and Maletta, G. (2000). Personality disorders in late life: understanding and overcoming the gap in research. *The American Journal of Geriatric Psychiatry*, **8**, 4–18.

3. Kroessler, D. (1990). Personality disorder in the elderly. *Hospital & Community Psychiatry*, **41**, 1325–9.

4. McCrae, R.R. and Costa, P.T. (1984). *Emerging lives, enduring dispositions*. Little Brown, Boston, MA.

5. Holroyd, S. and Rabins, P.V. (1994). Personality disorders. In *Principles of geriatric medicine and gerontology* (3rd edn) (eds. W.R. Hazzard, E.L. Bierman, J.P. Blass, W.H. Ettinger, and J.B. Hatter), pp. 1131–6. McGraw-Hill, NY.

6. Thompson, L.W., Gallagher, D., and Czirr, R. (1988). Personality disorder and outcome in the treatment of late-life depression. *Journal of Geriatric Psychiatry*, **21**, 133–46.

7. Hirschfeld, R.M.A., Klerman, G.L., and Clayton, P.J. (1983). Assessing personality: effects of the depressive state on trait measurement. *The American Journal of Psychiatry*, **140**, 695–9.

8. Reich, J., Noyes, R., Hirschfeld, R.M.A., *et al.* (1987). State and personality in depressed and manic patients. *The American Journal of Psychiatry*, **144**, 181–7.

9. Petry, S., Cummings, J.L., and Hill, M.A. (1990). Personality alterations in dementia of the Alzheimer type. *Archives of Neurology*, **45**, 1187–90.

10. Neary, D., Snowden, J., and Mann, D. (2005). Frontotemporal dementia. *Lancet Neurology*, **4**, 771–80.

11. Dian, L., Cummings, J.L., Petry, S., *et al.* (1990). Personality alterations in multi–infarct dementia. *Psychosomatics*, **31**, 415–19.

12. Cohen, B.J., Nestadt, G., Samuels, J.F., *et al.* (1994). Personality disorders in later life. A community study. *The British Journal of Psychiatry*, **165**, 493–9.

13. Grant, B.F., Hasin, D.S., Stinson, F.S., *et al.* (2004). Prevalence, correlates and disability of personality disorders in the United States: results from the national epidemiologic survey on alcohol and related conditions. *The Journal of Clinical Psychiatry*, **65**, 948–58.

14. Reich, J., Nduaguba, M., and Yates, W. (1988). Age and sex distribution of DSM–III personality cluster traits in a community population. *Comprehensive Psychiatry*, **29**, 298–303.

15. Fogel, B.S. and Westlake, R. (1990). Personality disorder diagnoses and age in inpatients with major depression. *The Journal of Clinical Psychiatry*, **51**, 232–5.

16. Molinari, V. (1993). Personality disorders and relapse rates among geropsychiatric inpatients. *Clinical Gerontologist*, **14**, 49–52.

17. Molinari, V., Ames, A., and Essa, M. (1994). Prevalence of personality disorders in two geropsychiatric inpatient units. *Journal of Geriatric Psychiatry and Neurology*, **7**, 209–15.

18. Molinari, V. and Marmion, J. (1993). Personality disorders in geropsychiatric outpatients. *Psychological Reports*, **73**, 256–8.

19. Abrams, R.C. and Horowitz, S.V. (1996). Personality disorders after age 50: a meta–analysis. *Journal of Personality Disorders*, **10**, 271–81.

20. Regier, D.A., Farmer, M.E., Rae, D.S., *et al.* (1988). One–month prevalence of mental disorders in the United States. *Archives of General Psychiatry*, **45**, 977–86.

21. Robins, L.N. (1984). Lifetime prevalence of specific psychiatric disorders in three sites. *Archives of General Psychiatry*, **41**, 949–58.

22. Weiss, J.M. (1973). The natural history of antisocial attitudes– what happens to psychopaths? *Journal of Geriatric Psychiatry*, **6**, 236–42.

23. Arboleda–Florez, J. and Holley, H.L. (1991). Antisocial burnout: an exploratory study. *Bulletin of the American Academy of Psychiatry and the Law*, **19**, 173–83.

24. Elliott, F.A. (1992). Violence, the neurologic contribution: an overview. *Archives of Neurology*, **49**, 595–603.

25. Gray, A., Jackson, A.N., and McKinlay, J.B. (1991). The relation between dominance anger and hormones in normally aging men: results from the Massachusetts Male Aging Study. *Psychosomatic Medicine*, **53**, 375–85.

26. Nestadt, G., Romanoski, A.J., Chahal, R., *et al.* (1990). An epidemiologic study of histrionic personality disorder. *Psychological Medicine*, **20**, 413–22.

27. Baron, M., Given, R., Asnis, L., *et al.* (1983). Age of onset in schizophrenia and schizotypal disorder. *Neuropsychobiology*, **10**, 199–204.

28. Abrams, R.C., Rosendahl, E., and Card, C. (1994). Personality disorder correlates of late and early onset depression. *Journal of the American Geriatric Society*, **42**, 727–31.

29. Devanand, D.P., Turret, N., and Moody, B.J. (2000). Personality disorder in elderly patients with dysthymic disorder. *The American Journal of Geriatric Psychiatry*, **8**, 188–95.

30. Moran, P., Stewart, R., Brugha, T., *et al.* (2007). Personality disorder and cardiovascular disease: results from a national household survey. *The Journal of Clinical Psychiatry*, **68**, 69–74.

31. Mann, A.H. (1981). The twelve–month outcome of patients with neurotic illness in general practice. *Psychological Medicine*, **11**, 535–50.

# 8.5.7 Suicide and deliberate self-harm in elderly people

Robin Jacoby

## Introduction

Although in some countries suicide rates in young males have risen dramatically in the last decade or so, suicide in old age is important because rates in older people, especially those over 74, are still proportionately higher in most countries of the world where reasonably reliable statistics can be obtained.[1] For example, in 2004 in Lithuania where suicide incidence is currently the highest, the overall rate in males per 100 000 total population was 70.1, but in men over 74 the rate was 80.2. In the United States, where suicide is neither especially common nor rare, in 2002 the overall rate for males per 100 000 total population was 17.9, but 40.7 in men over 74. Rates for older women are nearly always much lower than for their male counterparts.

A second reason for the importance of suicide in old age is that the proportion of older people in the population is rising worldwide. Indeed, the increase in developing countries is likely to be even greater than in developed countries. Although rates vary from year to year and birth cohort to cohort, it is highly likely that unless suicide prevention becomes a great deal more effective than at present, more and more older people will kill themselves in the coming years.

As with younger people, completed suicide in old age may be seen as part of a continuum from suicidal thinking through deliberate self-harm (which does not lead to death), to completed suicide. An added component within this continuum for older people is that of 'indirect self-destructive behaviour', such as refusal to eat and drink or 'turning one's face to the wall' which is clearly intended to hasten death. Finally, although this section does not deal with euthanasia and related issues, assisted suicide in people with terminal illness such Alzheimer's disease and cancer may also be seen as part of the suicide continuum.

## Suicidal thinking in community-dwelling elderly people

A number of studies have explored this issue. Fleeting thoughts of suicide or the idea that life is not worth living occur in up to about 15 per cent of community-dwelling older people,[2] but serious consideration of suicide is very much less.[3] It is those older people with mental disorders, mostly depressive, who show a higher frequency of thoughts that life is not worth living and harbour ideas of committing suicide. It seems logical to suppose, therefore, that depressed elders should be the target of suicide prevention strategies.

## Indirect self-destructive behaviour

Unlike the young, some elderly people have the possibility open to them of behaving passively in such a way as to hasten death. This may happen either by refusing medical treatment essential to maintain life, or simply by declining to eat and drink—'turning one's face to the wall'. As regards the latter, many people, especially non-medical, believe that this is reasonable behaviour akin to so-called 'rational suicide', and court rulings have sanctioned it. There is no doubt that there are several cases in which a person's right to refuse treatment or nutrition, for example during the terminal phase of cancer, should and would be respected. However, it has been argued that many of such cases suffer from undiagnosed but treatable depressive illnesses. Some support for this point of view was provided by a questionnaire study of more than 1000 residential and nursing home administrators in the United States.[4] Cognitive impairment, loss events, refusing medication, food, and drink, loneliness, feeling rejected by families are all risk factors for indirect suicidal behaviour in residential homes.[5] It is wise, therefore, that no one should be permitted to turn his or her face to the wall before assessment for the presence of a treatable depressive disorder.

## Deliberate self-harm

### Incidence

It is less possible to make a clear distinction between deliberate self-harm (DSH) and completed suicide in older than younger people. DSH at all ages has been quite extensively studied, but for obvious reasons mainly in hospital samples, and it is possible that several cases are undetected in the community. Broadly speaking the incidence curve for DSH is highest for the young and declines with age, whereas that for completed suicide rises with age. By the same token suicidal intent behind acts of DSH in older people is significantly greater than in younger adults.[6] In clinical practice it is therefore wise to consider deliberate self-harm in those over 75 as failed suicide.

### Sex

As with completed suicide, rates for DSH differ quite widely from country to country. As with younger attempters, females outnumber males at a raw number ratio of approximately 3:2, but the *proportionate* gender ratio is approximately unity because fewer males survive into old age. Contrast this with completed suicide where men clearly outnumber women.

### Methods

Deliberate drug overdose is the favoured method for DSH at all ages in Western countries; in some others, corrosive poisons or detergents are used. The most common types of drug for overdose are benzodiazepines, analgesics, and antidepressants. After drugs, self-cutting is the next most frequent method.

### Psychiatric diagnosis

Older people are more likely to be assigned a psychiatric diagnosis after DSH, about half suffering from major depressive disorder, up to about a third from alcohol abuse, and under 10 per cent from other disorders.[7] Only about 10 per cent have no psychiatric diagnosis at all. Alcohol abuse together with depressive disorder augments the risk of DSH in older people. The status of cerebral organic disorder is uncertain because selection bias in reported case series reduces comparability. However, mild cognitive impairment and a co-morbid depressive disorder have been considered risk factors, and should be borne in mind by the clinician, if only on common-sense grounds. Personality factors have been implicated in DSH in older people, but research data are too poor and too few to make reliable statements on the subject.

### Risk factors

Risk factors for deliberate self-harm in elderly people include: physical illness; widowhood and divorce or separation from a cohabitee; social isolation and loneliness (not the same thing); or simply living alone.[6,7] Unresolved grief, usually after death of a spouse, is a commonly found risk factor. The threat of transfer to a nursing home is, unsurprisingly, a precipitant of deliberate self-harm, although once an elderly patient is transferred to institutional care the risk of an overdose or some other attempt at suicide is reduced, probably because of lower access to the means and higher supervision. Surprisingly perhaps, terminal illness is not commonly found in older patients who attempt suicide but fail, although hitherto undiagnosed but treatable physical disorders are sometimes revealed.

In keeping with the fact that more older suicide attempters are assigned a psychiatric diagnosis than younger ones is the fact that about 50 to 90 per cent, depending on the case series, undergo some form of psychiatric treatment as a result of the act of deliberate self-harm. Although fewer older people commit DSH than younger ones (about 5 per cent compared with 12 per cent) the risk of subsequent completed suicide is higher, compared with people of all ages (about 7 per cent compared with 3 per cent). Individual risk factors for later successful suicide include being male, having a prior psychiatric history, divorce, and current treatment for a persistent depressive illness.[6,8]

## Completed suicide

### Rates

The point has already been made in the opening paragraph of this chapter that suicide rates are still highest in the oldest old in most countries. Men outnumber women by about three or four to one in most countries; the exception being rural China.[1] However, suicide rates in the old have in fact been declining in many industrialized countries over the past 25 years, whilst those in young males have been rising—a reminder of the maxim that rates in all groups can and do vary over time and between countries, so that general conclusions about suicide should always take context into account. The reasons for incidence variations are discussed elsewhere, but socio-economic conditions and access to means play their part with the old as well as younger suicide victims.

Suicide at all ages is associated with divorce, widowhood, and single marital status. Widowers are more likely to kill themselves than widows, which has relevance for old age psychiatry, since in the overall population there are more old widowers than young ones.

### Methods

Methods of suicide chosen by older people depend to a great extent on availability. In the United States, firearms are used by the majority of older men who kill themselves.[9] Shooting is also commonly chosen in Australia and Finland. In the United Kingdom, which has more stringent firearms control, drug overdose, especially in women and frequently with combination analgesics, hanging (especially in men), suffocation, or jumping from tall structures are preferred methods.[10] In Japan hanging, in Hong Kong jumping from one of the many very high buildings, and in Sri Lanka organophosphate poisoning are the commonest means in use.

### Planning

Suicide in older persons is marked by careful planning and about half of the victims leave a note to indicate why or to confirm that they have killed themselves.[10] Suicide pacts are generally rare, but half of those that do occur involve people over 65. A previous history of a suicide attempt (DSH) is found in about a third of those older people who kill themselves.

### Psychiatric diagnosis

Studies, including case-control, in the United States, Scandinavia, and the United Kingdom have found that 70 per cent of older suicide victims suffer from a mental illness, most commonly a major depressive disorder at the time they die.[11–14] Chronic symptoms of depression and a first depressive illness in later life are associated with a greater risk of suicide. Untreated or inadequately treated depressive illness is also found more commonly in elderly suicides. By contrast with younger suicide victims, alcohol and drug abuse rates are lower in elderly people, although co-morbid depression and alcohol abuse do occur more frequently than by chance. Schizophrenia or schizophrenia-like disorders are found less commonly in older than younger suicides. Similarly, cerebral organic impairment or dementia are infrequent and even absent from some series of cases. There has been more recent interest in the role of personality in suicide in older people. In various studies obsessional or anankastic traits which researchers have called 'low openness to experience' have been shown to predispose to suicide.[14,15]

### Co-morbid physical illness

Co-morbid physical illness is, on common-sense grounds alone, likely to be a risk factor for suicide in older people and this has been confirmed in a number of studies.[16–18] Also, older people are much more likely to have visited their primary care doctor in the month prior to killing themselves than are younger suicide victims, and furthermore more likely to complain of physical than mental symptoms. Nevertheless, suicide to bring about the premature ending of a terminal illness or the avoidance of pain, although found to be a factor in studies of a variety of specific diseases, is not as common as one might imagine.

### Social risk factors

Social risk factors for suicide in old age have been found to include: isolation and poor social integration; lack of a person to confide in; and concerns over dependence or a move from home to residential care.[13,18–20] Bereavement by itself is no more of a risk factor in older than the younger suicides, but a grief reaction prolonged for more than a year has been found to increase the risk.

## Risk assessment

The study of suicide at any age is primarily for the purpose of prevention. In older people this means that, episodes of deliberate self-harm need to be considered as serious, even and perhaps especially when they do not appear to be so. A quantitatively small overdose of a relatively less lethal drug is frequently no indication of the seriousness of suicidal intent. Primary care doctors should be aware of the suicide risk in those attending with physical disorders, especially where the patient's complaints seem to be out of proportion to the actual evidence of disease. Nor is the identification of a physical illness a reason to relax vigilance over suicide risk. Dismissal of an older person's wish to die as 'rational' is probably wrong in the great majority of cases, but in any case should never be done before a thorough assessment of the mental state concentrating in particular on depressive disorder. Anxiety is frequently so prominently a presenting symptom of depressive disorder in elderly people, that other manifestations, such as suicidal thinking, may be overlooked. Whilst elderly people respond well to antidepressant medication, many live alone. Thus, a prescription for perhaps a month of treatment might be an enhancement of suicide risk. It is therefore prudent either to arrange close supervision or administration of medication by a carer rather than the patient themselves, or for no more than a week's supply to be dispensed at a time. Pharmacists may be willing to assist in this by providing proprietary boxes with compartments for each dose.

## Further information

Harwood, D. (2008). Suicide in older persons. In *The Oxford textbook of old age psychiatry* (eds. R. Jacoby, C. Oppenheimer, T. Dening, and A. Thomas) Chapter 29 iii. Oxford University Press, Oxford.

Hawton, K. and van Heeringen, K. (eds.) (2000). *The international handbook of suicide and attempted suicide.* Wiley and Sons, Chichester.

Pirkis, J. and Burgess, B. (1998). Suicide and recency of health care contacts: a systematic review. *The British Journal of Psychiatry*, 173, 462–74.

## References

1. http://www.who.int/mental_health/prevention/suicide/country_reports/en/index.html

2. Kirby, M., Bruce, I., Radic, A., *et al.* (1997). Hopelessness and suicidal feelings among the community dwelling elderly in Dublin. *Irish Journal of Psychological Medicine*, 14, 124–7.

3. De Leo, D., Cerin, E., Spathonis, K., *et al.* (2005). Lifetime risk of suicide ideation and attempts in an Australian community: prevalence, suicidal process, and help-seeking behaviour. *Journal of Affective Disorders*, 86, 215–24.

4. Osgood, N.J. and Brant, B.A. (1990). Suicidal behavior in long-term care facilities. *Suicide & Life-threatening Behavior*, 20, 113–22.

5. Draper, B., Brodaty, H., Low, L.F., *et al.* (2002). Self-destructive behaviors in nursing home residents. *Journal of the American Geriatrics Society*, 50, 354–8.

6. Hawton, K. and Harriss, L. (2006). Deliberate self-harm in people aged 60 years and over: characteristics and outcome of a 20-year cohort. *International Journal of Geriatric Psychiatry*, 21, 572–81.

7. Draper, B. (1996). Attempted suicide in old age. *International Journal of Geriatric Psychiatry*, 11, 577–87.

8. Hepple, J. and Quinton, C. (1997). One hundred cases of attempted suicide in the elderly. *The British Journal of Psychiatry*, 171, 42–6.

9. Kaplan, M.S., Adamek, M.E., Geling, O., *et al.* (1997). Firearm suicide among older women in the US. *Social Science & Medicine*, 44, 1427–30.

10. Harwood, D.M.J., Hawton, K., Hope, T., *et al.* (2000). Suicide in older people: mode of death, demographic factors, and medical contact before death. *International Journal of Geriatric Psychiatry*, 15, 746–3.

11. Conwell, Y., Duberstein, P.R., Cox, C., *et al.* (1996). Relationships of age and axis I diagnoses in victims of completed suicide: a psychological autopsy study. *The American Journal of Psychiatry*, 153, 1001–8.

12. Waern, M., Runeson, B.S., Allebeck, P., *et al.* (2002). Mental disorder in elderly suicides: a case-control study. *The American Journal of Psychiatry*, 159, 450–5.

13. Beautrais, A.L. (2002). A case-control study of suicide and attempted suicide in older people. *Suicide & Life-threatening Behavior*, 32, 1–9.

14. Harwood, D.M.J., Hawton, K., Hope, T., *et al.* (2001). Psychiatric disorder and personality factors associated with suicide in older people: a descriptive and case-control study. *International Journal of Geriatric Psychiatry*, 16, 155–65.

15. Duberstein, P.R., Conwell, Y., and Caine, E.D. (1994). Age differences in the personality characteristics of suicide completers: preliminary findings from a psychological autopsy study. *Psychiatry*, 57, 213–24.

16. Conwell, Y., Lyness, J.M., Duberstein, P., *et al.* (2000). Completed suicide among older patients in primary care practices: a controlled study. *Journal of the American Geriatrics Society*, 48, 23–9.

17. Waern, M., Rubenowitz, E., Runeson, B., *et al.* (2002). Burden of illness and suicide in elderly people: a case-control study. *British Medical Journal*, 324, 1355–7.

18. Harwood, D.M.J., Hawton, K., Hope, T., *et al.* (2006). Life problems and physical illness as risk factors for suicide in older people: a descriptive and case-control study. *Psychological Medicine*, 36, 1265–74.

19. Turvey, C.L., Conwell, Y., Jones, M.P., *et al.* (2002). Risk factors for late-life suicide: a prospective, community-based study. *The American Journal of Geriatric Psychiatry*, 10, 398–406.

20. Duberstein, P.R., Conwell, Y., Conner, K.R., *et al.* (2004). Poor social integration and suicide: fact or artefact? A case-control study. *Psychological Medicine*, 34, 1331–7.

## 8.5.8 Sex in old age

John Kellett and Catherine Oppenheimer

### Introduction

A Darwinian sees man as devoted to reproducing himself. The decline of fertility with age makes one question the biological purpose of sexuality in the senium. Is it simply the remains of a once useful behaviour, a vestigial characteristic? The fact remains that sexual interest and sexual activity, both as sources of enjoyment and as important components of pair bonding, continue among men and women even into extreme old age. However, as Alex Comfort memorably remarked, 'old people give up sex for the same reasons that they give up cycling—general infirmity, fear of looking ridiculous, no bicycle'.[1] Or, more soberly: the common obstacles to the continued enjoyment of sex in old age are illness, attitudes, and demography.

### Surveys of sexuality in old age

A comprehensive discussion of surveys in this field can be found in Bouman.[2] These vary widely in their focus, setting, methods, and target age groups. The details are of great interest but only the main themes and a few illustrative examples can be described here.

#### Methodology

As with all surveys, one has to consider what factors influenced the selection (and self-selection) of the responders. In general, participants in these studies tend to be better educated and more liberal in their attitudes than their contemporaries; and important groups, such as people with chronic illness, may be under (or over) represented, depending on the setting of the survey.

#### Cross-sectional and longitudinal studies

Attempts to assess the effects of ageing on sexuality by surveying different age-groups at a single point in time are vulnerable to *cohort effects*—the sexual experience of those brought up before the Second World War is different from that of people whose childhood was in the 1950s, and need have nothing to do with age. Longitudinal studies are demanding and costly, but they reveal the effects of ageing more clearly, and they also allow individual patterns, stable over time, to be identified. For example, the series of studies conducted at Duke University showed that although the *prevalence* of sexual interest and activity in both men and women decreases with age, *individual* patterns of sexuality tend to be stable until some event (such as illness or loss of a partner) disrupts the pattern.[3]

### Sexual interest and sexual pleasure

There is more to sex than actual intercourse, especially in old age. A consistent finding is that in both sexes interest in sex is more resistant to ageing than is sexual activity, even when non-coital activity is included. For example, in a cross-sectional study of volunteer respondents aged 80 or over, living in a residential home in the United States,[4] 88 per cent of the men and 71 per cent of the women enjoyed daydreams and fantasies about sex, 82 per cent of the men and 61 per cent of the women engaged in touching and caressing, while 63 per cent of the men and 30 per cent of the women had sexual intercourse 'at least sometimes'. Janus and Janus[5] surveyed 2765 subjects in the United States by questionnaire, supplemented by 125 interviews. They found less reduction of activity in the older groups than had been found in earlier surveys, probably because they did not confine the question to coitus. In every age group men thought that they were more active than 3 years previously, but women, particularly those over 50, noted a decline. Unlike earlier studies foreplay was discussed, and the authors concluded that older men gain greater pleasure and experience more intimacy and warmth after coitus than younger men.

### Obstacles to continued sexual activity

The commonest reasons given by people for a decline in their accustomed level of sexual activity were illness, and the loss of their partner.[3] Interestingly, women (but not men) also gave illness of their partner as a reason. This may reflect the traditional male role in initiating sexual activity, and also perhaps the fact that husbands tend to be older (therefore more at risk of illness) than their wives. For example, in a Swedish community study of 85-year olds,[6] participation in sexual intercourse was reported by 10 per cent of married women but only 1 per cent of the unmarried women, and by 22 per cent of married men compared to 13 per cent of the unmarried men. The rates for sexual interest (as opposed to activity) were higher: 46 and 37 per cent for married and unmarried men respectively; 24 and 15 per cent for married and unmarried women.

### Attitudes to sexuality

Attitudes towards sexuality in old age—as revealed in responses to systematically varied vignettes—have become generally more positive over the last half-century, among both younger and older people.[2,7] Probably this is true also of professional attitudes, and where this matters most is among the staff caring for older people in institutional settings. The evidence suggests that care staff who are older, better educated and have had vocational training, and who have more experience of caring, are likely to be more open to the sexual needs of their residents. However as Bouman[2] points out, the same cannot be said of health policies and strategy. Government guidance on the care of older people has ignored their sexuality, and in most official surveys and policies on sexual issues, people aged 60 or more are excluded from consideration.

### Demography

With increasing life-expectancy many marriages continue well into the 9th decade of one or both partners. Divorce has now overtaken death as the main cause for the ending of a marriage, though this does not necessarily mean increasing numbers of people left single in old age. Many older people experience second or third marriages (or cohabitations), and the age gap between the partners in these new relationships tends to be larger than that between partners still in their first marriage. The complex effects on family structure of these different social trends are analysed by Harper.[8] She shows that married older people have higher levels of health, social participation, and life satisfaction than those not married, and they live longer; while divorced men (compared to women, and to widowers) are the most disadvantaged in those respects. To this we can add (based on the survey data mentioned above) that in old age married people also enjoy greater opportunities than the unmarried for sexual expression.

## Sexual orientation

Much less is known and written about the sexual lives of older people who are not heterosexual in their orientation. Despite the prevailing trend in Western societies towards valuing diversity, most older homosexual people in their earlier lives will have feared—or faced—stigma, discrimination, even the threat of criminal procedure, and may still face such discrimination. Further discussion of this important group of people can be found in Bouman.[2]

## Sexuality and dementia

The effect of dementia on sexual interest and activity is unpredictable. Most often it is associated with a decline in interest, but sometimes (probably in less than 10 per cent of cases) a person with dementia may become more sexually demanding, or may lose the ability to judge when the expression of sexual interest is unwanted or out of place.[2,9] The effect of the patient's dementia on the spouse is also difficult to predict. In some couples the physical relationship continues as an important expression of their affection, support, and concern for each other. More commonly, sexual activity declines. For example, Wright[10] followed a group of couples in which one partner had dementia, alongside a control group of couples without dementia. Only 27 per cent of the afflicted couples continued sexual contact over the 5 years after diagnosis, compared to 82 per cent of the control couples.

Patients with dementia who have altered sexual behaviour, or who can no longer make reliable judgments about potentially sexual social situations, become vulnerable to misunderstanding, exploitation, or censure. In marriages the impact of these changes is often borne alone by the spouse, who also keeps them hidden from others. But people with dementia who live alone or who go into institutional care (even if only temporarily, into hospital perhaps) are not so protected, and clinical staff may be asked to intervene—to control behaviour that has offended or is harmful to others, or to reduce risk to a vulnerable patient. It may be crucial to establish whether such a patient is making an autonomous choice (for example, to engage in sexual contact with a fellow resident) or whether their failure of understanding is being exploited; and Lichtenberg and Strzepek[11] describe a helpfully structured approach to this question.

## Normal sexual function in old age

The normal human sexual response cycle and the physiology of sexual intercourse are described in Chapter 4.11.1 in this textbook. These descriptions hold true for sexually active older people, although age does bring some relatively minor physical changes (see Table 8.5.8.1, based on data from Masters and Johnson[12])—changes experienced by some but not necessarily by all. The most noticeable of these are probably the much longer refractory period in older men (the interval which follows ejaculation before renewed erection is possible), and the oestrogen-dependent changes in vaginal tissue and lubrication in older women. However, according to the self-reports of older sexually active people, the capacity for sexual pleasure and the quality of orgasms are not at all affected by age.

## Sexual dysfunction in old age

The range of sexual dysfunctions is discussed in detail in Chapter 4.11.2 in this textbook. In old age, as mentioned earlier, physical illnesses and their treatments assume increasing importance in curtailing the normal sexual activity and interest of an established couple. Likewise, with ageing, the balance between psychological and physical factors in the causation of a sexual problem, tips towards the physical. An example of this is erectile dysfunction, where a notable increase in research into the physiology of penile erection has led to a number of effective physical treatments, especially relevant to erectile problems associated with illnesses common in old age (such as diabetes and vascular disorders).[13,14] However, a clearer understanding of the physical components of a problem does not diminish the importance of psychological factors. Myocardial infarction, probably accompanied by hypertension and atherosclerosis, provides a good example. After the infarction the couple may misperceive the breathlessness of orgasm as cardiac distress, and they may need encouragement to resume sexual relations which may reduce the risk of further infarction.[15] Even a hospital admission interrupts the couple's sexual routine which may then be difficult to resume.

Some of the most common physical causes of sexual dysfunction are listed in Tables 8.5.8.2, 8.5.8.3, and 8.5.8.4.

**Table 8.5.8.1** Physical changes of ageing

| | Male | Female |
|---|---|---|
| Retained | Nil | Nipple erection<br>Clitoral tumescence and retraction |
| Reduced | Penile and nipple erection<br>Testicle elevation<br>Power of ejaculation<br>Rectal contractions | Vaginal lubrication and expansion<br>Uterine elevation<br>Bartholin gland secretion<br>Orgasmic contractions |
| Lost | Flush<br>Scrotal swelling<br>Re-erection<br>Ejaculatory inevitability<br>Prostate contractions | Breast engorgement<br>Flush<br>Swelling of labia majora |
| Other | Refractory period >24 h | |

**Table 8.5.8.2** Medical factors affecting sexual function

| Drugs reducing sexual drive | Drugs reducing testosterone | Drugs blocking physical arousal |
|---|---|---|
| Dopamine antagonists | Digoxin | Thiazide diuretics |
| Major tranquillizers | Cimetrdine | Some β-blockers |
| Metaclopamide | Cyproterone | |
| 5-HT$_2$ agonists–SSRIs except nefazodone, trazodone, fluvoxamine | Finasteride | |
| Benzodiazepines | Oestrogens Progesterone | |

## Treatment of sexual problems in old age

The treatment of sexual dysfunction is founded on a comprehensive understanding of the problem. It begins with listening. Perhaps this is a statement of the obvious—except that the emotional power of sexuality makes it hard for patients and their partners to speak about sex, and for others to listen properly. Sexual histories are rarely taken as a routine part of the assessment of older people,[2] and even when patients disclose a sexual problem, their doctor may shrink from embarking on an exploration of the difficulty. Yet there is good evidence that opening up communication about a sexual problem—not only between clinician and patient but also (helped by the clinician) between sexual partners—forms a large part of successful treatment, and sometimes may be all that is needed. Even patients attending a specialized clinic may be satisfied by receiving assessment and information, without necessarily wanting active treatment.[13]

Sexual problems come to the notice of many different medical and surgical specialties (gynaecology, urology, genitourinary medicine, diabetology, endocrinology) who have expertise in the physical treatments now available, and sometimes also in the psychological and relationship components of the dysfunctions that they treat. In other cases the psychiatrist may be helping the couple to work with a physical treatment that one of them is receiving, and to make the most of the improvements in sexual function that it offers.

Behavioural treatment for sexual dysfunction, first described by Hunter,[16] was developed by Masters and Johnson.[17] Their *Sensate focus exercise* (see Chapter 4.11.2) is a simple behavioural technique that can be very effective in helping couples in whom sexual intercourse has become (for whatever reason) difficult, painful, or disappointing, and who have then retreated from all pleasurable physical contact with each other. In this technique attention is removed from intercourse (in fact intercourse is forbidden), and instead the focus is put on renewing the partners' pleasure in mutual touch and caressing for its own sake.

**Table 8.5.8.3** Surgical procedures affecting sexual function

Transurethral prostatectomy leads to retrograde ejaculation
Pararectal surgery damages nervi erigentes
Indwelling catheters and pessaries
Mutilation affecting body image
Surgery to genitalia

**Table 8.5.8.4**  Diseases affecting sexual function

| |
|---|
| Diabetes |
| Myxoedema, pituitary tumours |
| Neurofibromatosis, paralysis, myotonia dystrophica, autonomic neuropathy |
| Peyronie's disease |
| Malignancy and infections of genitalia and prostate, vaginal fistulas |
| Liver failure leading to higher oestrogens |
| Arthritis |
| Hypertension, vascular diseases, myocardial infarction |
| Respiratory distress |
| Depression, schizophrenia, cortical dementias |

There is little scope for pharmacological treatment of most sexual difficulties arising in old age, other than erectile dysfunction.[13,14] Hormonal treatments are no longer thought to be helpful except where deficiencies have been clearly demonstrated. The commonest hormonal treatment in old age is probably the use of oestrogen (topically) in dyspareunia. Treatment of hypersexuality and sexual aggression in the context of dementia is difficult: pharmacological methods have been reviewed by Series and Degano.[18]

## Conclusion

Ageing brings increasing diversity. This certainly applies to sexual behaviour. Those who work in the field of old age psychiatry can help their patients by understanding this diversity, making it safe and acceptable for patients to talk about whatever sexual concerns they have, and helping them in the acquisition of all the information they need. Sex in old age is not the frightening imperative of the teenager, but it can still contribute greatly to the quality of life.

## Further information

Bouman, W.P. (2008). Sexuality in later life. In *The Oxford textbook of old age psychiatry* (eds. R. Jacoby, C. Oppenheimer, T. Dening, and A. Thomas) (chapter 37). Oxford University Press, Oxford.

Gott, M. (2005). *Sexuality, sexual health and ageing*. Open University Press, Maidenhead, Berkshire.

Greengross, W. and Greengross, S. (1989). *Living, loving and ageing. Sexual and personal relationships in later life*. Age Concern England, Mitcham, Surrey.

Leiblum, S.R. and Rosen, R.C. (eds.) (2000). *Principles and practice of sex therapy*. The Guildford Press, New York.

Warner, J. (2000). Sexuality in dementia. In *Dementia* (2nd edn) (eds. J. O'Brien, D. Ames, and A. Burns), pp. 267–71. Arnold, London.

## References

1. Comfort, A. (1980). *Practice of geriatric psychiatry*. Elsevier, New York.
2. Bouman, W.P. (2008). Sexuality in later life. In *The Oxford textbook of old age psychiatry* (eds. R. Jacoby, C. Oppenheimer, T. Dening, and A. Thomas) (chapter 37). Oxford University Press, Oxford.
3. George, L.K. and Weiler, S.J. (1981). Sexuality in middle and later life; the effects of age, cohort and gender. *Archives of General Psychiatry*, **38**, 919–23.
4. Bretschneider, J.G. and McCoy, N.L. (1988). Sexual interest and behavior in healthy 80- to 102-year olds. *Archives of Sexual Behavior*, **17**, 109–29.
5. Janus, S.S. and Janus, C.L. (1993). *The Janus report on sexual behavior*. Wiley, New York.
6. Skoog, J. (1996). Sex and Swedish 85-year olds. *The New England Journal of Medicine*, **334**, 1140–1.
7. Gott, M. and Hinchliff, S. (2003). How important is sex in later life? The views of older people. *Social Science & Medicine*, **56**, 1617–28.
8. Harper, S. (2008). Sociological approaches to age and ageing. In *The Oxford textbook of old age psychiatry* (eds. R. Jacoby, C. Oppenheimer, T. Dening, and A. Thomas) (chapter 2). Oxford University Press, Oxford.
9. Haddad, P.M. and Benbow, S.M. (1993). Sexual problems associated with dementia: part 1. Problems and their consequences. *International Journal of Geriatric Psychiatry*, **8**, 547–51.
10. Wright, L.K. (1998). Affection and sexuality in the presence of Alzheimer's disease: a longitudinal study. *Sexuality and Disability*, **16**, 167–79.
11. Lichtenberg, P.A. and Strzepek, D.M. (1990). Assessment of institutionalized dementia patients' competencies to participate in intimate relationships. *The Gerontologist*, **30**, 117–20.
12. Masters, W. and Johnson, V. (1966). *Human sexual response*. Churchill, London.
13. Melman, A. and Christ, G.J. (2002). The hemodynamics of erection and the pharmacotherapies of erectile dysfunction. *Heart Disease*, **4**, 252–64.
14. Trost, L., Kendirci, M., and Hellstrom, W.J.G. (2006). Erectile dysfunction in the aging man: current options for treatment. *Aging Health*, **2**, 71–86.
15. Kellett, J. (1987). Treatment of sexual disorder: a prophylaxis for major pathology? *Journal of the Royal College of Physicians*, **21**, 58–60.
16. Hunter, J. (1782). *Venereal disease*. London.
17. Masters, W.H. and Johnson, V.E. (1970). *Human sexual inadequacy*. Little Brown, Boston.
18. Series, H. and Degano, P. (2005). Hypersexuality in dementia. *Advances in Psychiatric Treatment*, **11**, 424–31.

# Special features of psychiatric treatment for the elderly

## Catherine Oppenheimer

## Introduction

Three themes underlie the topics in this chapter.

### Old age is a time of multiple problems

Physical, psychological, and social problems often occur together, linked by chance or causality in the life of the old person. Very rarely can one problem be dealt with in isolation, and many different sources of expertise may be engaged with a single individual. Therefore good coordination between different agents is essential in old age psychiatry, both for the individual patient and in the overall planning of services.

### Clear boundaries between 'normality' and 'disease' are rare in old age

Many of the pathologies characteristic of old age are gradual in onset and degenerative in nature, and more due to failures in processes of repair than to an 'external foe', so the distinction between disease and health is often quantitative rather than qualitative. 'Normality' becomes a social construct with fluid borderlines, containing the overlapping (but not identical) concepts of 'statistically common' and 'functionally intact'. Thus the popular perception of normal old age includes the 'statistically common' facts of dependence and failing function, whereas 'intactness' (excellent health and vigorous social participation) is seen as remarkable rather than the norm. But the boundaries of 'old age' are also socially constructed—in developed countries good health at the age of 65 would nowadays be regarded as a normal middle-aged experience, whereas superb health at 95 would still be something noteworthy.

Since some degree of physical dependence, forgetfulness, and vulnerability to social exclusion is expected in old age, meeting those needs is also regarded as a 'normal' demand on families and community agencies such as social services, rather than the responsibility of health care providers. As the severity of the needs increases, however, so also does the perceived role of health professionals, both as direct service providers and in support of other agencies.

### Lack of competence is common in old age

Because of the high prevalence of cognitive impairment in old age (especially among the 'older old'), questions frequently arise as to the competence of patients to make decisions. Older people who cannot manage decisions alone may come to depend increasingly on others for help; or, resisting dependence, they become vulnerable through neglect of themselves or through the injudicious decisions they make. When an incompetent person is cared for by a spouse or family member, the danger of self-neglect or of ill-considered decisions is lessened, but instead, there are the risks of faulty decisions by the caregiver (whether through ignorance or malice), and also risks to the health of the caregiver from the burden of dependence by the incompetent person. Legal mechanisms, differing from one country to another, exist to safeguard the interests of incompetent people.

These three themes will be developed further, and with them the following special topics:

1 multiple problems: including sleep disorders in old age, medication in old age psychiatry, and psychological treatments in old age psychiatry;

2 blurred boundaries of normality: including the role of specialist services and support between agencies;

3 incapacity and dependence: including balancing the needs of patients and caregivers, abuse of older people, ethical issues, and medico-legal arrangements for safeguarding decisions.

## Multiple problems

### Sleep disorders in old age

Useful reviews of this topic may be found in Anconi-Israel and Ayalon,[1] Sivertsen and Nordhus,[2] and Mosimann and Boeve.[3] More detailed general discussion of sleep and its disorders will be found in Chapters 4.14.1–4.14.4 of this textbook.

#### (a) Normal changes with age

With age, the architecture of sleep changes—in fact, most of the change occurs before the age of 60. Sleep is divided into shorter periods interspersed with wakefulness or brief arousals, there is a decrease in total sleep time and in sleep efficiency (the ratio of time asleep to time in bed), and there is less stage 4 (deep) and more stage 1 and 2 (shallow) sleep, without an increase in the proportion of rapid-eye-movement (REM) sleep. This change in sleep architecture is conventionally associated with changes in circadian rhythms with age, such as decreased amplitude and phase length of these rhythms (but see Monk[4] for a critical review).

Many people adapt to these changes, but others find the altered pattern distressing. Thus the borderline between normal and problematic sleep is blurred, because subjective assessments of sleep quality are not necessarily matched by objective measures (such as polysomnography); consequently the definition of 'insomnia' hinges not only on features of night-time sleep, but on impaired functioning in the daytime.

### (b) Comorbidity

The majority of healthy older people have no complaints about their sleep, but there is a strong association between poor sleep and other health problems, and sleep problems make a material contribution to the impaired quality of life suffered by people with comorbid illness. In a study of patients in primary care,[5] a positive answer to even one question about sleep ('do you feel excessively sleepy during the day?') predicted the quality of life related to physical or mental health problems. Attention to improving sleep in these patients can improve their well-being, but too often the sleep problem is missed in the general assessment of the patient. Impaired sleep can have serious consequences: it is associated with symptoms of anxiety and depression, an increased risk of falls, and diminished memory and cognitive functioning.[1]

### (c) Causes of disordered sleep

These include the following:

1 **Environmental causes**: e.g. a strange bed, noise, cold or heat, or loss of a familiar bed companion (e.g. through bereavement).

2 **Physical causes**: sleep can be broken by pain, stiffness (e.g. Parkinson's disease or arthritis), limb movement (restless legs syndrome, periodic movements of sleep), breathlessness (cardiac failure or sleep apnoea), the need to urinate (prostatic disease or urinary tract infection), eating too close to bedtime, or dehydration (e.g. voluntary restriction of fluids to prevent nocturia).

3 **Medication**: alcohol, especially if taken to relieve anxiety or to assist sleep (since the rapid metabolism of alcohol leads to rebound anxiety and wakefulness), and antidepressants such as selective serotonin reuptake inhibitors (**SSRIs**) can cause wakefulness or nightmares. Information on the numerous other medications which may impair sleep can be found in Anconi-Israel and Ayalon.[1]

4 **Psychological causes**: for example, anxiety, depression, hypomania, and paranoid illness. Often a sleep problem is triggered initially by a physical cause, but is then maintained by the patient's anxiety about wakefulness.

5 **Sleep in dementia**: changes in sleep rhythm in dementia are similar to those of normal old age, but often more severe: daytime drowsiness or napping, difficulty in falling asleep at night, decreases in slow wave sleep and in rapid-eye-movement sleep. However, another common cause of sleep impairment is the use of benzodiazepines or major tranquillizers to treat behaviour disturbances: the patient may end up drugged in the day and wakeful at night. A partial remedy may be to create an overriding diurnal rhythm (e.g. by attendance at day care or a programme of physical activity in the day), together with the minimal use of medication at night. Patients in institutional care are particularly likely to be deprived of the normal cues for circadian rhythms: quiet and darkness at night, bright daylight in the morning, and physical activity in the day. On the other hand

sleep time may be strikingly increased in dementia, especially in vascular dementia where it may be part of the apathy that is common in that disease.

### (d) The parasomnias

The parasomnias that are common in old age are obstructive sleep apnoea (or sleep-disordered breathing); restless legs syndrome and periodic limb movements in sleep; and REM sleep behaviour disorder (RBD). They may range in severity from troublesome to severely disabling, and accurate recognition is important for all of them, because of the consequences both to the patients and to their bed partners if their diagnosis and treatment are missed. Further details can be found in the sources mentioned above,[1,3] but RBD warrants some further discussion here. This disorder is defined as an 'intermittent loss of the muscle atonia normally present during REM sleep, and episodes of elaborate motor activity associated with dream mentation'.[6] Typically, in the early hours the patient (usually male) shouts, thrashes around, and may attack his bed partner, without waking, and without any recollection of the episode when he does wake later. The importance of this condition lies in the fact that it is very distressing, and possibly dangerous, for the bed partner; it can often be treated effectively (with clonazepam); and it is strongly associated with the development (sometimes after a very long latent period, of a decade or more) of neurodegenerative disease—especially Lewy body dementia, Parkinson's disease, or multisystem atrophy—the alpha-synucleopathies.[6,7]

### (e) Management of sleep disorders
#### (i) Psychological methods

These are now the methods of choice with insomnia in older adults.[2,8] Trials comparing psychological with pharmacological treatment, and with a combination of the two, show equivalent effects in the short-term, but a longer-term advantage to the psychological methods. More importantly, it has also been shown that in secondary insomnia ('insomnia occurring when a psychiatric condition, a medical condition, a non-insomnia sleep disorder, or a medication appears to precipitate and then appears to maintain insomnia') it is not necessary to wait until the primary condition has been resolved: the insomnia can usually be effectively treated in its own right, and even if it is not completely cured, valuable improvements can be achieved.[8] Likewise, psychological methods can be used to help in withdrawing medication in hypnotic dependent insomnia.[9]

The methods used have generally been 'multicomponent behavioural treatments'. The components include:

◆ Relaxation training

◆ Stimulus control (requiring the patient to leave the bedroom if they are not sleeping)

◆ Sleep restriction and sleep compression (using a fixed time for getting up, progressively shortening the time in bed until it matches the time asleep)

◆ Cognitive restructuring (modifying the pre-sleep thinking patterns, which in insomnia usually include negative thoughts about the effects of sleep loss, and the use of worry and self-blame as an attempted strategy for controlling thoughts[10])

◆ Sleep hygiene education (advice on the effects of tea, coffee, exercise, etc on sleep)

Such treatment packages need not be dependent on sources of specialist expertise: Sivertsen and Nordhus[2] discuss the feasibility of treating insomnia psychologically within primary care.

### (ii) Treatment of sleep problems in dementia

When cognitive impairment makes psychological treatment difficult, pharmacological treatment may be necessary. Benzodiazepines (probably temazepam for preference) must be used very cautiously; they are dangerous in ambulant patients, though less so for a patient who is no longer mobile. Sedating antidepressants (e.g. trazodone) can be used instead. An atypical antipsychotic may be appropriate if there is severe anxiety and suspiciousness (sometimes of delusional intensity) of the carer at night.

The sleep problems of the carer of a patient with dementia also need to be taken very seriously. The carer may benefit from the psychological measures outlined above, and can institute some of the measures (such as sleep hygiene) on behalf of the patient. Insomnia in a caregiver, caused by the wakefulness of the person cared for, can lead to rapid breakdown of the support system. If the patient's sleep problem cannot be resolved then it is essential to give the carer the opportunity for uninterrupted sleep at times, through arranging residential respite care, a night-sitter, or some other form of relief.

## The use of medication in old age psychiatry

Specific uses of medication for the various psychiatric disorders occurring in old age are dealt with in the relevant chapters. Here, three general principles will be discussed:

- medication as an experimental trial
- stopping medication
- compliance and concordance.

### (a) Medication as an experimental trial

Starting medication for any condition ought to be treated as the test of a hypothesis. There should be a plan, shared with the patient, setting out the following:

1 how long the trial will last before a decision is made that the treatment is unsuccessful and should be ended;

2 which target symptoms will be monitored, and what records should be kept (by the patient or caregiver);

3 when progress will be reviewed;

4 what side-effects might be developing and which of these should alert the patient to stopping the drug and contacting the doctor;

5 what will follow if the trial succeeds;

6 what will be tried instead if the trial fails.

This watchful approach to medication is particularly important for people with dementia. Often the patient's confusion, lack of insight, and communication difficulties mean that a tentative diagnosis has to be based on scanty information. For example, disturbed behaviour in a patient in a nursing home may be due to depression, but the patient cannot describe the depressive symptoms. Clues to the diagnosis may come from the care staff (e.g. 'She never jokes with us now'), and an empirical trial of an antidepressant may result in a resolution of the symptoms. However, the trial must be set up carefully and medication not thoughtlessly continued for months without review, merely because no one has asked whether it is helpful or not.

### (b) Stopping medication

The decision to withdraw medication can be as valuable and informative as the decision to start it, and documentation of the reasons for the decision is equally important (though often neglected). In delirium, medication may be contributing to the problem, particularly where a cocktail of medications has been built up over time—improvement after withdrawal of a drug gives valuable guidance for a future episode. Also, patients reaching the terminal stages of dementia should have their medication gradually decreased, to test whether it is still needed: drugs prescribed at an earlier stage to control behavioural syndromes are rarely, if ever, required for the entire course of the disease.

However, there are also reasons for being cautious about stopping medication. Some drugs have important withdrawal effects (e.g. paroxetine and benzodiazepines). Medication that has been used prophylactically may seem to be unnecessary while the patient is well, but when the drug is withdrawn the need for it is revealed. For example, a patient can remain well for years on an antidepressant following a severe depressive episode, or on a low dose of antipsychotic after a schizophrenic illness—until well-intentioned withdrawal of the drug, however carefully monitored, precipitates the return of the illness.

### (c) Compliance and concordance

The word 'compliance' appears to imply that patients must be obedient in following instructions; but nowadays patients are seen more as partners in their own treatment, for which the word 'concordance' (when the partnership is successful) is more apt. The same principle of partnership in treatment decisions applies to older people, wherever possible. However, in addition to willingness to participate there needs to be the ability to do so, which in older people is often impaired by physical causes (such as arthritic hands which cannot open child-proof packaging, or poor vision which misreads instructions), and by psychological causes, especially memory loss and temporal disorientation. Therefore patients will often need help in maintaining their concordance with treatment, through suitable packaging and memory aids (such as calendar boxes), or through supervision or administration of the tablets by others. Families may take a long time to notice that their parent or grandparent, who has taken medication reliably for years, has started to miss or duplicate doses.

It is important to understand the feelings of a caregiver who takes responsibility for the medication prescribed for a patient with dementia, especially where it is being used to control behaviour. Anything prescribed on an 'as-needed' basis should be very carefully explained. The caregiver may be afraid of provoking the difficult behaviour by offering the medication, or conversely of overdosing her relative into stupor, or she may feel guilty about meeting her *own* needs by giving drugs to another. Such feelings make it hard for a caregiver to judge objectively when discretionary medication should be used.

## Psychological treatments in old age

Many older people prefer a 'talking treatment' to medication, and there is increasing evidence of the success of psychological interventions with cognitively intact older people.[11] Brief focused interventions are particularly suitable.

However, even mild cognitive impairment, too slight to amount to dementia but enough to interfere with grasp and retention, may hamper psychological treatment. For example, such a patient being treated psychologically for anxiety may try hard to cooperate with her therapist, only to be made more anxious as she fails to remember the instructions, or to put them into practice, and so the sense of failure she feels elsewhere in her life is reinforced.

The principles of supportive psychotherapy and problem-solving are always relevant, both on their own or in conjunction with medication: providing 'unconditional positive regard' for the patient; accepting a degree of dependence by the patient, while limiting its consequences; setting appropriate expectations so that the patient is not unnecessarily exposed to a sense of failure; openly facing realities that cannot be altered (such as loss, disability, and death); helping to think through practical problems as they arise.

Family and systems therapy[12] has a particular role in old age psychiatry, because it explicitly recognizes the patient in his or her social context. Although family therapy requires special training, the principles of a family approach can be adopted by all those working with older people.

When patients are cognitively impaired, psychological approaches generally focus more on the interaction between the patient and the caregivers, who can be helped to understand the patient and the reasons for her behaviour, as well as their own actions and the reciprocal effects that these have on her. For example, reminiscence therapy helps professionals to respond to patients as 'whole people' with individual lives, as well as helping patients to reconnect with their former identities, and to recover some of the confidence they took for granted in the past.

Therapies based on music, dance, drama, art, and sensory stimulation are also important in old age.[13] They can help patients, individually or in groups, to express feelings and thoughts, bypassing the impairments of verbal skills which come with dementia.

## The blurred boundaries of 'normality'

We consider two examples of the way in which 'normality' is not clearly defined in old age.

First, social expectations allow for increasing dependency in the old, and many people have personalities better suited for protective relationships than for solitude and independence. People who have struggled with anxiety and loneliness in middle age can experience the onset of physical dependence as a kind of relief: now they can allow themselves to be looked after. What was a dysfunctional personality structure in earlier life becomes adaptive in old age. In contrast, the person who has always jealously guarded his or her personal boundaries will find the adjustment to disability very hard. Determined refusal to accept necessary help converts a 'normal' preference for independence into a problem for others.

The second example concerns the idea of death. For a younger person to say that they were waiting for death would prompt a psychiatrist to look for evidence of a depressive illness. In old age this way of thinking may be found in someone with no disorder of mood, with the ability to enjoy life, and with a rational appreciation of life's inevitable limits. But even in old age, to see nothing valuable in one's future might be a sign of depression.

## The role of specialist services and cooperation between agencies

This topic is dealt with more fully in the succeeding chapter (see Chapter 8.7).

The difficulty in separating the normal from the pathological, and in deciding when specialist intervention is required, is reflected at a structural level in shaping the responsibilities of the different bodies involved in the welfare of older people. Help required by older people can range from the simplest of neighbourly assistance to the full resources of specialist hospital care. As people live longer, despite some morbidity, the demand for care increases. The response to this demand is shaped by many different factors: market forces, public concern, private enterprise, voluntary or charitable groups which spring up to fill perceived gaps, and governments acting to remedy abuse or to limit demand on state-funded services. The divisions of responsibility are arbitrary, and people fall between services as often as within them. Systems change. For example, in the United Kingdom older people with permanent disability (especially dementia) used to be cared for in state-funded hospitals, but this care has now become the responsibility of independent-sector nursing homes, with means-tested financial support from the social security system.

The scope of specialist services for older people extends beyond the treatment of established illness. They have a role in the prevention and early detection of illness, in supporting and educating other service providers and in collaborating with other agencies in strategic planning. This span of interest can be represented as a pyramid (Fig. 8.6.1). The peak of the pyramid represents those requiring the scarcest and most intensive specialist services, and the base represents the population at large. In the middle are the people who need day care, support at home, social support, and help in primary care.

Between a population base of, say 20 000 older people and an inpatient provision of, say 10 beds lies the range of people to whom psychiatric services can offer significant help without assuming total responsibility for care. It is essential that the different agencies interact effectively and overlap their care, rather than leaving patients to negotiate their way from one island of provision to another.

Key components of such a 'mixed economy of care' should include:

1 A system for prompt and accurate assessment of people's needs which leads to offers of appropriate help, including reassessment. Assessment for specialist psychiatric care should be both 'generic' (using the skills that all disciplines share) and specific (using the particular skills of medicine, nursing, occupational therapy, etc.).

2 A clear understanding by staff working in the various agencies of what their tasks will be, and good training that will allow them to carry these out with confidence and satisfaction. When non-specialist care breaks down, it is usually because the carer do not expect to have to deal with the problem which faces them.

3 Systems ensuring that people are not obliged to make frequent and abrupt transfers between one setting and another as their disabilities increase. Assessment must therefore include prediction of future need; and each provider should offer a degree of

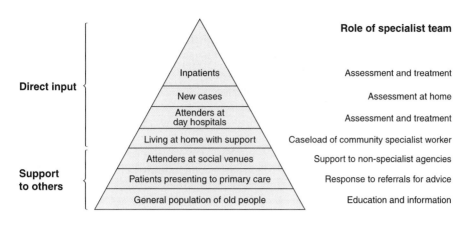

**Fig. 8.6.1** The span of old age psychiatry services.

flexibility, to encompass people who will soon need what they provide, and others whose needs are greater than the norm. For some people, a change of setting as their condition progresses—for example, from a sheltered flat to care in a nursing home—will be inevitable, so care systems must have ways of making transitions as smooth as possible.

## Loss of capacity and dependence on help

Mutual helpfulness is an accepted part of marital and family relationships. Family members often adapt unquestioningly to an older person's increasing dependence until the emotional pressures, or the adjustments they have to make in their day to day lives, become severe.

The 'needs of caregivers' are part of the currency of discussion amongst service providers. But people in everyday life do not necessarily perceive themselves that way: they think of themselves as simply participating in a normal aspect of family life. Younger people who have duties to their work, partner, and children—duties which conflict with the needs of their parents—may be readier to seek professional help than are the ageing spouses of a failing partner. Spouses often view caring as an intrinsic part of their lifelong relationship, and may resent offers from outside as an intrusion upon their privacy.

On the other hand, relationships can have malign as well as protective aspects, and sometimes the dependent partner in a caring relationship suffers more disadvantages than benefits. In extreme cases, abuse can occur.

### Abuse of older people

This is much better understood now than a few decades ago, although systematic study is difficult because of the varieties of abuse or exploitation that arise, the ambivalent relationships that surround them, and the concealment often practised by abusers and victims alike.[14] Abuse can occur in any circumstances, any class, and any relationship, from blood ties and friendships to professional and commercial relations. Nevertheless pointers to risk have been identified (Table 8.6.1).

Typically, the victim is disabled, often but not always with a dementing illness, perhaps with impaired communication, and is unrewarding to look after. Typically, the abuser is also impaired in

**Table 8.6.1** Some risk factors for abuse in old age

| Victim | Abuser | Relationship |
|---|---|---|
| Female | Family member in | Previous relationship – |
| Aged over 75 | caregiver role | not close, |
| Physically dependent | Psychiatric history | ambivalent, mutually |
| Cognitively impaired | History of abuse as a | abusive |
| Socially isolated | child | Role reversal |
| (lacking external | Substance misuse | Power reversal |
| support) | Financial dependence | Lack of problem- |
| Sensory impairment | on victim | solving skills in the |
| Incontinence | Dependence for | relationship |
| Abusive or | housing on victim | Forced proximity |
| unrewarding to | Overburdened by | Mutual dependence |
| caregiver | caregiver role | |
| Ready to adopt sick | Unsupported, or | |
| role | rejecting support | |

Reproduced from Fisk, J. Abuse of the elderly. In *Psychiatry in the elderly* (2nd edn.) (eds. R. Jacoby and C. Oppenheimer), copyright 1997, with permission from Oxford University Press.

some way, isolated from support (often by refusal rather than the absence of offers of help), and may abuse alcohol. There may have been a long history of ambivalence or of mutual aggression between abuser and victim, or the victim's illness may have reversed a power relationship that previously operated (damagingly) in the opposite direction. The intention of the abuser is sometimes clearly to do harm. In other cases the abusive behaviour seems to be an impulsive response to emotional pressures which the abusers are poorly equipped to deal with because they do not understand them properly, do not know how to share the burden with others, or are overwhelmed by the patient's need for care. The abuse may range from a single assault by a caregiver, who is immediately horrified by what he or she has done, to systematic cold-blooded persecution. Abuse may be physical, emotional, psychological, sexual, or financial.[15]

Where harm to a vulnerable person is suspected, there is an obligation to report it to the appropriate authority—in the United Kingdom, the local social services. Sometimes they in turn will involve the police and a criminal prosecution may follow. But frequently the problem can be dealt with in other ways, such as arranging a different form of care for the vulnerable person. The emphasis will be on reducing and managing risk, and on enhancing the quality of life of the person concerned. Difficult ethical issues arise when an elderly couple both suffer from dementia and one of them (often the husband) insists on continuing to care alone for his wife, unaware of the loss of his competence to do so. For a time, professional staff will try to support both partners in their wish to remain together at home, and to mitigate the effects of the inadequate care by the husband. But at some point the professional duty may need to shift from supporting, to taking over legal responsibility for the neglected person—though the displacement of the caregiving spouse in this way is distressing for everyone concerned.

## Ethical problems in old age psychiatry

The same classical principles of bioethics (beneficence, non-maleficence, autonomy, and confidentiality)[16] apply in old age psychiatry as in other age groups, but with differences in emphasis.[17] Since older people can rarely be considered in isolation, ethical principles have to be applied with the whole system in mind, and professionals often have ethical obligations to more than one person at a time.

### (a) Values

In old age, as in youth, we should seek to produce benefit and not harm—but identifying which of these is which may be more difficult in old age. Death is usually thought of as harm, but sometimes may be regarded as a blessing. Therefore it is essential to understand what the patient, rather than the professional, sees as beneficent, and the patient's right to name the value that they set on something must be respected. Some older people would prefer their assets to go to their descendants rather than being spent on their own care at the end of their lives—but the state sets limits to such self-denial.

### (b) Ambivalence

Impairments of thinking and communication can complicate ethically observant professional practice. People of all ages may have ambivalent feelings, or say things which seem belied by their actions, but this is particularly common among older people with cognitive impairment. Perhaps memory failure causes decisions to be swayed by feelings of the moment, so that decisions are not consistently maintained; and cognitive difficulty in marshalling complex information means that weighing alternative possible outcomes to a decision is much harder.

An illustration may make this clearer.

---

**Case study:** A woman with early cognitive impairment lives alone in the house where she brought up her children. She loves her house and garden, and tells her daughters that she never wants to live anywhere else, and she is convinced that she needs no help from them. At night, however, she becomes anxious and confused, and telephones her daughters, asking them why they 'haven't come home yet' and begging them not to abandon her.

---

Does the night or the day reveal her 'true wishes' better? Which should guide the decisions of her family, and of the professionals whose help they seek? Possibly, her considered daytime thoughts and her anxious actions at night are tapping different areas of her experience—the daytime communication reflects her aspirations and her lifetime self-perception, while her telephoning at night reflects the immediacy of her feelings and needs. Our duty is to give weight to both kinds of communication, helping the patient herself to understand what they mean, and to offer her the real-life opportunity (rather than theoretical discussion) of testing out the options she needs to consider.

### (c) Giving information and safeguarding information

Ethical obligations here include truth telling, giving information to patients about themselves, and protecting patients' information from others.

'Loss of insight' is a feature of dementia, but good insight is also dependent on sound information. A person who is making significant errors, or beginning to fail in self-care, should not be left in ignorance of what is happening to them. In fact, public knowledge nowadays about Alzheimer's disease is so much greater that sufferers often recognize the early signs themselves. They are entitled to an open discussion with their doctors, in which full information is put before them. (Relatives often shy away from such open disclosure, although when asked in surveys what they would wish for themselves, they tend to say that they would rather be told).

When it comes to disclosing information about a patient to the people involved in his or her care, the arguments are different. It is generally accepted that better care must depend on the best information, and it is normal for information to be shared between members of a clinical team, where the members share also in the duty of confidentiality to their patient. But in old age it is harder to know where to set these boundaries—both as regards information that should be protected, and as regards recognition of who is a team member. For example, senior staff in some residential homes, strictly preserving confidentiality, may not share information about the residents with the untrained care staff. However, if they know nothing about a resident's former life, caregivers will tend to respond to her as 'a bundle of needs' rather than as a real person; and if she cannot tell her own story, others must do it for her. This is much better recognized now than it used to be, and homes may ask families to construct a diary or album of a resident's life, with photographs, mementos, and recollections by different relatives. The diary also acts as a memory prompt and trigger for enjoyable conversations between resident and caregiver, and it creates a domain of shared information about individuals within the institution.

### (d) Autonomy

Healthy people strongly value the freedom to make their own decisions, to pursue their own aims, and to determine the course of their own lives. The onset of a physical illness may constrain this freedom, but people should still have as much influence as possible over decisions about their illness and its consequences.

Psychiatric disorder is different, because it may affect the powers by which that freedom is exercised, and may lead to decisions which would never have been made in health. From this comes the need, universally recognized although taking different legal forms in different countries, to set external controls over the decisions of people when they are mentally ill. Such legal controls are typically based on acute functional illness as the paradigm case. This gives them an 'all or nothing' character, envisaging hospital treatment of an illness capable of being relieved, so allowing patients to resume their autonomy when they recover their health.

This legal model is not really suited to cognitive impairment and its effect on decision-making in old age. The illness will not get better, and patients are unlikely to give (as they might with an acute illness) later 'retrospective informed consent' to the treatment. The emphasis therefore has to be much more on **minimal necessary interference**— on setting up protective frameworks, in which as much autonomy as possible can be exercised; on supporting patients at home or in homely settings, rather than bringing them into a hospital where no effective treatment can be given; and on gathering the information (both from patients and from those who know them best) which will enable professional decisions to reflect the wishes that the patient would have expressed, had they been able to do so.

Looking after cognitively impaired patients requires us to try constantly to maximize the opportunity for autonomous decisions, while also being very clear when a patient lacks the capacity to engage with a more complex issue. At such times, the responsibility for the decision must be openly and seriously taken by others. Trying to circumvent the problem by concealment and persuasion is a greater affront to autonomy than is an honest explanation to the patient of the reasons why a decision has been taken out of his hands.

## Medico-legal issues

'Doctors and lawyers have common responsibilities to ensure the protection of people who are incapable of deciding matters for themselves, and to promote the choice of those who can and should regulate their own lives. The careful assessment of whether individuals have or lack capacity is essential to protect their rights'.[18]

The legal framework in England and Wales for both financial and welfare decision-making where capacity is in doubt has been transformed by the Mental Capacity Act 2005, which came into force in April 2007. Some general principles of the Act are worth discussing here: more detail can be found in Lush.[19]

'Capacity' is a legal rather than a medical concept (see Chapter 11.1). Every adult is presumed to have full capacity, and a loss of capacity must be proved in relation to the particular decision being made: capacity is 'decision-specific'. For example, a person may *have* the capacity to choose another person to act for her in the management of her affairs, while *lacking* the capacity to manage those affairs herself. Although the final decision on capacity is made by the courts, they look to doctors to advise on whether a mental disorder has affected the individual's ability to make a particular decision or to carry out a specific task.

### (a) Assessing capacity

The Act states that a person lacks capacity if ' . . . he is unable to make a decision for himself . . . because of an impairment of, or disturbance in, the functioning of the mind or brain'. Such a person lacks capacity in relation to a particular decision if he cannot:

- understand the information about the decision
- retain the information
- use or weigh the information in the process of making the decision
- communicate the decision

The information that he must understand should include the consequences of deciding one way or another, and of making no decision. The information must be retained only for long enough to allow a decision to be made, therefore memory loss does not automatically remove capacity. The focus of this test of capacity is on the *process* of decision-making: the Act explicitly states that 'a person is not to be treated as unable to make a decision merely because he makes an unwise decision'.

### (b) Acting on behalf of a person who lacks capacity

Anyone acting on behalf of an incapacitated person must do so in the 'best interests' of that person. The action or decision in question should be delayed if there is a chance that the person may regain capacity; every effort should be made to enable them to participate in the decision-making process; the decision-maker should take into account the person's past and present wishes, beliefs, values, and feelings, especially any that had been written down when they had the capacity; the views of families, carers and anyone else interested in their welfare should be sought; and the least restrictive method for achieving the intended purpose should be chosen. The obligation to act in a person's best interests, and the protection from legal liability if they do so without negligence, extends to anyone carrying out acts of treatment and care, such as physical assistance, doing shopping, giving medical treatment, or nursing care.

### (c) Lasting power of attorney

A person with capacity can choose to appoint someone to act on their behalf (their 'attorney'). The power to act continues to be valid even after the 'donor' loses capacity, provided that the document giving the power has been registered with the Public Guardian (a newly created statutory office, replacing the former Court of Protection). The donor can give authority to his attorney to take both financial decisions *and* decisions relating to his health and welfare, provided that he is shown to lack the capacity to make those decisions himself at the relevant time. The attorney has the duty to act in accordance with the principles of the Mental Capacity Act 2005 and the guidance of its Code of Practice, and must act in the best interests of the donor.

### (d) Advance decisions to refuse treatment

The Mental Capacity Act 2005 also provides a framework and safeguards for a person who wishes to decide in advance what treatments should be withheld if they lose capacity in future. Advance decisions to refuse life-sustaining treatment have to be explicit, in writing, signed, and witnessed.

### (e) Driving

A common problem concerns the ability of older patients with early cognitive impairment to drive safely.[20] Scores on simple cognitive tests (e.g. the Mini-Mental State Examination) are very poorly correlated with driving ability, except where there is severe and obvious impairment. No quick objective test of driving skills has yet been devised. A worried but competent patient can often be reassured by booking an hour with a driving instructor. Loss of the freedom to drive represents such a loss of independence and enjoyment, and such a blow to self-esteem, that advice to give up driving may be strenuously resisted. On the other hand, families and professionals are conscious of potential risks to the public even if the patient denies these risks. Legally, the position in England and Wales is straightforward: individuals have a duty to notify the Driving and Vehicle Licensing Authority (DVLA) if they have an illness which might impair their ability to drive. A doctor must tell the patient who has such an illness that they are under an obligation to inform the DVLA; if it seems that this advice has been ignored, the doctor has an obligation to inform the DVLA himself—the duty of confidentiality is overruled by that requirement. Thereafter, the DVLA will arrange for the patient to receive an independent medical examination, and it is the DVLA which decides whether the driving licence should be withdrawn. If the patient fails to attend the medical examination (whether through forgetfulness or lack of insight), the licence is automatically withdrawn.

## Further information

Baldwin, C. (2005). *Making difficult decisions. The experience of caring for someone with dementia.* Alzheimer's Society, Gordon House, 10 Greencoat Place, London SW1P 1PH. (ISBN 1 872874 94 0).

Alzheimer's Society website: www.alzheimers.org.uk.

Ballard, C.G., O'Brien, J., James, I., *et al.* (2001). *Dementia: management of behavioural and psychological symptoms.* Oxford University Press, Oxford.

Herr, J.J. and Weakland, J.H. (1979). *Counseling elders and their families—practical techniques for applied gerontology.* (Springer series on adulthood and aging, Vol. 2). Springer, New York.

Jacoby, J., Oppenheimer, C., Dening, T., *et al.* (eds.) (2008). *The Oxford textbook of old age psychiatry.* Oxford University Press, Oxford.

## References

1. Anconi-Israel, S. and Ayalon, L. (2006). Diagnosis and treatment of sleep disorders in older adults. *The American Journal of Geriatric Psychiatry*, **14**, 95–103.
2. Sivertsen, B. and Nordhus, I.H. (2007). Management of insomnia in older adults. *The British Journal of Psychiatry*, **190**, 285–6.
3. Mosimann, U.P. and Boeve, B.F. (2008). Sleep disorders in older people. In *The Oxford textbook of old age psychiatry,* Chapter. 36. (eds. R. Jacoby, C. Oppenheimer, T. Dening, and A. Thomas). Oxford University Press, Oxford.
4. Monk, T.H. (2005). Aging human circadian rhythms: conventional wisdom may not always be right. *Journal of Biological Rhythms*, **20**, 366–74.
5. Reid, K.J., Martinovich, Z., Finkel, S., *et al.* (2006). Sleep: a marker of physical and mental health in the elderly. *The American Journal of Geriatric Psychiatry*, **14**, 860–6.
6. Uchiyama, M., Isse, K., Tanaka, N., *et al.* (1995). Incidental Lewy body disease in a patient with REM sleep behaviour disorder. *Neurology*, **45**, 709–12.
7. Ferini-Strambi, L., Fantini, M.L., Zucconi, M., *et al.* (2005). REM sleep behaviour disorder. *Neurological Sciences*, **26**, Part s3, s186–s92.
8. Nau, S.D., McCrae, C.S., Cook, K.G., *et al.* (2005). Treatment of insomnia in older adults. *Clinical Psychology Review*, **25**, 645–72.
9. Morin, C.M., Colecchi, C., Stone, J., *et al.* (1999). Behavioral and pharmacological therapies for late-life insomnia. *The Journal of the American Medical Association*, **281**, 991–9.
10. Zwi, R., Shawe-Taylor, M., and Murray, J. (2005). Cognitive processes in the maintenance of insomnia and co-morbid anxiety. *Behavioural and Cognitive Psychotherapy*, **33**, 333–42.
11. Wilkinson, P. (2008). Psychological treatments. In *The Oxford textbook of old age psychiatry*, Chapter 18i to iii (eds. R. Jacoby, C. Oppenheimer, T. Dening, and A. Thomas). Oxford University Press, Oxford.
12. Asen, E.K. (2008). Systemic interventions with older adults and their families. In *The Oxford textbook of old age psychiatry*, Chapter 18iv (eds. R. Jacoby, C. Oppenheimer, T. Dening, and A. Thomas). Oxford University Press, Oxford.
13. Evans, S. and Garner, J. (eds.) (2004). *Talking over the years. A handbook of dynamic psychotherapy with older adults.* Brunner-Routledge, Hove and New York.
14. Eastman, M. (1984). *Old age abuse.* Age Concern England, Mitcham.
15. Fisk, J. (1997). Abuse of the elderly. In *Psychiatry in the elderly* (2nd edn) (eds. R. Jacoby and C. Oppenheimer), pp. 736–48. Oxford University Press, Oxford.
16. Beauchamp, T.L. and Childress, J.F. (1989). *Principles of biomedical ethics* (3rd edn). Oxford University Press, New York.
17. Oppenheimer, C. (1999). Ethics in old age psychiatry. In *Psychiatric ethics* (3rd edn) (eds. S. Bloch, P. Chodoff, and S.A. Green). Oxford University Press, New York.
18. British Medical Association. (1995). *Assessment of mental capacity: guidance for doctors and lawyers.* British Medical Association, London.
19. Lush, D. (2008). The legal framework in the British Isles for making decisions on behalf of mentally incapacitated people. In *The Oxford textbook of old age psychiatry*, Chapter 43 (eds. R. Jacoby, C. Oppenheimer, T. Dening, and A. Thomas). Oxford University Press, Oxford.
20. O'Neill, D. (2008). Driving and psychiatric illness in late life. In *The Oxford textbook of old age psychiatry*, Chapter 43 (eds. R. Jacoby, C. Oppenheimer, T. Dening, and A. Thomas). Oxford University Press, Oxford.

# The planning and organization of services for older adults

Pamela S. Melding

## Introduction

When does an individual become an older adult? When they show signs of ageing? When they retire from work? When their health becomes frail? When they feel old? When society says they are old? Any of these indicators could define an 'older person' anywhere between 40 and 90 plus years! However, it was for statistical simplicity that many jurisdictions chose the chronological age of 65 to mark the change in status from mature adulthood to 'older person', mainly to establish an age for expected retirement and entitlement to certain benefits, including access to geriatric health services. When this arbitrary discriminator was instituted in the mid-twentieth century, 70 years was a good lifespan for most people. However, over the past 50 years, life expectancy steadily increased and is currently advancing at 6 weeks per annum, boosting the overall number of adults over 65 years and, particularly the over 80 years cohort.[1] Increasing life expectancy, due to improved health care and lowering birth rates, is causing worldwide 'population ageing'. This phenomenon will affect all health and mental health services in future years.

Already, health care resource and cost implications of population ageing for health services are enormous. Older adults occupy about two-thirds of general hospital medical, surgical, and orthopaedic beds; they are the greatest users of primary care and prescription medicines. Internationally, late-life illness takes up a considerable proportion of government or insurance funded health care budgets. As an example of the enormous costs involved, in 2003/2004, the United Kingdom's NHS spent around 43 per cent (£16.471 billion) of its hospital and community health services budget on people over the age of 65, and the cost of community and residential care for older people was 44 per cent (£7.38 billion) of all social welfare budgets.[2] These figures will rise dramatically over the next decades.

Mental Health Services have been slow to anticipate that population ageing will also increase the need for psychiatric services for older people. In many areas of the world, services are scarce, sporadic, or sub-standard. Even in developed nations, there is considerable variation in availability from one area to another. In the past decade, practically all OECD countries have promoted policies of de-institutionalization and community-based care for the elderly, in response to rising cost pressures associated with population ageing, plus a requirement to improve satisfaction for increasingly knowledgeable and assertive consumers, by providing better quality in all health services for older adults, including mental health.[3]

## The need for services for older adults
### Epidemiology

Whilst most people aspire to longevity, it can be a mixed blessing. Living longer increases risk of developing chronic degenerative diseases of body and brain, which can precipitate mental illness, possibly for the first time in life. Psychiatry services for older adults see a full range of new and chronic psychiatric disorders. However, the commonest new threats to mental health in late life are affective disorders and dementia.[4] Healthy, community-dwelling older adults are generally resilient, with a prevalence of major depressive illness of about 3 per cent, but studies of people in residential care find significant depressive symptoms in 14–42 per cent,[5] and in populations over 80 years, about 40 per cent.[6] Depression occurs in 15 to 40 per cent of medical inpatients[7] and in approximately 35.9 per cent of patients in geriatric rehabilitation units.[8] Among the many aetiological contributors to mental health problems in late life, physical illness and poor health are major risk factors, particularly for depression,[9] the risk increasing with disability.[10] Co-morbid physical disorders can mask depression or impede management with psychotropic medications. Although, pure anxiety disorders reduce in late life to about 1 per cent in community-dwelling older adults, anxiety co-morbid with other psychiatric disorders, particularly depression, is more common at approximately 4 per cent. Older people with anxiety disorders are high users of health care resources and may initially present with physical symptoms.[11] Affective disorders are often multi-dimensional, their treatment complicated, and frequently, they need joint management with geriatric colleagues.

Dementia affects 5–7 per cent of people at 65 and 20 per cent of those over age 80 years. By 2040, the number of people with the disorder will double in the developed countries of Europe and North America.[12] Older adults with dementia are an exemplar of consumers who require multi-disciplinary management. While geriatricians manage the majority of patients, those who exhibit behavioural and psychological symptoms of dementia (BPSD), approximately one-third, do best with additional specialist psychiatric expertise and management.[13] People with dementia can live for many years as their disorder progresses, requiring increasing levels of support from family, social workers, nurses, residential care providers, and other community health care workers in addition to psychiatry services.

## Why are specialist services required?

As indicated above, mentally or physically frail older adults have complex needs and frequently require a broad, multi-disciplinary approach in several domains, (a domain being a broad area of specialist services i.e. mental health, geriatrics, primary care, social services, etc.). This can be difficult to achieve if provision is by disjointed services. In many places in the world, lack of specialist services requires generic mental health services to treat older adults with dementia, depression, or other mental illnesses but this practice risks medical needs being unnoticed, or unappreciated. Frail older adults can find the experience of inpatient care in units with younger psychotic patients frightening and unacceptable. There are also different perspectives for working-age and geriatric psychiatry. Many working-age services promote a recovery model whereas care of older adults focuses on maintaining function, improving quality of life and paying more attention to the spiritual, environmental, and social influences on mental health. In addition, there is greater need to involve the social and family network of mentally frail elderly people than there is for working-age adults. For older adults, specialist services, with close collaboration with geriatricians and other geriatric providers, are preferred for optimal management.

## Principles of good service delivery for older adults

Optimal service delivery starts by establishing the principles that services wish to adopt. These should govern the ethos of service delivery. For the World Health Organization (WHO), the mnemonic CARITAS (Latin for Compassion) summarizes a global consensus on specific values required for good service delivery for psychiatry of old age.[14] These principles, championed over many years by many international pioneers of mental health services for older adults, assert that optimal services are:

- **Comprehensive**

    They take all aspects of the patient's physical, psychological, and social needs and wishes into account i.e. are *patient-centred*.

- **Accessible**

    They minimize the geographical, cultural, financial, political, and linguistic obstacles to obtaining care.

- **Responsive**

    They act promptly and appropriately to a wide variety of patient needs.

- **Individualized**

    They focus on each person in her/his family and community context aiming, wherever possible, to maintain and support the person within her/his home environment.

- **Transdisciplinary**

    They optimize the contributions of people with a range of personal and professional skills and facilitate collaboration with voluntary and other agencies.

- **Accountable**

    They accept responsibility for assuring the quality of the service delivered, monitoring this in partnership with patients and their families. They are ethically and culturally sensitive.

- **Systemic**

    They work flexibly with all available services to ensure continuity of care.

Summarizing, good services provide *patient-centred* care with *easy access to a comprehensive range of services* delivered by *multi-disciplinary personnel* working in a *collaborative, responsive, respectful, and accountable* way.

## Patient-centred care

The UK National Frameworks for Older People[15] and most OECD health administrations promote patient-centered care as a major means of improving quality of services and consumer satisfaction. Whilst most health professionals believe that they already practice patient-centred care, many patients would not agree. Predominantly, health systems for older people, particularly hospital-based, are far from patient-centered, being mostly organized around clinician or administrative requirements rather than patient needs. Patients encounter rigid appointment times, lack of evening or night services, inflexible boundaries between departments, inconvenient visiting hours, limited or expensive parking, and silo'd funding streams. Access or contact processes are obscure or difficult, information is inadequate, multiple assessments take place, and poor coordination between providers leads to treatment omissions or errors. Notably, older adults and their caregivers consider having multiple referrals to different specialists or providers and frequently repeating the same history to be a waste of time and resources.[16]

Consumer appraisals of their experience of services often result in common themes. Many experience poor communication—provider to patient, provider to caregiver, and provider to provider. Another common topic is lack of flexibility in developing management plans capable of involving several domains and dimensions of care (a dimension is a subset of a specialist domain, i.e. depression, dementia, continence, or mobility). As many elderly people have difficulties with mobility, or live far from services, transportation is another major issue.

In contrast, patient-centered services emphasize smoothing the progress of the patient 'journey' through the health system, eliminating duplication, matching care plans to patient needs, and generally making a demanding experience easier for the patient and their family. Unsurprisingly, the concept is appealing to patients and families. Increasingly, consumers, and their advocates, want to contribute to service planning, delivery, and evaluation.[17] So, what do older people want from their health care providers? Older people value their independence and being involved in the decision-making for their own care plans. Most want to remain in their own homes for as long as possible, but if that is detrimental for them, they want the right to relinquish decision-making, in various degrees, to other parties such as family members or their clinicians. They expect providers to treat them as an individual, to preserve their dignity, and to elicit and respect their preferences. Above all, they wish to be appropriately informed.[18] These desires are appropriate to all health care delivery for older adults, not just mental health. As most of us hope to grow old, we can empathize with these wishes. Perhaps we need to remember that in planning and organizing services for older adults, we are potentially designing them for ourselves. The quality of care required is what we would be happy with, if we ever become clients.

## Comprehensive and integrated services

Patient-centered care is more achievable with comprehensive or integrated services. The terms comprehensive and integrated are not interchangeable. A comprehensive service is one with a full range of inpatient and community services available within the same domain. An integrated service is one with a single point of entry capable of providing care plans that incorporate interventions and support in multiple domains and specific dimensions of care. Integrated services are characterized by a single point of entry, case management, geriatric, psychogeriatric and social assessments, and have multi-disciplinary teams.[3] They should have a seamless joining together of the various components of service, encompassing 'systemness' without diminishing component part identities.[19] Integration of different organizations is much easier if there are common administrative processes and financial systems. However, many mental health organizations have reporting and funding structures separate from other older adults' services (e.g. The Mental Health Trusts in the United Kingdom). Quasi-integration can be achieved by building effective *functional* links with a wide variety of health care professionals outside mental health e.g. primary care, geriatrics, acute medical and surgical care, social care, community health care, and non-clinical resources. For these collaborations to work, it is essential that bureaucratic processes enable easy transfer of funding and information across different entities and do not thwart clinicians' efforts to implement care plans for patients.

Integrated services are potentially more efficient as they should reduce duplication of assessments or investigations and service gaps. Currently, the majority of well-established services for older adults provide comprehensive rather than integrated services,[20] the latter being more ideology than practice, although this might be slowly changing. Research indicates that integrated care can delay institutionalization, reduce costs, and has benefits in consumer satisfaction[3] but is insufficient, as yet, to demonstrate that integrated services are more effective in achieving better health outcomes.

### (a) The place of the common geriatric assessment (CGA)

An important tool for assisting integration is the common geriatric assessment (CGA). Different disciplines all have their own styles and foci for assessment but, despite individual differences, it is useful to have some common information for all teams and multidisciplinary groups, regardless of who takes the main responsibility for the patient.[21] Advocacy for the comprehensive geriatric assessment (CGA) covering all the main domains and dimensions of physical illness, mental health, disability, and social assessment, is increasing internationally, notwithstanding a lack of research on their effectiveness in improving health outcomes. They aim to save a patient from multiple repetitions of the same information.[16] To be useful, CGAs require personnel to work across professional and agency barriers, which can have benefits in creating relationships with allied colleagues, essential for developing integrated services. There needs to be agreement amongst the providers as to the applicability of the information required, agreed processes by which the CGA generates onward referral to the appropriate domains of care

and procedures for updating and review. In some jurisdictions, (e.g. United Kingdom) CGAs or single assessment processes (SAPs) are mandatory for all older adults' services, in others, i.e. New Zealand and Australia, they are being trialed with a view to future obligatory use. SAPs and CGAs vary in their comprehensiveness and can aim at different levels, e.g. screening, proactive assessment, primary care, or secondary care services. They provide useful background information common to a range of providers but are not a substitute for specialized clinical assessment.

### (b) The 'core business' of mental health services for older adults

Irrespective of whether a mental health service for older adults is part of a comprehensive or integrated system, their 'core *business*' is the:

- Diagnosis and management of new cases of mental illness arising in late life, often associated with the ageing process.
- Treatment of mental illness complicating physical illness and disability.
- Management of older adults with long-term mental illness complicated by ageing.
- Education and support for caregivers of older adults with mental illness.

Most psychiatry for older adults is about the management of chronic illness and care, rather than cure, is usually the main priority. An adaptation of the 5As model for patient-centred chronic illness management[22] is useful to describe the 'core *tasks*' of patient-centered psychiatry of old age. They are:

- Assessment of multiple care needs
- Advice on diagnosis and options for management
- Agreement with patient and caregiver on a care plan
- Assistance with implementation of care plan
- Assertive follow-up when needed

The 'core areas of *expertise*' for specialist services for older adults are the:

- Treatment of affective and psychotic disorders in late life
- Assessment of neurocognitive disorders and the management of the behavioural and psychological symptoms of dementia (BPSD)
- Rehabilitation of long-standing, chronic psychiatric disorders in patients whose disorder is complicated by physical illness or ageing
- Management of delirium in medically ill or complicating dementia
- Liaison with families, caregivers, and community providers

## Core components of psychogeriatric service delivery

### The evidence base for the 'core components'

Working with mentally ill older adults involves a variety of locations i.e. the patient's own residence, medical and surgical wards in a general hospital, psychiatry inpatient facilities, residential care facilities, outpatient clinics, outreach clinics, geriatric rehabilitation units, or day hospitals. Several models of services for older adults have evolved over the past 30 or 40 years, shaping a degree of accord amongst clinicians on what are 'core components'. The evidence for these has been systematically reviewed by Draper and Low.[23] (See Table 8.7.1.)

## Community old age psychiatry services

The lynchpin of geriatric psychiatry services is the community-based assessment and case management team. The community team model originated from the closure of the mental hospitals and the move into community-care in the 1980–90s. Their focus is domiciliary assessment and management. This offers the clinician opportunities to observe patients in their own environment, and promotes optimal cognitive functioning by decreasing stress for the individual. Home assessment avoids the sometimes-perceived stigma of attending a psychiatric clinic and eliminates transportation difficulties, as well as allowing ready access to family members or other caregivers. Treatment for most patients can take place at their residence (own home or nursing home), reducing reliance on inpatient or residential care. The model has proven to be efficient and highly acceptable to consumers and caregivers.

A typical multi-disciplinary team consists of at least one psychiatrist, psychiatric nurses, clinical psychologists, social workers, occupational, and other therapists plus support and administration staff. A psychiatrist traditionally leads a multi-disciplinary team but not necessarily so. As a whole, the team should be able to address the biopsychosocial, therapeutic, and psychoeducational requirements of a wide range of disorders and intervention settings. Team members case-manage depending upon their own special skills and expertise. Working collaboratively, with appropriate training, good supervision, and well-designed protocols and communication systems enhances the multi-disciplinary team. Some of the most effective teams are 'interdisciplinary' who develop flexible working patterns characterized by a non-hierarchical structure, and shared decision-making. They facilitate lateral communication between team members, and free exchange of ideas to develop optimal treatment and support management plans as a group. The evidence for community-delivered specialized multi- or interdisciplinary psychogeriatric assessment and management teams is strong and indicates consistently better outcomes than 'usual care' of primary care or generic mental health management.

## Inpatient units

Inpatient units vary from the specialized older person's assessment, treatment, and rehabilitation (ATR) unit, similar to their geriatric counterparts, to dedicated beds in geriatric wards, or donated beds in working-age mental health units. Preferably, a specialized inpatient unit is purpose built or has the functionality to separate patients with functional and organic disorders, as each group has different clinical features, nursing needs, disabilities, and requirements for care plans. The evidence for specialized inpatient psychogeriatric units is positive but as there have been few random controlled trials (RCTs), it is less robust than the evidence for

**Table 8.7.1** Level of evidence and study qualities for areas of service delivery

| Area | No. of studies reviewed | No. of controlled trials | Quality range,* range (low) 0–1 (high) | Mean rating of quality | Level of evidence of effectiveness |
|---|---|---|---|---|---|
| Psychogeriatric day hospitals | 10 | 0 | 0.43–0.82 | 0.57 | Level IV (particularly depression) |
| Community old age psychiatry services | 24 | 7 | 0.79–0.94 | 0.87 | Level I for multi-disciplinary psychogeriatric teams, level IV for adult psychiatry teams |
| Integrated hospital and community-care | 4 | 2 | 0.71–0.82 | 0.76 | Level II for psychogeriatric services post-discharge care, no evidence for geriatric medical services (level I) |
| Primary care collaborations | 3 | 2 | 0.89–0.94 | 0.92 | Level II |
| Older people in general adult psychiatric wards | 6 | 0 | 0.51–0.67 | 0.59 | Level IV |
| Acute psychogeriatric wards | 23 | 0 | 0.43–0.78 | 0.61 | Level III-2 |
| Hospital medical services | 6 | 2 | 0.82–0.90 | 0.89 | Level II for prevention of delirium without dementia, no evidence for other mental health outcomes (level 1) |
| Combined psychogeriatric and medical wards | 3 | 0 | 0.52–0.53 | 0.52 | Level IV |
| Hospital-based CL psychogeriatric service delivery | 7 | 3 | 0.62–0.90 | 0.79 | Level II effectiveness for reducing costs and length of stay |
| Long-term psychogeriatric care | 11 | 0 | 0.58–0.71 | 0.66 | Level III-2 |
| Psychogeriatric outreach to long-term care | 8 | 6 | 0.73–0.95 | 0.84 | Level II for liaison style outreach services, Level III-2 for consultation style |
| Overall | 108 | 25 | 0.62–0.95** | 0.85** | |

*If ≥2 controlled trials in service area, quality range reported for RCTs only, otherwise reported for all studies. **overall mean and range reported for controlled trials only.
(Reproduced from Draper, B. Melding, P. and Brodaty, H. (2005) Psychogeriatric Services Delivery: An international perspective, copyright 2005, with permission from Oxford University Press.)

community teams. Nevertheless, what evidence exists points to specialized psychogeriatric units having better outcomes for psychogeriatric patients than working-age mental health, or geriatric medical units.[23] Scientific evaluation of combined psychogeriatric and geriatric medical wards is inadequate but expert clinical opinion considers them useful in the management of co-morbid medical and psychiatric illness.

## Consultation and liaison

Hospital-based consultation and liaison (CL) services are important components because of the high number of mental disorders in the physically ill, general hospital populations. However, while the evidence is relatively good for CL outcomes such as hospital stays and costs, it is only modestly positive for mental health outcomes.[24] Notwithstanding, in recent years, older adults' CL services have outreached from the general hospital to provider organizations in the community. The evidence for these liaison services, usually provided by community teams to psychogeriatric long-term care facilities and voluntary organizations, is relatively good.[23]

## Day Hospitals

Day Hospitals, originally attached to the old psychiatric institutions, have mostly devolved into community facilities and many United Kingdom psychiatrists of old age consider them indispensable.[25] Specialist day hospitals provide care for people with moderate and severe needs, including people with functional mental illnesses such as depression, anxiety, and schizophrenia, who may need specific support with daily activities and people with moderate to severe dementia. The Day Hospital allows hospital level treatment while allowing patients to remain living in their own residence. The evidence for their effectiveness, while positive, is sparse. As they are less common, they are not as revered in other parts of the world as much as they are in the United Kingdom. Day Hospitals need to be differentiated from Day Centres, managed by the voluntary or welfare sectors, which usefully provide social activities to keep the patient involved with their community and much needed respite for caregivers.

## Residential care

An elderly person unable to support themselves in their own home needing daytime or 24 h supervision requires a resident caregiver or residential care facility. A community may have a range of residential care facilities managed by a variety of agencies such as local authorities, voluntary organizations, for-profit or not-for-profit religious and welfare organizations in the independent sector. These non-government organizations (NGOs) provide care homes for older adults who need support because of physical or mental frailty but not to the extent of requiring hospital level care. Many of the residents have some cognitive impairment and, unsurprisingly, a relatively high number of patients have complicating depression and/or psychosis. Residential care homes vary markedly in their ability to support older adults with mental health problems. Evidence from The Netherlands[26] and Australia[27] indicates that mental health enhanced care in the form of regular psychogeriatric team liaison to these residential facilities has beneficial outcomes for patients for example less inpatient stays, less psychotropic medication, and improvement in depression and psychosis.

## Long-term care

Progressive de-institutionalization since the 1980s saw the transfer of many long-stay, public sector beds, for patients with dementia or intractable mental illness, to community-based nursing homes or hospitals. These facilities were generally smaller, more home-like and provided additional activities for the residents than traditional long-term care did. The change required many old age psychiatry services to collaborate with independent sector stakeholders and evolve outreach and liaison models of care with the new long-term residential care facilities. This paradigm shift for service delivery was beneficial for patient outcomes.[23]

Disturbed behaviour resulting from dementia (BPSD) can be severe enough for patients to need Specialized Care Units (SCUs). Examples are in Italy, France (CANTOUs), Tasmania (ADARDS unit), and London (Domus units). Such units have a small number of beds, well-trained staff with high staff to patient ratios and access to ongoing specialized psychogeriatric team care. When compared with traditional psychogeriatric ward patients, unsurprisingly, those in a specialized care unit, show improvements in cognition, self-cares, activity participation, and behaviour. The key elements to success appear to be training staff to anticipate and recognize mental health problems and close liaison with specialist mental health teams.

## Respite care

The community-care model relies on family, rather than professionals to attend to most of the needs of a mentally frail, elderly person. This is demanding, difficult work for caregivers who usually have other responsibilities of family, home, and jobs. The main focus of respite care is to give lay caregivers a break from caring every few weeks, so they may continue to provide care and thus delay the need for permanent nursing home care as long as possible. Respite can be in the patient's own home, by providing a 'live-in' professional caregiver, or in hospital or a residential care facility for a week or two, every couple of months, allowing the family caregiver to take a holiday. Whilst seeming an admirable concept, the effectiveness of respite care is doubtful and there is little evidence that it has a significant effect on caregivers' burden, psychiatric status or physical health, or on patients' cognition, function, physical health, or rate of institutionalization.[28] Respite care, even when available, may be poorly utilized. Caregiver barriers to using respite care include guilt, financial reasons, cultural attitudes, and fear of stigma. Access barriers include unavailability, lack of publicity about services, long waiting lists, and poor identification of at-risk caregivers. Patient barriers include severe problem behaviours, immobility, incontinence, wandering, and inability to communicate.[29]

## Primary care collaborations

Despite older adults forming the majority of patients seen by general practitioners (GPs), they detect and treat less than half the number of older adults with mental disorders.[30] Short consultation times, with a concentration on physical symptoms, with few patients presenting explicitly with mental health complaints, plus a reluctance of older adults, especially men, to express psychological distress to their GP, leads to under-recognition of mental disorders in older adults. Depression may be erroneously attributed to loneliness or ageing and early dementia overlooked. Primary care practitioners also make fewer decisions to treat or refer patients to specialist services and often preferred to monitor, or defer decisions.[31]

Mere cooperation between mental health services and primary care seems insufficient to improve matters. Collaborations such as mental health enhanced primary care looks more promising. Education of primary care nurses in recognition of mental disorders and use of screening instruments might be useful to improve identification of mental disorders.[31] Even better is the idea of 'embedding' nurses, who have the skills necessary to identify health problems and coordinate care for older adults, into primary care practices. One experimental scheme in New Zealand, 'The Coordinators of Services for the Elderly' (COSE project) works within a primary care small group of practices to coordinate care of the practices' elderly patients across health, mental health, community, and accident services. An RCT of the COSE project over usual care significantly demonstrated that patients in the COSE arm were less likely to be hospitalized, their residential care was delayed and morbidity reduced.[32]

The primary care physician is crucial to patient care from start to finish, not only in identifying people who are at risk but also for any post hospital discharge care as the majority of patients seen by specialist services eventually return to primary care for ongoing management, in conjunction with their family caregivers. Even if patients or their caregivers can self-refer to secondary services, it is important not to bypass the general practitioner, who has awareness of the patient's overall health care and context.

## Special components of services

### Memory clinics

The substantial growth in numbers of memory clinics, over the past 10–15 years, was stimulated by the licensing of cholinesterase inhibitor drugs for Alzheimer's disease.[33] Memory clinics offer a range of services from assessment of cognition to specialized treatment of memory problems. Dedicated memory services can improve diagnostic expertise and lessen stigma for the patient. Usefully, they often focus on education of patients and caregivers as well as monitoring medications. However, the concept of a 'memory clinic' flies in the face of the trend towards community-based services and integration with local services. Furthermore, the intervention base is often very narrow. Very few studies provide any evidence of increased mental health gain over other psychogeriatric services, but there is some evidence that the attention, communication, and counselling offered increases consumer satisfaction.[34]

### Older adults with intellectual handicap

People with intellectual handicap are also living longer and they are at particular risk for developing dementia. Over 55 per cent of people with Down's syndrome between the ages of 60–70 have Alzheimer type dementia, which often begins to emerge in midlife rather than old age. Consequently, the intellectually handicapped older person has complex care needs that require dementia, mental health, and learning disability services to work together assiduously.[2]

### Older prisoners

An often forgotten group is ageing prisoners, who are also increasing in number. Older prisoners have increased risk for depression and other mental health problems. Long-serving older prisoners may develop dementia and require the special challenge of care delivery whilst incarcerated. Specialist services for older prisoners are scarce and, if available, usually provided by visiting community assessment and treatment services in conjunction with local forensic psychiatry services.

### Younger people with dementia

Early onset dementia is fortunately rare but when it occurs, it is devastating. The patients usually have family responsibilities with young children, jobs, and financial commitments. Early onset dementia usually has a more accelerated course and genetically related family members may be concerned for themselves or their offspring. Diagnosis is often delayed for younger people so considerable distress and problems have usually built up before they reach services. Their management needs may also be different as they are usually physically fitter and they may require more structured activities than their older counterparts do, but need similar levels of supervision. Appropriate services for younger people who develop dementia are often scarce and the patients may fall into an under-resourced gap between working-age and older adults' services.

### Academic units

Although there has been a growth in the number of geriatric psychiatry academic units and positions worldwide, they are still under-represented in universities worldwide. They are important providers of under and postgraduate teaching and research.

## Planning to commissioning

Commissioning is 'the process of specifying, securing, and monitoring services to meet the needs of a population at a strategic level'.[2] Proposed services require a 'business case' with the place of an intended service clearly demonstrated in the overall schemata of health provision for a population. Demonstration of the need for services and projections of likely demand is necessary and the chief scientific tools available to identify these are epidemiology, demography, and utilization studies.

Epidemiology predicts the likely problems in a population and demography the characteristics of the population that could increase risk. The older the population, the more likely it will have a high prevalence of dementia requiring services. An important demographic to consider when planning services is the socio-economic status of a population. Low socio-economic status increases the likelihood of poor physical health, poor functionality and deprivation causes stress, leading to poverty of control over one's life, low self-esteem, anxiety, insecurity, and depression.[35] Also important is the number of immigrant residents. Ethnic elders are more likely to have earlier social disadvantage compounding in later life into a multiple jeopardy of social disadvantage, poorer physical health, and mental health problems.[36]

Whilst epidemiological studies may predict potential need, and demographics highlight areas of possible risk, not all people with problems will demand services. Demand or utilization is considerably less than the potential need as predicted from the demographical and epidemiological data. International research consistently shows similar demand patterns. About half of identified patients obtain treatment from a health care provider. Only 10–16 per cent reaches specialist mental health services, and primary care treats about 30–40 per cent. For older adults utilization is even less than for working-age adults.[37] Stigma can have a detrimental effect on willingness to access services[38] as may cultural barriers.[36] For individuals, utilization of mental health services is more likely if the disorder is severe, is adversely affecting the family or social network, or the patient is female.

Services are usually commissioned based on expected demand rather than predicted need. Demand often increases, outstripping supply once services are available and information about them permeates into the community. Resource review on a regular basis as demand rises is necessary.

Commissioning new or revised services involves stocktaking of available resources for older adults. Often these are inequitable, with urban areas enjoying a range of services that rural areas lack. Despite unique individualities of different countries of the world, some characteristics tend to be true of all rural communities. They tend to be older and poorer than urban populations with a higher percentage of females.[39] Stoical older adults living in rural areas have a high tolerance of distress and are often reluctant to seek help from mental health services.[40] Consequently, rural populations are even more vulnerable for late-life mental health disorders, yet outreach services are usually infrequent, and primary care limited. Some countries with very large rural areas, for example United States, Canada, Africa, Australia, and New Zealand commission novel methods of outreach, such as flying doctor services.

Ideally, service planning should be in conjunction with key stakeholders, that is consumers, other geriatric services and providers, including NGOs. For optimal patient-centred mental health care for older adults to be effective, individual specialist hospital services need to work with general practitioners and other community providers. Attention to administrative pathways and funding structures that promote collaboration between providers is important. Commissioning strategies that propose integration of existing services need to recognize that, whilst the end result *may* be beneficial to patients, the process *will* cause enormous upheaval and distress among the workforce involved, particularly if there is decommissioning or amalgamation of duplicate services.

Service development is contingent on there being a skilled, educated workforce. A development plan needs to consider the specialist disciplines required, based on expected case mix and work loads, staff availability, recruitment and retention, morale, job satisfaction, and very importantly, training issues. Clinical services have important roles in teaching and training ongoing professional development and in clinical evaluation, and systems research. These tasks can also be important means of cross-fertilization, dissemination of ideas between related services, teams, and disciplines. Involvement of different disciplines in undergraduate or postgraduate teaching programmes including psychiatry trainees can be useful for disseminating a broader perspective to prospective health professionals intending to work with older adults.

A vital aspect of commissioning is monitoring, that is, the methods of service review and evaluation. This is important for continuing quality initiatives and research but also to provide evidence for review and future commissioning of even better services.

## Conclusion

Worldwide, population ageing is driving the development of mental health services for older adults. Finite resources, burgeoning costs, expanding therapeutic repertoires, and increasing consumer interest in involvement in health care is challenging health organizations to develop effective, efficient, and economic patient-centred services for older adults. Fundamentally, the quality of services is dependent on health personnel working with their patients and other providers, towards shared aims of improving health outcomes and quality of life. Clinicians' adaptability, flexibility, responsiveness, availability for patients, and willingness to collaborate are the keys to success in developing future services for older adults.

## Further information

Draper, B., Melding, P., and Brodaty, H. (eds.) (2005). *Psychogeriatric service delivery: an international perspective*. Oxford University Press, Oxford, New York.

Department of Health and Care Services Improvement Partnership. (2005). *Everybody's business. Integrated mental health services for older adults: a service development guide*. www.everybody'sbusiness.org.uk

World Health Organization. (1997). *Organization of the care and the psychiatry of the elderly*. World Health Organization, Geneva.

Melding, P. and Draper, B. (eds.) (2001). *Consultation liaison geriatric psychiatry*. Oxford University Press, Oxford, New York.

## References

1. Draper, B., Melding, P., and Brodaty, H. (2005). Preface. In *Psychogeriatric service delivery*, pp. 4–13. Oxford University Press, Oxford, New York.

2. Department of Health, Care Services Improvement Partnership. (2005). *Everybody's business. Integrated mental health services for older adults: a service development guide*. Older people and disability division, Directorate of Care Services, Department of Health, London.

3. Johri, M., Beland, F., and Bergman, H. (2003). International experiments in integrated care for the elderly: a synthesis of the evidence. *International Journal of Geriatric Psychiatry*, **18**(3), 222–35.

4. Riedel-Heller, S.G., Busse, A., and Angermeyer, M.C. (2006). The state of mental health in old-age across the 'old' European Union—a systematic review. *Acta Psychiatrica Scandinavica*, **113**(5), 388–401.

5. Djernes, J.K. (2006). Prevalence and predictors of depression in populations of elderly: a review. *Acta Psychiatrica Scandinavica*, **113**(5), 372–87.

6. Zarit, S., Femia, E., Gatz, M., et al. (1999). Prevalence, incidence and correlates of depression in the oldest old: the OCTO study. *Aging & Mental Health*, **3**(2), 119–28.

7. Gareri, P., Ruotolo, G., Curcio, M., et al. (2001). Prevalence of depression in medically hospitalized elderly patients. *Archives of Gerontology and Geriatrics*, **33**(Suppl.), 183–9.

8. Shah, D.C., Evans, M., and King, D. (2000). Prevalence of mental illness in a rehabilitation unit for older adults. *Postgraduate Medical Journal*, **76**(893), 153–6.

9. Cole, M.G. and Dendukuri, N. (2003). Risk factors for depression among elderly community subjects: a systematic review and meta-analysis. *The American Journal of Psychiatry*, **160**(6), 1147–56.

10. Braam, A.W., Prince, M.J., Beekman, A.T.F., et al. (2005). Physical health and depressive symptoms in older Europeans: results from EURODEP. *The British Journal of Psychiatry*, **187**(1), 35–42.

11. Flint, A.J. (2005). Generalised anxiety disorder in elderly patients: epidemiology, diagnosis and treatment options. *Drugs & Aging*, **22**(2), 101–14.

12. Ferri, C., Prince, M., Brayne, C., et al. (2005). Global prevalence of dementia: a Delphi consensus study. *Lancet*, **366**(9503), 2112–17.

13. Brodaty, H., Draper, B., and Low, L.F. (2003). Behavioural and psychological symptoms of dementia: a seven-tiered model of service delivery. *Medical Journal of Australia*, **178**(5), 231–4.

14. World Health Organization. (1997). *Organization of the care and the psychiatry of the elderly.* World Health Organization, Geneva.

15. Department of Health. (2001). *National service framework for older people.*

16. Stevenson, J. (1999). *Comprehensive assessment of older people. Kings fund rehabilitation programme. Developing rehabilitation opportunities for older people.* Kings Fund, London.

17. Dening, T. and Lawton, C. (1998). The role of carers in evaluating mental health services for older people. *International Journal of Geriatric Psychiatry,* **13**(12), 863–70.

18. Robb, G. and Seddon, M. (2006). Quality improvement in New Zealand healthcare. Part 6: keeping the patient front and centre to improve healthcare quality. *The New Zealand Medical Journal,* **119**(1242), U2174.

19. Melding, P. (2005). Integrating service delivery and quality of care. In *Psychogeriatric service delivery* (eds. B. Draper, P. Melding, and H. Brodaty), pp. 251–80. Oxford University Press, Oxford, New York.

20. Challis, D., Reilly, S., Hughes, J., *et al.* (2002). Policy, organisation and practice of specialist old age psychiatry in England. *International Journal of Geriatric Psychiatry,* **17**(11), 1018–26.

21. Stevenson, J. (1999). *Comprehensive assessment of older people. Kings fund rehabilitation programme. Developing rehabilitation opportunities for older people.* Kings Fund, London.

22. Sheridan, S.L., Harris, R.P., and Woolf, S.H.A. (2004). Shared decision making about screening and chemoprevention: a suggested approach from the U.S. preventive services task force. *American Journal of Preventive Medicine,* **26**(1), 56–66.

23. Draper, B., and Low, L.F. (2005). Evidenced-based psychogeriatric service delivery. In *Psychogeriatric service delivery: an international perspective* (eds. B. Draper, P. Melding, and H. Brodaty), pp. 75–122. Oxford University Press, Oxford, New York.

24. Draper, B. (2001). Consultation liaison geriatric psychiatry. In *Geriatric consultation liaison psychiatry* (eds. P. Melding and B. Draper), pp. 3–34. Oxford University Press, Oxford, New York.

25. Hoe, J., Ashaye, K., and Orrell, M. (2005). Don't seize the day hospital! Recent research on the effectiveness of day hospitals for older people with mental health problems. *International Journal of Geriatric Psychiatry,* **20**(7), 694–8.

26. Depla, M., Pols, J., De Lange, J., *et al.* (2003). Integrating mental health care into residential homes for the elderly: an analysis of six Dutch programs for older people with severe and persistent mental illness. *Journal of the American Geriatrics Society,* **51**(9), 1275–9.

27. Brodaty, H., Draper, B., Millar, J., *et al.* (2003). Randomized controlled trial of different models of care for nursing home residents with dementia complicated by depression or psychosis. *The Journal of Clinical Psychiatry,* **64**(1), 63–72.

28. Flint, A. (1995). Effects of respite care on patients with dementia and their caregivers. *International Psychogeriatrics,* **7**, 505–17.

29. Brodaty, H. and Gresham, M. (1992). Prescribing residential care for dementia- effects, side-effects, indications and dosage. *International Journal of Geriatric Psychiatry,* **7**, 357–62.

30. Speer, D. and Schneider, M. (2003). Mental health needs of older adults and primary care: opportunity for interdisciplinary geriatric team practice. *Clinical Psychology: Science and Practice,* **10**(1), 85–101.

31. Watts, S.C., Bhutani, G.E., Stout, I.H., *et al.* (2002). Mental health in older adult recipients of primary care services: is depression the key issue? Identification, treatment and the general practitioner. *International Journal of Geriatric Psychiatry,* **17**(5), 427–37.

32. Parsons, M., Anderson, C., Senior, H., *et al.* (2007). *ASPIRE: Assessment of Services Promoting Independence and Recovery in Elders.* University of Auckland, Auckland.

33. Lindesay, J., Marudkar, M., van Diepen, E., *et al.* (2002). The second Leicester survey of memory clinics in the British Isles. *International Journal of Geriatric Psychiatry,* **17**, 41–7.

34. Jolley, D., Benbow, S.M., and Grizzell, M. (2006). Memory clinics. *Postgraduate Medical Journal,* **82**(965), 199–206.

35. Marmot, M. (2005). Social determinants of health inequalities. *Lancet,* **365**(9464), 1099–104.

36. Silveira, E.R.T. and Ebrahim, S. (1998). Social determinants of psychiatric morbidity and well-being in immigrant elders and whites in east London. *International Journal of Geriatric Psychiatry,* **13**(11), 801–12.

37. Wang, P.S., Lane, M., Olfson, M., *et al.* (2005). Twelve-month use of mental health services in the United States: results from the National Comorbidity Survey Replication. *Archives of General Psychiatry,* **62**(6), 629–40.

38. Brodaty, H., Cathy, T., Claire, T., *et al.* (2005). Why caregivers of people with dementia and memory loss don't use services. *International Journal of Geriatric Psychiatry,* **20**(6), 537–46.

39. Allan, D. and Cloutier-Fisher, D. (2006). Health service utilization among older adults in British Columbia: making sense of geography. *Canadian Journal on Aging,* **25**(2), 219–32.

40. Judd, F., Jackson, H., Komiti, A., *et al.* (2006). Help-seeking by rural residents for mental health problems: the importance of agrarian values. *The Australian & New Zealand Journal of Psychiatry,* **40**(9), 769–76.

# SECTION 9

# Child and Adolescent Psychiatry

**9.1 General issues** *1589*

9.1.1 Developmental psychopathology and classification in childhood and adolescence *1589*
Stephen Scott

9.1.2 Epidemiology of psychiatric disorder in childhood and adolescence *1594*
E. Jane Costello and Adrian Angold

9.1.3 Assessment in child and adolescent psychiatry *1600*
Jeff Bostic and Andrés Martin

9.1.4 Prevention of mental disorder in childhood and other public health issues *1606*
Rhoshel Lenroot

**9.2 Clinical syndromes** *1612*

9.2.1 Neuropsychiatric disorders *1612*
James C. Harris

9.2.2 Specific developmental disorders in childhood and adolescence *1622*
Helmut Remschmidt and Gerd Schulte-Körne

9.2.3 Autism and the pervasive developmental disorders *1633*
Fred R. Volkmar and Ami Klin

9.2.4 Attention deficit and hyperkinetic disorders in childhood and adolescence *1643*
Eric Taylor

9.2.5 Conduct disorders in childhood and adolescence *1654*
Stephen Scott

9.2.6 Anxiety disorders in childhood and adolescence *1664*
Daniel S. Pine

9.2.7 Paediatric mood disorders *1669*
David Brent and Boris Birmaher

9.2.8 Obsessive–compulsive disorder and tics in children and adolescents *1680*
Martine F. Flament and Philippe Robaey

9.2.9 Sleep disorders in children and adolescents *1693*
Gregory Stores

9.2.10 Suicide and attempted suicide in children and adolescents *1702*
David Shaffer, Cynthia R. Pfeffer, and Jennifer Gutstein

9.2.11 Children's speech and language difficulties *1710*
Judy Clegg

9.2.12 Gender identity disorder in children and adolescents *1718*
Richard Green

**9.3 Situations affecting child mental health** *1724*

9.3.1 The influence of family, school, and the environment *1724*
Barbara Maughan

9.3.2 Child trauma *1728*
David Trickey and Dora Black

9.3.3 Child abuse and neglect *1731*
David P. H. Jones

9.3.4 The relationship between physical and mental health in children and adolescents *1740*
Julia Gledhill and M. Elena Garralda

9.3.5 The effects on child and adult mental health of adoption and foster care *1747*
June Thoburn

9.3.6 Effects of parental psychiatric and physcial illness on child development *1752*
Paul Ramchandani, Alan Stein, and Lynne Murray

9.3.7 The effects of bereavement in childhood *1758*
Dora Black and David Trickey

**9.4 The child as witness** *1761*
Anne E. Thompson and John B. Pearce

**9.5 Treatment methods for children
and adolescents** *1764*

9.5.1 Counselling and psychotherapy for children *1764*
John B. Pearce

9.5.2 Psychodynamic child psychotherapy *1769*
Peter Fonagy and Mary Target

9.5.3 Cognitive behaviour therapies for
children and families *1777*
Philip Graham

9.5.4 Caregiver-mediated interventions
for children and families *1787*
Philip A. Fisher and Elizabeth A. Stormshak

9.5.5 Medication for children and
adolescents: current issues *1793*
Paramala J. Santosh

9.5.6 Residential care for social reasons *1799*
Leslie Hicks and Ian Sinclair

9.5.7 Organization of services for children and
adolescents with mental health problems *1802*
Miranda Wolpert

9.5.8 The management of child and adolescent
psychiatric emergencies *1807*
Gillian Forrest

9.5.9 The child psychiatrist as consultant
to schools and colleges *1811*
Simon G. Gowers and Sian Thomas

# General issues

## Contents

9.1.1 Developmental psychopathology and classification in childhood and adolescence
Stephen Scott

9.1.2 Epidemiology of psychiatric disorder in childhood and adolescence
E. Jane Costello and Adrian Angold

9.1.3 Assessment in child and adolescent psychiatry
Jeff Bostic and Andrés Martin

9.1.4 Prevention of mental disorder in childhood and other public health issues
Rhoshel Lenroot

## 9.1.1 Developmental psychopathology and classification in childhood and adolescence

Stephen Scott

### Introduction

Classification schemes of psychiatric disorders in childhood and adolescence have to take into account three particular features. Firstly, the individual is continually changing and growing. Sound knowledge is therefore required of the normal range of development and its limits. For example, some fears may be normal in a 5-year-old but abnormal in an 8-year-old. Once identified, it is helpful to decide if abnormalities are due to *delay in* or *deviance from* the usual pattern of development. The implications of each differ, and should be classified differently. Secondly, the majority of childhood mental health problems arise from an excess of behaviours exhibited by many young people, such as aggression or dieting.

They are seldom due to qualitatively distinct phenomena of the kind more often seen in adult conditions, such as hearing voices or hanging oneself. Consequently choosing a cut-off point to make a categorical entity from a dimensional construct is more often used in child psychiatry. This is inevitably an arbitrary process (albeit informed by empirical criteria), which may lead to loss of information, and may be held to be labelling the child unnecessarily. That dimensions can be interchanged with categories does not necessarily mean they are unhelpful—after all, day and night are useful terms yet the boundary between them is continuous and arbitrary. Psychiatrists in particular may be criticized for 'medicalizing' a child's difficulties by talking about disorders or diagnoses, whereas other professionals and parents may prefer to see them as understandable variations in child development, and prefer to call them 'emotional and behavioural difficulties'. However, diagnoses are a quick way to convey a lot of information that dimensions may not. Thus to only say a child is at an extreme of an antisocial behaviour dimension does not necessarily convey the association with specific reading retardation and ADHD, which could be (and often are) consequently missed.

Thirdly, children's difficulties nearly always arise in the context of relationships within the family. More often than in adulthood, some or all, of the problem may appear to be the result of the functioning of the family, rather than in the individual child who may merely be reacting to the situation. For example, a child who is disobedient and shouts in class may simply be behaving the way his parents do at home. A classification system will be stronger if it can take family functioning into account—it will have a greater chance of capturing clinically important causal and therapeutic considerations.

A valid and useful classification system will need to take into account these features and be based on a thorough understanding of normal development and how it can go wrong, rather than merely include static descriptions of presumed pathological states. The term of *developmental psychopathology* was coined in the early 1980s to denote the scientific study of how abnormalities can be understood in terms of processes underpinning human development.[1,2] There are now journals and books incorporating the term into their titles.[3,4] Many disciplines are relevant, from embryology and genetics to social learning theory and criminology. Developmental psychopathology, besides studying the impact of pathogenic influences on pathways through life, such as the way the monoamine oxidase-A (MAOA) genotype interacts with an abusive upbringing to cause conduct disorder,[5] or how specific reading retardation leads to low self-esteem, also investigates protective mechanisms, such as the ameliorating effect of high IQ on the propensity to juvenile offending, or the beneficial effect of a trusting and caring relationship with an adult on the impact of childhood abuse. This chapter aims to show how findings from developmental psychopathology have informed current classification systems, and what challenges remain.

## General issues

### Change over time

Because mental processes and behaviour change as a child develops, it is not always clear whether the same diagnoses should be applied across the age range. Thus a highly aggressive toddler may throw himself screaming onto the floor in daily tantrums, whereas a highly aggressive teenager may assault old ladies and rob them. Do they suffer from the same disorder? ICD 10 holds that they do—both meet criteria for conduct disorder, which is defined in terms of antisocial behaviour that is excessive for the individual's age, and that violates societal norms and the rights of others. DSM IV-R on the other hand has two separate diagnoses, oppositional-defiant disorder for the younger case, and conduct disorder for the older. However, as both diagnoses have similar correlates and there is a strong continuity from one to the other, the validity of the division is questionable. Yet current adult psychiatric schemes have no diagnosis at all to apply to antisocial behaviour, unless it is part of a personality disorder.

The extent to which adult criteria should be applied to children requires good empirical data. In the case of obsessive–compulsive disorder, the phenomenology is remarkably similar in childhood, so there is no problem. However, for depression the picture is rather different. Currently, ICD 10 and DSM IV-R have few emotional disorder categories specific to childhood, and they are mostly subtypes of anxiety. Mood disorders are diagnosed according to adult criteria, with the consequence that surveys of depression find prevalence rates close to zero under 8 years of age. Yet there are miserable children who cry frequently, say they are unhappy, look sad, and are withdrawn.[6] However, they usually sleep and eat reasonably well, and their mood fluctuates during the day, with spells when they sometimes appear more cheerful. Should they not be allowed a diagnosis? ICD 9 had a category for 'disturbance of emotions specific to childhood and adolescence, with misery and unhappiness', and such children suffer impairment.[7] Follow-up studies of prepubertal children referred with this picture showed a moderately increased risk of adult type depression later on, whereas adolescents with depressive symptoms had a higher risk of adult depression.[8] Genetic studies show that symptoms of depression in prepubertal children are predominantly due to environmental influences, whereas after puberty genetic influences become more important.[9] Finally, tricyclics are not effective in childhood but are effective in adults. This example shows that misery in younger children has some phenomenological features and external correlates in common with adult depression but also several differences, so the current approach which makes a comprehensive yet parsimonious classification system for all ages loses validity.

In contrast, there is continuing reluctance to diagnose personality disorders in childhood. This may be because they are often seen as a life sentence of a noxious, untreatable condition, in distinction to the general hope that there is opportunity for 'growing out of' conditions in childhood, or treatment for them. However, with perhaps the most destructive personality type, dissocial, there is growing evidence that the combination of antisocial behaviour and callous-unemotional traits is well established by the age of seven. Moreover, this combination of childhood characteristics has a far higher heritability than antisocial behaviour without callous-unemotional traits.[10]

### Validity

Categories need to be distinct not only in terms of the phenomena used to define them, but, crucially, also in terms of external criteria. Even if categories can be reliably distinguished, if external criteria are the same, then one is likely to be dealing with two variants of the same condition. An analogy would be the difference between black and white cats.

Typical validating criteria in child psychiatry derived from developmental psychopathology are:

1 *Epidemiological data*, such as age of onset and sex ratio. Forty years ago 'childhood psychosis' was a unitary classification, but work showing the clear difference in age of onset helped validate the distinction between autism and schizophrenia, which seldom co-occur. Disruptive disorders occur four times more commonly in boys, whereas emotional disorders are commoner in girls.

2 *Long-term course.* Most childhood disorders show reasonable *homotypic continuity*, that is they stay the same. Some show *heterotypic continuity*, so that for example, some cases of childhood hyperactivity end up as antisocial adults. This does not necessarily invalidate the category, but requires explanation.

3 *Genetic findings.* If individuals with distinct categorical diagnoses have relatives with different disorders, this helps validate the distinction. This has confirmed the validity of several diagnostic categories, but not all. For example, it has not held for the many specific subtypes of anxiety disorder in ICD 10, whose validity is questionable. Genetic studies can also clarify the scope of symptom clusters. For example, family studies of autism have revealed a broader phenotype in relatives of probands,[11] so that new disorders may need to be considered, which encompass only one of the original three constituent domains of classical autism, namely social relatedness, communication problems, and repetitive and stereotyped behaviours.

The hunt is now on for specific genes associated with particular psychiatric disorders. Thus dopamine receptor and transporter genes are reliably associated with Attention Deficit Hyperactivity Disorder,[12] but unless (i) the gene always leads to the disorder and (ii) all cases of the disorder are caused by the gene, particular genotypes are unlikely to be used to validate diagnostic categories.

4 *Psychosocial risk factors.* The association between institutional upbringing with many changes of carer and reactive attachment disorder is so strong that it has been made a requirement for diagnosis in ICD 10. Conduct disorders are strongly associated with discords at home, whereas autistic disorders are not. However, most psychosocial risk factors are less specific in their associations, and so are only modestly helpful as validating criteria.

5 *Neuropsychological tests.* The hyperkinetic syndrome is clearly distinguishable from conduct disorder on tests of attention such

as the continuous performance task. Recently, there has been considerable progress in showing that one of the core deficits in autism is failure on 'theory of mind' tests of ability, to see another person's point of view, which non-autistic children, with comparable levels of intellectual disability, can do.

6 *Medical investigations.* There have been many failed attempts in this field, including biochemical markers of adolescent depression and endocrine markers of aggression. However, the advent of functional neuroimaging is allowing exciting relatively non-invasive pictures of children's brains to be built up, and reliable findings are beginning to emerge, for example in ADHD.[13] In future these may well be helpful validators for classification.

### Reliability

This is a prerequisite for validity, and most categories have reasonable inter-rater and test–retest values, once investigators are trained up. Where there are many overlapping categories, as in current definitions of the many varieties of anxiety disorders, or personality disorders, inter-rater reliability falls.[14]

### Effect of informant and instrument

Traditionally information is obtained from parents and the child, and is then combined by the clinician on a case-by-case basis. However, the need for consistent diagnostic rules that is imposed by a 'menu-driven' approach can prove difficult, since the weight given to a particular informant may best vary according to condition. Thus, if a parent says a child has symptoms of conduct disorder but the child denies it, the parent is more likely to be right and the child may be covering up or ashamed. However, if the parent says the child is not depressed but the mental state examination of the child reveals otherwise, it is the parent who may be ignorant of their child's true state. Such difficulties reduce the validity of interviews which use invariant combination rules. Further, in genetic studies, the heritability of a condition may vary greatly according to which informant is believed. Thus in the Virginia Twin study, conduct disorder was 69 per cent heritable according to the information derived from the mother interview, 36 per cent using information from the child, and only 27 per cent using information from the father.[15] Studies such as these underline the need for clinically sensitive ways of combining information, and the use of multi-informant, multi-method ascertainment of information. Statistical techniques such as latent variable analysis may help reduce measurement error, but may build in unwarranted assumptions which distort the raw data.

Structured interviews, which accept the respondent's reply, do not require lengthy training or clinically informed investigators, and so are popular in epidemiological surveys. However, the quality of information differs little from that obtained by questionnaire,[16] and often has a high false-positive and false-negative rate in comparison to semi-structured interviews. Direct observation, although expensive, often provides the most reliable and valid information for assessment of disruptive disorders.

### Comorbidity

There are many artefactual reasons for comorbidity appearing high, such as Berkson's bias[17] in clinical samples (where not all cases get referred, the chance of referral will be related to the *combined* likelihood of referral for each condition separately), or overlapping criteria, or artificial subdivision of syndromes. However, even after taking these possible sources of error into account, comorbidity is marked for child psychiatric disorders. In a meta-analysis of community samples,[18] the odds ratio for anxiety with either Attention Deficit Hyperactivity Disorder (ADHD) or conduct disorder is 3, for anxiety and depression 8, and ADHD and conduct disorder 10. Rates are even higher in clinical samples. True comorbidity may arise through several mechanisms:[19] (i) shared risk factors (e.g. early deprivation may lead to oppositional-defiant disorder and an attachment disorder), (ii) overlap between risk factors (thus a depressed mother may pass on a genetic liability to depression in her son and provide inconsistent discipline which predisposes him to conduct disorder), (iii) one disorder creating an increased risk for the other (e.g. conduct disorder leading on to drug dependency), or (iv) the comorbid pattern constitutes a meaningful syndrome (e.g. depressive conduct disorder, described below under combined categories).

## Some classification schemes

### A simple scheme with three main groups of disorders

A simple but well researched, valid way of grouping child disorders 'lumps' them into three groups, which are helpful to hold in mind when considering specific diagnoses:

**Emotional disorders** including anxiety, depression, phobias, somatization, and obsessive–compulsive disorder; **disruptive disorders** including conduct disorder and hyperactivity; and **developmental disorders** including intellectual disability, the autistic spectrum, language and reading delays, and enuresis and encopresis.

Comorbidity within each grouping is very common, but only occurs across groups in a minority of cases. External criteria validating the differences between these groups are given in Table 9.1.1.1.

**Table 9.1.1.1** Validating criteria for main diagnostic groupings

|  | Emotional disorders | Disruptive disorders | Developmental disorders |
|---|---|---|---|
| Age of onset | over 8 | under 8 | under 3 |
| Sex ratio | commoner in girls after puberty | commoner in boys | commoner in boys |
| Family size | normal | large | normal |
| Family history | anxiety and depression increased | criminality increased | related disorders may be increased |
| Socio-economic status | normal | lower | normal |
| IQ | normal | lower range of normal | normal or low, sometimes very low |
| Specific delays | absent | present in a third | common |
| Neurological signs | absent | uncommon | common |
| Cause | mixed, sometimes mainly genetic | mixed, sometimes mainly environmental | often mainly genetic |

## Current schemes: ICD 10 and DSM IV-R

The DSM IV-R and ICD 10 committees worked closely together and strove to have names and criteria that are as close as possible. However, there are some general differences.

### (a) 'Picture-fitting' versus 'menu-driven' approaches

Firstly, as in adulthood, ICD 10 has one set of 'clinical descriptions and diagnostic guidelines' and a separate set of 'diagnostic criteria for research'. The former comprises general descriptions of disorders requiring a qualitative matching of case characteristics with the scheme, a 'picture-fitting' approach which is similar to the way clinicians practise. The latter comprises lists of symptoms with explicit criteria detailing the number and permutation required for diagnosis, a 'menu-driven' approach. DSM IV-R has only the latter. It has advantages in increased reliability, but is relatively cumbersome so that many clinicians do not bother to apply the criteria rigorously. Even for the simpler DSM III criteria, a study found that whilst trained researchers achieved kappa values of 0.83, 0.80, and 0.74 for attention deficit disorder, conduct disorder, and emotional disorder, the comparable figures for United States clinicians in regular practice were 0.30, 0.27, and 0.27, which are seriously low.[20]

A further disadvantage of the 'menu-driven' approach arises in cases where although the clinician believes a diagnosis is present because of the severity of symptoms, their number is insufficient to meet criteria. For example, consider the following youth: he repeatedly mugs old ladies, sets fires frequently, often argues, is often spiteful or vindictive, has unusually severe tantrums, and has no friends or job because of his behaviour. According to ICD 10 research diagnostic criteria (or DSM IV-R criteria) he has no diagnosis, as he has two but not three symptoms of conduct disorder, and three but not four symptoms of oppositional-defiant disorder. However, according to ICD 10 'diagnostic guidelines' he easily meets the requirements for conduct disorder since 'any category, if marked, is sufficient'.

### (b) Multiple diagnoses

A second difference between ICD 10 and DSM IV-R is in multiple diagnoses. ICD 10 encourages the selection of one diagnosis that closest fits the picture, assuming that differences are due to a variation upon the typical theme. DSM IV-R (and the closely linked ICD 10 research criteria) encourage selection of as many diagnoses as criteria are met. Problems arise with this approach when symptoms are common to two disorders, for example irritability contributes to affective disorders and to conduct disorders, so double coding is more likely. Since comorbidity is very common in clinical practice, multiple coding is frequent using a 'menu-driven' approach so that it begins to approach a dimensional system and to lose the advantages of categorization.

The pros and cons of each approach will vary according to whether extra information is conveyed by the second diagnosis. Where there is good evidence of the validity of common comorbid conditions, ICD 10 has combined categories. Thus the external validating characteristics of 'depressive conduct disorder' are similar to those of pure conduct disorder, with no increase of affective disorders in individuals, nor in their relatives, followed up to adulthood. Double coding would convey erroneous information about the depressive aspect. 'Hyperkinetic conduct disorder', on the other hand, is characterized by more severe neuropsychological deficits than occur in either condition alone, and by worse psychosocial outcome in adulthood. Double coding would not convey the poor prognosis.

### (c) Multiaxial framework

The ICD 10 has a multiaxial framework for psychiatric disorders in childhood and adolescence[21] which will be described here. DSM IV-R uses a somewhat different multiaxial framework, which is applicable for disorders arising at all ages. It will not be described here except as a contrast to ICD 10. Each axis except the last (psychosocial impairment) is coded independently of the apparent causal contribution to the psychiatric syndrome. This avoids tricky decisions about causality and allows conditions to be recognized and clinical needs addressed.

#### (i) Axis one: clinical psychiatric syndromes

Criteria for particular diagnoses are described in the relevant chapters of this text.

#### (ii) Axis two: specific disorders of development

These include speech and language, reading, spelling, and motor development. In DSM IV-R they are included in Axis one. However, having a separate axis helps to ensure that they are not overlooked. This can easily happen, for example, in children with conduct disorder, where the antisocial behaviour tends to command attention, while in fact one-third of the children also have specific reading retardation (dyslexia), which if untreated worsens the prognosis.[22] It very desirable to administer standardized psychometric tests in order to characterize specific disorders of development.

#### (iii) Axis three: intellectual level

The categories are no intellectual disability (IQ 70 or over), mild intellectual disability (50–69), moderate intellectual disability (IQ 35–49), severe intellectual disability (IQ 20–34), and profound intellectual disability (IQ under 20). In DSM IV-R personality disorders are also included on the axis.

Subtyping intellectual disability gives a good example of substantial differences which arise when categories are imposed on top of a dimensional construct. If all children with an IQ below 50 are taken together (often together also called severe), and compared with those having an IQ of 50–70 (mild), major differences emerge on independent validating criteria, as shown in Table 9.1.1.2.

From the table it will be seen that there are major differences between the categories on fronts as varied as brain pathology and life expectancy. There is no particular psychiatric pattern arising in children with intellectual disability, rather the incidence of all disorders is raised, so that in those with IQ under 50, fully one half have a psychiatric disorder.[23]

#### (iv) Axis four: associated medical conditions

All medical conditions should be coded. A few have specific associations with psychiatric disorders, for example tuberous sclerosis predisposes to autism, Cornelia de Lange syndrome to self-injury; Down syndrome on the other hand protects against autism but often leads to presenile dementia. Even where there is no specific disorder, congenital syndromes are often characterized by a particular pattern of behaviour. The study of these *behavioural phenotypes* is a discipline in its own right.

#### (v) Axis five: associated abnormal psychosocial conditions

These include a range of pyschosocial hazards, from abnormal intrafamilial relationships such as physical or sexual abuse, to mental disorders in other family members, distorted intrafamilial communication patterns, abnormal upbringing, e.g. in an institution,

**Table 9.1.1.2** Characteristics of children with severe versus mild intellectual disability

|  | Severe retardation | Mild retardation |
|---|---|---|
| *Definition* | IQ under 50 | IQ 50–70 |
| *Social functioning* | Invariably marked impairment | Many have minor or no impairment |
| *Cause* | Organic pathology in majority | Usually no organic cause evident |
| *Family history* | Parents and siblings usually of normal intelligence | Parents and siblings often at lower levels of intelligence |
| *Background* | Fairly equal distribution across SES levels. Neglect at home unlikely | Much commoner at lower SES levels. Neglect at home more likely |
| *Appearance* | Dysmorphic features often evident | Normal appearance |
| *Medical complications* | Physical handicap common (e.g. cerebral palsy). Major health problems frequent. Life expectancy shortened. Fertility low | Physical handicap uncommon. Health in normal range. Life expectancy normal. Fertility little impaired |
| *Psychiatric complications* | Severe and pervasive disorders such as hyperactivity, autism, and self-injury especially common. Presentation of disorders often altered, mental state may be difficult to determine | Disorders similar in type to those found in children without MR, but occur more frequently. Form of disorders and mental state examination similar to children without retardation |

acute life events, and chronic interpersonal stress arising from difficulties at school. Each is coded dimensionally on a three point scale. As the number of psychosocial adversities goes up, the rate of psychiatric disorders increases.[24] Conduct disorder is particularly associated with poor immediate psychosocial environments. As with other axes, abnormalities are coded irrespective of apparent cause. This is particularly relevant since while perhaps 20 years ago the mechanism was thought to be directly environmental, in the last 10 years good evidence has been collected to show that some environmental characteristics of the home are genetically mediated.[25] For example, the association between lack of books in the home and poor child reading is partly mediated through parents with lower IQ buying fewer books.

*(vi) Axis six: global social functioning*

Here a judgement is made on a nine point dimensional scale ranging from superior social functioning to profound and pervasive social disability. Unlike other axes, ratings of disability are not independent, but have to be judged as due to a psychiatric or developmental disorder on axes one to three. Thus impairment arising from adverse circumstances cannot be coded—it must arise from intraindividual factors. This rule therefore excludes recognition of psychosocial interventions which aid functioning, from reduction of parental Expressed Emotion to changing schools. DSM IV-R studies often use the Children's Global Assessment scale,[26] an adaptation of the Global Assessment of Functioning (GAF) used in adults. An advantage of the CGAS is that it is rated without

impairment having to be caused by psychiatric disorder. A disadvantage is that psychiatric symptoms, rather than impairment alone, contribute to the rating.

**(d) Should impairment of social function be part of psychiatric diagnosis?**

In general, ICD 10 and DSM IV-R do not require impairment of social functioning to be present in order to make a diagnosis. There are exceptions, thus in DSM IV-R, oppositional-defiant disorder *does* require impairment. With many qualitatively distinct adult disorders, having no impairment criterion makes sense, so that a person experiencing the delusions and hallucinations characteristic of schizophrenia, but able to go to work and form relationships while on neuroleptics still has schizophrenia. But should a child who says he is afraid of dogs and crosses to the other side of the pavement on seeing one, but otherwise functions well, be deemed to suffer from a phobia? If impairment criteria are not applied, very high rates of disorder are obtained in epidemiological surveys. This lacks credibility with the general public, who may then dismiss all psychiatric problems in children, and is unrealistic for clinicians and health planners, who would not see most of the identified individuals as cases needing treatment. For example, a large epidemiological survey[27] found that using DSM III criteria, 50 per cent of children and adolescents had a diagnosis. However, when an impairment criterion was added, the figure came down to 18 per cent. This would appear to be a much more realistic figure. However, it could be argued that social impairment is too constraining, and for example would exclude an adolescent who is fairly depressed but able to function. The term *impact* can be used to include subjective distress as well as impairment, and is gaining in popularity among many child psychiatrists.[28]

## Falling through the cracks: children with social impairment but no diagnosis

Diagnostic systems have to be practically useful above all. If they are overinclusive, the risk is that there are too many categories, which have poor reliability and high overlap. If on the other hand they are too exclusive, the risk is that there will be many individuals suffering from problems which are not encompassed by the scheme. In one thorough survey, 9.4 per cent had no diagnosis but significant impairment.[29] Across a variety of 'caseness' measures, the individuals were as disturbed as those with a diagnosis. Many of the difficulties were around relationships with parents and siblings, and arguably, such children who have symptoms associated with psychosocial impairment should be regarded as suffering from a psychiatric disorder.

## Conclusion

Classification of child psychiatric conditions has advanced enormously in the last 20 years. There is a much stronger empirical basis to support current schemes, which are grounded in the many scientific disciplines that contribute to developmental psychopathology. Nonetheless there are considerable obstacles to overcome if DSM V and ICD 11 are to be major steps forward.

## Further information

To access the journal *Development and Psychopathology*, visit http://journals.cambridge.org/action/displayJournal?jid=DPP

Cicchetti, D. and Cohen, D. (eds.) (2003). *Developmental psychopathology* (2nd edn). Wiley, New York.

Taylor, E. and Rutter, M. (2008). Classification. In *Rutter's child and adolescent psychiatry* (5th edn) (eds. M. Rutter, D. Bishop, D. Pine, *et al.*). Blackwell, Oxford.

Goodman, R. and Scott, S. (2005). *Child psychiatry* (2nd edn). Blackwell, Oxford.

To access the official website discussing issues around DSM IV criteria, visit http://www.dsmivtr.org/index.cfm and regarding ICD 10 visit http://www.who.int/classifications/icd/en/

## References

1. Cicchetti, D. (1984). The emergence of developmental psychopathology. *Child Development*, **55**, 1–7.

2. Rutter, M. (1988). Epidemiological approaches to developmental psychopathology. *Archives of General Psychiatry*, **45**, 486–95.

3. To access the journal *Development and Psychopathology*, visit http://journals.cambridge.org/action/displayJournal?jid=DPP

4. Cicchetti, D. and Cohen, D. (eds.) (2003). *Developmental psychopathology* (2nd edn). Wiley, New York.

5. Kim-Cohen, J., Caspi, A., Taylor, A., *et al.* (*2006*). MAOA, maltreatment, and gene-environment interaction predicting children's mental health: new evidence and a meta-analysis. *Molecular Psychiatry*, **11**, 903–13.

6. Puura, K., Tamminen, T., Almqvist, F., *et al.* (1997). Should depression in young children be diagnosed with different criteria? *European Child & Adolescent Psychiatry*, **6**, 12–19.

7. Costello, E.J., Mustillo, S., Erkanli, A., *et al.* (2003). Prevalence and development of psychiatric disorders in childhood and adolescence. *Archives of General Psychiatry*, **60**, 837–44.

8. Harrington, R., Fudge, H., Rutter, M., *et al.* (1990). Adult outcomes of childhood and adolescent depression—I. Psychiatric status. *Archives of General Psychiatry*, **47**, 465–73.

9. Scourfield, J., Rice, F., Thapar, A., *et al.* (2003). Depressive symptoms in children and adolescents: changing aetiological influences with development. *Journal of Child Psychology and Psychiatry, and Allied Disciplines*, **44**, 968–76.

10. Viding, E., Blair, R.J.R., Moffitt, T.E., *et al.* (*2005*). Evidence for substantial genetic risk for psychopathy in 7-year-olds. *Journal of Child Psychology and Psychiatry, and Allied Disciplines*, **46**, 592–7.

11. Rutter, M. (2000). Genetic studies of autism: from the 1970s into the millennium. *Journal of Abnormal Child Psychology*, **28**, 3–14.

12. Thapar, A., O'Donovan, M., and Owen, M.J. (2005). The genetics of attention deficit hyperactivity disorder. *Human Molecular Genetics*, **14**, R275–82.

13. Rubia, K., Smith, A.B., Brammer, M.J., *et al.* (2005). Abnormal brain activation during inhibition and error detection in medication-naive adolescents with ADHD. *The American Journal of Psychiatry*, **162**, 1067–75.

14. Thomsen, P., Jorgensen, J., and Nedergaard, N. (1992). ICD-10: a field study in a Danish child psychiatric unit. *European Psychiatry*, **7**, 287–91.

15. Eaves, L., Silberg, J., Meyer, J., *et al.* (1997). Genetics and developmental psychopathology: 2. The main effects of genes and environment on behavioral problems in the Virginia twin study of adolescent behavioral development. *Journal of Child Psychology and Psychiatry, and Allied Disciplines*, **38**, 965–80.

16. Boyle, M., Offord, D., Racine, Y., *et al.* (1997). Adequacy of interviews vs checklists for classifying childhood psychiatric disorder based on parent reports. *Archives of General Psychiatry*, **54**, 793–9.

17. Berkson, J. (1946). Limitations of the application of fourfold table analysis to hospital data. *Biometrics*, **2**, 47–53.

18. Angold, A., Costello, E., and Erkanli, A. (1999). Comorbidity. *Journal of Child Psychology and Psychiatry, and Allied Disciplines*, **40**, 57–87.

19. Rutter, M. (1997). Comorbidity: concepts, claims and choices. *Criminal Behaviour and Mental Health*, **7**, 265–85.

20. Prendergast, M., Taylor, E., Rapoport, J., *et al.* (1988). The diagnosis of childhood hyperactivity: a US-UK cross-national study of DSM-III and ICD-9. *Journal of Child Psychology and Psychiatry, and Allied Disciplines*, **29**, 289–300.

21. World Health Organization. (1996). *Multiaxial classification of child and adolescent psychiatric disorders*. Cambridge University Press, Cambridge.

22. Trzesniewski, K., Moffitt, T., Caspi, A., *et al.* (2006). Revisiting the association between reading achievement and antisocial behaviour: new evidence of an environmental explanation from a twin study. *Child Development*, **77**, 72–88.

23. Stromme, P. and Diseth, T. (2000). Prevalence of psychiatric diagnoses in children with intellectual disability: data from a population-based study. *Developmental Medicine and Child Neurology*, **42**, 266–70.

24. Appleyard, K., Egeland, B., van Dulmen, M., *et al.* (2005). When more is not better: the role of cumulative risk in child behavior outcomes. *Journal of Child Psychology and Psychiatry, and Allied Disciplines*, **46**, 235–45.

25. Braungart, J., Fulker, D., and Plomin, R. (1992). Genetic influence of the home environment during infancy: a sibling adoption study of the HOME. *Developmental Psychology*, **28**, 1048–55.

26. Shaffer, D., Gould, M., Brasic, J., *et al.* (1983). A children's global assessment scale (CGAS). *Archives of General Psychiatry*, **40**, 1228–31.

27. Bird, H., Yager, T., Staghezza, B., *et al.* (1990). Impairment in the epidemiological measurement of childhood psychopathology in the community. *Journal of the American Academy of Child and Adolescent Psychiatry*, **29**, 796–803.

28. Goodman, R. and Scott, S. (2005). *Child psychiatry* (2nd edn). Blackwell, Oxford.

29. Angold, A., Costello, E., Farmer, E., *et al.* (1999). Impaired but undiagnosed. *Journal of the American Academy of Child and Adolescent Psychiatry*, **3**, 129–37.

## 9.1.2 **Epidemiology of psychiatric disorder in childhood and adolescence**

E. Jane Costello and Adrian Angold

Epidemiology is the study of patterns of disease in human populations.[1] Patterns are non-random distributions, and patterns of disease distribution occur in both time and space. Whenever we observe a non-random distribution, we have the opportunity to identify causal factors that influence who gets a disease and who does not. For example, we observe that depression rises rapidly after puberty in girls, but not to the same extent in boys.[2] This non-random distribution in time suggests that there may be something about puberty in girls that is causally related to depression.[3] An example of disease distribution in space can be seen in the Methods for the Epidemiology of Child and Adolescent Mental Disorders (MECA) study of five sites in the United States and Puerto Rico.[4] Although the prevalence of psychiatric disorders was fairly similar across sites, the likelihood that a psychiatric diagnosis was accompanied by significant functional impairment was much higher in children at the mainland sites than in Puerto Rico. This offers the opportunity to study between-site differences that might result in differences in the level of impairment caused by psychiatric disorders. The task of epidemiology is to understand these observed patterns in time and space, and to use this understanding as a basis for the prevention and control of disease.

Epidemiological medicine has both similarities to and differences from clinical medicine. Like clinical medicine, epidemiology is an action-oriented discipline, whose goal is intervention to prevent and control disease. Scientific knowledge about the cause and course of disease is another common goal. Epidemiology also reflects clinical medicine in using two methods of attack on disease: *tactical* methods, concerned with the practical and administrative problems of disease control at the day-to-day level, and *strategic* methods, concerned with finding out what causes disease so that new weapons of prevention and control can be engineered.[5,6] Thus, for example, in their tactical or public health role epidemiologists can be found reporting on the prevalence of adolescent drug abuse, the social burden (including cost) that drug abuse creates, and the best ways to control its spread, while others working at the strategic level might be exploring the science underlying environmental constraints on gene expression.

Epidemiology diverges from clinical medicine to the extent that it concentrates on understanding and controlling disease processes in the context of the *population at risk*, whereas the primary focus of clinical medicine is the *individual* patient. This does not mean that epidemiology is not concerned with the individual; on the contrary, it is very much concerned with understanding the individual's illness and the causes of that illness. The difference lies in the frame of reference. Put crudely, clinical medicine asks: 'What is wrong with this person *and how should I treat him or her?*' Epidemiology asks: 'What is wrong with this person and *what is it about him or her that has resulted in this illness?*' Why is this child depressed, but not her brother? If her mother is also depressed, is the child's depression a cause, a consequence, or an unrelated, chance co-occurrence? Such questions immediately set the individual child within a frame of reference of other children, or other family members, or other people of the same sex or race or social class.

Sampling, or selecting the population within which to count cases, is of central importance in epidemiology. Counting cases is an important first step towards measuring the social burden caused by a disease, and the effectiveness of prevention. For most diseases, however, simply counting the number of individuals presenting for treatment will produce estimates that are seriously biased by referral practices, ability to pay, and other factors. This is a big problem in child psychiatry because parents, teachers, and pediatricians all serve as 'gatekeepers' to treatment.[7] Community-based data are needed to measure the extent of need, and the unmet need, for prevention or treatment. Methods for assessing psychiatric disorders in the general population are discussed in another chapter. However, it is worth noting that methods for assessing disorder, whether they take the form of interviews, questionnaires, or neuropsychiatric tests, can only be as good as the taxonomy they are designed to operationalize. Current instruments mainly use scoring algorithms that turn the responses into diagnoses based on the DSM-IV or ICD-10 taxonomies. If these taxonomies do not mirror the 'reality' of psychiatric disorder then the results of using interviews or questionnaires based on them will in turn be faulty.

## Estimating the burden of child and adolescent psychiatric disorders

In a world of scarce health care resources, it is important to understand the size of the burden to the community caused by these disorders. Burden, in terms of numbers affected, impact on the individual, and cost to the community, is a crucial factor in the battle for resources for treatment and prevention.

Attempts to reduce the burden of mental illness must, of necessity, pay attention to the early years. It is becoming increasingly clear that most psychiatric disorders have their onset before adulthood, and that many should be regarded as chronic or relapsing disorders. For example, the National Comorbidity Survey Replication, a representative population sample of over 9000 adults aged 18 and over in the United States,[8] found that, of the 46.4 per cent of all participants reporting one or more psychiatric disorders during there lifetime, half reported onset by age 12, and three-quarters by age 24.[9] Since we can expect a lot of forgetting of early episodes by older participants,[10] it is likely that onset in childhood is even more common than this.

If the burden of mental illness begins to be felt in childhood, it is important to know the extent of the problem so that we can begin to plan for treatment and prevention. Unfortunately, the data on which to build such estimates are very sparse. We have to rely on a national prevalence study of psychiatric disorders in the United Kingdom, and another of a large area of Brazil, together with a few national or large community surveys using symptoms scales, and a handful of diagnosis-based studies in smaller community samples, some of them longitudinal. Questionnaire-based surveys are not very useful for measuring prevalence, because they tend to define 'caseness' in terms of a certain percentage of the sample with high scores; a method that predefines prevalence.

In the past decade the United Kingdom has carried out a national prevalence study,[11,12] conducted by the Office for National Statistics, with funding from the Department of Education and other agencies. The primary purpose was to produce prevalence estimates of conduct, emotional, and hyperkinetic disorders, as well as pervasive developmental disorder, eating disorders, and tic disorders, using both ICD-10 and DSM-IV criteria. The second aim was 'to determine the *impact* or *burden* of children's mental health. *Impact* covers the consequences for the child; *burden* reflects the consequences for others'.[13] (p. 185). Third, the study measured service use. A stratified random sampling plan for England, Scotland, and Wales produced a sample of 10 438 children aged 5 to 15. Parent and child were interviewed using the Development and Well-Being Assessment (DAWBA),[14] a computer-assisted lay interview that uses a 'best-estimate' approach to diagnosis, in which responses recorded by lay interviewers are evaluated by clinicians. The first interview wave, conducted in 1999,[13] was followed by a questionnaire mailed 18 months later to all 'cases' with a diagnosis at Time 1, and a one-in-three random sample of non-cases. A second interview of all those completing questionnaires at Time 2, and all others who were cases at Time 1, was completed in 2002.[15] By weighting the responses to account for the various selection factors and for non-response, Meltzer and colleagues developed estimates of prevalence (i.e. the presence of a disorder at the Time 1 interview), of incidence (new cases between the two interviews), and of persistence.

The UK study found that almost one child in 10 (9.5 per cent) aged 5 to 15 had a psychiatric disorder based on the ICD-10 classification system. Prevalence was higher in adolescents (11.2 per cent at 11 to 15) than in children (8.2 per cent at 5 to 15), and in boys (11.4 per cent than girls 7.6 per cent). Conduct disorders were the most common (5.3 per cent), followed by anxiety disorders (3.8 per cent). Depression was rare in both sexes and all age groups

(0.9 per cent over all), as were hyperkinetic disorders (1.4 per cent). Seven per cent of previously unaffected children developed a psychiatric disorder in the 3 years between the interviews. Four per cent developed a new emotional disorder (anxiety and/or depression), and 5 per cent a behavioural and/or hyperkinetic disorder. More girls developed emotional disorders, and more boys developed behavioural disorders. Persistence, measured as the presence of the same diagnosis the years apart, was higher for behavioural disorders (43 per cent) than for emotional disorders (about one in four).

## Factors affecting prevalence estimates

It is not a simple matter to compare the British prevalence rates with those from other countries, because there are few large studies, and the age ranges do not overlap. A study of youth age 7 to 14 in south-eastern Brazil, which used the same diagnostic interview but the DSM-IV taxonomy, found an overall prevalence of 12.7 per cent. Although prevalence estimates were slightly different from those reported by the UK study, the relative ordering was the same. Behavioural disorders were again the most common (7 per cent), followed by anxiety disorders (5.2 per cent) and ADHD (1.8 per cent). Once again, depression was rare (1.0 per cent). Other studies from around the world[16] usually generate prevalence rates of around 20 per cent. This puts the British and Brazilian studies at the low end of the range. However, there are many factors other than the 'true' rate of psychiatric disorder (if there is any such thing) that affect a published prevalence rate. The most important of these are:

1 *The time frame of the diagnostic measure.* Questions can be asked about symptoms occurring 'now', 'in the past month', 'in the past 3, 6, or 12 months', or 'ever'. Clearly, if recall is accurate the latter questions will elicit more symptoms than the former. Unfortunately, recall is not always accurate. Prevalence rates are higher from interviews with longer time frames, but not as much higher as would be consistent with accurate recall. For example, The National Comorbidity Study Replication, based on a nationally representative sample of adults in the United States, found that the lifetime prevalence of any disorder was 46.4 per cent, while the 12-month prevalence was 26.2 per cent. This means that 26.2 per cent /46.4 per cent = 56.5 per cent of all cases across the lifespan were present in the past 12 months. This could be explained in several ways: (i) there was an epidemic of psychiatric disorders in the 12 months before the survey; (ii) over half of all psychiatric diseases are chronic; once they occur they remain active for the rest of life; (iii) many early episodes are forgotten, and people report the onset of the most recent episode as the first occurrence of the disorder. In the absence of any evidence for (i), some combination of (ii) and (iii) seems the most likely explanation. We have evidence that the reliability with which children and adults recall the first occurrence of a symptom falls dramatically after 3 months,[17] and recommend concentrating on symptoms occurring in the past 3 months if a fairly reliable estimate is sought.

In general, when comparing prevalence rates from different reports it is important to bear in mind the time frame. In a comparison of reported rates of child and adolescent depression published since the 1970s, we found that the time frame of the interview accounted for most of the variance, compared with

taxonomy (DSM-III, DSM-IIIR, DSM-IV, ICD-9, ICD-10), diagnostic interview, or birth cohort.[2]

2 *The number and nature of the informants.* For several decades now clinicians and epidemiologists alike have recommended collecting information about a child from a range of informants: the parents, siblings, teachers, and peers, as well as the child. Most diagnostic instruments, whether questionnaires or interviews, exist in forms for diverse informants, with scoring algorithms that allow a diagnosis to be made on the basis of one informant or more. In the latter case, most follow the rule that clinicians generally observe, of counting a symptom as present if reported by any informant, rather than expecting agreement among informants, which rarely occurs.[18] Rates of psychiatric disorder will vary with the number of informants, and also depending on which informants report on which diagnoses. For example, across repeated assessments of 1420 children and adolescents, only 26 per cent of those with a diagnosis from the child interview also had one from the parent interview, and only 22 per cent of those with a diagnosis based on the parent interview had one from the child interview. This was statistically a highly significant level of agreement (OR 5.4, 95 per cent; CI 3.6, 7.9; $p$ <.0001), but nevertheless only 13.5 per cent of cases were reported by both informants. Readers of epidemiological studies need to decide for themselves how much the number and type of informant matters in judging the accuracy of a prevalence estimate of a specific disorder. For example, parents often do not know much about their children's drug use, while young children themselves generally have little insight into their own hyperactivity, and teachers seldom notice children's depression. Prevalence rates based solely on these informants would be likely to be quite low.

3 *The age and sex of the subjects.* The prevalence rates of different disorders vary markedly by age, sex, and age-by-sex across childhood and adolescence. For example, a meta-analysis of 26 studies of child and adolescent depression[2] estimated the prevalence of adolescent depression (5.6 per cent) as twice that of childhood depression (2.9 per cent), and that of adolescent girls (5.9 per cent) as significantly higher than that of adolescent boys (4.6 per cent). Figure 9.1.2.1 shows prevalence rates of any psychiatric disorder (dotted lines) from a representative population sample of 1420 youth assessed regularly between ages 9 and 21. It is clear that prevalence, even when measured over time in the same subjects, varies markedly with age. This is because some of the common disorders of childhood, such as functional enuresis and encopresis, ADHD, and separation anxiety, diminish as children grow up, but then later on the problems of adolescence and young adulthood, such as drug abuse and depression, take their place. Between about 11 and 14, when the disorders of childhood have faded and those of adulthood not yet appeared, relatively few children have disorders. Prevalence rates will also differ depending on the distribution of males and females in the sample. Boys are significantly more likely to have developmental disorders, enuresis and encopresis, and ADHD in the early years, and drug abuse in the later years. Although girls are more vulnerable to depression after puberty,[19] this does not have a large effect on the overall prevalence of psychiatric disorder.

4 *The inclusion of measures of functional impairment.* Most DSM-IV and ICD-10 diagnoses require that to be clinically significant, symptoms must have a harmful effect on patients' ability to

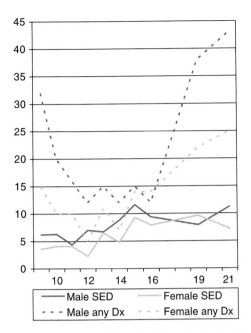

**Fig. 9.1.2.1** (solid lines) shows the effect of applying a functioning criterion to diagnoses. It has the effect of flattening the U-shaped curve and revealing a doubling of psychiatric disorder with age, from around 5 per cent at age 9–10 to 10 per cent at age 21. This gradual increase is seen in both boys and girls.

function in their normal environments.[20] There is a wide range of measures of functional impairment,[20] and many diagnostic interviews employ measures of impairment as part of their diagnostic algorithms.

The inclusion or exclusion of a measure of impairment can make a dramatic difference to prevalence estimates. For example, version 2.3 of the Diagnostic Schedule for Children, a widely used interview for youth and parents, uses two measures of impairment. First, if a symptom is reported further questions are asked about whether it affects the child's functioning. Second, the interviewer scores the child on the Global Assessment Scale,[21] which rates the child's overall level of function from 0 to 100. Table 9.1.2.1 shows the impact on the prevalence of any anxiety disorder of including or excluding either or both of these measures of impairment, using data from a multi-site epidemiological study.[21] When no measure of impairment was used almost 40 per cent of subjects received an anxiety diagnosis. With both criteria applied at their most rigourous level, the prevalence of anxiety was cut to 3.2 per cent.

# Future directions in the epidemiology of child and adolescent psychiatric disorders

Up to this point, the role of epidemiology has been mainly a descriptive one, addressing the basic questions: how many? who? where? when? However, child psychiatry is changing, and epidemiology will change as well. The goal is now to understand how risk exposure and vulnerability change over the life course, and how the requirements of 'normal' development shape the types of psychopathology that emerge if these requirements are not met. The term 'developmental epidemiology', first coined by Kellam in the 1970s,[22] is useful to describe what epidemiology is doing these days.

In this section we describe some rapidly growing research areas that will contribute to the next generation of studies, and will contribute to the shift from 'child psychiatric epidemiology' to 'developmental epidemiology'. We discuss the future under five headings: longitudinal research, genetic epidemiology, life course epidemiology, intergenerational epidemiology, and prevention science.

## Longitudinal research

Although there have been many longitudinal developmental studies, some of them beginning at birth (or even before), longitudinal studies of psychiatric disorders had to await the development of appropriate technology; specifically, data collection methods that validly and reliably translated the psychiatric taxonomy into instruments that could be used repeatedly with the same subjects. Several of these have become available in the past 20 years.[23]

There are now several research groups that have used their longitudinal data to look at continuities and discontinuities in mental illness from childhood into adolescence and beyond. Some of the longitudinal studies have followed their subjects into adulthood.[16] These are beginning to show indications of continuity of disorder across childhood and adolescence,[24] and between temperamental characteristics in early childhood and the onset of psychiatric disorders in late adolescence and young adulthood.[25]

## Genetic epidemiology

There have been two revolutions in genetic epidemiology in the past two decades that will have a tremendous impact on psychiatry in the next decade.

### (a) Psychiatric–behavioural genetics

The first revolution occurred when the methods of psychiatric epidemiology were applied to behavioural genetics. Psychiatric interviews

**Table 9.1.2.1** Effect of different rules for defining impairment on the per cent prevalence of any anxiety disorder (parent or child interview) using the DISC 2.3

| | Diagnosis without diagnosis-specific impairment criteria | | | | Diagnosis with diagnosis-specific impairment criteria | | | |
| --- | --- | --- | --- | --- | --- | --- | --- | --- |
| | Criteria only | CGAS < = 70 (mild) | CGAS < = 60 (moderate) | CGAS < = 50 (severe) | Criteria only | CGAS < = 70 (mild) | CGAS < = 60 (moderate) | CGAS < = 50 (severe) |
| Any anxiety diagnosis | 39.5 | 18.5 | 9.6 | 4.3 | 20.5 | 13.0 | 7.2 | 3.2 |

(Reproduced from D. Shaffer *et al.* The NIMH diagnostic interview schedule for children version 2.3 (DISC 2.3): description, acceptability, prevalence rates, and performance in the MECA study, *Journal of the American Academy of Child and Adolescent Psychiatry*, **35**, 865–77, copyright 1996, American Acadamy of Child and Adolescent Psychiatry, Lippincott Willams & Wilkins.)

DISC = Diagnostic Interview Schedule for Children. CGAS = Children's Global Assessment Scale.

like those described earlier were used in studies with genetically informative designs, such as twin, adoption, family, and migrant studies. For the first time, researchers examined categorical disorders such as depression, in ways that approximate clinical diagnosis. Furthermore, behavioural geneticists began to take seriously, issues of sampling, so that they could talk about the contribution of genes to disease in the population as a whole, rather than in highly selected families or groups. There have also been some longitudinal studies looking at how genes can have different effects at different developmental stages.[26]

### (b) Molecular genetics

The second genetic revolution occurred when it became feasible to apply the methods of molecular genetics to epidemiologic samples. This development opens up the opportunity to use not only twin or adoption studies but a wide range of singleton samples to test theories about candidate genes for specific symptoms. Even more exciting is the new opportunity to use the treasure house of data from longitudinal studies to test for gene–environment interactions. Such studies can answer questions about which genes interact with which environmental factors, and at what developmental stage.[27,28]

### Life course epidemiology

Life course epidemiology is the study of long-term effects on chronic disease risk, of physical and social exposures, during gestation, childhood, adolescence, young adulthood, and later adult life. It includes studies of the biological, behavioural, and psychosocial pathways that operate across an individual's life course, as well as across generations, to influence the development of chronic diseases.[29]

Life course epidemiology has developed a special concern with 'the "embodiment" of social phenomena into the biological'[30] encapsulated in the concept of 'health inequalities'. This concern arose historically from work showing that mortality from many diseases is spread unequally across the population and that these differences in risk can be linked to social inequalities that often go back to infancy or even to the parental generation. This body of work has had enormous significance for international thinking about social policy and is having a direct effect on the allocation of public resources in the United Kingdom and elsewhere.

### Intergenerational epidemiology

A life course approach to epidemiology intertwines biological and social transmission of risk across generations, recognizing that geographical and secular characteristics may be unique to one cohort of individuals.[31,32]

Experiences of the previous generation can operate at many different levels of generality. They may be specific to the mother–child dyad (e.g. the effect of drug use during pregnancy), or may affect everyone living in a certain neighborhood (e.g. poverty, or exposure to an environmental toxin). All mothers and children maybe affected by a particular event, such as a period of famine or disease, or children may be affected by their mother's developmental stage (e.g. children of teen mothers or elderly mothers). Models for intergenerational research have recently appeared[33] and statistical methods have become more tractable.

### Prevention science

Prevention science uses theory about the causes of disease to generate interventions, which when tested provide information not only about the effectiveness of the intervention, but also about the aetiology of the disease. Epidemiology traditionally divides prevention into thee categories, depending on the mean level of risk in the population of concern. Programmes available to all, like clean water, car seat belts, and parental leave programmes, are examples of *primary* or *universal* prevention. For example, the 'Just Say No' drug abstinence programme was introduced as a primary prevention for all children in school, designed to stop drug use before it began. Unfortunately, the results were neutral if not negative.[34] On the other hand, primary prevention with both children[35] and *families*[36] can be both effective, and suggest aetiologic pathways that could be explored in further research.

Secondary intervention *programmes* are based on high-risk children, schools, or communities. Many of them are both theory-driven and scientifically sound. A good example of a secondary intervention that yields insights for epidemiology is the 'Fast Track' programme for aggressive children in grade school. This was based on clearly articulated theory about cognitive difficulties that could interact with environmental risk to produce aggressive behaviour in socially ambiguous situations.[37] Hostile attributional bias was indeed found to be a partial mediator of the effect of the intervention on reductions in aggressive behaviour.

Once children have developed clinically defined psychiatric disorders, interventions tend at present to focus on clinical treatment rather than tertiary *prevention*. Tertiary prevention programmes are rare. One example of proven effectiveness is Multisystemic Therapy.[38] Given the early onset of most psychiatric disorders, this is clearly a vitally important area for future work.

## Conclusions

This chapter has covered a lot of ground; from the first stirrings of understanding about childhood psychiatric disorders to the possibility of using molecular genetics to identify gene–environment interactions that can generate psychiatric disorder. There are fuzzy boundaries between epidemiology and developmental psychopathology, life course epidemiology, genetic epidemiology, services research, and clinical psychiatry. It will be important to keep these boundaries pervious, to share a common language where possible, and to learn and use one another's methods.

## Further information

Meltzer, H., Gatward, R., Goodman, R., et al. (1999). *The mental health of children and adolescents in Great Britain*. Office for National Statistics, London.

Meltzer, H., Gatward, R., Corbin, T., et al. (2003). *Persistence, onset, risk factors and outcomes of childhood mental disorders*. Office for National Statistics, London.

## References

1. Kleinbaum, D.G., Kupper, L.L., and Morgenstern, H. (1982). *Epidemiologic research: principles and quantitative methods*. Van Nostrand Reinhold, New York.

2. Costello, E.J., Erkanli, A., and Angold, A. (2006). Is there an epidemic of child or adolescent depression? *Journal of Child Psychology and Psychiatry, and Allied Disciplines, 47*, 1263–71.

3. Angold, A., Costello, E.J., and Worthman, C.M. (1998). Puberty and depression: The roles of age, pubertal status, and pubertal timing. *Psychological Medicine, 28*, 51–61.

4. Shaffer, D., Fisher, P.W., Dulcan, M., *et al.* (1996). The NIMH diagnostic interview schedule for children (disc 2.3): Description, acceptability, prevalences, and performance in the meca study. *Journal of the American Academy of Child and Adolescent Psychiatry, 35*(7), 865–77.

5. Earls, F. (1980). Prevalence of behavior problems in 3-year-old children: a cross- national replication. *Archives of General Psychiatry, 37*, 1153–7.

6. Susser, M. (1973). *Causal thinking in the health sciences: concepts and strategies in epidemiology.* Oxford University Press, New York.

7. Horwitz, S.M., Leaf, P.J., and Leventhal, J.M. (1998). Identification of psychosocial problems in pediatric primary care. *Archives of Pediatrics & Adolescent Medicine, 152*, 367–71.

8. Kessler, R.C., Berglund, P., Demler, O., *et al.* (2005). Lifetime prevalence and age-of-onset distributions of DSM-IV disorders in the national comorbidity survey replication. *Archives of General Psychiatry, 62*(6), 593–602.

9. Insel, T.R. and Fenton, W.S. (2005). Psychiatric epidemiology: it's not just about counting anymore. *Archives of General Psychiatry, 62*, 590–2.

10. Giuffra, L.A. and Risch, N. (1994). Diminished recall and the cohort effect of major depression: a simulation study. *Psychological Medicine, 24*, 375–83.

11. Ford, T., Goodman, R., and Meltzer, H. (2003). The British child and adolescent mental health survey 1999: the prevalence of DSM-IV disorders. *Journal of the American Academy of Child and Adolescent Psychiatry, 42*, 1203–11.

12. Meltzer, H., Gatward, R., Goodman, R., *et al.* (2003). Mental health of children and adolescents in Great Britain. *International Review of Psychiatry, 15*(1–2), 185–7.

13. Meltzer, H., Gatward R., Goodman, R., *et al.* (1999). *The mental health of children and adolescents in Great Britain.* Office for National Statistics, London.

14. Goodman, R., Ford, T., Richards, H., *et al.* (2000). The development and well-being assessment: Description and initial validation of an integrated assessment of child and adolescent psychopathology. *Journal of Child Psychology and Psychiatry, 41*, 645–56.

15. Meltzer, H., Gatward, R., Corbin, T., *et al.* (2003). *Persistence, onset, risk factors and outcomes of childhood mental disorders.* Office for National Statistics, London.

16. Costello, E.J. and Angold, A. (2006). Developmental epidemiology. In *Theory and method* (eds. D. Cicchetti and D. Cohen), pp. 41–75. Wiley, Hoboken.

17. Angold, A., Erkanli, A., Costello, E.J., *et al.* (1996). Precision, reliability and accuracy in the dating of symptom onsets in child and adolescent psychopathology. *Journal of Child Psychology and Psychiatry, 37*, 657–64.

18. Achenbach, T.M., McConaughy, S.H., and Howell, C.T. (1987). Child/adolescent behavioral and emotional problems: implications of cross-informant correlations for situational specificity. *Psychological Bulletin, 101*, 213–32.

19. Angold, A. and Costello, E.J. (2006). Puberty and depression. In *Child and adolescent psychiatric clinics of north America* (eds. G. Zalsman and D.A. Brent), pp. 919–37. Saunders, Philadelphia.

20. Canino, G., Costello, E.J., and Angold, A. (1999). Assessing functional impairment and social adaptation for child mental health services research: a review of measures. *Journal of Mental Health Services Research, 1*, 93–108.

21. Shaffer, D., Gould, M.S., Brasic, J., *et al.* (1983). A children's global assessment scale (CGAS). *Archives of General Psychiatry, 40*, 1228–31.

22. Kellam, S.G., Ensminger, M.E., and Turner, R.J. (1977). Family structure and the mental health of children. *Archives of General Psychiatry, 34*, 1012–22.

23. Angold, A. and Fisher, P.W. (1999). Interviewer-based interviews. In *Diagnostic assessment in child and adolescent psychopathology* (eds. D. Shaffer, C. Lucas, and J. Richters), pp. 34–64. Guilford Press, New York.

24. Costello, E.J., Mustillo, S., Erkanli, A., *et al.* (2003). Prevalence and development of psychiatric disorders in childhood and adolescence. *Archives of General Psychiatry, 60*, 837–44.

25. Caspi, A., Henry, B., McGee, R.O., *et al.* (1995). Temperamental origins of child and adolescent behavior problems: From age three to fifteen. *Child Development, 66*(1), 55–68.

26. Rutter, M. (2002). The interplay of nature, nuture, and developmental influences. *Archive of General Psychiatry, 59*, 996–1000.

27. Caspi, A., McClay, J., Moffitt, T.E., *et al.* (2002). Role of genotype in the cycle of violence in maltreated children. *Science, 297*, 851–4.

28. Foley, D.L., *et al.* (2004). Childhood adversity, monoamine oxidase A genotype, and risk for conduct disorder. *Archives of General Psychiatry, 61*, 738–44.

29. Ben-Shlomo, Y. and Kuh, D. (2002). A life course approach to chronic disease epidemiology: conceptual models, empirical challenges and interdisciplinary perspectives. *International Journal of Epidemiology, 31*, 285–93.

30. Krieger, N. (2001). Theories for social epidemiology in the 21st century: an ecosocial perspective. *International Journal of Epidemiology, 30*, 668–77.

31. Cairns, R.B., Elder, G.H., and Costello, E.J. (1996). *Developmental science*, Vol. 20. Cambridge University Press, New York.

32. Stein, Z., Susser, M., Saenger, G., *et al.* (1975). *Famine and human development: the dutch hunger winter of 1944–45.* Oxford University Press, New York.

33. Rossi, A.S. (1989). A life-course approach to gender, aging, and intergenerational relations. In *Social structure and aging* (eds. K.W. Schaie and C. Schoder), pp. 207–36. Erlbaum, Hillsdale, NJ.

34. Lynam, D.R., Milich, R., Zimmerman, R., *et al.* (1999). Project dare: No effects at 10-year follow-up. *Journal of Consulting and Clinical Psychology, 67*(4), 590–3.

35. Kellam, S.G., Koretz, D., and Moscicki, E. (1999). Core elements of developmental epidemiologically based prevention research. *American Journal of Community Psychology, 27*, 463–82.

36. Costello, E.J., Compton, S.N., Keeler, G., *et al.* (2003). Relationships between poverty and psychopathology: a natural experiment. *The Journal of the American Medical Association, 290*, 2023–9.

37. Dodge, K.A., Pettit, G.S., and Bates, J.E. (1994). Socialization mediators of the relation between socioeconomic status and child conduct problems. *Child Development, 65*, 649–65.

38. Henggeler, S.W., Schoenwald, S.K., Pickrel, *et al.* (1994). *Treatment manual for family preservation using multisystemic therapy.* South Carolina Health and Human Services Finance Commission, Columbia, SC.

# 9.1.3 Assessment in child and adolescent psychiatry

Jeff Bostic and Andrés Martin

The goals of assessment of a child/adolescent are to (1) detect psychopathology and its impacts on the child's functioning in family, school, and peer domains, (2) allow appropriate intervention targets to be identified and prioritized; and (3) identify relevant variables, including family or school factors that may influence treatment adherence.

## Distinctive aspects of the psychiatric assessment in children

1 Parents (or other adults) ordinarily initiate and pursue the evaluation of the child for diverse reasons. Adult expectations for the child sometimes exceed the child's abilities, or the adult's own parenting or teaching style may be a poor fit with this child. Some adults may seek treatment to alter the child to remedy this poor fit.

2 Children may not be receptive to changing their behaviour. Children may attribute problems to others and be unable to accept their contribution to an identified problem. The psychiatric assessment of children requires attention to what the child wishes would change.

3 Young children may not trust unfamiliar adults (including clinicians), and adolescents may perceive the clinician as another adult imposing expectations or judgements. Multiple informants[1] are often needed to identify the child's functioning in school, home, and peer domains, to identify the child's areas of strength on which the clinician can build, and to identify others (peers or adults) able to introduce or reinforce more adaptive skills or behaviours.

4 Most DSM-IV-TR diagnoses were defined amongst adult samples.[2] Efforts to consider where a particular child fits on the depressed mood, anxiety, and aggression axes, for example, requires attention to developmental differences in symptom expression.

5 The ability of the clinician to forge alliances with the child, the parent, and outside entities is essential. A breach in any of these relationships can impede treatment. Parental permission should be obtained to contact and collaborate with relevant parties.

## Content of the clinical interview

### Reason for referral

Who initiated this referral, their motivations, and what changes they seek is vital. Expectations of various parties may collide and must be reconciled for effective treatments to be implemented. For example, the school may seek changes in parental discipline, while parents may expect the evaluation to yield additional school services.

### History of problem(s)

Parents often experience intense pain while recounting the deterioration or anguish of their child. Clinicians should provide parents an opportunity to describe the evolution of the problem, attending to the context in which symptoms emerged and occur, changes in frequency and intensity of symptoms, and their current progression. The clinician should inquire directly about the *functions* of problem behaviours, including secondary gains (e.g. tantrums diminish chore requirements, etc.). The clinician should clarify whether symptoms are specific to one functional domain or whether they pervade multiple areas of the child's functioning at home, school, and with peers.

### Past problems

Significant past symptoms impairing the child should be identified. It is especially important to understand whether symptoms have been persistent since early childhood, are intermittent, or represent deterioration from a previously better level of functioning.

### Comorbid problems

Clinicians should inquire about disorders often seen in tandem. For example, bipolar disorder in children is often associated with previous attention deficit hyperactivity disorder.[3] Screening instruments (such as those selectively available free of cost at websites such as www.schoolpsychiatry.org) can be useful to provide comprehensive information about less conspicuous symptoms.

### Substance use history

Clinicians should inquire about the child's exposure to and use of tobacco, alcohol, and illicit substances. Children may perceive that substances alleviate their distress (e.g. anxiety, depression) and 'self-medicate.' Clarifying impacts of substances on symptoms may yield intervention points attractive to the child.

### Previous treatment(s)

Chronological assessment of past treatments may reveal strategies adaptable to the current problem. Past treatment history may suggest treatment modalities (in)tolerable to this patient (and family). Medication trials, counselling, hospitalizations, or alternative treatments should be explored.

### Developmental history

Parents may vary in their recollection of their child's attainment of developmental milestones. Review of earlier videotapes of the child may improve the reliability and completeness of reports regarding the sequence of the child's growth.

The child's development regulating *sleep, eating,* and *toileting* should be investigated. Attained skills may suddenly be lost, sometimes signalling the importance of emotional events at particular times. Eating behaviour has become complicated as both hunger and obesity increase risks of psychopathology.[4,5]

*Psychomotor development* includes standing, walking, running, throwing, hopping, and playing sports or musical instruments. How the child fares at sports may clarify psychomotor skills. Fine motor and gross motor skills may not be congruent.

*Cognitive development* refers to the child's acquisition of thinking skills. Specific inquiry concerning speech development, reading, writing, and math skill progression may reveal global or specific difficulties.

*Interpersonal development* refers to how the child interacts with others, particularly family members and other children and adults.

Stability of relationships, numbers of friends, types of activities shared, and expectations of peers often reveal sources of difficulty or maladaptive patterns.

*Emotional development* and *temperament* reveal the child's capacity to recognize his or her own mood state and to self-soothe or regulate negative affect. Prevailing moods can be described by parents, who may also detail past suicidality, irritability, specific fears and anxieties, and conditions associated with the child's happiness and pleasure.

The child's *moral development* indicates whether conscience or moral values are too lax, too harsh, overly focused on particular areas, or uneven and out of proportion to daily events. The child's ability to recognize impacts of decisions on others, and to acknowledge and correct mistakes provides clarity about the child's strengths and limitations. The child's religious and cultural/ethical views and practices also shape this area, and may guide treatment interventions.

*Trauma* may impact or even arrest development. Investigation of actual events (such as documented abuse), but also of events perceived traumatic by the child and family may shed important light on the child's behaviours and patterns of relating to others. Events surrounding the trauma, disclosures to others, and reactions of adults are also important for the clinician to recognize and address.

*Harmful behaviour*, towards self or others, may reveal important developmental progressions that warrant intervention. Head-banging may reveal sensory disturbances, thoughts or comments about death may reveal suicidality, and self-harmful acts such as self-mutilation or cutting may reveal primitive coping mechanisms.[6] Harmful acts towards animals or people may indicate needs for monitoring while other diagnostic or treatment interventions occur.

### Family history

Few psychiatric disorders appear transmitted exclusively genetically. Many parents fear that their other child may be destined to suffer psychopathology when a family member manifests a disorder, so clarification of contributions to expression of disorders can reduce unwarranted fear, guilt, and distress. Please refer to Chapter 6.3.8 for more information on assessment of family functioning.

*Divorce, separation, and single-parent* family circumstances may stress all family members. Even when parents part amicably, children may attempt to reunite family members. Children may exhibit symptoms even years after separations as they enter different developmental phases.[7]

*Adoption* may be a positive event for the child, and adoption warrant tactful attention by the clinician, including age at adoption of the child and biological parents, the involvement with biological parents, the child's understanding of the adoption, and how the adoption is discussed at home.

### Medical history

Pregnancy complications, birth difficulties, hospital stays, and medical illnesses requiring treatments (e.g. asthma, diabetes) should be investigated, as they increase the child's risk for psychopathology.[8] Inquiry into emergency room visits or surgeries can shed light on the child's fears, or parental over/underprotectiveness. Allergies should be ascertained, as well as responses or side effects to medications, including naturopathic or homeopathic agents.

### Child strengths/weaknesses

*Interests, hobbies, and talents* of the child should be obtained from the child and parents. Parents may have aspirations the child does not share, or the child may have fantasies beyond apparent abilities. In most cases, though, the child will have some identifiable interests or abilities that serve as potential points of connection with peers and adults (including clinicians).

### The child's media diet

Children are exposed to television, music, videos, electronic games, cell phones, e-mail and instant messaging, personal digital assistants, etc. It is important to clarify which media the child uses, how much time each day is spent with these various media, and what consequences these media have on the child (e.g. in response to watching action TV show the child becomes more violent versus has developed interest in Asian food through watching cooking programmes).[9] The degree of parental awareness and appropriate limit-setting regarding TV, video games, and instant messaging may warrant intervention.

### Mental status examination (MSE)

The MSE must be adjusted for children (see Fig. 9.1.3.1). The MSE includes a clinical description of the child's appearance, mood, sensorium, intelligence, and thought content and process. Much of the MSE takes place implicitly as the clinician interacts and observes the child during the child and family interviews.

## Structure of the clinical interview

### Preparatory phase of the child interview

Unlike regular pediatric check-ups, the psychiatric evaluation usually occurs because of prominent symptoms often perceived as embarrassing by the parents or the child. A phone call before the interview by the clinician or staff can clarify the structure of the interview, the collaboration anticipated to devise solutions, and the opportunity for parents to provide any confidential information to the clinician.

### The parent interview

The parent interview can be complicated by parental ambivalence about having a child evaluated by a psychiatrist, fears of loss of control or criticism, or parental shame or embarrassment about perceived parenting faults. The clinician should remain sensitive throughout the interview to parent vulnerabilities. Techniques to help parents overcome such obstacles during the interview are summarized in Fig. 9.1.3.2.

### The developmentally sensitive clinical interview of the child

The interview process and wording of questions must be tailored to fit with the child's understanding.[10] The child may not understand terms necessary to answer questions accurately. The child may also provide misleading answers to shield other family members, to protect against acknowledging some perceived failing, or to address circumstances if the child fears it might entail placement out of the home. Please refer to Chapter 9.1.1 for more specific information for obtaining reliable information during the child interview.

| Category | Components | What to Assess |
|---|---|---|
| Appearance | Physical Appearance | Gender; ethnicity; age (actual and apparent); cleanliness and grooming, hair/clothing style, presence of physical anomalies, indicators of self-care and parental attentiveness |
| | Manner of Relating to Clinician and Parents | Ease of separation from parent, guardedness, defiance, eagerness to please, flirtatiousness |
| | Activity Level | Psychomotor retarded to agitated, sustained or episodic, goal-oriented or erratic; coordination, unusual postures or motor patterns (e.g., tics, stereotypies, compulsions, catatonia, akathisia, dystonia, tremors) |
| | Speech | Fluency (including stuttering, cluttering, speech impediments), rate, volume, prosody |
| Mood | Current Affect | Predominant emotion and range (constricted to labile) during the interview, and appropriateness to content (e.g., giggles while talks about sibling's illness); intensity; lability |
| | Persisting Mood | Predominant emotion over days/weeks; whether current affect unusual or consistent with mood; whether mood reactive to situations or same across range of situations |
| | Coping Mechanisms and Regulation of Affect | How child manages conflict or distress, age-appropriateness of responses to and dependency on parents; sexual interests, impulses, aggression; control or modulation of urges (finding alternative or socially appropriate means of satisfying urges); how deals with frustration or when anxious |
| Sensorium | Orientation | Self (name), place (town, State), time (awareness of morning, day of week, month, year varies by age), situation (why at this appointment) |
| Intellect/ Cognition | Attention | Need for repeating, how long sustained on activity, degree to which child shifts from activity to activity, distractibility (to outside noises, etc.) |
| | Memory | Immediate (repeat numbers, names back), short-term (recall 3 objects at 2 and 5 minutes), long-term (recall events of past week) |
| | Intelligence; Fund of Knowledge | Age-appropriate recognition of letters, vocabulary, reading, counting, computational skills; age-appropriate knowledge of geography, history, culture (celebrities, sports, movies, etc.); concrete to abstract thinking, ability to classify and categorize |
| | Judgment | Best assessed after rapport established, as initially minimization or denial more common); what would do if found stamped envelope next to mailbox, fire started in theater, say if saw man with big feet |
| | Insight | Ability to see alternative explanations, others' points of view; locus of control (internal v. external); defense mechanisms |
| Thought | Process: *Coherence* | Logical, goal-directed, circumstantial or tangential (consider age-appropriateness), looseness of associations, word salad (incoherent, clanging, neologisms) |
| | Process: *Speed* | Mutism, poverty of thought (long latency, thought blocking), poverty of content (perseveration), racing thoughts, flight of ideas |
| | Perceptions | Altered bodily experiences (depersonalization, derealization), misperception of stimulus (illusion), no stimulus (hallucination: auditory [psychosis > PTSD > organic causes], visual [substance use, delirium], olfactory (neurological, seizure disorder] gustatory [from medicine side effects]) |
| | Content | Obsessions (ego-dystonic), delusions (ego-syntonic), thoughts of harm to self or others (magical thinking, or fears at night often age appropriate) |

**Fig. 9.1.3.1** The mental status examination in children.

1 Forming a clinical alliance with parents
  (a) Facilitating Narrative History
      Open-ended questions allow parents control, and can be followed with narrow questions to fill in needed details. Using the parent's own words can help parents feel heard.
  (b) Finding Common Themes/Patterns
      Inquiry into problems or conflicts the child has with other adults, peers, or unfamiliar others may illuminate patterns of the child's behavior that play out in a variety of settings, decreasing parents' anxiety that they alone provoke the child's problem.
  (c) Finding Good Intentions Gone Awry
      Parents may feel ashamed of past parenting efforts done in desperation. Acknowledging the parent's good intention leading to a misguided effort can diminish self-reproach. For example, a parent's harsh response often belies a fear about the child's future behavior, so identifying the fear and then examining alternative responses can be productive).
  (d) Partnering with Parents (Clinician as "partner" in decision-making process)
      Clinicians increasingly serve as partners, outlining several appropriate treatments, risks, and side effects, and helping parents to choose and invest in preferred treatments. If parents propose treatments the clinician regards as unhealthy or unproven, the clinician can identify potential risks of such treatments to minimize risks to the child.
  (e) Clarifying Expectations of the Evaluation
      Parents sometimes have unrealistic fantasies about what the evaluation will accomplish. Inquiring early about what the parent hopes will be accomplished by this evaluation can reveal such expectations and fantasies, which the clinician can realistically address. For example, parents may believe the evaluation can definitively prove the child had been abused by someone. At the other extreme, parents may fear that the clinician will tell them that their child will never be normal, will require institutionalization, or ultimately harm others.
2 Eliciting Sensitive Information
  (a) Providing the Parent Opportunities to Convey Sensitive Information
      Apprising parents of times and methods to convey information can provide appropriate mechanisms for sharing of information.
  (b) Revisiting Sensitive Information at Safer Points
      If parents resist disclosing information, the clinician should not force answers (as they are more likely to be inaccurate or incomplete), but rather proceed to less distressing information.
  (c) Explaining the Purpose of Sensitive Information
      Some parents may need to understand the underlying reasons for inquiring about personal information. For example, the clinician may need to explain the need to inquire about relatives to clarify genetic contributions to the child's difficulties.
  (d) Describing How Sensitive Information Will Be Reported
      Parents are sometimes fearful that details of embarrassing past parental personal problems may be included in reports to be seen by others. Parents may fear that marital conflict information might be used to alter custody arrangements, or symptoms in a report that could jeopardize their child's future educational or occupational pursuits. Clarifying that general information will be provided ("history of substance abuse on maternal side") rather than specifics and that parents will be able to review reports whose release they authorize can diminish resistance to sharing sensitive information.
3 Handling Discrepant Reports
  (a) Contextualizing Points of View
      Differences between observers' descriptions of a child's behavior have several potential sources. For example, teachers sometimes report very different presentations than parents. Examining what precipitates the child's problem, and how it expresses itself in different environments may allow clinicians to borrow effective strategies across environments without "blaming" adults.
  (b) Aligning Different Perspectives
      When parents or adults exhibit conflict during the psychiatric evaluation, the clinician may continue to refocus adults to the child's needs. For example, the clinician may encourage "middle ground" approaches to increase consistency between environments.

**Fig. 9.1.3.2** Parent interview techniques.

## The child's understanding of the psychiatric interview

The child and parent are usually seen together at the beginning of the child psychiatric interview to put the child at ease. Once comfortable, the child usually can tolerate the parents leaving the room. Transitional objects (books, electronic devices from home) may ease these transitions. Inquiring about what the child believes parents, teachers, or other adults want to be different as a result of this interview often elucidates what the child recognizes about others' perspectives, and also facilitates the child projecting thoughts or fantasies about this evaluation.

*Adolescents* sometimes fear parents will skew the interview by telling their 'version' first to get the clinician to side against the adolescent.[11] Meeting briefly with the parent and adolescent to clarify objectives, and then meeting with the adolescent alone at length may enhance an alliance with an adolescent. During this initial segment the clinician can clarify the plan to meet alone with parents after meeting with the adolescent to review birth history, developmental milestones, and family.

Adolescents may resist answering questions or participating. Clinicians can identify the adolescent's priorities and side with those that are reasonable, or identify what the adolescent needs to do to satisfy parents so that the adolescent no longer needs to see a psychiatrist. Clinicians may also decrease resistance by inquiring first about the adolescent's interests, strengths, musical preferences, rather than focusing on their 'problems,' as adolescents are developmentally struggling with their identity, and may resist fitting into the 'psychiatric patient' category.

## Developmentally sensitive techniques for the psychiatric interview

Four categories of techniques are commonly employed in these interviews. *Engagement* techniques are often required to put the child at ease so that the child will provide accurate clinical information. *Projective* techniques allow the child to reveal underlying themes or issues which cannot be verbalized directly. *Direct questioning* techniques clarify particular points needed to distinguish disorders, contributions to the child's problems, and intervention options. *Interactive* techniques clarify how the child relates to, as well as accepts or integrates input from, others.

### Techniques to engage the child

Child psychiatrists often provide toys or objects for patients in the waiting room and office. Toy figures, puppets, and 'relationship-oriented' toys may ease the child into the interview. Generic toy figures are usually preferable, since they are more likely to evoke the child's specific themes and concerns rather than 'scripts' based on TV shows or movies. Tasks framed as 'games' or active (e.g. drawing a house or family) often help the child transition into the psychiatric interview. By allowing the child to direct the content, the interviewer can follow the sequence of the child's concerns, note themes that emerge, and observe the points at which a child avoids or shifts to a new topic.

With *adolescents*, efforts to indicate familiarity with contemporary adolescent tastes (music, movies, terms, etc.) can be perceived ingenuine by the adolescent. Instead, clinicians may inquire about current interests, musical preferences, and current adolescent values from a curious, 'help me understand it' perspective, rather than from one of 'trying to be hip.' Manipulable items (squeeze balls, modelling clay, finger cuffs, cards, etc.) may allow adolescents a socially acceptable option for keeping their hands busy so that the interview feels less like an interrogation.

### Projective techniques

Projective techniques may help the child express concerns indirectly, so that anxiety about significant fears, telling family secrets, or betraying loyalties is minimized. Common projective techniques include having the child draw a picture of him- or herself or family doing something. For pictures of the child, body details including sizes of appendages or body parts and articulation (fingers, toes), relative size of the figure to the page, and frequent erasures can all reveal underlying issues of anxiety, perceived agency to address difficulties, or needs to control the environment. Depictions of the self as non-human, grotesque, imbued with super powers, or of the opposite gender may provide clues about the child's self-image and underlying wishes. The relative size and placement or omission of family members in a family drawing may illuminate the child's feelings about family relationships. Aggressive or sexual themes may be revealed in drawings.

Verbal projective techniques can similarly yield important information. Asking what animal or character (TV/movie star, cartoon, superhero) the child would most like to be, or whom the child would take along to a deserted island, or asking what the child

would do with three magic wishes often allow underlying issues to emerge. Wishes may reveal basic needs, such as food or a safe place to live, or longings for parents to reunite or for the return of a departed friend. Wishes sometimes reveal specific desires, such as 'not to have tics anymore,' or 'never to get teased.' Very general or altruistic wishes, such as 'world peace' or 'to live in a big house with lots of money' warrant further exploration, such as 'Are there particular fights you would especially like to stop?' or 'Who else would live there?' and 'What would you do first with lots of money?'

Projective techniques may help *adolescents* to reveal and share emotionally significant concerns with the clinician. Inquiries into favourite, or most disliked, movies, television characters, political or historical figures, musicians or artists, or sports figures, all allow elaboration of the teenager's ideas in displacement. Adolescents less distrustful of the clinician may readily speak about their own social longings or anxieties regarding friends at school. Adolescent resistances are often revealed by reluctance to divulge names of friends, or even questions about why the clinician needs to know this information. If resistance is detected, questions about what the adolescent most admires about a character, or what the adolescent imagines this character would do in given situations may reveal the adolescent's perceptions. Asking the adolescent about the different cliques or groups at school and his or her relationship to them provides useful information about the teen's self-image. Similarly, questions about what the adolescent sees as fair or would most like to change about school or the world often reveals underlying concerns and issues.

### Direct questioning

Direct questioning can specify symptoms or events, clarify how the child sees the world and functions within it, and follow-up on material from other parts of the evaluation. Asking the child to describe friends ('Tell me about your best friend.'), siblings, or parents, is preferable to 'Do you get along with your brother?' Open-ended questions such as 'What sorts of things make you mad/afraid/happy?' and 'What do you daydream about?' are similarly preferable to 'Do you get mad?' or 'Do you ever daydream?'

Anchoring direct questions to major events may help children provide more accurate answers. For example, 'Did that happen before or after your birthday?' or 'How has that (problem) been since school ended?' improve respondent accuracy.

Substance abuse, sexuality, and risky behaviours are often assessed through direct questions. The clinician can use simple questions, such as 'Substance use?' that allow significant latitude, and then focus in further, contingent on the child's responses. For example, the clinician may hear 'No, I don't do any of that anymore,' which could then be followed by 'What led to that decision?' and then proceed back to when and what substances were used. Similarly, sexuality can be assessed by gentle direct questions that do not prematurely close off response options, such as 'Have you had romantic feelings towards another? How did that go?' (rather than 'Have you had a boyfriend yet?'). Adolescents may fear the interviewer will be disapproving, so questions like 'romantic feelings towards anyone' are preferable to 'are there any girls you like?'[12] Finally, direct inquiries into risky behaviours (stealing, vandalism, assaults, gambling, etc.) often require general questions such as 'Have you done anything that you now look back on and think was dangerous?' before proceeding to specific questions (e.g. 'Have you ever stolen anything? Have you ever been beaten up?

Beat up someone else?'). Suicidal risk behaviours may be minimized or trivialized, so additional questions to examine fantasies about impacts of the suicide on family and friends or value contradictions may be needed to clarify suicidality risks.[13]

### Interactive techniques

Throughout, the clinician observes how the child relates to another person and what feelings or reactions this child elicits. How the child reacts to a new person, sustains interactions, and terminates the interview often reveal patterns important in the child's larger social life. The clinician can evaluate more complex social interactions during transitions ('It's time to put these toys up in the box.') and during games. Short games (tic tac toe) are useful since the clinician can quickly detect the child's response to winning, tying, and losing.

*Adolescents* employ more complex patterns, often specific to a subgroup to which they now belong, so clarifying what clothing symbols represent, meanings of confusing terms, and values espoused by subgroups can clarify how the adolescent relates to others. The clinician should observe provocative comments, often used to titrate space between the clinician and the adolescent, or to reject others first.

### Concluding the interview

Ending collaboratively increases the likelihood that the child will feel positive about subsequent encounters with clinicians, including treatment. Questions such as 'Are there other things that would be important for me to know about what you're like or how things have been for you?' or 'What else have I not asked about that is important?' facilitate this process.

The child may be curious about what the clinician will say and to whom. The interview is one piece of a larger evaluation, so the clinician may need to clarify that other testing, conversations with others, or additional meetings may be needed. Discussing findings (including treatment recommendations) with parents is usually advisable since parents may disagree with the clinician's conclusions or resist suggested interventions (e.g. medication, school placement, etc.).

Confidentiality is one of the most challenging issues surrounding child psychiatric interviews, especially with adolescents. Describing to the adolescent what will be told to specific others is helpful, as well as what information will not be revealed (e.g. specific details about substance abuse or sexual behaviours). Parents and the child should be told explicitly that confidentiality does *not* extend to situations that pose a clear danger to the child or others. In cases where dangerous content emerges (e.g. the child describes obtaining bullets to frighten a peer), the clinician should clarify with the child *how* they will tell appropriate others, preferably together.

## Neuropsychological testing

Patients may have subtle or complicated difficulties processing certain types of information. Consultation with a pediatric neuropsychologist may clarify appropriate tests to address persisting diagnostic questions. Clinicians should recognize that young patients may not be 'interested' in testing tasks, so scores should be interpreted cautiously, with input from the person who did the testing, when the clinician discusses findings with families.

## Laboratory evaluation in the child psychiatric evaluation

Few definitive clinical tests identify specific child psychiatric disorders. Laboratory testing remains useful when symptoms and physical findings suggest a particular disorder. Collaboration with the primary pediatric care provider may guide decisions about possible further medical consultations (e.g. audiometric, genetic, neurological, speech, etc.) or diagnostic tests (e.g. blood tests, neuroimaging, sleep studies).

### Testing in specific childhood disorders

Laboratory testing yields findings that alter the working diagnosis in approximately 1 per cent of cases, and the yield for laboratory abnormalities, without the presence of other supportive physical findings, remains less than 5 per cent.[14] Laboratory tests commonly considered are summarized in Table 9.1.3.1. Specialized technologies, such as positron emission tomography (PET), single photon emission computerized tomography (SPECT), functional

**Table 9.1.3.1** Laboratory tests to consider in childhood psychiatric disorders

| Lab test | Disorder | | | | | |
| --- | --- | --- | --- | --- | --- | --- |
| | MR/PDD | Mood | Psychosis | OCD tics | Substance abuse | Eating disorders |
| Chromosomal testing | X | | X | | | |
| Wood's (UV) lamp | X | | | | | |
| Monospot | | X | | | | |
| Thyroid | | X | X | | | X |
| Lyme titre | | | X | | | |
| CBC | X | X | X | | X | X |
| Serum chemistry | X | X | X | | X | X |
| Lead level | X | | | | | |
| Throat culture antistreptolysin O antibody (ASO), antideoxyribonuclease B titres | | | | X | | |
| Urine drug screen | | X | X | | X | |
| Cerebrospinal fluid analysis | | X | X | | | |
| Neuroimaging | | | X | | | |
| EEG | X | | | | | |

MRI (fMRI), and brain electrical activity mapping (BEAM) remain attractive research tools at this time in child psychiatry.

## Further information

Recommended Websites:

www.aacap.org: the home site for American child psychiatry; includes current practice parameters for various psychiatric disorders.

www.schoolpsychiatry.org: rating scales, school interventions for psychiatric symptoms.

Baron, I.S. (2004). *Neuropsychological evaluation of the child.* Oxford, New York.

Martin, A. and Volkmar, F.R. (eds.) (2007). *Lewis's child and adolescent psychiatry: a comprehensive textbook* (4th edn). Lippincott, Williams, & Wilkins, Philadelphia.

Mash, E.J. and Barkley, R.A. (eds.) (2007). *Assessment of childhood disorders* (4th edn). Guilford, New York.

Rutter, M. and Taylor, E.A. (eds.) (2002). *Child and adolescent psychiatry* (4th edn). Blackwell, Oxford.

## References

1. Ferdinand, R.F., Hoogerheide, K.N., van der Ende, J., *et al.* (2003). The role of the clinician: three-year predictive value of parents', teachers' and clinicians' judgment of childhood psychopathology. *Journal of Child Psychology and Psychiatry, and Allied Disciplines,* **44**(6), 867–76.

2. Patel, V., Flisher, A.J., Hetrick, S., *et al.* (2007). Mental health of young people: a global public-health challenge. *Lancet,* **369**(9569), 1302–13.

3. Masi, G.P.G., Millepiedi, S., Mucci, M., *et al.* (2006). Developmental differences according to age at onset in juvenile bipolar disorder. *Journal of Child and Adolescent Psychopharmacology,* **16**(6), 679–85.

4. Weinreb, L., Wehler, C., Perloff, J., *et al.* (2002). Hunger: its impact on children's health and mental health. *Pediatrics,* **110**(4), e41.

5. Vila, G., Zipper, E., Dabbas, M., *et al.* (2004). Mental disorders in obese children and adolescents. *Psychosomatic Medicine,* **66**(3), 387–94.

6. King, R.A., Ruchkin, V.V., and Schwab-Stone, M. (2003). Suicide and the continuum of adolescent self destructiveness: is there a connection? In *Suicide in children and adolescents* (eds. R.A. King and A. Apter). Cambridge University Press, Cambridge.

7. Wallerstein, J.S. and Blakeslee, S. (2000). *The unexpected legacy of divorce: a 25 year landmark study.* Hyperion, New York.

8. Indredavik, M.S., Vik, T., Heyerdahl, S., *et al.* (2004). Psychiatric symptoms and disorders in adolescents with low birth weight. *Archives of Disease in Childhood. Fetal and Neonatal Edition,* **89**(5), F445–50.

9. Pataki, C., Bostic, J.Q., and Schlozman S. (2005). The functional assessment of media in child and adolescent psychiatric treatment. *Child and Adolescent Psychiatric Clinics of North America,* **14**(3), 555–70.

10. Lewis, M. (ed.) (1991). *Psychiatric assessment of infants, children, and adolescents.* Williams and Wilkins, Baltimore.

11. King, R.A. and Schowalter, J.E. (2004). The clinical interview of the adolescent. In *Textbook of child and adolescent psychiatry* (3rd edn) (eds. J.A. Wiener and M.K. Dulcan), pp. 113–16. American Psychiatric Publishing, Washington, DC.

12. King, R.A. (1997). Practice parameters for the psychiatric assessment of children and adolescents. American Academy of Child and Adolescent Psychiatry. *Journal of the American Academy of Child and Adolescent Psychiatry,* **36**(Suppl. 10), 4S–20S.

13. Galvin, M.R., Fletcher, J., and Stilwell, B.M. (2006). Assessing the meaning of suicidal risk behavior in adolescents: three exercises for clinicians. *Journal of the American Academy of Child and Adolescent Psychiatry,* **45**(6), 745–8.

14. Challman, T.D., Barbaresi, W.J., Katusic, S.K., *et al.* (2003). The yield of the medical evaluation of children with pervasive developmental disorders. *Journal of Autism and Developmental Disorders,* **33**(2), 187–92.

## 9.1.4 Prevention of mental disorder in childhood and other public health issues

Rhoshel Lenroot

### Introduction

Over the last two decades advances in psychiatric classification systems and screening tools have allowed the global and national burden of mental disorder to be described with the first large-scale epidemiologic studies. The World Health Organization's *World Health Report 2001* estimated that over 450 million individuals suffer from mental disorders, and that psychiatric disorders ranked as 5 of the top 10 causes of disability in the global population.[1] Studies specifically of psychiatric disorders in children report that between 3 per cent and 18 per cent of children have a clinically significant psychiatric disorder, a number far exceeding those with access to treatment.[2] A recent study which included data on age of onset found that 50 per cent of psychiatric disorders had their onset by age 14, and 75 per cent by age 24.[3] Treatment on this scale is unlikely to ever be feasible, even if available methods were more effective and less risky than those currently available. Preventing mental health disorders from occurring is an alternative to decrease the extent of this public health problem. However, if a key characteristic of prevention is acting prior to onset of a disorder, the early age of onset for most mental disorders indicates intervention must occur during long before adulthood.

Neuroscience has contributed evidence that longitudinal trajectories of brain development are affected by a combination of genetic and environmental factors. Neuroimaging studies have shown dynamic changes in brain structure and function continuing through childhood and adolescence, and geneticists have found that gene expression is highly dependent on environmental conditions. These findings imply that the brain is still highly plastic during childhood and adolescence. This may confer greater vulnerability to long-term effects of insults from trauma, substance abuse, or other adverse influences than in adulthood, but also the potential for lifelong beneficial effects from early positive interventions.

Growing interest in the possibilities afforded by research into prevention in children's mental health stimulated a series of large-scale reports and initiatives beginning in the early 1990s.[4–7] Advances in epidemiology, developmental psychopathology, and prevention science have converged to provide a framework to guide and evaluate prevention programmes. This chapter will discuss basic principles of public health and preventive medicine with application to mental health disorders in children and adolescents.

### Public health and prevention: history and basic concepts

The goal of public health is the prevention of disease and promotion of health in communities. The World Health Organization has defined *health* as 'a state of physical, mental and social well-being and not merely the absence of disease or infirmity',[8] and *mental health* as 'a state of well-being in which the individual realizes his or her own abilities, can cope with the normal stresses of life, can work productively and fruitfully, and is able to make a contribution to his or her community'.[1] Public health differs from clinical medicine in that it addresses health-related matters on the level of populations rather than individuals. Public health activities include assessment of the health status and risk factors within a community through epidemiology, and population-focused interventions such as supporting the practice of preventive medicine, health education and behavioural modifications, creating and enforcing measures to maintain a healthy environment, and working to increase support for public health initiatives within the political sphere. In countries without universal access to health care public health offices may also act as providers of medical treatment for individuals without other means of access.[9]

Communities have acted to support the health of their members throughout history.[10] Common concerns for most societies have included control of epidemics, public sanitation, and promotion of personal hygiene, although the forms of public health interventions have varied depending on societal values, conceptions of the causes of ill health, and available resources. The health risks posed by the large-scale urban poverty and overcrowding associated with the industrial revolution helped to stimulate the growth of modern public health organizations, whose concerns eventually broadened to include issues such as workplace safety and regulation of the production of foods and medicines. Public health interventions changed to reflect advances in the understanding of disease processes, for example moving from general notions of the value of sanitation to focusing on specific infectious agents. Measures such as widespread vaccination and regulation of sanitary conditions have been so effective in developed countries that the focus of public health in these areas has shifted to chronic disorders such as heart disease and hypertension. Although emotional and behavioural issues have always been a concern of communities, systematic intervention to prevent mental disorders has lagged behind other disorders, in large part because of the lack of consensus regarding the nature of these problems or even how to classify them. A key factor in the advances in public mental health of the past several decades has been progress in epidemiology of mental health disorders.[9]

## Epidemiology in public mental health

### Incidence and prevalence

Epidemiology provides information about the *incidence* of a condition, meaning the number of new cases, which arise during a certain period of time, and its *prevalence*, meaning how many individuals have the condition during a certain period. The goal of prevention is to decrease a condition's incidence, i.e. prevent new cases from occurring, while successful treatment results in the decrease of the prevalence. Mental health disorders have presented challenges to epidemiology on several levels. In order to determine how many cases of a certain condition exist within the population, it is necessary to know how to define a case, but this is far from straightforward in the realm of mental health. Classification of medical disorders tends to evolve from symptom-based to mechanism-based as the links between a specific pathophysiology and the observed signs and symptoms are established. The lack of knowledge about the mechanisms producing cognitive and behavioural symptoms means that classification of mental disorders still relies

upon descriptions of constellations of symptoms. *The International Classification of Disease version 10(ICD-10)*,[11] and its United States counterpart *the Diagnostic and Statistical Manual TR-IV (DSM-TR-IV)*,[12] are the results of iterative attempts by experts in the field to create meaningful classifications of psychiatric disorders based upon such observations in conjunction with applicable considerations of length and severity of illness, age of onset, and risk factors. This work has provided the standardized terminology that made possible the first large-scale epidemiologic descriptions of mental disorders. However, problematic issues pertinent to epidemiology remain, including questions regarding the relative merits of categorical versus dimensional classification systems; how to interpret the high rate of comorbidities for several disorders; and how best to account for individuals who have subthreshold symptoms, including how to determine the starting point of a disorder. It is not uncommon for individuals who have come to meet criteria for a mental health disorder such as schizophrenia or depression to have had a preceding period of subthreshold 'prodromal' symptoms, but healthy individuals also have occasional subthreshold symptoms that resolve without intervention. Unfortunately this differentiation often cannot be determined except retrospectively, despite the fact that there may be different implications for epidemiologic and preventive efforts.

The question of how symptoms change over time gains additional relevance when attempting to describe the epidemiology of mental health disorders in children and adolescents. As described in more detail elsewhere in this volume,[13] the science of developmental epidemiology has arisen as a response to the recognition that mental disorders may manifest in different ways over the lifespan, and that certain types of symptoms at one age may indicate that an individual is at high risk for developing a different disorder at a later stage of maturation. Risk factors may also have differing impact depending on an individual's developmental stage. Function may appear impaired if children are developing slowly in comparison with their peers, and it must be decided when this is normal variation and when it should be considered pathological. An additional layer of complexity in epidemiology in paediatric populations is the incorporation of information from additional informants such as parents and/or teachers, and determining how to evaluate the relationship of symptoms to particular contexts.

### Risk factors

Epidemiology is also used to assess for the presence of risk factors. *Fixed risk factors* are those that cannot be altered, such as genotype. *Malleable risk factors* are susceptible to intervention, such as exposure to lead-based paint or domestic violence. *Causative risk factors* are those with known relationships to a particular outcome, and are of particular interest to prevention because they represent potential points of intervention. *Protective factors* instead decrease the risk of an adverse outcome. *Resilience* is a term used to describe an individual's ability to do well despite exposure to a typically high-risk situation.

Effective intervention to decrease risk factors or increase protective factors requires determining how these factors relate to each other and to the targeted health issues. The ultimate goal is a chain of causative steps leading from risk factor to outcome, but epidemiological data itself may provide sufficient guidance for action. One of the most famous examples of this was John Snow's identification of tainted drinking water from a particular well as the root of a cholera epidemic in London, which he did based solely on epidemiological observations. Removal of the pump handle stopped the epidemic and proved that exposure was a causative risk, decades before the bacteria itself was identified. We are currently in a similar situation to Snow in regards to connecting risk factors to mechanisms for many mental health disorders, with the additional complication that mental health disorders are typically associated with combinations of a large number of individually modest potential risk factors.

Risk factors can be classified in terms of how they relate to each other and to the specified outcome,[14] and thus what type of intervention if any is appropriate. *Mediating* risk factors are those which explain how or why another factor affects the outcome; for example, the phenylketonuria enzyme *mediates* the effects of the phenylketonuria gene on IQ.[14] Although all causal factors are mediators, the reverse is not true, and experimental conditions are generally necessary to demonstrate that a particular mediator plays a causal role. A *moderating* risk factor instead specifies under what conditions or for whom another risk factor will affect outcome. Moderating risk factors describe populations that have differing responses to a given exposure, and may also represent potential sites of intervention to prevent an adverse outcome by reducing vulnerability or increasing resilience. A *proxy* risk factor, also called a *pseudocorrelation*, is one that itself does not strongly predict outcome but is highly correlated to a risk factor that does. *Overlapping* risk factors are those that arise from the same underlying construct and are observed to equally predict outcome, be highly correlated with each other and not stand in a specific temporal relationship; these can often be combined into a single factor. *Independent* risk factors conversely are unrelated to each other; they both predict outcome but without correlation or temporal precedence.

## Theoretical models in prevention

The identification of risk factors and their interpretation evolves together with theoretical models for the causes and treatments of health problems. The fundamental model used throughout public health and epidemiology is that of *host-agent-environment*, in which the *host* is the person affected or at risk, the *agent* is the direct cause of disease, and the *environment* includes external factors which affects the host's vulnerability to the agent and the vector by which the agent reaches the host. While this model was first developed for infectious disease, it has been expanded to include other types of chronic non-infectious disorders.[10] Examples of pathogenic agents in the latter case include nutrition, chemicals, and genes; host factors include age, sex, and lifestyle; while social or economic issues are among those potentially affecting the environment. Another dimension that has gained increased attention in psychopathology is the actual transaction between the individual and environment—for example, the features of the way a child and parent interact. Intervening to remove risk factors from multiple domains simultaneously can potentially provide the most effective outcome.

Incorporating development into this model adds many challenges. The fields of developmental science and developmental psychopathology arose to create as a framework for the integration of information from developmental epidemiology, neuroscience, genetics, psychology, psychiatry, sociology, and other disciplines in order to better understand the complex interplay of factors affecting the health of an individual throughout their lifespan.[15] Major contributions from work in this area have been establishing the importance of interactions between genes and environment in determining the trajectory of development, rather than attributing mental health outcome to being due entirely to one factor or the other, and the dialectical nature of the relationship between the developing individual and their environment. The recognition of the importance of context in development has led to an elaboration of the different overlapping systems, or *ecologies*[16] that a child resides within and which present unique risks and opportunities for intervention.

Risk factors may be generalized, such as malnutrition and poverty, or more disease-specific, such as exposure to a particular toxin. Many risk factors will tend to occur together, and often risk factors have a non-linear relationship to outcomes; i.e. one or two may not significantly affect outcome, while as the number goes above a certain level risk increases sharply for a number of disorders. An additional complexity in developmental psychopathology is the presence of multicausality and multifinality. Multiple risks or disease processes may produce similar behavioural phenomena, while specific risk factors may be associated with a wide range of clinical presentations. Tracing causal paths and determining what are the factors that are mediating and moderating the relationships between risks and outcomes depends upon the ability to follow the impact of specific interventions over time.

## The prevention research cycle and evidence-based prevention

Although direct experimentation on human subjects to establish causality among the risk factors affecting developmental trajectories is not in itself ethically feasible, suitably designed longitudinal controlled trials of preventive interventions can address the same goals.[17] Recognition of the value of considering prevention research as an iterative process led to the formulation of the *preventive research cycle*.[4] The steps in the cycle are: (i) identification of the problem or disorder and the size of its impact on a community; (ii) review of relevant information, particularly regarding relevant risk and protective factors available data from existing preventive research programmes; (iii) design, conduct, and analysis of pilot studies, including replication at multiple sites; (iv) implementation of larger-scale trials which will provide additional information about which populations may be more or less appropriate, and how the intervention does when scaled up in size; and (v) large-scale implementation and ongoing evaluation.

The randomized clinical trial, in which individuals or discrete communities are randomly assigned to receive either the intervention under investigation, a different intervention, or no intervention at all, continues to be a gold standard for determining whether a prevention programme itself is responsible for observed changes and thus to establish causality. Only a randomized clinical trial can determine if the intervention actually results in prevention, i.e. evidence that new cases did not develop that otherwise would have. Some trials, particularly those for populations in which some symptoms may already be present, result in decrease of those subsyndromal symptoms. While this is not without value, it is more strictly considered treatment than prevention.

The ability to make a convincing case for the value of a preventive intervention is particularly important because investing in prevention is asking an individual or community to devote resources towards a problem that has not yet occurred. Standards for evidence-based preventions have been explicitly identified to help with design and evaluation of studies, including criteria for when there is sufficient grounds to move along the research cycle from pilot studies to large-scale field trials and final dissemination.[18] The recommendations provide guidance for appropriate statistical methodology and design, and emphasize the need for replication in independent samples, adequate provision of training materials for non-research personnel as the scope of the project grows, and ongoing data collection after dissemination to inform communities and researchers about the impact of the intervention and direct the next iteration. They also differentiate between *effectiveness*, defined as showing a positive result in pilot studies under highly controlled circumstances, and *efficacy*, indicating a programme is also able to produce results in the less-optimal conditions associated with larger-scale trials.

## Types of preventive interventions

Once it has been determined that a particular problem is present, and pertinent risk and protective factors have been identified, it is necessary to determine what type of intervention is most likely to be effective. Two broad distinctions are applicable to any intervention. The first, as implied by the host-agent-environment model, is whether to address the individual, their environment, or both. The second distinction concerns which portions of the population potentially at risk are to be addressed.[19]

### Primary, secondary, and tertiary prevention

The first widely used public health prevention categories were proposed by the Chronic Disease Commission in 1957, who classified prevention as being primary, secondary, or tertiary.[20] *Primary prevention* is aimed at the normal population and defined as efforts aimed at decreasing the incidence of new cases, such as preventing access to contaminated water supplies as illustrated by the case of John Snow. *Secondary prevention* is targeted towards individuals who already show early signs of disease or disorder, with the aim of decreasing the prevalence of already established cases. *Tertiary prevention* attempts to minimize the degree of morbidity associated with an established illness, through decreasing its duration or associated disability. Such definitions were a crucial step in designing interventions to focus on a specific population and problem and take into account specific characteristics of that situation. However, classifying prevention by the disease stage may require a greater understanding of how risks related to disorders than is possible for many conditions.

### Universal, selected, and indicated prevention

An alternative classification system based upon risk–benefit considerations for preventive interventions was introduced by Gordon in 1983[21] and disseminated through the seminal *Institute of Medicine* report in 1994.[4] Gordon proposed that the benefit of a prevention programme could be assessed by comparing an individual's risk of developing a disorder with the risk or cost of the associated intervention. In his system, prevention is classified as *universal*, *selected*, or *indicated*, depending on the degree of identified risk. *Universal prevention* is applied to everyone in a defined population, and the associated interventions are optimally low risk, low cost, and may be administered by individuals who possess relatively little specialized training. However, universal prevention spends resources on a large number of individuals who would not have become ill in any case. *Selective intervention* is aimed at individuals at above-average risk for a disorder, and anticipates a commensurately higher cost and intensity of intervention. Finally, *indicated prevention* is for individuals who are showing early signs of a disorder or exhibit biological markers indicating risk; the acceptable cost and risk here would again be higher to reflect the increased need of the individual.

There are areas of similarity between the two systems, which has led to some confusion. The populations and goals of primary and universal prevention are comparable, but selected and indicated groups indicate individuals at increasing levels of risk but who do not yet meet criteria for a disorder, whereas secondary and tertiary address issues related to different stages of having a disorder.

### Comparison of prevention and health promotion

An alternate conceptualization of how to proactively intervene to improve outcomes is *health promotion*, defined as measures to increase likelihood of wellness as a positive quality rather than limiting efforts to decreasing risks for a negative outcome.[5] From a practical standpoint it overlaps largely with universal prevention, but the theoretical foundations and targeted outcomes differ. Although few would disagree with the potential benefits of promoting health in the community, health promotion has not always been included within the scope of prevention policy due to concerns that it may dilute efforts towards risk prevention that are characterized by more clearly definable and measurable outcomes. Others have argued that in view of the complex pathways of developmental psychopathology, a less-specific approach is more consonant with our existing knowledge, and may actually be more effective over the long run to create resilience against a broader range of disorders.[22]

## Effective preventive interventions for children's mental health

The degree of implementation of preventive measures for mental health disorders in children and adolescents depends largely on how convincingly specific risk factors can be demonstrated which are malleable to politically and economically feasible actions. For example, realization of the adverse effects of prenatal alcohol exposure on neurodevelopment resulted in widespread public education efforts. Other toxins such as lead-based paint have also been the focus of education and regulations to decrease children's exposure. Vaccination programmes have significantly reduced mental disorders associated with infectious diseases such as rubella, and programmes have been put in place to decrease risks from accidents through measures such as use of car seats and bicycle helmets.

For conditions where the core risk factors are less clearly defined progress has been slower, but enough data has accrued over the past two decades of systematic prevention trials to be able to begin to assess the effectiveness of preventive interventions in this context. The scope of the current chapter does not allow a detailed description, and the reader is referred to relevant chapters for specific disorders within this text, as well as general reviews and meta-analyses available elsewhere.[4,5,16,19]

## Health promotion

A recent report by the World Health Organization summarized globally relevant general risk factors and the state of evidence for specific interventions to promote mental health and resilience.[6] Social, environmental, and economic factors have a major impact on mental health. Increasing attention is also being paid to *social capital*, a concept which broadly refers to aspects of social organization and community norms that facilitate the ability of individuals to work together for mutual benefit. General measures for health promotion include improving nutrition, housing, access to education and economic security, as well as strengthening community networks, reducing exposure to violence, decreasing substance abuse, and intervention to help with recovery from disasters. Risks for children's mental health from the proximal family environment include adverse maternal behaviour during pregnancy, such as substance abuse, child abuse, parental mental illness, and domestic violence, and may be addressed with measures such as home-visiting programmes for pregnant women and new mothers and pre-school programmes.

While the benefits of such general health promotion activities seems highly plausible, rigorous evidence of their effects on mental health allowing quantification for cost-benefit questions is difficult to come by and currently patchy, especially for larger-scale interventions. Reasons for this include the length of time necessary to see the results of these interventions, which may be much longer than the policy environment which fostered them; the large samples necessary, which may range from difficult to impossible to randomize appropriately, and the lack of funding for this type of information-gathering. Here in particular naturalistic 'experiments' may be of aid, in which populations exposed to changes in risk factors or social policies are closely monitored for the impact on health outcomes.

## Prevention

The practical implementation of universal preventive measures overlaps largely with health promotion, despite the differences in their theoretical background and aims. Universal prevention programmes have the significant advantage of not conferring stigma upon participants, but their benefits are difficult to quantify due to the generally small effect sizes and consequent large samples necessary,[23] and they by definition devote significant resources to individuals who likely would not have had problems regardless. Universal prevention programmes with evidence of benefit have been developed for issues such as conduct disorder, anxiety, and depression. These have been primarily school-based, focusing on classroom behavioural management, social skills training, and cognitive strategies to help children learn prosocial behaviours and cope with stressful situations. Some programmes adopt a multimodal approach which includes parents. Universal approaches to decrease substance abuse have had mixed results. Educational techniques have shown clear success in increasing the knowledge base regarding risks of substance abuse, but impact on actual usage has been harder to demonstrate outside of more comprehensive programmes targeting multiple types of risk.[16]

Preventive measures for selected populations become more specific to individual disorders. Children at risk for conduct disorder often come from impoverished environments with high rates of exposure to violence, substance abuse, and weak family and community structures. Secondary preventions in these settings accordingly rely more strongly on multimodal interventions which include the family. Children with a depressed parent are at increased risk for depression, and secondary interventions in this case may include treatment of the depressed parent in addition to cognitive therapies for the child. Stress related to difficult transitions such as parental death, divorce, or unemployment are also significant risk factors for children, and have been effectively addressed with courses of cognitive group therapy.

Indicated prevention measures, for children with early symptoms or biological markers of a disorder, have the narrowest scope and generally the clearest evidence of effectiveness. A seminal study in the prevention of depression was performed by Clarke and colleagues,[24] who showed that cognitive therapy in adolescents with subsyndromal symptoms of depression and a depressed parent could reduce the incidence of new cases of depression compared to a control group. Schizophrenia has become a target of preventive medicine through studies showing that treatment of adolescents with early symptoms of psychosis may delay onset of a full psychotic break.[25] Multimodal interventions have also been shown to be effective for children and adolescents already showing signs of increased aggressive or antisocial behaviour.

Common themes in 'best-practice' mental health prevention programmes have included the need for multimodal approaches which simultaneously address both the child and components of the environment, and the increased durability of improved outcomes when interventions are maintained for significant lengths of time. Many programmes focus on reduction of proximal risk factors rather than mental health disorders themselves as a more feasible outcome measure, although when possible it is optimal to incorporate both. When preventive research began to stratify interventions into universal, selected, and indicated, it was originally predicted that the lowest-risk individuals would benefit the most from universal-level interventions. It was instead found that higher-risk children actually showed the greatest response, supporting the development of tiered systems in which children who did not benefit adequately from universal measures could also be referred for secondary and indicated levels.

In general, meta-analyses have found that preventive programmes in mental health for selected and indicated populations have small to moderate effect sizes, similar to those seen in other areas of medicine. Anxiety and depression have shown the most consistent responses. Universal programmes have not shown significant effectiveness in meta-analyses of controlled trials, which is understandable given the necessary sample sizes, but has led to debate regarding the justification of their claim on scarce resources. Another concern is that most research has been carried out at the level of pilot studies, with much less available from large-scale trials or fully disseminated programmes. What information is available shows a tendency for a fall off in effectiveness when moving to larger-scale implementation. This suggests a need to spend more attention from the earliest stages on issues relating to dissemination such as adapting programmes for existing community infrastructure. Early collaboration with the members of the targeted community also helps to ensure relevance of a programme and consequent participation; for example parenting classes, while potentially valuable, may not attract individuals preoccupied with issues, such as safety or securing transportation. Finally, the issue of how to transfer preventive programmes into different settings requires much more extensive attention. Most prevention research has been done in a few of the more affluent nations, primarily the United States, United Kingdom, Canada, Australia, and countries in northern Europe. Little is known about how to transfer programmes or which programmes may be suitable for other less-affluent areas.

## Conclusion

Enormous progress has been made in recognizing the scope of mental health problems for children around the world, and in developing the theoretical framework needed to address decreasing this burden in a systematic fashion. Technological advances in neuroimaging, genetics, and computational biology are providing the tools to start describing the biological processes underlying the complex course of development, and have renewed appreciation of the role of the environment in determining how a genetic heritage is expressed.

However, rapid technological change is also altering the environment of children and their families at an unprecedented rate, and what kinds of challenges to public health these changes may present is not yet fully understood. What is becoming clear is that as technological advances increase the range of available health care treatments, along with the potential cost, the choices for societies between spending limited resources on treatment or prevention will have to become increasingly deliberate.

A substantial body of work has demonstrated that prevention in mental health can be effective, but those who would benefit the most from preventive interventions are often not those with the political or economic resources to make them a priority. While the potential interventions to prevent mental health disorders in children are constrained by the knowledge and resources available, what is actually done depends upon the social and political values of individual communities and nations.[9] It is to be hoped that as our understanding of these disorders grows, public policies to prevent the development of mental health disorders in children will become as commonplace a responsibility for modern societies as the provision of clean drinking water.

## Further information

UK. *National Health Service Guide for Child and Adolescent Mental Health*: http://www.bma.org.uk/ap.nsf/Content/Childadolescentmentalhealth

*World Health Organization webpage for mental disorders*: http://www.who.int/topics/mental_disorders

U.S. *substance abuse and mental health services administration: clinical preventive services in substance abuse and mental health update: from Science to services* http://www.samhsa.gov/publications/allpubs/SMA04-3906/i.asp

*Society for prevention research*: http://www.preventionresearch.org

## References

1. WHO. (2001). *The world health report 2001: mental health: new understanding, new hope*. World Health Organization, Geneva.
2. Costello, E.J., Egger, H., and Angold, A. (2005). 10-year research update review: the epidemiology of child and adolescent psychiatric disorders: I. Methods and public health burden. *Journal of the American Academy of Child and Adolescent Psychiatry*, **44**(10), 972–86.
3. Kessler, R.C., Berglund, P., Demler, O., *et al.* (2005). Lifetime prevalence and age-of-onset distributions of DSM-IV disorders in the National Comorbidity Survey Replication. *Archives of General Psychiatry*, **62**(6), 593–602.
4. Mrazek, P.B. and Haggerty, R.J. (1994). *Institute of Medicine (U.S.). Committee on prevention of mental disorders, United States. Congress. Reducing risks for mental disorders: frontiers for preventive intervention research*. National Academy Press, Washington, DC.
5. WHO. (2004). *Prevention of mental disorders: effective interventions and policy options summary report*. World Health Organization, Geneva.
6. WHO. (2004). *Promoting mental health: concepts, emerging evidence, practice*. World Health Organization, Geneva.
7. HMSO. (1992). *The health of the nation: a summary of the strategy for health in England*. HMSO, London.
8. WHO. (2001). *Basic documents*. World Health Organization, Geneva.
9. Detels, R. (2002). *Oxford textbook of public health* (4th edn). Oxford University Press, Oxford, New York.
10. Tulchinsky, T.H. and Varavikova, E. (2000). *The new public health: an introduction for the 21st century*, In (eds. K. Rhoshel, and M.D. Lenroot). *Child Psychiatry Branch*, National Institute of Mental Health, pp. 5–54. Academic Press, San Diego.
11. World Health Organization. (1993). *The ICD-10 classification of mental and behavioural disorders: diagnostic criteria for research*. World Health Organization, Geneva.
12. American Psychiatric Association. (2000). *Task force on DSM-IV. Diagnostic and statistical manual of mental disorders: DSM-IV-TR* (4th edn). American Psychiatric Association, Washington, DC.
13. Costello, F.J and Angold, A. (2009). *Epidemiology of psychiatric disorder in Chilood and adolecence*. In *New Oxford Textbook od Psychiatry* (2nd edn.) (eds. M.G. Gelder, N.C. Andreasen, J.J. López-I bor Jr, and J.R. Geddes)
14. Kraemer, H.C., Stice, E., Kazdin, A., *et al.* (2001). How do risk factors work together? Mediators, moderators, and independent, overlapping, and proxy risk factors. *The American Journal of Psychiatry*, **158**(6), 848–56.
15. Rutter, M. and Sroufe, L.A. (2000). Developmental psychopathology: concepts and challenges. *Development and Psychopathology*, **12**(3), 265–96.
16. Greenberg, M.T., Domitrovich, C., and Bumbarger, B. (2001). The prevention of mental disorders in school-aged children: current state of the field. *Prevention & Treatment*, **4**(1), 1–62.
17. Coie, J.D., Watt, N.F., West, S.G., *et al.* (1993). The science of prevention. A conceptual framework and some directions for a national research program. *The American Psychologist*, **48**(10), 1013–22.
18. Flay, B.R., Biglan, A., Boruch, R.F., *et al.* (2005). Standards of evidence: criteria for efficacy, effectiveness and dissemination. *Prevention Science: The Official Journal of the Society for Prevention Research*, **6**(3), 151–75.
19. Durlak, J.A. and Wells, A.M. (1997). Primary prevention mental health programs for children and adolescents: a meta-analytic review. *American Journal of Community Psychology*, **25**(2), 115–52.
20. Commission on Chronic Illness. (1957). *Chronic illness in the United States*. Harvard University Press, Cambridge, MA.
21. Gordon, R.S., Jr. (1983). An operational classification of disease prevention. *Public Health Reports*, **98**(2), 107–9.
22. Cowen, E.L. and Durlak, J.A. (2000). Social policy and prevention in mental health. *Development and Psychopathology*, **12**(4), 815–34.
23. Cuijpers, P. (2003). Examining the effects of prevention programs on the incidence of new cases of mental disorders: the lack of statistical power. *The American Journal of Psychiatry*, **160**(8), 1385–91.
24. Clarke, G.N., Hornbrook, M., Lynch, F., *et al.* (2001). A randomized trial of a group cognitive intervention for preventing depression in adolescent offspring of depressed parents. *Archives of General Psychiatry*, **58**(12), 1127–34.
25. McGorry, P.D., Yung, A.R., Phillips, L.J., *et al.* (2002). Randomized controlled trial of interventions designed to reduce the risk of progression to first-episode psychosis in a clinical sample with subthreshold symptoms. *Archives of General Psychiatry*, **59**(10), 921–8.

# 9.2

# Clinical syndromes

## Contents

9.2.1 Neuropsychiatric disorders
James C. Harris

9.2.2 Specific developmental disorders in childhood
and adolescence
Helmut Remschmidt and Gerd Schulte-Körne

9.2.3 Autism and the pervasive
developmental disorders
Fred R. Volkmar and Ami Klin

9.2.4 Attention deficit and hyperkinetic disorders
in childhood and adolescence
Eric Taylor

9.2.5 Conduct disorders in
childhood and adolescence
Stephen Scott

9.2.6 Anxiety disorders in
childhood and adolescence
Daniel S. Pine

9.2.7 Paediatric mood disorders
David Brent and Boris Birmaher

9.2.8 Obsessive–compulsive disorder and
tics in children and adolescents
Martine F. Flament and Philippe Robaey

9.2.9 Sleep disorders in children and adolescents
Gregory Stores

9.2.10 Suicide and attempted suicide in
children and adolescents
David Shaffer, Cynthia R. Pfeffer, and
Jennifer Gutstein

9.2.11 Children's speech and language
difficulties
Judy Clegg

9.2.12 Gender identity disorder in
children and adolescents
Richard Green

*Note* Substance abuse is considered in Part 4, Section 4.12. Aspects relevant to young people are considered within the chapters of this section.

## 9.2.1 Neuropsychiatric disorders

James C. Harris

### The developmental perspective

Developmental neuropsychiatry addresses the neurobiological basis of behaviour in infants, children, and adolescents with neurodevelopmental disorders and in those with brain damage occurring during the developmental period. As a field, it includes the aetiology, diagnosis, and treatment of behavioural, emotional, interpersonal, and psychiatric disorders.[1, 2] The parent's response, adjustment to, and involvement in treatment is a critical element in outcome.

The developmental neuropsychiatrist utilizes a developmental perspective that focuses on the developing person who is active, socially oriented, and emerging rather than passively responding to the environment. The adaptive plasticity of the developing nervous system to change is emphasized, and the essential role of environmental experience in brain development is acknowledged. When working with the affected child, an effort is made to provide the supports needed to facilitate the mastery of age-appropriate developmental tasks always keeping in mind the child's individual capacities and strengths.

### Scope of developmental neuropsychiatry

The scope of developmental neuropsychiatry is broad[2] and includes the following.

1 Neurodevelopmental disorders that are described in other chapters of this book, including attention-deficit and hyperactivity disorders (Chapter 9.2.4), pervasive developmental disorders and childhood-onset schizophrenia (Chapter 9.2.3), obsessive–compulsive disorder and Tourette's syndrome (Chapter 9.2.8), and specific developmental disorders (Chapter 9.2.2).

2 Neurogenetic disorders, both cytogenetic and metabolic, with behavioural phenotypes, several of which are also reviewed in Chapter 10.4.

3 Teratogenic exposure from both organic and inorganic toxins. In these instances, behavioural dysfunction may result from gestational substance abuse with alcohol and other substances or exposure to inorganic metals.

4 Endocrinopathies.

5 Traumatic brain injury.

6 Other neurological disorders (e.g. epilepsy).

## Clinical features

### Neurodevelopmental disorders

Developmental psychopathology applies developmental concepts to the study of neurodevelopmental disorders. The relationship of disordered to non-disordered behaviour is considered, as are the early origins of maladaptive behaviours that may not appear in clinical form until adolescence or adulthood. Knowledge of normal development is utilized to study children whose development is atypical, in order to understand the natural history of their disorder and establish the developmental trajectory of that particular condition. Conversely, the investigation of such deviant behaviour associated with a particular disorder is considered in regard to our understanding of normal development. For example, attention-deficit hyperactivity disorder has been investigated as a disorder of executive functions of the prefrontal cortex, and autistic disorder as a disorder of social cognition and communication. In both instances, new knowledge about brain functions has been derived from these formulations. Among the neurodevelopmental disorders, the age of recognition varies, multiple causes are involved, and many transformations in behaviour may occur in determining their complex course. The goal is to understand the mechanisms and processes through which risk factors lead to the emergence of a disorder. Disordered behaviour is not viewed as a static condition, but is considered as part of a dynamic transactional engagement. Behaviour and development are viewed within a social context, and the transactional nature of interactions is considered from infancy through adulthood to understand these processes.

Attention-deficit hyperactivity disorder, pervasive developmental disorders, obsessive–compulsive disorder, Tourette's syndrome, and childhood-onset schizophrenia are developmental neuropsychiatric disorders under active investigation and each is reviewed in the respective chapters. Their developmental psychopathology is investigated by addressing the origins and course of individual patterns of behavioural maladaptation in each of these disorders and determining their genetic bases, thought to be complex, and involving more than one gene. Information derived from genetics, developmental psychology, clinical psychology, psychiatry, sociology, physiological sciences, neurosciences, and epidemiology is included in the description of each of these disorders.

The interrelationship of the various child neuropsychiatric disorders is an important consideration. Disorders may be risk factors for other conditions, so that attention-deficit disorder may be a risk factor for conduct disorder. In this instance, the child's behaviour affects the adult and the transactional interactions between child and adult may result in further disruptive behaviours. Moreover, there may be a developmental basis for disorders whose full presentation is not evident until later in life, as is the case with schizophrenia—generally considered to be a disorder of late adolescence or early adult life, but with origins in the developmental period.[3] Some disorders may have co-occurring diagnoses that influence their outcome, as in Tourette's syndrome, where co-occurring conditions may determine the behavioural presentation. In Tourette's syndrome, obsessive–compulsive symptoms may be an aspect of 'pure' Tourette's syndrome, while co-occurring disruptive behaviour may be secondary to co-occurring attention-deficit disorder. Social and behavioural dysfunction in children with Tourette's syndrome is largely ADHD-specific. Children with TS alone have a different social-emotional profile.[4–6] Compulsive behaviours may not only interfere with the normal routines for the affected child but also become particularly problematic for their impact on other family members.

### Neurogenetic syndromes with behavioural phenotypes

Particular patterns of behaviour, temperament, and psychopathology may be associated with specific chromosomal and genetic disorders.[2,5,7–9] The term 'behavioural phenotype' was introduced by Nyhan in 1972[7,10] to describe patterns of unusual behaviour that are so characteristic that they suggest a specific neurogenetic disorder. Nyhan described stereotypical patterns of behaviour occurring in syndromic fashion in sizeable numbers of affected individuals with a given syndrome, and observed that these patterns seemed self-programmed. In these children, he proposed that it is reasonable to hypothesize that their behaviours are associated with an abnormal neuroanatomy and that such stereotypical patterns of unusual behaviour could reflect the presence of structural deficits in the central nervous system. Recent developments in the neurosciences provide a means to investigate the biological bases of behavioural phenotypes. Behavioural assessments, neuropsychological testing, and neuroimaging procedures, carried out in well-characterized genetic syndromes, are being utilized to understand pathways from genes to cognition and complex behaviours in these conditions.

Comprehensive study of children with different neurogenetic disorders may increase our appreciation for the relative contribution of genetic variables in the pathogenesis of specific, affective, and behavioural disorders. Behavioural phenotypes have been studied most extensively in Down syndrome (language),[11] fragile X syndrome (gaze aversion, hyperkinesia, autistic-like behaviour),[12] Williams syndrome (sociability, hyperverbal behaviour, and visuospatial deficits),[13,14] Lesch–Nyhan syndrome (compulsive self-injury and aggression),[15–17] and Prader–Willi syndrome (hyperphagia, obsessive–compulsive behaviour).[13,18,19] The number of identifiable behavioural phenotypes is growing with careful observations of behaviours in neurogenetic disorders.[8,9] Besides behaviours, particular temperamental features have also been considered in these disorders. However, when studying temperament, the appropriate measures must be chosen. For example, when Down syndrome, proposed to be linked to a particular temperament, was studied using temperamental clusters of easy temperament, slow to warm-up, and difficult temperament, Gunn et al.[20] demonstrated both easy and difficult temperament in children with Down syndrome; therefore, a typical temperamental pattern among these three categories was not demonstrated. However, when a more comprehensive assessment was carried out in other syndromes[21] (that included the personality factors of extraversion, agreeableness, conscientiousness, emotional stability, and openness, along with motor activity and irritability), specific personality phenotypes were identified. These were differentially related to parental behaviours and family context in Prader–Willi, fragile X, and Williams syndromes. Moreover, isolated special abilities, as in calculation and in music,[22] are recognizable that might be considered as phenotypes and linked to the proposed modular organization of the central nervous system. Finally, physical and behavioural phenotypes are not only identified in neurogenetic syndromes but also in those caused by environmental events, such as intrauterine exposure to alcohol: namely, the foetal alcohol syndrome. Because alcoholism is a familial disorder, there may vulnerability to its effects resulting in a severe presentation in some individuals and less severe presentation in others.[23]

Both traditional Mendelian laws of inheritance (Lesch–Nyhan syndrome) and non-traditional inheritance have been identified in conditions with behavioural phenotypes. Among the non-traditional forms of inheritance are triplet repeat amplification (fragile X syndrome), microdeletion or contiguous gene deletion (Williams syndrome), imprinting (Prader–Willi syndrome), transcriptional derepression (Rett's syndrome), and excessive gene dosage (Down syndrome). A key finding is the recognition that mutations of single genes can lead to complex behavioural symptoms, especially if the affected protein is essential for the expression or processing of multiple 'downstream' genes.

Behavioural phenotypes are also discussed in relation to intellectual disability in Chapter 10.5.1.

### Neurobehavioural teratology

Neurobehavioural teratology investigates abnormal development of the nervous system and of cognition and complex behaviour that results from prenatal environmental insults. Neurobehavioural research addresses the prevalence of cognitive behavioural disorders in exposed individuals and the consequences of the brain insult on other developing brain systems, to identify risks for functional or behavioural deficits. Investigators focus on cognitive behavioural deficits and their underlying anatomy and embryology. Assessment emphasizes not only IQ but also neuropsychological profiles, because learning disability or difficulty in visuomotor integration may be evident in children who function in the low to average range of general mental ability.

The natural history of intrauterine drug exposure on motor, cognitive, emotional, and social behaviour is an area of growing concern. Multiple drug exposures during pregnancy are common among substance-abusing mothers. Of syndromes associated with intrauterine substance abuse, alcohol abuse has been studied the most extensively. Subsequently, retinoids, anticonvulsants (lithium, tegretol, and valproic acid), and the selective serotonin-reuptake inhibitors have also been studied. Other teratogens do not lead to major malformations of the nervous systems but they do compromise its integrity (for example, lead, heroin, methadone), and are associated with neurotoxic damage or effects on neurochemical systems.

The greatest period of vulnerability to drugs in a human pregnancy is during the period of embryogenesis (days 14 to 60). During embryogenesis, many neurobehavioural teratogens (for instance, retinoids and ethanol) produce syndromes with abnormalities that involve craniofacial, neural, and major organ systems. Behavioural abnormalities without detectable physical abnormality can occur when the insult occurs during the foetal period.

The extent of malformation is stage-specific and dose-dependent, with outcomes ranging from death with malformation, malformation and survival, effects on growth, and cognitive–neuropsychological or behaviour disorder. The same exposure to alcohol needed to produce cognitive behavioural change in the foetal period would generally cause malformation if it occurred during embryogenesis. The term 'developmental toxicology' is sometimes used if the insult occurs in the postnatal period.

There may be a genetic vulnerability that influences the extent of expression of response to environmental toxins in an individual. A common family of regulatory genes is involved in the formation of structures of the face, head, hindbrain, parts of the heart, and thymus gland, all of which share a common origin from neural crest cells (anterior neural tube). These regulatory genes, known as HOX genes, provide rules for assembling various structures and for determining particular anatomical segments.[24] Homozygous HOXA1 mutations have been shown to disrupt human brainstem, inner ear, cardiovascular and cognitive development. Because the retinoid family is involved in controlling these HOX genes,[25] a similar pattern is produced by excessive retinoid administration, as in hypervitaminosis of vitamin A (retinol). Moreover, the enzyme alcohol dehydrogenase functions in the metabolism of both retinol and ethanol so that intoxicating levels of ethanol can competitively inhibit the metabolism of retinol and impact brain development. Thus, both genetic and teratogenetic agents may produce similar developmental abnormalities. Understanding these mechanisms helps to understand how an abnormal facial appearance may suggest an abnormal brain.

## Foetal alcohol spectrum disorder syndrome

Foetal alcohol syndrome is one of the most commonly recognized causes of intellectual disability; one that is preventable if recommended guidelines regarding alcohol use are followed by mothers.[26]

### Clinical features

Children with the full foetal alcohol syndrome demonstrate prenatal and postnatal growth deficiency, microcephaly, infantile irritability, mild to moderate intellectual disability, and a characteristic facial appearance.[23] The extent of the abnormality depends on the time of maximal exposure to alcohol and the dose. Approximately half of those affected have co-ordination problems, are hypotonic, and have attention deficits. Between 20 and 50 per cent have other birth defects, including eye and ear anomalies and cardiac anomalies. Those children who do not show growth retardation or congenital anomalies may show more subtle changes, such as attention problems, disruptive behaviour, reduced speed of information processing, motor clumsiness, speech disorders, fine motor impairment, and learning problems, especially in mathematics.[23,27] These findings have been documented in a prospective longitudinal study of the effects of prenatal alcohol exposure on a birth cohort of 500 offspring who were selected from 1529 consecutive pregnant women in prenatal care in community hospitals.[28] Dose-dependent effects are most clear from the neurobehavioural status of subjects when regular neurodevelopmental evaluations are carried out from birth to age 14 years. The more subtle abnormalities are referred to as 'foetal alcohol effects', or alcohol-related neurodevelopmental disorder. The full range of disabilities is described as foetal alcohol spectrum disorder.[27]

Subjects with average to above-average IQ may demonstrate neuropsychological deficits in complex attention, verbal learning, and executive functioning. Disruptive behaviour, attention-deficit disorder, anxiety disorder, and communication disorder have been described[29,31,33] in children with foetal alcohol syndrome and foetal alcohol spectrum disorder who test in the low normal range and in the moderate to severe range of intellectual disability.

### Behavioural phenotype

The behavioural phenotype is characterized by problems in cognitive functioning, academic problems in arithmetic, difficulty with abstractions, understanding cause and effect, and generalizing from one situation to another. Thus, inattention, poor concentration, impaired judgement, memory deficits, and problems in abstract reasoning are characteristic. Behavioural problems related to impulsivity and hyperactivity makes them vulnerable to later diagnoses of oppositional defiant and conduct disorder.[27,30]

### Natural history

Foetal alcohol spectrum disorder is not only a childhood disorder; the cognitive and behavioural effects and psychosocial problems may persist throughout adolescence into adulthood.[28,33] Although the facial features are not as distinctive after puberty and the growth deficiency is not as apparent as in the younger child, the central nervous system effects do persist throughout life. Approximately 50 per cent of those affected function as intellectually disabled persons. Moreover, adaptive behavioural problems in communication skills and in socialization are apparent in those with foetal alcohol spectrum disorder whose intelligence test scores are in the normal range.

Poor judgement, attention problems, distractibility, difficulty in recognizing common social cues, and problems in modulating mood continue as characteristic features. Family environmental problems often continue as risk factors for behavioural problems if there is a lack of stability in family life. In one follow-up study[34] that used structured interviews with non-intellectually disabled affected subjects, the most common diagnoses were alcohol or drug dependence, mood disorders, and personality disorders (especially passive aggressive or antisocial). Further follow-up is needed to investigate the mechanisms involved in these psychiatric presentations, and particularly in determining the pathways leading to alcoholism.

### Epidemiology

Foetal alcohol syndrome is a common cause of neuropsychiatric disorders, with a worldwide incidence of approximately 1.9 in 1000 live births. When foetal alcohol syndrome and alcohol-related neurodevelopmental disorder are considered together, the combined rate in one study conducted in the United States was 9.1 in 1000.[35] Despite its frequency and severity, the syndrome may go unrecognized because physicians may not systematically enquire about alcohol use and may not recognize the spectrum of the effects of prenatal alcohol exposure on neurodevelopment.

### Aetiology

The amount and pattern of alcohol consumption and the trimester of use during pregnancy, especially if during critical periods of brain development, are major factors in determining outcome.

Binge drinking patterns with high blood concentrations are especially deleterious. Rapid changes in alcohol concentrations in the blood and central nervous system cause apoptotic damage (cell degeneration) in developing neurons and other cells in rat models.[36] Microcephaly is commonly reported in foetal alcohol syndrome and suggests an underdevelopment of the brain. Neuropathological studies demonstrate the underdevelopment or absence of the corpus callosum and enlarged lateral ventricles. Dendritic changes have been observed in animals with prenatal exposure to alcohol; these changes were correlated with decreased learning ability. Magnetic resonance imaging studies have documented brain abnormalities in foetal alcohol syndrome, particularly in midline frontal structures such as the corpus collosum.[37,38] Research to identify specific polymorphisms contributing to foetal alcohol spectrum disorder is at an early stage. Polymorphisms of only one of the genes for the alcohol dehydrogenase enzyme family, the ADH1B, have been demonstrated to contribute to vulnerability.[39]

### Treatment

#### (a) Evidence

Mothers of children with foetal alcohol syndrome who drank more alcohol and drank excessively early in gestation have more severe clinical features. Alcohol use in late pregnancy is primarily associated with prematurity and infants who are small for gestational age, rather than with the full foetal alcohol syndrome. Because of these risks, treatment must begin with prevention.[32] There is no clearly agreed safe dose of alcohol for pregnant women. Because there is no known safe amount of alcohol consumption during pregnancy, it is recommended that women who are pregnant or who are planning a pregnancy abstain from drinking alcohol. Special efforts for educating women of child-bearing age are required that highlight the harmful effects of alcohol; identified children must be referred for early educational services.

#### (b) Management

A comprehensive treatment programme begins with parental acknowledgement of the aetiology of foetal alcohol syndrome or spectrum disorder and treatment for the parent, as indicated, for alcohol misuse and abuse. Parental counselling should include discussion of the physical and behavioural phenotype. The family should be advised about the need for special educational programmes and assisted in behavioural management. Family therapy is often required to help family members cope with the developmental disorder. Appropriate educational and behavioural treatment resources are needed to address the social deficits, particularly in those cases where disruptive behaviour, attention-deficit disorder and mood disorders are identified.

Foetal alcohol syndrome is also considered as a cause of intellectual disability in Chapter 10.4.

## Gestational substance abuse

### Opiates

Exposure to heroin and methadone ranges from a neonatal withdrawal syndrome to less predictable long-term outcomes.[40] An impoverished environment may have disproportionate adverse effects on methadone-exposed children when compared to unexposed children.[41] Methadone effects have been associated with increased body tension, poor motor co-ordination, and delay in motor skills acquisition.[42] However, the effects on mental development are less clear, but they do affect the child-rearing environment. Since methadone exposure produces an increased vulnerability to the effects of poor parent–infant relationships, these relationships require careful monitoring.

## Cocaine

Cocaine is a central nervous system stimulant that inhibits nerve conduction in the peripheral nervous system. Cocaine is metabolized primarily through the plasma cholinesterase system, with the primary metabolic product being benzoylecgonine. Since cocaine rapidly crosses the placenta by simple diffusion, foetal peak blood levels are reached as quickly as 3 min.[43] Having crossed the placenta in the foetus, cocaine has the same direct actions on the foetal cardiovascular system as seen in the maternal system. These cardiac changes involve the direct effects of cocaine, as well as indirect effects such as foetal hypoxia. Cocaine may lead to placental dysfunction (via vasocontracture effects), structural changes (via vascular compromise), and neurobehavioural abnormalities (via postsynaptic junction neurotoxicity).

Infant gestational age, birth weight, head circumference, and length have been found to be decreased in affected infants, and low birth weight is a frequent finding in studies of the offspring of cocaine-using women. In addition to abnormal growth patterns, congenital anomalies involving the genitourinary tract, heart, and central nervous system as well as limb-reduction abnormalities have been reported. A potential mechanism for all these anomalies appears to be interruption of the intrauterine blood supply, with subsequent disruption of embryonic development. Although approximately 25 to 30 per cent of infants exposed to cocaine *in utero* may have physical difficulties, overall neurobehavioural problems may be more common, and most apparent in early infancy and childhood.[40, 44] In one large study, at age 4 years, prenatal cocaine exposure was not associated with lower full-scale, verbal, or performance IQ scores but was associated with an increased risk for specific cognitive impairments. A better home environment was associated with IQ scores for cocaine-exposed children that are similar to scores in non-exposed children. Although irritability and problems in state regulation are reported in infants and impulsive behaviour in pre-school children, these behaviours diminish over time with behavioural and psychosocial interventions.[45] Child abuse is closely linked to substance abuse.

## Treatment

These findings suggest that careful attention be paid to the postnatal home-rearing environment of children who are exposed to drugs *in utero*. Overall, the treatment programme must take into account physical and psychological change secondary to intrauterine drug use as well as the postnatal nurturing environment. Both substance use and psychiatric disorder in the parents must be considered, because parents with attention-deficit disorder and mood disorders may themselves self-medicate with cocaine. Without early intervention, special school programmes, behavioural management programmes, and a structured day programme will be necessary. Ongoing parent training is also required.[40, 42]

## Endocrinopathies
### Congenital hypothyroidism

Congenital hypothyroidism is associated with intellectual disablity and may be associated with decreased motor activity at birth, hoarse cry, and difficulty with feeding. It is rarely diagnosed at birth from clinical assessment alone, but it is recognized from newborn screening tests with confirmation by measurement in blood samples. Symptoms of hypothyroidism may not be clearly detected until the second month of life. The overall prevalence is 1 in 4000 live births. Neurological and learning disorders associated with untreated congenital hypothyroidism include attention-deficits, hearing loss, speech defects, ataxia, and abnormal muscle tone.[46] Rapid diagnosis in infancy is essential to prevent these complications. Without treatment, severe neurological dysfunction ensues. With initiation of oral thyroid hormone treatment (levothyroxine in a single daily dose of 8 to 10 μg/kg per day) in the first 6 weeks of life, IQ is in the normal range. If treatment is delayed until 3 to 6 months, IQ drops to an average of 75, and, if initiated after 6 weeks, to an IQ of 55 or less. Rearing environment is important in long-term outcome. Despite early treatment there still may be enduring cognitive and motor deficits in young adults.[47]

## Traumatic brain injury

Traumatic brain injury is defined as physical damage or impairment in function of the brain as a consequence of the application of acute mechanical force. Other causes of brain injury result from birth trauma, poisoning, or asphyxia. Traumatic brain injury is a major cause of death and disability among children, adolescents, and young adults, and is one of the most common causes of chronic brain syndromes in childhood. Traumatic head injury is common and becoming increasingly more so.

### Clinical features
#### (a) Cognitive and behavioural

The most common long-term outcomes of traumatic brain injury are cognitive and behavioural changes. Immediately after emerging from a coma, the child will be unable to form new memories. The time, from the accident to the time when new memories emerge, is referred to as post-traumatic amnesia. The length of coma and the duration of post-traumatic amnesia are especially important in regard to the extent of cognitive recovery. Moreover, there is a strong inverse relationship between subsequent IQ and duration of coma. The persistence of cognitive deficits is correlated with the duration of post-traumatic amnesia; the more persistent deficits follow more than 3 weeks of post-traumatic amnesia. Persistent verbal memory impairment is reported as long as 10 years after injury in up to one-quarter of those studied. Psychiatric symptoms in adults occurs more often following focal frontal-lobe traumatic brain injury than injury to other cerebral areas. In children, Rutter[48,49] reported behavioural disinhibition after severe closed traumatic brain injury characterized by over-talkativeness, ignoring social conventions, impulsiveness, and poor personal hygiene.

#### (b) Psychiatric

Psychiatric outcomes can be divided into those that occur during the early phases of recovery and those that occur later. The earliest psychiatric sequelae are found before the termination of post-traumatic amnesia. During this time, behavioural and affective symptoms are linked to the neurological presentation. The most common psychiatric diagnosis is delirium. Symptoms include short attention span, agitation, hallucinations, and disturbances in the sleep–wake cycle.

Subsequent occurrence of post-traumatic psychiatric symptoms is linked to the severity of the injury, its location, the child's behavioural and emotional features prior to the accident, and the psychosocial interactions of the family members during the recovery phases. The more severe the traumatic brain injury, the greater the likelihood of psychiatric sequelae. All children in one prospective study of severely injured children who had premorbid psychiatric conditions showed post-traumatic psychiatric disorders.[50,51] Moreover, over half the children in this group who had no premorbid symptoms prior to the accident had developed psychiatric symptoms during a 28-month, follow-up period. The greatest premorbid risks for psychiatric disorder were previous difficulties with impulse control and disruptive behaviour. In addition, a prior history of family dysfunction increased the risk for later symptomatology. The range of disorders includes attention-deficit hyperactivity disorder,[52] disruptive behaviour[53] post-traumatic mood disorders (both depressive and manic symptoms), post-traumatic stress disorder,[54] and family dysfunction.[55, 56] Transient psychotic features may occur. Hallucinations tend to be less bizarre and more concrete than the typical hallucination in schizophrenia. Moreover, head injury in childhood may accelerate the expression of schizophrenia in families where there is strong genetic predisposition[57] Injuries involving focal frontal-lobe dysfunction are associated with impulsive aggression and behavioural dyscontrol,[58] most often following focal orbitofrontal injury. The rate of actual aggression is less than often assumed. When forensic issues are considered regarding violent behaviour each case should be evaluated individually taking into account the type of head injury and other risk factors especially a history of physical abuse.

## Classification—types of traumatic brain injury

Neurological damage associated with head trauma can be produced in several ways. Traumatic brain injury is classified as open or closed; these types differ in the pattern of injury and neurobehavioural outcome. Open refers to penetration of the skull, as in a depressed skull fracture or bullet wound, the extent depending on the regions damaged by contusion or cerebral oedema. Closed head injury results from acceleration and deceleration of the brain within the hard skull; this often leads to contusion of the brain from a sudden impact and may result in subarachnoid haemorrhage. Different parts of the brain have different densities, and therefore shearing stresses that develop during rapid brain movement cause injury. Furthermore, compression of blood vessels against the falx cerebri or tentorium may result in infarction of the areas, which these blood vessels supply. Penetrating traumatic brain injury causes specific and direct loss of neural tissue.

## Epidemiology

It is estimated that 185 children per 100 000 from infancy to 14 years of age and 295 per 100 000 adolescents and young adults aged between 15 and 24 are hospitalized each year for traumatic brain injury.[59] The risk is highest among the 15- to 19-year-olds where the rate is 550 per 100 000.[60] The incidence in paediatric populations is similar to that in adults. In the United Kingdom the rates for those under 16 years is approximately 45 000, with about 300 deaths each year.[61] A mortality rate of 10 per 100 000 makes head trauma a major cause of death in children, but the death rate is still less than that in adults. There is no difference in the death rate between boys and girls before the age of 5 years, but after this age males are four times more likely to die than females. Approximately 90 per cent of head injuries are mild.[61] Falls and transport injuries make-up the majority of cases. Inflicted traumatic brain injury from physical abuse is a growing concern especially of repeated injuries. A US statewide population based study found the incidence of inflicted traumatic brain injury to be 17 per 100 000 person-years in the first 2 years of life with the highest incidence in infants during their first year (30/100 00). The rate was higher in boys than girls.[62]

## Aetiology

The causes of traumatic brain injury are different depending on the age of the child. The incidence is twice as high in males as in females, and children who live in poor psychosocial circumstances are at greater risk. Traumatic brain injury from child abuse occurs in infancy: in the pre-school years the most common cause is falls; in early elementary school, it is pedestrian accidents. From 10 to 14 years of age there is an increase in sports and bicycle accidents, but by 15 years motor vehicle accidents and violent assault are the most common. Risk factors include poverty, single-parent homes, congested living arrangements, and a parental history of psychiatry disorder.

A common complication of traumatic brain injury is cerebral oedema, but there are other complications such as infection and haematoma formation both inside and outside the brain. These complications result in neurological deficits that may be extensive. Furthermore, compensatory mechanisms that are involved in recovery from head trauma may alter brain function. A child who has suffered a traumatic brain injury is likely to experience both neurological and psychiatric difficulties depending on the brain regions involved. Multiple mechanisms lead to psychological symptom formation—both psychosocial and physiological factors are involved.

## Course and prognosis

The level of consciousness, degree of somatic injury, extent and duration of post-traumatic amnesia, severity of head injury, and degree of neurocognitive dysfunction in the early post-trauma period are important in determining outcome. Children who experience severe traumatic brain injury usually follow a predictable postoperative course.[48] As previously noted, landmarks for recovery are associated with the time of emergence from coma and the time of emergence from post-traumatic amnesia. The emergence from coma is most often defined as the point at which the patient is able to follow simple verbal commands. Concurrently, visual tracking of objects in the environment may be observed.

Post-traumatic amnesia ends when the child is able to form new memories. The frequency of post-traumatic amnesia is probably related to concurrent injury to the temporal lobes associated with the head trauma. However, older memories may be recalled that do not involve the temporal lobe. The hippocampus has a central role in the formation of new memories. Besides recovery from post-traumatic amnesia, another form of memory loss-retrograde amnesia-for events that took place before the accident, typically becomes shorter and shorter during the recovery process. It is important to remember that children with severe head trauma will rarely have specific memories of the accident itself. Overall, the most important milestones in recovery for future outcome are the length of coma and the duration of post-traumatic amnesia.

### Treatment

#### (a) Evidence

Most mild head injury and post concussive problems will resolve without treatment. When there are ongoing symptoms, parents and teachers must adjust expectations depending on the extent of injury. Complete recovery of all brain functions following severe brain injury is rarely accomplished. Still, if recovery is defined as a reduction in impairments in behavioural and physiological functions over time then changes do occur so that, typically, there is recovery of function together with a fair amount of substitution of function. Mechanisms include resolution of brain swelling (oedema), resolution of damage to other brain regions damaged through shock (diaschisis), changes in the structure of the nervous system (plasticity), and regrowth of neural tissue (regeneration). The extent of recovery depends on the severity of the injury, the number of times injured, the age at the time of injury, premorbid cognitive status, extent to which loss functions can be subsumed under other systems, integrity of other parts of the brain, individual brain structures, motivation, emotional considerations, and the quality of rehabilitation programme.[63, 64]

Although children and adolescents tend to have a better outcome after severe traumatic brain injury than those over the age of 21, the adult brain has greater plasticity than previously considered. Despite this general rule, children who are younger than 7 years may have a worse outcome since they may be at increased risk of child abuse as a cause of injury which may be particularly traumatic. Furthermore, younger children may have a worse outcome based on the global effects of trauma on the developing brain. The duration of recovery of significant neuropsychological, behavioural, and emotional deficits may last several years following injury. These higher cognitive deficits lead to the major disability observed with traumatic brain injury.

#### (b) Management

Partial recovery of function can and does occur over time, not only in children but also in adults. Intervention through retraining and the use of cognitive memory aids is targeted to improve areas of cognitive functioning such as memory, attention, language, and perception.[63] Even though partial recovery does occur after various types of brain injury, there is variability in the extent of recovery.

### Possibilities for prevention

The most important primary injury prevention activities focus on teaching safe behaviour, the use of seat belts in cars, and wearing helmets when riding horses, bicycles, or motorcycles. Once an injury has occurred both anticipatory guidance, which teaches the family and child what to expect, and preventive intervention strategies are necessary. Early and focused rehabilitation procedures coupled with medication for associated psychiatric disorder,

behaviour management, supportive therapy for families, and appropriate school programmes are necessary to prevent behavioural and psychiatric complications.

## Epilepsy

Epilepsy refers to recurrent seizures that are idiopathic (of unknown aetiology) or due to congenital or acquired brain lesions. Epilepsy is the symptomatic expression of brain pathology or disordered brain function and is not a disease in itself. The symptom complex is episodic and associated with an excessive self-limiting neuronal discharge. The seizure is a frightening experience for parents and they require support and guidance. Epilepsy impacts the whole family and can create problems for all family members.[65]

### Clinical features and clinical course

Complex partial seizures involving the temporal and frontal lobe is the most common condition where complex neurological and psychiatric symptoms are seen in the same person. Complex symptoms include behavioural automatisms, perceptual alterations, changes in affect and memory, distorted thinking, and hallucinations[66] Forms occurring in infancy and childhood include temporal lobe epilepsy, frontal-lobe epilepsy, infantile spasms, Lennox–Gastaut syndrome, Landau–Kleffner syndrome, and benign focal epilepsy.[67]

Children with partial seizures and electroencephalographic evidence of frontal involvement have more severe formal thought disorders and deficits in communication discourse than those with temporal involvement. Because these seizures are rare in children, reports of symptoms are primarily found in case reports. For example, Saygi et al.[68] and Stores et al.[69] have described sexual disinhibition, pressured and tangential speech, screaming, aggression, disorganized behaviour, and nightmares in affected children.

Frontal-lobe epilepsy should be considered if there are episodes of brief sudden unresponsiveness without loss of consciousness. These episodes occur with continued understanding of spoken language and clonic or tonic motor phenomena involving the face and arms bilaterally. Laughing, crying, pedalling movements, and sexual automatisms may also suggest this diagnosis. A normal electroencephalograph does not rule out the diagnosis. Left frontal hypometabolism on positron-emission tomography scanning or reduced cerebral blood flow to the frontal area, although not diagnostic, support this diagnosis.

The Lennox–Gastaut syndrome is characterized by early onset of intractable seizures and bilateral slow spike-wave complexes on the EEG.[70] The onset is typically between the ages of 1 and 7 years. The seizure pattern includes tonic, generalized tonic–clonic, atypical absence, atonic, and myoclonic seizures. Approximately half of children with the Lennox–Gastaut syndrome test as intellectually disabled. Marked language delay, overactivity, and irritability are characteristic. However, these behavioural symptoms may improve with seizure control. Ultimately, the diagnosis is based on the characteristic EEG finding of interictal slow spike-wave discharges in children with the early onset of poorly controlled seizures and a developmental disorder. In some instances, there is prolonged minor status epilepticus. Such episodes may last for several weeks during which the child engages in a variety of everyday activities but is socially unresponsive, aggressive, less articulate, and has minor twitching of the face and hands. This presentation must be differentiated from a psychiatric disorder.

## Classification

Classification of epileptic seizures utilizes both clinical and electroencephalographic features.[71] The current classification divides seizures into two categories: partial and generalized. Partial seizures involve one cerebral hemisphere, in part or totally. They begin focally, although they may become generalized. Consciousness is preserved but cognitive functions may be transiently impaired: for example, speech may be impaired if the dominant hemisphere is affected. Partial seizures are further subdivided into those with simple or complex symptomatology. In children, simple complex seizures are most often simple motor or sensory phenomena. Complex partial seizures usually begin in temporal or frontal-lobe structures. It is this group that is particularly important to psychiatrists.

## Diagnosis and differential diagnosis

Epilepsy is a clinical rather than a laboratory diagnosis, and diagnostic errors most commonly occur due to inadequate history and physical examination. The accuracy of diagnosis has improved with the establishment of a universally agreed upon classification. In some instances there may be confusion between sleep arousal disorders and epilepsy.[72]

The differential diagnosis includes complex partial seizures of temporal lobe origin and pseudoseizures. Frontal-lobe complex partial seizures differ from those of temporal lobe origin in that the amnesia of frontal-lobe seizures is more pronounced than the extent of loss of consciousness. Moreover, frontal-lobe involvement is associated with unilateral or bilateral tonic posturing and pedalling movements, partial and not complete loss of consciousness, and eye and head deviation to the contralateral side. In complex partial seizures of temporal lobe origin, oroalimentary and repetitive hand automatisms, and looking around are characteristic. Lastly, sensory, gustatory, or olfactory hallucinations in frontal-lobe epilepsy must be differentiated from psychotic disorders such as schizophrenia and manic psychosis.

The distinction between true seizures and pseudoseizures can be difficult. Children with pseudoseizures commonly also have true seizures. Emotional dysphoria can precipitate true seizures and many children with chronic seizures have psychiatric diagnoses. Frontal-lobe seizures may be confused with pseudoseizures. Frontal complex partial seizures differ from pseudoseizures in that pseudoseizures have a gradual onset and longer duration, while frontal-lobe seizures start slowly and last less than 1 min. Pseudoseizures include thrusting or rolling movements rather than the rhythmic flexion and extension clonic movements seen in frontal-lobe epilepsy. Still, it may be difficult to distinguish pseudoseizures[73] and video and electroencephalograph monitoring with depth electrodes may be necessary to definitively diagnose frontal-lobe epilepsy.

Other features differentiating pseudoseizures are as follows:

1 The seizure occurs when the child is observed, but not when alone.

2 The seizures are gradual rather than of sudden onset.

3 Uncontrolled flailing occurs, rather than true tonic–clonic movements.

4 The seizure is accompanied by histrionics, with screaming and shouting.

5 Painful stimuli are avoided during an attack;

6 There is a sudden cessation of the seizure, with immediate return to an alert and responsive state.

7 There is absence of paroxysmal discharge during an attack on electroencephalography.[73]

## Epidemiology

The incidence of epilepsy ranges from 0.7 to 1.1 per cent of the general population. It is the most common of the neurological diseases diagnosed in children.[67] Approximately 50 per cent of all cases of epilepsy begin during the childhood years and about 5 per cent of children will experience repeated epileptic seizures without a known extracerebral cause. In addition, about 3 per cent of children will have febrile convulsions that are usually benign and accompany a febrile illness. The great majority of these children, approximately 98 per cent, do not go on to develop true epilepsy. Other causes include hypoglycaemic seizures in children with diabetes. In some instances, as in tuberous sclerosis complex, cognitive impairment and autistic regression with onset in the first year of life, are linked to epilepsy; and in others there is a late onset of language disorder as in the Laudau–Kleffner syndrome.

The British Child and Adolescent Mental Health Survey[74] canvassed over 10 000 children and adolescents and identified 0.7 per cent of 5–15 year olds with a diagnosis of epilepsy. Among them there was an increased prevalence of emotional, behavioural, and relationship problems within families and among peers.

## Aetiology

Advances in understanding epilepsy in childhood have come from the newer medical technologies. Recognition of a typical spike-wave pattern has led to the identification of benign focal epilepsy. CT scanning and high-resolution magnetic resonance imaging (**MRI**) have led to the recognition of mesial temporal sclerosis, tuberous sclerosis, neuroblast migrational disorders, and small temporal lobe tumours. Positron-emission tomography scanning can demonstrate lesions undetected by MRI, such as focal lesions in patients with hypsarrhythmia. Advances in surgical procedures have decreased the risks associated with callosotomies and hemispherectomies used for catastrophic seizures. New understanding about neurotransmitters involved in the production and inhibition of seizures has led to advances in seizure medications.

Epileptic seizures are the result of an imbalance between inhibitory [(γ-aminobutyric acid (**GABA**) and excitatory (glutamate)] neurotransmitter systems. Neuronal hyperexcitability leading to seizures may result from decreased inhibition or increased excitation.[75] Epilepsy has its highest incidence in childhood, suggesting that the immature brain is more vulnerable to seizures than the mature brain—a finding that is borne out by animal studies. Decreased inhibition or increased excitation may result in neuronal excitability and seizures.[75] The specific mechanisms responsible for this imbalance remain uncertain. However, it is known that the binding of GABA to $GABA_A$ receptors opens a chloride channel (ionophore) leading to a flux of chloride ions and consequent membrane hyperpolarization: it is also known that there are fewer $GABA_A$ high-affinity receptors in immature animals. Similarly, there are maturational differences in the development of major ionotrophic receptors in excitatory systems and in the activation of *N*-methyl-d-aspartate receptors. In younger animals this results in larger excitatory postsynaptic potentials. It remains a puzzle why certain seizure types are age-specific in their onset.[76]

Epilepsy syndromes may have a genetic basis.[77] Gene localization for five epilepsy syndromes with Mendelian inheritance are recognized, and localization has been suggested in three epilepsies with complex inheritance. Those epilepsies with a single gene inheritance include symptomatic epilepsies with associated diffuse brain dysfunction and idiopathic epilepsies, where the seizures are the primary brain abnormality. Idiopathic single gene epilepsies include benign, familial neonatal convulsions. To date four autosomal-dominant forms of epilepsy have been described. Most genes discovered to be involved in human epilepsies encode subunits of ion channels, both voltage-gated and ligand-gated.[77] Molecular genetic studies are expected to lead to the discovery of other epilepsy genes. Investigation of animal models of epilepsy is continuing.

The aetiology of temporal lobe seizures includes mesial temporal sclerosis, tumours, and cortical dysplasia. The younger the child, the less frequent is mesial temporal sclerosis. Other factors linked to aetiology are proposed: temporal lobe hypoperfusion and hypometabolism in Landau–Kleffner syndrome, and diffuse cortical and subcortical hypoperfusion in Lennox–Gastaut syndrome.

### Course and prognosis

Early-onset epilepsies are associated with cognitive, behavioural, and communication disorders. Moreover, there is evidence that both clinical and subclinical epilepsy may result in developmental deviance, which has led to earlier and more aggressive treatment to try to prevent these impairments. Psychosocial factors are important in impairment. One prospective study evaluated 220 adults with childhood-onset seizures[78] up to age 35. The majority of subjects were free of seizures as adults, but were at risk for social and educational problems. When compared with random control subjects, those with epilepsy demonstrated correlations between neurological and cognitive impairment and social deficits. Those with epilepsy only (100 subjects) had a fourfold risk of psychiatric disorder. The authors reported social adjustment problems, competence problems, and reduction in marriage rate and fertility. Psychotic disorders occur significantly more frequently in people with epilepsy than in the general population with prevalence rates ranging from 2 to 8 per cent; the prevalence varying with the type of seizure disorder.[79]

### Management

Cognitive and behavioural findings suggest the importance of early intervention to prevent negative outcomes. The behavioural and psychiatric problems should be treated with the same approach used in children who are neurologically intact and include educational, family, and pharmacological approaches. The indications and choice of psychiatric drugs is similar; epilepsy is not a strong contraindication for the use of neuroleptic or antidepressants, even though some of these medications may increase the frequency of seizures. Dexedrine may be the treatment of choice for hyperkinetic behaviour because it may increase the seizure threshold. Although caution is needed in those with more severe neurological involvement, there is no strong evidence for an increased risk for neuroleptic-induced tardive dyskinesia. When there are behavioural problems one must consider the behavioural effects associated with

anticonvulsant medications.[80] In some instances, reducing the dose or changing the medication may be helpful and this should be discussed with the referring physician.

The major drugs used for treatment include carbamazepine, valproic acid, gabapentin, vigabatrin, and topiramate. These medications are used for the various forms of epilepsy described above including temporal lobe seizures and Lennox–Gastaut syndrome. Lamotrigine is also used, but with caution because severe dermatological side-effects may occur. In some instances, temporal lobectomy has been successful in the control of behavioural dysfunction and illogical thinking when performed in children with intractable temporal lobe seizures. In tuberous sclerosis complex the seizure medication vigabatrin may be helpful (and more so than corticosteroids) for infantile spasms.[81]

### Possibilities for prevention

A developmental perspective is indicated as there is increasing evidence of there being a developmental period during which a structure or function can be developed most completely.[82] For example, in tuberous sclerosis complex the cognitive impairment and autistic regression may be approached by way of early drug therapy and, in some instances, by the surgical removal of tubers.[83] Thus a developmental understanding of epilepsy is now crucial in treatment planning. Research is continuing to clarify why, in some instances, epilepsy may have a severe developmental impact and in other instances be more benign. With greater understanding of genetic mechanisms appropriate family counselling will be needed, and perhaps, new drug treatments may emerge. An important treatment goal is to prevent adverse psychosocial outcome by correct diagnosis, early intervention for seizures, continual assessment for cognitive and behavioural disorders, appropriate schooling, as well as effective family support, guidance, and therapy. Careful prospective follow-up studies are needed to demonstrate which interventions are most appropriate to specific types of epilepsy.

## Further information

Harris, J. (ed.) (1998). *Developmental neuropsychiatry: the fundamentals.* Oxford University Press, New York.

Harris, J. (ed.) (1998). *Developmental neuropsychiatry: assessment, diagnosis and treatment of the developmental disorders.* Oxford University Press, New York.

## References

1. Harris, J. (1998). *Developmental neuropsychiatry: the fundamentals.* Oxford University Press, New York.

2. Harris, J. (1998). *Developmental neuropsychiatry: assessment, diagnosis and treatment of the developmental disorders.* Oxford University Press, New York.

3. Rapoport, J.L., Addington, A.M., Frangou, S., *et al.* (2005). The neurodevelopmental model of schizophrenia: update 2005. *Molecular Psychiatry*, **10**, 434–49.
   Harris, J. (2006). *Intellectual disability: understanding its development, causes, classification, evaluation, and treatment.* Oxford University Press, New York.

4. Spencer, T., Biederman, J., Harding, M., *et al.* (1998). Disentangling the overlap between Tourette's disorder and ADHD. *Journal of Child Psychology and Psychiatry*, **39**, 1037–44.

5. Carter, A.S., O'Donnell, D.A., Schultz, R.T., *et al.* (2000). Social and emotional adjustment in children affected with Gilles de la Tourette's

syndrome: associations with ADHD and family functioning. Attention deficit hyperactivity disorder. *Journal of Child Psychology and Psychiatry*, **41**, 215–23.

6. Rizzo, R., Curatolo, P., Gulisano, M., *et al.* (2007). Disentangling the effects of Tourette syndrome and attention deficit hyperactivity disorder on cognitive and behavioral phenotypes. *Brain and Development*, **29**, 413–20.

7. Flint, J. (1998). Behavioral phenotypes: conceptual and methodological issues. *American Journal of Medical Genetics*, **81**, 235–40.

8. Skuse, D.H. (2000). Behavioural phenotypes: what do they teach us? *Archives of Diseases of Childhood*, **82**, 222–5.

9. O'Brien, G. and Yule, W. (eds.) (1995). *Behavioural phenotypes. Clinics in developmental medicine*, No. 138. MacKeith, London.

10. Nyhan, W. (1972). Behavioral phenotypes in organic genetic disease. Presidential address to the society for pediatric research, May 1, 1971. *Pediatric Research*, **6**, 1–9.

11. Chapman, R.S. and Hesketh, L.J. (2000). Behavioral phenotype of individuals with Down syndrome. *Intellectual Disability and Developmental Disability Research Reviews*, **6**, 84–9.

12. Hagerman, R.J. (1999). Clinical and molecular aspects of fragile X syndrome. In *Neurodevelopmental disorders* (ed. H. Tager-Flusberg), pp. 27–42. MIT Press, Cambridge, MA.

13. Cassidy, S.B. and Morris, C.A. (2002). Behavioral phenotypes in genetic syndromes: genetic clues to human behavior. *Advances in Pediatrics*, **49**, 59–86.

14. Howlin, P., Davies, M., and Udwin, O. (1998). Syndrome specific characteristics in Williams syndrome: to what extent do behavioral patterns extend into adult life? *Journal of Applied Research in Developmental Disabilities*, **32**, 129–41.

15. Lesch, M. and Nyhan, W.L. (1964). A familial disorder of uric acid metabolism and central nervous system function. *The American Journal of Medicine*, **36**, 561–70.

16. Harris, J.C. (1998). Lesch–Nyhan disease. In *Developmental neuropsychiatry: assessment, diagnosis and treatment of the developmental disorders* (ed. J.C. Harris), pp. 306–19. Oxford University Press, New York.

17. Schretlen, D.J., Ward, J., Meyer, S.M., *et al.* (2005). Behavioral aspects of Lesch-Nyhan disease and its variants. *Developmental Medicine and Child Neurology*, **47**, 673–7.

18. Holland, A.J., Whittington, J.E., Butler, J., *et al.* (2003). Behavioural phenotypes associated with specific genetic disorders: evidence from a population-based study of people with Prader-Willi syndrome. *Psychological Medicine*, **33**, 141–53.

19. Dykens, E.M. and Kasari, C. (1997). Maladaptative behavior in children with Prader–Willi syndrome, Down syndrome and non-specific intellectual disability. *American Journal of Intellectual disability*, **102**, 228–37.

20. Gunn, P., Berry, P., and Andrews, R.J. (1981). The temperament of Down's syndrome in infants: a research note. *Journal of Child Psychology and Psychiatry*, **22**, 189–94.

21. van Lieshout, C.F.M., DeMeyer, R.E., Curfs, L.M.G., *et al.* (1998). Family contexts, parental behaviour, and personality profiles of children and adolescents with Prader–Willi, fragile-X, or Williams syndrome. *Journal of Child Psychology and Psychiatry*, **39**, 699–710.

22. Miller, L.K. (1999). The savant syndrome: intellectual impairment and exceptional skill. *Psychological Bulletin*, **125**, 31–46.

23. Hoyme, H.E., May, P.A., Kalberg, W.O., *et al.* (2005). A practical clinical approach to diagnosis of fetal alcohol spectrum disorders: clarification of the 1996 institute of medicine criteria. *Pediatrics*, **115**, 39–47.

24. Tischfield, M.A., Bosley, T.M., Salih, M.A., *et al.* (2005). Homozygous HOXA1 mutations disrupt human brainstem, inner ear, cardiovascular and cognitive development. *Nature Genetics*, **37**, 1035–7.

25. Glover, J.C., Renaud, J.S., and Rijli, F.M. (2006). Retinoic acid and hindbrain patterning. *Journal of Neurobiology*, **66**, 705–25.

26. American Academy of Pediatrics. (2000). Committee on substance abuse and committee on children with disabilities. Fetal alcohol syndrome and alcohol-related neurodevelopmental disorders. *Pediatrics*, **106**(2 Pt 1), 358–61.

27. Nash, K., Rovet, J., Greenbaum, R., *et al.* (2006). Identifying the behavioural phenotype in fetal alcohol spectrum disorder: sensitivity, specificity and screening potential. *Archives of Womens Mental Health*, **9**, 181–6.

28. Streissguth, A.P., Barr, H.M., Sampson, P.D., *et al.* (1994). Prenatal alcohol and offspring development: the first fourteen years. *Drug and Alcohol Dependence*, **36**, 89–99.

29. Olson, H.C., Streissguth, A.P., Sampson, P.D., *et al.* (1997). Association of prenatal alcohol exposure with behavioral and learning problems in early adolescence. *Journal of the American Academy of Child and Adolescent Psychiatry*, **36**, 1187–94.

30. Steinhausen, H.C., Willms, J., Metzke, C.W., *et al.* (2003). Behavioural phenotype in foetal alcohol syndrome and foetal alcohol effects. *Developmental Medicine and Child Neurology*, **45**, 179–82.

31. O'Malley, K.D. and Nanson, J. (2002). Clinical implications of a link between fetal alcohol spectrum disorder and attention-deficit hyperactivity disorder. *Canadian Journal of Psychiatry*, **47**, 349–54.

32. Mukherjee, R.A., Hollins, S., and Turk, J. (2006). Fetal alcohol spectrum disorder: an overview. *Journal of the Royal Society of Medicine*, **99**, 298–302.

33. Streissguth, A.P. and O'Malley, K. (2000). Neuropsychiatric implications and long term consequences of foetal alcohol spectrum disorders. *Seminars in clinical neuropsychiatry*, **5**, 177–90.

34. Barr, H.M., Bookstein, F.L., O'Malley, K.D., *et al.* (2006). Binge drinking during pregnancy as a predictor of psychiatric disorders on the structured clinical interview for DSM-IV in young adult offspring. *The American Journal of Psychiatry*, **163**, 1061–5.

35. Sampson, P.D., Streissguth, A.P., Bookstein, F.L., *et al.* (1997). Incidence of fetal alcohol syndrome and prevalence of alcohol-related neurodevelopmental disorder. *Teratology*, **56**, 317–26.

36. Ikonomidou, C., Bittagau, P., Ishimaru, M.J., *et al.* (2000). Ethanol induced apoptotic neurodegeneration and fetal alcohol syndrome. *Science*, **287**, 1056–60.

37. Bookstein, F.L., Streissguth, A.P., Sampson, P.D., *et al.* (2002). Corpus callosum shape and neuropsychological deficits in adult males with heavy fetal alcohol exposure. *Neuroimage*, **15**, 233–51.

38. Spadoni, A.D., McGee, C.L., Fryer, S.L., *et al.* (2007). Neuroimaging and fetal alcohol spectrum disorders. *Neuroscience and Biobehavioural Reviews*, **31**, 239–45.

39. Warren, K.R. and Li, T.K. (2005). Genetic polymorphisms: impact on the risk of fetal alcohol spectrum disorders. *Birth Defects Research A Clinical and Molecular Teratology*, **73**, 195–203.

40. Chiriboga, C.A. (2003). Fetal alcohol and drug effects. *The Neurologist*, **9**, 267–79.

41. Hans, S.L. (1989). Developmental consequences of prenatal exposure to methadone. *Annals of the New York Academy of Sciences*, **562**, 195–207.

42. Rosen, T.S. and Johnson, H.L. (1985). Long-term effects of prenatal methadone maintenance. *NIDA Research Monograph*, **59**, 73–83.

43. Stewart, D.J., Inaba, T., and Lucassen, M. (1979). Cocaine metabolism: cocaine and norcocaine hydrolysis by liver and serum esterases. *Clinical Pharmacology and Therapeutics*, **25**, 464–8.

44. Chasnoff, I.J. (1992). Cocaine, pregnancy, and the growing child. *Current Problems in Pediatrics*, **22**, 302–21.

45. Singer, L.T., Minnes, S., Short, E., *et al.* (2004). Cognitive outcomes of preschool children with prenatal cocaine exposure. *The Journal of the American Medical Association*, **291**, 2448–56.

46. New England Congenital Hypothyroidism Collaborative. (1990). Elementary school performance of children with congenital hypothyroidism. *The Journal of Pediatrics*, **116**, 27–32.

47. Oerbeck, B., Sundet, K., Kase, B.F., *et al.* (2003). Congenital hypothyroidism: influence of disease severity and L-thyroxine treatment on intellectual, motor, and school-associated outcomes in young adults. *Pediatrics*, **112**, 923–30.

48. Rutter, M. (1981). Psychological sequelae of brain damage in children. *The American Journal of Psychiatry*, **138**, 1533–44.

49. Brown, G., Chadwick, O., Shaffer, D., *et al.* (1981). A prospective study of children with head injuries. III: psychiatric sequelae. *Psychological Medicine*, **11**, 63–78.

50. Max, J.E., Koele, S.L., Smith, W.L. Jr, *et al.* (1998). Psychiatric disorders in children and adolescents after severe traumatic brain injury: a controlled study. *American Academy of Child and Adolescent Psychiatry*, **37**, 832–40.

51. van Reekum, R., Bolago, I., Finlayson, M.A., *et al.* (1996). Psychiatric disorders after traumatic brain injury. *Brain Injury*, **10**, 319–27.

52. Max, J.E., Schachar, R.J., Levin, H.S., *et al.* (2005). Predictors of secondary attention-deficit/hyperactivity disorder in children and adolescents 6 to 24 months after traumatic brain injury. *Journal of the American Academy of Child and Adolescent Psychiatry*, **44**, 1041–9.

53. Max, J.E., Lindgren, S.D., Knutson, C., *et al.* (1998). Child and adolescent traumatic brain injury: correlates of disruptive behaviour disorders. *Brain Injury*, **12**, 41–52.

54. Max, J.E., Castillo, C.S., and Robin, D.A. (1998). Posttraumatic stress symptomatology after childhood traumatic brain injury. *The Journal of Nervous and Mental Disease*, **186**, 589–96.

55. Max, J.E., Castillo, C.S., and Robin, D.A. (1998). Predictors of family functioning after traumatic brain injury in children and adolescents. *Journal of the American Academy of Child and Adolescent Psychiatry*, **37**, 83–90.

56. Wade, S.L., Taylor, H.G., Drotar, D., *et al.* (1998). Family burden and adaptation during the initial year after traumatic brain injury in children. *Pediatrics*, **102**, 110–16.

57. AbdelMalik, P., Husted, J., Chow, E.W., *et al.* (2003). Childhood head injury and expression of schizophrenia in multiply affected families. *Archives of General Psychiatry*, **60**, 231–6.

58. Brower, M.C. and Price, B.H. (2001). Neuropsychiatry of frontal lobe dysfunction in violent and criminal behaviour: a critical review. *Journal of Neurology, Neurosurgery, and Psychiatry*, **7**, 720–6.

59. Kraus, J.F. and Nourjah, P. (1988). The epidemiology of uncomplicated brain injury. *The Journal of Trauma*, **28**, 1637–43.

60. Kraus, J.F., Fife, D., and Conroy, C. (1987). Pediatric brain injuries: the nature, clinical course, and early outcomes in a defined United States population. *Pediatrics*, **79**, 501–7.

61. Middleton, J.A. (2001). Practitioner review: psychological sequelae of head injury in children and adolescents. *Journal of Child Psychology and Psychiatry*, **42**, 165–80.

62. Keenan, H.T., Hooper, S.R., Wetherington, C.E., *et al.* (2007). Neurodevelopmental consequences of early traumatic brain injury in 3-year-old children. *Pediatrics*, **119**, e616–23.

63. Limond, J. and Leeke, R. (2005). Practitioner review: cognitive rehabilitation for children with acquired brain injury. *Journal of Child Psychology and Psychiatry*, **46**, 339–532.

64. Rosen, C.D. and Gerring, J.P. (1986). *Head injury: educational reintegration*. College Hill Press, Boston, MA.

65. Ellis, N., Upton, D., and Thompson, P. (2000). Epilepsy and the family: a review of current literature. *Seizure*, **9**, 22–30.

66. Aicardi, J. (1992). *Diseases of the nervous system in children*. Clinics in developmental medicine, No. 115/118. MacKeith Press, London.

67. Guerrini, R. (2006). Epilepsy in children. *Lancet*, **367**, 499–524.

68. Saygi, S., Katz, A., Marks, D.A., *et al.* (1992). Frontal lobe partial seizures and psychogenic seizures: comparison of clinical and ictal characteristics. *Neurology*, **42**, 1274–7.

69. Stores, G., Zaiwalla, Z., and Bergel, N. (1991). Frontal lobe complex partial seizures in children: a form of epilepsy at particular risk of misdiagnosis. *Developmental Medicine and Child Neurology*, **33**, 998–1009.

70. Stephani, U. (2006). The natural history of myoclonic astatic epilepsy (Doose syndrome) and Lennox-Gastaut syndrome. *Epilepsia*, **47**(Suppl. 2), 53–5.

71. Commission on Classification and Terminology of the International League Against Epilepsy. (1989). Proposal for revised classification of epilepsies and epileptic syndromes. *Epilepsia*, **30**, 389.

72. Stores, G. (1991). Confusions concerning sleep disorders and the epilepsies in children and adolescents. *The British Journal of Psychiatry*, **158**, 1–7.

73. Stores, G. (1999). Practitioner review: recognition of pseudoseizures in children and adolescents. *Journal of Child Psychology and Psychiatry*, **40**, 851–7.

74. Davies, S., Heyman, I., and Goodman, R. (2003). A population survey of mental health problems in children with epilepsy. *Developmental Medicine and Child Neurology*, **45**, 292–5.

75. Scott, R.C. and Neville, G.R. (1998). Developmental perspectives on epilepsy. *Current Opinion in Neurology*, **11**, 115–18.

76. Holmes, G.L. (1997). Epilepsy in the developing brain: lessons from the laboratory and clinic. *Epilepsia*, **38**, 12–30.

77. Berkovic, S.F., Mulley, J.C., Scheffer, I.E., *et al.* (2006). Human epilepsies: interaction of genetic and acquired factors. *Trends in Neuroscience*, **29**, 391–7.

78. Jalava, M., Sillanpaa, M., Camfield, C., *et al.* (1997). Social adjustment and competence 35 years after onset of childhood epilepsy: a prospective controlled study. *Epilepsia*, **38**, 708–15.

79. Kanner, A.M. and Dunn, D.W. (2004). Diagnosis and management of depression and psychosis in children and adolescents with epilepsy. *Journal of Child Neurology*, **19**(Suppl. 1), S65–72.

80. Mula, M., Monaco, F., and Trimble, M.R. (2004). Use of psychotropic drugs in patients with epilepsy: interactions and seizure risk. *Expert Review of Neurotherapeutics*, **4**, 953–64.

81. Chiron, C., Dumas, C., Jambaque, I., *et al.* (1997). Randomized trial comparing vigabatrin and hydrocortisone in infantile spasms due to tuberous sclerosis. *Epilepsy Research*, **26**, 389–95.

82. Neville, B. (1998). The reemergence of critical periods of development. *Current Opinion in Neurology*, **11**, 89–90.

83. Bebin, E., Kelly, P., and Gomez, M. (1993). Surgical treatment for epilepsy in cerebral tuberous sclerosis. *Epilepsia*, **34**, 651–7.

## 9.2.2 Specific developmental disorders in childhood and adolescence

Helmut Remschmidt and Gerd Schulte-Körne

### Introduction

The term 'specific developmental disorders' includes a variety of severe and persistent difficulties in spoken language, spelling, reading, arithmetic, and motor function. Skills are substantially below the expected level in terms of chronological age, measured intelligence, and age-appropriate education and cannot be explained by any obvious neurological disorder or any specific adverse psychosocial or family circumstances. As the deficits are quite substantial, analogies were initially made to neurological concepts and disorders such as word-blindness, alexia, aphasia, and apraxia, thus giving rise to the notion that neurological deficits are the aetiological basis of these disorders. Since this could not be demonstrated, the next step was to define the disorders in a more functional way,

**Table 9.2.2.1** Specific developmental disorders: a comparison of ICD-10 and DSM-IV NOS, not otherwise specified

| ICD-10 | DSM-IV |
| --- | --- |
| Specific developmental disorders of speech and language (F80) | Communication disorders |
| Specific speech articulation disorder (F80.0) | Expressive language disorder (315.31) |
| Expressive language disorder (F80.1) | Mixed receptive–expressive language disorder (315.31) |
| Receptive language disorder (F80.2) | Phonological disorder (315.39) |
| Acquired aphasia with epilepsy (Landau–Kleffner syndrome) (F80.3) | Stuttering (307.0) |
| Other developmental disorders of speech and language (F80.8) | Communication disorder NOS (307.9) |
| Specific developmental disorders of scholastic skills (F81) | Learning disorders |
| Specific reading disorder (F81.0) | Reading disorder (315.00) |
| Specific spelling disorder (F81.1) | Mathematics disorder (315.1) |
| Specific disorder of arithmetical skills (F81.2) | Disorder of written expression (315.2) |
| Specific disorder of scholastic skills (F81.3) | Learning disorder NOS (315.9) |
| Other developmental disorders of scholastic skills (F81.8) | |
| Specific developmental disorder of motor function (F82) | Motor skills disorder |
| | Developmental co-ordination disorder (315.4) |
| Mixed specific developmental disorders (F83) | |

taking into account not only psychometric testing but also psychosocial risk factors and the quality of schooling and education.

Today, numerous findings support the validity of the diagnostic concept of specific developmental disorders. These disorders and pervasive developmental disorders have the following features in common (ICD-10)[1]:

◆ An onset that invariably appears during infancy or childhood.

◆ An impairment or delay in the development of functions that are strongly related to biological maturation of the central nervous system.

◆ A steady course that does not involve the remissions and relapses that tend to be characteristic of many mental disorders.

Thus the term 'specific developmental disorders' reflects the fact that the deficits are circumscribed and relatively isolated against the background of an otherwise undisturbed psychological functioning.

## Classification

In the multiaxial classification of child and adolescent psychiatric disorders,[2] specific developmental disorders are classified on the second axis named 'Specific disorders of psychological development', whereas pervasive developmental disorders are classified on the first axis (clinical psychiatric syndromes).

Based on the history and course of the disorders, two types can be distinguished:

◆ Disorders in which a phase of previously normal development has occurred prior to manifestation of the disorder. This, for example, applies to the Landau–Kleffner syndrome.

◆ An additional condition in which the abnormality was present from birth. This is especially true for autism. Autism is classified in the category 'pervasive developmental disorders', which are discussed elsewhere.

In DSM-IV,[3] nomenclature is somewhat different, but generally includes disorders identical or similar to those in ICD-10.

In DSM-IV, 'communication disorders' correspond to 'specific developmental disorders of speech and language'. However, they also include stuttering, which is not included in the corresponding category of ICD-10.

'Learning disorders' (DSM-IV) is the category that corresponds to specific developmental disorders of scholastic skills, and 'motor skills disorder' to 'specific disorders of motor function'.

Table 9.2.2.1 shows the terminology used in both classification systems. The headlines of the two systems correspond; however, the subcategories show some differences.

Figure 9.2.2.1 shows a decision tree which includes the three main areas of dysfunction and addresses diagnosis and differential diagnosis.

## Specific developmental disorders of speech and language

The main characteristic of these disorders is a disturbance of language acquisition from the early stages of development. The disturbance, however, is not directly attributable to neurological or speech mechanism abnormalities, sensory impairments, intellectual disability, or environmental factors.[1]

There are three main problems in distinguishing these disorders from the normal state and other conditions:

1 **Differentiation from the normal state**: the disorders must be distinguished from normal speech and language development, bearing in mind the great variations seen in the normal pattern. To make the diagnosis, the disorder must clearly be clinically significant, which can be determined by four main criteria: severity, course, pattern, and associated problems.

2 **Differentiation from intellectual disability (mental retardation)**: the degree of speech and language dysfunction must always be considered with respect to the child's cognitive level.

3 **Differentiation from disorders due to sensory impairment or impairments of the central nervous systems**: speech and language disorders resulting from severe deafness, specific

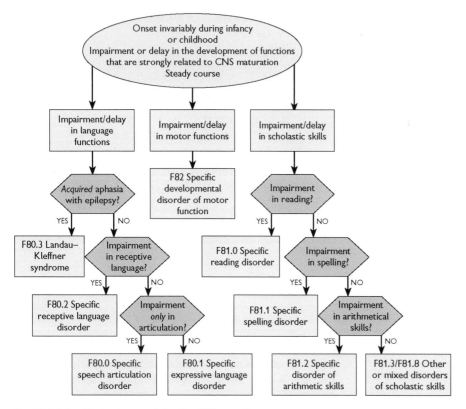

**Fig. 9.2.2.1** Specific developmental disorders. CNS, central nervous system.

neurological impairments, or structural brain abnormalities are not classified in the category of specific developmental disorders of speech and language.

## Specific speech articulation disorder

### (a) Clinical features

The main feature of the disorder is the child's failure to use speech sounds appropriate for his or her mental age, while other language skills are within the normal range. Difficulties include errors in sound production and use, especially substitution of one sound for another. Difficulties in speech sound production usually interfere either with academic achievement or social communication. There are several degrees of severity reaching from mild or no impairment of speech intelligibility to completely incomprehensible speech. Sound substitutions are considered less severe than sound omissions. The sounds most frequently misarticulated are those acquired later during speech development (l, r, s, z, th, ch). However, consonants and vowels that range early in the development sequence may be affected in younger children.

It is very important to relate the misarticulations to normal development. At the age of 4 years, errors in speech and sound production are very frequent, but children are usually understood even by strangers. At 6 to 7 years of age, most speech sounds can be adequately reproduced, and by the age of 11 to 12, children should be capable of almost all speech sounds.

### (b) Classification

In ICD-10, speech articulation disorder (F80.0) is classified in the category 'Specific developmental disorders of speech and language'. The counterpart in DSM-IV is the category 'Phonological disorder'

(315.39), classified in the category 'Communication disorders' (see Table 9.2.2.1).

### (c) Diagnosis and differential diagnosis

The leading feature, the age-appropriate misarticulation of speech sounds with the result that others have difficulties in understanding the child, usually allows one to diagnose the disorder. There are three types of symptoms that can be observed: substitutions, omissions, and distortions of speech sounds. The diagnosis should only be made if the severity of misarticulation is outside the limits of the normal variation for the child's mental age. Further requirements are that non-verbal intelligence and expressive and receptive language skills should be within the normal range.

Differential diagnoses include intellectual disability, hearing impairment, or other sensory deficits or severe environmental deprivation.

### (d) Epidemiology

Moderate to severe developmental articulation disorders can be found in 2 to 3 per cent of 6- and 7-year-old children, with less severe disorders even more frequent. The frequency of occurrence falls to 0.5 per cent by the time children are 17 years old (DSM-IV).

### (e) Aetiology

As it has been demonstrated that the disorder runs in families, it is assumed that genetic factors are important for its manifestation.

### (f) Course and prognosis

The prognosis is favourable if no other associated features such as hearing impairment, neurological conditions, cognitive impairments, or psychosocial problems are present. However, the course varies depending on the severity and the above-mentioned associated features.

### (g) Treatment

Treatment is necessary and appropriate if the child is handicapped in his or her everyday life and cannot be understood by parents, siblings, or other persons. The focus of the therapy depends on whether speech articulation disorder is an isolated phenomenon or if other impairments or dysfunctions are present (e.g. developmental disorder of motor functions). If it is an isolated phenomenon, functional speech therapy can be carried out on the principle that mispronounced sounds should not be repeated when correcting them, but substituted by the correctly pronounced sound.[4] It is advisable to carry out this kind of therapy before the child enters school. If other disorders are present, a comprehensive therapeutic programme that includes speech therapy needs to be developed.

## Expressive language disorder

### (a) Clinical features and classification

The main feature of this disorder is that the child's ability to use expressive spoken language is reduced below the mental age appropriate level, while language comprehension ranges within normal limits. Abnormalities in articulation may co-occur.

In ICD-10, the following symptoms are considered important for diagnosis (ICD-10, p. 237)[1]:

◆ delay of the development of expressive language (e.g. absence of single words by the age of 2 years, failure to generate simple two-word sentences by 3 years)

◆ restricted vocabulary development

◆ overuse of a small set of general words

◆ difficulties in selecting appropriate words and word substitutions

◆ short utterance length and immature sentence structure

◆ syntactical errors, especially omissions of word endings or prefix

◆ misuse of or failure to use grammatical features such as prepositions, pronouns, articles, and verb and noun inflexions.

The DSM-IV criteria requires measures of expressive language development being substantially below those obtained from standardized measures of both non-verbal intellectual capacity and receptive language development, interference with academic or occupational achievement, and the exclusion of mixed receptive–expressive disorder and pervasive developmental disorders.

### (b) Diagnosis and differential diagnosis

The diagnosis is made by clinical observation, with special emphasis on expressive language functions and the use of individually administered standardized tests of expressive language. The differential diagnosis should rule out mixed receptive–expressive language disorder (DSM-IV), characterized by an impairment of receptive language functions. Autistic disorder may also involve expressed language impairment, but autism can be distinguished by characteristic communication impairments. Finally, intellectual disability and sensory impairments (e.g. hearing impairment or other sensory deficits) need to be ruled out, as well as severe environmental deprivation. The diagnosis is confirmed using intelligence tests, audiometric tests, neurological investigations, and a careful history. Finally, acquired aphasia needs to be ruled out.

This can be done by assessing any medical condition that may have caused the disorder.

### (c) Epidemiology

In the absence of thorough epidemiological studies, estimates suggest that between approximately 3 and 5 per cent of children may be affected by expressive language disorder of the developmental type. The acquired type seems to be less common.

### (d) Aetiology

DSM-IV distinguishes two types of expressive language disorders: the developmental type and the acquired type. In the developmental type, impairment of expressive language begins at a very early age and is not associated with neurological factors, while the acquired type occurs after a period of normal development and is caused by neurological or general medical conditions (e.g. head trauma, encephalitis). It is assumed that the developmental type is caused by genetic factors that influence language development.

### (e) Course and prognosis

The course depends on the type of disorder (developmental or acquired type) and severity. Usually, the disorder can be diagnosed by the age of 3 years, while milder forms are often only detected later. According to DSM-IV,[3] approximately half of the children appear to outgrow the developmental type of expressive language disorder, while the other half have persistent difficulties. The outcome of the acquired type depends on the severity and location of the brain pathology.

### (f) Treatment

As causal treatment is not possible, treatment measures are based on general principles that have been found to be useful and effective in clinical practice.

1 The first step is to explain clearly to parents the nature of the disorder and the fact that several other disturbances manifested by the child may be a result of the child's communication deficit.

2 The best time to commence speech therapy depends upon the severity of the disorder, the child's cognitive and motivational structure, and other disorders that might be present. Instead of treating children too early (e.g. before the age of 3 years), offering advice and guidance to the parents is extremely important.

3 Treatment itself concentrates on teaching language skills using techniques such as imitation and modelling. The therapist should focus interventions selectively on the areas of difficulty, thus increasing the child's phonological repertoire. Non-verbal communication techniques may be used if verbal communication is substantially impaired. But the therapist should always make sure that non-verbal communication does not dominate the verbal one.

4 In therapeutic programmes, everyday situations are now preferred to very structured programmes. This is because many therapists found that therapeutic progress during sessions was not transferred to everyday life situations. During structured treatment sessions the children are taught to give correct answers to questions that have nothing to do with their situation in everyday life, and it is now thought that structured language training may prevent them using language according to their needs.[5]

5 Alternative communication, such as sign language, should only be used if the child suffers from severe auditory comprehension deficits. The use of a sign language, however, is no longer regarded as an obstacle to the improvement of expressive language skills.[6]

## Receptive language disorder

### (a) Clinical features and classification

This disorder is characterized by the child's inability or reduced ability to understand language in a way appropriate for his or her mental age. As expressive language production depends on language comprehension; expressive language is also profoundly disturbed and abnormalities in word-sound production can be observed.

The diagnostic guidelines of ICD-10 include the following features:

◆ failure to respond to familiar names (in the absence of non-verbal clues) by the first birthday

◆ inability to identify at least a few common objects by 18 months

◆ failure to follow simple, routine instructions by the age of 2 years

◆ inability to understand grammatical structures (e.g. questions, comparatives)

◆ lack of understanding of the more subtle aspects of language (tone of voice, gestures, etc.).

Owing to the disturbances in both receptive and expressive functions, the disorder is called 'receptive–expressive language disorder' in DSM-IV. The diagnostic criteria require scores of both receptive and expressive language development substantially below those obtained from standardized measures of non-verbal intellectual capacity, interference with academic or occupational achievement, and exclusion of pervasive developmental disorders.

### (b) Diagnosis and differential diagnosis

Diagnosis is based on three factors: a careful history taken from the child's parents, a thorough clinical investigation including neurological assessment and detailed speech and language assessment, and standardized tests measuring expressive and receptive language functions.

Differential diagnosis should rule out expressive language disorder (which is the case in the presence of language comprehension), specific speech articulation disorder, in which the receptive and expressive language functions are unimpaired, autism (which can be distinguished by the typical communication disturbance), intellectual disability, sensory deficits, and severe environmental deprivation. These disorders can be excluded by intelligence tests, audiometric tests, neurological investigations, and taking a history.

### (c) Epidemiology

Owing to the absence of epidemiological studies, the frequency with which the disorder occurs can only be estimated. According to estimations, the disorder occurs in up to 3 per cent of school-age children and is probably less common than expressive language disorder.

### (d) Aetiology

As in other developmental language disorders, there is evidence that genetic factors play the most important role in aetiology.[7]

The frequent association of disturbed language acquisition with adverse psychosocial factors in the family does not contradict a primarily genetic cause, as many children who grow up under these circumstances show entirely normal developmental patterns of speech and language skills.[8]

### (e) Course and prognosis

The long-term prognosis is poor. Only half the patients in the sample studied by Rutter *et al.*[9] had normal conversational skills when they were in their twenties, and there was a decline in non-verbal IQ from childhood to adulthood. The course again depends on the type (developmental or acquired) and severity of the disorder. The disorder is usually detected before the age of 4 years, but earlier in severe cases. The prognosis is poorer than in expressive language disorder. As far as the acquired type is concerned, the prognosis varies depending on severity, location of brain pathology, the child's age, and the level of language development prior to the disorder.

### (f) Treatment

Treatment is generally undertaken along the same lines as in expressive language disorders. However, owing to the nature of the disorder, all factors that facilitate language comprehension should especially be encouraged. Non-verbal forms of communication such as sign language can be helpful.

## Acquired aphasia with epilepsy (Landau–Kleffner syndrome)

### (a) Clinical features and classification

The Landau–Kleffner syndrome is a rare disorder characterized by receptive and expressive language impairment and epileptic seizures, but retained general intelligence, and manifestation after a period of normal development, including language development. The onset of the disorder typically occurs between 3 and 7 years of age and is accompanied by paroxysmal electroencephalographic abnormalities, mainly bilateral spikes in the posterior temporal and parietal regions and epileptic seizures in about 80 per cent of cases.[10] The loss of language may occur gradually over a period of months or abruptly within a few days or weeks.

Aphasia usually starts with receptive language problems occurring together with the characteristic electroencephalographic changes, followed by expressive language difficulties. Usually, the first sign is the impairment of receptive language functions with difficulties in auditory comprehension. During the manifestation period, symptomatology is variable: some children become mute, others express jargon-like sounds, and some produce misarticulations and have difficulties in word fluency. During the manifestation period, emotional and behavioural symptoms are common; they can be regarded as a reaction to the loss of language functions and appear as anxiety reactions, acting-out behaviour, and aggression.

In DSM-IV, the condition is classified in the category mixed receptive–expressive language disorder, acquired type.

### (b) Diagnosis and differential diagnosis

The diagnosis can be based upon a detailed history of the child's development, assessment of language functions, careful neurological assessment, and by electroencephalography. The differential diagnosis includes other types of acquired aphasia without epileptic seizures and electroencephalographic abnormalities, and disintegrative disorders of childhood such as dementia infantilis Heller (Heller's syndrome) (see Chapter 9.2.2).

### (c) Epidemiology

The prevalence of the disorder is unknown.

### (d) Aetiology

The aetiology is unknown. There is, so far, no indication of any genetic cause. Clinical characteristics suggest that an encephalitis might be considered a causal mechanism. The electroencephalographic changes and the seizures are thought to cause the language and the behavioural and emotional problems.

### (e) Treatment

So far, three different approaches to treatment have been undertaken:

1 Anticonvulsant treatment (mainly with carbamazepine): the frequency of seizures can be reduced to some extent with this medication, but paroxysmal electroencephalographic changes are not substantially influenced.

2 Corticosteroids have also been administered,[11] but the benefits remain unclear.

3 Finally, surgical treatment by bilateral temporal transection has been attempted.[12,13]

## Specific developmental disorders of scholastic skills

'Specific developmental disorders of scholastic skills' (ICD-10) or 'Learning disorders' (DSM-IV) include disorders characterized by one or more significant impairments in acquisition of reading, spelling, or arithmetical skills. ICD-10 suggests that the category 'Mixed disorder of scholastic skills' (F81.3) be used as an ill-defined, but necessary, category in which arithmetical and reading or spelling skills are significantly impaired, although not because of general intellectual disability or inadequate schooling.

The disorders classified in the category 'Specific developmental disorders of scholastic skills' (**SDDSS**) resemble specific disorders of speech and language. As in these latter disorders, normal patterns of skill acquisition are disturbed and detectable at an age when these functions are required. The disorders are not due to a lack of opportunity to learn or a consequence of brain trauma or disease, but represent a specific type of dysfunction in cognitive processing. The dysfunction affects specific skills, which can be distinguished from the cognitive functions that are usually in the normal range. As in other specific developmental disorders, the condition is more common in boys than in girls.

ICD-10 notes five difficulties regarding diagnosis and differential diagnosis:

1 differentiation of the disorder from normal variations in scholastic achievement (this problem applies to all specific developmental disorders and was discussed in relation to specific developmental disorders of speech and language);

2 consideration of the normal developmental course;

3 interference with learning and teaching;

4 underlying abnormalities in cognitive processing;

5 uncertainties over the best way of subdifferentiating SDDSS.

Based on these considerations, the following diagnostic guidelines for all SDDSS have been suggested (ICD-10):

◆ **Clinically significant degree of impairment:** this is judged on the basis of severity (e.g. occurrence in less than 3 per cent of school children), developmental precursors (e.g. speech or language disorder in preschool years), and associated problems (e.g. inattention).

◆ **Specific impairment not explained solely by intellectual disability or by lesser impairments in general intelligence:** for this requirement to be met, individually administered and standardized IQ scholastic achievement tests are obligatory to demonstrate that the child's level of achievement is substantially below the expected level compared to a child of the same mental age and IQ.

◆ **Developmental nature of the impairment:** this must be demonstrated by the presence of the disorder during the early years of schooling and by exclusion of impairment acquired later. The child's history of school progress is decisive in this respect.

◆ **Absence of external factors that could explain the impairment:** SDDSS are thought to be mainly based on factors intrinsic to the child's development, and not due to inadequate schooling or any other environmental factors such as absence from school or educational discontinuities. However, such conditions may occur, making the diagnostic process difficult.

◆ **Exclusion of visual and hearing impairments:** by definition, SDDSS do not occur as a result of impairment of sensory function, such as visual or hearing impairment.

The main differential diagnostic task is distinguishing SDDSS from neurological disorders (e.g. alexia, aphasia, agraphia, apraxia) or impairments that also could influence the development of scholastic skills (e.g. emotional disorder). In cases of normal child development prior to the manifestation of a defined neurological disorder, differential diagnosis is not difficult. However, if minor neurological signs (soft signs) were diagnosed previously, independent of any defined disorder, and the findings persist, it may be difficult to distinguish recent symptoms from previous ones. In such cases, associated disorders or symptoms should be classified separately in the appropriate neurological section of the classification systems.

### Specific reading disorder

The ICD-10 classification system distinguishes between 'Specific reading disorder' and 'Specific spelling disorder'. In DSM-IV, 'Specific reading disorder' is distinguished from 'Disorder of Written Expression'. The latter is not identical with the ICD-10 category 'Specific spelling disorder', insofar as that disorder excludes children whose sole problem is one of handwriting.

#### (a) Clinical features and classification

The main feature of this disorder is a specific and significant impairment in the development of reading skills, which is not solely accounted for by mental age, visual acuity problems, or inadequate schooling.[1]

Other functions may also be affected:

◆ word recognition

◆ reading comprehension skills

◆ oral reading skills

◆ performance of tasks requiring reading

In many cases, spelling difficulties continue into adolescence and persist in adulthood, even when reading skills improve considerably. The history of children with specific reading disorder frequently reveals a specific developmental disorder of speech and language. Symptoms of these disorders may still be present at elementary school when the specific reading disorder is first diagnosed. Additional frequently associated problems include poor school attendance and problems with social adjustment.

The DSM-IV criteria for reading disorder state that reading achievement as measured by standardized tests should be substantially below the expected level and that the disturbance should interfere with academic achievement or activities of daily living that require reading skills.

### (b) Diagnosis and differential diagnosis

The diagnosis is made on the basis of the ICD-10 and/or DSM-IV criteria, which are similar. The ICD-10 diagnostic guidelines require the following:

◆ A reading performance below the level that is expected on the basis of age, general intelligence, and school placement. For clinical purposes, usually 1.5 standard deviations below the expected level is regarded as a requirement for the diagnosis. For research purposes, two standard deviations are used.

◆ Performance to be assessed by individually administered standardized tests of reading accuracy, latency, and comprehension.

◆ Errors demonstrated in oral reading skills and deficits in reading comprehension. Errors in oral reading include:

   (a) omissions, substitutions, distortions, or additions of words or parts of words;

   (b) slow reading rate;

   (c) false starts, long hesitations, or 'loss of place' in text, and inaccurate phrasing;

   (d) reversals of words in sentences or of letters within words.

Deficits in reading comprehension include:

   (a) an inability to recall facts that have been read;

   (b) inability to draw conclusions or interferences from material that has been read;

   (c) use of general knowledge as background information, rather than of information from a particular story, to answer questions about a story that has been read.

### (c) Comorbidity and associated features

It is important to analyse the features of the disorder with a longitudinal perspective. Thus, several associated disorders can be observed: emotional problems during the early school years; hyperactivity and conduct disorders in later childhood and adolescence. Additional frequent features include low self-esteem, adjustment problems at school, and problems in peer relationships. In about 40 per cent of children with reading and/or spelling disorder, other disorders of clinical relevance are present. After finishing school, this rate decreases to 30 per cent, which includes a high proportion of antisocial behaviour and delinquency.[14]

### (d) Epidemiology

Specific reading and spelling disorder occur in about 4 per cent of 8- to 10-year-old children, when defined as two standard deviations below non-verbal IQ.[15,16] By using a wider definition, the rates are approximately 7 to 8 per cent, with a predominance of boys (2:1).

### (e) Aetiology

Currently, four main aetiological factors have been discussed:

1 genetic influences;

2 deficits in central information processing;

3 general psychosocial factors;

4 specific learning conditions.

Familial clustering in dyslexia was recognized a few years after the first description of the disorder by Hinselwood in 1895. A child with an affected parent has a risk of between 40–60 per cent of developing dyslexia.[17] This risk is increased when other family members are also affected. There is estimated to be a 3 to 10-fold increase in the relative risk for a sibling ($\lambda_s$), with an increase in $\lambda_s$ being observed when stricter criteria are applied.[18]

Twin studies have confirmed that genetic factors are substantially responsible for the familial clustering of dyslexia. It is generally accepted that the proportion of inherited factors involved in the development of dyslexia is between 40–80 per cent, the highest estimates being reported for the phenotype dimensions word reading (up to 58 per cent) and spelling (70 per cent).[19] Whereas shared environmental effects are low for word reading, for with reading, and spelling correlated traits, for example, phonological awareness, shared environmental is substantially higher at about 14 per cent. Based on genome-wide linkage analyses nine candidate gene regions (DYX1-9) could be identified. Most replicated are two regions, 6p22, and 15q21. More recently, four candidate genes, DCDC2, KIAA0319, ROBO1, and DYX1C1 were identified by systematic association analyses. All these genes play a functional role in neuronal migration making them promising candidate genes for dyslexia. However, a functional relevant mutation has not been identified yet.[19]

The hypothesis of deficits in central information processing is based on behavioural and neuroimaging studies that identified cognitive processes that are impaired in dyslexics individuals. These are impaired visual processing, auditory processing, speech perception, phonologic processing, orthographic processing, and motor coordination.[20] The mainstream hypothesis is a phonological processing deficit supported by longitudinal, intervention, and brain imaging studies. Among the latter, the importance of left hemispheric specialization has been widely discussed in the literature, either suggesting maturational lag of the left hemisphere or a structural deficit in white and grey matter.[20]

General psychosocial factors may also play a role in the manifestation of specific reading and spelling disorder. However, the influence seems to be rather marginal. The same applies, more or less, to the special learning condition, because severe deficits in schooling are excluded by definition as a main cause of these disorders. However, given a genetic predisposition for specific reading or spelling disorder, poor learning conditions at school and at home may contribute to the manifestation of these disorders. In summary, the different factors responsible for the manifestation of specific reading and specific spelling disorder can be best understood in terms of a vulnerability model, in which several genetic predispositions, on the one hand, and general psychosocial factors and special learning conditions, on the other, interact with one another.

### (f) Course and prognosis

More than 40 longitudinal follow-up studies have shown similar results:

◆ There is a high persistence of reading and spelling problems, phonological difficulties, and slowness in word recognition.[23,24]

◆ Retarded readers make poorer progress than backward readers.[25]

◆ On the other hand, considerable progress is possible in oral reading and reading comprehension.[26]

As far as schooling is concerned, a substantial proportion of children with specific reading disorder remain behind the school level of their age group. However, there is a difference regarding social background. Children from middle-class homes more frequently show a positive educational outcome compared with children from socially disadvantaged homes.[27]

An epidemiological study in Germany[16] showed that only 3 per cent of children with specific reading disorder were able to attend high school and more than 50 per cent remained at the lowest normal school level. At the age of 18, the rate of unemployment was three times as high as in a normal control group.

### (g) Treatment

As mentioned above, treatment is difficult because the disorder tends to persist. Nevertheless, the following principles have been found to be useful:

1 Treatment should start as early as possible in order to avoid a sense of failure and low self-esteem.

2 The treatment should focus on individual instruction and teaching sessions in basic phonetic and other skills such as reading, spelling, and writing. This needs to be done in an age-appropriate way based on the principles of learning theory and starting at a very low level to avoid disappointment and a sense of failure. There are several programmes used in different countries based on these principles, sometimes using computers.

3 Although very popular methods based on training basic perceptual skills like figure-ground discrimination, tone discrimination, temporal auditory processing have not been proven by empirical studies.

4 Even when feelings of failure and, consequently, low self-esteem are present, the instruction in basic skills is the appropriate approach. The child's psychological and learning situation deserves special attention. Psychotherapeutic measures alone are not successful.

5 Parental support is extremely important. Therefore, the parents should not only be educated in detail about the disorder, but also encouraged to listen to their children reading from school books. This has been shown to be a successful approach.[28]

6 There is no specific medication to improve reading and spelling skills, but there is some indication that stimulants may be helpful for poor readers who simultaneously suffer from attention-deficit hyperactivity disorder.

## Specific spelling disorder

### (a) Clinical features

In ICD-10, the main characteristic of this disorder is a specific and significant impairment in the development of spelling skills in the absence of a history of specific reading disorder, which is not solely accounted for by low mental age, visual acuity problems, or inadequate schooling. The children have difficulties in spelling orally and writing words correctly. For this diagnosis, the following criteria are required (ICD-10):

◆ The spelling performance of the child should be significantly below the expected level regarding age, general intelligence, and school placement. This has to be assessed individually by administration of a standardized spelling test.

◆ The reading skills should be within the normal range and there should be no history of preceding reading difficulties.

◆ The spelling difficulties should not be due to grossly inadequate teaching, to sensory deficits, or to neurological disorders or dysfunctions. They should not be acquired, either as a result of neuropsychiatric or any other disorders.

In DSM-IV, there is no category that corresponds exactly to the ICD-10 category 'Specific spelling disorder'. The DSM-IV category that most closely resembles 'Specific spelling disorder' is 'Disorder of written expression', as defined by measured writing skills substantially below the expected level, interference with academic achievement, and, in the case of a sensory deficit, writing skills greater than the difficulties usually associated with sensory deficits.

It is uncertain whether a pure spelling disorder as described in ICD-10 actually exists or whether spelling skills usually overlap with other functions that constitute scholastic skills. It is, however, possible to assess the different functions separately, as several studies show.

### (b) Diagnosis and differential diagnosis

The diagnosis is made according to the criteria mentioned above and by the administration of standardized spelling tests.

## Specific disorders of arithmetical skills

### (a) Clinical features

The main clinical feature of this disorder (also called dyscalculia) is a specific impairment in arithmetical skills that cannot be explained on the basis of general intellectual disability or inadequate schooling. Dyscalculia is a difficulty in learning and remembering arithmetic facts and executing calculation procedures, with immature problem-solving strategies, long solution times, and high error rates.[29] A number of different skills may be impaired, as understanding or naming mathematical terms, operations, or concepts, and decoding written problems into mathematical symbols.

The impairment affects basic computational skills of addition, subtraction, multiplication, and division, whereas other functions such as reading and writing or motor skills are within the normal range (except in mixed disorder of scholastic skills). The arithmetical difficulties vary, but in most cases include the following features (ICD-10):

◆ difficulties in understanding the concepts underlying arithmetical operations

◆ difficulties or lack of understanding of mathematical terms or signs

◆ difficulties in recognizing numerical symbols

◆ difficulties in carrying out arithmetical manipulations

◆ difficulties in aligning numbers or symbols when performing calculations

◆ poor spatial organization of arithmetical calculations

◆ reduced ability to learn multiplication tables satisfactorily.

The diagnosis is made according to ICD-10 (Specific disorders of arithmetical skills) or DSM-IV criteria (Mathematics Disorder) and the diagnostic guidelines. The ICD-10 guidelines require the following criteria:

◆ The child's arithmetical performance should be significantly below the expected level on the basis of age, general intelligence, and school placement, assessed by an individually administered standardized arithmetical test.

◆ Reading and spelling skills should be within the normal range expected for the child's mental age, also tested by an individually administered standardized test.

◆ The difficulties in arithmetical skills should not be mainly due to grossly inadequate teaching or the direct effects or defects of visual, hearing, or neurological functions and should not be acquired as sequelae of neurological, psychiatric, or other disorders.

The DSM-IV criteria follow the same principles as with other specific developmental disorders. Required criteria include mathematical ability substantially below the expected level, interference with academic achievement, and in the case of a sensory deficit, the difficulties in mathematical ability greater than the difficulties usually associated with sensory deficits.

### (b)  Diagnosis and differential diagnosis

The diagnosis is made according to the above-mentioned criteria in the ICD-10 and DSM-IV systems. Differential diagnosis must rule out acquired arithmetical disorder (acalculia), arithmetical difficulties associated with a reading or spelling disorder, and arithmetical difficulties as a result of inadequate teaching.

### (c)  Epidemiology

It is estimated that between 3 and 6 per cent of all schoolchildren suffer from a specific arithmetical disorder.[30] The sex ratio is approximately equal, in some studies girls are found to be more often affected than boys.[31] An important correlate of maths disorder is dyslexia. It is estimated that 40 per cent of dyslexics also have maths disorder.[31]

### (d)  Aetiology

Dyscalculia has not been studied with the same intensity as dyslexia. Therefore, knowledge about aetiology, course, and outcome is limited.

Numerical abilities, including arithmetic, are mediated by areas in the parietal lobe. In functional imaging studies performed during mental calculation tasks, a pattern of bilateral activation in the prefrontal, premotor, and parietal cortices has been observed.[32] Neuropsychological evidence indicates that numerical processing is localized to the parietal lobes bilaterally, in particular the intra-parietal sulcus[33] and is independent of other abilities. A reduced volume of grey cortical matter in dyscalculic individuals was found in the sulcus intraparietalis of the left hemisphere.[34,35]

There have been a few studies into genetic contributions to mathematical cognitive ability. Most have studied the possible genetic aetiology of mathematics disorder, at least partly because of its comorbidity with reading disorder.[36]

Results from twin studies were consistent with a genetic basis for mathematics disorder whether combined with reading disability or not and estimates of high heritability of mathematical ability were obtained in a sample of twins with normal intelligence ascertained for reading disability and family samples.[37,38]

So far developmental dyscalculia is likely to be the result of the failure of these brain areas to develop normally and can best be defined as a deficit in the representation or processing of specifically numerical information.[39]

A substantial proportion of children with specific disorder of arithmetical skills have associated emotional problems and difficulties in social interactions. It is not quite clear whether these difficulties are secondary complications of the specific difficulties of arithmetical skills.

### (e)  Course and prognosis

As a matter of fact, specific disorder of arithmetical skills is only diagnosed at the end of the first year or the beginning of the second year of elementary school, because of the necessity of these skills at that time. Especially in cases when the disorder is associated with a high IQ, children may initially compensate for the difficulties with the result that the dysfunction is discovered only in the third year of elementary school or later. According to some studies,[40,41] children with specific disorder of arithmetical skills show poor visuospatial abilities and also have difficulties in complex and motor tasks. Share et al.[42] compared these results with their own. Deficits of right hemisphere functioning were found, but only in boys. These results suggest that boys and girls with specific disorder of arithmetical skills should be studied separately. A further interesting result is the association of the disorder with anxiety.[43] This association is more pronounced in those children in whom arithmetical skills are substantially impaired compared with relatively good reading and spelling skills.

### (f)  Treatment

The treatment of specific disorders of arithmetical skills follows the same general lines as treatment of specific reading disorder. All treatment components have to focus on the training of skills that are impaired in a way that keeps the child motivated. Treatment strategies should focus on the mathematical disability itself or the mathematics anxiety with which the disorder is frequently associated. In many cases, both facets need to be included in the treatment programme. When treating the mathematical disability according to the child's individual profile of impairment, four aspects should be emphasized: semantic memory, procedural difficulties, visuospatial difficulties, and difficulties with mathematical problem-solving.[44] Mathematics anxiety requires a more psychotherapeutic approach using relaxation techniques, with the aim of reducing anxiety prior to and during maths lessons in order to avoid a sense of failure.

## Mixed disorders of scholastic skills

In ICD-10, this is specified as an ill-defined and inadequately conceptualized, but necessary residual, category of disorders in which both arithmetical and reading or spelling skills can be significantly impaired, and in which the disorder cannot be explained in terms of general intellectual disability or inadequate schooling. This category covers disorders that meet the criteria of 'Specific disorder of arithmetical skills' (F81.2) and either 'Specific reading disorder' (F81.0) or 'Specific spelling disorder' (F81.1). As has been explained earlier, in the case of a mixed disorder of scholastic skills, it is specific arithmetical disorder that seems to dominate both in severity and with respect to associated psychopathological features.

# Specific developmental disorder of motor function

## Clinical features and classification

Many children to whom this category applies, were previously diagnosed as having 'minimal brain dysfunction'. This term is no longer used. The essential clinical features of the disorder include the following (ICD-10):

♦ An impairment of motor coordination that is significantly below the expected level on the basis of age and general intelligence assessed by an individually administered and standardized test.

♦ The difficulties in coordination should already have been present early in development.

♦ They should not be acquired and not be a direct result of deficits of vision or hearing or of any neurological disorder.

Variability of fine or gross motor coordination is great. The milestones of motor development are usually delayed. In many cases, there is an association with speech difficulties, especially articulation. Parents usually report that the child was slow in learning to sit, run, hop, climb stairs, and ride a bicycle. Many children also have difficulties in learning to tie shoelaces, fasten and unfasten buttons, and throw or catch balls. Some children may be generally clumsy in fine and gross movements others tend to have their main difficulty with fine movements and coordination. In many cases, drawing skills are also impaired and the child's difficulties are particularly obvious during ball games, which require a considerable amount of gross motor coordination.

The DSM-IV criteria are similar, and emphasize a substantial backlog of motor coordination, significant interference with academic achievement, and require general medical conditions and pervasive developmental disorders to be ruled out.

There is growing evidence that specific developmental disorders of motor function are a quite heterogeneous group that needs to be subclassified.[45]

## Diagnosis and differential diagnosis

Diagnosis is made according to the criteria and guidelines in ICD-10 and DSM-IV. Differential diagnosis should rule out specific neurological disorders, which can be done with a careful history and neurological examination, pervasive developmental disorders, which can be distinguished by the criteria of these disorders, or attention-deficit hyperactivity disorder. The latter can be distinguished by their pronounced distractibility and impulsivity rather than impairment of motor coordination.

## Epidemiology

According to an estimation in DSM-IV about 6 per cent of 5- to 11-year-old children suffer from the disorder.

## Aetiology

There are two main factors said to be responsible for the aetiology, genetic influences and brain damage. As far as genetic influences are concerned, there are no valid studies that confirm this assumption. Regarding brain damage, the question arises whether early brain damage can result in a specific impairment of motor functions, while other functions are within normal limits.[46–48] As this appears very unlikely, comorbidity with other disorders should be considered the norm and specificity regarded as the exception.[49]

## Course and prognosis

The few follow-up studies have shown that children who suffer from the disorder between 5 and 10 years of age show a high persistence of motor problems in adolescence. Almost all children who were identified as having had motor difficulties at elementary school, had similar problems as teenagers.[50–52]

## Treatment

Treatment measures should focus on two main facets: the difficulties and impairments in the different motor functions, and the associated social and emotional difficulties. The first facet requires an active functional treatment of motor functions focusing on the child's individual difficulties. Programmes are available for this kind of treatment, which is usually carried out by physiotherapists and occupational therapists.[53]

In treating the second facet, therapists are confronted with the child's insecurity, which is a direct result of motor difficulties, poor body scheme, avoidance reactions of peers and classmates, and frequent feelings of inferiority and a low self-esteem.[54] These associated problems need to be addressed in psychotherapy, in addition to programmes that focus solely on training motor functions.

## Further information

Butterworth, B. (2004). *Dyscalculia guidance helping pupils with specific learning difficulties in Maths.* Nelson Publishing Company, London.

Snowling, M. and Stackhouse, J. (2006). *Dyslexia, speech and language: a practitioner's handbook* Whurr Publishers, West Sussex.

Bishop, D. (2000). *Speech and language impairments in children: causes, characteristics, intervention and outcome.* Taylor and Francis, Philadelphia, PA.

## References

1. World Health Organization. (1992). *International statistical classification of diseases and related health problems*, 10th revision. WHO, Geneva.

2. World Health Organization. (1996). *Multiaxial classification of child and adolescent psychiatric disorders.* Cambridge University Press, Cambridge.

3. American Psychiatric Association. (1994). *Diagnostic and statistical classification of diseases and related health problems* (4th edn). American Psychiatric Association, Washington, DC.

4. Böhme, G. (1980). *Therapie der Sprach-, Sprech- und Stimmstörungen.* Fischer, Stuttgart.

5. Webster, A. and McConnell, C. (1987). *Children with speech and language difficulties.* Cassell, London.

6. Bishop, D.V.M. (1994). Developmental disorders of speech and language. In *Child and adolescent psychiatry* (eds. M. Rutter, E. Taylor, and L. Hersov), pp. 546–68. Blackwell, London.

7. Bishop, D.V.M. (1987). The causes of specific developmental language disorder ('developmental dysphasia'). *Journal of Child Psychology and Psychiatry*, **28**, 1–8.

8. Paul, R. (1992). Language and speech disorders. In *Developmental disorders: diagnostic criteria and clinical assessment* (eds. S.R. Hooper, G.W. Hynd, and R.E. Mattison), pp. 209–38. Erlbaum, Hillsdale, NJ.

9. Rutter, M., Mawhood, L., and Howlin, P. (1992). Language delay and social development. In *Specific speech and language disorders in children* (eds. P. Fletcher and D. Hall), pp. 63–78. Whurr, London.

10. Aicardi, J. (ed.) (1992). *Diseases of the nervous system in childhood. Clinics in developmental medicine, No. 115/118.* McKeith Press, London.

11. Lerman, P. and Lerman-Sagie, T. (1989). Early steroid therapy in Landau–Kleffner syndrome. *Advances in Epileptology*, **17**, 330–2.

12. Morrell, F., Whisler, W.W., and Bleck, T.P. (1989). Multiple subpial transsection: a new approach to the surgical treatment of focal epilepsy. *Journal of Neurosurgery*, **70**, 231–9.

13. Nass, R., Heier, L., and Walker, R. (1993). Landau–Kleffner syndrome: temporal lobe tumor resection results in good outcome. *Paediatric Neurology*, **9**, 303–5.

14. Esser, G. and Schmidt, M.H. (1993). Die langfristige Entwicklung von Kindern mit Lese-Rechtschreibschwäche. *Zeitschrift für Klinische Psychologie*, **22**, 100–16.

15. Rutter, M., Tizard, J., and Whitmore, K. (1970). *Education, health and behaviour.* Longmans, London.

16. Esser, G. and Schmidt, M.H. (1994). Teilleistungsstörung und depression. *Kindheit und Entwicklung*, **3**, 157.

17. Schulte-Körne, G. (2001). Annotation: genetics of reading and spelling disorder. *Journal of Child Psychology and Psychiatry*, **42**, 985–97.

18. Ziegler, A., König, I.R., Deimel, W., *et al.* (2005). Developmental dyslexia—recurrence risk estimates from a German bi-center study using the single proband sib pair design. *Human Heredity*, **5**, 136–43.

19. Schumacher, J., Hoffmann, P., Schmäl, C., *et al.* (2007). Genetics of dyslexia: the evolving landscape. *Journal of Medical Genetics*, **44**, 289–97.

20. Démonet, J.F., Taylor, M.J., and Chaix, Y. (2004). Developmental dyslexia. *Lancet*, **363**, 1451–60.

21. Satz, P. and Sparrow, S. (1970). Specific developmental dyslexia: a theoretical formulation. In *Specific reading disability: theory and method* (eds. D.J. Bakker and P. Satz), pp. 41–60. Rotterdam University Press.

22. Masland, R.L. (1975). Neurological bases of correlates of language disabilities: diagnostic implication. *Acta Symbolica*, **6**, 1–34.

23. Finucci, J.M. (1986). Follow-up studies of developmental dyslexia and other learning disabilities. In *Genetics and learning disabilities* (ed. S.D. Smith), pp. 97–121. Taylor and Francis, Philadelphia, PA.

24. Spreen, O. (1988). Prognosis of learning disability. *Journal of Consulting and Clinical Psychology*, **56**, 836–42.

25. Rutter, M., Tizard, J., Yule, W., *et al.* (1976). Isle–of–Wight studies 1964–1974. *Psychological Medicine*, **6**, 313–32.

26. Bruck, M. (1990). Word recognition skills in adults with childhood diagnosis of dyslexia. *Developmental Psychology*, **26**, 439–54.

27. Clay, M. (1985). *The early detection of reading difficulties* (3rd edn). Heinemann, Tadworth, Surrey.

28. Hewison, J. (1988). Long-term effectiveness of parental involvement in reading: a follow-up to the Haringey Reading Project. *British Journal of Educational Psychology*, **58**, 184–90.

29. Geary, D.C. (1993). Mathematical disabilities: cognitive, neuropsychological, and genetic components. *Psychological Bulletin*, **114**, 345–62.

30. Gross-Tsur, V., Manor, O., and Shalev, R.S. (1996). Developmental dyscalculia: prevalence and demographic features. *Developmental Medicine and Child Neurology*, **38**, 25–33.

31. Lewis, C., Hitch, G.W., and Walker, P. (1994). The prevalence of specific arithmetic difficulties and specific reading difficulties in 9 to 10 year–old boys and girls. *Journal of Child Psychology and Psychiatry*, **35**, 283–92.

32. Dehaene, S., Spelke, E., Pinel, P., *et al.* (1999). Source of mathematical thinking: behavioral and brainimaging evidence. *Science*, **284**, 970–4.

33. Dehaene, S., Piazza, M., Pinel, P., *et al.* (2003). Three parietal circuits for number processing. *Cognitive Neuropsychology*, **20**, 487–506.

34. Isaacs, E.B., Edmonds, C.J., Lucas, A., *et al.* (2001). Calculation difficulties in children of very low birthweight: a neural correlate. *Brain*, **124**, 1701–7.

35. Levy, L.M., Reis, I.L., and Grafman, J. (1999). Metabolic abnormalities detected by 1H-MRS in dyscalculia and dysgraphia. *Neurology*, **53**, 639–41.

36. Light, J.G. and DeFries, J.C. (1995). Comorbidity of reading and mathematics disabilities—genetic and environmental etiologies. *Journal of Learning Disability*, **28**, 96–106.

37. Plomin, R. and Kovas, Y. (2005). Generalist genes and learning disabilities. *Psychological Bulletin*, **131**, 592–617.

38. Schulte-Körne, G., Ziegler, A., Deimel, W., *et al.* (2006). Interrelationship and familiality of dyslexia related quantitative measures. *Annals of Human genetics*, **70**, 1–16.

39. Landerl, K., Bevan, A., and Buttherworth, B. (2004). Developmental dyscalculia and basic numerical capacities: a study of 8-9-year-old students. *Cognition*, **93**, 99–125.

40. Rourke, B.P. and Finlayson, M.A.J. (1978). Neurophysiological significance of variations in pattern of academic performance: verbal and visuo-spatial abilities. *Journal of Abnormal Child Psychology*, **6**, 121–33.

41. Rourke, B.P. and Fuerst, D.R. (1991). *Learning disabilities and psychosocial functioning: a neuropsychological perspective.* Guilford Press, New York.

42. Share, D.L., Moffitt, T.E., and Silva, P.A. (1988). Factors associated with arithmetic-and-reading disability and specific arithmetic disability. *Journal of Learning Disabilities*, **21**, 313–20.

43. Lansdown, R. (1978). Retardation in mathematics: consideration of multifactorial determination. *Journal of Child Psychology and Psychiatry*, **19**, 181–5.

44. Geary, D.C. (1994). *Children's mathematical development. Research and practical applications.* American Psychological Association, Washington, DC.

45. Hoare, D. (1994). Subtypes of developmental coordination disorder. *Adapted Physical Activity Quarterly*, **11**, 158–69.

46. Caron, D. and Rutter, M. (1991). Co-morbidity in child psychopathology: concepts, issues, and research strategies. *Journal of Child Psychology and Psychiatry*, **32**, 1063–80.

47. Henderson, S.E., Barnett, A.L., and Henderson, L. (1994). Visuo-spatial difficulties and clumsiness. On the interpretation of conjoint deficits. *Journal of Child Psychology and Psychiatry*, **35**, 961–9.

48. Powell, R.P. and Bishop, D. (1992). Clumsiness and perceptual problems in children with specific language impairment. *Developmental Medicine and Child Neurology*, **34**, 755–65.

49. Henderson, S.E. and Barnett, A.L. (1988). Developmental movement problems. In *Perspectives on the classification of specific developmental disorders* (eds. J. Rispens, T.A. van Yperen, and W. Yule), pp. 209–30. Kluwer Academic, Dordrecht.

50. Knuckey, N.W. and Gubbay, S.S. (1983). Clumsy children: a prognostic study. *Australian Paediatric Journal*, **19**, 9–13.

51. Losse, A., Henderson, S.E., Elliman, D., *et al.* (1991). Clumsiness in children—do they grow out of it? A ten-year follow-up study. *Developmental Medicine and Child Neurology*, **33**, 55–68.

52. Cantell, M.H., Smyth, M.M., and Ahonen, T.P. (1994). Clumsiness in adolescents: educational, motor a nd social outcomes of motor delay detected at five years. *Special Issue of Adapted Physical Activity Quarterly*, **11**, 115–29.

53. Schoemaker, M.M., Hijlkema, M.G.J., and Kalverboer, A.F. (1994). Physiotherapy for clumsy children: an evaluation study. *Developmental Medicine and Child Neurology*, **36**, 143–55.

54. Kalverboer, K.F. (1998). On the relevance of specific classifications of disorders with particular focus on DCD, developmental coordination disorder. In *Perspectives on the classification of specific developmental disorders* (eds. J. Rispens, T.A. van Yperen, and W. Yule), pp. 265–78. Kluwer Academic, Dordrecht.

# 9.2.3 Autism and the pervasive developmental disorders

Fred R. Volkmar and Ami Klin

## Introduction

The pervasive developmental disorders (PDDs) are characterized by patterns of deviance and delay in social-communicative development in the first years of life, which are associated with restricted patterns of interest or behaviour. The prototypic PDD is childhood autism; other conditions included in the PDD class in ICD-10[1] include Rett's syndrome, childhood disintegrative disorder, Asperger's syndrome, and atypical autism. Except for one additional category in ICD-10 (hyperkinetic stereotyped movement disorder), the disorders included in ICD-10 and DSM-IV[2] are essentially identical. In this chapter each of these conditions will be reviewed in terms of their clinical features, definition, epidemiology, course, and aetiology; final sections of the chapter address aspects of treatment and prevention for the group of disorders as a whole (Box 9.2.3.1).

## Childhood autism

Autism was first recognized by Kanner[3] in his report of 11 children with 'autistic disturbances of affective contact'. He emphasized two essential diagnostic features: autism and difficulties with change; but he also noted atypical language (when language was present at all). He used Bleuler's term 'autistic' to convey the children's social isolation. Although children with autism had undoubtedly been previously observed,[4] it was Kanner's particular genius to so precisely describe the condition. False leads for research arose since the term autism introduced an unintended confusion with schizophrenia. Also, Kanner assumed that the children had normal intellectual potential. Subsequently, it became clear that autism and schizophrenia were distinct and that autism was often associated with intellectual disability.[5] Although describing autism as inborn, Kanner mentioned that parents were very well educated and successful. In turn this led to the idea, common during the 1950s, that autism might somehow result from deviant patterns of care by unusually successful parents. A large body of evidence shows that this is most certainly not the case.[6] It is clear that families of children with autism come from all social classes and circumstances[7] and that the original impression had been the result of referral bias.

### Clinical features

Social deficits of a particular type remain a hallmark of autism. The nature of this deficit varies, somewhat, over time but remains a

| **Box 9.2.3.1** The pervasive developmental disorders |
| :--- |
| Childhood autism/autistic disorder |
| Rett's disorder |
| Childhood disintegrative disorder |
| Asperger's disorder |
| PDD-NOS/atypical autism |

source of great disability to the affected individual throughout life.[8] In younger and more impaired individuals there may be little interest in social interaction; less impaired individuals may come to a passive acceptance of social interaction while older and more cognitively able individuals are more likely to seem highly eccentric and one-sided.[9] Difficulties are observed in the use of eye contact or other non-verbal social cues, in social emotional reciprocity and empathy, in activities involving shared interests with others, and with peer relationships (see Table 9.2.3.1). As Rutter[10] suggested, these problems do not simply reflect cognitive impairment, which is present in about 60 per cent of individuals affected. Abnormalities in communication (not only in language) are also observed. In a substantial minority (perhaps 30 per cent) of cases, the child never acquires the capacity for communicative speech; among individuals who do talk, various unusual features of language are observed such as echolalia, idiosyncratic language, deficits in prosody, and pronoun reversal.[11] Deficits in pragmatic language are particularly striking. As with the social disturbance, the deficits observed are not solely due to intellectual disabilities. Various unusual behaviours are subsumed under the term 'resistance to change'. These behaviours include literal resistance to change ('insistence on sameness'), stereotyped and repetitive motor mannerisms, strict adherence to non-functional routines, and interest in non-functional parts of objects. Various other features may be observed, such as unusual sensitivities to aspects of the environment and attachments to unusual objects.

### Definition

In the 1950s and 1960s there was disagreement about autism, e.g. was it a form of schizophrenia or psychosis? Gradually evidence began to accumulate that suggested the role of central nervous system dysfunction in pathogenesis—for example, high risk for developing seizures. Differences in clinical features, onset and course, and family history also supported the distinctiveness of autism apart from childhood schizophrenia.[12,13] By 1978, there was a substantial body of work on the validity of autism. Rutter synthesized this in his influential definition of autism,[10] which required the presence of patterns of delay and deviance in the areas of social and language development that were not simply the result of developmental delay along with the group of unusual behaviours subsumed under Kanner's term 'insistence on sameness'. Onset before 30 months of age was required. In ICD-9[14] infantile autism was still termed a psychotic condition but by 1980 the highly influential DSM-III[15] appeared and recognized autism as a condition apart from schizophrenia, including it in a new class of disorders—the pervasive developmental disorders. The latter term has been the topic of some debate, although a better term has yet to be proposed and, in any case, the term PDD has now come into general usage in both DSM and ICD.[16,17]

The name chosen in DSM-III ('Infantile autism') was consistent with Kanner's original report but reflected a lack of developmental orientation; these concerns were addressed in DSM-III-R,[18] which provided a detailed, and more developmentally oriented, set of diagnostic guidelines. Unfortunately, this definition proved overly inclusive and it became apparent that additional work would be needed. Further impetus was given to this effort by pending changes in ICD-10[1] and DSM-IV. Accordingly, an international field trial was undertaken.[19] Based on the results of this field trial

**Table 9.2.3.1** ICD-10 criteria for childhood autism (F84.0)

A. Abnormal or impaired development is evident before the age of 3 years in at least one of the following areas:

   1 receptive or expressive language as used in social communication;

   2 the development of selective social attachments or of reciprocal social interaction

   3 functional or symbolic play

B. A total of at least six symptoms from (1), (2), and (3) must be present, with at least two from (1) and least one from each of (2) and (3)

   1 Qualitative impairment in social interaction is manifested in at least two of the following areas:

     (a) failure adequately to use eye-to-eye gaze, facial expression, body postures, and gestures to regulate social interaction

     (b) failure to develop (in a manner appropriate to mental age, and despite ample opportunities) peer relationships that involve a mutual sharing of interests, activities, and emotions

     (c) lack of socio-emotional reciprocity as shown by an impaired or deviant response to other people's emotions; or lack of modulation of behaviour according to social context; or a weak integration of social, emotional, and communicative behaviours

     (d) lack of spontaneous seeking to share enjoyment, interests, or achievements with other people (e.g. a lack of showing, bringing, or pointing out to other people objects of interest to the individual)

   2 Qualitative abnormalities in communication in at least one of the following areas:

     (a) delay in or total lack of development of spoken language that is not accompanied by an attempt to compensate through the use of gestures or mime as an alternative mode of communication (often preceded by a lack of communicative babbling)

     (b) relative failure to initiate or sustain conversational interchange (at whatever level of language skill is present), in which there is reciprocal responsiveness to the communications of the other person

     (c) stereotyped and repetitive use of language or idiosyncratic use of words or phrases

     (d) lack of varied spontaneous make-believe play or (when young) social imitative play

   3 Restricted, repetitive, and stereotyped patterns of behaviour, interests, and activities are manifested in at least one of the following:

     (a) an encompassing preoccupation with one or more stereotyped and restricted patterns of interest that are abnormal in content or focus; or one or more interests that are abnormal in their intensity and circumscribed in nature though not in their content or focus

     (b) apparently compulsive adherence to specific non-functional routines or rituals

     (c) stereotyped and repetitive motor mannerisms that involve either hand or finger flapping or twisting or complex whole-body movements;

     (d) preoccupations with part-objects or non-functional elements of play materials (such as their odour, the feel of their surface, or the noise or vibration they generate)

C. The clinical picture is not attributable to the other varieties of pervasive developmental disorders; specific developmental disorder of receptive language (F80.2) with secondary socio-emotional problems, reactive attachment disorder (F94.1), or disinhibited attachment disorder (F94.2); mental retardation (F70–F72) with some associated emotional or behavioural disorders; schizophrenia (F20.-) of unusually early onset; and Rett's syndrome (F84.12).

Taken from Disorders of psychological development (*criteria for research*), pp. 154–5. © World Health Organization, www.who.int

autism is defined (see Table 9.2.3.1) on the basis of characteristic problems in three areas: social interaction, communication and play, and restricted patterns of interest. By definition, autism must be present by the age of 3 years. ICD-10 provides for various ways in which a diagnosis of atypical autism can be made—for example, because of failure to meet age of onset or behavioural criteria. Data on this system suggest that it has good agreement with the diagnoses of experienced clinicians, avoids the problem of the overdiagnosis of autism in the most mentally handicapped persons, and has reasonably good reliability.

### Epidemiology and demographics

Over 40 epidemiological studies of autism and related conditions have been conducted with prevalence estimates ranging from 0.7 per 10 000 to 72.6 per 10 000.[20] In his recent 2005 review, Fombonne notes that prevalence rates are negatively correlated with sample size and there is an apparent trend for increased rates over time. Various considerations (including changes in definition) complicate the interpretation of increased rates. In this review, Fombonne suggests that a reasonable estimate of prevalence is

13 per 10 000 (Box 9.2.3.2). Although higher rates of 1 in 150 are reported if broad definitions are used.

---

**Box 9.2.3.2** Epidemiology of autism and related conditions

Autism. . . . . . . . . . . . . . . . . . . . . . . . . . . . .13 per 10 000

Rett's disorder. . . . . . . . . . . . . . . . . . . . . . . . 1 per 10 000 girls

Childhood disintegrative disorder . . . . . . .1.9 per 100 000

Asperger's syndrome . . . . . . . . . . . . . . . . . . . . 4 per 10 000

PDD-NOS/atypical autism . . . . . . . . . . . . . . .1 per 150

Source: Cohen, D.J. and Volkmar, F.R. (eds.) (2005) *Handbook of autism and pervasive developmental disorders* (3rd edn.) Wiley, New York.

---

A number of studies, including both epidemiological and clinically referred samples, report higher rates of autism in boys than in girls (typically 3.5:1 or 4:1). This ratio varies with IQ level, i.e. females with autism who have IQs in the normal range are probably

20 times less common than males.[21] The explanation for this sex difference remains unclear. It is possible that the degree of insult required to produce autism in females must be greater than for males, but other hypothesis have been raised. Ethnic and cultural differences have been little studied.[20,22]

## Course and prognosis

Although childhood autism is a chronic disability, there is some suggestion that with early intervention and remediation outcome is improving.[23] For example, the number of individuals with either a 'good' or 'fair' outcome is now about 50 per cent—a noteworthy increase since 1980.[24] However, even in the highest functioning individuals marked social problems persist.

Changes in the degree of social relatedness, communication, and self-help skills are observed with increases in developmental level. Seizure disorders are observed in up to 25 per cent of individuals and may have their onset at any point, but adolescence and early childhood are particularly common times.[25] Factors that predict long-term outcome include the presence of some communicative speech by the age of 5 or 6 years, and non-verbal intellectual level.

## Aetiology

Early interest centred on the possibility that experiential factors might somehow cause autism, but a host of research findings suggests that this is not the case. Rather, a fundamental disturbance in the central nervous system is implicated.

### (a) Psychological factors

Disabilities affecting attentional mechanisms, arousal, sensory deficits, memory management, and complex information processing, among others, have been proposed as 'primary' deficits underlying the social impairment in autism. Although each of these helps us understand some aspects of the condition, none has, as yet, provided a more comprehensive account of the condition as a whole.[26] Among the most influential recent theories attempting to do that is the hypothesis that posits a lack of a central drive for coherence in children with autism, with the consequent focus on dissociated fragments of their environment rather than integrated 'wholes', leading to a fragmentary and overly concrete experience of the world.[27] Another cognitive account of autism posits that the commonly found difficulties in abstracting rules, inhibiting irrelevant responses, shifting attention, and profiting from feedback as well as in maintaining relevant information 'on-line'—the so-called 'executive functions'—underlie the social, communicative, and behavioural disabilities in autism.[28] Although both these theories—'weak central coherence' and 'executive dysfunction'—provide insightful new views of well-known clinical features, neither phenomena can be seen as specific to autism relative to other developmental disorders.

Probably the most influential current cognitive hypothesis focuses on mechanisms directly impacting on social understanding. This view, the 'theory of mind' hypothesis, posits that autism is caused by the child's inability to attribute mental states such as beliefs and intentions to others. Devoid of this ability, individuals with autism are thought to be unable to infer the thoughts and motivations of others, thus failing to predict their behaviour and adjust their own actions accordingly, which results in a lack of reciprocity in communication and social contact.[29] Although more than 50 studies have documented such deficits in autism, there are still many limitations to this hypothesis. For example, more able individuals with autism do exhibit 'theory of mind' skills—and yet may be totally unable to utilize this capacity in their spontaneous social adjustment. Such phenomena suggest that factors other than a cognitive understanding of mental phenomena are required for a person to meet the demands of everyday social life. For example, the 'enactive mind' hypothesis focuses on early emerging and highly conserved mechanisms of socialization that precede the advent of mentalizing abilities, and which culminate in the development of joint attention and perspective taking skills.[30] Of great interest in the past few years has been the confluence of experimental psychological paradigms and functional neuroimaging studies focusing on the same constructs. This new trend is leading to new insights into brain systems subserving basic social mechanisms such as gaze behaviour, face processing, social-affective responses, and thinking about other people's intentions and beliefs,[31] all of which are greatly compromised in autism.

### (b) Biological factors

The importance of biological factors in the pathogenesis of autism is suggested by several lines of evidence. Autism has been associated with a host of medical conditions; but the absence of population data and rigorous diagnostic assessment makes such associations difficult to interpret. For example, early reports suggested an association with congenital rubella, but this now seems questionable given the diagnostic dilemmas and the observation that 'autistic-like' features diminish over time.[32] Gillberg[33] argues that medical conditions may be associated with autism in as many as one-third of the cases, but Rutter and colleagues[34] suggest that a more reasonable figure would be roughly 10 per cent of all cases. The strongest associations are with fragile X syndrome and tuberous sclerosis—both conditions having a strong genetic component (Box 9.2.3.3).

---

**Box 9.2.3.3** Medical conditions associated with autism

Seizure disorder (epilepsy)
Fragile X syndrome
Tuberous sclerosis

---

Fragile X syndrome is an X-linked intellectual disability syndrome involving a mutation characterized by a triplet repeat of cytosine–guanine–guanine (CGG) that may amplify with succeeding generations. It is associated with a characteristic facial appearance, enlarged testicles, intellectual disability, and some autistic features. Early reports suggesting high rates of fragile X in autism have now been modified; fragile X affects perhaps 1 to 2 per cent of all individuals with autism.[20]

The autosomal dominant disorder tuberous sclerosis is characterized by abnormal tissue growth, or benign tumours (hamartomas), in the brain and in other organs. The condition, which may affect 1 in 10 000 individuals, is variably expressed; the phenotype ranges from minor skin problems or seizures to severe intellectual disability with intractable seizures. The rate of this condition in autism (0.4–2.8 per cent) is significantly increased.[20]

Autism is a strongly genetic condition. Studies of monozygotic and dizygotic twins revealed much higher levels of concordance for monozygotic relative to dizygotic twin pairs, but also elevated rates of concordance in dizygotic twins relative to population rates.[35] General studies suggest that the recurrence risk of autism in siblings is in the order of between 2 and 10 per cent—which is a substantial increase in risk over population rates. There also appear to be higher rates of social and language problems and rigid patterns of behaviour in siblings and close relatives, raising the possibility that what is inherited is a broader phenotype reminiscent of autism but which also may reflect a more general predisposition to developmental difficulties. Recent work also suggests elevated rates of anxiety and mood disorders in family members. Specific modes of inheritance remain unclear. It now appears that several interacting genes are probably involved in the pathogenesis of autism. Efforts are underway to identify susceptibility genes and trace their impact on brain development. Although several studies have shown increased rates of pre-, peri-, and neonatal complications in children with autism, it is possible that some of these difficulties may reflect a genetic vulnerability in the child or that there may be an interaction of genetic and perinatal factors.[35] A recent report has noted the presence of placental abnormalities in pregnancies of children with autism.

Attempts have been made to identify neuropathological and neuroanatomical correlates of autism. Areas of interest have included the cortical areas responsible for language and social interaction (frontal and temporal lobes) as well as the neostriatum and cerebellum.[36] The report of reduced cerebellar size in the neocerebellar vermal lobules VI and VII has not proven readily replicable. Some individuals with autism have enlarged brains and head sizes, with some evidence that abnormal growth occurs in the first 2 years of life.[37] Neuropathological studies have suggested possible cellular changes in areas of the brain such as the hippocampus and amygdala and changes in the cytoarchitecture of the brain, e.g. in the arrangement of cortical 'minicolumns'.

Various neurotransmitter systems have been studied. Probably the most robust finding has been the observation that about one-third of the children with autism have increased peripheral levels of serotonin. This finding is not specific to autism and its significance remains unclear.[38] Studies of other neurotransmitters such as dopamine produced inconsistent findings. The possible involvement of dopamine is suggested by the high levels of stereotyped behaviours in autism—behaviours, which can be induced in animals by the administration of agents (stimulants) that affect levels of dopamine in the brain. Agents such as the neuroleptics, which block dopamine receptors, are effective in reducing the stereotyped and hyperactive behaviours of many autistic children. Another hypothesis has centred on the possible role of endogenous opioids, in that overproduction of such compounds might lead to social withdrawal and unusual sensitivities and behaviours. This has led to the administration of opioid antagonists such as naltrexone in autism; unfortunately results have been disappointing. Studies of the immune system in autism have been relatively uncommon and findings inconsistent.

## Rett's syndrome

In 1966, Andreas Rett described an unusual syndrome in girls characterized by a history of initial normal development, subsequent head growth deceleration, and the development of specific clinical findings such as breathing difficulties, movement problems, and some features suggestive of autism.[39] His findings were replicated and extended by Hagberg and colleagues.[40] As more

extensive information became available it became clear that the more 'autistic-like' phase of Rett's syndrome was relatively brief, but this was a major rationale for its inclusion in the PDD class.[41]

### Clinical features

Early pre- and perinatal histories are generally unremarkable in Rett's syndrome, as is very early development. Usually within the first or second year of life development begins to slow or actually regress and various motor problems—including characteristic hand-washing stereotypies start to develop.[42] A significant loss of developmental skills occurs and head growth decelerates.[40] The potential for misdiagnosis of autism is greatest during this time; during school age developmental regression often stabilizes and children are more socially responsive. As individuals with Rett's syndrome approach adolescence they are frequently subject to increased spasticity, scoliosis, loss of ambulation, bruxism, hyperventilation, areophagia, apnoea, and seizures.[43] Although debated,[44] the inclusion of Rett's syndrome in the PDD class reflects an awareness of the confusion with autism and the importance of including the condition somewhere.[41]

### Definition

Various diagnostic criteria for Rett's syndrome have been developed.[45] As presently defined in ICD-10 (see Table 9.2.3.2) the condition develops after some months of normal development; head circumference is normal at birth but begins to decelerate between 5 and 48 months. Characteristic midline hand-wringing or hand-washing stereotypies develop and purposeful hand movements are lost.

### Epidemiology and demographics

Prevalence estimates range from 1 per 12 000 to 1 per 23 000 females; cases are observed in all racial and ethnic groups.[46,47] Rett's syndrome may account for one-quarter to one-third of progressive developmental disabilities among females.[46] A small number of cases have now been reported in males.

### Course and prognosis

Various clinical stages of the condition have been identified.[42] Early developmental losses may be subtle initially but become more marked with time. Purposeful hand movements are often then lost, as are speech skills. Ataxia and gait abnormalities are noted in those

**Table 9.2.3.2** ICD-10 criteria for Rett's syndrome (F84.2)

A. There is an apparently normal prenatal and perinatal period and apparently normal psychomotor development through the first 5 months and normal head circumference at birth.

B. There is a deceleration of head growth between 5 months and 4 years and loss of acquired purposeful hand skills between 5 and 30 months of age that is associated with concurrent communication dysfunction and impaired social interactions and the appearance of poorly co-ordinated/unstable gait and/or trunk movements.

C. There is severe impairment of expressive and receptive language, together with severe psychomotor retardation.

D. There are stereotyped midline hand movements (such as hand-wringing or 'hand-washing') with an onset at or after the time when purposeful hand movements are lost.

Taken from Disorders of psychological development (*criteria for research*), pp. 154–5.
© World Health Organization, www.who.int

patients who had acquired the ability to walk, unusual breathing patterns (hyperventilation and/or apnoea), and seizures may also be observed. While social and communication skills may improve in middle childhood motor problems are more pronounced. During the final phase (roughly after age 10) progressive scoliosis and spasticity are observed, while cognitive function stabilizes and seizure activity may diminish. There is a dearth of information on adults with the condition. There does appear to be an increased risk of sudden death due to seizures and/or respiratory difficulties.[48]

### Aetiology

Rett[39] originally speculated that the condition might be associated with high peripheral ammonia levels, but this was incorrect. Recent work identified mutations in the MeCP2 gene as the cause of Rett syndrome in most cases; this gene has a major role in regulating various genes during brain development.[49]

## Childhood disintegrative disorder

Shortly after the turn of the twentieth century a special educator working in Vienna, Theodor Heller,[50] reported children who had a period of several years of normal development prior to a marked regression with loss of skills in multiple areas and minimal recovery. He initially termed the condition dementia infantilis; subsequently it has been referred to as Heller's syndrome, disintegrative psychosis, or childhood disintegrative disorder.[51] Once it develops the condition is indistinguishable from autism,[52] but it is accorded separate diagnostic status since it appears distinctive in terms of onset and course.

### Clinical features

In this condition an 'autistic-like' clinical picture develops after a prolonged period of normal development.[50] More than 100 cases have now been reported; the condition is rare but probably under-diagnosed.[51] Essential clinical features include a relatively long period of normal development followed by a marked developmental regression and development of various 'autistic-like' features; onset is typically between the ages of 3 and 4 years.

Onset can be relatively abrupt or more gradual, and a premonitory phase of non-specific anxiety or agitation may be observed. Parents often note associations between the onset of the condition and various psychosocial or medical events but such associations are probably correlational rather than causative.[53] Once established it resembles autism.[52] Given the behavioural similarity to autism, it might be argued either that the condition does not warrant separate diagnostic recognition or that the condition is inevitably the result of an association with some progressive medical condition. However, the pattern of onset is quite distinctive, the outcome appears to be even worse than in autism, and usually even with very intensive medical evaluations no general medical condition accounting for the regression is identified.[52]

### Definition

Criteria for the disorder are listed in Table 9.2.3.3. By definition the disorder cannot coexist with autism or another other explicitly defined pervasive developmental disorder, schizophrenia, elective mutism, or the syndrome of acquired aphasia with epilepsy.

### Epidemiology and demographics

Epidemiological data are quite limited. Some limited data suggest a prevalence rate of 1 in 100 000. Initially cases seemed to be equally

**Table 9.2.3.3** ICD-10 criteria for other childhood disintegrative disorder (F84.3)

A. Development is apparently normal up to the age of at least 2 years. The presence of normal age-appropriate skills in communication, social relationships, play, and adaptive behaviour at age 2 years or later is required for diagnosis.

B. There is a definite loss of previously acquired skills at about the time of onset of the disorder. The diagnosis requires a clinically significant loss of skills (not just a failure to use them in certain situations) in at least two of the following areas:
  1 expressive or receptive language
  2 play
  3 social skills or adaptive behaviour
  4 bowel or bladder control
  5 motor skills.

C. Qualitatively abnormal social functioning is manifested in at least two of the following areas:
  1 abnormalities in reciprocal social interaction (of the type defined for autism)
  2 qualitative abnormalities in communication (of the type defined for autism)
  3 restricted, repetitive, and stereotyped patterns of behaviour, interests, and activities, including motor stereotypes and mannerisms
  4 a general loss of interest in objects and in the environment.

D. The disorder is not attributable to the other varieties of pervasive developmental disorder; acquired aphasia with epilepsy (F80.6); elective mutism (F94.0); Rett's syndrome (F84.2); or schizophrenia (F20.-).

Taken from Disorders of psychological development (criteria for research), pp. 154–5 © World Health Organization, www.who.int

distributed between males and females, but it now seems likely that cases of Rett's syndrome may have been included in early case series. Recent reviews have noted a preponderance of males.[20]

### Course and prognosis

In about 75 per cent of cases the deterioration reaches a plateau, in that there is no further loss of skills, but subsequent gains tend to be minimal. Thus the child who previously was normally socially related, spoke in full sentences, and was toilet-trained becomes indifferent to social interaction, loses all expressive language and toilet skills, and remains mute and relatively low functioning.[52] In the remainder of cases there is more limited recovery, for example the child regains the capacity to speak but only in single words or only echoes language. If a progressive metabolic or neuropathological process is present, the developmental progression may continue until death ensues; such cases often have a later onset.[54] Life expectancy otherwise appears to be normal. In a very small number of cases significant recovery has been noted.

### Aetiology

Various lines of evidence suggest the importance of neurobiological factors in pathogenesis. Occasionally medical conditions such as the neurolipidoses, metachromatic leukodystrophy, Addison–Schilder's disease, and subacute sclerosing panencephalitis are associated with the condition. Rates of electroencephalographic abnormalities and seizure disorders are of roughly the same frequency as seen in autism.

# Asperger's syndrome

The condition known as Asperger's syndrome was described by a paediatrician with interest in intellectual disability, Hans Asperger,[55] who reported on four boys with marked social problems, unusual perseverative interests, and motor clumsiness but with seemingly good verbal and cognitive abilities. Like Kanner, Asperger used the word autism (autistic psychopathy) to describe this condition. His concept, however, had points of difference, as well as similarity, to autism. For example, verbal abilities tended to be an area of strength, concerns typically did not arise until later in the preschool period, and there was a tendency for the condition to run in families—particularly in fathers. Lorna Wing's[56] report of Asperger's work and publication of a series of cases brought wider attention to the diagnostic concept. The validity of this condition, particularly apart from higher-functioning autism, remains the topic of much debate. A major complication has been the marked differences in definition of the conditions and its potential overlap with other diagnostic concepts (e.g. schizoid personality,[57] non-verbal learning disabilities,[58] semantic–pragmatic disorder,[59] and right hemisphere learning problems).[60] As a result, the literature on this condition is difficult to interpret, although areas of potential differences from autism have been identified, such as neuropsychological profiles[61] and family history.[62]

## Clinical features

This condition is characterized by impairments in social interaction and restricted interests and behaviours as seen in autism. However, the child's early development is marked by lack of any clinically significant delay in spoken or receptive language, cognitive development, self-help skills, and curiosity about the environment. Consistent with Asperger's[55] original report, all-absorbing and intense circumscribed interests as well as motor clumsiness are typical, but are not required for diagnosis. The validity of this condition, apart from high-functioning autism and PDD not otherwise specified (PDD-NOS) is controversial. Available research is difficult to interpret given the markedly different ways in which the diagnostic concept has been used. Differences are more likely to be noted relative to autism if a rather stringent diagnostic approach is used. Evidence for external validity of the condition relative to autism includes differences in neuropsychological profiles, patterns of comorbidity, and family history.

Persons with Asperger's syndrome often exhibit a somewhat eccentric social style rather than the more passive or aloof style noted in autism; for example, they may engage others in very one-sided conversations about their area of special interest. They maybe overly reliant on rigid rules for social interaction and may fail to 'see the forest for the trees' in social matters (e.g. an appreciation of exactly when the usual rules do not apply is as important as when they do). Their social oddity and lack of flexibility is a source of much disability.

While early speech-communication skills are apparently normal, certain aspects of communication become more deviant over time. Prosody may be poor, rate of speech may also be unusual, or it may have a somewhat disorganized, tangential, and circumstantial quality. The issue of whether such persons are at increased risk for thought disorder and psychosis remains unresolved, but some part of this impression probably reflects communication problems.

It is rather typical for patients to amass considerable factual information about their topic of interest, which they pursue with great intensity; Asperger originally observed that family life may revolve around the topic of special interest. He also suggested that motor clumsiness was present and, although not required for the diagnosis, there is often a history of motor delay and persistent motor awkwardness—for instance, the child may talk before he walks, have trouble fastening fastener, catching a ball, learning to ride a bicycle, engaging in cursive handwriting, and may also display stiffened gate.

Differences in neuropsychological profiles have been reported.[63] A stringent diagnostic approach may suggest areas of relative strengths (auditory and verbal skills and rote learning) and weakness (visuomotor and visuoperceptual skills); this pattern differs from that observed in higher-functioning individuals with autism[64] and the heritability of social difficulties may be even greater in Asperger's syndrome than in autism.[62]

Interest in the condition has revolved around the possibility that it might represent a transition between autism and other disorders such as schizophrenia. Associated conditions have included depression, anxiety and other mood problems, violence, and other psychotic conditions.[63] Unfortunately, almost all of this literature rests on case reports; controlled studies are needed.

## Definition

The ICD-10 criteria for Asperger's syndrome are given in Table 9.2.3.4. As presently defined the social deficit is the same as in autism. In contrast to autism, however, early language, cognitive, and other skills develop typically early in life. By definition, the case does not meet the criteria for childhood autism. Miller and Ozonoff[65] note that several aspects of the current definition can be problematic; Asperger consistently felt that the syndrome he described differed from Kanner's autism (1979). Thus the current definition almost certainly will be refined (or discarded) in future editions of ICD and DSM.

**Table 9.2.3.4** ICD-10 criteria for Asperger's syndrome (F84.4)

A. There is no clinically significant general delay in spoken or receptive language or cognitive development. Diagnosis requires that single words should have developed by 2 years of age or earlier and that communicative phrases be used by 3 years of age or earlier. Self-help skills, adaptive behaviour, and curiosity about the environment during the first 3 years should be at a level consistent with normal intellectual development. However, motor milestones may be somewhat delayed and motor clumsiness is usual (although not a necessary diagnostic feature). Isolated special skills, often related to abnormal preoccupations, are common, but are not required for the diagnosis.

B. There are qualitative abnormalities in reciprocal social interaction (criteria as for autism).

C. The individual exhibits an unusual intense circumscribed interest or restricted, repetitive, and stereotyped patterns of behaviour interests and activities (criteria as for autism; however, it would be less usual for these to include either motor mannerisms or preoccupations with part-objects or non-functional elements of play materials).

D. The disorder is not attributable to other varieties of pervasive developmental disorder; simple schizophrenia; schizotypal disorder; obsessive-compulsive disorder; anankastic personality disorder; reactive and disinhibited attachment disorders of childhood.

Taken from Disorders of psychological development (criteria for research), pp. 154–5
© World Health Organization, www.who.int

### Epidemiology and demographics

Estimates of prevalence vary markedly depending on the stringency of the definition used. A stringent approach to diagnosis would suggest a rate in the order of 1 in 2000 or so, but a much less stringent approach may yield one in several hundred.[66]

Asperger[55] originally reported the condition only in boys, although Wing reported on girls with the condition. There does appear to be a male predominance in the order of 20 to 1; similar sex ratios are observed in autism not associated with intellectual disability.

### Course and prognosis

Asperger's original[55] impression was of favourable long-term prognosis.[67] Many individuals can attend regular school with some additional support; unfortunately such children may be seen as eccentric and are often prime targets for being victimized. Better verbal skills can mislead educators about the child's vulnerability in other areas, and difficulties academically may be misattributed to wilful non-compliance. There is the impression that these individuals are capable of greater degrees of personal and occupational self-sufficiency than those with autism, but definitive data are lacking. It does appear that the social difficulties persist into adulthood.[68]

### Aetiology

Although the cause of Asperger's syndrome remains unknown, the report of high rates of the condition in family members and the reports of occasional familial associations with autism suggests the potential importance of genetic factors. Neurobiological information on the condition is limited. The potential association of the condition with specific neuropsychological profiles is of some interest.

## Atypical autism/PDD not otherwise specified

Recent editions of both ICD and DSM have included a 'subthreshold' category (termed either atypical autism or pervasive developmental disorder not otherwise specified—PDD-NOS). In some ways, this notion has historical links to earlier diagnostic concepts.[23] In practice, the term atypical autism in ICD-10 and the term PDD-NOS in DSM-IV refer to what is a residual diagnostic category. ICD-10 provides the possibility for various forms of special coding—for example, failure to meet the onset criteria for autism, failure to meet developmental/behavioural criteria, or failure to meet both.

Research on this diagnostic category has been less advanced than that for other disorders—no doubt reflecting the problems intrinsic to 'subthreshold' disorders. Several attempts have recently been made to identify potential subgroups within the rather heterogeneous disorder, but none has yet achieved general acceptance. Various attempts have been made to identify specific subgroups within this broader category.[69] It is sometimes the case that social and/or communicative skills are relatively preserved but the child exhibits unusual sensitivities, affective responses, and thought processes. It is likely that the term presently encompasses a number of conditions, which may be identified in the future.

## Differential diagnosis

Autism and related PDDs must be differentiated from each other, from the specific developmental disorders (e.g. of language), from intellectual disability not associated with PDD, and from other conditions. In intellectual disability not associated with PDD, social and communicative skills are typically on a par with the child's overall intellectual ability. Diagnostic differentiation can be most challenging in persons with severe and profound intellectual disability where assessment is more difficult and stereotyped movements common. Occasionally language and other specific developmental disorders may be confused with autism/PDD. Usually, however, the child's social abilities are preserved and the child is very communicative non-verbally. Schizophrenia rarely has its onset in childhood and almost never before the age of 5 years.

On occasion, selective mutism or social anxiety disorder may be confused with a PDD (particularly PDD-NOS/atypical autism). However, in selective mutism the child can speak in some situations. Similarly, children with anxiety in social situations will usually not exhibit the other symptoms characteristic of autism/PDD. The unusual behaviour and interests of children with obsessive–compulsive disorder may be taken to suggest autism or PDD, but social and language-communication skills are preserved.

In considering the differential diagnosis of conditions that present with regression it is important to review carefully previous diagnostic evaluations. Occasionally, progressive neuropathological conditions may have their onset in childhood. In the Landau–Kleffner syndrome (acquired aphasia with epilepsy) social skills should be relatively preserved even in the face of an extensive aphasia.

Sometimes children who have experienced marked neglect may present with social difficulties, initially suggesting autism or PDD. However, in reactive attachment disorder the history of severe neglect is observed and, as the name of the condition implies, social deficits should remit substantially if an appropriate and nurturing environment is provided.

## Treatment

Over the past decade a relatively substantial body of research on treatment of autism has appeared. Recent summaries of this work are available.[70] Much of this work relates to behavioural and educational interventions although a body of well-controlled studies of psychopharmacological agents has appeared as well.[71]

Children with autism and other PDDs generally require an intensive and highly structured intervention programme. More able children may be able to tolerate regular classroom situations, with appropriate support, but more impaired children often need higher levels of teacher supervision and a more intensive classroom setting.[72] For lower-functioning children areas of priority include the ability to tolerate adult guidance and intrusion, to follow routines, to develop communicative abilities, and move from associative to more conceptual learning strategies.[73] The classroom setting can be important, as children with PDD can be readily distracted by extraneous stimuli. The tendency of such children to rely on routines can be used effectively to help promote more systematic learning. Generalization of skills learned is particularly important since the child may have difficulties in applying skills learned in new settings. Speech and communication are a critically important aspect of any intervention programme.[11] Techniques to foster communication through non-verbal means such as sign language, picture-exchange, visual schedules, and other augmentative methods can be very helpful to non-verbal children.[74] The use of such methods does not preclude, and in fact may foster, the use of spoken communication.

Behaviour modification techniques are helpful in increasing the frequency of desired behaviours while simultaneously diminishing problem behaviours. Typically, a functional analysis of the target behaviour is initially performed, and then a plan developed for prompting or decreasing the behaviour.[73] While there is general agreement that children with autism/PDD profit from a behaviourally based intervention, there is more controversy over the degree to which progress can be made; for instance, there have been some claims for dramatic improvement and even 'cures' of autism.

Neuroleptics have been the most intensively studied psychopharmacological agents in this population, and there have been several well-designed double blind, placebo-controlled trials.[71] The main mechanism of action appears to be dopamine-receptor blockade. The agents may reduce maladaptive behaviours such as stereotypies,[75] but side effects include sedation, irritability, and movement problems (including tardive dyskinesia). Recently, interest has centred on the newer atypical neuroleptics.[76]

## Management

Goals for treatment include promoting learning and reducing behaviours that interfere with learning. Treatment is best based on a comprehensive view of the child and his or her strengths and areas of need. A structured and individualized intervention programme is needed. Various professionals such as speech pathologists, special educators, occupational and physical therapists may be involved.[72,73] Goals for intervention will vary depending on developmental level, life circumstance, and clinical context—for example, vocational factors will be more important during adolescence, and for individuals with conditions like Rett's syndrome the efforts of other professionals (orthopaedists and respiratory therapists) may be needed.

For higher functioning and older individuals the acquisition and generalization of social skills are particularly important. The use of rehearsal and social scripts may be indicated. Teaching must be explicit and can include modelling and rehearsal within individual instruction and small group settings, with the use of naturalistic settings to encourage generalization whenever possible. For higher functioning students, including those with Asperger's syndrome, this can include explicit analyses of challenging social situations, videotaping for self-observation, role playing, and the use of individualized social stories.[77]

There is no evidence that unstructured psychotherapy is useful in autism and related conditions. Structured and supportive psychotherapy may be appropriate for some carefully selected, higher-functioning individuals, particularly if it focuses on explicit problem-solving strategies for frequently troublesome situations.

Pharmacotherapy interventions are not curative, but they may provide considerable help with specific problematic symptoms.[71] The best evidence relates to the atypical neuroleptics but data on other agents are less substantive. The balance of potential benefits and risks should be considered, and informed consent obtained from parents or, whenever possible, the affected child.

Mood stabilizers and antidepressants have sometimes been used, given the increase in affective lability, anxiety, and depression in individuals with autism and PDDs. However, the response to antidepressants has been somewhat variable. Lithium and other mood stabilizers are sometimes used clinically, particularly if there is a strong family history of bipolar disorder, but there have been few controlled studies of these agents.

Selective serotonin-reuptake inhibitors (SSRIs) were of initial interest in autism, given the repeated reports of high group levels of peripheral serotonin in this population as well as of the high levels of repetitive behaviours observed in this group (i.e. reminiscent of those seen in obsessive–compulsive disorder). Several reports have suggested that, at least in adults, these agents may be helpful in lowering the levels of obsessive–compulsive-like behaviours, although activation is sometimes observed; Studies of children have been less frequent, but there is some suggestion that they may also respond.[71]

Various other agents have been used in autism, including anxiolytics, β-blockers, clonidine, and naltrexone. Unfortunately, it is difficult to draw firm conclusions from the limited data available, but at present the clinical efficacy of these agents is not well established in this population. Surprisingly few studies have systematically evaluated the use of stimulants in autism. However, the observation that these agents induce stereotyped behaviours in animals would suggest their potential for increasing levels of stereotyped behaviours.

## Prevention

At present information on the prevention of autism and related PDDs is clearly quite limited. Apart from the association with two strongly genetic conditions (fragile X syndrome and tuberous sclerosis) no specific biological markers for autism have yet been found although some promising leads for early screening or children at risk (i.e. siblings) have appeared. It is likely that early diagnosis may change dramatically in the not so distant future as potential susceptibility genes are identified or are combined with innovative approaches to screening—this will have potentially major importance since there is some suggestion that early intervention may significantly improve outcome.

## Further information

www.autism.fm. Regularly updated website with links to other sites.

Quackwatch www.quackwath.com. Information about non-conventional treatments.

Jacobson, J.W., Foxx, R.M., and Mulick, J.A. (2005). *Controversial therapies for developmental disabilities: fad, fashion and science in professional practice*. Lawrence Erlbaum Associates, Mahwah, NJ. A comprehensive guide to nonconventional treatments.

Center for disease control—autism related information: http://www.cdc.gov/ncbddd/dd/ddautism.htm This website provides basic information for physicians (including early warning signs of autism) in both English and Spanish.

Federal autism research networks website: www.autismresearchnet.work.org provides links to US federally funded autism research projects.

## References

1. World Health Organization. (1992). *International statistical classification of diseases and related health problems* (10th revision). WHO, Geneva.

2. American Psychiatric Association. (1994). *Diagnostic and statistical classification of diseases and related health problems* (4th edn). American Psychiatric Association, Washington, DC.

3. Kanner, L. (1943). Autistic disturbances of affective contact. *Nervous Child*, **2**, 217–50.

4. Treffert, D. (1989). *Extraordinary people*. Bantam, New York.

5. Rutter, M. (1970). Autistic children: infancy to adulthood. *Seminars in Psychiatry*, **2**, 435–50.

6. Rutter, M., Bailey, A., Simonoff, E., *et al.* (1997). Genetic influences in autism. In *Handbook of autism and pervasive developmental disorders* (2nd edn) (eds. D.J. Cohen and F.R. Volkmar), pp. 370–87. Wiley, New York.

7. Schopler, E., Andrews, C.E., and Strupp, K. (1979). Do autistic children come from upper-middle-class parents? *Journal of Autism and Developmental Disorders*, **9**, 139–52.

8. Carter, A.S., Davis, N.O., Klin, A., *et al.* (2005). Social development in autism. In *Handbook of autism and pervasive developmental disorders* (3rd edn) (eds. F.R. Volkmar, R. Paul, A. Klin, and D.J. Cohen), pp. 312–34. Wiley, New York.

9. Wing, L. (1997). Syndromes of autism and atypical development. In *Handbook of autism and pervasive developmental disorders* (2nd edn) (eds. D.J. Cohen and F.R. Volkmar), pp. 148–72. Wiley, New York.

10. Rutter, M. (1978). Diagnosis and definition of childhood autism. *Journal of Autism and Childhood Schizophrenia*, **8**, 139–61.

11. Tager-Flusberg, H., Paul, R., and Lord, C. (2005). Language and communication in autism. In *Handbook of autism and pervasive developmental disorders* (3rd edn) (eds. F.R. Volkmar, R. Paul, A. Klin, and D.J. Cohen), pp. 335–64. Wiley, New York.

12. Kolvin, I. (1971). Studies in the childhood psychoses. I. Diagnostic criteria and classification. *The British Journal of Psychiatry*, **118**, 381–4.

13. Rutter, M. (1972). Childhood schizophrenia reconsidered. *Journal of Autism and Childhood Schizophrenia*, **2**, 315–37.

14. World Health Organization. (1977). *International statistical classification of diseases and related health problems* (9th revision). WHO, Geneva.

15. American Psychiatric Association. (1980). *Diagnostic and statistical classification of diseases and related health problems* (3rd edn). American Psychiatric Association, Washington, DC.

16. Volkmar, F.R. and Cohen, D.J. (1991). Debate and argument: the utility of the term pervasive developmental disorder. *Journal of Child Psychology and Psychiatry*, **32**, 1171–2.

17. Rutter, M. and Schopler, E. (1992). Classification of pervasive developmental disorders: some concepts and practical considerations. *Journal of Autism and Developmental Disorders*, **22**, 459–82.

18. American Psychiatric Association. (1987). *Diagnostic and statistical classification of diseases and related health problems* (3rd edn, revised). American Psychiatric Association, Washington, DC.

19. Volkmar, F.R., Klin, A., Siegel, B., *et al.* (1994). Field trial for autistic disorder in DSM-IV. *The American Journal of Psychiatry*, **151**, 1361–7.

20. Fombonne, E. (2005). Epidemiological studies of pervasive developmental disorders. In *Handbook of autism and pervasive developmental disorders* (3rd edn) (eds. F.R. Volkmar, R. Paul, A. Klin, and D.J. Cohen), pp. 42–69. Wiley, New York.

21. Volkmar, F.R., Szatmari, P., and Sparrow, S.S. (1993). Sex differences in pervasive developmental disorders. *Journal of Autism and Developmental Disorders*, **23**, 579–91.

22. Schopler, E. (2005). Cross-cultural program priorities and reclassification of outcome research methods. In *Handbook of autism and pervasive developmental disorders* (3rd edn) (eds. F.R. Volkmar, R. Paul, A. Klin, and D.J. Cohen), pp. 1174–91. Wiley, New York.

23. Howlin, P. (2005). Outcomes in autism spectrum disorders. In *Handbook of autism and pervasive developmental disorders* (3rd edn) (eds. F.R. Volkmar, R. Paul, A. Klin, and D.J. Cohen), pp. 201–21. Wiley, New York.

24. Howlin, P. and Goode, S. (1998). Outcome in autism and related conditions. In *Autism and pervasive developmental disorders* (ed. F.R. Volkmar), pp. 209–41. Cambridge University Press, New York.

25. Volkmar, F.R. and Nelson, D.S. (1990). Seizure disorders in autism. *Journal of the American Academy of Child and Adolescent Psychiatry*, **29**, 127–9.

26. Volkmar, F.R., Lord, C., Bailey, A., *et al.* (2004). Autism and pervasive developmental disorders. *Journal of Child Psychology and Psychiatry*, **45**, 1–36.

27. Happé, F. (2005). The weak central coherence account of autism. In *Handbook of autism and pervasive developmental disorders* (3rd edn) (eds. F.R. Volkmar, R. Paul, A. Klin, and D.J. Cohen), pp. 640–9. Wiley, New York.

28. Ozonoff, S., South, M., and Provencal, S. (2005). Executive functions. In *Handbook of autism and pervasive developmental disorders* (3rd edn) (eds. F.R. Volkmar, R. Paul, A. Klin, and D.J. Cohen), pp. 606–27. Wiley, New York.

29. Baron-Cohen, S. (1995). *Mind blindness*. MIT Press, Cambridge, MA.

30. Klin, A., Jones, W., Schultz, R.T., *et al.* (2003). The enactive mind—from actions to cognition: lessons from autism. *Philosophical Transactions of the Royal Society of London. Series B, Biological Sciences*, **358**, 345–60.

31. Schultz, R.T. (2005). Developmental deficits in social perception in autism: the role of the amygdala and fusiform face area. *International Journal of Developmental Neuroscience*, **23**, 125–41.

32. Chess, S. (1977). Follow-up report on autism in congenital rubella. *Journal of Autism and Childhood Schizophrenia*, **7**, 69–81.

33. Gillberg, C.L. (1992). The Emanuel Miller Memorial Lecture 1991. Autism and autistic-like conditions: subclasses among disorders of empathy. *Journal of Child Psychology and Psychiatry*, **33**, 813–42.

34. Rutter, M., Bailey, A., Bolton, P., *et al.* (1994). Autism and known medical conditions: myth and substance. *Journal of Child Psychology and Psychiatry*, **35**, 311–22.

35. Rutter, M. (2005). Genetic influences and autism. In *Handbook of autism and pervasive developmental disorders* (3rd edn) (eds. F.R. Volkmar, R. Paul, A. Klin, and D.J. Cohen), pp. 425–52. Wiley, New York.

36. Minshew, N.J., Sweeney, J.A., Bauman, M.L., *et al.* (2005). Neurologic aspects of autism. In *Handbook of autism and pervasive developmental disorders* (3rd edn) (eds. F.R. Volkmar, R. Paul, A. Klin, and D.J. Cohen), pp. 473–514. Wiley, New York.

37. Hazlett, H.C., Poe, M., Gerig, G., *et al.* (2005). Magnetic resonance imaging and head circumference study of brain size in autism: birth through age 2 years. *Archives of General Psychiatry*, **62**, 1366–76.

38. Anderson, G.M. and Hoshino, Y. (2005). Neurochemical studies of autism. In *Handbook of autism and pervasive developmental disorders* (3rd edn) (eds. F.R. Volkmar, R. Paul, A. Klin, and D.J. Cohen), pp. 453–72. Wiley, New York.

39. Rett, A. (1966). Uber ein eigenartiges hirntophisces Syndröm bei hyperammonie intramuscular Kindersalter. *Wein Medizinische Wochenschrift*, **118**, 723–6.

40. Hagberg, B., Aicardi, J., Dias, K., *et al.* (1983). A progressive syndrome of autism, dementia, ataxia, and loss of purposeful hand use in girls: Rett's syndrome, report of 35 cases. *Annals of Neurology*, **14**, 471–9.

41. Rutter, M. (1994). Debate and argument: there are connections between brain and mind and it is important that Rett syndrome be classified somewhere. *Journal of Child Psychology and Psychiatry*, **35**, 379–81.

42. van Acker, R., Loncola, J.A., and van Acker, E.Y. (2005). Rett syndrome: a pervasive developmental disorder. In *Handbook of autism and pervasive developmental disorders* (3rd edn) (eds. F.R. Volkmar, R. Paul, A. Klin, and D.J. Cohen), pp. 126–64. Wiley, New York.

43. Trevathan, E. and Adams, M.J. (1988). The epidemiology and public health significance of Rett syndrome. *Journal of Child Neurology*, **3**(Suppl.), S17–20.

44. Gillberg, C. (1994). Debate and argument: having Rett syndrome in the ICD-10 PDD category does not make sense. *Journal of Child Psychology and Psychiatry*, **35**, 377–8.

45. Rett Syndrome Diagnostic Criteria Work Group. (1986). Diagnostic criteria for Rett syndrome. *Annals of Neurology*, **23**, 125–8.

46. Hagberg, B. (1985). Rett's syndrome: prevalence and impact on progressive severe mental retardation in girls. *Acta Paediatrica Scandinavica*, **74**, 405–8.

47. Kozinetz, C.A., Skender, M.L., MacNaughton, N., *et al.* (1993). Epidemiology of Rett syndrome: a population-based registry. *Pediatrics*, **91**, 445–50.

48. Hagberg, B. (1989). Rett syndrome: clinical peculiarities, diagnostic approach, and possible cause. *Pediatric Neurology*, **5**, 75–83.

49. Kaufmann, W.E., Johnston, M.V, and Blue, M.E. (2005). MeCP2 expression and function during brain development: implications for Rett syndrome's pathogenesis and clinical evolution. *Brain & Development*, **28**(Suppl. 1), S77–87.

50. Heller, T. (1908). Dementia Infantilis. Zeitschrift fur die Erforschung und Behandlung des Jugenlichen. *Schwachsinns*, **2**, 141–65.

51. Volkmar, F.R. and Rutter, M. (1995). Childhood disintegrative disorder: results of the DSM-IV autism field trial. *Journal of the American Academy of Child and Adolescent Psychiatry*, **34**, 1092–5.

52. Volkmar, F.R., Koenig, K., and State, M. (2005). Childhood disintegrative disorder. In *Handbook of autism and pervasive developmental disorders* (3rd edn) (eds. F.R. Volkmar, R. Paul, A. Klin, and D.J. Cohen), pp. 70–87. Wiley, New York.

53. Rutter, M. (1985). Infantile autism and other pervasive developmental disorders. In *Child and adolescent psychiatry—modern approaches* (eds. M. Rutter and L. Hersov), pp. 545–66. Blackwell, London.

54. Corbett, J. (1987). Development, disintegration and dementia. *Journal of Mental Deficiency Research*, **31**, 349–56.

55. Asperger, H. (1944). Die 'autistichen Psychopathen' intramuscular Kindersalter. *Archive für Psychiatrie und Nervenkrankheiten*, **117**, 76–136. [Translated by U. Frith in U. Frith (ed.) (1991). *Autism and Asperger syndrome*, pp. 37–92. Cambridge University Press, New York.]

56. Wing, L. (1981). Asperger's syndrome: a clinical account. *Psychological Medicine*, **11**, 115–29.

57. Wolff, S. and Barlow, A. (1979). Schizoid personality in childhood: a comparative study of schizoid, autistic and normal children. *Journal of Child Psychology and Psychiatry*, **20**, 29–46.

58. Rourke, B. (1989). *Nonverbal learning disabilities: the syndrome and the model.* Guilford Press, New York.

59. Bishop, D.V. (1989). Autism, Asperger's syndrome and semantic-pragmatic disorder: where are the boundaries? *British Journal of Disorders of Communication*, **24**, 107–21.

60. Ellis, H.D., Ellis, D.M., Fraser, W., *et al.* (1994). A preliminary study of right hemisphere cognitive deficits and impaired social judgments among young people with Asperger syndrome. *European Child and Adolescent Psychiatry*, **3**, 255–66.

61. Klin, A., Volkmar, F.R., Sparrow, S.S., *et al.* (1995). Validity and neuropsychological characterization of Asperger syndrome: convergence with nonverbal learning disabilities syndrome. *Journal of Child Psychology and Psychiatry*, **36**, 1127–40.

62. Klin, A., Pauls, D., Schultz, R., *et al.* (2005a). Three diagnostic approaches to Asperger syndrome: implications for research. *Journal of Autism and Developmental Disorders*, **35**, 221–34.

63. Klin, A., McPartland, J., and Volkmar, F.R. (2005b). Asperger syndrome. In *Handbook of autism and pervasive developmental disorders* (3rd edn) (eds. F.R. Volkmar, R. Paul, A. Klin, and D.J. Cohen), pp. 88–125. Wiley & Sons, New York.

64. Lincoln, A., Courchesne, E., Allen, M., *et al.* (1988). Neurobiology of Asperger syndrome: seven case studies and quantitative magnetic resonance imaging findings. In *Asperger syndrome or high functioning autism?* (eds. E. Schopler, G.B. Mesibov, and L.J. Kunc), pp. 145–66. Plenum, New York.

65. Miller, J.N. and Ozonoff, S. (1997). Did Asperger's cases have Asperger disorder? A research note. *Journal of Child Psychology and Psychiatry*, **38**, 247–51.

66. Fombonne, E. (2003). The prevalence of autism. *The Journal of the American Medical Association*, **289**, 87–9.

67. Asperger, H. (1979). Problems of infantile autism. *Communication*, **13**, 45–52.

68. Tsatsanis, K. (2003). Outcome research in Asperger syndrome and autism. *Child and Adolescent Psychiatric Clinics of North America*, **12**, 47–64.

69. Towbin, K. (2005). Pervasive developmental disorder not otherwise specified. In *Handbook of autism and pervasive developmental disorders* (3rd edn) (eds. F.R. Volkmar, R. Paul, A. Klin, and D.J. Cohen), pp. 165–200. Wiley, New York.

70. National Research Council. (2001). *Educating children with autism.* National Academy Press, Washington, DC.

71. Scahill, L. and Martin, A. (2005). Psychopharmacology. In *Handbook of autism and pervasive developmental disorders* (3rd edn) (eds. F.R. Volkmar, R. Paul, A. Klin, and D.J. Cohen), pp. 1102–21. Wiley, New York.

72. Handleman, J.S., Harris, S.L., and Martins, M.P. (2005). Helping children with autism enter the mainstream. In *Handbook of autism and pervasive developmental disorders* (3rd edn) (eds. F.R. Volkmar, R. Paul, A. Klin, and D.J. Cohen), pp. 1029–42. Wiley, New York.

73. Schreibman, L. and Ingersoll, B. (2005). Behavioral interventions to promote learning in individuals with autism. In *Handbook of autism and pervasive developmental disorders* (3rd edn) (eds. F.R. Volkmar, R. Paul, A. Klin, and D.J. Cohen), pp. 882–96. Wiley, New York.

74. Prizant, B.M. and Wetherby, A.M. (2005). Critical issues in enhancing communication abilities for persons with autism spectrum disorders. In *Handbook of autism and pervasive developmental disorders* (3rd edn) (eds. F.R. Volkmar, R. Paul, A. Klin, and D.J. Cohen), pp. 925–45. Wiley, New York.

75. Research Units on Pediatric Psychopharmacology Autism Network. (2002). A double blind, placebo-controlled trial of risperidone in children with autistic disorder. *The New England Journal of Medicine*, **347**, 314–21.

76. McDougle, C.J., Scahill, L., Aman, M.G., *et al.* (2005). Risperidone for the core symptom domains of autism: results from the study by the autism network of the research units on pediatric psychopharmacology. *The American Journal of Psychiatry*, **162**, 1142–8.

77. Marans, W., Rubin, E., and Laurent, A. (2005). Addressing social communication skills in individuals with high-functioning autism and Asperger syndrome: critical priorities in educational programming. In *Handbook of autism and pervasive developmental disorders* (3rd edn) (eds. F.R. Volkmar, R. Paul, A. Klin, and D.J. Cohen), pp. 977–1002. Wiley, New York.

# 9.2.4 Attention deficit and hyperkinetic disorders in childhood and adolescence

Eric Taylor

## Introduction

The concept of ADHD arose from neurological formulations, but does not entail them, and the modern definition simply describes a set of behavioural traits. The historical evolution of the concept was described by Schachar.[1] It began with the idea that some behavioural problems in children arose, not from social and familial adversity, but from subtle changes in brain development. The term 'minimal brain dysfunction (MBD)' was often applied, and covered not only disorganized and disruptive behaviour but other developmental problems (such as dyspraxias and language delays) presumed to have an unknown physical cause. MBD, however, stopped being a useful description when studies of children with definite and more-than-minimal brain damage made it plain that they showed a very wide range of psychological impairment, not a characteristic pattern (see Harris, this volume); and therefore it was invalid to infer the presence of brain disorder from the nature of the psychological presentation.

The successor to the concept of MBD was attention deficit and hyperactivity: defined, observable behaviour traits without assumption of cause. 'Attention Deficit/Hyperactivity Disorder' (ADHD) in DSM-IV, and 'Hyperkinetic Disorder' in ICD-10, describe a constellation of *overactivity, impulsivity* and *inattentiveness*. These core problems often coexist with other difficulties of learning, behaviour or mental life, and the coexistent problems may dominate the presentation. This coexistence, to the psychopathologist, emphasizes the multifaceted nature of the disorder; to the sociologist, a doubt about whether it should be seen as a disorder at all; to the developmentalist, the shifting and context-dependent nature of childhood traits. For clinicians, ADHD symptoms usually need to be disentangled from a complex web of problems. It is worthwhile to do so because of the strong developmental impact of ADHD and the existence of effective treatments. Public controversy continues, but professional practice in most countries makes ADHD one of the most commonly diagnosed problems of child mental health.

## Clinical features

### Overactivity

The idea of overactivity refers simply to an excess of movement. It is not totally dependent on context and cannot be reduced to non-compliance: physical measures of activity level have indicated that it is higher in children with ADHD than in controls, even during sleep.[2] It is, however, partly dependent upon context: it is often inhibited by a novel environment, creating a pitfall for the inexperienced diagnostician who may exclude it incorrectly because it is not manifested during observation at a first clinic visit. It may not be evident in situations where high activity is expected, such as the games field. The key situations where it is evident are familiar to the child and where calm is expected, such as visiting family friends, attending church, mealtimes, homework and—often the most troublesome—at school, during class.

### (a) Impulsivenes

Impulsiveness means action without reflection—often described as a failure to 'stop and think'. The term covers premature, unprepared and poorly timed behaviours—such as interrupting others, and giving too little time to appreciate what is involved in a school task or a social situation.

### (b) Inattentiveness

Inattentiveness means disorganized and forgetful behaviour: short-sequence activities, changing before they are completed, with a lack of attention to detail and a failure to correct mistakes. All these are behavioural observations, not psychological constructs. At a cognitive level, 'Attention deficit' is a rather poor descriptor; the performance of affected children does not fade with time on a task any more than that of ordinary people and the presence of irrelevant information ('distractors') does not worsen their performance disproportionately to that of other people.[3] There are cognitive changes of a different kind (see 'Aetiology' below); but the diagnosis of inattentiveness depends on descriptions and observations of behaviour rather than on tests of performance.

Many other behavioural changes characterize some children with ADHD. They are, for instance, often irritable and their emotions can flash very rapidly when provoked. They may sleep badly (and this in turn can contribute to poor concentration). They can be aggressive to other people and non-compliant to authority. They can also be charming, humourous, inquisitive and intuitive. None of these, however, are either constant in ADHD or confined to those with ADHD. They are worth noting, but they do not make the diagnosis.

## Classification

Attention Deficit/Hyperactivity Disorder in DSM-IV is defined as the presence of a number, above a cut-off, of behaviours considered to reflect the cardinal features described above to a degree that is developmentally inappropriate and gives rise to some impairment in more than one setting (e.g. school and home).[4] Overactive and impulsive behaviours are considered together as a single construct of 'hyperactivity-impulsiveness', and for convenience the combined dimension will be referred to in this chapter as 'hyperactivity'. Examples of inattentive behaviour are added together and form a separate dimension. There are therefore three subtypes: hyperactive-impulsive, inattentive and combined.

The same problems characterize the ICD-10 definition of 'Hyperkinetic Disorder' (HD),[5] but with added requirements: especially, that all three cardinal features are present, pervasively across home, school and other situations. HD is therefore, in effect, a subtype of ADHD.[6, 7] The subtypes of hyperkinetic disorder are based on the presence or absence of conduct disorder—and indeed the presence of conduct disorder is an important factor with which to reckon in the course.

## Diagnosis

Description of the symptoms makes them sound easy to recognize, and indeed the problems are usually very salient, disruptive to other people, and common causes of referral to health and special education services. Nevertheless, there are pitfalls in the diagnosis, making it necessary for a specialist assessment to be undertaken before the diagnosis is given.

## Ambiguous criteria

The behavioural problems, described in outline above, are translated into detailed criteria in DSM-IV and ICD-10, and some of them can be ambiguous. For example, 'does not follow instructions' is a DSM item intended to imply that instructions are forgotten or not attended to; but the behaviour can also be shown for reasons of wilfulness and therefore a part of oppositional/defiant disorder. Careful description or witnessing the behaviours complained of is necessary.

## Confusion of cardinal and associated features

Many behavioural problems—such as temper tantrums, sleeplessness, aggression and disobedience to adult authority—are common in children with ADHD, and may be the key reasons for presentation. It is easy to make the mistake of diagnosing ADHD when only disruptive behaviour is present. Much of the confusion comes from the way impulsiveness is operationalized in the diagnostic schemes. Behaviours, such as calling out in class and interrupting others, can indeed come from a difficulty in holding oneself back; but they can also represent deliberate flouting of the rules, and in a London survey of 6- to 8-year-old boys they were as common in non-hyperactive but defiant children as in the hyperactive.[8] Direct observation can usually make the distinction—watching either the children tackling tasks requiring them to stop and think in the clinic, or their natural behaviour in the classroom. Inattentive behaviour also helps to make the diagnosis of ADHD and is less confounded by oppositionality.

### (a) Reliance on non-expert judgements

The behaviours of ADHD are continuously distributed in the population (see 'Epidemiology'). The level that is considered normal or acceptable will vary from one culture to another and from one rater to another. To be diagnosed, they should be excessive not only for the child's age but also for the developmental level; and this demands considerable familiarity with the usual range of variation. The diagnostician will acquire this in the course of training and experience; experienced teachers will be excellent judges; but inexperienced or overstressed parents may identify the problems at a low level of hyperactive behaviour, or suppose that an abnormal level is only to be expected in childhood. It is usually helpful to obtain a detailed behavioural account rather than rely on an overall judgment of 'overactivity' or 'failure to concentrate'. Contradiction between sources may occur, and leads to arguments between parents and teachers. This may be due to different expectations, the emotional relationship of raters with the child, or children behaving very differently in contexts that vary in the demands placed on the children. The clinician needs to understand the full context of the way involved adults describe the child.

### (b) Problems of recognition in the presence of coexistent problems

It is commonplace for children whose problems meet the criteria for ADHD to show other patterns of disturbance as well. This is often, confusingly, called 'comorbidity' – confusing because it

assumes that the other pattern is a distinct disorder, which is only one of the explanations for coexistent problems. Clinicians need to understand the relationships for two reasons; so that they do not make or miss the diagnosis of ADHD; and so that they can make good strategies for treating ADHD in the presence of other disorders and other disorders in the presence of ADHD (see 'Treating Complex cases', below).

### (c) Conduct and oppositional disorders

The commonest association and the best researched is with conduct and oppositional disorders. Nearly half the children with hyperactive behaviour in a community survey showed high levels of defiant and aggressive conduct as well; but the associations of the two problems were different, with hyperactivity (but not conduct problems) being associated with delays in motor and language development.[8] Genetic research indicates higher heritability for hyperactivity than for defiant and aggressive behaviour; but there are some genetic influences that are common to both.[9] Hyperactivity is more responsive to stimulant medication than are less hyperactive forms of conduct problem.[10]

When both ADHD and conduct problems are present, then the combined diagnosis ('hyperkinetic conduct disorder' in ICD-10) shows the associations of both disorders. ADHD is therefore not to be diagnosed by the absence of conduct disorder features, but by the clear presence of the core problems of inattentivess and disorganization.

### (d) Tourette disorder and multiple tics

A different kind of differential is presented by children with Tourette disorder. Their motor restlessness may indeed represent the coexistence of ADHD, but can result directly from tics. If a child's tics are very frequent and there are a large number of them, then their repetitive and stereotyped nature may not be apparent and they may be seen simply as restless fidgetiness. Again, direct observation of the pattern of overactivity is the key. When there is doubt, videorecording the child and subsequent slow-motion review may make repetitive patterns evident.

### (e) Autism spectrum disorders

Children with autism have clear and characteristic impairments of language, communication, and social development. Spectrum disorders, however, can raise diagnostic challenges. Children with ADHD alone often show language delays (usually of an expressive nature with over-simple utterances, by contrast with the receptive difficulties and idiosyncratic patterns of autism). Their attention difficulties may make them unresponsive to the overtures of others in a way that can simulate the social obliviousness of people in the spectrum of autism, and they are often friendless—not because of lack of interest in others but because of the capacity of hyperactive behaviour to irritate other people. Indeed, attention problems can extend to perseverativeness on certain activities such as video games that may be mistaken for the restricted interests of autism. All these factors can lead to ADHD being mistaken for autism, but the reverse can happen too. There are other reasons for overactive behaviour in autism. First, stereotyped patterns of driven overactivity can be seen: they are not disorganized or impulsive and are often made worse by change and novelty (which usually reduce the overactivity of ADHD). Second, episodic bursts of extreme activity can be seen and may be best regarded and treated as catatonic. Third, akithisia may result from neuroleptic medication, or irritable restlessness from anticonvulsants, and it will be necessary to establish a clear history that ADHD has been a persistent trait.

#### (f) Attachment disorders

Reactive attachment disorder (RAD) may share with ADHD a disinhibited style of relating to other people (an unreserved but shallow making of social contact). Children with RAD, however, tend to be controlling rather than disorganized, and vigilant rather than inattentive; and inattention and impulsiveness are not cardinal features of RAD; so it is not difficult to recognize both patterns when present in an individual child. The confusion in practice often comes from theoretical misconceptions. Those caring for neglected or abandoned children may consider that the diagnosis of ADHD cannot be accurate because the cause of the children's problems is clearly to be found in their early deprivation. The causal pathway may indeed be that of neglect (though genetic inheritance and fetal exposure to toxins also need considering); but ADHD is a descriptive category, not an explanatory one. If the pattern of ADHD is present it still needs recognizing—not least because the cause of the ADHD behaviour does not seem to determine the response to stimulant medication, and children who have encountered neglect or abnormal early attachment may still have their ADHD problems reduced by medication.[10]

#### (g) Bipolar disorders

Both ADHD and manic conditions are characterized by overactivity, overtalkativeness, a sensation of whirling thoughts, and often by irritable mood. The distinction is made by the presence in bipolar disorder of episodicity, euphoria, and grandiosity. A suggestion that these distinguishing features are not in fact present in childhood bipolar disorder has naturally led to great overlap between the expanded childhood bipolar diagnosis and ADHD with poor emotional regulation, and further research will be needed to clarify whether there is a distinction.

In all these differential diagnoses, the principle is to establish that the child shows not only overactive behaviour, but the specific pattern of ADHD. Experienced judgement may be required, and the practice of diagnosing on the basis of questionnaire scores alone risks overidentification.

In adult life, there are still more possibilities for misdiagnosis. The commonest reasons for uncertainty are in distinguishing from atypical bipolar disorder and the effects of substance misuse. 'Personality disorder' is sometimes applied; and indeed ADHD shares with personality disorders a long-standing trait quality, but can also be a more precise way of describing the difficulties presented. Differentiation from the normal range of variation can be difficult in the absence of clear standards. The task of the diagnostician is harder when adults are presenting for the first time if only self-report is available; the self-description of hyperactivity may be a form of self-depreciation.

### Methods of recognition

#### (a) Rating scales and informant interviews

Questionnaire ratings by parents or teachers are very useful for screening purposes, and in group studies they give a fairly good discrimination between people with a clinical diagnosis of ADHD and controls from the ordinary population.[11] Many are available[12,13] and the most famous are those from Conners, which yield several different scoring systems; and derivatives such as the Iowa Conners, the SWAN and SNAP scales.[14] They do however leave a fair number of individuals misclassified, and are not suitable as the sole means of establishing a diagnosis. A detailed interview with parents establishes what actual behaviours are the basis for ratings, allows professional judgement to be included, and remains the most informative single method.

#### (b) Psychiatric interview

Interview with the child is valuable for the observation of attention and social interaction that it yields, and for understanding a child's view of their predicament. Children, however, are not good witnesses about their own concentration and impulse control, and even affected adults are not good at describing themselves in these terms. The experience of ADHD is usually one of suffering the reactions evoked from other people, or an experience of repeated failure. Adults often describe an experience of whirling and interrupted thoughts (in the absence of manic features); and some children will say the same, especially if treatment has enabled them to make a comparison with another way of being.

#### (c) Investigating underlying causes

Assessment needs not only to distinguish ADHD from related disorders, but to consider whether the ADHD pattern may result from remediable causes. The anamnestic history is by far the most productive investigation. It should include whether hearing problems have been excluded by previous testing (and, if not, an expert assessment should be arranged), and any injuries or diseases are potentially damaging the brain. The strengths and weaknesses of the family environment need to be assessed; they may dictate the choices of treatment. Physical examination should be sufficient to detect congenital anomalies, skin lesions, and motor abnormalities that can be the pointers to a neurological cause. Psychometric assessment is desirable whenever there are problems at school, both to generate an idea of developmental level against which the 'developmental inappropriateness' of behavioural symptoms can be judged, and to detect barriers to learning that may be the reason for inattentiveness. Special physical investigations are not routinely necessary. EEG often yields evidence of immaturity, but this does not advance assessment much and is not routinely indicated. It is valuable in the investigation of epilepsy and in the rare cases when deterioration of function suggests the possibility of a degenerative disorder. Blood tests should be planned only on the basis of history and examination, but may include tests of thyroid function, lead (in high-lead areas) chromosomal integrity (including fragile-X probe) when there is other evidence of developmental delay, and specific DNA tests when there is clinical suspicion of a phenotype such as that of Williams syndrome.

### Epidemiology

Prevalence estimates vary widely; but most of the variation between studies comes from differences in definition[6] A community survey in London of more than 2000 6–8-year-old boys found a continuum of severity on rating scales: at each successively higher level of hyperactive behaviour there were successively fewer number of children[8] The genetic evidence also supports a continuum: in a population-based twin study, the influences on hyperactive behaviour were similar over the whole range of variation.[15] Estimates of prevalence are therefore critically dependent upon the cut-off point chosen.

Two major influences on the cut-off are the diagnostic criteria applied and the cultural attitudes of raters. Attention Deficit/Hyperactivity Disorder has a rate in the school age population usually given at about 5 per cent, but varies from 2.4 to 9 per cent[6,16] probably depending on how rigorously 'impairment' is defined. The ICD-10 diagnosis of Hyperkinetic disorder yields rates around 1 to 2 per cent of the school age population.[6,17] Sex differences are marked: population surveys suggest that 2–3 boys are affected for every girl.[18]

The frequency of hyperactive behaviour in the population, at least as indexed by rating scales in surveys, has not been increasing over the last two decades.[19] By contrast, there have been large increases in the frequency with which hyperactivity as a medical condition has in practice been recognized—most obviously evidenced by a great increase in the rates of stimulant prescription between 1995 and 2005 in the UK (Wong et al, in submission) and a continuing increase in the USA.[20] The studies suggest that stimulant medication is given for about 3 children per 1000 in the UK (i.e. about 12 per cent of those in the community meeting ADHD criteria with impairment) and about 40 per 1000 in the USA. It is likely that health service organization plays a part in determining recognition. In the USA survey, a diagnosis of ADHD was more likely to have been made for children whose families Carried Health Insurance.[20] In a UK survey, children with high hyperactivity as rated by teachers and parents seldom received a diagnosis, with the main filter coming at the level of recognition by primary health care services.[21]

In adult life, those who were hyperactive as children still have an elevated rate of hyperactivity and related social impairment (reviewed systematically by Faraone et al.).[22] Indeed, a cross-sectional population survey of adults described a surprisingly high prevalence rate of about 4 per cent, with a high rate of co-existent psychological morbidity.[23] More evidence is needed on the extent of the adult problem. It is however clear that a substantial number of adults, who were not diagnosed in childhood, may be affected, and an increasing number are presenting for the first time to adult services.

## Aetiology

### Genetic inheritance

Genetic influences are strong: Twin studies suggest a heritability around 80 per cent, making it one of the psychological disorders most strongly influenced by genetic inheritance,[24,25] and adoptive family studies concur in emphasizing the strength of association with biological relatives.[26] Indeed, several DNA variants in genes coding for relevant proteins have now been identified and replicated.[27] In particular, the genes coding for the dopamine D4 and D5 receptors, the dopamine transporter, SNAP25 (affecting synaptosomal protein), the serotonin 1b receptor and the serotonin transporter have all been associated with ADHD by more than one group of investigators. Several kinds of caution are, however, needed in interpreting these findings. The odds ratios are all quite small (between 1.1 and 1.5), no polymorphism so far found is either necessary or sufficient; it is possible that there are subtypes of ADHD with different genetic influences[28]

Current research continues to seek more associated genes, especially by genome scans and positional cloning and to emphasize the likely importance of gene-environment interactions.

Individual studies have reported that the risk alleles for genes in the dopamine system magnify the effects on the foetus of maternal smoking and alcohol consumption during pregnancy,[29,30] and catechol o-methyl transferase (COMT) of low birth weight[31]

### Environment

Environmental influences are reviewed by Taylor & Warner Rogers.[32] There are associations with several kinds of adversity in fetal and early postnatal life; and genetic factors may influence the exposure to some hazards (e.g. to lead, via playing in contaminated areas) as well as their impact. Many of the insults have generalized effects on brain development and can also lead to low IQ.

### Prenatal

The prenatal factors implicated include smoking and drinking in pregnancy,[33] cocaine,[34] maternal stress during pregnancy,[35] anticonvulsant use[36] and the factors causing very low birth weight.[37] For some of these, there is experimental evidence for a harmful effect in animals. Smoking, for example, has high biological plausibility: the substances inhaled have an effect in animal models, and there is a dose-response relationship in human studies.[38] It is important to recognize these risk factors in assessing a referred child, because one may be able to prevent a subsequent child from suffering the same injury. Interpretation of a positive history, however, is not straightforward, because of the likely effects of genetic influences as well. There is no doubt of the existence of the fetal alcohol syndrome, nor that it can include ADHD symptoms, but the effect of lesser degrees of exposure is uncertain. Apparent associations could be magnified by gene-environment correlations. Maternal drinking may be influenced by the same genes that influence ADHD; the genes and the pregnancy toxin may be handed down together. Knopic et al.[39] investigated this by studying the offspring of mothers who were identical twins yet differed in whether they had a history of alcohol abuse: ADHD was common in both groups: the suggestion was that the genes were more important than the presumed exposure to alcohol.

### Postnatal

In postnatal life, the best defined risks are at extreme levels of misfortune. Head injury and brain disease have to be severe before they have a causative effect; minor injury is often a result of hyperactivity rather than a cause.[32] Children who experienced extreme deprivation in the orphanages of Romania showed increased rates of pervasive and persistent overactivity and inattention in later childhood, even though they had been adopted into English families before the age of 4 years.[40] Minor degrees of psychological adversity have not been shown to cause ADHD (though they may well be associated with coexistent conduct disorder). Indeed, the twin studies that show genetic influences can also be used to distinguish between the environment that all children in the family share (such as a chaotic family life style or the use of television), and the environmental influences that affect one child but not another; only the latter play a part.

Diet is often blamed for hyperactivity. There is some truth in it, but the effects seem to be modest. The main evidence comes from therapeutic trials (see under 'Treatment') which indicate that a range of foodstuffs can be harmful for individual children – including cow's milk, wheat flour, eggs, and artificial colourings and additives. Individual idiosyncrasies seem more important than a damaging effect of the substances on everyone. Experimental trial, however, giving colourings including tartrazine to an unselected population of preschool children, suggests that the substances have a small but measurable adverse effect on behaviour across the whole range and so ought to be seen as mildly toxic.[41]

## Pathogenesis

The effect of these aetiological influences on the developing brain is being clarified by the neuroimaging possibilities being created by magnetic resonance and other non-invasive techniques. Several brain areas are smaller in ADHD than controls.[42] The difference persists through adolescence into adult life and is more marked in those who have never received medication than those who have. The areas most affected—frontal, striatal and cerebellar—are involved in self-organizational abilities that fail in those with ADHD.

At a neuropsychological level, there have been extensive comparisons between young people referred for, and diagnosed with ADHD in the USA and age-matched controls without psychopathology. 'Executive function'—which has become a broad and ill-defined term for psychological processes by which people modify their responsiveness to stimuli or the organization of their responses—has received special attention and is reviewed by Willcutt et al.[43] In general summary, many such functions show significant differences between ADHD and controls, but the effect sizes are modest and do not suggest that research has yet hit on either a fundamental deficit or on a means of diagnosis to replace behavioural description.

Motor inhibition and cognitive inhibition have received particular attention, deriving from the behavioural observation that children with ADHD can be described as 'disinhibited', and from an influential suggestion by Barkley[44] that failures of inhibitory process could underlie the other cognitive deficits – such as inefficient planning ahead, and poor self-control by internal language. There is not much doubt that experiments reliably produce poor performance in ADHD on tests of suppressing motor responses.[45] Indeed, functional neuroimaging has found that people with ADHD, as a group, show less activation of brain structures involved in response suppression, even when they are performing at a satisfactory level on a simple test.[46] There is more uncertainty about whether this form of impulsiveness does indeed derive from deficits in inhibition or from other kinds of psychological alteration, such as reluctance to put effort into planning responses of any kind, or to be patient during a period of waiting. This last idea, 'delay aversion', has been elaborated and tested[47] and suggests that some children with hyperactive behaviour are still capable of delaying a response when appropriate provided that the length of time they have to wait for the reward is controlled. A head-to-head comparison of inhibition failure action (in a 'stop' test) and delay aversion (in a test of delaying gratification) has been carried out, with the result that either test on its own produced a moderate distinction between ADHD and controls, but combining the two resulted in a much better discrimination, with sensitivity and specificity around 80 per cent.[48]

The clinical applicability of the extensive research investment in psychological testing is rather small. The tests have for the most part lacked either standardization or establishment of test–retest reliability; the interpretation of an individual child's score, accordingly, lacks quantitative support. There are a few tests of related abilities that have normative values with age standardization (e.g. the Tests of Everyday Attention for Children: TEACH). Their place in practice is not to make a diagnosis of ADHD, but to suggest which of several possible cognitive weaknesses apply in the individual child. In principle, useful advice for education could follow from such testing; but evaluations—of the uptake by teachers, of the advice or the impact on the child—are lacking.

## Course and prognosis

### First 3 years

A 'difficult temperament' in early childhood includes overactivity and poor self-regulation, and can have a harmful effect on parent–child relationships; but the concept of inattentiveness is hard to apply at this age and the diagnosis would be insecure.

### Age 3–6

ADHD behaviours are clearly recognizable by this age, and there is a strong likelihood of persistence into the school years.[49] Parent training is an effective intervention (see 'Treatment') and should be available for parents with children at risk, without waiting for formal diagnosis.

### Age 7–11

School and peer demands make ADHD behaviours impairing; the tolerance of families and the culture at large help to determine whether ADHD is seen as a problem; and this is a very common age for referral and diagnosis. Hyperactivity (as opposed to inattentiveness alone) becomes important in generating aggressive and antisocial behaviour and delinquency.[50] The extent to which there is a poor social outcome may depend upon genetic influences,[51,52] on environmental influences such as a hostile home atmosphere,[53] and on gene–environment interactions (a COMT gene polymorphism together with a low birth weight predicted the development of antisocial symptoms in those with ADHD).[31]

### Age 12–18

During adolescence, there is a maturing in the abilities of self-control, and some children with ADHD will lose their problems; but the demands for self-control rise as well, and so the children are still more impulsive and inattentive than their peers and four times as likely to merit a psychiatric diagnosis.[54] Indeed, about half of cases diagnosed in childhood will retain the full diagnosis in adolescence.[55]

Those who continue to show hyperactivity are at risk for other problems, notably aggressive and antisocial behaviour and delinquency,[50] and motor traffic accidents.[56]

### Adult life

By adult life, most will no longer meet full diagnostic criteria for ADHD; but, equally, most will retain some functional impairment related to hyperactivity.[22] This should imply a falling prevalence, but survey of adults has found high rates (about 4 per cent).[23] Some part of this discrepancy may derive from adults developing impairment for the first time; they may have had ADHD symptoms as children, but the symptoms were not impairing, and have only become impairing when adult life imposes responsibility and high expectations.

The implications for practice are that from childhood to early adult life, and perhaps longer, severe levels of hyperactivity and inattentiveness should be seen as potentially chronic disability; and that intervention should not target only the core symptoms but also the surrounding tangle of adverse personal relationships and educational failure.

## Treatment evaluations

### Medication

There have been many trials of central nervous stimulants (especially methylphenidate, with some work on dexamfetamine and pemoline) and atomoxetine. A systematic review was undertaken by NICE (National Institute for Clinical Excellence).[57] Sixty-five trials met quality criteria and were assessed. Quantitative review indicated heterogeneity among the trials, so a meta-analysis was not attempted; but there was no doubt about the superiority of methylphenidate, atomoxetine, and dexamfetamine to placebo. Economic analyses were undertaken and were not very robust, but suggested that all three gave acceptable cost per Quality-Adjusted Life Year. All three should be in clinical use, with the decision regarding which product to use to be based on comorbidity, adverse effects, compliance, potential for drug diversion, and individual preferences with differences in cost as a secondary consideration.

Several proprietary preparations of methylphenidate have appeared that offer an extended release through the day; they differ in the physics of their delivery systems and therefore in their speed of onset and duration of action. Banaschewski *et al.*[58] made a systematic review of trials on them and on atomoxetine, which also has a sustained effect through the day. They indicated that the effect size of extended-release methylphenidate preparations was comparable to that of immediate-release—around 0.8–1.1 SD; but, not surprisingly, the effect of an 8-hour preparation was somewhat smaller than that of a 12 preparation on parent ratings, though similar on teachers' ratings of child behaviour. The effect size of atomoxetine was around 0.6 SD.

Most studies have been carried out on children and adolescents of school age. In children under 6 years, the limited trial evidence suggests that stimulants are more effective than placebo in reducing hyperactivity and the level of stress in family relationships[59] The safety of the drugs in this age group is uncertain. For adults, enough randomized controlled trials have appeared for stimulants and atomoxetine that meta-analysis has been possible, with the conclusion that they are more effective than placebo.[58,60]

### Psychological evaluations

Behaviour therapy has received several trials, but no satisfactory systematic review has yet appeared. Miller *et al.*[61] attempted one, but decided to exclude most of the trials because they did not meet the quality criteria that were imposed. Nevertheless, reasonably good effect sizes have been reported in randomized trials comparisons for the comparisons of behaviour modification programmes (usually delivered on an individual family basis) with no treatment or treatment as usual.[62,63] Group programs of parent training—which typically include supportive education in behavioural management—are also effective, perhaps particularly for preschool children.[64,65] Cognitive therapy, by contrast, has been disappointing in trials.[66]

### Elimination diets

Several trials of eliminating foods that seem to be incriminated for an individual child, followed by double-blind administration of those foods in experimental design, have found that the identified foods can worsen that child's behaviour more than a placebo.[67] The implication, as for food effects on disorders such as eczema, is of idiosyncratic intolerances so that each child needs investigating individually. This is troublesome for families, and perhaps only applicable to younger children whose diet is still under parental control.

### Drug vs. psychosocial intervention

There has been controversy over the relative merits of medication and behaviour therapy. In the USA, the debate has been sharpened by a perceived over-prescription of drugs and led to a large-scale random-allocation non-blind trial.[68] The trial compared rather idealized versions of: medication (with very careful and systematic monitoring of dose and response), behaviourally oriented psychosocial therapy (delivered with high intensity and a combination of approaches to teachers, parents and the young people themselves), both interventions given together, and a 'treatment as usual' policy of referring back to community agencies (which usually resulted in medication). At the prime outcome point—14 months after randomization—the outcome for those given the research style of medication was better than those given behavioural treatment only and considerably better than those given treatment as usual, even when that included medication. Adding medication to behaviour therapy improved the outcome for the primary measures of hyperactive behaviour; adding behaviour therapy to medication did not—but did yield better control of aggression at home, improvement in the overall sense of satisfaction of parents, lower medication dosage, and a higher rate of very good outcomes. These improvements in the combination treatment were real, but very expensive to achieve, and it remains uncertain whether such benefits could be matched by behaviour therapy delivered under the constraints of ordinary practice. The marked superiority of careful medication to other forms of intervention did not persist at later follow-up points. At 2 and 3 years after the start of the trial, those who had been allocated to all arms of the trial showed rather similar outcomes. None were untreated, and all groups showed less hyperactivity than at the beginning of the trial, so the finding should not lead to therapeutic nihilism. The likely reasons for the waning of the medication effect are that the drug loses its effect, stops being taken, or depends upon careful and skilled adjustment of dosage in the longer term.

## Management

### Psychoeducation

Unlike most psychiatric conditions, a diagnosis of ADHD is often sought by parents and welcomed by them. The image, of being a physically caused neurological disease, is often perceived as a relief from the stigma of mental disorder. On the other hand, the media controversy over whether it is a 'real' disorder, and over the use of controlled drugs, leaves some parents confused and fearful.

Assessment on the principles above will have led to an individual formulation of the nature and causes of the impairment. Extended explanation is worthwhile in the longer term. An over-simple description in terms of a chemical deficiency in the brain may seem a useful starting point but can lead to unrealistic expectations for treatment and frustration with the doctor or, worse, with the child. A model of chronic disability is in keeping with the evidence from longitudinal studies; but needs to be modulated by the good outcome for some children, the improvement for most, and the ability of warm and encouraging parenting to reduce the risks of antisocial behaviour in later childhood and adolescence.[53]

Children's understanding of their problems is also worth a good deal of effort. Little research has so far addressed the issue, but it is important to their ability to cope. They need to know that their problem is understood, that treatments are available, that they can influence their outcome by their own actions, and that the people around them understand all this and can be encouraging. Positive role models are useful: some successful sports stars, performers, politicians and business people have outed themselves as having, and sometimes using, ADHD. Explanations need to be repeated as the young people mature and expect a fuller and more interactive discussion.

Explanation is often needed by teachers as well. They may need to revise their expectations of the level of challenge with which the child can cope; and for some frustration can lead to antagonism towards the child's family. If they already see ADHD as a neurological disease, then the frequent observations of changeability in the children, and of ability to cope sometimes with difficult tasks, may make them reject a neurological cause—and with it the diagnosis and the validity of drug treatment. They may need to know that physical and psychological factors can both enter into the child's presentation and that the effect of medication does not depend on the aetiology.[10]

After explanation comes basic advice on helping the children's development. The first steps with parents are to establish whether there is already a framework of frequent warm interactions and effective ways of giving instructions and following up children's actions with consistent patterns of reward or loss of reward. If this does not already exist, then a parent training group is often helpful. Both a supportive atmosphere and the teaching of skills in behaviour modification seem to be necessary. The target behaviours for modification are often the ones most troublesome to parents—disobedience and aggression—rather than restlessness or inattentiveness specifically.

Liaison with schools should include advice on the severity of the problem and the intensity and nature of extra help that will be required. Teachers will often be able to share good practice in classroom management. One of the principles is to maintain good stimulus control, for instance by having the affected child at the front of the class under the teacher's eye. Another is to find opportunities for the children to let off physical energy (they can sometimes be used as messengers between classrooms) and to learn in short chunks. Variety and interest in the material to be learned or understood is useful. Transitions between activities in the classroom are often the time for children to become disorganized, and the child with ADHD should be the first to change activity with the teacher's supervision. Individual attention is probably the most effective resource in the classroom, but it is also very demanding: a classroom assistant may help to achieve it. Star charts for younger children and token economy systems for older ones are often recommended, but usually depend upon the system used for the rest of the class.

## Specific interventions

When straightforward advice is not enough, then the two best-evaluated treatment approaches are *behaviour modification* and *medication management*. The choice of which to start with will depend on several conclusions from the assessment: the severity of the problem (with more severe problems responding preferentially to medication rather than behaviour therapy[7] the availability of treatment; the willingness and ability of parents (or teachers) to engage in psychological intervention; the urgency of the problem (with medication affording a more rapid change); and the wishes of the family. Whichever approach is taken first, the other should be available without undue delay if the response is below expectation.

### (a) Behaviour modification

The principles of behaviour modification do not differ from those used in other kinds of behaviour problem (e.g. 62). Target behaviours should be clearly specified and monitored; the antecedents and consequences of the behaviours should be understood and modified as appropriate; clear schemes of reward and punishment should be established, understood by the child, and applied consistently. There are, in addition, some modifications to suggest for the specific needs that come from the nature of ADHD. The rapid delay-of-reward gradient calls for contingencies to be applied with particular attention to speed. For example, a kitchen timer can be set for an appropriate length of activity depending upon the individual child (for instance, 5 min application to homework, or 30 min spent free of aggression to siblings). When the timer sounds, an obvious reward (such as a token) is given within a very few seconds. The reward may swiftly lose its reinforcing quality with repetition, so frequent changes in the reward (or the backup to a token) are needed. Impairment in error correction may make it all the more necessary to be explicit and swift in explaining to the child which of their behaviours has earned the reward, or its loss. Response cost (such as loss of tokens) is usually advocated in conjunction with the reward scheme.

### (b) Medication

Prescription of medicines can be guided by published schemes (e.g.[13]). Specialist assessment is highly desirable when problems are at the level that warrants medication—not because the treatment is specially risky, but because it is important that remediable causes and associated conditions are not overlooked. The first choice of medicine is usually methylphenidate. If immediate-release is chosen, then one usually begins with doses, three times a day about 5 mg to 10 mg, depending on the child's weight. If there are no adverse effects, then the dose is increased upwards (probably weekly) until there is a good response, or adverse effects become troublesome, or the ceiling of 0.7 mg/kg/dose is reached—whichever comes first. If an extended-release preparation is chosen, then a similar policy is followed of starting at a low level (e.g. 10–20 mg as a single dose) and titrating in the light of response.

The choice of immediate—or extended—release preparation should be discussed with the family. School children often have a strong preference for a single tablet to be taken in the morning before school, so as to avoid stigmatization. Schools should also be part of the decision making, because of the organizational problems for them of maintaining secure storage and accurate administration. On the other hand, advantages of immediate-release include lower cost and the possibility of accurate control of the profile of action through the day.

Individual variation in drug response is considerable, so good monitoring is a key to achieving good effects. A simple rating scale such as the abbreviated Conners is suitable: a short scale is more likely to be completed than a long one. The wide variety of presentations means that key problems for the individual child may not be included on a standard scale. An individualized scale can therefore be constructed as part of the assessment and used as the prime outcome measure. Ratings by teachers are particularly important, but communication problems can mean that their voice is not heard. If the dose is set only by the level seen as optimal by the parents, then there is a danger of over-treatment. The child's behaviour will be seen at home in the mornings and evenings of schooldays, i.e. at times when the blood level of medication is lower than during school hours. The best dose for mornings and evenings may then lead a child being over-controlled and unspontaneous during school hours. Internet feedback from class teacher can be quick and accessible, but care is needed to maintain confidentiality. Telephone monitoring is useful, especially to allow frequent adjustments in the initial phase of setting dosage, but cannot replace individual contact.

Physically, blood pressure and height and weight need regular checks; mentally, the examiner should be alert to the possibilities that agitation, depression, loss of spontaneity and perseveration can appear as a result of medication and not only as part of the condition.

Under some circumstances, atomoxetine is the medication of first choice. It is not a controlled drug, and does not maintain an illicit market, so it may be preferred if there is a substance-misusing family member. The media controversy over the use of stimulants has entailed that atomoxetine may be acceptable to some families who reject 'Ritalin'. It may also be preferred in the presence of Tourette disorder and perhaps of high levels of anxiety. Children who have failed to respond to a stimulant may nevertheless show a good response to atomoxetine. The balance of adverse effects is somewhat different and atomoxetine may therefore be preferred when, for example, insomnia has resulted from stimulants or is a major problem in itself. The action of atomoxetine may take some weeks to appear, and close titration is not recommended. Rather, a test dose around 0.5 mg/kg is given (in case adverse effects appear even on a small dose), and is followed after a week by an increase to 1.2 mg/kg.

## Treatment in comorbid conditions

In general, and as considered in 'Diagnosis' above, the cluster of ADHD symptoms is similar whether or not co-existent disorders are present. The principles are for the most part the same as when treating uncomplicated ADHD. In the most frequent combination—of ADHD and conduct disorder—stimulant treatment can reduce antisocial problems as well as the core of ADHD[57] and is often worth trying even before conduct disorder is addressed.

### (a) Anxiety

In the combination of ADHD and anxiety states, there is some trial evidence that the superiority of stimulant to placebo is less than in ADHD without anxiety.[10,69] There may need to be particular attention to monitoring both problems in establishing the correct dose level, and atomoxetine will sometimes be chosen. The reasons for anxiety should be sought and corrected.

### (b) Pervasive developmental disorders

When an autism spectrum disorder is also present, then treatment of ADHD with stimulants is possible, but particular attention needs to be given to the possibility of exacerbating social withdrawal and repetitive patterns of behaviour, and monitoring these should be given a priority as high as detecting the desired effects. The RUPP Autism Network[70] treated 72 cases in a design with a 1-week test period, 4 weeks randomized crossover, and 8 weeks of continued treatment for those who responded well. Methylphenidate produced a better reduction of hyperactive behaviour than did placebo. The most satisfactory dose level was a modest 0.25 mg/kg.

### (c) Substance misuse

In the presence of substance misuse, many clinicians are wary of prescribing the potentially misusable stimulants. There may be too much hesitation. People with ADHD taking stimulants show lower rates of substance misuse than those who do not take prescribed medication.[71]

### (d) Epilepsy

The presence of epilepsy raises extra needs in assessment before treatment. In poorly controlled epilepsy, ADHD symptoms may be the direct result of very frequent small seizures ('absence status' at the extreme) or of very frequent seizures at night, so ambulant and sleeping EEGs are useful. In less extreme cases, brief lapses of attention can be the result of minor seizures causing transient cognitive impairment; simultaneous recording of EEG with behaviour observation and/or psychological test performance is the best way of getting the answer. Anticonvulsant medications can also cause disturbances of attention and irritability; the clues come from high blood levels of anticonvulsants, low folate levels, polypharmacy, and a temporal relationship between drug changes and hyperactivity or inattention. Once these are excluded, then treatment of ADHD can proceed as usual. Methylphenidate, it has been copied from textbook to textbook, can worsen epilepsy. I have not been able to find empirical evidence for this, do not find that it matches with clinical experience and regard methylphenidate as safe in controlled epilepsy. Atomoxetine has had numerous reports of seizures following its use, but very few of first seizures. In uncontrolled epilepsy, and especially where there is a risk for status epilepticus, I prefer to use dexamfetamine.

## Review after a satisfactory response

When a child has responded well to the first treatment chosen, a specialist's review of the case is in order.

Is the improvement sufficient? Impulsiveness and inattentiveness may not have disappeared entirely; but the goal should be that they are no longer impairing. If the problems are still more than minor, then the other main intervention should be explored.

What has happened to any co-existent disorders: are they satisfactorily resolved or is further treatment or referral indicated?

Has the improvement led to different understanding of the child? Old habits of reacting to the children or setting expectations for them may need to be modified. At home, parents may well have found that they set disciplinary sanctions at a high level when the need was to have an impact on an inattentive person. Those sanctions may be too severe, for a person who is now more responsive to reward and punishment and lead to distress or discouragement.

At school, there may be opportunities for normalizing the curriculum. Social skills learning, which may have been abandoned in the past because of the child's failure to profit, may now be well worth another try.

Does the child understand the nature of the improvement? This, like the nature of the disability, will need discussing in different ways as the child matures. The initial reaction may well be one simply of relief at being out of trouble. If, however, medicines are seen as a tablet 'to make me good', this attitude may lead to a rejection of medicine in adolescence when rejecting other aspects of adult authority. There are usually many decisions to make about medication—whether to take it during the school holidays and at weekends, whether to vary the dose in line with environmental demands, and whether to continue taking it even though indulging in alcohol or cannabis. There is every reason to involve the child as an active agent in these decisions and to help them to learn from the consequences.

For how long should the treatment continue? Scientific study has not given a secure answer to this question, and individual decision making is needed. Periodic spells off medication—perhaps for a fortnight every two years—is a good way of deciding whether it is still needed. These are also good times for the patient to review why he is taking it, and perhaps to seek the reactions of others to his state off medication.

Are there satisfactory follow-up arrangements? Shared care between primary care and the specialist service is the ideal, with physical monitoring (perhaps 6-weekly) and minor dose adjustments carried out in primary care, and psychological monitoring and strategy decisions about therapy (perhaps 6-monthly) carried out by the specialist team.

### Review in refractory cases

A case can be considered refractory when the problems are still impairing after the exhibition of methylphenidate (or dexamfetamine), atomoxetine and behavioural therapy.

There are several reasons for failure at the first line, of which failure to follow treatment is the commonest. If behaviour modification was the first line tried, and the child was too hyperactive for it to be adequately delivered, then it may well be worth another try in combination with medication, even if the medication alone was not obviously successful. If medication was not taken, then the reason may have been stigma and careful discussion may allow a more successful attempt. Public controversy about ADHD and medication has been intense for decades and has not been resolved by increasing knowledge. It is right for there to be strong debate, not least because the issues raised—of whether it is legitimate to make changes in one's learning and social abilities through physical methods—arise in many other areas of public concern. Unfortunately, however, some journalism accuses parents and teachers of bad faith, in pretending a physical cause to disguise failings in parental childrearing or inadequacies in schools. This is understandably disquieting for children and those around them. Involvement with a user group can help to maintain a positive attitude to overcoming disability, and counter some of the noxious attitudes expressed in some of the media.

Another reason for failure of medication is the appearance of adverse effects, either precluding the treatment or limiting the dose to subtherapeutic levels. Symptomatic treatment of adverse reactions is often possible.

*Appetite loss* can result from stimulants (and less commonly from atomoxetine). This will often disappear towards the end of the day, as the medication is cleared from the body, so increased intake in the evenings (or at weekends or other holidays from stimulant medication) is often enough to prevent faltering in growth.

*Insomnia* is a frequent complaint, but should be carefully recorded at baseline as it often precedes medication. The commonest problem to result from stimulants is a delay in settling and falling asleep. Sleep hygiene measures can help, for instance, a planned deceleration of activity towards bedtime (perhaps in a place other than the bedroom, to avoid conditioning the bedroom environment to wakefulness); a reduction in light intensity (including sitting farther away from the television or computer screen); and prescription of melatonin shortly before settling. A switch from stimulants to atomoxetine may be needed.

*Tics* can be worsened or produced by stimulants. Some people find that mild tics are a price worth paying for the beneficial actions, or not even notice them; but they can be disfiguring and stigmatizing. A switch to atomoxetine will often be the first action; or the combination of methylphenidate with clonidine may be useful in both reducing tic severity and reducing the necessary dose of methylphenidate.

Treatment can also fail because the initial assessment was incomplete and set the wrong targets for therapy. Another disorder may have masqueraded as ADHD (see 'Diagnosis') and a failure to respond should raise the index of suspicion for the presence of autistic or hypomanic overactivity. (The converse, however, does not hold; a response to methylphenidate does not make the diagnosis of ADHD, because qualitatively similar changes can be seen when ordinary children receive a stimulant, vide Rapoport *et al.*)[72] A variant of this comes when ADHD was present, but not the main problem, and the main problem perceived by parents or teachers is not drug-sensitive.

When the above reasons for failure to respond to treatment have been considered and dealt with, then the psychiatrist should consider some of the wide variety of unlicensed medications that have been shown effective in randomized controlled trials.

Some noradrenergic agents (clonidine, guanfacine), may act to stimulate presynaptic autoreceptors and may downregulate noradrenergic activation. They can be useful when there is a great deal of agitation as part of the symptom pattern (e.g. in autism). They do not, however, improve the cognitive aspects of inattentiveness.

Modafinil has effects in reducing hyperactivity and may enhance cognition as well. A licence has been applied for, but was interrupted by the possible emergence of skin disorders as a complication.

Tricyclic antidepressants (e.g. imipramine, protriptyline) and some other antidepressants (bupropion, but not SSRIs) are more effective than placebo in reducing hyperactivity; their effect often wanes after a few weeks or months, but they can be useful for short periods, e.g. to allow a period off stimulants in a child with a growth problem.

Monoamine oxidase inhibitors also reduce hyperactivity; they are in general unsafe for use in children, partly because of the difficulty in maintaining dietary restrictions, but the reversible MAOIs such as meclobomide are somewhat safer and could be considered. Nicotine patches can be considered for their combination of cognitive and behavioural effects, but quite often produce nausea and local irritation.

Risperidone and other atypical neuroleptics are often used, especially in intellectually impaired populations, but have not been evaluated for the treatment of ADHD. Their power, and the reason they are prescribed, is in the symptomatic reduction of severely aggressive and agitated behaviour rather than the improvement of attentive and reflective behaviour. Clarity of indication is therefore important, and their benefits should be set against the many hazards.

Some efficacious drugs have been contraindicated because of rare but severe, adverse effects: pemoline after reports of liver failure, desipramine because of cardiac toxicity. In general, the use of unlicensed or unevaluated drugs should be embarked on only by prescribers with specialist experience, who obtain carefully informed consent and monitor appropriately. The most effective medication protocol yet evaluated was that of the MTA approach (see above), in which stimulants were sufficient for about 90 per cent of cases and there was little recourse to the second line of drugs.

## Treatment in adult life

A key problem in current knowledge is that of making an accurate diagnosis when adults present for the first time. Adults may be mistaken in identifying themselves (see above); but their recall of their childhoods is a reasonably reliable predictor of their parents' ratings.[73] Self-report scales have emerged[74, 75] but are not yet fully validated. The account of somebody who knows the patient well—perhaps a spouse or a partner—is very desirable, but does of course need interpreting in the light of their own interests in a diagnosis.

Psychosocial treatment for adults is not yet well evaluated. In principle, adults ought to have greater capacities for cognitive and other self-instructional approaches. Young and Bramham[76] provide a useful guide. Simply the giving of a diagnosis comes as a relief to some who have puzzled over the reasons for their failures, and can liberate problem-solving approaches.

Treatment with stimulant drugs and atomoxetine has been evaluated by several randomized controlled trials in adults (reviewed by Faraone *et al.* and Banaschewski *et al.*).[58,60] The drugs are efficacious. Only atomoxetine has a licence in Europe, and that only when treatment was started in childhood; but it does not seem reasonable to withhold a therapy because it was unavailable to the person earlier. Their use follows similar principles to those described above for children, and Asherson[77] provides a guide.

In conclusion, this chapter has presented a picture of ADHD and its severe form, hyperkinetic disorder, as disabilities that change with development and are often accompanied by other problems that can mask it or themselves be masked by it. They are rewarding challenges for diagnosis and treatment in adulthood as well as during childhood and adolescence.

## Further information

The National Institute of Mental Health (NIMH) Website: http://www.nimh.nih.gov/health/topics/attention-deficit-hyperactivity-disorder-adhd/index.shtml

The National Attention Deficit Disorder Information and Support Service (ADDISS) Website: www.addiss.co.uk

Eric, T. (ed.) (2007). *People with Hyperactivity: Understanding and Managing Their Problems.* Mac Keith Press.

## References

1. Schachar, R. (1986). Hyperkinetic syndrome: Historical development of the concept. In *The Overactive Child* (ed. E. Taylor), Clinics in Developmental Medicine No. 97. MacKeith Press/Blackwells, London.

2. Porrino, L.J., Rapoport, J.L., Behar, D., *et al.* (1983). A naturalistic assessment of the motor activity of hyperactive boys. I. Comparison with normal controls. *Archives of General Psychiatry,* **40**, 681–7.

3. Sergeant, J.A. (2005). Modeling attention-deficit/hyperactivity disorder: A critical appraisal of the cognitive-energetic model. *Biological Psychiatry,* **57**, 1248–55.

4. American Psychiatric Association (2000). *Diagnostic and Statistical Manual of Mental Disorders version IV text revision.* American Psychiatric Association, Washington, DC.

5. World Health Organization (1992). *The ICD-10 classification of mental and behavioural disorders: Clinical descriptions and diagnostic guidelines.* Geneva, World Health.

6. Swanson, J.M., Sergeant, J., Taylor, E., *et al.* (1998). Attention Deficit Hyperactivity Disorder and Hyperkinetic Disorder. *The Lancet,* **351**, 429–33.

7. Santosh, P.J., Taylor, E., Swanson, J., *et al.* (2005). Refining the diagnoses of inattention and overactivity syndromes: A reanalysis of the Multimodal Treatment study of attention deficit hyperactivity disorder (ADHD) based on ICD-10 criteria for hyperkinetic disorder. *Clinical Neuroscience Research,* **5**, 307–14.

8. Taylor, E., Sandberg, S., Thorley, G. *et al.* (1991). *The epidemiology of childhood hyperactivity. Maudsley Monograph No. 33.* Oxford University Press, Oxford.

9. Nadder, T.S., Rutter, M., Silberg, J.L., *et al.* (2002) Genetic effects on the variation and covariation of attention deficithyperactivity disorder (ADHD) and oppositional-defiant disorder/conduct disorder (Odd/CD) symptomatologies across informant and occasion of measurement. *Psychological Medicine,* **32**(1), 39–53.

10. Taylor, E. A., Schachar, R., Thorley, G., *et al.* (1987). Which boys respond to stimulant medication? A controlled trial of methylphenidate in boys with disruptive behaviour. *Psychological Medicine,* **17**, 121–43.

11. Green, M., Wong, M., Atkins, D., *et al.* (1999). *Technical Review Number 3: Diagnosis of Attention-Deficit/Hyperactivity Disorder.* Rockville, MD: Agency for Health Care Policy and Research, US Department of Health and Human Services, AHCPR Publication 99-0050.

12. Stein, M.T., and Perrin, J.M. (2003). Diagnosis and treatment of ADHD in school-age children in primary care settings: a synopsis of the AAP Practice Guidelines. *Pediatrics in Review,* **24**, 92–8.

13. Taylor, E., Döpfner, M., Sergeant, J., *et al.* (2004). European clinical guidelines for hyperkinetic disorder - first upgrade. *European Child and Adolescent Psychiatry,* **13**(Suppl 1), 17–30.

14. Conners, C.K. (1997) Conners' ADHD/DSM-IV Scales (CADS). www.mhs.com

15. Gjone, H., Stevenson, J., and Sundet, J.M. (1996). Genetic influence on parent-reported attention-related problems in a Norwegian general population twin sample. *Journal of the American Academy of Child and Adolescent Psychiatry,* **35**, 588–96.

16. Ford, T., Goodman, R., Meltzer, H. (2003). The British Child and Adolescent Mental Health Survey 1999: the prevalence of DSM-IV disorders. *Journal of the American Academy of Child and Adolescent Psychiatry,* **42**(10), 1203–11.

17. Meltzer, H., and Gatward, R. (with Goodman, R., and Ford, T.) (2000). *Mental health of children and adolesdents in Great Britain,* London, The Stationery Office.

18. Heptinstall, E., and Taylor, E. (2002). Sex differences and their significance. In *Hyperactivity and Attention Disorders of Childhood* (ed. S. Sandberg). Cambridge University Press, Cambridge.

19. Collishaw, S., Maughan, B., Goodman, R., *et al.* (2004). Time trends in adolescent mental health. *Journal of Child Psychology and Psychiatry,* **45**, 1350–62.

20. CDC (2003). *Prevalence of Diagnosis and Medication Treatment for Attention-Deficit/Hyperactivity Disorder*. Center for Disease Control http://www.cdc.gov/mmwr/preview/mmwrhtml/mm5434a2.htm

21. Sayal, K., Taylor, E., Beecham, J., *et al.* (2002). Pathways to care in children at risk of attention-deficit hyperactivity disorder. *British Journal of Psychiatry*, **181**, 43–8.

22. Faraone, S.V., Biederman, J., and Mick, E. (2006). The age-dependent decline of attention deficit hyperactivity disorder: a meta-analysis of follow-up studies. *Psychological Medicine*, **36**, 159–65.

23. Kessler, R.C., Adler, L., Barkley, R., *et al.* (2006). Prevalence of adult ADHD in the United States: results from the National Comorbidity Survey Replication (NCS-R). *American Journal of Psychiatry*, **163**, 716–23.

24. Asherson, P., Kuntsi, J., and Taylor, E. (2005). Unravelling the complexity of attention-deficit hyperactivity disorder: a behavioural genomic approach. *British Journal of Psychiatry*, **187**, 103–5.

25. Thapar, A., O'Donovan, M., and Owen, M.J. (2005a). The genetics of attention deficit hyperactivity disorder. *Human Molecular Genetics*, **14**, R275–R282.

26. Sprich, S., Biederman, J., Crawford, M.H., *et al.* (2000). Adoptive and biological families of children and adolescents with ADHD. *Journal of the American Academy of Child and Adolescent Psychiatry*, **39**, 1432–37.

27. Faraone, S.V., Perlis, R.H., Doyle, A.E., *et al.* (2005). Molecular genetics of attentiondeficit/hyperactivity disorder. *Biological Psychiatry*, **57**, 1313–23.

28. Todd, R.D., Sitdhiraksa, N., Reich, W., *et al.* (2002). Discrimination of DSM-IV and latent class attention-deficit/hyperactivity disorder subtypes by educational and cognitive performance in a population based sample of child and adolescent twins. *Journal of the American Academy of Child and Adolescent Psychiatry*, **41**, 820–8.

29. Kahn, R.S., Khoury, J., Nichols, W.C., *et al.* (2003). Role of dopamine transporter genotype and maternal prenatal smoking in childhood hyperactive-impulsive, inattentive, and oppositional behaviors. *Journal of Pediatrics*, **143**, 104–10.

30. Brookes, K., Mill, J., Guindalini, C., *et al.* (2006) A common haplotype of the dopamine transporter gene associated with attention deficit/hyperactivity disorder and interacting with maternal use of alcohol during pregnancy. *Archives of General Psychiatry*, **63**, 74–81.

31. Thapar, A., Langley, K., Fowler, T., *et al.* (2005b). Catechol O-methyltransferase gene variant and birth weight predict early-onset antisocial behavior in children with attention-deficit/hyperactivity disorder. *Archives of General Psychiatry*, **62**, 1275–78.

32. Taylor, E., and Warner-Rogers, J. (2005). Practitioner review: Early adversity and developmental disorders. *Journal of Child Psychology and Psychiatry*, **46**, 451–67.

33. Linnet, K.M., Dalsgaard, S., Obel, C., *et al.* (2003). Maternal lifestyle factors in pregnancy risk of attention deficit hyperactivity disorder and associated behaviors: Review of the current evidence. *American Journal of Psychiatry*, **160**, 1028–40.

34. Linares, T.J., Singer, L.T., Kirchner, H.L., *et al.* (2006). Mental health outcomes of cocaine-exposed children at 6 years of age. *Journal of Pediatric Psychology*, **31**, 85–97.

35. O'Connor, T.G., Heron, J., Golding, J., *et al.* (2003). *Maternal antenatal anxiety and behavioural/emotional problems in children: A test of a programming hypothesis.*

36. Steinhausen, H.C., Losche, G., Koch, S., *et al.* (1994). The psychological-development of children of epileptic parents. I. Study design and comparative findings. *Acta Paediatrica*, **83**, 955–60.

37. Bhutta, A.T., Cleves, M.A., Casey, P.H., *et al.* (2002). Cognitive and behavioral outcomes of school-aged children who were born preterm - A meta-analysis. *Journal of the American Medical Association*, **288**, 728–37.

38. Thapar, A., Fowler, T., Rice, F., *et al.* (2003). Maternal smoking during pregnancy and attention deficit hyperactivity disorder symptoms in offspring. *American Journal of Psychiatry*, **160**, 1985–89.

39. Knopik, V.S., Heath, A.C., Jacob, T., *et al.* (2006). Maternal alcohol use disorder and offspring ADHD: disentangling genetic and environmental effects using a children-of-twins design. *Psychological Medicine*, **36**, 1461–71.

40. Kreppner, J.M., O'Connor, T.G., and Rutter, M. (2001). Can inattention/overactivity be an institutional deprivation syndrome? *Journal of Abnormal Child Psychology*, **29**, 513–28.

41. Bateman, B., Warner, J.O., Hutchinson, E., *et al.* (2004) The effects of a double blind, placebo controlled, artificial food colourings and benzoate preservative challenge on hyperactivity in a general population sample of preschool children. *Archives of disease in childhood*, **89**(6), 506–11.

42. Castellanos, F.X., Lee, P.P., Sharp, W., *et al.* (2002). Developmental trajectories of brain volume abnormalities in children and adolescents with attention-deficit/hyperactivity disorder. *Journal of the American Medical Association*, **288**, 1740–48.

43. Willcutt, E.G., Doyle, A.E., Nigg, J.T., *et al.* (2005). Validity of the executive function theory of attention-deficit/hyperactivity disorder: A meta-analytic review. *Biological Psychiatry*, **57**, 1336–46.

44. Barkley, R.A. (1997). Behavioral inhibition, sustained attention, and executive functions: Constructing a unifying theory of ADHD. *Psychological Bulletin*, **121**, 65–94.

45. Castellanos, X., Sonuga-Barke, E.J.S., Tannock, R., *et al.* (2006). Characterising Cognition in ADHD: Beyond Executive Dysfunction. *Trends in Cognitive Science*, **10**, 117–23.

46. Rubia, K., Smith, A.B., Brammer, M.J., *et al.* (2005). Abnormal brain activation during inhibition and error detection in medication-naive adolescents with ADHD. *American Journal of Psychiatry*, **162**, 1067–75.

47. Sonuga-Barke, E.J. (2005). Causal models of attention-deficit/hyperactivity disorder: from common simple deficits to multiple developmental pathways. *Biological Psychiatry*, **57**, 1231–8.

48. Solanto, M.V., Abikoff, H., Sonuga-Barke, E.J.S., *et al.* (2001). The ecological validity of measures related to impulsiveness in AD/HD. *Journal of Abnormal Child Psychology*, **29**, 215–28.

49. Lahey, B.B., Pelham, W.E., Loney, J., *et al.* (2004). Three-year predictive validity of DSM-IV attention deficit hyperactivity disorder in children diagnosed at 4–6 years of age. *American Journal of Psychiatry*, **161**, 2014–20.

50. Farrington, D.P. (1995). The Twelfth Jack Tizard Memorial Lecture. The development of offending and antisocial behaviour from childhood: key findings from the Cambridge Study in Delinquent Development. *Journal of Child Psychology & Psychiatry*, **36**, 929–64.

51. Faraone, S.V. (2004). Genetics of adult attention-deficit/hyperactivity disorder. *Psychiatric Clinics of North America*, **27**, 303–21.

52. Mill, J., Caspi, A., Williams, B.S., *et al.* (2006). Prediction of heterogeneity in intelligence and adult prognosis by genetic polymorphisms in the dopamine system among children with attention-deficit/hyperactivity disorder: Evidence from 2 birth cohorts. *Archives of General Psychiatry*, **63**, 462–9.

53. Rutter, M., Maughan, B., Meyer, J., *et al.* (1997). Heterogeneity of antisocial behavior: Causes, continuities, and consequences. In *Motivation and delinquency* (ed. D. W. Osgood), (pp. 45–118). Lincoln, NE: University of Nebraska Press; and *Nebraska Symposium on Motivation*, **44**, 45–118.

54. Taylor, E., Chadwick, O., Heptinstall, E., *et al.* (1996). Hyperactivity and conduct problems as risk factors for adolescent development. *Journal of the American Academy of Child and Adolescent Psychiatry*, **35**, 1213–26.

55. Klein, R.G., and Mannuzza, S. (1991). Long-term outcome of hyperactive children: a review. *Journal of the American Academy of Child and Adolescent Psychiatry*, **30**, 383–7.

56. Barkley, R.A., Fischer, M., Edelbrock, C.S., *et al.* (1990). The adolescent outcome of hyperactive children diagnosed by research criteria: I. An 8-year prospective follow-up study. *Journal of the American Academy of Child and Adolescent Psychiatry*, **29**, 546–57.

57. NICE (National Institute for Health and Clinical Excellence). (2005). *Methylphenidate, atomoxetine and dexamfetamine for the treatment of*

*attention def cit hyperactivity disorder in children and adolescents.* http://www.nice.org.uk/page.aspx?o=TA013

58. Banaschewski, T., Coghill, D., Santosh, P., *et al.* (2006). Long-acting medications for the hyperkinetic disorders: A systematic review and European treatment guideline. *European Child and Adolescent Psychiatry.* [Epub ahead of print]

59. Kratochvil, C.J., Egger, H., Greenhill, L.L., *et al.* (2006). Pharmacological management of preschool ADHD. *Journal of the American Academy of Child and Adolescent Psychiatry,* **45**, 115–18.

60. Faraone, S.V., Spencer, T., Aleardi, M., *et al.* (2004). Meta-analysis of the efficacy of methylphenidate for treating adult attention-deficit/hyperactivity disorder. *Journal of Clinical Psychopharmacology,* **24**, 24–9.

61. Miller, A., Lee, S.K., Raina, P., *et al.* (1998). *A review of therapies for attention-deficit/hyperactivity disorder.* Ottawa, ON: Canadian Coordinating Office for Health Technology Assessment.

62. Barkley, R.A., Edwards, G., Laneri, M., *et al.* (2001). The efficacy of problem-solving communication training alone, behaviour management training alone, and their combination for parent-adolescent conflict in teenagers with ADHD and ODD. *Journal of consulting and clinical psychology,* **69**(6), 926–41.

63. Pelham, W.E., Gnagy, E.M., Greiner, A.R., *et al.* (2000). Behavioral versus behavioral and pharmacological treatment in ADHD children attending a summer treatment program. *Journal of abnormal child psychology,* **28**(6), 507–25.

64. Sonuga-Barke, E.J.S., Daley, D., Thompson, M., *et al.* (2001). Parent-based therapies for preschool attentiondeficit/hyperactivity disorder: A randomized, controlled trial with a community sample. *Journal of the American Academy of Child and Adolescent Psychiatry,* **40**, 402–8.

65. Bor, W., Sanders, M.R., and Markie-Dadds, C. (2002). The effects of the Triple P-Positive Parenting Program on preschool children with co-occurring disruptive behavior and attentional/hyperactive difficulties. *Journal of Abnormal Child Psychology,* **30**, 571–87.

66. Gittelman-Klein, R., and Abikoff, H. (1989) The role of psychostimulants and psychosocial treatments in hyperkinesis. In *Attention def cit Disorder: Clinical and basic research* (eds. T. Sagvolden and T. Archer), Lawrence Erlbaum, Hillsdale NJ, pp. 167–180.

67. Schab, D.W., and Trinh, N.H.T. (2004). Do artificial food colors promote hyperactivity in children with hyperactive syndromes? A meta-analysis of double-blind placebo-controlled trials. *Journal of Developmental and Behavioral Pediatrics,* **25**, 423–34.

68. MTA Cooperative Group. (1999). A 14-month randomized clinical trial of treatment strategies for attention-deficit/hyperactivity disorder. Multimodal Treatment Study of Children with ADHD. *Archives of General Psychiatry,* **56**, 1073–86.

69. Buitelaar, J.K., Van der Gaag, R.J., Swaab-Barneveld, H., *et al.* (1995). Prediction of clinical response to methylphenidate in children with attention-deficit hyperactivity disorder. *Journal of the American Academy of Child and Adolescent Psychiatry,* **34**, 1025–32.

70. Research Units on Pediatric Psychopharmacology Autism Network. (2005). Randomized, controlled, crossover trial of methylphenidate in pervasive developmental disorders with hyperactivity. *Archives of General Psychiatry,* **62**, 1266–74.

71. Wilens, T.E., Faraone, S.V., Biederman, J., *et al.* (2003). Does stimulant therapy of attention-deficit/hyperactivity disorder beget later substance abuse? A meta-analytic review of the literature. *Pediatrics,* **111**, 179–85.

72. Rapoport, J.L., Buchsbaum, M.S., Weingartner, H., *et al.* (1980). Dextroamphetamine. Its cognitive and behavioral effects in normal and hyperactive boys and normal men. *Archives of General Psychiatry,* **37**, 933.

73. Ward, M.F., Wender, P.H., and Reimherr, F.W. (1993). The Wender Utah Rating Scale: An aid in the retrospective diagnosis of childhood attention deficit hyperactivity disorder. *American Journal of Psychiatry,* **150**, 885–90. Erratum in, **150**, 1280.

74. Conners, C.K., Erhardt, D., Sparrow, E., *et al.* (1998). In *CAARS Adult ADHD Rating Scales.* New York, NY, Multi Health Systems Inc.

75. Brown, T.E. (1996). In *Brown Attention-Deficit Disorder Scales,* San Antonio, The Psychological Corporation.

76. Young, S., and Bramham, J. (2007). *ADHD in Adults: A Psychological Guide to Practice.* Chichester, UK, John Wiley & Sons.

77. Asherson, P. (2005). Clinical assessment and treatment of attention deficit hyperactivity disorder in adults. *Expert Review of Neurotherapeutics,* **5**, 525–39.

## 9.2.5 Conduct disorders in childhood and adolescence

Stephen Scott

### Introduction

The term conduct disorder refers to a persistent pattern of antisocial behaviour in which the individual repeatedly breaks social rules and carries out aggressive acts which upset other people. It is the commonest psychiatric disorder of childhood across the world, and the commonest reason for referral to child and adolescent mental health services in Western countries. Antisocial behaviour has the highest continuity into adulthood of all measured human traits except intelligence. A high proportion of children and adolescents with conduct disorder grow up to be antisocial adults with impoverished and destructive lifestyles; a significant minority will develop antisocial personality disorder (psychopathy). The disorder in adolescence is becoming more frequent in Western countries and places a large personal and economic burden on individuals and society.

### Relation to other disorders

Conduct disorder is one of the two *disruptive disorders* of childhood, (also known as *externalizing disorders*); the other is the hyperkinetic syndrome (ICD 10), a more severe form of attention-deficit hyperactivity disorder (ADHD, DSM IV-R). Conduct disorder and the hyperkinetic syndrome are distinct disorders but often co-occur. As discussed in Chapter 9.1.1 on classification, disruptive disorders can be distinguished on a number of criteria from the other main grouping of child psychiatric conditions, the *emotional disorders* (also known as *internalizing disorders*). For example, unlike emotional disorders, disruptive disorders are commoner in boys, the socially disadvantaged, children from large families, and where there is parental discord.

Juvenile delinquency is a legal term referring to an act by a young person who has been convicted of an offence which would be deemed a crime if committed by an adult. Most, but not all, recurrent juvenile offenders have conduct disorder. In this chapter the term conduct disorder is used as defined by ICD 10 diagnostic criteria; the term conduct problems will be used for less severe antisocial behaviour.

### Social problem or medical diagnosis?

Infringement of the rights of other people is a requirement for the diagnosis of conduct disorder. Since the manifestations include a failure to obey social rules despite apparently intact mental state and social capacities, many have seen the disorder as principally socially determined. They therefore believe the responsibility for its cause and elimination lies with people who can influence the socialization process, such as parents, schoolteachers, social service departments, and politicians. Due to the impossibility of their seeing all cases, there is some debate within child and adolescent psychiatry as to whether doctors and mental health professionals should be involved in any but the most complex presentations.[1] Some have argued that involvement of medical personnel carries the risk of their becoming agents of social control through the misapplication of diagnostic labels, which may lead to abuses of the kind seen in some totalitarian regimes.

However, advances in the last decade have shown there are substantial genetic and biological contributions to conduct disorder, and in some cases the symptoms may be responsive to medication. Work in the last 25 years mainly from the field of child and adolescent mental health has clarified many of the mechanisms contributing to the development and persistence of antisocial behaviour, and has led to the development of effective treatments. As yet these are not being widely used with the children and adolescents who need them. Therefore psychiatrists need to be able to contribute to the planning and delivery of an appropriate service.

## Clinical features

Aggressive and defiant behaviour is an important part of normal child and adolescent development which ensures physical and social survival. Indeed, parents may express concern if a child is too acquiescent and unassertive. The level of aggressive and defiant behaviour varies considerably amongst children, and it is probably most usefully seen as a continuously distributed trait. Empirical studies do not suggest a level at which symptoms become qualitatively different, nor is there a single cut-off point at which they become impairing for the child or a clear problem for others. There is no hump towards the end of the distribution curve of severity to suggest a categorically distinct group who might on these grounds warrant a diagnosis of conduct disorder.

Picking a particular level of antisocial behaviour to call conduct disorder is therefore necessarily arbitrary. For all children, the expression of any particular behaviour also varies according to child age, so that for example physical hitting is at a maximum at around 2 years of age but declines to a low level over the next few years. Therefore any judgement about the significance of the level of antisocial behaviour has to be made in the context of the child's age. Before deciding that the behaviour is abnormal or a significant problem, a number of other clinical features have to be considered:

- Level: severity and frequency of antisocial acts, compared with children of the same age and gender
- Pattern: the variety of antisocial acts, and the setting in which they are carried out
- Persistence: duration over time
- Impact: distress and social impairment of child; disruption and damage caused to others.

### Change in clinical features with age

The type of behaviour seen will depend on the age and gender of the individual.

*Younger children*, say from 3 to 7 years of age, usually present with general defiance of adults wishes, disobedience of instructions, angry outbursts with temper tantrums, physical aggression to people especially siblings and peers, destruction of property, arguing, blaming others for things that have gone wrong, and a tendency to annoy and provoke others.

In *middle childhood*, say from 8 to 11, the above features are often present but as the child grows older, stronger, and spends more time out of the home, other behaviours are seen. They include: swearing, lying about what they have been doing, stealing of others belongings outside the home, persistent breaking of rules, physical fights, bullying of other children, cruelty to animals, and setting of fires.

In *adolescence*, say from 12 to 17, more antisocial behaviours are often added: cruelty and hurting of other people, assault, robbery using force, vandalism, breaking and entering houses, stealing from cars, driving and taking away cars without permission, running away from home, truanting from school, extensive use of narcotic drugs.

Not all children who start with the type of behaviours listed in early childhood progress on to the later, more severe forms. Only about half continue from those in early childhood to those in middle childhood[2]; likewise only about a further half of those with the behaviours in middle childhood progress to show the behaviours listed for adolescence. However, the early onset group are important as they are far more likely to display the most severe symptoms in adolescence, and to persist in their antisocial tendencies into adulthood. Indeed over 90 per cent of severe, recurrent adolescent offenders showed marked antisocial behaviour in early childhood. In contrast, there is a large group who only start to be antisocial in adolescence, but whose behaviours are less extreme and who tend to desist by the time they are adults.

### Girls

Severe antisocial behaviour is less common in girls who are less likely to be physically aggressive and engage in criminal behaviour, but more likely to show spitefulness, emotional bullying (such as excluding children from groups, spreading rumours so others are rejected by their peers), frequent unprotected sex leading to sexually transmitted diseases and pregnancy, drug abuse, and running away from home.

### Pattern and setting

Prognosis is determined by the frequency and intensity of antisocial behaviours, the variety of types, the number of settings in which they occur (e.g. home, school, and in public), and their persistence. For general populations of children, the correlation between parent and teacher ratings on the same measures is only 0.2 to 0.3, so that there are many children who are perceived to be mildly or moderately antisocial at home but well behaved at school, and vice versa. However, for more severe antisocial behaviour, there are usually manifestations both at home and at school.

### Impact

At home the child often is subject to high levels of criticism and hostility, and sometimes made a scapegoat for a catalogue of family misfortunes. Frequent punishments and physical abuse are not uncommon. The whole family atmosphere is often soured and siblings also affected. Maternal depression is often present, and families who are unable to cope may, as a last resort, give up the child to be cared for by the local authority. At school, teachers may take a range of measures to attempt to control the child and protect the other pupils, including sending the child out of the class, sometimes culminating in permanent exclusion from the school. This may lead to reduced opportunity to learn subjects on the curriculum and poor examination results. The child typically has few if any friends, who get fed up with their aggressive behaviour. This often leads to exclusion from many group activities, games, and trips, so restricting the child's quality of life and experiences. On leaving school the lack of social skills, low level of qualifications, and presence of a police record make it harder to gain employment.

## Classification

The ICD-10 classification has a category for conduct disorders, F91. The *Clinical descriptions and diagnostic guidelines*[3] state:

> Examples of the behaviours on which the diagnosis is based include the following: excessive levels of fighting or bullying; cruelty to animals or other people; severe destructiveness to property; firesetting; stealing; repeated lying; truancy from school and running away from home; unusually frequent and severe temper tantrums; defiant provocative behaviour; and persistent severe disobedience. Any one of these categories, if marked, is sufficient for the diagnosis, but isolated dissocial acts are not. (p. 267)

An enduring pattern of behaviour should be present, but no time frame is given and there is no impairment or impact criterion stated.

The ICD-10 *Diagnostic criteria for research*[4] differ, requiring symptoms to have been present for at least 6 months, and the introductory rubric indicates that impact upon others (in terms of violation of their basic rights), but not impairment of the child, can contribute to the diagnosis. The research criteria take a menu-driven approach whereby a certain number of symptoms have to be present. 15 behaviours are listed to consider for the diagnosis of **Conduct Disorder**, which usually but not exclusively apply to older children and teenagers. They can be grouped into four classes:

### (a) Aggression to people and animals

- often lies or breaks promises to obtain goods or favours or to avoid obligations

- frequently initiates physical fights (this does not include fights with siblings)

- has used a weapon that can cause serious physical harm to others (e.g. bat, brick, broken bottle, knife, gun)

- often stays out after dark despite parenting prohibition (beginning before 13 years of age)

- exhibits physical cruelty to other people (e.g. ties up, cuts, or burns a victim), and

- exhibits physical cruelty to animals.

### (b) Destruction of property

- deliberately destroys the property of others (other than by firesetting) and

- deliberately sets fires with a risk or intention of causing serious damage).

### (c) Deceitfulness or theft

- steals objects of non-trivial value without confronting the victim, either within the home or outside (e.g. shoplifting, burglary, forgery).

### (d) Serious violations of rules

- is frequently truant from school, beginning before 13 years of age

- has run away from parental or parental surrogate home at least twice or has run away once for more than a single night (this does not include leaving to avoid physical or sexual abuse)

- commits a crime involving confrontation with the victim (including purse-snatching, extortion, mugging)

- forces another person into sexual activity

- frequently bullies others (e.g. deliberate infliction of pain or hurt, including persistent intimidation, tormenting, or molestation), and

- breaks into someone else's house, building, or car.

To make a diagnosis, three symptoms from this list have to be present, one for at least 6 months. There is no impairment criterion. There are three subtypes: *conduct disorder confined to the family context* (F91.0), *unsocialized conduct disorder* (F91.1, where the young person has no friends and is rejected by peers), and *socialized conduct disorder* (F91.2, where peer relationships are normal). It is recommended that age of onset be specified, with *childhood onset type* manifesting before age 10, and *adolescent onset type* after. Severity should be categorized as *mild*, *moderate*, or *severe* according to number of symptoms *or* impact on others, e.g. causing severe physical injury, vandalism, theft.

For younger children, say up to 9 or 10 years old, there is a list of eight symptoms for the subtype known as **Oppositional Defiant Disorder** (F91.3):

1 has unusually frequent or severe temper tantrums for his or her developmental level

2 often argues with adults

3 often actively refuses adults' requests or defies rules

4 often, apparently deliberately, does things that annoy other people

5 often blames others for his or her own mistakes or misbehaviour

6 is often touchy or easily annoyed by others

7 is often angry or resentful

8 is often spiteful or resentful.

To make a diagnosis of the oppositional defiant type of conduct disorder, four symptoms from *either* this list *or* the main conduct disorder 15 symptom list have to be present, but no more than two from the latter. Unlike the main variant, there is an impairment criterion: the symptoms must be amaladaptive and inconsistent with the developmental level (p. 161).

Where there are sufficient symptoms of a comorbid disorder to meet diagnostic criteria, the ICD-10 system discourages the application of a second diagnosis, and instead offers a single, combined category. There are two major kinds: mixed disorders of conduct and emotions, of which **Depressive Conduct Disorder** (F92.0) is the best researched; and **Hyperkinetic Conduct Disorder** (F90.1). There is modest evidence to suggest these combined conditions may differ somewhat from their constituent elements.

The DSM IV-R system[5] follows the ICD-10 research criteria very closely and does not have separate clinical guidelines. The same 15 behaviours are given for the diagnosis of conduct disorder 312.8, with almost identical wording. As for ICD-10, three symptoms need to be present for diagnosis. Severity and childhood or adolescent onset are specified in the same way. However, unlike ICD-10, there is no division into socialized/unsocialized, or family context only types, and there *is* a requirement for the behaviour to cause a clinically significant impairment in social, academic, or social functioning. Comorbidity in DSM IV-R is handled by giving as many separate diagnoses as necessary, rather than by having single, combined categories.

In DSM IV-R, oppositional defiant disorder is classified as a separate disorder on its own, and not as a subtype of conduct disorder. Diagnosis requires four symptoms from a list of eight behaviours which are the same as for ICD-10, but unlike ICD-10, all four have to be from the oppositional list, and none may come from the main conduct disorder list. It is doubtful whether oppositional defiant disorder differs substantially from conduct disorder in older children in any associated characteristics, and the value of designating it as a separate disorder is arguable. In this article, the term conduct disorder will henceforth be used as it is in ICD-10, to refer to all variant including oppositional defiant disorder.

## Differential diagnosis

Making a diagnosis of conduct disorder is usually straightforward but comorbid conditions are often missed. The differential diagnosis may include:

1 *Hyperkinetic syndrome/Attention-deficit hyperactivity disorder.* These are the names given by ICD-10 and DSM IV-R respectively for similar conditions, except that the former is more severe. For convenience the term *hyperactivity* will be used here. It is characterized by impulsivity, inattention, and motor overactivity. Any of these three sets of symptoms can be misconstrued as antisocial, particularly impulsivity which is also present in conduct disorder. However, none of the symptoms of conduct disorder are a part of hyperactivity so excluding conduct disorder should not be difficult. A frequently made error however, is to miss comorbid hyperactivity when conduct disorder is definitely present. Standardized questionnaires are very helpful here, such as the Strengths and Difficulties Questionnaire, which is brief, and just as effective at detecting hyperactivity as much longer alternatives.[6]

2 *Adjustment reaction to an external stressor.* This can be diagnosed when onset occurs soon after exposure to an identifiable psychosocial stressor such as divorce, bereavement, trauma, abuse, or adoption. The onset should be within 1 month for ICD-10, and 3 months for DSM IV-R, and symptoms should not persist for more than 6 months after the cessation of the stress or its sequelae.

3 *Mood disorders.* Depression can present with irritability and oppositional symptoms but unlike typical conduct disorder mood is usually clearly low and there are vegetative features; also more severe conduct problems are absent. Early manic depressive disorder can be harder to distinguish, as there is often considerable defiance and irritability combined with disregard for rules, and behaviour which violates the rights of others. Low self-esteem is the norm in conduct disorder, as is a lack of friends or constructive pastimes. Therefore it is easy to overlook more pronounced depressive symptoms. Systematic surveys reveal that around a third of children with conduct disorder have depressive or other emotional symptoms severe enough to warrant a diagnosis.

4 *Autistic spectrum disorders.* These are often accompanied by marked tantrums or destructiveness, which may be the reason for seeking a referral. Enquiring about other symptoms of autistic spectrum disorders should reveal their presence.

5 *Dissocial/antisocial personality disorder.* In ICD-10 it is suggested a person should be 17 or older before dissocial personality is considered. Since at age 18 most diagnoses specific to childhood and adolescence no longer apply, in practice there is seldom difficulty. In DSM IV-R conduct disorder can be diagnosed over 18 so there is potential overlap. A difference in emphasis is the severity and pervasiveness of the symptoms of those with personality disorder, whereby all the individual's relationships are affected by the behaviour pattern, and the individual's beliefs about his antisocial behaviour are characterized by callousness and lack of remorse.

6 *Subcultural deviance.* Some youths are antisocial and commit crimes but are not particularly aggressive or defiant. They are well adjusted within a deviant peer culture that approves of recreational drug use, shoplifting, etc. In some localities a third or more teenage males fit this description and would meet ICD-10 diagnostic guidelines for socialized conduct disorder. Some clinicians are unhappy to label such a large proportion of the population with a psychiatric disorder. Using DSM IV-R criteria would preclude the diagnosis for most youths like this due to the requirement for significant impairment.

## Multiaxial assessment

ICD-10 recommends that multiaxial assessment be carried out for children and adolescents, while DSM IV-R suggests it for all ages. In both systems axis one is used for psychiatric disorders which have been discussed above. The last three axes in both systems cover general medical conditions, psychosocial problems, and level of social functioning respectively; these topics will be alluded to below under aetiology. In the middle are two axes in ICD-10, which cover specific (Axis two) and general (Axis three) learning disabilities respectively; and one in DSM IV-R (Axis two) which covers personality disorders *and* general learning disabilities.

Both specific and general learning disabilities are essential to assess in individuals with conduct problems. Fully a third of children with conduct disorder also have specific reading retardation[7] defined as having a reading level two standard deviations below that predicted by the person's IQ. While this may in part be due to lack of adequate schooling, there is good evidence that the cognitive deficits often precede the behavioural problems. General learning disability (mental retardation) is often missed in children with conduct disorder unless IQ testing is carried out. The rate of conduct disorder rise several-fold as IQ gets below 70.

# Epidemiology

Between 5 per cent and 10 per cent of children and adolescents have significant persistent oppositional, disruptive, or aggressive behaviour problems.[8,9] With respect to historical period, a modest rise in diagnosable conduct disorder over the second half of the twentieth century has also been observed comparing assessments of three successive birth cohorts in Britain.[10] There is a marked social class gradient.[9] With respect to ethnicity, youth self-reports of antisocial behaviours, and crime victim survey reports of perpetrators' ethnicity show an excess of offenders of black African ancestry. Importantly, Hispanic Americans in the United States of America and British Asians in the United Kingdom do not tend to show an excess of offending compared to their white counterparts.

## Sex differences in prevalence

The sex ratio is approximately 2:5 males for each female overall, with males further exceeding females in the frequency and severity of behaviours. On balance, research suggests that the causes of conduct problems are the same for the sexes, but males have more conduct disorder because they experience more of its individual-level risk factors (e.g. hyperactivity, neurodevelopmental delays). However, recent years have seen increasing concern amongst clinicians about treating antisocial behaviour amongst girls.[11]

# Developmental subtypes

## Life-course persistent versus adolescence-limited

There has been considerable attention paid to the distinction between conduct problems that are first seen in early childhood versus those that start in adolescence[2] and these two subtypes are encoded in the DSM-IV. Early onset is a strong predictor of persistence through childhood, and early onset delinquency is more likely to persist into adult life. Those with early onset differ from those with later onset in that they have lower IQ, more attentional and impulsivity problems, poorer scores on neuropsychological tests, greater peer difficulties and they are more likely to come from adverse family circumstances.[2] Those with later onset become delinquent predominantly as a result of social influences such as association with other delinquent youths. Findings from the follow-up of the Dunedin cohort support relatively poorer adult outcomes for the early onset group in domains of violence, mental health, substance abuse, work, and family life.[2] However the 'adolescence-limited' group were not without adult difficulties. As adults they still engaged in self-reported offending, and they also had problems with alcohol and drugs. Thus, the age-of-onset subtype distinction has strong predictive validity, but adolescent onset antisocial behaviours may have more long-lasting consequences than previously supposed, and so both conduct problems warrant clinical attention.

# Aetiology

## Individual-level characteristics

### (a) Identified genotypes

The search for specific genetic polymorphisms is a very new scientific initiative, and little has yet been accomplished. The most-studied candidate gene in relation to conduct problems is the MAOA promoter polymorphism. The gene encodes the MAOA enzyme, which metabolizes neurotransmitters linked to aggressive behaviour. Replicated studies show that maltreatment history and genotype interact to predict antisocial outcome.[12]

### (b) Perinatal complications and temperament

Recent large-scale general population studies have found associations between life-course persistent type conduct problems and perinatal complications, minor physical anomalies, and low birth weight.[13] Most studies support a biosocial model in which obstetric complications might confer vulnerability to other co-occurring risks such as hostile or inconsistent parenting. Smoking in pregnancy is a statistical risk predictor of offspring conduct problems,[13] but a causal link between smoking and conduct problems has not been established. Several prospective studies have shown associations between irritable temperament and conduct problems.[14]

### (c) Neurotransmitters

In general the findings with children have not been consistent.[15] For example, in the Pittsburgh Youth cohort, boys with long-standing conduct problems showed downward changes in urinary adrenaline level following a stressful challenge task, whereas prosocial boys showed upward responses. However other studies have failed to find an association between conduct disorder and measures of noradrenaline in children.[15] It should be borne in mind that neurotransmitters in the brain are only indirectly measured, most measures of neurotransmitter levels are crude indicators of activity, and little is known about neurotransmitters in the juvenile brain.

### (d) Verbal deficits and autonomic reactivity

Children with conduct problems have been shown consistently to have increased rates of deficits in language-based verbal skills.[16] The association holds after controlling for potential confounds such as race, socio-economic status, academic attainment, and test motivation. Children who cannot reason or assert themselves verbally may attempt to gain control of social exchanges using aggression; there are likely also to be indirect effects in which low verbal IQ contributes to academic difficulties which in turn mean that the child's experience of school becomes unrewarding, rather than a source of self-esteem and support.

A low resting pulse rate or slow heart rate has been found consistently to be associated with antisocial behaviour, and a meta-analysis of 40 studies suggested it is the best replicated biological correlate of antisocial behaviour.[17] Other psychophysiological indicators show that antisocial and psychopathic boys are also slowest to show a skin-conductance response to aversive stimuli.[17] The explanation for the link between slow autonomic activity and antisocial behaviour remains unclear.

### (e) Information-processing and social cognition

Dodge proposed the leading information-processing model for the genesis of aggressive behaviours within social interactions.[18] The model hypothesises that children who are prone to aggression focus on threatening aspects of others' actions, interpret hostile intent in the neutral actions of others, and are more likely to select and to favour aggressive solution to social challenges. Several studies have demonstrated that aggressive children make such errors of social cognition.[18]

## Risks outside the family

### (a) Risks in the neighbourhood

It has long been assumed that bad neighbourhoods have the effect of encouraging children to develop conduct problems. Many parents strive to secure the best neighbourhood and school for their child that they can afford. Although it is obvious that some local areas have higher crime rates than others, it has been difficult to document any direct link between neighbourhood characteristics and child behaviour, for a number of reasons. For example, neighbourhood characteristics were conceptualized in overly simple structural-demographic terms such as percentage of non-white residents or percentage of single-parent households. Moreover, research designs could not rule out the alternative possibility that families whose members are antisocial tend to selectively move into bad neighbourhoods. A new generation of neighbourhood research is addressing these challenges, and suggests that the neighbourhood factors that are important include social processes such as 'collective efficacy' and 'social control', do influence young children's conduct problems, probably by supporting parents in their efforts to rear children.

### (b) Peer influences

Children with conduct problems have poorer peer relationships than non-disordered children in that they tend to associate with children with similar antisocial behaviours, they have discordant interactions with other children, and experience rejection by non-deviant peers. Three processes have been identified, namely that children's antisocial behaviours lead them to have peer problems, deviant peer relationships lead to antisocial behaviours, and thirdly some common factor leads to both.[19]

## Risks within the family

### (a) Concentration of crime in families

Fewer than 10 per cent of the families in any community account for more than 50 per cent of that community's criminal offenses, which reflects the coincidence of genetic and environmental risks. There is now solid evidence from twin and adoption studies that conduct problems assessed both dimensionally and categorically are substantially heritable.[20] However, knowing that conduct problems are under some genetic influence is less useful clinically than knowing that this genetic influence appears to be reduced, or enhanced, depending on interaction with circumstances in the child's environment. Several genetically sensitive studies have allowed interactions between family genetic liability and rearing environment to be examined. Both adoption and twin studies have reported an interaction between antisocial behaviour in the biological parent and adverse conditions in the adoptive home that predicted the adopted child's antisocial outcome, so that the genetic risk was modified by the rearing environment.

### (b) Family poverty

There is an association between severe poverty and early childhood conduct problems. Early theories proposed direct effects of poverty related to strains arising from the gap between aspirations and realities, and from lacking opportunity to acquire social status and prestige. Subsequent research has indicated that the association between low income and childhood conduct problems is indirect, mediated via family processes such as marital discord and parenting deficits.

### (c) Parent–child attachment

Parent–child relationships provide the setting for the development of later social functioning, and disruption of these attachment relationships, for example through institutional care, is associated with subsequent difficulties in relating. Thus, conduct problems might be expected to arise from infant attachment difficulties. One study found that ambivalent and controlling attachment predicted externalizing behaviours after controlling for baseline externalizing problems[21]; disorganized child attachment patterns seem to be especially associated with conduct problems. Although it seems obvious that poor parent–child relations in general predict conduct problems, it has yet to be established whether attachment difficulties as measured by observational paradigms have an independent causal role in the development of behaviour problems; attachment classifications could be markers for other relevant family risks.

### (d) Discipline and parenting

Patterns of parenting associated with conduct problems were delineated by Patterson in his seminal work *Coercive Family Process*.[22] Parents of antisocial children were found to be more inconsistent in their use of rules, to issue more, and unclear, commands, to be more likely to respond to their children on the basis of mood rather than the characteristics of the child's behaviour, to be less likely to monitor their children's whereabouts, and to be unresponsive to their children's prosocial behaviour. Patterson proposed a specific mechanism for the promotion of oppositional and aggressive behaviours in children. A parent responds to mild oppositional behaviour by a child with a prohibition to which the child responds by escalating his behaviour, and mutual escalation continues until the parent backs off thus negatively reinforcing the child's behaviour. The parent's inconsistent behaviour increases the likelihood of the child showing further oppositional or aggressive behaviour. In addition to specific tests of Patterson's reinforcement model there is ample evidence that conduct problems are associated with hostile, critical, punitive, and coercive parenting.[23]

In considering the role of coercive processes in the origins or maintenance of conduct problems, we need to consider possible alternative explanations, (i) that the associations reflect familial genetic liability towards children's psychopathology and parents' coercive discipline, (ii) that they represent effects of children's behaviours on parents, and (iii) that coercive parenting may be a correlate of other features of the parent/child relationship or family functioning that influence child behaviours. There is considerable evidence that children's difficult behaviours do indeed evoke parental negativity. The fact that children's behaviours can evoke negative parenting does not however mean that negative parenting has no impact on children's behaviour. The E-risk longitudinal twin study of British families examined the effects of fathers' parenting on young children's aggression.[24] As expected, a prosocial father's *absence* predicted more aggression by his children. But in contrast, an antisocial father's *presence* predicted more aggression by his children, and his harmful effect was exacerbated the more time each week he spent taking care of the children.

### (e) Exposure to adult marital conflict and domestic violence

It is likely that family processes other than parenting skills and quality of parent–child attachment relationships have a role. Many studies have shown that children exposed to domestic violence between adults are subsequently more likely to themselves become aggressive. Cummings and Davies[25] proposed that marital conflict influences children's behaviour because of its effect on their regulation of emotion. For example a child may respond to frightening emotion arising from marital conflict by down-regulating his own emotion through denial of the situation. This in turn may lead to inaccurate appraisal of other social situations and ineffective problem-solving. Repeated exposure to family conflict is thought to lower childrens' thresholds for psychological dysregulation, resulting in greater behavioural reactivity to stress.[25] Children's aggression may also be increased by marital discord because children are likely to imitate aggressive behaviour modelled by their parents. Through parental aggression children may learn that aggression is a normative part of family relationships, that it is an effective way of controlling others, and that aggression is sanctioned, not punished.

### (f) Maltreatment

Physical punishment is widely used, and parents of children with conduct problems frequently resort to it out of desperation. Overall, associations between physical abuse and conduct problems are well established.[15] In the Christchurch longitudinal study, child sexual abuse predicted conduct problems, after controlling for other childhood adversities.[26] Links with conduct problems are not however straightforward. The risk for conduct problems does not apply equally to all forms of physical punishment. The E-risk longitudinal twin study was able to compare the effects of corporal punishment (smacking, spanking) versus injurious physical maltreatment using twin-specific reports of both experiences.[27] Results showed that children's genetic endowment accounted for virtually all of the association between their corporal punishment and their conduct problems. This indicated a 'child effect', in which children's bad conduct provokes their parents to use more corporal punishment, rather than the reverse. Findings about injurious physical maltreatment were the opposite. There was no child effect provoking maltreatment and moreover, significant effects of maltreatment on child aggression remained after controlling for any genetic transmission of liability to aggression from antisocial parents.

### From risk predictor to causation

Associations have been documented between conduct problems and a wide range of risk factors. A variable is called a 'risk factor' if it has a documented predictive relation with antisocial outcomes, whether or not the association is causal. The causal status of most of these risk factors is unknown; we know what statistically predicts conduct-problem outcomes, but not how or why. Establishing a causal role for a risk factor is by no means straightforward, particularly as it is unethical to experimentally expose healthy children to risk factors to observe whether those factors can generate new conduct problems. There is no one solution to the problem, although the use of genetically sensitive designs and the study of within-individual change in natural experiments and treatment studies have considerable methodological advantages for suggesting causal influences on conduct problems.

### Course and prognosis

Of those with early onset conduct disorder (before eight) about half persist with serious problems into adulthood. Of those with adolescent onset, the great majority (over 85 per cent) desist in their antisocial behaviour by their early twenties.

Many of the factors which predict poor outcome are associated with early onset (Table 9.2.5.1).

To detect protective factors, children who do well despite adverse risk factors have been studied.

**Table 9.2.5.1** Factors predicting poor outcome

| Onset | Early onset of severe problems, before 8 years of age |
|---|---|
| Phenomenology | Antisocial acts which are severe, frequent, and varied |
| Comorbidity | Hyperactivity and attention problems |
| Intelligence | Lower IQ |
| Family history | Parental criminality; parental alcoholism |
| Parenting | Harsh, inconsistent parenting, with high criticism, low warmth, low involvement, and low supervision |
| Wider environment | Low-income family in poor neighbourhood with ineffective schools |

These so-called 'resilient' children, however, have been shown to have lower levels of risk factors, for example a boy with antisocial behaviour and low IQ living in a rough neighbourhood but living with supportive, concerned parents. Protective factors are mostly the opposite end of the spectrum of the same risk factor, thus good parenting, high IQ are protective. Nonetheless there are factors which are associated with resilience independent of known adverse influences. These include a good relationship with at least one adult, who does not necessarily have to be the parent; a sense of pride and self-esteem; and skills or competencies.

### Adult outcome

Studies of groups of children with early onset conduct disorder indicate a wide range of problems not only confined to antisocial acts, as shown in Table 9.2.5.2.

What is clear is that not only are there substantially increased rates of antisocial acts, but that the general psychosocial functioning of children with conduct disorder grown up is strikingly poor. For most of the characteristics shown in Table 9.2.5.2, the increase

**Table 9.2.5.2** Adult outcome

| Antisocial behaviour | More violent and non-violent crimes, e.g. mugging, grievous bodily harm, theft, car crimes, fraud |
|---|---|
| Psychiatric problems | Increased rates of antisocial personality, alcohol and drug abuse, anxiety, depression and somatic complaints, episodes of deliberate self-harm and completed suicide, time in psychiatric hospitals |
| Education and training | Poorer examination results, more truancy and early school leaving, fewer vocational qualifications |
| Work | More unemployment, jobs held for shorter time, jobs low status and income, increased claiming of benefits and welfare |
| Social network | Few if any significant friends, low involvement with relatives, neighbours, clubs, and organizations |
| Intimate relationships | Increased rate of short-lived, violent cohabiting relationships; partners often also antisocial |
| Children | Increased rates of child abuse, conduct problems in offspring, children taken into care |
| Health | More medical problems, earlier death |

compared to controls is at least double for community cases who were never referred, and three to four times for referred children.[18]

## Pathways

The path from childhood conduct disorder to poor adult outcome is neither inevitable nor linear. Different sets of influences impinge as the individual grows up and shape the life-course. Many of these can accentuate problems. Thus a toddler with an irritable temperament and short attention span may not learn good social skills if he is raised in a family lacking them, and where he can only get his way by behaving antisocially and grasping for what he needs. At school he may fall in with a deviant crowd of peers, where violence and other antisocial acts are talked up and give him a sense of esteem. His generally poor academic ability and difficult behaviour in class may lead him to truant increasingly, which in turn makes him fall further behind. He may then leave school with no qualifications and fail to find a job, and resort to drugs. To fund his drug habit he may resort to crime, and once convicted, find it even harder to get a job. From this example, it can be seen that adverse experiences do not only arise passively and independently of the young person's behaviour; rather, the behaviour predisposes them to end up in risky and damaging environments. Consequently, the number of adverse life events experienced is greatly increased.[28] The path from early hyperactivity into later conduct disorder is also not inevitable. In the presence of a warm supportive family atmosphere it is far less likely than if the parents are highly critical and hostile.

Other influences can however steer the individual away from and antisocial path. For example, the fascinating follow-up of delinquent boys to age 70 by Laub and Sampson[29] showed that the following led to desistence: being separated from a deviant peer group; marrying to a non-deviant partner; moving away from a poor neighbourhood; military service which imparted skills.

## Treatment

### Evidence-based treatments

Proven treatments include those which singly or in combination address (i) Parenting skills, (ii) Family functioning, (iii) Child interpersonal skills, (iv) Difficulties at school, (v) Peer group influences, and (vi) Medication for coexistent hyperactivity.

### (a) Parenting skills

*Parent management training* aims to improve parenting skills. There are scores of randomized controlled trials showing that it is effective for children up to about 10 years old.[30] They address the parenting practices identified in research as contributing to conduct problems. A more detailed account is given by Scott.[30] Typically, they include five elements:

#### (i) Promoting play and a positive relationship

In order to cut into the cycle of defiant behaviour and recriminations, it is important to instil some positive experiences for both sides and begin to mend the relationship. Teaching parents the techniques of how to play in a constructive and non-hostile way with their children helps them recognize their needs and respond sensitively. The children in turn begin to like and respect their parents more, and become more secure in the relationship.

#### (ii) Praise and rewards for sociable behaviour

Parents are helped to reformulate difficult behaviour in terms of the positive behaviour they wish to see, so that they encourage wanted behaviour rather than criticize unwanted behaviour. For example, instead of shouting at the child not to run, they would praise him whenever he walks quietly; then he will do it more often. Through hundreds of such prosaic daily interactions, child behaviour can be substantially modified. Yet some parents find it hard to praise, and fail to recognize positive behaviour when it happens, with the result that it become less frequent.

#### (iii) Clear rules and clear commands

Rules need to be explicit and constant; commands need to be firm and brief. Thus shouting at a child to stop being naughty doesn't tell him what he *should* do, whereas for example telling him to play quietly gives a clear instruction which makes compliance easier.

#### (iv) Consistent and calm consequences for unwanted behaviour

Disobedience and aggression need to be responded to firmly and calmly, but for example putting the child in a room for a few minutes. This method of timeout from positive reinforcement sounds simple but requires considerable skill to administer effectively. More minor annoying behaviours such as whining and shouting often respond to being ignored, but again parents often find this hard to achieve in practice.

#### (v) Reorganizing the child's day to prevent trouble

There are often trouble spots in the day which will respond to fairly simple measures. For example, putting siblings in different rooms to prevent fights on getting home from school; banning TV in the morning until the child is dressed; and so on.

Treatment can be given individually to the parent and child which enables live feedback in light of the parent's progress and the child's response. Alternatively, group treatments with parents alone have been shown to be equally effective.[31] Trials show that parent management training is effective in reducing child antisocial behaviour the short-term, with moderate to large effect sizes of 0.5 to 0.8 standard deviations, and there is little loss of effect at 1 or 3 year follow-up.[32]

### (b) Family functioning

*Functional Family Therapy, Multisystemic Therapy,* and *Treatment Foster Care* aim to change a range of difficulties which impede effective functioning of teenagers with conduct disorder. Functional family therapy addresses family processes which need to be present such as improved communication between parent and young person, reducing interparental inconsistency, tightening up on supervision and monitoring, and negotiating rules and the sanctions to be applied for breaking them. Functional family therapy has been shown to reduce reoffending rates by around 50 per cent.[33] Other varieties of family therapy have not been subjected to controlled trials for young people with conduct disorder or delinquency, so cannot be evaluated for their efficacy.

In multisystemic therapy,[34] the young person's and family's needs are assessed in their own context at home and in their relations with other systems such as school and peers. Following the assessment, proven methods of intervention are used to address difficulties and promote strengths. Multisystemic therapy differs from most types of family therapy such as the Milan or systemic approach as usually practised in a number of regards. Firstly, treatment is delivered in the situation where the young lives, e.g. at home. Secondly, the therapist has a low caseload (4–6 families) and the team is available 24 h a day. Thirdly, the therapist is responsible for ensuring appointments are kept and for making change happen—families cannot be blamed for failing to attend or 'not being ready' to change. Fourthly, regular written feedback on progress towards goals from multiple sources is gathered by the therapist and acted upon. Fifthly, there is a manual for the therapeutic approach and adherence is checked weekly by the supervisor. Several randomized controlled trial attest to the effectiveness, with reoffending rates typically cut by half and time spent in psychiatric hospitalization reduced further.[34]

Treatment foster care is another way to improve the quality of encouragement and supervision that teenagers with conduct disorder receive. The young person lives with a foster family specially trained in effective techniques; sometimes it is ordered as an alternative to jail. Outcome studies show useful reductions in reoffending.[35]

### (c) Anger management and child interpersonal skills

Most of the programmes to improve child interpersonal skills derive from cognitive behaviour therapy. A typical example is the *Coping Power* Programme.[36] This and other programmes have in common, in training the young person to:

i) slow down impulsive responses to challenging situations by stopping and thinking,

ii) recognize their own level of physiological arousal, and their own emotional state,

iii) recognize and define problems,

iv) develop several alternative responses,

v) choose the best alternative based on anticipation of consequences,

vi) reinforce himself for use of this approach.

Over the longer-term they aim to increase positive social behaviour by teaching the young person to:

i) learn skills to make and sustain friendships,

ii) develop social interaction skills such as turn-taking and sharing,

iii) express viewpoints in appropriate ways and listen to others.

Typically, given alone, treatment gains with interpersonal skills training are good within the treatment setting, but only generalize slightly to 'real-life' situations such as the school playground. However, when they are part of a more comprehensive programme which has those outside the young person reinforcing the approach, they add to outcome gains.[36]

### (d) Difficulties at school

These can be divided into learning problems and disruptive behaviour. There are proven programmes to deal with specific learning problems such as specific reading retardation, such as. reading recovery. However, few of the programmes have been specifically evaluated for their ability to improve outcome in children with conduct disorder, although trials are in progress. Preschool education programmes for high risk populations have been shown to reduce arrest rates and improve employment in adulthood (see below).

There are several schemes for improving classroom behaviour, which vary from those which stress improved communication such as 'circle time', and those which work on behavioural principles or are part of a multimodal package. Many of these schemes have been shown to improve classroom behaviour, and some specifically target children with conduct disorder.[37]

### (e) Peer group influences

A few interventions have aimed to reduce the bad influence of deviant peers. However, a number attempted this through group work with other conduct disordered youths, but outcome studies showed a *worsening* of antisocial behaviour. Current treatments therefore either see youths individually try to steer them away from deviant peers, or work in small groups (say 3–5 youths) where the therapist can control the content of sessions. Some interventions place youths with conduct disorder in groups with well-functioning youths, and this has led to favourable outcomes.[38]

### (f) Medication for coexistent hyperactivity

Where there is comorbid hyperactivity in addition to conduct disorder, several studies attest to a large (effect size of 0.8 standard deviations or greater) reduction in both overt and covert antisocial behaviour,[39] both at home and at school. However, the impact on long-term outcome is unstudied.

## Management

Engagement of the family is particularly important for this group of children and families as dropout from treatment is high, at around 30–40 per cent. Practical measures such as assisting with transport, providing childcare, holding sessions in the evening, or at other times to suit the family will all help. Many of the parents of children with conduct disorder may themselves have difficulty with authority and officialdom and be very sensitive to criticism. Therefore the approach is more likely to succeed if it is respectful of their point of view, does not offer overly prescriptive solutions, and does not directly criticize parenting style. Practical homework tasks increase changes, as do problem-solving telephone calls from the therapist between sessions.

Parenting interventions may need to go beyond skill development to address more distal factors which prevent change. For example, drug or alcohol abuse in either parent, maternal depression, and a violent relationship with the partner are all common. Assistance in claiming welfare and benefits and help with financial planning may reduce stress from debts.

A multimodal approach is likely to get larger changes. Therefore involving the school in treatment by visiting and offering strategies for managing the child in class is usually helpful, as is advocating for extra tuition where necessary. If the school seems unable to cope despite extra resources, consideration should be given to moving the child to a different school which specializes in the management of behavioural difficulties. Avoiding antisocial peers and building self-esteem may be helped by getting the child to attend after school clubs and holiday activities.

Where parents are not coping or a damaging abusive relationship is detected, it may be necessary to liaise with the social services department to arrange respite for the parents or a spell of foster care. It is important during this time to work with the family to increase their skills so the child can return to the family. Where there is permanent breakdown, long-term fostering, or adoption may be recommended.

## Opportunities for prevention

Conduct disorder should offer good opportunities for prevention since:

1 it can be detected early reasonably well,

2 early intervention is more effective than later,

3 there are a number of effective interventions.

In the United States of America, a number of comprehensive interventions based on up to date empirical findings are being carried out. Perhaps the best known is Families and Schools Together.[40] Here the most antisocial 10 per cent of 5–6 year olds in schools in disadvantaged areas were selected, as judged by teacher and parent reports. They were then offered intervention which was given for a whole year in the first instance and comprised:

i) weekly parent training in groups with videotapes

ii) an interpersonal skills training programme for the whole class

iii) academic tutoring twice a week

iv) home visits from the parent trainer

v) a pairing programme with sociable peers from the class.

Almost 1000 children were randomized to receive this condition or controls, and the project has cost over $50 million. However, so far, preliminary reports of outcome have been limited with no improvement of antisocial behaviour at home on questionnaire measures and modest improvements in the classroom. There are a number of possible reasons for the smaller effects compared to those obtained in trials with clinically referred populations. The motivation of families may be less as they don't perceive they have a problem; starting levels of antisocial behaviour are lower, so there is not so far to go to reach normal levels; and keeping up the quality of the intervention across several sites is harder. It remains to be seen whether longer-term effects will be greater.

In the United States of America, preschool education programmes for disadvantaged children have shown good outcomes in small demonstration projects, but replication on a larger scale has generally proved rather disappointing. In the United Kingdom, the government stressed the importance of helping parents of children in the first 3 years of life and put substantial resources (£540 million) into *SureStart* centres in specifically targeted high risk neighbourhoods to support parenting. Early evaluation of outcome showed no change on 24 of 25 variables; maternal acceptance of the child was the only measured outcome to change, child antisocial behaviour did not.[41] Separate from conduct disorder prevention but related is crime prevention, which can include reducing the opportunities for antisocial behaviour by tighter policing, reducing access to drugs and guns, and so on.

## Conclusion

Much is known about the risk factors leading to conduct disorder and effective treatments exist. The challenge is to make these available on a wide scale, and to develop approaches to prevention which are effective and can be put into practice at a community level.

## Further information

To access the US Federal Government's site National Youth Violence Prevention Resource Center which has recent research findings, visit http://www.safeyouth.org/scripts/index.asp

To access the US Surgeon Generals' thorough report on youth violence, visit http://www.surgeongeneral.gov/library/youthviolence/

Bloomquist, M.L. and Schnell, S.V. (2002). *Helping children with aggression and conduct problems: best practices for intervention.* Guilford Press, New York.

Connor, D.F. (2002). *Aggression and antisocial behaviour in children and adolescents: research and treatment.* Guilford Press, New York.

Essau, C. (2003). *Conduct and oppositional defiant disorders: epidemiology, risk factors and treatment.* Lawrence Erlbaum Associates, Mahwah, New Jersey.

## References

1. Vostanis, P., Meltzer, H., Goodman, R., *et al.* (2003). Service utilisation by children with conduct disorders: findings from the GB national study. *European Child & Adolescent Psychiatry,* **12**, 231–8.

2. Moffitt, T.E. (2006). Life-course-persistent versus adolescence-limited antisocial behaviour. In *Developmental psychopathology: risk, disorder, and adaptation,* Vol. 3 (2nd edn) (eds. D. Cicchetti and D.J. Cohen), pp. 570–98. John Wiley, Hoboken, NJ.

3. World Health Organization. (1992). *The ICD-10 classification of mental and behavioural disorders: clinical descriptions and diagnostic guidelines.* World Health Organization, Geneva.

4 World Health Organization. (1993). *The ICD-10 classification of mental and behavioural disorders—diagnostic criteria for research.* World Health Organization, Geneva.

5. American Psychiatric Association. (2000). *Diagnostic and statistical manual of mental disorders—DSM IV-R* (4th edn), text revision. American Psychiatric Association, Washington, DC.

6. Goodman, R. and Scott, S. (1999). Comparing the strengths and difficulties questionnaire and the child behaviour checklist: is small beautiful? *Journal of Abnormal Child Psychology,* **27**, 17–24.

7. Trzesniewski, K., Moffitt, T., Caspi, A., *et al.* (2006). Revisiting the association between reading achievement and antisocial behaviour: new evidence of an environmental explanation from a twin study. *Child Development,* **77**, 72–88.

8. Angold, A. and Costello, E.J. (2001). The epidemiology of disorders of conduct: nosological issues and comorbidity. In *Conduct disorders in childhood and adolescence* (eds. J. Hill and B. Maughan). Cambridge University Press, Cambridge.

9. Green, H., McGinnity, A., Meltzer, H., *et al.* (2005). *Mental health of children and young people in Great Britain.* TSO, London.

10. Collishaw, S., Maughan, B., Goodman, R., *et al.* (2004). Time trends in adolescent mental health. *Journal of Child Psychology and Psychiatry,* **45**, 1350–62.

11. Pullatz, M. and Bierman, K.L. (2004). *Aggression, antisocial behaviour, and violence among girls: a developmental perspective.* Guilford Press, New York.

12. Kim-Cohen, J., Caspi, A., Taylor, A., *et al.* (2006). MAOA, maltreatment, and gene-environment interaction predicting children's mental health: new evidence and a meta-analysis. *Molecular Psychiatry,* **11**, 903–913.

13. Brennan, P.A., Grekin, E.R., and Mednick, S.A. (2003). Prenatal and perinatal influences on conduct disorder and serious delinquency. In *Causes of conduct disorder and delinquency* (eds. B. Lahey, T.E. Moffitt, and A.Caspi), pp. 319–44. Guilford Press, New York.

14. Keenan, K. and Shaw, D.S. (2003). Starting at the beginning: exploring the etiology of antisocial behaviour in the first years of life. In *Causes of conduct disorder and delinquency* (eds. B. Lahey, T.E. Moffitt, and A.Caspi), pp. 153–81. Guilford Press, New York.

15. Hill, J. (2002). Biological, psychological and social processes in the conduct disorders. *Journal of Child Psychology and Psychiatry,* **43**, 133–64.

16. Lynam, D.R. and Henry, W. (2001). The role of neuropsychological deficits in conduct disorders. In *Conduct disorders in childhood and adolescence* (eds. J. Hill and B. Maughan). Cambridge University Press, Cambridge.

17. Ortiz, J. and Raine, A. (2004). Heart rate level and antisocial behaviour in children and adolescents: a meta-analysis. *Journal of the American Academy of Child and Adolescent Psychiatry*, **43**, 154–62.

18. Dodge, K. (2006). Translational science in action: hostile attributional style and the development of aggressive behaviour problems. *Development and Psychopathology*, **18**, 791–814.

19. Coie, J.D. (2004). The impact of negative social experiences on the development of antisocial behaviour. In *Children's peer relations: from development to intervention* (eds. J.B. Kupersmidt and K.A. Dodge), pp. 243–67. American Psychological Association, Washington, DC.

20. Moffitt, T.E. (2005). Genetic and environmental influences on antisocial behaviours: evidence from behavioural-genetic research. *Advances in Genetics*, **55**, 41–104.

21. Moss, E., Smolla, N., Cyr, C., *et al.* (2006). Attachment and behaviour problems in middle childhood as reported by adult and child informants. *Development and Psychopathology*, **18**, 425–44.

22. Patterson, G.R. (1982). *Coercive family process*. Castalia Publishing Company, Eugene, OR.

23. Rutter, M., Giller, H., and Hagell, A. (1998). *Antisocial behaviour by young people*. Cambridge University Press, Cambridge.

24. Jaffee, S.R., Moffitt, T.E., Caspi, A., *et al.* (2003). Life with (or without) father: the benefits of living with two biological parents depend on the father's antisocial behavior. *Child Development*, **74**, 109–26.

25. Cummings, E.M. and Davies, P. (2002). Effects of marital conflict on children: recent advances and emerging themes in process-oriented research. *Journal of Child Psychology and Psychiatry*, **43**, 31–64.

26. Fergusson, D.M., Horwood, L.J., and Lynskey, M.T. (1996). Childhood sexual abuse and psychiatric disorder in young adulthood. II. Psychiatric outcomes of childhood sexual abuse. *Journal of the American Academy of Child and Adolescent Psychiatry*, **35**, 1365–74.

27. Jaffee, S.R., Caspi, A., Moffitt, T.E., *et al.* (2004). The limits of child effects: evidence for genetically mediated child effects on corporal punishment, but not on physical maltreatment. *Developmental Psychology*, **40**, 1047–58.

28. Champion, L., Goodall, G., and Rutter, M. (1995). Behavioural problems in childhood and stressors in early adult life: a 20 year follow-up of London school children. *Psychological Medicine*, **25**, 231–46.

29. Laub, J. and Sampson, R. (2003). *Shared beginnings, divergent lives: delinquent boys to age 70*. Harvard University Press, Cambridge, MA.

30. Scott, S. (2008). Parenting programs. Chapter in *Rutter's child and adolescent psychiatry* (5th edn) (eds. M. Rutter, D. Bishop, D. Pine, *et al.*). Blackwell, Oxford.

31. Scott, S., Spender, Q., Doolan, M., *et al.* (2001). Multicentre controlled trail of parenting groups for child antisocial behaviour in clinical practice. *British Medical Journal*, **323**, 194–7.

32. Scott, S. (2005). Do parenting programmes for severe child antisocial behaviour work over the longer term, and for whom? 1 year follow up of a multi-centre controlled trial. *Behavioural and Cognitive Psychotherapy*, **33**, 1–19.

33. Alexander, J.F., Holtzworth-Munroe, A., and Jameson, P.B. (1994). The process and outcome of marital and family therapy research: review and evaluation. In *Handbook of psychotherapy and behaviour change* (eds. A. E. Bergin and S. Garfield), pp. 595–630. Wiley, New York.

34. Curtis, N.M., Ronan, K.R., and Borduin, C.M. (2004). Multisystemic therapy: a meta-analysis of outcome studies. *Journal of Family Psychology*, **18**, 411–19.

35. Eddy, J.M., Whaley, R.B., and Chamberlain, P. (2004). The prevention of violent behavior by chronic and serious male juvenile offenders: a 2-year follow-up of a randomized clinical trial. *Journal of Emotional and Behavioral Disorders*, **12**, 2–8.

36. Lochman, J.E. and Wells, K.C. (2004). The coping power program for preadolescent aggressive boys and their parents: outcome effects at the 1-year follow-up. *Journal of Consulting and Clinical Psychology*, **72**, 571–8.

37. Durlak, J. (1995). *School-based prevention programs for children and adolescents*. Sage, Thousand Oaks, CA.

38. Feldman, R. (1992). *The St Louis experiment: effective treatment of antisocial youths in prosocial peer groups. Preventing antisocial behaviour* (eds. J. McCord and R. Tremblay), pp. 233–52. Guilford Press, New York.

39. Connor, D.F., Glatt, S.J., Lopez, I.D., *et al.* (2002). Psychopharmacology and aggression. I. A meta-analysis of stimulant effects on overt/covert aggression-related behaviors in ADHD. *Journal of the American Academy of Child and Adolescent Psychiatry*, **41**, 253–61.

40. Conduct Problems Prevention Research Group. (1992). A developmental and clinical model for prevention of conduct disorder. *Development and Psychopathology*, **4**, 509–27.

41. Belsky, J., Melhuish, E., Barnes, J., Leyland, A., and Romanuik, H. (2006). Effects of sure start local programmes on children and families: early findings from a quasi-experimental, cross sectional study. *British Medical Journal*, **332**, 1476–9.

# 9.2.6 **Anxiety disorders in childhood and adolescence**

Daniel S. Pine

## Introduction

The term 'fear' refers to the brain state evoked by dangerous stimuli that are avoided because they are capable of harming the organism. The term 'anxiety', in contrast, refers to the brain state evoked by 'threats', stimuli that signal the *possibility* of danger at some point in the near future. Fear and anxiety represent adaptive responses to overt dangers and threats, in that these responses typically reduce the potential for harm to the organisms. Anxiety *disorders* represent conditions where the level of fear is maladaptive either because it leads to clinically significant distress or impairment in function. These effects can result from the production of an anxiety response in a situation not perceived as dangerous by healthy people or by the production of an extreme anxiety response in a situation that healthy people would find mildly anxiety provoking.

The current chapter summarizes recent research on paediatric anxiety disorders. A focus on developmental aspects of anxiety is important since most clinically impairing forms of anxiety typically begin during childhood.[1] Moreover, childhood anxiety disorders show associations with a range of adult psychopathologies beyond anxiety, including most prominently various mood disorders. This fact has stimulated considerable debate concerning the degree to which childhood anxiety disorders reflect early manifestations of adult anxiety disorders. Separation anxiety disorder (SAD) represents the only specific anxiety disorder that primarily occurs in children and adolescents but not adults. Two other disorders frequently co-occur with SAD, social phobia (SOPH), and generalized anxiety disorder (GAD). The current chapter focuses specifically on these three conditions. The chapter also reviews in somewhat less detail data for specific phobia (SPH), a typically minimally impairing condition, and panic disorder (PD), a condition that occurs primarily in adults.[1] Other chapters review material for conditions that frequently co-occur with these five anxiety disorders. This includes major depression (see Chapter 9.2.7), obsessive–compulsive disorder (Chapter 9.2.8), and trauma-related disorders (Chapters 9.3.2). Material on SAD, SOPH, GAD, SPH, and PD are reviewed in three sections. The first, most detailed, section reviews clinical features of these disorders, including typical presentations and diagnosis. The second somewhat briefer section reviews pathophysiology, and the final section briefly reviews therapeutics.

# Clinical features

## Clinical presentation

Children presenting with symptoms of anxiety typically manifest signs of various disorders. In fact, in the clinical setting, presentation with a 'pure' form of anxiety is relatively rare. This suggests that current classifications group children into categories that are unlikely to represent distinct pathophysiologies. Nevertheless, while the current nosology is likely to change as understandings of pathophysiology advance, current classification schemes remain quite useful in that they facilitate communication among individuals working with a child and allow clinicians to draw on research in therapeutics using a common diagnostic system. The current section describes clinical presentation of five specific anxiety disorders, as defined in the fourth edition of the *Diagnostic and Statistical Manual* (DSM-IV). These definitions are similar to those used in the 10th edition of the *International Classification of Disease* (ICD-10), although ICD-10 provides single diagnosis for children with multiple anxiety disorders, whereas and DSM-IV provides multiple diagnoses.

### (a) Separation anxiety disorder

The key feature of SAD involves presentation of anxiety related to fear that harm will befall an attachment figure. In severe forms, SAD typically presents with avoidance of situations, such as school, where separation is required. The term 'school phobia' had been used on occasion for these presentations, but current approaches no longer use this term. Symptoms of SAD often are severe at night, leading many children to refuse to sleep alone or at friends' homes. Considerable research examines the relationship between childhood SAD and adult panic disorder.

### (b) Social phobia

The key features of SOPH involve intense fear or anxiety in situations where the individual is scrutinized. This presents either as extreme form of pervasive shyness or as extreme fear in particular social situations, such as during class presentations. SOPH can also be classified as a 'generalized subtype', indicating that most social situations are feared. The condition can markedly interfere with function by leading children to avoid important academic exercises that must be performed in social settings or by markedly impacting on social development. This effect on social relationships has led to some controversy concerning the boundaries between SOPH and pervasive developmental disorders (PDD). Classically, this distinction can be made based on the presence of language dysfunction and stereotypic behaviour in PDD but not SOPH. Considerable research examines the relationship between late-childhood SOPH and early-childhood temperament.

### (c) Generalized anxiety disorder

The key feature of GAD involves a pervasive sense of worry about various events or circumstances. For example, children with GAD frequently worry about their competence, as might manifest on school or athletic performances. These worries are associated with other symptoms, such as muscle tension or other somatic complaints, irritability, and trouble sleeping. Because children with SAD and SOPH also present with worry, clinicians face difficulties when attempting to determine if worries reflect aspects of these disorders or another problem. GAD is diagnosed only when worries cannot be accounted for by another diagnosis. Considerable research examines the relationship between GAD and major depressive disorder (MDD).

### (d) Specific phobia

The key feature of SPH involves fear of a specific stimulus or object. SPH can manifest to a range of objects, such as potentially dangerous animals or natural scenarios, and SPH can be categorized into one of five types, based on the content of the fear. Children rarely present for clinical care when they suffer from SPH in the absence of another anxiety disorder, despite the fact that SPH does present relatively commonly in pure forms in the community. This suggests that SPH typically is associated with relatively mild degrees of distress and impairment, unless SPH is associated with another anxiety disorder.

### (e) Panic disorder

The key feature of PD involves spontaneous panic attacks. The term 'panic attack' refers to crescendo paroxysms of severe anxiety that occur suddenly and are associated with somatic and cognitive sensations, such as rapid heart beat, shortness of breath, and a strong desire to flee. Panic attacks occur in many situations and with various clinical syndromes. The key feature of PD is that at least some of these attacks occur in the absence of any cue or trigger. As such, the patient cannot attribute the attack to fear of any specific circumstance. PD virtually never occurs prior to puberty, and the disorder is also very rare before adulthood.

## Assessment

The assessment for anxiety involves input from multiple sources. Clearly obtaining information directly from the patient is vital. Children with anxiety disorders may be reluctant to report the precise nature of their fears. As a result, adults may be unaware of vital symptoms. On the other hand, children also often show reluctance to acknowledge their anxiety, either because they are unaware of their degree of incapacitation or because they are highly embarrassed about their symptoms. In this instance, adults provide vital information concerning specific objects or situations that might be feared by children or adolescents.

Various forms of standardized assessment are available for paediatric anxiety.[2] This includes rating scales that can be directly completed by parents, teachers, or children, as well as scales that are completed by clinicians based on their interview of the child and parent. Moreover, standardized observational batteries typically are used for the assessment of temperament, in very young children, that relate to anxiety disorders in older children. Temperament also can be measured by parent or self-report.[3] In general, while high scores on various rating scales does provide some indication regarding the presence of an anxiety disorder, structured psychiatric interviews, completed by a trained clinician, represents the gold standard for arriving at a diagnosis.

## Prevalence and demographics

As a group, paediatric anxiety disorders probably represent the most common form of developmental psychopathology. It is difficult to provide precise data concerning their overall prevalence, as the rate of anxiety disorders is highly variable across studies, most likely due to variations in assessment. Rates of anxiety disorders are unusually sensitive to even subtle changes in assessments of impairment.[4] In general, overall lifetime rates of paediatric anxiety probably fall in the 10–20 per cent range.[5] Rates of individual disorders vary with age. Thus, SAD represents the most common condition, with prevalence typically in the 5 per cent range, before puberty, whereas GAD and SOPH become more prevalent during adolescence, again with rates in the 5 per cent range. Rates of SPH are highly variable, depending on the stringency of impairment criteria, with some estimates surpassing 20 per cent. As noted above, PD is very rare before late adolescence.

In terms of demography, anxiety disorders show a strong female predominance. This gender difference manifests for all of the conditions examined here, and, unlike data for MDD, it emerges before puberty. While the overall rate of anxiety disorders changes relatively little from childhood to adolescence, the nature of disorders does change. Thus, SAD is most common in young children, whereas SOPH is most common in adolescence. Data concerning associations with social class appear somewhat mixed. While some inconsistent reports note higher rates among individuals in the relatively lower social strata, the data appear most consistent for SPH, with weaker or absent associations in other conditions.[1] Consistent with weak relationships, recent work suggests that abrupt changes in family economics do not lead to changes in rates of anxiety disorders, despite strong associations with changing rates of other disorders.[6]

### Comorbidity

Data concerning comorbidity reveal distinct trends in the clinic relative to the community, most likely due to the effects of referral biases on data from the clinic. Thus, in the clinic, paediatric anxiety disorders have been linked to virtually every form of psychopathology. This includes mood disorders, behaviour disorders, attention deficit hyperactivity disorder, and substance use disorders. In the community, however, associations appear particularly strong with a more restricted group of conditions. The most common comorbidity represents associations with other anxiety disorders, with odds ratios typically appearing in the three-to-five range.[1] Associations between SOPH and GAD appear particularly strong in this work. Comorbidity with mood disorder, particularly MDD, is only slightly weaker than comorbidity among the anxiety disorders.[7] Other forms of psychopathology show far weaker associations.

### Clinical course

Paediatric anxiety disorders predict an increased risk for a range of adverse psychiatric outcomes in adults. This includes most prominently risk for adult anxiety disorders and MDD.[1,8] In general, children and adolescent with one or another anxiety disorder face a two- to five-fold increased risk for adult anxiety or MDD. These relationships reflect the fact that most adults with various forms of mood or anxiety disorder show the initial signs of their problem during childhood or adolescence, manifest as a paediatric anxiety disorder. However, the overall magnitude of these longitudinal relationships between paediatric anxiety and any form of adult psychopathology appears somewhat weaker than longitudinal relationships for other developmental psychopathologies, such as the behaviour disorders.[9]

Relatively few studies consider the long-term outcome of the specific paediatric anxiety disorders. In the few studies that do examine this issue, the overall weight of the evidence suggests that risk for poor outcome is similar among all paediatric anxiety disorders.[5] However, some inconsistent data do note specific associations among individual child and adult disorders. For example, some evidence documents a particularly strong association between paediatric GAD and adult MDD,[1] though studies following adolescents into their 30s suggest a comparable risk for MDD in adolescent SOPH.[8] Similarly, some studies note an association between childhood SAD and adult PD, but the overall weight of the evidence does not provide strong support for this link.[10] Finally, some inconsistent evidence also suggests that the outcome of paediatric SPH appears relatively good, as compared with other anxiety disorders.

## Pathophysiology

### Neuroscience and fear

Work on the pathophysiology of anxiety disorders benefits from a wealth of research examining brain regions involved in fear and anxiety among rodents and non-human primates.[11] Data also document strong cross-species parallels in the effects of threats and danger on behaviour, physiology, and information processing. This suggests that neural circuits implicated in fear and anxiety among rodents or non-human primates are likely involved in fear and anxiety among humans.

Basic science work delineates a distributed neural circuit engaged by various forms of dangerous or threatening stimuli. This includes stimuli recognized as dangerous through learning, as classically studied in the 'fear conditioning' paradigm, whereby a neutral conditioned stimulus is paired with an aversive unconditioned stimulus.[12] This also includes stimuli innately recognized as dangerous, even in the absence of prior training.[13] Finally, work in immature rodents and non-human primates demonstrates strong developmental influences on the neural circuitry associated with both learned and innate fears.[11] Specifically, in immature relative to mature organisms, both genetic and environmental manipulations show the capacity to exert more robust, long-standing effects on anxiety and fear-related behaviours as well as the underlying neural circuitry mediating these behaviours.

Figure 9.2.6.1 illustrates the core components of the underlying circuitry associated with fear and anxiety. The amygdala represents a hub in the fear circuit. As shown in Fig. 9.2.6.1, this collection of nuclei lies within the medial temporal lobe, where it receives input from various sensory cortices as well as brain-stem monoamine systems, and where it sends output to the hypothalamus and other structures that orchestrate the organism's response to danger. While some debate continues concerning the precise role played by the amygdala in fear, the structure has been implicated in both learned and innate fears as well as various positive-valence emotions. Some data suggest that the amygdala plays a vital role in regulating attention when organisms learn to associate neutral stimuli with salient events.

Fear and anxiety represent complex states that reflect influences from other brain regions beyond the amygdala. Figure 9.2.6.1 shows the location of two particularly important regions. Thus, the hippocampus also plays a role in fear and anxiety, with data most clearly implicating this brain region in the representation of spatial

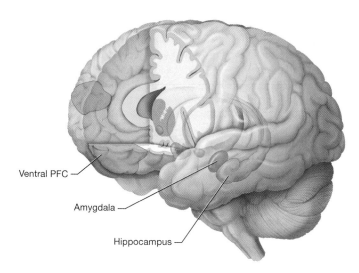

**Fig. 9.2.6.1** Displays key anatomical components of brain circuitry engaged when various organisms encounter threats or dangers. Functional aspects of this circuitry show strong cross-species conservation, and Figure 9.2.6.1 depicts the location in the human brain of three particularly important neural structures: the ventral prefrontal cortex (PFC), amygdala, and hippocampus.

contexts associated with threat. As shown in Fig. 9.2.6.1, the hippocampus lies posterior to the amygdala in the medial temporal lobe. Various components of the prefrontal cortex (PFC) also are involved in fear and anxiety. As shown in Fig. 9.2.6.1, particularly strong associations occur with ventral PFC, including both lateral and medial expanses. PFC is thought to play a regulatory role for fear and anxiety responses, serving to delineate the temporal context where fear and anxiety are either necessary or not appropriate, given the organism's goals.

### Familial aggregation and genetics

Most complex behaviours, including fear and anxiety, represent phenomena that result from influences of both genes and the environment. The associations of genes and the environment with anxiety can be examined directly with behavioural indicators of anxiety or psychiatric diagnosis. Alternatively, these associations can be examined with constructs beyond symptoms that show closer relationships to brain function. The term 'endophenotype' has been used to describe such underlying constructs linked to both disorders and their underlying risks.[14]

Family studies consistently demonstrate strong associations among various anxiety disorders in parents and anxiety disorders in their children. More than 10 studies show that children born to parents with PD, SOPH, or GAD face a two- to four-fold increased risk for anxiety disorders.[5] As with data from longitudinal studies, some non-specificity emerges in other family studies. Children born to parents with MDD even in the absence of anxiety face the same elevated risk for paediatric anxiety as children born to parents with anxiety disorders. These data are consistent with a wealth of data among adults documenting strong familial associations.[15]

These findings on familial aggregation might reflect the effects of either genes or the environment. Data from twin and adoption studies suggest that genes account for approximately 40 per cent of the risk for anxiety both among children and adults.[5,15] Much like for longitudinal and family aggregation studies, twin studies suggest pathophysiologic similarities in the genetics of anxiety and depression. In particular, GAD and MDD appear to share many of the same genes.[16] In terms of specific genes, the field has only begun to examine associations with specific paediatric anxiety disorders. While considerable enthusiasm pertains to research on serotonin-related genes, this enthusiasm emerges predominantly from studies in adults.[11]

The effects of genes on risk for paediatric anxiety are not thought to moderate overt symptomatic expressions. Rather, genes, either as main effects or through interactions with the environment, are hypothesized to produce disruptions in the underlying function of the neural circuit illustrated in Fig. 9.2.6.1. These disruptions are expected to produce perturbations in physiologic regulation and information processing functions, examples of endophenotypes for paediatric anxiety disorders. Work on endophenotypes in paediatric anxiety disorders generally focus on three related profiles.

First, considerable work examines variations in children's temperaments, as they relate to both parental histories of anxiety as well as children's risk for anxiety, manifest later in life. This work shows that children who react with fear and hesitation in novel social scenarios face a high risk for anxiety.[3] This temperamental classification is known as 'behavioural inhibition'. Some evidence suggests that these associations pertain particularly strongly to the association with later-life SOPH.

Second, other work examines associations with variations in physiologic or cognitive responses to various threats. While various forms of fear and anxiety produce robust changes in autonomic physiology, inconsistent data document strong associations between individual differences in anxiety among humans and the magnitude of these physiological responses. Particularly interest focuses on between-group differences in conditioned physiologic reactions, but findings in this area appear weak and inconsistent.[17] Some of the strongest findings emerge from research on the startle response. This defensive reflex shows strong cross-species similarities in the degree to which it can be modulated by the presence of a threat. In general, adult anxiety disorders are characterized by enhanced startle in some contexts, though data in paediatric anxiety disorders appear inconsistent. Moreover, children born to parents with either PD or MDD also show enhanced startle responses under some circumstances.[18,19] Other work focuses on biases in various cognitive processes, such as attention and memory, where associations with specific disorders generally appear stronger than for studies of physiology. Here some work suggests that perturbations in face processing predict both risk for anxiety and the presence specifically of paediatric SOPH.[20]

Finally, perturbations in respiration have been linked most convincingly to the diagnosis of PD.[21] Data among adults show these respiratory perturbations aggregate within families. Moreover, findings in children and adolescents show that respiratory perturbation is associated with SAD but not other paediatric anxiety disorders, such as SOPH. Given evidence of familial aggregation between parental PD and childhood SAD, these data suggest that respiratory perturbation may confer a familial risk for panic disorder. Nevertheless, data examining respiratory function in offspring of PD patients are not consistent with this possibility.[22]

### Stress

Work in animal models demonstrates strong relationships between exposure to various forms of physical or emotional stress and individual differences in anxiety or fear.[11] These associations appear particularly strong in juvenile organisms. For studies among children and adolescents, strong associations also emerge with various measures of stress including either stress that occurs within the family or in other social contexts.[23] Nevertheless, it remains unclear the degree to which these association reflect specific connections with anxiety, given that stress is associated with a range of other psychopathologies besides anxiety.[24] Moreover, considerable heterogeneity exists in terms of the relationship between stress and anxiety, given that some individuals exposed to extreme stress are resilient, whereas other individuals exposed to mild stress develop anxiety. At least some of these individual differences are though to reflect the influences of genes on underlying neural circuitry, such that the development of paediatric anxiety reflects influences of gene–environment interactions.[11]

### Brain imaging

Through studies of brain imaging, it is now possible to examine associations between paediatric anxiety disorders and perturbations in brain structure or function. Relatively few brain-imaging studies have examined paediatric anxiety disorders, and the few studies that do focus on neural structures depicted in Fig. 9.2.6.1.

Without question, the amygdala stands as the most frequently investigated brain structure in paediatric anxiety. Two studies examine amygdala morphometry in paediatric anxiety disorders, with one of these studies reporting reduced volume and the other reporting enlarged volume, both focusing mostly on children with GAD.[25,26] Such inconsistencies are consistent with mophometry studies in adults, where inconsistent evidence of amygdala enlargement or reduction emerges across a range of studies. Two other studies use functional magnetic resonance imaging (fMRI) to examine amygdala function in paediatric anxiety disorders.[27,28] Here, the findings are more consistent, much like in a larger series of studies in adults. Specifically, both studies reported enhanced amygdala activation in paediatric GAD, consistent with data in adult SOPH, MDD, as well as post-traumatic distress disorder or behavioural inhibition. Finally, imaging work focused on other structures documents abnormalities with less consistency. This includes structural and functional studies of the PFC and hippocampus.[5]

## Therapeutics

A range of approaches has been suggested as useful in the treatment of paediatric anxiety disorders. The current chapter restricts considerations to a review of modalities studied with the randomized controlled trial (RCT). Two modalities have been studied in sufficient detail to provide conclusions on efficacy: cognitive behavioural psychotherapy treatment (CBT) and selective serotonin reuptake inhibitors (SSRIs). The data for these two treatments are reviewed in most detail, whereas other treatments are mentioned only briefly.

CBT relies on the principles of extinction, whereby an individual with an anxiety disorder undergoes exposure to a feared object or situation while relying on cognitive techniques taught as part of the therapy. In general, CBT is easiest when a child presents with a relatively specific set of fears and worries that allow the therapist to work with the child to create a fear hierarchy. The child then gradually undergoes exposure to situations on this hierarchy that are increasingly anxiety provoking. More than 10 studies use an RCT design to examine the efficacy of CBT, and the overwhelming majority of these document strong efficacy.[5] Nevertheless, most of these studies compare CBT to a wait-list control condition, a condition that may actually be aversive. The few RCTs of CBT using more suitable control conditions generally find weaker advantages for CBT. These studies suggest that CBT is a viable treatment option for any of the anxiety disorders considered in this chapter.

Five RCTs examine the efficacy of one or another SSRI in paediatric anxiety disorders, all using placebo control.[5] As with the data for CBT, this work provides strong justification for using SSRIs, in that robust treatment effects emerge. Moreover, these studies rely on placebo, a more credible control than in the CBT studies relying on wait-list comparison. Thus, the strength of the evidence supporting efficacy is probably somewhat greater in SSRIs than it is for CBT. Nevertheless, serious concerns about the safety of SSRIs emerged in 2002, due to the suggestion that SSRIs were associated with an increased risk over placebo for suicidal thoughts or behaviour. This ultimately led the Food and Drug Administration to place a 'black box' warning on the use of SSRIs in children, a warning recently extended to adults aged 25 and younger. Given these concerns, CBT probably represents the most reasonable first-line treatment for paediatric anxiety disorders. Among children who either cannot complete a course of CBT or who fail to respond to CBT, SSRIs represent an eminently reasonable treatment.

A range of other treatments have been considered for paediatric anxiety disorders. These include both psychotherapies, such as dynamically oriented therapy, and medications, such as various non-SSRI antidepressants or benzodiazepines. Due to either the dearth of data on efficacy or concerns with safety, all of these treatments should be considered third-line options, after CBT and SSRIs.

## Conclusions

The current chapter reviews data for paediatric anxiety disorders in three sections. The longest section reviews clinical characteristics of these disorders. This section describes the clinical features, demography, and outcome of paediatric anxiety disorders, the most common class of mental syndrome afflicting children and adolescence. The first section is followed by a shorter section focused on pathophysiology. Here, data on neural circuits implicated in anxiety are reviewed most comprehensively. Finally, treatment is briefly reviewed in the third section. More detailed considerations of therapeutics for a range of paediatric psychiatric disorders can be found in section 9.5. This includes a discussion of both psychotherapies and medication.

## Further information

Costello, E.J., Egger, H.L., and Angold, A. (2005). The developmental epidemiology of anxiety disorders: phenomenology, prevalence, and comorbidity. *Child and Adolescent Psychiatric Clinics of North America*, **14**, 631–48, vii.

Kagan, J., Snidman, N., McManis, M., *et al.* (2001). Temperamental contributions to the affect family of anxiety. *The Psychiatric Clinics of North America*, **24**, 677–88.

Pine, D.S. (2007). Research review: a neuroscience framework for pediatric anxiety disorders. *Journal of Child Psychology and Psychiatry, and allied disciplines*, **48**, 631–48.

Pine, D.S. and Klein, R.G. (2008). Anxiety disorders. In *Rutter's Child and Adolescent Psychiatry* (5th edn) (eds. M. Rutter, D. Bishop, D.S. Pine, et al.). Blackwell Publishing, Oxford.

## References

1. Pine, D.S., Cohen, P., Gurley D., *et al.* (1998). The risk for early-adulthood anxiety and depressive disorders in adolescents with anxiety and depressive disorders. *Archives of General Psychiatry*, **55**(1), 56–64.

2. Brooks, S.J. and Kutcher, S. (2003). Diagnosis and measurement of anxiety disorder in adolescents: a review of commonly used instruments. *Journal of Child and Adolescent Psychopharmacology*, **13**(3), 351–400.

3. Perez-Edgar, K. and Fox, N.A. (2005). Temperament and anxiety disorders. *Child and Adolescent Psychiatric Clinics of North America*, **14**(4), 681–706, viii.

4. Shaffer, D., Gould, M.S., Fisher, P., *et al.* (1996). Psychiatric diagnosis in child and adolescent suicide. *Archives General of Psychiatry*, **53**(4), 339–48.

5. Pine, D.S. and Klein, R.G. (2008). Anxiety disorders. In *Rutter's child and adolescent psychiatry* (5th edn) (eds. M. Rutter, D. Bishop, D.S. Pine, *et al.*). Blackwell Publishing, Oxford.

6. Costello, E.J., Compton, S.N., *et al.* (2003). Relationships between poverty and psychopathology: a natural experiment. *The Journal of the American Medical Association*, **290**(15), 2023–9.

7. Angold, A., Costello, E.J., Erkanli A. (1999). Comorbidity. *Journal of Child Psychology and Psychiatry*, **40**(1), 57–87.

8. Beesdo, K., Bittner, A., Pine, D.S., *et al.* (2007). Incidence of social anxiety disorder and the consistent risk for secondary depression in the first three decades of life. *Archives of General Psychiatry*, **64**(8), 903–12.

9. Pine, D.S. (2002). Treating children and adolescents with selective serotonin reuptake inhibitors: how long is appropriate? *Journal of Child and Adolescent Psychopharmacology*, **12**(3), 189–203.

10. Aschenbrand, S.G., Kendall, P.C., Webb, A., *et al.* (2003). Is childhood separation anxiety disorder a predictor of adult panic disorder and agoraphobia? A seven-year longitudinal study. *Journal of the American Academy of Child and Adolescent Psychiatry*, **42**(12), 1478–85.

11. Gross, C. and Hen, R. (2004). The developmental origins of anxiety. *Nature Reviews. Neuroscience*, **5**(7), 545–52.

12. LeDoux, J.E. (2000). Emotion circuits in the brain. *Annual Review of Neuroscience*, **23**, 155–84.

13. Davis, M. (1998). Are different parts of the extended amygdala involved in fear versus anxiety? *Biological Psychiatry*, **44**(12), 1239–47.

14. Gottesman, I.I. and Gould, T.D. (2003). The endophenotype concept in psychiatry: etymology and strategic intentions. *The American Journal of Psychiatry*, **160**(4), 636–45.

15. Hettema, J.M., Neale, M.C., Kendall K.S., *et al.* (2001). A review and meta-analysis of the genetic epidemiology of anxiety disorders. *The American Journal of Psychiatry*, **158**(10), 1568–78.

16. Silberg, J.L., Rutter, M., Eaves L. (2001). Genetic and environmental influences on the temporal association between earlier anxiety and later depression in girls. *Biological Psychiatry*, **49**(12), 1040–9.

17. Lissek, S., Powers, A.S., McClure, E.B., *et al.* (2005). Classical fear conditioning in the anxiety disorders: a meta-analysis. *Behaviour Research and Therapy*, **43**, 1391–424.

18. Merikangas, K.R., Avenevoli, S., Dierker L., (1999). Vulnerability factors among children at risk for anxiety disorders. *Biological Psychiatry*, **46**(11), 1523–35.

19. Grillon, C., Warner, V., Hille J., *et al.* (2005). Families at high and low risk for depression: a three-generation startle study. *Biological Psychiatry*, **57**(9), 953–60.

20. Pine, D.S., Klein, R.G., Roberson-Nay, R., *et al.* (2005a). Face emotion processing and risk for panic disorder in youth. *Journal of the American Academy of Child and Adolescent Psychiatry*, **44**, 664–72.

21. Klein, D.F. (1993). False suffocation alarms, spontaneous panics, and related conditions. An integrative hypothesis. *Archives of General Psychiatry*, **50**(4), 306–17.

22. Pine, D.S., Klein, R.G., Roberson-Nay, R., *et al.* (2005b). Response to 5% carbon dioxide in children and adolescents: relationship to panic disorder in parents and anxiety disorders in subjects. *Archives of General Psychiatry*, **62**(1), 73–80.

23. Pine, D.S. and Cohen, J.A. (2002). Trauma in children and adolescents: risk and treatment of psychiatric sequelae. *Biological Psychiatry*, **51**(7), 519–31.

24. Wood, J.J., McLeod, B.D., Sigman, M., *et al.* (2003). Parenting and childhood anxiety: theory, empirical findings, and future directions. *Journal of Child Psychology and Psychiatry, and allied disciplines*, **44**, 134–51.

25. De Bellis, M.D., Casey, B.J., Dahl R.E., *et al.* (2000). A pilot study of amygdala volumes in pediatric generalized anxiety disorder. *Biological Psychiatry*, **48**(1), 51–7.

26. Millham, M.P., Nugent, A.C., Drevets, W.C., *et al.* (2005). Selective reduction in amygdala volume in pediatric generalized anxiety disorder: a voxel-based morphometry investigation. *Biological Psychiatry*, **57**, 961–6.

27. Thomas, K.M., Drevets, W.C., Dahl, R.E., *et al.* (2001). Amygdala response to fearful faces in anxious and depressed children. *Archives of General Psychiatry*, **58**(11), 1057–63.

28. McClure, E.B., Monk, C.S., Nelson E.E., *et al.* (2007). Abnormal attention modulation of fear circuit function in pediatric generalized anxiety disorder. *Archives of General Psychiatry*, **64**(1), 97–106.

## 9.2.7 Paediatric mood disorders

David Brent and Boris Birmaher

In this chapter, we describe the nosology and epidemiology of paediatric unipolar and bipolar disorders, risk factors and predictors of course, and the evidence base for pharmacological and psychosocial treatments. We conclude this chapter by suggesting areas for future research.

### Clinical picture

Mood disorders may be classified on three dimensions: (a) severity; (b) course; and (c) presence or absence of mania/hypomania.[1] Depressed children and adolescents may not describe their mood as sad, but instead as, 'grouchy', 'bored', 'having no fun', or 'empty'.[2] The most severe depressive condition is major depression, which requires at least 2 weeks of a depressed, sad, bored, or anhedonic mood for most of the time, and four additional depressive symptoms involving impairment in concentration, suicidal thoughts, difficulty making decisions, impaired sleep and appetite, guilt, and a decreased sense of self-worth (Box 9.2.7.1). Patients with depressive symptoms, but whose clinical picture is below the threshold for major depression (so-called minor depression or depression NOS) can still show significant impairment.[3] Dysthymic disorder is more chronic and intermittent than major depression, with periods of depression interspersed with normal mood, but with duration of at least 1 year (Box 9.2.7.2). Adjustment disorder with depressed

---

**Box 9.2.7.1** Criteria for the diagnosis of a major depressive episode

A. Five (or more) of the following symptoms have been present during the same 2-week period and represent a change from previous functioning; at least one of the symptoms is either (1) depressed mood or (2) loss of interest or pleasure.

*Note*: Do not include symptoms that are clearly due to a general medical condition, or mood-incongruent delusions or hallucinations.

1 Depressed mood most of the day, nearly every day, as indicated by either subjective report (e.g. feels sad or empty) or observation made by others (e.g. appears tearful). *Note*: In children and adolescents, can be irritable mood.

2 Markedly diminished interest or pleasure in all, or almost all, activities most of the day, nearly every day (as indicated by either subjective account or observation made by others).

3 Significant weight loss when not dieting or weight gain (e.g. a change of more than 5 per cent of body weight in a month), or decrease or increase in appetite nearly every day. *Note*: In children, consider failure to make expected weight gains.

4 Insomnia or hypersomnia nearly every day.

5 Psychomotor agitation or retardation nearly every day (observable by others, not merely subjective feelings of restlessness or being slowed down).

6 Fatigue or loss of energy nearly every day.

7 Feelings of worthlessness or excessive or inappropriate guilt (which may be delusional nearly every day (not merely self-reproach or guilt about being sick).

8 Diminished ability to think or concentrate, or indecisiveness, nearly every day (either by subjective account or as observed by others).

9 Recurrent thoughts of death (not just fear of dying), recurrent suicidal ideation without a specific plan, or a suicide attempt or a specific plan for committing suicide.

B. The symptoms do not meet criteria for a Mixed Episode (see p. 365).[1]

C. The symptoms cause clinically significant distress or impairment in social, occupational, or other important areas of functioning.

D. The symptoms are not due to the direct physiological effects of a substance (e.g. a drug of abuse, a medication (or a general medical condition (e.g. hypothyroidism).

E. The symptoms are not better accounted for by bereavement, i.e. after the loss of a loved one, the symptoms persist for longer than 2 months or are characterized by marked functional impairment morbid preoccupation with worthlessness, suicidal ideation, psychotic symptoms, or psychomotor retardation.

(Modified from APA (2000), *Diagnostic and statistical manual of mental disorders* (4th edn), American Psychiatric Association Press, Washington, DC.)

---

**Box 9.2.7.2** Criteria for the diagnosis of dysthymic disorder

A. Depressed mood for most of the day, for more days than not, as indicated either by subjective account or observation by others, for at least 2 years. *Note*: In children and adolescents, mood can be irritable and duration must be at least 1 year.

B. Presence, while depressed of two (or more) of the following:

1 poor appetite or overeating

2 insomnia or hypersomnia

3 low energy or fatigue

4 low self-esteem

5 poor concentration or difficulty making decisions

6 feelings of hopelessness

C. During the 2-year period (1 year for children or adolescents) of the disturbance, the person has never been without the symptoms in Criteria A and B for more than 2 months at a time.

D. No Major Depressive Episode (see p. 356)[1] has been present during the first 2 years of the disturbance (1 year for children and adolescents); that is the disturbance is not better accounted for by chronic Major Depressive Disorder, or Major Depressive Disorder, In Partial Remission. *Note*: There may have been a previous Major Depressive Episode provided there was a full remission (no significant signs or symptoms for 2 months) before development of the dysthymic disorder. In addition, after the initial 2 years (1 year in children or adolescents) of dysthymic disorder, there may be superimposed episodes of Major Depressive Disorder, in which case both diagnoses may be given when the criteria are met for a Major Depressive Episode.

E. There has never been a Manic Episode (see p. 362),[1] a Mixed Episode (see p. 365),[1] or a Hypomanic Episode (see p. 368),[1] and criteria have never been met for Cyclothymic Disorder.

F. The disturbance does not occur exclusively during the course of a chronic Psychotic Disorder, such as Schizophrenia or Delusional Disorder.

G. The symptoms are not due to the direct physiological effects of a substance (e.g. a drug of abuse, a medication) or a general medical condition (e.g. hypothyroidism).

H. The symptoms cause clinically significant distress or impairment in social, occupational, or other important areas of functioning.

(Modified from APA (2000), *Diagnostic and statistical manual of mental disorders* (4th edn), American Psychiatric Association Press, Washington, DC.)

---

mood is a milder and self-limited disturbance of mood that follows a significant life stressor (Box 9.2.7.3).

The presence of clinically significant manic or hypomanic symptomatology suggests bipolar spectrum disorder. The symptomatology of mania can be thought of as the mirror image of depression, with mood characterized by elation or grandiosity. Mania is associated

**Box 9.2.7.3** Criteria for the diagnosis of adjustment disorder with depressed mood

A. The development of emotional or behavioural symptoms in response to an identifiable stressor(s) occurring within 3 months of the onset of the stressor(s).

B. These symptoms or behaviours are clinically significant as evidenced by either of the following:

1 marked distress that is in excess of what would be expected from exposure to the stressor

2 significant impairment in social or occupational (academic) functioning

C. The stress-related disturbance does not meet the criteria for another specific Axis I disorder and is not merely an exacerbation of a pre-existing Axis I or Axis II disorder.

D. The symptoms do not represent bereavement.

E. Once the stressor (or its consequences) has terminated, the symptoms do not persist for more than an additional 6 months.

(Modified from APA (2000), *Diagnostic and statistical manual of mental disorders* (4th edn), American Psychiatric Association Press, Washington, DC.)

with clear impairment, whereas hypomania, while associated with a change in functioning, does not always result in impairment per se. Bipolar individuals, especially in the paediatric age group, frequently do not show the classic distinct alternating manic and depressive periods found in adult bipolar patients. Instead they may either experience depression and manic symptoms simultaneously, so-called mixed episodes, or alternations of mania and depression that may occur within a month, a week, or even a day, e.g. rapid cycling.[4] Common symptoms of paediatric bipolar disorder are pressure of speech, increased energy, and decreased need for sleep. Risk-taking behaviour showing poor judgement (e.g. gambling, hypersexuality, excessive spending) and joking and excessive humour are very specific for paediatric bipolar disorder, but less common in paediatric samples. While irritability is a common symptom of paediatric bipolar disorder, it is very non-specific and is commonly found in many other conditions, such as depression, oppositional defiant disorder, and attention deficit disorder. The DSM-IV requires a relatively long duration of mania (7 days) and hypomania (4 days) in order to meet criteria. Many paediatric patients may show the same symptom pattern but have very rapid cycling and therefore, do not meet these criteria. If altered function is present, such patients should receive a diagnosis of Bipolar Disorder NOS. Bipolar NOS is a common diagnosis for children with manic symptoms because very often, paediatric bipolar illness does not fulfil the duration criteria for mania, in part due to the frequency of rapid cycling conform to the classic adult patterns of distinct patterns of mania and depression.[4] However, in children and adolescents, Bipolar disorder NOS does not appear to be different from Bipolar I or II with regard to impairment, rate of comorbid disorders, response to treatment, or family history of bipolar disorder, and many patients with BP-NOS upon longitudinal follow-up go on to develop BP-I or BP-II disorders.[4]

Individuals who have had a history of full mania plus major depression receive a diagnosis of Bipolar I disorder, those with hypomania plus major depression receive a diagnosis of Bipolar II disorder, and those with hypomania and dysthymia receive a diagnosis of cyclothymic disorder (see Boxes 9.2.7.4 and 9.2.7.5).

While some in the field continue to raise questions about the validity of the diagnosis of paediatric bipolar disorder, the convergent evidence from longitudinal and high-risk studies is that there it is the essentially an earlier manifestation of the same illness as is found in adults, is highly familial, and shows a chronic and consistent course.[4,5]

## Differential diagnosis

### Attention deficit hyperactive disorder (ADHD) and disruptive disorders

Patients with ADHD, oppositional disorder, and conduct disorder are often irritable, show a low frustration tolerance, and can become demoralized due to school failure and peer rejection. However, in the absence of true depression, their mood will be restored as soon as the source of their frustration has been remedied. While both ADHD and depression are associated with poor concentration, the age of onset of ADHD is usually earlier than in mood disorders. Patients with ADHD have other accompanying difficulties such as hyperactivity and impulsivity that are part of the depressive picture. Conversely, depressed patients will show changes in sleep, energy level, appetite, mood, and self-worth that are not part of the picture of ADHD. The symptoms of ADHD, such as poor concentration, hyperactivity, and impulsivity can also be seen in bipolar disorder but patients with ADHD rarely have concomitant hypersexuality, grandiosity, and decreased need for sleep.[4,5] However, hypersexuality may also be seen in victims of sexual abuse, but in contrast with the hypersexuality of bipolar disorder, is not accompanied by clinically significant grandiosity, pressure of speech, increased energy, and diminished need for sleep. Often, the diagnostic difficulty is not simply distinguishing between disruptive and mood disorders, but in the proper attribution of shared symptoms in patients with comorbidity, as is very often the case. When patients have both mood disorder and ADHD, usually the ADHD antedates the mood disorder. A diagnosis of a mood disorder can only be made when the shared symptoms, such as impaired concentration become worse in association with depressed or manic mood.

### Anxiety disorders

Patients with anxiety disorder may also become quite dysphoric, but when the anxiogenic situation is removed, normal mood frequently ensues. Anxiety is a frequent antecedent of paediatric depression and bipolar disorder.[5,6] Symptoms that are shared between disorders, such as difficulty with sleep, or impaired concentration, are attributed to the mood disorder only if they become worse with the onset of a depressed or manic mood state. Panic disorder is often comorbid with paediatric bipolar disorder.[5] However, it is important to distinguish between the symptoms of panic disorder, that are prominently somatic and associated with thoughts and feelings of dread, and rapid cycling and a mixed state, which are marked with mood instability and the presence of simultaneous, or rapidly alternating depressive and manic symptoms.

---

**Box 9.2.7.4** Criteria for the diagnosis of bipolar disorder

A. Currently (or most recently) in a Manic Episode (see p. 362).[1]

B. There has previously been at least one Major Depressive Episode (see p. 356),[1] Manic Episode (see p. 362),[1] or Mixed Episode (see p. 365).[1]

C. The mood episodes in Criteria A and B are not better accounted for by Schizoaffective Disorder and are not superimposed on Schizophrenia, Schizophreniform Disorder, Delusional Disorder, or Psychotic Disorder Not Otherwise Specified.

Past or current history of a Manic Episode is characterized by:

A. A distinct period of abnormally and persistently elevated, expansive, or irritable mood, lasting at least 1 week (or any duration if hospitalization is necessary).

B. During the period of mood disturbance, three (or more of the following symptoms have persisted (four if the mood is only irritable) and have been present to a significant degree:

1 inflated self-esteem or grandiosity

2 decreased need for sleep (e.g. feels rested after only 3 h of sleep)

3 more talkative than usual or pressure to keep talking

4 flight of ideas or subjective experience that thoughts are racing

5 distractibility (i.e. attention to easily drawn to unimportant or irrelevant external stimuli)

6 increase in goal-directed activity (either socially, at work or school, or sexually) or psychomotor agitation

7 excessive involvement in pleasurable activities that have a high potential for painful consequences (e.g. engaging in unrestrained buying sprees, sexual indiscretions, or foolish business investments)

C. The symptoms do not meet criteria for a Mixed Episode (see p. 365).[1]

D. The mood disturbance is sufficiently severe to cause marked impairment in occupational functioning or in usual social activities or relationships with others, or to necessitate hospitalization to prevent harm to self or others, or there are psychotic features.

E. The symptoms are not due to the direct physiological effects of a substance (e.g. a drug of abuse, a medication, or other treatment) or a general medical condition (e.g. hyperthyroidism).

*Note:* Manic-like episodes that are clearly caused by somatic antidepressant treatment (e.g. medication, electroconvulsive therapy, light therapy, should not count toward a diagnosis of Bipolar I disorder.

(Modified from APA (2000), *Diagnostic and statistical manual of mental disorders* (4th edn), American Psychiatric Association Press, Washington, DC.)

---

**Box 9.2.7.5** Criteria for the diagnosis of cyclothymic disorder

A. For at least 2 years, the presence of numerous periods with hypomanic symptoms (see p. 368)[1] and numerous periods with depressive symptoms that do not meet criteria for a Major Depressive Episode. *Note*: In children and adolescents, the duration must be at least 1 year.

B. During the above 2-year period (1 year in children and adolescents), the person has not been without the symptoms in Criterion A for more than 2 months at a time.

C. No Major Depressive Episode (p. 356),[1] Manic Episode (p. 362),[1] or Mixed Episode (see p. 365)[1] has been present during the first 2 years of the disturbance.

*Note*: After the initial 2 years (1 year in children and adolescents) of Cyclothymic Disorder, there may be superimposed Manic or Mixed Episodes (in which case both Bipolar I disorder and Cyclothymic Disorder may be diagnosed) or Major Depressive Episodes (in which case both Bipolar II disorder and Cyclothymic Disorder may be diagnosed).

D. The symptoms in Criterion A are not better accounted for by Schizoaffective Disorder and are not superimposed on Schizophrenia, Schizophreniform Disorder, Delusional Disorder, or Psychotic Disorder Not Otherwise Specified.

E. The symptoms are not due to the direct physiological effects of a substance (e.g. a drug of abuse, a medication) or a general medical condition (e.g. hyperthyroidism).

F. The symptoms cause clinically significant distress or impairment in social, occupational, or other important areas of functioning.

(Modified from APA (2000), *Diagnostic and statistical manual of mental disorders* (4th edn), American Psychiatric Association Press, Washington, DC.)

---

### Substance abuse

The use of marijuana, alcohol, or opiates can mimic the symptoms of depression, such as difficulty with concentration, motivation, low energy, and dysphoria. Amphetamine and cocaine abuse can mimic mania. Depressed and bipolar patients are at greatly increased risk of abusing substances, so that the presence of substance abuse does not rule out a mood disorder or vice versa, but in fact, should raise the suspicion of possible comorbidity.

### Eating disorder

Patients with a restricting eating disorder who are nutritionally compromised may show symptoms that overlap with depression, including decreased appetite, low energy, and sad mood. Often the sadness is found in patients with anorexia who are being forced to gain or maintain weight against their will. A diagnosis of depression, unless there is a clear historical precedent that antedates the eating disorder, should only be made when the nutritional status of the patient has been normalized. Bulimic disordered patients often have difficulties with impulse control that need to be differentiated from bipolar disorder.

## Borderline personality disorder

Although there is evidence that borderline personality disorder can be reliably diagnosed in adolescents,[7] diagnostic convention requires that this diagnosis only be applied for adults. Still, there is general agreement that many adolescents, particularly those with mood disorders, have 'borderline features', such as mood lability, impulsivity, suicidal thoughts and behaviour, chaotic interpersonal relationships, and risky behaviour that has a high likelihood of resulting in personal harm. Others have argued that borderline personality disorder is really a form of bipolar spectrum disorder, although family studies have not confirmed this.[5] Instead, the high degree of overlap between personality disorder and bipolar disorder suggests that care be taken in not attributing symptoms that more appropriately are associated with a lifelong personality style to bipolar disorder. Conversely, in the presence of a clear and unremitting paediatric mood disorder, personality disorder should not be diagnosed.

## Psychosis

Although rare in childhood, incipient schizophrenia can present with sad and detached mood, sleep disturbance, and social withdrawal. Psychotic symptoms that evolve in schizophrenia are more likely to be mood-incongruent. In contrast, psychosis in depression and bipolar disorder is more often, but not always, mood-congruent.[2,5] This is a diagnosis that often can only be made upon careful longitudinal follow-up. Since psychosis is often seen in youth with mood disorders, and schizophrenia is rare at this age group, any child or adolescents with psychosis needs to be carefully assessed for the presence of a mood disorder, particularly bipolar illness.

## Comorbidity

Comorbidity is the rule, rather than the exception.[8] Anxiety disorder frequently antedates paediatric depression and bipolar disorder, with common precursors being social phobia and panic disorder, respectively. ADHD is frequently comorbid with both conditions. Substance abuse is often a complication of mood disorder, although this condition in turn lengthens episodes and increases the risk for recurrence.

## Medical comorbidity

Medications used to treat epilepsy, inflammatory bowel disease, and rheumatic and allergic disease can have profound effects on mood. Corticosteroids can induce depression or mania. Phenobarbital is associated with depression, as is use of interferon.[9] Moreover, systemic aspects of the diseases themselves may increase the risk for depression, in epilepsy, asthma, diabetes, and thyroid illness. Oral contraceptives can also result in mood changes.

## Descriptive epidemiology

The point prevalence of major depression in around 1–2 per cent in prepubertal samples, and between 3–8 per cent in adolescent samples.[10] The prevalence of bipolar disorder is around 1 per cent in paediatric populations, although the rate of 'soft' bipolar disorder, which has some, but not all of the core features of bipolar disorder, has been reported to be as high as 5 per cent in some adolescent samples.[11] The male to female ratio is around 1:1 for prepubertal depression, but increases to around 1:3 for depression after puberty. In contrast, the males and females have similar risk for bipolar disorder, regardless of pubertal status. The increased rate of depression after puberty is accounted for almost entirely by the increased risk in females, and may be related to changes in estradiol and testosterone associated with puberty.[12] Prepubertal major depression is an admixture of two subtypes: one is highly familial, with a high risk for recurrence and for eventual paediatric mania, and the second with comorbid with disruptive disorders, a low risk for depressive recurrence, an association with parental criminality, substance abuse, and family discord, and a course more similar to conduct disorder than to mood disorder.[13] A clear clinical syndrome of depression has been reported in children as young as aged 3, particularly in those young children with a family history of mood disorders.[14]

## Course

Paediatric mood disorders tend to be both chronic and recurrent. While prepubertal depression comorbid with conduct disorder is likely not to be recurrent, studies of child-onset depression with a family history of depression show high rates of recurrence, with risks of recurrence of 40 per cent in 2 years, and over 70 per cent within 5 years.[2] The average length of a depressive episode is around 4–6 months in community samples, and 6–8 months in clinical samples.[15] The duration of dysthymic disorder is much longer, on average, around 5 years, according to one careful longitudinal study.[2] In patients with comorbid dysthymic disorder and depression, so-called double depression, the risk for prolonged episodes and recurrence are both very high.[2] Longer episodes are also predicted by comorbidity with substance abuse, conduct disorder, or anxiety disorder, family conflict, and parental depression.[10,16]

Paediatric bipolar disorder does not often present with 'classic' periods of alternating depression and mania. Instead, such patients frequently present with either a mixed state, e.g. simultaneous occurrence of depression and mania, or rapid cycling, with brief and alternating periods of depression and mania.[4] In comparing the course of paediatric and adult bipolar patients, paediatric bipolar patients have many more episodes per year, and spend less time in remission.[4] Consistent with these longitudinal observations are findings from adult pedigrees that age of onset in bipolar disorder appears to be familial, and that earlier age of onset is associated with higher rates of drug abuse, alcohol abuse, rapid cycling, and suicide attempts.[17] Much of the impairment in paediatric bipolar disorder is associated with depressive symptoms that often never completely remit. As noted above, the adult criteria requiring 1 week and 4 days for mania and hypomania, respectively, may be overly stringent, insofar as a fairly high proportion (25 per cent) of patients below those criteria, so-called bipolar NOS, go on in longitudinal follow-up to develop clear Bipolar I or II disorder and 20 per cent of those with BP-II go on to develop BP-I within 2 years of follow-up.[4] A longer period to recovery is predicted by longer duration of mood disorder, rapid cycling or mixed episode, psychosis, and lower SES.[4]

Children and adolescents who present with a unipolar depressive disorder are at increased risk for developing a bipolar disorder, both in comparison to children without a mood disorder, and to individuals whose mood disorder has its onset in adulthood. Young depressed patients with a family history of bipolar disorder, who present with psychotic symptoms, and/or pharmacologically induce mania or hypomania are at increased risk for developing paediatric bipolar disorder.[5,18] According to one pharmacoepidemiological study, the younger the depressed patient, the higher the risk for pharmacologically induced mania, although there was no standardized, direct assessment of manic behaviour.[19] Additionally, one study suggests that paediatric bipolar patients with comorbid ADHD tolerate amphetamine as well as non-bipolar children with ADHD.[20]

## Sequelae

The most dreaded consequent of paediatric mood disorders is suicide. A unipolar depression conveys a 10–60-fold increased risk of suicide; nearly 80 per cent of adolescent suicide attempters have some form of a mood disorder.[21] Suicide attempts may be even more frequent in paediatric bipolar disorder, with almost one-third of clinical samples showing a lifetime history of a suicide attempt. Studies in adults and adolescents that have assessed for bipolar disorder find that as many as 10–20 per cent of all suicides have some form of bipolar spectrum disorder.[21] Correlates of suicidal behaviour in both unipolar and bipolar disorder include earlier age of onset, history of abuse, comorbid disruptive and substance abuse disorders, hopelessness, mood lability, and chronic and unremitting course.[21]

Other sequelae of untreated depression include educational and occupational under-attainment, interpersonal difficulties, obesity, cardiovascular disease, and alcohol and substance abuse. The effect of depression on body mass index (BMI) appears to be independent of treatment effects.[22]

## Aetiology

Both unipolar and bipolar disorders have a strong genetic component. The child of a unipolar depressed parent is at around 2–4 times the risk of the population to develop a depressive disorder; this is even higher in children of parents with earlier onset (<age 20) and recurrent depression.[23] Twin studies indicate that around 50 per cent of the variance in familial transmission of depressive symptoms is explained by heritable factors, and that the liability of depression and to anxiety may be co-transmitted.[6] There is some evidence that adolescent onset depression is more highly heritable than prepubertal depression.[24]

Bipolar disorder has an even stronger genetic component, with a bipolar parent conveying at least an 8-fold increased risk of bipolar spectrum disorder in children; twin studies suggest that heritable factors account for 70–80 per cent of the variance in familial transmission.[23] High-risk studies of both unipolar depression and bipolar disorder show the transmission of a wider phenotype, with increased rates of anxiety disorder being most prominent in both the offspring of depressed and bipolar parents.[5,25]

Genetic linkage studies are beginning to converge on specific regions associated with depression and anxiety, with other regions implicated in bipolar disorder.[23] Linkage studies for early onset, recurrent depression suggest that there may be sex-specific linkage sites.[23]

The serotonin transporter promoter gene has a 44 bp insertion/deletion, with the latter resulting in less vigorous transcription. Several studies have now shown an interaction between stressful life events and the less functional form of the transporter gene with regard to an increased risk for depression in adolescents and young adults.[26] brain-derived neurotrophic factor (BDNF) is a gene that appears to protect the hippocampus system from the neurotoxic effects of stress. A three-way interaction between maltreatment, the less functional 5HTTLPR allele, and the met allele of the BDNF gene has been found with regard to risk for depression in children and adolescents.[27] An association between the val66 form of BDNF and early onset depression has been reported.[28]

Genetic linkage studies have also identified regions of interest for bipolar disorder, although paediatric bipolar disorder per se has not been studied. In aggregate, linkage studies converge on chromosomal regions 6q and 8q.[23,29] Certain phenotypes of bipolar disorder have been reported, such as 'lithium responsiveness', 'alcoholism/suicidal behaviour', and 'psychosis', with distinct areas of familial aggregation and linkage.[17] Geller et al.[30] has reported in an association study of paediatric bipolar families that val66 form of BDNF is associated with the disease.

Structural changes in depression have been reported, with the most widely replicated result being changes in the anterior cingulated, an area associated with emotion regulation, in both bipolar and unipolar familial depression.[31]

Paediatric bipolar subjects, compared to healthy controls, show decreased grey matter in the dorsolateral prefrontal cortex (DLPFC), cingulate cortex, and amygdale.[32] Diffusion tensor imaging and magnetic resonance spectroscopy both point to alterations in axonal development and organization in the superior frontal (decreased white matter) and DLPFC regions (decreased levels of n-acetyl aspartate), respectively.[33,34]

# Neurocognitive factors and emotion regulation

## Depression

Depressed children and adolescents, relative to normal controls, show greater attention to, and distraction by sad stimuli, whereas normal controls are more likely to be distracted by happy stimuli.[35] Depressed adolescents are more vulnerable to the effects of rumination and sad mood induction[35] Depressed children and adolescents may show less activation of reward-related circuitry when participating in a reward paradigm.[36] These findings are consistent with earlier research showing that tendency to pessimism and rumination were risk factors for the onset of depressive symptoms, especially when confronted with stressful life events.[35] Functional neuroimaging studies find alterations in amygdala activation to threat and other cognitive tasks, although the direction is not consistent across studies.[37,38]

There is evidence that these tendencies may be present prior to the development of a mood disorder. The young children of mothers with a history of childhood onset depression (COD) show greater evidence of physiological distress (e.g. poor heart rate recovery after disappointment, resort to more passive waiting and less active distraction than normal controls, and show less efficient cognitive processing when confronted with an affectively laden cognitive task.[39,40] Positive reward anticipation, however, moderated the relationship between parent early onset depression and child internalizing symptoms.[41]

The extent to which negative affective bias, and difficulty with active coping is intrinsic versus learned is still unclear. Mothers with early onset depression are less responsive to their children's expression of distress, tend to endorse and promote fewer emotion regulation strategies for their children, whereas maternal accuracy of recognition of their child's emotional state was protective against child psychopathology.[42–44] Taken together, these findings support a role in helping parents teach their children emotion regulation strategies such as distraction, emphasis on positive reward, and active coping as a means of preventing or treating depression.[45]

## Bipolar disorder

There is growing consensus that paediatric bipolar disorder is associated with difficulty with attention, verbal and visuospacial memory, executive function, set-shifting, and recognition of facial expressions.[32] In some studies, these findings are present regardless of current mood state or medication[46] and some of these findings are present in the unaffected, high-risk offspring of adults with bipolar disorder.[47] Bias towards threat, and less activation of areas involved in emotion regulation in the face of frustration have also been reported.[32] Many of these findings are also reported in unipolar depression, and therefore, a direct comparison of these two conditions is needed.

Functional neuroimaging data are consistent with these findings, with greater activation of reward-related circuitry (e.g. caudate and thalamus) and greater activation of inhibitory areas (e.g. DLPFC, anterior cingulated) when performing working memory tasks and viewing negatively valenced pictures compared to healthy controls.[32]

## Neuroendocrine/sleep

Neuroendocrine studies suggest that alterations in serotonergic and noradrenergic neurotransmission are associated with early onset unipolar depression.[48] There are no clear findings with regard to cortisol regulation and depression, although hypersecretion of cortisol close to the time of sleep has been reported to be related to adolescent depression.[49] While subjective sleep complaints are common in child and adolescent depression, polysomnographic studies have not consistently shown the decreased REM latency associated with depression that has been reported in adults.[50]

## Environmental risk factors

Environmental factors can also influence the onset and expression of paediatric mood disorders, often interacting with a genetic diathesis. Early abuse and neglect is a profound risk factor for depression, especially in interaction with a positive family history for mood disorder and certain genetic polymorphisms.[26,27,51] Family discord, substance abuse, and criminality are associated with depression in children from families at low familial risk for depression.[52] Maternal-child conflict shows a birectional relationship over time with regard to both parental and child mood disorder.[53] A history of abuse is associated with an earlier age of onset and more prolonged and unremitting course in bipolar disorder.[54] Loss of a parent, close friend, or sibling is associated with an increased risk of depression in those children and adolescents with a pre-existing depressive diathesis.[55] Conversely, a positive connection to family, school, and a pro-social peer group, can, in cross sectional studies, protect against depression and other health risk behaviours.[56]

## Assessment and monitoring

The properties of different assessment tools of mood disorder were recently reviewed.[57,58] The most common interview-based assessment for the severity of depression is the Children's Depression Rating Scale, Revised (CDRS-R), a 17-item rating scale. Commonly used self-rating measures are the Children's Depression Inventory for children and early adolescents, the Beck Depression Inventory (for adolescents and adults), the Reynolds Adolescent Depression Scale, the Center for Epidemiological Studies, Depression Scale (CES-D), and the Mood and Feelings Questionnaire (MFQ). The CDI shows treatment sensitivity, but does not distinguish well between anxiety and depression, and the CES-D does not have an item about suicidal ideation. The main advantage of the MFQ is that it has a short form for screening, has been validated in both community and clinical sites, has a parent form (so does the CDI), and can be used for both children and adolescents.

Two interview-based methods for monitoring the level of mania are the Young Mania Rating Scale and the Mania Rating Scale from the K-SADS.[4] The advantage of the latter is that it can be taken from one of the most commonly used diagnostic interviews for children and adolescents. A self-report for mania also shows promise, but has not yet been used in clinical trials.[5]

## Treatment and prevention

### Depression

Practice guidelines recommend that the initial treatment for mild-to-moderate depression be support, education, and one of two forms of psychotherapy (cognitive behaviour therapy [CBT] or interpersonal therapy [IPT]). For patients who eschew psychotherapy, or who live in a region where specific indicated forms of psychotherapy are not available, antidepressant medication is an appropriate approach. Guidelines agree that for more severe depression, combination of antidepressant medication and psychotherapy are ideal, although the data are mixed on this point (reviewed below).[59,60]

Because depression is a chronic and recurrent illness, a long-term approach should be taken to the management of child and adolescent depression. Therefore, after symptomatic relief, treatment should be continued for at least 6–12 months, since there is evidence that without psychotherapy booster sessions or continued medication treatment, there is a substantially increased risk of relapse or recurrence.[59]

There is strong and convergent evidence for the efficacy of CBT for adolescent depression in clinical samples, and for child depression in symptomatic volunteers,[59,61] with a relatively modest effect size ($d = 0.34$) relative to a waitlist condition or a comparison treatment. While some studies in clinical samples showed superiority of CBT to credible alternative treatments, the largest and most comprehensive study of the treatment of adolescent depression found that CBT was no better than placebo with regard to acute clinical response (43 per cent versus 35 per cent).[62] In that study, CBT was more efficacious than placebo in those with higher incomes (>$75 000) and with higher levels of cognitive distortion.[63] While the response rate for combination (of medication and CBT) treatment was not different than for medication alone (71 per cent versus 61 per cent), combination resulted in a more rapid response and greater likelihood of remission (37 per cent versus 20 per cent) than medication alone.[63] However, studies of combination treatment for depression have been inconsistent. The addition of CBT to antidepressant treatment, both in primary care, and to the management of moderately to severely ill depressed patients failed to improve outcome over antidepressant treatment alone.[64,65] A more recent study of depressed adolescents who did not respond to an adequate initial trial of an antidepressant found that the combination of medication and CBT resulted in a higher rate of improvement among subjects than medication alone.[66]

Interpersonal therapy is a well-established treatment for adult depression, and more recently has been shown to be superior to waitlist control, clinical management, and treatment as usual.[61] This treatment has been demonstrated to be superior to treatment as usual in a community setting, as well.[59] Other forms of treatment that show promise are attachment-based therapy and family psycho-education, but have not yet been replicated by other groups.[59]

A group CBT approach that has been used for the treatment of depression,[67] has been adapted for the prevention of depression. In adolescents with subsyndromal depression, the group CBT resulted in a lower risk of onset of major depression than in the treatment usual group.[67] This approach was extended to the adolescent offspring of depressed parents. Adolescents, in addition to having parents with a history of depression needed to have had a prior depressive episode or subsyndromal symptoms. In an initial clinical trial and one 4-site replication, the intervention resulted in a 2–5-fold lower risk for new-onset depression.[68] The presence of current depression in the caregiver moderated the effectiveness of the CBT intervention, with children of parents with current depression failing to show an effect from the intervention. Weissman *et al.*[69] recently demonstrated that treatment of maternal depression resulted in symptomatic improvement in their children, particularly with regard to internalizing symptoms. A family psychoeducational approach has been shown to improve communication and support with regard to depression in a family member, although there was no difference in the incidence of depression in this approach versus a comparison educational treatment.[70]

The selective serotonin reuptake inhibitors (SSRIs) form the mainstay of medication management of depression. Fluoxetine is the only medication that is approved by the Food and Drug Administration (FDA) and the Medicines and Health care Regulatory Agency (MHRA) for use in paediatric depression, because it has the strongest evidence of efficacy (http://www.fda.gov and http://www.mhra.gov.uk). Other medications for which there is some evidence of efficacy are citalopram, sertraline, and venlafaxine, although for each of these medications, there is some evidence that these agents are more efficacious for adolescent than for child-onset depression.[71] In contrast, fluoxetine shows similar efficacy for both children and adolescents. Tricyclic antidepressants have been shown to be ineffective for children and adolescents with depression.[72] One possible exception is clomipramine, that has been demonstrated, when given IV to reverse chronic and refractory depression.[73] While there are no controlled trials, buproprion is commonly used for paediatric depression, and in open trials shows evidence of efficacy.[74] One small controlled study suggests that omega-3 fatty acids may be efficacious for the relief of child depression.[75]

Children and adolescents metabolize several of the antidepressants more quickly (e.g. citalopram, sertraline) compared to adults, and so equal or higher doses may be required in order to achieve a similar effect.[76] There has been little work in pharmacogenetics in paediatric populations, although one study has replicated adult findings showing that the less functional form of the serotonin transporter gene is associated with a less vigorous response to an antidepressant.[77]

The use of SSRIs increased steadily over the past decade, but enthusiasm for their use on the part of both families and clinicians has been curtailed by recent reports of an association between antidepressant use and the occurrence of spontaneously-reported suicidal adverse events (i.e. new-onset or worsening suicidal ideation or an attempt), which resulted in the FDA issuing a black box warning about this side effect. The FDA conducted a meta-analysis that showed on average that around 4 per cent of the drug-treated and 2 per cent of those on placebo developed a suicidal adverse event.[78] In the subset of studies where suicidal ideation was measured systematically, there was no difference in suicidality by treatment condition, with a trend towards a protective effect in the medication group. A more recent meta-analysis, using random- rather than fixed-effects modelling and including more studies that were not available at the time of the FDAs analysis also found an increased risk, although the estimates of the risk difference for suicidal ideation and behaviour were 0.7 per cent rather than 2 per cent.[71] In this meta-analysis, the benefits of antidepressants were also assessed, and in the case of depression, around 11 times more individuals showed clinical improvement than developed these suicidal adverse events, suggesting a favourable risk-benefit ratio for the use of antidepressants, given careful clinical monitoring.

For patients who have been treated with psychotherapy or medication, addition of a complementary modality (e.g. psychotherapy or medication) is indicated. Family discord should be addressed by family therapy, and parental depression should be identified and referred for treatment. Failure to respond at that point suggests the need to try a second SSRI, followed by either venlafaxine or bupropion. A recent study comparing depressed adolescents who did not respond to an adequate trial with an SSRI found that a switch to second SSRI was as efficacious as a switch to venlafaxine.[66] Augmentation is indicated if a patient shows a partial but palpable response but still is symptomatic, whereas those who have not responded at all should be tapered and switched to another medication.[79] There have been no clinical trials of augmentation in paediatric depressed subjects, but placebo-controlled trials in adults support the use of augmentation of SSRI treatment with lithium, T3, and bupropion.[80] Also, for depression with a seasonal component, light therapy has been shown to be efficacious in psychiatric clinical trials.[81]

## Paediatric bipolar disorder

Because paediatric bipolar disorder is rarer than unipolar depression and because of the previous controversy about diagnosis, there has only recently been increased attention paid to its treatment. Best practice guidelines are based upon downward extension of experience in adults, as well as a handful of clinical trials, but the field is changing very rapidly, and it is expected that these guidelines will change in parallel.[82] Paediatric bipolar disorder has intrinsic in it a paradox: the most functionally impairing aspect of the condition is depression, but treatment of depression may induce mania. Therefore, treatment of paediatric bipolar disorder must be viewed as the prevention of future episodes, with an emphasis on mood stabilization, and not just on the relief of acute symptoms, important as that may be in the short-run. This idea that one needs to take medication in order to stay well, as compared to achieve symptomatic relief, is one that is difficult for children and adolescents to grasp, and therefore needs to be an important target of ongoing management.

## Acute management of mania

*Emergent* mania represents a true emergency, as it can result in risky behaviour with irreversible consequences. One key to the control of mania is to restore sleep, since sleep deprivation increases mania in a vicious cycle. Most commonly, for the acute control of mania, practitioners use atypical neuroleptics such as risperdone, olanzapine, and quetiapine, which have been shown to be more efficacious than placebo in reducing manic symptoms.[82] Quetiapine has also been shown, in one study, to be superior to divalproex in reducing manic symptoms and achieving both response and remission, whereas lithium and divalproex were shown to have similar efficacy. An open trial comparing the efficacy of three mood stabilizers for achieving clinical response in paediatric bipolar disorder found that divalproex was somewhat more efficacious (ES = 0.58) compared to either lithium or carbamazepine (ESs = 0.38). Oxcarbazepine, a metabolite of carbamazepine, on the other hand, was found to be no better than placebo in achieving stabilization. Both for the management of psychotic symptoms and mania, the combination of a mood stabilizer such as lithium or divalproex and a neuroleptic appears to be more efficacious in producing remission than a mood stabilizer alone.[82]

## Acute management of depression

For the treatment-naïve patient, the first step in the management of the depressed bipolar patient is treatment with a mood stabilizer.[5,82] Open trials show that divalproex and lithium are relatively efficacious as mood stabilizers, with carbamazepine being efficacious, but less so than either of the former two agents. In adults, atypical neuroleptics are also being established as mood stabilizers with potency equal to lithium and divalproex, although with very concerning side effects of rapid weight gain. Once a therapeutic blood level of divalproex or lithium has been attained patients often will experience a relief of their depression. Sometimes alteration in the dosage, either an increase or a decrease, can bring further symptomatic relief. If a patient is still experiencing significant depressive symptoms, then an antidepressant can be added, but very carefully. Some data from adult studies suggests that bupropion may result in fewer manic break throughs than other antidepressants but those data do not exist yet in children. Lamotrigine has been shown in adults to provide prophylaxis against future depressive episodes, but is not helpful for the treatment of acute depression; this has not yet been investigated in children, except in open trials.[82]

## Medical management

The medications used for mood stabilization all have systemic and potentially very serious side effects. The atypical neuroleptics cause rapid weight gain; therefore weight, a lipid profile, fasting blood sugar, and waistline should be carefully monitored. One preliminary study suggests that concomitant treatment with metformin may attenuate weight gain.[83] Hypoprolactinaemia and galactorrhoea are also consequences of neuroleptic use. Lithium is associated with thyroid disease (usually hypothyroidism), which if undetected can affect mood and treatment reponse. Lithium also can impair kidney function, resulting in an inability to concentrate urine, reduced glomerular fitration rate, and proteinuria. Therefore, renal function should be assessed prior to treatment and annually with a creatinine clearance and a 24 h urine for protein should be obtained at baseline and annually. Divalproex can have toxic effects on the hemopoetic system and the liver, both of which must be carefully monitored. Lamotrigine is rarely associated (0.5 per cent) with Stevens–Johnson syndrome, a disease of mucous membranes that can be potentially life-threatening.

## Psychotherapeutic management

Patient and parent education and support are essential, including the importance of medication adherence, keeping regular sleep habits, avoidance of caffeine and other substances, and ability to recognize subtle signs of a shift in mood. Some specific forms of psychotherapy that target family process and emotion regulation have been developed.[84] Family focused treatment (FFT) has been used successful for adult bipolar disorder and results in fewer depressive episodes and better overall functioning. Pilot studies indicate what appear to be similar effects for adolescent bipolar disorder. A family psychoeducational approach also shows promise for improving adherence and reducing the risk of relapse.[85] Two other approaches that have been piloted but not yet tested in randomized clinical trials are the application of CBT to paediatric bipolar disorder, which includes family education, emotion regulation, self-monitoring, and social skills training, and the adaptation of dialectic behaviour therapy (DBT) to adolescent bipolar disorder.[86,87]

# Future directions

With regard to both conditions, it is important to try to understand neural circuitry and identify potential intermediate phenotypes, such as emotion dysregulation or impaired executive functioning, which are trait markers for risk for these disorders. The identification of intermediate phenotypes then opens up great opportunities for monitoring treatment response, identifying youth at risk for the disorder, and conducting genetic studies on less complex phenotypes that are more likely to yield definitive results.

While there have been great strides in the treatment of depression, it is difficult to predict who is going to respond to what treatment, and also, who is most likely to experience side effects such as increased suicidal ideation. Pharmacogenetics and monitoring of biomarkers may hold promise for improving matching of patient to treatment. The best approaches to continuation and maintenance have only been addressed for the simplest cases (e.g. uncomplicated episode with patient having a successful response to fluoxetine.[88]

Almost every aspect of treatment in paediatric bipolar disorder requires further study, including the best approach to the management of mania, depression, and mixed state, testing the role of various promising psychosocial approaches, and identifying pharmacogenetic and biomarker predictors of treatment response.

While major depression has been described in high-risk children as young as age 3,[14] it is less clear what are the earliest manifestations of paediatric bipolar disorder. Ongoing longitudinal and high-risk studies will help to clarify the answer to this question in coming years, and may then provide the basis for preventive interventions.

# References

1. APA. (2000). *Diagnostic and statistical manual of mental disorders* (*DSM-IV-TR*) (4th edn). American Psychiatric Association, Washington, DC.
2. Kovacs, M. (1996). Presentation and course of major depressive disorder during childhood and later years of the life span. *Journal of the American Academy of Child and Adolescent Psychiatry*, **35**, 705–15.
3. Fergusson, D.M., Horwood, L.J., Ridder, E.M., *et al.* (2005). Subthreshold depression in adolescence and mental health outcomes in adulthood. *Archives of General Psychiatry*, **62**, 66–72.
4. Birmaher, B. and Axelson, D. (2006). Course and outcome of bipolar spectrum disorder in children and adolescents: a review of the existing literature. *Development and Psychopathology*, **18**, 1023–35.
5. Pavuluri, M.N., Birmaher, B., and Naylor, M.W. (2006). Pediatric bipolar disorder: a review of the past 10 years. *Journal of the American Academy of Child and Adolescent Psychiatry*, **44**, 846–71.
6. Kovacs, M. and Devlin, B. (1998). Internalizing disorders in childhood. *Journal of Child Psychology and Psychiatry, and Allied Disciplines*, **39**, 47–63.
7. Becker, D.F., Grilo, C.M., Edell, W.S., *et al.* (2002). Diagnostic efficiency of borderline personality disorder criteria in hospitalized adolescents: comparison with hospitalized adults. *The American Journal of Psychiatry*, **159**, 2042–7.
8. Angold, A., Costello, E.J., and Erkanli, A. (1999). Comorbidity. *Journal of Child Psychology and Psychiatry, and Allied Disciplines*, **40**, 57–87.
9. Birmaher, B., Dahl, R.E., Perel, J., *et al.* (1996). Corticotropin-releasing hormone challenge in prepubertal major depression. *Biological Psychiatry*, **39**, 267–77.
10. Lewinsohn, P.M., Rohde, P., and Seeley, J.R. (1998). Major depressive disorder in older adolescents: prevalence, risk factors, and clinical implications. *Clinical Psychology Review*, **18**, 765–94.
11. Lewinsohn, P.M., Klein, D.N., and Seeley, J.R. (1995). Bipolar disorders in a community sample of older adolescents: prevalence, phenomenology, comorbidity and course. *Journal of the American Academy of Child and Adolescent Psychiatry*, **34**, 454–63.
12. Angold, A., Costello, E.J., Erkanli, A., *et al.* (1999). Pubertal changes in hormone levels and depression in girls. *Psychological Medicine*, **29**, 1043–53.
13. Harrington, R., Rutter, M., and Fombonne, E. (1996). Developmental pathways in depression: multiple meanings, antecedents, and endpoints. *Development and Psychopathology*, **8**, 601–16.
14. Luby, J.L., Heffelfinger, A.K., Mrakotsky, C., *et al.* (2003). The clinical picture of depression in preschool children. *Journal of the American Academy of Child and Adolescent Psychiatry*, **42**, 340–8.
15. Birmaher, B., Arbelaez, C., and Brent, D. (2002). Course and outcome of child and adolescent major depressive disorder. *Child and Adolescent Psychiatric Clinics of North America*, **11**, 619–37.
16. Brent, D.A. and Birmaher, B. (2006). Treatment resistant depression in adolescents: recognition and management. *Child and Adolescent Psychiatric Clinics of North America*, **15**, 1015–34.
17. Potash, J.B. (2007). Carving chaos: genetics and the classification of mood and psychotic syndromes. *Harvard Review of Psychiatry*, **14**, 47–63.
18. Geller, B., Zimerman, B., Williams, M., *et al.* (2001). Bipolar disorder at prospective follow-up of adults who had prepubertal major depression disorder. *The American Journal of Psychiatry*, **158**, 125–7.
19. Martin, A., Young, C., Leckman, J.F., *et al.* (2004). Age effects on antidepressant-induced manic conversion. *Archives of Pediatrics & Adolescent Medicine*, **158**, 773–80.
20. Scheffer, R.E., Kowatch, R.A., Carmody, T., *et al.* (2005). Randomized, placebo-controlled trial of mixed amphetamine salts for symptoms of comorbid ADHD in pediatric bipolar disorder after mood stabilization with divalproex sodium. *The American Journal of Psychiatry*, **162**, 58–64.
21. Bridge, J.A., Goldstein, T.R., and Brent, D.A. (2006). Adolescent suicide and suicidal behavior. *Journal of Child Psychology and Psychiatry, and Allied Disciplines*, **47**, 372–94.
22. Pine, D.S., Goldstein, R.B., Wolk, S., *et al.* (2001). The association between childhood depression and adulthood body mass index. *Pediatrics*, **107**, 1049–56.
23. Craddock, N. and Forty, L. (2006). Genetics of affective (mood) disorders. *European Journal of Human Genetics*, **14**, 660–8.
24. Silberg, J., Rutter, M., Meyer, J., *et al.* (1996). Genetic and environmental influences on the covariation between hyperactivity and conduct disturbance in juvenile twins. *Journal of Child Psychology and Psychiatry, and Allied Disciplines*, **37**, 803–16.
25. Weissman, M.M., Wickramaratne, P., Nomura, Y., *et al.* (2005). Families at high and low risk for depression: a 3-generation study. *Archives of General Psychiatry*, **62**, 29–36.
26. Caspi, A., Sugden, K., Moffitt, T.E., *et al.* (2003). Influence of life stress on depression: moderation by a polymorphism in the 5-HT gene. *Science*, **301**, 386–9.
27. Kaufman, J., Yang, B.Z., Douglas-Palumberi, H., *et al.* (2006). Brain-derived neurotrophic factor-5-HTTLPR gene interactions and environmental modifiers of depression in children. *Biological Psychiatry*, **59**, 673–80.
28. Strauss, J., Barr, C.L., George, C.J., *et al.* (2005). Brain-derived neurotrophic factor variants are associated with childhood-onset mood disorder: confirmation in a Hungarian sample. *Molecular Psychiatry*, **10**, 861–7.
29. McQueen, M.B., Devlin, B., Faraone, S.V., *et al.* (2005). Combined analysis from eleven linkage studies of bipolar disorder provides strong evidence of susceptibility loci on chromosomes 6q and 8q. *American Journal of Human Genetics*, **77**, 582–95.
30. Geller, B., Badner, J.A., Tillman, R., *et al.* (2004). Linkage disequilibrium of the brain-derived neurotrophic factor Val66Met polymorphism in children with a prepubertal and early adolescent bipolar disorder phenotype. *The American Journal of Psychiatry*, **161**, 1698–700.
31. Todd, R.D. and Botteron, K.N. (2001). Family, genetic, and imaging studies of early-onset depression. *Child Adolescent Psychiatric Clinics of North America*, **10**, 375–90.
32. Dickstein, D.P. and Leibenluft, E. (2006). Emotion regulation in children and adolescents: boundaries between normalcy and bipolar disorder. *Development and Psychopathology*, **18**, 1105–31.
33. Adler, C.M., Adams, J., DelBello, M.P., *et al.* (2006). Evidence of white matter pathology in bipolar disorder adolescents experiencing their first episode of mania: a diffusion tensor imaging study. *The American Journal of Psychiatry*, **163**, 322–4.
34. Sauri, R.B., Stanley, J.A., Axelson, D., *et al.* (2005). Reduced NAA levels in the dorsolateral prefrontal cortex of young bipolar patients. *The American Journal of Psychiatry*, **162**, 2109–15.
35. Kyte, Z. and Goodyer, I. (2005). The neurobiology of social cognition and its relationship to unipolar depression. In *The cognitive neuroscience of social behaviour* (eds. A. Easton and N.J. Emery), pp. 257–90. Psychology Press, New York.
36. Forbes, E.E., May, C., Siegle, G.J., *et al.* (2006). Reward-related decision-making in pediatric major depressive disorder: an fMRI study. *Journal of Child Psychology and Psychiatry, and Allied Disciplines*, **47**, 1031–40.
37. Roberson-Nay, R., McClure, E.B., Monk, C.S., *et al.* (2006). Increased amygdala activity during successful memory encoding in adolescent major depressive disorder: an fMRI Study. *Biological Psychiatry*, **60**, 966–73.
38. Thomas, K.M., Drevets, W.C., Whalen, P.J., *et al.* (2001). Amygdala response to facial expressions in children and adults. *Biological Psychiatry*, **49**, 309–16.
39. Silk, J.S., Shaw, D.S., Skuban, E.M., *et al.* (2006). Emotion regulation strategies in offspring of childhood-onset depressed mothers. *Journal of Child Psychology and Psychiatry, and Allied Disciplines*, **47**, 69–78.

40. Perez-Edgar, K., Fox, N.A., Cohn, J.F., *et al.* (2006). Behavioral and electrophysiological markers of selective attention in children of parents with a history of depression. *Biological Psychiatry*, **60**, 1131–8.

41. Silk, J.S., Shaw, D.S., Forbes, E.E., *et al.* (2006). Maternal depression and child internalizing: the moderating role of child emotion regulation. *Journal of Clinical Child and Adolescent Psychology*, **35**, 116–26.

42. Garber, J., Keiley, M.K., and Martin, N.C. (2002). Developmental trajectories of adolescents' depressive symptoms: predictors of change. *Journal of Consulting and Clinical Psychology*, **70**, 79–95.

43. Shaw, D.S., Schonberg, M., Sherrill, J., *et al.* (2006). Responsivity to offspring's expression of emotion among childhood-onset depressed mothers. *Journal of Clinical Child and Adolescent Psychology*, **35**, 490–503.

44. Sharp, C., Fonagy, P., and Goodyer, I.M. (2006). Imagining your child's mind: psychosocial adjustment and mothers' ability to predict their children's attributional response styles. *British Journal Developmental Psychology*, **24**, 197–214.

45. Kovacs, M., Sherril, J., George, C.J., *et al.* (2006). Contextual emotion-regulation therapy for childhood depression: description and pilot testing of a new intervention. *Journal of the American Academy of Child and Adolescent Psychiatry*, **45**, 892–903.

46. Pavuluri, M.N., Schenkel, L.S., Aryal, S., *et al.* (2006). Neurocognitive function in unmedicated manic and medicated euthymic pediatric bipolar patients. *The American Journal of Psychiatry*, **163**, 286–93.

47. Gotlib, I.H., Traill, S.K., Montoya, J.J., *et al.* (2005). Attention and memory biases in the offspring of parents with bipolar disorder: indications from a pilot study. *Journal of Child Psychology and Psychiatry, and Allied Disciplines*, **46**, 84–93.

48. Ryan, N.D. (1998). Psychoneuroendocrinology of children and adolescents. *The Psychiatric Clinics of North America*, **21**, 435–41.

49. Forbes, E.E., Williamson, D.E., Ryan, N.D., *et al.* (2006). Peri-sleep-onset cortisol levels in children and adolescents with affective disorders. *Biological Psychiatry*, **59**, 24–30.

50. Bertocci, M.A., Dahl, R.E., Williamson, D.E., *et al.* (2005). Subjective sleep complaints in pediatric depression: a controlled study and comparison with EEG measures of sleep and waking. *Journal of the American Academy of Child and Adolescent Psychiatry*, **44**, 1158–66.

51. Kaufman, J., Birmaher, B., Perel, J., *et al.* (1998). Serotonergic functioning in depressed abused children: clinical and familial correlates. *Biological Psychiatry*, **44**, 973–81.

52. Nomura, Y., Wickramaratne, P.J., Warner, V., *et al.* (2002). Family discord, parental depression, and psychopathology in offspring: ten-year follow-up. *Journal of the American Academy of Child and Adolescent Psychiatry*, **41**, 402–9.

53. Frye, A.A. and Garber, J. (2005). The relations among maternal depression, maternal criticism, and adolescents' externalizing and internalizing symptoms. *Journal of Abnormal Child Psychology*, **33**, 1–11.

54. Leverich, G.S. and Post, R.M. (2006). Course of bipolar illness after history of childhood trauma. *Lancet*, **367**, 1040–2.

55. Brent, D.A., Moritz, G., and Liotus, L. (1996). A test of the diathesis-stress model of adolescent depression in friends and acquaintances of adolescent suicide victims. In *Severe stress and mental disturbance in children* (ed. C.R. Pfeffer), pp. 347–60. American Psychiatric Press, Inc., Washington, DC.

56. Borowsky, I.W., Ireland, M., and Resnick, M.D. (2001). Adolescent suicide attempts: risks and protectors. *Pediatrics*, **107**, 485–93.

57. Myers, K. and Winters, N.C. (2002). Ten-year review of rating scales. II. Scales for internalizing disorders. *Journal of the American Academy of Child and Adolescent Psychiatry*, **41**, 634–59.

58. Dierker, L., Albano, A.M., Clarke, G.N., *et al.* (2001). Screening for anxiety and depression in early adolescence. *Journal of the American Academy of Child and Adolescent Psychiatry*, **40**, 929–36.

59. Birmaher, B. and Brent, D. (in press). Work group on quality issues. Practice parameters for the assessment and treatment of children and adolescents with depressive disorders. *Journal of the American Academy of Child and Adolescent Psychiatry*.

60. National Institute for Health and Clinical Excellence (NICE). (2005). *Depression in children and young people. Identification and management in primary, community, and secondary care.* NICE, London.

61. Weisz, J.R., McCarty, C.A., and Valeri, S.M. (2006). Effects of psychotherapy for depression in children and adolescents: a meta-analysis. *Psychological Bulletin*, **132**, 132–49.

62. March, J.S., Silva, S., Petrycki, S., *et al.* (2004). Fluoxetine, cognitive-behavioral therapy, and their combination for adolescents with depression. Treatment for Adolescent Depression Study (TADS) randomized controlled trial. *The Journal of the American Medical Association*, **292**, 807–20.

63. March, J., Silva, S., Vitiello, B., *et al.* (2006). The Treatment for Adolescents with Depression Study (TADS): methods and message at twelve weeks. *Journal of the American Academy of Child and Adolescent Psychiatry*, **45**, 1393–403.

64. Clarke, G., Debar, L., Lynch, F., *et al.* (2005). A randomized effectiveness trial of brief cognitive-behavior therapy for depressed adolescents receiving antidepressant medication. *Journal of the American Academy of Child and Adolescent Psychiatry*, **44**, 888–98.

65. Goodyer, I., Dubicka, B., Wilkinson, P., *et al.* (2007). Selective serotonin reuptake inhibitors (SSRIs) and routine specialist care with and without cognitive behaviour therapy in adolescents with major depression: randomised controlled trial. *British Medical Journal*, **335**, 106–7.

66. Brent, D.A., Emslie, G.J., Clarke, G.N., *et al.* (2007). Treatment of SSRI-Resistant Depression in Adolescents (TORDIA): a test of treatment strategies in depressed adolescents who have not responded to an adequate trial of a Selective Serotonin Reuptake Inhibitor (SSRI). Presented at NCDEU 47th Annual Meeting, Boca Raton, FL.

67. Rohde, P., Lewinsohn, P.M., Clarke, G.N., *et al.* (2005). The adolescent coping with depression course: a cognitive-behavioral approach to the treatment of adolescent depression. In *Psychosocial treatments for child and adolescent disorders: empirically based strategies for clinical practice* (eds. E.D. Hibbs and P.S. Jensen), pp. 219–37. Washington, DC.

68. Clarke, G.N., Hornbrook, M., Lynch, F., *et al.* (2001). A randomized trial of a group cognitive intervention for preventing depression in adolescent offspring of depressed parents. *Archives of General Psychiatry*, **58**, 1127–34.

69. Weissman, M.M., Pilowsky, D.J., Wickramaratne, P.J., *et al.* (2006). Remissions in maternal depression and child psychopathology: a STAR*D child report. *The Journal of the American Medical Association*, **295**, 1389–98.

70. Beardslee, W., Gladstone, T.R.G., Wright, E.J., *et al.* (2003). A family based approached to the prevention of depressive symptoms in children at risk: evidence of parental and child change. *Pediatrics*, **112**, e119–e31.

71. Bridge, J., Iyengar, S., Salary, C.B., *et al.* (2007). Clinical response and risk for reported suicidal ideation and suicide attempts in pediatric antidepressant treatment: a meta-analysis of randomized controlled trials. *The Journal of the American Medical Association*, **297**, 1683–96.

72. Hazell, P., O'Connell, D., Heathcote, D., *et al.* (1995). Efficacy of tricyclic drugs in treating child and adolescent depression: a meta-analysis. *British Medical Journal*, **310**, 897–901.

73. Sallee, F.R., Vrindavanam, N.S., Deas-Nesmith, D., *et al.* (1997). Pulse intravenous clomipramine for depressed adolescents: double-blind, controlled trial. *The American Journal of Psychiatry*, **154**, 668–73.

74. Daviss, W.B., Perel, J.M., Brent, D.A., *et al.* (2006). Acute antidepressant response and plasma levels of bupropion and metabolites in a

pediatric-aged sample: an exploratory study. *Therapeutic Drug Monitoring*, **28**, 190–8.

75. Nemets, H., Nemets, B., Apter, A., *et al.* (2006). Omega-3 treatment of childhood depression: a controlled, double-blind pilot study. *The American Journal of Psychiatry*, **163**, 1098–100.

76. Findling, R.L., McNamara, N.K., Stansbrey, R.J., *et al.* (2006). The relevance of pharmacokinetic studies in designing efficacy trials in juvenile major depression. *Journal of Child and Adolescent Psychopharmacology*, **16**, 131–45.

77. Kronenberg, S., Apter, A., Brent, D., *et al.* (in press). Serotonin transporter (5HTT) polymorphism and citalopram effectiveness and side effects in children with depression and anxiety disorders. *Journal of Child and Adolescent Psychopharmacology*.

78. Hammad, T.A., Laughren, T., and Racoosin, J. (2006). Suicidality in pediatric patients treated with antidepressant drugs. *Archives of General Psychiatry*, **63**, 332–9.

79. Hughes, C.W., Emslie, G.J., Crismon, L., *et al.* (1999). The Texas children's medication algorithm project: report of the Texas consensus conference panel on medication treatment of childhood major depressive disorder. *Journal of the American Academy of Child and Adolescent Psychiatry*, **38**, 1442–54.

80. Brent, D. and Birmaher, B. (2006). Treatment resistant depression in adolescents: recognition and management. *Child and Adolescent Psychiatric Clinics of North America*, **15**, 1015–34.

81. Swedo, S.E., Allen, A.J., Glod, C.A., *et al.* (1997). A controlled trial of light therapy for the treatment of pediatric seasonal affective disorder. *Journal of the American Academy of Child and Adolescent Psychiatry*, **36**, 816–21.

82. McClellan, J., Kowatch, R., and Findling, R.L. (2007). Work group on quality issues. Practice parameter for the assessment and treatment of children and adolescents with bipolar disorder. *Journal of the American Academy of Child and Adolescent Psychiatry*, **46**, 107–25.

83. Klein, D.J., Cottingham, E.M., Sorter, M., *et al.* (2006). A randomized, double-blind, placebo-controlled trial of metformin treatment of weight gain associated with initiation of atypical antipsychotic therapy in children and adolescents. *The American Journal of Psychiatry*, **163**, 2072–9.

84. Miklowitz, D.J. (2006). A review of evidenced-based psychosocial interventions for bipolar disorder. *The Journal of Clinical Psychiatry*, **67**, 28–33.

85. Fristad, M.A. (2006). Psychoeducational treatment for school-aged children with bipolar disorder. *Development and Psychopathology*, **18**, 1289–306.

86. Pavuluri, M.N., Graczyk, P., Henry, D., *et al.* (2004). Child- and family-focused cognitive behavioral therapy for pediatric bipolar disorder: development and preliminary results. *Journal of the American Academy of Child and Adolescent Psychiatry*, **43**, 528–37.

87. Goldstein, T.R., Axelson, D.A., Birmaher, B., *et al.* (2007). Dialectical behavior therapy for adolescent with bipolar disorder: a one year open trial. *Journal of the American Academy of Child and Adolescent Psychiatry*, **46**, 820–30.

88. Emslie, G.J., Heiligenstein, J.H., Hoog, S.L., *et al.* (2004). Fluoxetine treatment for prevention of relapse of depression in children and adolescents: a double-blind, placebo-controlled study. *Journal of the American Academy of Child and Adolescent Psychiatry*, **43**, 1397–405.

## 9.2.8 Obsessive–compulsive disorder and tics in children and adolescents

Martine F. Flament and Philippe Robaey

### Introduction

Although obsessive–compulsive disorder (**OCD**) has long been considered as a disorder of adulthood, the early child psychiatric literature contains famous descriptions of typical cases. At the beginning of the twentieth century, Janet reported on a 5-year-old with classical obsessive–compulsive (**OC**) symptoms, and Freud described in his adult patients obsessional behaviours dating back from childhood, while speculating on the strong constitutional influence in the choice of these symptoms. In the 1950's, Kanner noted the resemblance and sometimes the association between compulsive movements and tics, and Despert described the first large series of obsessive–compulsive children, noting the preponderance of males and the children's perception of the abnormality and undesirability of their behaviours.

Tics have been described since antiquity, but the first systematic reports are those of Itard, in 1825, and Gilles de la Tourette, in 1885. Both noted the association between tic disorders and OC symptoms, and speculated on the hereditary nature of the syndrome.

For the last two decades, there has been a tremendous growth of interest and research on OCD and tic disorders. Significant advances have occurred regarding the phenomenology, epidemiology, genetics, neurophysiology, pathogenesis, and treatment of both disorders. The frequent association of OCD and/or tic disorders with other neuropsychiatric disorders, as well as the increasing evidence coming from in-vivo neuroimaging studies, have led to a fascinating aspect of current neurobiological research—the possible localization of brain circuits mediating the abnormal behaviours. Of all paediatric psychiatric disorders, OCD and tic disorders now appear as model neurobiological disorders to investigate the role of genetic, neurobiological, and environmental mechanisms that interact to produce clinical syndromes of varying severity.

### Clinical features

#### Obsessive–compulsive disorder

Obsessions are persistently recurring thoughts, impulses, or images that are experienced as intrusive, inappropriate, and distressing, and that are not simply excessive worries about realistic problems. Compulsions are repetitive behaviours or mental acts that a person feels driven to perform according to a rigidly applied rule, in order to reduce distress or to prevent some dreaded outcome. Obsessions and compulsions are egodystonic, i.e. there are considered by the subject himself as irrational or unrealistic, and are, at least partly, resisted. Children and adolescents with OCD may hide their symptoms, or will only allow them to appear at home, or in the presence of family members, suggesting partial voluntary control.

The clinical presentation of OCD during childhood and adolescence has been documented in various cultures, with clinical series reported from the U.S., Japan, India, Israel, Denmark, and Spain. Typically, children and adolescents with OCD experience multiple obsessions and compulsions, whose content may change over time. The most frequent obsessions in young people include fear of dirt or germs, of danger to self or a loved one, symmetry or exactness, somatic, religious and sexual obsessions. The most common compulsions consist of washing rituals, repeating, checking, touching, counting, ordering, and hoarding. Generally, compulsions are carried out to dispel anxiety and/or in response to an obsession (e.g. to ward off fear of harm). However, some obsessions and rituals involve an internal sense that 'it does not feel right' until the thought or action is completed, and certain children with OCD may be unable to specify the dreaded event that the compulsive rituals are intended to prevent, beyond a vague premonition of something bad happening. Simple compulsions, such as repetitive touching or symmetrical ordering, may even lack any discernable ideational component, and may be phenomenologically indistinguishable from complex tics. Several symptom dimensions have been identified in OCD, which could suggest possible aetiologic heterogeneity. Based on the symptom categories of the Children's Yale-Brown Obsessive–Compulsive Scale (CY-BOCS, the most widely used symptomatic measure in paediatric OCD research,[1]) Stewart et al.[2] identified four distinct factors, using principal components analysis: (1) symmetry/ordering/repeating/checking; (2) contamination/cleaning/aggressive/somatic; (3) hoarding; and (4) sexual/religious symptoms. These symptom dimensions are congruent with those described in similar studies of adults with OCD, suggesting fairly consistent covariation of OCD symptoms through the developmental course.

## Tics

Tics are sudden, rapid, non-rhythmic, stereotyped, repetitive movements (motor tics) or sounds (vocal tics). They may mimic simple or more complicated fragments of normal motor or vocal behaviours, which are misplaced in context. Tics vary greatly in nature, location, number, intensity, forcefulness, and frequency.[4,5] Common simple motor tics are neck jerking, eye blinking, elevation of shoulders, mouth movements. Common simple vocal tics include throat clearing, sniffing, sucking air, grunting, snorting, humming, or barking. Complex motor tics may combine simple tics, and involve facial movements, jumping, gyrating, touching, kicking, grooming behaviours, or echokinesis (repeating someone else's movement). They may appear to be purposive in character, as brushing hair back, or suddenly rotating on one foot to make a 360-degree turn. In a small fraction of cases, the complex motor tics are self-injuring behaviours, which may be potentially dangerous. Complex verbal tics include the repetition of what was just heard (echolalia) or said (palilalia), or socially inappropriate utterances (coprolalia), even disguised through sign language. The specific tic repertoire of an individual typically changes over time with no predictable course, but complex tics are rare in the absence of simple tics. Tics often occur in discrete unpredictable bouts over the course of a day, separated by tic-free intervals. The combination of bouts over different time scales explains why globally tics wax and wane over time.

Tics are suggestible, as indicated by their transient reappearance when they are recalled. They are also suppressible, as they can generally be willfully held back for brief periods of time. Tics are preceded by an inner tension, an urge to move or utter that may build-up during suppression. Suppressing tics requires mental effort and may accentuate inattention; conversely, attentional problems decrease the ability to suppress tics, and are associated with more severe tics. Various premonitory sensory urges have been reported to prompt the tics, together with feelings of inner conflicts over whether and when to yield to these urges. Sensory urges include focal tension, pressure, tickling, cold, warmth, paresthesias, and generalized inner tension or anxiety. They usually arise in the part of the body involved in the subsequent motor act, and completing the tic seems to yield a temporary relief of the urge. Also, various auditory and visual cues, highly selective for each individual, can elicit tics, and some patients are extremely sensitive to these external cues, as in echo phenomena. Excitement and fatigue typically worsen tics, which are often more frequent and forceful when the individual is alone. Activities requiring fine motor skills and attention improve tics. Although much diminished, tics can occur during sleep, unlike many other movement disorders.

Children and adolescents with tic disorders may present a broad array of associated behavioural difficulties, including OC symptoms, disinhibited speech or conduct, impulsivity, distractibility, and motor hyperactivity.[5] The presence of motor and/or phonic tics can be associated with difficulties in self-esteem, self-definition, family life, peer acceptance or relationships, and school performance.

## Age of onset

The age at onset of OCD appears bimodal.[6] Prepubertal onset is associated with a male preponderance and an increased risk for tic disorders, including Tourette's disorder. A second peak of onset occurs at or after puberty. Overall, the mean age at onset of OCD in children and adolescents have ranged from 9 years in referred subjects[7] to 12.8 years in a community sample.[8]

The median onset age for simple motor tics is between 4 and 6 years.[9] Phonic or vocal tics usually appear several years after the onset of motor tics, in most cases between 8 and 15 years. Many young children are completely oblivious of their tics, or experience them as wholly involuntary. Premonitory urges typically show up several years after the onset of the tics, on average around 10 years of age. Suppressibility of tics developmentally precedes awareness of premonitory urges, but may get easier as awareness increases.[10]

## Sex ratio

In community-based samples of adolescents with OCD, there are approximately equal numbers of males and females, while in most studies of referred children and youth with OCD, males outnumber females by 2:1 or 3:1.[11]

Most studies show that the prevalence of tics is higher among boys than girls, with a ratio of 6–8:1 in clinic-based samples, and about 2:1 in community-based studies.[12] The sex ratio generally increases with tic duration and severity. Thus, in one study, the ratio of boys to girls was 1.6:1 for motor tics present for 1-2 consecutive months, increasing to 7.5:1 when tics were present for 2 non consecutive months, or more than 3 months.[13]

## Comorbidity

In referred children and adolescents with OCD, the frequency of a diagnosis of any tic disorder ranges from 17 per cent to 40 per cent, and that of Tourette's disorder from 11 per cent to 15 per cent.[14]

Conversely, one study found that 29 per cent of Tourette's disorder patients displayed OC behaviours.[15] In longitudinal studies, about 50 per cent of children and adolescents with Tourette's disorder develop OC symptoms or OCD by adulthood,[16] whereas, in a follow-up study of children and adolescents initially treated for OCD, nearly 60 per cent were found to have a lifetime history of tics that ranged from simple, mild, and transient tics to Tourette's disorder, for which the rate was 11 per cent.[17] On the basis of personal or family history of tics, a distinction has been proposed between 'tic-related OCD' and 'non-tic-related OCD', under the assumption that the two forms might differ in terms of clinical phenomenology, neurobiological concomitants, and responsiveness to pharmacological interventions.[18] Tic-related OCD appears to have an earlier onset, and to occur more frequently in boys than in girls. The need to touch or rub, blinking and staring rituals, worries over symmetry and exactness, a sense of incompleteness, and intrusive aggressive thoughts and images, are significantly more common in tic-related OCD, whereas contamination worries and cleaning compulsions are more frequent in patients with non-tic-related OCD.

The overall lifetime psychiatric comorbidity in children and adolescents with OCD is about 75 per cent, both in referred and in community cases. The most common conditions comorbid with OCD are affective disorders, with prevalence ranging across studies from 8 per cent to 73 per cent for mood disorders, and from 13 per cent to 70 per cent for anxiety disorders.[19] While occurring less frequently in non-referred subjects, a high rate of disruptive behaviour disorders—attention deficit/hyperactivity disorder (ADHD) and oppositional defiant disorder—has been reported in subjects seen in paediatric OCD clinics. In girls, OCD can be comorbid to anorexia nervosa.

Less than 10 per cent of clinically referred children and adolescents with Tourette's disorder do not have another morbid condition. About 55 per cent also have ADHD, and more than a third have anger control problems.[9] Rage attacks in response to minimal provocation, lasting from a few minutes to an hour and usually followed by remorse, as well as an increased vulnerability for drug abuse, depression, and antisocial behaviour, are primarily observed when comorbid ADHD is present. Globally, comorbidity of Tourette's disorder increases in adolescence, but more markedly for OCD and anxiety disorders in those without ADHD. Individuals with Tourette's disorder have consistently shown difficulties with fine motor control and visual motor integration, as well as impairment in procedural or habit-based learning. Sleep is often disturbed, with increased short lasting motor activity, especially in non-REM sleep, compared to healthy controls.

## Classification

Both DSM-IV and ICD-10 define OCD, regardless of age, by obsessions and/or compulsions, which are described, at some point during the course of the disorder, as excessive or unreasonable (criterion B), and are severe enough to cause marked distress or to interfere significantly with the person's normal routine, or usual social activities or relationships. The specific content of the obsessions or compulsions cannot be restricted to another Axis I diagnosis, such as an eating disorder, a mood disorder, or schizophrenia. The DSM-IV adds that the disturbance is not due to the direct physiological effects of a substance or a general medical condition.

The ICD-10 allows subclassification of forms with predominant obsessions, predominant compulsions, or mixed symptoms. In DSM-IV, the only difference in diagnostic criteria between children and adults appears in criterion B; although most children and adolescents actually acknowledge the senselessness of their symptoms, the requirement that insight is preserved is waived for children.

In both DSM-IV and ICD-10, tic disorders are divided into four categories, according to duration of the symptoms, and presence of vocal tics in addition to motor tics: Tourette's disorder, chronic motor or vocal tic disorder, transient tic disorder, and tic disorder not otherwise specified (NOS). Transient tic disorder is defined by single or multiple motor and/or vocal tics that occur many times a day, nearly everyday for at least 4 weeks, but for no longer than 12 consecutive months. In chronic motor or vocal tic disorder, either motor or vocal tics, but not both, have been present at some time during the illness. In Tourette's disorder, both multiple motor and one or more vocal tic have to be present, although not necessarily concurrently. Both Tourette's disorder and chronic motor or vocal tic disorder have a duration of more than 1 year, with no tic-free period of more than 3 months. All tic disorders must have onset before age 18 years. In all, the disturbance causes marked distress or significant impairment in social, occupational, or other important areas of functioning, and is not due to the direct physiological effects of a substance (e.g. stimulants), or a general medical condition. The ICD-10 recognizes that there is an immense variation in the severity of tics. At the one extreme of the continuum, the presence of transient tics, at some time during childhood, is near-normal. At the other extreme, Tourette's disorder is an uncommon, chronic, and incapacitating disorder.

## Diagnosis and differential diagnosis

In ICD-10, it is stated that OCD cannot be diagnosed if the patient meets Tourette's disorder criteria, while both diagnoses may be given simultaneously in DSM-IV. Unlike tics, compulsions are aimed at neutralizing the anxiety resulting from an obsession, and/or they are performed according to rules that must be applied rigidly. However, both compulsive rituals and complex tics may be preceded by premonitory urges, which persist until the action is completed. In individuals with both Tourette's disorder and OCD, these symptoms are sometimes so closely intertwined that efforts to distinguish them would be futile.

From a developmental perspective, pathological OC behaviours and thoughts differ from normal childhood rituals, mainly by their emotional context and their use of maladaptive versus adaptive cognitive and behavioural strategies.[20] Developmental childhood rituals are part of learning new skills, and accompanied by expressions of positive affect and interest. They are most intense in 4- to 8-year-olds, stress rules about daily life, help the child master anxiety, and enhance the socializing process. In contrast, perseverative behaviours in OCD are not goal-oriented, they are accompanied by a burdened, anxious affect, provoke frustration, are incapacitating and painful, and promote social isolation and regressive behaviour.

OCD must be distinguished from other anxiety disorders and, in some cases, from autism or schizophrenia. In phobias, subjects are preoccupied by their fears only when confronted to the phobogen stimuli, and, in separation anxiety disorder, fear of harm to parents or loved ones are part of persistent worries and behaviours which are not criticized by the child. Stereotyped movements and ritualistic behaviours are frequent in intellectual disability and autism, but they convey no particular intentionality, and the child does not try to resist them. In schizophrenia, there are erroneous belief systems in several areas, but the subject does not criticize them and does not consider the subsequent behaviours to be abnormal.

Tics should be differentiated from other types of abnormal movements which can occur in numerous congenital or acquired neurological and neuropsychiatric disorders (Sydenham's chorea, encephalitis, Huntington disease, tuberous sclerosis, neuroacanthocytosis, Wilson's disease, head trauma, mental retardation, autism). The term of secondary tics or Tourettism has been applied to these disorders, and the abnormal movements can be choreiform movements, dystonic movements, myoclonic movements, spasms, or stereotypies. Some medications such as central nervous system stimulants (methylphenidate, amphetamine, pemoline, cocaine), antihistaminic and anticholinergic drugs, antiepileptics (carbamazepine, phenytoin), antipsychotics, and opioids may also produce or exacerbate tics.[21] The distinction between tic disorders and other disorders with abnormal movements is based on anamnesis, family history, observation, and neurological examination, which is usually normal in tic disorders. Specific diagnostic tests may be required to confirm neurological or exogenous causes.

## Epidemiology

Tics might be one of the most common behavioural problems in childhood, but estimates of the prevalence of tic disorders greatly vary because of differences in the methods used (e.g. parental report versus direct observation), differences in the populations surveyed (e.g. age and sex distribution), and the transient nature of tics. Surveys among school-age children indicate that up to 18 per cent of boys, and 11 per cent of girls manifest frequent 'tics, twitches, mannerisms or habit spasms'. Race and socio-economic status do not seem to influence the frequency of tics. There are virtually no general population studies of transient tic disorder or chronic motor or vocal tic disorder. For Tourette's disorder, most population-based surveys yield prevalence estimates in the range of 5–10 per 10,000, with children being more likely to be identified than adults, and males more than females.[22, 13] In a study amongst all inductees into the Israeli Defence Force over 1 year, the point prevalence of Tourette's disorder was 4.9 per 10 000 males and 3.1 per 10 000 females, and the prevalence of OCD was elevated in those with Tourette's disorder (41.7 per cent vs. 3.4 per cent in others).[23] One longitudinal study assessed the presence of tics and OCD in an epidemiological sample of individuals followed from childhood to adulthood.[24] The prevalence of tics was 17.7 per cent at age 1–10 years, decreasing to 2–3 per cent in adolescence; childhood tics were associated with increased rates of OCD in adolescence; in adolescents with tics, the presence of comorbid OCD predicted persistence of tics into early adulthood.

There has been only one survey on the prevalence of OCD in children (5- to 15-year old), indicating an overall prevalence of OCD at 0.25 per cent, with an exponential increase as a function of age, from 0.026 per cent in 5–7 year olds to 0.63 per cent in 13–15 year olds.[25] In adolescents, epidemiological studies using strict diagnostic criteria and structured clinical interviews have been conducted in several parts of the world, estimating the prevalence of juvenile OCD between 1 and 4 per cent. In the largest study to date (N=5 596 high-school students), the lifetime prevalence of OCD in adolescents was estimated to 1.9 (±0.7) per cent, and none of the identified cases had been previously diagnosed.[8] In a later study,[26] the point prevalence of OCD was 3.6 (±0.7) per cent, decreasing to 1.8 per cent when excluding those individuals with only obsessions; among the OCD cases, there was a significant elevation of tic disorders (Tourette's disorder 5 per cent, chronic multiple tics 10 per cent, transient tics 10 per cent). In two longitudinal studies following cohorts of children in the community up to the age of 18 years, the prevalence for OCD ranged from 1.2 to 4 per cent.[27, 28] Thus, it appears that OCD might be as frequent in adolescents as it is in adults (see Chapter 4.8).

## Aetiology
### Psychological factors

Psychological theories of OCD have encompassed psychoanalytic as well as more general non-psychodynamic etiological approaches, focusing alternatively on volitional, intellectual, and/or emotional impairment. Freud's famous patient, the Rat Man, has been seen as a paradigm of a psychologically determined illness, illustrating the central role of anal sadistic concerns with control, ambivalence, magical thinking, and the salience of defenses such as reaction formation, intellectualization, isolation, and undoing. Freud also provided fascinating speculations on the similarity between OC phenomena, children's games, and religious rites. Later, Anna Freud stated that 'obsessional outcomes are promoted by a constitutional increase in the intensity of the anal-sadistic tendencies probably as the result of inheritance combined with parental handling'. However, despite the beautifully described dynamics of obsessional symptoms, most illustrative of unconscious processes, the psychoanalysts have also pointed out the extreme difficulty in treating OCD with classical analytic treatment.

Even though psychological factors are insufficient to cause Tourette's disorder, tic behaviours have long been identified as stress-sensitive, and temporally associated with important events in the lives of children. In a prospective study over 2 years, children and adolescents with Tourette's disorder and/or OCD experienced significantly more psychosocial stressors than did healthy controls, and the level of psychosocial stress was a significant predictor of future tic and OC symptoms severity.[29]

### Biochemical factors

Although a variety of biological aetiologies have been proposed in OCD since the 19th century, modern neurobiological theories began with the clinical studies showing that clomipramine and other serotonin reuptake inhibitors (**SRIs**) had a unique efficacy in treating the disorder. This inspired a 'serotoninergic hypothesis' of OCD (see Chapter 4.8). In children, the involvement of the serotonin system in the pathophysiology of OCD is supported by one study in which improvement of OC symptoms during clomipramine treatment was closely correlated with pretreatment platelet serotonin concentration,[30] and reports of decreased density of the platelet serotonin transporter in children and adolescents with OCD but not in those with Tourette's disorder.[31] However, the delayed and incomplete action of serotonergic drugs, suggesting multiple effects on other neurotransmitters as well, and numerous biochemical studies of OCD patients and controls have not yet indicated a single biochemical abnormality as a primary etiological mechanism in OCD.

In Tourette's disorder, multiple neurochemical systems have been implicated by pharmacological and metabolic studies, but a primary disturbance in the dopaminergic system is supported by the tic suppressing effect of dopamine receptor antagonists (see below). Post-mortem studies have shown an increase in the number of presynaptic dopamine transporter sites in the striatum and the frontal cortex of individuals with Tourette's disorder. PET/SPECT studies have demonstrated greater binding to dopamine transporter sites in both the caudate and putamen nuclei,[32] increased dopamine release by psychostimulants in the putamen,[33] and an association between density of dopamine receptors in the caudate and severity of tics.[34] The 'tonic-phasic hypothesis' proposes both a hyperresponsive spike-dependent (phasic) dopaminergic system (possibly related to an alteration in afferent cortical inputs), and a reduction in tonic dopamine levels (possibly secondary to an overactive dopamine transporter system), that would upregulate pre- and postsynaptic dopamine receptors and further increase the phasic-tonic unbalance. There is also some evidence for the role of serotonin in tic disorders, notably a study showing that reduced serotonin transporter binding correlated with vocal tics and OC symptoms.[35]

## Genetic factors

In both OCD and Tourette's disorder, twin and family studies provide strong evidence that genetic factors are involved in the vertical transmission of vulnerability within families. The average concordance rate in monozygotic twins is 65 per cent for OCD,[36] and 53 per cent for Tourette's disorder.[37] Family studies have consistently found higher rates of OCD and tic disorders in probands with paediatric OCD, as well as higher rates of tic disorders and OCD in those with tic disorders. Thus, Lenane et al.[38] investigating 147 first-degree relatives of children and adolescents with OCD found that 44 per cent of the families had a positive history of tics in at least one first-, second-, or third-degree relative. Conversely, Pauls et al.[39] reported that the prevalence rates of OCD and tic disorders were significantly greater among the first-degree relatives of 100 probands with OCD (10.3 per cent and 4.6 per cent, respectively) than among relatives of psychiatrically unaffected subjects (1.9 per cent and 1.0 per cent). These findings suggested that Tourette's disorder and some forms of OCD could be variant expressions of the same underlying genetic factors.

Results from two genome-wide scans have been reported,[40,41] with the strongest linkage peaks being on chromosome 2 for Tourette's disorder (p=0.00004), and chromosome 3 for OCD (p=0.0002); there were also regions that showed moderate evidence for linkage to both disorders. In early-onset OCD, family-based evidence for association at several serotonin system genes (SCL6A4, HTR1B, HTR2A) and brain-derived neurotropic factor (BDNF) has been reported in some studies, and the association seemed stronger in subjects with tic disorders associated with OCD.[42] There is also preliminary evidence for an association between OCD and two glutamate genes, the glutamate transporter gene (SLC1A1), and a glutamate receptor gene (GRIN2B).[43] A complementary approach involving examining rare cases of cytogenetic abnormalities

co-segregating with Tourette's and related disorders has pointed to regions on chromosomes 3p, 7q, 8q, 9p, and 18q.[44]

Thus, as suggested by earlier family studies, OCD and Tourette's disorder might have both shared and distinct susceptibility genes involved in their etiology. It is likely that epigenetic and non genetic factors may also contribute to phenotypal heterogeneity. A range of prenatal and perinatal events have been suggested as risk factors for increased tic severity, including lower birth weight, in utero exposure to caffeine, alcohol or tobacco, and maternal stress.[45] As the basal ganglia are especially sensitive to hypoxia, it is possible that factors associated with transient hypoxia could increase the risk for Tourette's disorder in those with a genetic vulnerability.

## Dysfunction of frontal–subcortical circuits

It has been known for a long time that OC symptoms could be associated with neurological disorders of motor control, including Tourette's disorder, Huntington's disease, Parkinson's disease, as well as traumatic or infectious lesions of the basal ganglia.[46] Conversely, in both adults and children with typical OCD, an increased frequency of soft neurological signs has been reported.[47] Since the era of neuroimaging, numerous studies have consistently found that the ventral prefrontal cortical (VPFC) regions, such as orbital prefrontal cortex and anterior cingulate cortex, the striatum, the basal ganglia and the thalamus were basic brain structures involved in the pathophysiology of OCD. These studies have generally identified abnormally high metabolic activity and/or blood flow in the orbital cortex and the head of the striatal caudate nucleus in untreated OCD subjects at rest, compared to various control populations.[48,49] Furthermore, the same two regions, as well as the thalamus to which each projects, have shown further increase in activity during OC symptom provocation. In several functional neuroimaging studies of patients with childhood onset OCD, measures of VPFC and striatal activity correlated positively with OCD symptom severity and treatment response.[50,51] Some studies have also indicated that the anatomy of the caudate, putamen and globus pallidus could differ between paediatric OCD patients and controls,[52] especially in cases of paediatric autoimmune neuropsychiatric disorders associated with streptococcal infections (PANDAS).[53] Although most studies have implicated the VPFC in the pathogenesis of OCD, recent investigation suggests a role for the dorsolateral prefrontal cortex (DLPFC) as well. Thus, one study found a significant increase in N-acetyl-aspartate (NAA), a neuronal marker of activity, in the left DLPFC of unmedicated paediatric OCD patients compared to controls.[54]

Recent MRI studies found that the volume of the caudate nucleus is decreased in both children and adults with Tourette's disorder, whereas the volume of putamen and globus pallidus nuclei are primarily reduced in adults with the disorder.[55] This is consistent with a study comparing monozygotic twins discordant for tic expression, in which caudate nuclei volumes were smaller in the more severely affected co-twin.[56] In addition, subjects with Tourette's disorder were found to have larger volumes in dorsal prefrontal and parieto-occipital regions.[57] Although no association was found between tic severity and the volumes of the basal ganglia, ratings of worst-ever tic severity were associated with larger orbito-frontal and parieto-occipital regions. In one recent study, cortical and subcortical hyperintensities that are considered as a subclinical manifestation of small-vessel disease, were significantly more abundant in children and adolescents with Tourette's disorder, OCD or ADHD than in healthy controls.[58] These results support a primary disturbance of the cortico-striato-pallidal-thalamo-cortical circuit, especially the projection into or out of the striatum. The small reduction of the caudate (about 5 per cent) may represent a marker for Tourette's disorder, and larger prefrontal cortex would likely result from the ability to suppress tics. Although tics are highly heritable, non genetic factors appear to contribute to these brain differences.

### Autoimmune factors

For the last decade, clinical and research interest has grown in an autoimmune model of OCD and/or tic disorders, which could apply to a subgroup of subjects whose disorder begins abruptly during childhood. An association was first reported between acute onset OCD and Sydenham's chorea, a childhood movement disorder associated with rheumatic fever, which is thought to result from an antineuronal antibody-mediated response to group A beta-haemolytic streptococcus (GABHS), directed at portions of the basal ganglia.[59] OCD, or some of its symptoms, have been reported in 70 per cent of Sydenham's chorea cases.[60, 61] Furthermore, in the absence of the neurological symptoms of Sydenham's chorea, post-streptococcal cases of childhood-onset OCD, tics and/or other neuropsychiatric syndromes have been described under the acronym of paediatric autoimmune neuropsychiatric disorders associated with streptococcal infections (PANDAS). Swedo et al.[6] defined this novel group of patients using five diagnostic criteria: presence of OCD and/or tic disorder, prepubertal onset, episodic course of symptom severity, abrupt onset or dramatic exacerbations of symptoms temporally associated with GABHS infections (as evidenced by positive throat culture and/or elevated anti-GABHS titers), and association with neurological abnormalities (motoric hyperactivity or adventitious movements, such as choreiform movements or tics). An antigen labelled D8/17, on the surface of peripheral blood mononuclear cells has been shown to be a marker for the genetic tendency to generate abnormal antibodies to GABHS. Two independent groups of researchers have found a greater expression of the D8/17 antigen in the B lymphocytes of patients with childhood-onset OCD or Tourette's disorder compared with healthy controls, indicating that the presence of the D8/17 antigen may serve as a marker of susceptibility for OCD or tics.[62, 63]

## Course and prognosis

Several follow-up studies of subjects treated for OCD during childhood or adolescence have looked at the outcome of the disorder in early adulthood.[11] All studies demonstrate the continuity of the diagnosis of OCD from childhood to adulthood: when subjects are still symptomatic, the main diagnosis is almost invariably OCD, although comorbid disorders are frequent, especially mood and/or anxiety disorders. Spontaneous course is most often marked by a waxing and waning severity of the disorder, whereas remissions under treatment can be followed by relapses, even after long periods of time. In the early studies in which subjects had received no or non-specific treatment, the recovery rate was poor (13–30 per cent). By the time patients had access to specific treatment with SRIs and/or cognitive behavioural therapy (CBT), recovery rates increased to 55–65 per cent, although many of the symptom-free subjects at follow-up were still taking medication. A meta-analysis analyzed 16 studies that followed paediatric OCD patients between 1 and 15 years.[64] The overall remission rate (not fulfilling criteria for subthreshold or full OCD) was 40 per cent, with pooled mean persistence rates of 41 per cent for full OCD. Poor prognostic factors included a poor initial treatment response, and comorbid psychiatric illness.

In the majority of cases, tics are transient (present for less than 12 months), or wax and wane in severity with periods of exacerbation of an average duration of 9 weeks. The course of worst-ever tic severity usually falls between 7 and 14 years of age, which also includes the period when tics are most variable (10–12 years). By the end of the second decade, there is usually a steady decline in tic severity. However, adults who are able to suppress tics may be left with distracting urges, and a significant minority (15–30 per cent) continues to have severe tics into adulthood.[65] Despite substantial problems in childhood, the majority of patients with Tourette's disorder grow up to become well socially integrated and economically independent adults. However, as much as 25 per cent have persistent mental health problems. In those, tic severity fluctuates, and psychiatric co-morbidities (ADHD, other disruptive behaviour problems, OCD, mood and anxiety disorders, learning problems) are often the main determinants of global outcome. Poorer prognoses are also associated with comorbid developmental disorders, chronic physical illness, unstable or unsupportive family environment, social difficulties, or exposure to psychoactive drugs such as cocaine.[5]

## Treatment

### Evidence

The treatment of paediatric OCD has changed dramatically over the past 20 years, with two modalities being empirically shown to ameliorate the core symptoms of the disorder: CBT and pharmacological treatment with SRIs. In Tourette's disorder, $D_2$ dopamine antagonists have been used with relative success since the 1960s, and CBT techniques are being increasingly scrutinized.

### Cognitive behavioural treatment

The cognitive behavioural model of OCD posits that compulsions function to reduce fear, and are subsequently reinforced by fear reduction, which prevents normal habituation and realistic appraisal of the threat value of feared stimuli. Techniques incorporating exposure and ritual prevention are designed to break this cycle by exposing the individual to feared situations, while simultaneously reducing compulsive behaviours.[66] Discussion of obsessive thoughts, and other irrational beliefs, is often part of the exposure exercises but these informal cognitive techniques are used to support exposure rather than to replace it. The CBT of youth with OCD generally involves a three-stage approach, consisting of information gathering, therapist-assisted graded exposure with response prevention, and homework assignments.[67] Anxiety management training plays an adjunctive role. For children with predominantly internalizing symptoms, treatment also includes relaxation and cognitive training. Families need to be involved, to varying extents according to individual situations. CBT is usually implemented with 13 to 20 weekly individual or family sessions, and homework assignments. Partial responders or nonresponders may require more frequent sessions, and out-of-office therapist-assisted training.

**Table 9.2.8.1** Controlled studies of pharmacological or psychological treatment in paediatric OCD

| Study, Year | N (age), Study duration | Drug (daily dose), Study design | Outcome | % Improvement from baseline on active treatment for OC symptoms |
|---|---|---|---|---|
| Flament et al., 1985 | 19 (6–18 yr), 5 wk | CMI (mean 141 mg) Crossover vs. PBO | CMI > PBO at 3–5 wk | 22–44 % |
| Leonard et al., 1989 | 47 (7–19 yr), 5 wk | CMI (mean 150 mg) Crossover vs. DES | CMI > DES at 3–5 wk | 19–44 % |
| DeVeaugh-Geiss et al., 1992 | 60 (10–17 yr), 8 wk | CMI (75–200 mg) Parallel vs. PBO | CMI > PBO at 3–8 wk | 34–37 % |
| Riddle et al., 1992 | 14 (8–15 yr), 8 wk | FLX (20 mg) Crossover vs. PBO | FLX > PBO at 8 wk | 33–44 % |
| March et al., 1998 | 187 (6–17 yr), 12 wk | SER (mean 167 mg) Parallel vs. PBO | SER > PBO at 3–12 wk | 21–28 % |
| Riddle et al., 2001 | 120 (8–17 yr), 10 wk | FLV (50–200 mg) Parallel vs. PBO | FLV > PBO at 1–10 wk | 21–25 % |
| Geller et al., 2001 | 103 (7–17 yr), 13 wk | FLX (mean 40 mg) Paralell vs. PBO | FLX > PBO at 7–13 wk | 25–49 % |
| Liebowitz et al., 2002 | 43 (8–17 yr), 16 wk | FLX (mean 64 mg) Parallel vs. PBO | FLX > PBO at 16 wk | 42 % |
| Geller et al., 2004 | 203 (7–17 yr), 10 wk | PAR (mean 30 mg) Parallel vs. PBO | PAR > PBO at 2–10 wk | 47–65 % |
| Barrett et al., 2004; 2005 | 77 (7–17 yr), 14 wk | Randomized parallel study ICBFT vs. GCBFT vs. control condition | ICBFT and GCBFT > control condition at 14 wk | 65 % for ICBFT 60 % for GCBFT |

CMI: clomipramine; DES: desipramine; FLV: fluvoxamine; FLX: fluoxetine; PAR: paroxetine; PBO: placebo; SER: sertraline
ICBT: individual cognitive behavioural treatment, GCBT: group cognitive behavioural treatment

A number of open trials, and four controlled studies (see Tables 9.2.8.1 and 9.2.8.2), have documented the beneficial effects of CBT, alone or in combination with pharmacotherapy, for children and adolescents with OCD, with improvement measured on the CY-BOCS scores ranging from 25 per cent to 67 per cent. In the first controlled study by Barrett et al.,[68] 88 per cent of youth treated with individual cognitive behavioural family treatment (CBFT), and 76 per cent of those treated with group CBFT showed clinically significant improvement, as compared to no improvement for any patients in the waitlist condition. Treatment gains were maintained at 12- to 18-month follow-up, with a total of 70 per cent of participants in individual therapy, and 84 per cent in

**Table 9.2.8.2** Comparative studies of cognitive behavioural treatment and pharmacological treatment in paediatric OCD

| Study, Year | N (age), Study duration | Drug (daily dose), Study design | Outcome | % Improvement / Remission for OC symptoms |
|---|---|---|---|---|
| De Haan et al., 1998 | 22 (8–18yr), 12 wk | CMI CMI (25–200 mg) vs. BT | BT > CMI | Improvement from baseline BT: 59.9 % CMI: 33.4 % |
| POTS Team 2004 | 112 (7–17yr), 12 wk | SER (mean 150 mg) vs. PBO vs. CBT vs. Combi (CBT+SER) 3-site study, Parallel design | Combi > CBT = SER > PBO effect size: 1.4 (Combi), 0.97 (CBT), 0.67 (SER) | Improvement from baseline Combi: 53 %; CBT: 46 %; SER: 30 %; Placebo: 15 % Remission post-treatment (CY-BOCS<10) Combi: 53.6 %; CBT: 39.3 % SER: 21.4 %; PBO: 3.6 % |
| Asbahr et al., 2005 | 40 (9–17 yr), 12 wk F/U: 9 mo | SER (mean 137 mg) vs. GCBT | Significant improvement on CY-BOCS with both GCBT and SER Relapse during F/y: 50% (SER), 5 % (GCBT) | NR |

BT: behavioural treatment; CBT: cognitive behavioural treatment; CMI: clomipramine; Combi: combination treatment; F/U: follow-up; GCBT: group cognitive behavioural treatment; NR: not reported; PBO: placebo; POTS: paediatric obsessive–compulsive disorder treatment study; SER: sertraline group therapy diagnosis-free at follow-up, and no significant difference between the two treatment modalities.[69] More evidence for the efficacy of CBT in the treatment of paediatric OCD comes from three studies that have compared CBT to pharmacotherapy and/or their combination (see below).

Behavioural techniques play an important role in the treatment of tics, although generally as adjunctive to medication. In a model of operant conditioning, ticking relieves unpleasant premonitory sensations, which reinforces the maintenance of tics. Habit reversal (HR) is based on awareness training regarding the premonitory urges, followed by training a competing response (a movement that involves the same muscle group as the tic) after the first sensation that a tic is about to occur. The response must be temporally contingent on each occurrence of the urge, but using a muscle group related or unrelated to the tic may not be crucial for tic suppression. Relaxation, self-monitoring, contingency training for positive reinforcement of not ticking, and social support are used as ancillary components of HR. An extension of HR is exposure and response prevention (ERP): after the urge, the patient suppresses the tic voluntarily, which should lead to its extinction. Both techniques have been showed to yield relatively large effect size (1.06 to 1.42) in reducing tic severity at post-treatment[70] and long-term follow-up.[71] A recent review of the literature[72] concluded that the use of HR to treat tics can currently be classified as a 'well established' treatment, and that of ERP as a 'probably efficacious' treatment. Contrary to initial fears, these behavioural techniques have no negative consequences, such as substitution of the targeted tics, or post-suppression rebound or worsening due to increased awareness of premonitory urges.

## Psychopharmacological treatment

In the past 25 years, a number of randomized, controlled clinical trials (summarized in Table 9.2.8.1) have been conducted in children and adolescents with OCD demonstrating, as in adults, the selective and unique efficacy of the SRIs in the short-term and long-term treatment of the disorder.[67,73–79] Results have consistently shown that: the antiobsessional action of the SRIs is independent of the presence of depressive symptoms at baseline; their antiobsessional action takes longer to appear than their antidepressant action; the therapeutic response occurs gradually over a few weeks to a few months; final response is most often partial, with a mean reduction of OC symptoms from baseline to post-treatment ranging from 19 per cent to 44 per cent across measures and across studies.[80] Geller et al.[81] conducted a meta-analysis of 12 randomized, controlled medication trials in children and adolescents with OCD (total N=1044), demonstrating that all serotonergic medications were highly significantly superior to placebo, with consistent findings across studies but a modest overall effect (the pooled standard mean difference between active drug and placebo was only 0.46). Clomipramine was statistically superior to the specific serotonin reuptake inhibitors (SSRI), but temporal trends might, at least, partly explain this apparent superiority: the clomipramine trials were conducted earlier in time when no other treatment was available, while the patient population included in subsequent controlled trials have changed over the years with increased availability of pharmacological alternatives. No head-to-head paediatric studies of clomipramine versus an SSRI have been conducted. The recommended daily dosages for SSRIs in the treatment of paediatric OCD are shown on Table 9.2.8.3.

**Table 9.2.8.3** Recommended daily dosages of serotonin reuptake inhibitors for the treatment of paediatric OCD

| Medication | Starting Dose[a] | Initial Targeted Dose[b,c] | Maximal Dose[b] |
|---|---|---|---|
| Citalopram | 10 mg | 40 mg | 60 mg |
| Escitalopram | 5 mg | 20 mg | 20 mg |
| Fluoxetine | 10 mg | 40 mg | 80 mg |
| Fluvoxamine | 25 mg | 200 mg | 300 mg |
| Paroxetine | 10 mg | 40 mg | 60 mg |
| Sertraline | 25 mg | 100 mg | 200 mg |
| Clomipramine | 10 mg | 150 mg | 250 mg |

[a] these doses should be given for about one week, that is about the time necessary to achieve steady state for these drugs, with the exception of fluoxetine. This would ensure that no agitation or increased anxiety is triggered by the medication.

[b] for subjects weighing at least 50 kg; for smaller individuals, a weight-proportional regimen should be used

[c] according to side effects and response

A few studies, summarized in Table 9.2.8.2, have compared pharmacological treatment to CBT or their combination for children and adolescents with OCD.[82–84] In the U.S. 12-week paediatric OCD treatment study (POTS; N=112), the combined treatment with CBT and sertraline had the best rate of clinical remission (53.6 per cent vs 39.3 per cent on CBT alone, 21.4 per cent on sertraline alone, and 3.6 per cent on placebo); the remission rate for the combined treatment was not statistically different from that in the CBT only condition.[83] In Asbahr et al.[84] study, both group CBT and sertraline induced a significant improvement in OC symptoms, but after a 9-month post-treatment follow-up period, subjects in the group CBT condition had a significantly lower rate of symptom relapse. A few case reports have also indicated that the addition of CBT to pharmacotherapy can allow successful withdrawal from medication.

The use of clomipramine can entail anticholinergic side effects (dry mouth, dizziness, headache, tremor, fatigue, constipation, sweating, dyspepsia, sexual dysfunction), which may not abate over time and even increase with ascending titration.[85] Clomipramine can cause tachycardia and prolongation of the QT and QTc intervals, and ECG monitoring is recommended.[86] Risks of toxicity also include seizures, and rare cases of sudden death have been reported in children taking tricyclic antidepressants.[87] Although less frequent and less disturbing that the secondary effects of clomipramine, the most commonly described adverse effects of the SSRIs include gastro-intestinal (nausea, constipation, abdominal pain), and central nervous system complaints (headache, tremor, drowsiness, akathisia, insomnia, disinhibition, agitation).[88] The possible induction of mania can also be of concern. Although not commonly reported in clinical trials, the eventual occurrence of sexual side effects should be reviewed with adolescents, since these may impact adherence to treatment. Recent reports of possible growth suppression associated with the SSRIs suggest that monitoring of height may also be advisable.[89] A recent concern, highly visible in the media, has been a possibly increased risk for suicidal thoughts, self-harm and/or harm to others, in youth treated with the SSRIs. However, no individual OCD study has documented a significantly increased risk for suicidal ideation or behaviour on a SSRI compared to placebo. In pooled analyses of the controlled studies conducted in youth with OCD and other anxiety disorders, behavioural side effects variously labelled as activation, akathisia, disinhibition, impulsivity, and hyperactivity have appeared, but there was no evidence for a significant increase in the relative risk of suicidal thoughts or behaviours.[90] In a recent review of 27 trials of antidepressants in participants younger than 19 years (including six trials for treatment of OCD), there was an increased risk difference of suicidal ideation/suicide attempts across trials and across indications for drug versus placebo, but no completed suicide, and the benefits of antidepressants appeared much greater than the risk.[91] In any case, rigorous clinical monitoring for suicidal ideation and other potential indicators for suicidal behaviour remains advised in youth treated with the SSRIs.

The mainstay of treatment for Tourette's disorder has been traditional antipsychotics, i.e. the potent dopamine (D2) postsynaptic blockers haloperidol and pimozide.[92] The usual starting dose is 0.25 mg/day of haloperidol or 1 mg/day of pimozide. Increments (0.5 mg haloperidol or 1 mg pimozide) may be added at 7 to 14 days intervals, up to 1–4 mg/day for haloperidol and 2–8 mg/day for pimozide. Atypical antipsychotics have also been used for the treatment of tics, and differences in efficacy appear to be related to their relative potency of dopamine blockade. Risperidone has been shown to be superior to placebo,[93,94] and equally effective to pimozide,[95,96] at doses ranging from 1 to 3 mg/day (starting dose, 0.25–0.50 mg). The specific D2 receptor-blocking agents, tiapride and sulpiride, have been commonly used for the treatment of tics in Europe in doses ranging from 15–500 mg/day and 200–1000 mg/day, respectively, but they are not available in the U.S. The use of traditional antipsychotics is limited by a range of side effects, both in the short term (parkinsonism, dystonia, dyskinesia, and akathisia) and in the long term (tardive dyskinesia). The newer antipsychotics appear to have a lower frequency of neurological side effects in the short term, and a lower relative risk of tardive dyskinesia, but weight gain, hyperlipidemia and diabetes are of growing concern. Among the antipsychotics used in the treatment of tics, pimozide is the most likely to be associated with prolonged QTc interval, although this is a rare occurrence at therapeutic doses. An ECG is recommended before starting treatment, during the dose-adjustment phase, and annually during ongoing treatment. Patients should also be informed that the risk for cardiac conduction abnormalities may increase when pimozide is combined with drugs that inhibit cytochrome P450 3A4 isoenzyme (e.g. macrolide antibiotics, SSRIs, etc.).[97]

Clonidine is an antihypertensive agent (α-2-adrenergic agonist) that has been shown effective for treatment of tic disorders, presumably via acute and chronic downstream effects on dopamine. Clinical trials indicate an average 25–35 per cent reduction in symptoms over 8 to 12 weeks. Clonidine seems especially useful in improving attention problems and ameliorating complex motor tics. Treatment must be started at a low dose (0.05 mg in the morning), and slowly increased to 0.15–0.30 mg per day, given in several doses throughout the day. The major side effects are sedation, hypotension, dizziness, and a decrease of salivatory flow; blood pressure and pulse should be measured at baseline and monitored during dose adjustment, and patients and families should be educated about the potential for rebound increases in blood pressure, tics, and anxiety upon abrupt discontinuation.[98] Guanfacine is another α-adrenergic antihypertensive that has entered into clinical practice. Given the added disability attributable to ADHD in children and adolescents with tic disorders, a treatment combining an α-2 agonist and a stimulant may produce better outcomes than either alone. Recent studies suggest that the acute onset or worsening of tic symptoms among patients receiving stimulants may be simply an expression of the spontaneous time course of tics and comorbid ADHD.[99] Atomoxetine is a selective norepinephrine reuptake inhibitor that reduces significantly ADHD symptoms, and may also improve tics.

## Management

As described above, OCD and tic disorders are frequently chronic, and most treatments, notably medication, are suspensive but not curative. Therefore, when defining a treatment plan, clinicians should be aware that they embark on a long-lasting task.

CBT is generally favoured as the initial treatment of choice for OCD, especially in milder cases without significant comorbidity, whereas presence of comorbid depression, anxiety, disruptive behaviour, or insufficient cognitive or emotional ability to cooperate in CBT, are indications for including an SRI in the initial treatment. However, youth who have OCD and comorbid conditions may not be as responsive to SSRIs for OCD, as shown in Geller *et al.*[100] study, in which the response rate was 75 per cent in the non-comorbid OCD group, but significantly lower when OCD was comorbid with ADHD (56 per cent), tic disorder (53 per cent), or oppositional defiant disorder (39 per cent); comorbid OCD may also be more vulnerable to relapse with SSRI discontinuation. Although the SSRIs are indicated for OCD, depression, and anxiety disorders, which make them an ideal first drug teatment when OCD is comorbid with an affective disorder, monitoring for the emergence of manic symptoms is required. The treatment of OCD comorbid with ADHD using stimulants may present a challenge because theoretical concerns exist that stimulants may increase obsessional symptoms. However, it is common clinical practice to combine a SSRI (or CMI) with a psychostimulant.[101]

Similar to adult patients, at least one third of young people with OCD prove refractory to treatment, and many 'responders' exhibit only partial response.[11] For children and adolescents who do not seem to benefit from SRI treatment, the first steps are (i) to reevaluate the diagnosis and associated features, and (ii) to review the adequacy of the dose, duration, and compliance with medication. Then, for many youth with a partial response to pharmacotherapy, further improvement may be obtained by adding a concurrent CBT intervention. Furthermore, if a first SSRI trial fails to produce an adequate response, pharmacological algorithms generally recommend switching to a second SSRI. Considering that these drugs all inhibit the 5-HT transporter, the first drug can be discontinued abruptly, and the second initiated at a dose in the middle of its therapeutic range. Because of its longer half-life, if fluoxetine has been the first treatment, it could be stopped abruptly, but the second SSRI must be titrated slowly. If two or three successive trials of SSRIs have failed, clomipramine is generally considered as the next option. Given that it has a half-life in the same range as most of the other SRIs, no time should be wasted in the substitution, unless a switch from fluoxetine is carried out.

Very few drug augmentation or combination strategies have been tested for youth with treatment-resistant OCD. The addition of risperidone to various SRI agents (clomipramine, sertraline, fluoxetine, paroxetine) has been reported in a series of OCD adolescents with no comorbid tic disorder, with only modest benefits.[102] The combination of an SSRI with clomipramine takes advantage of the pharmacokinetic and pharmacodynamic interactions of these medications, but it is important to monitor for adverse effects, particularly cardiovascular side effects, and the possible emergence of a serotonin toxic syndrome. Combining two SSRIs is a common clinical practice, despite the risk for drug interaction, since all SSRIs inhibit cytochrome P-450, and combinations may result in increased blood levels of each SSRI.

If short-term treatment with a SSRI often leaves OCD youth with residual symptoms, over an extended period of SSRI treatment, they may experience greater improvement. Three long-term (1–2 years) open studies have documented continued improvement after the acute phase, but at a much slower rate, with fluvoxamine, sertraline, and citalopram. Similarly, in two continuation studies of clomipramine (4–12 months), treatment continued to be effective and well tolerated. There are hardly any data on the doses of SRIs that should be used in treatment prolongation, versus those used in the acute treatment phase. It would thus be prudent to maintain the regimen that produced the maximal improvement in the acute treatment. The most recent guidelines for adult patients recommend a minimum treatment of one to two years, followed by a gradual taper to, first, avoid discontinuation phenomena and, second, monitor patients for a possible deterioration.[103] In youth, it is particularly recommended to choose a period free of stress (e.g. summer vacation) for tapering medication, and to provide alternative psychological support (CBT, education on relapse risk and management) for the period of discontinuation.

Although tics are a common childhood problem, only a small minority of cases find their way to clinics. Given the waxing and waning nature of tic disorders, usual therapeutic practice will initially focus on careful clinical observation, along with educational and supportive interventions, and pharmacological treatments are held in reserve. The decision about whether and how to treat will depend on the primary diagnosis, and the degree of interference with the child's development and functioning. Most simple tics occurring in the absence of severe functioning impairment respond to a simple explanation of the mechanisms. In case of comorbidity with a mood and anxiety disorder, it is not uncommon to see improvement in tic severity after successful treatment of the affective disorder with a SSRI.[104] When tics are responsible of functional impairment, the decision to use medication follows careful assessment and identification of target symptoms, that are interfering in the patient's quality of life. The selection of medication is based on a balance of risks and benefits, and in order not to expose the subject to excessive unwanted side effects, pharmacological treatment should not aim at complete disappearance of tics. For tics of moderate severity, clonidine or guanfacine may be considered as the first line treatment given their safety margin, and an expected 30 per cent decrease in tic severity may be sufficient. For tics in the marked or severe range, however, more potent medications, such as antipsychotics, that decrease tics severity by 35–60 per cent should be considered, despite the increased risk of adverse effects. In addition, patients with tic disorders and their families should be cautioned about both licit and illicit drug use, since sympathomimetic agents ranging from decongestants through speed and cocaine, markedly exacerbate tics.

For children and adolescents with OCD and comorbid tic disorder, the SSRIs alone might have little anti-obsessional effect, and there are reports suggesting that fluvoxamine and fluoxetine may exacerbate or even induce tics in some patients. The adult literature, and a few case reports of children and youth with OCD and comorbid tic disorder suggest that combined treatment with a SRI and a low dose of risperidone or another atypical antipsychotic is a reasonable option.[105] Using data from the POTS study, March et al.[106] found that tic disorders appeared to adversely impact the outcome of medication management of paediatric OCD, in contrast to CBT outcomes which were not differentially impacted.

Therapeutically, the finding of possible autoimmune cases of OCD and tic disorders raises the clinical possibility that immunosuppressant treatments might be effective, and a few experimental studies have been conducted. A double-blind, placebo-controlled study in resistant cases of PANDAS supported the efficacy of both plasma exchange and intravenous immunoglobulin compared to a sham condition at one month, and the effects were maintained after 1 year for 82 per cent of subjects with follow-up assessment.[107] In another study antibiotic prophylaxis with penicillin or azithromicin was administered for 12 months to a group of children with PANDAS; compared to the year prior to entry in the study, significant decreases were observed in the number of streptococcal infections, and the number of neuropsychiatric exacerbations with both prophylactic treatments.[108] There is preliminary evidence for the efficacy of CBT in OCD cases of the PANDAS phenotype.[109] However, it is still unknown what percentage of children with OCD may be part of the PANDAS subgroup, and neither immunosuppressant nor antibiotic treatments are to be used for such cases out of the context of board-approved research protocols. Nevertheless, children with abrupt onset or exacerbation of OC and/or tic symptoms require careful consideration of medical illnesses including upper respiratory tract infections during the preceding months, to be promptly treated if present. A throat culture and antistreptolysin O or antistreptococcal DNAase B titers may be considered to assist in diagnosing a GABHS infection.[101]

Even if they are less efficacious alone, other treatment modalities should not be neglected. The effectiveness of psychotherapy per se—apart from behavioural and cognitive interventions—on OCD and tic disorders has not been demonstrated, but the symptoms may have a profound impact on the life of subjects affected, and traditional psychotherapeutic approaches may be useful to help children and adolescents address the intrapsychic conflicts that may affect or result from their illness. Some families become extensively involved in participating in compulsive rituals or reassuring obsessional worries, others become mired in gruelling angry struggles with their symptomatic child. Work with families on how to manage the child's symptoms, cope with the stress and family disruption that often accompanies OCD and tic disorders, and participate effectively in behavioural or pharmacological treatment is crucial. Most cognitive behavioural approaches of paediatric OCD include the involvement of a parent in some therapeutic sessions, and it is noteworthy that the Barrett et al.[68] study, which actively involves the family in the child's treatment, reports improvement in the highest range of outcomes among CBT studies. In children with tic disorders, oppositional, defiant, and disruptive behaviours are common, and parenting skill training may be an important adjunctive to treatment. For cases of very incapacitating OCD, there is some empirical evidence that milieu therapy in an inpatient setting may be a useful resource. Finally, the growing availability, in many countries, of family support and advocacy groups for patients with OCD and tic disorders may be most useful to alleviate the discouragement and incomprehension created by these disorders, and give access to appropriate treatment resources.

## Possibilities for prevention

At present, there is no known preventive strategy individually targeted at either OCD or tic disorders. However, early intervention and comprehensive treatment, as long as needed, is certainly the best way to prevent severe incapacitation, and achieve complete recovery in some cases. Even when response to successive treatment efforts is less than optimal, the improvement in function and quality of life may be considerable. In families with one or several cases of OCD or tic disorders, clinicians should be attentive to the onset of similar symptoms in children and siblings, and treat cases of newly occurring disorder early and vigorously. Although this might concern only a fraction of patients, evidence of the onset or exacerbation of OCD or tics associated with streptococcal exposure warrants standard antibiotic treatment and ongoing monitoring for recurrent infection.

## Conclusion

Paediatric OCD is the disorder, in child psychiatry, whose clinical picture most closely resembles its adult counterpart. Despite a relative diversity, the symptom pool is remarkably finite, and very similar to that seen in older individuals. Prevalence, comorbidity, and response to behavioural and drug treatment also appear similar across the lifespan. For tic disorders, there is continuity between child and adult presentations, but the disease is much more prone to resolve spontaneously, or to be less disruptive in adulthood. Both OCD and tics occur more often in males than in females, and are likely to be linked to an array of neurobiological abnormalities, many of which remain to be understood.

Invaluable benefits can now be obtained from available behavioural and pharmacological treatments, but complete remission remains uncertain and long-term management may be required. Thus, the treatment of OCD and tics in children and adolescents remains a clinical challenge. It requires careful assessment of the targeted symptoms and, in many cases, comorbidity; attention to the quality of the child's functioning at home and with peers; use of specific CBT interventions, which are not readily available (or accessible) in all communities; patience and caution in the choice and adjustment of medication; and vigilance in watching potential side effects. Given the possible chronicity of OCD and/or tic disorders, and their changing patterns in severity and impact over the childhood and adolescent years, optimal treatment generally requires a long-term ongoing relationship with the child and family.

Current conceptualizations of OCD and tic disorders have been shaped by advances in systems neuroscience and functional in vivo neuroimaging. Continued success in these areas should lead to the targeting of specific brain circuits for more intensive research. This should include testing novel pharmacological agents, tracking treatment response using neuroimaging techniques, and possibly investigating circuit-based therapies using deep-brain stimulation for refractory cases. The identification of the PANDAS subgroup of patients, with an abrupt onset and dramatic exacerbations, certainly brings new insights into the pathophysiology of OCD and tic disorders, and may lead to new assessment and treatment strategies. The increasing evidence for susceptibility genes in OCD and tic disorders will also doubtless point to new therapeutic directions. Furthermore, it is likely that many of the empirical findings used in research on paediatric OCD and tic disorders will be relevant to a better understanding of both normal development, and other disorders of childhood onset.

## Further information

Obsessive Compulsive Foundation. Available at: http://www.ocfoundation.org
Tourette Syndrome Association. Available at: http://www.tsa-usa.org/index.html
Tourette syndrome online. Available at: http://www.tourette-syndrome.com/default.htm

## References

1. Scahill, L., Riddle, M.A., McSwiggin-Hardin, et al. (1997). Children's Yale-Brown Obsessive-Compulsive Scale: reliability and validity. *Journal of the American Academy of Child and Adolescent Psychiatry*, **36**, 844–52.
2. Stewart, S.E., Rosario, M.C., Brown, T.A., et al. (2007). Principal component analysis of obsessive-compulsive disorder symptoms in children and adolescents. *Biological Psychiatry*, **61**(3), 285–91.
3. Comings, D.E., and Comings, B.G. (1985). Tourette syndrome: clinical and psychological aspects of 250 cases. *American Journal of Human Genetics*, **37**, 435–50.
4. Leckman, J.F., Bloch, M.H., Scahill, L. et al. (2006). Tourette Syndrome: The Self Under Siege. *Journal of Child Neurology*, **21**, 642–49.
5. Leckman, J.F., and Cohen, D.J. (1994). Tic disorders. In *Child and adolescent psychiatry. Modern approaches* (3rd edn) (ed. M. Rutter, E. Taylor and L. Hersov), pp. 455–66. Blackwell Science, Oxford.
6. Swedo, S., Leonard, H.L., Mittleman, B., et al. (1998). Pediatric autoimmune neuropsychiatric disorders associated with streptococcal infections (PANDAS): clinical description of the first 50 cases. *American Journal of Psychiatry*, **155**, 264–71.
7. Riddle, M.A., Scahill, L., King, R., et al. (1990). Obsessive compulsive disorder in children and adolescents: phenomenology and family history. *Journal of the American Academy of Child and Adolescent Psychiatry*, **29**, 766–72.
8. Flament, M.F., Whitaker, A., Rapoport, J.L., et al. (1988). Obsessive compulsive disorder in adolescence: an epidemiological study. *Journal of the American Academy of Child and Adolescent Psychiatry*, **27**, 764–71.
9. Burd, L., Freeman, R., Klug, M., et al. (2006). Variables associated with increased tic severity in 5,500 participants with Tourette Syndrome. *Journal of Developmental & Physical Disabilities*, **18**(1), 13–24.
10. Banaschewski, T., Woerner, W. and Rothenberger, A. (2003). Premonitory sensory phenomena and suppressibility of tics in Tourette syndrome: developmental aspects in children and adolescents. *1: Dev Med Child Neurol*, **45**(10), 700–703.
11. Flament, M.F. and Cohen, D. (2000). Child and adolescent obsessive compulsive disorder. In *Obsessive-Compulsive Disorder: WPA Series Evidence and Experience in Psychiatry – Volume Four* (eds. M. Maj, N. Sartorius), John Wiley & Sons, Chichester, England, pp. 147–83.
12. Burd, L., Kerbeshian, J., Wikenheiser, M., et al. (1986). Related Articles, Links A prevalence study of Gilles de la Tourette syndrome in North Dakota school-age children. *Journal of the American Academy of Child Psychiatry*, **25**(4), 552–3.
13. Snider, L.A., Seligman, L.D., Ketchen, B.R., et al. (2002). Tics and problem behaviors in schoolchildren: prevalence, characterization, and associations. *Pediatrics*, **110**(2 Pt 1), 331–6.

14. Geller, D.A., Biederman, J., Griffin, S., *et al.* (1996). Comorbidity of obsessive–compulsive disorder with disruptive behaviour disorders. *Journal of the American Academy of Child and Adolescent Psychiatry*, **35**, 1637–46.

15. Kano, Y., Ohta, M., and Nagai, Y. (1998). Clinical characteristics of Tourette syndrome. *Psychiatry and Clinical Neuroscience*, **52**, 51–7.

16. Leckman, J.F. (1993). Tourette's syndrome. In *Obsessive compulsive related disorders* (ed. E. Hollander), pp. 113–37. American Psychiatric Press, Washington, DC.

17. Leonard, H.L., Lenane, M.C., Swedo, S.E., *et al.* (1992). Tics and Tourette's disorder. A 2-to 7-year follow-up study of 54 obsessive–compulsive children. *American Journal of Psychiatry*, **149**, 1244–51.

18. Leckman, J.F., McDougle, C.J., Pauls, D.L., *et al.* (2000). Tic–related vs non-tic related obsessive compulsive disorder. In *Obsessive compulsive disorders: contemporary issues in treatment* (ed. W.K. Goodman, J.D. Maser, and M.V. Rudorfer), pp. 43–68. Erlbaum, Hillsdale, NJ.

19. Geller, D.A., Biederman, J., Jones, J. *et al.* (1998). Is juvenile obsessive-compulsive disorder a developmental subtype of the disorder? A review of the pediatric literature. *Journal of the American Academy of Child and Adolescent Psychiatry*, **37**(4), 420–27.

20. Pollock, R. and Carter, A. (1999). The familiar and developmental content of obsessive-compulsive disorder. *Child Adoles Psychiatry*, **33**, 2–15.

21. Kumar, R., and Lang, A. (1997). Secondary tic disorders. *Neurologic Clinics of North America*, **15**, 309–30.

22. Scahill, L., Tanner, C. and Dure, L. (2001). The epidemiology of tics and Tourette syndrome in children and adolescent, in Tourette Syndrome and Associated Disorders. *Advances in Neurology Seriews*, **85**, 261–71.

23. Apter, A., Pauls, D., Zohar, A.H., *et al.* (1993). An epidemiologic study of Gilles de la Tourette in Israel. *Archives of General Psychiatry*, **50**, 734–38.

24. Peterson, B.S., Pine, D.S., Cohen, P. *et al.* (2001). Prospective, longitudinal study of tic, obsessive compulsive, and attention-deficit/hyper activity disorders in an epidemiological sample. *Journal of the American Academy of Child and Adolescent Psychiatry*, **40**, 685–95.

25. Heyman, I., Fombonne, E., Simmons, H., *et al.* (2001). Prevelence of obsessive-compulsive disorder in the British Nationwide Survey of Child Mental Health. *British Journal of Psychiatry*, **179**, 324–9.

26. Zohar, A.H., Ratzosin, G., Pauls, D.L., *et al.* (1992). An epidemiological study of obsessive-compulsive disorder and related disorders in Israeli adolescent. *Journal of the American Academy of Child and Adolescent Psychiatry*, **31**, 1057–61.

27. Reinherz, H.Z., Giaconia, R.M., Lefkowitz, E.S., *et al.* (1993). Prevalence of psychiatric disorders in a community population of older adolescents. *Journal of the American Academy of Child and Adolescent Psychiatry*, **32**, 369–77.

28. Douglass, H.M., Moffitt, T.E., Reuven, D., *et al.* (1995). Obsessive–compulsive disorder in a birth cohort of 18-year-olds: prevalence and predictors. *Journal of the American Academy of Child and Adolescent Psychiatry*, **34**, 1424–31.

29. Lin, H., Katsovich, L., Ghebremichael, M. *et al.* (2007). Psychosocial stress predicts future symptom severities in children and adolescents with Tourette syndrome and/or obsessive-compulsive disorder. *JF. 1: Journal of Child Psychology and Psychiatry, and Allied Disciplines*, **48**(2), 157–66.

30. Flament, M.F., Rapoport, J.L., Murphy, D.L., *et al.* (1987). Biochemical changes during clomipramine treatment of childhood obsessive compulsive disorder. *Archives of General Psychiatry*, **44**, 219–25.

31. Sallee, F.R., Richman, H., Beach, K., *et al.* (1996). Platelet serotonin transporter in children and adolescents with obsessive–compulsive disorder or Tourette's syndrome. *Journal of the American Academy of Child and Adolescent Psychiatry*, **35**, 1647–56.

32. Serra-Mestres, J., Ring, H.A., Costa, D.C. *et al.* (2004). Related Articles, Links Dopamine transporter binding in Gilles de la Tourette syndrome: a [123I]FP-CIT/SPECT study. *Acta Psychiatr Scand*, **109**(2), 140–6.

33. Singer, H.S., Szymanski, S., Giuliano, J. *et al.* (2002). Elevated intrasynaptic dopamine release in Tourette's syndrome measured by PET. *1: American Journal of Psychiatry*, **159**(8), 1329–36.

34. Wong, D.F., Singer, H.S., Brandt, J. *et al.* (1997). D2-like dopamine receptor density in Tourette syndrome measured by PET. *1: Journal of Nuclear Medicine*, **38**(8), 1243–7.

35. Heinz, A., Knable, M.B., Wolf, S.S. *et al.* (1998). Tourette's syndrome: [I-123]beta-CIT SPECT correlates of vocal tic severity. *1: Neurology*, **51**(4), 1069–74.

36. Rasmussen, S.A., and Tsuang, M.T. (1984). The epidemiology of obsessivecompulsive disorder. *Journal of Clinical Psychiatry*, 45, 450–7.

37. Price, R.A., Kidd, K.K., Cohen, D.J., *et al.* (1985). A twin study of Tourette syndrome. *Archives of General Psychiatry*, **42**, 815–20.

38. Lenane, M. (1989). Families in obsessive-compulsive disorder. Rapoport, J. L. Obsessive-compulsive disorder in children and adolescents. Washington DC: American Psychiatric Press, pp. 237–49.

39. Pauls, D., Alsobrook, J., Goodman, W., *et al.* (1995). A family study of obsessive–compulsive disorder. *American Journal of Psychiatry*, **152**, 76–84.

40. Tourette Syndrome International Consortium for Genetics (1999). A complete genome screen in sib-pairs affected with Gilles de la Tourette syndrome. *American Journal of Human Genetics*, **65**, 1428–36.

41. Merette, C., Brassard, A., Potvin, A., *et al.* (2000). Significant linkage for Tourette syndrome in a large French Canadian family. *American Journal of Human Genetics*, **67**, 1008–13.

42. Dickel, D.E., Veenstra-VanderWeele, J., Chiu Bivens, N., *et al.* (2007). Association studies of serotonin system candidate genes in early-onset obsessive-compulsive disorder. *Biological Psychiatry*, **61**, 322–9.

43. Arnold, P.D., Sicard, T., Burroughs, E., *et al.* (2006). Glutamate transporter gene SLC1A1 associated with obsessivecompulsive disorder. *Archives of General Psychiatry*, **63**(7), 769–76.

44. State, M., Greally, J.M., Cuker, *et al.* (2003). Epigenetic abmormalities associated with a chromosome 18(q21–q22) inversion and a Gilles de la Tourette syndrome phenotype. *Proceedings of the National Academy of Sciences of the United States of America*, **100**, 4684–9.

45. Mathews, C.A., Bimson, B., Lowe, T.L., *et al.* (2006). Association between maternal smoking and increased symptom severity in Tourette's syndrome. *Reus VI. 1: American Journal of Psychiatry*, **63**(6), 1066–73.

46. Rapoport, J.L. (1989). The neurobiology of obsessive compulsive disorder. *Journal of the American Medical Association*, **260**, 2888–90.

47. Flament, M.F., Koby, E., Rapoport, J.L., *et al.* (1990). Childhood obsessive–compulsive disorder: a prospective follow–up study. *Journal of Child Psychology and Psychiatry*, **31**, 363–80.

48. Baxter, L.R. (1998). Functional imaging of brain systems mediating obsessive-compulsive disorder. In *Neurobiology of Mental Illness* (eds. *E.J. Charney, E.J. Nestler, B.S. Bunney*), 534–47.

49. Evans, D.W., Lewis, M.D. and Iobst, E., (2004). The role of the orbitofrontal cortex in normally developing compulsive-like behaviors and obsessive-compulsive disorder. *Brain and cognition*, **55**, 220–34.

50. Baxter, L.R., Jr., Schwatrz, J.M., Bergman, K.S., *et al.* (1992). Caudate glucose metabolic rate changes with both drug and behavior therapy for obsessive-compulsive disorder. *Archives of General Psychiatry*, **49**, 681–9.

51. Swedo, S.E., Pietrini, P., Leonard, H.L., *et al.* (1992) Cerebral glucose metabolism in childhood on-set obsessive compulsive disorder. Revisualization during pharmacotherapy. *Archives of General Psychiatry*, **49**, 690–4.

52. Szeszko, P.R., MacMillan, S., McMeniman, M., *et al.* (2004). Brain structural abnormalities in psychotropic drug-naïve pediatric patients with obsessive-compulsive disorder. *Journal of the American Academy of Child and Adolescent Psychiatry*, **161**, 1049–56.

53. Giedd, J.N., Rapoport, J.L., Garvey, M.A., *et al.* (2000). MRI assessment of children with obsessive-compulsive disorder or tics associated with

streptococcal infection. *Journal of the American Academy of Child and Adolescent Psychiatry,* **157**, 281–3.

54. Russell, A., Cortese, B., Lorch, E., *et al.* (2003). Localized functional neurochemical marker abnormalities in dorsolateral prefrontal cortex in pediatric obsessive-compulsive disorder. *Journal of child and adolescent psychopharmacology,* **13**, S31–S38.

55. Peterson, B.S., Thomas, P., Kane, M.J., *et al.* (2003). Basal Ganglia volumes in patients with Gilles de la Tourette syndrome. *Archives of General Psychiatry,* **60**(4), 415–24.

56. Hyde, T., Aaronson, B., Randolph, C., *et al.* (1992). Relationship of birth weight to the phenotypic expression of Gilles de la Tourette's syndrome in monozygotic twins. *Neurology,* **42**, 652.

57. Peterson, B.S., Staib, L., Scahill, L. *et al.* (2001b). Regional brain and ventricular volumes in Tourette syndrome. *Archives of General Psychiatry,* **58**(5), 427–40.

58. Amat, J.A., Bronen, R.A., Saluja, S. *et al.* (2006). Increased number of subcortical hyperintensities on MRI in children and adolescents with Tourette's syndrome, obsessive-compulsive disorder, and attention deficit hyperactivity disorder. *American Journal of Psychiatry,* **163**(6), 1106–08.

59. Rapoport, J.L., and Fiske, A. (1998). The new biology of obsessive compulsive disorder: implications for evolutionary psychology. *Perspectives in Biology and Medicine,* **41**, 159–75.

60. Swedo, S.E., Leonard, H.L., Schapiro, M.B., *et al.* (1993). Sydenham's chorea: physical and psychological symptoms of St Vitus Dance. *Pediatrics,* **91**, 706–13.

61. Asbarh, F.R., Negrao, A.B., Gentil, V., *et al.* (1998). Obsessive-compulsive and related symptoms in children and adolesdents with rheumatic fever with and without chorea: a prospective 6-month study. *American Journal of Psychiatry,* **155**, 1122–4.

62. Murphy, T., Goodman, W., Fudge, M., *et al.* (1997). B lymphocyte antigen D8/17: a peripheral marker for childhood onset obsessive-compulsive disorder and Tourette's syndrome? *American Journal of Psychiatry,* **154**, 402–7.

63. Swedo, S.E., Leonard, H., Mittleman, B., *et al.* (1997). Identification of children with pediatric autoimmune neuropsychiatric disorders associated with streptococcal infections by a marker associated with rheumatic fever. *American Journal of Psychiatry,* **154**, 110–12.

64. Stewart, S.E., Gellar, D.A., Jenkie, M., *et al.* (2004). Long-term outcome of pediatric obsessive-compulsive disorder: a meta-analysis and qualitative review of the literature. *Acta Psychiatrica Scandinavica,* **110**(1), 4–13.

65. Bruun, R.D., and Budman, C.L., (1993). The natural history of Gilles de la Tourette's syndrome. In *Handbook of Tourette's syndrome and related tic and behavioural disorders* (ed. R. Kurlan). Dekker, New York.

66. March, J.S., Franklin, M., Nelson, A., *et al.* (2001). Cognitive-behavioral psychotherapy for pediatric obsessive-compulsive disorder. *Journal of clinical child psychology,* **30**(1), 8–18.

67. March, J.S. and Mulle, K. (1998). OCD in Children and Adolescent. *A Cognitive-Behavioral Treatment Manual.* New York, Guilford Press.

68. Barrett, P.M., Healy-Farrell, L. and March, J.S. (2004). Cognitive-behavioral family treatment of childhood obsessive-compulsive disorder: a controlled trial. *Journal of the American Academy of Child and Adolescent Psychiatry,* **43**(1), 46–62.

69. Barrett, P., Farrell, L., Dadds, M., *et al.* (2005). Cognitive-behavioral family treatment of childhood obsessive-compulsive disorder: long-tern follow-up and predictors of outcome. **44**(10), 1005–14.

70. Verdellen, C., Keijsers, G., Cath, D., *et al.* (2004). Hoogduin Exposure with response prevention versus habit reversal in Tourettes's syndrome: a controlled study, *Behaviour Research and Therapy,* **42**, 501–11.

71. O'Connor, K.P., Brault, S., Robillard, J., *et al.* (2001). Stip Evaluation of a cognitive-behavioural program for the management of chronic tic and habit disorders. *Behaviour Research and Therapy,* **39**, 667–81.

72. Cook, C.R. and Blacher, J. (2007). Evidence-Based Psychosocial Treatments for Tic Disorders. *Clinical Psychology: Science and Practice,* **14**(3), 252–67.

73. Flament, M.F., Rapoport, J.L., and Kilts, C. (1985). A Controlled Trial of Clomipramine in Childhood Obsessive Compulsive Disorder. *Psychopharmacology Bulletin,* **21**(1), 150–152.

74. Leonard, H.L., Swedo, S.E., Rapoport, J.L., *et al.* (1989). Treatment of Obsessive-Compulsive Disorder With Clomipramine and Desipramine in Children and Adolescents. A Double-Blind Crossover Comparison. *Archives of General Psychiatry,* **46**(12), 1088–92.

75. DeVeaugh-Geiss, J., Moroz, G., Biederman, J., *et al.* (1992). Clomipramine Hydrochloride in Childhood and Adolescent Obsessive-Compulsive Disorder–a Multicenter Trial. *Journal of the American Academy of Child and Adolescent Psychiatry,* **31**(1), 45–9.

76. Riddle, M.A., Scahill, L., King, R.A., *et al.* (1992). Double-Blind, Crossover Trial of Fluoxetine and Placebo in Children and Adolescents With Obsessive-Compulsive Disorder. *Journal of the American Academy of Child and Adolescent Psychiatry,* **31**(6), 1062–69.

77. Riddle, M.A., Reeve, E.A., Yaryura-Tobias, J.A., *et al.* (2001). Fluvoxamine for Children and Adolescents With Obsessive-Compulsive Disorder: a Randomized, Controlled, Multicenter Trial. *Journal of the American Academy of Child and Adolescent Psychiatry,* **40**(2), 222–9.

78. Liebowitz, M.R., Turner, S.M., Piacentini, J., *et al.* (2002). Fluoxetine in Children and Adolescents With OCD: a Placebo-Controlled Trial. *Journal of the American Academy of Child and Adolescent Psychiatry,* **41**(12), 1431–38.

79. Geller, D.A., Wagner, K.D., Emsile, G., *et al.* (2004). Paroxetine Treatment in Children and Adolescents With Obsessive-Compulsive Disorder: a Randomized, Multicenter, Double-Blind, Placebo-Controlled Trial. *Journal of the American Academy of Child and Adolescent Psychiatry,* **43**(11), 1387–96.

80. Flament, M.F., Geller, D. and Blier, P. (2007). Specifi cities of treatment in pediatric obsessive-compulsive disorder. *CNS Spectrum,* **12**(2), 43–57.

81. Geller, D.A., Biederman, J., Stewart, S.E., *et al.* (2003a). Which SSRI? A meta-analysis of pharmacotherapy trials in pediatric obsessivecompulsive disorder. *American Journal of Psychiatry,* **160**(11), 1919–28.

82. De Haan, E., Hoogduin, K.A., Buitleaar, J.K., *et al.* (1998). Behavior Therapy Versus Clomipramine for the Treatment of Obsessive-Compulsive Disorder in Children and Adolescents *Journal of the American Academy of Child & Adolescent Psychiatry,* **37**(10), 1022–9.

83. Pediatric OCD Treatment Study (POTS). (2004) Cognitive behavior therapy, setraline, and their combination for children and adolescents with obsessive-compulsive disorder: the Pediatric OCD Treatment Study (POTS) randomized controlled trial. *JAMA,* **292**(16), 1969–76.

84. Ashbar, F.R., Castillo, A.R., Ito, L.M., *et al.* (2005). Group cognitive-behavioral therapy versus setraline for the treatment of children and adolescents with obsessivecompulsive disorder. *Journal of the American Academy of Child and Adolescent Psychiatry,* **44**(11), 1128–36.

85. Blier, P., Habib, R. and Flament, M.F. (2006). Pharmacotherapies in the management of obsessive-compulsive disorder. *Canadian Journal of Psychiatry,* **51**(7), 417–30.

86. Leonard, H.L., Meyer, M.C., Swedo, S.E. *et al.* (1995). Electrocardiographic changes during desiprime and clomipramine treatment in children and adolescents. *Journal of the American Academy of Child and Adolescent Psychiatry,* **34**(11), 1460–8.

87. Varley, C.K. (2001). Sudden death related to selected tricyclic antidepressants in children: epidemiology, mechanisms and clinical implications. *Pediatric Drugs,* **3**(8), 613–27.

88. Hammerness, P.G., Vivas, F.M. and Gellar, D.A. (2006). Selective serotonin reuptake in pediatric psychopharmacology: a review of the evidence. *Journal of pediatrics,* **148**(2), 158–65.

89. Nilsson, O., Jakobsen, A.M., Bernhardt, P., *et al.* (2004). Importance of vesicle proteins in the diagnosis and treatment of neuroendocrine tumors. *Annals of the New York Academy of Sciences,* **1014**, 240–83.

90. Hammad, T.A., Laughren, T. and Racoosin, J. (2006). Suicidality in pediatric patients treated with antidepressant drugs. *Archives of General Psychiatry*, **63**(3), 332–9.

91. Bridge, J.A., Iyengar, S., Salary, C.B., *et al.* (2007). Clinical response and risk for reported suicidal ideation and suicide attempts in pediatric antidepressant treatment: a meta-analysis of randominzed controlled trials. *JAMA*, **297**(15), 1683–96.

92. Shapiro, E., Shapiro, A.K., Fulop, G., *et al.* (1989). Controled study of haloperidol, pimozide, and placebo for the treatment of Gilles de la Tourette's syndrome. *Archives of General Psychiatry*, **46**, 722–30.

93. Dion, Y., Annable, L., Sandor, P., *et al.* (2002). Risperidone in the treatment of tourette syndrome: a double-blind, placebo-controlled trial. *Journal of Clinical Psychopharmacology*, **22**, 31–9.

94. Scahill, L., Leckman, J.F., Schultz, R.T., *et al.* (2003). A placebo-controlled trial of risperidone in Tourette syndrome. *Neurology*, **60**, 1130–5.

95. Bruggemann, R., van der Linden, C., Buitelarr, J.K., *et al.* (2001). Risperidone versus pimozide in Tourette's syndrome: a comparative double-blind parrallel group study. *Journal of Clinical Psychaitry*, **62**, 50–56.

96. Gilbert, D.L., Batterson, J.R., Sethuraman, G., *et al.* (2004). Tic reduction with risperidone versus pimozide in a randomized, doubleblind, crossover trial. *Journal of the American Academy of Child and Adolescent Psychiatry*, **43**, 206–14.

97. Desta, Z., Kerbusch, T. and Flockhart, D.A. (1999). Effect of clarithromycin on the pharmacodynamics of pimozide in healthy poor and extensive metabolizers of cytochrome P450 2D6 (CYP2D6). *Clinical pharmacology and therapeutics*, **65**, 10–20.

98. American Academy of Child and Adolescent Psychiatry (1997). Practice parameters for the assessment and treatment of children, adolescents, and adults with attention-deficit hyperactivity disorder. *Journal of the American Academy of Child and Adolescent Psychiatry*, **36**, 85S–121S.

99. Tourette Syndrome Study Group (2002). Treatment of ADHD in children with tics: a randomized controlled trial. *Neurology*, **58**, 527–36.

100. Geller, D.A., Biederman, J., Stewart, S.E. *et al.* (2003b). Impact of Comorbidity on Treatment Response to Paroxetine in Pediatric Obsessive-Compulsive Disorder: Is the Use of Exclusion Criteria Empirically Supported in Randomized Clinical Trials? *Journal of Child and Adolescent sychopharmacology*, **13** (Supplement 1), S19–S29.

101. American Academy for Child Adolescent Psychiatry (1998). Practice parameters for the assessment and treatment of children and adolescents with obsessive-compulsive disorder. *Journal of the American Academy of Child and Adolescent Psychiatry*, **37**(10), 27S–45S.

102. Thomsen, P.H. (2004). Risperidone augmentation in the treatment of severe adolescent OCD in SSRI-refractory cases: a case series. *Annals of Clinical Psychiatry*, **16**(4), 201–7.

103. Baldwin, D.S., Anderson, I.M., Nutt, D.J., *et al.* (2005). Evidence based guidelines for the pharmacological treatment of anxiety disorders: recommendations from the British Association for Psychopharmacology. *Journal of psychopharmacology*, **19**, 567–96.

104. Reinblatt, S., Walkup, J.T. (2005). Psychopharmacological treatment of pediatric anxiety disorders. *Child and Adolescent Psychiatric Clinics of North America*, **14**, 877–908.

105. Fitzgerlad, K.D., MacMaster, F.P., Paulson, L.D., *et al.* (1999). Neurobiology of childhood obsessive-compulsive disorder. *Child and Adolescent Psychiatric Clinics of North America*, **8**(3), 533–75.

106. March, J.S., Franklin, M.E., Leonard, H., *et al.* (2007). Tics moderate treatment outcome with sertraline but not cognitive-behavior therapy in pediatric obsessive-compulsive disorder. *Biological Psychiatry*, **61**(3), 344–7.

107. Perlmutter, S.J., Leitmen, S.F., Garvey, M.A., *et al.* (1999). Therapeutic plasma exchange and intravenous immunoglobulin for obsessivecompulsive disorders in childhood. *Lancet*, **354**, 1153–8.

108. Snider, L.A., Lougee, L., Slattery, M., *et al.* (2005). Antibiotic prophylaxis with azithromycin or penicillin for childhood-onset neuropsychiatric disorders. *Biological Psychiatry*, **57**(7), 788–92.

109. Storch, E.A., Murphy, T.K., Geffken, G.R., *et al.* (2006). Cognitive-behavioral therapy for PANDAS-related obsessive-compulsive disorder: findings from a preliminary waitlist controlled open trial. *Journal of the American Academy of Child and Adolescent Psychiatry*, **45**(10), 1171–8.

# 9.2.9 Sleep disorders in children and adolescents

Gregory Stores

## Introduction

It was argued in Chapter 4.14.1 that sleep disorders medicine should be viewed as an integral part of psychiatry, whatever the age group of patients, because of the various close connections between sleep disturbance and psychological disorders seen in clinical practice. This is certainly the case regarding child and adolescent psychiatry in view of the high rates of psychiatric disorder of which sleep disturbance is often a part, and also the frequent occurrence of sleep disorders in young people with potentially serious developmental effects of a psychological and sometimes physical nature. The temptation to view children's sleep disorders as merely transitory problems, mainly in infancy, encountered by many parents and of no lasting or serious significance, should be resisted. This may be true for some families but is frequently not the case in others.

The following account summarizes sleep disorders in childhood and adolescence. *Familiarity is assumed with the earlier accounts of sleep disorders in adults (4.14.1), including the introduction to that section which covers basic aspects of sleep and other fundamental issues.*

## Sleep and sleep disorders in children compared to adults

In spite of the fact that much has now been discovered about the special characteristics of sleep disorders occurring at an early age, very little of this information has found its way into the training of paediatricians, child and adolescent psychiatrists, psychologists, or other professionals involved in the care of children. This must mean that many treatment and preventive possibilities are missed.

The solution does not lie simply in extending the practice of adult sleep disorders medicine to children. Children are not miniature adults and they need special approaches reflecting their many differences from older patients. These differences extend from basic features of sleep to various aspects of sleep disorders.

### Sleep physiology

Profound changes take place during childhood in basic sleep physiology although many are complete by about 6–12 months of age. In general, there is a progression towards differentiation and organization of conventionally defined sleep states, shorter sleep time, less napping, less slow wave sleep (**SWS**), and longer sleep cycles.

Specific aspects of particular clinical importance are as follows:

♦ Typical sleep duration (including naps) at different ages as shown in Table 9.2.9.1.

**Table 9.2.9.1** Average sleep requirements at different ages

| Term birth | 17 h |
|------------|------|
| 1 year | 14 h |
| 2 years | 13 h |
| 4 years | 12 h |
| 10 years | 10 h |
| Adolescence | 9 h plus* |

*Many adolescents are thought to obtain far less sleep than this.

◆ The body clock controlling (amongst other processes) the circadian sleep–wake cycle has become established by about 6 months.

◆ Rapid eye movement (**REM**) sleep is prominent in early infancy, perhaps reflecting its role in brain maturation and early learning, and possibly explaining why sleep is fragile at this stage.

◆ In comparison, by early childhood **SWS** is especially pronounced. This predisposes children of that age to arousal disorders (e.g. sleepwalking) which arise from **SWS**.

◆ Between about 5 years and puberty, overnight sleep is especially sound and alertness is maximal during the day. Various conditions causing excessive daytime sleepiness in adults (e.g. narcolepsy) may not have this effect in children because of this increased alertness. However, overnight sleep may become extended.

◆ In contrast, adolescence is characterized by an increase in daytime sleepiness. The amount of **SWS** decreases, the sleep phase is physiologically delayed and, with the onset of puberty, there is no longer the decrease in physiological sleep requirements seen progressively at earlier ages. The combination of these factors and strong influences to stay up late (especially at weekends but perhaps also during the week) for social and recreational purposes frequently causes unsatisfactory sleep–wake patterns.

## Parental influences

The influence of parents is seen throughout children's sleep disorders medicine.

◆ Especially in the case of young children, parents' perceptions usually determine whether there is a sleep problem. The same sleep pattern or behaviour may be a problem to one family but not another. Factors influencing parental attitudes include their expectations, family and cultural practices (e.g. regarding parents and children sleeping together), and their own emotional state. Sometimes parents can be reassured that what they think is a serious problem about their child's sleep is, in fact, within the normal range. The view taken of the situation might be the result of parental psychiatric illness needing attention in its own right; children of mothers with an affective illness have been shown to have an increased rate and severity of sleep problems although the nature of the connection is debatable.

◆ Conversely, parents may not seek help for their child's sleep when they ought to do. They may be unaware of the problem, indifferent, or they may mistakenly believe that the child's sleep problem is inevitable and untreatable. This mistaken view is sometimes expressed by parents of children with a learning disability (intellectual disability) whose sleep problems can be particularly severe yet amenable to treatment.

◆ Parental practices are commonly the reason why a child's sleep problem develops or is maintained. Early child-rearing practices determine sleep–wake patterns which can be delayed or disrupted by over-conscientious night-time feeding in infancy, failure to set limits on bedtime activities, or inconsistency (see later). Sleep disorders of physical origin may be complicated in these ways and exacerbated. It follows that treatment of many sleep disorders relies heavily on correcting parenting practices.

◆ Sometimes parents are not motivated to improve their child's sleep for reasons that may be difficult to influence. For example, a child's presence in the parental bed may be welcome by one partner as a means of distancing himself or herself from the other at night. Families of handicapped children may lose their extra state financial allowance if their child's sleep problems are successfully treated.

◆ The child's basic attitude to sleeping is also influenced by its parents. Wider cultural factors are important but, within westernized societies, the child's attitudes to going to sleep and being separated from its parents at night are strongly influenced by their ability to settle the child without being anxious about the separation. Children depend on their parents to provide positive attitudes to sleeping and to avoid negative associations such as disputes, punishment, and rejection.

◆ Especially in the early years, most children need their parents' help in coping with night-time separation from them, and the potentially frightening experience of the dark or their own thoughts and fantasies. Infants need the comfort of physical contact. Toddlers are helped by bedtime routines and comforting 'transitional objects', and encouragement to become 'self-soothing' so that they can fall asleep without their parents' presence and attention (see later). Parents' ability to provide such help depends on their personality and sensitivity and mental state and perhaps their cognitions about their child's sleep based partly on their own experiences in childhood. Hopefully, older children and adolescents become increasingly independent.

## Effects on parenting and the family

The effects of a child's persistent sleep disturbance on family life, including its possible influence on parenting skills, is another important dimension.

◆ Mothers of children with a learning disability and severe sleep problems are reported to be more irritable, concerned about their own health, and less affectionate towards their children, with less control and increased use of punishment compared with mothers of such children without sleep problems. Similarly, associations have also been suggested between sleeplessness in toddlers in the general population and family problems, including marital discord and possibly physical abuse of the child.

◆ Family tensions are likely to increase when diagnosis of the child's sleep disorder is delayed or inaccurate, or when effective treatment is not provided.

◆ Some reports have suggested that successful treatment of the child's sleep problems generally leads to improvement in the mother's mental state, confidence in her own parenting ability, her relationship with the child, and also the child's behaviour. Wider aspects of family function, including effects on siblings, have received little attention.

## Developmental effects of sleep disturbance

◆ These parental and wider family issues indicate ways in which a child's psychological and social development can be affected by persistent sleep disturbance. In addition, children can be distressed by their experience of sleep disorder phenomena. Examples include night-time fears (which may be intense) alarming hypnagogic imagery, or sleepwalking and sleep (night) terrors which can be embarrassing, especially if they occur away from home. Excessive daytime sleepiness often leads to educational problems and can produce extreme reactions such as the denial, aggression or depression described in narcolepsy, or accidents and substance abuse in adolescence.

◆ In addition to these largely indirect ways in which a child's sleep disorder may have psychological effects, sleep disturbance can produce direct effects on mood, behaviour, and cognitive function. The developmental consequences might become severe if not arrested at an early age.

◆ Adolescents appear to be at particular risk of sleep loss and its possible psychological consequences, i.e. depressed mood, anxiety, behaviour problems, alcohol abuse, and even attempted suicide, as well as lower academic performance. The causal relationship between sleep loss and these problems, however, have yet to be fully established. The same is true of the outcome of attempts to correct this sleep loss by various means.

◆ Even impairment of physical growth is associated with sleep disturbance. Failure to thrive is a recognized possible consequence of early onset obstructive sleep apnoea (**OSA**) and possibly other severe and persistent sleep disturbance, perhaps as a result of reduced slow wave sleep (**SWS**) with which the production of growth hormone is closely linked.

◆ Other possible physical consequences of sleep disruption includes impaired immunity and endocrine disorders.

## Patterns of occurrence of sleep disorders

◆ Some sleep behaviours which are developmentally usual in children are abnormal in adults and require investigation. Examples are bedwetting and repeated napping. Certain sleep disorders are seen exclusively in children (e.g. sleeplessness caused by infantile colic). Others, such as settling problems and confusion arousals, occur primarily in children (see later).

◆ Sleeplessness caused mainly by child-rearing practices is particularly common in early childhood. That attributable to the delayed sleep phase syndrome (see later) is considered to be particularly common in adolescence.

◆ Many of the parasomnias (such as headbanging, sleepwalking, or sleep terrors) are more common in childhood where, generally, they represent a temporary developmental phase without pathological significance. The same behaviours in adults might be more likely to be manifestations of psychological problems requiring exploration.

◆ Some sleep disorders thought to be confined to adulthood are now recognized in children. While much attention has been paid to OSA in adults, it is now thought that at least 2 per cent of children have this condition to some degree. Restless leg syndrome (**RLS**) and periodic limb movements in sleep (**PLMS**) are now known to occur not uncommonly in children. The RLS may explain some cases of 'growing pains'. PLMS has been implicated as a cause of poor quality sleep resulting (as in other forms of sleep disturbance) with daytime attention deficit hyperactivity disorder (**ADHD**) type of symptoms. Narcolepsy starts by the age of 15 years in at least one-third of cases. Even REM sleep behaviour disorder (once thought to be confined to elderly males), or something similar, has been reported in children and adolescents.

## Manifestations of sleep disorders

◆ The clinical features of basically the same sleep disorder can be very different in children compared with older people. The overall behavioural effects of excessive sleepiness in adults are a reduction of physical and mental activity. In contrast, its effects in young children can be increased activity with irritability, tantrums, or other behavioural difficulties. Some examples of ADHD are thought to be the result of sleep disorders (OSA, PLMS, or circadian sleep–wake rhythm disorder) with improvement in the difficult behaviour following treatment of the sleep disorder.

◆ OSA illustrates the important differences between children and adults, not only in the clinical manifestations of a particular sleep disorder but also in the underlying cause and treatment needs. Similarly the many manifestations of narcolepsy in childhood may be very far removed from the classical narcolepsy syndrome in adults, at least in its fully developed form. The same sleep disorder may also show different physiological features according to age. Diagnostic criteria (e.g. for OSA and narcolepsy) derived from polysomnographic (PSG) studies in adults do not necessarily apply in children and may well need modification.

## Misinterpretation of children's sleep disorders

Chapter 4.14.1 contains an account of the fundamental issue that, especially if clinicians are unfamiliar with the manifestations and consequences of the many sleep disorders now documented in the second edition of the International Classification of Sleep Disorders (ICSD-2), there is a serious risk that these disorders will be misconstrued as something else (or even overlooked completely). The examples given include a number of particular relevance to practice in child psychiatry and paediatrics.[1]

## Treatment and prognosis

◆ Because of the aetiological differences discussed earlier, especially parental involvement, treatment often needs to be very different in children compared to adults. Appropriate behavioural approaches usually entail alterations to parenting practices designed to be acceptable and feasible in each individual family. Other forms of treatment, including chronobiological measures (such as adjustment of sleep schedules from the delayed sleep phase syndrome in adolescence) usually require considerable parental involvement. The same is true of the general sleep hygiene principles described in Chapter 4.14.2. Explanation and (where appropriate) reassurance for the child and parents is an essential part of any treatment and may be effective in their own right without the need for more specific measures. As in adults, medication has a limited part to play overall.

♦ An optimistic point of view can be taken of the treatment of most children's sleep disorders because children's sleep is usually more amenable to change than that of adults where the factors underlying the sleep problem may well have become well established and complicated, as in many cases of chronic insomnia. However, treatment needs to be chosen carefully and implemented properly, and parents' confidence in the recommended measures, and their willingness and ability to play their part in treatment, are an important determinant of success or failure. In some instances, it is not possible to implement a treatment programme for the child until parents themselves have been helped (e.g. by treatment for a depressive illness) or problems in the family as a whole have been resolved.

## Assessment

The various means by which sleep disorders might generally be detected and assessed are described in Chapter 4.14.1. These subjective and objective approaches need to be modified for use with children because of the involvement of parents, developmental factors, and the differences between children and adults regarding clinical manifestations and diagnostic criteria.

The detection of sleep problems can be improved by routinely asking basic screening questions as part of the history-taking in any child:

♦ Does the child have difficulty getting to sleep or staying asleep?

♦ Is there excessive sleepiness during the day?

♦ Are there episodes of abnormal behaviour or experiences at night?

Positive answers to any of these questions call for a detailed sleep history.

### Sleep history and general review

This is the cornerstone of sleep assessment. Unfortunately, history-taking schedules are usually perfunctory in the attention they pay to sleep and its possible disorders. Parents and also the child (if old enough) should be interviewed and the reasons for any disparities considered. Sometimes sibs or teachers can provide important additional information. The main aspects that should be covered are as follows:

♦ Current sleep problems and their evolution.

♦ Past treatments and their effects.

♦ Review of the child's current 24 h sleep–wake cycle (see Table 9.2.9.2) in order to determine in particular

  (a) duration of sleep

  (b) quality of sleep (continuous or disrupted)

  (c) timing of sleep

  (d) features suggestive of specific sleep disorders (e.g. breathing difficulty or jerking limbs).

♦ Sleep environment and arrangements.

♦ Development of the child's sleep patterns and problems.

**Table 9.2.9.2** Review of child's 24 h sleep–wake pattern (modified according to child's age)

| |
|---|
| **Evening** |
| Time of evening meal |
| Other evening activities |
| **Going to bed** |
| Preparation for bed, by whom |
| Time of going to bed |
| Reluctance to go at required time, parents' reactions |
| Fears, rituals |
| Wanting to sleep with someone, other comforts |
| Time taken to fall asleep, other experiences during that period |
| **When asleep** |
| Wakings, frequency, causes ability to return to sleep |
| Episodic events, exact nature, timing, frequency |
| Other behaviours during sleep, e.g. snoring, restlessness, bedwetting |
| Parents' reaction to night-time events |
| **Waking** |
| Wakes spontaneously or needs to be woken up |
| Time of final waking |
| Total duration of sleep period |
| Longest period of uninterrupted sleep |
| On waking: preoccupations, mood, feeling of being refreshed, other experiences |
| Difficulty getting out of bed, time of getting out of bed |
| **Daytime** |
| Sleepiness, naps |
| Lethargy |
| Mood |
| Overactivity |
| Concentration and performance |
| Other unusual episodes |

♦ General review of possible sleep symptoms.

♦ Family history of sleep disorder or other conditions.

A **sleep questionnaire** completed by parents before the interview can provide a useful outline account of these and other aspects.[2]

Additional parts of the overall review of children with a sleep problem that are important in order to identify possible contributory factors are as follows:

♦ Developmental history including developmental delays, illnesses, or significant events at school or within the family.

♦ Review of physical health.

♦ Physical examination.

♦ Assessment of behaviour and emotional state.

♦ Family history and circumstances.

Following the initial consultation, a **sleep diary**, kept over a period of 2 or more weeks, can be particularly useful. This provides a more complete and balanced view than that obtained especially from fraught parents likely to give a distorted or unbalanced retrospective account.

### Special investigations (see also Chapter 4.14.1)

These depend on the nature of the sleep problem:

♦ Indications for PSG are essentially the same as for adults.

- The use in children of multiple sleep latency tests (**MSLT**) as an objective measure of sleepiness is hampered by the absence of good normative data at different ages. However, in school-aged children, about 16–18 min to fall asleep is considered normal; less than this might indicate significant daytime sleepiness which is also indicated by falling asleep in three or more of the naps. Nevertheless, in the presence of sleep disorders usually characterized by excessive sleepiness, MSLT results can be normal in late childhood because of the naturally enhanced daytime wakefulness at that age.

- **Actigraphy**, which provides information unobtrusively on basic sleep–wake patterns, is well established for children of all ages.

- **Other possible measures** include toxic screening and the special tests mentioned earlier in Chapter 4.14.1.

## Children at special risk of sleep disturbance

The prevalence of children's sleep disorders is not known with any accuracy, even for those which are severe and persistent. A number of methodological problems make it difficult to collect accurate figures and no really vigorous attempt has yet been made to overcome them. It seems that 20–30 per cent of children from infancy to adolescence have sleep problems that are considered significant by them or their parents.

The occurrence of sleep problems exceeds this overall rate considerably in various categories within the general population as a whole, and also in certain clinical subgroups. Determining the exact nature and cause of the sleep problems in these high risk groups (and also in any other affected children), with a view to successful treatment, is important because of the possible adverse effects on the child in a family that have just been discussed. Behavioural sleep problems probably predominate throughout these high risk groups but sleep disorders of a different nature may well be encountered instead or as well as those of behavioural origin.

### Children in the general population

- Reference was made earlier to the fact that children in general appear to be particularly prone to different types of sleep disorders at certain ages of development i.e. early infancy, early childhood, and adolescence.

- Adverse psycho-social circumstances are also associated with increased risk of childhood sleep problems. The importance of such factors as the degree of organization in family life, parental concern, child-rearing practices, and the mental health of parents was stressed earlier. High rates of various sleep problems, as well as other psychological difficulties, have been reported in homeless children.

### Children with psychiatric disorders

High rates of sleep disturbance have been described in child psychiatric groups in general compared with other children, and in specific psychiatric disorders.

- Various sleep problems, including panic attacks, have been described in **anxious children** in general including those with **panic disorders**. Similarly, many types of sleep problem (including nightmares and other disturbed nocturnal episodes, excessive daytime sleepiness, and bedwetting) have been reported to be particularly frequent in **traumatized children** including those who have suffered burn injury, abuse, or road traffic accidents. Treatment of the sleep disturbance has appeared to improve their emotional state but further research is needed to asses the therapeutic contribution of specific treatment for the sleep disorder as part of the overall care of the traumatized children.

- Difficulty in sleeping is the main complaint in children and in adolescents with severe **depressive disorders** but many complain of excessive sleepiness, possibly because of difficulty getting to sleep and/or poor quality sleep.

- Parental reports of sleep problems in children with **ADHD** are very common. Parental impressions can be distorted but preliminary objective evidence also suggests that persistent sleep disturbance is common and sometimes important as the primary cause (or a significant contributory factor) rather than simply a consequence of ADHD. It was mentioned earlier that ADHD symptoms have sometimes been attributed to definitive sleep disorders in which sleep quality is impaired, with improvement in ADHD symptoms following treatment of the sleep disorder. Preliminary studies of sleep physiology or other objective aspects of sleep in children have also produced evidence of sleep abnormalities. Even where ADHD is attributable to other factors, sleep disruption is likely to worsen a child's behaviour, meriting treatment in its own right wherever possible.

- **Other psychiatric disorders** in which different types of sleep disturbance is reported to be prominent are autism (including circadian sleep–wake rhythm disorders and Asperger's syndrome, tic disorders including Tourette syndrome (sleeplessness and parasomnias), and obsessive–compulsive disorders (poor quality sleep).

Sleep complaints are also prominent in the chronic fatigue syndrome. As mentioned earlier, disruption by frequent awakenings (not obviously attributable to daytime inactivity) has been described in teenagers with this condition suggesting that daytime symptoms might be at least partly attributable to poor quality sleep. Occasionally Munchausen's syndrome by proxy have come to light in the form of parental complaints of a sleep disturbance. Reports of the sleep of conduct disordered children are in keeping with the expectation that their sleep is disturbed because of their adverse or disorganized home and social circumstances, and general way of life.

- Apart from psychiatric disorders themselves, **medications** used in their treatment may affect sleep. Stimulant medication for ADHD appears to cause sleeping difficulties in some children but some children with ADHD may settle to sleep more readily even if their medication is given later in the day because this improves their bedtime behaviour. See Chapter 4.14.1 for other possible medication effects on sleep.

### Children with a learning disability or other neurological disorder

Particularly high rates of sleep disturbance has been consistently reported in children with a **learning disability**. The disturbance is often severe, poorly managed and, therefore, persistent.

- Sleep problems in this group are often behavioural in origin (largely attributed to parenting practices), arising from often understandable over-permissiveness, inconsistency, or parents' inability to set limits on their child's behaviour because of their own emotional state or excessive demands on their time. Other physical sleep problems include some chronic physical conditions. OSA features prominently in various specific learning difficulty conditions such as Down syndrome, the mucopolysaccharidosis and fragile X syndrome. Epilepsy can also play an important role as well as other co-morbid conditions.

♦ Sleep problems are also widely reported in children with **neuro-degenerative disorders**, e.g. Rett's syndrome and other neurological disorders such as head injury. Again, behavioural factors might be partly the reason, although interference with sleep mechanisms also seems likely, at least in the advanced stages of the disease.

### Children with other chronic physical illness

Acute physical illnesses disturb sleep but only for the duration of the illness in most cases. By comparison, chronic illnesses are commonly complicated by long-standing sleep disturbance caused in various ways (see Chapter 4.14.1 for medical causes of sleep disorder some of which apply to paediatric cases).

## Main sleep problems: sleeplessness

The second edition of the International Classification of Sleep Disorders was outlined in Chapter 4.14.1. The following selective account of sleep disorders in children and adolescents is organized according to the three main types of sleep complaint: sleeplessness, excessive sleepiness, and the parasomnias. Childhood psychiatric and medical conditions in which sleep disturbance is a prominent feature has already been mentioned. Emphasis is placed on the differential diagnosis of sleep complaints and also on points of particular relevance to psychiatric practice.

The breakdown of problems and disorders according to age should not be interpreted too strictly as there is overlap between the different age groups. In addition to specific treatments mentioned for particular sleep disorders, the promotion of adequate sleep, regular sleep habits, and the other sleep hygiene principles referred to in Chapter 4.14.1 are important. Evidence for the effectiveness of psychological treatments for sleeplessness in children is reviewed in detail elsewhere.[3]

### Infants

Ways of preventing or dealing with babies' sleep problems are rarely taught to parents or prospective parents, with the result that many suffer needless sleep loss and distress because the child does not sleep well. It is important to encourage good sleep habits from the start to avoid bad sleep habits later on. There are certain general guidelines for achieving this, admitting that babies vary temperamentally in their response to recommendations and parents vary in their ability to adhere to them. The main basic principles are as follows:

♦ Establishing a consistent 24 h routine, including a bedtime routine that provides cues that is timed to go to sleep.

♦ Not prolonging night-time feeding beyond the age (about 6 months) when the baby's body clock has developed enough to confine feeding to daytime.

♦ Teaching the baby to fall asleep alone so that when he or she wakes in the night (a natural occurrence at all ages) it will be possible to fall asleep again without requiring parental attention ('**self-soothing**').

♦ Establishing a clear difference in the infant's experience between day and night to help to develop his/her body clock which controls sleep and wakefulness.

♦ Ensuring the environment is conducive to sleep.

Safety measures to reduce the risk of the infant coming to harm at night from suffocation, or other breathing problems associated with sudden infant death syndrome (**SIDS**), should also be part of parent education about sleep.[4] Main recommendations are: having the infant sleep on his/her back and on a firm mattress that will not obstruct breathing, ensuring that his or her face cannot be covered during the night, ensuring the bedroom is smoke free, and avoiding co-sleeping if either parent has consumed alcohol or has taken medication or other substances with a sedative affect. Also, the baby should not be overheated at night.

### Toddlers and pre-school children

About 30 per cent of children of this age present a problem of recurrently not going to bed at the required time, and/or waking repeatedly at night and demanding their parents' attention including coming into their bed. Medical factors must be excluded but the usual explanations are behavioural especially:

♦ Anxiety about separating from parents at night

♦ Unhelpful associations with going to bed, e.g. stimulating activities within the bedroom, threats, or recriminations

♦ Inadequate limit setting on bedtime or night-time behaviour

♦ Failure to require self-soothing ways of coping with night waking.

Behavioural methods of treating these problems can be very effective, even in severe and long-standing cases, including children with developmental disorders such as learning disability or autism, providing the treatment programme is implemented properly. The main methods used include graded changes and desensitization rather than leaving the child to cry (a quickly effective measure but one which is unacceptable to many parents).

### School-age children

Some of the causes of sleeplessness in pre-school children still apply in older children but other factors become more relevant with increasing age:

♦ **Night-time fears** are common from very early childhood onwards although, in keeping with cognitive development, the content of the fears changes from aspects of the immediate environment (e.g. shadows or noises) through imaginary objects (ghosts, monsters) or the dark, to more realistic and specific fears concerning the child's own health. Such fears are usually transient and require only reassurance and comfort until they cease.

In some children the fears are so intense and persistent that they reach phobic proportions and need special attention. The cause of the fear should be investigated. The night-time fear might be one aspect of an anxiety state, including post-traumatic stress disorder in which case the child might also suffer from nightmares.

The content of the fear or nightmare might be revealing, suggesting abuse, for example. Other sleep disturbances (e.g. alarming hypnagogic hallucinations) may be the cause of the night-time fears. The child's reluctance to go to bed because he or she is genuinely afraid must be distinguished from pretending to be afraid as a delaying tactic.

Behavioural treatment is said to be very effective in cases of severe night-time fears. The child with night-time fears should be helped by positive associations with bedtime and by not going to bed so early that he or she lies awake in a fearful state.

◆ Even without night-time fears, a child will be unable to settle to sleep if **bedtime is too early**. Like some adults and even other species, children often have an evening period of intense wakefulness and activity before they begin to relax in preparation for sleep. A child is physiologically unable to sleep if put to bed in this 'forbidden zone'. Instead the sequence of events leading up to bedtime should be arranged so that the child goes to bed when 'sleepy tired'.

◆ **Worry and anxiety** about daytime matters such as school progress may cause difficulty in getting to sleep or staying asleep. The original source of concern may no longer exist but the difficulty falling asleep may persist because the child has developed the habit of lying awake in bed in an agitated state ('conditioned insomnia'). Sympathetic discussion of the child's worries, attention to the source of concern if possible, and ways of helping the child to relax at night, are generally thought to help. More specific psychiatric measures will be needed if the child has an anxiety or depressive disorder, or if there is evidence of serious problems within the family.

◆ '**Childhood onset insomnia**' or '**idiopathic insomnia**' refers to a lifelong difficulty sleeping not attributable to environmental, emotional, or medical factors and therefore of constitutional origin. The condition is usually diagnosed retrospectively in adult life.

◆ **Early morning waking** (i.e. when a child habitually wakes very early, does not return to sleep, and is noisy or demands attention) can be very distressing to parents, and disruptive to the whole family. In pre-school children, early waking may be the result of excessive or otherwise inappropriate napping, but at a later age the problem may be part of the advanced sleep phase syndrome. In this disorder the child's bedtime and sleep onset is so early that his or her sleep requirements have been met well before other members of the family wake in the morning. Gradual resetting of the child's sleep onset time is required.

In older children and adolescents early morning wakening may be part of an anxiety or depressive disorder. Otherwise, the child may have been woken too early by noise or other environmental factors which intrude into his or her sleep.

## Adolescents

High rates of insomnia have been consistently reported in adolescents. The change from the highly efficient sleep of pre-pubertal children to less satisfactory sleep in adolescence was mentioned earlier, including the biological influences in this change. The psychological and social demands and stresses of adolescence further conspire to disrupt sleep patterns. Worries, anxiety, and depression are commonly quoted reasons for not being able to sleep at this age. Nicotine, alcohol, and caffeine-containing drinks, as well as illicit drug use, are additional possible influences.

Difficulty getting off to sleep is often part of the delayed sleep phase syndrome which is reported to be particularly common in adolescence. In this condition (which will be considered further in relation to excessive sleepiness as this is often the major complaint) there is a physiological inability to go to sleep until much later than the required time because of a shift in the sleep phase. The adolescent's reluctance to go to bed earlier (or the bedtime struggles of parents with younger children with this disorder) are often misinterpreted as 'difficult' behaviour. Instead of recriminations and attempts to set limits, the timing of the sleep phase needs to be reset by so-called chronotherapeutic means.

# Main sleep problems: excessive daytime sleepiness

Despite the evidence that it is a common problem,[5] sleepiness remains neglected in child and adolescent psychiatry and in paediatrics:

◆ Part of the explanation is that sleepiness is not usually viewed as a medical problem by parents, teachers, and children themselves, the symptoms being misperceived as laziness or disinterest. Otherwise, they may be interpreted as depression or even limited intelligence.

◆ Another difficulty is that excessive sleepiness can take various forms including prolonged overnight sleep or inappropriate periods of sleep during the day.

◆ Extreme degrees of sleepiness will cause a reduction of activity at any age, but lesser degrees in children may produce irritability, over-activity, restlessness, poor concentration, impulsiveness, or aggression. Explanations of such behaviours other than sleep loss or disturbance (such as ADHD) are more likely to be considered, as mentioned earlier.

◆ A high level of daytime alertness in older pre-pubertal children may be sufficient to offset a tendency to sleep, providing a different clinical picture of sleepiness but not seen at a younger or older age.

Because of these problems of recognition, the prevalence of excessive sleep in children and adolescents is not known. Clearly, it is not rare in view of the range of underlying conditions causing it, many of which are individually quite common.

It is important to establish that the problem really is excessive sleepiness. 'Tiredness' is an ambiguous term: ideally, sleepiness should be distinguished from fatigue or lethargy, without necessarily the need to sleep, for which different explanations are likely including physical illnesses, such as anaemia or endocrine disorders in which other signs are usually present. Occasionally, excessive sleepiness with long periods in bed or at home is simulated in order to escape from a difficult situation. Detection of such cases requires very careful clinical evaluation and assessment and possibly PSG.

Excessive sleepiness is mainly a problem in older children and (especially) adolescents. Many teenagers complain about excessive sleepiness but it has been claimed that very many more than those who seek help are likely to be suffering from chronic sleep deprivation or '**sleep debt**'. As mentioned earlier, the adverse effects of this are thought to be wide-ranging from underperformance at school, college or work, to road traffic accidents and other mishaps, as well as antisocial behaviour.[6] Sometimes the situation is complicated by the use of stimulants to stay awake, and alcohol or sedative drugs to get to sleep.

The differential diagnosis of excessive sleepiness can be considered in terms of three main categories of cause: insufficient sleep, disturbed sleep, and an increased need for sleep (Table 9.2.9.3).

### Insufficient sleep

The combination of late-night social activities or staying up late for study, and having to get up early for school or college reduces the number of hours many adolescents sleep to below that needed for satisfactory daytime functioning. Difficulty getting off to sleep at night and recurrent waking makes the problem worse (or may be sufficient in themselves to reduce or seriously impair sleep). The result is considerable difficulty getting up in the morning, irritability, emotional liability, lethargy, tiredness, or actually falling asleep during the day.

Correction of the problem of late-night social activities requires a change of lifestyle or other measures which may be difficult to achieve without there being strong motivation to do so. The ideal solution is an agreed, co-operative effort on the part of both the young person and parents.

More specific measures will be needed if the habit of going to bed late has developed into a disturbance of the circadian sleep–wake cycle. This may take the form of irregular sleep–wake schedules or, more usually, the **delayed sleep phase syndrome (DSPS)** which deserves special mention because it is common, especially in adolescents, and potentially very disruptive.

The time at which children fall asleep may become delayed during a period of illness, or because of protracted bedtime disputes about going to bed. In adolescents the problem arises from habitually staying up late for social or other reasons, especially at weekends or during holidays. After a time (the length of which varies with the

**Table 9.2.9.3** Differential diagnosis of excessive sleepiness in older children and adolescents

| |
|---|
| **Insufficient sleep** |
| Late-night activities combined with getting up early |
| Insomnia |
| Erratic sleep–wake patterns |
| Delayed sleep-phase syndrome |
| **Disturbed sleep at night** |
| Sleep-related upper airway obstruction |
| Recreational drugs (caffeine, alcohol, nicotine) |
| Illicit drugs (including withdrawal) |
| Medical and psychiatric disorders |
| Other sleep disorders (frequent parasomnias, periodic limb movements in sleep) |
| **Increased need for sleep** |
| Narcolepsy |
| Idiopathic central nervous system hypersomnia |
| Depression |
| Substance abuse |
| Neurological disease |
| Kleine–Levin syndrome (intermittent sleepiness) |
| Menstruation-related hypersomnia (intermittent sleepiness) |

individual) the sleep phase becomes physiologically delayed with the result that it becomes impossible to go to sleep earlier by choice, in spite of feeling tired and having been awake for a long time. Entreaties to go to bed at a sensible time and get up on time for school are likely to be ineffective.

The diagnostic features of DSPS are persistently severe difficulty getting to sleep, uninterrupted sound sleep, great difficulty getting up for school or work, and sleepiness and under-functioning especially during the first part of the day, giving way to alertness in the evening and early hours. The abnormal sleep pattern is maintained by sleeping in very late when able to do so at weekends and during holidays.

Treatment consists of gradually and consistently changing the sleep phase to an appropriate time. This can be achieved by slowly advancing the sleep phase (e.g. by 15 min a day) where the phased delay is about 3 h or less. More severe forms of the disorder require progressive sleep phase delay in 3 h steps ('round the clock'). Additional measures to maintain the improved sleep schedule include early morning exposure to bright light and firm agreement with the adolescent to maintain the new pattern of social activities and sleep. The place of melatonin remains unclear in view of the many uncertainties about its use and potential hazards, including possible adverse affects on reproductive physiology.

Achieving and maintaining an improved sleep–wake schedule by these means may not be easy. The difficulties are compounded if there is a vested interest in maintaining the abnormal sleep pattern, for example to avoid school ('**motivated sleep phase delay**'). The presence of psychological problems, including depression, may well make successful treatment less likely. 'Conditioned insomnia' may appear similar to DSPS but its origins and treatment are different.

### Disturbed nocturnal sleep

Daytime sleepiness, despite apparent normal time asleep at night, suggests that the restorative quality of sleep is impaired. Poor quality sleep can result from frequent awakenings or less obvious arousals including brief subclinical interruptions (or 'fragmentation') of sleep. Sleep may be disturbed by the following:

♦ Excessive caffeine, alcohol, or nicotine (combinations are particularly hazardous), and illicit drug use and withdrawal.

♦ Medical and psychiatric disorders in childhood, and some of their treatments.

♦ Other sleep disorders: frequent parasomnias are likely to be obvious but periodic limb movements in sleep (now considered to be more important in childhood than previously thought) are much more subtle in their effects on sleep continuity.

♦ Sleep-related respiratory problems, including OSA. This condition merits some emphasis because of its widespread occurrence: at least 2 per cent of children in the general population are affected with a peak onset at 2 to 6 years. The prevalence is much higher than this in various learning disability syndromes such as Down syndrome, as mentioned earlier.

There are important differences between OSA in children and OSA in adults. The typical adult with OSA is an obese middle-aged male who snores very loudly, under-functions during the day and usually responds to continuous positive airway pressure (CPAP) treatment at night.

◆ In contrast, most children with OSA are not obese, the usual causes are large tonsils and adenoids (the removal of which can be beneficial), the sex ratio is equal and, whereas adults have prolonged obstructive apnoeas, children often have partial airway obstruction with hypoventilation, actual apnoea events being less frequent and shorter. As already mentioned, the result may be over-activity and other disruptive behaviour rather than obvious sleepiness during the day.

Clinical assessment is the cornerstone of recognizing OSA.

◆ Night-time signs suggesting the diagnosis are combinations of snoring (although only about one in five children who snore most nights have this condition), other noises suggesting breathing difficulties during sleep, paradoxical chest–abdomen respiratory movements, unusual sleeping positions including neck extension, very restless sleep, profuse sweating, nocturnal enuresis, and sudden distressing awakenings during the obstructive event. There is also a higher incidence of other parasomnias but for reasons that are unclear.

◆ Daytime features include mouth breathing and adenoidal facies, headache and bad mood on wakening, and the behaviour problems already mentioned.

◆ Physical examination may reveal the anatomical cause of the obstruction (usually enlarged tonsils and adenoids). Radiological studies are required in the more complicated cases. PSG with respiratory measures is needed to assess the severity of the obstruction and the effects on blood gases during sleep which may be greater than suspected from clinical findings.

Treatment is essential to counter or prevent physical and psychological complications. This usually consists of adenotonsillectomy or, much less commonly, other measures such as CPAP depending on the individual case.

### Disorders involving an increased tendency to sleep

This occurs where prolonged or otherwise excessive sleep is an intrinsic part of the condition, rather than a consequence.

### (a) Narcolepsy

Narcolepsy is a neurological disorder mainly affecting REM sleep physiology. It is not the rarity once supposed; prevalence in the United States has been estimated at 4–9 per 10 000.

Onset has occurred by adolescence in a high number of cases but the diagnosis is often not made for several years. The reasons for this are that symptoms may be subtle in their early stages, concealed, misinterpreted as laziness or psychological disorder such as depression or conversion disorder, or overshadowed by the child's extreme emotional reaction to the condition. Especially because of its many manifestations in childhood, narcolepsy is a good illustration of how a sleep disorder can be misconstrued as another type of clinical condition, especially when familiarity with the field of children's sleep disorders is limited.[7]

The clinical presentation of early narcolepsy is very variable and some time usually elapses before the classic combination of daytime sleep attacks, overnight sleep disruption, cataplexy, hypnagogic hallucinations, and sleep paralysis develop if, indeed, it does at all. In young patients the first sign may consist of no more than prolonged overnight sleep.

It is appropriate to consider narcolepsy in any young person who is excessively sleepy during the day without an obvious explanation, but repeated clinical and PSG assessment may be required at intervals before a definite diagnosis can be made, including its distinction from other forms of sleepiness such as the group of conditions known as **idiopathic CNS hypersomnia**. The demonstration of low CSF levels of the neuropeptide hypocretin (orexin) is now considered diagnostic of narcolepsy. The PSG features of narcolepsy in adults, which are described elsewhere (Chapter 4.14.3) do not necessarily apply in the childhood stage of the condition.

Narcolepsy is a persistent and disturbing condition for which careful treatment with medication together with ancillary measures, as well as much support and advice about education, career, and psycho-social matters, are required. Other aspects of diagnosis and management are discussed in Chapter 4.14.3.

### (b) Kleine–Levin syndrome

This also usually begins in the teenage years with periods of excessive sleepiness alternating with periods of normality. The sleepy episodes are associated (in its classical form) with overeating, hypersexuality, and other disturbed behaviours which are often bizarre and out of character. It is also frequently mistaken for a psychological disorder or other medical conditions. The condition should be distinguished from other causes of intermittent sleepiness in young people such as substance abuse, major depressive disorder (in which the sleepiness is much less marked), menstruation-related hypersomnia, and certain neurological disorders.

## Main sleep problems: parasomnias

This category of sleep disorders is described in Chapter 4.14.4 in relation to adult psychiatry. The present account emphasizes aspects of the parasomnias of particular importance in childhood and adolescence when, collectively, they are more common than in adult life. Frequently, parasomnias cause parents much concern and they appear to be the subject of considerable diagnostic confusion and delay. As in older patients, different types of parasomnia may co-exist. A detailed account of parasomnias in young patients is available elsewhere.[8]

The following general points about childhood parasomnias have clear implications for clinical practice.

◆ Precise diagnosis is important as different parasomnias may well need contrasting types of treatment. Accurate diagnosis depends principally on a detailed account of the subjective and objective sequence of events from the onset of the episode to its resolution, as well as the circumstances in which the episode occurs, including its timing. Audio–visual recording (including the use of home video systems) can be very informative. Only occasionally is PSG required, although this can be instructive where clinical evaluation is inconclusive and, sometimes, where there is the possibility that another type of sleep disorder co-exists.

◆ The more dramatic forms of parasomnia seem to be a particular cause of diagnostic confusion and imprecision, and also quite possibly unnecessary concern about their psychological significance as most are benign.

◆ Especially when the range and manifestations of sleep disorders is not appreciated, parasomnias (and other sleep disorders) may well be misinterpreted as other physical or psychological conditions.

◆ A child may have more than one kind of parasomnia or, indeed, more than one sleep disorder (e.g. arousal disorders associated with obstructive sleep apnoea).

◆ As many childhood primary parasomnias remit spontaneously within a few years, children and parents can often be reassured about the future, although protective measures (e.g. in severe headbanging or sleepwalking) may be required in the meantime.

◆ Specific treatment, including medication, is needed in only a minority of cases of primary parasomnia but is likely to be required for the underlying disorder in many of the secondary parasomnias.

◆ Research information on this point is limited, but a primary parasomnia might be symptomatic of a psychological problem if it is very frequent, unusually late in onset or persistent, or associated with a traumatic experience.

◆ Parasomnias may lead to psychological complications if the child is frightened, embarrassed, or otherwise upset by the experience, or because of the reactions of other people to the episodes.

### Primary parasomnias

◆ Sleep-related **rhythmic movement disorders** such as head-banging, occur in many young children, almost always remitting spontaneously by 3 to 4 years of age. Although alarming to parents, they are usually of no psychological significance (unlike daytime headbanging associated with severe neurodevelopmental disorder). However, protective measures, such as padding the cot-sides, may be needed.

◆ **Hypnagogic** (sleep onset) and **hypnopompic** (on waking) hallucinations are common and may be frightening to the child.

◆ Parents are often distressed to witness **confusional arousals**, **agitated sleepwalking**, or **sleep terrors** which are a form of '**partial arousal disorder**' common in young children (see Chapter 4.14.4 for an account of arousal disorders). The degree of agitation and confused behaviour may be extreme, suggesting that the child is suffering in some way. In fact, in arousal disorders the child remains asleep and unaware of the events. Understandable attempts to arouse the child and provide comfort should be discouraged, as this may cause real distress. Although violence during sleep is described mainly in sleepwalking adults, such behaviour can occur in children.

◆ The term 'nightmare' is sometimes used misleadingly for any form of dramatic parasomnia. **True nightmares** (frightening dreams) are common. If frequent and associated with intense bedtime fears, they may indicate an anxiety disorder and their content may suggest a cause.

◆ **Nocturnal enuresis** is very common, affecting about 5 per cent of 7-year-olds at least once a week. Delayed maturation often seems to be the explanation, but physical or psychological factors may be involved, especially where previous bladder control is lost. Behavioural treatment can be very effective.

### Secondary parasomnias

**Nocturnal epileptic seizures** are not uncommon in children and must be distinguished from primary parasomnias because of their different significance, and also the investigation and treatment they require. Seizures which are behavioural in manifestation are the most likely to be misdiagnosed as non-epileptic, for example benign centro-temporal (Rolandic) epilepsy of childhood and nocturnal frontal lobe seizures both of which are closely related to sleep.

**Other parasomnias**, which are part of medical or psychiatric disorders and which may be encountered in patients of any age, include nocturnal asthmatic attacks with accompanying distress, those associated with OSA or gastro-oesophageal reflux, panic attacks, nocturnal disturbance that is part of the post-traumatic stress disorder, and dissociative states. Simulated parasomnias, shown by PSG to be enacted during wakefulness, can sometimes occur in children.

## Further information

Stores, G. (2008). *Sleep problems in children and adolescents: the facts*. Oxford University Press, Oxford.

Stores, G. and Wiggs, L. (2001). *Sleep disturbance in children and adolescents with disorders of development: its significance and management*. Clinics in Developmental Medicine No. 155. Mac Keith Press, London.

## References

1. Stores, G. (2007). Clinical diagnosis and misdiagnosis of sleep disorders. *Journal of Neurology, Neurosurgery and Psychiatry*, **78**, 1293–7.
2. Owens, J.A., Spirito, A., and McQuinn, M. (2000). The children's sleep habits questionnaire. Psychometric properties of a survey instrument for school-aged children. *Sleep*, **23**, 1043–51.
3. Kuhn, B.R. and Elliot, A.J. (2003). Treatment efficacy in pediatric sleep medicine. *Journal of Psychosomatic Research*, **54**, 587–97.
4. Fleming, P., and Blair, P.S. (2007). Sudden infant death syndrome. *Sleep Medicine Clinics*, **2**, 463–76.
5. Fallone, G., Owens, J.A., and Deane, J. (2002). Sleepiness in children: clinical implications. *Sleep Medicine Reviews*, **6**, 287–306.
6. Dahl, R.E. and Lewin, D.S. (2002). Pathways to adolescent health: sleep regulation and behavior. *Journal of Adolescent Health*, **31**, 175–84.
7. Stores, G. (2006). The protean manifestations of childhood narcolepsy and their misinterpretation. *Developmental Medicine and Child Neurology*, **48**, 307–10.
8. Stores, G. (2007). Parasomnias of childhood and adolescence. *Sleep Medicine Clinics*, **2**, 405–17.

# 9.2.10 Suicide and attempted suicide in children and adolescents

David Shaffer, Cynthia R. Pfeffer, and Jennifer Gutstein*

## Introduction

Suicidal behaviour is a matter of great concern for clinicians who deal with the mental health problems of children and adolescents. The incidence of suicide attempts reaches a peak during the mid-adolescent years, and mortality from suicide, which increases steadily through the teens, is, in many countries, one of the leading causes of death at that age.

## Historical review

Until the late 1950s, knowledge about youth suicide was drawn from unrepresentative case reviews, reviews of the demography of suicide drawn from death certificate data, and speculation about dynamics. The late 1950s saw the first systematic psychological autopsy study among adults that demonstrated the importance of psychiatric disorder as a proximal cause of most suicides.[1] This was followed by similar studies on children and adolescents,[2–5] confirming the association in adolescence. Starting in the mid-1960s, the incidence of suicide in young males began to rise in many countries.[6] The rate of increase eventually stabilized in the late 1980s and, in many countries, is now showing signs of falling.[7] These changes stimulated efforts to develop methods of preventing youth suicide.[8–11]

A good deal is now known about which teenagers commit suicide, less about who attempts it, and very little about the optimal management of suicidal adolescents. The number of randomized controlled trials designed to assess different forms of treatment is exceedingly small, and many suggestions for clinical management are based on anecdotal accounts rather than on findings from well-designed experimental trials.

## Clinical features

### Completed suicide

Completed suicide occurs most commonly in older adolescents, and, although it can also occur in children as young as 6 years of age, it is excessively rare before puberty.[7] Psychological-autopsy studies have shown that about 90 per cent of adolescent suicides occur in individuals with a pre-existing psychiatric disorder, often present for several years.[3–5] In teenagers, the most common disorders are some form of mood disorder, substance and/or alcohol abuse, often comorbid with a mood disorder in boys over age 15, and anxiety disorders.[3,4] At a trait level, many suicide completers have been noted to be irritable, impulsive, volatile, and prone to outbursts of aggression. However, this pattern of behaviour is by no means universal, and anxious suicides have usually shown no evidence of prior behavioural, academic, or social disturbances.[3]

Although some adolescents—predominantly girls suffering from a major depressive disorder—appear to have thought about suicide for some time before death, most adolescent suicides appear to impulsively follow a recent stress event, such as getting into trouble at school or with a law-enforcement agency; a ruptured relationship with a boy- or girlfriend; or a fight among friends. In many instances, these stress events can be seen as a by-product of their underlying psychiatric disorder.[12]

It also appears that a completed suicide can be precipitated—in a presumably already suicidal youth-by exposure to news of another person's suicide, or by reading about or viewing a suicide portrayed in a romantic light in a book, magazine, or newspaper.[13]

About a third of completed suicides have made a previous known suicide attempt, more commonly girls and those who suffered from a mood disorder.[3] Completed suicide must be distinguished from autoerotic asphyxia, which is rare in teenagers.[3] Suicide pacts, common between middle-aged or elderly married couples and/or other family members, are similarly rare in adolescents, but are not unknown.[3]

## Non-lethal suicidal behaviour

### (a) Suicidal ideation

Suicidal ideation includes thoughts about wishing to kill oneself, making plans of when and where, and having thoughts about the impact of one's suicide on others. Such thoughts may occur without great significance among young children, who may not appreciate that suicide may result in irreversible death.[14] However, appreciation of the finality of death should not be a factor in judging the seriousness of suicidal ideation. Suicide threats made by young children and adolescents most often involve a threat to jump out of a window, to run into traffic, or to stab himself or herself.

### (b) Attempted suicide

The most common profile of a teenaged attempter is a 15- to 17-year-old girl who has taken a small- or medium-sized overdose of an over-the-counter analgesic or medication taken by another family member. The behaviour is usually impulsive and occurs in the context of a dispute and humiliation with family or a boyfriend.[15] The clinical features most strongly associated with suicide attempts are irritability, agitation, threatening, violent, or psychotic behaviour, and a persistent wish to die.[16]

Groups in whom suicide attempts appear to be common include runaways,[3] children who have been exposed to physical and sexual abuse, and homosexual teenagers.[17] However, study-design issues make it unclear whether this is because of a high rate of psychopathology or substance abuse in these groups or because of some factor that specifically predisposes to suicidal behaviour.

A subset of non-fatal suicidal behaviour involving ingestion with a non-lethal intent is sometimes referred to as parasuicide. However, intent is difficult to gauge retrospectively, and not all teenagers are aware of the lethalness of an ingestion, so that this term carries with it a risk of complacency and is probably best avoided in teenagers.

## Assessment

### Suicide attempts

Assessment of a suicide attempt involves an evaluation of the short-term risk for suicide and attempt repetition, and an assessment of the underlying diagnosis or other promoting factors. If the child or teenager has been referred to as an ideator, it is important to determine whether they are contemplating or have secretly attempted suicide.

Repeated attempts, attempts by unusual methods (other than ingestions or superficial cutting), medically serious attempts, and attempts where the patient has taken active steps to prevent discovery all increase the risk for further attempts or death.[18,19] Children and adolescents systematically overestimate the lethality of different suicidal methods, so that a child with a significant degree of suicidal intent may fail to carry out a lethal act.[20–22]

The mental states leading to suicidal behaviour include anticipatory anxiety, pessimism, or hopelessness, as well as paranoid or other cognitive distortions arising from an underlying psychiatric diagnosis.[23] Inappropriate coping styles (e.g. impulsivity or catastrophizing) in response to external stress may also contribute to the behaviour. Motivating feelings may include the wish to effect a change in interpersonal relationships, to rejoin a dead relative, to avoid an intolerable situation, to get revenge, or to gain attention.[22]

## Classification of associated diagnoses

### Suicide

Psychiatric diagnoses commonly associated with a suicide include depression, bipolar disorder, substance abuse, conduct disorder, and overanxious and panic disorders.[3–5] Although the rate of suicide in schizophrenics is high, because of the rarity of the condition, it accounts for very few suicides.

### Suicide attempts

Recurring suicidal behaviour has been associated with hypomanic personality traits and cluster B personality disorders.[22] A history of impulsivity, mood lability, with rapid shifts from brief periods of depression, anxiety, and rage to euthymia and/or mania—associated with transient psychotic symptoms, including paranoid ideas and auditory or visual hallucinations-is associated with a risk for further suicide attempts and is compatible with the diagnosis of borderline personality disorder. Many of these symptoms are also features of bipolar mood disorder.

## Epidemiology

### Completed suicide

#### (a) Age

In the United States, the age-specific mortality rate from suicide for 10- to 14-year-olds was 1.6 per 100 000 in 1997.[24] This age group accounts for 7 per cent of the population but only 1 per cent of all suicides, and most of these occur in 12- to 14-year-olds.

The comparable figures for 15- to 19-year-olds are about six times higher. The suicide rates at this age in the United States and Canada in 1997 were 9.5 per 100 000 and 12.86 per 100 000 respectively.[7] The proportion of suicides that occur in this age group is about the same as its representation in the general population.

Suicide rates for 15- to 24-year-olds in some other English-speaking countries were 11.0 for males and 2.2 for females in the United Kingdom (1995), 16.0 in Australia (1995), and 26.1 in New Zealand (1997) (all per 100 000 population).[7]

#### (b) Gender

In the United States and most other countries, male suicides outnumber female suicides among 15- to 24-year-olds by a ratio of 4:1. In China and Cuba, the suicide rate is higher in females than in males.[7]

#### (c) Cultural and ethnic differences

Rates of suicide vary considerably in different cultural and national groups.[7] Possible reasons include variable access to lethal methods, different degrees of social support, integration, or group adherence, or the influence of religious beliefs or spirituality.[25–27] In some instances, the differences may be a function of geography rather than culture. Contagion within isolated groups may determine differences in rates.

#### (d) Secular changes

From 1964 to 1995, the suicide rate in the United States and Canada among 15- to 19-year-old males increased almost three-fold, and similar increases were reported in Australia, New Zealand, and the

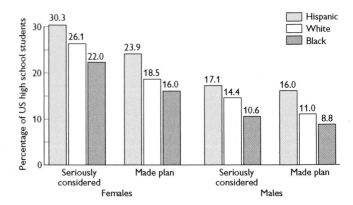

**Fig. 9.2.10.1** Youth risk behaviour survey: prevalence of suicidal ideation in teenagers in the previous 12-month period (1997) broken down into gender and ethnicity. (Reproduced from Centers for disease control (1998). Attempted suicide among high-school students–US, 1997. Morbidity and Mortality weekly Report, **47**, 47–9, copyright 1998, centers for Disease Control and Prevention, US.)

United Kingdom.[7] In most of these countries, there was little change in the female rate or in the rate amongst 10- to 14-year-olds. Fluctuations in the suicide rate appear to be real, rather than due to any methodological artefact (e.g. changes in reporting practices). The most plausible reason for the increase in suicidal behaviour among teenage boys is an increase in alcohol and substance use in the youth population.[3] The reasons offered for the recent decline in suicide rates include lowered substance- and alcohol-use rates among the young and more effective diagnosis and treatment.[28]

## Attempted suicide

There is a strong inverse relationship between attempted suicide and age. A large epidemiological survey of four suicide-related behaviours (ideation, plan, gesture, and attempt) in the United States has shown a significantly higher rate of all four behaviours in the youngest age group (15–24 years).[29] This study also compared rates of these four behaviours across two decades (1990–1992 and 2001–2003). It found that rates did not decrease, despite a dramatic increase in pharmacologic treatment.

Suicide attempts in adolescents are at least twice as common in females as males (see Figs 9.2.10.1 and 9.2.10.2). Considerable ethnic variation is seen in the United States, with, for unknown

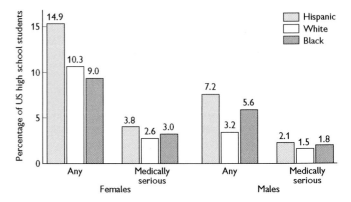

**Fig. 9.2.10.2** Youth risk behaviour survey: prevalence of suicide attempts in teenagers in the previous 12-month period (1997) broken down into gender and ethnicity. (Reproduced from Centers for disease control (1998). Attempted suicide among high-school students–US, 1997. Morbidity and Mortality weekly Report, **47**, 47–9, copyright 1998, centers for Disease Control and Prevention, US.)

reasons, Hispanic high-school students having twice the rate of black or white teenagers.[30]

## Aetiology

### Completed suicide

#### (a) Psychiatric disorders

The most important risk factor for suicide is a psychiatric disorder.[3] Controlled studies of completed suicide suggest similar risk factors for boys and girls,[3,h31] but with marked differences in their relative importance[3–5] (Table 9.2.10.1). In girls, major depression is the most powerful risk factor, which, in some studies, increases the risk of suicide 12-fold; followed by a previous suicide attempt, which increases the risk approximately three-fold. In boys, a previous suicide attempt is the most potent predictor, increasing the rate over 30-fold. It is followed by depression (12-fold increase), disruptive behaviour (two-fold increase), and substance abuse (increasing the rate by just under two-fold).[3]

#### (b) Psychosocial stressors

Stressful life events often precede a suicide and/or suicide attempt.[12] They are rarely a sufficient cause in suicide, and their importance seems to lie in their action as a precipitant of stress in young people who are at risk by virtue of their psychiatric condition. Family discord, lack of family warmth, and a disturbed parent-child relationship are commonly associated with types of child and adolescent psychopathology, but these factors do not play a more important role in suicide.[12]

#### (c) Cognitive factors

Perceptions of hopelessness, negative views about one's own competence, poor self-esteem, a sense of responsibility for negative events, and the immutability of these distorted attributions may contribute to the 'hopelessness' repeatedly found to be associated with suicidality.[18,19]

#### (d) Biology

Biological factors, specifically dysregulation of the serotonergic system, are common in adult suicides.[32] Dysregulation is manifested by low levels of serotonin metabolites in central nervous system fluids, low concentrations of presynaptic serotonergic receptors, and dense concentrations of postsynaptic receptors. Such serotonin abnormalities have been localized to the ventrolateral prefrontal cortex and brainstem of suicide victims and attempters (in postmortem positron-emission tomographic studies as well as in *in vivo* biological challenges).[33] Serotonin may inhibit extreme fluctuations of mood and reactivity, and the vulnerability to suicide of individuals with these biological abnormalities may be mediated by impulsivity and emotional volatility. As the ventral prefrontal cortex plays a role in behavioural inhibition, it is conceivable that serotonin irregularities in this area make it more difficult for a suicidal individual to control his suicidal impulses.[33] The frequency with which these biological findings occur in adolescent suicide attempters is not yet clear, and studies to demonstrate the precise behavioural correlates of serotonin dysregulation profiles are still lacking. Nordstrom *et al.*[34] have suggested that knowing the biological status of suicide attempters may have a practical value, in that low 5-hydroxyindole acetic acid concentrations in cerebrospinal fluid examined shortly after a suicide attempt may differentiate between suicide attempters who will commit suicide or repeat the attempt within a year and those who will not. The biology of suicidal behaviour is considered more fully in chapter 4.15.3

**Table 9.2.10.1** Psychiatric diagnoses in child and adolescent suicides

|  | Martunnen *et al.*[5] | | | Shaffer *et al.*[6] | | | Brent *et al.*[4] | | |
|---|---|---|---|---|---|---|---|---|---|
| Country | Finland | | | USA | | | USA | | |
| Area | National | | | Greater New York | | | Western Pennsylvania | | |
| Period | 1987–1988 | | | 1984–1986 | | | 1984–1994 | | |
| N | 53 | | | 120 | | | 140 | | |
| Age | 13–19 | | | <20 | | | 13–19 | | |
| Percentage girls | 17 | | | 21 | | | 15 | | |
| Control group | None | | | Matched community | | | Matched community | | |
| Diagnostic system | DSM-IIIR | | | DSM-III | | | DSM-III | | |
|  | **Males** | **Females** | **All** | **Males** | **Females** | **All** | **Males** | **Females** | **All** |
| Any diagnosis (%) | 93 | 100 | 94 | 90 | 92 | 91 | 82 | 81 | 82 |
| Any mood disorder (%) | 48 | 67 | 51 | 60 | 68 | 61 | 43 | 71 | 47 |
| Substance abuse (%) | 27 | 44 | 30 | 42 | 12 | 35 | 35 | 24 | 34 |
| Conduct/antisocial/ disruptive disorder (%) | 18 | 11 | 17 | 54 | 36 | 50 | 35 | 10 | 31 |
| Any anxiety disorder (%) | 2 | 11 | 4 | 27 | 28 | 27 | 13 | 24 | 14 |
| Schizophrenia (%) | 5 | 11 | 6 | 3 | 4 | 3 | — | — | — |
| Past suicide attempt | 27 | 67 | 34 | 28 | 50 | 33 | 37 | 62 | 41 |

### (e) Imitation

Evidence has accumulated indicating that suicide in vulnerable teenagers can be precipitated by exposure to real or fictional accounts of suicide, such as intense media coverage of a real suicide or the fictional representation of a suicide in a popular film or television programme. The risk is especially high in the young, and lasts for approximately 2 weeks.[13] The phenomenon of suicide clusters is also presumed to be related to imitation.

"Cybersuicide," or a tendency for internet sites such as Bebo or MySpace" to encourage suicide pacts or to increase completed or attempted suicide in vulnerable adolescents, has become an increasing concern. This concern is based on multiple case reports from Japan, Wales, and the United States. These have captured substantial media attention. As yet no objective empirical data have been amassed to determine if there is a causal relationship between internet use and youth suicide.

One hypothetical model for how biological and social factors fit together is illustrated in Fig. 9.2.10.3.

In a longitudinal study of a large African-American community in the United States, Juon and Ensminger[35] found risk factors for suicidal behaviour in African-Americans to be very similar to those found in Caucasians (depression, substance use, and a number of family variables).

## Course and prognosis

### Natural history

Little is known about the natural history of suicidal behaviour, but early-onset suicidal behaviour in prepuberty predicts suicidal behaviour in adolescence[36,37] and an early-onset major depressive disorder is associated with suicidal behaviour in adolescence and adulthood.[38] Attempts to predict, at the time of the first attempt, which adolescents are likely to repeat their suicidal behaviour have been unsuccessful.[22]

## Emergency treatment

Because of the need to respond to a suicidal crisis, it is desirable to offer treatment within a service-delivery system that includes inpatient and outpatient settings, acute crisis work, stabilization, extended management, and follow-up care and monitoring.

**Outpatient treatment** should be used when the child or adolescent is unlikely to act on suicidal impulses, when there is sufficient support at home, and when there is someone who can take action if the adolescent's behaviour or mood deteriorates. Children and adolescents should never be discharged from an emergency or care service without the child's or adolescent's caretaker having been interviewed (see Box 9.2.10.1) to ensure that firearms and/or lethal medications will be made inaccessible to the child. Unless this advice is given, parents will rarely, on their own initiative, take the necessary precautions. Before discharge, the clinician must have a good understanding of the amount of support that will be available for the child or adolescent if he or she is discharged home.

**Acute psychiatric inpatient care** should be reserved for patients for whom intensive surveillance and intervention are considered essential-as in the presence of active suicidal ideation and intent or when the youngster is unable to commit to not carrying out a suicidal act, when the youth is unpredictable, impulsive, agitated, or psychotic, or if there is a lack of support and supervision in the

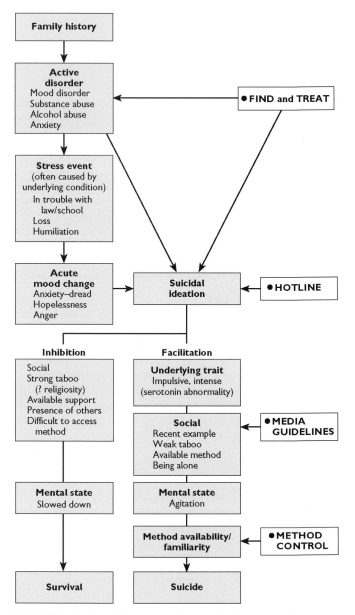

**Fig. 9.2.10.3** How do suicides occur and how can they be prevented?

home. There is no evidence that exposure to other suicidal psychiatric inpatients increases the risk of suicidal behaviour. Determining when a patient is ready for discharge from the hospital or crisis centre will usually include an evaluation of the severity of existing suicidal ideation and intent. Implicit coercions (e.g. telling patients that discharge will be delayed until they can state that they are not suicidal) should be avoided.

Treatment compliance may be improved by offering definite, closely spaced, follow-up appointments, being flexible in arranging appointments if a crisis should arise, and reminding the family and patient by telephone or note about the next appointment. If an appointment is missed, the patient and parent should be contacted. Hopeless and depressed children and adolescents, who may be not be able to commit to a lengthy treatment process, may be better engaged by offering short-term treatment plans with defined intervention goals. While offering confidentiality for some issues,

> **Box 9.2.10.1** Checklist before discharging an adolescent who has attempted suicide
>
> Before discharging a patient from the emergency room or crisis centre, always:
> - Check that *firearms* and lethal *medications* have been secured or removed
> - Check that there is a *supportive person* at home
> - Check that a *follow-up appointment* has been scheduled

it is essential that the clinician communicate to the patient that, if they feel that suicidal thinking or behaviour is imminent, such information will be shared with the parents.

## Contracts

A written or verbal 'no-suicide' contract is commonly negotiated at the start of treatment in the hope that it will improve treatment compliance and reduce the likelihood of further suicidal behaviour.[39] In its usual form, the child or adolescent promises not to engage in suicidal behaviour without first informing the parents, therapist, or other responsible adult when he or she has thoughts of suicide or plans to commit suicide. No empirical studies have evaluated the efficacy of a contract, and contracts should be seen as no more than adjuncts to the management of patients with low intent. Even if the patient agrees to such a contract, suicide risk may persist. It should also be appreciated that a 'no-suicide' contract may lessen a patient's communication of stress and dysphoria, decrease the potential for developing a therapeutic alliance, and impair risk management. As mentioned above, coercive communications should be avoided, because these may encourage deceit and defiance.

## Specific psychotherapies

Working with suicidal children and adolescents is best done by a clinician who is available, has skill and training in managing suicidal crises, relates to the patient in an honest and consistent way, and can convey a sense of optimism and activity. Given these personal attributes, the therapist may use various models of psychotherapy, although relatively few empirical studies have evaluated their efficacy.

### (a) Cognitive behavioural therapy

Cognitive hbehavioural therapy is effective in depressed teenagers,[40] but its value for suicidal adolescents has not been demonstrated.[23] Brent *et al.*[23] modified the approach for depressed adolescents. The treatment comprized 12 to 16 once-weekly sessions, followed by a 6-month booster phase of monthly or bimonthly sessions. It included a psychoeducational manual about mood disorders, training to monitor and modify automatic thoughts, assumptions, and beliefs, training in more assertive and direct methods of communicating, and help in conceptualizing alternative solutions to problems. Meetings with parents were sometimes held to augment the treatment, and psychopharmacology was used adjunctively if depressed adolescents had not improved after 4 to 6 weeks of pharmacotherapy.

Brent's study provides no evidence of the efficacy of cognitive-behavioural therapy for teenagers who had made a suicide attempt who were not included in this study.

### (b) Dialectical behavioural therapy

Dialectical behavioural therapy (**DBT**) is the only form of psychotherapy that has been shown in a randomized control trial to reduce suicidality in adults with borderline personality disorder.[41] This treatment is based on a biosocial theory in which suicidal behaviours are considered to be maladaptive solutions to painful negative emotions that also have affect-regulating qualities and elicit help from others.[41]

The treatment involves developing problem-oriented strategies to increase distress tolerance, emotion regulation, interpersonal effectiveness, and the use of both rational and emotional input to make more balanced decisions. It usually involves individual and group sessions over the course of a year, although an untested modification for adolescents (DBT-A) is designed to take 12 weeks.[42] It involves the participation of a relative who is charged to improve the home environment and to teach other relatives how to model and reinforce adaptive behaviours for the adolescents.

### (c) Family therapy

As indicated above, family discord, poor communication, disagreements, lack of cohesive values and goals, and irregular routines and activities are common in suicidal children and adolescents who often feel isolated within the family. Family intervention aims to decrease such problems, improve family problem-solving and conflict resolution, and reduce blame directed at the suicidal child or adolescent. Family-based cognitive therapy aims to reframe the family's understanding of their problems, to alter the family's maladaptive problem-solving techniques, and to encourage positive family interactions. Psychoeducational approaches can help parents clarify their understanding of childhood and adolescent suicidal behaviour, identify changes in mental state that may herald a repetition, and reduce the extent of expressed emotion or anger.[31]

## Psychopharmacological interventions

In meta-analyses of adult studies, lithium maintenance treatment greatly reduces (8.6-fold) the recurrence of suicide attempts in adults with bipolar or other major affective disorders. Further, when lithium is discontinued there is a seven-fold increase in the rate of suicide attempts and a nine-fold increase in the rates of suicide.[43] Other mood stabilizers, such as valproate and carbamazepine, are also widely used to treat bipolar disorders in children and adolescents; although their efficacy has yet to be empirically demonstrated. Depressed suicidal children and adolescents with a history of bipolar disorder should first be treated with a mood stabilizer before receiving an antidepressant.

Studies in depressed adults have found that the selective serotonin reuptake inhibitor (**SSRI**) antidepressants reduce suicidal ideation, and also reduce the frequency of suicide attempts in non-depressed patients with cluster B personality disorders with a past history of suicide-attempt behaviour.[44] In contrast to the highly lethal potential of tricyclic antidepressants when taken in overdoses, SSRIs have low lethal potential. In a controlled trial of the depot neuroleptic flupenthixol, Montgomery and Montgomery[45] noted a significant reduction in suicide-attempt behaviour in adults who had made numerous previous attempts. Similar studies have yet to be conducted for adolescents.

In the past decade, there has been much controversy over whether the SSRI antidepressants can induce suicidal ideation and/or behaviour. A number of case reports appeared in 1990 describing patients who had developed suicidal preoccupations after starting treatment with fluoxetine. These reports were not supported by meta-analyses and re-analyses of large SSRI-treatment trials of depressed, bulimic, or anxious patients.[46,47] The conclusion was reached that suicidal ideation is a common feature of depression and that the prevalence in SSRI-treated depressives was no greater than expected.

However, one reanalysis of the data presented in certain of these studies suggested that new ideation was significantly more common in SSRI-treated depressed patients who had not previously reported suicidal ideation. Further, in a naturalistic challenge study, Rothschild and Locke[48] were able to reinduce suicidal ideas in a small series of patients who had first experienced ideation after starting treatment with fluoxetine. These patients had also experienced akathisia as a complication of fluoxetine treatment, and a relationship between suicidality and fluoxetine-induced akathisia has been noted by others.

Several meta-analyses have shed some additional light on this complex issue. A British meta-analysis of 702 clinical trials involving 87,650 adult patients documented a two-fold increase in suicide attempts in patients receiving SSRIs as compared to placebo.[49] An American meta-analysis of pediatric patients used data from 23 trials involving 4582 patients.[50] This study also found an increased risk of suicidality in patients taking SSRIs, after controlling for the risk associated with suffering from depression. Both British and American regulatory agencies now require warnings about suicidal risks associated with SSRIs. (See also chapter 9.5.5)

At this stage, the wisest course of action is for the practitioner to be particularly observant during the early stages of fluoxetine treatment of a depressed adolescent, to systematically enquire about suicidal ideation before and after treatment is started, and to be especially alert to the possibility of suicidality if SSRI treatment is associated with the onset of akathisia.

One must be careful about the risk of inducing suicidal ideation or behaviour through psychopharmacological activation or disinhibition. Clinicians should be cautious about prescribing medications that may reduce self-control, such as the benzodiazepines, and phenobarbitone (phenobarbital). These drugs also have a high lethal potential if taken in overdose. Montgomery[51] noted that benzodiazepines may disinhibit some individuals who then become aggressive and attempt suicide and that there are suggestions of similar effects from the antidepressants, maprotiline and amitriptyline, the amphetamines, and phenobarbitone. Amphetamines or other stimulant medication should only be prescribed when treating suicidal children and adolescents with attention-deficit hyperactivity disorder.

# Possibilities for prevention
## Community-based suicide prevention

The principal public health approaches to suicide prevention have been as follows:

- crisis hotlines
- method control
- media counselling to minimize imitative suicide

- indirect case-finding by educating potential gatekeepers, teachers, parents, and peers to identify the 'warning signs' of an impending suicide
- direct case-finding among high-school or college students or among the patients of primary practitioners by screening for conditions that place teenagers at risk for suicide
- training professionals to improve the recognition and treatment of mood disorders.

### (a) Crisis hotlines

Although crisis hotlines are available almost everywhere in the United States, research so far has been fairly limited and has failed to show that they impact on the incidence of suicide.[52] Possible reasons for this include the fact that actively suicidal individuals (males and individuals with an acute mental disturbance) do not call hotlines because they are acutely disturbed, preoccupied, or intent on not being deflected from their intended course of action. It also seems that the large majority of callers are females, whereas males are at the greatest risk for suicide, that crisis lines are often busy and there may be a long wait before a call is answered so that callers disconnect, and that the advice that individuals receive on calling a hotline may be stereotyped, inappropriate for an individual's needs, and perceived as unhelpful by the caller.

While each of these deficiencies is potentially modifiable, to date there have been no systematic attempts to do so. Research studies in this area have been sparse and are sorely needed.

### (b) Method restriction

Method preference varies by gender and by nationality. In the United States, the most common method for committing suicide is by firearm, and it has been suggested that reducing firearm availability will reduce the incidence of suicide. However, in a natural experiment in the United Kingdom, when self-asphyxiation with coal gas became impossible after the introduction of natural gas, the decline in the suicide rate was marked but short-lived. There is, as yet, no good evidence that reducing access to firearms by gun-security laws has a significant impact on suicides attributable to such, although they do impact on accidental and homicidal deaths from firearms.[53]

### (c) Media counseling

The United States Centers for Disease Control have issued sensible guidelines for reporters and editors, pointing to the risks of exaggerated or prominent coverage of youth suicide in general, and of the risks in focusing attention on an individual suicide.[11] These sensible guidelines should be known to child clinicians who are engaged in public-health practice, even though there is, as yet, no good evidence that their application is effective in reducing the suicide rate.

### (d) Indirect case-finding through education

Controlled studies have failed to show that classes for high-school students about suicide increase students' help-seeking behaviour when they are troubled or depressed.[54] On the other hand, there is evidence that previously suicidal adolescents are perturbed by exposure to such classes.[51] Such educational programmes seem, therefore, to be both an ineffective mode of case-finding and to carry with them an unjustified risk of activating suicidal thoughts. Educational approaches in schools are dsicussed further in chapter 4.15.4

### (e) Direct case-finding

If asked in a non-threatening way, adolescents will provide accurate information about their own suicidal thoughts and/or behaviours.[21] Therefore a sensible approach to suicide prevention is to systematically screen 15- to 19-year-olds (the age group at greatest risk) for previous suicide attempts, recent serious suicidal preoccupations, depression, or complications of substance or alcohol use. Youths identified in this way should be referred for evaluation and, if necessary, treatment.

### (f) Training primary care physicians and gatekeepers in the recognition and treatment of mood disorders

Preliminary and, as yet, unreplicated studies in Sweden[55] suggest that education of primary practitioners to identify the characteristics of mood disorders better and to treat these effectively produced a significant reduction in suicide and suicide-attempt rates in women. Because the optimal treatment of adolescent depression is not as well understood as that of adult depression, this is an option that may prove to be useful, but further work is needed.

## Further information

Bridge, J.A., Goldstein, T.R. and Brent, D.A. (2006). Adolescent suicide and suicidal behaviour. *Journal of Child Psychology and Psychiatry* **47**, 372–94.

Hawton, K., Rodham, K. and Evans, E.(2006). *By their own hand: deliberate self harm and suicidal ideas in adolescents.* London, Jessica Kingsley

Hawton, K., & Fortune, S. (2008). Suicidal behaviour and deliberate self-harm. In *Rutter's Child and Adolescent Psychiatry*, (eds. M. Rutter, D. Bishop, D. Pine, S. Scott, J. Stevenson, E. Taylor, and A. Thapar) 5th Edition. pp. 647–68. Blackwell, Oxford.

## References

1. Robins, E.R., Murphy, G.E., Wilkinson, R.H., *et al.* (1959). Some clinical considerations in the prevention of suicide based on a study of 134 successful suicides. *American Journal of Public Health*, **49**, 888–99.

2. Shaffer, D. (1974). Suicide in childhood and early adolescence. *Journal of Child Psychology and Psychiatry*, **15**, 275–91.

3. Shaffer, D., Gould, M.S., Fisher, P., *et al.* (1996). Psychiatric diagnosis in child and adolescent suicide. *Archives of General Psychiatry*, **53**, 339–48.

4. Brent, D.A., Baugher, M., Bridge, J., *et al* (1999). Age- and sex-related risk factors for adolescent suicide. *Journal of the American Academy of Child and Adolescent Psychiatry*, **38**, 1497–1505.

5. Martunnen, M.J., Aro, H.M., Henriksson, M.M., *et al.* (1991). Mental disorders in adolescent suicide DSM-III-R axes I and II diagnoses in suicides among thirteen- to nineteen-year-olds in Finland. *Archives of General Psychiatry*, **48**, 834–9.

6. Shaffer, D. and Hicks, R. (1993). The epidemiology of child and adolescent suicide. In *The epidemiology of childhood disorders* (ed. B. Pless), pp. 339–68. Oxford University Press, New York.

7. World Health Organization (1996). *World health statistics annual.* WHO, Geneva.

8. Taylor, S.J., Kingdom, D., and Jenkins, R. (1997). How are nations trying to prevent suicide? An analysis of national suicide prevention strategies. Review. *Acta Psychiatrica Scandinavica*, **95**, 457–63.

9. Ministry of Youth Affairs, Ministry of Health, Te Puni Kokiri (Ministry of Maori Development) (1999). *In our hands: New Zealand youth suicide prevention strategy.* New Zealand Ministry of Health, Wellington.

10. Commonwealth Department of Health and Family Services, Mental Health Branch (1997). *Youth suicide in Australia: the national youth suicide prevention strategy.* Australian Government Publishing Service, Canberra.

11. Center for Diseases Control Prevention Guidelines, United States of America (1994). Programs for the prevention of suicide among adolescents and young adults. *Morbidity and Mortality Weekly Report*, **43**, 1–18.

12. Gould, M.S., Fisher, P., Parides, M., *et al.* (1996). Psychosocial risk factors of child and adolescent completed suicide. *Archives of General Psychiatry*, **53**, 1155–62.

13. Gould, M.S. and Shaffer, D. (1986). The impact of television movies: evidence of imitation. *New England Journal of Medicine*, **315**, 690–4.

14. Cuddy–Casey, M. and Orvaschel, H. (1997). Children's understanding of death in relation to child suicidality and homicidality. *Clinical Psychology Review*, **17**, 33–45.

15. Schmidtke, A., Bille–Brahe, U., DeLeo, D., *et al.* (1996). Attempted suicide in Europe: rates, trends and sociodemographic characteristics of suicide attempters during the period 1989–1992. Results of the WHO/EURO Multicentre Study on Parasuicide. *Acta Psychiatrica Scandinavica*, **93**, 327–38.

16. Fergusson, D.M. and Lynskey, M.T. (1995). Suicide attempts and suicidal ideation in a birth cohort of sixteen-year-old New Zealanders. *Journal of the American Academy of Child and Adolescent Psychiatry*, **34**, 1308–17.

17. Remafedi, G., French, S., Story, M., *et al.* (1998). The relationship between suicide risk and sexual orientation: results of a population-based study. *American Journal of Public Health*, **88**, 57–60.

18. Beck, A.T., Weissman, A., Lester, D., *et al.* (1974). The measurement of pessimism: the Hopelessness Scale. *Journal of Consulting and Clinical Psychology*, **42**, 861–5.

19. Beck, A.T., Kovacs, M., and Weissman, A. (1979). Assessment of suicide intention: the Scale for Suicide Ideation. *Journal of Consulting and Clinical Psychology*, **47**, 343–52.

20. Pfeffer, C.R., Conte, H.R., Plutchik, R., *et al.* (1979). Suicidal behavior in latency-age children: an empirical study. *Journal of the American Academy of Child Psychiatry*, **18**, 679–92.

21. Safer, D.J. (1997). Self-reported suicide attempts by adolescents. *Annals of Clinical Psychiatry*, **9**, 263–9.

22. Hawton, K. (1986). *Suicide and attempted suicide among children and adolescents.* Sage, Beverly Hills, CA.

23. Brent, D.A., Holder, D., Kolko, D., *et al.* (1997). A clinical psychotherapy trial for adolescent depression comparing cognitive, family, and supportive therapy. *Archives of General Psychiatry*, **54**, 877–85.

24. National Center for Health Statistics (2000). *Death rates for 72 selected causes by 5-year age groups, race, and sex, 1979–1997*, pp. 485–90. Centers for Disease Control, Atlanta, GA. (Website: http://www.cdc.gov/nchs/datawh/statab/unpubd/mortabs.htm)

25. Neeleman, J. and Wessely, S. (1999). Ethnic minority suicide: a small area geographical study in south London. *Psychological Medicine*, **29**, 429–36.

26. Neeleman, J., Wessely, S., and Lewis, G. (1998). Suicide acceptability in African- and white Americans: the role of religion. *Journal of Nervous and Mental Disease*, **186**, 12–16.

27. Neeleman, J., Halpern, D., Leon, D., *et al.* (1997). Tolerance of suicide, religion and suicide rates: an ecological and individual study in 19 Western countries. *Psychological Medicine*, **27**, 1165–71.

28. Carlsten, A., Allebeck, P., and Brandt, L. (1996). Are suicide rates in Sweden associated with changes in the prescribing of medicines? *Acta Psychiatrica Scandinavica*, **94**, 94–100.

29. Kessler, R., Berglund, P., Borges, G., *et al.* (2005) Trends in Suicide Ideation, Plans, Gestures, and Attempts in the United States, 1990-1992 to 2001-2003. *Journal of the American Medical Association*, **293**, 2487–95.

30. Centers for Disease Control (1998). Attempted suicide among high–school students–United States, 1997. *Morbidity and Mortality Weekly Report*, **47**, 47–9.

31. Brent, D.A., Poling, K., McKain, B., *et al.* (1993). A psychoeducational program for families of affectively ill children and adolescents. *Journal of the American Academy of Child and Adolescent Psychiatry*, **32**, 770–4.

32. Mann, J.J. and Stoff, D.M. (1997). A synthesis of current findings regarding neurobiological correlates and treatment of suicidal behavior. *Annals of the New York Academy of Sciences*, **836**, 352–63.

33. Arango, V., Underwood, M.D., and Mann, J.J. (1997). Biologic alterations in the brainstem of suicides. *Psychiatric Clinics of North America*, **20**, 581–93.

34. Nordstrom, P., Samuelsson, M., Asberg, M., *et al.* (1994). CSF 5–HIAA predicts suicide risk after attempted suicide. *Suicide and Life Threatening Behavior*, **24**, 1–9.

35. Juon, H.S. and Ensminger, M.E. (1997). Childhood, adolescent, and young adult predictors of suicidal behaviors: a prospective study of African-Americans. *Journal of Child Psychology and Psychiatry and Allied Disciplines*, **38**, 553–63.

36. Pfeffer, C.R., Klerman, G.L., Hurt, S.W., *et al.* (1991). Suicidal children grow up: demographic and clinical risk factors for adolescent suicide attempts. *Journal of the American Academy of Child and Adolescent Psychiatry*, **30**, 609–16.

37. Pfeffer, C.R., Klerman, G.K., Hurt, S.W., *et al.* (1993). Suicidal children grow up: rates and psychosocial risk factors for suicide attempts during follow-up. *Journal of the American Academy of Child and Adolescent Psychiatry*, **32**, 106–13.

38. Harrington, R., Bredenkamp, D., Groothues, C., *et al.* (1994). Adult outcomes of childhood and adolescent depression. III: Links with suicidal behaviours. *Journal of Child Psychology and Psychiatry and Allied Disciplines*, **35**, 1309–19.

39. Drye, R., Goulding, R., and Goulding, M.E. (1973). No-suicide decisions: patient monitoring of suicide risk. *American Journal of Psychiatry*, **130**, 171–4.

40. Clarke, G.N., Rohde, P., Lewinsohn, P.M., *et al.* (1999). Cognitive-behavioral treatment of adolescent depression: efficacy of acute group treatment and booster sessions. *Journal of the American Academy of Child and Adolescent Psychiatry*, **38**, 272–9.

41. Linehan, M.M. (1993). *Cognitive behavior therapy of borderline personality disorder*. Guilford, New York.

42. Miller, A.L., Rathus, J.H., Linehan, M.M., *et al.* (1997). Dialectical behavior therapy adapted for suicidal adolescents. *Journal of Practical Psychiatry and Behavioral Health*, **3**, 78–86.

43. Tondo, L., Jamison, K.R., and Baldessarini, R.J. (1997). Effect of lithium maintenance on suicidal behavior in major mood disorders. *Annals of the New York Academy of Sciences*, **836**, 339–51.

44. Letizia, C., Kapik, B., and Flanders, W.D. (1996). Suicidal risk during controlled clinical investigations of fluvoxamine. *Journal of Clinical Psychiatry*, **57**, 415–21.

45. Montgomery, S.A. and Montgomery, D. (1982). Pharmacological prevention of suicidal behaviour. *Journal of Affective Disorders*, **4**, 291–8.

46. Fava, M. and Rosenbaum, J.F. (1991). Suicidality and fluoxetine: is there a relationship? *Journal of Clinical Psychiatry*, **52**, 108–11.

47. Beasley, C.M., Jr., Dornseif, B.E., Bosomworth, J.C., *et al.* (1991). Fluoxetine and suicide: a meta–analysis of controlled trials of treatment for depression. *British Medical Journal*, **21**, 685–92.

48. Rothschild, A.J. and Locke, C.A. (1991). Reexposure to fluoxetine after serious suicide attempts by three patients: the role of akathisia. *Journal of Clinical Psychiatry*, **52**, 491–3.

49. Fergusson, D., Doucette, S., Glass, K.C., *et al.* (2005). Association between suicide attempts and selective serotonin reuptake inhibitors: systematic review of randomized controlled trials. *British Medical Journal*, **330**, 396–402.

50. Hammad, T.A., Laughren, T., Racoosin, J., *et al.* (2006). Suicidality in Pediatric Patients Treated with Antidepressant Drugs. *Archives of General Psychiatry*, **63**, 332–9.

51. Montgomery, S.A. (1997). Suicide and antidepressants. *Annals of the New York Academy of Sciences*, **29**, 329–38.

52. Shaffer, D., Garland, A., Gould, M., *et al.* (1988). Preventing teenage suicide: a critical review. *Journal of the American Academy of Child and Adolescent Psychiatry*, **27**, 675–87.

53. Cummings, P., Grossman, D.C., Rivara, F.P., *et al.* (1997). State gun safe storage laws and child mortality due to firearms. *Journal of the American Medical Association*, **278**, 1084–6.

54. Shaffer, D., Vieland, V., Garland, A., *et al.* (1990). Adolescent suicide attempters: response to suicide-prevention programs. *Journal of the American Medical Association*, **264**, 3151–5.

55. Rihmer, Z., Rutz, W., and Pihlgran, H. (1995). Depression and suicide on Gotland: an intensive study of all suicides before and after a depression–training programme for general practitioners. *Journal of Affective Disorders*, **35**, 147–52.

## 9.2.11 **Children's speech and language difficulties**

Judy Clegg

### Introduction

Speech and language difficulties have a significant impact on the lives of children and their families. This chapter will give an overview of the types of speech and language difficulties children present with and how these are generally classified and diagnosed. Specific Language Impairment (SLI) and speech and language difficulties associated with child psychiatric disorder, specifically disorders of attention and selective mutism will be a focus. The life course of children with speech and language impairments will be described through childhood, adolescence, and adult life. Current management approaches will be presented and evaluated and strategies for effective communication considered.

### Clinical features

#### Typical speech and language development

It is remarkable how quickly and easily most children progress through the typical stages of speech and language development to become competent communicators by the age of 5 years. Much is known about how children acquire speech and language and when these skills are achieved.[1] Children need to be competent communicators prior to starting school, as learning is dependent on adequate speech and language abilities. At school entry age, children are expected to be able to speak clearly, to understand and use complex grammatical structures, to use language for a range of communicative reasons from requesting to negotiating and predicting, to take part confidently in conversations with both children and adults and to have a knowledge of letter names and sounds and to read some single words. The acquisition of these speech and language skills will enable the child to access the educational curriculum where learning is dependent on both verbal and written language. If children are not competent in these skills then they will experience significant difficulties in their learning from the start of their school career.

## Features of speech and language difficulties

Speech and language development can be affected by hearing impairment, visual impairment, general learning disability, epilepsy, and specific syndromes of learning disability such as Down's syndrome, and Fragile X syndrome. In these examples, speech and language difficulties are usually attributed to and explained by an aetiological cause. However, speech and language difficulties do occur in the absence of an obvious identifiable cause and are therefore considered as a specific impairment, e.g. SLI.

Prevalence rates of speech and language difficulties vary and are dependent on the criteria used to define and classify them. Law et al.[2] report prevalence rates in children as high as 24.6 per cent whereas rates for SLI are much lower between 3 and 7 per cent.[3] Importantly, speech and language difficulties can persist over time and often have a negative impact on the child's education and general well-being.

### (a) Speech difficulties

A speech difficulty reduces a child's intelligibility and may result in speech sounds being omitted, substituted with another sound or distorted. Speech difficulties can be evident when a child says single words, sentences, and participates in conversation. The physical articulation of speech sounds is affected by physiological and structural abnormalities, such as cleft lip/palate, and neurological impairments leading to dysarthria characterized by weakness and/or in-coordination of the speech musculature system. There is another group of children who have phonological speech difficulties. These children have an intact speech musculature system but have not managed to acquire all the speech sounds of their language and so can only use a limited range, which subsequently limits their intelligibility.

### (b) Language difficulties

Language difficulties can involve problems in the development of both comprehension and production.

#### (i) Vocabulary difficulties

Restricted word knowledge and poor development of the understanding of word meanings result in small vocabularies. Some children have impoverished vocabularies but other children can have specific word finding or retrieval difficulties. Here, the child knows the word he wants to say but is unable to retrieve it accurately and quickly. This is usually evident by 'searching' behaviours where the child may substitute the word for a related word, use a filler word such as 'thingy' or 'stuff', gesture the word instead of saying it or say the first sound of the word but not the rest. For example,

ICE SKATING: 'I can't do that thing . . . erm . . . you know . . . where you put sharp shoes on . . . I always fall over'.
PLUM: 'well, I don't really like that one which smells like soil and is purple and juicy'

These problems may not only be due to lexical difficulties but also problems retrieving the right phonological sounds of the word. Cognitive impairments in information processing, specifically short-term and phonological working memory have been associated with problems in vocabulary learning.[4]

#### (ii) Syntax difficulties

Children often have difficulties in their understanding and use of syntax and as a consequence find it very difficult to not only understand language but also to construct sentences in order to use language to communicate effectively, for example giving a narrative where past events are described and future events predicted. Common problems are learning how to use inflections to mark different tenses and understanding as well as constructing complex sentences such as passives. The child in the following example has lots of syntax difficulties as well as word finding difficulties and it is clear how this affects his ability to convey verbal information. The correct forms the child is attempting are shown in brackets.

'They erm . . . was . . . erm . . . goed to make (made) some vegetable circles (pizzas) and rolls (they rolled) it (the dough) out because that's what you do first and he was reading the menu (recipe) as well and then they is erm . . . erm . . . erm . . . printing (cut) them out and then they put them in the oven because they'll taste crunchy (to cook) and then erm . . . then they took them out of the oven so they be . . . er . . . get . . . cool down (could cool down) and then you would take (ate) them'.

#### (iii) Social communication difficulties

Children with speech and language difficulties often show associated problems in social communication behaviours, also referred to as pragmatics. These can be both verbal and non-verbal and include difficulties with eye contact, initiation, turn taking, interaction, sharing, requesting, and responding. Higher level social communication abilities can also be affected such as inferring information, giving the listener adequate information and self-monitoring. Ultimately, these can all hinder effective communication between the child and others and also expose the child to negative social experiences, particularly with their peers. For some children, the social communication difficulties may be an intrinsic part of a developmental disorder where speech and language difficulties are evident, for example children with autistic spectrum disorders. In other children, it is important to note that these behaviours can develop as a secondary consequence of poor communication skills due to the speech and language difficulty.

## Classification

Speech difficulties can occur in isolation without the presence of language difficulties. Language difficulties can also occur without the presence of speech difficulties but often speech and language difficulties co-occur together. Children can have difficulties with both language comprehension and language production.

Within child psychiatry, both the ICD-10[5] and DSM-IV[6] systems categorize developmental speech and language difficulties. However, there is little robust empirical evidence to support the subtyping of speech and language difficulties. Children are usually classified according to whether the speech and language difficulty is specific, i.e. cognitive development is age appropriate and if there are any co-morbid aetiological or functional explanations. Descriptions of the type of speech and language difficulty involve identifying how the speech and language system is disrupted, describing the levels of impairment, and how this is impacting on the child's communication and their access to learning.

# Diagnosis and differential diagnosis

## Descriptions of developmental speech and language disorders

Children's language is said to be 'delayed' when their language abilities are behind those expected for their chronological age and 'impaired' or 'disordered' when a language delay does not resolve and the child continues to experience significant and severe problems. Several established diagnoses of developmental speech and language disorders are described below:

### (a) Cleft lip and palate

A cleft/lip palate results from the incomplete fusion of the hard or soft palate in the embryonic stages of development. A cleft palate can be accompanied by a cleft lip or either one can occur independently. In the United Kingdom, cleft lip/palate is repaired in the first few months of life. However, some children can be left with fistulas and velopharyngeal incompetency, which significantly affects speech development and intelligibility. Children with cleft lip/palate receive speech and language therapy from birth onwards. At birth the focus of attention is primarily on feeding and then the development of speech and language.

### (b) Dysarthria

Dysarthria is a speech disorder due to neurological impairment which affects how the speech musculature system functions. Children with cerebral palsy often have dysarthria, which makes their speech slow, weak, and uncoordinated. There may be a mild, slight slurring of speech to profound dysarthria where a child cannot produce any intelligible sounds or words. Children with moderate and severe dysarthria have shallow breathing which is insufficient to sustain speech and/or a low-pitched voice, nasal speech, and a reduced range of vowels and consonants that can be produced accurately.

### (c) Developmental phonological disorder

Unlike cleft lip/palate and dysarthria, phonological speech disorders involve the child's developing speech sound or phonological system. The child's speech is difficult to understand because the child makes speech sound errors which are either due to the speech sound system developing more slowly or in an atypical way and this is not a result of obvious structural, sensory, or neurological impairments. Often, there are systematic patterns of errors in the child's speech, for example the child always replaces the 's' sound with a 'd' sound. Auditory processing and discrimination skills have been implicated in the development and maintenance of this disorder. Over time, phonological disorders often resolve with speech and language therapy input. However, for some children they are severe and do persist into adult life.

### (d) Childhood apraxia of speech (CAS)

This developmental speech disorder is characterized by both speech and non-speech behaviours. The speech sound errors are inconsistent and are accompanied with oral movement difficulties in drooling, feeding, and blowing. Reduced early verbal behaviours such as babbling are often evident. CAS often co-occurs with motor apraxia but for some children, only speech and oral movements are affected. There is some debate as to the existence of CAS as there is no obvious cause although both neuromotor planning and the organization of the child's phonological system have been implicated. CAS is often a label given to children where the speech disorder has persisted despite intervention and oral non-speech movements are affected. See Dodd[7] for a detailed review of children's speech disorders.

### (e) Fluency disorders

Although classified under speech disorders, stuttering is not an articulatory or phonological difficulty. There are no structural abnormalities and the child usually has a typically developing phonological system. Core stuttering behaviours include part-word or whole-word repetitions, revisions, pauses, blocks, sound prolongations, and obvious struggling behaviours such as jerky head movements. Secondary behaviours result from the stuttering and generally help the individual to avoid stuttering. For example, circumlocution where the speaker substitutes a word he knows he will stutter on for an easier word and environmental control such as avoiding the use of the telephone or talking to certain people. Fluency disorders are often identified in young children before the age of 5 years although many children experience a period of normal non-fluency usually between the ages of 2 and 5 years, which is not severe and resolves spontaneously.

### (f) Learning disability

Level of cognitive ability is the strongest predictor of language ability and therefore language development is certainly affected in learning disability. The sequence of language development is similar to that found in typical development but with mild to moderate to severe and profound delay. A child with a profound learning disability may never develop an intent to communicate whereas another child may have established an intent but no verbal language and uses some signs or symbols to communicate instead. For children with mild and moderate learning disability, language abilities plateau with no further improvement, usually in adolescence at a level below the child's chronological age.

It should be noted that specific patterns of speech and language development have been identified in specific syndromes of learning disability. Down's syndrome is characterized by superior vocabulary development to grammatical development and children with William's syndrome often appear as competent communicators but do have significant language learning problems. Speech and fluency problems are common in learning disability and vary according to the aetiology of the learning disability. For example, conductive hearing loss and articulatory speech problems occur where there is cranio-facial involvement.

### (g) Acquired childhood aphasias

Acquired aphasias refer to a loss or deterioration in language ability after a period of typical language development. The child acquires language but then loses these language abilities, usually between 3 and 7 years of age. Causes of childhood aphasia include open and closed head injury, cerebrovascular lesions, cerebral infections, cerebral tumours, and epilepsy. Landau Kleffner (first described by Landau and Kleffner in 1957)[8] is an acquired aphasia where language deteriorates after a period of typical language development and the deterioration in language is usually, although not always accompanied with a seizure disorder. Receptive language is severely affected with expressive language problems as well, often word finding difficulties. See Lees[9] and Deonna[10] for a complete review.

# Specific language impairment (SLI)

Specific language impairment (SLI) is a term used to describe language impairment (and additional speech impairment) where there is no identifiable medical, neurological, sensory, or functional cause and where cognitive ability measured by non-verbal intelligence (IQ) is within the normal range. Therefore, there is a discrepancy between language and cognitive ability with the exclusion of any obvious causes for the language impairment. Diagnosis of SLI according to exclusionary and discrepancy criteria is dependent on standardized language and cognitive psychometric assessments. However, there is continuing debate regarding which criteria to use to establish a meaningful discrepancy between language and cognition. ICD-10,[5] for example adopt a strict criteria of language skills at least two standard deviations below the level expected for the child's chronological age and language skills at least one standard deviation below the child's level of non-verbal IQ. More liberal criteria advocates a non-verbal IQ of 75 or above with language abilities often only one SD below the mean. Proponents of liberal criteria claim that more stringent criteria may fail to identify children who are at risk of poor long-term outcomes. However, liberal criterion may identify children who simply perform at the lower end of the normal distribution of language ability. It should be recognized that different criteria are used. Although the diagnosis of SLI stipulates good cognitive ability, some specific cognitive deficits in phonological memory, verbal, and visuo-spatial memory and symbolic play are evident and thought to underpin the language impairment.

SLI is considered to affect 3–7 per cent of all children.[3] The use of the exclusionary and discrepancy criteria to define SLI means that as a group, children with SLI are very heterogenous with impairments in many areas of language. Although useful, attempts to subtype SLI[11] have not yet proved clinically robust. However, children with SLI are considered to show disproportionate difficulties in vocabulary and syntax compared to other aspects of language.

## (a) Aetiology of SLI

Research in SLI primarily focuses on trying to establishing a cause. SLI is a heritable disorder and much research is underway to try and establish the genetic basis.[12,13] SLI is of particular interest to researchers because of the unusual dissociation between cognitive and language ability and whether this dissociation is explained by innate modular theories of language acquisition or more general cognitive processing deficit theories. Some attempt has been made to identify genetic markers of SLI such as a phonological memory deficit[12] which stems from the research into general cognitive processing deficits as underlying SLI and a specific tense marking deficit[14] or a syntax representational deficit[15] which argues for the disruption of innate modular components of language.

## (b) Diagnostic overlaps between SLI and autistic spectrum disorders (ASD)

### (i) Pragmatic language impairment

Autism and autistic spectrum disorders (ASD) are discussed extensively in Chapter 9.2.2 of this text. Language and communication difficulties are central to both SLI and ASD. However, the fundamental difference between these disorders is the severity and pervasiveness of the social communication impairment. In SLI, social communication difficulties are considered secondary to the language impairment where children with speech and language difficulties will have problems in developing appropriate social communication skills. In ASD, the social communication impairment is an intrinsic part of the disorder and does not develop as a secondary consequence of a speech and language impairment. Due to the increase in the identification of ASD and the use of the autistic spectrum many more children with milder difficulties are being diagnosed with ASD. This has led to some researchers proposing that there are overlaps between SLI and ASD.

Semantic–pragmatic disorder was first described in the 1980s as a subtype of SLI[16,17] and was a label used to describe children with comprehension problems, echolalia, behaviour difficulties, and difficulty with non-literal language, semantics and pragmatics. At the time, these children were not considered as autistic. However, the increasing use of the autistic spectrum led to debates about whether semantic–pragmatic disorder exists as a separate category of SLI or whether it should be included on the autistic spectrum.[18,19] The crucial issue was whether the social impairment was intrinsic to the language disorder or a secondary consequence of the language disorder. To address this, researchers have attempted to show differences in pragmatic abilities between children with SLI, ASD, and typically developing children. For example, Bishop and Norbury[19] identified a subgroup of SLI children who show a profile of Pragmatic Language Impairment (PLI). These children showed inappropriate behaviours across aspects of social communication including initiating conversations, understanding subtle aspects of language such as humour and sarcasm, adapting their communication to different contexts, understanding and using non-verbal communication, and engaging in conversations about specific interests. Importantly, these children did not show the non-verbal repetitive behaviours typically characteristic of autism. Overall it is argued[19] that there are continuities between autism and specific language impairment but not all children with pragmatic impairments have autism. Therefore, pragmatic language impairment alone should not be used to make diagnoses of autistic spectrum disorders. It is recognized that there are conflicting opinions about the increasing evidence that indicates continuity between disorders that have traditionally been regarded as distinct from one another. However, assessment should consider whether a child's social communication difficulties are being compounded by language difficulties as amelioration of the language difficulties may improve the child's social communication.

## (c) Associations between language and behaviour in child psychiatric disorders

Children with primary psychiatric disorders often have a history of developmental problems which can include speech and language delay. Children with primary speech and language disorders are at greater risk of developing behaviour difficulties than children without speech and language disorders. Various mechanisms have been put forward to try and explain this association. These include common antecedents such as low intelligence and deprivation,[20] environmental factors where language stimulation is negatively affected by poor parent–child interactions or the child's inability to attend to the language stimulus,[21] the psychosocial rejections and academic failure experienced by children with communication impairments affecting their self-confidence and self-esteem and therefore their subsequent emotional behaviour development,[22–24] and a neurodevelopmental abnormality or immaturity as a shared underlying cause.[25,26] Although the simplicity of these mechanisms is appealing, identifying, and differentiating them is certainly complex.

More recently studies have shown that children with primary psychiatric disorders can have undetected speech and language disorders.[27,28] ADHD is one of the most commonly reported psychiatric disorders associated with speech and language difficulties.[29] In ADHD, language difficulties consist of both receptive and expressive problems[30] and pragmatic language difficulties[31,32] such as excessive talking and poor topic maintenance. Although studies have not identified a distinct profile of speech and language difficulties in ADHD, they should be considered in assessment and management.

It has been hypothesized that these undetected speech and language disorders somehow play a role in the development and maintenance of the psychiatric disorder and even that the psychiatric disorder is secondary to the undetected speech and language disorder (see mechanisms above). There is very limited evidence available to specify what the associations are and importantly, it may be that referral practices play a role where the psychiatric problem takes priority and the child is referred to mental health services first. In the United Kingdom SLT and mental health services are usually very separate and it is not common that SLTs work in mental health services. The identification of previously undetected speech and language disorders in the studies above are really the late identification of pre-existing difficulties. Nevertheless, management of childhood psychiatric disorders should consider if speech and language difficulties are a factor in the child's behaviour as they may have an impact on how the child is managed, particularly with respect to participation in verbal therapies and education.

### (c) Selective mutism

This childhood disorder is described as the persistent refusal to talk in certain social situations despite being able to talk in other situations. The most common pattern is talking at home but not at school and the refusal to talk cannot be better accounted for by a communication disorder or difficulties in understanding and using spoken language. Pervasive developmental disorder or psychotic disorder should also be excluded. The mutism must last for more than a month (this cannot be the first month of school) and interfere significantly with educational progress, social communication with others, and occupational achievement. In the case of a bilingual child, it is suggested that the mutism should persist for at least 6 months and be present in both the first and second language before diagnosis.[33]

Selective mutism is rare and as a result only a limited number of studies reporting the epidemiology of this disorder are available. Prevalence figures estimate a prevalence of approximately 0.75 to 0.80 per cent [34,35] and it is slightly more common in girls[36] with an onset between the ages of 3 and 5 years.[34] Although there is no clear consensus to explain the cause(s) of the disorder, social phobia, and anxiety are certainly involved. Co-morbidity with behaviour problems, communication difficulties and developmental delay are also found which indicates that a multi-factorial aetiology is the best explanation. Data regarding the long-term outcomes is scarce but there are indications that with early intervention improvements are made but often children are still left feeling uncomfortable in some speaking situations.

### (d) Intervention for selective mutism

Intervention approaches include pharmacology, cognitive behaviour therapy, family therapy, psychodynamic therapy, and speech and language therapy. Although some success with fluoxetine has been reported[37] this has not been widely replicated. A behavioural approach considers the disorder as learned behaviour and techniques including contingency management, shaping and stimulus fading, systematic desensitization, and self-modelling are advocated. Family therapy aims to identify whether there are difficulties in family relationships that are contributing to the mutism and attempts to work with the whole family to foster more positive relationships. Psychodynamic approaches involve techniques of play therapy and art therapy to identify the underlying reasons for the mutism and to help the child to express the possible unconscious conflicts he is experiencing. Although children with selective mutism are expected to have good speech and language skills, several studies have reported a high incidence of speech and language difficulties such as articulation and expressive and receptive language difficulties.[38,39] In these circumstances, speech and language therapy is used as a valuable adjunct to the other approaches. Speech and language therapy aims to facilitate the child's communication rather than resolving the underlying causes of the mutism. Therapists work with the child to desensitize him/her to communicating with others by considering the child's communication environment and the communication load of the tasks he is expected to engage in. A hierarchy of stages is followed from easy to hard speech tasks within easy to hard speaking situations. A multi-modal perspective incorporating a combination of the above approaches is advocated. The combination of family involvement with cognitive behavioural, speech and language, psychodynamic and family involvement meet the multi-factorial needs of this disorder. See Cohan *et al.*[40] for a detailed review of the efficacy of the different intervention approaches described. Although social anxiety is the predominating feature of selective mutism, the resulting lack of communication is challenging. Several strategies to facilitate communication with these children are presented and these can easily be incorporated into other intervention approaches:

- Check that there are no speech and language difficulties that may be contributing to the mutism. For some children, although early speech and language difficulties may have resolved the child may still feel under confident in their talking.

- One-to-one settings are most comfortable and try and include the familiar person, (usually the primary carer) who the child communicates regularly with in your interventions to start with. After a while the child may be able to manage this setting without the familiar person. This process may have to be repeated to encourage the child to talk in another setting.

- Encourage and accept non-verbal communication such as head nods, writing, drawing, and gesture as well as verbal communication. Non-verbal communication is easier than talking for most of these children.

- Follow a hierarchy of verbal communication from easy to hard, most children find whispering and talking quietly easier than loud talking.

- Consider the complexity of the task the child is expected to engage in. Questions, which are factual or only require a yes or no response are much less confrontational than questions, which ask the child about their feelings or opinion.

Further management considerations are detailed in Johnson and Wintgens.[41]

## Course and prognosis

### Life course and outcomes

An interest in the long-term outcomes of children with speech and language difficulties has emerged fairly recently. Historically, it was considered that primary speech and language difficulties resolved over time with no implications for other areas of development. This is certainly not true and much more is now known about the developmental trajectories through childhood, adolescence, and into adult life. Generally, children with speech and language difficulties continue to show difficulties not only in communication but in cognition, behaviour, educational attainment, and psychosocial functioning. This section will focus on the life course and outcomes of children with profiles of primary speech and language difficulties where there is no cognitive deficit. Cognitive ability is a powerful predictor of development, and therefore the outcomes of children with speech and language difficulties associated with cognitive delay are usually attributed to level of IQ rather than the specific speech and language difficulties themselves.

### The impact of a speech and language impairment over the lifespan

Speech and language impairment leads to impoverished communication skills, which certainly impact on other areas of development. The developmental trajectories of children with primary speech and language impairment show impaired receptive and expressive language development in later childhood, adolescence, and even adult life. Cognition, as measured by non-verbal IQ has been shown to fluctuate and even deteriorate over time, particularly in adolescence and later life. Research to date suggests that any deterioration is temporary and resolves but much more needs to be known about this.[42,43] Children with speech and language difficulties are more likely to experience emotional and behavioural problems (see earlier section). During the course of childhood, the risk of developing emotional and behavioural problems seems to increase with obvious negative implications for other areas of development and functioning. There is a possible association between SLD and the development of antisocial behaviour in early adult life. At the age of 19 years participants with SLD in a Canadian community sample did not show high levels of aggression but did have higher rates of arrests and convictions.[26]

The increase in social and behaviour problems may be the result of communication and interaction problems young people experience in conjunction with the increasing social and academic demands placed on them. However, it is hard to disentangle cause and effect when so many variables interact. Socio-economic status (SES), learning ability, and type of educational placement no doubt also make a contribution. Therefore, SES and IQ are probably implicated in the development of social and behavioural difficulties as well as the speech and language impairment. In adult life, severe mental health conditions such as schizophrenia, depression, and personality disorder have been linked with early histories of and persisting severe speech and language impairment.[44]

There are strong associations between speech, language, and literacy development and in fact, speech and language are fundamental in learning to read and write. In order to learn, children need to be competent communicators when they start school. Language is the medium through which children are expected to learn and literacy is dependent on identifying and discriminating speech and letter sounds. Children with persisting speech and language difficulties are at risk for literacy problems and subsequent low academic achievement. Children with speech and language difficulties find it much harder to learn to read and write than children without speech and language difficulties. Educational attainment is dependent on literacy and therefore these children are very disadvantaged. Studies measuring educational attainment using Standard Assessment Tests (SAT) have found that children with speech and language difficulties gain significantly lower SAT scores than controls.[45] In older individuals, attainment at GCSE and A level is also affected. Children with speech and language difficulties are often bullied by their peers and can be targets for victimization.[46] Studies suggest that this is due to their odd communication particularly difficulties with social communication behaviour. Unclear speech is also a significant factor. In adult life, high levels of social maladaption and poor psychosocial functioning were found in adults in their mid 30s with SLI. Employment, relationships, independent living, and health were all significantly and negatively affected.[44] See Clegg[47] for a full review.

### Identification of children at risk

There are variations in outcomes and not all children with speech and language impairment are at risk of later negative outcomes. Issues of variability and risk and resilience are not yet fully understood. Risk factors for poor outcomes in later life are the severity of the initial impairment, involvement of receptive language, low IQ, and low SES. Resilience factors are the presence of pure speech difficulties only, high IQ, high SES, and access to specialist support. A critical age hypothesis[48] proposes that any speech and language difficulties that impact on a child's communication after 5 years should be considered as significant and prioritized for intervention.

Speech and language difficulties should not be underestimated in terms of their impact on children's lives. With respect to clinical management, the risk factors should be considered in identifying those children at particular risk. In the United Kingdom, there is specialist educational provision now available that provides post-16 years provision for some young adults to try and reduce negative outcomes, e.g. supporting individuals to gain further qualifications and to enter the work place. Information about long-term outcomes can certainly inform the individuals themselves, their families, and other professionals about prognoses and how best to support individuals to meet their learning and other needs effectively.

## Management

Speech and language therapists (SLTs) work in education, health, and social care, voluntary organizations and independent practice. A SLT is an important member of the interdisciplinary team and will lead on the assessment, differential diagnosis, intervention with, and management of individuals with communication and swallowing disorders. In recent years due to the shift to inclusion, many paediatric SLTs now work in schools with educational professionals as part of the school team. This enables the SLT to contribute to statements of special education needs, formulating independent learning plans (ILP), and delivering the curriculum to make it accessible for children with speech and language difficulties. SLTs also work in community services such as the government Sure Start programme, primary and secondary health care, e.g. acute hospital settings and community clinics, specialist health services, e.g. child development centres and education, e.g. from preschool, mainstream and special schools/resourced provision. The inclusion of SLTs in Child and Adolescent Mental Health Services (CAMHS) is increasing but this is not consistent across the United Kingdom. However, there is now recognition that the SLT can have a valuable role within the CAMHS[49,50] in terms of the identification of any communication difficulties and the subsequent impact on mental health and offering intervention that will help to ameliorate the communication difficulty and facilitate communication. Within CAMHS, a SLT may be employed in a specialist unit, child psychiatry outpatient service, or other. Differential diagnoses are usually made in collaboration with the team and a SLT will use a combination of formal and informal assessment. Formal assessment consists of using measures that compare the child's speech and language abilities with abilities that are expected for the child's chronological age. Various types of assessments are available criterion referenced, standardized, developmental scales, and observational. Intervention may be direct, i.e. individual or as part of a group or indirect, i.e. through working with the family or in the context of the child's classroom and school.

## Identification of speech and language difficulties in children

The following checklist may be helpful when working with young school age children in identifying speech and language difficulties and initiating referral to speech and language therapy services.

### (a) Speech

1 Is the child's speech difficult to understand?
2 Does the child miss out sounds from words?
3 Is the child less intelligible when speaking in sentences than in single words?
*If yes*, to one or more of the above then speech difficulties are evident and referral to speech and language therapy is advised.

### (b) Comprehension

1 Can the child follow and engage in conversations with both children and adults?
2 Can the child carry out verbal instructions correctly or does he need lots of prompting?
3 Can the child understand a range of concepts such as time and space?
*If no*, to one or more of the above then comprehension difficulties are evident and referral to speech and language therapy is advised.

### (c) Production

1 Does the child have a wide range of vocabulary?
2 Can the child use more complex sentences such as the 'the boy ran for the bus because he was late' rather than the boy was late and ran for the bus?
3 Is the child able to give a narrative of a past and future event?
4 Does the child frequently say non-specific words such as 'stuff' or 'thingy' or hesitate when talking?

*If no* to 1 to 3 and yes to 4 then production difficulties are evident and referral to speech and language therapy is advised.

### (d) Social communication

1 Is the child willing to participate in conversations and does he enjoy this?
2 When the child talks, is it meaningful and relevant to the conversation and/or situation?
3 Does the child use appropriate verbal and non-verbal communication behaviours?
*If no* to one or more of the above the social communication difficulties are evident and referral to speech and language therapy is advised.

### (e) Education and social activities

1 How is the child functioning at school?
2 Is the child able to access and participate in a range of social activities?
3 Are the speech and language difficulties long standing and persisting beyond the age of 5 years?
If the child is struggling to meet the demands of school and presents with persisting speech and language difficulties then this is a cause of concern for later development and outcomes. Referral to speech and language therapy is advised.

## General principles for working with children with speech and language difficulties

It may be useful to consider these general principles when working with children with speech and language difficulties

1 Consider your own communication and adapt it to:

  ◆ Offer forced choice answers.

  ◆ Break up long instructions and sentences into short steps.

  ◆ Slowdown delivery and use pauses.

  ◆ Use short simple sentences with familiar vocabulary and avoid ambiguous language.

  ◆ Use visual strategies such as pictures, real objects, and symbols to support spoken language.

  ◆ Remember that children with spoken speech and language difficulties will also have written language difficulties.

2 It is always challenging when you are unable to understand what a child is saying to you. While there is no perfect solution, the following strategies will help:

  ◆ Reassure the child that you are interested in what they are trying to tell you.

  ◆ Be honest and say that you don't understand but also make it clear which parts you did and did not understand.

  ◆ Offer a choice of possible answers to the child, as this will reduce the number of choices available to you to guess from.

  ◆ Ask the child to show you something to help or can the child describe it to you or point to it or draw it.

  ◆ If these are still not successful, reassure the child that you are interested in what they are trying to tell you and that you will try again later.

# Further information

Speake, J. (2004). *How to identify and support children with speech and language difficulties*. LDA, Cambridge, UK.

This is a useful text, which describes children's speech and language difficulties and offers practical strategies for assessment and management.

*www.afasic.org.uk*

Afasic is a UK charity that offers information and advice to children with speech and language difficulties and their families as well as professionals working in this area.

*www.ican.org.uk*

ICAN is a UK charity that funds specialist educational provision for children and adolescents with severe speech and language difficulties as well as offering information and advice.

*www.rcslt.org*

The Royal College of Speech and Language Therapists (RCSLT) is the professional body for practicing speech and language therapists in the UK. Information about speech and language therapy services is available on this website.

# References

1. Buckley, B. (2003). *Children's communication skills. From birth to five years*. Routledge, London, UK.
2. Law, J., Boyle, J., Harris, F., *et al.* (2000). The relationship between the natural history and prevalence of primary speech and language delays: findings from a systematic review of the literature. *International Journal of Language & Communication Disorders*, **35**, 165–88.
3. Tomblin, J.B., Records, N., Buckwalter, P., *et al.* (1997). Prevalence of specific language impairment in kindergarten children. *Journal of Speech, Language, and Hearing Research*, **40**, 1245–60.
4. Gathercole, S., Service, E., Hitch, G., *et al.* (1999). Phonological short term memory and vocabulary development: further evidence on the nature of the relationship. *Applied Cognitive Psychology*, **13**, 65–77.
5. World Health Organization (WHO). (1993). *Mental disorders: a glossary and guide to their classification in accordance with the 10th revision of the international classification of diseases (ICD 10)*. World Health Organization, Geneva.
6. American Psychiatric Association. (1994). *Diagnostic and statistical manual of mental disorders* (4th edn) (DSM-IV). American Psychiatric Association, Washington, DC.
7. Dodd, B. (2005). *Differential diagnosis and treatment of children with speech disorders*. Whurr, London, UK.
8. Landau, W.M. and Kleffner, F. (1957). Syndrome of acquired aphasia and convulsive disorder in children. *Neurology*, **7**, 523–30.
9. Lees, J. (2005). *Children with acquired aphasias* (2nd edn). Whurr Publishers, London.
10. Deonna, T. (2004). Acquired epileptic aphasia (AEA) or Landau-Kleffner syndrome: from childhood to adulthood. In *Speech and language impairments in children. Causes, characteristics, intervention and outcome* (eds. D.V.M. Bishop and L.B. Leonard). Psychology Press, Hove, UK.
11. Rapin, I. and Allen, D. (1983). Developmental language disorders: nosologic considerations. In *Neuropsychology of language, reading, and spelling* (ed. U. Kirk), pp. 155–84. Academic Press, New York.
12. Bishop, D.V.M., Laws, G., Adams, C.V., *et al.* (2006). Distinct genetic influences on grammar and phonological short-term-memory deficits: evidence from 6-year-old twins. *Genes, Brain and Behaviour*, **5**, 158–69.
13. Marcus, G.F. and Fisher, S.E. (2003). FOXP2 in focus: what can genes tell us about speech and language? *Trends in Cognitive Sciences*, **7**, 257–62.
14. Rice, M. (2000). Grammatical symptoms of specific language impairment. In *Speech and language impairments in children. Causes, characteristics, intervention and outcome* (eds. D.V.M. Bishop and L.B. Leonard). Psychology Press, Hove, UK.
15. Van der Lely, H.K.J. (2005). Domain-specific cognitive systems: insight from grammatical-specific language impairment. *Trends in Cognitive Sciences*, **9**(2), 53–9.
16. Bishop, D.V.M. and Rosenbloom, L. (1987). Classification of childhood language disorders. In *Language development and disorders: clinics in developmental medicine* (eds. W. Yule and M. Rutter). Mackeith Press, London.
17. Rapin, I. and Allen, D. (1987). Developmental dysphasia and autism in pre-school children: characteristics and subtypes. *Proceedings of the first international symposium on specific speech and language disorders in children*. Association for All Speech Impaired Children, London.
18. Bishop, D.V.M. (2004). Pragmatic language impairment: a correlate of SLI, a distinct subgroup, or part of the autistic continuum? In *Speech and language impairments in children. Causes, characteristics, intervention and outcome* (eds. D.V.M. Bishop and L.B. Leonard). Psychology Press, Hove, UK.
19. Bishop, D.V.M. and Norbury, C.F. (2002). Exploring the borderlands of autistic disorder and specific language impairment: a study using standardised diagnostic instruments. *Journal of Child Psychology and Psychiatry*, **43**, 917–29.
20. Cantwell, D.P. and Baker, L. (1977). Psychiatric disorder in children with speech and language retardation. *Archives of General Psychiatry*, **34**, 583–91.
21. Prizant, B., Audet, L., Burke, G., *et al.* (1990). Communication disorders and emotional/behavioural disorders in children and adolescents. *Journal of Speech and hearing research*, **55**, 179–92.
22. Gertner, B.L., Rice, M.L., and Hadley, P.A. (1994). Influence of communicative competence on peer preferences in a preschool classroom. *Journal of Speech and Hearing Research*, **37**, 913–23.
23. Howlin, P. and Rutter, M. (1987). The consequences of language delay for other aspects of development. In *Language development and disorders* (eds. J. Yule and M. Rutter). Mackeith Press, Oxford, UK.
24. Redmond, S.M. and Rice, M.L. (1998). The socio-motional behaviours of children with SLI: social adaptation of social deviance? *Journal of Speech, Language, and Hearing Research*, **41**, 588–700.
25. Beitchman, J.H. (1985). Speech and language impairment and psychiatric risk: toward a model of neurodevelopmental immaturity. *Symposium on Child Psychiatry*, **8**, 721–35.
26. Brownlie, E.B., Beitchman, J.H., Escobar, M., *et al.* (2004). Early language impairment and young adult delinquent and aggressive behaviour. *Journal of Abnormal Child Psychology*, **32**, 453–67.
27. Cohen, N.J., Barwick, M.A., Horodezky, N.B., *et al.* (1998). Language achievement and cognitive processing in psychiatrically disturbed children with previously identified and unsuspected language impairments. *Journal of Child Psychology and Psychiatry*, **39**, 865–77.
28. Gilmour, J., Hill, B., Place, M., *et al.* (2004). Social communication deficits in conduct disorder: a clinical and community service. *Journal of Child Psychology and Psychiatry*, **45**, 967–78.
29. Tirosh, E. and Cohen, A. (1998). Language deficits in ADD: a prevalent co-morbidity. *Journal of Child Neurology*, **13**, 493–97.
30. Oram, J., Fine, J., Okamoto, C., *et al.* (1999). Assessing the language of children with attention deficit hyperactivity disorder. *American Journal of Speech-Language Pathology*, **8**, 72–80.
31. Kim, O.H. and Kaiser, A.P. (2000). Language characteristics of children with ADHD. *Communication Disorders Quarterly*, **21**, 154–65.
32. Tannock, R., Purvis, K.L., and Schachar, R. (1993). Narrative abilities in children with attention deficit hyperactiviy disorder. *Journal of Abnormal Child Psychology*, **21**, 103–17.

33. Toppleberg, C.O., Tabors, P., Coggins, A., *et al.* (2005). Differential diagnosis of selective mutism in bilingual children. *Journal of the American Academy of Child and Adolescent Psychiatry*, **44**, 592–5.

34. Cline, T. and Baldwin, S. (1994). *Selective mutism in children*. Singular, San Diego, CA.

35. Bergman, R.L., Piacentini, J., and McCracken, J.T. (2002). Prevalence and description of selective mutism in a school-based sample. *Journal of the American Academy of Child and Adolescent Psychiatry*, **41**, 938–46.

36. Cunningham, C.E., McHolm, A., Boyle, M.H., *et al.* (2004). Behavioural and emotional adjustment, family functioning, academic performance, and social relationships in children with selective mutism. *Journal of Child Psychology and Psychiatry*, **45**, 1363–72.

37. Dummit, E., Klein, R.G., Tancer, N.K., *et al.* (1996). Fluoxetine treatment of children with selective mutism: an open trial. *Journal of the American Academy of Child and Adolescent Psychiatry*, **35**, 615–21.

38. Steinhausen, H.C. and Juzi, C. (1996). Elective mutism: an analysis of 100 cases. *Journal of the American Academy of Child and Adolescent Psychiatry*, **35**, 847–56.

39. Baltaxe, C.A.M. (1994). *Communication issues in selective mutism*. Paper presented at the American Speech-Language-Hearing Association Convention, New Orleans.

40. Cohan, L., Chavira, D.A., and Stein, M.B. (2006). Practitioner review: psychosocial interventions for children with selective mutism: a critical evaluation of the literature from 1990–2005. *Journal of Child Psychology and Psychiatry*, **47**, 1085–97.

41. Johnson, M. and Wintgens, A. (2006). *Selective mutism resource manual*. Speechmark Publishing, Oxon, UK.

42. Botting, N. (2005). Non-verbal cognitive development and language impairment. *Journal of Child Psychology and Psychiatry*, **46**, 317–26.

43. Botting, N. (2006). The interplay between language and cognition in typical and atypical development. In *Language and social disadvantage: theory into practice* (eds. Clegg, J. and J. Ginsborg). Wiley, London.

44. Clegg, J., Hollis, C., Mawhood, L., *et al.* (2005). Developmental language disorders—a follow up in later adult life. Cognitive, language and psycho-social outcomes. *Journal of Child Psychology and Psychiatry*, **46**, 128–49.

45. Nathan, L., Stackhouse, J., Goulandris, N., *et al.* (2004). Educational consequences of developmental speech disorder: key stage I national curriculum assessment results in English and Mathematics. *The British Journal of Educational Psychology*, **74**, 173–86.

46. Conti-Ramsden, G. and Botting, N. (2004). Social difficulties and victimisation in children with SLI at 11 years of age. *Journal of Speech, Language and Hearing Research*, **47**, 145–61.

47. Clegg, J. (2006). Speech and language difficulties and later life chances. In *Language and social disadvantage: theory into practice* (eds. Clegg, J. and J. Ginsborg). Wiley, London.

48. Bishop, D.V.M. and Edmundson, A. (1987). Language impaired 4-year olds: distinguishing transient from persistent impairment. *Journal of Speech and Hearing Disorders*, **52**, 156–73.

49. Clegg, J. and Hartshorne, M. (2004). Speech and language therapy in hyperactivity: a United Kingdom perspective in complex cases. *Seminars in Speech and Language*, **25**, 263–71.

50. Law, J. and Garret, Z. (2004). Speech and language therapy: its potential role in CAMHS. *Child & Adolescent Mental Health*, **9**, 50–5.

## 9.2.12 **Gender identity disorder in children and adolescents**

Richard Green

### Variance in psychosexual development

Psychosexual development of sex-typed behaviours spans a broad mix of the elements that comprise 'masculinity' and 'femininity'. The possibility for variation is extensive. Among males, there are boys and men whose stereotypical masculinity may pose problems in mental health and criminality. They are not the focus here. Rather, here it is the marked deviation from the mean towards the 'non-masculine' or 'feminine' extreme. That pattern can also cause clinical concern and constitutes gender identity disorder (**GID**) as manifested in childhood. For females, conventional 'tomboyism' is not the focus here, but rather the extreme that can cause clinical concern and constitutes GID.

### Epidemiology

No epidemiological studies exist of GID in children. Prevalence can be estimated only roughly from indirect sources. Two items on the Child Behaviour Checklist[1] are consistent with components of the diagnosis. They are 'behaves like opposite sex' and 'wishes to be of opposite sex'. Among 4- to 5-year old boys, not clinically referred for behavioural problems, about 1 per cent of parents answer in the affirmative that their child 'wishes to be the opposite sex'. For ages 6 to 7 it drops to near zero, but rises to 2 per cent at age 11. For girls, the highest rate was 5 per cent at ages 4 to 5, but less than 3 per cent for other ages. With respect to 'behaves like opposite sex', among the boys the rate was 5 per cent and among girls 11 per cent for all ages. However, these data do not indicate any longitudinal aspect of the reported behaviour, and do not detail the behaviour.[2]

An alternative source of estimation looks to the percentage of adults believed to be homosexually oriented. From this population the percentage of homosexual men and women who typically report childhood cross-gender behaviour is used for the estimate. If the rate of exclusive homosexuality is 3 to 4 per cent for men and 1.5 to 2 per cent for women,[3] with perhaps half of homosexual men and women recalling childhood cross-gender behaviour,[4,5] the estimate of childhood cross-gender behaviour is about 3 per cent for boys and under 1 per cent for girls. However, this estimate suffers from problems of retrospective recall and poor comparability between surveys of adults. Further, the recalled behaviour may not have constituted GID.

A disparate sex ratio is evident in referral rates with GID. Four to five boys to one girl are referred. One reason may be greater parental concern over cross-gender behaviour in boys and the greater stigmatizing peer group response to 'sissiness' than to 'tomboyism'. An alternative explanation is that, as with most atypical patterns of sexuality, there is a higher ratio of males to females reflecting a common intrinsic predisposition among males.

### Clinical picture

Children with GID differ from other children, including those who merely are not conventionally masculine or feminine as boys or girls. Their behaviours are typical of other-sex children. Not only do they express a wish to be the other sex, at least in earlier years before they may learn not to verbalize it, but also their dressing preferences, peer group preferences, toy preferences, game preferences, and perhaps their physical mannerisms are those of the other sex.[6]

The picture of GID in children as described in DSM-IVTR,[7] can manifest, in part, by the repeatedly stated desire to be of the other sex: in boys by a preference for dressing in girls' or women's clothing or simulating female attire from available materials, and in girls an insistence on wearing stereotypically masculine clothing with refusal to wear traditional girls' clothing. In role playing, as in make-believe play or imitating media characters, there is a strong preference by the child for other-sex roles. There is also a strong preference for toys generally identified with the other sex, such as Barbie dolls by boys. The peer group is composed primarily or exclusively of other-sex children. Pictures drawn are generally of other-sex figures. There may be cross-sex physical mannerisms. Concurrently, there is an avoidance of traditionally sex-typed activities. Criteria in ICD-10 are similar.[8]

The diagnosis of GID in girls can be more problematic than in boys. This is because 'tomboyism' is a more common part of paediatric psychosexual development than 'sissyness'. There is, however, a distinction between GID in girls and tomboyism. Typical tomboys do not insist that they want to be boys and will wear girls' clothes from time to time, will have both girls and boys as playmates, and will not work to present themselves as young boys.

Substantial cross-gender behaviours are generally manifest in the third or fourth year. Although they are believed by parents and perhaps professional advisors to be a passing phase, at least with those children, seen clinically they endure into school years. Most children are evaluated at about age 7 or 8, when parents become increasingly concerned that the 'passing phase' is not passing and negative reactions by the peer group are enhanced, causing the child social distress.[6]

## Aetiology

Understanding the aetiology of GID considers typical influences on early psychosexual development in male and female children.

### Early sex differences

Very early behavioural differences are evident between males and females. There may be recognition of the 'like me', 'not like me' dichotomy of one's sex. When boys and girls aged between 10 and 18 months were shown pictures of faces of infants of the same and other-sex, males looked at faces of males longer and females looked at faces of females longer. This 'like me', 'not like me' dichotomy is also interpretable in the study in which two male and two female 1-year-old children were placed at the four corners of a room and permitted, one at a time, to crawl to any other child. Children more often crawled to a child of the same sex.[9,10]

In early play patterns, boys and girls may differ. When 12-month-old children were observed with their fathers in a waiting room, boys were more likely to handle 'forbidden' objects such as trays and vases.[11] The 1-year-old's toy preferences may also differ, with girls preferring soft toys and dolls and boys preferring transportation toys and robots.[12,13]

Preference for mother or father appears to discriminate boys and girls early. When 2- to 3-year-old children were asked which parent

in an adjoining room they would prefer to play a game with, or to build with using blocks, or make a sketch with, both boys and girls preferred their father. At 4 years, girls shifted to mother but boys stayed with father.[14]

When children aged between 2 and 3 years were observed in a free play setting, boys were more aggressive toward peers and showed more rough-and-tumble play. When paired in a test play situation with a boy, girls showed more passive behaviour, i.e. standing or sitting quietly and watching their partner play.[15]

The preference for a same-sex peer group emerges early. When 3.5- to 4.5-year-olds were shown pairs of photographs of boys and girls and asked to select the children with whom they would prefer playing, boys preferred boys and girls preferred girls.[16]

Children become aware of sex role stereotypes early. At 2 years of age, boys believe that boys like to play with cars and help their father, 3-year-olds believe that boys like to build things and that only boys like to play with trains. They also believe that girls like to play with dolls, help mother, and cook dinner. Girls are also seen as more likely to say 'I need help'.[17]

The peer group influences psychosexual development. In mixed-gender peer groups, boys more often receive positive responses for masculine activities than girls receive for feminine activities. Boys seem more responsive to peer pressure, in that they will discontinue feminine activities more rapidly than girls will discontinue masculine activities when they are the target of negative responses from either boys or girls.[18]

These findings suggest that if sex-typed attributes emerge in psychosexual development of typical children shortly after the basic dichotomization of 'like me', 'not like me', or male/female, then the first two components of gender identity are consolidated early: (a) the basic sense of male or female; (b) masculine or feminine gender role. The age at which they consolidate coincides with the emergence of significant cross-gender identity and behaviour as seen in the GID of childhood.

### Parental influences

Fathers, when observed with 12-month-old children, were more likely to present their sons with trucks rather than dolls, whereas daughters were given both trucks and dolls equally. However, among those children who were given dolls, boys played with them less.[19]

Mothers of young children have been observed with infant actor/actress babies (Baby X experiments). Some of these stranger infants are cross-dressed or given cross-sex names. The perceived sex of the infant influences the mother's behaviour. Children believed to be boys, whether they were or not, were more likely to be encouraged to physical action. Infants believed to be girls were more likely to be given a doll, whereas male infants were more likely to be presented with a football.[20]

None of these findings of early sex differences have been systematically observed with children followed up years later to determine whether early variation from the more common patterns are associated with later variation in psychosexual development.

In our prospective research of several dozen cross-gender behaving boys and conventionally masculine boys,[21] more mother-son shared time was not found in the group of feminine (prehomosexual) versus masculine boys. There was substantial variability in the extent to which mothers and sons were emotionally close. However, with respect to father-son experiences, feminine boys shared less time with their fathers in their first years when compared with the contrast group of conventionally masculine boys or with their masculine preheterosexual brothers. There was an inverse relationship between the extent of father-son shared time in the first years and later Kinsey score of sexual orientation. Less father-son time was associated with a higher (more homosexual) score.

Identifying the 'chicken and egg' here is problematic. Possibly, boys with a feminine identification who prefer feminine-type activities are less interesting to their fathers. This would lead to father-son distancing. In many of the families, this was the case. However, the finding that early father absence or father-son alienation was associated with cross-gender behaviour was not invariable. Further, there are families in which the mother and father relate comfortably with children and in which GID manifests itself.

## Hormonal influences

Evidence for hormonal influences on psychosexual development derives primarily from studies of the intersexed. Girls with congenital virilizing adrenal hyperplasia who produce an excess of androgen beginning prenatally are more rough-and-tumble in childhood play behaviours and less interested in doll play. They are more likely to be considered tomboys.[22] However, less evidence exists for a deficiency in prenatal androgen for boys with cross-gender behaviours.[23–25] Prenatal sex hormone levels are important theoretically, in that to the extent they influence sex-typed behaviour, such as rough-and-tumble or doll play, they may influence peer group composition. They may influence the labelling of the child as 'sissy' or 'tomboy', and may place the child on an atypical developmental track.

Seminal studies of the intersexed in the 1950s indicated that the sex of assignment in the first 2 to 3 years of life was the critical variable in establishing the basic concept of sexual identity as male or female. This was irrespective of gonadal status, hormonal status, internal reproductive structures, and, to some extent, genital configuration.[26] These studies have been criticized on the ground that with the anatomically intersexed the prenatal endocrine status has not been normal.[27] Thus recent interest has focused on individuals believed to have had normal prenatal development but who shortly after birth were nevertheless reassigned to live in the other-sex role, as well as those with a prenatal abnormality.

In one widely publicized case, one male of a pair of monozygotic twins suffered penectomy through circumcision trauma in the first year of life and was reassigned to live as a girl alongside the boy co-twin at about 23 months of age. Although earlier reports indicated that the reassigned twin was adjusting successfully to life as a girl,[28] more recent follow-up revealed that the individual reverted to living as a male in late adolescence, had undergone phalloplasty, and married a female.[29] The other case involves a male infant who also underwent penectomy from circumcision trauma and was assigned to live as a girl, earlier, in the seventh month. That individual was reported to be living as a woman and is bisexual in orientation.[30] One explanation for the discrepancy in the two reports is that the first child was reassigned as a female later than the time during which basic identity of male or female may be set. Both reports, however, suggest a prenatal influence on sexual orientation.

Children born with cloacal exstrophy also provide evidence for prenatal factors influencing gender identity, irrespective of postnatal socialization. Prenatal sex steroid levels are thought to be normal. However, the genital area of these infants, if chromosomally male is so malformed, that there is little prospect of male genital reconstruction. Therefore, many are socialized as girls. Reports from the US reveal a high rate of rejection of living as girls and transition to living as boys.[31] However, an early report from the UK does not indicate female gender role rejection.[32]

The enzyme deficiency of 5-alpha reductase is another clinical example of competing influences of prenatal sex steroids and postnatal socialization. Without this enzyme testosterone is not converted to dihydrotestosterone, needed prenatally to virilize the genitalia. At birth these chromosomal males with intra-abdominal testes appear to be girls based on their external genitalia. Traditionally, they have been raised as girls. Then, at puberty, they do not feminize but rather their clitoris grows substantially to resemble a phallus and there is no gynecomastia. Most then adopt a male role.[33] Debate continues whether this facility to live as heterosexual men is the product of prenatal testosterone or the extensive body virilization and social pressures to live as men. Long-term study of children where the testes are removed before puberty will provide further information.

## Longitudinal aspects of atypical early development

Beginning in the late 1960s, the author conducted a prospective study of several dozen boys with extensive cross-gender identification and behaviour.[6] Most of these boys would today be diagnosed with GID, although at the time the diagnosis had not yet entered into the diagnostic nomenclature. These boys were evaluated periodically and assessments continued until late adolescence or young adulthood for two-thirds. At that time, three-quarters of the boys were homosexual or bisexual. One was gender dysphoric. In contrast, a demographically matched group of boys with conventional boyhood behaviours was heterosexual at outcome.[34] More recent follow-up studies at another program reveal a higher minority percentage of cross-gender children remaining gender dysphoric but with the majority homosexually oriented.[35]

These prospective studies are consistent with retrospective reports by adult transsexual males and homosexual males. Many transsexuals recall extensive cross-gender identification and behaviours in childhood. Often, however, these are not documentable because of the length of time from onset to description and the difficulty of corroboration. Several studies have interviewed adult gay men and lesbian women with respect to gender-typed behaviours in childhood. Typically, more extensive cross-gender behaviours are reported than by groups of heterosexual men and women. These retrospective studies of men and women are consistent cross-culturally.[4,5]

Of theoretical and practical import is the overlap in childhood gender behaviours between retrospective reports given by transsexuals and homosexuals, and in the prospective study of cross-gendered boys. Because transsexualism and homosexuality in the adult male are quite different, the question is: Why should there be such an overlap?

One possibility is that the two groups are relatively similar in earlier years, but that different life circumstances promote more comfort for one group continuing to live as males. Treatment intervention to change cross-gender behaviour may be decisive. Transsexuals were rarely treated as children. Different prevalence rates may also be key. Whereas the incidence of transsexualism may be one in 10 000 males,[36] the incidence of homosexuality may be 3 or 4 per cent.[3] Thus if there are overlapping behaviours between the two in early years, probability would predict that the vast majority of cross-gendered males will emerge as homosexual, rather than transsexual. However, this does not explain the behavioural overlap between prehomosexual boys and pre-transsexual boys who will later be sexually attracted only to females (the latter living as lesbian women after sex reassignment surgery).

## Gender identity and mental disorder

GID of childhood was introduced into the DSM in 1980. Its inclusion derived from the prospective study of cross-gender behaving boys described above, with the present author also being a member of the nomenclature committee. The criteria for a set of behaviours being included in the DSM was that a condition be experienced subjectively as distressing and that it constitute a social disadvantage. GID of childhood met the criteria because of the distress the children experienced in consequence of being either male or female and the peer group stigmatization that flowed from their behaviours.

In the past decade, there has been increasing controversy over whether GID of childhood should remain in the list of disorders. In the same period in which GID of childhood was introduced, homosexuality was removed. As our prospective study revealed that a substantial majority of boys with GID matured into homosexual men, to some critics the inclusion of GID was seen as a backdoor through which homosexuality reentered the list of disorders. A response to this concern is that when the subjective distress of being male or female present in children with GID disappears the person no longer has a disorder, whether a heterosexual or homosexual adult. On the other hand, when the distress of being male or female persists, the diagnosis remains GID as seen in adolescence or adulthood, commonly termed transsexualism.

Inclusion of GID for children in the list of disorders is also seen by some critics as perpetuating sex stereotyping in society, and demanding that children conform to traditional masculine/feminine behaviours. A response to this is that the diagnosis is not made merely for gender non-conformity but only when the child is unhappy being male or female, and where the child's behaviours are so atypical that there is substantial adverse reaction from the peer group.

## Initial assessment

In the initial assessment of children with suspected GID, the professional should attempt to engage both parents as well as the child. Frequently there is reluctance by one parent, usually the father, to attend. However, this is a family matter, and the clinician needs to gain impressions of the parent-child relationship, the parent-parent relationship, and the child's behaviour from both parents as well as the child.

Assessment is directed towards understanding whether the behaviours described represent a normal variant of psychosexual development. Does the child overtly express dissatisfaction being the sex to which he or she was born? Is there a marked skewing of gender-typed behaviours towards those of other-sexed children or is there some mix? How long has there been cross-gender behaviour? What have parental reactions been to it initially and

more recently? What is the child's response when parents attempt to frustrate the cross-gender toy or clothing preferences, if such attempts have been made? What time availability is there for each parent with the child? What do they do together? Are there other persons, for example grandparents or teachers, who may be reinforcing cross-gender behaviours? What are the parental concerns, both in the short and long term, with respect to the significance of the behaviours? Are there other behavioural or medical problems in addition to the gender identity issue?

## Treatment

Typically, three principal targets are set for intervention with GID in children. First, the children are unhappy being the sex to which they were born; second, they are experiencing substantial peer group alienation; third, there is conflict with one or both parents in consequence of their atypical behaviour. A principal intervention strategy is helping the child understand that the world of gender is not necessarily black and white, but that greys exist as well. Boys can understand that not all boys need to be good athletes or rough-and-tumblers, and that boys can be sensitive and creative. Girls do not have to be boys to participate in rough-and-tumble play and sports. Children do not need to conform arbitrarily to all sex-typed attributes to remain in their birth sex role. To the extent this can be internalized, the path to transsexualism may be blocked.

The peer group of children with GID can be expanded to include children of both sexes. Parents may have to make efforts, particularly with cross-gendered boys, to find boys of their son's age who will enjoy non-athletic non-rough-and-tumble companionship, perhaps engaging in board games or computer games together. Similarly, girls with GID who are very athletically motivated may find girls who are also athletically inclined, and not just boys to play with. Children who develop comfort in socializing with both boys and girls may experience enhancement of same-sex identification.

Cross-gendered boys are notably alienated from their fathers and intervention can promote their relationship by finding mutually enjoyable activities. This may serve as a source of same-sex identification in the child, will enhance the quality of the parent-child relationship, and will be a positive outcome irrespective of its influence on later sexual identity.

Very few adult transsexuals had entered into any treatment intervention to address GID during childhood. Children with GID referred for evaluation or treatment may, as a product of that concern by parents, and/or professional intervention, have that route to transsexualism diverted. However, there is no empirical support for intervention directed at emerging sexual orientation. There is no evidence that a specific type of 'treatment' in childhood has any effect on outcome on that dimension of gender identity.[34] Parents should understand that if they are concerned about the ultimate sexual orientation of their child, that is a long time ahead. For the immediate period the child is unhappy who he or she is, is experiencing conflict with the peer group, and may be having difficulties at home with at least one parent. These are concerns that should be addressed.

### Cross-gender living by children

In recent years, some children with GID have been permitted to live as children of the other sex. Their parents consider that the strong preference by their child for the dress, activities, and companionship of the other sex with aversion to conventional sex-typed activities, along with the stated preference for being the other sex, argues for the child expressing its gender needs. Complexities of this decision include integrating it into the child's school and neighborhood environment.

Typically, children with GID experience peer group stigma and domestic conflict in consequence of their gender identity. Reduction of conflicts could enhance self-esteem. This social experiment should provide information on whether the longer-term status of the children differs from the children with GID not permitted cross-gender living, most of whom mature into homosexual adults and a minority into transsexual adults.

## Early adolescent gender identity disorder

GID continuing into adolescence merges with GID of adulthood. Management issues address the young teenager's continuing gender dysphoria and the consequent social problems. There may be peer group alienation. Depression may develop. School avoidance may develop. Awareness of sexual attraction to same-sex persons may be an additional source of conflict. Parents may be unaware of their teen's GID.

GID in adolescents presents medical, legal, and ethical dilemmas for clinicians. The somatic changes of puberty are very distressing to these young teenagers. And for those who will ultimately progress to adult GID or transsexualism, these changes may pose substantial obstacles to effective 'passing' in their desired gender role. The latter is especially true for males as the voice deepens, facial hair sprouts, and skeletal proportions masculinize. For females, menses are especially troublesome, though not visible, and breast development, especially when prominent, is very distressing.

Clinical recognition of these issues has led to an innovative program for some young teens with GID. This is a trial period of putting puberty on hold and possibly a later cross-sex hormone induced puberty. In the Netherlands, treatment may consist of administering a gonadotrophin releasing hormone agonist (GnRH analogue) at Tanner Stage 2-3 to block secretion of sex steroids that promote pubertal changes. This could be at age 12–14. Depending on the clinical picture of gender identity, at age 16, cross-sex steroids may be administered, or the analogue withdrawn so that endogenous puberty continues.[37] UK practice disfavors analogue treatment prior to Tanner Stage 4 or 5 after substantial pubertal changes. In the early experience of the Dutch treatment program, no patients who have commenced hormonal treatments prior to age 18 have regretted the decision to live as a person of the other sex. Although there is concern that a couple of years of gonadal steroid suppression could predispose to osteoporosis, this concern remains theoretical.

Legally, there is no age barrier to a minor consenting to a medical intervention in the United Kingdom, providing that there is sufficient understanding of the implications of the treatment.[38] At 16 years, adolescents are presumed competent to consent to medical treatment..

The psychiatric management dilemma here is predicting which gender dysphoric adolescents will mature into adult transsexuals, and which will be able to live in the gender role expected from birth, perhaps as homosexual adult men and women.

## Further information

Zucker, K.J. (2008) Gender identity disorder. In *Child and Adolescent Psychiatry* (5th edn.) (eds. M. Rutter and E. Taylor). Blackwell, Oxford.

## References

1. Achenbach, T. and Edelbrook, C. (1981). Behavioral problems and competencies reported by parents of normal and disturbed children aged four through sixteen. *Monographs of the Society for Research in Child Development*, 46.
2. Zucker, K. and Green, R. (1996). Gender identity disorders in children and adolescents. In *Child and adolescent psychiatry* (2nd edn) (ed. M. Lewis), pp. 611–22. Williams and Wilkins, Baltimore, MD.
3. Diamond, M. (1993). Homosexuality and bisexuality in different populations. *Archives of Sexual Behavior*, **22**, 291–310.
4. Whitam, F. and Mathy, R. (1986). *Male homosexuality in four societies: Brazil, Guatemala, the Philippines and the United States*. Praeger, New York.
5. Whitan, F. and Mathy, R. (1991). Childhood cross-gender behavior of homosexual females in Brazil, Peru, the Philippines and the United States. *Archives of Sexual Behavior*, **20**, 151–70.
6. Green, R. (1974). *Sexual identity conflict in children and adults*. Duckworth, London; Basic Books, New York. reprinted by Penguin, Baltimore, MD, 1975.
7. American Psychiatric Association (2000). *Diagnostic and statistical manual of mental disorders* (4th edn, *Text revision*). American Psychiatric Association, Washington, DC.
8. World Health Organization. (1992). *International Classification of Diseases and Related Health Problems*.10. Geneva.
9. Lewis, M. and Weinraub, M. (1974). Sex of parent × sex of child. In *Sex differences in behavior* (ed. R. Friedman, R. Richart, and R. Vande Wiele), pp. 165–89. Wiley, New York.
10. Michalson, L., Brooks, J., and Lewis, M. (1974). Peers, parents, people. Cited in Lewis, M. (1975). Early sex differences. *Archives of Sexual Behavior*, **4**, 329–35.
11. Maccoby, E. and Jacklin, C. (1980). Sex differences aggression. *Child Development*, **51**, 964–80.
12. Fagot, B. (1974). Sex differences in toddlers' behavior and parental reaction. *Developmental Psychology*, **10**, 554–8.
13. Jacklin, C., Maccoby, E., and Dick, A. (1973). Barrier behavior and toy preference. *Child Development*, **44**, 196–200.
14. Lynn, D. and Cross, A. (1974). Parent preference of preschool children. *Journal of Marriage and the Family*, **36**, 555–9.
15. Jacklin, C. and Maccoby, E. (1978). Social behavior at thirty-three months in same-sex and mixed-sex dyads. *Child Development*, **49**, 557–69.
16. Strayer, F. (1977). Peer attachment and affiliative subgroups. In *Ethological perspectives on pre-school social organization* (ed. F. Strayer). Research Memo 5, Department of Psychology, University of Quebec.
17. Kuhn, D., Nash, S., and Brucbern, L. (1978). Sex role concept of two and three-year-olds. *Child Development*, **49**, 445–51.
18. Fagot, B. (1977). Consequences of moderate cross–gender behavior in preschool children. *Child Development*, **49**, 459–65.
19. Snow, M., Jacklin, C., and Maccoby, E. (1983). Sex-of-child differences in father-child interaction at one year of age. *Child Development*, **54**, 227–32.
20. Sidorowicz, L. and Lunney, G. (1980). Baby X revisited. *Sex Roles*, **6**, 67–73.
21. Green, R. (1987). *The 'sissy boy syndrome' and the development of homosexuality*. Yale University Press, New Haven, CT.
22. Ehrhardt, A. and Baker, S. (1974). Fetal androgens, human central nervous system differentiation and behavior sex differences.

In *Sex differences in behavior* (eds. R. Friedman, R. Richart, and R. van de Wiele), pp. 33–51. Wiley, New York.

23. Yalom, I., Green, R., and Fisk, N. (1973). Prenatal exposure to female hormones: effect on psychosexual development in boys. *Archives of General Psychiatry*, **28**, 554–61.

24. Kester, P., Green, R., Finch, S., *et al.* (1980). Prenatal female hormone administration and psychosexual development in human males. *Psychoneuroendocrinology*, **5**, 269–85.

25. Hines, M. and Kaufman, F. (1994). Androgen and the development of human sex–typical behavior. *Child Development*, **65**, 1042–53.

26. Money, J., Hampson, J., and Hampson, J. (1955). An examination of some basic sexual concepts: the evidence of human hermaphroditism. *Bulletin of the Johns Hopkins Hospital*, **97**, 301–19.

27. Diamond, M. (1965). A critical evaluation of the ontogeny of human sexual behavior. *Quarterly Review of Biology*, **40**, 147–75.

28. Money, J. and Ehrhandt, A. (1972). *Man and woman, boy and girl*. Johns Hopkins Press, Baltimore, MD.

29. Diamond, M. and Sigmundson, H. (1997). Sex reassignment at birth. Long–term review and clinical implications. *Archives of Pediatric and Adolescent Medicine*, **15**, 298–304.

30. Bradley, S., Oliver, G., Chesnick, A., *et al.* (1998). Experiment of nature: ablatio penis at 2 months, sex reassignment at 7 months

and a psychosexual follow–up in young adulthood. *Pediatrics*, **102**, 9–21.

31. Reiner, W. and Gearhart, J. (2004). Discordant gender identity in some genetic males with cloacal exstrophy assigned to female sex at birth. *New England Journal of Medicine*, **350**, 333–41.

32. Carmichael, P., Schober, J., Hines, M. *et al.* (2003). Abstract, International Academy of Sex Research, Bloomington, IN.

33. Imperato-McGinley, J., Guerrero, L., Gautier, T. *et al.* (1974). Steroid 5 alpha reductase deficiency in man, an inherited form of male psuedohermaphrodism. *Science*, **186**, 1213–1215.

34. Green, R. (1987). The 'Sissy Boy Syndrome' and the Development of Homosexuality. Yale University Press, New Haven.

35. Zucker, K. (2005). Gender identity disorder in children and adolescents. Annual Review of Clinical Psychology, **1**, 467–492.

36. Kestersen, P., Gooren, L., and Magers, J. (1996). An epidemiological and demographic study of transsexuals in The Netherlands. *Archives of Sexual Behavior*, **25**, 589–600.

37. Delemarre-van de Waal, H., Cohen-Kettenis, P. (2006). Clinical management of gender identity disorder in adolescents. European Journal of Endocrinology. Online via www.eje.online.org.

38. Gillick v West Norfolk and Wisbeck Area Health Authority (1986). AC 112.

## 9.3

# Situations affecting child mental health

## Contents

9.3.1 The influence of family, school,
and the environment
Barbara Maughan

9.3.2 Child trauma
David Trickey and Dora Black

9.3.3 Child abuse and neglect
David P. H. Jones

9.3.4 The relationship between physical and mental
health in children and adolescents
Julia Gledhill and M. Elena Garralda

9.3.5 The effects on child and adult mental
health of adoption and foster care
June Thoburn

9.3.6 Effects of parental psychiatric and
physcial illness on child development
Paul Ramchandani, Alan Stein, and Lynne Murray

9.3.7 The effects of bereavement in childhood
Dora Black and David Trickey

## 9.3.1 The influence of family, school, and the environment

Barbara Maughan

### Introduction

Like adult disorders, most child psychiatric problems are now regarded as multifactorially determined: both genetic and environmental factors play a role in their development. This chapter provides an overview of some of the key environmental elements in that equation. Subsequent chapters discuss risks for specific disorders; the focus here is on the more general issues that arise when considering the effect of environmental influences on the onset or persistence of psychopathology in childhood.

### Environments and development

As in all aspects of child psychiatry, a developmental perspective is crucial when considering environmental risks. Some developmental periods may be especially sensitive for neurodevelopment, and show heightened effects of environmental insults. In addition, key sources of environmental influence change with age, and the meaning and impact of events will vary with the child's stage of cognitive, emotional, and social development. The family is the central source of early environmental influences, charged as it is in most societies with prime responsibility for the care, nurture, and socialization of the young. As children develop, so their social worlds expand; childcare and school settings take on increased importance, as do relationships with friends and peers. Throughout, each of these proximal contexts is shaped by influences from the wider culture and society. Any comprehensive assessment of a child's environment needs to take each of these types and levels of influence into account.

### Nature-nurture interplay

At one time, causal associations between adverse experiences and childhood disorder were assumed to run in just one direction. Today, it is clear that the situation is vastly more complex. Children are not simply passive recipients of experience; they influence, as well as being influenced by, those around them, and they play an active role in constructing and interpreting their social worlds.[1] Even very young infants influence the nature of their interactions with caregivers, and children's capacities for shaping and selecting their experiences increase as they mature. The temperamentally difficult child is likely to evoke more negative responses from parents; when parents themselves are under stress, or find it hard to maintain consistency, troublesome child behaviours can play a key role in fuelling harsh or punitive responses. Delinquent adolescents may seek out delinquent peers, who further encourage their antisocial activities. Associations between environmental factors and disorder often involve complex reciprocal patterns of effects.

Some of the evocative effects of children's behaviour will reflect heritable traits.[2] The advent of behaviour–genetic studies in child psychiatry has provided important insights into environmental as well as genetic risks. Genetic analyses have shown, for example, that many ostensibly 'environmental' factors include some element of genetic mediation.[3] Parents provide children not only with their environments but also with their genes, so that in biologically related families, nature and nurture are inevitably interwoven. Musical parents will encourage their children to enjoy music, buy them a violin, and may also pass on musical talents. In a similar way, anti-social parents may rear children in hostile and punitive environments, provide models of antisocial behaviour, and also pass on genes that predispose to disruptive behaviours. In all likelihood, genes and environments will often be *correlated* in this way.

Genetically informative studies have also highlighted other key mechanisms in ***gene-environment interplay***.[4] First, environments may *moderate* genetic influences, such that the heritability of some traits may vary systematically with qualities of the environment. Second, genetic factors may contribute to *differential sensitivity to environmental risks*. Research has consistently shown marked individual differences in children's responses to all but the most severe forms of psychosocial adversity. As yet, reasons for these differences are not well understood. They may reflect variations in the severity of exposure; individual differences in resilience or coping strategies, or in environmental sources of protection; or variations in vulnerability. Genetic predispositions clearly constitute one source of such vulnerability, and several examples of gene x environment interactions have now been documented. Finally, pre-clinical studies provide clear evidence that environments can influence *gene expression* through *epigenesis;* as yet, the extent to which processes of this kind apply in humans is unknown.

### Risk variables and risk mechanisms

Identifying environmental factors that show links with children's adjustment is only the first step in understanding *how* they function to increase risk for disorder. A variety of different mechanisms has been proposed here. Some may run through the effects of stress on the biological substrate. Exposure to aggression and hostility may influence children's cognitive processing, leading to the development of negative cognitive sets and attributional biases. In a related way, disrupted early attachments are argued to affect the psychological structures needed for later relationship formation. Adverse experiences may lead to direct increases in negative emotionality, disruptive behaviours, and impulsiveness, or to negative interactional styles that impact on social relationships. And finally, stress may affect children's self-concepts, or compromise their coping skills in ways that increase the risks for disorder. Any given environmental risk may be associated with a number of risk mechanisms, and the processes involved in the persistence of disorder may differ from those involved in its onset.

## Family influences

### Pre- and early post-natal development

Some vulnerability to psychopathology is laid down in foetal development. The potential for adverse effects of maternal substance use on the developing foetus have been known for many years; much recent attention has focussed on associations between prenatal cigarette smoking and risk for externalizing disorders in offspring. In addition, current estimates suggest that as much as 15 per cent of the load of childhood emotional/behavioural problems may be attributable to exposure to maternal anxiety and stress in pregnancy. Though the mechanisms involved here remain to be elucidated, there is speculation that these effects may reflect foetal programming of stress response systems akin to those posited in studies of early life influences on risk for cardiovascular disease.

Post-natally, as children progress from the complete dependence of infancy to increasing independence, they need stable and secure family relationships to provide emotional warmth, responsiveness, and constructive discipline. The influential work of Bowlby[5] and others has shown that a child's need to be attached to others is a basic part of our biological heritage. Infants become increasingly socially responsive over the first 6 months of life. At 6 to 8 months of age they begin to form selective attachments to particular individuals; they seek proximity to these attachment figures if distressed or frightened, and protest if the person they are attached to leaves. In evolutionary terms, these behaviours function to provide protection for the infant, and to reduce anxiety and distress.

Almost all infants—even those neglected or maltreated by their carers—develop attachment relationships of this kind. Their quality varies, however, depending on characteristics of the parent, the child, and the mesh between the two. Infants who have received sensitive and responsive care tend to show ***secure*** attachment patterns; ***insecure*** attachments are more likely to develop when parents themselves are stressed or unsupported, and are unresponsive to their children. Two main types of insecure attachment have been identified: avoidant attachments (associated with rejecting or highly intrusive parental care) and resistant–ambivalent patterns (associated with inconsistent or unresponsive parenting). More recently, a third disorganized category has been described, in which infants show a variety of contradictory behaviours after brief separations, and often appear confused, depressed, or apprehensive. This seems especially associated with parental behaviours that are frightening, unpredictable, or abusive.

Attachment theorists argue that the quality of these early relationships may have long-term implications. Though not entirely resistant to change, infants' attachment patterns do tend to be stable over time. Some of this stability may reflect continuity in the quality of family care. In addition, attachment theory proposes that early attachment experiences are internalized in internal working models of self and others, which function as templates for future relationship formation. Children who have experienced responsive early care come to expect others to be caring and reliable; those who have been ignored or rejected develop less positive expectancies of others, of relationships, and of themselves. Later in development, new relationships may be created in line with these expectancies.

Although many aspects of these models await confirmation, securely attached infants are known to go on to be more sociable and co-operative in their social relationships, and to show more positive affect and self-esteem. Insecurely attached infants show less positive relationships, and are at some increased risk for psychopathology. Taken alone, attachment security in infancy is only a weak predictor of global functioning in early adulthood, suggesting that early attachment experiences work with and through other experiences—including peer relationships, later family experiences, and eventually mature intimate relationships—to contribute to later functioning. In addition, both ICD-10 and DSM-IV recognize two varieties of attachment disorders: non-attachment with emotional withdrawal, typically associated with abuse, and non-attachment with indiscriminate sociability, most usually observed when children have been exposed to repeated changes of caretaker or institutional care. Although as many as 40 per cent of infants receive insecure attachment classifications, these more severe forms of attachment disorder are rare.

## Family relationships and parenting

Many other aspects of family life and relationships, and of parenting styles and behaviours, have been examined for their impact on children's development. Research on families emphasizes the complexity of family relationships; each dyadic relationship is influenced by other relationships in the family, and normative transitions in family life—the birth of a sibling, or mother starting work—reverberate to affect all family members.[6] Relationships with parents and siblings change as children develop, and both these, and specific aspects of parenting, may impact on risks for disorder.

The implications of the most severely compromised parenting, involving abuse or neglect, are examined in Chapter 9.3.3, and family-based risks for individual childhood disorders are discussed in detail in the chapters dealing with each specific condition. In general, these reflect four broad themes:

◆ discordant, dysfunctional relationships between parents, or in the family system as a whole;

◆ hostile or rejecting parent-child relationships, or those markedly lacking in warmth;

◆ harsh or inconsistent discipline;

◆ ineffective monitoring and supervision.

Within this broad pattern, differential treatment of siblings is known to increase conflict between children, and may have important implications for psychopathology. In addition, outcomes are markedly poorer when children face multiple family-related risks.

Family life can also provide important sources of protective influences for children facing life events and other stressors. Cohesion and warmth within the family, the presence of one good relationship with a parent, close sibling relationships, and the nature of parental monitoring and supervision have all been found to show protective influences of this kind.

## Parent and family characteristics

Psychopathology in parents is associated with increased risks of emotional and behavioural problems in children. Recent estimates suggest that as many as 60 per cent of the children of parents with major depression will develop psychiatric problems in childhood or adolescence, and their risks of affective disorder are increased fourfold. Psychosis, alcohol and drug abuse, and personality disorders in parents are also associated with increased risks of disorder in offspring, and parental criminality is a strong risk factor for conduct problems and delinquency.

In most instances, these links will reflect a complex interplay between genetic and environmental effects. Disorder in parents is frequently associated with disturbed marital relationships, and parental psychopathology may also impair parenting capacities. Depressed mothers, for example, are less sensitive and responsive to their infants, and attend less, and respond more negatively, to older children. Alcohol and drug abuse and major mental disorders in parents may impair parenting in more wide-ranging ways. When parents are antisocial, effects may also be mediated through the endorsement of antisocial attitudes and social learning.

Young maternal age is associated with increased risk for child and adolescent conduct problems. In part, these associations are likely to reflect the educational and social disadvantages that predict very early parenthood; in part, the poor social conditions and lack of support faced by many young mothers; and in part, less than optimal parenting styles. Delinquency is also associated with large family size. Once again, the more proximal risks involved are likely to be complex: parental supervision may be less effective in large families, and opportunities to 'learn' from delinquent siblings higher. Beyond this, family size shows few consistent links with childhood disorder. Only children are not at increased psychiatric risk, and they share with other first-borns some small advantages in terms of cognitive development. Birth order also appears to have few implications for behavioural adjustment, although youngest children show some increased rates of school refusal.

## Changing family patterns

Recent decades have seen massive changes in the pattern of many children's family lives. The most obvious markers are the dramatic increases in rates of divorce, single parenthood, and step-family formation, along with major increases in maternal employment. In the years immediately after the Second World War, just 6 per cent of British couples divorced within 20 years of marriage. By the mid-1960s that figure had increased four-fold, and divorce rates continued to rise into the 1980s. For most children, parental divorce will be followed by a period in a single-parent household; for a substantial minority, further family transitions will mean that they become part of a step family. In the early years of the 21st century more than 10 per cent of UK families with dependent children were step-families, and approaching a quarter of children lived in single parent households.

## Parental divorce

There is now extensive evidence that divorce is associated with negative consequences for children.[7] Psychological and behavioural distress are common, especially in the period immediately following divorce; more severe disturbance is not. Boys in particular are at increased risk for conduct problems. Educational attainments and motivation are often compromised, and subsequent relationships may also be affected. As they approach adulthood, children of divorce move into close relationships earlier than their peers, but also experience higher risks of relationship breakdowns.

Events both before and after the separation seem central in understanding these effects. Longitudinal studies, for example, have shown that children in divorcing families often show disturbed behaviour well before their parents separate. Exposure to the discord and conflict that frequently precede divorce thus seem to be key components of risk. After separation, problematic relationships between parents may continue, and the parents' own distress may compromise their capacity to respond sensitively and consistently to their children's needs. Many families face a sharp decline in economic circumstances after divorce, and for many children their parents' separation may involve house moves, school changes, and other disruptions to their established social networks. Each of this constellation of factors may contribute to subsequent outcomes.

## Single parents and step families

Research on the effects of growing up in single-parent and step families illustrates the complexity of family-related influences.[8]

Overall, children in single-parent and step families show higher mean levels of emotional and behavioural problems than those in non-divorced two-parent families; they also have an increased probability of health problems and educational underachievement. But there are also marked differences within each family type and associations between the quality of mother–child relationships and children's adjustment is similar across family settings. In addition, single-parent and reconstituted families often differ from stable two-parent families in a plethora of other ways; in particular, they are much more likely to face economic pressures, poor social support, and higher levels of maternal depression. Once these variations and the degree of negativity in family relationships are taken into account, family type *per se* shows few consistent links with children's adjustment.

## Peer influences

Beyond the family, relationships with peers are now recognized to provide a unique and essential contribution to children's social, emotional, and cognitive development.[9] By the end of the pre-school period most children have at least one reciprocated friendship. In childhood and adolescence, peers take on increasing importance; in middle childhood, more than 30 per cent of children's social interactions are with peers, and adolescents are estimated to spend more than twice as much time with peers than they do with parents or other adults. The functions of friendship change with development, expanding to encompass companionship and stimulation, help and sharing, social and emotional support and intimacy.

With friends and peers children acquire skills, attitudes, and experiences that contribute to many aspects of their adaptation. By the same token, children who have poor social skills, or who are rejected or neglected by peers, are at risk of a range of adverse outcomes including poor school performance, school drop-out, and psychiatric disorder. Social rejection may increase children's feelings of loneliness, reduce supports that can buffer against stressors, and also mean that isolated children miss out on important social learning experiences. Since many children with psychiatric disorders also show difficulties in relationships with peers, processes of this kind may well compound their problems. In adolescence, affiliations with behaviourally deviant peers have attracted particular interest as correlates of conduct disorder and delinquency. Here, reciprocal influences have been demonstrated: aggressive disruptive children are more likely to associate with deviant peers, but relationships with peers also show an independent effect on both the onset and persistence of delinquency.

## Child care and schooling

By the late 1990s approaching 50 per cent of mothers in the UK returned to full- or part-time work before their infants reached one year of age. This major increase in early maternal employment has prompted extensive research on the impact of alternative childcare on children's development. Recent evidence[10] suggests that multiple features of early care need to be considered in assessing effects. Higher child-care *quality* (as indexed by features such as sensitive and responsive care-giving, and cognitive and language stimulation), is associated with improved performance on tests of cognitive, language, and early academic skills, and with more prosocial skills and fewer behaviour problems, By contrast, higher *quantity* of child care (as indexed by hours per week in any kind of non-maternal care), is associated with some increased risks of problem behaviours in both the preschool and early school years.

School life then brings its own demands and challenges. Starting and changing schools are significant, sometimes troublesome, events for children; although most young children adapt well, a significant minority show some disturbance when they start school, and both attainment levels and self-perceptions are affected for many young adolescents after the transition from primary to secondary school. Tests and examinations rank high on children's lists of fears, and levels of psychological distress are elevated at times of major examinations. Although fears of this kind are not generally severe, they do show links with clinically significant symptoms. Bullying is a further problem especially associated with the school context. Self-report surveys suggest that over 15 per cent of young children experience some bullying at school, mostly unknown to parents or teachers. Although rates fall with age, up to 5 per cent of adolescents continue to face bullying in secondary school. Persistently victimized children have identifiable characteristics, with histories of anxious insecure behaviours and social isolation often beginning before they started school; bullying then increases their risks of adjustment problems.

Like families, schools differ in their atmosphere and social climate, and these variations show an independent impact on children's academic progress and behaviour. In part, these variations reflect differences in initial pupil intakes. In addition, they show systematic links with organizational characteristics of schools. Schools with more positive outcomes are characterized by purposeful leadership, constructive classroom management techniques, an appropriate academic emphasis, and consistent but not oversevere sanctions. In relation to behavioural outcomes, the composition of pupil groupings may also be influential. Young children are more likely to become aggressive if placed in highly aggressive classes, and risks of delinquency are increased in secondary schools where intakes include large proportions of less able children. For some severely disadvantaged groups, however, schooling may offer an important source of positive experiences. Experimental studies of preschool programmes, for example, have shown important long-term gains in terms of reduced risks of delinquency and unemployment many years after participants left school.

## Wider social and environmental influences

### Poverty and social disadvantage

Poverty and social disadvantage are most strongly associated with deficits in children's cognitive skills and educational achievements.[11] In the behavioural domain, disruptive behaviours also show links with family poverty. Effects appear to be more marked for boys than for girls, and seem to be stronger in childhood than in adolescence. Intermittent hardship is associated with some increased risk for conduct problems, but the impact is most marked for children in families facing persistent economic stress. Most current evidence suggests that these effects are indirect. Poverty imposes stress on parents, and reduces the supports available to them; these in turn increase the risks of harsh or coercive parenting, and reduce parents' emotional availability to their children's needs. Some studies suggest that relative deprivation—the perception that one is disadvantaged by comparison with others—may be more important than income levels *per se*.

## Neighbourhood and community contexts

Rates of childhood disorder vary in different neighbourhoods and communities. Urbanization is frequently associated with increased risks of disorder, and rates may be especially high in chronically disadvantaged inner-city neighbourhoods. In early childhood, many of these effects seem to be indirect; neighbourhood disadvantage increases stress on families, and these in turn largely account for associations with children's difficulties. In severely disadvantaged settings, however, even quite young children may be directly exposed to community violence, and in adolescence, neighbourhood influences may be mediated through associations with delinquent peers.

## Multiple stressors

For many children, exposure to these differing types of adversity will covary. Stressed families frequently live in poor neighbourhoods, where schools are under pressure and peer groups deviant. Early epidemiological findings suggested that isolated single risks have relatively little impact on disorder, but that rates rise sharply when risk factors combine. More recently, studies have shown that child, sociocultural, parenting, and peer-related risks each add uniquely to the prediction of behaviour problems. In addition, the total number of risks a child faces explains further variance in outcomes.

## Secular trends in disorder and psychosocial risks

Finally, it is important to consider how psychosocial risks may impact on overall levels of disorder. There is now clear evidence that rates of many adolescent disorders—including depression, suicide, alcohol and drug use, and delinquency—have risen since the Second World War.[12] Since it is implausible that changes in the gene pool could occur so rapidly, environmental risk factors must be implicated. Some of these may overlap with risks for individual differences in disorder, but others may be quite distinct. Based on an extensive review of available evidence, Rutter and Smith[12] concluded that a variety of factors are likely to be implicated:

1 increased rates of family breakdown, with their associated effects on the disruption of relationships and exposure to conflict and discord;

2 a change in the meaning of adolescence, with prolonged education and economic dependence on parents occurring alongside increased autonomy in other spheres;

3 a possibly increased disparity between young people's aspirations and the opportunities available to meet them;

4 increased alcohol consumption and illegal drug use;

5 changing social attitudes to acceptable behaviour, possibly enhanced by influences from the mass media.

Other specific factors may affect rates of juvenile crime. In particular, the increasing commercialization of youth culture, providing more goods to steal, may have coincided with diminished surveillance and increased situational opportunities for property crime.

## Further information

Clarke-Stewart, A. and Dunn, J. (2006). *Families count: effects on child and adolescent development.* Cambridge University Press, Cambridge.

Rutter M. (2005). Environmentally mediated risks for psychopathology: Research strategies and findings. *Journal of the Amrican Academy of Child and Adolescent Psychiatry,* **44**, 3–18.

## References

1. Lytton, H. (1990). Child and parent effects in boys' conduct disorder: a reinterpretation. *Developmental Psychology,* **5**, 683–97.

2. Scarr, S. and McCartney, K. (1983). How people make their own environments: a theory of genotype–environment effects. *Child Development,* **54**, 424–35.

3. Plomin, R. and Bergeman, C.S. (1991). The nature of nurture. Genetic influences on 'environmental' measures. *Behavioural and Brain Sciences,* **14**, 373–86.

4. Rutter, M., Moffitt, T., and Caspi, A. (2006). Gene–environment interplay and psychopathology: Multiple varieties but real effects. *Journal of Child Psychology and Psychiatry,* **47**, 226–61.

5. Bowlby, J. (1988). *A secure base: clinical applications of attachment theory.* Routledge, London.

6. Dunn, J. (1994). Family influences. In *Development through life: a handbook for clinicians* (eds. M. Rutter and D.F. Hay), pp. 112–31. Blackwell Science, Oxford.

7. Rodgers, B. and Pryor, J. (1998). *Divorce and separation: the outcomes for children.* Joseph Rowntree Foundation, York.

8. Dunn, J., Deater-Deckard, K., Pickering, K., *et al.* (1998). Children's adjustment and prosocial behaviour in step–, single-parent, and non-stepfamily settings: findings from a community study. *Journal of Child Psychology and Psychiatry,* **39**, 1083–95.

9. Rubin, K.H., Bukowski, W., and Parker, J.G. (1998). Peer interactions, relationships, and groups. In *Handbook of child psychology,* Vol. 3 *Social, emotional and personality development* (ed. N. Eisenberg), pp. 619–700. Wiley, New York.

10. NICHD Early Child Care Research Network (2006). Child-care effect sizes for the NICHD Study of Early Child Care and Youth Development. *American Psychologist,* **61**, 99–116.

11. Duncan, G.J. and Brooks-Gunn, J. (ed.) (1997). *Consequences of growing up poor.* Russell Sage, New York.

12. Rutter, M. and Smith, D.J. (1995). *Psychosocial disorders in young people: times trends and their causes.* Wiley, Chichester.

## 9.3.2 Child trauma

David Trickey and Dora Black

## Children's reactions to traumatic events

This chapter will focus on the impact on children of traumatic events other than child abuse or neglect, which are covered in Chapter 9.3.3. According to the DSM-IV-TR definition of post-traumatic stress disorder (PTSD), traumatic events involve exposure to actual or threatened death or injury, or a threat to physical integrity. The child's response generally involves an intense reaction of fear, horror, or helplessness which may be exhibited through disorganized or agitated behaviour. Terr suggested separating traumatic events into type I traumas which are single sudden events and type II traumas which are long-standing or repeated events.[1]

If the traumatic event includes bereavement, the reactions may be complicated and readers should consult Chapter 9.3.7 to address the bereavement aspects of the event.

Following a traumatic event, children may react in a variety of ways (see Chapters 4.6.1 and 4.6.2 for the adult perspective on reactions to stressful and traumatic events). Many show some of the symptoms of post-traumatic stress disorder—re-experiencing the event (e.g. through nightmares, flashbacks, intrusive thoughts, re-enactment, or repetitive play of the event), avoidance and numbing (e.g. avoidance of conversations, thoughts, people, places, and activities associated with the traumatic event, inability to remember a part of the event, withdrawal from previously enjoyed activities, feeling different from others, restriction of emotions, sense of foreshortened future), and physiological arousal (e.g. sleep disturbance, irritability, concentration problems, being excessively alert to further danger, and being more jumpy). In young children the nightmares may become general nightmares rather than trauma-specific. Other reactions to trauma in children are:

- becoming tearful and upset or depressed
- becoming clingy to carers or having separation anxiety
- becoming quiet and withdrawn
- becoming aggressive
- feeling guilty
- acquiring low self-esteem
- deliberately self-harming
- acquiring eating problems
- feeling as if they knew it was going to happen
- developing sleep disturbances such as night-terrors or sleepwalking
- dissociating or appearing 'spaced out'
- losing previously acquired developmental abilities or regression
- developing physical symptoms such as stomach aches and headaches
- acquiring difficulties remembering new information
- developing attachment problems
- acquiring new fears
- developing problems with alcohol or drugs.

Such problems may individually or in combination cause substantial difficulties at school and at home. The reactions of some children will diminish over time; however, for some they will persist, causing distress or impairment, warranting diagnosis, and/or intervention. Research predicting which children will be more likely to be distressed following a traumatic event suffers from a number of methodological flaws. However, factors which are often identified as constituting a risk for developing PTSD across a number of studies include: level of exposure, perceived level of threat and peri-traumatic fear, previous psychological problems, family difficulties, co-morbid diagnoses, subsequent life events, and lack of social support.

### Diagnosis of PTSD

Both DSM-IV-TR and the ICD-10 diagnostic classification of PTSD are appropriate for use with adults and although children from 8 years old do display similar symptoms to adults[2] there are some developmental differences particularly in younger children.[3] Alternative diagnostic criteria for pre-school children have therefore been developed, which draw on reports by carers and include more behavioural symptoms such as loss of developmental skills, and development of new fears or anxiety.[4]

### Other diagnoses

Careful assessment is required to make an accurate differential diagnosis. According to DSM-IV-TR, PTSD can only be diagnosed 1 month after the event, prior to that a diagnosis of acute stress disorder (ASD) may be appropriate. Whereas ICD-10 PTSD can be diagnosed within the first month, and the acute stress reaction is reserved to describe a disturbance that resolves rapidly. If the event is not of sufficient severity to meet the criteria for PTSD and the reaction does not last more than 6 months after the stressor has ceased, then a diagnosis of adjustment disorder may be appropriate. Recovery may take longer for children if their parents continue to suffer from symptoms of PTSD which may constitute a chronic source of stress which may in turn prolong the symptoms of the child. Further information on these diagnoses from an adult perspective can be found in Chapters 4.6.1–4.6.5.

Other diagnosable disorders may result from traumatic events, and may be present singularly or co-morbidly with PTSD; 60 per cent of children with PTSD have a co-morbid mental health diagnosis.[5] According to Fletcher's meta-analysis, common co-morbid diagnoses are: anxiety disorders, depression, alcohol and drug abuse in adolescents, and attention deficit hyperactivity disorder (ADHD).[2]

### Assessment

As with other psychiatric disorders, the best assessment can be made by integrating information from a number of sources such as an interview of the parent/carer alone, an interview of the family together, information from school, and information from psychological measures (see below). Careful consideration should be given to which members of the family will be involved in any interviews so as to avoid exposing previously unaffected children to the traumatic details of the event. Sometimes children try to 'protect' their carers from distress by under-reporting their symptoms of trauma, it is therefore also essential to interview the child on their own where possible.[6]

In order to assess what elements of the child's current functioning and distress may be a result of the traumatic event, and those that may pre-date it, it is important to gain as full a picture as possible of their developmental history and their pre-morbid functioning. Reports from teachers and other professionals may be particularly useful in this respect.

On assessment, some account of the traumatic event is necessary so that the clinician can gain an understanding of what exactly was experienced. Furthermore, it is helpful to give the sense that the clinician can bear to hear a story which the child and family may have been avoiding to tell for some time. However, this must be balanced against the child's understandable avoidance of the memory. There is little point gaining a full account of the event during the assessment, if the child becomes so distressed that they do not return for treatment. Pynoos and Eth offer a structure for conducting such an initial assessment which begins with a projective drawing and storytelling. It then proceeds to discussion of the actual event and its impact, followed by closure.[7] If the assessment has included talking about the traumatic event the child and family may become very distressed, and it may be necessary to invest some time in winding down the session, so that the family does not leave overly distressed. This will increase the likelihood of them engaging in the treatment process, which is likely to involve thinking through the event—something which they often do not intuitively want to do.

Assessment includes asking about the motivation for the contact with the service. Unlike many other problems, families with traumatized children may not simply present at the service in order to effect a change in their child's symptoms. They may be asking for advice following a traumatic event to try and prevent problems from appearing later by ensuring that they are 'doing the right thing', or they may be seeking an assessment for the purpose of compensation or other legal purposes.

### Psychological instruments

A number of questionnaires and diagnostic interviews are available to assist in the assessment of PTSD. Such instruments cannot replace a clinical interview, but may assist by strengthening clinical opinion and giving a reliable and valid indication of perceived symptom severity or frequency. This can give an indication of the impact of an event, can raise hypotheses which can be further investigated (e.g. screening for possible presence of PTSD which can then be further assessed) and if repeated after treatment can help to measure change. Ohan and colleagues reviewed those measures used in research studies that have adequate psychometric properties.[8] The best diagnostic instrument is the children's PTSD inventory. This is a structured diagnostic interview, the psychometric properties of which are good and have been published in peer-reviewed journals.[9,10] The Children's Revised Impact of Events scale[11] is a useful self-report questionnaire of 13 items appropriate for children aged 8 years and above. It has good screening properties[12] and is freely available from the Children and War Foundation's website (see below). Similarly Foa's Child PTSD Symptom scale (CPSS) is a 24-item self-report questionnaire designed for children aged 8 years and above. It is emerging as having good psychometric properties.[13] The CPSS has the advantage of specifically assessing the symptoms of PTSD from the DSM-IV-TR, and unlike most other self-report measures, it also addresses the important question of the impact of the symptoms on the child's functioning.

## Evaluation of treatments

An increasing amount of evidence indicates that trauma-focussed cognitive behavioural therapy (TF-CBT) is the treatment of choice for PTSD.[14] Much of the evidence is from studies of children with PTSD as a result of child sexual abuse. Dalgleish and colleagues summarize the evidence thus; 'The current take-home message from this nascent literature therefore is that CBT appears to have well-established efficacy in treating a range of post-traumatic stress responses following sexual abuse, with preliminary evidence in favour of this form of intervention following other types of trauma'.[15] Consequently, TF-CBT is the only intervention recommended by the United Kingdom's National Institute for Health and Clinical Excellence (NICE) for the treatment of children and young people with PTSD.[6]

Family therapy and psychodynamic psychotherapy as stand alone therapies for children with PTSD are not currently supported by the same level of evidence as TF-CBT. However, there is evidence to illustrate the importance of involving parents or carers in treatment where appropriate.[16] Psychodynamic psychotherapy may have some contribution to the treatment of traumatized children[17] and clinical experience indicates this to be true particularly in children with co-morbid diagnoses or where the traumas are multiple and prolonged (type II) such as in war and civil conflicts, and have led to failures of basic care.

Eye Movement Desensitisation and Reprocessing (EMDR) has proven to be effective with adults and has increasingly been used with children.[18] It shows promise for use with children and young people, but it has not yet established the same level of evidence as TF-CBT.[6]

The available evidence does not currently support the use of medication to treat PTSD in children or young people,[6] although medication may be necessary to treat any co-morbid conditions such as depression, ADHD, or sleep problems.

## Management

### Trauma-focussed cognitive behavioural therapy (TF-CBT)

'Processing' of an event involves bringing the event to mind and thinking it through often by talking, writing, or playing. This enables the memory to be stored as an ordinary narrative memory which is under the child's control, rather than as the vivid sensory information of the original event which is prone to being involuntarily re-experienced. Furthermore, processing enables a more helpful meaning to be attributed to the event; so whilst it may well be thought of as 'terrifying' and 'unfortunate', it no longer colours the way that *everything* in the child's world, including him or herself is seen.

Many children will process difficult and traumatic experiences naturally, often with the help of those around them such as their carers. Some may take a little while to do so. However, bringing up the memory may initially trigger the fear or distress of the original event, so some children avoid thinking about it, which in turn prevents processing.[19] Similarly the adults around the child may try to protect either themselves or the child from further distress by not discussing the event and so opportunities to enable the child to process it may be missed through avoidance by proxy. Therefore some children will not manage to process the event without professional help.

TF-CBT for traumatized children and families involves enabling the child or young person to bring the traumatic event to mind within the safe environment of therapy. This is akin to *exposure* to the memory, which enables the memory to be processed. *Cognitive restructuring* involves enabling the child to alter their unhelpful negative view of themselves or the world, which is based on the event, to a more helpful and realistic one. Cognitive behavioural therapy for children is further described in Chapter 9.5.3, Stallard provides excellent resources in the form of a workbook,[20] and Cohen offers a comprehensive description of the treatment of trauma and traumatic grief.[21]

Younger children with PTSD may not be able to make use of TF-CBT in the same way that older children can, and their treatment is likely to involve much more family work and ensuring that they learn that their environments are safe through re-assurance and stability.[22]

### Early interventions

There continues to be much debate about the value of early intervention (i.e. within the first month). Research to date does not support the use of single session debriefing,[23] however, there may be value in the provision of practical and emotional support in the immediate aftermath, together with some education of what reactions can be expected. Development of a culture where the child is permitted, or encouraged to talk about the event (e.g. within the family or within the school) may protect against the development of PTSD.[24] Early trauma-focussed cognitive behavioural therapy may be offered to older children with the most severe symptoms[6] which may be completed in groups (e.g.[25]). There may be a role for EMDR in the early stages following a traumatic event, although this has yet to receive empirical support.

## Further information

Dyregrov, A. (2006). *Grief in Children: a handbook for adults*, (2nd edn) London, Jessica Kingsley Publishers.

Salmon, K. and Bryant, B.A. (2002). Posttraumatic stress disorder in children. The influence of developmental factors. *Clinical Psychology Review*, **22**, 163–88.

The National Child Traumatic Stress Network. An American based network that provides excellent resources for parents, schools, the media, and professionals. www.nctsnet.org

The Children and War Foundation. This is a charity which aims to improve the care of children affected by war and disaster. Two professional groups, the Center for Crisis Psychology in Bergen, Norway and the Institute of Psychiatry in London, UK, have been instrumental in setting up this foundation. Copies of the Children's Revised Impact of Events scale (CRIES), the Depression Self-rating Scale for Children and the Revised Children's Manifest Anxiety scale (RCMAS) are available free from the website in various languages. www.childrenandwar.org

## References

1. Terr, L.C. (1991). Childhood traumas: an outline and overview. *The American Journal of Psychiatry*, **148**(1), 10–20.
2. Fletcher, K.E. (1996). Childhood post-traumatic stress disorder. In *Child psychopathology* (eds. E.J. Marsh and R. Barkley), pp. 242–76. Guilford Press, New York.
3. Salmon, K. and Bryant, R.A. (2002). Posttraumatic stress disorder in children. The influence of developmental factors. *Clinical Psychology Review*, **22**(2), 163–88.
4. Scheeringa, M.S., Zeanah, C.H., Myers, L., *et al.* (2003). New findings on alternative criteria for PTSD in preschool children. *Journal of the American Academy of Child and Adolescent Psychiatry*, **42**(5), 561–70.
5. AACAP. (1998). Practice parameters for the assessment and treatment of children and adolescents with posttraumatic stress disorder. *Journal of the American Academy of Child and Adolescent Psychiatry*, **37**(Suppl. 10), 4S–26S.
6. NICE. (2005). *The management of PTSD in adults and children in primary and secondary care*. National Clinical Practice Guideline 26. Gaskell & BPS.
7. Pynoos, R.S. and Eth, S. (1986). Witness to violence: the child interview. *Journal of the American Academy of Child and Adolescent Psychiatry*, **25**(3), 306–19.
8. Ohan, J.L., Myers, K., and Collett, B.R. (2002). Ten-year review of rating scales. IV: scales assessing trauma and its effects. *Journal of the American Academy of Child and Adolescent Psychiatry*, **41**(12), 1401–22.
9. Yasik, A.E., Saigh, P.A., Oberfield, R.A., *et al.* (2001). The validity of the children's PTSD inventory. *Journal of Traumatic Stress*, **14**(1), 81–94.
10. Saigh, P.A., Yasik, A.E., Oberfield, R.A., *et al.* (2000). The children's PTSD inventory: development and reliability. *Journal of Traumatic Stress*, **13**(3), 369–80.
11. Smith, P., Perrin, S., Dyregrov, A., *et al.* (2003). Principal components analysis of the impact of event scale with children in war. *Personality and Individual Differences*, **34**, 315–22.
12. Perrin, S., Meiser-Stedman, R., and Smith, P. (2005). The children's revised impact of event scale (CRIES): validity as a screening instrument for PTSD. *Behavioural and Cognitive Psychotherapy*, **33**(4), 487.
13. Foa, E.B., Johnson, K.M., Feeny, N.C., *et al.* (2001). The child PTSD symptom scale: a preliminary examination of its psychometric properties. *Journal of Clinical Child Psychology*, **30**(3), 376–84.
14. Stallard, P. (2006). Psychological interventions for post-traumatic reactions in children and young people: a review of randomised controlled trials. *Clinical Psychology Review*, **26**(7), 895–911.
15. Dalgleish, T., Meiser, S.R., and Smith, P. (2005). Cognitive aspects of posttraumatic stress reactions and their treatment in children and adolescents: an empirical review and some recommendations. *Behavioural and Cognitive Psychotherapy*, **33**(4), 459.
16. Cohen, J.A. and Mannarino, A.P. (1998). Factors that mediate treatment outcome of sexually abused preschool children: six- and 12-month follow-up. *Journal of the American Academy of Child and Adolescent Psychiatry*, **37**(1), 44–51.
17. Trowell, J., Kolvin, I., Weeramanthri, T., *et al.* (2002). Psychotherapy for sexually abused girls: psychopathological outcome findings and patterns of change. *The British Journal of Psychiatry*, **180**(3), 234.
18. Tufnell, G. (2005). Eye movement desensitization and reprocessing in the treatment of pre-adolescent children with post-traumatic symptoms. *Clinical Child Psychology and Psychiatry*, **10**(4), 587.
19. Meiser-Stedman, R. (2002). Towards a cognitive-behavioral model of PTSD in children and adolescents. *Clinical Child and Family Psychology Review*, **5**(4), 217–32.
20. Stallard, P. (2002). *Think good—feel good: a cognitive behaviour therapy workbook for children and young people*. John Wiley and Sons Ltd., Chichester.
21. Cohen, J.A., Mannarino, A.P., and Deblinger, E. (2006). *Treating trauma and traumatic grief in children and adolescents*. Guilford Press, New York.
22. Scheeringa, M.S. (1999). Treatment for posttraumatic stress disorder in infants and toddlers. *Journal of Systemic Therapies*, **18**(2), 20–31.
23. Stallard, P., Velleman, R., Salter, E., *et al.* (2006). A randomised controlled trial to determine the effectiveness of an early psychological intervention with children involved in road traffic accidents. *Journal of Child Psychology and Psychiatry*, **47**(2), 127–34.
24. Dyregrov, A. (2001). Early intervention—a family perspective. *Advances*, **17**(3), 168–74.
25. Giannopolou, I., Dikaiakou, A., and Yule, W. (2006). Cognitive-behavioural group intervention for PTSD symptoms in children following the Athens 1999 earthquake: a pilot study. *Clinical Child Psychology and Psychiatry*, **11**, 543–53.

# 9.3.3 Child abuse and neglect

David P. H. Jones

## Introduction

Child abuse and neglect (child maltreatment) is a combination of a consensus about what comprises unacceptable child rearing/care, together with what children have a right to be free from. This is made explicit in the United Nations Convention on the Rights of the Child,[1] which sets out basic rights and standards for judging children's welfare, including, but not limited to, maltreatment. It incorporates both maltreatment of children within families and that arising from wider social influences, including child labour and sexual exploitation, and children in war zones.[1]

Maltreatment affects the healthy and normal course of development. It causes deviation from an expected trajectory, preventing the developing child's negotiation of sequential tasks and disrupting normal transaction between different facets of development.[2] Therefore maltreatment is the very antithesis of adequate child care and rearing, posing a major public health threat.[3]

Adequate rearing of the young is such a fundamental activity that the state must be concerned with the overall welfare of children within its society; in family settings where they are normally brought up, and in schools, hospitals, and residential settings.

While the Convention provides a framework, several states have developed a children's ombudsman, with wide-ranging powers to oversee the status of children's welfare and to tackle obstacles to it.

There are laws within each society to regulate the care and welfare of children, specifying the consequences if children are maltreated. In England and Wales, the Children Acts 1989, and 2004 address the overall welfare of children, including those deemed in need of extra help and support, and provide a legislative structure for those children who are at risk of, or are actually being, significantly harmed (child maltreatment).

Countries vary in their response to child maltreatment. In the United States, any professional who has reason to suspect that a child is being maltreated is legally required to inform the local child welfare agency (mandatory reporting). Some countries in Europe (e.g. Belgium and Holland) have a system whereby child-maltreatment concerns are dealt with confidentially, through health and social care supportive systems, rather than through primarily legal methods. The United Kingdom lies between these extremes, but relatively closer to the United States model than to the 'confidential doctor' system. Whatever system is in place, it is clear from the scope of the problem of child maltreatment that multidisciplinary working is a core requirement.

A developmental-ecological model is the most useful conceptual framework, which draws together the various factors known to contribute or be associated with the predisposition, occurrence, course and effects of child maltreatment.[3,4] It incorporates individual and interpersonal factors, family influences, immediate neighbourhood ones, together with broader social influences on child rearing and care. However, these layers of increasing social complexity, which surround the individual child, are not static. In addition to transactions between factors, there are important influences historically, and subsequent to any maltreatment, which have an impact on outcome. This inclusive conceptual framework enables genetic and environmental factors to be integrated in a manner that can inform clinical assessment and intervention.

# Types of maltreatment

Identification of different types of maltreatment may be necessary for social and legal purposes, but epidemiologically, co-occurrence of varieties of maltreatment is more usual than singularity.[3,5] Official registers often record predominant type or that perceived to be the most serious. This knowledge is one of several methodological problems that affect confidence in research findings. However separate types are retained here, for descriptive purposes, while encouraging the reader to consider likely overlap in individual cases.

# Epidemiology

Accurate figures for incidence and prevalence are bedevilled by ascertainment and recording difficulties, including secrecy and shame which are often associated. These influences are illustrated by the wide gulf between incidence and prevalence rates.[3]

Incidence rates increase from reported cases to higher rates obtained from representative community samples. The incidence of significant violence to children varies between 50 to 90 per thousand across cultures in community samples, and dropping to the mid-20s per thousand for cases known to professionals working with children. Cases known to social welfare agencies departments only comprise a minority of these. However, officially reported maltreatment ranges from 2 to 12 per thousand in England, North America and Australia. Neglect is commonest (34 to 59 per cent of cases); physical abuse (15 to 28 per cent); sexual (10 to 28 per cent); and emotional (7 to 34 per cent).

Most prevalence figures for each of physical, emotional and neglect range between 5 and 10 per cent. The equivalent rate for contact sexual abuse is 10 per cent (15 per cent of girls; 5 per cent of boys). Children with a disability are three times more likely to be maltreated.[3]

Life-threatening maltreatment rates have remained relatively constant, currently 0.1 to 2.2/1000 children in industrialized countries, rising to two to three times this in low to mid-income countries. Children are at their most vulnerable during infancy and neonatal periods.

# Child sexual abuse

## Definition and clinical features

This is defined as sexual activities which involve a child and an adult, or a significantly older child. There are two elements: the sexual activities and the abusive condition.[6] Contact sexual activities include penetrative acts (e.g. penile, digital, or object penetration of the vagina, mouth, or anus) and non-penetrative acts (e.g. touching or sexual kissing of sexual parts of the child's body, or through the child touching sexual parts of the abuser's body). Non-contact sexual activities include exhibitionism, involving the child in making or consuming pornographic material, or encouraging two children to have sex together.

The abusive condition is founded on the premise that children cannot generally give consent to sex, because of their dependent condition. Consent can be difficult to assess in older children or if there is a small age gap between abuser and abused. Considering whether exploitation has occurred can aid this decision: it comprises misuse of authority or age differentials through deceit, unreasonable persuasion, coercion, or overt force.

Half the sexual abuse cases coming to the attention of welfare agencies involve penetration or orogenital contact. The proportion is less in community samples, because reported cases tend to be more serious in nature.

Abuse perpetrated by a caretaking adult normally consists of increasingly severe sexual contact over time, with parallel increases in coercion and threats to the child if the 'secret' is disclosed. As the physical acts and psychological climate worsen, so the child's reluctance to disclose the predicament deepens.

## Diagnosis

The most common presentation is through a statement from the child.[7] Unless the child is responded to sympathetically at this point, they may be reluctant to reveal the full nature of their plight. More than half of those who are abused do not disclose the fact, especially if they are male.

Less commonly the child's behaviour can draw attention to abuse, particularly if the child shows sexual behaviour problems, either directed towards themselves or towards other children. However, behaviour and emotional difficulties are normally non-specific, occurring in about two-thirds of children. Older children and adolescents show behaviour difficulties which are unexpected for themselves or their peer group, including substance abuse, suicide attempts, running away from home, or becoming unpredictably out of control. Not surprisingly, high rates of prior sexual abuse are noted among young people involved in prostitution.

Medical presentations do occur, for instance venereal diseases, evidence of acute assault, or an otherwise unexplained pregnancy.

Prior to investigation, one-third of reported cases are already known to child welfare agencies for other reasons. Children are more likely to disclose their predicament if they have first made a spontaneous statement to someone before being interviewed by professionals.

Child psychiatric services may assist social workers interviewing children and young people with a psychiatric disorder, or very young children. Other specialists should be enlisted for those with communication problems and learning difficulties. The aim of interviewing is to help a child describe their predicament whilst avoiding suggestion.[8] Child psychiatry also has a role to play in providing psychological treatments for symptomatic children and working with disturbed families.

Screening for the possibility of child sexual abuse increases recognition in both adult and child populations, revealing information that can be essential for psychiatric management. Adult services have a role to play in addressing psychiatric problems in family members, including treatment for paraphilias, often in conjunction with the probation service or other specialized provision.

## Aetiological and background factors

### (a) Characteristics of abused children

Sexual abuse affects children of both sexes and all ages. The most common age when children are abused is between the ages of 7 and 13 years, but up to one-quarter of reported cases comprises the under-fives. Race and socio-economic status are not major risk factors, but there are increased rates of sexual abuse among children living with parents who are emotionally unavailable, psychiatrically disturbed, violent, or who abuse alcohol or drugs.[9] Children from lower socio-economic groups are over-represented in child protection samples, but in adult retrospective surveys there is a weaker link with economic status. Children who have been in substitute care are at higher risk.

Girls are more than twice as likely to be victimized. Boys are less likely to be reported or discovered to have been abused during their childhood. Compared with girls, boys are more likely to be older when first victimized and to be abused by someone from outside the immediate family, and more likely to be abused by women or by offenders who are known to have abused other children. The risk of sexual abuse is almost doubled for children with a disability.[10]

### (b) Characteristics of abusers

Most abusers are male, but up to 10 per cent of children are abused by a female, though this figure is higher when the victim is male. Of abusers, 70 to 90 per cent are known to the child, with family members comprising between a third and a half of those who abuse girls, and between 10 and 20 per cent of abusers of boys.

Up to one-third of children are abused by a person who is under 18 years of age. **Young abusers** are, on average, 14 years old, while their victims are 7 years old and usually known to them.[11] The abusers lack social skills and assertiveness, and show impulse-control problems, learning difficulties, and clinical depression. Their home environments are characterized by instability, family violence, and sexual problems in their parents. Parental loss or separation is common among adolescent abusers.

Between 20 and 50 per cent of abusers have a history of childhood sexual abuse themselves. Physical abuse histories are even more common, together with deprivation and periods of substitute care in childhood. These characteristics are common among other offenders for non-sexual abuse offences, and thus do not explain the aetiological pathways through which some young people and adults develop a pathway of sexual attraction or desire to sexually assault a child. Marshall and Barbaree[12] have drawn together psychological, biological, and social factors into an integrated theory of aetiology.

Abusers typically deny sexual abuse allegations. Even measures of penile tumescence in response to childhood imagery are unlikely to discriminate a denying abuser from a falsely accused man. Some psychological features are common among abusers but are unlikely to be definitive, prior to any admission of guilt.[13] The demarcation between intrafamilial and extrafamilial abusers is less sharp than originally thought, and mixed abusers are relatively common.

### (c) Family aspects

Up to half of all cases are abused by someone outside the family. In the majority of these extrafamilial cases the abuser is known to the child and in a position of trust, either providing care or supervision, or involved in an educational or recreational activity with the child. Among within-family cases, the original stereotype-of a closed family with a controlling abusive father and mother who is collusive with her husband's abuse of her child-has been demonstrated to be inaccurate. Although such a pattern may be seen, a variety of family styles of functioning occur. However, investigators have found that families containing sexual abuse victims are less cohesive, more disorganized, and permit less healthy expression of emotion than comparison families.[14] These differences may pre-date the onset of sexual abuse or be a consequence of its occurrence.[9] Nonetheless, the observations are important for intervention purposes.

Support from non-abusive adult carers (usually mothers) in terms of belief, protection, and help for children to understand their victimization, is positively linked with the children's response to their experience.[15] This is important for assessment and intervention purposes, because there is a significant link between sexual abuse and markers of parent-child relationship difficulties, such as emotional unavailability, interparental conflict, parental mental health, and substance abuse problems.

### (d) Course and prognosis

A wide range of psychological sequelae in childhood and adult life are associated with prior childhood sexual abuse (Table 9.3.3.1).[9,15] However, these are linked with the effects of both the quality of the family environment at the time of abuse, and the nature of subsequent life events.[16] In particular, factors such as family disharmony and violence, existence of other forms of abuse and neglect, and parental mental health difficulties, in addition to subsequent events, such as losses through death or separation, combined with the child's own method of coping with the abuse and ameliorative effects of positive school or social relationships, all contribute to outcome.

About one-third of children are symptom free. Approximately 10 per cent of children show worsening symptoms over time, including depression and post-traumatic symptoms. While effects on personality and social relationships can be disabling during development, other children are relatively unaffected.[16,17]

**Table 9.3.3.1** Impairments and problems associated with childhood sexual abuse

|  | Childhood impairment | Adult impairment |
|---|---|---|
| Affective symptoms | Fears<br>PTSD<br>Depression | Anxiety<br>PTSD<br>Depression |
| Behaviour problems | Conduct disorder<br>Sexualized behaviour<br>Self-destructiveness<br>Hyperactivity | Aggressive conduct<br>Self-destructiveness<br>Alcohol/substance abuse |
| Cognitive functioning | Educational problems<br>Language difficulties | Educational<br>underachievement |
| Personality and social adjustment | Self-esteem<br>Attachment<br>Peer relationships | Pregnancy under 19 years<br>Sexual aggression<br>Prostitution<br>Parenting problems<br>Somatization<br>Personality disorder<br>Revictimization<br>Sexual problems |

# Physical abuse

## Definition and clinical features

Physical abuse is the physical assault of a child by any person having custody, care, or charge of that child. It includes hitting, throwing, biting, inducing burns or scalds, poisoning, suffocating, and drowning.[3] In the United States and United Kingdom physical chastisement of children is commonplace, leading to problems of definition. In other parts of Europe and in some Eastern cultures physical chastisement is regarded as unacceptable. Legal definitions in the United States and Western Europe normally link physical acts to observable harm. However, for research and clinical purposes an endangerment-based definition is preferable, because of the widely different sequelae resulting from similar assaults.[18] Failure to prevent injury or suffering is preferably considered a manifestation of neglect. Other definition problems include the frequency or repetitiveness of the acts, their severity, and whether intent to harm should be included. In addition, developmental factors affect the recognition of abuse and possibly its definition also—a smack to the head of an 8-year-old, although unacceptable, will have significantly different consequences from that to an 8-month-old.

The distinction between accidental injury, non-accidental injury, and specific medical diseases is sometimes straightforward (e.g. particular types of fractures, burns, or bruising) but difficult diagnostic dilemmas do occur. It is important to resolve these dilemmas so that the way forward for psychiatric assessment and treatment can be clarified.[19]

The 'battered child syndrome' refers to young children with multiple bruises, skeletal injuries, and head injuries, often accompanied by neglect, malnutrition, and fearfulness, whose parents deny responsibility.[20]

## Diagnosis and recognition

Physical abuse is detected through the observation of physical injuries without an alternative non-abusive explanation.[19]

Less commonly, a direct account comes from a child or a witness, or through confession by a parent or carer. Usually, the diagnosis is based upon a discrepancy between the physical findings and the history provided. The history may be insufficient or simply improbable. When an explanation is forthcoming, trigger events or developmental challenges are common—for example, persistent crying in infancy, problems of toileting or feeding among toddlers, or issues of discipline in later childhood. In adolescents, conflict surrounding independence may coincide with parental midlife crises. Not all physical abuse can be related to loss of control, however, and the assessor has to consider planned or even sadistic activities, such as scalding, burning, or torture.

There may have been previous episodes of similar or lesser concern, for which adequate explanations were unavailable at the time. Delay in presenting the child for medical attention is not a reliable diagnostic feature; neither is the apparent absence of parental concern nor their unreasonable behaviour at presentation.

## Aetiology and background factors

### (a) Child characteristics

Physical abuse occurs at all ages, although biological sequelae are more severe in infancy. There is no association with ethnic group, but a strong one with low socio-economic status among the under-fives, becoming weaker throughout childhood and disappearing by adolescence.[21] Children with developmental disabilities have a raised risk.[10] Associations with low birth weight, prematurity, or physical ill health disappear once parental and social variables are controlled for. Boys under 5 years of age are more likely to be abused, whereas girls are at greater risk in childhood overall.

### (b) Abuser characteristics

Young maternal age at the time of the child's birth is linked with abuse, but generally the effect of age is overshadowed by low socio-economic status and high social stress.[21] Physical abusers of young children are likely to be female, but male abusers predominate during adolescence. They are more likely to be single parents and to have large numbers of closely spaced children. Their educational level, but not necessarily their intelligence, is lower; they are, however, more likely to be unemployed. Most physical abuse is perpetrated by parents, but others who adopt a caretaking role become increasingly significant in the abuse of older children.

Abusive parents are more likely to have had a childhood history of abuse themselves. However, regarded prospectively, 70 per cent of abused children do not abuse their own children.[22] Non-repeaters are more likely to have enjoyed social support from a partner, had a positive relationship with an adult during childhood, and to have received psychological help during adolescence. In addition, they have a more balanced and coherent perspective about their childhood experiences than those who show intergenerational continuity of parenting problems. The quality of attachment relationships between parents and children shows continuity, rather than the specific type of abuse. Hence, physically abused children have an increased risk of perpetrating both physical and sexual abuse when they become parents themselves.

Frank psychiatric disorder is relatively infrequent among abusers, but studies of physical abuse fatalities underline their importance in a minority of cases.[23] Personality difficulties and disorders are more common, however. Hostile adults with poor impulse control, low self-esteem, antisocial and aggressive personalities, with accompanying mood disorder are more likely to abuse. These abusers have disrupted social relationships and inadequate coping responses in a wide range of domains. They are frequently socially isolated, alienated, and have disharmonious relationships with neighbours and relatives. For these adults, potentially protective supportive relationships with friends and relatives are inhibited.[3,21]

Abusive parents have maladaptive ideas about their children. They tend to have high expectations for their children's development and behaviour, perceiving it to be deviant when objectively it is not. They are more likely to believe in the appropriateness of strict physical discipline, and to hold negative views and perceptions about their children. They show limited attention to their children, less positive affect, and respond with aversion, anger, or irritation to their children's bids for care or attention, as well as to their positive behaviours, when compared with non-maltreating parents. Physically, abusers show heightened arousal to both child stimuli and non-child-related stressors.[3,21]

#### (c) Family aspects

Families in which physical abuse occurs are more likely to support mutually abusive coercive communications and interactions than controls. Partner abuse and domestic violence is relatively more common, combined with pervasive hostility and decreased cohesion. Discussion, positive displays of affection, and encouragement of prosocial behaviours are less common than in non-maltreating families.[3,21]

The quality of attachment between child and parent is significantly linked with physical abuse, especially when combined with high levels of social stress, low socio-economic status, and negative parental family attitudes and behaviours. Although infant temperament can be associated with maltreatment it probably only does so if combined with other risk factors, such as parent–child attachment problems, parental attitudes, and family difficulties of the sort described above. Clinicians have long observed that individual children can be perceived negatively by parents, without objective evidence, particularly if the child represents a particular issue or problem for the parent.

### Course and prognosis

Some physically abused children have neurological and other physical sequelae as a result of their injuries.[4] Educational difficulties are consistently found on follow-up. The children are less attentive to social cues and less skilful at managing personal problems and more likely to attribute a hostile motivation to their peers, compared with non-abused children, at the age of 5. Their capacity for empathic concern with the everyday problems of their peers becomes blunted. Not surprisingly therefore, chronic oppositional and aggressive behaviour is the most consistently documented childhood outcome. These children range from the socially withdrawn and avoidant, to those who demonstrate fear, anger, and aggression. These features are linked both to the physical abuse and the family context of pervasive aggression and conflict.[3]

The children's attachments to their caretakers are anxious and insecure. Children view themselves negatively, and show increased rates of both depression and anxiety throughout childhood. Long-term exposure results in a constellation of reactions characterized by pervasive denial by the child, an apparent repression or dissociation of memories, relative indifference to pain or distress, episodes

of rage directed towards self or others, and an unremitting sadness. Male victims may develop a characteristic hypervigilance.[21]

The major health consequences of physical abuse in childhood have become clarified.[3] The causal connection between physical abuse and later psychological and physical health problems is underlined through clear links between early age of onset, and severity of maltreatment and subsequent severity of psychological and physical ill effects in teenage and adult years. Further, physical abuse cases embedded within violent families and associated with accompanying neglect have relatively worse outcomes, psychosocially and in physical health. Approximately 20 to 30 per cent of physically abused children develop conduct problems in teenage years, starting earlier and displaying more violence than their non-abused counterparts. They are at increased risk of running away from home, and are overrepresented among young homeless children in inner cities. Childhood physical abuse is associated with subsequent substance abuse problems, self-destructive behaviour and suicidality, depression, teenage pregnancy and poor physical health outcomes. Genetic factors mediate the association between physical abuse and later antisocial behaviour and, probably, affective disorder too.[3]

## Child neglect

### Definition and clinical features

Neglect refers to the underprovision of the child's basic needs, both physical and psychological. Most cases comprise omissions of care by parents and others in the parental role. However, institutional neglect also occurs, mainly in the form of collective caretaking failure—for example, residential children's homes in the United Kingdom, orphanages and nurseries in Eastern Europe, and neglect of care by educational establishments.[3]

Definition problems include whether neglect should include the apparent impact on the child and/or the degree to which it was intended.[3] There are cultural variations in what might be perceived as neglect. The practice of putting young children into separate bedrooms, while considered normal practice in much of Western Europe, would be considered frankly neglectful in some Eastern cultures.

Notwithstanding these definition problems, four main types can be identified: physical, supervisory, cognitive, and emotional neglect. Neglect can occur first during the prenatal period, for example through maternal substance abuse, and may be observed throughout childhood. **Physical** neglect includes inadequate nutrition, clothing, shelter, but also exclusion and abandonment. This is the most common form of neglect reported to welfare agencies in North America, Australia and Western Europe. **Supervisory** involves inadequate parental overview, relative to the child's needs, for developmental needs of the child, but also employing unsafe alternative carers, and failure to use available health care. **Emotional** neglect includes insufficient parental affection, and inattention to the child's cues, which has been termed 'psychological unavailability'.[24] **Cognitive** is insufficient parental responsiveness, attention and speech, but also denying access to education opportunities.

### Diagnosis and presentation

Although most reported cases involve younger children, neglect occurs at all ages. Many cases are followed for years before being finally identified by professionals. Non-organic failure to thrive can precipitate earlier recognition. Otherwise neighbours, relatives, or school teachers report the child's plight to protection agencies, by which time the effects are severe and neglectful caretaking entrenched. Recognition may also come about through the child's presentation with developmental delay, language problems, school non-attendance, inadequate medical or dental care, or with significant psychological difficulties. Conclusions about neglect need to be linked with the individual's developmental needs. Additionally neglect must be distinguished from the effects of poverty. Conclusions are assisted by using multiple sources of information; from the children themselves, caregivers, reviewing longitudinal case records, direct observation and standardized measures.[3]

## Aetiological and background factors

### (a) Characteristics of neglectful parents

Neglectful parents are likely to be poor, have multiple difficulties, and display what has been described as the apathy-futility syndrome. Parents show immature personality characteristics, with low self-esteem, impulsivity, and an inability to plan or demonstrate choice in such important areas as adult partners, having children, or employment. Neglectful parents frequently hold inaccurate or unrealistic expectations about their children's development or behaviour. Neglect may derive from parental psychiatric illness such as schizophrenia, depression, or drug or alcohol abuse.

### (b) Characteristics of neglected children

Neglected infants have anxious, disorganized attachments with their caretakers. Later in childhood they are more aggressive than comparison children, though less so than physically abused children. Neglected toddlers show non-compliance and become easily frustrated, later developing low self-esteem and self-assertiveness and showing less flexibility or self-control. Both in preschool and school they lack persistence and enthusiasm, and become socially isolated.

### (c) Family aspects

Child neglect is normally embedded within broader family insularity, lack of cognitive stimulation, affection or emotional nurturing between its members, and significant household disorganization. Neglectful parents are likely to be unresponsive to both their infants and older children, showing a paucity of prosocial positive behaviours, less interactions and stimulation, and more negative behaviours than controls. Even though there is a strong link with poverty, parents who neglect children stand out among their equally materially impoverished neighbours.

## Course and prognosis

The seeds for the neglected child's long-term difficulties with social interaction, relationships, and educational progress can be observed in infancy. Neglected children tend towards passiveness and helplessness under stress. They show significant developmental delays, especially language problems, attention-seeking behaviour, and superficial displays of affection, as well as conduct problems, persistent defiance, and hostile behaviour. Studies of children who as infants were subjected to psychologically unavailable caretaking reveal persisting difficulties with anger, non-compliance, low frustration tolerance, little enthusiasm or persistence for tasks, poor impulse control, relative rigidity, and lack of creativity. Similar negative developmental outcomes have been reported to occur

following non-organic failure to thrive in infancy, especially where combined with physical neglect, leading to long-term cognitive delay and poor educational attainment. Children who as infants experienced psychologically unavailable parenting do even worse than physically abused children, showing a greater number of emotional problems, inattention, social withdrawal, and unpopularity with other children.[24]

# Psychological maltreatment

## Definition and clinical features

Emotional abuse (better termed 'psychological maltreatment') refers to those interactions with children that have the potential to damage the child psychologically, given his or her particular developmental needs.[3] Four broad groupings of acts are described: the need for psychological safety and security; for acceptance and positive regard; for age appropriate autonomy, and sufficient opportunities to explore environment and extra familial relationships. Included within **psychological safety** are exposure to domestic violence, threats of injury, suicide or abandonment, and discipline through intimidation. Within **acceptance and self-esteem** are verbal and non-verbal negativity, active rejection, ridiculing, inappropriate expectations and undermining. **Age appropriate autonomy** includes both inappropriate responsibility giving and prohibiting age appropriate socialization and placing a child in a reversed parental role. **Restriction** includes restrictive confinement and isolation.

Psychological maltreatment may be direct toward the child, or operate indirectly, for example through the child witnessing domestic violence, or observing parental involvement in antisocial activities. It may occur in institutional settings as well as within families. The overlap with neglect is evident from the list of acts of omission and commission listed above.

## Diagnosis and recognition

Recognition may occur when other kinds of maltreatment are discovered, or when domestic violence is revealed. It may also occur when a child is noted to be living with, and/or providing care for a parent with mental or physical illness, personality disorder or substance abuse. Sometimes recognition follows a child's referral to developmental or mental health clinic, or through the reported observations of neighbours or professionals (e.g. teachers, police). Diagnosis requires detailed history, with examples, direct observations of parent-child interactions, and interviews with older children. Standardized data gathering schemas may assist diagnosis.

## Aetiological and background factors

### (a) Characteristics of abused children

Reports of emotional abuse in children become more frequent throughout childhood into adolescence. Reported cases are more likely to be linked with lower socio-economic status. There is no particular link with racial or ethnic groups. Psychological maltreatment is frequently integral to other forms of maltreatment and so distinguishing different aetiological factors and consequences is complex.

### (b) Characteristics of abusers

Although not systematically studied, this probably varies according to the mixture of subtypes present, and whether any other kinds of abuse or neglect coexist.

### (c) Course and prognosis

Psychological maltreatment in infancy has a very poor outlook (see discussion of neglect). Much less is known about the outcome of different mixtures of psychological maltreatment identified during childhood and adolescence. There are indications that the degree and extent of psychological maltreatment is a better predictor of case outcome than the extent of any coexisting physical or sexual abuse, thus underlining its importance to the developing person's mental health.

## Fabricated or induced illness (Munchausen syndrome by proxy)

### Definition and key elements

Fabricated or induced illness (FII) is where a parent or carer feigns an impression or induces a state of ill health in a child whom they are looking after. The key elements are parental falsification or deceit, and a triangular interaction between parent, child, and health professional, in which the doctor is misled by the parent, some parental need is met, and the child harmed (directly or indirectly). The harm occurs through: verbal fabrication of symptoms/signs; falsification of reports or specimens; or through inducing ill health (either actively or by withholding essential substances).[25]

### Diagnosis

The presentation can be in any bodily system, but common forms are fabricated epilepsy, non-accidental poisoning, apparent life-threatening events in infancy (either directly induced suffocation, or fabricated), or multi-system disorders (e.g. gastrointestinal and renal problems).

The diagnosis of fabrication is almost always undertaken by paediatricians, whose awareness of the possibility of fabricated signs or symptoms is now much greater and leads to an earlier diagnosis than when first described by Meadow.[26]

There are several elements to the phenomenon:

1 the harm caused to the child through fabrication;

2 the impact on the child's development, both physically and emotionally;

3 the psychological status of the fabricator.

Psychological services are especially involved in (2) and (3)—assessing the child's developmental status, and considering the mental state of the fabricator and assessing family dynamics. Differentially, factitious illness by proxy needs to be distinguished from parental overanxiety or exaggeration, or frank malingering, though sometimes FII contains elements of all these.[25]

### Epidemiology

The annual incidence among children in the United Kingdom has been calculated to be 0.5 per 100 000, but for those under 1 year it is 2.8 per 100 000.

### Aetiological and background factors

#### (a) Characteristics of abused children

The majority of children are under 5 years of age, with boys and girls equally represented. Affected infants are likely to have feeding problems; withdrawal and hyperactivity are seen in school-age children, whereas adolescents may develop somatization themselves. Up to three-quarters of the children show evidence of other fabrications, or of physical abuse and neglect.

#### (b) Abuser characteristics

Most fabricators are female—79 per cent of whom have a somatization disorder themselves and half have a personality disorder, particularly so among fabricators who induce illness. Most abusers deny responsibility, at least initially.

#### (c) Family characteristics

Unusually, families are often intact, though 40 per cent have serious marital problems. Child-parent attachment difficulties are common, and other siblings in the family may be affected. Typically, fathers are not involved in family life.

### Course and prognosis

Affected children may be damaged by the abuse itself, while mortality is between 5 and 10 per cent. About 20 per cent are reabused, though not necessarily in the same way as the original FII. Emotional harm, conduct problems, and educational difficulties occur in half the children on follow-up.

## Prevention of maltreatment

Reducing the incidence and recurrence of child maltreatment are crucial initiatives, because of the resultant ill effects[27] and difficulty in instituting effective treatments, quite apart from the humanitarian prerogative. Family support—and education concerning parenting, child development, and the management of problems—has a positive impact on parental attitudes and knowledge as well as on observed behaviour. Significant effects on children's behaviour, cognitive outcome, and child maltreatment rates are less clear. Preventive efforts have more impact upon physical abuse than on neglect.[28]

Brief interventions are beneficial for low-risk parents, whereas more intensive approaches are needed for higher risk groups. High-risk groups include deprived, impoverished parents, young mothers, and those with a personal history of childhood abuse themselves. However, for a prevention approach to be effective it must be personalized to the needs of the individual families and include outreach components for the most negative and hard to access parents.[28] Including males, whether resident or occasional visitors, is crucial to maintaining and sustaining improvements in parenting and child care. Equally, effective programmes are more likely to be valued by the parents themselves, underlining the importance of matching the skills of staff and the contents of programmes with the families' specific needs.[29,30] Similarly, programmes must be culturally sensitive if they are to be effective and accepted by parents. Interventions are most effective when they impact upon a broad network of influences and relationships, ranging from those of the immediate family to broader neighbourhood and social influences on children's welfare.[3] Furthermore, primary, secondary and tertiary prevention approaches need to be integrated and carefully planned within each area.[31]

Sexual abuse prevention is probably ineffective when aimed at enhancing children's capacity to protect themselves.[28] On the other hand, programmes which include parents (and increase their capacity to keep their children safe) and incorporate antibullying tactics are much more likely to be effective, although this probably stems from increasing disclosure of early sexually abusive actions rather than primary prevention.[28] Additionally, broader social initiatives to reduce child sexual abuse within schools and institutions are essential to a comprehensive area strategy.[27,31]

# Intervention and psychological treatment

## Treatments

Psychological treatments have been developed for different types of maltreatment, notwithstanding contemporary appreciation that co-occurrence of types of maltreatment is common place. Effective treatments for physical and sexual abuse are reasonably well established.

Interventions with empirical support are principally behavioural, and cognitive behavioural ones.[3] These are normally structured and emphasize skill building to overcome emotional distress and behavioural disturbance in children and parents. Trauma-focussed, cognitive behavioural therapies are significantly superior to family and general therapeutic treatments for both physical and sexual abuse. These treatments combine psycho-education, exposure therapy, cognitive procedures and restructuring as well as behavioural management. Children are also assisted with emotional recognition and regulation and attention to maladaptive ideas. Other empirically supported interventions include child parent psychotherapy (blending psychodynamic and cognitive behavioural components).

Psychological treatments in neglect have concentrated on improving parenting skills and sensitivity through direct encouragement of positive interactions in feeding, play, general care, combined with individual therapy for parents themselves.[3] Parallel psychiatric treatment of parental mental health problems, such as depression or substance abuse is also important, although there is debate about whether such treatments should precede or be delivered subsequent to treatments focussed on parenting. There has been some support for therapeutic day treatment programmes and multisystemic therapy for neglect.

Psychiatric interventions for psychological maltreatment have not been subject to empirical evaluation thus far. In the meantime it seems reasonable to focus on improving sensitivity and responsiveness within parent child relationships (through direct work and feedback), together with family based work, and individual work with parents who have been subject to deprived or abusive backgrounds themselves.

Treatments for FII are sparse, but combinations of treatments for neglect and psychological maltreatment, combined with behavioural management of somatization appears promising.[3]

## Management

### (a) Guiding principles[3,32]

The first priority is to establish the **child's safety** and/or freedom from neglect. This may require separation of child and abuser. Those cases involving neglect or psychological maltreatment may be managed through verifiable agreement, and providing services designed to promote the child's welfare within the family. Interdisciplinary planning and coordination will be essential in order to achieve this.

Interventions must be focused primarily on the **child's welfare**, rather than other objectives such as adult treatment or family preservation. Interventions should also focus on the child's **physical and emotional safety**, and be **developmentally focused**, while simultaneously tackling **parenting problems**. A developmental focus involves adapting treatments to a child's age and developmental status, and taking into account any developmental impairment. Additionally, it is essential that treatment approaches comprehensively address those developmental processes affected by maltreatment, i.e. affect regulation, attachment, the evolving self system, and peer relationships.[5]

Approaches to parenting problems range from interventions with parents individually, those focused specifically on parent child dyads, through to more broadly based social support services, including day attendance at family centres designed to improve parenting care, the use of family support workers, harnessing neighbourhood supports and other parents prepared to assist new parents at risk, and parenting classes. Services to improve family conflict resolution and parental management of hostility and aggression may also be needed for a comprehensive approach to tackling parenting problems. Parents with mental health problems need to be psychiatrically evaluated to see whether treatment could assist overall case management. Sexually abusive behaviour or physical violence perpetrated by adults may be amenable to psychiatric intervention. Persistently dangerous abusers need to be identified and child safety assured.

Further, interventions should specifically address the **child's experience** of maltreatment and any moral or legal dimensions to this. Interventions should not focus solely on maltreatment itself, but equally address any **general mental health issues**. They should also aim to **prevent future difficulties** as well as addressing current problems. Supportive and **nonabusive parents and carers** should be part of the intervention and incorporated into treatment plans. Obtaining **parental acknowledgement and recognition** of their part in maltreatment is an important part of successful interventions. Parental acknowledgement may be achieved through education and discussion, and through treatment approaches designed to alter hostile or neglectful views and attributions held by parents. First choice interventions should be those with the highest level of **empirical support**. Generally, interventions should involve school and **local networks** of child professionals in a systemic fashion. A systemic perspective is helpful with respect to all families. Sensitive working across disciplinary boundaries requires knowledge of **local** family justice system and child protection **working practices**.

### (b) Case planning

When deciding what to do in the individual case, treatment may have to address several aspects of abuse and neglect, because co-occurrence of maltreatment type is common. Safety is of paramount consideration. There is little value in starting treatment if the child remains unsafe. This will require multidisciplinary or multiagency co-operation in order to develop a comprehensive plan for child and family. Even where intensive treatments are unavailable, psycho-educational approaches are helpful for all abused children. In reality, most maltreated children receive no systematic therapeutic intervention.

The majority of treatment approaches combine intervention for the child with adult treatment and often family based work. Supportive work with non-abusive carers is of proven value. In planning this, however, it must be remembered that failure to protect a child is harmful and dangerous for the child's future too. In addition, in one family there may be more than one maltreating carer, e.g. abuse by one adult carer and neglect by another.

Effectiveness of intervention is gauged through several dimensions. For example, child safety, improved carer availability and sensitivity for the child, whether the child has overcome effects of trauma, psychological symptom reduction, improved peer relationships, speech and language catch up and educational progress. Improvements in family functioning which are sensitive to interventions include; reduced conflict and violence, improved communication and emotional expression, changes to disturbed attachment patterns and improved child to parent attachment, and greater warmth in parent/child relationships. In addition, effectiveness may be gauged through target mental health objectives for individual carers, e.g. reduction in parental depression or improvements in anger management.

Developmental considerations will also contribute to evaluation of effectiveness. For example, a shorter timescale is appropriate for younger children in view of their developmental needs; and greater than average improvement in parenting may be needed for children with impairments or disabilities.

Risk management is a central issue for mental health practitioners when providing interventions in maltreatment cases, and underlines the need for systemic awareness and well-developed interdisciplinary practice. Risk factors for occurrence are reviewed elsewhere.[3] Recurrence risk has been the focus of systematic review[33], and narrative overview, using an eco-developmental perspective and identifying risk elevating as well as lowering factors.[34] Nonetheless, multiplicity of relevant factors as well as complexity of transactions in individual cases render actuarial approaches to risk management an unrealistic aspiration at this point. In its place, an approach that has been characterized as structured professional judgment appears the most appropriate.[35] Key risk elevating factors for recurrence include: domestic violence, child neglect, cases where there had been previous maltreatment, and parents with mental health disorders. A structured approach to risk management entails an approach to data gathering, diagnostic formulation and subsequent decision making that rests explicitly on available evidence about risk factors for recurrence.[34]

### (c) Ethical and legal considerations

Decisions as to whether to share sensitive information with other professionals will be guided by child welfare and safety considerations, which are paramount, and override adult consent withheld. Sometimes children request confidentiality, in situations where their safety is potentially compromised. Normally, explaining to children why information must be shared, and involving them enables their trust to be maintained even where there is initial disagreement.

Generally, patient information will need to be shared during multidisciplinary planning meetings, but agreement can usually be made to respect confidentiality, except to the degree necessary to assure child safety. Many cases will involve family justice systems, which normally require overview of progress. Practitioners will need to provide reports for planning meetings and family courts, in order to contribute to safe care.

### (d) Long term

Mental health effects may present at different points in the life course, particularly at key times of developmental change, e.g. at a first romantic relationship, or when becoming a parent. If possible, such possible future difficulties should be noted in a person's medical record, to facilitate future intervention. As part of an area's comprehensive prevention approach, new parents with a history of childhood maltreatment should be offered extra support, as they are a vulnerable group for parenting problems (although it is important to stress that discontinuity of parenting problems is more common than continuity).

## Further information

### Web sites

California Evidence-based Clearinghouse for Child Welfare. http://www.cachildwelfareclearinghouse.org/
Every Child Matters. http://www.everychildmatters.gov.uk/
International Society for the Prevention of Child Abuse and Neglect. http://www.ispcan.org/
National Society for the Prevention of Cruelty to Children. http://www.nspcc.org.uk/Inform/informhub_Wda4993.html

## References

1. World Health Organization. (2002). *World report on violence and health*. Geneva: World Health Organization.
2. Cicchetti, D. (1989). How research on child maltreatment has informed the study of child development: perspectives from developmental psychopathology. In *Child maltreatment; theory and research on the theory and causes of child abuse and neglect* (ed. D. Cicchetti and V. Carlson), pp. 377–431. Cambridge University Press, Cambridge.
3. Jones, D P H. (2008). Child maltreatment. In *Rutter's child and adolescent psychiatry* (5th edn) (ed. M. Rutter, D. Bishop, D. Pine, *et al.*). Blackwell, Oxford.
4. Cicchetti, D. and Toth, S. (1995). A developmental psychopathology perspective on child abuse and neglect. *Journal of the American Academy of Child and Adolescent Psychiatry*, **34**, 541–65.
5. Leventhal, J. (2007). Children's experiences of violence: some have much more than others. *Child Abuse and Neglect*, **31**, 3–6.
6. Finkelhor, D. (1994). Current information on the scope and nature of child sexual abuse. *Future of Children*, **4**, 31–53.
7. Jones, D.P.H. (1997). Assessment of suspected child sexual abuse. In *The battered child* (5th edn) (ed. R. Helfer, R. Kempe, and R. Krugman), pp. 296–312. University of Chicago Press, Chicago.
8. Jones, D.P.H. (2003). *Communicating with vulnerable children: a guide for practitioners*. Gaskell, London.
9. Berliner, L., and Elliott, D. (2002). Sexual abuse of children. In *The APSAC handbook on child maltreatment* (eds. J. Myers, L. Berliner, J. Briere, *et al.*), pp. 55–78. Sage, London.
10. Westcott, H.L., and Jones, D.P.H. (1999). Annotation: the abuse of disabled children. *Journal of Child Psychology and Psychiatry*, **40**, 497–506.
11. Vizard, E., Monck, E., and Misch, P. (1995). Child and adolescent sex abuse perpetrators: a review of the research literature. *Journal of Child Psychology and Psychiatry*, **36**, 731–56.
12. Marshall, W., and Barbaree, H. (1990). An integrated theory of the aetiology of sex offending. In *Handbook of sexual assault* (ed. W. Marshall, D. Laws, and H. Barbaree), pp. 257–75. Plenum Press, New York.
13. Becker, J. (1994). Offenders: characteristics and treatment. *Future of Children*, **4**, 176–97.
14. Madonna, P., Van Scoyk, S., and Jones, D.P.H. (1991). Family interactions within incest and non-incest families. *American Journal of Psychiatry*, **148**, 46–9.
15. Jones, D.P.H., and Ramchandani, P. (1998). *Child sexual abuse—informing practice from research*. Radcliffe Medical Press, Oxford.

16. Glaser, D. (2008). Child sexual abuse. In *Rutter's child and adolescent psychiatry* (5th edn) (ed M. Rutter, D. Bishop, D. Pine, *et al.*). Blackwell, Oxford.

17. Rind, B., Tromovitch, P., and Bauserman, R. (1998). A meta-analytic examination of assumed properties of child sexual abuse using college samples. *Psychological Bulletin*, **124**, 22–53.

18. National Research Council (1993). Scope of the problem. In *Understanding child abuse and neglect*, pp. 78–105. National Academy Press, Washington, DC.

19. Johnson, C. (2002). Physical abuse: accidental versus intentional trauma in children. In *The APSAC handbook on child maltreatment* (ed. J. Myers, L. Berliner, J. Briere, *et al.*), pp. 249–68. Sage, London.

20. Kempe, C.H., Silverman, F.N., Steele, B.F., *et al.* (1962). The battered child syndrome. *Journal of the American Medical Association*, **181**, 17–24.

21. Kolko, D. (2002). Child physical abuse. In *The APSAC handbook on child maltreatment* (ed. J. Myers, L. Berliner, J. Briere, *et al.*), pp. 21–54. Sage, London.

22. Kaufman, J., and Zigler, E. (1989). The intergenerational transmission of child abuse. In *Child maltreatment; theory and research on the theory and causes of child abuse and neglect* (ed. D. Cicchetti, and V. Carlson), pp. 129–50. Cambridge University Press, Cambridge.

23. Jones, D.P.H., and Lynch, M.A. (1998). Diagnosing and responding to serious child abuse. *British Medical Journal*, **317**, 484–5.

24. Erickson, M., and Egeland, B. (2002). Child neglect. In *The APSAC handbook on child maltreatment* (ed. J. Myers, L. Berliner, J. Briere, *et al.*), pp. 3–20. Sage, London.

25. Jones, D.P.H., and Bools, C.N. (1999). Factitious illness by proxy. In *Recent advances in paediatrics* (ed. T. David), pp. 57–71. Churchill Livingstone, Edinburgh.

26. Meadow, S.R. (1997). Munchausen's syndrome by proxy: a hinterland of child abuse. *Lancet*, **ii**, 232–5.

27. Daro, D., and Cohn Donnelly, A. (2002). Child abuse prevention: accomplishments and challenges. In *The APSAC handbook on child maltreatment* (ed. J. Myers, L. Berliner, J. Briere, *et al.*), pp. 431–48. Sage, London.

28. Wolfe, D., Reppucci, N., and Hart, S. (1995). Child abuse prevention: knowledge and priorities. *Journal of Clinical Child Psychology*, **24** (Supplement), 5–22.

29. Cox, A. (1998). Preventing child abuse: a review of community based projects. II: Issues arising from reviews and future directions. *Child Abuse Review*, **7**, 30–43.

30. Leventhal, J. (2005). Getting prevention right: maintaining the status quo is not an option. *Child Abuse and Neglect*, **29**(3), 209–13.

31. MacMillan, H.L., MacMillan, J.H., Offord, D.R., *et al.* (1994). Primary prevention of child physical abuse and neglect: a critical review—part I. *Journal of Child Psychology and Psychiatry*, **35**, 835–56.

32. Saunders, B.E., Berliner, L., Hanson, R.F. (eds.) (2004). *Child Physical and Sexual Abuse: guidelines for treatment (Final Report: January 15, 2003)*. Charleston, SC; National Crimes Victims Research and Treatment Center.

33. Hindley, N., Ramchandani, P., and Jones, D.P.H. (2006). Risk factors for recurrence of maltreatment: a systematic review. *Archives of Disease in Childhood*, **91**(9), 744–52.

34. Jones, D.P.H., Hindley, N., and Ramchandani, P. (2006). Making plans: assessment, intervention and evaluating outcomes. In *The Developing World of the Child* (eds, J. Aldgate, D. Jones, W. Rose, *et al.*) (Chap 15, pp 267–86). London: Jessica Kingsley.

35. Douglas, K.S., and Kropp, P.R. (2002). A prevention-based paradigm for violence risk assessment: Clinical and research applications. *Criminal Justice and Behavior*, **29**(5), 617–58.

## 9.3.4 The relationship between physical and mental health in children and adolescents

Julia Gledhill and M. Elena Garralda

### Introduction

The link between physical and psychological disorder in children and adolescents is well established. Children with chronic illness are at increased risk of emotional and behavioural disorders. In addition, repeated presentations with physical symptoms may represent underlying psychological distress or psychiatric disorder.

Because of the inextricable links between young people and the family in which they live, it is inappropriate to consider symptoms in an index child in isolation. The effects of symptomatology on family functioning, parent, and sibling relationships should be considered. This may have important aetiological and prognostic significance.

### Associations between physical and psychological symptoms

There are various ways in which physical and psychological disorders are related; these are summarized in Table 9.3.4.1.

In this chapter we shall consider the following:

- The psychiatric consequences of physical illness
- Helping the dying child and his or her family
- The effects of psychiatric disorder on the course and outcome of physical illness
- Aspects of assessment and treatment intervention

**Table 9.3.4.1** Associations between physical and psychological symptoms

| Nature of association | Examples |
| --- | --- |
| Psychiatric consequences of physical illness and treatment | *Organic*: acute confusional state, psychosis induced by brain disorder *Functional*: adjustment disorder after diagnosis of diabetes, specific needle phobia in young child with cancer receiving chemotherapy |
| Effects of psychiatric disorder on physical illness | Depression delaying the mobilization of a child following partial limb amputation after severe meningococcal disease, oppositional-defiant disorder affecting treatment adherence in diabetes |
| Physical complications of psychiatric problems e.g. deliberate self-harm, substance abuse | Liver failure following paracetamol overdose |
| Psychiatric disorders or psychological distress presenting with physical symptoms | Aches and pains in school age children, reduced physical well-being in adolescent depression, somatoform pain disorder, dissociative disorder |

◆ Somatization and somatoform disorders, with a particular focus on recurrent abdominal pain, dissociative/conversion disorder, and chronic fatigue syndrome

# Psychiatric aspects of chronic physical illness

## Chronic physical illness and the risk of psychiatric disorder

Chronic physical illness in children, defined as disorders that last at least 1 year and are associated with persistent or recurrent handicap, affects about 4 per cent of children in Western countries.[1] This encompasses a broad spectrum of disorders including more common problems such as eczema, asthma, diabetes, epilepsy, and less prevalent conditions such as cystic fibrosis and cancer. Many children successfully adapt to living with a chronic illness, but it can be associated with a number of different types of stresses for children and their families.

The stress of chronic illness may operate at several levels. In addition to the presence of the illness itself, diagnostic and treatment procedures may be painful or have undesirable side-effects—changes in physical appearance such as alopecia, scars, and obesity may lead to difficulties in peer relationships. The demands of treatment such as dietary restrictions in diabetes may be difficult. The illness, together with hospital attendance for treatment, may lead to a considerable interruption to schooling as well as a reduced ability to participate in leisure activities and socialize with peers.

Although the majority of children and families successfully adapt to these stresses, children with chronic physical illness have a slightly increased risk for the development of associated psychiatric disorders. Specific factors related to the child and the illness have been shown to contribute to the likelihood of developing psychiatric disturbance and to influence the nature of the psychiatric disorder that develops (Table 9.3.4.2).[2]

### (a) Nature of the physical disorder

Much of the increased prevalence of psychiatric disorder in children with chronic physical illness is accounted for by those with disorders affecting the brain, especially when epilepsy is involved.[3] They have a three-fold increased risk of psychiatric disorder over general population rates. The risk in young people with a chronic physical illness that does not involve the brain is considerably lower and only slightly increased over general population expectations.[3] The excess of psychopathology in children with brain anomalies may be attributable to the direct effects of organic pathology on behaviour, or may be mediated by the greater physical disability that frequently accompanies brain damage. Associated intellectual impairment may also be an important contributory factor.

**Table 9.3.4.2** Factors related to the risk of psychiatric disorder and the form of its presentation

| |
|---|
| Nature of physical disorder (whether brain involvement) |
| Stage of illness (whether acute stresses involved) |
| Severity of illness |
| Degree of life threat |
| Psychosocial risk and protective factors in family |
| Age (developmental stage) |
| Effects of illness and treatment procedures |

Whilst this dichotomy between disorders involving and not involving the brain is useful, there is little specificity in the behavioural pattern that may be attributable to intracerebral pathology. As a possible exception, children with brain dysfunction such as epilepsy or cerebral palsy may be more likely to exhibit externalizing disorders such as hyperactivity.[3] Psychiatric disorders in this group of children may be persistent, with 70 per cent still experiencing difficulties at 4-year follow-up. Overactivity, restlessness, and inattention are the best predictors of persistence.

For conditions not affecting the brain, the development of psychiatric disorder seems most likely to be linked with the accumulation of generic stress factors and family changes common to living with a chronic illness. These include life stresses such as hospitalization and daily difficulties such as specific dietary requirements and disruption of family routines.[4] A broad spectrum of psychiatric presentations are associated and these are not specific to the nature of the underlying disease processes. Children with nonneurological physical illnesses are more prone to developing emotional symptoms and eating anomalies as opposed to antisocial behaviour. Eating anomalies may arise from an emphasis on diet and a concern about poor appetite in the families of many children with chronic illnesses. Maternal anxiety may focus on feeding, especially in preschool children. The specificity of the relationship with emotional disorders is of interest. Physical illness in the child can generate family and social stresses and changes that are known risk factors for the development of emotional disorders in children. This includes mood disorders in parents and overinvolved and overprotective parenting.[2]

### (b) Stage of the illness

Disorder at the time of initial diagnosis is not uncommon and is frequently short lived. In one study, 36 per cent of 8- to 13-year-olds with newly diagnosed insulin-dependent diabetes mellitus developed an adjustment disorder (most commonly dominated by depressive symptoms) within the first 3 months of diagnosis; 50 per cent had recovered within 2 months.[5] Similarly, in patients with chronic renal failure, psychological problems were reported in 60 per cent of children at the time of starting dialysis. One year later, after stabilization of their physical condition, the prevalence of disturbance was reduced to 21 per cent.[6] It is very likely therefore that in many children with chronic physical illness, psychiatric disorders are most frequently transitory adjustment disorders to stressful times in the illness.

### (c) Severity of illness/degree of life threat

More severe physical disorders and those constituting a greater degree of life threat are associated with a higher risk of psychiatric disturbance. In children with end-stage chronic renal failure, those with more severe disorders (on hospital haemodialysis) have been found to have more psychiatric disorder than those not yet requiring dialysis.[7] More severely affected diabetic children and adolescents with a history of hospitalization for ketoacidosis in the previous year are more likely to exhibit psychiatric disorder than a control group of outpatients also with insulin-dependent diabetes mellitus.[8] Posttraumatic stress disorder (which by definition requires acknowledgement of perceived life threat), and high levels of post-traumatic stress symptoms have been found in children and parents up to a year after admission to Paediatric Intensive Care Units[9]; (a much higher proportion than following admission to general paediatric wards), and up to 10 years after treatment for childhood cancer.[10]

The link between illness severity and risk of psychosocial impairment may vary with the setting in which it is examined. Less severe physical impairment has been shown to be associated with a higher risk of behavioural problems in the school setting.[7] Teachers may be less aware of the presence of an underlying physical disorder in this group who have less visible physical signs, and may make less allowance for these children than for those with a more overt disorder.

### (d) Psychosocial risk and intrafamilial protective factors

When a physically ill child develops psychological symptoms, these are frequently attributed by families and professionals to the presence of the illness and its stresses. It is important not to neglect consideration of other predisposing factors (i) within the child, for example genetic vulnerability, temperamental characteristics, (ii) in the family such as marital disharmony, lack of open communication, maternal mental illness affecting parenting, and (iii) within the broader social environment such as bullying at school and poor peer relationships. These factors contribute to child psychopathology in ill as well as in healthy children. Conversely, protective factors such as secure parent–child attachments, increased family social support in response to the physical diagnosis, as well as sensitive paediatric management of hospitalizations and stressful medical procedures may reduce the risk of developing psychiatric disorder.

### (e) Age (developmental stage)

Manifestations of psychological distress in ill children vary with each developmental stage. Preschool children have fewer cognitive resources to cope with discomfort and stressful medical procedures and are likely to rely on maternal support and distraction to cope with illness. Between 4 and 7 years of age, children may believe that illness has been caused by something bad they have done and that they should be punished.[4] Clinginess to parents, fearfulness, sleep difficulty, and oppositional–defiant behaviour are seen in preschool children. The need for repeated painful procedures, for example with cancer chemotherapy, can lead to the development of specific needle phobia.

For school-age children, school life is a key aspect of their adjustment to illness. Return to school after cancer chemotherapy can be associated with the development of school phobia, loneliness, and social isolation. School absence and having to catch up with school work, teasing, or even bullying, especially of children who look different, may also occur and contribute to lowered self-esteem and the risk of affective disturbance. Cognitive development in adolescence allows a greater understanding about the implications of chronic illness and the realities of death; depression occurs more frequently in this age group. Adolescents may begin to challenge and experiment with their treatment; they may fail to come to outpatient appointments or attend erratically. There may also be a decline in compliance with medical advice and adherence to treatment regimens.[4] For example, diabetics may not follow dietary advice or pay reduced attention to their insulin regimen and monitoring of blood sugars leading to poorer diabetic control. Adherence may be influenced by family factors; poorer metabolic control is associated with less family cohesion and a parenting style that is perceived as critical and negative.[11] Adolescents aged 13–18 years with diabetes and co-morbid internalizing disorders, and discharged from hospital, have been found to be at greater risk of readmission up to 2 years later. This relationship was not found for younger children, suggesting that greater parental control of diabetes management (as is usual for younger children) may ameliorate the potential for psychiatric disorder to affect treatment adherence.[12]

The way in which psychiatric disorder presents may influence its perceived significance to health professionals and the likelihood of psychiatric referral. Presentations with behavioural disturbances such as screaming, struggling, panicking, or a failure to comply with treatment are more likely to precipitate referral than internalizing disorders such as depression.

## Effects on parents and siblings

Whilst most families successfully adjust to the presence of a child with chronic illness in the family, this may act as a risk factor for psychological disorder. The incidence of marital break-up is not increased, but there are reports of increased marital distress. Interparental conflict may not be directly expressed but instead diverted to excessive worry and focus on the illness, which can be very stressful for the child.[13] In parallel with the heightened short-term psychological difficulties found in ill children immediately following diagnosis, a similar temporal pattern of disorder has been reported for parents and siblings. Most research has focused on mothers, who often undertake the practicalities of caring for a sick child. They may need to stop work themselves, leading to increased social isolation and a reduction in extra-familial support.[14] Fathers and mothers often cope differently with the diagnosis; mothers tend to react by emotional release, whereas fathers are more likely to withdraw and concentrate on practicalities.[14] Higher rates of maternal psychiatric treatment and negative affect have been found in families with a chronically ill child. The risk of maternal depression is greater for mothers of children with chronic as compared with newly diagnosed epilepsy; the burden of illness may impede parenting capacity and contribute to the development or maintenance of psychopathology in the children.[13] Siblings may resent both the extra attention an ill brother or sister is receiving, and repeated separations from parents during periods of hospitalization. Their psychological adjustment is related to the degree of functional impairment[15] and recent physical health of their ill sibling, the extent to which family life is disrupted by the illness, and the psychosocial support available. The need for improved communication with healthy siblings has been identified.

One disorder which highlights the complexities of interaction between living with a chronic illness and its effect on family members is AIDS. Vertical transmission from an infected mother to her unborn child has decreased in the last 10 years but there has been an increase in the number of adolescents with the virus due to survival of children with perinatally acquired HIV into adolescence in addition to adolescents acquiring the virus through other means. For many children with HIV, infection is also present in other family members, often the mother. Families have to cope with the disease itself and its treatment, the stresses of chronic illness which include an uncertain prognosis and the possibility of death as well as having to negotiate the stigma and social isolation that frequently accompany the diagnosis. Caregivers who are HIV positive themselves report poorer physical and emotional health compared with non-infected caregivers; this is associated with greater psychosocial impairment in the children—a higher risk of internalizing problems such as anxiety and depression, more externalizing problems e.g. oppositional behaviour and poorer academic functioning. Disclosure of the diagnosis to affected children is often avoided; reasons include parental unease discussing their own HIV infection, fear of stigma, beliefs that the child is not emotionally ready to cope with the information and parents' own distress.[16] Children (aged 6–16) who are not told their diagnosis have been reported as having more internalizing problems than those informed.

## Management

In the absence of rigorous treatment research in this area, the most important tenet of the psychological care of children with physical illness is based on good clinical practice, with clear and consistent communication between paediatricians, child psychiatrists and their multi-disciplinary teams. This allows early detection and intervention for psychological disorder.

Child psychiatrists frequently work closely with paediatric colleagues to assist in identifying young people at risk for psychiatric disorder, to provide assessment and treatment when indicated, and to give support and advice with regard to diagnosis and management. Many paediatric units have regular weekly psychosocial ward rounds where professionals both from within the hospital and from the community—representing paediatrics, child and adolescent psychiatry teams, social work, and education—can meet to discuss the progress of the child from each perspective.

A full psychiatric assessment involving the child and the family will be carried out in referred cases. This needs to be preceded by a careful explanation to families about the reasons why a psychiatric consultation has been sought.

Important information about premorbid concerns and the child's level of functioning may be obtained from schools, social workers, and other professionals involved with the family.

Specific psychiatric diagnoses should be treated appropriately. Children may develop acute confusional disorders associated with intracerebral infection or febrile illness. Manipulation of the ward environment to ensure: clear differentiation between night and day, that familiar toys are nearby, close family members are in attendance, and developmentally appropriate explanations are given to the child about where they are and what is happening, may help considerably. If behaviour is too difficult for staff to safely manage and is interfering with treatment, sedative medication may be needed and should be discussed with paediatricians.

Children with adjustment disorders may be helped by psychological interventions. Management may include ways of decreasing existing stresses or helping individuals to adjust to them. Possible interventions include supportive counselling, individual therapy using cognitive behavioural principles, and family therapy.

When there is a chronically ill child in the family, parents often find it difficult to maintain the usual boundaries. For example, disciplining an ill child may be associated with parental guilt; this can lead to increasing anxiety for children who exhibit increasingly oppositional behaviour in an effort to test the boundary limits. Discussion regarding parenting techniques in the context of these feelings may be helpful. Parents also tend to increase their protective responses to ill children and show more overinvolved parenting. If excessive it may impede the child's development, but to a modest degree it may be helpful and advantageous.

Systematic desensitization together with relaxation and distraction techniques may be used to treat a specific needle phobia.

This needs to be carried out in collaboration with ward staff taking account of associated psychopathology, for example, oppositional behaviour, a generalized anxiety state, or an adjustment reaction. Treatment of the associated problems can often obviate the need for direct phobic treatment. When indicated, the latter's success is likely to be dependent on external changes that reduce anticipatory anxiety. These might include minimizing the time the child needs to wait for treatment and ensuring that more experienced members of the medical team are responsible for cannula insertion.

Generalized symptoms of anxiety are not uncommon in parents and children and may be manifested in different ways, for example, a young child may resume bed-wetting, a school-age child may become intensely distressed by being away from his parents, adolescents may experience difficulties sleeping, and anxious parents may become agitated with ward staff. Regular explanations from staff about the child's condition and treatment may help to alleviate this anxiety. Communication difficulties within the family may contribute to anxiety and be helped by family meetings where difficulties can be shared. Relaxation and distraction techniques together with cognitive behavioural interventions may also be of benefit. If symptoms are intense and interfering with physical treatment, anxiolytic medication may be indicated.

Antidepressant medication may be considered for children and adolescents with a depressive episode. This should be discussed with the medical team to minimize drug interactions and side-effects that may exacerbate the physical condition of the patient.

Treating children with severe illness who may be receiving distressing and painful treatment can arouse intense emotions in the most experienced of paediatric staff. Regular meetings with mental health professionals may help them to process some of these feelings and prevent them impeding patient care.

## Prognosis of psychiatric disorder in children with chronic physical illness

Many of the psychological difficulties experienced by chronically ill children are short lived and do not continue into adult life. Overall, studies indicate that psychiatric outcome is not severely compromised in the majority of adult survivors. Persistence of disorder is related to the severity of childhood psychological symptoms (the more severe being more likely to last), persistence of physical symptoms into adulthood,[17] and to the presence of physical disorder affecting the brain (Table 9.3.4.3).

The form of psychiatric symptomatology in childhood and adulthood may also be different; for example, cystic fibrosis sufferers, aged 8–15, have been found to report more eating related symptoms whereas symptoms of anxiety and depression are more prevalent in the adult group. With regard to cystic fibrosis, a consistent association between disease severity in adulthood and psychiatric disorder has not been shown. However, increased disease severity in childhood is associated with lower educational attainment;

**Table 9.3.4.3** Factors associated with persistence of psychosocial dysfunction into adulthood

| |
|---|
| Severity of childhood symptoms |
| Persistence of *physical* symptoms into adulthood |
| Physical disorder involving the brain |

in adulthood, employment is associated with both higher academic achievement and less depressive symptoms.[18]

Many studies suggest that by adulthood, most survivors of childhood cancer are indistinguishable from the general population with regard to psychosocial outcome. However, more detailed analysis suggests that factors such as age at diagnosis, site of the tumour, and nature of treatment (e.g. cranial irradiation) may influence cognitive and psychological outcome. For children and adolescents up to age 18 diagnosed with brain tumours, cognitive deficits and psychosocial problems increased with age and time since diagnosis.[19] As survival has increased, adults are exposed to the chronic toxic effects of treatment such as endocrine abnormalities, cardiac or pulmonary problems, and infertility. Follow-up of childhood cancer survivors, to a mean age of 28, revealed that current physical functioning, including pain, was associated with suicidality even after accounting for treatment and depression variables. Younger age at diagnosis, longer time since diagnosis, and cranial irradiation were also important risk factors.[20] Survivors of acute lymphoblastic leukaemia and Wilms' tumour did not show increased psychopathology as adults but had more difficulties with interpersonal functioning and day-to-day coping.[21]

Individuals with intracerebral pathology maintain high levels of disorder in adulthood, especially with regard to behaviour and social isolation. By contrast, patients with congenital heart disease surgically corrected in childhood, are not at increased risk of psychiatric disorder as adults.

Although young adults with end-stage chronic renal failure report more episodes of psychiatric disturbance than healthy matched controls before 17 years, they do not necessarily have increased psychopathology in late adolescence and adulthood. In common with survivors of other chronic childhood disorders,[17] the majority of adult renal patients are reported as functioning well socially, but they are more likely than age-matched controls to be living with their parents, to have less school qualifications, higher rates of unemployment, and fewer intimate relationships outside the family.

## Care of the dying child

Children at different developmental stages differ in their understanding of death. They gradually acquire components of the death concept; between 9 and 11 years of age, most children have reached a full understanding, acknowledging that it is permanent, inevitable, and universal. However, experience of serious illness and death interacts with the stage of understanding, so that children aged 5 or younger may have a more mature understanding and exhibit symptoms of anxiety about death. There is evidence that even young children with terminal illness are aware that they are dying, although they may not tell anyone that they know.[22]

Parents (and professionals) often find it difficult to talk about death with children. This is likely to interfere with coping for the whole family. Families with an open pattern of communication do better psychologically.[22] Mental health professionals may have a role in facilitating this discourse, promoting parents' confidence, and competence in communicating with their children. This will help the whole family to begin the process of mourning.

Children need information, reassurance, an opportunity to express their feelings, and adults with whom they can do so. As children lack the vocabulary of adults they may often exhibit their distress by behavioural changes, for example, bed-wetting, difficulty sleeping, and school refusal. Children and their siblings faced with death need clear, simple, and truthful explanations. They should not be pushed to talk, nor frightened with excessive medical detail.

Dying and grieving lead to a whole range of distressing feelings. This is part of a normal process, and mental health professionals can help their colleagues and families to acknowledge that this upset is acceptable.

Bereaved children frequently model their grief experience on what they perceive as being acceptable in the family, and an overt denial of upset by parents may lead to psychological difficulties in the child. The issue of whether to involve siblings after the death of the child in funerals or graveside visits often arises. If children are prepared for what to expect, involvement can be helpful in enabling them to acknowledge that a change has taken place and other people are feeling as sad as they are.[22]

Mothers are involved in nursing and caring for their dying children. They report an excess of depression, problems of helplessness, and a fear of being unable to cope with the child dying. Parents may feel that they can never fully recover from the loss of a child. Fathers tend to report more difficulties with feeling left out of the ill child's life and then with worry about their spouse being too preoccupied with the dead child. The effects of a child's death on family life can be traced even years after the death.[22] Formal follow-up after bereavement may help to identify those families and individuals experiencing psychological reactions that may benefit from more intensive support.

## The effects of psychiatric disorder on the course and outcome of physical illness

Psychological disorder, as well as being a consequence of both acute and chronic physical ill-health, may also have an impact on the course of physical illness.

An increasingly recognized disorder in this respect is post-traumatic stress disorder. Sudden physical trauma, such as burns and road traffic accidents, are examples of antecedents. Victims of road traffic accidents between 5 and 18 years of age, particularly those who experience high levels of distress immediately after the accident, are at greatest risk of exhibiting post-traumatic stress symptoms 3 months later.[23] Such responses may be contributed to not only by the accident itself but also by the medical procedures that take place on arrival in hospital. Surgical collars, intravenous infusions, and monitoring equipment can be associated with intense fear.[23] Children with acute severe sepsis such as meningococcal disease admitted to paediatric intensive care units are also at risk of developing similar symptoms.[24] In turn, these reactions can have an effect on the child's ability to co-operate with future hospital attendance, medical, and surgical interventions. Stress reactions may be ameliorated, to some extent, by the provision of age-appropriate information about what has happened and what is going to happen.

The diagnosis and treatment of such disorders may be impeded by the fact that follow-up for young people may not be at the admitting hospital. Burns units and paediatric intensive care facilities are often at tertiary centres some distance from the patient's home. General practitioners and local paediatricians have a role to play in assessing how the family is coping, specifically regarding symptoms of post-traumatic stress. Child psychiatry involvement may be appropriate if psychological treatment is required both during admission and at follow-up. Cognitive behavioural interventions with individual children and families may be used to alleviate symptoms.

Affective symptoms, particularly depression and anxiety, are not uncommon following an acute medical admission and may interfere with physical treatment. For example, an adolescent admitted to paediatric intensive care with meningococcal disease requiring a partial limb amputation could develop a depressive disorder. Symptoms of despair and hopelessness coupled with a lack of interest and energy may impede the physiotherapy programme, delay mobilization, and hospital discharge. Paediatric staff need to be alert to such potential sequelae and to have child psychiatric colleagues readily available for assessment and treatment.

Exacerbation of chronic illnesses such as asthma can be precipitated by emotional disturbance; adolescents aged 11–17 with anxiety or depressive disorders reported more asthma symptoms in the previous 2 weeks than young people without these affective diagnoses.[25] Adjunctive psychological treatments such as family therapy have been shown to lead to an objective improvement in airways disease,[26] compliance, and reduced hospital admissions.[27]

## Somatization and somatoform disorders

### Disorders presenting with functional physical symptoms and somatization

'Functional' somatic symptoms with no obvious organic explanation are frequent in childhood. Children have a limited vocabulary for expressing their emotions and often communicate their distress by means of physical symptoms. Somatization refers to this process. In some cases these symptoms become persistent with associated functional impairment; this may lead to consultation. The definitions of somatization disorder (one of the somatoform disorders) used in ICD-10 and DSM-IV are too stringent for children (in that diagnosis requires multiple physical symptoms over years). Other disorders (namely somatoform pain disorder, dissociative/conversion disorder, and neurasthenia) are seen in children and adolescents. The risk factors for somatization in this population are shown in Table 9.3.4.4.

**Table 9.3.4.4** Risk factors for somatization in children and adolescents

| Individual: | Personal experience of physical illness |
| | Enhanced focus on physical sensations |
| | Somatic attributions |
| | Conscientious, vulnerable, sensitive, anxious personalities with particular concerns about peer relationships |
| | High achievement orientation |
| Family: | Physical health problems |
| | Psychiatric problems |
| | Parental somatization |
| | Emotional overinvolvement |
| | Limitations in the ability to communicate about emotional issues |
| Environment: | Life stresses e.g. school, teasing or bullying, academic pressure |

### Aches and pains and somatoform pain disorder

Aches and pains (often abdominal pains and headaches) are a common manifestation in young children. Between 2 and 10 per cent of children in the general population have problems in this area. Mothers assess the child's symptomatology with specific regard to whether the child is 'pretending', 'upset', or 'ill' and generally respond appropriately. They recognize that children may experience symptoms as a result of stress or use them to avoid something they find difficult.

Abdominal pain commonly leads to a general practitioner consultation and may account for 10 per cent of new appointments with paediatricians. In only a few of these cases is serious organic pathology found. Lack of identifiable organic pathology does not imply a psychogenic aetiology. The latter is rather supported by evidence that psychological events influence the symptoms.

Children who somatize tend to have a family history of physical ill-health and parental illness. In some cases there are also psychosocial difficulties in the family. There is an association with stressful life events. Co-morbid internalizing disorders (depression and anxiety) are commonly present.[28]

In adolescence, headaches become a prominent symptom, peaking in prevalence at 12 years of age. As with abdominal pain in younger children, they are frequently preceded by physical or psychological precipitants, such as academic or social stresses in school or difficulties at home. Headaches lead to absence from school but are not associated with underachievement. A family history of migraine is common.

As defined in ICD-10, in persistent somatoform pain disorder, severe distressing pain occurs in association with emotional conflict or psychosocial problems that are sufficient to allow the conclusion to be drawn that they are the main causative influences. The result is usually a marked increase in support and attention, either personal or medical.

In trying to best manage severely affected children, close collaboration between paediatricians and child psychiatrists is helpful. The lack of demonstrable organic pathology should be communicated and professionals should help the family to make the link between physical symptoms and psychological precipitants with the help of a written diary if necessary. It is important to reduce the attention given to the physical symptoms in order to decrease the resulting functional handicap. Early return to school together with the resumption of normal activities should be encouraged. The short-term prognosis for presentations to medical services is good, with 75 per cent of children recovering within several months.

### Dissociative/conversion disorder

Children and adolescents present as if having a physical disorder affecting voluntary motor or sensory functioning, although none can be found; the symptoms correspond to the patient's idea of physical disorder, which may not coincide with physiological or anatomical principles. Aetiologically, the disorder is believed to arise largely unconsciously and to represent an escape from an unbearable personal conflict. It usually manifests in adolescence and is more common in girls. The most common presentation is neurological with disturbance of motor function such as weakness of legs, paralysis of a limb, or bizarre gait. Multiple symptoms often occur.

Premorbid psychopathology in the child and family are often absent, although perfectionistic and conscientious traits with concerns about academic performance and a child and family focus on high achievement have been noted. Overconcern with physical health and illness often characterize these families; frequently there is a family history of physical health problems. Families often present as being close, but communication, particularly regarding emotions, may be limited.

It is assumed children develop conversion disorders as an unconscious means of escaping a situation with which they cannot cope. This includes intolerably high academic expectations (often the child's own), unresolved family conflict, and, in a minority of cases, sexual abuse. The disorder is often precipitated by minor physical illness and may also occur in children with identified organic pathology, for instance the development of pseudoseizures in an individual with epilepsy.

The majority of these patients are managed by paediatricians. After investigations have excluded organic pathology and a psychogenic contribution is suspected, this needs to be communicated to the family. The shift from physical to psychological factors may be difficult for the family to accept; information may need to be conveyed slowly 'at a pace the family can cope with'. A collaborative approach between paediatricians and child psychiatrists is important. A persistent focus on physical aetiology may be unhelpful but in management it is more useful to focus on the handicap caused by specific symptoms rather than on their cause by introducing a programme of rehabilitation and physiotherapy directed at these features, including school attendance. Psychotherapeutic work, both individually and with the family, may help the family understand the factors maintaining the child's symptoms and explore any identified stressors or conflicts. Time can also be spent helping families to consider alternative strategies they may use to cope with future conflicts.

### Chronic fatigue syndrome (neurasthenia in ICD-10)

This is operationally defined as disabling physical fatigue of over 6 months' duration, unexplained by primary physical or psychiatric causes. There are often other unexplained somatic symptoms and a strong belief by the patient and their family that the aetiology is physical.[29] It might be considered as one of the somatoform disorders, as similarities are shared with regard to aetiology and management.

There is no firm evidence that chronic fatigue syndrome results from a specific viral infection but a physical illness is often the precipitating factor. There is frequently a family history of physical illness and a preoccupation with physical symptoms. Parents invariably attribute the symptoms to an organic aetiology. Children tend to be described as high achieving and perfectionistic, as well as sensitive, vulnerable and anxiety-prone; onset can be temporally related to transitions at school, for example transfer to secondary school. Depressive mood changes are common and on assessment depressive disorder is found in one-third of cases.[29]

Chronic fatigue syndrome can be extremely disabling. A self-perpetuating cycle is set up whereby fatigue and the resultant inactivity lead to loss of muscle bulk and deterioration in physical fitness. Activity becomes increasingly difficult and is avoided, leading to a further deterioration in physical ability. An essential focus of treatment is to disrupt this cycle.

Management is often multi-disciplinary including paediatricians, physiotherapists, school teachers, and child psychiatrists. A clear explanation of the results of physical investigations and the fact that no serious organic pathology has been found is important.

Focusing on improving symptoms, as opposed to debating aetiology, is most helpful. Helping the family to shift from a purely physical model to one that includes psychological factors in maintaining symptoms may be difficult and needs to be negotiated slowly. In particular, enabling them to see the disorder as an interaction between physical, social, and emotional factors can be useful.

Treatment ingredients usually include a graded exercise programme, a progressive return to school, and work with the family to facilitate engagement and address factors that may be impeding recovery. Antidepressants may be useful for co-morbid depressive disorder. There is an evidence base for both cognitive behaviour therapy (CBT) and graded exercise in adults and one study which demonstrates the effectiveness of CBT in adolescents.[30]

### Treatment of functional symptoms and somatoform disorders in children and adolescents: research evidence

There are few satisfactory controlled studies on the effects of treatment for childhood somatization. Most work on children with somatoform disorders has been based on small groups with severe problems, and the management advice outlined above is derived from the conclusions of experienced clinicians and open-treatment case reports. However, there is some evidence from controlled studies indicating the efficacy of a cognitive behavioural family intervention for recurrent abdominal pains in children.[31] For hospitalized children with severe, recurrent abdominal pain, parental attribution of symptoms to psychological factors facilitated resolution.[32] The superiority of relaxation training over placebo in reducing migraine attacks has been shown.

### Outcome of functional somatic symptoms and somatoform disorders

Of adults with a childhood history of abdominal pains, 50 per cent have recurrent symptoms in adult life despite a pain-free period in adolescence; they also have an increased prevalence of psychiatric disorders (particularly anxiety disorders).[33] Childhood conversion disorder is generally associated with a good outcome; recovery is usually complete by 3 months. When children (9–16 years) were followed up 4 years after a conversion disorder from which 85 per cent had recovered, 35 per cent had a mood or anxiety disorder; affective disorder was higher (100 per cent) in the minority who had failed to recover as compared with 23 per cent in those who were better.[34] In young people with chronic fatigue syndrome, recovery or marked improvement in symptoms can be expected in 50–75 per cent of cases in the short to medium term. School non-attendance may be over a year and time to full recovery 3 years or more. There are indications of an increased likelihood for the development of psychiatric disorder after recovery.[35]

## Concluding remarks

Somatic and psychological symptoms are intimately linked. Changes in physical health can affect psychiatric outcome. Conversely, emotional distress may affect adherence to treatment, and it is sometimes expressed through physical symptoms. Awareness of this interplay is important and should be mirrored by a close working relationship and close communication between paediatricians and child psychiatrists.

## Further information

Shaw, R.J. and DeMaso, D.R. (2006). *Clinical manual of pediatric psychosomatic medicine.* American Psychiatric Publishing Inc.

Rutter, M., Bishop, D., Pine, D., *et al.* (eds.) (2008). *Rutter's child and adolescent psychiatry* (5th edn). Blackwell Publishing, Oxford.

## References

1. Cadman, D., Boyle, M., Szatmari, P., *et al.* (1987). Chronic illness, disability and mental and social well being: findings of the Ontario child health study. *Pediatrics*, **79**, 805–12.

2. Garralda, M.E. and Palanca, M.I. (1994). Psychiatric adjustment in children with physical illness. *British Journal of Hospital Medicine*, **52**, 230–4.

3. Rutter, M., Tizard, J., and Whitmore, K. (eds.) (1970). *Education, health and behaviour.* Longmans, London.

4. Eiser, C. (1993). *Growing up with a chronic disease. The impact on children and their families.* Jessica Kingsley, London.

5. Kovacs, M., Feinberg, T.L., Paulauskas, S., *et al.* (1985). Initial coping responses and psychosocial characteristics of children with insulin-dependent diabetes mellitus. *Journal of Pediatrics*, **106**, 827–34.

6. Wass, V.J., Barratt, T.M., Howarth, R.V., *et al.* (1977). Home dialysis in children. *Lancet*, **1**, 242–6.

7. Garralda, M.E., Jameson, R.A., Reynolds, J.M., *et al.* (1988). Psychiatric adjustment in children with chronic renal failure. *Journal of Child Psychology and Psychiatry*, **29**, 79–90.

8. Liss, D.S., Waller, D.A., Kennard, B.D., *et al.* (1998). Psychiatric illness and family support in children and adolescents with diabetic ketoacidosis: a controlled study. *Journal of the American Academy of Child and Adolescent Psychiatry*, **37**, 536–44.

9. Rees, G., Gledhill, J., Garralda, M.E., *et al.* (2004). Psychiatric outcome following paediatric intensive care unit (PICU) admission: a cohort study. *Intensive Care Medicine*, **30**, 1607–14.

10. Kazak, A.E., Alderfer, M., Rourke, M.T., *et al.* (2004). Posttraumatic stress disorder (PTSD) and posttraumatic stress symptoms (PTSS) in families of adolescent childhood cancer survivors. *Journal of Pediatric Psychology*, **29**, 211–19.

11. Fiese, B.H. and Everhart, R.S. (2006). Medical adherence and childhood chronic illness: family daily management skills and emotional climate as emerging contributors. *Current Opinion in Pediatrics*, **18**, 551–7.

12. Garrison, M.M., Katon, W.J., and Richardson, L.P. (2005). The impact of psychiatric comorbidities on readmissions for diabetes in youth, *Diabetes Care*, **28**, 2150–4.

13. Rodenburg, R., Meijer, A.M., Dekovic, M., *et al.* (2005). Family factors and psychopathology in children with epilepsy: a literature review. *Epilepsy and Behaviour*, **6**, 488–503.

14. Mastroyannopoulou, K., Stallard, P., Lewis, M., *et al.* (1997). The impact of childhood non-malignant life-threatening illness on parents: gender differences and predictors of parental adjustment. *Journal of Child Psychology and Psychiatry*, **38**, 823–9.

15. Sharpe, D. and Rossiter, L. (2002). Siblings of children with a chronic illness: a meta-analysis. *Journal of Pediatric Psychology*, **27**, 699–710.

16. Steele, R.G., Nelson, T.D., and Cole, B.P. (2007). Psychosocial functioning of children with AIDS and HIV infection: review of the literature from a socioecological framework. *Journal of Developmental and Behavioural Pediatrics*, **28**, 58–69.

17. Pless, I.B., Cripps, H.A., Davies, J.M.C., *et al.* (1989). Chronic physical illness in childhood: psychological and social effects in adolescence and adult life. *Developmental Medicine and Child Neurology*, **31**, 746–55.

18. Burker, E.J., Sedway, J., and Carone, S. (2004). Psychological and educational factors: better predictors of work status than $FEV_1$ in adults with cystic fibrosis. *Pediatric Pulmonology*, **38**, 413–18.

19. Poggi, G., Liscio, M., Galbiati, S., *et al.* (2005). Brain tumours in children and adolescents: cognitive and psychological disorders at different ages. *Psycho-oncology*, **14**, 386–95.

20. Recklitis, C.J., Lockwood, R.A., Rothwell, M.A., *et al.* (2006). Suicidal ideation and attempts in adult survivors of childhood cancer. *Journal of Clinical Oncology*, **24**, 3852–7.

21. Mackie, E., Hill, J., Kondryn, H., *et al.* (2000). Adult psychosocial outcomes in long-term survivors of acute lymphoblastic leukaemia and Wilms' tumour: a controlled study. *Lancet*, **355**, 1310–14.

22. Black, D. (1998). Coping with loss. The dying child. *British Medical Journal*, **316**, 1376–8.

23. Di Gallo, A., Barton, J., and Parry-Jones, W.L. (1997). Road traffic accidents: early psychological consequences in children and adolescents. *The British Journal of Psychiatry*, **170**, 358–62.

24. Shears, D., Nadel, S., Gledhill, J., *et al.* (2005). Short-term psychiatric adjustment of children and their parents following meningococcal disease. *Pediatric Critical Care Medicine*, **6**, 39–43.

25. Richardson, L.P., Lozano, P., Russo, J., *et al.* (2006). Asthma symptom burden: relationship to asthma severity and anxiety and depression symptoms. *Pediatrics*, **118**, 1042–51.

26. Gustaffson, P.A., Kjellman, N.I.M., and Cederblad, M. (1986). Family therapy in the treatment of severe childhood asthma. *Journal of Psychosomatic Research*, **30**, 369–74.

27. Godding, V., Kruth, M., and Jamart, J. (1997). Joint consultation for high-risk asthmatic children and their families, with paediatrician and child psychiatrist as co-therapists: model and evaluation. *Family Process*, **36**, 265–80.

28. Campo, J.V., Bridge, J., Ehmann, M., *et al.* (2004). Recurrent abdominal pain, anxiety and depression in primary care. *Pediatrics*, **113**, 817–24.

29. Garralda, M.E. (1996). Somatisation in children. *Journal of Child Psychology and Psychiatry*, **37**, 13–33.

30. Stulemeijer, M., de Jong, L.W.A.M., Fiselier, T.J.W., *et al.* (2005). Cognitive behaviour therapy for adolescents with chronic fatigue syndrome: randomized controlled trial. *British Medical Journal*, **330**, 14.

31. Robins, P.M., Smith, S.M., Glutting, J.J., *et al.* (2005). A randomized controlled trial of a cognitive-behavioural family intervention for pediatric recurrent abdominal pain. *Journal of Pediatric Psychology*, **30**, 397–408.

32. Crushell, E., Rowland, M., Doherty, M., *et al.* (2003). Importance of parental conceptual model of illness in severe recurrent abdominal pain. *Pediatrics*, **112**, 1368–72.

33. Plunkett, A. and Beattie, R.M. (2005). Recurrent abdominal pain in childhood. *Journal of the Royal Society of Medicine*, **98**, 101–6.

34. Pehlivantürk, B. and Unal, F. (2002). Conversion disorder in children and adolescents. A 4 year follow-up study. *Journal of Psychosomatic Research*, **52**, 187–91.

35. Garralda, M.E. and Chalder, T. (2005). Practitioner review: chronic fatigue syndrome in childhood. *Journal of Child Psychology and Psychiatry*, **46**, 1143–51.

---

## 9.3.5 The effects on child and adult mental health of adoption and foster care

June Thoburn

### Introduction: mapping the terrain

Adoption and foster care are important 'solutions' to identified problems or risks, but potentially they are also contributors to problem behaviours or emotional difficulties. In their problem-solving role, they are seen as potential solutions, not only to actual or future mental health problems of children, but also to the adverse effects of involuntary childlessness.

This chapter concentrates on the impact of adoption and foster care on the children placed, but their role in problem solution or problem generation for adults is also touched on. Adoption is more often than not a satisfactory way of meeting the need to become parents for those childless couples who succeed in having a child placed with them (a tiny minority of the involuntary childless). It is very rarely a solution to the problems of a parent who gives up a child for adoption whether voluntarily or involuntarily. Studies of adults who relinquished children indicate that the reaction to the loss of their child may be associated with moderate distress or may lead to a long-term grief reaction, which in turn will potentially harm children subsequently born to that parent. One must also note that some parents who lose a child to adoption or foster care are themselves children, sometimes not yet in their teens, whose needs are often overlooked in the interests of providing for the infant.

Fostering and adoption started as very similar processes, diverged in Europe and North America in the first half of this century, and are now much closer together again. The 'total severance' model of legal adoption—the type that most people in Europe, the United States, and Australasia immediately recognize—has a short history. In the United Kingdom it was not until the passing of the 1958 Adoption Act that secrecy became the norm. The 'sealing' of birth information started in the United States around 1948 but it was not until 1991 that Alabama 'sealed' its adoption records.[1] This experiment of totally closed adoption was short-lived, and many countries have introduced legislation to allow adult adoptees and/ or birth relatives to access identifying information that allows them to seek each other out.[2] 'Open' adoptions, in which some degree of contact between the adopters, the birth parents, and the children is maintained after placement, are increasingly common.

As countries have become richer, the need to place children for adoption has diminished and the number of infants placed at the request of their parents has fallen well short of the 'demand' of those wishing to start a family through adoption. In consequence, it has been possible to encourage potential adopters to 'stretch' their notions of parenthood, and to place older children, those with disabilities, and those with behavioural or emotional problems with adoptive parents as well as with foster parents. The main remaining difference between adoption and foster care is that the majority of children placed in foster homes live there for comparatively short periods before returning to their families of origin. They are best seen as supplementary rather than substitute parents, although in all 'first world' countries long-term or 'permanent' foster care is an important option for a minority of those entering public care, especially in those countries (the majority) who rarely use adoption as a route out of care.

Adoption and foster care will impact on the mental health of the children in different ways, which may be considered along six main dimensions (see Box 9.3.5.1). The dimensions interact differently for different children. An infant placed from an Asian country might be adopted by childless relatives in Europe and have had a positive early experience of parenting, or might have experienced very adverse early nurturing and be adopted by strangers of a different ethnic origin. The child placed at six may have had good care from one or both parents until some traumatic event led to the need for an adoptive placement, or the child may have been seriously maltreated and had several placements before finally joining a substitute family.

## The nature of the evidence on the impact of adoption and fostering on mental health

The actual or potential problems most obviously associated with child placement are those resulting from separation and loss. Brodzinsky et al.[3] have made significant contributions to our understanding of the psychology of adoption. Put simply:

> . . . for later-placed children, the loss of family or surrogate family connections is overt, often acute, and sometimes traumatic. In contrast, for children placed as infants, loss is, of necessity, more covert, emerging slowly as the youngster begins to understand the magnitude of what has happened. . . . In addition, there may be loss of a clear sense of genealogical connections and, in the case of transracial and inter-country adoption, loss of cultural, ethnic, and racial ties.

The impact of loss will also vary with the child's temperament, and the work of Rutter,[4] and of others who have written on 'resilience', are important sources. A 'born worrier' will go through life wondering what there was about him or her that was not worth keeping, and no amount of positive parenting will make this angst go away; a resilient child will shrug away the past and make the best of even not particularly good parenting by the substitute parents.

It is important, before considering the research findings, to take note of the limitations of our knowledge on the long-term outcomes of foster care and adoption. Turning first to the characteristics of the children, studies of family placement often include both infants and older children, those with emotional difficulties and those without. Some studies of foster care include children placed temporarily alongside others placed permanently, and in some US studies the term 'foster care' includes all children in out-of-home placements (for family placements the term 'foster family care' is used).

At the other end of the process a broad range of 'outcome' measures is used[5] and 'success' rates vary depending on the measures used and the length of time between placement and reported outcome. The well-being of the young adult (using a range of standardized instruments) is the most reliable outcome measure but more often 'output' measures are used. (Was the child placed? Was legal adoption completed? Was a satisfactory reunion with the birth parents achieved during childhood or as an adult?). Measures of satisfaction of the different members of the adoptive family are also used. Unsurprisingly, therefore, reported 'success' rates have varied between below 50 per cent and around 95 per cent.

---

**Box 9.3.5.1** Dimensions of family placement

- The age of the child at placement.

- The degree of disturbance of the child prior to placement.

- The nature of attachments with birth family members and short-term foster carers.

- (For those in foster care) the duration of placements, the frequency with which they occur, and whether the child returns to the same foster carers on each occasion.

- (In the case of adoption) whether the child is adopted within the family (step-parent or relative adoptions), by foster carers to whom the child is already attached, or by parents not known previously (stranger adoption).

- Whether or not the child is adopted or fostered by parents of the same cultural and ethnic background or country of origin.

---

The placement process that researchers seek to evaluate is extremely complex. When, as with adoption or permanent fostering, the aim is for the child's life chances to be improved by their becoming fully a part of the new family, it becomes impossible to unpick the very many variables that will have had an impact on the mental health of the young person between placement at 6 weeks and maturity at around 26. (There is some evidence that adopted people move towards emotional maturity at a slower pace—not surprisingly with at least two extra hurdles to surmount: that of separation and loss, and that of making sense of their adoptive identity). In longitudinal studies, if numbers are large enough, it is possible to control for the major variables such as age at placement, disability, and emotional or behavioural problems at the time of placement. However, the many aspects of parenting, and the nature of any therapeutic input may all have had an impact on the placement. The researchers may seek the opinions of parents and children as to what they found helpful, but clear causal relationships between outcomes and variables such as parenting styles, models of social work practice, and therapy cannot be claimed.

In summary, whilst researchers have, for many years, sought to bring academic rigour to their studies, family placement remains an 'untidy' subject. The more complex the placement circumstances and the longer the timescale, the more difficult it is to attribute success to any one factor, type of placement, or model of intervention.

## A review of the research evidence on outcomes

The above section explains why, although there are some random controlled trials of treatment approaches and of short-term foster care models, the literature contains more research syntheses of the different aspects of family placement[5–10] than 'classical' systematic reviews. The findings from the large volume of quantitative and qualitative research will be summarized under the broad headings of time-limited foster care placements and placements made with the intention that the child will become a full part of the adoptive or foster family. The emphasis will be on the second group, which will be further subdivided into placements of infants and placements of older children.

### Time-limited placements

In general terms, short-term foster care is used along with other services in an attempt to improve family functioning so that the child may benefit from increased stability in the family home or as a short-term crisis intervention measure. The aims of short-term fostering can be summarized as: temporary care; emergency care; assessment; treatment and 'bridging'—to independence or between placements following placement break down.[7]

Generally short-term placements used as part of family support are successful in that few placements actually break down and most parents express satisfaction with the service. This is especially so if the placement follows careful preparation for the child, the birth parents, and the foster parents and if those who need a series of placements return to the same foster family. Several UK researchers have found that a 'keep them out of care at all costs' attitude tends to prevail in child welfare agencies, thus leading to too many ill-planned and ill-matched emergency placements, which in turn lead to placement break down and to unnecessary moves in care.

Testa and Rolock[11] conclude broadly positively from an overview of treatment foster care research in the United States, and

Fisher and Chamberlain[12] report better outcomes for very troubled children in multi-systemic treatment foster care than for a 'service as usual' group. (These approaches involve placement with specially recruited, trained, and financially rewarded foster carers on a time-limited basis. Intensive multi-agency support is provided to the parents, foster carers, and children.) Though placement stability remains a problem, behavioural improvements are reported and these schemes are well rated by most of the young people and their foster carers. Some researchers report a problem of 'over-staying', but this should perhaps be reframed as a success, in that some young people settle in so well that, against the odds, the task-centred foster family becomes a 'secure base' and the foster parents continue to provide support to the young people as they move into adult life.

Associations have been found in some studies between positive child outcomes and practitioners who facilitate good contact between the birth parents, foster carers, and the child; provide support to the foster carers and the birth parents; and take a multi-agency approach to treatment of the child and parents before, during, and after placement.

### Adoption and long-term foster-family placement

Whilst, in the United Kingdom and North America, adoption is considered to be the major placement option for most young children who cannot remain with their birth parents, opinion is divided (often along country lines) as to the importance of long-term foster family care as a placement of choice. Practice also varies in different countries in respect of placement with relatives. In most countries it is the exception rather than the rule for relatives to adopt (foster care, guardianship, or informal arrangements being preferred) whereas in the United States legal adoption by relatives tends to be encouraged.[13]

#### (a) Outcomes for children placed as infants

The largest volume of research on the long-term outcome of adoption concerns children placed 'voluntarily' as infants. However, inevitably, the practice referred to in these studies is already dated by the time the long-term outcomes can be measured some 20 years or so after the child was placed. Although some may have been born to mothers who had poor antenatal care, few of these early-placed children will have experienced neglect or maltreatment. However, with the growth of inter-country adoptions, studies of infants placed more recently are more likely to include substantial numbers of children who have experienced adverse conditions during their early months. It is likely that disruption rates will be higher than they have been in the past.

#### (b) The impact of placement in the short-term

An important source of detailed information on short-term outcomes of infant placements is the longitudinal study by Rutter et al.[14] which compares young Romanian children placed with British families with a cohort of English infants placed in 'stranger' adoptive families. Reactions to placement of the English infants who had generally good postnatal care are predictable in the light of knowledge about child development, attachment, separation, and loss. Those placed quickly settle with no obvious signs of stress; those with adverse early experiences including institutionalization (most of the Romanian infants) also appear to settle well if placed in their early months. Those placed when older than 6 months are more likely to show stress reactions at the loss of a carer to whom they are beginning to be attached, or to show adverse reactions resulting from early maltreatment, neglect, or institutionalization.

### (c) Signs of stress during childhood

The more robust studies of the mental health of adopted infants in their middle years and early adolescence are those that prospectively follow them as they grow-up. The conclusion drawn from these studies is that children placed with substitute families as infants tend to do better at each stage than non-adopted peers living in the generally adverse environments in which the children were likely to have lived had they remained with their birth parents.

All studies have found that, even for those with poor antenatal and birth history or who experience adverse circumstances in their early months, subsequent physical and cognitive development is generally good. However, children adopted as infants appear to be at a slightly higher risk of experiencing problems in their social, emotional, and behavioural development compared with other children raised in similar socio-economic circumstances. This is particularly the case with adopted boys. Information from longitudinal studies is supplemented by studies of clinical populations, such as those whose parents seek psychiatric help for them. Rates of maladjustment appear to be higher around the age of 11, and decrease as the children move into later adolescence. Some studies report that adopted children are more vulnerable on some measures of behavioural and emotional development than others, including an inability to settle, restlessness, a tendency to lie or fantasize, and difficulties in getting on with their peers and teachers. Low self-esteem and feelings of insecurity are also more likely to be present amongst children in their middle years and adolescence.

### (d) Long-term outcomes

There is a lack of recently published quantitative studies of the well-being of adults adopted as infants. Summaries of the research[3,6,7] report that few of those placed as infants (around 5 per cent) will leave their adoptive families before the age of 18, in circumstances of conflict, which can be described as 'adoption break downs'. Qualitative studies have reported that around 80 per cent of both adopters and adoptees express broad satisfaction with the growing-up experience. Howe[15] uses in-depth interviews with the parents of adult adoptees to analyse the mental health problems that have persisted into adulthood and reports that, when more serious problems do emerge, the issue of adoptive identity often underlies a range of presenting symptoms. Also, amongst the over 80 per cent of adults who are generally satisfied with the experience of growing-up adopted are some who continuously or episodically have a sense of unease around questions of identity and the reasons why their birth parents 'gave them up' for adoption.[2] The most authoritative recent research on long-term outcomes is the Swedish cohort study of Lindblad et al.[16] These authors compared population data on nearly 6000 inter-country adopted adults (mostly placed when under the age of 5) with their non-adopted peers. They note that whilst there were more similarities than differences, the adopted children were more likely than peers brought up in similar circumstances to have psychiatric problems, including substance abuse, and there was a higher suicide rate.

In summary, when well-being and mental ill-health are the outcome measure used, adults who were adopted as infants tend to be healthier, have higher IQ scores, lower rates of criminal behaviour, and fewer psychiatric symptoms than non-adopted peers from similar backgrounds to those into which they were born and to be broadly similar to those brought up by birth parents living in similar circumstances to the adopters. However, the larger scale studies that allow for the control of the many intervening variables tend to lack detail on the children's experiences of family life and of any therapeutic interventions. It is therefore unclear whether any differences can be associated with adoption *per se* or with the more advantaged home circumstances of the adopted children.

### (e) Children placed when past infancy

Researchers and clinicians tend to agree that beyond 6 months of age, the risks of moving children increase, and the older the child at placement, the more likely it is that there will be difficulties in the child's behaviour, which increase the risk of placement break down. Some delays in placement are caused by incompetence or poor practice. However, the main reason for delay in placement (sometimes referred to as 'drift') is contested legal proceedings. In most countries it is only possible in extreme circumstances to place a child for adoption without the consent of the birth parents, although adoption by long-term foster carers they have lived with for some years sometimes occurs. In the United Kingdom, United States, and Canada it is not uncommon for parental consent to be dispensed with by court order, but human rights legislation and the attempts at reunification mean that few children are placed from care before the age of 6 months. International adoptions tend to be delayed because of the search within the country of origin for an in country placement, or because of legal formalities.

### (f) Medium-term outcomes

Many of the children placed when older bring problems with them into placement, to which may be added those discussed earlier, which are specifically associated with being adopted or fostered. For those placed from overseas, the difficulties are those commonly associated with institutionalization and privation of affection and consistent care. For a large proportion of those placed from care, the problems are those associated with maltreatment or neglect, including attachments with parent figures that may have been anxious, ambivalent, or avoidant, followed by the loss of those attachment figures. They may also have been separated from siblings and experienced multiple changes of carer.

Rushton and Dance[17] provide detailed accounts of the behaviour of 133 English children placed when over the age of 5. Eight years after placement, 19 per cent of the children had left their placements and only just over half of the 99 continuing placements were in the 'continuing/happy' group. Behaviours their parents had difficulty managing included over-activity, aggression, and destructiveness.

### (g) Longer-term outcomes for late-placed children

Whilst some children placed in positive environments that provide committed and loving parenting and stability will recover from the adverse effects of early significant harm, developmental recovery cannot be anticipated in all cases. From a longitudinal study of over 1100 'hard-to-place' children placed in adoptive or permanent foster families not previously known to them, Thoburn[18] found that one in five of the placements had disrupted between 2 and 6 years after placement. There was a strong and statistically significant association between disruption and the age at placement (see Fig. 9.3.5.1). Of those aged between 7 and 8 years at placement, one in five experienced placement break down; this proportion rose to almost one in two for those placed between the ages of 11 and 12. The graph is less stable for teenagers, in part because numbers are smaller and statistics less reliable, and in part because families are

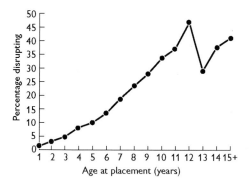

**Fig 9.3.5.1** Age at placement and percentage of placements disrupting. (Reproduced from J. Thoburn, Evaluating placement: survey findings and conclusions. In *Permanent family placement: a decade of experience* (eds. J. Fratter, J. Rowe, and J. Thoburn), pp. 34–57, copyright 1991, Brirish Agencies for Adoption & Fostering (BAAF), London.)

more likely to 'hang on in' if they know the young person can be helped to leave home 'respectably' in a year or so. More recently, Rushton and Dance[17] found that the placements that disrupted did so between 6 months and 7 years after placement (a mean of 34 months). Rushton and Dance[17] followed up 90 children placed for adoption when aged at least three for an average of 7 years. Seventeen per cent of placements had disrupted (mostly before adoption was finalized), and for a third of those still in placement, there were many problems, which were often getting worse. Festinger followed up for 4 years 516 American children placed from care at a mean age of 2 years. The lower disruption rate (10 per cent) when compared to the UK studies may be explained by the younger age at placement and also by the fact that roughly half were adopted by relatives. She reported that many of the parents in the continuing placements reported difficulties and unmet needs.

## Variables about the child and pre-placement history

Researchers and clinicians concur that, in addition to age at placement, variables relating to the child's behaviour and emotional well-being at the time of placement are most strongly associated with better or worse outcomes. These in turn are linked with biography, including experiences of early parenting and multiple caregivers. Having experienced early abuse or neglect has been found to be independently associated with less positive outcomes, whilst more positive outcomes are reported even for late-placed children who had formed a good-enough attachment with a parent or other main carer during the first few years of life.

Thoburn *et al.*[20] found that children of minority ethnic origin, whether placed with a family of the same or a different ethnic origin, were no more likely to experience break down than white children placed with white families. However, qualitative studies note that parents of a different ethnic and cultural background to the child have extra hurdles to overcome in the parenting process, and that some are unable to bring the child up to feel pride in his or her heritage, culture, and appearance, with consequent problems for self-esteem and identity.

### Variables about the adoptive or foster families

Early studies reported an association between less positive outcomes and there being a 'home-grown' child younger or close in age to the placed child, but these have not been replicated more recently. The age of the adopters, whether they are single or in a partnership, experienced parents or childless, have not been consistently found to be significantly associated with placement break down. Two in-depth prospective studies of long-term foster care[21] and adoption[22] conclude that those new parents do best who can empathize with both the child and the family of origin, who enjoy a challenge, who have the skills to help the child with disabilities or emotional problems, and who, for older-placed children, can give out love even if the child gives little back and can find pleasure in tiny 'successes'.

Brodzinsky *et al.*[3] identify the importance of adopters treading a fine line between understanding and accepting the difference between parenting by adoption and parenting by birth, but not overemphasizing the difference.

### Variables about placement practice and therapy

Few of the studies involving large enough numbers for statistical analysis look for statistically significant associations between outcome and placement practice or therapeutic interventions.

The child who remains for longer than a few weeks in temporary foster care is especially vulnerable to placement break down or moves made for bureaucratic reasons. Once settled in a planned long-term placement, when variables such as age at placement and behavioural difficulties are controlled for, break down rates for older-placed children are similar for children placed for adoption or in permanent foster families. Placements with relatives, and temporary foster placements confirmed as permanent (through adoption, guardianship, or administrative decision), have been found in most studies to have higher success rates that 'stranger' placements. Qualitative studies indicate that most children gain a sense of security from the legal status of adoption, but some can feel trapped and resentful, especially if they lose contact with birth relatives they want to see.[19,20,21,23]

Chapters by US and UK researchers in a book on birth family contact[24] indicate that post-placement contact, in itself, does not adversely impact on the attachment process, and that it can help new parents and children to be more comfortable in talking about adoption issues. For children placed when older, remaining in face-to-face contact with a birth parent, relative, or sibling, and being placed with a sibling, have been associated in several studies with more successful outcomes. However, this contact needs to be carefully managed and can sometimes be harmful to the child and to the stability of the placement.

## The role of the psychiatrist

Child or adult psychiatrists will become involved in child placement work because they are asked to provide therapy for a child, young person, or adult who has been placed for adoption or in foster care, or for a teenager or adult who has lost a child to adoption. Whether working with task-centred or permanent carers, the special challenges of this different form of family life have to be acknowledged and incorporated into the therapeutic processes. It is for this reason that the need for specialist child mental health services for children in care or placed for adoption is now recognized, which adapt the full range of effective therapeutic approaches to the special needs of the adoptive or foster family. Barth and colleagues[25] have noted that adoptive parents tend to prefer attachment-based therapies to the parent-training approaches that have been demonstrated to be effective with non-adoptive families.

They hypothesize that in part this is because adopters believe that their special issues are better understood by the clinicians using these therapies, but they point to some potentially harmful effects of some of these methods, which can be experienced by the child as intrusive and coercive. Some clinicians who use attachment theories in their work also challenge the validity of some of these methods.[26,27]

Psychiatrists are often consulted about the advisability of adoption or a return to the birth parents or relatives. The message from research is that adoption and foster care will be better for most children than being left with parents who can not be helped to provide them with safe and loving care. However, they are not without risks, which have to be carefully weighed for each child, and the first step must always be to try to improve the quality of parenting in the birth family. At first sight, the break down rates for the placement of older children (now the majority of those needing placement) may appear discouraging. However, given their many difficulties, it should be welcomed that as many as 50 per cent of 11-year-old children, and more of those below that age, do find permanent substitute families. If permanent out-of-home placement does become necessary, the inherent risks demand the provision of the highest quality services provided for as long as needed.

## Further information

**For those who wish to pursue these issues in more depth look at references:**

- ◆ 1, 2, 21, 22, 23 if you are providing therapy for a teenager or adult suffering the harmful effects of losing a child to adoption or foster care

- ◆ 7, 8, 10, 11, 12 on therapeutic and task-centred foster care

- ◆ 6, 9, 14, 15, 16, 17, 18, 19 to help with the decision-making process on substitute family placement options

- ◆ 2, 20, 21, 22, 23, 24 on birth family contact

- ◆ 3, 4, 14, 17, 21, 22, 25, 26, 27 on therapeutic approaches and methods when working with troubled children and their adoptive or foster families.

## References

1. Carp, E.W. (2004). *Adoption politics: bastard nation and ballot initiative 58*. Kansas University Press, Lawrence.
2. Triseliots, J., Feast, J., and Kyle, F. (2005). *The adoption triangle revisited. A study of adoption, search, and reunion experiences*. BAAF, London.
3. Brodzinsky, D.M., Smith, D.W., and Brodzinsky, A.B. (1998). *Children's adjustment to adoption: developmental and clinical issues*. Sage, Thousand Oaks, CA.
4. Rutter, M. (1999). Resilience concepts and findings: implications for family therapy. *Journal of Family Therapy*, **21**, 119–44.
5. Bullock, R., Courtney, M., Parker, R., *et al.* (2006). Can the corporate state parent? *Children and Youth Services Review*, **28**, 1344–58.
6. Quinton, D. and Selwyn, J. (2006). Adoption: research, policy and practice. *Child and Family Law Quarterly*, **18**(4), 459–77.
7. Sellick, C., Thoburn, J., and Philpot, T. (2004). *Success and failure in permanent family placement*. Hants, Avebury, Aldershot.
8. Sinclair, I. (2005). *Fostering now: messages from research*. Jessica Kingsley, London.
9. Thoburn, J. (2003). The risks and rewards of adoption for children in the public care. *Child and Family Law Quarterly*, **15**(4), 391–402.
10. Wilson, K., Sinclair, I., Taylor, C., *et al.* (2004). *Fostering success: an exploration of the research literature in foster care*. SCIE, London.
11. Testa, M.F. and Rolock, N. (1999). Professional foster care: a future worth pursuing? *Child Welfare*, **LXXVIII**(1), 109–24.
12. Fisher, P. and Chamberlain, P. (2000). Multi-dimensional treatment foster care. *Journal of Emotional and Behavioural Disorders*, **8**(3), 155–64.
13. Festinger, T. (2002). After adoption: dissolution or permanence? *Child Welfare*, **LXXXI**(3), 515–33.
14. Rutter, M. and the English and Romanian Adoptees (ERA) Study Team. (1998). Developmental catch–up and deficit, following adoption after severe global early privation. *Journal of Child Psychology and Psychiatry*, **39**, 465–76.
15. Howe, D. (1997). Parent-reported problems in 211 adopted children. *Journal of Child Psychology and Psychiatry*, **38**(4), 401–11.
16. Lindblad, F., Hjern, A., and Vinnerljung, B. (2003). Inter-country adopted children as young adults-a Swedish cohort study. *The American Journal of Orthopsychiatry*, **73**, 190–202.
17. Rushton, A. and Dance, C. (2004). The outcomes of late permanent placements. *Adoption & Fostering*, **28**(1), 49–58.
18. Thoburn, J. (1991). Evaluating placements: survey findings and conclusions. In *Permanent family placement: a decade of experience* (eds. J. Fratter, J. Rowe, and J. Thoburn), pp. 34–57. BAAF, London.
19. Selwyn, J. and Quinton, D. (2005). Stability, permanence and outcomes: foster care and adoption compared. *Adoption and Fostering*, **28**(4), 6–16.
20. Thoburn, J., Norford, L., and Rashid, S.P. (2000). *Permanent family placement for children of minority ethnic origin*. Jessica Kingsley, London.
21. Beek, M. and Schofield, G. (2004). *Providing a secure base in long-term foster care*. BAAF, London.
22. Neil, E. (2003). Understanding other people's perspectives: tasks for adopters in open adoptions. *Adoption Quarterly*, **6**(3), 3–30.
23. Timms, J. and Thoburn, J. (2006). Your shout! Looked after children's perspectives on the Children Act 1989. *Journal of Social Welfare and Family Law*, **28**(2), 153–70.
24. Neil, E. and Howe, D. (2004). *Contact in adoption and permanent foster care: research, policy and practice*. BAAF, London.
25. Barth, R.P., Crea, T.M., John, K., *et al.* (2005). Beyond attachment theory and therapy: towards sensitive evidence-based interventions with foster and adoptive families in distress. *Child and Family Social Work*, **10**(4), 257–68.
26. Dozier, M. (2003). Attachment-based treatment for vulnerable children. *Attachment and Human Development*, **5**, 253–7.
27. Prior, V. and Glaser, D. (2006). *Understanding attachment and attachment disorders. Theory, evidence and practice*. Jessica Kingsley, London.

# 9.3.6 Effects of parental psychiatric and physical illness on child development

Paul Ramchandani, Alan Stein, and Lynne Murray

## Introduction

A broad range of physical and psychiatric illnesses commonly affect adults of parenting age. For example, approximately 13 per cent of women are affected by depression in the postnatal period, and the prevalence of depression in parents of all ages remains high. Many parents will also experience severe physical illness: breast cancer affects approximately 1 in 12 women in the United Kingdom, about a third of whom have children of school age. Worldwide HIV has an enormous impact on adults of parenting age. In some parts of sub-Saharan Africa up to 40 per cent of women attending antenatal clinics are HIV positive. Many of these parental disorders are associated with an increased risk of adverse emotional and social development in their children, and in some cases cognitive development and physical health are also compromized. It must be emphasized that a significant proportion of children at high risk do not develop problems and demonstrate resilience,[1] and, many parents manage to rear their children well despite their own illness. Nonetheless these risks represent a significant additional impact and burden of adult disease (both physical and psychiatric) that is often overlooked.

This chapter reviews the current state of evidence regarding selected examples of psychiatric and physical conditions, from which general themes can be extracted to guide clinical practice. Some of the key mechanisms whereby childhood disturbance does or does not develop in conjunction with parental illness are considered, and strategies for management and intervention reviewed.

## Parental psychiatric illness

There is now reasonable evidence to suggest that most types of psychiatric disorder affecting parents are associated with an increased risk of difficulties for their children. There are some differences in risk by type of disorder; however, there are also some commonalities, suggesting that some of the mechanisms may be shared. Children's disorders may resemble those of their parents[2,3] but there is also evidence of a much broader range of problems, including adverse effects on children's social, emotional, cognitive and physical development. In the following section we will focus on parental depression, schizophrenia, eating disorders, alcoholism and substance abuse, and anxiety, but similar issues apply for other disorders not considered here.

### Depression

Depression in either parent is associated with an increased risk of child psychopathology and other developmental difficulties, with the risks continuing into adulthood.[3] The longest running longitudinal study[4] found that, as well as a three-fold increase in major depressive disorder, the adult offspring of depressed parents had increased rates of anxiety disorders and substance dependence, as well as greater social impairment and physical health impairment. There has been a large body of research focusing on depression affecting mothers in the postnatal period, with studies demonstrating that infants and children have an increased risk of emotional and behavioural problems.[5] Some studies have suggested that children's cognitive development may also be affected, although the results from studies are not consistent.[6] Similarly, there is a suggestion that boys may be more affected than girls in early childhood. As the children enter adolescence an increased risk of mood and anxiety disorders emerges.[7] More recently research in developing countries has shown an association between postnatal depression and an increased risk of physical health problems in infants such as poor growth and diarrhoel illness.[8]

Much less work has been done on depressed fathers, although consistent evidence is now beginning to emerge of an independent effect of paternal depression on children's development.[9] The overall impact may be less than that of maternal depression, and there are also conjoint effects to consider, as depression in one parent can often co-occur with depression or another psychiatric disorder in the other parent. Similarly there may be protective effects if one parent remains well.[10]

While genetic factors clearly play an important role in the transmission of risk from parents to children, environmental factors, and the interactions that occur between genetic and environmental factors, also have substantial influence.[11,12] In the case of depression, the core symptoms of low mood, loss of interest and low energy can have a significant impact on parenting capacity and parent-child relations. These include a parent's capacity to be responsive, consistent, and warm when interacting with their children, particularly in the first few years of life. For example, depressed mothers may be less vocal, less positive, and less spontaneous than controls, more negative, unsupportive, and intrusive, and have more difficulty in communicating and listening to their young children.[13, 14]

Depression in either parent is strongly associated with marital discord.[15] This may play a key role in mediating the effects of parental depression and may be a more proximal predictor of child outcomes than depression.[13] The way in which conflicts are resolved may be very important and depressed parents are likely to use less effortful strategies, such as withdrawal. Children are generally more at risk as they are exposed to an increased number of risk factors, and children whose parents are depressed are particularly at risk if they are also socio-economically disadvantaged.

The direction of effects is not all from parent to child, and temperamental and behavioural factors in the child may also contribute to increasing family discord, parental psychiatric disturbance, and parenting impairments, and ultimately to disturbances in parent-child attachment. Infant irritability and poor motor control, measured before the onset of any maternal depression at 10 days postpartum, increase the risk that a mother will become depressed.[16] The influence of parental depression on child development thus represents a complex bidirectional interaction between individual vulnerability (which may be genetic), influences of depression on parenting characteristics, parent–child relationships, the wider context of the parental relationship, and other aspects of social disadvantage.

### Schizophrenia

Parents with a diagnosis of schizophrenia have a greatly increased risk of having children who later develop schizophrenia themselves. Risks to child development are identified from birth, with an increased likelihood of obstetric complications, not fully accounted for by maternal behaviour during pregnancy, or by genetic risk.[17] During childhood, prior to the onset of any psychiatric symptoms, attentional problems similar to those found in adult schizophrenic patients have been identified and these problems not only persist into adulthood, but attentional problems have been identified as key neurobiological indicators of risk for subsequent schizophrenia or other psychopathology in adolescence and young adulthood.[18]

Social difficulties with peers and teachers are found in many longitudinal studies of children with schizophrenic parents,[19] although not necessarily to a greater extent than in children with parents suffering from affective disorder and a higher IQ can be protective. Social relationship problems and associated thought disorder may become more marked in adolescence and seem to be predicted by attentional problems.[18] As young adults, children of schizophrenic parents are at high risk for schizotypal behaviour, although this broader range of difficulties does not necessarily distinguish them from parents with affective illness.

A pattern of disturbed communication has been described in families with a schizophrenic parent,[20] but the importance of these interactions in explaining long-term outcomes has been questioned.

Overall, cognitive and attention difficulties appear to be largely associated with specific brain abnormalities linked with schizophrenia, but other kinds of childhood problems are probably influenced more by the general family disruption associated with a parent who requires hospital admission and who may have difficulties with employment and other social relationships beyond the family.

## Eating disorders

Eating disorders occur commonly among women of child-bearing age.[21] Studies have raised concern that mothers' attitudes and behaviours regarding food and body shape, may influence their children's feeding, and ultimately the children's own attitudes to body shape and eating.[22] Children are particularly vulnerable at two stages of development—infancy and adolescence. During infancy feeding and mealtimes take up a significant part of the day and provide important times for close communication between parents and children. A Scandinavian study has indicated that failure to thrive may be a risk in the first year amongst women with a history of anorexia nervosa.[23] One controlled observational study of 1-year-old children of mothers with eating disorders found that the mothers were intrusive with their infants during both mealtimes and play, and they expressed more negative emotion and conflict during mealtimes than controls, and allowed their children less autonomy.[24] Furthermore, infant weight was independently and inversely related to mealtime conflict.[25] Follow up studies of children of mothers who have experienced eating disorders in the postnatal period indicate that in middle childhood they are more likely than control children to value themselves by body shape and weight, and to use dietary restriction.[22, 26]

During adolescence children become more aware of societal pressures and develop increasing interest in body shape and attractiveness while preoccupied with their own concerns about food, body shape, and weight. Children may model themselves on their parents, and parents may influence their adolescent children directly by expressing attitudes towards their children's weight, shape, and eating habits. However, it should be emphasized that, in common with most parent psychopathology, the children of parents with eating disorders are not invariably adversely affected. Some parents manage well and their children develop without apparent problems.

## Alcoholism and substance abuse

A substantial body of evidence has been amassed on the effects of parental alcoholism and substance abuse.[27] They are wide ranging, identifiable throughout development, and work has highlighted the importance of the social effects on the child in addition to physical and psychological outcomes.[28] Both genetic and environmental factors seem to be involved.

The impact of maternal alcoholism on the developing child can be found from the prenatal period.[29] Present in 0.01 to 0.03 per cent of normal births, foetal alcohol syndrome appears in 5.9 per cent of births of alcoholic women. There is also considerable evidence that infants exposed prenatally to heroin and cocaine are at increased risk of a number of developmental difficulties which may persist throughout childhood.[30]

Studies of outcome consistently describe impaired cognitive and social development in children of alcoholics and heroin users.[27,30] An increased risk of attention-deficit hyperactivity disorder, attention problems, and impulsivity in children of alcoholics is the most consistent finding. Children of drug abusers may also be more aggressive and have fewer friends and are at risk for criminality, depression, anxiety, and somatic problems. Children of alcoholics have an increased risk of becoming alcoholics themselves and, similarly, children of drug abusers also have an increased risk of drug abuse in adolescence, although many are resilient and do not develop similar problems themselves.

Social factors such as poverty and social isolation are known to influence child development adversely and it has been difficult to differentiate between the effects of the disorder and the associated adversity. Substance abuse in the parent may lead to impaired parenting and an impoverished social environment, leaving children vulnerable to neglect or abuse and contributing to impaired social and cognitive functioning, psychopathology, substance abuse, and delinquency but the relative impact of each factor has yet to be resolved. Studies have identified deficits in parenting behaviour and, in particular, neglect and harsh discipline.[31] Divorce and marital conflict are also more likely and there is evidence of assortative mating, all of which are likely to compound the risk for the children.

Stressful life events, and in particular those related to family conflict, have proved to be important in accounting for the link between paternal alcoholism and alcohol use in their offspring.[32] Overall, clinicians have emphasized a family perspective when conceptualizing the multiple levels of stress and vulnerability associated with parental alcoholism and opiate abuse and the need to enhance social supports for the family.[30]

## Anxiety disorders

There is less information about children whose parents have anxiety disorders but there appears to be a considerable degree of specificity in the familial transmission of anxiety disorder.[33] One study showed a two-fold increased risk of anxiety disorders among offspring of parent probands compared with offspring of substance abusers or controls.[34] However, they are also at risk of other kinds of problems such as depression.[35]

In a search for the mechanism of transmission, it has been suggested that children at risk for developing anxiety disorders have a temperamental vulnerability characterized by behavioural inhibition and autonomic reactivity, identifiable in infancy by an increased startle response.[36,37] The question of the relative influence of genetic or environmental factors does suggest a lesser genetic component for anxiety disorders,[38] and a developing line of research has led to a number of aspects of parenting behaviour of parents with anxiety being considered important, including over-protection and the limiting of children's opportunities to develop new skills[39]. There appear to be some specific differences by type of anxiety disorder with, for example, mothers with social phobia demonstrating characteristic patterns of modelling of anxiety by the parent, and failure to provide encouragement/opportunities for child autonomy.[40]

Recent lines of research have also explored possible risks in utero to the developing foetus. Children exposed to maternal anxiety in utero are at an increased subsequent risk of behavioral problems. This increased risk appears to persist through childhood, leading to suggestions that the mechanism may be in part mediated through an antenatal effect on the HPA axis of the developing foetus.[41] More research is needed to clarify the mechanisms but it is clear that children whose parents have anxiety disorders are at risk of developing psychiatric disturbance themselves.

## Parental physical illness

Many families experience chronic parental illness and paradoxically, as treatment techniques improve illnesses may extend over longer time periods, which may have greater impact on family members including children. There have been limited reports about the impact of physical parental illness on children, however the importance of this area is beginning to be recognized, particularly in relation to parental cancer, and also HIV.[42] Similar associated difficulties can arise with many other parental illness, particularly chronic ones such as diabetes. However we will here confine our comments to parental cancer and HIV, and the general issues that these conditions illustrate for the developing child.

### Cancer

Parental cancer is likely to be associated with depression and marital difficulties, both risk factors for the child. The balance of evidence indicates that their children are at increased risk of developing psychological disturbance.[43] The impact of parental cancer on family communication and child outcomes may vary according to the child's developmental level, their gender, the presence of disability in the child, and the parent's level of psychological distress and marital discord.[44]

A recent review[45] found that adolescents who had a parent with cancer had higher levels of emotional disturbance, than a normal population sample, but younger children were not consistently found to exhibit higher rates of problems, although some studies suggest this. Children's own responses to their predicament are likely to affect their eventual adjustment. Problem-focused or active coping affects the stressors (e.g. seeking information, positive reinterpretation of stressful events) and is expected to be more adaptive while emotion-focused coping (e.g. venting emotions, denial, apathy) draws attention away from the stressors but may place children at risk for anxiety and depression.[46] Health professionals may need to assist parents in recognizing and coping with their children's distress when it is present. Specifically, communication about the parental illness and how the children feel appears to be crucial to children's coping.[47] The levels of anxiety and distress amongst the children are related to whether they are told about the illness and the quality of the communication with the parents, with informed children having lower levels of anxiety than those who are uninformed.[44]

### HIV status and AIDS

Women of child-bearing age account for an increasing number of sufferers of HIV/AIDS in the developing world and there is now increasing evidence that their children are at increased developmental risk, even if the children are not HIV positive themselves.[43] Young children may have fewer problems[48] but those of school age are at risk for externalizing and internalizing problems, lower social skills, and academic achievement difficulties.[49] Maternal depression is relatively common amongst women diagnosed with HIV during pregnancy,[50] and the impact of this on their caregiving capabilities may be one of the key mechanisms by which children are affected. Given the enormity of the HIV pandemic and possible parallels with other common infectious diseases such as Malaria and TB, there is serious need for further research in this specific field.

### Summary of mechanisms

Some of the key mechanisms by which increased risk for child disturbance is transmitted from ill parents to their children have been described above. In cases of psychiatric disorder the link may in part reflect genetic transmission, but clearly a considerable amount of the variance is accounted for by environmental mechanisms and

a number of such mechanisms have been proposed.[5,11] Most of these can apply equally to parental physical or psychiatric illness. First, parental illness may interfere with parental functioning and parent-child interactions, for example where a parent becomes withdrawn or preoccupied and relatively unavailable to the child. Second, a number of family and environmental factors such as marital/family discord and severe housing or associated economic deprivation are associated with mental illness and these constitute risks in their own right, as well as sometimes being a direct consequence of the parental disorder (for example, parental depression leading to increased marital conflict, although the reverse direction of causality can also occur). Third, in rarer instances parental symptoms may impinge directly on the child, for example where the parent incorporates a child into the core symptomatology such as a delusion or an obsession. Finally, it should not be assumed that influences are unidirectional. Child characteristics such as early temperamental difficulties or behavioural problems may influence the outcome of parental illness, particularly in the case of depression.[3] Child characteristics such as coping style, intellectual ability, or sociability may be particularly important in explaining resilience.

## Implications—responding to a parent in clinic and preventive interventions

As the influences of parental illness on children's development become better understood there is increasing recognition of the potential importance of addressing parent-child links. This is both in making better enquiry about child welfare when a parent is seriously ill, but also enquiring about parental health when a child presents with a disorder such as depression (e.g. NICE guidance on depression in children and young people[51]) Two particular areas will be considered here; when a parent presents with a serious illness (psychiatric or psychological) and potential intervention strategies with high-risk groups who may or may not be presenting to health services.

When parents with serious physical or psychological illness are seen as outpatients, especially if they are subsequently admitted to hospital, it should be routine to enquire about children—their ages, developmental and scholastic progress, child care arrangements, and family support. In the limited time available, it makes most sense to enquire about the areas most likely to be affected by the parental disorder.[52] For example, where a parent with depression has young children, enquiry could focus on the level of care that the parent feels able to provide to the children, the feelings that the parent has for their children, and the presence of any marital or family discord, as well as the available support. These questions obviously require sensitive handling, as parents can easily feel blamed for any effect that they perceive their illness may have had on their children. In many cases provision of appropriate support and treatment to the parent will have a sufficiently beneficial effect for the whole family that no further intervention is required, (for example, findings from a recent large randomized controlled trial identify improvements in children's outcomes when their mother's depression is treated.[53]) However it is crucial to ask and make at least this preliminary assessment. Close collaboration with the primary care team, including the family's general practitioner, is of considerable importance. The general practitioner's involvement may be critical, both in terms of potential treatment and support for the family, and also as a source of knowledge of the wider family system, and the resources available to the family.

In those cases where a child is more severely affected (either directly by a parent's illness or by other related factors), consideration should be given to including relevant children's services, either Child and Adolescent Mental Health Services (CAMHS) or children's care services. Close collaborative relationships between child and adult mental health services clearly ease potential joint working, and should be the norm. Communication with, and the close involvement of, the family's general practitioner, can also contribute to a plan to benefit the whole family system.

In those cases where a parent has a chronic illness and the clinician gets to know them over a period of time, it can be helpful to ask about children's understanding and knowledge of the parental illness and the extent to which it has been discussed within the family. These issues will need to be carefully and sensitively handled. Families have a range of ways in which they communicate and it is important not to compound the parent's problems by making them feel their illness is harming their children. As far as inpatients are concerned, it is important that facilities should be available for children visiting and, unless specifically contraindicated, regular contact should be encouraged, and appropriate play and other materials should be available. Discussions should be held with the patient and/or relatives about child-care arrangements, and the patient and family need to be helped to think about providing the child with an appropriate explanation about parental health and absence.

Communication either about the parental illness or the associated discord may help to alleviate some of the risks for childhood problems.[44] Studies of marital disruption and divorce have found that children cope better with marital conflict when they are given some explanation or told that the conflict has been resolved.[54] Children often feel left out and, without knowledge of the parental illness, they may be particularly likely to attribute any family conflict or disruption to themselves in their effort to understand the changes taking place. Intervention, including working with family communication, can have significant positive effects if well handled. Some guidelines are available.[55,56]

Less work has been conducted in families where the parent is physically ill, although reports of treatment once the family members are experiencing problems are providing some ways forward.[45] Parents may consciously avoid disclosure because of the questions they anticipate from their children, particularly about death. Communication in this context is not only a matter of disclosure of the illness but a starting point for ongoing discussion and questions, without which children may be at increased risk.[57] The most important role of support services may be to rehearse with parents the kinds of questions that might occur and how they could respond, a strategy which may also facilitate discussion of the ill parent's anxieties.

## Prevention

Beyond the scope of the individual parent and family in clinic there have been a number of studies which have examined the possibility of preventative intervention in high-risk groups. This is most often conducted in the context of parental depression. One series of intervention studies with children of parents with major depression has shown marked improvement in family functioning and child outcome.[58] These interventions have taken a variety of formats, but all include a component of psycho-education directed to

the whole family. However, in another trial, the involvement of parents in a group programme for adolescent offspring of parents with depression did not show any additional benefit.

Some preventive intervention can clearly be accomplished earlier. In infancy it is possible to promote the development of secure parent–child attachment, which should be protective even if the parental illness is chronic. Maternal sensitivity can be enhanced using videotaped mother-child interactions, which can increase the rate of secure attachment in at-risk families.[59] In the case of maternal eating disorders there is now some encouraging evidence for the effectiveness of video feedback treatment to enhance maternal responsivity to the infant, and to decrease mother-infant conflict.[60] A recent review of treatments for mothers and infants in the context of maternal depression found that treatment of maternal depression alone did not appear to mitigate the impact of the depression on the child. However, a number of different mother-infant psychotherapies did appear to confer benefit on mother child interaction and child outcome. However, much work remains to be done.[61]

## Conclusions

In conclusion, children of parents with physical or psychiatric illness are at risk of a wide range of developmental and psychiatric difficulties, although not all will develop problems. Future work should be directed to developing and evaluating ways of providing support so that parents can best manage their illnesses and to prevent or mitigate any negative effects on their children.

## Further information

The SCIE parental mental health network (www.scie.org.uk/mhnetwork/resources.asp)

The Children of Parents with a Mental Illness (COPMI) (www.aicafmha.net.au/copmi/index.html)

## References

1. Rutter. M. (1990). Psychosocial resilience and protective mechanisms. In *Risk and protective factors in the development of psychopathology* (eds. J. Rolf, A.S. Masten, D. Cicchetti, K.H. Neuchterlein, and S. Weintraub), pp. 181–214. Cambridge University Press, New York.
2. Bernstein, G.A. and Borchardt, C.M. (1991). Anxiety disorders of childhood and adolescence: a critical review. *Journal of the American Academy of Child and Adolescent Psychiatry*, **30**, 519–32.
3. Downey, G. and Coyne, J.C. (1990). Children of depressed parents: an integrative review. *Psychological Bulletin*, **108**, 50–76.
4. Weissman MM, Wickramaratne P, Nomura Y, *et al.* (2006). Offspring of depressed parents: 20 years later. *American Journal of Psychiatry*, **163**(6), 1001–8.
5. Murray, L. and Cooper, P. (2003). Intergenerational transmission of affective and cognitive processes associated with depression: infancy and the preschool years. In *Unipolar Depression: a Lifespan Perspective* (ed. I. Goodyer), pp. chapter 2. Oxford University Press, Oxford.
6. Sohr-Preston, S.L. and Scaramella, L.V. (2006). Implications of timing of maternal depressive symptoms for early cognitive and language development. *Clinical Child and Family Psychology Review*, **9**(1), 65–83
7. Halligan, S.L., Murraym, L., Martins, C., *et al.* (2007). Maternal depression and psychiatric outcomes in adolescent offspring: a 13-year longitudinal study. *Journal of Affective Disorders*, **97**, 145–54.
8. Rahman, A., Iqbal, Z., Bunn, J., *et al.* (2004). Impact of maternal depression on infant nutritional status and illness: a cohort study. *Archives of General Psychiatry*, **61**, 946–52.
9. Ramchandani, P., Stein, A., Evans, J., *et al.* (2005). Paternal depression in the postnatal period and child development: a prospective population study. *Lancet*, **365**(9478), 2201–5.

10. Kahn, R.S., Brandt, D. and Whitaker, R.C. (2004). Combined effect of mothers' and fathers' mental health symptoms on children's behavioral and emotional well-being. *Archives of Pediatrics and Adolescent Medicine*, **158**(8), 721–9.

11. Rutter, M. (2007). Gene-environment interdependence. *Development Science*, **10**(1), 12–8.

12. Kim-Cohen, J., Moffitt, T.E., Taylor, A., *et al.* (2005). Maternal depression and children's antisocial behavior: nature and nurture effects. *Archive of General Psychiatry*, **62**(2), 173–81.

13. Stein, A., Gath, D.H., Bucher, J., *et al.* (1991). The relationship between post–natal depression and mother–child interaction. *British Journal of Psychiatry*, **158**, 46–52.

14. Murray, L., Fiori-Cowley, A., Hooper, R., *et al.* (1996). The impact of postnatal depression and associated adversity on early mother-infant interactions and later infant outcome. *Child Development*, **67**(5), 2512–26.

15. Cummings, E. M., Keller, P. S., and Davies, P. T. (2005). Towards a family process model of maternal and paternal depressive symptoms: exploring multiple relations with child and family functioning. *Journal of Child Psychology and Psychiatry and allied disciplines*, **46**(5), 479–89.

16. Murray, L., Hipwell, A., Hooper, R., *et al.* (1996). Cognitive development of 5 year old children of postnatally depressed mothers. *Journal of Child Psychology and Psychiatry*, **37**, 927–35.

17. Sacker, A., Done, D.J., and Crow, T.J. (1996). Obstetric complications in children born to parents with schizophrenia: a meta–analysis of case–control studies. *Psychological Medicine*, **26**, 279–87.

18. Dworkin, R.H., Lewis, J.A., Cornblatt, B.A., *et al.* (1994). Social competence deficits in adolescents at risk for schizophrenia. *Journal of Nervous and Mental Disease*, **182**, 103–8.

19. Weintraub, S. (1987). Risk factors in schizophrenia: the Stony Brook High–Risk Project. *Schizophrenia Bulletin*, **13**, 439–50.

20. Greenwald, D.F. and Harder, D.W. (1994). Outcome predictors in a longitudinal study of high-risk boys. *Journal of Consulting and Clinical Psychology*, **50**, 638–43.

21. Fairburn, C. G., and Harrison, P. J. (2003). Eating disorders. *Lancet*, **361**(9355), 407–16.

22. Stein, A., Woolley, H., Cooper, S., *et al.* (2006). Eating habits and attitudes among 10-year-old children of mothers with eating disorders. A longitudinal study. *British Journal of Psychiatry*, **189**, 324–9.

23. Brinch, M., Isager, T., and Tolstrup, K. (1988). Anorexia nervosa and motherhood: reproduction pattern and mothering behaviour of 50 women. *Acta Psychiatrica Scandinavica*, **77**, 611–17.

24. Stein, A., Woolley, H., Cooper, S.D., *et al.* (1994). An observational study of mothers with eating disorders and their infants. *Journal of Child Psychology and Psychiatry*, **35**, 733–48.

25. Stein, A., Murray, L., Cooper, P., *et al.* (1996). Infant growth in the context of maternal eating disorders and maternal depression: a comparative study. *Psychological Medicine*, **26**, 569–74.

26. Jacobi, C. Agras, W.S. and Hammer, L. (2001). Predicting children's reported eating disturbances at 8 years of age. *Journal of American Academy of Child and Adolescent Psychiatry*, **40**, 364–72.

27. Lieberman, D. (2000). Children of alcoholics: an update. *Current Opinion in Pediatrics*, **12**(4), 336–340.

28. Burns, E.C., O'Driscoll, M., and Wason, G. (1996). The health and development of children whose mothers are on methadone maintenance. *Child Abuse Review*, **5**, 113–22.

29. Nordberg, L., Rydelius, P.–A., and Zetterstrom, R. (1994). Parental alcoholism and early child development. *Acta Paediatrica*, **83** (Suppl. 404), 14–18.

30. Hogan, D.M. (1998). The psychological development and welfare of children of opiate and cocaine users: review and research needs. *Journal of Child Psychology and Psychiatry*, **39**, 609–20.

31. Famularo, R., Kinscherff, R., and Fenton, T. (1992). Parental substance abuse and the nature of child maltreatment. *Child Abuse and Neglect*, **16**, 475–83.

32. Hill, S.Y. and Hruska, D.R. (1992). Childhood psychopathology in families with multigenerational alcoholism. *Journal of the American Academy of Child and Adolescent Psychiatry*, **31**, 1024–30.

33. Biederman, J., Petty, C., Faraone, S. V., *et al.* (2006). Effects of parental anxiety disorders in children at high risk for panic disorder: A controlled study. *Journal of Affective Disorder*, **94**, 191–7.

34. Merikangas, K.R., Dierker, L.C., and Szatmari, P. (1998). Psychopathology amongst offspring of parents with substance abuse and/or anxiety disorders: a high risk study. *Journal of Child Psychology and Psychiatry*, **39**, 711–20.

35. Warner, V., Mufson, L., and Weissman, M. (1995). Offspring at high risk for depression and anxiety: mechanisms of psychiatric disorder. *Journal of the American Academy of Child and Adolescent Psychiatry*, **34**, 786–97.

36. Grillon, C., Dierker, L., and Merikangas, K.R. (1997). Startle modulation in children at risk for anxiety disorders and/or alcoholism. *Journal of the American Academy of Child and Adolescent Psychiatry*, **36**, 925–32.

37. Kagan, J., Reznick, J., and Snidman, N. (1987). The physiology and psychology of behavioral inhibition in children. *Child Development*, **58**, 1459–73.

38. Gordon, J. A., and Hen, R. (2004). Genetic approaches to the study of anxiety. *Annual review of neurosciences*, **27**, 193–222.

39. Wood, J.J., McLeod, B.D., Sigman, M., *et al.* (2003). Parenting and childhood anxiety: theory, empirical findings, and future directions. *Journal of Child Psychology and Psychiatry*, **44**, 134–51.

40. Murray, L. Cooper, P. Cresswell, C. *et al.* (2007). The effects of maternal social phobia on mother-infant interactions and infant social responsiveness. *Journal of Child Psychology and Psychiatry*, **48**, 45–52.

41. O'Connor TG, Ben-Shlomo Y, Heron J, *et al.* (2005). Prenatal anxiety predicts individual differences in cortisol in pre-adolescent children. *Biological Psychiatry*, **58**(3), 211–7.

42. Stein, A., Krebs, G., Richter, L., *et al.* (2005). Babies of a pandemic. *Archives of Disease in Childhood*, **90**, 116–8.

43. Welch, A.S., Wadsworth, M.E., and Compas, B.E. (1996). Adjustment of children and adolescents to parental cancer. *Cancer*, **77**, 1409–18.

44. Kroll, L., Barnes, J., Jones, A., *et al.* (1998). Cancer in parents: telling children. *British Medical Journal*, **316**, 880.

45. Visser, A., Huizinga, G. A., van der Graaf, W. T., *et al.* (2004). The impact of parental cancer on children and the family: a review of the literature. *Cancer Treat Rev*, **30**(8), 683–94.

46. Compas, B.E., Worsham, N.L., Ey, S., *et al.* (1996). When mom or dad has cancer. II. Coping, cognitive appraisals, and psychological distress in children of cancer patients. *Health Psychology*, **15**, 167–75.

47. Forrest, G., Plumb, C., Ziebland, S., *et al*, (2006). Breast cancer in the family—children's perceptions of their mother's cancer and its initial treatment: qualitative study. *British Medical Journal*, **332**, 998–1003.

48. Black, M.M., Nair, P., and Harrington, D. (1994). Maternal HIV infection: parenting and early child development. *Journal of Pediatric Psychology*, **19**, 595–616.

49. Forehand, R., Steele, R., Armistead, L., *et al.* (1998). The Family Health Project: psychosocial adjustment of children whose mothers are HIV infected. *Journal of Consulting and Clinical Psychology*, **66**, 513–20.

50. Rochat, T.J., Richter, L.M., Doll, H.A., *et al.* (2006). Depression among pregnant rural South African women undergoing HIV testing. *Journal of the American Medical Association*, **295**(12), 1376–8.

51. National Institute for Health and Clinical Excellence (NICE). (2005). *Depression in children and young people: identification and management in primary, community and secondary care*. London: National Collaborating Centre for Mental Health

52. Rutter, M. (1989). Psychiatric disorder in parents as a risk factor for children. In *Prevention of mental disorder, alcohol and other drug use in children and adolescents*. (eds. D Schaffer, I. Phillips, and N.B. Enger), pp. 157–189. Office for Substance Abuse, Rockville, MD.

53. Weissman, M., Pilowsky, D. J., Wickramaratne, P. J., *et al.* (2006). Remissions in maternal depression and child psychopathology. A STAR*D-Child Report. *Journal of the American Medical Association*, **295**(12), 1389–98.

54. Cummings, E.M. and Davies, P.T. (1998). *Families, conflict, and conflict resolution: the children's perspective*. Guilford Press, New York.

55. Falkov, A. (ed.) (1999). *Crossing bridges: training resources for working with mentally ill parents and their children.* Pavilion Publications, Brighton.
56. Beardslee, W. (2004). *When a parent is depressed.* Little, Brown and company:USA.
57. Rotheram–Borus, M.J., Draimin, B.H., Reid, H.M., *et al.* (1997). The impact of illness disclosure and custody plans on adolescents whose parents live with AIDS. *AIDS*, **11**, 1159–64.
58. Beardslee, W.R., Gladstone, T.R., Wright, E.J., *et al.* (2003). A family-based approach to the prevention of depressive symptoms in children at risk: evidence of parental and child change. *Pediatrics*, **112**(2), e119–131.
59. Van Zeijl, J., Mesman, J., Van IJzendoorn, M.H., *et al.* (2006). Attachment-based intervention for enhancing sensitive discipline in mothers of 1- to 3-year-old children at risk for externalizing behavior problems: a randomized controlled trial. *Journal of Consulting and Clinical Psychology*, **74**(6), 994–1005.
60. Stein, A., Woolley H, Senior R, *et al.* (2006). Treating disturbances in the relationship between mothers with eating disorders and their infants: a randomized controlled trial. *American Journal of Psychiatry*, **163**(5), 899–906.
61. Nylen, K.J., Moran, T.E., Franklin, C.L., *et al.* (2006). Maternal depression: a review of relevant treatment approaches for mothers and infants. *Infant Mental Health Journal*, **27**(4), 327–43.

# 9.3.7 The effects of bereavement in childhood

Dora Black and David Trickey

## Introduction

Bereavement is not an illness in itself, although it may cause illness or predispose to one. The reaction to the loss of a loved one may lead to temporary or long-term psychological distress and/or loss of function, and may occasion consultation with the general practitioner and referral to mental health professionals.

During the first two years of life, through instinctive behaviours which are modified by experience, infants and their main carers develop an attachment. This bond between a child and his caretaker(s) ensures the child's survival, enables his or her optimum physical, intellectual, and emotional development, and in due course ensures the survival of the species. The nature of the attachment between infant and carer(s) influences the way in which children come to view their social world; the pattern of attachment developed in the first two years of life often remains stable and is associated with the way in which children relate to other people later in their life. Attachment behaviour has been observed across different species and has obvious benefits for survival. However, part and parcel of attachment for the child is distress at separation. Infants who develop a secure attachment can gradually tolerate longer periods of separation from their carer and any distress is rapidly assuaged when they are re-united with their carer. When considered within the context of attachment theory, it is inevitable that permanent separation (e.g. through bereavement) will cause distress for the bereaved. Parkes reviews the body of attachment research and offers a comprehensive description of attachment with particular reference to its role in understanding the impact of loss.[1]

The DSM-IV-TR has a classification for 'Bereavement' (V62.82) differentiating it from 'Major depressive disorder' (296.2) which, unless the symptoms are severe, is generally not diagnosed until 2 months after the loss. ICD-10 has no separate classification for bereavement and suggests the use of 'Adjustment disorders' (F43.2) for temporary reactions to life-events, and 'Death of a family member' (Z63.4) for normal bereavement reactions not exceeding 6 months in duration.

In industrialized countries between 1.5 and 4 per cent of children are orphaned of at least one parent in childhood. Premature deaths in the parenting years may be due to illness, accident, war, civil conflict, natural and man-made disasters and the incidence of these are all higher in developing countries. It is estimated by UNICEF that, in some developing countries, 21 per cent of children are orphaned of at least one parent; with HIV AIDS responsible for up to three-quarters of the deaths.[2]

## Reactions to the death of a parent
### Research studies

It is generally accepted that loss of a parent in childhood is associated with harmful psychological consequences, however it is difficult to tease out the independent effects of adverse circumstances before the death, the loss itself and the subsequent disruption to the child's life, including the possibility of compromised parenting post-bereavement[3,4]. Most published research about bereaved children describes small-scale uncontrolled studies carried out on children and adolescents referred to mental health facilities. Dowdney comprehensively reviews the research examining the psychological impact of being bereaved of a parent in childhood. She concludes that despite methodological weaknesses, certain findings consistently emerge: 'Children do experience grief, sadness, and despair following parental death. Mild depression is frequent, and can persist for at least a year after parental death'. Bereaved children commonly exhibit a range of psychological symptoms that may not constitute a specific disorder, but the severity of which is likely to warrant referral to a specialist service for one in five bereaved children.[5]

### Long-term effects of bereavement

There continues to be debate about a possible link between being bereaved of a parent as a child, and mental health as an adult. The debate is complicated by methodological weaknesses in studies, inconsistent results and difficulty in isolating the impact of experiences which may precede or follow the loss. Any long term consequences of parental bereavement can be mitigated by the subsequent provision of adequate parenting[6,7]. Furthermore, studies in behavioural genetics are increasing the understanding of how genetic endowment interacts with environmental hazards to lead to the presence or absence of mental health problems.[8]

### Cultural and religious issues

Reactions to loss are biologically based and are therefore likely to transcend cultural differences, although culture may modify their expression.[3] Religious beliefs about what happens after death can be confusing to young children at the stage of concrete thinking and need to be presented taking account of their developmental stage. A helpful text[9] gives guidance on religious and cultural differences in the conceptualization of death.

### Developmental issues

Young children react to the absence of a parent by developing an anxiety or depressive reaction, often expressed somatically (regression in acquired control, anorexia, insomnia), but young children cannot distinguish temporary from permanent loss[3,10]. Research consistently demonstrates that children ordinarily do not develop a full understanding of the concepts of death before the age of 7 years, although younger children of 4 years and above can understand it with appropriate help.[11]

Pre-pubertal schoolchildren can be helped more easily to comprehend the reality of death, especially if they are given an opportunity to see for themselves the cessation of function. In cultures where viewing the body is the norm, there may be fewer misconceptions about death among children, but this should not be undertaken where the body is mutilated.[12] Although difficult to substantiate scientifically, clinical literature suggests that attending the funeral helps the grieving process.[5]

For adolescents the death of a parent may come at a time when they are freeing themselves from dependence and may have been in conflict with the parent who subsequently dies, leaving the young person with feelings of guilt and anger. Suicidal feelings are more likely to be acted upon if part of a depressive reaction. Adolescents are more able to sustain sad affects and express grief directly, but they may also react with behavioural and academic difficulties.

The reader is referred to Dyregrov for a more comprehensive description of common reactions to bereavement in childhood.[13]

Children and adolescents with learning difficulties may be at higher risk for developing psychological problems following bereavement, because of their cognitive difficulty in understanding the components of the concept of death and because of their greater dependency.[14] Everatt and Gale provide a helpful review of the available research and draw implications for bereaved children with learning disabilities.[15]

### Traumatic bereavement

As with adults, children who witness horrific events involving the death or severe injury of people close to them, or upon whom they are dependent, are at risk of developing post-traumatic stress disorder (see Chapter 9.3.2). Traumatic symptomatology can impede the resolution of grief through mourning as for mourning to proceed, the child has to summon up an image of the dead person. However, if when she/he tries to imagine the deceased, a frightening picture appears or she/he experiences again the helplessness or terror he felt at the time of the death, she/he will tend to avoid recalling the person and thus will not be able to grieve for her/him. Similarly, children whose parents die through suicide or homicide are more likely to have difficulties. In such cases, not only is the nature of the death traumatic and more difficult to make sense of, but there is often an unhelpful media interest and, social support systems that would ordinarily be available may find the circumstances of the death unbearable. If there is a body at all it may be disfigured or its release to the relatives may be delayed the investigation or the authorities and mementoes or suicide notes may be retained by the authorities. Children who have been traumatized by experiencing the sudden, violent, or horrific death of someone close to them are unlikely to benefit from bereavement counselling or therapy until the post-traumatic stress symptoms have been treated[16,17].

### Other losses

Much of our knowledge of the impact of bereavement on children and young people is drawn from research on children bereaved of a parent. Other losses have been less well studied; however reactions may be similar depending upon the relationship between the child and the deceased. The death of a grandparent, particularly if he or she lived with the child or carried out caretaking functions, can be devastating to child and parents. Sibling death carries a high morbidity for the survivors, but this can be mitigated by preparation for the death when possible and by participation in community rituals.[18] Adolescents losing a sibling often deny the finality and universality of death, even when these concepts are well established prior to the death.[19] The losses of friends, of pets, or of homes, whilst eliciting sadness, are less likely to provoke pathological grief reactions provided that the child is supported by parents and other adults who are not themselves withdrawn in grief. However, adolescents are affected by the suicide of a friend. A controlled study found that there was a higher incidence of depression than in a matched population sample, although the incidence of attempted suicide was no higher.[20]

### Evaluation of treatments

Many of the adverse sequelae of childhood bereavement can be modified or prevented by an intervention before the death or shortly afterwards. In a controlled study, a brief family intervention 2 months after the death of a parent significantly reduced children's morbidity at 1 year post-bereavement. The differences between the treatment and the control group were no longer significant at 2 year follow up, but some of the more affected children had been lost to follow-up, making comparison difficult. But even if by 2 years the effect of the intervention is no longer significant, there is an argument for intervening to relieve symptoms and reduce suffering in the short and medium term.[21] Schut & Stroebe's most recent review concludes that, although in the general adult population a bereavement intervention is more effective for those with more complicated grief reactions, 'children are likely to be a special case, perhaps benefiting from primary intervention.' (A primary intervention is one which is open to all bereaved people rather than targetted at those who are at risk of difficulties such as following traumatic death, or those experiencing complicated reactions.).[22]

### Management

Children whose symptoms reach the threshold for a diagnosable psychiatric disorder require a careful clinical assessment to determine the most appropriate treatment, and other sections detail the appropriate interventions for disorders such as depression (Chapter 9.2.7), anxiety (Chapter 9.2.6) or Post-traumatic Stress Disorder (PTSD: Chapter 9.3.2). Some studies have found that parents report fewer symptoms in their bereaved children than the children do themselves; this means that it is important in research and clinical practice to interview the children individually if possible.[5]

Children bereaved of a carer urgently need to be looked after and will transfer their attachment to a new caretaker who is available for them and responsive to them. Supporting a widowed parent in his or her grief, and enabling the process of mourning to occur by providing practical help (child care, financial advice, etc.), may be as important as counselling in helping the children. It may be also appropriate to offer support, supervision and guidance to other adults involved in the child's life such as teachers and religious leaders.

The therapeutic elements of appropriate interventions include the promotion of communication within the family about the dead parent, the promotion of mourning through reminiscing, the appropriate expression of feelings, and making sense of the death. An overview of techniques used directly with children and young people is provided by Stokes.[23] Techniques for use with children, many of which can be done in groups, include:

◆ Using art and story-telling

◆ Writing letters to the deceased

◆ Creating memory boxes to store reminders of the deceased

◆ Rituals (such as lighting candles, releasing balloons)

◆ Making something that represents different aspects of the person (e.g. salt statues of different colours)

◆ Playing games which encourage children to open up

◆ Role playing

As with all direct interventions with children, the choice of which techniques to use depends upon the child factors such as age and intelligence, the therapist's or counsellor's training, skill, and experience, the nature of the therapeutic relationship and the organizational context. These interventions can be provided by carefully selected, well-trained and well-supervized volunteers. As part of an intervention, young children may require help to understand what has happened to the deceased by offering a careful and sensitive explanation of what death means in straight-forward biological terms ensuring that the child understands what they are being told. They may also need help to recognize, understand and cope with sad affects both in themselves and in the surviving family members.

Given the indications that problems may develop much later, a useful intervention strategy should include follow-up appointments after any time-limited intervention. Children who have been prepared for the death of a family member have been shown to fare better, in terms of anxiety levels, than those who have not.[24]

## Conclusion

Bereavement in childhood, particularly the loss of a parent, represents a significant adversity, although the majority of bereaved children do not develop anything other than transient symptoms. Nevertheless, there is evidence that a brief preventive intervention can reduce subsequent morbidity. Children, who lose a parent through suicide, homicide, accident, or disaster, especially if they have witnessed the death, are at high risk of developing post-traumatic stress disorder and other psychiatric disorders and their treatment needs should be assessed by mental health professionals.

## Further information

Dyregrov A (1991). *Grief in children: a handbook for adults.* London, Jessica Kingsley Publishers.

Cohen JA, Mannarino AP, Deblinger E (2006). *Treating Trauma and Traumatic Grief in Children and Adolescents.* New York, The Guilford Press.

Various useful resources for professionals, parents, carers and bereaved young people and children are provided by the UK child bereavement charities: The Child Bereavement charity (www.childbereavement.org. uk) and Winston's Wish (www.winstonswish.org.uk).

*Help is at Hand: A resource for people bereaved by suicide and other sudden, traumatic death.* This booklet is published by the National Health Service in the UK, and provides particularly good advice for parents of suddenly bereaved children. www.dh.gov.uk/assetroot/04/13/90/07/04139007.pdf

## References

1. Parkes, C.M. (2006). *Love and Loss: The Roots of Grief and its Complications.* London and New York, Routledge.

2. UNICEF (2006). *Africa's Orphaned and Vulnerable Generations: Children Affected by AIDS.* Geneva: UNICEF, UNAIDS and PEPFAR.

3. Bowlby, J. (1980). *Attachment and Loss.* London, Hogarth Press.

4. Rutter, M. (1972). *Maternal Deprivation Reassessed.* Harmondsworth, Penguin.

5. Dowdney, L. (2000). Annotation: Childhood Bereavement Following Parental Death. *Journal of Child Psychology and Psychiatry,* **41,** 819–30.

6. Harrington, R. (1999). Unproven assumptions about the impact of bereavement on children. *Journal of the Royal Society of Medicine,* **92,** 230–3.

7. Bifulco, A., Harris, T., and Brown, GW. (1992). Mourning or early inadequate care? Re-examining the relationship of maternal loss in childhood with adult depression and anxiety. *Developmental Psychopathology,* **4,** 433–49.

8. Lau, J.Y.F., Rijksdijk, F.V., Gregory, A.M., *et al.* (2008). Pathways to childhood depressive symptoms: The role of social cognitive and genetic risk factors. *Developmental Psychology,* **43,** 1402–14.

9. Parkes, C.M., Laungani, P., and Young, B. (eds.) (1997). *Death and bereavement across cultures.* London, Routledge.

10. Furman, E. (1974). *A child's parent dies.* New Haven, CT, Yale University Press.

11. Slaughter, V. (2005). Young children's understanding of death. *Australian Psychologist,* **40**(3), 179–86.

12. Cathcart, F. (1988). Seeing the body after death (editorial). *British Medical Journal,* **297,** 997–8.

13. Dyregrov, A. (2008). *Grief in children: a handbook for adults (2nd edn).* London, Jessica Kingsley Publishers.

14. Kloeppel, D., and Hollins, S. (1989). Double Handicap: mental retardation and death in the family. *Death Studies,* **13,** 31–8.

15. Everatt, A., and Gale, I. (2004). Children with learning disabilities and bereavement: A review of the literature and its implications. *Educational and Child Psychology,* **21**(3), 30–40.

16. Cohen, J.A., Mannarino, A.P., and Deblinger, E. (2006). *Treating Trauma and Traumatic Grief in Children and Adolescents.* New York, The Guilford Press.

17. Harris-Hendriks, J., Black, D., and Kaplan, T. (2000). *When Father Kills Mother.* Second edition. London, Routledge.

18. Pettle, M.S., and Lansdown, R. (1986). Adjustment to the death of a sibling. *Archives of Diseases of Childhood,* **61**(3), 278–83.

19. Hogan, N., and DeSantis, L. (1996). Adolescent sibling bereavement. In *Handbook of adolescent death and bereavement* (eds. C. Corr, D. Balk), pp. 173–95. New York, Springer.

20. Brent, D., Perper, J., Moritz, G., *et al.* (1992). Psychiatric effects of exposure to suicide among the friends and acquaintances of adolescent suicide victims. *Journal of the American Academy of Child and Adolescent Psychiatry,* **31,** 629–39.

21. Black, D., and Urbanowicz, M.A. (1987). Family intervention with bereaved children. *Journal of Child Psychology and Psychiatry,* **28,** 467–76.

22. Schut, H., and Stroebe, M. (accepted for publication). Interventions to Enhance Adaptation to Bereavement: A Review of Efficacy Studies. *The Lancet.*

23. Stokes, J.A. (2004). *Then, now and Always.* Cheltenham, Winston's Wish.

24. Rosenheim, E., Reicher, R. (1985). Informing children about a parent's terminal illness. *Journal of Child Psychology and Psychiatry,* **26,** 995–8.

## 9.4

# The child as witness

Anne E. Thompson and John B. Pearce

## Introduction

In the last 20 years, many societies have paid greater attention to children's rights and the importance of protecting children from abuse. As perpetrators of abuse have been tried in court, so more children have been called as witnesses. From being described as 'the most dangerous of all witnesses', children have become recognized to be able to provide valuable and credible testimony in the correct circumstances. Many jurisdictions are now making allowances for children so that their testimony can be delivered in court as fully and accurately as possible. It is no longer tenable to dismiss the capacity of a child to be a witness in court simply because of their age. **Children may be less reliable, as reliable, or more reliable than adult witnesses, depending on a variety of developmental and environmental factors.**

## Developmental considerations for children as witnesses

### Memory is immature below the age of 12

In the first 3 years of life recall is via preverbal memory (sometimes called eidetic memory), which allows early events to be recalled visually but not in words. Preverbal memory is very accurate but is largely lost around the age of 3 years as language develops. This form of memory remains longer in children who have delayed language development. The loss of this early form of memory explains why **adults do not usually have conscious memories from the first 3 years of life**. It is only around the age of 3 years that experiences begin to be memorized in 'explicit memory', which is accessed by verbal recall.[1] Memories laid down in explicit memory are organized according to hierarchical cognitive structures formed by the child's past experiences of the world. In young children, this organization is rudimentary. This means that new memories are stored with little selection or adaptation to reflect preconceptions, and **in younger children the retrieval of stored memories from poorly organized mental representations is difficult**. External prompts and cues help children recall more fully but in court witnesses are not generally allowed to be 'led' by questioning.

Younger children are more likely than older children to forget information over time. **By the age of 12 years, children are generally considered to have the same capacities to lay down memories and recall information as adults**.

Surprisingly, children's **immature memories can sometimes actually improve the quality of information provided in witness statements**. For example, events may be memorized without being influenced by the prejudices that affect adult perceptions, and seemingly trivial details may be memorized by a child whose primitive cognitive schemas allow incoming sensory information to be memorized unselectively.[2] However, cognitive **immaturity more often acts as a barrier to children giving their testimonies fully and accurately**, especially when they are asked to talk about what they remember, rather than being allowed to communicate by behaviour or play.

### Children's expectations of adults in conversation influence testimony

By the age of 6 years, many children are using the syntax and grammar of adults in their spoken language. However, their vocabulary is still limited and they are **easily confused by sophisticated or complex speech**. A particularly important aspect of language development for child witnesses is the role played by children and adults in conversational partnerships. **Children are used to being co-operative partners when talking with adults**. They attempt to please by providing answers to questions, even if they do not know the answer or have not understood the question.[3] Young children rarely answer 'I don't know' to a question they are uncertain about and prefer to give a false 'yes' or 'no'. This willingness to provide an answer is probably encouraged by the frequent experience of being 'tested' by adults who already know the answers to the question (for example, 'Look at this picture! Can you see the duck?' or 'How many sweets am I holding?'). As children expect adults to know the answers to their questions, and if a question is repeated, children may change the answer they gave in the assumption that the questioner feels it to be wrong. **The readiness of young children to please adults in conversation no doubt adds to their suggestibility.**

## Young children are particularly suggestible

The suggestibility of children as witnesses has been a major concern in legal arenas. Modern research does not endorse the stereotype of the child witness as being highly suggestible. However, there is clear evidence that both children and adults are prone to suggestion at times, and that **pre-school children are particularly vulnerable to this**. The necessity to avoid suggesting information or answers to a child has led to the development of guidelines for interviewing child witnesses in several jurisdictions.

## Immature moral development is not always a problem

According to Kohlberg's seminal description of children's moral development, children below 10 years of age operate with 'pre-conventional morality' and evaluate events according to whether the child themselves will gain reward or avoid punishment. Only after this age do children develop 'conventional morality' and begin to be motivated by the approval of other people and society. Therefore, **only older child witnesses have a full understanding of their moral obligations in court**. However, young children, who may hold concrete worldviews such as 'bad people must be punished' as moral imperatives, may be strongly motivated to tell the truth in court.

## Children do not lie more than adults, but their lies are more easily detected

Contrary to popular belief, children above the age of 3 years have no more difficulty than adults in distinguishing fact from fantasy. Neither do children tell more lies than adults (although children's lies are more often unconvincing and therefore more easily discovered). **Children and adults are motivated to lie for similar reasons.**[4] The two motives for lying, which may particularly influence child witnesses asked to testify in cases of child abuse, are fear of personal recrimination and a wish to protect those to whom a child feels loyal.

## Immature sense of time and short attention span influence testimony

**Before 8 years of age, children do not generally have a clear sense of time.** Young children therefore often have a muddled recollection of the timing of events and they may have difficulty saying how many times an event occurred. Similarly, **children below this age have short attention spans,** and readily become bored or overwhelmed by prolonged questioning. Both of these developmental limitations can cause difficulties in the preparation of witness statements when a child appears in court.

## Traumatic memories may be recalled with more or less clarity

Many of the events child witnesses are called upon to remember were unpleasant and frightening at the time. These events will have been experienced in a state of high emotional arousal. Clinical experience suggests that **emotional arousal can either enhance or diminish recalled information**. For example, extremely traumatic events such as watching a parent being killed can be remembered by child witnesses in a series of highly accurate and detailed visual images that persist in memory over time. By contrast, some children process potentially overwhelming experiences using a variety of psychological defense mechanisms, which limit the amount and

**Table 9.4.1** Guidelines for interviewing child witnesses

- Allowing a child to talk freely without being questioned maximizes the chances of accurate recall
- Questioning children may elicit additional information but lessen accuracy
- Accuracy is greatest when children give their statements as soon as an event occurred
- Children's accounts are most likely to be accurate when they tell the story for the first time
- Children are less likely to give a full account if they feel under pressure from the interviewer
- Younger children may attempt to please an interviewer by providing information even if it is untrue

accuracy of material available in explicit memory. The psychological trauma associated with the witnessed event and the emotional state of the child during subsequent recall are both likely to have an influence on a child's capacity to give evidence in court.

# Environmental considerations for children as witnesses

## Skilled interviewing is essential

Because of their developmental immaturity, child witnesses face many disadvantages in the legal system, but these can be substantially offset by a skilled interviewer. Not only must an interviewer facilitate a child to say as much as he or she can remember, but the interview must be conducted so that its process and content will be considered to be acceptable evidence by the court.[5] Psychological research guides the practice of interviewing child witnesses. Some principles are outlined in Table 9.4.1.

## Helpful adjustments to legal standards and courtroom process

Many jurisdictions have now made allowances for the developmental and emotional needs of children appearing in court as witnesses. Some legal systems have **relaxed their rules of evidence** where children are concerned so that hearsay evidence (in other words, reports from other people about what a child said or did) may be admissible and lawyers may be allowed to ask child witnesses leading questions. The detrimental effect of extreme stress on children's abilities to give accurate and credible evidence in court is well recognized. A variety of actions have therefore been taken by courts to make a child witness's appearance in court less stressful. The **courtroom may be rearranged to be less formal** and professionals may not wear gowns or wigs. The public may be excluded from courtrooms. Means of **preventing the child from having to face the accused** such as the use of screens or a live video-link to the child in a separate room may be used. Although many professionals agree that children generally find giving evidence by video-link less stressful than giving their entire evidence in open court, there is concern that the child's testimony may have less impact on a jury when viewed on video.[6]

## Child witnesses need extra support in the courtroom

There is no doubt that **children find appearing in court a stressful event**. Typical concerns of child witnesses are shown in Table 9.4.2. Feelings of anxiety, confusion, humiliation, embarrassment, and the fear of retaliation or of not being believed

**Table 9.4.2** Children giving evidence are often concerned about[7]

◆ People shouting at them in court
◆ Not understanding the questions
◆ Not being believed
◆ Giving 'wrong' answers
◆ Speaking in front of strangers
◆ Crying while giving evidence
◆ Needing to go to the toilet

(Reproduced from Hamilton, C. Working with young people: legal responsibility and liability, pp. 102–6, copyright 2005, The Children's Legal Centre.)

are common. The stress of appearing in court may be a further trauma for a child who was first traumatized by witnessing or experiencing the alleged crime in question. Some children report that although giving evidence was stressful, they also derived some satisfaction from playing their part in bringing a perpetrator to justice.

Anxiety created by the unfamiliarity of the surroundings and a lack of knowledge about what is happening in the courtroom can be addressed by **preparing child witnesses for their appearance in court**. Preparation often involves visiting the courthouse, receiving age-appropriate written information about the court process, and having the opportunity to ask questions. Ideally, the professional who prepares the child should be available to attend court with the child on the day of the trial. Some helpful information for child witnesses is shown in Table 9.4.3.

### Receiving therapy prior to being a witness

Many child witnesses have been traumatized by witnessing or experiencing the alleged crime to which they will testify. Some of these children will develop emotional or behavioural problems as a result of the trauma and will be referred to child and adolescent mental health services. Treatment of trauma-related symptoms usually involves recounting the past experiences in a therapeutic setting. At this point **a conflict of interests arises between the needs of the child as a patient and as a witness**. The psychotherapeutic treatment of traumatized children centres on eliciting the child's subjective truth by the therapist using a variety of means to encourage communication. Within the legal system, the child's recollection of events must be examined in a neutral setting to determine the objective truth, while the rights of both the accused and the witness are protected. Therapy is seen as potentially detrimental to child witnesses because of the potential for their recollections

**Table 9.4.3** A child appearing as a witness in court should know that[7]

◆ They have not done anything wrong
◆ They should always tell the truth
◆ They can take time to answer a question
◆ They should speak to the judge as clearly as possible
◆ Its OK to answer a question by saying 'I don't know' or 'I don't remember'
◆ Its OK to answer a question by saying 'I don't understand'
◆ They must not guess or make up an answer

(Reproduced from Hamilton, C. Working with young people: legal responsibility and liability, pp. 102–6, copyright 2005, The Children's Legal Centre.)

to be altered by repetition or suggestion. The very fact that a child needs psychiatric help may be used to discredit the child as a witness in the eyes of the jury.

If a child witness clearly requires psychological or psychiatric treatment and cannot wait for many months until the trial is over for the treatment to begin, mental health professionals should discuss the child's needs with a representative of the legal service. **The therapy may be allowed to proceed with some restrictions about what can be discussed**. The therapist should be prepared to be called to court themselves in order to give evidence about the nature of their work. **The court will want to be satisfied that the child has not been coached by the therapist or told about information given by other witnesses.**

### Children's testimony is worth hearing

The status of child witnesses has improved considerably in the last 20 years. Modern psychological research shows that although most children under 3 years of age lack the cognitive capacities to be competent witnesses, many older children are able to produce useful evidential information provided they are questioned competently. To make full use of what children can remember, they need to be allowed to talk in a comfortable setting, guided by professionals who are sensitive to developmental issues and aware of legal constraints. Child witnesses have often been traumatized by their experience. It is important that further distress caused by appearing in court is kept to a minimum and that children who need therapeutic help to deal with their trauma are not denied access to this in the pre-trial period.

## Further information

www.childrenslegalcentre.com

www.victimsupport.org.uk

http://www.homeoffice.gov.uk/justice/what-happens-at-court/being-a-witness

http://www.homeoffice.gov.uk/documents/achieving-best-evidence/guidance-witnesses.pdf

## References

1. Fundudis, T. (1997). Young children's memory: how good is it? How much do we know about it? *Child Psychology and Psychiatry Review*, **2**, 150–8.
2. Terr, L.C. (1986). The child psychiatrist and the child witness: traveling companions by necessity, if not by design. *Journal of the American Academy of Child Psychiatry*, **25**, 462–72.
3. Ceci, S.J. and Bruck, M. (1993). Suggestibility of the child witness: a historical review and synthesis. *Psychological Bulletin*, **113**, 403–39.
4. Flin, R. and Spencer, J.R. (1995). Annotation: children as witnesses—legal and psychological perspectives. *Journal of Child Psychology and Psychiatry*, **36**, 171–89.
5. Saywitz, K. and Camparo, L. (1998). Interviewing child witnesses: a developmental perspective. *Child Abuse and Neglect*, **22**, 825–43.
6. Williams, G.A. (1998). Video technology and children's evidence: international perspectives and recent research. *Medicine and Law*, **17**, 263–81.
7. Hamilton C. (2005). *Working with young people: legal responsibility and liability*, pp. 102–6. The Children's Legal Centre, Colchester.

# 9.5

# Treatment methods for children and adolescents

## Contents

9.5.1 Counselling and psychotherapy for children
John B. Pearce

9.5.2 Psychodynamic child pscyhotherapy
Peter Fonagy and Mary Target

9.5.3 Cognitive behaviour therapies
for children and families
Philip Graham

9.5.4 Caregiver-mediated interventions
for children and families
Philip A. Fisher and Elizabeth A. Stormshak

9.5.5 Medication for children and
adolescents: current issues
Paramala J. Santosh

9.5.6 Residential care for social reasons
Leslie Hicks and Ian Sinclair

9.5.7 Organization of services for children and
adolescents with mental health problems
Miranda Wolpert

9.5.8 The management of child and
adolescent psychiatric emergencies
Gillian Forrest

9.5.9 The child psychiatrist as consultant
to schools and colleges
Simon G. Gowers and Sian Thomas

## 9.5.1 Counselling and psychotherapy for children

John B. Pearce

### Introduction

There is a remarkable lack of high quality research to support an evidence base for counselling and psychotherapy for children.
And the words 'psychotherapy' and 'counselling' are so non-specific that they should always be clarified in more detail. Nevertheless, these approaches are used frequently in child mental health. While most psychotherapeutic approaches are based on work with adults it is important to note that there are marked differences between children and adults. In spite of these obvious differences, psychotherapy for children is usually based on techniques used for adults. However, psychotherapy that may work perfectly well for adults has to be modified to accord with the developmental level of each child.

### Definitions

We each have a mental image of 'a child'. Often this is a stereotypical child aged about 5 to 10 years old. But the word 'childhood' covers the whole period from birth to adulthood, and of course every adult is also somebody's child. In this chapter **the term 'child' will be used to refer to anyone who is not an adult**, but who has matured sufficiently to develop a clear concept of themselves as individuals and of the nature of the real world around them. The ability to distinguish fact from fantasy is an important prerequisite for psychotherapy. This develops as a gradual process with an important stage at around 2.5 years of age when children normally start to refer to themselves as 'I' for the first time. Another stage occurs around 7 to 8 years of age when children develop a clear understanding of time and of the real world. If the therapist ignores these developmental issues it is likely that treatment will be harmful rather than helpful.

Psychotherapy is a very general term that implies treatment of mental dysfunction by psychological rather than physical methods. The aim is to improve function by changing cognition and emotions through the therapeutic relationship, by means of language, play, art, or drama. Dynamic child psychotherapy can be defined as a highly specialized technique where the primary aim is to explore a child's conscious and unconscious thoughts, feelings, and conflicts in such a way that inner resources become strengthened and enabled. It is child-led so that the child is able to follow and explore his or her own agenda, thus helping the child to make sense of the world and to find his or her own solutions to problems and dilemmas. Therapy is mediated by language, which can either be verbal or non-verbal and may use play or creative activities such as drawing, painting, and modelling. Counselling children is very similar, but the therapist usually takes a more passive role than in psychotherapy and would not be so concerned with the interpretation of unconscious processes. Cognitive behaviour therapy on the other hand is a highly structured approach focused on challenging false cognitions in order to change behaviour and emotions. It is an approach that can be rather easily adapted to children and made sufficiently enjoyable to engage their interest and cooperation.

## Differences from adult psychotherapy

A number of **interesting paradoxes and dilemmas** occur when treating children with psychotherapy (Table 9.5.1.1). For example, who should give consent for treatment. Should it be the child, a parent, both parents, or all three? Clearly, this depends on the age and understanding of the child, and each case should be approached in a way that puts the child's needs first. It is generally best to obtain consent from the child and both parents. Any other arrangement is likely to lead to problems at some stage. Psychotherapy and counselling are traditionally non-directive and patient-led, but children, unlike most adults, need to be given some direction otherwise they become easily lost and confused. They cannot be expected to find their own solutions without guidance and support. Most psychotherapeutic approaches for adults are based on coming to terms with and finding explanations for problems that are rooted in the past. However, children are still busy making their past, and their main focus of concern and interest is the present and the immediate future. A further dilemma in child psychotherapy concerns the management of the transference relationship between therapist and patient, which is a reflection of the parent–child relationship. A high degree of trust has to be established to use transference effectively. At the same time, it could be argued that it is not really appropriate for young children to develop high levels of trust and dependence on a therapist whom they only meet briefly in very artificial circumstances. Thus any interpretation of the transference relationship in child psychotherapy must be done carefully and with a good understanding of the subtle complexities of a child's dependency on the parent.

Adult psychotherapy is usually based on a single theoretical model that explains mental mechanisms. Children, however, benefit from the freedom to experiment with a number of different models of their inner world and to learn how to use these ideas in a flexible and constructive way. The use of a single-theory therapy in child psychotherapy is best avoided.

## Counselling and psychotherapy

There are undoubtedly differences between child psychotherapy and counselling, but they are difficult to define precisely. This may

**Table 9.5.1.1** Differences between children and adults in relation to therapy

Consent for treatment usually given by parent/carer rather than child

Child may nor understand or want therapy

Children need more help with problem solving than adults

Therapy should be relatively more directive and instructive

Problems tend to be rooted in present or recent past

Therapy should be mostly enjoyable for child to benefit

Transference is complicated because children live with and need parents/carers

Different approaches needed at various stages of development

Children are developing and changing quickly so therapy needs to do this too

be because there is a continuum of therapeutic interventions, from advice and guidance at one end of a therapeutic spectrum through more specific counselling and psychotherapeutic techniques to intensive child psychoanalysis at the other end. Counselling children requires a high level of skill, but less theory and technique than in psychotherapy, and it is focused primarily on normal reactions to abnormal events.

Psychotherapy is directed more at psychopathology than normal reactions to stress. It is therefore essential to know about the normal range of children's responses to life events. For example, a 5-year-old child whose mother has just died will grieve differently from a 10-year-old child, because at 5 years of age most children have not yet developed a clear concept of death. Grief in a 5-year-old is most strongly influenced by the way the adults around the child react to the death, whereas a grieving 10-year-old child, although responsive to guidance from the adults around, will also have his or her own unique way of coping with grief. As a general rule, the younger the child the more important it is to consider the attitude and mental state of the parents.

## Other psychotherapies

Dynamic psychotherapy based on the theories of Sigmund Freud and his daughter Anna Freud,[1] Melanie Klein,[2] and others has been the mainstay of individual child therapy. More recently, Virginia Axline[3] adapted the ideas that Carl Rogers[4] applied to counselling (trust, genuineness and understanding) and developed 'play therapy' as a specific technique for children. Subsequently, brief psychotherapy and interpersonal therapy have grown out of the need to update psychodynamic methods. Various forms of cognitive therapy are now increasingly used for children, although they were originally developed for the treatment of adults by Beck.[5] These therapies focus on a problem-solving approach to resolve current issues, rather than on resolving unconscious conflicts based in the past.

## Natural emotional healing

Counselling and psychotherapy have been used with increasing frequency to help children cope with traumatic events such as death, divorce, abuse, illness, and so on. It is arguable whether this trend is at all helpful. Fortunately, the human psyche is remarkably resilient and there are powerful healing processes that take time, which in most cases achieve a satisfactory result. There are similarities between the way the body and mind respond to trauma and a strong correspondence between the natural healing processes that accompany both physical and emotional trauma. The initial healing process starts with a brief period where no pain or distress is felt whatever the cause of the trauma, and this is often accompanied by disbelief that such a thing could have happened. This first phase of shock and 'denial' is then replaced by the full impact of what has happened and is accompanied by high levels of physical or emotional pain. During the second phase the pain may be so severe that it interferes with everyday life, but this stage is usually over within 2 weeks. In the third stage, the healing process continues for a period of up to 6 weeks when the emotional or physical wound is normally healed sufficiently for the traumatized person to be able to return to everyday life, albeit with continuing pain and discomfort at times. The final phase of the healing process then continues over the next 6 to 12 months, leaving a scar that will always remain.

Routine counselling following traumatic events carries the risk of interfering with this normal healing process. Psychotherapy could also be misused to check that all is well, rather like opening up a wound unnecessarily, which will only serve to delay the healing process and might even introduce a secondary 'infection'. The parallel between physical and emotional healing provides some guidelines as to when and how counselling and psychotherapy should be used, as well as the dangers that can occur when they are misused.

## The use of play in therapy

The fact that **children are still developing language and communication skills** means that play is often useful as a method of communicating in a therapeutic way with children. Play is essential for normal development. It helps children to develop a repertoire of responses and encourages behavioural flexibility. The main developmental stages of play need to be appreciated if it is to be used in an effective way in either counselling or psychotherapy (see Table 9.5.1.2).

Children will play with almost anything, and so the choice of play materials for use in psychotherapy requires careful thought. It is best to select toys that encourage imagination and creativity. It is important to remember that the type of play equipment provided will actually constrain the way the child plays. For example, there is a limit to what cars or toy animals can do. Similarly, a set of family dolls may have their usefulness restricted if there are not enough of them to represent all the key figures in the child's life. A thoughtful and appropriate choice of toys and play materials including drawing, modelling, and painting equipment can make the difference between the success and failure to engage a child in therapy.

Children's play can be a pointer to what is going on in the child's mind (either conscious or unconscious), but it can also mislead. A child's play will only give a very general indication of what the child thinks and feels and will not provide precise information. Perhaps the best way of viewing the use of play in therapy is that it is an aid to communication—and no more than that.

## The treatment setting

There are a number of steps that can be taken to make the treatment setting more beneficial for the child and help to create a relaxed atmosphere. How the therapy and the therapist are introduced to the child is of some importance. The attitude of the therapist is undoubtedly more important than the way the therapy room is organized and the more anxious and tentative the introduction,

**Table 9.5.1.2** The development of children's play

| Age | Type of play |
| --- | --- |
| 12–18 months | Symbolic play (e.g. block of wood is a car) |
| 18 months–3 years | Imaginary play (e.g. blocks become a family) |
| 3–7 years | Imaginary friends in 30 per cent of children |
| 5–7 years | Rule-governed make-believe games |
| 7 years onwards | Imagination founded much more strongly on the real world |

the more uneasy the child will be. There are no hard and fast rules about the duration or frequency of the treatment session. It is best to arrange it to suit the child. Some children find more than 20 min with an adult extremely difficult to cope with whatever their age. Many children find the formal structure of therapy quite stressful and it may help to put the child at ease by talking about unimportant issues before the session itself begins. Anxiety can also be reduced by organizing the sessions to be as predictable as possible in place and time. Making it clear to children that the therapeutic time is specially for them and that they are the focus of all their therapist's attention can also motivate children to be more co-operative and to be less wary.

## The treatment process

Each child's experiences of distress must always be considered in the context of the child's family circumstances, the child's stage of development, and his or her temperamental characteristics. It follows that the therapeutic approach needs to be individually tailored and adjusted for each child. Nevertheless, it is possible to arrive at some general guidelines that will assist in treatment. The concern, interest, and supportive attitude of the therapist is central to the treatment process, since it is the interaction between the child's need and the adult's response that establishes the transference relationship.

The start of the first session is particularly important because it sets the tone for the future treatment. The child should know the role that the therapist has and what the aims of the treatment are. Something needs to be said about the limits to behaviour in the session and the nature and degree of confidentiality. It is important to remember that complete confidentiality cannot be assured. For example, the therapist may be presented with information that concerns the health or safety of the child as in the case of abuse, where information has to be disclosed for the benefit of the child.

The timing and number of sessions needs to be agreed at this stage. Therefore it is often a good idea to suggest a limited number of sessions in the first instance, together with an agreement to review whether or not further sessions are required. This type of introduction helps children to feel their needs are being taken seriously, especially if they are actively involved in the process. Sessions should start and finish on time and the links between the present and any previous sessions should be clarified.

Most children will remember their treatment experience for many years to come—if not for the rest of their lives. The child who feels uncomfortable, embarrassed, and misunderstood is likely to retain a memory that is painful and unhelpful. On the other hand, if the therapeutic experience was positive, where the therapist was seen as supportive, encouraging, and understanding, the memory is likely to be one that the child returns to again and again for emotional strength and support.

## Different approaches to psychotherapy

There is a wide variety of jargon associated with various types of psychotherapy. Each approach has its own 'language' and associated special techniques. However, there is no evidence that any one method is better than another, and it would appear that the personal preference of the professional involved is more important in determining which approach is used rather than the characteristics of the child. Whichever approach is used it is likely that there will be the same common themes in the focus of treatment. Common themes include dealing with feelings of anxiety and insecurity, difficulties in relationships, low self-esteem, and a feeling of failure. These emotions are often generated by difficulties with aggression, jealousy, sexuality, and death.

### A focus on the past versus the present

The child comes to psychotherapy with a range of problems rooted in the past. A decision has to be made whether to focus the therapy on trying to understand and come to terms with the past, or to consider how a child might best cope with what is actually happening in the here and now. **The danger** in concentrating primarily on the past is that it may interfere with the child's ability to cope with the present and plan for the future. While it is important to learn from what has happened in the past, children tend to learn more from what is happening in the present in their daily lives. Understanding how their emotional stress was generated in the first place may not lead to a resolution or to a greater ability to deal with current problems. It is generally helpful to start therapy with an acknowledgement of what has happened in the past and a consideration of how that might affect what is happening in the present. In a few cases it may be helpful to focus more on the past, but only if the child has clearly become preoccupied with a particular issue from the past and is unable to move on. Normal development moves on so rapidly during childhood that any fixation with the past can have serious consequences, thus every effort needs to be made to promote and sustain developmental progress.

### Theory vs. common humanity

While it is undoubtedly helpful to have a theoretical framework within which treatment can take place, the observation that different psychotherapeutic approaches for the same type of problem can be equally effective suggests that the precise theoretical framework underpinning treatment may not be that important. The basic human qualities of kindness, trust, caring and understanding are perhaps the most important qualities in psychotherapy. It is not an unusual experience for therapists to find that their early cases turn out to be the most successful, which is probably due to the enthusiasm and therapeutic optimism of the new therapist. It is clearly important to hold on to these therapeutic qualities as one becomes more experienced.

### Supportive counselling vs. in-depth psychoanalysis

It is easy to assume that the more intensive the psychotherapy and the more it explores the deep unconscious world, the more effective it must be. Clearly there is no reason why this should be the case. For example, one would not expect a surgeon to cut deeper for greater effect or a physician to prescribe more medication than is necessary. This would only increase the adverse effects of the treatment. It is not difficult to see that regular psychoanalysis two or three times per week could be quite disruptive to family life merely as a result of the time commitment alone. There are also other potential problems for children who are treated with intensive psychoanalysis over a period of years, as this may delay or shape a child's development in an unhelpful way. On the other hand, it might be equally inappropriate to commence supportive counselling for a child who is deeply disturbed and whose need for

loving care and protection is not being met. These primary and basic needs must always be given priority.

### Cognitive therapy vs. psychoanalytically based psychotherapies

There has been an increased interest in cognitive therapy and cognitive behaviour therapy, where the emphasis is much more on the here and now and the behavioural consequences of abnormal thought patterns. The techniques used in cognitive therapy for anxiety and depressive disorder are described in Chapters 6.3.2.1 and 6.3.2.3 respectively. The only modification that is required for their use in children is to adapt them to the developmental stage and the level of cognitive ability that the child has reached. Cognitive therapy has a theoretical advantage for use in children in that its focus is more on the present and the future, in contrast to most psychoanalytically based psychotherapy. Its approach is strongly based on learning new ways of coping. Cognitive therapy is pragmatic and active rather than passive and reflective, making it generally more appropriate for the needs of younger children. Unfortunately, there is as yet limited evidence to support the theoretical underpinning of the various cognitive models of childhood disorders.

### Limit setting vs. free expression

It is a common dilemma to know how much freedom children should be allowed to express themselves. Some children appear to enjoy pushing the limits to see how far they can go. Other children appear too inhibited and need encouragement to express themselves. Part of the art of child therapy is to strike a comfortable balance between control and freedom. Children gain nothing from disruptive and destructive behaviour, even if they normally tend to be quiet and inhibited. Indeed, they rapidly develop overwhelming feelings of anxiety and insecurity if they do not feel sufficiently contained. It is essential that the therapist retains a very clear notion of what behaviour is acceptable and what is not. It is therefore the therapist's responsibility to set the scene and establish the boundaries of acceptable behaviour within the therapeutic context. Should the child go beyond the limit then a warning should be given, and if the child persists it is quite acceptable to end the session early or at least until the disruptive behaviour has stopped. The therapist's reaction to bad behaviour should make it quite clear that it is unacceptable. However, the emotional response should be neutral or sad, in much the same way that one might behave in a shoe shop when a desirable new shoe does not fit as expected.

### Closeness vs. distance

It is natural for an adult to be physically much closer to younger children and then to become more distant as they grow older. For example, it is quite natural for an adult to hold the hand of a 3- or 4-year old and to physically guide the child. On the other hand, any physical contact with a teenager can easily be misconstrued and is likely to be most unwelcome. In addition to the developmental perspective, every child has its own preferred degree of closeness or distance from other people. The task of the therapist is to judge what is right for each occasion. It is absolutely essential that the therapist must always avoid intruding into the child's space in any way that could be construed as abusive. This may prove difficult where children are unsure of their boundaries and seek out physical contact (in cases of sexual abuse, children may seek out sexual contact). However, to maintain an artificial physical or emotional distance can be perceived as disinterest or even rejection by some children. To achieve a comfortable level of emotional warmth and physical closeness in therapy is obviously a very important matter, but a relaxed approach in the therapeutic relationship is generally best.

### Individual vs. group therapy

There are no agreed guidelines to determine which child would benefit from an individual or from a group approach to psychotherapy. Some children, however, find the emotional intensity of undivided adult attention too much to cope with and learn better from others in a group situation. As the selection of cases for group psychotherapy tends to be determined by the therapist's skills, there is no clear evidence that one approach is better than any other. Nevertheless, there is a growing literature on group therapy for children and an increasing interest in this method of treatment if only because the cost per case is likely to be less.

## Practical issues in child psychotherapy

### Involving parents and the school

The younger the child, the more helpful it is to involve the parents in treatment. How this is managed will depend to some extent on the resources available. It is generally best for separate therapists to work with the child and with the parents. However, there will usually be occasions when it is helpful for the child's therapist to have some direct contact with the parents as a way of monitoring progress and keeping a link between the therapy sessions and the child's real world. As children grow older they tend to become increasingly inhibited by the involvement of their parents, so it is helpful to check with the young person how they would like the contact with their parents to be organized. All children should be considered in the context of the family and the school because so many risk factors are associated with these environments. Parental support for the treatment is a critical factor in a successful outcome. Equally, it is possible for parents to undermine treatment by their negative comments or overintrusiveness after each session.

The extent to which a child's school should be involved needs to be carefully considered on an individual basis. Although it is best to have the full co-operation of the school, this may not be possible.

### Confidentiality and record-keeping

Confidentiality in relation to the individual therapy sessions is clearly important, but it should not dominate. The most vital issue is that the children feel safe in what they say and do during the session. They need to know that there is a reasonable level of confidentiality. However, there are obvious exceptions to the general rule of confidentiality: for example, in cases of child abuse or criminal activity, or in cases where the child may be at risk from harming itself. A suitable compromise is to indicate to the child that their session would be treated as confidential, but there may be occasions when it is best to inform their parents or somebody else about important information that was given during the session. This would only occur after discussion between the therapist and the child—the overarching rule is that it must be in the best interest of the child.

There is obviously a need for accurate record-keeping for each session, partly to keep track of the therapeutic process and also for medico-legal purposes. It is unnecessary to include the more detailed recording of the therapeutic process in the official notes if the record is purely for training purposes. These training notes then remain the property of the therapist and must be kept at the same level of security as the official notes.

### Failure to attend

If there is a genuine and legitimate reason why a child is unable to attend for a therapy session then little or no importance needs be attached to this. On the other hand, if therapy sessions are cancelled repeatedly, cancelled with inadequate excuses, or simply not attended it is essential for the therapist to question whether therapy is actually achieving the original stated goal. Factors such as family disadvantage, parental stress, and the severity of the child's problems all increase the likelihood of failing to complete therapy successfully. It is all too easy to either blame the carers or to rationalize failure to attend as being some problem in the child, rather than an issue that could be due to the therapist. Of course, one good reason for failure to attend is that the child no longer needs to. It is usually unhelpful to send out repeated appointments that are not attended. A reasonable compromise is for one reappointment to be made, then if this is failed for a letter to be sent to the carers or to an older teenager asking them to contact you if further sessions are thought necessary. Occasionally, if treatment is at a very critical stage or if there is high level of concern about the child, it would then be appropriate for more effort to be put into arranging a further appointment.

### Individual and cultural issues

A child's sociocultural background needs to be taken into account when planning therapy. Temperament, age, gender, and intellectual ability are also important factors to be considered. Ethnicity, on the other hand, is probably not that significant an issue. Some children enjoy, and benefit from, the freedom to express themselves openly and with little constraint; others need direction and structure if they are to resolve psychological problems. There is no point in trying to fit the child to the therapy rather than the other way round. One factor that supersedes all cultural and individual factors is that children generally wish to enjoy themselves and to have a good time. They are pleasure-seeking beings who, unlike most adults, see no benefit from the experience of pain and distress of therapy.

### Ending therapy

Bringing therapy to a satisfactory conclusion is more likely to happen if the treatment was well set up in the first place and if achievable goals were agreed. Because it is so easy for therapy to lose its focus, it is helpful to consider how and when the treatment will be concluded at the same time as setting it up. Even if treatment goals have not been achieved it should still be possible to end the therapy on a positive note, identifying areas where self-knowledge has been increased and anything that has been positive in the therapeutic relationship.

## Training and supervision

The objectives of training in psychotherapy are primarily to do with increasing knowledge and understanding of the issues that arise during psychotherapeutic treatment, many of which have been referred to above. It is essential for this to be underpinned by a sound knowledge of child development, but less important for therapy to be founded in any particular psychodynamic theory. The key training method in psychotherapy is the conduct of therapy under supervision. Choosing a supervisor and the role of that supervisor are critically important issues for the trainee therapist, since the relationship between supervisor and trainee mirrors that of the therapist and client even if there is a clear understanding that the purpose of the supervision is not intended to be therapeutic. Most therapists find that supervision continues to be helpful even after they are 'trained'.

## Measures of effectiveness and outcome

There is a lack of high quality research to support an evidence base for counselling and psychotherapy for children. One of the main difficulties in conducting research is in the selection of an adequate control group. Reviews of psychotherapeutic treatments indicate a general improvement in children that persists for many months after the intervention. However, it seems likely that the theoretical basis for the psychotherapeutic approach is less important than the caring and supportive relationship that develops between the child and the therapist.

## Further information

Fitzgerald, M. (1998). Child psychoanalytic psychotherapy. *Advances in Psychiatric Treatment*, **4**, 18–24.

Jacobs, W.J. (2002). Individual and group therapy. In Child and Adolescent Psychiatry (4th edn) (ed M. Rutter, E. Taylor), pp. 983–97. Blackwell Science, Oxford.

Rutter, M., Bishop, D. Pine, D., *et al.* (eds.)(2008). *Rutters's Child and Adolescent Psychiatry* (5th edn.). Blackwell, Oxford.

Roth, A.D. and Fonagy, P. (2005). What works for whom? A critical review of psychotherapy research. Guilford Press. New York.

### Useful web sites

www.youngminds.org.uk
www.psychnet-uk.com
www.babcp.com
www.rcpsych.ac.uk

### References

1. Freud, A. (1974). *Introduction to psychoanalysis.* Hogarth Press, London.
2. Klein, M. (1932). *The psychotherapy of children.* Hogarth Press, London.
3. Axline, V. (1969). *Play therapy.* Ballentine Books, New York.
4. Rogers, C. (1951). *Client centred therapy in current practice: implications and theory.* Houghton Mifflin, New York.
5. Beck, A.T. (1976). *Cognitive therapy and emotional disorders.* International Universities Press. New York.

---

## 9.5.2 Psychodynamic child psychotherapy

Peter Fonagy and Mary Target

## Introduction

Psychodynamic psychotherapy for children is based on a range of assumptions concerning mental functioning that have gradually evolved over the past 100 years out of the theories of Sigmund Freud. As these assumptions have been widely reviewed, we need to provide only a very brief introduction here.

Psychodynamic child clinicians assume that:

(a) The child's presenting difficulties may usefully be seen in terms of thoughts, feelings, wishes, beliefs, and conflicts. This entails the assumption that mental disorders can meaningfully be understood as specific organizations of a child's conscious or unconscious mental states.

(b) To understand conscious experiences, we need to consider non-conscious narrative-like experiences, analogous to conscious fantasies, which powerfully affect behaviour, affect regulation, and the capacity to handle the social environment. Modern neuroscience, with fMRI studies that show cortical response reflecting processing to meaning in the absence of awareness and non-conscious motivation,[1] has put the existence of an unconscious beyond debate.

(c) Intense relationship experiences are represented in the mind as structures of interpersonal interaction, and are aggregated across time before coming to form a schematic mental structure, which is often represented metaphorically as a neural network. Within many models, self-other relationship representations are also considered the organizers of emotion, as feeling states are seen as coming to characterize particular patterns of self-other and interpersonal relating (e.g. sadness and disappointment at the anticipated loss of a person).[2]

(d) Inevitably, wishes, affects and ideas will at times be in conflict with one another. The psychodynamic therapeutic approach sees such conflicts as key causes of distress and the lack of a sense of safety. Adverse environments either increase the intensity of conflict or fail to equip the child with the capacity to resolve such incompatibilities through mental work.[3] They may also set the child on a developmental trajectory in which the normal development of key psychological capacities is undermined, thereby reducing the child's competence to resolve mental conflict.[4] For this reason, while reviewers of psychodynamic psychotherapy often contrast conflict and development-focussed approaches, the reality of developmental trajectories means that the conflict and deficit often come together.[5]

(e) The child's mental mechanisms for dealing with intrapsychic conflict include defence mechanisms that distort mental representations in order to reduce conflict and unpleasure.[6] Such self-serving distortions of mental states relative to an external or internal reality are frequently demonstrated experimentally and have become accepted.[7–10] Classification of defences has frequently been attempted,[11,12] often as a method for categorizing individuals or mental disorders,[13,14] but few of these approaches have stood the test of time or achieved general acceptance.

(f) Behaviour may be understood in terms of 'complex meanings', that is, mental states that are not explicit in action or within the awareness of the person concerned. Thus, symptoms of disorders are classically considered as condensations of conflicting wishes together with the failed defence against conscious awareness of those wishes. Therapy is an effort to seek *personal* meaning,[15] and to elaborate and clarify implicit meaning structures—a process that may turn out to be the essence of psychodynamic psychotherapy—rather than to give the patient insight in terms of any particular meaning structure.

(g) A relationship with a supportive and respectful empathic adult will benefit the young person, not least by enhancing their own understanding and emotional responsiveness. The nature of the relationship with psychodynamic therapists varies across therapies—from the highly transferential and fantasy oriented[17] to the quite practical and supportive,[18] although most therapies contain elements of both.[19] Establishing an attachment relationship with a clinician (i.e. with an interested, understanding, and respectful adult) may be a new experience for some young people[20] and is believed to trigger a basic set of human capacities for relatedness that appears therapeutic, apparently almost regardless of content.[21–27] The child's relationship with the therapist often appears to become the vehicle for disowned aspects of the child's thoughts and feelings, creating a process termed transference, which enables the psychoanalytic clinician to understand the child's representation of relationships and his or her feelings about them.[28]

## Background

The roots of child psychoanalysis lie in Freud's observation of young children, most notably of the young Anna Freud's wishful dream for strawberries,[29] his grandson's separation game,[30] and his case study of Little Hans, a 5-year old with a phobic disorder who was treated by his physician father under Freud's supervision.[31]

Play therapy, incorporating both an insight-oriented interpretive approach and the developmental assistance perspective, was introduced by Hermine Hug-Helmuth.[32] Thereafter, two women, in strong opposition but frequently making reference to each other, established the field: Anna Freud[33] and Melanie Klein.[34]

Klein's approach was to regard children's play as essentially the same as free association with adults; that is, motivated by unconscious fantasy and activated by the relationship with the therapist (transference). The child's anxiety required verbalization (interpretation) if it was to be addressed. The focal point of therapy was the verbalization of anxieties concerning destructive and sadistic impulses, whilst the child's external relationships (with parents, teachers, etc.) were seen as peripheral and irrelevant.

A key construct was the notion of projective identification.[35] This term referred originally to the infantile tendency to project unwanted aspects of the self on to another person. The clinician, by understanding the child's perception of her as a person, could gain valuable insights about conflictual aspects of the child's experience of himself. Bion[36] described how the 'container's' capacity to understand and accept the projections could be critical both to successful therapy and to normal development. More recently, Kleinian child analysts have been less likely to offer early interpretations of deeply unconscious material; defences beyond projective identification are more commonly considered.[17,37]

Strongly influenced by Melanie Klein, Donald Winnicott firmly endorsed her emphasis on the impact of the first years of life on childhood psychopathology.[3] However, he also introduced new techniques (e.g. drawing) and various theoretical innovations, including the identification of a transitional space between self and other where the subjective object and the truly objective object could simultaneously be recognized.[38] The notion of transitional space, an intermediate area between the intrapsychic and the interpersonal, was critical to the development of an interpersonal[39,40] and intersubjectivist[41] approach within psychoanalysis.

Along this continuum, Anna Freud was perhaps most concerned with the child's developmental struggle with a social as well as an internal environment. Her background as a teacher may have led her to be as concerned with children's actual external circumstances as with their unconscious worlds.[42] Her focus was restricted to complications and conflicts arising from the child's libidinal impulses and, unlike Melanie Klein, she rarely focussed on innate aggression. The interpretation of defence was central to her technique.[43] Her approach paid careful attention to limitations on the child's cognitive capacities (ego functioning) and had as its explicit aim the restoration of the child to a normal developmental path.[44] Her concern with normal development led her to evolve a model of pathology as a disturbance of normal developmental processes, and she developed a systematic analysis of such anomalies using the concept of developmental lines.[45] Her propositions are in many respects consistent with modern developmental psychopathology.[46] Developmental help is aimed at facilitating the forward movement of the psychological processes that underpin social cognition and interpersonal function, and which include mentalization, impulse control and emotion regulation, symbolization and the use of metaphor, and the capacity for play.[47,48] Notwithstanding the curious historical fact that Anna Freudian, Kleinian, and Winnicottian approaches all originated in London, the Anna Freudian approach came to dominate child therapy in the United States,[49] whereas in the United Kingdom and in Latin America Melanie Klein's approach proved more popular.[50] Two comprehensive and detailed histories of the field have been provided.[51,52]

## Techniques

Techniques of child therapy differ considerably depending on the degree of pathology manifested by the child. Two sets of technique may be distinguished: those with single diagnosis, usually involving anxiety, are offered what most would recognize as 'classical' forms of psychodynamic, insight-oriented therapy. Those with multiple diagnoses, severe behavioural problems and/or emergent personality disorders[53] require a different psychodynamic treatment approach. These will be discussed separately.

### Principal features of 'classical' technique

Child psychotherapy involves the elaboration of distorted and, to a lesser or greater extent, non-conscious mental representations. The therapist, using the child's verbalizations, non-verbal play, and other behaviours, aims to provide a rational understanding of the child's non-conscious thoughts, feelings, and expectations. This understanding may encompass and integrate earlier modes of the child's thinking into a more mature, age-appropriate framework.[54] With young children, the treatment involves the use of toys, play, and any device that helps to engage the children in a process of self-exploration. The therapist works to elaborate the children's understanding of their emotional responses, their unconscious concerns about their body, and the way their symptoms might link together anxieties about relationships, including non-conscious aggressive or sexual thoughts and other conflictual feelings in relation to the parents, siblings, and peers.

The techniques used by the child therapist go beyond interpretive interventions and were usefully enumerated by Paulina Kernberg.[55] She delineated: (i) *supportive interventions*, which are aimed at addressing the child's anxiety and increasing the child's sense of competence and mastery through the provision of information, reassurance, empathy, and suggestions (ii) *facilitative statements*, which seek chiefly to maintain the therapeutic relationship with the child by reviewing, summarizing or paraphrasing the child's communications and (iii) *clarifications*, which review and summarize the child's communication, and which usually involve relabelling communication or behaviour. Clarifications also serve to focus the child's attention on certain patterns in his behaviour indicative of unconscious determination.

Interpretation may centre on: (i) the content of the child's communications (ii) the contents that the child systematically omits from verbalization (iii) the child's non-verbal behaviour (iv) the nature of the child's play, including the roles that he or she tends to assign to himself and to the therapist (v) the child's current emotional state, particularly sadness, anxiety, or guilt, and; (vi) dreams that the child recounts in his sessions. While the therapist may be able to link the child's therapeutic material to past experiences with attachment figures, such reconstructive interpretations are rare in child therapy. It is only gradually that the therapist hopes to be able to generate an emotionally meaningful understanding of the impact of past experiences on current anxiety and conflict.

Paulina Kernberg[55] distinguished between three types of child therapeutic interpretation. First and most common are interpretations of defences, which aim to show the child how it protects itself from thoughts, feelings, and actions that it considers unacceptable. For example, the therapist may draw the child's attention to repeated examples of self-denigration, and hint at his anxiety about being thought boastful; this serves a dual function in both bringing to the child's awareness what he is protecting himself from and also in prompting him to find alternative strategies to cope with warded off ideas. Second are interpretations that address the child's unconscious wishes, which are themselves thought to underpin behaviour. Frequently, these interpretations are made following interpretations of defences. Finally, child therapists might address the child's past experiences. The therapy may reveal traumatic experiences, and some therapists consider it helpful to bring these memories into consciousness. It should be noted that current psychodynamic theory in no way assumes that addressing such trauma directly is essential to cure. Far more important in terms of therapeutic progress is addressing the distorted relationship representations that are sequelae to early trauma.[56]

Whatever the interpretation, the child therapist aims to address the child's anxiety and how other emotions relate to it. Thus, destructive wishes would most likely be taken up in connection with the child's anxiety about his or her angry feelings. Child therapeutic technique also demands that the child's attempt actively to struggle with these wishes be clearly acknowledged. Interpretations are ideally tied to a highly specific context, such as the child's experience of anxiety associated with his anger that an ungenerous but otherwise valued therapist will not give him a special treat for his birthday.

An important part of child therapeutic work involves the child's parents. Some of this work is psychoeducational; in particular, parents often need guidance on appropriate, uncritical, warm, and playful methods of child rearing. Discussion of the child's symptoms may enable parents to gain greater awareness of the child's difficulties and how their own representation of the child may be distorted.[57]

## Psychodynamic technique with complex childhood disturbances

The child psychotherapeutic approach has been extended to apply not only to so-called neurotic disorders, but also to the understanding and treatment of borderline, narcissistic, delinquent, and conduct disordered youngsters, as well as schizoid and even psychotic children.[53] The classical psychoanalytic approach as outlined above has clear limitations with these children: anxiety may not be accessible; there may be little evidence of conflict/of the child's struggle with wishes; defences may be hard to identify, and the child may be developmentally inaccessible to insight. Taking these issues into consideration, we have suggested that a dramatic modification of child psychotherapeutic technique may be in order[19] based on what Anna Freud called 'developmental help'. We have described this intervention in detail,[58] and colleagues in the Netherlands have elaborated and researched this form of therapy.[59]

Essentially, the therapist begins by performing mental functions of which the child is incapable, or by showing the child ways of performing these functions until he or she can take over and do it himself. These interventions are used with pathologies traditionally defined as ego defects, deficiencies in relationships, or developmental disturbances—pathologies understood here as mental process disturbances. These techniques have sometimes been labelled remedial education or ego-support, but, broadly, the therapist's aim is to free the mental processes from inhibition and to aid in the development of these processes. The therapist achieves this by: (i) providing a safe place and relationship within which the child can dare to change or wish to be different (ii) making up for some deficits in the parenting that the child has received by providing him with the missing elements (iii) stimulating delayed or stunted developmental processes by drawing the child's attention to what is missing, and encouraging his interest and desire to function better and (iv) using interpretations not to uncover the source of his difficulties but to help the child understand the extent and impact of his problems, his contribution to his developmental difficulties, and to confront the role played by his environment. The main foci of these modified forms of child therapeutic intervention are six-fold:

(a) *The enhancing of reflective processes*; that is, the understanding of how mental states (beliefs, desires, wishes, and emotions) determine human behaviour. This is achieved by encouraging the observation and labelling of both physical and psychological experiences in the immediate situation. It is assumed that, regardless of cause, the final common pathway of most personality disorders is a dramatic impairment of reflective function.[60]

(b) *The enhancing of impulse control* by identifying and helping the child to exercise ways in which impulses may be channelled into socially acceptable forms of behaviour. The therapist may initially have to control this herself by 'setting limits'. She tells the child what he may and may not do during the sessions, explaining that she will not let him hurt her or himself, or damage things in the room.

(c) *Affect regulation* is an important aim of developmental work. It can be assisted by the verbalization and labelling of affect, and by explaining to the child possible reasons for his feelings; for example, that his aggressive attacks are reactions to his sense of being threatened and endangered.

(d) The elaboration of strategies involving symbolization and metaphor for *enhancing cognitive self-regulation*. The therapist demonstrates her own capacities for reflection and the moderation of experience through mental representation rather than physical action or coercion.

(e) Focussing the child's awareness on *the mental states of others*. This is achieved initially by focussing interventions around the child's perception of the therapist's mental states, which can be a precursor to reflective processes in relation to the self.

(f) Developing the child's *capacity for play*, initially with physical objects, then with another person and, ultimately, with ideas. Play is not simply the creation of a pretend world but has the aim of creating a safe opportunity for alternative meanings of the child's experiences to emerge. This can show the child how his habitual ways of thinking and feeling represent but one of multiple ways of construing reality. Perhaps more importantly in this context, he can experience adults relating to him, as perhaps they have not often related to him before.

While the child therapist working with such severely disturbed children is still 'working in the transference', in the sense that the child's feelings about the therapist remain central, this is no longer thought to entail the displacement of feelings and ideas from one person to another, e.g. from the parent to the therapist. Rather, the clarification of the child's feelings about the therapist may be the most effective route towards assisting the child to acquire a reflective capacity. In this way, the therapist conveys that the child's affect can be understood and managed by another person.

## Indications, contraindications, and the selection of procedures

There is general agreement on the indications for child psychotherapy.[61] These have traditionally included: (i) high IQ and verbal ability (ii) supportive environment (iii) conflict-related pathology (iv) adequate internal and external object relations and (v) the presence of anxiety. Contraindications include: (i) pervasive developmental disorder (ii) psychosis (iii) major deficiencies in psychological capacities and (iv) family constellations incompatible with adherence to treatment, for example, chaotic home environments or psychologically severely disturbed parents.

As described above, however, by substantially modifying traditional technique, child therapists have successfully worked with populations beyond this restricted group,[62] treating children with a variety of psychological deficiencies.

One way of conceptualizing the difference between the needs of the two groups is by using the classical distinction between mental representations and mental processes in cognitive science.[63] Classical techniques primarily impact on the organization and shape of the child's mental representations of self-other relationships.[64] By contrast, developmental help for the more severely disordered group aims at developing the function of mental processes, which may have been defensively distorted in early development,[65] by strengthening and supporting the patient's adaptive

defences and helping them to label and verbalize their thoughts and feelings.

The distinction between classical technique and developmental help is a heuristic one. In reality, all child therapeutic treatments involve both, but it is nevertheless suggested that developmental help is essential for the effective treatment of severe disturbances, whilst it remains an 'optional extra' for children with neurotic disturbances.

## Managing treatment

### Starting treatment

At the beginning of psychodynamic child therapy, the therapist's aim is to communicate that: (i) sessions have the purpose of expressing thoughts and feelings through play and words and (ii) the therapist is trying to help the child make sense of his experience so that he can master his inner turmoil in a more effective manner. Children are generally able to develop a therapeutic alliance in the context of an empathic, respectful, non-exploitative relationship with an adult. A similar collaboration is established with the parents, and early meetings also allow the child therapist to acquire relevant information and assess family interactional patterns that may be relevant to the child's treatment. In early sessions, the therapist attempts to interest the child in meaning and to link mental states to activity by using child's play to address the child's understanding of momentary anxieties, and to explain that his struggles, thoughts, and feelings may be explored through his verbalizations and behaviour.[66] Children who are able to use therapy tend to respond to these interventions with an enhancement of the therapeutic alliance, showing greater freedom in their play and verbalizations. It is important to note that the same process of relationship building characterizes other individual therapies such as cognitive behaviour therapy (CBT).[23]

### The middle phase

The middle phase of child therapy is expected to focus on the systematic use of transference interpretations and the initiation of the 'working through' process. The development of the transference is facilitated by a therapeutic structure that emphasizes regularity, consistency, and the specialness of the hour of therapy.[67] The child's play is 'interpreted', but normally these interpretations are kept within the context of the play situation. Clinical experience suggests that interpreting the play in reference to the child's 'real' feeling only serves to disrupt the child's communication.[68]

The major themes in children's lives are often expressed in the therapeutic relationship. Internal working models of attachment relationships, for example, will come to colour the child's relationship with the therapist,[69] be that a pattern of reluctance in forming trusting relationships (avoidant/dismissing) or excessive anxieties about separation and sometimes angry preoccupation with the therapist's thoughts and feelings (resistant/preoccupied). This, of course, opens up the possibility of correcting distortions and mastering conflicts and associated anxieties. The child gains information (insight) in a relational context that elaborates his understanding of his experience, provides him with a way of coping with thoughts and feelings that make him feel uncomfortable and interrupts maladaptive interactions.[70] Progress is often slow, and regression and progression tend to alternate as children struggle to face these anxieties without undue repression. Yet, gradually, given a capacity for the symbolic transformation of experience, they are able to bring their experience of internal and external worlds into play and can therefore internalize the therapeutic attitude to solving their problems. Of course, development is helpful too in this regard.[71]

### The ending of treatment

Indications for the termination of long-term child psychotherapy are both external and internal to the therapy. External indications are not restricted to symptomatic improvement, but include considerations of changes in family interaction and peer relationships. Relational changes indicate a capacity to use caretakers, teachers, and others as sources of protection, guidance, comfort, and models of identification. In general, the therapist seeks evidence that the child has returned to the path of normal development, can cope effectively with stress and conflict, and can respond with greater freedom to adaptive demands coming both from within and without.

There are also indications from the child that the therapy may be ended. Some were enumerated by Paulina Kernberg[72] as follows: (i) the therapist finds more opportunities for interpretation than for confrontation (ii) the child manifests more reflectiveness and the capacity to make interpretations (iii) there is greater freedom, expressiveness, and pleasure in play (iv) there is insight and humour and (v) the child assumes responsibility for his own actions.

The end of psychodynamic therapy often generates anxiety and can bring a temporary reactivation of symptoms and the re-emergence of dysfunctional patterns of interaction within the family. As the therapy creates an attachment relationship, its termination may be an essential part of resolving attachment-related concerns (e.g. fear of abandonment, rejection). Mourning the anticipated loss of the therapy and the therapist may well be an essential part of a successful ending to treatment. Other issues may involve children's disappointments—with themselves, with the unfulfilled promise of the therapy, and with adults who do not measure up to their expectations. Research and clinical experience suggests, however, that as this turmoil subsides, progress continues to be made after the end of treatment.[57,73,74]

## Efficacy

The most comprehensive survey of outcome studies specifically concerned with psychodynamic treatment was undertaken by Kennedy[75] as part of a project sponsored by the British Association of Child Psychotherapists—although there are other comprehensive reviews of treatment of children[76–80] and of psychosocial interventions limited to 'evidence-based treatments'.[81,82] The general reviews highlight that research of psychodynamic treatment in the field of child therapy has lagged behind the evaluation of other approaches.

There are relatively few randomized controlled trials of psychodynamic psychotherapy.[83–88] All but one of these trials contrasted individual child psychotherapy with another (evidence-based) treatment. In addition, several studies employed quasi-randomized methods of assignment, such as postcode[89] or therapist vacancy.[90,91] Six studies reported on findings with matched comparison groups.[92–96] A further two studies reported non-matched control groups.[97,98] Two further studies used an untreated but poorly matched control sample.[99,100] In addition, there are a number of open trials of child psychotherapy employing no comparison groups.[101–107] Three studies used an experimental, single-case methodology.[108–110]

Considering studies of the common disorders of childhood separately, Muratori and colleagues[91] contrasted the efficacy

of 11 weeks of psychodynamic therapy to treatment as usual in 58 children with depression and anxiety. At 2-year follow-up, 34 per cent of the treated group were in the clinical range on symptomatic measures, compared to 65 per cent of the controls. Treatment effects increased during the 2-year follow-up period (the so-called 'sleeper effect'), including a move into the non-clinical range for the average child with internalizing problems (in the psychodynamically treated group only).[90] It is encouraging that psychodynamic psychotherapy patients sought mental health services at a significantly lower rate than those in the treatment as usual comparison condition over the 2-year follow-up period.

In a multi-centred European trial,[88] moderate childhood depression was shown to be accessible to a brief individual psychodynamic psychotherapy. At 7-month follow-up, none of the moderately to severely depressed young people met criteria, which is comparable to children treated with a combination of fluoxetine and CBT.[111] The presence of anxiety/dysthymia signalled particular suitability for individual treatment, whilst comorbidity with oppositional defiant disorder (ODD) or conduct disorder (CD) contraindicated it. These children, however, appeared to do better with family based approaches that were also psychodynamic in orientation. A classic study, and for many years one of the only studies that considered the issue of intensity of psychological therapy, focussed on specific learning difficulties as a target of therapy.[93,112] Boys in middle childhood with serious reading problems benefited significantly from psychodynamic psychotherapy. There was a dose-response relationship over the 2-year treatment period. Children who received more intensive help (more sessions per week) benefited most from the therapy in terms of self-esteem, the capacity to form relationships, and the capacity to work, including frustration tolerance. Particularly interesting is the multi-centred randomized trial of the treatment of sexually abused girls treated in individual psychotherapy and psychoeducational group therapy.[87] Trowell et al.[87] randomized 71 sexually abused girls to either 30 sessions of individual psychoanalytic psychotherapy or 18 sessions of group psychotherapy with psychoeducational components. These young people presented with a range of psychiatric problems, most commonly post-traumatic stress disorder (PTSD) and depression. Psychodynamic treatment was somewhat superior to psychoeducation, but the difference was not as marked as might be expected. Superiority was particularly evident in relation to PTSD and generalized anxiety disorder (GAD). Depression, however, was relatively less likely to improve, as was separation anxiety. A subsequent report underscored the importance of the mother's support for the therapy as a predictor of improvement in the children and the benefit that the mothers gained in terms of their own mental health from the child's treatment.[113]

A chart review of the outcome of 763 cases in child psychotherapy has been carried out at the Anna Freud Centre in London.[103] While this retrospective methodology has severe limitations, the study reached a number of fairly robust conclusions, that need to be explored further in controlled, prospective investigations. The main findings were:

(a) Attrition was low compared to reports of other treatment approaches.

(b) Children with pervasive developmental disorders (e.g. autism) or intellectual disability did not do well, even with prolonged, intensive treatment. Children with serious disruptive disorders also had relatively poor outcomes.

(c) Younger children improved significantly during psychodynamic treatment, and gained additional benefit from 4–5 weekly sessions.

(d) Anxiety disorders, particularly specific rather than pervasive symptoms, were associated with a good prognosis, even if the primary diagnosis was of a different type, e.g. disruptive disorder.

(e) Children with emotional disorders and/or severe or pervasive symptomatology responded very well to intensive treatment (4–5 sessions per week), but did not show satisfactory rates of improvement in non-intensive psychotherapy.

(f) Predictors of improvement varied considerably between subgroups of the full sample, and, by subdividing the sample according to diagnostic group and developmental level, it was possible to predict a majority of the variance in outcome within the subgroups.

## Limitations of the psychotherapeutic approach

The empirical status of all psychodynamic approaches remains controversial. The body of rigorous research supporting psychodynamic therapies for adults for most disorders remains limited, particularly relative to research supporting pharmaceutical treatments and even other psychosocial approaches such as CBT.[80] There are both practical and theoretical difficulties to mounting trials of dynamic therapies, and these go some way to explaining the lack of evidence (e.g. identifying suitable control groups for long-term intensive treatments, difficulties in operationalizing the treatment methods, the expense of mounting trials sufficiently powered to yield information on what treatments are appropriate for which disorder, the failure to tightly manualize psychodynamic treatments, etc.). Those who argue for continued investment in this approach (correctly in our view) point to the limitations of the evidence base supporting CBT[114] or pharmacological approaches.[115] Ultimately, however, such a negative case cannot persuade policy makers and funders, and, without intense research on the effectiveness of the method deeply rooted in and shaped by psychological models of pathology, the long-term survival of this orientation is not assured.[116] This is not to say that the techniques that have evolved as part of this approach will not survive (they are effective, and clinicians, being pragmatic people, will continue to discover and use them), but they will be increasingly absorbed into alternative models, and the unique approach pioneered by Freud and outlined in this chapter might not continue. Child therapists thus face formidable challenges to their clinical and theoretical convictions, to their professional status, and, as evidence-based medicine and managed care relentlessly expand their control over reimbursement and deny payment for child therapy, to their livelihood. If child psychotherapy is to have a future, its unique effectiveness for specific childhood disorders must be demonstrated in randomized controlled trials. We believe that children with severe disorders of personality and multiple psychiatric diagnoses are indeed well suited to and dramatically benefit from a psychotherapeutic approach. Such faith, however, now requires support from empirical investigations.

## Further information

Fonagy, P., Target, M., and Gergely, G. (2004). Psychoanalytic perspectives on developmental psychopathology. In *Developmental psychopathology* (2nd edn) (eds. D. Cicchetti and D.J. Cohen), pp. 504–54. Guilford Press, New York.

Kennedy, E. (2004). *Child and adolescent psychotherapy: a systematic review of psychoanalytic approaches*. North Central London Strategic Health Authority, London.

Lanyado, M. and Horne, A. (2006). *A question of technique*. Routledge, London.

## References

1. Pessiglione, M., Schmidt, L., Draganski, B., *et al.* (2007). How the brain translates money into force: a neuroimaging study of subliminal motivation. *Science*, **316**, 904–6.

2. Kernberg, O.F. (2005). Unconscious conflict in the light of contemporary psychoanalytic findings. *The Psychoanalytic Quarterly*, **74**, 65–81; discussion 327–63.

3. Winnicott, D.W. (1965). *The maturational process and the facilitating environment*. Hogarth Press, London.

4. Freud, A. (1965). *Normality and pathology in childhood: assessments of development*. International Universities Press, Madison, CT.

5. Fonagy, P. and Target, M. (2003). *Psychoanalytic theories: perspectives from developmental psychopathology*. Whurr, London.

6. Freud, A. (1936). *The ego and the mechanisms of defence*. International Universities Press, New York, 1946.

7. Blagov, P.S. and Singer, J.A. (2004). Four dimensions of self-defining memories (specificity, meaning, content, and affect) and their relationships to self-restraint, distress, and repressive defensiveness. *Journal of Personality*, **72**, 481–511.

8. Jorgensen, R.S., Frankowski, J.J., Lantinga, L.J., *et al.* (2001). Defensive hostility and coronary heart disease: a preliminary investigation of male veterans. *Psychosomatic Medicine*, **63**, 463–9.

9. Lyons-Ruth, K. (2003). Dissociation and the parent-infant dialogue: a longitudinal perspective from attachment research. *Journal of the American Psychoanalytical Association*, **51**, 883–911.

10. Shamir-Essakow, G., Ungerer, J.A., Rapee, R.M., *et al.* (2004). Caregiving representations of mothers of behaviorally inhibited and uninhibited preschool children. *Developmental Psychology*, **40**, 899–910.

11. Kaye, A.L. and Shea, M.T. (2000). Personality disorders, personality traits, and defense mechanisms. In Task force for the handbook of psychiatric measures (edn). *Handbook of psychiatric measures*, pp. 713–49. American Psychiatric Association, Washington, DC.

12. Vaillant, G.E. (1992). *Ego mechanisms of defense: a guide for clinicians and researchers*. American Psychiatric Association Press, Washington, DC.

13. Bond, M. (2004). Empirical studies of defense style: relationships with psychopathology and change. *Harvard Review of Psychiatry*, **12**, 263–78.

14. Lenzenweger, M.F., Clarkin, J.F., Kernberg, O.F., *et al.* (2001). The inventory of personality organization: psychometric properties, factorial composition, and criterion relations with affect, aggressive dyscontrol, psychosis proneness, and self-domains in a nonclinical sample. *Psychological Assessment*, **13**, 577–91.

15. Holmes, J. (1998). The changing aims of psychoanalytic psychotherapy: an integrative perspective. *International Journal of Psychoanalysis*, **79**, 227–40.

16. Allen, J.G. and Fonagy, P. (eds.) (2006). *Handbook of mentalization-based treatment*. Wiley, New York.

17. O'Shaughnessy, E. (1988). W. R. Bion's theory of thinking and new techniques in child analysis. In *Melanie Klein today: developments in theory and practice: mainly practice*, Vol. 2 (ed. E.B. Spillius), pp. 177–90. Routledge, London.

18. Kennedy, H. and Moran, G. (1991). Reflections on the aims of child psychoanalysis. *The Psychoanalytic Study of the Child*, **46**, 181–98.

19. Bleiberg, E., Fonagy, P., and Target, M. (1997). Child psychoanalysis: critical overview and a proposed reconsideration. *The Psychiatric Clinics of North America*, **6**, 1–38.

20. Hurry, A. (ed.) (1998). *Psychoanalysis and developmental theory*. Karnac, London.

21. Daniel, S.I. (2006). Adult attachment patterns and individual psychotherapy: a review. *Clinical Psychology Review*, **26**(8), 968–84.

22. Fonagy, P. and Bateman, A.W. (2006). Mechanisms of change in mentalization-based treatment of BPD. *Journal of Clinical Psychology*, **62**, 411–30.

23. Kazdin, A.E., Marciano, P.L., and Whitley, M.K. (2005). The therapeutic alliance in cognitive-behavioral treatment of children referred for oppositional, aggressive, and antisocial behavior. *Journal of Consulting and Clinical Psychology*, **73**, 726–30.

24. Krupnick, J.L., Sotsky, S.M., Simmens, S., *et al.* (1996). The role of the therapeutic alliance in psychotherapy and pharmacotherapy outcome: findings in the National Institute of Mental Health Treatment of Depression Collaborative Research Program. *Journal of Consulting and Clinical Psychology*, **64**, 532–9.

25. PDM Task Force. (2006). *Psychodynamic diagnostic manual*. Alliance of Psychoanalytic Organizations, Silver Spring, MD.

26. Safran, J.D. and Muran, J.C. (2000). *Negotiating the therapeutic alliance*. Guilford Press, New York.

27. Wynn Parry, C. and Birkett, D. (1996). The working alliance: a re-appraisal. *British Journal of Psychotherapy*, **12**, 291–9.

28. Kernberg, P. and Chazan, S.E. (1991). *Children with conduct disorders: a psychotherapy manual*. Basic Books, New York.

29. Freud, S. (1900). The interpretation of dreams. In *The standard edition of the complete psychological works of Sigmund Freud*, Vols. 4 and 5 (ed. J. Strachey), pp. 1–715. Hogarth Press, London.

30. Freud, S. (1920). Beyond the pleasure principle. In *The standard edition of the complete psychological works of Sigmund Freud*, Vol. 18 (ed. J. Strachey), pp. 1–64. Hogarth Press, London.

31. Freud, S. (1909). Analysis of a phobia in a five-year-old boy. In *The standard edition of the complete psychological works of Sigmund Freud*, Vol. 10 (ed. J. Strachey), pp. 1–147. Hogarth Press, London.

32. Hug-Helmuth, H. (1921). On the technique of child analysis. *International Journal of Psychoanalysis*, **2**, 287–303.

33. Freud, A. (1946). *The psychoanalytic treatment of children*. Imago Publishing, London.

34. Klein, M. (1932). *The psycho-analysis of children*. Hogarth Press, London.

35. Klein, M. (1946). Notes on some schizoid mechanisms. In *Developments in psychoanalysis* (eds. M. Klein, P. Heimann, S. Isaacs, and J. Riviere), pp. 292–320. Hogarth Press, London.

36. Bion, W.R. (1959). Attacks on linking. *International Journal of Psychoanalysis*, **40**, 308–15.

37. Williams, G. (1997). *Internal landscapes and foreign bodies*. Duckworth, London.

38. Winnicott, D.W. (1971). *Playing and reality*. Tavistock, London.

39. Altman, N., Briggs, R., Frankel, J., *et al.* (2002). *Relational child psychotherapy*. Other Press, New York.

40. Mitchell, S.A. (1997). *Influence and autonomy in psychoanalysis*. Analytic Press, Hillsdale, NJ.

41. Trevarthen, C.A., Aitken, K.J., Vandekerckhove, M., *et al.* (2006). Collaborative regulations of vitality in early childhood: stress in intimate relationships and postnatal psychopathology. In *Developmental psychopathology: developmental neuroscience*, Vol. 2 (2nd edn) (eds. D. Cicchetti and D.J. Cohen), pp. 65–126. Wiley, New York.

42. Edgcumbe, R. (2000). *Anna Freud: a view of development, disturbance and therapeutic techniques*. Routledge, London.

43. Miller, J.M. (1996). Anna Freud. *The Psychoanalytic Study of the Child*, **51**, 142–71.

44. Freud, A. (1981). *A psychoanalytic view of developmental psychopathology*. International University Press, New York.

45. Freud, A. (1963). The concept of developmental lines. *The Psychoanalytic Study of the Child*, **18**, 245–65.

46. Cicchetti, D. and Cohen, D.J. (eds.) (2006). *Developmental psychopathology*, Vols. 1–3 (2nd edn). John Wiley & Sons, New York.

47. Fonagy, P., Edgcumbe, R., Moran, G.S., *et al.* (1993). The roles of mental representations and mental processes in therapeutic action. *The Psychoanalytic Study of the Child*, **48**, 9–48.

48. Fonagy, P. and Target, M. (1998). Mentalization and the changing aims of child psychoanalysis. *Psychoanalytic Dialogues*, **8**, 87–114.

49. Garber, B. (2001). Freud's impact on therapeutic work with children. *Annual of Psychoanalysis*, **29**, 133–43.

50. Rustin, M. (1999). The training of child psychotherapists at the Tavistock clinic: philosophy and practice. *Psychoanalytic Inquiry*, **19**, 125–41.

51. Geissmann, C. and Geissmann, P. (1998). *The history of child psychoanalysis*. Routledge, London.

52. Housman, A. (1997). *The history of child psychoanalysis*. Routledge, London.

53. Bleiberg, E. (2001). *Treating personality disorders in children and adolescents: a relational approach*. Guilford Press, New York.

54. Abrams, S. (1988). The psychoanalytic process in adults and children. *The Psychoanalytic Study of the Child*, **43**, 45–261.

55. Kernberg, P.F. (1995). Child psychiatry: individual psychotherapy. In *Comprehensive textbook of psychiatry* (6th edn) (eds. H.I. Kaplan and B.J. Sadock), pp. 2399–412. Williams & Wilkins, Baltimore, MD.

56. Fonagy, P. and Target, M. (1997). Perspectives on the recovered memories debate. In *Recovered memories of abuse: true or false?* (eds. J. Sandler and P. Fonagy), pp. 183–216. Karnac Books, London.

57. Sandler, J., Kennedy, H., and Tyson, R. (1980). *The technique of child psychoanalysis: discussions with Anna Freud*. Harvard University Press, Cambridge, MA.

58. Fonagy, P., Edgcumbe, R., Target, M., *et al.* (Unpublished manuscript). *Contemporary Psychodynamic Child Therapy: Theory and Technique*.

59. Verheugt-Pleiter, A.J.E., Zevalkink, J., and Schmeets, M.G.J. (eds.) (in press). *Mentalizing in child therapy: guidelines for clinical practitioners*. Karnac Books, London.

60. Bateman, A.W. and Fonagy, P. (2004). *Psychotherapy for borderline personality disorder: mentalization based treatment*. Oxford University Press, Oxford.

61. Dowling, A.S. and Naegele, J. (1995). Child and adolescent psychoanalysis. In *Psychoanalysis: the major concepts* (eds. B.E. Moore and B.D. Fine), pp. 26–44. Yale University Press, New Haven, CT.

62. Fonagy, P. and Target, M. (1996a). A contemporary psychoanalytical perspective: psychodynamic developmental therapy. In *Psychosocial treatments for child and adolescent disorders: empirically based approaches* (eds. E. Hibbs and P. Jensen), pp. 619–38. APA and NIH, Washington, DC.

63. Mandler, G. (1985). *Cognitive psychology. An essay in cognitive science*. Lawrence Erlbaum Associates, Hillsdale, New Jersey.

64. Sandler, J. and Rosenblatt, B. (1962). The concept of the representational world. *The Psychoanalytic Study of the Child*, **17**, 128–45.

65. Fonagy, P., Moran, G.S., Edgcumbe, R., *et al.* (1993). The roles of mental representations and mental processes in therapeutic action. *The Psychoanalytic Study of the Child*, **48**, 9–48.

66. Coppolillo, H.P. (2002). Use of play in psychodynamic psychotherapy. In *Child and adolescent psychiatry: a comprehensive textbook* (3rd edn) (ed. M. Lewis), pp. 992–8. Lippincott, Williams & Wilkins, Philadelphia.

67. Yanof, J.A. (1996). Language, communication, and transference in child analysis. I. Selective mutism: the medium is the message. II. Is

child analysis really analysis? *Journal of the American Psychoanalytic Association*, **44**, 100–16.

68. Fonagy, P. and Target, M. (1996b). Playing with reality. I. Theory of mind and the normal development of psychic reality. *International Journal of Psycho-Analysis*, **77**, 217–33.

69. Slade, A. (2000). The development and organization of attachment. *Journal of the American Psychoanalytic Association*, **48**, 1147–74.

70. Lewis, M. (2002). Intensive individual psychodynamic psychotherapy: the therapeutic relationship and the technique of interpretation: the use of play in psychodynamic therapy. In *Child and adolescent psychiatry: a comprehensive textbook* (3rd edn) (ed. M. Lewis), pp. 984–92. Lippincott, Williams & Wilkins, Philadelphia.

71. Ritvo, R.Z. and Ritvo, S. (2002). Psychodynamic psychotherapy. In *Child and adolescent psychiatry: a comprehensive textbook* (3rd edn) (ed. M. Lewis), pp. 974–84. Lippincott, Williams & Wilkins, Philadelphia.

72. Kernberg, P.F. (1991). Termination in child psychoanalysis: criteria from within the sessions. In *Saying goodbye: a casebook of termination in child and adolescent analysis and therapy* (eds. A.G. Schmulker), pp. 321–37. Analytic Press, Hillsdale, NJ.

73. Kolvin, I., MacMillan, A., and Wrate, R.M. (1988). Psychotherapy is effective. *Journal of the Royal Society of Medicine*, **81**, 261–6.

74. Muratori, F., Picchi, L., Casella, C., *et al.* (2002). Efficacy of brief dynamic psychotherapy for children with emotional disorders. *Psychotherapy and Psychosomatics*, **71**, 28–38.

75. Kennedy, E. (2004). Child and adolescent review of psychotherapy: A systematic review of psychoanalytic approaches. North Central London Strategic Health Authority, London.

76. Fonagy, P., Target, M., Cottrell, D., *et al.* (2002). *What works for whom? A critical review of treatments for children and adolescents.* Guilford, New York.

77. Kazdin, A.E. (2000). *Psychotherapy for children and adolescents: directions for research and practice.* Oxford University Press, Oxford.

78. Kazdin, A.E. (2003). Psychotherapy for children and adolescents. *Annual Review of Psychology*, **54**, 253–76.

79. Kazdin, A.E. (2004). Psychotherapy for children and adolescents. In *Bergin and Garfield's handbook of psychotherapy and behavior change* (5th edn) (ed. M. Lambert), pp. 543–89. Wiley, New York.

80. Roth, A. and Fonagy, P. (2004). *What works for whom? A critical review of psychotherapy research* (2nd edn). Guilford Press, New York.

81. Hibbs, E.D. (ed.) (2004). *Psychosocial treatments for child and adolescent disorders: empirically based strategies for clinical practice* (2nd edn). American Psychological Association, Washington DC.

82. Weisz, J.R. (2004). *Psychotherapy for children and adolescents: evidence-based treatments and case examples.* Cambridge University Press, Cambridge.

83. Robin, A.L., Siegel, P.T., Moye, A.W., *et al.* (1999). A controlled comparison of family versus individual therapy for adolescents with anorexia nervosa. *Journal of the American Academy of Child and Adolescent Psychiatry*, **38**, 1482–9.

84. Sinha, U.K. and Kapur, M. (1999). Psychotherapy with emotionally disturbed adolescent boys: outcome and process study. *NIMHANS Journal*, **17**, 113–30.

85. Smyrnios, K.X. and Kirkby, R.J. (1993). Long-term comparison of brief versus unlimited psychodynamic treatments with children and their parents. *Journal of Consulting and Clinical Psychology*, **61**, 1020–7.

86. Szapocznik, J., Rio, A., Murray, E., *et al.* (1989). Structural family versus psychodynamic child therapy for problematic Hispanic boys. *Journal of Consulting and Clinical Psychology*, **57**, 571–8.

87. Trowell, J., Kolvin, I., Weeramanthri, T., *et al.* (2002). Psychotherapy for sexually abused girls: psychopathological outcome findings and patterns of change. *The British Journal of Psychiatry*, **180**, 234–47.

88. Trowell, J., Rhode, M., Miles, G., *et al.* (2003). Childhood depression: work in progress. *Journal of Child Psychotherapy*, **29**, 147–69.

89. Moran, G., Fonagy, P., Kurtz, A., *et al.* (1991). A controlled study of the psychoanalytic treatment of brittle diabetes. *Journal of the American Academy of Child and Adolescent Psychiatry*, **30**, 926–35.

90. Muratori, F., Picchi, L., Bruni, G., *et al.* (2003). A two-year follow-up of psychodynamic psychotherapy for internalizing disorders in children. *Journal of the American Academy of Child and Adolescent Psychiatry*, **42**, 331–9.

91. Muratori, F., Picchi, L., Casella, C., *et al.* (2001). Efficacy of brief dynamic psychotherapy for children with emotional disorders. *Psychotherapy and Psychosomatics*, **71**, 28–38.

92. Fonagy, P. and Target, M. (1994). The efficacy of psychoanalysis for children with disruptive disorders. *Journal of the American Academy of Child and Adolescent Psychiatry*, **33**, 45–55.

93. Heinicke, C.M. and Ramsey-Klee, D.M. (1986). Outcome of child psychotherapy as a function of frequency of sessions. *Journal of the American Academy of Child Psychiatry*, **25**, 247–53.

94. Reid, S., Alvarez, A., and Lee, A. (2001). The Tavistock autism workshop approach. In *Autism-the search for coherence* (eds. J. Richer and S. Coates), pp. 182–92. Jessica Kingsley, London.

95. Target, M. and Fonagy, P. (1994a). The efficacy of psychoanalysis for children with emotional disorders. *Journal of the American Academy of Child and Adolescent Psychiatry*, **33**, 361–71.

96. Target, M. and Fonagy, P. (1994b). The efficacy of psychoanalysis for children: developmental considerations. *Journal of the American Academy of Child and Adolescent Psychiatry*, **33**, 1134–44.

97. Apter, A., Bernhout, E., and Tyano, S. (1984). Severe obsessive compulsive disorder in adolescence: a report of eight cases. *Journal of Adolescence*, **7**, 349–58.

98. Boston, M. and Lush, D. (1994). Further considerations of methodology for evaluating psychoanalytic psychotherapy with children: reflections in the light of research experience. *Journal of Child Psychotherapy*, **20**, 225–9.

99. Lush, D., Boston, M., and Grainger, E. (1991). Evaluation of psychoanalytic psychotherapy with children: therapists' assessments and predictions. *Psychoanalytic Psychotherapy*, **5**, 191–234.

100. Target, M. and Fonagy, P. (2002). The long-term follow-up of child analytic treatments (AFC3). In *An open door review of outcome studies in psychoanalysis* (2nd edn) (ed. P. Fonagy), pp. 141–6. International Psychoanalytic Association, London.

101. Baruch, G. (1995). Evaluating the outcome of a community-based psychoanalytic psychotherapy service for young people between 12 and 25 years old: work in progress. *Psychoanalytic Psychotherapy*, **9**, 243–67.

102. Baruch, G., Fearon, P., and Gerber, A. (1998). Evaluating the outcome of a community-based psychoanalytic psychotherapy service for young people: one year repeated follow-up. In *Rethinking clinical audit* (eds. R. Davenhill and M. Patrick), pp. 157–82. Routledge, London.

103. Fonagy, P. and Target, M. (1996c). Predictors of outcome in child psychoanalysis: a retrospective study of 763 cases at the Anna Freud Centre. *Journal of the American Psychoanalytic Association*, **44**, 27–77.

104. Petri, H. and Thieme, E. (1978). Katamnese zur analytischen psychotherapie im kindes und jugendalter. *PSYCHE*, **1**, 21–54.

105. Vilsvik, S.O. and Va2glum, P. (1990). Teenage anorexia nervosa: a 1 to 9 year follow up after psychodynamic treatment. *Nord Psykiatr Tidsskr*, **44**, 249–55.

106. Winkelmann, K., Hartmann, M., Neumann, K., *et al.* (2000). Stability of therapeutic outcome after child and adolescent psychoanalytical therapy. *Praxis Kinderpsychol Kinderpsychiatr*, **49**, 315–28.

107. Zelman, A.B., Samuels, S., and Abrams, D. (1985). IQ changes in young children following intensive long-term psychotherapy. *American Journal of Psychotherapy*, **39**, 215–27.

108. Fonagy, P. and Moran, G.S. (1990). Studies on the efficacy of child psychoanalysis. *Journal of Consulting and Clinical Psychology*, **58**, 684–95.

109. Lush, D., Boston, M., Morgan, J., *et al.* (1998). Psychoanalytic psychotherapy with disturbed adopted and foster children: a single case follow-up study. *Clinical Child Psychology and Psychiatry*, **3**, 51–69.

110. Moran, G.S. and Fonagy, P. (1987). Psychoanalysis and diabetic control: a single case study. *British Journal of Medical Psychology*, **60**, 357–72.

111. Goodyer, I., Dubicka, B., Wilkinson, P., *et al.* (2007). Selective serotonin reuptake inhibitors (SSRIs) and routine specialist care with and without cognitive behaviour therapy: randomised controlled trial. *British Medical Journal*, **335**, 142–6.

112. Heinicke, C.M. (1965). Frequency of psychotherapeutic session as a factor affecting the child's developmental status. *The Psychoanalytic Study of the Child*, **20**, 42–98.

113. Rushton, A. and Miles, G. (2000). A study of a support service for the current carers of sexually abused girls. *Clinical Child Psychology and Psychiatry*, **5**, 411–26.

114. Westen, D., Novotny, C.M., and Thompson-Brenner, H. (2004). The empirical status of empirically supported psychotherapies: assumptions, findings, and reporting in controlled clinical trials. *Psychological Bulletin*, **130**, 631–63.

115. Whittington, C.J., Kendall, T., Fonagy, P., *et al.* (2004). Selective serotonin reuptake inhibitors in childhood depression: systematic review of published versus unpublished data. *Lancet*, **363**, 1341–5.

116. Gabbard, G.O., Gunderson, J.G., and Fonagy, P. (2002). The place of psychoanalytic treatments within psychiatry. *Archives of General Psychiatry*, **59**, 505–10.

# 9.5.3 **Cognitive behaviour therapies for children and families**

Philip Graham

## Introduction

Cognitive behaviour therapy (CBT) is derived from both behavioural and cognitive theories. Using concepts such as operant conditioning and reinforcement, behavioural theories treat behaviour as explicable without recourse to description of mental activity. In contrast, mental activity is central to all concepts derived from cognitive psychology. Both sets of theories have been of value in explaining psychological disorders and, in the design of interventions they have proved an effective combination.

Central to that part of cognitive theory that is relevant to CBT is the concept of 'schemas', first described in detail by Jean Piaget.[1] A schema is a mental 'structure for screening, coding, and evaluating impinging stimuli'.[2] The origin of mental schemas lies in the pre-verbal phase when material is encoded in non-verbal images that, as the child's language develops, gradually become verbally labelled. They form part of a dynamic system interacting with an individual child's physiology, emotional functioning, and behaviour with their operation depending on the social context in which the child is living. There are similarities but also differences between schemas and related concepts in psychoanalysis, such as Freudian 'complexes' and Kleinian 'positions'.

Schemas can be seen as organized around anything in the child's world, especially objects, beliefs, or emotions. They develop from past experience. The processing of new information in relation to such schemas can usefully be seen as involving the evaluation of discrepancies between information that is received and information that is expected. If there is a discrepancy, (the information not corresponding with that expected), then during the coding process information may be distorted so that it no longer creates discomfort, or, more adaptively, it may be incorporated into a modified schema.

## Cognitive development

The theory of cognitive development that Piaget constructed on the basis of an immense amount of experimental work was characterized by stages of development. He described characteristic features of the sensori-motor (0–2 years), pre-operational (2–7 years), concrete operational (7–12 years), and formal operational (12 years onwards) stages. Before the end of a stage is reached the child is incapable of showing more advanced thinking. In particular, the child's thinking before the concrete operational stage is characterized by egocentricity and an inability to take the perspective of another person. Abstract reasoning is not possible for the child until the formal operational stage is reached.

Even though Piaget's views of the limitations of the cognitive abilities of young children have been strongly criticized especially on the grounds that he was judging egocentricity on the basis of findings obtained in highly artificial situations, Piaget remained a dominant influence in cognitive psychology and education throughout the twentieth century. It is now widely accepted that, although obviously young children are less competent than those in middle childhood and these are less competent than adolescents, cognitive competence advances much more rapidly than Piaget described and the social context in which a child's competence is investigated has a much more profound influence on performance than he allowed. Children do a great deal better in naturalistic circumstances than when they take part in experiments. Further, coaching can improve performance to a level not previously obtainable. For example, it has been shown that, with preliminary training, 3-year-old children understand that drawings of thought bubbles can represent what people think. They can distinguish between thoughts and actions, recognize that thoughts are subjective and that two people can have different thoughts about the same events.[3]

Investigation of the development of the 'theory of mind' held by children has revealed that between 3 and 4 years they begin to realize that other children can be deceived by appearances and hold false beliefs they themselves do not hold. This shows that, given the right circumstances, children of this young age are able to 'de-centre' and are not necessarily limited by egocentricity. By the age of 8 years children have such stable concepts of their own self-esteem that they are capable of reliably completing self-esteem questionnaires about their own feelings and performance in comparison to other children.[4] Some schemas in young children are however relatively unstable, gradually increasing in stability as they get older. For example, it has been shown that attributional style (the tendency to attribute adverse events either to the self or to external circumstances) does not become stable until early adolescence, though it may be identified earlier if the events are particularly salient to the child in question.[5]

It has been hypothesized[6] that maladaptive schemas developed during childhood are responsible for the formation and maintenance of adult psychopathology. Building on this model, a therapeutic approach (schema-focused therapy) based on the identification of particular maladaptive schemas has been proposed for adults. Subsequently Stallard and Rayner[7] have developed a schema questionnaire that builds on adult work to identify such maladaptive schema in 11 to 16-year-old school children.

## Technique and management in the paediatric age group

Although there are certain common principles, CBT does not involve, as will be seen, a single approach that can be applied across all disorders; it is better seen as a family of approaches with certain core elements in common. In adults the type of disorder and the individual circumstances of the patient will determine the choice of therapeutic methods. In children and adolescents the cognitive level of the patient will also need to be taken into account. Though the age of the child will give some indication of the cognitive level of the child, there is wide variation in competence amongst children of the same age. Further, the therapist may use the skills of an educationist to bring the child's competence up to a level at which the child can more actively participate in therapy. Kendall[8] suggests indeed that one of the therapeutic roles that the therapist should adopt is that of *educator*, who needs communication skills to assist children to learn to think for themselves.

## Behaviour therapy or CBT?

In principle, the decision as to whether to include a cognitive component in therapy depends on whether the clinical formulation incorporates cognitive distortions or biases. In practice, because of their cognitive limitations CBT is rarely used in children under the age of 7 years. Treatment in children younger than 7 years is predominantly behavioural, with the cognitive component limited to coping self-talk. Conditioning approaches to the treatment of feeding and sleeping problems as well as enuresis and encopresis usually have a very small or no significant cognitive component.

In some conditions such as anxiety disorders, especially specific phobias, where desensitization and reinforcement approaches are widely used in adults, the use of a mainly behavioural approach does not reduce effectiveness. A cognitive component may nevertheless be incorporated because the CBT principles of collaboration, openness, and guided discovery, usually less marked when purely behavioural approaches are applied, are advantageous to the patient.

### Aids to cognitive tasks

Where experience with adults suggests that cognitive tasks add significantly to the effectiveness of treatment, as in depressive disorders and problems of social relationships, even young people in early adolescence will usually be able to co-operate as well as adults. The cognitive treatment of younger children with these conditions may be helped by the use of age-adapted techniques.[9]

For example, card-sorting *games* have been devised to help children distinguish between thoughts, feelings, and situations. *Puppets* can be used to facilitate discussion as part of the assessment process, to model alternative ways the child might cope with difficult situations and to engage the child in rehearsal and practice of new skills. *Story telling* can provide an insight into the child's inner world; they provide a way of externalizing and accessing the child's cognitions, allow an opportunity to challenge the child's assumptions, introduce the child to more positive ways of coping, and can be used to model success and help the child gain more functional assumptions and beliefs.

### Working with parents

Parents play many roles in the delivery of CBT to children and adolescents. To begin with, even up to mid-adolescence, it is nearly always parents who identify the behaviour and emotional problems that lead to advice being sought. They are the people most likely to press for psychological help. It is they who have to persuade often reluctant children and adolescents to attend and participate in a service that their offspring may fear, not without reason, will result in stigmatization.

They are then likely to play a major part in the assessment process. From mid- to late adolescence, the patient or client will be the main source of information, but before that it is the parents and teachers who will often provide most relevant information. If treatment is proposed it is they who need to give consent, though their child will also need to assent if the therapy is to have any chance of succeeding.

Once treatment planning has begun, the part that parents play will depend very much on the age of the child or adolescent, the diagnosis, family circumstances (especially the quality of the relationships between parents and child), and the degree to which the assessment has revealed that the parents as well as being the main carers are also involved in the origin and maintenance of the problem. Most explanatory theories of anxiety disorders in children, for example, point to the ways in which parents can provide inappropriately anxious models for imitation by their children. In a small scale study it has been shown that changing parental attributions can, in itself, result in improvements in problem behaviour scores on a questionnaire.[10] Parents may also be seen as clients in their own rights in parallel sessions, as co-therapists or as facilitators of therapy for their children. Therapists dealing with adolescent offspring are often in a difficult position *vis-à-vis* parents in that they will wish to encourage autonomy and independent decision-making in the child or adolescent, while needing the parents to monitor homework, encourage further attendance, and provide information on progress.

The involvement of parents also brings ethical dilemmas. There are three main areas of ethical concern.[11] The therapist often has to balance the different viewpoints of parents and children, a particular problem in the management of oppositional and conduct disorders where children often fail to acknowledge the existence of problems that are causing distress to their parents. There is frequently need to address family issues such as marital conflict that are clearly relevant yet not the reasons why the child has been brought for treatment. Finally, there is the need to achieve genuine collaboration with parents, making explicit their role as co-therapists. This is made easier if children are also actively involved as fellow collaborators, taking responsibility for progress and being encouraged to make suggestions for alternative approaches. A collaborative stance may however not be possible if it becomes clear that there are child protection issues with one or both parents involved in maltreatment of their children. Wolpert and her colleagues provide a useful checklist for clinicians to help assess how far they are attempting to balance different viewpoints in issues involving different family members and promoting collaboration.

### Failure to engage and failure to respond

In adolescents, lack of motivation for change is often a major impediment to engagement in therapy. Not only is there often a failure to recognize the importance of a problem, to accept the need for change or to appear to understand why change is necessary, but there may also be an absence of the level of self-belief, self-confidence, or self-efficacy that is necessary before hopeful steps can be taken in the right direction. In these circumstances techniques of motivational interviewing will help the therapist to achieve engagement.[12]

The reasons for non-response to CBT in adults have been discussed by Kingdon et al.[13] Common problems include unsuitability for treatment possibly arising from misdiagnosis, resistance to treatment, an inadequate number of sessions, difficulties in the therapeutic relationship and the presence of concurrent social and/or physical pathology. Non-response in children and adolescents arises from similar issues, with, additionally, complicating problems arising from negative parental attitudes and behaviour.

## Anxiety disorders

### Cognitive distortions and deficits

A characteristic constellation of cognitive deficits and distortions underlies the presence of anxiety disorders in children and adolescents. A central feature is the exaggerated perception of threat arising from an inability to assess accurately the seriousness of danger. Thus a deficit in perceptual competence results in cognitive distortion. The characteristic nature of the threat involved will depend to a considerable degree both on the stage of cognitive development of the child and on the social demands that are encountered during that particular phase of life. Pre-school children are most likely to be threatened by separation from parents; children aged 5 to 12 years by feared situations at school and adolescents by social situations as well as wider concerns such as environmental pollution. Certain fears and phobias such as fear of spiders and snakes appear more biologically based and are present through childhood to adolescence.

These cognitive deficits and distortions both result in and are maintained and increased by abnormal levels of physiological arousal and by behavioural avoidance of the feared situations. Autonomic arousal produces symptoms such as dry mouth, palpitations, and abdominal pain and these may be misinterpreted as implying serious threatening illness. Panic attacks may be catastrophized and taken to mean that death is imminent. Avoidance of feared situations such as separation from parents in younger children, refusal to go to school in older children or to social events such as parties in adolescence prevent cognitive testing of the reality of the supposed threat and reinforce the cognitive distortion.

The fact that anxiety disorder is partly genetically determined means that children suffering from this condition have an increased risk of having anxious parents. Such parents are likely to model anxious behaviour, especially in the way they show over-protection to their children. Anxious children are therefore likely to be exposed to social learning situations at home that will increase the risk of avoidance of feared situations. Gene-environment interactions ensure that many parents who cannot bear to be separated from their children or who are anxious every time they leave the house will transmit their fears to their children both directly and indirectly. In adolescence, anxious young people may selectively choose shy, inhibited friends who reinforce their sense of unrealistic threat.

### Techniques of assessment and intervention

The assessment of children with anxiety disorders by a cognitive behaviour therapist focuses on the identification of cognitive deficits and distortions and the manner in which they are currently being reinforced, especially by avoidant behaviour. Nevertheless it is important that before enquiry is made along these lines a full history is taken of the development of anxious symptoms, the presence of other symptomatology, the situations that increase and reduce anxiety, the presence of anxiety in parents, sibs, and friends, and the measures that have already been taken, especially by parents, to improve the condition. Skilled assessment involves listening to the anxious preoccupations of both children and parents sympathetically and without any hint of criticism.

There are a number of systematic cognitive approaches to the reduction of anxiety in children of which the most widely used is the four-step coping or FEAR plan, in which F = **F**eeling frightened (awareness of anxiety symptoms such as somatic aches and pains), E = **E**xpecting bad things to happen (awareness of negative self-talk), A = **A**ttitudes and actions that can help (problem-solving strategies), and R = **R**esults and rewards (rewarding for success, dealing with failure).[14] The 'Cool Kids' programme is generally similar but puts more emphasis on parent involvement.[15] When parents show significant levels of anxiety themselves, effectiveness of treatment is enhanced if parental anxiety management is included as part of treatment.[16] A self-help book for parents broadly based on the same principles provides a practical approach to the management of anxiety, using the so-called COPE programme.[17]

Treatment begins with one or two psycho-educational sessions in which the child and parent(s), together or separately, are given information about the way anxiety develops and is maintained, the manner in which the body shows anxiety (somatic symptoms), and the effects of avoidant behaviour and exposure to feared situations. It is important that these sessions are interactional with the child being encouraged to talk spontaneously about, for example, how he or she experiences somatic symptoms. The next few sessions involve children engaging in an exercise to identify their own negative thoughts, to test them against reality and to develop positive thinking in situations that have previously triggered anxiety. This will usually need to be done in imagination before it is tried out using 'graded exposure' in real situations. There are advantages in teaching relaxation techniques before the child embarks on exposure to feared situations. The use of imagery, such as the 'stepladder' approach to a hierarchy of feared situations may also be helpful. When the child makes progress, as is usually the case, rewards such as outings or other treats may be built in to the procedure.

Therapists vary in the degree to which they involve parents in management. The therapy can be delivered in a family context, parents can be seen separately from children, parents may not be seen at all, or the therapy may only be delivered to parents. Some centres use a group approach, with one or two therapists providing a group experience for parents and anxious children who go through the stages of treatment together and benefit from learning of each others' experiences. Some programmes have now been developed for use via the Internet with minimal personal contact with the child and family. Some therapists combine CBT with the use of medication, generally not anxiolytic agents because of the risk of dependency, but tricyclics or selective serotonin reactive inhibitors.

### Evaluation of effectiveness and efficacy

A systematic review of the effectiveness of CBT for anxiety disorders in childhood and adolescence identified 10 randomized controlled trials that met inclusion criteria.[18] The outcome measure used was the remission of anxiety disorder. The remission rate was higher in the CBT groups (56.5 per cent) than in the control groups (34.8 per cent). The pooled odds ratio was 3.3 (CI = 1.9–5.6). The authors of this review conclude that CBT definitely provides benefit to children and adolescents with anxiety disorder, but that there is a lack of information concerning the value of CBT in younger children and that there are virtually no satisfactory studies comparing effectiveness with alternative treatments.

There is contradictory evidence concerning the importance of involving parents in therapy. Some[19,20] find little or no benefit, while others[21,22] find a trend towards benefit. A pilot study has found benefit from a programme that did not involve children directly but only involved parents seen in a group, who applied what they had learned in the group in managing the situations in which their children showed anxiety at home. Information on the use of therapy delivered via the Internet is limited, but those that exist suggest that Internet treatment is highly acceptable to families, creates minimal dropout and is effective when added to clinic treatment.[23] Dropout from more conventional treatment is likely to be high in single-parent families, ethnic minority families, and where anxiety levels are not conspicuously high.[24] There is evidence that the presence of co-morbid disorders does not reduce the efficacy of CBT.[25] The addition of antidepressants may increase the efficacy of CBT, especially in the treatment of school refusal.[26] Limited findings from long-term studies suggest that treatment benefits from the delivery of CBT to anxious children are maintained over at least 6 years.[27]

There is also evidence from controlled studies for the effectiveness of interventions, especially the FRIENDS programme[28] in the prevention of anxiety and depression in early adolescence. Stallard et al.[29] have shown how this programme can be delivered successfully by school nurses.

These evaluative studies have provided most encouraging findings for the effectiveness of CBT in this condition. However the findings also make clear that CBT, while producing worthwhile and persistent benefits in most children and adolescents with anxiety disorders, is not effective in a significant number of cases and in a significant number of others it is only partially effective. It is also less effective in socially disadvantaged groups. Finally, most evaluative studies have been carried out in highly specialist

centres and there is a lack of evidence for their value in everyday practice.[18]

## Depressive disorders

### Cognitive distortions and deficits

The classical signs of depressive disorders, such as chronic misery and unhappiness, lack of interest in food, and motor retardation, may be seen as early as the first year of life. Infants and young children who show such symptomatology may well suffer depressive experiences similar to those of older people though in the pre-verbal phase there is no reliable method available to confirm this possibility. Awareness of feeling states develops towards the end of the second year of life.[30] By 2 to 3 years children realize that there can be a variety of personal reasons for an emotional reaction. By 4 years there is some consensus about the kind of situations that will provoke the common emotional reactions, including fear, sadness, and anger.[31] By 5 or 6 years a child is capable of understanding the concept of stability of mood, 'always being unhappy or just now and again', and by 7 or 8 years concepts of shame and guilt are understood at least in simplified form. Enduring and relatively stable negative attributions about the self become possible at around this age and the concept of death as a permanent state is established. By 13 to 14 years, emotional experiences of adult intensity occur and mature cognitions about different mood states will have been attained. Although the above account relates stage of development to chronological age, there is wide variation in the ages at which cognitive competence is gained. Further, the settings in which children are questioned or encouraged to express themselves freely and spontaneously, for example in play situations will greatly influence their capacity to show their abilities.

The cognitive model underlying CBT approaches to children and adolescents does not differ from that with adults. It is assumed that thoughts are the primary experience of depression and that depressed mood is secondary. Dysfunctional assumptions, including low feelings of self-worth, self-blame for events in the past, and hopelessness about the future are present either as stable features of a depressive personality or as a reaction to adverse experiences, real or imagined. Depressed children and adolescents systematically distort their experience to match their beliefs about themselves. At some point, these negative thoughts are automatically experienced without reflection. Increasingly situations are avoided because of a fear of negative outcomes. Therapy involves identifying and reality testing these negative thoughts. In addition the patient is encouraged to enter into activities that will be rewarding and disconfirm pessimistic assumptions.

### Techniques of assessment and intervention

Initial assessment will involve taking a full history of the development of symptoms and the factors that reduce or exacerbate them, the child's functioning in different settings, and an account of family relationships. If the child is taken on for CBT, a typical approach[32] begins with the establishment of symptom status by the use of questionnaires such as the Children's Depression Inventory[33] in young patients and the Mood and Feelings Questionnaire[34] in adolescents. The goals of therapy are then discussed in a collaborative manner with emphasis on what the child or young person wishes to achieve. The proposed therapeutic approach is then explained together with the importance of homework outside the therapy sessions. An indication of the number of sessions likely to be required, usually 12–16, is given. In early sessions an account of the child's current daily activities is obtained. Adolescents are helped to keep a diary of their activities and moods. In a form of 'affective education' a check is made on the vocabulary the child uses to describe feelings and links are then established between the child's mood and the activities he or she is undertaking.

During the next sessions, in collaboration with the child, homework is planned that aims to increase activity to the level previously undertaken. Emphasis is placed on the resumption of everyday activities rather than offering treats or special occasions. At this point a problem-solving approach may be indicated. This begins with problem definition, followed by brain-storming a number of different solutions. The outcomes for different solutions are discussed and a plan developed to achieve what seems to be a satisfactory outcome. Homework involves attempts to implement the plan while keeping a record of progress and how this has influenced mood.

At least from early adolescence it will usually be possible to introduce self-monitoring procedures, in which the child identifies and notes his level of mood in relation to the thoughts he is experiencing. The child is encouraged to imagine different situations and to record how each situation makes him feel. The child is encouraged to continue this process at home, recording what happens so that his experience can be discussed in the next session. This process is accompanied by self-evaluation training, a form of cognitive restructuring in which children learn to evaluate themselves in a more positive manner. They are encouraged to consider the evidence for having a poor opinion of themselves and then to examine carefully more positive alternative explanations. This process may be expected to reduce negative automatic thoughts.

### Evaluation of effectiveness and efficacy

A comprehensive evidence-based review of controlled evaluation of cognitive behavioural psychotherapy for children and adolescents with depressive disorders[35] identified 12 studies that fulfilled methodological criteria. Most reported positive outcome for CBT post-treatment and at short-term follow-up. However, studies with longer follow-up periods from 9 months to 2 years found that a sizable percentage of subjects continued to report significant depressive symptoms or a recurrence of their depressive illness.

More recently the results of a major multi-centre trial, the Treatment of Adolescent Depression study (TADS) have been reported. In this study 479 adolescents, aged 12 to 17 years with depressive disorders were allocated randomly to a combination of fluoxetine and CBT, fluoxetine alone, CBT alone and an inert pill placebo. After 12 weeks of treatment the effects of combination therapy were clearly superior to either form of monotherapy and greatly superior to pill placebo. Fluoxetine alone was superior to CBT alone and to placebo, but CBT alone was not superior to placebo. On the other hand, fluoxetine alone was accompanied by higher rates of suicidal events and this did not occur in the combined group. It seemed therefore that CBT protected against the suicidality linked to fluoxetine use. The investigators concluded that the combination treatment produced the best outcomes.[36]

The published evidence mainly relates to children and adolescents with mild or moderate depressive disorders. There is some indication both from the TADS described and from other evidence that more severe depressive disorders do not respond as well or perhaps not at all to CBT alone.[37]

Attempts to use CBT to prevent depression in adolescents have met with varied success. One universal school-based approach found no difference at 2 to 4-year follow-up in children who received a teacher-administered cognitive behavioural intervention compared with a control group.[38] In contrast, positive effects were found for a CBT intervention targeting 13–18-year-old children of parents with depressive disorders.[39] Application of the Resourceful Adolescent Programme has also been shown to produce promising results in preventing depression in younger adolescents.[40]

## Conduct disorder

### Cognitive distortions and deficits

Both young children with oppositional disorders and adolescents with more severe conduct disorders show characteristic cognitive distortion in their thinking. They recall inaccurately high rates of hostile cues in social situations and when neutral remarks and movements are made by their peers, they see these as hostile.[41] In competitive situations with peers they exaggerate the aggressive behaviour of others and underestimate their own aggressiveness. These distorted attributions lead them into aggressive behaviour which then triggers angry behaviour from peers so that the originally neutral environment does indeed become more hostile.

Aggressive children and adolescents also have difficulties in problem-solving, both in experimental and naturalistic situations. They prefer rapid action-orientated solutions to those that require reflective thinking before any action is taken. Underlying this tendency to prefer rapid, aggressive solutions is the fact that their social goals relate more to the need for dominance and revenge than for affiliation.[42]

Parents of aggressive children also show cognitive distortions that are of relevance to the way they discipline their children.[43] This is of relevance both to the understanding and the management of childhood conduct disorders. For example, it has been shown that mothers of children with conduct disorder tend to attribute their children's difficult behaviour to deliberate wilfulness that is not within their children's capacity to control. They perceive themselves as helpless in the face of their children's behaviour. These cognitive distortions prevent them from acting effectively as parents, for example by drawing firm boundaries between acceptable and unacceptable behaviour.

### Techniques of assessment and intervention

Until the early 1980s there were really no effective, evidence-based psychological interventions for children and adolescents with conduct disorder. Since that time a number of moderately effective psychological measures have been developed. All of these, including the cognitive behavioural techniques described below are only likely to be successful if they are combined with psychosocial measures directed towards the family as well as with appropriate education. All approaches require preliminary assessment of the child and family to identify the severity of the disorder and the possible presence of co-morbid disorders as well as to determine suitability for the approach envisaged.

Cognitive approaches to conduct disorder have been summarized by Lochman *et al.*[44] *Problem-solving skills training (PSST)* has been developed for children aged 7 to 13 years. The programme is delivered over 25 sessions.[45] The group leaders teach problem-solving skills such as generating multiple solutions to a problem and reflecting on the different consequences of the alternatives. The skills are applied to interpersonal situations with teachers, parents, peers, and siblings. Parent participation is a major component of the training, with parents observing the sessions and acting as co-therapists in supervising the use of the new skills in the home.

*The Anger Coping and Coping Power Programme* is a school-based prevention programme delivered in group sessions to 13–14-year-old children.[46] The group sessions focus on enhancing emotional awareness, anger management training, attribution retraining and perspective-taking, social problem-solving and social skills training, behavioural and personal goal-setting, and handling peer pressure.

*Multi-system therapy* was designed as a multi-level intervention for 12 to 15-year-olds with multiple, severe antisocial problems.[47] Highly trained and closely supervised psychologists manage individualized programmes in the home setting. A variety of treatment approaches, including parent training, family therapy, school consultation, and individual therapy are employed in association with social measures such as helping lone mothers to find employment are used. The aim is to achieve change in one area before targeting another.

*Functional Family Therapy* combines family systems and cognitive behavioural approaches. The programme begins with an engagement and motivation phase in which the therapist addresses maladaptive beliefs in the family system thus aiming to increase expectations for change, reduce negativity and blaming, build respect for individual differences and develop a strong alliance between family members and the therapist. Practical behavioural interventions are designed to produce change and this is followed by a generalization phase in which the family is encouraged to interact effectively with the various systems in the community with which it is in contact.

*Parent Management Training Programmes* usually involve parents of young children with oppositional or conduct disorders. They derive from work originally carried out by Patterson and his colleagues at the Oregon Social Learning Center. His findings established the importance of coercive parental behaviour in the development of childhood aggression. Many treatment programmes have been based on their work,[48,49] which focus on ways of reducing parental coerciveness, often in group settings. Parents are taught to pinpoint problem behaviours, to apply positive reinforcement when their children's behaviour is more appropriate and to learn problem-solving and negotiating techniques. It has been suggested that the incorporation of a cognitive component into parent training, using a 'thoughts, feelings, behaviour cycle' can improve effectiveness of this approach.[50]

### Evaluation of efficacy and effectiveness

All of the above programmes have been evaluated in controlled clinical trials and have been shown to be moderately effective.[51–53] However, virtually all the controlled studies have been carried out in highly resourced specialist centres. There is a conspicuous lack of studies of effectiveness carried out in routine clinical care.

# Attention deficit hyperactivity disorder (ADHD)

## Cognitive distortions and deficits

Children with ADHD show a range of cognitive deficits of attention and concentration with a strong predisposition to impulsivity, accompanied by explosive temperament and poor regulation of affect and impulses. Until recently these problems have been explained on the basis of deficits in one of two cognitive pathways. It has been proposed that there is a deficit in executive function, based on deficient inhibitory control arising from frontodorsal striatal brain networks.[54] Such failure of control results in deficits in self-monitoring, planning, attentional control, and executive skills. Stimulant medication remedies these deficits by increasing the activity of inhibitory pathways. Alternatively the condition has been attributed to disturbances in motivational processes, manifest as aversion to delay in gratification. More recently Sonuga-Barke,[55] has proposed that both these mechanisms are supported by the evidence and that there are two distinct but complementary neuro-developmental bases for ADHD which is thus, at least in the pre-school period, psychologically heterogeneous. As children get older and executive function matures, deficits in executive functions may become more prominent in affected children, especially in the areas of inhibition, set shifting, working memory, planning, and fluency.[56]

## Techniques of assessment and intervention

Information about children with suspected ADHD needs to be obtained from both parents and school teachers as the child is likely to behave differently in the two settings. Both interviews and rating scales should be used. Observation of the child can confirm the presence of ADHD, but cannot rule it out as some children who are clearly showing symptomatology both at home and in school may appear normal in the clinic. Although it is helpful to reach a diagnosis, increasingly treatment approaches are focusing on the presence of specific impairments rather than on the presence of symptoms.[57]

Three types of psychological interventions have been found of value: ensuring the child's environment is structured and, when the child is engaged in a task that there is an absence of extraneous, distracting stimuli; counselling to parents and teachers, and behavioural and/or cognitive behavioural approaches directed to the child.

In the classroom the child will benefit if seated close to the teacher, task demands are kept short and there are interspersed periods of physical exercise. Teachers should be helped to reduce negative interactions by focusing on positive reinforcement for appropriate behaviour however brief this might be. Short periods of timeout before potentially problematic situations get out of hand may reduce the number of painful, angry confrontations. Similar principles can be applied in the home situation with parents being helped to understand and act on the principles of the identification of antecedents that result in problematic behaviour which will then have consequences that either increase or reduce the likelihood of recurrence. Positive reinforcement can be provided in the form of star charts, tokens, or other rewards. Training of parents of children with ADHD follows similar lines to training of parents with children with conduct disorder (see above) and, of course, many children show co-morbid ADHD and conduct disorder.

Cognitive behavioural approaches generally aim to achieve increased self-control. Most approaches involve encouraging appropriate self-instruction. The child is taught separate steps of self-instruction ('Stop: What is the problem?—Are there possible plans?—What is the best plan?—Do the plan—Did the plan work?') This approach can be applied when the child is faced with cognitive tasks which would usually be tackled impulsively or to social situations that often result in confrontations, such as arguments with parents or friends.[58]

### Evaluation of effectiveness and efficacy

The delivery of behavioural treatment to children with ADHD presents particular problems. As a group they are slow to respond to conditioning procedures. Their distractibility and short attention span leads to problems in co-operation. Parents are likely to show similar behavioural and cognitive characteristics to their children, so collaboration of parents in treatment regimes may be problematic. The children's lack of reflectivity is a barrier to the use of cognitive approaches.

There is no good evidence that cognitive approaches alone are significantly effective in children with severe ADHD.[59] The most thorough evaluation of behavioural approaches to date is the Multi-modal Treatment of Attention-Deficit Hyperactivity Disorder (MTA) study carried out in the 1990s. The 579 children in the study were randomly allocated to one of three conditions: medication with stimulants, intensive behavioural treatment, and a combination of the two. The behavioural approach involved a parent training component, a two-part school intervention and an intensive summer treatment programme. It can therefore hardly be regarded as typical of psychological interventions applied in everyday clinical practice. There were slight advantages to combined treatment over medication alone. Behavioural treatments alone were much less effective for ADHD, though more useful for co-morbid anxiety disorders.[60] A 9-month follow-up revealed that the effectiveness of behavioural management approaches had been maintained over this period.[61] Interpretations of the findings of this study have been divergent. Re-analysis suggests that it may well be that medication alone or in combination with behavioural treatment is strongly indicated in severely affected children, while behavioural treatment and parent training are equally effective where impairment is mild or moderate.[58]

Parent training alone is effective in pre-school children with mild or moderately severe ADHD when delivered in a specialist setting, but is not when provided as part of routine primary care by non-specialist nurses.[62]

## Obsessive–compulsive disorders

### Cognitive distortions and deficits

The core cognitive distortion in children and adolescents with obsessive–compulsive disorder (OCD) is thought to lie, as it does with adult patients, in the appraisal of responsibility.[63] This is defined as 'the belief that one has power which is pivotal to bring about or prevent subjectively crucial negative outcomes'. Now we all do have responsibility for our actions; what makes patients with OCD different is that they take upon themselves quite unreasonable levels of responsibility. A 13-year-old might, for example, think 'I am responsible for making sure my mother does not die'.

This sense of responsibility leads to attempts both to suppress and to neutralize the unwelcome thoughts of responsibility.

'Neutralizing' is defined as voluntary activity intended to have the effect of reducing the perceived responsibility. 'If I tap on my glass three times before I drink from it, my mother will not die'. But neutralizing activities increase discomfiting cognitions and this leads to further neutralizing activity. Attempts to suppress the intrusive thoughts also increase the likelihood of their recurrence. An additional complicating feature of the cognitive distortion is that, in the mind of the child with OCD, thoughts become imbued with unrealistic or magical powers. It is enough just to have a thought for it to be translated into action, so-called 'thought-action fusion'. 'If I allow myself to think about my mother dying this will mean that she will die'.

In general the cognitive distortions made by children and adolescents with OCD are similar to those seen in adults. However in a study comparing the various components of OCD cognitions in children, adolescents and adults it was found that children experienced fewer intrusive thoughts and these were less distressing and less uncontrollable than those experienced by adolescents and adults.[64] On the other hand, cognitive processes of thought-action fusion, perceived severity of harm, self-doubt and cognitive control were similar across the three age groups.

### Techniques of assessment and intervention

The aim of cognitive therapy is to help the patient reach the view that obsessional thoughts, however distressing, are irrelevant to any activities that may be undertaken in the future. This is achieved by increasing the patient's sense of personal efficacy, predictability, controllability, and self-attributed likelihood of a positive outcome. The techniques used involve the conduct of tasks involving exposure to feared stimuli as well as response prevention, stopping the activities that reinforce the unwelcome thoughts.

The most widely applied treatment approach to OCD in children and adolescents is that developed by John March and his colleagues.[65] The treatment protocol involves 12 sessions of which the first two are spent on psycho-education and cognitive training and the next 10 sessions on exposure and response prevention with the first and last two sessions, as well as an intermediate session involving parents. The effectiveness of exposure depends on the fact that anxiety diminishes after repeated contact with a feared stimulus. Thus the anxiety of a child worried about germs will be reduced by prolonged contact with a surface the child thinks has germs on it. Encouraging parents not to provide reassurance to children who compulsively and repetitively demand it, removes reinforcement, and results in extinction of the behaviour. Some children become extremely distressed when their parents, on instruction, fail to provide such reassurance; more success is achieved by putting the child in control of reducing parents' inappropriate behaviour. Modelling and shaping behaviours are also helpful in giving the children or adolescents the skills to expose themselves to feared stimuli. Liberal use of rewards when the child behaves appropriately is also helpful in reinforcing desired behaviour.

### Evaluation of effectiveness and efficacy

The most informative findings on efficacy come from the Pediatric OCD Treatment study (POTS) Team.[66] 112 patients aged from 12 to 17 years, suffering from OCD were divided randomly into four groups: CBT alone, sertraline alone, combined sertraline, and CBT treatment and a pill placebo. Both sertraline alone and CBT alone were superior in outcome to pill placebo at 12 weeks after the beginning of treatment. But combined treatment was superior to both treatments administered separately with a clinical remission rate of 54 per cent, compared to 4 per cent for placebo.

Most studies report the results of individual treatment with children and adolescents, with limited input from parents. Initial findings suggest that for middle-school aged children, aged 8–14 years, CBT delivered with a stronger focus on parental involvement than is usually the case with adolescents is effective in reducing symptomatology[67] at least in the short-term. Success has also been reported for similar treatment provided in a group format. Group CBT is as effective as sertraline, and shows better results than sertraline at 9 months follow-up.[68] The presence of tics does not reduce the effectiveness of CBT in the treatment of OCD.[69] There are few studies investigating the longer-term effect of CBT on OCD. However it has been shown that improvement after both individual and group therapy is maintained for at least 18 months without attenuation.[70]

# Application of CBT for miscellaneous purposes

There are a number of other conditions and adverse psychosocial situations occurring in childhood and adolescence in which the use of CBT is an important component of management. For a further discussion of these conditions and their management, see other sections of this book.

## Chronic fatigue syndrome (CFS)

In this condition, characterized by severe fatigue and overwhelming exhaustion, with excessive sleepiness and a variety of other unexplained physical complaints, cognitive distortions involving an enhanced tendency to believe in the presence of disease in the absence of medical evidence (illness attribution), and deficits in the use of problem-solving techniques related to illness and disability have been identified.[71] The illness is not uncommon, occurring in around 2 per 1000, 11 to 15-year-olds. Rehabilitative methods, including the use of CBT have been found to be successful in adults and are also employed in the paediatric age group. A controlled clinical trial has found 10–17-year-olds with CFS to show greater improvement with CBT than a waiting list control group.[72]

## Substance abuse

Cognitive distortions in young people presenting with substance abuse commonly relate to denial they have a serious, ultimately life-threatening problem, unwillingness to believe that effective help is available, and lack of belief in their own self-efficacy to change their behaviour. There is increasing evidence from controlled clinical trials that cognitive behaviour therapies can achieve positive results.[73] Motivational interviewing preceding the use of CBT is important with many children and adolescents and this is likely to be particularly the case with those suffering from substance abuse.

## Eating disorders

Central features of both anorexia nervosa and bulimia nervosa include distorted cognitions about shape and weight. Cognitive behavioural

approaches used with adults with these conditions require modification when used with adolescents, with greater emphasis on involvement of parents.[74] While CBT is the most effective treatment for bulimia in older adolescents and adults,[75] family counselling is now established as the most effective intervention for anorexia nervosa in younger patients.[76]

## Post-traumatic stress disorder

This condition is characterized by disorders of thinking including repetitive, intrusive thoughts, phobic avoidance of the situation in which the individual was exposed to trauma, 'survivor guilt', and problems in concentration. CBT is the most effective, evidence-based technique in the management in both children and adolescents.[77,78]

## Non-organic pain

Abdominal pain and headache for which no physical cause can be found are commonly seen in primary health care. Although when these conditions occur it is often difficult to establish a psychological mechanism for the pain, it is reasonably well established that management based on CBT is the most effective approach. CBT is also effective in reducing pain from organic disease as well as in reducing distress when painful paediatric procedures are carried out. For a review of the use of CBT in the management of pain in childhood, see McGrath and Goodman.[79]

## Adverse psychosocial situations

Children and adolescents in adverse psychosocial situations are frequently troubled by distorted perceptions of their predicament. In particular, they may feel themselves responsible for the separation and divorce of their parents or that they have deserved the maltreatment, either physical or sexual, inflicted on them by adults who have abused them. CBT has a significant part to play in helping children adjust to parental separation and divorce.[80] It has also been shown to have demonstrable value when applied to victims of sexual abuse.[81]

# Further information

Graham, P. (2005). *Cognitive-behaviour therapy for children and families* (2nd edn). Cambridge University Press, Cambridge.

Stallard, P. (2005). *A clinician's guide to think good-feel good.* John Wiley, Chichester.

Kazdin, A. and Weisz, J. (2003). *Evidence-based psychotherapies for children and adolescents.* Guilford Press, New York.

# References

1. Piaget, J. (1970). Piaget's theory. In *Carmichael's manual of child psychology*, Vol. 1 (ed. P.H. Mussen), pp. 703–32. Wiley, New York.
2. Beck, A. (1964). Thinking and depression: 2. Theory and therapy. *Archives of General Psychiatry*, **10**, 561–71.
3. Wellman, H.M., Hollander, M., and Schult, C.A. (1996). Young children's understanding of thought bubbles and thoughts. *Child Development*, **67**, 768–88.
4. Hoare, P., Elton, R., Greer, A., *et al.* (1993). The modification and standardisation of the Harter self-esteem questionnaire with Scottish school children. *European Child & Adolescent Psychiatry*, **2**, 19–33.
5. Turner, J.E. and Cole, D.A. (1994). Developmental differences for cognitive diathesis in childhood depression. *Journal of Abnormal Child Psychology*, **22**, 15–32.

6. Young, E.J. (1990). *Cognitive therapy for personality disorders: a schema-focused approach.* Professional Resource Exchange, Sarasota, FL.

7. Stallard, P. and Rayner, H. (2005). The development and preliminary evaluation of a Schema Questionnaire for Children (SQC). *Behavioural and Cognitive Psychotherapy*, **33**, 217–24.

8. Kendall, P. (1991). *Child and adolescent therapy: cognitive-behavioral procedures*, p. 6. Guilford Press, New York.

9. Stallard, P. (2005). *A clinician's guide to think-good, feel-good.* John Wiley, Winchester.

10. Wilson, C. and White, C. (2006). A preliminary investigation of the effect of intervention on parental attributions and reported behaviour. *Behavioural and Cognitive Psychotherapy*, **34**, 503–7.

11. Wolpert, M., Doe, J., and Elsworth, J. (2005). Working with parents: ethical and practical issues. In *Cognitive behaviour therapy for children and families* (ed. P.J. Graham), pp. 103–20. Cambridge University Press, Cambridge.

12. Schmidt, U. (2005). Engagement and motivational interviewing. In *Cognitive behaviour therapy for children and families* (ed. P.J. Graham), pp. 67–83. Cambridge University Press, Cambridge.

13. Kingdon, D., Hansen, L., Finn, M., *et al.* (2007). When standard cognitive-behavioural therapy is not enough. *Psychiatric Bulletin*, **31**, 121–3.

14. Kendall, P., Chansky, T.E., Friedman, M., *et al.* (1991). Treating anxiety disorders in children and adolescents. In *Child and adolescent therapy* (ed. P.C. Kendell), pp. 131–64. Guilford Press, New York.

15. Allen, J.L. and Rapee, R.M. (2005). Anxiety disorders. In *Cognitive behaviour therapy for children and families* (ed. P.J. Graham), pp. 300–19. Cambridge University Press, Cambridge.

16. Cobham, V., Dadds, M., and Spence, S. (1998). The role of parental anxiety in the treatment of childhood anxiety. *Journal of Consulting and Clinical Psychology*, **66**, 893–905.

17. Dacey, J.S. and Fiore, L.B. (2000). *Your anxious child.* Jossey-Bass, San Francisco.

18. Cartwright-Hatton, S., Roberts, C., Chitsabesan, P., *et al.* (2004). Systematic review of the efficacy of cognitive behaviour therapies for childhood and adolescent anxiety disorders. *The British Journal of Clinical Psychology*, **43**, 421–36.

19. Heyne, D., King, N.J., and Tonge, B., *et al.* (2002). Evaluation of child therapy and caregiver training in the treatment of school refusal. *Journal of the American Academy of Child and Adolescent Psychiatry*, **41**, 687–95.

20. Nauta, M.H., Scholing, A., Emmelkamp, P.M., *et al.* (2003). Cognitive-behavioral therapy for children with anxiety disorders in a clinical setting: no additional effect of a cognitive parent training. *Journal of the American Academy of Child and Adolescent Psychiatry*, **42**, 1270–8.

21. Spence, S.H., Donovan, C., and Brechman-Toussaint, M. (2000). The treatment of childhood social phobia: the effectiveness of a social skills training-based, cognitive-behavioural intervention, with and without parental involvement. *Journal of Child Psychology and Psychiatry*, **41**, 713–26.

22. Wood, J.J., Piacentini, J.C., Southam-Gerow, M., *et al.* (2006). Family cognitive behavioral therapy for child anxiety disorders. *American Academy of Child and Adolescent Psychiatry*, **45**, 314–21.

23. Spence, S.H., Holmes, J.M., March, S., *et al.* (2006). The feasibility and outcome of clinic plus internet delivery of cognitive-behavior therapy for childhood anxiety. *Journal of Consulting and Clinical Psychology*, **74**, 614–21.

24. Kendall, P. and Sugarman, A. (1997). Attrition in the treatment of childhood anxiety disorders. *Journal of Consulting and Clinical Psychology*, **40**, 787–94.

25. Rapee, R.M. (2003). The influence of comorbidity on treatment outcome for children and adolescents with anxiety disorders. *Behaviour Research and Therapy*, **41**, 105–12.

26. Bernstein, G.A., Borchardt, C.M., Perwien, A.R., *et al.* (2000). Imipramine plus cognitive-behavioral therapy in the treatment of school refusal. *Journal of the American Academy of Child and Adolescent Psychiatry*, **39**, 276–83.

27. Barrett, P.M., Duffy, A.L., Dadds, M.R., *et al.* (2001). Cognitive-behavioral treatment of anxiety disorders in children: long-term (6-year) follow-up. *Journal of Consulting and Clinical Psychology*, **69**, 135–41.

28. Barrett, P., Farrell, L., Ollendick, T., *et al.* (2006). Long term outcomes of an Australian universal prevention program of anxiety and depressive symptoms in children and youth. *Journal of Clinical Child and Adolescent Psychology*, **35**, 403–11.

29. Stallard, P., Simpson, N., Anderson, S., *et al.* (2007). The friends emotional health programme: initial findings from a school-based project. *Child and Adolescent Mental Health*, **12**, 32–7.

30. Kagan, J. (1982). The emergence of self. *Journal of Child Psychology and Psychiatry*, **23**, 363–81.

31. Terwogt, M.M. and Stegge, H. (1995). Emotional behaviour and emotional understanding: a developmental fugue. In *The depressed child and adolescent: developmental and clinical perspectives* (ed. I.M. Goodyer), pp. 27–52. Cambridge University Press, Cambridge.

32. Harrington, R. (2005). Depressive disorders. In *Cognitive behaviour therapy for children and families* (ed. P.J. Graham), pp. 263–80. Cambridge University Press, Cambridge.

33. Kovacs, M. (1981). Rating scales to assess depression in school-aged children. *Acta Paedopsychiatrica*, **46**, 305–15.

34. Angold, A., Costello, E.J., Messer, S.C., *et al.* (1995). The development of a short questionnaire for use in epidemiological studies of depression in children and adolescents. *International Journal of Methods in Psychiatric Research*, **5**, 237–49.

35. Compton, S.N., March, J.S., Brent, D., *et al.* (2004). Cognitive-behavioral therapy for anxiety and depressive disorders in children and adolescents: an evidence-based review. *Journal of the American Academy of Child and Adolescent Psychiatry*, **43**, 930–59.

36. March, J., Silva, S., Vitiello, B., and TADS Team. (2006). The Treatment for Adolescents with Depression Study (TADS): methods and message at 12 weeks. *Journal of the American Academy of Child and Adolescent Psychiatry*, **45**, 1393–403.

37. Jayson, D., Wood, A.J., Kroll, L., *et al.* (1998). Which depressed patients respond to cognitive-behavioral treatment? *Journal of the American Academy of Child and Adolescent Psychiatry*, **37**, 35–9.

38. Spence, S.H., Sheffield, J.K., and Donovan, C.L. (2005). Long-term outcome of a school-based, universal approach to prevention of depression in adolescents. *Journal of Consulting and Clinical Psychology*, **73**, 160–7.

39. Clarke, G.N., Hornbrook, M., Lynch, F., *et al.* (2001). A randomized trial of a group cognitive intervention for preventing depression in the offspring of depressed parents. *Archives of General Psychiatry*, **58**, 1127–34.

40. Merry, S., McDowell, H., Wild, C., *et al.* (2004). A randomized placebo-controlled trial of a school-based depression prevention program. *Journal of the American Academy of Child and Adolescent Psychiatry*, **43**, 538–47.

41. Dodge, K.A. and Frame, C.L. (1982). Social cognitive biases and deficits in aggressive boys. *Child Development*, **53**, 620–35.

42. Lochman, J., Wayland, K., and White, K. (1993). Social goals: relationship to adolescent adjustment and to social problem solving. *Journal of Abnormal Child Psychology*, **21**, 135–51.

43. Baden, A.G. and Howe, G.W. (1992). Mother's attributions and expectancies regarding their conduct disordered children. *Journal of Abnormal Child Psychology*, **20**, 467–85.

44. Lochman, J., Phillips, N., McElroy, H., *et al.* (2005). Conduct disorders in adolescence. In *Cognitive behaviour therapy for children and families* (ed. P.J. Graham), pp. 443–58. Cambridge University Press, Cambridge.

45. Kazdin, A., Siegel, T., and Bass, D. (1992). Cognitive problem solving skills training and parent management in the treatment of antisocial

behavior in children. *Journal of Consulting and Clinical Psychology*, **60**, 733–47.

46. Lochman, J. and Wells, K. (2002). The coping power programme at the middle school transition. *Psychology of Addictive Behaviors*, **16**, S40–S54.

47. Henggeler, S. (1999). Multisystemic therapy: an overview of clinical procedures, outcomes and policy implications. *Child Psychology and Psychiatry Review*, **4**, 2–10.

48. Webster-Stratton, C., Hollinsworth, T., and Kolpacoff, M. (1989). The long-term effectiveness and clinical significance of three cost-effective training programs for families with conduct-problem children. *Journal of Consulting and Clinical Psychology*, **57**, 550–53.

49. Sanders, M., Markie-Dadds, C., Tully, L., *et al.* (2000). The triple-P Positive Parenting Program: a comparison of enhanced, standard and self-directed behavioral family intervention for parents of children with early onset conduct problems. *Journal of Consulting and Clinical Psychology*, **68**, 624–60.

50. White, C., McNally, D., and Cartwright-Hatton, S. (2003). Cognitively enhanced parent training. *Behavioural and Cognitive Psychotherapy*, **31**, 99–102.

51. Kazdin, A. and Wassell, G. (2000). Therapeutic changes in children, parents and families resulting from treatment of children with conduct problems. *Journal of the American Academy of Child and Adolescent Psychiatry*, **39**, 414–20.

52. Van de Wiel, N., Matthys, W., Cohen-Kettenis, P., *et al.* (2002). Effective treatments of school-aged conduct disordered children: recommendations for changing clinical and research practices. *European Child & Adolescent Psychiatry*, **11**, 79–84.

53. Scott, S., Spender, Q., Doolan, M., *et al.* (2001). Multicentre controlled trial of parenting groups for childhood antisocial behaviour. *British Medical Journal*, **323**, 194–8.

54. Sonuga-Barke, E. (2003). The dual pathway of AD/HD: an elaboration of neuro-developmental characteristics. *Neuroscience and Biobehavioral Reviews*, **27**, 593–604.

55. Sonuga-Barke, E. (2005). Causal models of attention-deficit/hyperactivity disorder: from common simple deficits to multiple developmental pathways. *Biological Psychiatry*, **57**, 1231–8.

56. Sergeant, J., Geurts, H., and Oosterlaan, J. (2002). How specific is a deficit of executive functioning in attention-deficit/hyperactivity disorder? *Behavior Brain Research*, **130**, 3–28.

57. Pelham, W.E. and Walker, K.S. (2005). Attention deficit hyperactivity disorder. In *Cognitive behaviour therapy for children and families* (ed. P.J. Graham), pp. 225–43. Cambridge University Press, Cambridge.

58. Taylor, E., Dopfner, M., Sergeant, J., *et al.* (2004). European clinical guidelines for hyperkinetic disorder—first upgrade. *European Child & Adolescent Psychiatry*, **13**(Suppl. 1), 7–30.

59. Abikoff, H. (1991). Cognitive training in ADHD children: less to it than meets the eye. *Journal of Learning Disabilities*, **24**, 205–9.

60. Jensen, P., Hinshaw, S., Swanson, J., *et al.* (2001). Findings from the NIMH Multimodal Treatment Study of ADHD (MTA): implications and applications for primary care providers. *Journal of Behavioral and Developmental Pediatrics*, **22**, 60–73.

61. Arnold, L., Chuang, S., Davies, M., *et al.* (2004). Nine months of multi-component behavioural treatment for ADHD and effectiveness of MTA fading procedures. *Journal of Abnormal Child Psychology*, **32**, 39–51.

62. Sonuga-Barke, E., Thompson, M., Daley, D., *et al.* (2004). Parent training for attention deficit/hyperactivity disorder: is it as effective when delivered as routine rather than as specialist care? *The British Journal of Clinical Psychology*, **43**, 449–57.

63. Salkovskis, P.M. and Kirk, J. (1997). Obsessive-compulsive disorder. In *Science and practice of cognitive behaviour therapy* (eds. D.M. Clark and C.G. Fairbairn), pp. 179–208. Oxford Medical Publications, Oxford.

64. Farrell, L. and Barrett, P. (2006). Obsessive-compulsive disorder across developmental trajectory: cognitive processing of threat in children, adolescents and adults. *The British Journal of Psychology*, **97**, 95–114.

65. March, J.S. and Mulle, K. (1998). *OCD in children and adolescents: a cognitive-behavioral treatment manual*. Guilford Press, New York.

66. Pediatric, O.C.D. Treatment Study (POTS) Team. (2004). Cognitive-behavior therapy, sertraline, and their combination for children and adolescents with obsessive-compulsive disorder: the Pediatric OCD Treatment Study (POTS) randomized controlled trial. *The Journal of the American Medical Association*, **292**, 1969–76.

67. Martin, J. and Thienemann, M. (2005). Group cognitive-behavior therapy with family involvement for middle-school-age children with obsessive-compulsive disorder. *Child Psychiatry and Human Development*, **36**, 113–27.

68. Asbahr, F., Castillo, A., Ito, L., *et al.* (2005). Group cognitive-behavioral therapy versus sertraline for the treatment of children with obsessive-compulsive disorder. *Journal of the American Academy of Child and Adolescent Psychiatry*, **44**, 1128–36.

69. Himle, J., Fischer, D., Van Etten, M., *et al.* (2003). Group behavioral therapy for adolescents with tic-related and non-tic-related obsessive compulsive disorder. *Depression and Anxiety*, **17**, 73–7.

70. Barrett, P., Farrell, L., Dadds, M., *et al.* (2005). Cognitive-behavioral family treatment of childhood obsessive-compulsive disorder: long-term follow-up and predictors of outcome. *Journal of the American Academy of Child and Adolescent Psychiatry*, **44**, 1005–14.

71. Garralda, E. and Chalder, T. (2005). Chronic fatigue syndrome in childhood. *Journal of Child Psychology and Psychiatry*, **46**, 1143–51.

72. Stulemeijer, M., De, J., Lieke, W., *et al.* (2005). Cognitive behaviour therapy for adolescents with chronic fatigue syndrome. *British Medical Journal*, **330**, 14.

73. Waldron, H. and Kaminer, Y. (2004). On the learning curve: the emerging evidence supporting cognitive-behavioral therapies for adolescent substance abuse. *Addiction*, **99**(Suppl. 2), 93–105.

74. Lock, J. (2002). Treating adolescents with eating disorders within the family context: empirical and theoretical considerations. *Child and Adolescent Psychiatric Clinics*, **11**, 331–42.

75. Thiels, C., Schmidt, U., Treasure, J., *et al.* (1998). Guided self-change for bulimia nervosa incorporating use of a self-care manual. *The American Journal of Psychiatry*, **155**, 947–53.

76. Eisler, I., Dare, C., Hodes, M., *et al.* (2000). Family therapy for adolescent anorexia nervosa: the results of a controlled comparison of two family interventions. *Journal of Child Psychology and Psychiatry*, **41**, 727–36.

77. Perrin, S., Smith, P., and Yule, W. (2000). The assessment and treatment of post-traumatic stress disorder in children and adolescents. *Journal of Child Psychology and Psychiatry*, **41**, 277–89.

78. Deblinger, E., Mannarino, A., Cohen, J., *et al.* (2006). A follow-up study of a multisite, randomized, controlled trial for children with sexual abuse-related PTSD symptoms. *Journal of the American Academy of Child and Adolescent Psychiatry*, **45**, 1474–84.

79. McGrath, P. and Goodman, P. (2005). Pain in childhood. In *Cognitive behaviour therapy for children and families* (ed. P.J. Graham), pp. 426–42. Cambridge University Press, Cambridge.

80. Herbert, M. (2005). Adjustment to parental separation and divorce. In *Cognitive behaviour therapy for children and families* (ed. P.J. Graham), pp. 170–83. Cambridge University Press, Cambridge.

81. Jones, D. and Ramchandani, P. (1999). *Child sexual abuse: informing practice from research*. Radcliffe Medical Press, Abingdon.

# 9.5.4 Caregiver-mediated interventions for children and families

## Philip A. Fisher and Elizabeth A. Stormshak

This chapter summarizes interventions that have been developed to address child and adolescent behaviour problems and externalizing disorders within the therapeutic milieu of the family. Although it has long been recognized that caregiver-mediated treatments can be employed to address children's problems, research with families in the past two decades has resulted in numerous systematic, theory-driven approaches that have been subjected to rigorous scientific evaluation and have been found to be effective at improving outcomes. Although no intervention is certain to work for every child and it is not possible to engage every family in the intervention process, caregiver-mediated interventions are among the most promising approaches currently available to practitioners.

In recent years, progress in the field of caregiver-mediated interventions has included an expansion of the evidence base supporting specific intervention practices for use with the general population, with high-risk segments of the population (e.g. children in foster care and children in Head Start settings), and with underserved populations (e.g. girls and racial/ethnic minorities). In addition, an increasing emphasis has been placed on the dissemination of proven interventions on large-scale bases within community settings in North America, Europe, and Australia. Evidence is currently being gathered to evaluate the impact of many of these large-scale dissemination efforts. The chapter that follows contains background information on the theoretical underpinnings of caregiver-mediated interventions to address child behaviour problems. Specific interventions that have been developed for children in specific age groups—prenatal through early childhood, the school-age period, and adolescence—are then described. Finally, we discuss adaptations that have been made to address issues of gender and cultural diversity within this field.

Before providing a background on caregiver-mediated interventions, a disclaimer is necessary. The term 'caregiver-mediated' is employed throughout this chapter, rather than the term 'family-mediated', to convey the sense that these interventions need not occur specifically within the context of the child's biological family. Recognition of the diversity of family types in which children are raised requires a shift from a nuclear family conceptualization to include multigenerational families, lesbian/gay/bisexual families, and other nontraditional family configurations. In addition, many children are reared in contexts that include no direct biological relatives. For instance, increasing numbers of children are reared in foster care. To a certain extent, this is indicative of the need to address and prevent child maltreatment and to provide services that allow children to remain in their biological families. In addition, it represents a positive development to the extent that many children who have previously been cared for in institutional settings are now being placed in community families, which have the potential to provide more adequate rearing environments than institutions. However, it is often the case that caregivers in these foster/adoptive families will require additional support services to improve outcomes for children. Thus, we have adopted the term caregiver-mediated interventions to reflect the spectrum of existing rearing environments.

## Background on caregiver-mediated interventions

There is no single predominant cause of the development of behaviour problems in an individual child. Rather, as is noted in Patterson *et al.*[1] research has implicated a broad array of factors that contribute to behaviours at virtually every level of analysis. From a *societal perspective*, factors such as poverty, discrimination, and unemployment have been implicated as contributing to higher rates of disruptive behaviour in children. In addition, children in various underprivileged contexts (e.g. children in foster care or with incarcerated parents) show higher rates of disruptive behaviour. *Neighbourhood factors* such as crowded living conditions and violence also appear to be associated with higher rates of behaviour problems. At the *individual level*, psychosocial and neurobiological factors have been associated with higher rates of behaviour problems. For example, poor social skills, and low cognitive functioning appear to be linked to the development of behaviour problems. Recent evidence also indicates that genetic factors play a role in whether or not a child develops externalizing behaviour.[2]

With this multitude of factors implicated in the development of disruptive behaviour, one might question why caregiver-mediated interventions have become so predominant. The answer is straightforward. In as much as children exist within the context of their families, caregivers exert the single largest influence on children's behavioural and developmental outcomes. Numerous longitudinal studies have shown that caregiver factors predict over and above individual-, neighbourhood-, and society-level variables in determining trajectories towards disruptive behaviour.[1] Moreover, randomized trials of caregiver-mediated interventions have provided information that manipulating caregiver behaviours (e.g. teaching them to use effective parenting strategies) is extremely powerful for improving child outcomes.[3] Thus, although child behaviour problems are multidetermined, the most direct method for improving child outcomes appears to be via the caregiver–child relationship.

The interventions that are described below are categorized by developmental epoch. It is also important to recognize that interventions exist across the spectrum of risk, including proven interventions to reduce problem behaviours in children with disruptive behaviour disorders and preventive efforts to deflect children from developing disruptive behaviour disorders. An overall synopsis of the interventions to be described is that they have shown great promise for addressing problems at a number of levels. Although a number of issues still confront the field, the progress that has been made in the last two decades has been remarkable in demonstrating that it is possible to address child behaviour problems through caregiver-mediated interventions.

### Prenatal and early childhood caregiver-mediated interventions

Caregiver-mediated interventions for the prenatal period through infancy and early childhood are generally oriented towards prevention. That is, rather than addressing concurrent problems with the child, they are based on the supposition that targeting known precursors of child problems is an effective way to prevent those problems. Among the most influential work in this area has been the home visitation programme developed and evaluated by Olds and colleagues to prevent antisocial behaviour in children.[4] This project involved a randomized control trial that included longitudinal data collection over more than 25 years.[5] A total of 400 pregnant women were enrolled in the original study according to one of the three following criteria: under 19 years of age, unmarried, or of low socioeconomic status. Those assigned to the intervention condition received an average of 9 home visits during pregnancy and an average of 23 home visits between birth and the child's second birthday. The home visits were conducted by nurses. The focus of visits was upon prenatal and neonatal maternal health behaviours, child care skills, and maternal life issues (e.g. education and employment).

Olds and colleagues reported 15-year outcomes for the children of the mothers in this study. Those in the intervention group reported fewer arrests than those in a comparison group.[6] In addition, among those in higher risk categories (as indicated by their mother being both low SES and unmarried at the time of the child's birth), youth in the intervention group reported lower rates of running away, arrests, criminal convictions and parole violations, and smoking and alcohol consumption than did youth in the comparison group. The authors concluded that this approach may be an effective means of preventing early-onset conduct disorder, which has been considered the more treatment-resistant and complex form of the disorder.[1] However, it is also noteworthy that, in subsequent randomized trial studies to examine how variations in the programme structure affect outcomes, the intervention was found to be less effective when paraprofessionals were used in place of nurses as home visitors.[7] More recently, and consistent with other evidence-based programmes, the emphasis of Olds and colleagues has shifted to a wide-scale dissemination of the intervention in community settings.[8] Within this context, emphasis has been placed on maintaining the programme's effectiveness by developing practices to ensure that the intervention is delivered with high fidelity to the original model.

It is important to recognize that not all caregiver-mediated preventive interventions for children in this age group have shown positive effects. For example, the Healthy Start programme was designed to prevent child abuse and neglect, using an initial screening process (usually in hospital settings) to identify families at risk for child maltreatment and employing a home-visitor model of service delivery for the intervention. Although modest positive effects were observed in individual sites implementing this programme, the overall results from a large-scale randomized trial of this intervention did not support the efficacy of the intervention.[9] A related problem in the evaluation of the Healthy Start programme was low rates of family participation. Of those recruited, many received very few home visitation sessions. With such low dosage rates, it can be difficult to determine whether the lack of positive intervention effects was due to a failure of the approach to impact targeted behaviours or was due to families receiving too little of the intervention for it to have been effective. Thus, as is true across the span of child development, it is important to consider what the critical elements of effective interventions are and to make sure that these are included in any intervention efforts.

## Caregiver-mediated interventions in the preschool years

The preschool years are marked by a number of important developmental changes. Dramatic increases in the use of language and physical mobility in addition to an increase in autonomous behaviour provide challenges for many parents. Preschool children need substantial support from parents and caretakers in socialization in their family and school environments. As a result, as with interventions in infancy, the majority of caregiver-mediated interventions at this age are focused on parenting, and the parent–child relationship.

Within the parenting literature, there are many different types of parenting skills that have been found to be important in promoting healthy child development. Typically, interventions include a dual focus on increasing positive parenting and decreasing negative parenting. Positive parenting usually refers to supportive, warm, involved parenting that includes praise, positive support, approval, and responsiveness to children and their needs.[10] Negative parenting usually refers to parenting deficits, including poor limit setting, inconsistency, verbal and physical aggression, and harsh discipline.[11]

Caregiver-based interventions at this age typically focus on building a strong positive parent–child relationship in addition to teaching specific behaviour management techniques to promote healthy child adjustment and prevent later problems. Although some programmes target at-risk children, such as Head Start children or those with early behaviour problems, there is some evidence that more severe child behaviour problems are related to more limited effects of parent training programmes.[12]

One of the more successful caregiver-based programmes for preschoolers, *The Incredible Years*, was developed by Webster-Stratton and colleagues.[13] This videotaped programme includes a number of salient parenting skills for preschoolers, starting with building a positive parent–child relationship, praise, and rewards and moving to limit setting, problem solving, and discipline. Randomized trial evaluations have suggested that this programme is effective when administered in group and individual settings.[14] Results have suggested that the programme improves parent–child interactions immediately post-test and 1 year later. The programme was subsequently expanded from basic parenting skills to include more advanced parenting, such as anger management, communication, and self-control skills, which is also effective at improving the parent–child relationship and reducing child behaviour problems at short-term follow-up. The advanced programme is able to deal effectively with parent–child problems and the mediators that might influence the parent's ability to effectively manage the child, including depression and the marital relationship. Overall, this parent training programme has been effective with a number of different age groups and populations, including preschool- and school-aged children as well as clinic-referred and community Head Start families.[15]

Other caregiver-mediated interventions involving preschoolers have also shown success at enhancing the parent–child relationship and decreasing child behaviour problems. For example, *Parent–Child Interaction Training (PCIT)* was originally developed for at-risk children enrolled in Head Start.[16] Training involved teaching parents effective play skills and positive interaction. The programme has been effective at reducing teacher ratings of behaviour problems 1 year after the intervention was completed. This approach has subsequently been used for other populations. For example, Chaffin *et al.* reported on the results of using *PCIT* to prevent child abuse among families with a history of child welfare system involvement.[17] The intervention significantly reduced future reports of maltreatment. Interestingly, an enhanced version of the intervention designed to provide individualized services to meet families' needs was no more effective than the original *PCIT* intervention.

Home visitation programmes in preschool have also shown promise as effective interventions. Head Start, for example, provides home-visiting services to all families in the programme. The goals of these visits are to work with families on meeting the Head Start performance standards in four areas: education, health–nutrition–mental health, social services, and parent involvement. Research has indicated that children who received home services have shown improvements in the parent–child relationship and early academic achievement compared to children and families who did not receive the home visits or parenting model.[18] Home-visiting programmes at this age also provide families with social support, self-efficacy, and a positive therapeutic relationship with the visitor. This relationship serves to enable parents to process and understand parenting and family histories that impede the development of successful parenting skills with their own child.

## Caregiver-mediated interventions in the school-aged years

As children move into the school years, they face a new set of challenges at home and in the school environment, including academic achievement, negotiating peer relationships, and the demands of teachers and the school context. At this age, children who have begun developing problems in the context of their families may generalize these problems to the school environment, which is associated with increased risk of later difficulties in addition to problems across multiple domains of functioning.[19] As a result, the transition to school serves as an important target of preventive intervention programmes.[20] Furthermore, school problems and peer difficulties may exacerbate problems in the home as parents struggle with issues such as homework completion and their child's social skills and changing peer network. Thus, effective interventions aimed at school-aged children must support families and parents through an emphasis on parent training and improving or maintaining academic achievement and positive peer relationships at school.

Although the emphasis on increasing positive parenting skills and decreasing negative parenting is typically maintained in interventions at this age and across development, additional components targeting academic achievement, learning and early literacy, and parent–school involvement are important aspects of comprehensive, caregiver-mediated interventions for school-aged children. There are multiple examples of comprehensive, caregiver-mediated prevention programmes that have been associated with positive outcomes for school-aged youth and families, including the *Families and Schools Together (FAST) Track* programme,[21] the *Linking the Interests of Families and Teachers (LIFT)* programme,[22] and the *Schools and Families Educating (SAFE) Children* programme.[23]

The *FAST Track* programme began in 1991 and targeted children in early elementary school at risk of developing later conduct disorder and delinquent behaviour problems.[21] Children and families received a multifocused intervention package targeting development across multiple domains, including peers, the school environment, academic achievement, and the family context. The family intervention integrated successful approaches to parent training regarding the development of school-aged children, including parent–school involvement and early reading.[21,24,25] Parents met in groups weekly during the first-grade year and bi-weekly in second grade. One hour of parent–child learning activity that emphasized positive parent–child interactions in a controlled environment and early literacy was also provided. Home visits and individualized programming were implemented to meet the special needs of families, such as stress management, marital problems, and maternal depression. The intervention continued through adolescence, with new components adapted to the changing development of children and families. Results of this programme indicated that it was successful at the end of first grade and third grade in improving outcomes across a number of different domains, including parenting and child peer relations, emotional understanding, and reading skills. Specifically, parents showed less physical discipline, more consistent and appropriate discipline, and more warmth and positive involvement in their child's school.[24,26,27]

The *LIFT* programme was designed as a preventive intervention for at-risk children to decrease the development of conduct problems and delinquency.[28,29] *LIFT* was designed for first- and fifth-graders living in at-risk neighbourhoods. Intervention components consisted of a school-based intervention focused on social skills and problem solving, a parent training group, a playground behavioural programme, and communication between parents and teachers. Creative intervention techniques were employed to increase parent participation in schooling; for example, a phone answering machine was installed in each classroom, and newsletters were sent home to parents about school *LIFT* activities. Parents could call in to the answering machine or leave messages for teachers at any time. This programme was successful at decreasing aggression on the playground and increasing positive behaviours with peers during the year following the intervention. Additionally, the programme was successful at decreasing negative parenting during observed mother–child interactions.[28]

The *SAFE Children* programme was administered within different schools in high-risk neighbourhoods in the Chicago area with a diverse group of families.[23] Youth were randomly assigned within classrooms to receive the intervention, which included parenting and academic tutoring components. The parenting component focused on disseminating information about child development, parenting, skill practice, and home assignments to increase parenting skills and on group problem solving around skills when parents needed additional assistance with implementation. The intervention targeted children during the transition to elementary school, based on developmental research and theory suggesting that transition points are key points for intervention.[30] The intervention significantly impacted academic performance and parental involvement in school, with additional outcomes for high-risk families that included higher parental monitoring and reductions in child behaviour problems.[23]

In summary, effective school-aged, caregiver-mediated interventions for families are multifocused, typically including foci on parenting skills and school success for children. The majority of successful interventions at this age combine a family component with additional interventions to support school adjustment (e.g. social skills training, academic tutoring). Clearly, interventions that target parenting, families, and other domains of children's functioning are the most efficacious interventions to administer during the transition to school.

## Caregiver-mediated interventions involving adolescents

By adolescence, many youth have achieved a degree of independence from their parents and are embedded in the culture of peers, school, and/or their community. The extent of adolescents' autonomy in today's world is such that there may be a temptation to consider addressing adolescent mental health problems in a different manner than those of younger children. However, among the interventions that have demonstrated the biggest impact for adolescents are those focused on youth in the context of their families.[31] The only difference between these programmes and those discussed for younger children is that there is an increased emphasis on parenting skills that are more relevant to adolescent youth, such as problem solving, helping your adolescent gain autonomy, and communication. Adolescents may be more active participants in the interventions that target this age group, attending family sessions and practicing the skills outside of the treatment at home or at school.

There have been a variety of programmes associated with positive outcomes for adolescent youth. At this age, effective interventions tend to be brief, family-centred approaches that teach parents the skills needed to parent effectively during adolescence. Caregiver-mediated interventions at this age may be delivered in the school context or in a community centre or clinic. Within the school context, several programmes have shown success at decreasing adolescent problem behaviour, including substance use over time.

The *Adolescent Transitions Program* (ATP) is a caregiver-mediated treatment for adolescent problem behaviour and substance use. Over the past 15 years, the *ATP* has been shown to be effective in a number of different randomized control trials with parents recruited from the community and schools.[32,33] The *ATP* curriculum focuses on building a positive parent–adolescent relationship, decreasing known risk factors at this age for problem behaviour (e.g. lack of parental monitoring), and increasing communication and listening skills. In the first series of research studies using the *ATP*, the intervention was delivered in a group format and was successful at reducing problem behaviour.[34] More recently, the *ATP* curriculum has been developed into a caregiver-mediated, tailored approach to treatment called the *Family Check-Up* (FCU).[31] The *FCU* is a preventative intervention based on a health maintenance model appropriate for at-risk and high-risk youth. The *FCU* incorporates the content from the *ATP* curriculum into a model that targets parent engagement in treatment. In the *FCU* model, families receive a comprehensive, ecological assessment, videotaped observation, and feedback using motivational interviewing to engage families in treatment. Across numerous randomized controlled intervention trials, the *FCU* has been shown to be effective at reducing teacher-reported risk behaviour, reducing arrest rates, increasing attendance and achievement at school, reducing substance use, and reducing antisocial behaviour.[35–37] Interestingly, these outcomes have been mediated by an increase in family management skills, including parental monitoring.[36]

There have been several other comprehensive, caregiver-mediated approaches to the treatment of adolescents that have also shown positive outcomes. Many of these models are school-based and preventive, focusing on at-risk and high-risk youth and families via group format from schools. Spoth et al.[38] examined outcomes associated with both the *Preparing for the Drug Free Years* programme[39] and the *Iowa Strengthening Families Program*.[40] Both of these parenting programmes have been hypothesized to reduce the initiation of substance use in the high school years and to reduce antisocial behaviour and were both strength based and focused on teaching parents the skills necessary to prevent adolescent problem behaviour. Schools were randomly assigned to deliver the interventions at the school level as universal programmes. Results suggested that these programmes were associated with decreases in the growth of substance use from 6th through 12th grade at the school level. Interestingly, both programmes were brief (up to seven sessions), and effects were found all the way up to 12th grade. These results are promising because they suggest that caregiver-mediated interventions in adolescence can be delivered as universal school-based curricula to decrease problem behaviour in the school population.

The intervention programmes discussed previously are appropriate for typically developing youth, at-risk youth, and high-risk youth. Unfortunately, adolescent youth who have had serious problems with behaviour since early childhood may need caregiver-mediated support that is more intensive and focused around their specific problems. One intervention programme that is particularly promising for high-risk youth is *Multidimensional Treatment Foster Care* (MTFC).[3] *MTFC* is an alternative to institutional treatment for youth with severe emotional and behavioural problems, including those involved with the juvenile justice system. Within the *MTFC* intervention model, youths are placed with foster parents who have received specialized training and who receive a high level of support and supervision from professional staff during the placement. The *MTFC* approach includes the use of highly structured behaviour management programmes as a component of the treatment plan implemented in the foster home. This structure provides the youth with the opportunity to practice the skills that the foster parents are attempting to develop while adjusting the youth's access to risky situations at a rate that matches the youth's progress in treatment.

While the youth is in foster care, his/her biological parents receive intensive behavioural parent training. As the youth shows signs of progress in the foster home, he/she is allowed home visits. The duration of these visits is gradually increased, until the child is ready to return home. An extensive aftercare programme ensures that gains are maintained following reunification.

The *MTFC* approach was evaluated via a randomized control trial and was found to reduce recidivism, especially in comparison to group care.[41–43] Moreover, Chamberlain and Reid reported that youth in the *MTFC* programme had lower incidences of substance use and less contact with delinquent peers than youth in institutional settings.[3] Subsequently, variations of the *MTFC* programme have been developed for a variety of populations, including preschoolers[44–46] and adolescent girls.[47]

## Mediators of intervention efficacy

There are many commonalities among the intervention programmes discussed in this chapter. First, each programme is grounded in developmental research and theory suggesting that families are central to the process of intervening in the mental health issues of children and adolescents. Transitions are critical times for intervention, including transitions to school and puberty.[48] Each programme is strength-based, focusing on increasing protective factors for children and reducing risks in the environment. Lastly, each programme is multifocused, targeting parenting skills and other important factors in a child's life that impact development (e.g. academic achievement).

The literature in this area has suggested some common themes in the mediators that impact the success of interventions for families. First, recruiting parents into treatment can be difficult.[49] Heinrichs *et al.* examined recruitment issues by examining participation in parent training groups in their sample of about 600 families using the *Triple P* parenting programme.[50] They were only able to recruit 31 per cent of low-income families into their parenting groups but were able to retain 77 per cent of families once they began treatment, which included the retention of high-risk families. Similarly, Brody *et al.* found that having more children in the household and youth risk-taking behaviour was related negatively to attendance and engagement in their parenting intervention.[51] Recruitment and attendance issues have been a constant struggle in parenting interventions and have led to the development of brief parenting interventions[52,53] and more tailored, individualized approaches to family treatment.[31] For many families, issues such as childcare, work schedules, and the time commitment required to attend parenting groups prohibit participation. In addition, a parent's interpersonal problems, such as depression and parental resources, can impact participation and outcomes associated with family-based interventions.[54,55]

Second, *culture* plays a key role in the efficacy of family interventions. Parenting skills are inextricably connected to cultural values. For example, racial differences are evident in the literature linking parenting practices to child behaviour problems.[56–58] In previous decades, there was an emphasis on cultural sensitivity within interventions targeting diverse groups. Currently, interventions must be not only culturally sensitive but also adapted to meet the needs of the community in which they are implemented.

Several interventions for families have attempted to address the issue of culture by providing ecologically valid and culturally sensitive interventions to ethnic minority groups in the United States. For example, the *Effective Black Parenting Program* integrated a cognitive behavioural parent training programme with information of relevance to inner-city African-American families, including discussions of traditional discipline (physical punishment) versus modern discipline (internalizing standards of behaviour).[59,60] Components such as helping the child deal with racism at school and positive communication about ethnicity were also included. This programme has been effective at changing parenting behaviour and child behaviour 1 year later.

Another example may be found in the work of Szapocznik and colleagues, who have developed a programme to engage Latino families in treatment that includes less traditional forms of engagement and more of an emphasis on the ecosystems of families and the cultural context. These researchers have hypothesized that resistance to change occurs during the initial stages of therapy and that traditional forms of engagement may not be successful within the Latino population. Instead, engagement includes joining and encouraging the family to participate in home visits and meetings with significant family members. This type of engagement strategy has been effective in retaining families in treatment with the final goal of reducing drug use and other problem behaviours in adolescence.[61–63] Although these programmes serve as examples of specific approaches to working with populations of different cultures, intervention research is just beginning to emphasize these differences and integrate approaches to culturally diverse families into more traditional caregiver training curriculums. More work in this area is clearly necessary, both inside and outside of the United States.

## Summary and conclusions

In this chapter, we have attempted to provide a framework for understanding caregiver-mediated, developmentally based interventions for parents and families and to provide examples of interventions that fall within that framework. As is noted previously, the field of caregiver-mediated interventions and the variety of interventions available is a much broader topic than has been addressed here. We hope that the information presented here serves both to inform about the specifics of certain interventions and to organize the study of the larger field.

## Further information

http://www.oslc.org/index.html

http://www.mtfc.com/index.html

http://cfc.uoregon.edu/

Dishion, T.J. and Stormshak, E.A. (2007). *Intervening in children's lives: an ecological, family-centered approach to mental health care.* APA Books, Washington, DC.

## References

1. Patterson, G.R., Reid, J.B., and Dishion, T.J. (eds.) (1992). *A social learning approach: 4. Antisocial boys.* Castalia, Eugene, OR.

2. Moffit, T.E. (2005). The new look of behavioral genetics in developmental psychopathology: gene–environment interplay in antisocial behaviors. *Psychological Bulletin*, **131**, 533–54.

3. Chamberlain, P. and Reid, J.B. (1998). Comparison of two community alternatives to incarceration for chronic juvenile offenders. *Journal of Consulting and Clinical Psychology*, **66**, 624–33.

4. Olds, D., Henderson, C.R., Tatelbaum, R., *et al.* (1988). Improving the life-course development of socially disadvantaged mothers: a randomized trial of nurse home visitation. *American Journal of Public Health*, **78**, 1436–45.

5. Olds, D. (2003). Reducing program attrition in home visiting: what do we need to know? *Child Abuse & Neglect*, **27**, 359–61.

6. Olds, D., Henderson, C.R., Cole, R., *et al.* (1998). Long-term effects of nurse home visitation on children's criminal and antisocial behavior: 15-year follow-up of a randomized controlled trial. *The Journal of the American Medical Association*, **280**, 1238–44.

7. Olds, D.L., Hill, P.L., O'Brien, R., *et al.* (2003). Taking preventive intervention to scale: the nurse-family partnership. *Cognitive and Behavioral Practice*, **10**, 278–90.

8. Olds, D.L. (2002). Prenatal and infancy home visiting by nurses: from randomized trials to community replication. *Prevention Science*, **3**, 153–72.

9. Duggan, A.K., McFarlane, E.C., Windham, A.M., *et al.* (1999). Evaluation of Hawaii's healthy start program. *The Future of Children*, **9**, 66–90.

10. Pettit, G.S., Bates, J.E., and Dodge, K.A. (1997). Supportive parenting, ecological context, and children's adjustment: a seven-year longitudinal study. *Child Development*, **68**, 908–23.

11. Campbell, S.B. and Ewing, L.J. (1990). Follow-up of hard to manage preschoolers: adjustment at age 9 and predictors of continuing symptoms. *Journal of Child Psychology and Psychiatry*, **31**, 871–89.

12. Ruma, P.R., Burke, R.V., and Thompson, R.W. (1996). Group parent training: is it effective for children of all ages? *Behavior Therapy*, **27**, 159–69.

13. Webster-Stratton, C. (1984). Randomized trial of two parent-training programs for families with conduct disordered children. *Journal of Consulting and Clinical Psychology*, **52**, 666–78.

14. Webster-Stratton, C. (1994). Advancing videotape parent training: a comparison study. *Journal of Consulting and Clinical Psychology*, **62**, 583–93.

15. Webster-Stratton, C. (1998). Preventing conduct problems in head start children: strengthening parenting competencies. *Journal of Consulting and Clinical Psychology*, **66**, 715–30.

16. Strayhorn, J.M. and Weidman, C.S. (1991). Follow-up one year after parent-child interaction training: effects on behavior of preschool children. *Journal of the American Academy of Child and Adolescent Psychiatry*, **30**, 138–43.

17. Chaffin, M., Silovsky, J.F., Funderburk, B., *et al.* (2004). Parent-child interaction therapy with physically abusive parents: efficacy for reducing future abuse reports. *Journal of Consulting and Clinical Psychology*, **72**, 500–10.

18. Peters, D.L., Bollin, G.G., and Murphy, R.E. (1991). Head start's influence on parental competence and child competence. In *Advances in reading and language research: a research annual: literacy through family, community, and school interaction*, Vol. 5 (ed. S.B. Silvern), pp. 91–123. Jai Press, Greenwich, CT.

19. Stormshak, E.A. and Bierman, K.L. (1998). Conduct Problems Prevention Research Group. The implications of four developmental patterns of disruptive behavior problems for school adjustment. *Development and Psychopathology*, **10**, 451–68.

20. Cicchetti, D. and Toth, S.L. (1992). The role of developmental theory in prevention and intervention. *Development and Psychopathology*, **4**, 489–93.

21. Conduct Problems Prevention Research Group. (1992). A developmental and clinical model for the prevention of conduct disorders: the FAST Track program. *Development and Psychopathology*, **4**, 509–27.

22. Reid, J.B., Eddy, J.M., Fetrow, R.A., *et al.* (1999). Description and immediate impacts of a preventive intervention for conduct problems. *American Journal of Community Psychology*, **27**, 483–517.

23. Tolan, P., Gorman-Smith, D., and Henry, D. (2004). Supporting families in a high-risk setting: proximal effects of the SAFEChildren preventive intervention. *Journal of Consulting and Clinical Psychology*, **72**, 855–69.

24. Conduct Problems Prevention Research Group. (1999). Initial impact of the FAST Track prevention trial for conduct problems. I. The high-risk sample. *Journal of Consulting and Clinical Psychology*, **67**, 631–47.

25. McMahon, R.J. and Slough, N. (1996). Conduct Problems Prevention Research Group. Family-based intervention in the FAST Track Program. In *Preventing childhood disorders, substance abuse, and delinquency* (eds. R.D. Peters and R.J. McMahon), pp. 90–110. Sage, Thousand Oaks, CA.

26. Conduct Problems Prevention Research Group. (2002). Evaluation of the first 3 years of the FAST Track prevention trial with children at high risk for adolescent conduct problems. *Journal of Abnormal Child Psychology*, **30**, 19–36.

27. Conduct Problems Prevention Research Group. (2004). The effects of the FAST Track program on serious problem outcomes at the end of elementary school. *Journal of Clinical Child and Adolescent Psychology*, **33**, 650–61.

28. Eddy, J.M., Reid, J.B., Stoolmiller, M., *et al.* (2003). Outcomes during middle school for an elementary school-based preventive intervention for conduct problems: follow-up results from a randomized trial. *Behavior Therapy*, **34**, 535–53.

29. Stoolmiller, M., Eddy, J.M., and Reid, J.B. (2000). Detecting and describing preventive intervention effects in a universal school-based randomized trial targeting delinquent and violent behavior. *Journal of Consulting and Clinical Psychology*, **68**, 296–306.

30. Kellam, S.G. and Rebok, G.W. (1992). Building developmental and etiological theory through thorough epidemiologically based preventive intervention trials. In *Preventing antisocial behavior: interventions from birth through adolescence* (eds. J. McCord and R. Tremblay), pp. 162–95. Guilford Press, New York.

31. Dishion, T.J. and Stormshak, E. (eds.) (2007). *Intervening in children's lives: an ecological, family-centered approach to mental health care*. APA Books, Washington, DC.

32. Dishion, T.J., Andrews, D.W., Kavanagh, K., *et al.* (1996). Preventive interventions for high-risk youth: the adolescent transitions program. In *Preventing childhood disorders, substance abuse, and delinquency* (eds. R.D. Peters and R.J. McMahon), pp. 184–214. Sage, Thousand Oaks, CA.

33. Dishion, T.J. and Kavanagh, K. (eds.) (2003). *Intervening in adolescent problem behavior: a family-centered approach*. Guilford Press, New York.

34. Dishion, T.J. and Andrews, D.W. (1995). Preventing escalation in problem behaviors with high-risk young adolescents: immediate and 1-year outcomes. *Journal of Consulting and Clinical Psychology*, **63**, 538–48.

35. Connell, A., Dishion, T.J., Jo, B., *et al.* (in press). An ecological approach to family intervention to reduce adolescent problem behavior: intervention engagement and longitudinal change. *Journal of Consulting and Clinical Psychology*.

36. Dishion, T.J., Nelson, S.E., and Kavanagh, K. (2003). The family check-up for high-risk adolescents: motivating parenting monitoring and reducing problem behavior. *Behavior Therapy*, **34**, 553–71.

37. Stormshak, E.A., Dishion, T.J., Light, J., *et al.* (2005). Implementing family-centered interventions within the public middle school: linking service delivery change to change in problem behavior. *Journal of Abnormal Child Psychology*, **33**, 723–33.

38. Spoth, R., Redmond, C., Shin, C., *et al.* (2004). Brief family intervention effects on adolescent substance initiation: school-level growth curve analyses 6 years following baseline. *Journal of Consulting and Clinical Psychology*, **72**, 535–42.

39. Catalano, R., Kosterman, R., Haggerty, K., *et al.* (1999). A universal intervention for the prevention of substance abuse: preparing for the drug free years. In *NIDA research monograph on drug abuse prevention through family interventions* (eds. R. Ashery, E. Robertson, and K. Kumpfer), pp. 130–59. National Institute on Drug Abuse, Rockville, MD.

40. Molgaard, V. and Spoth, R. (2001). Strengthening families program for young adolescents: overview and outcomes. In *Innovative mental health programs for children: programs that work* (eds. S.I. Pfeiffer and L.A. Reddy), pp. 15–29. Haworth Press, Binghamton, NY.

41. Chamberlain, P. (1990). Comparative evaluation of specialized foster care for seriously delinquent youths: a first step. *Community Alternatives: International Journal of Family Care*, **2**, 21–36.

42. Chamberlain, P. (ed.) (2003). The Oregon multidimensional treatment foster care model: features, outcomes, and progress in dissemination. *Cognitive and Behavioral Practice*, **10**, 303–12.

43. Chamberlain, P. and Friman, P.C. (1997). Residential programs for antisocial children and adolescents. In *Handbook of antisocial behavior* (eds. D.M. Stoff, J. Breiling, and J.D. Maser), pp. 416–24. John Wiley & Sons, New York.

44. Fisher, P.A., Burraston, B., and Pears, K.C. (2005). The early intervention foster care program: permanent placement outcomes from a randomized trial. *Child Maltreatment*, **10**, 61–71.

45. Fisher, P.A., Burraston, B., and Pears, K.C. (2006). Permanency in foster care: conceptual and methodological issues. *Child Maltreatment*, **11**, 92–4.

46. Fisher, P.A., Gunnar, M.R., Dozier, M., *et al.* (2006). Effects of a therapeutic intervention for foster children on behavior problems, caregiver attachment, and stress regulatory neural systems. *Annals of the New York Academy of Sciences*, **1094**, 215–25.

47. Leve, L.D., Chamberlain, P., and Reid, J.B. (2005). Intervention outcomes for girls referred from juvenile justice: effects on delinquency. *Journal of Consulting and Clinical Psychology*, **73**, 1181–5.

48. Coie, J.D., Watt, N.F., West, S.G., *et al.* (1993). The science of prevention: a conceptual framework and some directions for a national research program. *The American Psychologist*, **48**, 1013–22.

49. Gottfredson, D., Kumpfer, K., Polizzi-Fox, D., *et al.* (2006). The strengthening Washington, DC families project: a randomized effectiveness trial of family-based prevention. *Prevention Science*, **7**, 57–74.

50. Heinrichs, N., Bertram, H., Kuschel, A., *et al.* (2005). Parent recruitment and retention in a universal prevention program for child behavior and emotional problems: barriers to research and program participation. *Prevention Science*, **10**, 275–86.

51. Brody, G.H., Murry, V.M., Chen, Y., *et al.* (2006). Effects of family risk factors on dosage and efficacy of a family-centered preventive intervention for rural African-Americans. *Prevention Science*, **7**, 281–91.

52. Lim, M., Stormshak, E.A., and Dishion, T.J. (2005). A one-session intervention for parents of young adolescents: videotape modeling and motivational group discussion. *Journal of Emotional and Behavioral Disorders*, **13**, 194–9.

53. Stormshak, E.A., Kaminski, R., and Goodman, M.R. (2002). Enhancing the parenting skills of head start families during the transition to kindergarten. *Prevention Science*, **3**, 223–34.

54. Smith, K.E., Landry, S.A., and Swank, P.R. (2005). The influence of decreased parental resources on the efficacy of a responsive parenting intervention. *Journal of Consulting and Clinical Psychology*, **73**, 711–20.

55. Webster-Stratton, C. and Hammond, M. (1990). Predictors of treatment outcome in parent training for families with conduct problem children. *Behavior Therapy*, **21**, 319–37.

56. Deater-Deckard, K., Dodge, K.A., Bates, J.E., *et al.* (1996). Physical discipline among African-American and European-American mothers: links to children's externalizing behaviors. *Developmental Psychology*, **32**, 1065–72.

57. Florsheim, P., Tolan, P.H., and Gorman-Smith, D. (1996). Family processes and risk for externalizing behavior problems among African-American and Hispanic boys. *Journal of Consulting and Clinical Psychology*, **64**, 1222–30.

58. Lansford, J.E., Chang, L., Dodge, K.A., *et al.* (2005). Physical discipline and children's adjustment: cultural normativeness as a moderator. *Child Development*, **76**, 1234–46.

59. Alvy, K.T. and Marigna, M. (eds.) (1985). *Effective black parenting program: instructor's manual.* Center for Improvement of Child Caring, Studio City, CA.

60. Myers, H.F., Alvy, K.T., Arrington, A., *et al.* (1992). The impact of a parent training program on inner-city African-American families. *Journal of Community Psychology*, **20**, 132–47.

61. Coatsworth, J.D., Duncan, L., Pantin, H., *et al.* (2006). Patterns of retention in a preventive intervention with Hispanic and African American families. *The Journal of Primary Prevention*, **27**, 171–93.

62. Santisteban, D.A., Szapocznik, J., Perez-Vidal, A., *et al.* (1996). Efficacy of intervention for engaging youth and families into treatment and some variables that may contribute to differential effectiveness. *Journal of Family Psychology*, **10**, 35–44.

63. Szapocznik, J., Kurtines, W., Santisteban, D.A., *et al.* (1997). The evolution of a structural ecosystems theory for working with Hispanic families in culturally pluralistic contexts. In *Psychological interventions and research with Latino populations* (eds. J. Garcia and M.C. Zea). Allyn & Bacon, Boston, MA.

# 9.5.5 Medication for children and adolescents: current issues

Paramala J. Santosh

## Introduction

Problems of mental health and behaviour in children are multidisciplinary in nature and optimal treatment is often multimodal. This article focuses on aspects of psychopharmacology that has special relevance in children and adolescents, especially the recent controversies. In general, this article provides information about classes of medication and not detailed information about specific medicines. Treatment recommendations of the specific disorders have been dealt within the appropriate chapters.

The use of psychotropic medication in children is higher in the United States than in many other countries, and polypharmacy is common. About 1 per cent of overall medical consultations visits by children and adolescents in 2003–2004 in the US resulted in a second-generation antipsychotic (SGA) prescription. The majority of the visits involving antipsychotics were by Caucasian boys aged over nine years, visiting specialists, without private insurance, with a diagnosis of bipolar disorder, psychosis, depression, disruptive disorder, or anxiety.[1]

Pre-school (2 to 4 year olds) psychotropic medication use, between 1995 and 2001 increased across the US for stimulants, antipsychotics, and antidepressants, while the use of anxiolytics, sedatives, hypnotics and anticonvulsants remained stable across these years, suggesting non-psychiatric medical usage.[2] Ethnicity may influence differential prescription rates; for example, as compared to Caucasian youths, African-American youths are less likely to be prescribed psychotropic medications especially methylphenidate.[3]

## Information assisting psychopharmacological decision-making

Apart from a thorough diagnostic assessment, a full medical history including present, recent, and past prescribed and over-the-counter medication, response to treatment, and attitude towards interventions play a major role in deciding treatment. History of substance misuse needs to be elicited to ascertain potential medication-misuse liability and because certain medication significantly interact with illicit drugs. A family history of mental illness, suicide, substance abuse, neurological or medical conditions, especially early onset coronary artery disease, hyperlipidemias and diabetes, and specifically the response of family members to psychotropic medication are all important.

## Medication as a part of multimodal treatment package

Disorders that have an extended course, where emergence of new problems is common, require continuous, dynamic treatment planning and monitoring to ensure effectiveness of the current treatment. The treatment should stress multi-modal intervention and address co-morbid psychiatric disorders. Treatment plans should be individualized according to the pattern of target symptoms and strengths identified in the evaluation. A thorough functional analysis of problems or symptoms is central to pharmacological decision-making. Treatment should target situations in which symptoms cause the most impairment. Custom-designed target symptom scales or daily behavioural report cards are useful in monitoring treatment progress.

One way to conceptualize paediatric psychopharmacotherapy is the 'Symptom-based Approach' for core symptoms as follows:

♦ *Symptoms that require and are likely to respond to medication alone*: inattention, impulsivity, hyperactivity, tics, obsessions, psychotic symptoms, labile mood etc;

♦ *Symptoms less likely to respond to medication alone, requiring both medication and psychosocial interventions*: aggression, rituals, self-injury etc;

♦ *Symptoms that are unlikely to respond to medication that need specific remediation or rehabilitation*: skill deficits in academic, social, or sports domain.[4]

Psychosocial interventions may be required to address either primary or secondary relationship problems associated with the core deficits or to deal with co-morbidity.

## The 'art' of prescribing medication

Pharmacological interventions do not necessarily work exclusively because of their 'neurochemical' effects. Response to medication also includes the inherent 'placebo response' or 'expectancy effect' that prescribing can induce, as well as the effect of the 'therapeutic concordance' achieved through getting the agreement and acceptance of why the medication is being prescribed and also what is the expected response.

Parents as well as patients respond better when they feel understood, accept why treatment is necessary and are in agreement with the prescriber regarding the need for treatment. Simple strategies help this process: collaborating with parents, patients, school and care providers; giving a clear explanation of diagnoses, of why medication (with or without psychosocial interventions) is necessary; setting realistic expectations (for example, aiming for a 40–60 per cent reduction in anxiety symptoms in a child with multiple co-morbidity); keeping track of the larger systems of care at school and home; providing clear, appropriate information sheets, websites etc to obtain further information if needed; prioritizing and tracking target symptoms; asking them to 'opt in' to treatment after having weighed all the pros and cons, as opposed to them perceiving that they are being 'told' that they 'have to' start medication; using short telephone-based medication monitoring during the stabilization phase in order to pick up emerging side-effects and monitoring dosage accordingly; initiating medication using small doses and titrating it up over a period of 4 to 6 weeks, to identify the **minimum effective dose (MED)**, which is the minimum dose with which 'acceptable' improvement with minimal side-effects is achieved; involving school in monitoring symptoms regularly even if it means maintaining a school-home dairy; and willingness to change treatment if the expected outcome has not been achieved.

Domains that each therapy focusses on should be clearly documented and periodically evaluated. The designation of a case manager is essential for chronically disabled individuals to coordinate the wide range of services necessary for their care and to ensure periodic diagnostic reassessments.

## Developmental issues, pharmacokinetic and pharmacodynamic factors affecting pharmacotherapy in children

Generally, drug response may vary with age, weight, sex, disease state, absorption, distribution, metabolism, and excretion. Thus, developmental factors that influence these are important to consider. Although the extent of drug absorption for most medication is similar in children and adults, the rate of absorption may be faster in children and peak levels are reached earlier.[5]

Absorption is also dependent on the form in which it is administered, i.e. liquid versus tablet, and levels peak faster for liquid preparations. Generally speaking, hepatic metabolism is highest during infancy and childhood, 1 to 6 years, approximately twice the adult rate in pre-puberty at six to 10 years, and equivalent to adults by the age of 15.[5] This is clinically important as younger children may require higher mg/kg doses of hepatically metabolized medications than older children or adults.[6]

Adolescence is a period of particularly high ketosteroid levels, which have significant impact on brain neurotransmitter systems. A transient decrease in metabolism for some medication has been reported in a few months before puberty, which is believed to be due to the competition for hepatic enzymes with sex hormones.[7]

Fat distribution varies in children raising during year one then gradually falling until puberty and increasing with obesity. Substantial fat stores slow elimination of highly lipo-soluble drugs from the body (e.g. fluoxetine and pimozide).

Protein binding and volume of distribution affect the pharmacokinetics of medications. These parameters differ in children and have practical clinical implications such as the fraction of the drug that is active and unbound.[8] This is especially a factor when medicating children with eating disorders such as anorexia.

Overall, it is recognized due to the various factors covered in this article, non-pharmacological strategies are more effective in preschoolers. Pharmacotherapy in school-going children has a reasonable risk/benefit ratio and older adolescents behave more like adults. As patients mature, treatment plans often must be adapted to change according to the changing individual, family, and environmental conditions.

### Antidepressant efficacy

The poor antidepressant response in childhood depression may have its basis on differences in the hormonal milieu of the brain, and incomplete maturation of the neurotransmitter systems involved in the control of affect, inclusion of adolescents who will over time become bipolar, adolescents with depressive phenocopies, and possible differences in pharmacokinetics and pharmacodynamics. The more rapid hepatic metabolism of imipramine and amitriptyline results in noradrenergically active metabolites, shifting the ratio of the noradrenergic to serotonergic activity of these compounds in children to a ratio higher than that seen in adults. This activity shift is significant because the noradrenergic system does not fully develop both anatomically and functionally until early adulthood.[9,10]

### Cardiotoxicity

The maturation of vagal modulation of heart rate increases during the first decade of life, peaks sometime during the second decade, and declines gradually with age through the sixth decade of life. Sympathetic modulation follows a similar pattern, but rate of maturation of the two branches differ. Furthermore, there is considerable variation between individuals of similar age in autonomic maturation. The relative loss of vagal modulation associated with tricyclic antidepressants may be accentuated in some younger subjects because of these maturational factors, leading to cardiotoxicity.[11]

## Stimulants

Stimulants have been used for decades and good research evidence exists for their short-term use in ADHD. More recently, various stimulant delivery systems have been developed (the osmotic controlled-release system (OROS) – Concerta XL®; the wax-matrix-based beaded system – Metadate CD®; the patch release system – Daytrana®; etc) resulting in long-acting preparations which makes it possible to avoid medication needing to be administered in school. This once daily dosing schedule possibly reduces stigmatization and embarrassment. The release systems and preparation of stimulants (immediate release / slow release ratios) allow the tailoring of the long-acting preparations to suit the need of individual children.[12]

### Precautions with stimulants

Stimulants are contraindicated in schizophrenia, hyperthyroidism, cardiac arrhythmias, angina pectoris, glaucoma, or a history of hypersensitivity to drug. They can be used with caution in those with hypertension, depression, tics (or family history of Tourette's syndrome), pervasive developmental disorders or severe intellectual disability. Occasionally tics can be made worse with stimulants.

#### (a) Rebound effects

It consists of increased excitability, activity, talkativeness, irritability and insomnia beginning 4–15 h after a dose. It may be seen as the last dose of the day wears off or for up to several days after sudden withdrawal of high daily doses of stimulants. This may resemble a worsening of the original symptoms and is encountered frequently by clinicians. Management strategies include increased structure after school, addition of a smaller dose of medication in the late afternoon, use of long-acting formulations or the addition of clonidine or guanfacine to the regime.

#### (b) Seizures

Methylphenidate can be used in the presence of well-controlled epilepsy. If seizures worsen or emerge during treatment, methylphenidate should to be changed to dexamfetamine, which is supposed to increase seizure threshold.

#### (c) Growth retardation

The MTA study indicates that there is significant growth reduction with stimulant use.[13] It would be advisable not to start stimulants in children who are short and are biologically predisposed to short stature (e.g. short parental stature, growth hormone deficiency etc.).

#### (d) Cardiac problems

Stimulants may increase pulse rate and rarely can lead to increased blood pressure. Importantly, African-American male adolescents may be at a higher risk from mild chronic elevation in blood pressure on methylphenidate, needing more rigorous blood pressure monitoring for hypertension than their Caucasian counterparts.[14] After several reports of death of patients on Adderall®, there is currently a warning to clinicians to be aware of possible cardiac side effects, especially in the presence of known cardiovascular illness. The reported rates of sudden death on Adderall® do not exceed reported rates of sudden death on other stimulants or the base rate of sudden death per age group in general off medication.

#### (e) Abuse potential of stimulants

There is little evidence that substance misuse or dependence results from the prescription of stimulants for ADHD. Self initiated increase in dose by emotionally unstable adults with substance use disorders is possible and needs to be suspected in those who repeatedly claim to have lost medication or in parents who repeatedly insist that higher doses are necessary to control symptoms, when the child is functioning well in other settings. In such situations it may be better to use long-acting preparations such as Concerta XL®, as the delivery system makes it difficult to abuse. Other drugs that are useful in this setting are atomoxetine and bupropion.

#### (f) Psychotic symptoms

Post-marketting surveillance led to enhanced labelling warnings regarding psychosis, mania and hallucinations as adverse events (*http://www.fda.gov/ohrms/dockets/ac/06/minutes/2006-4210m_Mi nutes%20PAC%20March%2022%202006.pdf*). Many such drug-related psychiatric adverse events may be self-limited and resolve with drug cessation. Stimulants are better avoided in those who have a first degree relative with a psychotic disorder or in children who have psychotic or quasi-psychotic experiences.

## Non-stimulants

**Atomoxetine** is a non-stimulant noradrenaline reuptake inhibitor, which has a high affinity and selectivity for the noradrenaline reuptake site over serotonin and dopamine transporters. In extensive metabolizers (EMs), inhibitors of CYP2D6 e.g. *paroxetine, fluoxetine and guanidine* increase atomoxetine steady-state plasma concentrations. Atomoxetine is long acting and can be used once a day and does not result in rebound symptom worsening and has little potential for abuse. It does not worsen tics, anxiety or low mood and hence may be useful in some children with ADHD and co-morbid disorders.

#### (a) Precautions with atomoxetine

Atomoxetine is contraindicated in hepatic insufficiency/impairment, glaucoma, uncontrolled seizures or a history of hypersensitivity to drug. They can be used with caution in those with hypertension or with any condition that may predispose to it, tachycardia, cardiovascular problems in patients with congenital or acquired long QT or a family history of QT prolongation or with cerebrovascular disease.[15]

#### (b) Growth retardation

Acute treatment studies show that atomoxetine-treated patients lose some weight. Michelson *et al.* (2004)[16] reported a change of 2–3 percentiles in mean height, which appear to be similar to effects observed in stimulant-treated patients. Patients treated for extended periods should be monitored regularly.

#### (c) Seizure liability

A review of risks and benefits of atomoxetine in 2996 led to warnings on the risk of seizures when taking atomoxetine. It is not to be used in uncontrolled seizures and should be discontinued in those who develop seizures or who experience an increase in frequency of their seizures.

### (d) Cardiac problems

Atomoxetine increases noradrenergic tone and produces increased heart rate and small increases in blood pressure, which subsides on discontinuing atomoxetine. QT interval prolongation can occur but ECG monitoring is not necessary unless one suspects cardiac problems.

### (e) Suicidal risk

In September 2005, a 'black box' warning was added to the product labelling of atomoxetine as a result of an analyses that showed that suicidal ideation was more frequently observed in clinical trials among children and adolescents treated with atomoxetine (5/1357 [0.37 per cent]) compared to those treated with placebo (0/851 [0 per cent]) (*http://www.fda.gov/cder/foi/label/2007/021411s004s012s013s015s021lbl.pdf*). There was one suicide attempt in the atomoxetine treated group. No completed suicides occurred during these trials. There was, however, no evidence of increased suicidal thoughts in adults taking atomoxetine. Prescribers should monitor for signs of depression, suicidal thoughts or suicidal behaviour and refer for appropriate treatment if necessary.

### (f) Hepatic dysfunction

Reports indicate that atomoxetine can cause severe liver injury in rare cases. The spontaneous adverse event database search identified two cases that were probably associated with atomoxetine use as a cause or contributor to the event. One spontaneously reported case of liver injury (fulminant hepatitis) appeared probably related to atomoxetine therapy by positive re-challenge in a population exposure of about 2.2 million patients within the 2-year period (2002–2004) after approval which is likely to be an underestimate. Less severe liver dysfunction indicated by abnormal liver enzymes is more common and such reactions may occur several months after therapy is started and atomoxetine should be discontinued in patients with jaundice abnormal liver enzyme levels, which should be done upon the first symptom or sign of liver dysfunction (e.g. pruritus, dark urine, jaundice, right upper quadrant tenderness or unexplained 'flu-like' symptoms).

## Antidepressants

The pattern of antidepressant use in children and adolescents has changed significantly over the last couple of decades. Tricyclic antidepressants were predominantly being used for ADHD, enuresis, depression, and anxiety disorders during the eighties and early nineties. Over the last 10–15 years, this has changed to predominantly prescribing the newer antidepressants, especially for anxiety disorders and depression, despite little real evidence for its efficacy. Current data suggests that other than fluoxetine, no other antidepressant has evidence to clearly support its use in depression in children and adolescents.

### Tricyclic antidepressants

Tricyclic antidepressants include amitriptyline, desipramine, nortriptyline, imipramine, and clomipramine. Historically, they have been used as a second-line pharmacologic treatment for ADHD (though only as an off-licence drug), following stimulant

medications. Their use has declined in recent years due to concerns of cardiac arrhythmias and case reports of sudden death in the paediatric population. Drawbacks include potential cardiotoxicity, especially in pre-pubertal children, the danger of accidental or intentional overdose, troublesome sedation, anticholinergic side-effects, lowering seizure threshold and possibly declining efficacy over time.

### New generation antidepressants

Fluoxetine, sertraline, fluvoxamine, citalopram, escitalopram, and paroxetine are all specific serotonin reuptake inhibitors (SSRIs) while venlafaxine is a specific noradrenaline and serotonin reuptake inhibitor (SNRI) and reboxetine a specific noradrenaline reuptake inhibitor (SNI) and mirtazapine. Few trials exist in pre-pubertal children with these drugs; however, the data suggest that the SSRIs have reasonable efficacy in severe anxiety disorders such as OCD (fluoxetine, sertraline) but only fluoxetine is effective in depression. Theoretically, the SNIs may help managing symptoms of ADHD but little research evidence exists.

### Precautions with antidepressants

#### (a) Antidepressant-induced behavioural activation

Frequently children prescribed antidepressants (especially those with developmental disorders or intellectual disability) develop increased motor activity, restlessness, excitability and impulsivity. This usually occurs early in treatment and is often misconstrued as being a manic or hypomanic switch and wrongly treated as if the child had a bipolar disorder. This can be managed by reducing the dose and may need the cover of a benzodiazepine for a few days. This side-effect can be reduced by initiating antidepressants in vulnerable children in small doses (about a fourth of the final dose needed) and gradually increasing the dose over a few weeks.

#### (b) Antidepressant-related suicidal ideation and behaviour

It was realized two decades ago that imipramine was not effective in pre-pubertal major depression.[17] The Committee for Safety of Medicines (CSM) in December 2003 reviewed all the relevant trials with new generation antidepressants on remission, response to treatment, depression symptom scores, serious adverse events, suicide-related behaviour, and discontinuation of treatment because of adverse events and concluded that the evidence was adequate to establish effectiveness only for fluoxetine and contra-indicated all SSRIs (except fluoxetine) for depressed children (*http://www.mhra.gov.uk/home/groups/plp/documents/drugsafetymessage/con019472.pdf*).[18] This was then followed by the FDA asking for black box warnings on all SSRIs warning about the possibility of suicide-related behaviour as a side-effect in depressed children (*http://www.fda.gov/Cder/drug/antidepressants/SSRIPHA200410.htm*). It is currently advised that children or adolescents being started on or dose being increased of antidepressants should be monitored closely for emergence or worsening of suicidal ideation or behaviour.

## Antipsychotics

Recent years have witnessed increased antipsychotic treatment of children despite limited long-term safety data in children. Second generation antipsychotics (SGAs) are the most frequently prescribed ones; for example, risperidone, quetiapine, aripiprazole, olanzapine, ziprazidone, and amisulpiride.

*Risperidone* is the commonest atypical antipsychotic used in children and adolescents to manage psychoses and disruptive behaviour in autism. It is a potent dopamine D2 receptor blocker (hence reduces positive symptoms but produces hyperprolactinaemia) and 5HT-2A receptor blocker (enhances dopamine release in certain brain regions, thus reducing motor side effects and possibly improving cognitive and affective symptoms). The Research Units for Paediatric Psychopharmacology (RUPP) studies have shown that risperidone is effective in managing disruptive behaviours in autism spectrum disorders.[19] Apart from the side effects of sedation and weight gain, hyperprolactinaemia is common and a few develop extrapyramidal side effects such as tardive dyskinesia.

*Aripiprazole* is dopamine partial agonist or dopamine stabilizer, used in managing schizophrenia and bipolar disorder. The partial antagonism of D2 receptors reduces dopamine output when dopamine concentrations are high, thus improving positive symptoms and mediating antipsychotic actions. Blockade of 5HT-2A receptors may cause enhancement of dopamine release in certain brain regions, thus reducing motor side effects and possibly improving cognitive and affective symptoms. Actions at D3 receptors and partial agonism of 5HT-1A receptors could also theoretically contribute to aripiprazole's efficacy.[20] Even though symptoms may improve in the first week, it is recommended to wait for four to six weeks to determine efficacy due to the pharmacokinetics of the drug. The mean elimination half-life is 75 h of aripiprazole and 94 h for the major metabolite dihydro-aripiprazole and is primarily metabolized by CYP450 2D6 and CYP450 3A4. ketoconazole, fluvoxamine, and fluoxetine all increase plasma levels of aripiprazole, while Carbamazepine decreases plasma levels of aripiprazole. Early experience of aripiprazole suggests that it produces less weight gain, diabetes, or hyperlipidaemia, compared to the other SGAs. It is however less sedating and rather activating. Little published evidence exists currently on its use in managing non-psychotic disruptive behaviour in developmental disorders but clinical experience suggests that very small doses (2 to 5 mg per day) are sufficient.

*Quetiapine* is an effective SGA with moderate effect on weight, but usually needs to be taken at least twice daily because of relative weak receptor binding. *Ziprasidone* is being increasingly used and is the only SGA that is weight neutral, but has greater impact on cardiac rhythm and QTc interval. *Clozapine* is used in those with resistant psychoses or those with tardive dyskinesia, but can lead to neutropaenia, sialohorrea, and significant weight gain. *Olanzapine* is used less in children and adolescents because of the propensity to weight gain and metabolic syndrome. Evidence from adults suggests that Clozapine, Olanzapine, and low-potency conventional antipsychotics such as chlorpromazine are associated with increased risk of insulin resistance, hyperglycaemia, and type 2 diabetes mellitus.[21,22]

## Precautions with antipsychotics

### (a) Movement disorders

Tardive dyskinesia and extrapyramidal side-effects are more common with conventional antipsychotics. Ethnicity may be a risk factor for dyskinesia in children as African-American children appear to be more prone to tardive dyskinesia when compared to European-American children.[23] Aripiprazole or clozapine are useful in those who require antipsychotics but have developed tardive dyskinesia.

### (b) Weight gain and metabolic dysfunction

Weight gain is a serious side effect of SGAs and potential consequences of obesity include non-compliance with medication and significant morbidity and mortality.

### (c) Risk for SGA-induced metabolic dysfucntion

*High risk* – clozapine, olanzapine

*Moderate risk* – risperidone, quetiapine, sertindole

*Low risk* – amisulpiride, aripiprazole, ziprazidone

### (d) Baseline information before starting an SGA

Weigh the children and adolescents and track the BMI during treatment; get baseline personal and family history of obesity, dyslipidaemia, hypertension, and cardiovascular disease; children of parents with total cholesterol >24 mmol/l (parents with high BMI), and history of overt heart disease in parent or grandparent at age 55 or younger should be considered to be at high risk; get waist circumference at umbilicus, blood pressure, fasting plasma glucose, and fasting lipid profile.

### (e) Monitoring after starting an SGA

BMI monthly for three months then quarterly with blood pressure, fasting plasma glucose, fasting lipids within three months and then annually but earlier and more frequently for patients with diabetes or who have gained greater than 5 per cent of initial weight; treat or refer for treatment and consider switching to another atypical antipsychotic for patients who become overweight, obese, prediabetic, diabetic, hypertensive, or dyslipidaemic while receiving an atypical antipsychotic. Elevated fasting plasma triglyceride or increased insulin levels may be important signals of potential insulin resistance. Increased low density lipoprotein (LDL) cholesterol and decreased high density lipoprotein (HDL) cholesterol is associated with increased adiposity, especially visceral adiposity. Even in patients without known diabetes, one should be vigilant for the rare but life threatening onset of diabetic ketoacidosis, which always requires immediate treatment by monitoring for the rapid onset of polyuria, polydipsia, weight loss, nausea, vomiting, dehydration, rapid respiration, weakness, clouding of sensorium, and even coma.

## Treatment of SGA-induced metabolic dysfunction

Careful selection of treatments taking the metabolic-risk profile into account, preventative healthy lifestyle counselling, and regular monitoring of body composition and metabolic variables need to become clinical routine. Total caloric intake is more important than the content of the diet and motivational interviewing and cognitive behavioural techniques can be used to address unhealthy diet, physical inactivity and smoking. Clinically an effective method is to insist that the family (as opposed to only the child) go onto a healthy diet and activity schedule. In fact, informing the parents that they will also be weighed along with the child, helps address this issue effectively. Although preliminary, co-treatment with an SGA plus a mood stabilizer seems to be associated with a greater risk for age-inappropriate weight gain than treatment with one or even two mood stabilizers. A pilot study has shown Metformin therapy is safe and effective in decreasing weight gain, insulin sensitivity, and abnormal glucose metabolism in children aged 10 to 17 whose weight had increased by more than 10 per cent during less than one year of olanzapine, risperidone or quetiapine therapy.[24]

Developmentally appropriate monitoring guidelines[25] need to be implemented in routine clinical practice and the effectiveness of suggested behavioural and pharmacological interventions should be evaluated.

## Mood-stabilizers

Mood stabilizers are usually antiepileptics (except SGAs and lithium) and are used to treat epilepsy or bipolar disorders and occasionally mood lability. Commonly used mood stabilizers include carbamazepine, sodium valproate, lamotrigine, and lithium carbonate. Lithium use warrants regular blood level monitoring, which is often a problem in children. *Sodium valproate or valproic acid* is the most used mood stabilizer and has a reasonable evidence base for its use in bipolar disorder. It however should be used very cautiously, if at all, in girls of child-bearing age due to its teratogenic effects, as well as possible side effect of polycystic ovarian disease. Lamotrigine is a more recent addition and hence being discussed.

*Lamotrigine* works by inhibiting effects on sodium channels and stabilizes neuronal membranes and thereby moderates the release of excitatory amino acids such as glutamate and aspartate. Lamotrigine is especially useful when significant depressive symptoms exist in bipolar disorder.[26] It has a moderately long half-life, especially as monotherapy and can be given once or twice a day. When used with hepatic enzyme inducing medications such as phenytoin and carbamazepine, the half-life is reduced to 12 h. Valproic acid markedly increases the half-life of lamotrigine to 48 to 72 hand the concomitant use of these medications increases the likelihood of developing severe drug rashes including Steven–Johnson syndrome. Lamotrigine is to be started at very low doses (as low as 5 mg/day) and increased slowly over a couple of months. In general, the initiation of this drug requires great patience. Evidence for anti-manic effects is limited.

## Rapid tranquilization when managing severe maladaptive aggression in children and adolescents

Managing acute severe maladaptive aggression requires a quick functional analysis to identify the underlying cause – mood lability, mania, impulsivity, sensory trigger such as hypersensitivity to sound in autism, psychotic experience, autonomic arousal, anxiety or depression etc. The management involves:

- 'Talking down' as the first strategy.

- The patient should be offered the choice of having an oral medication before forcing parental medication.

- Oral medication – risperidone 0.5–1mg, or olanzapine 1–2.5 mg or lorazepam 0.5–1 mg.

- If the above fails, repeat giving either the antipsychotic or the benzodiazepine again in 30 min.

- If this fails, combine the antipsychotic and benzodiazepine after 30 min.

- If oral treatment is not accepted or has not helped, IV haloperidol 1–2 mg or IV diazepam 100–200 mcg/kg or IM haloperidol 1–2mg or IM lorazepam 50–100 mcg/kg can be used.

- The IV can be repeated after 10 min if not sufficient or the IM can be repeated after 30 min. Supportive staff and equipment are necessary as side-effects such as cardio-respiratory arrest can occur. *Maximum safe doses based on age and weight of the child or adolescent should not be exceeded over a 24-hour period.*

- Physical restraint and seclusion in safe environment may also be necessary.

- If **aggression is occurring in the context of a medical condition** (for example, cardiac delirium leading to pulling out catheters etc), midazolam 500 mcg/kg (max 15 mgs) can be used in the context of the medical setting.

## Pharmacological preparation for medical or surgical interventions in children and adolescents with intellectual disability or severe behavioural disorders

Children with intellectual disability or mental health problems should receive the same level of medical care if they are physically unwell, as normal children. As they may not be co-operative, often, physical investigations (for example, MRI or dental X-rays) are avoided or postponed, often leading to late interventions and poorer medical outcomes. If the procedure is a minor one, lasting a few minutes, oral midazolam can be used; if it requires longer or for more serious procedures, an anaesthetist could administer oral ketamine or another general anaesthetic. Simple strategies such as anti-emesis prophylaxis, removal of cannulas before they recover consciousness etc., help minimize difficulties.

## Conclusions

Paediatric pharmacovigilance for psychotropic agents are essential and more studies on efficacy in this population is necessary. Studies are urgently required in children and adolescents investigating the metabolic effects of individual medication, especially the SGAs and mood stabilizers, using sex and age adjusted measures of weight and body composition, including fasting blood work and blood pressure measurements, protective factors and long-term follow-up. Until such detailed data become available, it is safe to assume that paediatric populations are at least as or more vulnerable to adverse effects compared to adults. True long-term data is not available currently on most psychotropic agents. Evidence on treatment impact on co-morbid disorders, cost-effectiveness and impact on Quality of Life are sparse and urgently need to be addressed.

## Further information

Stahl, S. M. (ed.) (2008). *Essential Psychopharmacology* (3rd edn). Cambridge University Press, New York.

Osterheld J.R. and Shader, R.I. (1998). Cytochromes: A primer for child and adolescent psychiatrists. *Journal of the American Academy of Child and Adolescent Psychiatry*, **37**(4), 447–50.

Martin, A., Scahill, L., Charney, D. S., *et al*. (2003). *Paediatric Psychopharmacology—Principles and Update*. Oxford University Press, New York.

Prescribing unlicensed drugs or using drugs for unlicensed indication (1992). *Drugs and Therapeutic Bulletin*, **30**(25), 97–100.

# References

1. Aparasu, R.R. and Bhatara, V. (2007). Patterns and determinants of antipsychotic prescribing in children and adolescents, (2003–2004). *Current Medical Research and Opinion*, **23**(1), 49–56.

2. Zito, J.M., Safer, D.J., Valluri, S., *et al.* (2007). Psychotherapeutic medication prevalence in Medicaid-insured preschoolers. *Journal of Child and Adolescent Psychopharmacology*, **17**(2), 195–203.

3. Zito, M., Safer, D.J., DosReis, S., *et al.* (1998). Racial disparity in psychotropic medications prescribed for youths with Medicaid insurance in Maryland. *Journal of the American Academy of Child and Adolescent Psychiatry*, **37**, 179–84.

4. Santosh, P.J. and Baird, G. (1999). Psychopharmacotherapy in children and adults with intellectual disability. *Lancet*, **354**(9174), 233–42.

5. Bourin, M. and Couetoux du Tertre, A. (1992). Pharmacokinetics of psychotropic drugs in children. *Clinical Neuropharmacology*, **159**(1), 224A–5A.

6. Wilens, T.E., Biederman, J., Baldessarini, R.J., *et al.* (1992). Developmental changes in serum concentrations of desipramine and 2-hydroxydesipramine during treatment with desipramine. *Journal of the American Academy of Child and Adolescent Psychiatry*, **31**, 691–98.

7. Hughes, C. and Preskorn, S.H. (1989). Depressive syndromes in children and adolescents: diagnosis and treatment. *Annals of Clinical Psychiatry*, **1**, 109–18.

8. Paxton, J. and Dragunow, M. (1993). Pharmacology. In *Practitioner's Guide to Psychoactive Drugs for Children and Adolescents*, (eds. J. Werry and M. Aman), pp. 34–46. Plenum, New York.

9. Goldnan-Rakic, Patricia, S. and Brown, R.M. (1982). Postnatal development of monoamine content and synthesis in the cerebral cortex of rhesus monkeys. *Developmental Brain Research*, **4**, 339–49.

10. Thorn, G.W. and Lauler, D.P. (1972). Clinical therapeutics of adrenal disorders. *American Journal of Medicine*, **53**, 673–84.

11. Mezzacappa, E., Steingard, R., Kindlon, D., *et al.* (1998). Tricyclic antidepressants and cardiac autonomic control in children and adolescents. *Journal of the American Academy of Child and Adolescent Psychiatry*, **37**, 52–9.

12. Banaschewski, T., Coghill, D., Santosh, P., *et al.* (2006). Long-acting medications for the hyperkinetic disorders. A systematic review and European treatment guideline. *European Child & Adolescent Psychiatry*, **15**(8), 476–95.

13. Swanson, J.M., Elliott, G.R., Green hill, L.L. *et al.* (2007). Effects of stimulant indication on growth rates across 3years in the MTA follow-up. *J Am Acand Child Adolesce Psychiatry*, **46**, 1015–27.

14. Brown, R.T. and Sexson, S.B. (1989). A controlled trial of methyjphenidate in black adolescents. *Clinical Pediatrics*, (Phila) **27**, 74–81.

15. Unni, J.C. (2006). Atomoxetine. *Indian Pediatrics*, **43**(7), 603–6.

16. Michelson, D., Buitelaar, J.K., Danckaerts, M., *et al.* (2004). Relapse prevention in paediatric patients with ADHD treated with atomoxetine: a randomized, double-blind, placebo-controlled study. *Journal of the American Academy of Child and Adolescent Psychiatry*, **43**(7), 896–904.

17. Puig-Antich, J., Perel, J.M., Lupatkin, W., *et al.* (1987). Imipramine in prepubertal major depressive disorders. *Archives of General Psychiatry*, **44**(1), 81–9.

18. Whittington, C.J., Kendall, T., Fonagy, P. *et al.* (2004). Selective serotonin reuptake inhibitors in childhood depression: systematic review of published versus unpublished data. *Lancet*, **363**(9418), 1341–5.

19. McCracken, J.T., McGough, J., Shah, B., *et al.* (2002). Risperidone in children with autism and serious behavioural problems. *The New England Journal of Medicine*, **347**(5), 314–21.

20. Davies, M.A., Sheffler, D.J. and Roth, B.L. (2004). Aripiprazole: a novel atypical antipsychotic drug with a uniquely robust pharmacology. *CNS Drug Reviews*, **10**(4), 317–36.

21. American Diabetes Association. (2004). *Consensus development conference on antipsychotic drugs and obesity and diabetes. Diabetes Care*, **27**, 596–601.

22. Casey, D.E., Haupt, D.W., Newcomer, J.W., *et al.* (2004). Antipsychotic-induced weight gain and metabolic abnormalities: implications for increased mortality in patients with schizophrenia. *Journal of Clinical Psychiatry*, **65**(7), 4–18.

23. Wonodi, I., Reeves, G., Carmichael, D., *et al.* (2007): Tardive dyskinesia in children treated with atypical antipsychotic medications. *Movement Disorders*, **22**(12), 1777–82.

24. Klein, D.J., Cottingham, E.M., Sorter, M., *et al.* (2006): A randomized, double-blind, placebo-controlled trial of metformin treatment of weight gain associated with initiation of atypical antipsychotic therapy in children and adolescents. *American Journal of Psychiatry*, **163**(12), 2072–9.

25. Correll, C.U. and Carlson, H.E. (2006). Endocrine and metabolic adverse effects of psychotropic medications in children and adolescents. *Journal of the American Academy of Child and Adolescent Psychiatry*, **45**(7), 771–91.

26. Goldsmith, D.R., Wagstaff, A.J., Ibbotson, T., *et al.* (2004): Spotlight on lamotrigine in bipolar disorder. *CNS Drugs*, **18**(1), 63–7.

# 9.5.6 Residential care for social reasons

Leslie Hicks and Ian Sinclair

## Introduction

Residential care for the young is an elusive object of study. Provided in the past by establishments as diverse as workhouses, orphanages, and reformatories, it has no clear definition marking its boundaries with foster care or boarding education; at the same time it variously aims to shelter, classify, control, and reform and it has no agreed theory or body of values. The need for residential care, and the difficulties of providing it, vary with time and place; the issues it raises are quite different in Romania than they are in California, or were in Victorian England.

Given this diversity, any discussion of residential care needs to outline the context within which it was written. In the case of this chapter the context is provided by current British social policy. Although the focus is on residential care provided to young people by Children's Services in England for social reasons, the conclusions drawn are applicable to the rest of the United Kingdom. The issues raised by this provision have similarities in other parts of the developed world, in virtually all of which the use of residential care is declining.[1,2] This chapter is written against the background of this decline. Its aims are as follows:

♦ to describe the current characteristics of residential child care in England, and by extension in Great Britain

♦ to outline the problems that have led to its numerical decline

♦ to identify practices that should overcome or reduce these problems

♦ to discuss the role that residential care might play in future.

## The characteristics of residential care

In 1979, official statistics for England (the figures for Wales, Scotland, and Northern Ireland are published separately) showed that there were approximately 95 000 children in substitute care (mainly foster care and residential care). By 2006 this figure had dropped to 60 300. While for much of this time numbers in foster care were fairly constant, the numbers in residential care fell from 35 000 to 6 600.[3] The great bulk of residential care is directly provided by local authority social services departments (more recently Children's Services), although provision by the private sector is increasing.

These figures give, in some respects, a misleading impression of the numerical importance of homes. The turnover in them is quite rapid—roughly 60 per cent leave a home within 2 months of arrival and just under half the placements result from movements within the care system rather than the breakdown of community care. On average homes still see around three times the number of residents in a year than they accommodate at any one time.[4] A recent study found that residential care accounted for about 28 per cent of the time that children aged 12 or over spent in the care system.[5]

The basic characteristics of the local authority homes are well known. They are 'open' in the sense that the residents are expected to go out to school or work and are not restricted at other times. They are typically small, 50 per cent of them have five or fewer places and the average capacity is around six.[6] The buildings are not markedly institutional, although identifiable to the practised eye, are usually located near to where the residents are likely to live, and aim to take local young people. Staff are non-resident. Many care staff do not possess a recognized appropriate qualification and although government targets in the form of National Minimum Standards[7] aim to rectify this situation, progress towards these remains relatively slow. Homes have more staff than residents and research has shown substantial variation in the number of care hours delivered for each resident young person each week (between 37 and 254 h).[6]

Children enter the care system in Britain to be 'looked after' because of a temporary emergency (for instance hospital admission of the carer) or because of abuse, extremely problematic behaviour on the child's part, or a breakdown of family relationships. The main characteristics that distinguish residents from other users of substitute care are as follows:

◆ Age: 81 per cent of those who start their period of being 'looked after' in local authority homes were aged 10–15 over and about 15 per cent are aged 16 or 17. By contrast, 62 per cent of those entering foster care are under 10 years of age and only 2 per cent are aged 16 or 17.[8]

◆ Sex: the proportions of males and females in foster care are roughly equal, but nearly 60 per cent of those in residential care are male.

◆ Geographical location: some local authorities use residential care much more than others. In 2006 the proportions of 'looked after' adolescents in residential care varied from just under 3 per cent in one local authority to slightly over 24 per cent in another.[3]

◆ Behaviour: on average children in residential care exhibit more 'challenging' behaviour than do foster children, as reflected for example in educational performance, measures of psychiatric ill health, delinquency, and the likelihood of being imprisoned as an adult.[9,10]

One study[4] carried out as part of a major tranche of research on residential child care in England showed that residents had

relatively high levels of school exclusion, truancy, delinquency, violence towards adults and children, running away, risk-taking sexual behaviour, self-harm, and suicide attempts. Around two-thirds of residents entered 'care' for the first time as teenagers, generally because family relationships had broken down, and a further one-fifth entered because of abuse. They were unwilling to be fostered or seen as too disturbed for this. The great majority had previous placements in foster care, residential care, or with relatives.

The role of the homes was to return some as soon as possible to their families, attempt to improve the behaviour of others, or prepare them for independent living, and to keep a minority (around one-fifth) for the foreseeable future. Although there was some specialization, most homes attempted to fulfil all these roles and took all types of resident.

## Problems of residential care

Residential care lacks the moral basis that it formerly had; the disciplines and virtues required for successful group life are no longer seen as imperatives. The Children Act 1989 ensured that, except in rare circumstances, young people could no longer be 'looked after' simply on the grounds of delinquency when their own welfare and those of others are not at risk.

Theoretical uncertainty accompanies these moral shifts. The best-known texts on residential care are now around 25 years old and are dubiously relevant to the current situation where staff no longer live on the premises, and where there have been major changes in staffing, turnover of residents, clientele, and the size and purpose of homes. In any event, there was never a consensus about which theory should underpin treatment or training. Clear evidence for the efficacy of any approach has been lacking, whereas the evidence for the harmful effects of bad residential care has been clear—and frequently repeated on social work courses. Young people reach residential care as the culmination of a process that marks, and possibly even exacerbates, their social exclusion. Typically, they are disturbed, poorly supported by their families, and lack educational qualifications, a combination which makes it difficult for them to compete subsequently in the job market or to lead happy lives. Descriptions of residential care do not suggest that it mounts the determined attack on these problems that might have some chance of success.

There are particular problems for those young people who leave residential care to live independently. Residential homes have difficulty in retaining young people until such time as they are 'properly launched'. To do so would create problems related to cost and to creating a regime suitable at the same time for younger and older teenagers. This means that young people leave care when they are still vulnerable, to cope with lives that are lonely and difficult, at an age much younger than their better qualified and supported contemporaries leave home. Their transitions to the adult roles of getting an income, maintaining a home, and living with a partner are made earlier than those of others and compressed into a shorter period.[11] Unsurprisingly, they have a much higher chance than their contemporaries of becoming lone parents, unemployed, imprisoned, or homeless.[12,13]

In addition to these problems, there are often pragmatic difficulties.

◆ Residential care is very expensive; estimated costs are around £78 000 per place per year in local authority homes and around £87 000 in the non-statutory sector.[6] The system costs considerably more than foster care or preventive work.[14] Around 14 per cent of those who enter stay for prolonged periods and take up half the beds.

◆ Residential homes are prone to scandals involving sexual abuse, outbreaks of disorder, and suicidal behaviour.[4]

◆ Delinquency and running away are widespread within residential homes.[4]

◆ There is widespread bullying, sexual harassment, and personal unhappiness.[4]

Official reports[15] have emphasized the need to recruit a better trained workforce, and there are considerable efforts being made to raise standards in this respect.[16] However, the proportions of qualified staff remain low and studies that have looked for a relationship between the proportion of qualified staff and a measure of performance found no association.[4,6,13]

Contrary to common belief high staff ratios do not in themselves lead to better control in homes or better staff morale or better outcomes, although they do increase costs.[4,6,13]

## Improving the quality of residential care

If residential care is to overcome these problems, it will need to reduce the incidence of difficulties in the home and increase its influence after residents have left.

In terms of immediate impact, residential homes and schools vary widely in the morale of the staff, the incidence of delinquent behaviour and running away, the proportion of residents who avoid going to school, the relationships between staff and residents, and the degree to which the residents report that they are bullied, offered drugs, or feel part of a friendly establishment to which they are committed. These characteristics are far from fully accounted for by intake, and establishments which do 'well' in terms of one of them tend to do 'well' in terms of the others.[4,6,13]

These studies suggest the following conditions are required for managing homes that are successful in the short-term.

◆ The residential units are either small in size or consist of a large unit divided into small subunits. Such small establishments seem better able to combat the influence of delinquent residents.

◆ The units have clear aims, with which the manager of the home is in agreement.

◆ The manager of the home has a clear philosophy on how the young people can be helped, and the staff are in agreement with this outlook.

◆ The residential unit is not based close to the residents' homes. An emphasis on local placement makes it harder to combat the influence of local negative cultures or to maintain a clear focus.

The most recent of these studies[6] was able to demonstrate the link between these immediate outcomes for young people and the practice of managers of homes. Young people experienced better outcomes where managers were accepted as embodying good practice from within a clear ethos, had positive strategies for working with the behaviour and education of young people, and importantly, could enable staff to reflect and deploy these. Without this bedrock, the systems, procedures, and management targets advocated in reports on the residential system will fail. The basic principle is to establish a set of shared expectations and approaches and this is more easily done in a small well-led establishment with a cohesive staff group.

Unfortunately, the ability of homes to affect the behaviour of residents in the short-term implies that the environments to which residents go next are equally powerful. This has been shown to be the case and creates problems for homes in achieving long-term change. (Evidence on the short- and long-term impact of residential care is discussed in more detail elsewhere.[4,6,13]) Overcoming these problems requires the following:

◆ Reduction of delinquent and problematic behaviour in the home—as noted above these are influenced by the residential environment, and there is evidence that they lead to future delinquency.

◆ Encouraging educational achievement and those skills required for 'success' in subsequent life and that are relevant to the resident's subsequent environment—and are seen by the residents as being so.

◆ Working to improve family relationships so that the resident either goes back to an improved family situation or can turn for support to his or her family even though he or she is not living with them.

◆ Providing continuing back-up from the residential home or an aftercare scheme and practical support (e.g. relating to accommodation).

Success is probably more likely where the home operates on a number of fronts simultaneously: seeking to improve skills, learning and educational achievement, and the way the residents see themselves and also the environment to which the residents return.

## Future of residential child care

The case for residential care is essentially three-fold. First, it is able to tolerate behaviour that leads to foster-care placements, the main alternative at the moment, breaking down. Second, a number of young people choose it in preference to foster care. Third, it offers a major resource for adolescents, in preparation for adulthood, in providing supported accommodation, and for those who make a later entry to the care system, such as unaccompanied asylum seeking young people. Its future will depend, in part, on the degree to which other provisions can be developed that can match these advantages.

It seems likely that more alternative provision will be developed. Some intensive American fostering schemes do appear able to contain young people who are as challenging as those in British children's homes, and these schemes are being adapted to conditions in the United Kingdom. Some forms of fostering with outreach support from respite residential units are in their early stages of development. Remand fostering, 'crash pads', and occasional beds in family centres might provide for some young people currently accommodated briefly in children's homes. Supported lodgings could provide for some, particularly older adolescents who avoid foster care because they feel they cannot live in a family, or that it is time that they started to move out on their own. Boarding schools might provide for younger children who do not want to enter foster care because they feel it invites disloyalty to their family, or who enjoy the company of other teenagers.

The comparative advantages of these differing kinds of provision have not been evaluated and it is important that they should be.

The growth of alternative provision will allow the continuing reduction of the more traditional residential sector. It is also likely that the sector itself will change, with the current all-purpose children's home being replaced by more specialist provision that can focus upon clear goals. Research that could determine the shape of such provision is lacking and should be carried out. Possible models of provision include the following:

◆ Secure (namely, closed) provision—public opinion will not allow young people who have committed very serious crimes to remain in open conditions.

◆ Brief- to medium-term provision designed to allow time for young people to consider their situation and move on to new placements in a planned way—there is evidence that fostering placements made from residential care are less likely to disrupt, although it is not yet clear why this is.

◆ Medium-term provision designed to provide treatment—the case for such provision is that treatment involving a group can be more effective. Evidence for this is lacking, although the variations in the behaviour of residents in different establishments is evidence of the power of the group.

In addition to these kinds of residential care, there is a case for some long-stay accommodation in which groups of residents live together. Such provision would be similar to a large foster home or the former family group homes. There seems no reason why it should not work well. It would, however, need to be less generously staffed than current residential homes, otherwise there would be pressure to move residents on for purely economic reasons.

## Conclusions

Residential care is very different in different parts of the world. In the United Kingdom it is provided by small community-based homes, who work with an extremely complex and challenging clientele, and face problems associated with high costs, scandal, and frequently a lack of a clear rationale. Despite these difficulties there are wide variations in the performance of such homes, particularly in terms of their immediate impact. Outcomes after the residents have left are harder to influence. However, an approach which combines attention to the residents' education, behavioural problems, and family environment seems most likely to be effective. In the longer-term, the residential sector is likely to continue to shrink and the part that remains may well need to become more specialized. Research that could guide such developments is presently lacking and should be undertaken.

### Further information

Department of Health. (1998). *Children looked after away from home: messages from research.* Wiley, Chichester.

Sinclair, I. (2006). Residential care in the UK. In *Enhancing the well-being of children and families through effective interventions: international evidence for practice* (eds. C. McAuley, P. Pecora, and W. Rose). Jessica Kingsley, London.

### References

1. Gottesman, M. (ed.) (1991). *Residential child care: an international reader.* Whiting and Birch in association with FICE, London.

2. Colton, M. and Hellinckx, W. (eds.) (1993). *Child care in the EC.* Arena, Aldershot.

3. Department for Education and Skills. (2007). *Children looked after by local authorities, year ending 31 March 2006* (Internet only) Department for Education and Skills. http://www.dfes.gov.uk/rsgateway/DB/VOL/v000721/index.shtml

4. Sinclair, I. and Gibbs, I. (1998). *Children's homes: a study in diversity.* Wiley, Chichester.

5. Sinclair, I., Baker, C., Lee, J., et al. (2007). *The pursuit of permanence: a study of the English care system.* Jessica Kingsley, London.

6. Hicks, L., Gibbs, I., Byford, S., et al. (2007). *Managing children's homes: developing effective leadership in small organisations.* Jessica Kingsley, London.

7. Department of Health. (2002). *Children's homes national minimum standards and children's homes regulations.* The Stationery Office, London.

8. Department for Education and Skills. (2006). *Statistics of education: children looked after by local authorities, year ending 31 March 2005, Vol. 1: National Tables.* HMSO, Norwich.

9. Department for Education and Skills. (2006). *Care matters: transforming the lives of children and young people in care green paper.* The Stationery Office, Norwich.

10. Koprowska, J. and Stein, M. (2000). The mental health of looked after young people. In *Young people and mental health* (eds. P. Aggleton, J. Hurry, and I. Warwick). Wiley, Chichester.

11. Biehal, J., Clayden, J., Stein, M., et al. (1995). *Moving on: young people and leaving care schemes.* National Children's Bureau, London.

12. Anderson, I., Kemp, P.A., and Quilgars, D. (1993). *Single homeless people.* HMSO, London.

13. Berridge, D. and Brodie, I. (1998). *Children's homes revisited.* Jessica Kingsley, London.

14. Carr-Hill, R.A., Dixon, P., Mannion, R., et al. (1997). *A model of the determinants of children's personal social services.* Centre for Health Economics, University of York, York.

15. Utting, W. (1991). *Children in the public care.* HMSO, London.

16. Training Organisation for the Personal Social Services. (2003). *National occupational standards for registered managers (child care).* TOPSS, England.

## 9.5.7 Organization of services for children and adolescents with mental health problems

Miranda Wolpert

### Introduction

This chapter aims to guide the thinking of practitioners who might be involved in developing services to meet the needs of children and young people with mental health difficulties. Anyone involved in this challenging but vital endeavour will need to address the following questions:

◆ Who should the service be for?

◆ What sort of interventions should be provided?

◆ How should the service be structured?

◆ Who should the staff be?

◆ How can the service be made most accessible?

◆ How can service quality be ensured?

This chapter will look at each of these issues in turn to explore how each might best be approached.

## Who should the service be for?

Ever expanding conceptualization of mental health needs has meant that at least four groups of children are routinely referred to in the discussions about service development in this area:

1 Children and young people in difficult (and often terrible) circumstances

2 Children at risk of developing diagnosable mental health problems

3 Children with diagnosable mental health problems

4 Children with levels of impairment due to mental health issues that make it difficult for them to function within their community/culture

Lack of clarity when discussing the needs of the different groups can confuse service planning. In particular, it can result in the range of agencies that are all increasingly involved in collaborating in planning provision, talking at cross purposes. When resources are limited (as they generally are for these populations of children, even in the most economically developed countries of the world) it is likely that choices will need to be made about prioritizing between and within these groups. It is therefore vital to be clear at the outset which groups are seen as the priority for a given community and to achieve multi-agency agreement on this.

The needs of each of these groups in relation to service provision in this area is considered in turn below.

### Children in difficult circumstances

Definitions of 'difficult circumstances' vary with national context. The estimated 14 million AIDS orphans (concentrated largely in Africa) would fall into this category as would the 12 million children in the United States living below the poverty line along with all those children who are in contexts of war, famine, or abuse.[1] This group is likely to include those children with high and complex mental health needs who are the hardest to reach and who are a policy priority in many areas. However it may also include children who do not have specific mental health needs. Services need to ensure they are accessible to these groups where they do have mental health issues but specialist mental health services are unlikely to be the main provider of care for the majority of children in such circumstances.

### Children 'at risk'

Risk factors for developing diagnosable mental health problems include some aspect of difficult circumstances (such as violent environments, lack of warm family environments) but risk is also heightened by other individual and interpersonal factors such as: brain injury, low birth weight, poor parental mental health, low IQ, irritable temperament, family dysfunction, and the lack of a key supportive relationship with an adult. For children identified as 'at risk' the focus for mental health provision is likely to be on how

to enhance resilience. There may be key opportunities for intervention, such as when the child is born or at key transition points (such as starting school, changing school, leaving school, etc). There is an argument for targeting particular groups such as children of parents with mental health problems. However, evidence for the effectiveness of health promotion and prevention initiatives is still limited and there is some evidence that the promotion of resilience may best be achieved by agencies other than child mental health specialists, such as welfare sectors creating greater neighbourhood cohesion, perinatal services reducing risk of low birth weight and educational services implementing appropriate programmes to promote emotional well-being and support children in times of stress. It is likely that services should only put major resources into targeting 'at risk' children if they have sufficient resources to meet the needs of those children with existing problems.

### Children with diagnosable mental health problems

Epidemiological data from Europe and the United States suggests that around 10–20 per cent of children suffer from diagnosable mental health problems (using ICD-10 or DSM-IV criteria). There are indications of differences between countries, with slightly lower rates found in India and Norway, for example, and slightly higher in Brazil, Bangladesh, and Russia. However, not all of these children need direct service provision. Some diagnosable mental health problems may get better without intervention (such as depressions in mild form). For these reasons, amongst others (in particular the fact that not all current treatments are proven to do more good than harm—as will be discussed below), it is not advised to go down the route recently suggested by the American Psychiatric Association of screening all children in schools and treating all diagnosable difficulties.[2]

### Children with impairment due to mental health difficulties

It is children in this category who are likely to be the main target for specialist child mental health provision. The impact of significant and impairing mental health difficulties if not effectively treated can be substantial. Worldwide, suicide is the third leading cause of death amongst adolescents; major depressive disorder, often starting in adolescence, is associated with substantial psychosocial impairment; conduct disorders amongst children tend to persist into adult life and are reflected in later drug abuse, antisocial behaviour, and poor physical health. This group covers a wide variety of children and young people with problems ranging from bed-wetting to psychosis. It includes those with chronic and multiple difficulties and those with discrete and defined difficulties. It encompasses those with difficulties where there are known to be effective interventions and those presenting with problems where the best course of action is much less clear (as will be discussed below). It is this very mixed range of problems that child mental health services must address.

## Prioritizing needs

The way needs are prioritized in planning service provision will be heavily influenced by the context in which services are located. In some countries independent child mental health provision and unaffordable luxury when pitted against other basic needs. The World Health Organisation[3] has suggested that where resources are particularly limited, priority for funds for child mental health provision should be given to those children with existing difficulties which are:

◆ occur frequently (and/or have highest cost implications)

◆ cause a high degree of impairment

◆ have the greatest long-term care/cost consequences

◆ have an evidence base for treatment and (particularly in those countries with the most limited resources)

◆ where the difficulties can be dealt with in primary care or universal services such as schools or GPs.

In countries with greater resources, child mental health professionals' input can be conceptualized as being provided at universal, targeted, and specialist levels. This involves supporting and working alongside universal provision to promote emotional well-being whether in schools or via primary health care workers. Targeted provision aims to promote emotional well-being in those deemed either at most risk (group 2 above) or in most need (group 1 above) with the groups being determined by policy imperatives. Here specialist mental health professionals will work alongside workers from other sectors who take a lead in relation to the needs of these groups as a whole, such as social welfare workers and primary care staff. Specialist provision aims to intervene primarily with those with existing impairment due to mental health difficulties (group 4 above) and can be provided at a local community level, though for more rare and specialized resources may be provided at a regional ore even at a national level.

Weighing mental health promotion initiatives against interventions for those with existing impairments requires particularly careful thought. Whilst there is evidence that promotion programmes may sometimes promote emotional well-being, research to date has not proved that this will reduce levels of significant disturbance and thus impact on specialist services, nor that such programmes are necessarily the most effective approach. It therefore does not seem warranted at this stage to assume that investment in prevention can be done at the expense of investment in services for those with existing impairing mental health difficulties.

In planning response to 'need', it is also important to consider the potential negative and even harmful impact of increased specialist mental health services. Mental health professionals are frequently in danger of assuming that more specialist mental health provision is unquestionably an unalloyed good. The need for more provision must be set in the context of other (sometimes competing) 'needs', such as: the primary need of children to be nourished, sheltered, and protected; their need not to be stigmatized or miss education; and their need not to receive inappropriate, ineffective, or harmful treatment. At times an inappropriate mental health focus can be an unhelpful drain on resources. One documented example is when well-meaning voluntary groups entered a country following a disaster to provide 'interventions for PTSD' that were not linked to other relief efforts and actually interfered with and undermined key initiatives.[1] Whilst the costs of not providing effective specialist mental health inputs can be high, it is important to remember there are also costs to providing unhelpful services.

## What sort of interventions should be provided?

As yet, few services have been developed on the basis of considered evidence. Systems of care in CAMHS (as for many areas in health care) have historically been developed on the basis of beliefs, assertion, and innovation within the limits of given structures but with little reference to the slowly and tentatively emerging evidence base. The arguments for trying to promote evidence-based service development are compelling. Natural biases in reasoning mean that people tend to make decisions based more on things that fit their assumptive world view than those that challenge it and are more influenced by the charisma of those promoting a particular approach than by evidence for its effectiveness. When the evidence base is not used as the basis for service development, it makes it more likely that seemingly plausible but ineffective and/or harmful interventions may be introduced or continued and that new interventions that have been shown to do more good than harm may never be introduced.[4]

The evidence base in relation to child mental health interventions, whilst growing, is still limited both in extent and quality. Shortcomings include the sheer paucity of studies, the fact that most research is conducted in United States and there is lack of agreement over appropriate outcome measures. Even where interventions have been found to work in academic studies they are generally not as effective when applied in 'real life' settings. This difference may be due to differences in the populations of children seen, types of interventions made, and/or outcomes assessed. There is increasing evidence of the necessity of carefully implementing all aspects of a particular intervention if it is to be as helpful, and that lack of 'fidelity to model' may account for the lack of generalizability of some of the interventions. On the other hand, the role of non-specific factors such as therapeutic engagement, expectations of change and therapist warmth may need to be taken into account.[5]

Whilst bearing these limitations of the research evidence base in mind there is an emerging consensus in relation to some key interventions[6–8] and increasing attempts to develop guidance for practitioners based on the evidence in this area are being developed (e.g. National Institute of Clinical Excellence guidelines in England, American Psychiatric Association Practice parameters in the United States). Those interested in the detail of the sorts of interventions currently found by the evidence base to be most efficacious should go to these guidelines and may also be interested in attempts to summarize the evidence base[8, 9] (condenses current findings to inform the work of practitioners and others and is freely available via the internet).

It is hoped that as the evidence base develops, so should the sophistication with which it might be interrogated. For every intervention listed above as having 'good evidence' to support it, the following questions should be asked (modified from Kazdin[10], p. 113):

◆ What are the costs, risks, and benefits of this intervention relative to no intervention?

◆ What are the costs, risks, and benefits of this intervention relative to other interventions?

◆ What are the key components that appear to contribute to positive outcomes?

◆ What parameters can be varied to improve outcomes (e.g. including addition of other interventions, non-specific clinical skills, etc)?

◆ To what extent are effects of interventions generalizable across (a) problem areas, (b) settings, (c) populations of children, and (d) other relevant domains?

We are a long way from being able to answer these questions in relation to CAMHS currently but it is to be hoped that this will develop with time.

However, even as the evidence base grows from academic studies this must still be treated with caution. It is not suggested that findings from even the most rigorously undertaken randomized controlled trials can necessarily be applied wholesale to all individuals with similar problems. The full context of an individual's range of needs and circumstances must be taken into account and it is also hoped that understanding of the academic literature will be supplemented with a growing evidence base emerging from practitioners own routine evaluation of their own work (see discussion in 'ensuring service quality' section below).

## How should the service be structured?

If the evidence base for types of intervention is limited, this is even more so for types of organization.

The 'Fort Bragg Study' (and the subsequent Stark County Study) conducted by Bickman and colleagues in the United States warrants particular attention as they generated such high levels of interest and controversy. This study evaluated a large-scale system change project designed to improve outcomes by providing an unrestricted set of coordinated inputs from a range of services. Results were compared with other sites using traditional services. Information was collected on service use, cost, satisfaction, clinical, and functional data over the course of the 3-year study and at follow-up since. The study found greater access and increased rates of satisfaction and less use of inpatient services, but no differences in behavioural–emotional functioning overall and the cost was much greater at Fort Bragg. The subsequent Stark County Study also found that a multi-agency system for care led to no significant difference in clinical outcomes when compared with routine services. Bickman concluded 'the current national policy of large investments in systems of care infrastructure is unlikely to affect children in the manner intended . . . we need to focus on the services or treatments themselves to improve outcomes'.[11]

This conclusion has been hotly contested. Flaws in the study design, implementation, and interpretation have been highlighted. It was argued that services were overwhelmed in the early months and provided less effective interventions, that the researchers failed to take into account some of the positive outcomes on some of the measures used and so on. It has been suggested that there is evidence that 'wrap around services' (whereby a range of services are provided in a coordinated fashion to children and families based on their needs and not those of the services) do produce better outcomes and that the poor results above may have been due to lack of fidelity to this model.[12]

There is some evidence that shared understandings at the highest level and pooled budgets seem to be crucial to positive multi-agency collaboration. 'MHSPY' in the United States is an initiative that involves five public and two private agencies who have come together with blended funding to provide a coordinated focus on a group of 'at risk' and ill children and where outcomes look positive though lacking a control group or clear cost-effectiveness data as yet.

There is little evidence available currently to guide service developers as to the best way to structure services in relation to a number of other key issues, such as: what age of children should be seen by different services? Is it best to structure services around particular problems or around different age groups? What should be the balance between inpatient and outpatient provision? Whilst it is hoped that with time, more evidence will emerge in relation to these issues, it may be hypothesized that, here too, non-specific factors, may be relevant. Thus the leadership skills of the clinicians who establish a given service, the strength of their commitment in a particular shape of service, and the ability of key individuals to collaborate across whatever boundaries are inevitably created, may impact as much, if not more, than the specifics of different forms of service structure.

## Who should the staff be?

In terms of who the key staff should be who provide specialist mental health services for children, whilst there is much assertion and rhetoric as to what is the ideal workforce composition and an emphasis on multi-disciplinary and multi-agency team development wherever possible, there is, in fact, very little hard evidence as to what an ideal workforce should look like.

In many parts of the world specialist mental health professionals are in short supply, and there is an increasing focus on capitalizing on opportunities for mental health provision to piggyback on other sectors with more provision (such as HIV programmes in Africa or schools in many areas of the world). The potential contribution of paediatricians, primary care workers, and teachers is increasingly recognized, though care must be taken not to overload already stretched systems and research highlighting the importance of 'fidelity to model' (as discussed above) suggest that there may be a necessary threshold of amount of training combined with ongoing organizational support, for subsequent interventions to be effective.

## How can the service be made most accessible?

Attempts to make provision more accessible as well as less stigmatizing can include use of education and primary care workers, community and religious leaders, and family networks. There is evidence that linking with relevant belief systems of the community, such as ayurvedic treatment and yoga in parts of India, may be crucial, and that providing training for traditional healers may help increase child mental health capacity. The work of voluntary organizations can be a major source of innovation and energy and communities need to find ways for statutory services to learn from them. For example the walk in community centre, Empilwent in South Africa pioneered a more accessible drop in approach.

It could be argued that child mental health services have been slow on the whole to 'get out of the clinic' and in particular to embrace the impact of new technologies that might increase access. However some interesting innovations are developing. These range from mobile services such as the peripatetic child mental health team which travels across Germany providing follow-up on previously hospitalized young people, providing new consultations, and supervision of institutions for children[13] to increased use of telephone and text contact generally, and telephone helplines and websites specifically.

Telephone helplines such as 'Kids Help'[14] in Australia, 'Childline'[15] in the United Kingdom, and 'Parents Information

Service' (YoungMinds Parent Information Service)[16] in the United Kingdom, are often run by charities independent of statutory provision but it may be in the future that greater links can be made by such resources and more traditional services. 'Telefono Azzuro' of Italy shows the way these can be combined with other provisions.[13]

A range of websites have been developed by and for young people some of which allow for discussions between young people and others offer access to specialist advice and support (e.g. 'ru-ok.com').[17] The use of emails and text messaging to communicate between professionals and young people is now increasing as are the use of IT aids to assessment and treatment and the pace of innovation in this area is likely to accelerate sharply in the future.

## How can service quality be ensured?

The implementation of routine outcome evaluation is likely to be a crucial factor in ensuring service quality. There are increasing attempts to ensure routine outcome evaluation is in place. The CAMHS Outcome Research Consortium (CORC)[18] (chaired by the author) is collaboration between over half of all services across the United Kingdom who are implementing an agreed model of routine outcome and agreeing jointly ways to present the data in order to inform service providers and users and to help inform service developments (CORC).[8] The approach has parallels with that being employed in the United States and Australia. In all cases a small suite of measures is completed by service users and providers at initial contact and at some time(s) later. Increasingly models are being developed whereby individual practitioners evaluate outcomes over the course of treatment which can be immediately compared with outcomes from others with similar difficulties at the outset, allowing practitioners to get feedback about progress relative to others.

For child mental health service to institute routine outcome evaluation and to develop into self-reflective and learning organizations, requires functioning IT systems and an agreed core dataset.[19] There are now datasets for child mental health emerging in some countries.[20] But even in the most developed countries, the promise of coherent IT systems, remains more a hope than a reality. It is key that IT systems develop that are capable of supporting decision-making by providing easy access to information for practitioners so that they can get feedback on their work and learn accordingly.

There is an increasing emphasis on the importance of involvement of service users to inform service development priorities and to be part of any evaluation of services, to ensure quality. Some innovative models have been tried such as in Ohio which has created outcome systems from service user perspective and in parts of the United Kingdom where young people are trained as service evaluators though again the impact of these on quality of services in the future is yet to be researched.

## Conclusion

There is no one ideal model for organizing services, however some key principles can be identified:

1 It is helpful to start with an analysis of the range of anticipated needs, and to seek clarity as to the current priorities for a given community.

2 Where resources are limited, specialist mental health provision should be targeted foremost on those with greatest levels of impairment for whom there are the most effective interventions.

3 Implementation of effective models of prevention and promotion should be supported so far as resources allow and not at the expense of provision for those with existing difficulties.

4 The existing evidence base in relation to effective interventions and models of delivery should be seen as a starting point for practice, though the limitations of the evidence base should be held in mind.

5 Successful service development is likely to rest on collaboration across health, social care, and education—using pooled budgets where possible.

6 Good information gathering systems are needed that allow individual practitioners and managers to audit and review work.

7 Staff members should be encouraged to adapt their practice in the light of the emerging evidence from literature and their own outcomes rather than retaining allegiance to any one theoretical model or framework.

8 Collaborations between service providers that focus on developing best practice may be of help.

9 The input and involvement of service users may be of relevance in helping develop accessible and acceptable services.

10 Remember not all service developments are benign—always weigh up possible harm that may be caused as well as potential for good.

## Further information

Wolpert, M., Fuggle, P., Cottrell, D., *et al.* (2006). *Drawing on the evidence: advice for mental health professionals working with children and adolescents-revised version* (Child and Adolescent Mental Health Services Evidence Based Practice Unit-University College London) http://www.ucl.ac.uk/clinical-health-psychology/pdf Files/DotEBooklet2006.pdf

Wolpert, M. (2008). Organisation of services for children and adolescents with mental health problems. In *Rutter's child and adolescent psychiatry*, (eds. M. Rutter, D. Bishop, D. Pine, *et al.*) Blackwell, Oxford.

Goodman, R. and Scott, S. (2005). *Child psychiatry* (2nd edn). Blackwell, Oxford.

## References

1. World Health Organization. (2005). *Atlas: child and adolescent mental health resources. Global concerns: implications for the future.* World Health Organization, Geneva.

2. American Psychiatric Association. (2002). *Quality indicators-defining and measuring quality in psychiatric care for adults and children.* American Psychiatric Association.

3. World Health Organization. (2003). *Caring for children and adolescents with mental disorders: setting WHO directions.* World Health Organization, Geneva.

4. Gray, M.J.A. (2001). *Evidence-based healthcare: how to make health policy and management decisions.* Churchill Livingstone, Edinburgh.

5. Fonagy, P., Target, M., Cottrell, D., *et al.* (2002). *What works for whom? A critical review of treatments for children and adolescents.* Guilford Press, London.

6. Goodman, R. and Scott, S. (2005). *Child psychiatry* (2nd edn). Blackwell, Oxford.

7. Rutter, M., Tizard, J., and Whitmore, K. (1970). *Education, health and behaviour*. Longman, London.

8. Wolpert, M., Fuggle, P., Cottrell, D., *et al.* (2006). *Drawing on the evidence: advice for mental health professionals working with children and adolescents-revised version* (Child and Adolescent Mental Health Services Evidence Based Practice Unit-University College London) http://www.annafreudcentre.org/dote_booklet_2006.pdf

9. CAMHS publications, London. (2007). Choosing what's best for you. What scientists have found helps children and young people who are sad, worried or troubled. http://www.annafreudcentre.org/ebpu/choosing.pdf

10. Kazdin, A.E. (2004). Evidence-based psychotherapies for children and adolescents: strategies, strengths and limitations. In *Facilitating pathways: care, treatment and prevention in child and adolescent mental health* (eds. H. Remschmidt, M. Belfer, and I. Goodyer), pp. 103–18. Springer-Verlag, Berlin.

11. Bickman, L., Lambert, E.W., Andrade, A.R., *et al.* (2000). The Fort Bragg continuum of care for children and adolescents: mental health outcomes over 5 years. *Journal of Consulting and Clinical Psychology*, **68**(4), 710–6.

12. Bruns, E.J., Burchard, J.D., Suter, J.C., *et al.* (2005). Measuring fidelity within community treatments for children and families. In *Outcomes for children and youth with emotional and behavioral disorders and their families*, Vol. 2 (eds. M. Epstein, A. Duchnowski, and K. Kutash). Pro-ED, Austin, TX.

13. Remschmidt, H., Belfer, M., and Goodyer, I. (eds.) (2004). *Facilitating pathways: care, treatment and prevention in child and adolescent mental health*. Springer-Verlag, Berlin.

14. Kids Help Line. http://www.kidshelp.com.au/home_KHL.aspx?s=6

15. Childline. http://www.childline.org.uk/

16. YoungMinds' Parents Information Service. http://www.youngminds.org.uk/parents

17. RU-OK.Com. http://www.ru-ok.com/

18. CAMHS Outcome Research Consortium. (CORC). http://www.corc.uk.net

19. Wolpert, M., Bartholomew, R., Domb, Y., *et al.* (2005). *Collaborating to improve Child Mental Health Services. CAMHS outcome research consortium handbook. Version1.* CORC, London.

20. http://www.ic.nhs.uk/our-services/standards-and-classifications/dataset-list/camhs

## 9.5.8 The management of child and adolescent psychiatric emergencies

Gillian C. Forrest

*'Child' is used throughout this chapter to refer to anyone aged under 18, to avoid the repetition of 'child or young person'. 'His' and 'her' are used interchangeably.*

### Introduction

This chapter provides a practical approach to the management of psychiatric emergencies in children and adolescents. Such emergencies are challenging for a number of reasons. The professional resources available are usually very limited, and there is often confusion or even disagreement between professionals over what constitutes a psychiatric, as opposed to a social emergency. The parents or carers play a key role in the situation and need to be engaged and involved appropriately in the assessment and management; and issues of confidentiality and consent need to be taken into account. In addition, the psychiatrist may find himself or herself working in a variety of settings—the child's home, a hospital emergency department (A and E), a police station, a children's home, or residential school—where the facilities for assessing an angry, disturbed, or upset child may be far from ideal.

Most emergencies occurring in community settings involve externalizing behaviours: aggression, violence; deliberate self-harm, or threats of harm to self or others; or extreme emotional outbursts.[1,2] Some will involve bizarre behaviour which could be an indication of serious mental illness or intoxication by drugs or alcohol, or a combination of both. The emergency situation often arises in the context of acute family conflict or distress.

Frequently other agencies are involved before the psychiatrist is called in (for example, emergency room staff, social workers, or the police). The on-call psychiatrist needs to be familiar with or able to obtain immediate advice about his or her local child and adolescent psychiatric services, the local child protection and child care procedures, and with the relevant mental health and child care legislation.

*Vignette 1:*

A 12-year-old boy is in the police station, after attacking a neighbour and smashing a window. He punched a police officer when they tried to pacify him. He has refused to talk to the police, and is sweating and dishevelled, pacing up and down and muttering to himself. The police think he is psychotic. The neighbour is in the waiting room; his father has been called back from work.

After obtaining the history of the incident from the neighbour and the police, the psychiatrist interviewed the father. The boy had been diagnosed with an autistic spectrum disorder when he was 5. He was easily upset by any change of routine. His mother had gone away for a few days, leaving him in the care of a neighbour while his father was at work. This aggressive outburst was precipitated by the neighbour refusing to let him watch his favourite video. The boy calmed down with his father and a mental state assessment confirmed autistic features but no psychotic symptoms. The psychiatrist persuaded the neighbour and the police to drop charges and the boy was allowed to return home. The family were offered an out-patient appointment but declined this, and arrangements were made for his General Practitioner (GP) to review the situation in a few days' time.

*Vignette 2:*

A 15-year-old girl has locked herself in the bathroom at home with a carving knife and is threatening to cut her wrists. Her parents have been unable to persuade her to come out and are now distraught. The GP was called but she refuses to speak to him.†

When the psychiatrist arrived, he asked the family to withdraw so that he could talk to the girl through the bathroom door. She was very upset and described how she had been dumped by her boyfriend earlier that day, had had a row with her step-mother about a large phone bill, and now felt that she didn't want to live any more. The psychiatrist persuaded her to come out to talk things over with her parents. There was no evidence of a depressive disorder and after the psychiatrist helped the girl share her distress about her boyfriend with her

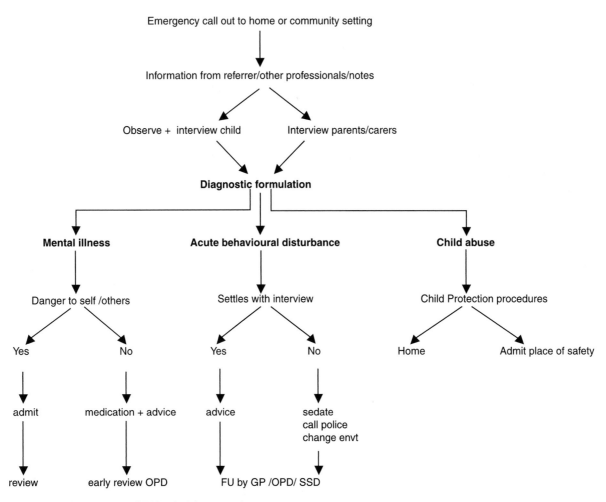

**Fig. 9.5.8.1** Flow chart of management of child and adolescent psychiatric emergencies.

parents, she calmed down. There was a history of one previous attempt at self-harm, also connected with peer relationship difficulties, and the psychiatrist felt that there were some underpinning issues around family communication. He offered the family an out-patient appointment to explore these further.

In the emergency situation, the role of the psychiatrist is to:

♦ assess the disturbed behaviour

♦ make a diagnostic formulation which distinguishes behaviour associated with mental illness from that which is a reaction to an upsetting event or situation

♦ produce a care plan to manage the situation safely and effectively in the short-term.

A step-by-step approach to the management of child and adolescent emergencies is described here. The management of deliberate self-harm is dealt with in Chapter 9.2.10.

## Step 1. Gathering information

Before attempting to assess the child and his or her family, it is very important to gather as much background information as possible about the incident or behaviour from any professionals who have

been directly involved. They may be able to give an accurate description of the child's behaviour and any incident which preceded it; or useful background information about the family. Take time to read any notes that are available; and talk to those involved (GP, police, paediatric staff, A and E staff, etc.).

## Step 2. Interview with the child/young person

Although this is described first, parents may expect to be seen before the child, or it may be preferable to talk to them first to gather background information (see Step 3).

A disturbed or upset child in this situation will be wary of any stranger, and the more out of control they are, emotionally and behaviourally, the more likely they are to be uncooperative initially. The psychiatrist needs to calmly establish that they have come to try and help the child, that they are non-judgemental and that they can be trusted. She should always ask to see the child alone, to establish a confidential relationship, and to be able to assess the child without the influence of parents.

Honest and open communication is essential, especially if there is any possibility of child protection issues. Often the child is terrified that they are going to be forcibly taken away from their home or family (a desperate and angry parent will often threaten this), and this fear may need to be addressed before the assessment can begin.

A useful approach is to say to the child: 'I'm Dr ..... I'm a psychiatrist who sees children and young people with all sorts of worries and troubles. I've come to see you now, to try and understand what this is all about, and see if I can find a way to help'.

If the child refuses to talk at this stage, they may be angry, mistrustful, or psychotically withdrawn. Patience is required to see if this can be overcome by convincing the child that you have come to listen to them and not to 'take them away'. Reflecting back to the child how you perceive their emotional state may also help. For example, the psychiatrist might say: 'You are obviously very upset and angry. I wonder what it is that's made you feel this way'. Sometimes children will choose to communicate by writing notes or drawing, rather than by using speech, and if the child is mute, the psychiatrist should try offering paper and pencil.

If the child remains violent and out of control and the behaviour is being reinforced by attention and anxiety, it will be necessary to ask everyone to withdraw for a while to give the child the chance to calm down on their own. If this still does not help to calm the situation, the psychiatrist will need to set some limits, which could include calling the police to regain control of the behaviour. Medication should only be considered as a last resort when all other strategies to deescalate the situation and calm the child have failed (see Step 5: Management of emergencies in community settings section).

When the child starts to be able to communicate with the psychiatrist, they can then be encouraged to give their account of what happened to precipitate the behaviour. As this is explored, it will be possible to assess the child's mental state (see Chapter 9.1.3) and to form an impression about whether this is mental illness, or whether the disturbed behaviour is the result of emotional turmoil secondary to relationship problems, family conflict, or other psychosocial issues. Further information from the parents or carers will be needed to clarify this.

If child abuse is suspected, an interview with the child alone is crucial. The psychiatrist will need to enquire about the possibility of physical and sexual abuse without using leading questions[3] (see Chapter 9.3.2). A good starting point is 'Has anyone ever hurt you or made you do anything you didn't like?' The child needs to understand that you may need to breach confidentiality in order to protect them from further harm. (see Consent and confidentiality section).

## Step 3. Interview with parents/carers

It is essential to see the parents or carers as part of the assessment, in order to fully understand the context of the crisis, and identify any relevant contributory factors. They may be seen first, or after the child's assessment, depending on the situation. It is often helpful to see the parents or carers on their own so that they can speak freely about their child.

These are the areas that will need covering:

♦ History of current episode/disturbance. Current medication?

♦ Previous emotional or behavioural problems.

♦ Brief developmental history: normal or unusual features? Learning difficulties? School and academic progress.

♦ Temperament; relationships with family/extended family members, other adults, peers.

♦ Family composition and history (parental separations/divorce; relationships mental and physical illness; recent life events).

During this interview, an assessment can be made of the family functioning; the parent's or carer's mental health, and their attitude to the child, and whether this seems to be playing a part in the current problem (e.g. high levels of family discord; rejecting, neglectful or hostile attitudes to the child; harsh parenting practices; parental depression, anxiety, drug or alcohol abuse).

*Vignette 3:*

A 10-year-old has been raging around his house for several hours, following an argument with his mother about going out with his friends. He has been smashing toys and kicking in doors and wrecking his bedroom. His single mother and 6-year-old sister are terrified and cowering in the sitting room.

The psychiatrist spoke calmly to the boy through the door, stating that he wanted to talk to him. The boy continued being aggressive and abusive and the psychiatrist then said he would give him 5 minutes to calm down and come out, otherwise the police would have to be called in to help. The boy did then manage to calm down and talked about his resentment of his mother's rules, and his angry feelings about the loss of his father, who had had little contact with him since leaving the family.

His mother told the psychiatrist that she and the boy's father had divorced a year ago, and there had been on-going disputes with her exhusband about money and his erratic contact with the children. Recently she had become depressed, and her son had become increasingly irritable and oppositional at home. She felt unable to control her boy's temper outbursts.

The mother agreed to see her GP about her depression, try and talk to her ex-husband about seeing the children on a regular basis, and attend the clinic with the children for some family counselling sessions. The boy appeared relieved that his mother was going to seek some help.

## Step 4. Making and sharing the diagnostic formulation

There should now be sufficient information available to make a diagnostic formulation. This will include the diagnostic category for the disturbed behaviour, the factors which led up to the acute disturbance; the factors which precipitated it, and the risk factors for continuing or recurring problems.

**The Three Ps:**

Predisposing Factors

Precipitating

Perpetuating

These factors may be present in the child herself (temperament, illness); in the family environment; at school or college; in the child's wider social environment (friends, neighbours; clubs, etc.); or any combination of these.

Apart from acute intoxication with drugs or alcohol, and deliberate self-harm, most child and adolescent psychiatric emergencies in the community fall into three categories:

♦ mental illness

♦ acute behavioural disturbance due to family/psychosocial factors

♦ child abuse

The psychiatrist should share his formulation with the child and parents/carers, using age-appropriate, and jargon-free language, to help their understanding of the events. Sometimes the parents or the child will need further discussions before a shared understanding between the psychiatrist and the family about the problems can be reached, and an acceptance of the proposed management/care plan by the family.

The formulation should also be shared with any other professionals present, as they may be needed to contribute to the immediate management plan, or even to take over the care of the child.

## Step 5. Management of emergencies in community settings (see Fig. 9.5.8.1)

### Mental illness

The emergency management of a child diagnosed with a mental illness will depend on the risk assessment. Is the child a danger to himself or others? If the psychiatrist considers this to be a high risk, then referral to inpatient care will be necessary to allow further assessment and treatment in a safe setting. Compulsory admission, using mental health legislation, may be required if the child or the parents refuse to cooperate with this plan (see Consent section). In some places, it may be possible to admit younger children to a paediatric ward for further observation and treatment. Where there are medical complications of a mental illness (for example, low output cardiac failure in severe anorexia nervosa), admission to a paediatric or medical ward will be needed.

If there is a low risk of any danger, and the child and family are cooperative, the psychiatrist can prescribe appropriate medication for the mental illness (see Chapter 9.5.5), give advice on the management of the symptoms in the short-term, and arrange for early follow-up and review in the outpatient clinic.

### Acute behavioural disturbance (no mental illness)

Very often, the situation is defused by the psychiatrist's assessment, and the child's behaviour settles. In this case, the psychiatrist will need to decide whether there is a high risk of further episodes. If not, she may simply give advice to the family about how to avoid or deescalate future situations, and inform the child's GP about the incident. However, if she has identified significant ongoing issues underpinning or precipitating the child's disturbed behaviour, she will need to give the family advice about how to try and deal with these. For example, if the child has difficulties with family conflict, the psychiatrist could recommend referral for outpatient family therapy or anger management; if stress at school was linked to the outburst, she might advise the parents to arrange a meeting with the child's teachers; or she could advise a parent to seek help for their own mental health problems (such as depression or addiction) or social problems such as overcrowding or financial difficulties.

If the disturbed and violent behaviour continues in spite of the psychiatrist's intervention, a decision must be made about how best to regain control of the situation. The police may need to be called in, to provide sufficient manpower to safely control the violent behaviour. It may be possible to change the environment by calling in significant other people (for example, another relative) who can calm the child. The use of medication needs very careful consideration.[4] Children may react paradoxically to sedatives and

tranquillizers, and the use of medications with the risk of respiratory suppression is not recommended unless life support equipment (and staff) is available. However, sometimes it may be possible to persuade a child to accept an appropriate dose of oral medication such as lorazepam or midazolam, and this may be beneficial.[5]

### Child abuse

Although it is not common for child abuse to present as a psychiatric emergency, nevertheless it is vitally important for any psychiatrist on call to be able to recognize this, and manage the situation according to local child protection procedures. If the child is making allegations of abuse, these will need to be discussed with the parents/carers, and then it will be necessary to consult with other professional colleagues (including the police, social services, or paediatric staff) to decide on how best to care for the child. The welfare of the child must always be paramount, even if this involves the child being taken to a place of safety such as a paediatric ward or to alternative accommodation while further investigations are carried out. Clear and accurate notes of all aspects of the assessment are vital as they may be needed for legal proceedings later. (The assessment of possible child abuse is considered further in Chapter 9.3.3.)

### Emergencies in paediatric/medical wards

Psychiatric assessment and advice is needed at times for children showing acutely disturbed behaviour on paediatric wards, as well as for deliberate self-harm.

The child may be acting bizarrely or aggressively. The psychiatrist will need to make a thorough assessment of the situation, including the background of the child and family and the medical aspects of the case. He will then need to assess whether the behaviour is part of the physical illness, (e.g. hypoglycaemia, hypoxia, delirium, pain), a primary mental illness (e.g. psychosis, somatoform reaction), the side effects of medication, or an acute behavioural reaction. Management will need to be discussed and agreed with the paediatric staff, and shared with the family if they are available. The psychiatric assessment and care plan should be carefully written up in the medical file to ensure continuity through shift changes of the ward staff.

The use of sedation needs to be given careful consideration, and used only if other strategies fail (such as finding out from the child the cause of any upset and talking it over; moving the child to a quieter setting; calling in the parent to help reassure or pacify the child). Oral lorazepam or midazolam are useful drugs of first choice.

If the primary problem is one of mental illness and the child cannot be cared for effectively and safely in a paediatric ward setting, bearing in mind the needs and safety of the other patients, then transfer to a psychiatric ward will need to be arranged as soon as possible.

Follow-up visits or phone calls to the ward will be needed, to make sure the child is improving or to reconsider the diagnosis or treatment.

Psychiatric problems in paediatric or medical wards are considered further in Chapter 9.3.4

## Step 6. Follow-up and communication with other professionals

Effective management of the emergency situation can be undermined by inadequate follow-up arrangements or poor communication between professionals and agencies. It is therefore very important that the on-call psychiatrist communicates with the child's general practitioner, the team providing routine care for the child, and any other relevant professional involved as soon as practicable, usually the following day. This will hopefully ensure that there is a seamless provision of care for the child and the family, and prevent or forestall future emergencies.

## Consent and confidentiality issues

### (a) Consent

Psychiatrists who assess and treat children and adolescents, like all mental health professionals, have a duty of care to ensure that the welfare of children is protected. They must also work within the limits of the laws of the land. This means that care and attention must be paid to the rights of children to consent to their treatment, while at the same time taking into account the circumstances, their mental capacity, their parents' views and the risks and necessity for treatment. In many cases, the sharing of information with the child and the family, and their involvement in the decision about the best care will ensure that an agreement can be reached. However, there are other occasions when either the child or their parents refuse to cooperate with treatment felt to be essential by the psychiatrist. If the child is refusing but the parents consent, it is usually possible to treat the child under parental consent, or for adolescents, to use other legal means (for example, the mental health legislation to allow the hospitalization and treatment of a mental disorder). If the child is consenting to treatment, but the parents refuse, care proceedings may need to be considered. If both child and parents are refusing treatment, the situation is very difficult and a second opinion on the need for treatment and legal advice may have to be obtained before anything further can be done.

### (b) Confidentiality

The confidentiality of the doctor–patient relationship, as mentioned in the Hippocratic Oath, is a fundamental prerequisite for patients being able to trust their doctor with sensitive information. However when working with children and adolescents, confidentiality is complicated by the need to share information with parents, in order for them to fulfil their responsibilities to their child, and also with the other agencies which may be involved in providing services for the child (education, social care, etc.). Children and their families should be informed of the scope of any promises of confidentiality at the beginning, and it is always good to ask for the child's or adolescents' consent to share information where this is necessary and in the best interests of the child. Breaches of confidentiality may be clinically or legally necessary (such as where an adolescent with a mental illness is exposing them self to risk, or when child abuse is suspected).

Tan et al.[6] provide a full discussion of these issues, and decision-making algorithms. Effective management of an emergency should result in the child receiving appropriate care and treatment, the parents having a greater understanding of the issues associated with the disturbed behaviour, and any other professionals feeling supported by the psychiatrist's advice and intervention. This will all reduce the likelihood of further emergency situations arising for that child and family.

## Further information

Jones, D.P.H. (2003). *Communicating with vulnerable children.* Gaskell, London.

## References

1. Halamandaris, P.V. and Anderson, T.R. (1999). Children and adolescents in the psychiatric emergency setting. *The Psychiatric Clinics of North America,* **22**(4), 865–74.
2. Stewart, C., Spicer, M., and Babl, F. (2006). Caring for adolescents with mental health problems: challenges in the emergency department. *Journal of Paediatrics and Child Health,* **42**(11), 726–30. DOI: 10.1111/j.1440-1754.2006.00959.x
3. Jones, D.P.H. (2003). *Communicating with vulnerable children.* Gaskell, London.
4. Sorrentino, A. (2004). Chemical restraints for the agitated, violent or psychotic paediatric patient in the emergency room; controversies and recommendations. *Current Opinion in Pediatrics,* **16**, 201–4.
5. Taylor, D., Paton, C., and Kerwin, R. (eds.) (2007). Rapid tranquillisation (RT) in children and adolescents. In *The Maudsley 2005–2006 prescribing guidelines 8E,* p. 226. Taylor and Francis Group, London and New York.
6. Tan, J.A.O., Passerini, G., and Stewart, A. (2007). Consent and confidentiality in clinical work with young people. *Clinical Child Psychology and Psychiatry,* **12**(2), 191–210. DOI: 10.1177/1359104507075921.

# 9.5.9 The child psychiatrist as consultant to schools and colleges

Simon G. Gowers and Sian Thomas

## Introduction

Those who provide public services for children and young people may have a role in the identification, prevention, and within reasonable parameters, the treatment of mental health problems. Social services and education in particular have a key responsibility to safeguard the physical and psychological health of children and identify potential areas of avoidable harm, including those which may develop within their institutions.

There is a well-recognized mismatch between the rates of child mental health problems identified in epidemiological studies and the number of children referred to child and adolescent mental health services (CAMHS). School staff will often be in the best position to identify unrecognized difficulties and also to help children and their families address prejudices associated with referral to CAMHS, though they may need training and help to do so.

The responsibilities of teachers have been confirmed by schools' inclusion within the broad concept of CAMHS in a number of countries. In the United Kingdom, the Health Advisory Service (now the Health and Social Care Advisory Service—HASCAS), proposed a model, subsequently adopted by the Department of Health of a tiered approach to service provision, in which schools, alongside primary medical care and social services formed the first Tier.[1] Within this model schools have been seen as offering unique opportunities to identify problems, provide simple assessments and refer up to more specialized tiers as judged appropriate and in negotiation with caregivers. Teachers though, often feel inadequately trained to fulfil this role and look to other professionals, including psychiatrists to advise and support them. Fortunately there are a number of professional roles, some employed within education and some outside, forming a bridge between education and mental health services. Some of these roles vary in their detail between countries, but most developed countries will have professionals (possibly with different titles) filling roles comparable to those in the United Kingdom.

It is important to note that CAMHS generally work as multidisciplinary teams, hence any support and liaison may be offered by a range of professionals and not exclusively by psychiatry. One of the HAS recommendations was the creation of a new professional group—the primary child mental health worker—with the particular aim of liaising between Tier 1 and Tier 2 services. The following are some of the professionals involved in the interface between child mental health and education:

### Primary child mental health worker

A practitioner, often with a mental health nursing background, employed either by education or CAMHS with the specific brief to liaise between the two in identifying children with mental health needs.

### Special educational needs coordinator (SENCO)

Employed by the school as a teacher, the role of the SENCO is primarily to develop effective ways of identifying and removing barriers to learning, which may result from intellectual retardation, physical, or mental health problems. Alongside primary child mental health workers they have a role in the identification, management, and referral of children as well as a responsibility to contribute to in-service training for teachers.

### Educational psychologist

Educational psychologists (EP) provide assessments of special educational needs. In the United Kingdom a consultation model has been adopted, whereby the Educational Psychologist meets with the person who has raised concerns as they are likely to be the person most motivated to bring about change. The new model recognizes that teachers are often skilled in assessing pupil attainment, learning styles, behaviour, strengths, and weaknesses. EPs have an important role in early identification and intervention and aim to promote child development and learning through the application of psychological theory using information gathered within a wider ranging context.

### Education welfare officer (EWO)

In the United Kingdom, each school has an EWO assigned, to provide a support service to families and schools to help them meet legal obligations related to a child's education. They work with parents/carers to monitor attendance, with schools to consider courses of action of benefit to poor school attendees and with other agencies (e.g. health, social services, police, and youth offending teams) to provide a suitable programme that will help the child return to full-time education.

### School nurse

An integral part of the school health team, the school nurse's responsibilities include supporting children with complex health needs, running immunization programmes, providing drop-in clinics, parenting programmes and bed-wetting clinics, assessing the health needs of every child on starting school, and providing health schemes for young people.

### Learning mentor

Learning mentors have a broad remit including supporting the safe and effective transition from primary to secondary school, supporting provision for pupils with special educational needs and developing a relationship with identified pupils, based on a trusting individual relationship.

### Connexions advisors

Primarily concerned with those in the 13–16 age range, connexions advisors offer one-to-one support and guidance similar to that previously carried out by careers officers. There is a strong emphasis on surveillance and monitoring. Young people who are seen to be 'at risk' of dropping out of education or who present behavioural problems are a priority for intervention. Personal advisers act as advocates, especially for those who are vulnerable or who have special needs.

### Teachers' training in mental health

Despite their responsibility for identifying mental health problems, teachers in many countries are offered little specific training in this area. In the United Kingdom, most post graduate certificate of education courses offer only a very small amount of time, perhaps as little as a half day to the teaching of special educational needs. A survey of SENCO'S training and their wish for further teaching about mental health issues[2] revealed a significant lack of training. Many had no training in 3 years. In contrast they showed a great willingness to receive more and welcomed liaison from CAMHS professionals. There have been a number of useful initiatives to improve teachers' experience including the National Healthy Schools Programme[3] which aimed to improve learning by reducing emotional and health inequalities using a whole school approach; this involved improving the emotional literacy not only of pupils but of staff and parents too.

## Developing a school liaison service

Establishing a liaison service between CAMHS and a school can have a number of benefits including:

- Early identification of child mental health problems
- Information sharing
- Monitoring and evaluation of treatment e.g. for attention-deficit hyperactivity disorder (ADHD)
- Establishing pathways of referral to higher tiers of service
- Offering school-based interventions for common problems
- Promoting the development of social skills and positive self-esteem.

The majority of CAMHS services do work with schools, the nature of the intervention ranging from consultation and support for school staff to direct work with children, including observation and assessment. However, joint working between CAMHS and schools has a record of patchiness across the United Kingdom, with a lack of key personnel often leading to a fragmented service.

Good examples of joint practice are characterized by secondments between organizations, shared working environments, a clear understanding of the different roles and expertise of team members, and a shared vision of joint working.

Where good practice is operating, schools are often faced with anxieties around short-term funding for specific projects, for example, the recent initiatives 'City Education Action Zones', 'Health Action Zones', and the 'Healthy Schools Standards'.

Schools in the United States tend to operate within multi-disciplinary settings and research suggests that these are effective in breaking down professional barriers and also addressing the stigma associated with a young person being referred to external agencies such as CAMHS.

The provision of a key mental health worker within the school facilitates better communication between services and helps develop a greater understanding of how the culture of a school operates. Integrated links between CAMHS and the local authority, educational psychologists, behaviour and emotional support teams, and education welfare promotes a cohesive and collaborative service for children.

### Practical issues

In order for a CAMHS service to establish an effective working link with a school, there are several issues to address:

#### (a) Gaining the cooperation of all the staff

Commitment of all staff (and indeed parents) rather than just one interested teacher is crucial. Effective prevention, treatment, and referral pathways require a 'whole school' approach.

#### (b) Negotiating realistic aims

Child mental health problems are common and often long-lasting; a realistic balance should be struck between prevention and management.

#### (c) Establishing a level of service

Both the school and CAMHS should be clear about who is providing the service, at what frequency and the expected level of commitment on both sides. There should be perceived benefits to the school and CAMHS. Does the service provide an urgent referral component or not? Who is the named contact?

#### (d) Confidentiality

Schools say that policies around sharing information act as barriers to effective joint working and so there is a need to determine a process whereby a joint strategy on confidentiality is agreed. At an individual level, young people can expect that private discussions on personal matters should be kept confidential unless they are told otherwise. However, teaching staff should not give unreserved assurances on confidentiality as these may have to be breached if the young person discloses information which leads an adult to believe that they or others are at risk. Sometimes the teacher will need to share information with others in the staff team in the young person's interests, or for supervision purposes. On occasions, (for example, where there is a serious risk of self-harm) it will be necessary to contact parents, but in these circumstances the young person should be told explicitly what has been shared with whom and why. Confidences should not be breached to other pupils.

#### (e) Pitfalls

There are several dangers of providing a mentoring/counselling service for the inexperienced teacher. Some of the commonest are: becoming over involved (emotionally and with time), giving unconditional guarantees of confidentiality, and dealing inappropriately with pupils concerns about another pupil. Obtaining advice or supervision from a more experienced member of the team or a CAMHS liaison worker is the most effective way of addressing these difficulties.

### What do teachers need to know?

#### (a) Education about mental health problems

Surveys suggest teachers want to understand the common presentations of mental health problems in childhood, how they affect children's behaviour, and their impact on learning. They are often uncertain about aetiology and prognosis. Where disorders have a genetic component to their aetiology, teachers often mistakenly believe that this diminishes the potential impact of school-based interventions. They like to understand the distinction between generalized and specific learning difficulties.

Distinguishing disorder from bad behaviour is especially complex, particularly when attempting to differentiate between what a child can't or won't do. This is commonly an issue with hyperactive children whose attention in school is poor.

#### (b) Identification/detection

Teachers benefit from guidance on the detection of disorders, by learning about common symptoms and behavioural phenotypes. They can be helped in this by being aware of groups at risk and by the use of screening instruments designed to be used in school. Commonly used measures include the Conners Teacher Rating scale (CTRS)[4] and the Strengths and difficulties questionnaires.[5]

#### (c) Interventions/treatments teachers can deliver in school

These may include simple counselling interventions, e.g. to address anxiety at exam times or supporting a child during parental separation or after a bereavement. The teacher's role may involve supporting the administration of medication within school (e.g. for hyperactivity). This treatment (and the child's motivation to take it) can be severely undermined if teachers do not support its use.

#### (d) Knowledge/understanding of treatments given by CAMHS

Many myths about child mental health problems and their treatment may be shared by teaching staff. These include the aims, benefits, and likely adverse effects of medication. Some will mistakenly believe, for example that drugs for hyperactivity are sedative and will turn a child into a 'zombie'. Stigmatizing attitudes to inpatient child psychiatry units may impair a child's rehabilitation after admission.

#### (e) Pathways of referral

Schools should be clear about which problems should be referred to which agency. For example, acute self-harm should be referred to the accident and emergency department of a general hospital, whilst child protection issues should be referred to social services.

### Specific issues posing a challenge for schools

A major concern for a school is how to manage disruptive disorders and their impact on other children. A disorder such as Tourette's syndrome will excite younger children and they will be easily distracted. Those whose attention is poor, who are more impulsive or who are low achievers are particularly vulnerable, whilst the subject may find their behaviour reinforced by their unexpected celebrity and status as the 'class clown'.

Appropriate behavioural management can be difficult to institute without it being punitive or unwittingly reinforcing. This applies to conduct problems and for example where teaching staff may offer lunchtime supervision of a child with an eating disorder.

It is often difficult to address minor self-harm sympathetically without reinforcing the behaviour. Similarly the wish to be sympathetic towards those with eating disorders may be tempered by concerns to avoid 'epidemic' dieting.

## The school's role in child protection

Schools in the United Kingdom have a responsibility to safeguard and promote the well-being of pupils under the Education Act of 2002[6] and, where appropriate, under the Children Act 1989.[7] Each school has a designated lead for child protection and if staff have concerns about the safety and well-being of a child they should report their concerns to them. The child protection lead will refer to the school Child Protection Policy and then directly to Children's Social Care services as necessary.

A guidance document 'safeguarding children and safer recruitment in education' was produced in the United Kingdom in 2006[8] and is a consolidated version of earlier guidance material. It focuses on the recruitment and selection processes, vetting checks, and duties for safeguarding and promoting the welfare of children in education. The document also forms a guide to inter-agency working. The guidance explains that a school should 'create and maintain a safe learning environment' and have the appropriate arrangements in place. Child protection arrangements, pupil health and safety, and bullying are all subject to statutory requirements. The guidance directs that if a child is the subject of an inter-agency child protection plan, the school should be involved with the preparation of that plan.

Through the delivery of personal, health, and social education (PHSE) the school may provide opportunities for children and young people to learn about keeping safe. Pupils should be taught to:

◆ Recognize and manage risk in different situations and then decide how to behave responsibly

◆ Judge what kind of physical contact is acceptable and unacceptable

◆ Recognize when pressure from others (including people they know) threatens their personal safety and well-being and develop effective ways of resisting pressure.

## School-based intervention strategies

### Primary prevention

A healthy school promotes physical and emotional health by providing accessible and relevant information and equipping pupils with the skills and attitudes to make informed decisions about their health. It understands the importance of investing in health to assist in raising levels of pupil achievement and improving standards. It also recognizes the need to provide both a physical and social environment that is conducive to learning.

The National Healthy School Standard was part of the Healthy Schools programme, led by the DFES and the Department of Health.[9] Launched in October 1999, it offered support for local programme coordinators and provided an accreditation process for education and health partnerships. It provided a model of partnership working between the health service and schools, with the aim of promoting a coherent and holistic message about the importance of a healthy lifestyle.

The standard covered four key themes:

◆ Personal, Health, and Social Education (PHSE).

◆ Healthy eating

◆ Physical activity

◆ Emotional health and well-being (including bullying)

PHSE is now included in many countries' teaching curricula. This provides education on social and emotional development and citizenship, including the individual's place in society, responsibility, and rights. In The United Kingdom, the PHSE syllabus now has sessions on mental health issues including the use of drugs and alcohol and the links between drug misuse and mental illness. It also covers self-harm and suicidal behaviour.

*Social and Emotional Aspects of Learning—(SEAL)* is a whole-curriculum framework for teaching social, emotional, and behavioural skills to primary school children in five areas: self-awareness, managing feelings, motivation, empathy, and social skills. In 2004, the scheme was piloted in 250 schools in 25 authorities in the United Kingdom with a subsequent planned extension to high schools.

### Secondary prevention

*Solution Oriented Schools (SOS)* is an approach used in many United Kingdom local authorities, comprising training and resources to support the whole-school promotion of positive behaviour. The focus is on establishing small steps that can be taken to resolve conduct problems, attendance issues, poor peer group interactions and negative attitudes to learning.

The approach invites staff to consider: 'What works in school?'. It encourages them to take a pragmatic approach; learning from what is working, leaving behind practice that is failing to pay-off, recognizing 'the problem' as the problem (not the child, teacher, or professional), and building on strengths that each individual brings. It stems from the principles of solution-oriented brief therapy which focuses on finding and creating solutions to a problem whilst spending little time on the problem itself.

*Circle time* was developed in the 1930s particularly for primary schools, as a forum for children to share views and concerns about issues arising in school (such as bullying) or outside (within the family or neighbourhood). It is still widely practised.

### Mobile phone, text, and Internet-based initiatives

A number of education authorities have developed pilot schemes using new technologies such as online counselling and support services. Various websites offer qualified counsellors and other support services. Services are confidential and young people book in for their session of online chat. In addition the young people can often access a Frequently Asked Questions area. Some sites have counsellors who can make referrals to CAMHS for the young people who access them.

Other initiatives include a pilot scheme in Wales in which pupils used mobile phones to text their school nurses for health advice. This short-term project ran in office hours, offered students instant help and provided those who might be wary of approaching adults with their problems face-to-face the chance to do so anonymously.

In Liverpool, *The Health and Education for Life Project (HELP)* was set-up in 2003, as an action research project that worked in schools to change pupils' attitudes towards mental health issues and to provide coping strategies.

## Meeting the needs of children with special educational needs

While most pupils with complex needs are educated in special schools, where the special needs of children can be met by a mainstream school, they are often taught in this setting. Attitudes to inclusion have changed over time. The latest draft guidance in the United Kingdom moves away from the inclusion drive of 2004 and advises councils that they should provide a 'range of provision' for children with special educational needs. The national curriculum requirements may often impact negatively on the experiences of a young person with specific learning needs; the challenge for teachers is to create a stimulating, engaging programme of study whilst still meeting the national requirements. The use of teaching assistants in a creative and well-planned way can facilitate the delivery of lessons in an inclusive setting. Ultimately, the needs of the individual child should be of primary concern in the inclusive–exclusive decision-making process.

Some special schools offer outreach to the mainstream, so that expertise can be shared and support given for inclusive practice. Some local authorities name specialist schools for each area to meet the needs for example, of autistic young people. Where a young person lives too far from the locality of the specialist school; the specialist school may adopt an advisory role.

Special schools attempt to offer a tailored and focussed response to the needs of specific groups of young people; it is arguable that a young person who has for example, high functioning Asperger's syndrome will feel more 'included' in a special school setting where his differences are less noticeable. The social exclusion that such a young person may experience in a mainstream setting can have detrimental effects on their progress. Successful inclusive education relies on a school approach that creates an inclusive culture; develops inclusive policies, and evolves inclusive practices.

Children and young people with emotional and behavioural difficulties (EBD) present a major challenge to schools attempting to become fully inclusive organizations. Through emotional literacy programmes such as SEAL, anger management groups, social skills, and self-esteem groups, schools can offer a variety of behavioural interventions that support an inclusive experience.

*Hospital schools or Medical Pupil Referral Units* offer education to young people who are unable to attend school because of medical needs. The term 'medical needs' includes those with mental illness; anxiety, depression, and school phobia. There is a strong emphasis on a strategic planning framework which ensures a continuum of provision; a focus on close liaison with all parties and the development of a robust reintegration plan.

The role of CAMHS within special education has a higher profile than in many mainstream educational provisions; children should all have statements of special educational need and therefore should be reviewed regularly. The reviews of children with a statement of emotional and social need or with autistic spectrum disorders (ASD) tend to require the involvement of a CAMHS worker; subsequently good relationships are developed through close and regular interactions with educationalists. CAMHS may offer consultation and advice or direct intervention with the child or group of children in a special educational setting.

## The psychiatrist as advisor to higher/further education

Recent years have shown a growing awareness of the unmet needs of students in higher education.[10] Although higher education institutions often have quite sophisticated pastoral and counselling provision in place, they may need to consult with mental health services regarding issues with specific students. The psychiatrist should be aware of the following particular issues in relation to this group:

♦ The vulnerability of young people living away from home for the first time.

♦ Recent expansions in student numbers. In a number of countries, greater training opportunities for young people have resulted in access to higher education no longer being restricted to those from privileged backgrounds. One adverse consequence of this otherwise desirable state of affairs is that those with greater risks (or indeed histories) of mental health problems may take up places at colleges and universities.

♦ Vocational courses. Some courses (such as medicine, nursing, and social work) may restrict those suffering with particular mental health problems. The psychiatrist may have a duty to report such issues as, for example, drug dependence. Related to this a student may be reluctant to disclose a problem which would have implications for continuing on their course.

♦ Interface/communication issues. Young people living away from home at college may be vulnerable to falling into any gap that might exist between child and adult services and between services local to their home and those at their college. Effective communication between service providers is of paramount importance.

♦ Confidentiality. Students are often concerned about confidentiality from their parents, their peers, and their college's academic staff. As with the examples given earlier in this chapter, confidences should only be breached on a strictly 'need to know' basis.

## Conclusions

As participation in education is almost universally compulsory for children, schools are in a unique position to offer prevention and identification of child mental health problems. Effective practice requires good liaison with CAMHS. There are a number of obstacles to effective working but recent times have seen a number of examples of good practice and policies to support these.

## Further information

Royal College of Psychiatrists. (2003). *Mental health of students in higher education. Council report CR112.* Royal College of Psychiatrists, London.
The National Healthy Schools Programme. www.healthyschools.gov.uk
Safeguarding Children. www.everychildmatters.gov.uk

## References

1. Health Advisory Service. (1995). *Together we stand: the commissioning, role and management of child and adolescent mental health services.* HMSO, London.

2. Gowers, S.G., Thomas, S., and Deeley, S.D. (2004). Can primary schools provide effective Tier 1 child mental health services? *Journal of Clinical Child Psychology and Psychiatry*, **9**(3), 419–25.

3. The National Healthy Schools Programme. www.healthyschools.gov.uk

4. Conners, C.K. (1973). Rating scales for use in drug studies with children [Special issue/Pharmacotherapy of Children]. *Psychopharmacology Bulletin*, **9**, 24–9.

5. Goodman, R. (2001). Psychometric properties of the strengths and difficulties questionnaire (SDQ). *Journal of the American Academy of Child and Adolescent Psychiatry*, **40**, 1337–45.

6. Department for Education. (2002). *Education Act*. HMSO, London.

7. Department of Health. (1991). *Children Act 1989; guidance and regulations*. Department of Health, London.

8. Safeguarding Children. www.everychildmatters.gov.uk

9. National Healthy Schools Standard. http://www.standards.dfes.gov.uk

10. Royal College of Psychiatrists. (2003). *The mental health of students in higher education. Council report CR112*. Royal College of Psychiatrists, London.

# SECTION 10

# Intellectual Disability (Mental Retardation)

**10.1 Classification, diagnosis, psychiatric assessment, and needs assessment** *1819*
A. J. Holland

**10.2 Prevalence of intellectual disabilities and epidemiology of mental ill-health in adults with intellectual disabilities** *1825*
Sally-Ann Cooper and Elita Smiley

**10.3 Aetiology of intellectual disability: general issues and prevention** *1830*
Markus Kaski

**10.4 Syndromes causing intellectual disability** *1838*
David M. Clarke and Shoumitro Deb

**10.5 Psychiatric and behaviour disorders among mentally retarded people** *1849*

10.5.1 Psychiatric and behaviour disorders among children and adolescents with intellectual disability *1849*
Bruce J. Tonge

10.5.2 Psychiatric and behaviour disorders among adult persons with intellectual disability *1854*
Anton Došen

10.5.3 Epilepsy and epilepsy-related behaviour disorders among people with intellectual disability *1860*
Matti Iivanainen

**10.6 Methods of treatment** *1871*
T. P. Berney

**10.7 Special needs of adolescents and elderly people with intellectual disability** *1878*
Jane Hubert and Sheila Hollins

**10.8 Families with a member with intellectual disability and their needs** *1883*
Ann Gath and Jane McCarthy

**10.9 The planning and provision of psychiatric services for adults with intellectual disability** *1887*
Nick Bouras and Geraldine Holt

# Classification, diagnosis, psychiatric assessment, and needs assessment

## A. J. Holland

## Introduction

The general principles developed during the latter part of the twentieth century and continued into the twenty-first century guiding support for people with intellectual disabilities remain those of social inclusion and the provision of services to enable people to make, as far is possible, their own choices and to participate as full citizens in society. These are articulated in national policy documents, such as the White Paper for England, 'Valuing people[1] and also at an international level in the UN Declaration on the rights of people with disability.[2] However, given that people with intellectual disabilities represent a highly complex and heterogenous group with very varied needs, in order for such objectives to be achieved, a range of community based support and interagency and interdisciplinary collaboration is required. It is acknowledged that people with intellectual disabilities experience considerable health inequalities with the presence of additional disabilities due to the presence of physical and sensory impairments and co-morbid physical and mental ill-health, much of which goes unrecognized, and also the occurrence of behaviours that impact on their lives and the lives of those supporting them.[3,4,5] In the twenty-first century, few would now challenge the objectives of social inclusion and community support. The tasks for Government and society are to provide special educational support in childhood and also support to the families of children with intellectual disabilities, and the necessary range of services to meet the social and health needs of this diverse group of people in their adult life. This includes enabling adults with intellectual disabilities to gain meaningful support or full employment and to exercise their rights as citizens and to participate fully in society. To achieve such objectives there is a need to be able to characterize the nature and level of need, to establish the presence and significance of co-morbid illnesses and/ or challenging behaviours, and to organize and provide support and services to meet such identified needs.

This complexity of need has meant that no single 'label', such as 'intellectual disability', can adequately describe this group of people.

What individuals have in common is a difficulty in the acquisition of basic living, educational, and social skills that is apparent early in life, together with evidence of a significant intellectual impairment. However, for some this may be of such severity that, for example, meaningful language is never acquired and there are very substantial care needs. For others, there is the presence of subtle signs of early developmental delay, and evidence of learning difficulties that only becomes clearly apparent at school when there is an expectation that more sophisticated skills will be acquired. The nature and extent of disability and of any functional impairments in general, distinguishing those people with intellectual disabilities from those with specific learning difficulties, such as dyslexia.

In infancy and early childhood, the reason for any apparent developmental delay needs to be established. This is primarily the responsibility of paediatric and clinical genetic services. Such information helps parents understand the reasons for their child's difficulties and may guide, in a limited way, an understanding of future needs and potential risks. Later in childhood, the nature and extent of a child's learning difficulties and a statement of special educational needs is the main task and later still, the main focus may be the assessment of longer-term social care needs. Throughout life, there may also be questions about a child's or adult's behaviour or mental state or the nature and extent of physical or sensory impairments and disabilities. The role of assessment is essentially to determine need and to inform the types of intervention and treatments, whether educational, medical, psychological, or social, which are likely to be effective and of benefit to the person concerned. Systems of classification provide useful frameworks for such assessments.

## Classification

The term 'classification' is unfortunate as it carries with it the stigma associated with previous legislation (e.g. Mental Deficiency Act, 1913) and the associated history of institutionalization consequent upon the eugenics movement at the beginning of the twentieth century.

However, systems of classification are an important way of organizing information and thereby enabling the reliable passing of that information to others and providing a framework to guide intervention. Whilst there are clear strengths to this process, any system of classification has serious limitations. It will tend to focus on a few particular characteristics to the potential exclusion of others, and none can impart a truly comprehensive picture. Methods of classification have inevitably changed over time in an attempt to better clarify the key issues and to minimize stigma that might be associated with any given label. However, the central principle of any system of classification is to bring order to knowledge in a manner that may then enable further advances or the instigation of interventions that previous research has shown to be effective. There is no single universal system—the system of classification used depends on the reasons for its use. These may be as diverse as being predominately administrative or for the purposes of guiding intervention and the use or not of specific treatments.

Classification systems also differ with respect to whether they are dimensional or categorical in nature. Intellectual disability illustrates this difference in that measures such as those obtained from IQ tests are clearly dimensional and continuous whereas labels such as 'intellectual disability' or the identification of particular syndromes are categorical. More recently such obvious categorical distinctions have begun to break down as the genetic basis for syndromes are more clearly elucidated. For example, in fragile X syndrome there is variation in the extent of the number of repeat sequences in the FMR-1 mutation, both within carrier and affected individuals that influence whether or not an intellectual disability is likely to be present.[6] Various different systems of classification are examined below and the relationship between assessment and classification is considered.

## Mental retardation (DSM-IV)

From January 1st 2007, the previously named American Association on Mental Retardation changed its name, replacing 'mental retardation' with the term 'intellectual and developmental disabilities'. This followed similar changes in other organizations. However, in DSM-IV[7] the term 'mental retardation' remains for the moment. This standard diagnostic system provides a framework for multiaxial diagnosis with Axis II for personality disorders and mental retardation. Table 10.1.1 summarizes the DSM-IV criteria for mental retardation. The focus is not primarily one of aetiology but rather of quantifying the extent of 'mental retardation' through defining the level of intellectual impairment and listing the range of possible adaptive functions that might be impaired. The definition makes explicit that the onset is in the developmental period and that mental retardation is the final common pathway of a number of potential aetiologies. Significant sub-average intellectual function is defined as an IQ of 70 or below (using standard IQ tests). The IQ is also used to help determine the level of mental retardation (mild, moderate, severe, or profound).

The use of such a multi-axial system recognizes the fact that intellectual disability is a disorder of development, which is separate from other mental disorders, such as mental illness (Axis I), general medical conditions (Axis III), and which may be associated with particular psychosocial and environmental problems (Axis IV). Thus, the process of formulation requires that all these broad domains be considered in arriving at an understanding of an individual's particular difficulties.

## International Classification of Functioning, Disability and Health (ICF)

In 2001, the World Health Organization published the International Classification of Functioning, Disabilities and Health (ICF).[8] This is a complete revision of the International Classification of Impairments, Disabilities, and Handicaps.[9] The latter classification was an advance at that time in that it had attempted to overcome the limitations of other methods of classification (particularly with respect to chronic disability) and, most importantly, aimed to guide intervention at several levels and in a more holistic manner than classification systems that were primarily focused on diagnosis, had been able to do. In this context, intellectual disabilities could be conceptualized at different levels. In the case of impairment, the organ system involved is that of the central nervous system. It is the impairment of this system for genetic, chromosomal, or environmental reasons that have primarily affected the acquisition of developmentally determined skills and the ability to learn. The associated disability is the effect of the impairment on a person's ability to learn and acquire new skills that come with development. The exact nature and extent of the disability may not only include the impact of an intellectual disability but also physical and sensory disabilities. The extent to which a given

**Table 10.1.1** Summary of the diagnostic criteria for mental retardation (DSM-IV)

A. Significant subaverage general intelligence
B. Significant limitations in adaptive functioning in at least two of the following:
  Communication
  Self-care
  Home living
  Social/interpersonal skills
  Use of community resources
  Self-direction
  Functional academic skills
  Work
  Leisure
  Health
  Safety
C. Onset before age 18 years of age

*Note*

- Significant subaverage intellectual functioning is defined as an IQ of about 70 or below. The choice of testing instrument should take into account the individual's socio-economic background, native language, and other associated handicaps
- Adaptive functioning refers to how effectively individuals cope with common life demands and how well they meet the standards of personal independence expected of someone in their particular age group, sociocultural background, and community setting. Adaptive behaviour may be influenced by individual and/or environmental factors including the presence or not of additional mental or physical disorders. Information on adaptive behaviour should be gathered from one or more independent sources
- The degree of severity of mental retardation may be specified on the basis of intellectual impairment taking into account other aspects of functioning
  Mild mental retardation: IQ level 50–55 to approximately 70
  Moderate mental retardation: IQ level 35–40 to 50–55
  Severe mental retardation: IQ level 20–25 to 35–40
  Profound mental retardation: IQ level below 20 or 25

impairment results in a loss of function (disability) may well be influenced by the extent and nature of interventions such as special education, or the correction of hearing loss through the use of a hearing aid. The final level, that of 'handicap', is a consequence of an interaction between the disability and the extent to which support is available or environmental adjustments made. It is a measure of disadvantage that can be ameliorated through, for example, the presence of carers to enable individuals to go out, or environmental modifications (e.g. wheelchair ramps) that diminish the impact of physical disabilities.

The ICF attempts to take classification further and to conceptualize 'disability' within the context of society as a whole, recognizing that everyone can experience disability at one time or other—the stated aim of the ICF is to 'mainstream the experience of disability and recognize it as a universal human experience'. The intent is to encourage those using the ICF to take into account more fully the social aspects of dysfunction and not to see disability as only a medical or biologically determined dysfunction. This means of classification aims to enable the recording of the environmental effects on an individual's functioning. The ICF itself is divided into two Parts. Part 1 is concerned with 'Functioning and Disability' and Part 2 is concerned with 'Contextual Factors'. Each of the two components are expressed in both positive and negative terms in order to emphasize what a person is able to do as well as what he/she is not able to do. The ICF is more complex and more comprehensive than the 1980 WHO system of classification attempting to provide a conceptual framework that forces a much wider understanding by bringing together more comprehensively social and biological models of disability. In doing so, it does what a sound formulation should do, moving from the limitations of a diagnosis to an understanding of the individual within a biological, social and environmental context. This is illustrated in the diagram in Fig. 10.1.1 taken from the ICF.

As with the 1980 'Impairments, Disabilities and Handicaps' means of classification, the ICF is seen as complementing other WHO classification systems, such as the ICD-10.[10] The ICD-10 is focused on disease and the ICF on 'components of health'. The latter, in doing so, provides an appropriate means for characterizing need and for ensuring that people with chronic disabilities have such needs met in the context of their individual human rights and also based on rights established through national legislation. However, as knowledge has increased, for example, about the nature and extent of physical and psychiatric co-morbidity affecting people with intellectual disabilities, so then has the need to use different and other relevant systems of classification increased.

Such different approaches provide the necessary frameworks for a rigorous and comprehensive formulation of a person's needs and to guide treatment of any identified co-morbid illness.

## Assessment

Assessment is a task that is undertaken to address specific questions and is informed by the relevant theoretical knowledge and conceptual framework. The type of assessment undertaken therefore, depends on the issue in question and in turn, on both the relevant theoretical background and the appropriate systems of classification, where they are required. The above systems of classification provide a broad framework for considering need. However, in the field of intellectual disabilities a truly holistic assessment will frequently require different theoretical perspectives because of the variability in and complexity of need. The precise form of any focussed assessment will depend on the reasons for undertaking the assessment. The nature of the assessment will vary considerably if it is primarily to determine a person's social care needs, as opposed to the reasons for a particular problematic behaviour. Even with the context of challenging behaviour, the assessments undertaken will vary. Increasingly, the skills expected of those working in community teams supporting people with intellectual disabilities is to be able to recognize what assessments are relevant and required and to be able to undertake such assessments in the community setting where the person with intellectual disability lives. For the sake of clarity, a distinction is made below between those assessments that are fundamentally directed at characterizing the persons, intellectual disability and those whose main focus is on psychiatric and behavioural aspects.

## Intellectual disability, its characterization and causes

The term intellectual disability is not in itself a diagnosis as it does not inform in any reliable way about aetiology, prognosis, or specific treatments. Rather, it refers to a clinical state that is developmental in origin and affects intellectual and social functioning. The diagnosis is the identification of the underlying cause for the observed developmental delay. The extent of early developmental delay can be measured against standardized developmental scales (e.g. Bayley or Griffiths Developmental Scales), and during childhood and adult life. There are also well-established specific assessments of intellectual, language, and functional abilities. These assessments provide a profile of a person or group of people that can be compared against the norms for age and a given population. Adaptive functioning has to be measured against what would be expected for a person of that age, and the social and cultural experiences of the person have to be taken into account. The Wechsler Scales for IQ, and the Vineland Adaptive Behaviour Scales[11] or the revised Adaptive Behaviour Scales of the American Association for Intellectual and Developmental Disabilities[12] for characterizing functioning are established instruments for the measurements of these abilities and for which there are normative data for comparison.

Possible single major causes for an intellectual disability are covered in more detail in a separate chapter and are mainly the province of paediatrics or clinical genetics. However, where there is clear evidence for developmental delay in childhood and for the person having an intellectual disability and no obvious cause has been previously established, further investigation is indicated. This will be informed by the clinical history and by physical

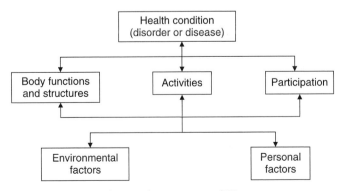

**Fig. 10.1.1** Interactions between the components of ICF.

examination (e.g. presence of a family history of similar disorder or not, evidence of the physical characteristics of a particular syndrome). As part of this process, the developmental history should also establish whether the developmental profile is not only characteristic of an intellectual disability but also whether the person meets criteria for having an autistic spectrum condition. This is important because of the high rates of autism within the population of people with intellectual disability and the implications such a diagnosis may have for the type of support.[13] Particularly where the person has evidence of dysmorphic physical characteristics, a moderate, severe or profound intellectual disability, and/or a family history of disability, chromosomal, biochemical, and/or molecular genetic studies may be indicated. With improving knowledge about the developmental differences and the different predispositions to specific co-morbidities that exist between genetically determined syndromes, establishing the cause of a person's intellectual disability is becoming increasingly important and may help inform psychiatric and psychological assessments.[14]

### (a) Assessments of index problem and psychiatric diagnosis

There have been significant advances in the conceptual models used to help understand the occurrence and maintenance of problem behaviours or abnormal mental states in people with intellectual disabilities. The following four approaches are particularly relevant and each of these perspectives needs to be considered in any assessment. First, applied behavioural analytical studies have demonstrated how the occurrence of behaviours, such as self-injurious behaviour, can be shaped in the context of particular environmental or individual setting conditions.[15] This approach attempts to identify the 'functions' of behaviours. Specific behaviour (e.g. self-injurious behaviour, aggressive outbursts etc.) may, for example, be identified as being attention-maintained or demand avoidant. Secondly, some behaviours may be a consequence of arrested development. In such cases the behaviour itself (e.g. repetitive checking) may be similar to that which occurs as part of typical childhood development but it has continued into adult life. Thirdly, the behaviours may be a manifestation of co-morbid physical or psychiatric disorder. For example, as a consequence of increasing irritability and agitation associated with depression[16] or consequent upon pain or some other physical distress. Fourthly, the abnormal mental state or behaviour may be associated with the cause of the person's developmental disability. This is increasing referred to as 'the behavioural phenotype' of a particular syndrome.[14] These different models of understanding are not necessarily mutually exclusive. For example, the behaviours and psychiatric problems that commonly affect people with Prader Willi syndrome includes examples of each of the above. The increased propensity to temper outbursts and to repetitive and ritualistic behaviours are likely to be partly a consequence of arrested development and to be partly re-inforced and modified depending on environmental contingencies, the over-eating behaviour is a direct consequence of the syndrome and, if obesity is not prevented, it can lead to physical illness that may present with changes in behaviour (e.g. sleep disorders), and those with one genetic form of the syndrome have a high risk for developing co-morbid affective psychotic illness.[17,18] In case of each of these examples, rather different approaches will be required, varying from environmental change to the possible prescription of medication to treat co-morbid psychiatric illness. Assessments should therefore be informed by

these different theoretical perspectives recognizing that similar 'behaviours' may have different aetiologies and that what predisposes to, precipitates, or maintains a particular behaviour and/or mental state may each be different. The challenge of assessment is to identify the developmental, biological, psychological, and social factors that relevant and the treatment/management implications.

In psychiatric practice, the referrals and the assessments are usually to determine the reasons for the occurrence of a particular maladaptive/challenging behaviour and/or apparent change in mental state or in cognitive and functional ability. The focus of the assessment is therefore to address these issues but, in doing so, it invariably requires an assessment of the developmental profile of the person concerned and consideration of the cause of any such disability. In principle, however, the psychiatric assessment of people with intellectual disability is not dissimilar to that undertaken in general child or adult psychiatry. The main differences are as follows:

1 Special care may have to be taken in assessing an individual's mental and cognitive state and whether this has changed over time and, where language development is impaired, a greater reliance may have to be placed on information from an informant;

2 a good developmental history is essential to map early development and the potential developmental origins of the individual's present state;

3 it is important to investigate the enabling and constraining aspects of a person's environment that facilitate or impinge on a person's life and thereby how environmental change might bring real benefit;

4 the possibility of multiple physical and mental health problems and the potential for complex interactions between the individual and his or her carers and the immediate and distant environment should be appreciated.

5 where co-morbidity is a possibility, evidence of a change in physical and mental state or behaviour or an exaggeration of previous states (e.g. obsessional behaviours) that might be indicative of the development of a physical or psychiatric illness must be enquired about. The development of physical illness may also manifest as behavioural change.

Psychiatric assessment is therefore invariably an iterative process, especially so with the uncertainties associated with the assessment of a person with an intellectual disability and the different conceptual models. In undertaking an assessment it can be helpful to draw a distinction between:

1 the characterization of the nature and extent of the person's intellectual disability and the identification of its aetiology;

2 the identification of the onset, nature and extent of additional problem behaviours or abnormal mental states;

3 the determination of the possible aetiological factors of the person's behaviour, such as whether there is a co-morbid psychiatric diagnosis or whether there are particular factors that might have predisposed to, precipitated and are now maintaining a particular behaviour or abnormal mental state.

A detailed history taking from both the person him- or herself and an informant covering both childhood development and the presenting problem, a mental state examination and where indicated a physical examination, direct observation, and often detailed record keeping of particular behaviours (depending on the reason for referral) by care staff over time are the key components of a comprehensive assessment. Where referrals are about the occurrence of problem behaviours, the assessments should include a description of the behaviour as well as an attempt to identify those factors that might increase or decrease the likelihood of the behaviour occurring. These will include the identification of those factors affecting the person him- or herself and those that are particular to the environment. Specifically from a psychiatric perspective, this includes the identification of psychiatric or physical illnesses, the relationship of the index behaviour to any change in mental state or, for example, the occurrence of seizures, as well as the possible contribution of the developmental disability to the problem. For example, the presence of autism may account for observed ritualistic and obsessional behaviours and might also help to make sense of a person's aggressive outbursts that staff observation and record keeping over time has shown occurs at times of unexpected change in routine or activity. Knowledge about the chronicity of a particular behaviour might influence the understanding of the likely contributory factors that give rise to that behaviour. If the behaviour is of recent onset then the role of recent life events or the possibility that the person has developed a mental or physical illness should be investigated. However, if the behaviour has been present since early childhood, psychological models of understanding may be more relevant.

In terms of assessment instruments, a clear distinction needs to be drawn between those that are essentially descriptive in nature and those that are investigating the potential aetiology of the index behaviour. The former include, for example, the Aberrant Behaviour Checklist[19] and the latter, which are based on particular theoretical models, may include, for example, the Psychiatric Assessment Schedule for Adults with Developmental Disorders[20] (a structured assessment of mental state) and the Motivational Assessment Scale[15] (a structured assessment of the possible 'functions' of particular behaviours).

### Mental state examination

Central to the practice of psychiatry in particular is the identification of specific mental phenomena that, when clustered together, are indicative of a specific psychiatric disorder. The gold standard for diagnoses are the diagnostic manuals ICD-10 and DSM-IV. Diagnostic criteria have also been modified to better fit what is observed when assessing people with intellectual disabilities. These have been based on the ICD-10, (DC-LD).[21] The process is two-staged and includes first a detailed history and mental state examination that establishes whether there has been a change in a person's mental state and if so, the characteristics of the change, and secondly, a comparison of these changes against diagnostic criteria to establish the presence or not of specific psychiatric disorders. Investigations may be necessary where there is uncertainty or other possible causes for what is observed need to be ruled out as part of the differential diagnosis.

For people with intellectual disabilities with spoken language, disorders such as schizophrenia present in similar ways to the general population, with the onset of the characteristic mental phenomena. [22] Similarly, disorders such as Alzheimer's disease can be diagnosed using very similar criteria, although the early features may be different.[23] In each of these examples, greater emphasis may have to be placed on informant observation, as some people with intellectual disabilities may have difficulty with concepts such as mood and with being able to describe the presence or not of abnormal mental phenomena.

The key to mental state examination and psychiatric diagnosis in people with intellectual disabilities is to be able to characterize the nature of any observed change. The assessment of mood, sleep, appetite, and concentration may be relatively easy as carers observe increasing distress, tearfulness, and agitation over time in the context of sleep and appetite changes, therefore giving rise to the suspicion of the presence of an affective disorder. Similarly, carers may observe personality and memory changes suggestive of dementia. The presence of hallucinations or delusions may have to be inferred by the development of odd behaviour that might reasonably be interpreted as responses to abnormal mental experiences, such as appearing to respond to auditory hallucinations. Family or other carers who have known the person for some time may well be able to describe more subtle mental state abnormalities such as a deterioration in a person's ability to express his or her thoughts indicating the possibility of thought disorder, or increasing perplexity or evidence of paranoid ideas. The interpretation of cognitive findings is more difficult because of the pre-existing intellectual impairments, but clear documentation of cognitive abilities is important as further deterioration or evidence of improvement over time can be very informative.

### Needs assessment

A full needs assessment brings together the identified social, emotional, and health needs of an individual, including an understanding of the wishes of the person and views of other people who are concerned for and involved in the support and care of that individual. This whole process has, over the last few years in both mental health and intellectual disability services, become more formalized through 'needs-led assessments' and sometimes through the 'care programme approach'. Person-centred planning is the process by which this information is brought together in a manner that directs the allocation of support and any necessary treatment interventions.[24]

Social services are in general responsible for undertaking assessments at key transitions (e.g. prior to the end of statutory education) or if there is evidence that need has changed. If the person lacks the capacity to express his or her view then the question of what is in the person's best interests should be determined. The balance that this process is attempting to achieve is to respect the wishes of the person concerned and to balance an adult's right to autonomy, on the one hand, versus the need for care and support, on the other. More recently, the critical importance of assessing a person's ability to make decisions about his or her own life and the pivotal role of a person's 'decision-making capacity' in achieving the correct balance between the respect for autonomy and the need for care and support has received more attention. Legislation has been enacted first in Scotland and more recently in England and Wales that provides the framework for intervention where the person concerned lacks the capacity to make the relevant decision for him/herself. The assessment of a person's decision-making capacity requires an evaluation of a person's ability to understand and use information relevant to the decision, retain and balance the necessary information and then to communicate a choice.[25]

Although there is clearly an overlap, it can be helpful to distinguish between social care, educational, and health-care needs. In the case of children, the need for special education and for family support are likely to be central, depending on the extent of the disability and any other associated disabilities. For adults, accommodation with an appropriate level of support, meaningful daytime occupation, and companionship and practical help according to need will be key. Systematic assessments provide a structured way to determine whether a low, medium, or high service environment will best meet an individual's needs. The types and range of services that need to be provided are covered in other chapters. Health-care needs will include the same as those of the general population but high rates of physical and sensory impairments, mental health and behavioural problems, and impairment in communication are all likely to give rise to additional needs. Particularly for those people with more severe intellectual disabilities and limited and/or no language, there is also a clear responsibility for carers to ensure a healthy lifestyle, health screening, and to help identify health-related problems when they do occur. Special help may be required to ensure access to both primary and secondary health-care services and to ensure the person understands what is happening to them. This will include questions of consent to health treatment and how a person with intellectual disabilities can be best helped to give maximally informed consent or at least be able to assent when it is in his or her best interests to do so. A structured process of assessment, paying attention to the cause of the intellectual disability and its associated problems and the extent and nature of other impairments, disabilities, and handicaps will minimize the risk that health-related problems might go unnoticed or that social care needs might be ignored.

## Further information

Emerson, E. (2001). *Challenging Behaviour: Analysis and intervention in people with severe intellectual disabilities.* Cambridge University Press, Cambridge.

Bouras, N. and Holt, G (eds.). (2007). *Psychiatric and Behavioural Disorders in Intellectual and Developmental Disabilities.* Cambridge University Press, Cambridge.

## References

1. Department of Health. *Valuing People: a new strategy for the 21st Century,* Department of Health, London
2. United Nations. (2007). *Convention on the Rights of People with Disabilities.*
3. Beange, H., McElduff, A., and Baker, W. (1995). Medical disorders of adults with mental retardation: a population study. *American Journal of Mental Retardation,* **99**, 595–604.
4. Cooper S.A., Smiley E., Morrison J., *et al.* (2007). Mental ill-health in adults with intellectual disabilities: prevalence and associated factors. *British Journal of Psychiatry,* **190**, 27–35.
5. Lowe, K., Allen, D., Jones, E., *et al.* (2007). Challenging behaviours: prevalence and topographies. *Journal of Intellectual Disabilities Research,* **51**, 625–36.
6. Verkerk, A., Pieretti, M., Sutcliffe, J.S., *et al.* (1991) Identification of a gene (FMR–1) containing a CGG repeat coincident with a breakpoint cluster region exhibiting length variation in fragile X syndrome. *Cell,* **65**, 905–14.
7. American Psychiatric Association (1994). *Diagnostic and statistical classification of diseases and related health problems* (4th edn). American Psychiatric Association, Washington, DC.
8. World Health Organization (2001). *International Classification of Functioning, Disability and Health (ICF).* World Health Organization, Geneva.
9. World Health Organization (1980). *International classification of impairments, disabilities and handicaps* (10th revision). World Health Organization, Geneva.
10. World Health Organization (1992). *International statistical classification of diseases and related health problems,* (10th revision). WHO, Geneva.
11. Sparrow, S., Ball, D., and Cicchetti, D. (1984). *Vineland Adaptive Behaviour Scale* (Interview Edition–Survey Version). American Guidance Association, Circle Pines, MN.
12. Nihara, K., Leland, H., and Lambert, N. (1993). *Adaptive Behavior Scales–Residential and Community* (2nd edn). Pro–Ed, Austin, TX.
13. Shah, A., Holmes, N., and Wing, L. (1982). Prevalence of autism and related conditions in adults in a mental handicap hospital. *Applied Research in Mental Retardation,* **3**, 303–17.
14. Editorial by Oliver, J..and Hagerman, R. (2007) Trends and challenges in behavioural phenotypes. *JIDR,* **51**, 649–52
15. Durrand, V.M. and Crimmins, D.B. (1988). Identifying the variables maintaining self-injurious behaviour. *Journal of Autism and Developmental Disorders,* **18**, 99–117.
16. Meins, W. (1995). 'Symptoms of major depression in mentally retarded adults' *Journal of Intellectual Disability Research,* **39**, 41–46.
17. Holland, A.J., Whittington, J.E. Butler, J., Webb, T., Boer, H and Clarke, D.J. (2003) Behavioural phenotypes associated with specific genetic disorders: evidence from a population-based study of people with Prader-Willi Syndrome. *Psychological Medicine,* **33**, 141–53
18. Boer, H., Holland, A.J., Whittington, J., Butler, J., Webb, T. and Clarke, D. (2002) Psychotic illness in people with Prader Willi Syndrome due to chromosome 15 maternal uniparental disomy *The Lancet,* **359**, 135–36.
19. Aman, M., *et al.* (1985). The Aberrant Behavior Checklist: a behavior rating scale for the assessment of treatment effects. *American Journal of Mental Deficiency,* **89**, 485–91.
20. Moss, S.C., *et al.* (1993). Psychiatric morbidity in older people with moderate and severe learning disability (mental retardation). Part 1: Developmental and reliability of the patient interview (the PAS-ADD). *British Journal of Psychiatry,* **163**, 471–80.
21. Cooper, S.-A., C. Melville, *et al.* (2003). 'Psychiatric diagnosis, intellectual disabilities and diagnostic criteria for psychiatric disorders for use with adults with learning disabilities/mental retardation (DC-LD)'. *Journal of Intellectual Disability Research,* **47**, 3–15.
22. Meadows, G., Turner, T., Campbell, L., *et al.* (1991). Assessing schizophrenia in adults with mental retardation. A comparative study. *British Journal of Psychiatry,* **158**, 103–5.
23. Ball, S.L., Holland, A.J., Huppert, F.A., *et al.* (2004).The modified CAMDEX informant interview is a valid and reliable tool for use in the diagnosis of dementia in adults with Down's syndrome. *Journal of Intellectual Disability Research,* **48**(6), 611–20.
24. Robertson, J., Emerson, E., Hatton, C. *et al.* (2007). Person-centred planning: factors associated with successful outcomes for people with intellectual disabilities. *Journal of Intellectual Disability Research,* **51**, 232–43.
25. Wong, J.G., Clare, I.C.H., Gunn, M.J., *et al.* (1999). Capacity to make health care decisions: Its importance in clinical practice. *Psychological Medicine,* **29** (2): 437–46.

# Prevalence of intellectual disabilities and epidemiology of mental ill-health in adults with intellectual disabilities

Sally-Ann Cooper and Elita Smiley

## Prevalence of intellectual disabilities

If intelligence quotient (IQ) was normally distributed in the population, with a mean of 100 and standard deviation of 15, then about 2 per cent of the population would have an IQ below 70. However, reported rates vary widely depending on the definition of intellectual disabilities used, the country and region of study, the time of the study, the age range and ethnicity of the population, and the method of population ascertainment.[1-3]

### Definition

ICD-10 and DSM-IV-TR definitions of intellectual disabilities are similar:

◆ significantly sub-average intellectual functioning (IQ below approximately 70; mental age less than 12 years);

◆ concurrent impairments in present adaptive functioning; diminished ability to adapt to the daily demands of the social environment;

◆ onset before the age of 18 years.

IQ is a continuous measure, so when basing a definition of intellectual disabilities upon it the threshold is arbitrary, and changes in threshold can have a large impact on prevalence. For example, in the past the American Association on Intellectual and Developmental Disabilities' criteria had an IQ threshold of 84. This was subsequently changed to 70 in 1973, and then to 70–75 in 1992. ICD-10 and DSM-IV-TR definitions are not statistical constructions; the requirement of impaired adaptive functioning may half estimated prevalence rates compared with a statistical definition. Furthermore, different methods to assess intelligence and adaptive behaviour can lead to different prevalence rates.

### Country and region

Prevalence of intellectual disabilities is reported to be much higher in developing than developed countries, due to socio-economic factors, although mild intellectual disabilities may possibly be less disadvantaging in non-literate societies. Iodine deficiency is the most common preventable cause of intellectual disabilities worldwide, and is indigenous in some regions of Asia and Africa. Exposure of populations to heavy metals and toxins can lower the average population IQ by a few points, hence some people who would otherwise have had low-average ability move into the intellectual disabilities range. Regions with a high level of consanguineous marriages can also have higher prevalence. For example, Tay-Sachs disease is prevalent amongst Ashkenazi communities, although premarital genetic counselling has markedly reduced it in the United States. The availability and sophistication of antenatal, perinatal, and neonatal care account for some differences between countries. Some studies show differences in ethnic groups, although the cultural suitability of the measures used may have contributed to these findings.

### Time

Prevalence varies with time, due to preventative measures, and social developments. In developed countries, an increase in prevalence was seen in the early 1960s, with falling prevalence thereafter, due to developments in neonatal care with increasing survival of very low birth weight infants. Down syndrome is the most common chromosomal disorder causing intellectual disabilities, and survival rates of neonates and children with Down syndrome have increased substantially in recent decades, primarily due to access to surgery for congenital heart disease. The widespread introduction of antenatal screening for Down syndrome might have been expected to reduce the population prevalence of Down syndrome through lowering birth rate, but rising maternal age at birth, and increasing life expectation counter this, and there appears to be little change in the population prevalence. The widespread introduction of antenatal screening for phenylketonuria in the 1960s, and congenital hypothyroidism in the 1970s has virtually eliminated intellectual disabilities due to these conditions in developed countries. Better living conditions, with individualized packages of support, and a political agenda for social justice and equality of access to health care and supports may all have contributed to the increasing life expectation for people with intellectual disabilities, although this is still lower than that of the general population. Increasing maternal age and increasing maternal alcohol consumption are expected to lead to higher birth rate of infants with foetal alcohol syndrome, and genetic causes of intellectual disabilities. Overall, there appears to have been little change in prevalence compared with 50 years ago.

## Age

Prevalence is higher in child than adult cohorts, and lower in older than younger adult cohorts, with the highest prevalence at around age 10 years. This is due to intellectual disabilities having been identified by this age, combined with an earlier age of death for persons with intellectual disabilities compared with the general population. Children with the mildest intellectual disabilities are likely to benefit from additional support for learning at school, but will develop skills and experience over time, such that some no longer meet criteria for intellectual disabilities in adulthood.

## Ascertainment

Reported prevalence varies with the methods of population ascertainment. For children, the ascertained prevalence doubled compared with case registers, when record linkage to education department data on educational attainments was included (giving an estimated prevalence of 1.4 per cent).[3] There was a disproportional increase in indigenous Australian children, who were possibly false positives. For adult populations, only a proportion with intellectual disabilities will be in contact with specialist health services for adults with intellectual disabilities. Ascertainment is higher when data is combined from primary health care, specialist health services, and social services, if the provision of day opportunities, supported work, respite care, funded support packages, and direct payments is considered. This is likely to identify almost all persons with moderate to profound intellectual disabilities, and adults with mild learning disabilities receiving support; it will not identify adults with IQ below 70 who no longer have impaired adaptive functioning (who therefore do not meet ICD-10 or DSM-IV-TR criteria for intellectual disabilities) and do not need support, or some people who receive all their support exclusively from unpaid carers. The assessment of IQ (culturally sensitive), adaptive functioning and support needs, plus medical assessment, of all individuals within a whole population or a representative sample would provide accurate prevalence data for that time point and area. However, this would be a substantial undertaking, in view of the tens or hundreds of thousands of participants required.

## Prevalence

There have been many studies of prevalence of intellectual disabilities. For the reasons above, there is substantial variation in reported prevalence in developed countries, varying from 2 to 85/1000 general population, and there are few robust studies in developing countries. Less variability is found between studies of moderate to profound intellectual disabilities. Given the variation, it is inappropriate to provide average figures from across the studies. Interpreting the literature, we suggest that prevalence of intellectual disabilities in the United Kingdom may be in the order of 9–14/1000

childhood population, and 3–8/1000 adult population, varying with time and geography. However, it should be noted that the figure of 2 per cent is frequently assumed. Intellectual disabilities are more prevalent in males than females, particularly amongst children, young- and middle-aged adults: the reported ratio varies between 1:1 and 2:1. At older age, the gender ratio equalizes due to greater life expectancy of women compared with men (mirroring the general population), and at extreme old age, women may even outnumber men. The distribution of level of intellectual disabilities varies with age, due to the shorter life expectancy of people with more severe intellectual disabilities. Mild intellectual disabilities are associated with socio-economic status. These issues are explored in greater depth elsewhere.[1,2]

# Prevalence and incidence of adult mental ill-health

Some genetic causes of intellectual disabilities have specific behavioural phenotypes. For example, Down syndrome confers protection from mania, and problem behaviours, whilst increasing risk for dementia, Prader Willi syndrome is associated with affective psychosis, and velo-cardio-facial syndrome increases risk for psychosis. Behavioural phenotypes are considered in greater depth in Chapter 10.4. In this section we consider mental ill-health of adults with intellectual disabilities of all causes.

## Study methodologies

Mental ill-health is thought to be commonly experienced by adults with intellectual disabilities. Many of the existing prevalence studies have methodological limitations, accounting for the wide discrepancy in reported prevalence which ranges from 7 to 97 per cent. Limitations have included biased sampling; reliance upon existing case-note information, or instruments designed as screening tools only; lack of information on the extent of detail within assessments, the instruments, or diagnostic criteria used; and population-based studies limited by small cohort sizes. Other limitations include failure to indicate whether rates are lifetime, point, or period prevalence; reporting combined prevalence for children and adults; reporting mental ill-health in total, but not describing nor being comprehensive as to what is, and what is not, included (particularly with regards to problem behaviours, autistic spectrum disorders, attention-deficit hyperactivity disorder, and anxiety disorders); and studying selected subgroups such as only adults with verbal communication skills. All of these points must be carefully considered when interpreting and drawing conclusions from the existing literature.

## Diagnostic criteria

Prevalence of mental ill-health varies, depending upon the diagnostic criteria employed. This is because many of the diagnostic categories within *The ICD-10 Classification of Mental and Behavioural Disorders: Diagnostic Criteria for Research* (DCR), and the DSM-IV-TR contain criteria that cannot be met due to the person's degree of intellectual disabilities and communication skills, and do not include other criteria that are important in this population. For these reasons, *Diagnostic Criteria for Psychiatric Disorders for Use with Adults with Learning Disabilities/Mental Retardation* (DC-LD) was developed for use specifically with this population. These, and other important diagnostic issues are explored in further depth elsewhere.[4]

## Prevalence

Population-based studies where participants received a psychiatric assessment are shown in the Table 10.2.1. [5-9] A high prevalence of mental ill-health was reported in all but Lund's study, which used assessment methods which would today be considered limited.[6] Point prevalence is higher than that observed in the UK general population. Specific types of mental ill-health with a higher prevalence compared with the general population including problem behaviours, autism, dementia, bipolar disorder, and psychoses. Dementia is part of the behavioural phenotype of Down syndrome, and also occurs three to four times more commonly amongst people with intellectual disabilities of other causes.[10,11] Bipolar disorder occurs at about double the prevalence of that reported for the general population. This is despite a high proportion of people (about 25 per cent) taking mood-stabilizing drugs (typically for epilepsy management). Depression is either more prevalent, or occurs at the same rate, depending upon the criteria used. Prevalence of non-affective psychotic disorders (including schizo-affective disorders) has consistently been reported to be higher than for the general population; a recent study found a point prevalence of 4.4 per cent including schizophrenia, in remission, or 4.0 per cent for psychosis, currently in episode. Problem behaviour is the most prevalent type of mental ill-health at 22.5 per cent (Consultant psychiatrist's opinion) or 18.7 per cent (DC-LD) in the most recent of the studies.[9]

Given the numerous biological, psychological, social, and developmental disadvantages experienced by adults with intellectual disabilities compared with the general population, a higher prevalence of mental ill-health is expected. The higher prevalence of bipolar disorder and of psychosis points to biological origins yet to be determined, and likely to be of relevance to the whole general population.

## Incidence

There has been limited study of the incidence of mental ill-health in adults with intellectual disabilities. Longitudinal studies in the general population have not included persons with moderate to profound intellectual disabilities, but have demonstrated the higher prevalence of symptoms of depression and anxiety in adults with mild intellectual disabilities compared with the general population.[12,13] A recent study of a population-based cohort of 651 adults with intellectual disabilities found that incidence varied, depending upon the criteria used.[14] According to the Consultant psychiatrists opinion, the 2-year incidence of mental ill-health (of all types, except specific phobias) was 16.3 per cent (12.6 per cent excluding problem behaviours, and 4.6 per cent for problem behaviours), giving a standardized incident ratio for common mental disorders of 1.87 (95 per cent CI = 1.51–2.28). The comparison general population data was broadly similar, but not identical in its classification. The episodes with most frequent incidence were affective disorders at 8.3 per cent, followed by problem behaviours. The incidence of episodes of psychosis over the 2-year period was 1.4 per cent, of which 0.5 per cent were first episodes of psychotic disorders, giving a standardized incidence ratio of 10.0 (95 per cent CI = 2.1–29.3). The rate of full remission from an episode of psychosis within the 2-year period was low, at 14.3 per cent. The authors concluded that the high point prevalence of mental ill-health is explained by both a high incidence and high level of enduring mental ill-health, with slightly more enduring than incident cases.

## Protective and vulnerability factors

Many of the factors that might afford protection from or increase vulnerability for mental ill-health are interrelated, for example level of ability, age, gender, and epilepsy. Few studies have attempted to tease these apart. Further work in this area is important, particularly as the pattern of related factors appears to differ from those found in the general population, suggesting that inferences cannot necessarily be drawn from general population data.

### Ability

The relationship between ability level and mental ill-health has variously been reported to be absent, present with higher prevalence of mental ill-health at lower ability levels, or present with higher prevalence of mental ill-health at higher ability levels; these differences are explained by the limitations in the previous literature, as described above. Recent reports suggest lower ability is associated with mental ill-health in general, and specifically with

**Table 10.2.1** Prevalence of mental ill-health among adults with intellectual disabilities

| Study | Sample size | Ability | Diagnostic criteria | Prevalence (%)* |
|---|---|---|---|---|
| Corbett (1979)[5] | 402 | Borderline-profound intellectual disabilities | ICD-8 | 46.3† |
| Lund (1985)[6] | 302 | Borderline-profound intellectual disabilities | Modified DSM-III | 28.1 |
| Cooper and Bailey (2001)[7] | 207 | Mild-profound intellectual disabilities | Modified DCR | 37.0 |
| Deb et al. (2001)[8] | 101 | Mild-moderate intellectual disabilities | ICD-10 | 14.4‡ |
| Cooper et al. (2007)[9] | 1023 | Mild-profound intellectual disabilities | Psychiatrists opinion<br>DC-LD<br>DCR<br>DSM-IV-TR | 40.9<br>35.2<br>16.6<br>15.7 |

*Excluding specific phobias.

†Excluding dementia.

‡Excluding problem behaviours, personality disorder, dementia, autism, alcohol problems, schizophrenia not in episode, and bipolar disorder not in episode.

problem behaviours, but not depression nor psychosis; and that lower ability also predicts incident problem behaviours.[6,7,9,14] However, diagnostic complexities may contribute to the lack of association between lower ability and some disorders.

### Age

The prevalence and incidence of dementia is higher with increasing age. Whilst it has been suggested that problem behaviours are more prevalent at younger ages, there is no consistent evidence to support this. Of the population-based studies quoted above, no relationship was found between age and mental ill-health.

### Gender

Autism and attention-deficit hyperactivity disorder are more common in males. Most studies have not otherwise found any association between gender and mental ill-health in this population, unlike the general population. A higher prevalence of problem behaviours has been reported in women,[8,9] but aggression has also been reported as more common in men[15]; these differences might possibly be due to whether the independent effects of gender and autism are investigated. Women have been reported to score higher than men on the 'affective/neurotic disorders' subdomain of a screening tool,[16] and to have a higher prevalence of mental ill-health,[9] and specifically depression; however, within the same cohort gender did not predict incident mental ill-health.[14]

## Epilepsy and other physical ill-health

There are conflicting findings regarding whether there is a relationship between epilepsy and mental ill-health in this population, with the interaction between level of ability and epilepsy and use of antiepileptic drugs possibly contributing. It remains unclear whether physical and mental ill-health are related.

### Life events

Associations have been demonstrated between preceding life events in adults with intellectual disabilities and scores for 'affective/neurotic disorders', and between life events and scores on the *Developmental Behaviour Checklist for Adults*.[17] A relationship has been reported with mental ill-health in general, and specifically with depression, but not psychosis, nor problem behaviours, nor incident mental ill-health (excluding problem behaviours),[9,14] but has been reported for incident problem behaviours.[14]

### Accommodation/support

Both prevalence and incidence of mental ill-health, and of problem behaviours, is related to living in a setting other than with family carers, and this is independent of past psychiatric history. This highlights the need for engagement between professionals, service managers, and paid carers.

### Deprived localities

Unlike for children, no relationship had been found between area-based measures of deprivation and mental ill-health in the adult population with intellectual disabilities, although there have been few investigations of this. It is possible that adults with intellectual disabilities may not have the same lifestyle characteristics as the general population living in the same area, due to being 'placed' in

areas dissimilar from those they originated from and within which they acquired life-long habits and preferences, and through ongoing important relationships with family members whose own views and actions may be of greater influence than those of their paid carers or local community. It may be that the biological, social, and developmental causes and consequences of intellectual disabilities far outweigh some of the factors of relevance to the general population, in the aetiology of mental ill-health. This requires further study.

### Smoking

As for the general population, smoking is associated with mental ill-health, and specifically with depression and psychosis.

### Other factors

Other factors which may be independently related to mental ill-health in this population include urinary incontinence (as in the general population), not being immobile, visual impairment (for psychosis, as for the general population), abuse, neglect and exploitation, and parental divorce during childhood. However, few studies have investigated these factors. Few people with intellectual disabilities use alcohol or cannabis, so it is not known if there is any relationship between these behaviours and mental ill-health in this population.

## Conclusions

- The prevalence of intellectual disabilities varies, depending upon definition, country, time, age range, and methods of population ascertainment. Reported rates vary substantially, and may be in the order of 9–14/1000 childhood populations, 3–8/1000 adult populations in developed countries, and higher in developing countries.

- Mental ill-health is more commonly experienced by adults with intellectual disabilities than the general population. Point prevalence is about 40 per cent, with problem behaviours being the most prevalent type.

- Dementia, problem behaviours, autism, bipolar disorder, and psychoses are more prevalent than for the general population.

- Incident mental ill-health is also greater than for the general population, at about 8 per cent per year. Common mental disorders and psychoses both have higher incidence than that for the general population.

- There is limited information on the protective and vulnerability factors for mental ill-health.

- Some factors related to prevalence and incidence of mental ill-health are similar to those found in the general population suggesting similar underlying causative mechanisms, but other factors differ, suggesting that inferences cannot necessarily be drawn from general population data and applied to the population with intellectual disabilities.

- Identifying high-risk groups within the population may allow for the provision of early interventions and supports, whilst some causative factors may be amenable to interventions to prevent or improve mental ill-health in this population. We need to gain a better understanding of these issues.

## Further information

NHS Health Scotland. (2004). *Health needs assessment report. People with learning disabilities in Scotland*. NHS Health Scotland, Glasgow.

Royal College of Psychiatrists. (2001). *DC-LD [diagnostic criteria for psychiatric disorders for use with adults with learning disabilities/mental retardation]*. Gaskell Press, London.

Smiley, E. (2005). Epidemiology of mental health problems in adults with learning disability: an update. *Advances in Psychiatric Treatment*, **11**, 214–22.

http://www.intellectualdisability.info/home.htm

## References

1. Leonard, H. and Wen, X. (2002). The epidemiology of mental retardation: challenges and opportunities in the new millennium. *Mental Retardation and Developmental Disabilities Research Reviews*, **8**, 117–34.

2. Roeleveld, N., Zielhuis, G.A., and Gabreëls, F. (1997). The prevalence of mental retardation: a critical review of recent literature. *Developmental Medicine and Child Neurology*, **39**, 125–32.

3. Leonard, H., Petterson, B., Bower, C., *et al.* (2003). Prevalence of intellectual disability in Western Australia. *Paediatric and Perinatal Epidemiology*, **17**, 58–67.

4. Cooper, S.-A. and Simpson, N. (2006). Classification and assessment of psychiatric disorders in adults with learning disability. *Psychiatry*, **5**, 306–11.

5. Corbett, J.A. (1979). Psychiatric morbidity and mental retardation. In *Psychiatric illness and mental handicap* (eds. F.E. James and R.P. Snaith), pp.11–25. Gaskell, London.

6. Lund, J. (1985). The prevalence of psychiatric disorder in mentally retarded adults. *Acta Psychiatrica Scandinavica*, **72**, 563–70.

7. Cooper, S.-A. and Bailey, N.M. (2001). Psychiatric disorders amongst adults with learning disabilities—prevalence and relationship to ability level. *Irish Journal of Psychological Medicine*, **18**, 45–53.

8. Deb, S., Thomas, M., and Bright, C. (2001). Mental disorder in adults with intellectual disability I: prevalence of functional psychiatric disorder among a community-based population aged between 16 and 64 years. *Journal of Intellectual Disability Research*, **45**, 495–505.

9. Cooper, S.-A., Smiley, E., Morrison, J., *et al.* (2007). Prevalence of and associations with mental ill-health in adults with intellectual disabilities. *The British Journal of Psychiatry*, **190**, 27–35.

10. Cooper, S.-A. (1997). High prevalence of dementia amongst people with learning disabilities not attributed to Down's syndrome. *Psychological Medicine*, **27**, 609–16.

11. Strydom, A., Livingston, G., King, M., *et al.* (2007). Prevalence of dementia in intellectual disability using different diagnostic criteria. *The British Journal of Psychiatry*, **191**, 150–7.

12. Maughan, B., Collishaw, S., and Pickles, A. (1999). Mild mental retardation: psychosocial functioning in adulthood. *Psychological Medicine*, **29**, 351–66.

13. Richards, M., Maughan, B., Hardy, R., *et al.* (2001). Long-term affective disorder in people with learning disability. *The British Journal of Psychiatry*, **170**, 523–7.

14. Smiley, E., Cooper, S.-A., Finlayson, J., *et al.* (2007). The incidence, and predictors of mental ill-health in adults with intellectual disabilities. Prospective study. *The British Journal of Psychiatry*, **191**, 313–19.

15. McClintock, K., Hall, S., and Oliver, C. (2003). Risk markers associated with challenging behaviour in people with intellectual disabilities: a meta-analytic study. *Journal of Intellectual Disability Research*, **47**, 405–16.

16. Taylor, J.L., Hatton, C., Dixon, L., *et al.* (2004). Screening for psychiatric symptoms: PAS-ADD Checklist norms for adults with intellectual disabilities. *Journal of Intellectual Disability Research*, **48**, 37–41.

17. Hamilton, D., Sutherland, G., and Iacano, T. (2005). Further examination of relationships between life events and psychiatric symptoms in adults with intellectual disability. *Journal of Intellectual Disability Research*, **49**, 839–44.

# Aetiology of intellectual disability: general issues and prevention

## Markus Kaski

## Causation

### The complexity of causes

Intellectual disability can follow any of the biological, environmental, and psychological events that are capable of producing a decline of cognitive functions. Some factors do not directly or inevitably cause intellectual disability but add to the effects of a previous primary cause. Genetic causes may be hereditary or non-hereditary, and may or may not produce specific syndromes. Some lead to inborn errors of metabolism.[1]

Neurological symptoms during the neonatal period are strongly associated with prenatal developmental disturbances. For example in maternal pre-eclampsia, placental insufficiency may lead to malnutrition, foetal asphyxia, intrauterine growth retardation and prematurity, and subsequently to perinatal problems including asphyxia, intracranial haemorrhage, hyperbilirubinaemia, and hypoglycaemia. It is important to detect these coexisting conditions, because their effects may add to or interact with those of the primary cause.[2]

*The biomedical cause* of intellectual disability may lead to *additional disorders or disabilities*, or may itself be progressive.[1–3] In fact, intellectual disability exists commonly with many other symptoms in a patient, for example with sensory problems, dysphasia, cerebral palsy, epilepsy, or autism. These additional factors affect *opportunities for gaining experiences necessary for development*. Activity may be restricted by sickness, or the effects of medication. Motor disability may reduce mobility, or cause dysphasia. Sensory impairment may restrict vision or hearing. These restrictions add to the effects of the primary cause and interact with environmental and emotional factors to retard the development of the individual.[1–4]

### How often do we know the cause(s)?

The various concepts of intellectual disability and its causes have led to *different epidemiological estimates*. The population at risk consists of survivors, but some figures include also all live born. Differences in the definition and detection of cases, the classification system used, the population studied, the timing of the study in relation to measures of the general population, the resources available for the study, and sources of the data make it difficult to compare both the frequency of persons with intellectual disability and the frequency of various causes obtained in different studies. However, a specific cause for intellectual disability can be identified for approximately 80 per cent for persons with severe intellectual disability (IQ <50, includes the groups of moderate, severe, and profound intellectual disability in ICD-10) and 50 per cent of persons with mild intellectual disability. The principal cause of intellectual disability is estimated to be prenatal in 50 to 70 per cent, perinatal in 10 to 20 per cent, and postnatal in 5 to 10 per cent of persons.[3–7] In general, knowledge of aetiologies is more accurate for people with severe intellectual disability than for those with mild intellectual disability.[8, 9]

## Classifying causes

The causes of intellectual disability may be classified according to the particular clinical entity, the causative agent or presumed cause, or the *timing of the causative factor*. The newer and more successful classification systems are based on timing.[10] The principle is biomedical in nature and it is intended to elucidate the *earliest factor* that has affected the development of the central nervous system. The discovery of the primary cause (or sequential causes) aids family counselling and may lead to identification of a preventable general risk.

Viewed in this way, diagnoses can be divided into six main groups according to the probable cause and the timing of damage to the central nervous system (Table 10.3.1)[11]:

♦ genetic causes;

♦ central nervous system malformations of unknown origin;

♦ external prenatal factors;

♦ disorders acquired in the paranatal* period;

♦ disorders acquired postnatally; and

♦ untraceable or unclassified causes.

*The paranatal period is defined as the period from 1 week before birth to 4 weeks after birth.

**Table 10.3.1** Aetiology based on the time and mechanism of the injury to the central nervous system and the history helping identification, timing, and diagnosis of intellectual disability

| Aetiology | History[a] |
|---|---|
| *Genetic causes*<br>Chromosomal disorders<br>Malformations due to microdeletion<br>Single-gene disorders<br>Multifactorial intellectual disability<br>Mitochondrial disorders | *Family history*<br>Family tree, intellectual disability, learning disabilities, neurological diseases, congenital anomalies, psychoses, consanguinity of parents, recurrent abortions, previous stillbirths, low parity or infertility, and parental ages |
| *CNS malformations of unknown origin*<br>Isolated malformation or malformation sequence of the CNS<br>Multiple malformations | *Family and gestational history* |
| *External prenatal factors*<br>Infections<br>Physical, chemical, and toxic agents<br>Maternal and gestational disorders<br>Other | *Gestational history*<br>Maternal infections of the TORCH group, HIV, radiation, trauma, chronic maternal diseases, drugs, pre-eclampsia, severe malnutrition, alcohol, bleeding, and abnormal intrauterine growth or fetal movements |
| *Paranatally acquired disorders*<br>Infections<br>Delivery problems<br>Other newborn complications | *Birth and neonatal history*<br>Gestational age, multiple pregnancy, birth order, placental abnormalities, labour or delivery complications/mode and duration, asphyxia, intracranial haemorrhage, trauma, 5-min Apgar scores, newborn weight, length and head circumference, infections, hypoglycaemia, hyperbilirubinaemia, neurological problems, and weight gain |
| *Postnatally acquired disorders*<br>Infections<br>Other damage to CNS<br>Psychosocial problems<br>Psychoses without family history | *Childhood history*<br>Feeding and sleeping patterns, nutrition, growth charts, developmental milestones, infections of CNS, head injuries, submersions, metabolic and endocrine disorders, vascular accidents or thromboses of cerebral veins, cerebral tumours, toxic agents, and psychosocial environment |
| *Untraceable or unclassified causes*<br>Pure non-familial<br>With CNS symptoms<br>Not classified | *History of associating conditions*<br>No history of adverse events or signs or history with CNS symptoms such as cerebral palsy, epilepsy, or autism in addition to mental retardation |

CNS, central nervous system; TORCH, toxoplasmosis–other infection–rubella–cytomegalovirus–herpes.

[a]Gives the time of the risk event or cause, or appearing time of the sign whose cause(s) may also be earlier.

## (a) Genetic causes

**Chromosomal disorders** include all intellectual disability caused by a proven chromosomal aberration or a clinically obvious chromosomal syndrome such as Down syndrome. However, chromosome analysis should be performed in Down syndrome because translocation, mosaicism, or other abnormalities are found in 5 per cent of cases. Chromosomal anomalies associated with intellectual disability account for up to 40 per cent of severe cases, and 10 to 20 per cent of mild cases.[3,6,12,13] However, the detection rates for chromosome abnormalities with the novel molecular karyotyping methods, such as micro**array**-based **c**omparative **g**enomic **h**ybridization (**array CGH**), range from 5 to 17 per cent in individuals with normal results from prior routine cytogenetic testing.[14] Array CGH has the ability to detect any genomic imbalance including deletions, duplications, aneuploidies, and amplifications.

**Malformations due to microdeletion** include many malformation syndromes whose causative agent is obscure. A new method of using DNA probes and fluorescence in situ hybridization has increased understanding of the causes of syndromes such as the Angelman, Cornelia de Lange, CATCH 22 (**c**ardiac defects, **a**bnormal face, **t**hymic hypoplasia, **c**left palate, and **h**ypocalcaemia) (velocardiofacial syndrome), Miller–Dieker, Prader–Willi, Rubinstein–Taybi, Smith–Magenis, Sotos, Williams, and Wolf–Hirschhorn syndromes. Parental imprinting modifies the expression of the genes involved in the Prader–Willi and Angelman syndromes.[12, 14–16]

**Subtelomeric deletions** or **chromosomal rearrangements** have been found in some persons with intellectual disability of hitherto unknown aetiology. Subtelomeric aberrations may explain up to 5 to 10 per cent of previously unknown causes.[13,15]

**Single-gene disorders** include states with intellectual disability in which the pedigree is highly suggestive of a single-gene origin. Some are caused by a mutant gene with simple Mendelian inheritance. Single-gene mutations may increase or diminish in frequency in areas with long-standing populations of the same origin, or in populations isolated by language or culture. For example, the so-called Finnish *disease heritage* includes 36 disorders, from which 10 manifest with central nervous symptoms and some others may have them.[17] Most of the specific disorders due to mutant gene have characteristic clinical phenotypic features, but there are a considerable number of non-syndromic individuals, especially in early infancy.[12,18,19]

*Autosomal dominant inheritance* causes tuberous sclerosis, myotonic dystrophy, Gorlin syndrome, neurofibromatosis I, Apert syndrome, Menkes syndrome, and Huntington's disease.

*Autosomal recessive inheritance* is the cause of most metabolic diseases with intellectual disability. These diseases include phenylketonuria, homocystinuria, maple syrup urine disease, aspartylglucosaminuria, mannosidosis, Salla disease, I-cell disease, mucopolysaccharidoses (except type II), neuronal ceroid lipofuscinoses, Tay–Sachs disease, metachromatic leucodystrophy, Smith–Lemli–Opitz syndrome, and Joubert syndrome.

*X-linked inherited disorders* include the fragile X, Aicardi, Lesch–Nyhan, Lowe, Norrie, and Coffin–Lowry syndromes, mucopolysaccharidosis II, Duchenne muscular dystrophy, α-thalassaemia intellectual disability syndrome, and Rett syndrome. The most common intellectual disability syndrome caused by mutation of a single gene is fragile X syndrome. The pattern of its inheritance is X-linked dominant with decreased penetrance.[17,19,20] The prevalence of the 24 other genes identified to date in the X chromosome is low.[20] Dystrophic myotony, fragile X syndrome, and Huntington's disease are caused by so-called *dynamic mutation* in which the length of the repeated sequence of three DNA bases can vary from generation to generation increasing the variability in the phenotype.[21] In Rett syndrome female inactivation of X chromosome may be skewed. It explains the existing of the syndrome in a male or the very mild phenotype in a female.[22] Epigenetic regulatory factors are also involved in the aetiology of Rett syndrome.[23]

**Mitochondrial disorders** are inherited in most cases due to mutations in the *nuclear genes* encoding proteins targeted to this organelle. Autosomal dominant, recessive, or X-linked inheritances are possible. In addition, mitochondrial dysfunction is shown among others in patients with fragile-X, Rett, and Wolf–Hirschhorn syndromes or autism. [24–27] *Mitochondrial DNA* (mtDNA) is inherited maternally. Sporadic deletions and duplications are also found (Kearns–Sayre syndrome, sporadic deletion or partial duplication in mtDNA). Examples of the maternally inherited (mtDNA) syndromes with central nervous symptoms are the MELAS (mitochondrial myopathy, encephalomyopathy, lactic acidosis, and stroke-like episodes), MERRF (myoclonus epilepsy with ragged red fibres), and NARP (neurogenic muscle weakness, ataxia, retinitis pigmentosa), FSFD (facio-scapulo-femoral muscular dystrophy, familial cerebellar ataxia, recurrent Reye syndrome, cerebral palsy with intellectual disability), and cytochrome c oxidase (COX) deficiency (deafness, myoclonic epilepsy, ataxia, and intellectual disability) syndromes. Nuclear genes are often involved in mitochondrial DNA depletion and Leigh syndromes, which are severe progressive diseases in early childhood.[11, 18, 21]

**Multifactorial** intellectual disability may be a state of *pure familial* intellectual disability or associated to some *multifactorially inherited* conditions, for example neural-tube defects. One or more first-degree relatives are also affected. Similar pervasive developmental disorders or childhood or other psychoses in one or more of first-degree relatives or otherwise strong family background suggest a polygenic component of intellectual disability.[12, 21]

### (b) Central nervous system malformations of unknown origin

Approximately 30 to 40 per cent of all malformations are *genetic* and 10 per cent have *exogenous* causes. The aetiology of the rest is unknown. The number included in this aetiological group decreases with more accurate diagnosis of genetic malformations, intrauterine infections, other teratogenic agents, or deficiencies of essential ingredients needed for the normal development.[28,29] The development of the central nervous system may be disturbed at the following stages[2,12,21,28,29]:

1 dorsal induction at the 3rd to 7th weeks of gestation, leading to anencephaly, encephalocele, meningomyelocele, or other neural-tube-closure defects;

2 ventral induction at the 5th to 6th weeks of gestation, causing prosencephalies and other faciotelencephalic malformations;

3 proliferation of the neurones at the 2nd to 4th month of gestation, leading to microcephaly or macrocephaly;

4 migration of the neurones at the 3rd to 5th month of gestation, causing gyrus anomalies and heterotopias;

5 organization of neurones from the 6th month of gestation to a year postpartum, leading to disturbances in the formation of dendrites and synapses;

6 myelination from 6th month of gestation to a year postpartum, disturbing the proliferation of oligodendrocytes and the formation of the myelin sheets.

The **malformation sequence** is a type of multiple malformation, which includes secondary anomalies caused by an earlier anomaly, for example equinovarus with meningomyelocele. **Multiple malformation syndromes** are caused by the disturbances in blastogenesis or organogenesis. Multiple malformation syndromes of unknown origin include some whose causes are unknown such as the Goldenhar and Kabuki syndromes, and research will show that some of these aetiologically unknown syndromes have a genetic cause.[30,31]

### (c) External prenatal factors

The nature of the impairments or malformations, and the severity of resulting intellectual disability appear to relate, at least partially, to the timing of the causative factor as discussed earlier. Also dosage may be important. Effects are most serious when the cause acts *early in embryonic development*; during blastogenesis or organogenesis, when it may result in *multiple malformations*. Effects on the central nervous system of *causes acting later* may be severe even though outward signs may be lacking. These causes include congenital infections such as rubella, cytomegalovirus, herpes simplex type 2, parvovirus, and HIV infection, as well as toxoplasmosis and syphilis. Exposure to medication and other substances such as hydantoin, lipid solvents, alcohol, cocaine, and other drugs can affect the developing foetus.[2,3,28,32,33]

*Maternal disorders* that may contribute to the causes of intellectual disability include maternal diabetes, arterial hypertension, placental insufficiency, pre-eclampsia, pre- and postmaturity, multiple pregnancy, and foetal growth retardation. In other cases no specific causes can be identified with certainty but available data strongly suggest a prenatal external cause of central nervous system impairment such as exposure to ionizing radiation or trauma.[2, 34]

### (d) Disorders acquired in the paranatal period

The effects of the last week of pregnancy extend to the neonatal period and are very important for the outcome of the newborn,[11,35] and combinations of the prenatal and postnatal factors are not rare. *Infections* are transmitted via placenta or the birth canal. They include neonatal septicaemia, pneumonia, meningitis, and encephalitis, which may lead by several mechanisms to neurological deficits, intellectual disability, and sometimes microcephaly, or in bacterial meningitides also to hydrocephalus. *Congenital infections* of herpes simplex and HIV as well as tertiary syphilis may manifest later. *Problems during delivery* may lead to asphyxia, intracranial haemorrhage, or other birth injuries and cause various symptoms of cerebral palsy and epilepsy. *Other newborn complications* include hypoglycaemia, hyperbilirubinaemia, and respiratory distress. Paranatal aetiologies may cause disorders of cognitive functions, as well as motor and sensory impairments.[2,35,36]

### (e) Disorders acquired postnatally

Improved postnatal care has reduced the frequency of these causes, which include *infections* such as meningitides and encephalitides.[37] Other causes of postnatal damage to the central nervous system include *toxic agents*, *vascular accidents*, *brain tumours*, *hypoxia*, *and traumas*. Traffic accidents, other traumas, submersions, and cerebral tumours are common causes of disability in childhood. Lead poisoning has been a problem in the United States, iodine deficiency in some regions of the world, and malnutrition almost worldwide.[38] *Psychosocial problems* causing intellectual disability are not as common as was thought in the past, partly because of better identification of medical factors.[39] Severe maternal mental or chronic physical illness, parental alcohol or drug abuse, and some consequences of poverty may be contributory causes leading to inadequate care and stimulation. *Deprived environments* are linked to other risks such as malnutrition, poor medical care, child abuse, usage of alcohol and other substances, and teenage pregnancies.[40]

### (f) Untraceable or unclassified causes

The aetiology of intellectual disability can be classified as unknown if the causative factor or timing of the brain damage cannot be established. ***Pure non-familial*** intellectual disability is the term used when there is no family history of intellectual disability and no signs and symptoms suggesting brain damage. It represents the extreme of normal variation. In the untraceable group, the second category is ***intellectual disability of unknown aetiology*** with other symptoms and signs of the central nervous system suggesting brain damage, but with no family history of intellectual disability and no identified malformations or dysmorphic features (see Table 10.3.1). Common examples are intellectual disability associated with cerebral palsy, epilepsy, or autism. Patients should not be assigned to the untraceable group if the diagnostic work-up is incomplete.[11] If so, the aetiology is still ***unclassified***.

### How to assess causes

*A comprehensive history* and a *careful physical examination* are essential for identifying and timing the causative factor(s). In everyday practice it is appropriate to assess the family history, embryological, and postnatal development, possible pathogenetic mechanisms, and the time of the exposure to the supposed agent (Table 10.3.1). The finding of *more than three minor malformations* suggests genetic or early developmental disorder provided that the same dysmorphic features are not found in close relatives.[41] Infants at risk for external prenatal causes, perinatal causes, or postnatally acquired disorders should be examined carefully for dysmorphic features which may indicate alternative or additional cause. The diagnosis usually becomes evident by working out the history and clinical signs. *Databases for analyses of dysmorphology*, symptoms, or other findings are useful aids in the search of an aetiological diagnosis.[42,43]

Ophthalmological and audiological *examinations* can be arranged and other necessary investigations carried out when suggested by the history and physical examination (Table 10.3.2).[2,4,11,12,18,21,37,38,41–43] *If the findings are in accordance with history* and a person has no congenital anomalies, further examinations are seldom needed. However, the possibility of a metabolic disorder should be kept in mind, especially as congenital anomalies or dysmorphic features may occur in people with metabolic disorders. *Metabolic studies* should be performed for every patient with *progressive symptoms. If the history and physical findings do not match*, or if there are congenital anomalies or more than three minor dysmorphic features, additional studies are needed.[41] Because more accurate diagnostic methods are being developed, it is useful to keep for each person *a dated chart of examinations* performed.[11]

**Prenatal diagnosis** may be indicated when there is a known parental balanced translocation, chromosomal aberration of a sibling, a known hereditable disorder in family, a multifactorial disorder such as neural-tube defect in the family, or the mother is elderly.

The gravidity can be detected by *ultrasound examination* at 6th to 8th gestation weeks. Many structural changes can be found from 11th to 15th weeks and confirmed by repeated examinations to 22nd gestation week, for example neural-tube defects. The *nuchal translucency in relation to crown-rump length and gestation week* can be measured during the 9th and 14th for detecting Down syndrome. Other general screening methods for Down syndrome are based on the *applicable markers from the serum of the mother* to the 10th to 14th and 15th to 18th gestation weeks.[44,45] According to the positive screening result or abnormal morphology finding in the ultrasound examination foetal karyotype or some other further examination may be indicated. The age-specific screening of foetal chromosomes is based on the significantly increased probability of a Down syndrome child among mothers aged 35 years or older.[12]

*The karyotype of a foetus* can be identified after the 10th week of gestation from a *chorionic villus sample*, or after 15th week gestation from the *cells of amniotic fluid*. A known single-gene disorder can also be searched from the chorionic villus sample by *DNA*,

---

**Table 10.3.2** Diagnostic examinations of intellectual disability

- Neurological, ophthalmological, audiological, cardiological, neuropsychological, etc., assessments

- Blood count, vacuolated lymphocytes, and thyroid function

- Antibodies, serology, and urine (TORCH, HIV)

- Radiographs of skull, vertebral column, chest, hands, feet, and long bones, and bone age

- Chromosomes: G-banding, high-resolution banding, and FISH array CGH

- FraX DNA, specific DNA tests, and other molecular genetic techniques

- Blood/urine: amino and organic acids, muchopolysaccharides, oligosaccharides, long- and very-long-chain fatty acids, Astrup, glucose, ammonia, lactate, pyruvate, uric acid, phytanic acid, carnitine, lead, copper, ceruloplasmin

- Fibroblast culture or white blood cell sample; specific enzymes

- Biopsies: muscle, skin, rectal

- Neurophysiological: EEG and evoked potentials

- Neuroimaging: cranial ultrasound, CT, MRI, MRS, functional MRI, SPECT, and PET

- Neuropathological examinations

---

TORCH, toxoplasmosis–other infection–rubella–cytomegalovirus–herpes; FISH, fluorescence in situ hybridization; MRI, magnetic resonance imaging; SPECT, single-photon emission CT; PET, positron emission tomography; MRS, magnetic resonance spectroscopy.

*enzyme, or other specific methods.* Cell cultures of few amniotic fluid cells can be used for karyotyping or diagnosing metabolic diseases, but it needs more time. Neural-tube defects, also the small ones, can be seen as elevated levels *of α-fetoprotein* in amniotic fluid. Sometimes a blood sample from the umbilical cord is needed after the 18th gestation week for confirmation of karyotype.

Prenatal diagnostic methods and identification of parental balanced translocations or aberrations in single gene are increasingly available. Microarray-based comparative genomic hybridization (array CGH), examination of foetal DNA or cells derived from maternal blood circulation, and preimplantation diagnoses becoming available for some diseases will change the prenatal diagnosing practice considerably.[12,21,46,47]

## Why knowledge of causation is important

*Intellectual disability is a confusing concept.* The people with intellectual disabilities have more differences than common features. Developmental delay may appear in different ages and with different degrees of severity in different children. The development of a child can come to a stop or can even regress. There is a multitude of confirmed causes of intellectual disability. Single aetiologies are rare and the clinical picture within the same aetiology and between different aetiologies can vary greatly. It is now possible to detect causes that until recently were unknown. Associated disabilities and chronic diseases are common and modify further the complex interplay of individual and environmental factors.

The factors believed to be related to the incidence and prevalence of intellectual disability, such as personal history and gender, the age and the marital status of the parents, the number of siblings, and the living conditions and the social situation of the family, as well as the neighbouring community, vary in persons with intellectual disability. *Attitudes to disabilities* may differ in different families and societies. The permanence of the cognitive impairment is difficult to accept. Insufficient or inadequate information or a prolonged diagnostic process may lead the family or the child to become fearful about the cause of the condition or to try and identify some reason for it. The way is then open for misunderstandings, feelings of guilt, or projections.[4,11,48]

*For the person with intellectual disability* a confirmed aetiology is the basis of a correct awareness of his or her own disability; the limitations set by the disability and the possibilities for learning and development. The clinical manifestations of some developmental disorders, such as phenylketonuria, galactosaemia, or hypothyroidism can be prevented or arrested by dietary management or hormonal replacement therapy. Knowledge of the prognosis increases awareness of associated disease and disabilities such as sensory impairments, communication disorders, motor and joint problems, epilepsy, and behavioural or psychiatric problems. Thus, aetiology aids the planning of follow-up, rehabilitation, education, and living arrangements.[4,11] Knowledge of aetiology is particularly important at the time of transition from childhood to adult services, helping to ensure continuity of provision and to avoid drop-out.

*For the family,* knowledge of causes helps to dispel wrong beliefs, self-blame, and anxieties. The parents and siblings may change their preconceived ideas about the disability. It helps the parents to adopt appropriate standards for bringing up their child, and for life as an adult. It helps them to become aware of the child's special needs.[4,11] Aetiologic diagnosis is the necessary basis of reliable genetic counselling and helps the parents and siblings in family planning.[12,48]

*In society* the knowledge of the aetiologies of intellectual disability increases the likelihood that its people will adopt positive attitudes towards the disabled. Both the society and its service providers need understanding of the causes of intellectual disability, their prevalence, and their prognoses when planning primary prevention, organizing services and education, optimizing environmental factors, or preparing relevant legislation. Society needs experts continuously alert to advances in scientific research to keep this knowledge up to date.

*When the causes are unknown,* prognosis is uncertain and the planning and provision of the services is difficult. The risks of discontinuities in service provision and of drop-outs increase. Because families have limited information they are more likely to develop wrong beliefs, self-blame, and projections. They have unrealistic expectations about alternative therapies.[12, 48]

## Prevention

### Primary prevention

*The identification of factors that contribute to intellectual disability, their removal or avoidance, and the protection of the population or individuals against them* are the main principles of primary prevention. Immunization and other measures to prevent rhesus incompatibility, congenital rubella, measles encephalitis, tuberculosis and other bacterial meningitides, prionic diseases, and the provision of folic acid around the time of conception to prevent neural-tube defects have been successful preventive measures.[2,37]

Primary prevention includes *good medical follow-up, the identification and prompt removal of, or effective intervention in,* at-risk situations during pregnancy, delivery, the neonatal period, and childhood. Avoidable causes include intrauterine and perinatal infections due to many sexually transmitted diseases, and fetal alcohol spectrum disorders (FASD).[49] Lead intoxication, iodine deficiency, accidents in the home, and traffic accidents are preventable.[2,36,38] The primary prevention of genetic disorders has not been possible, although the disorder, the chromosomal aberration, or some associated abnormality can sometimes be identified.[21,29,44] However, all the means of the secondary prevention are available, and pregnancies may be terminated after counselling. Screening tests can identify some parents who are carriers.[48] The preimplantation diagnosis could give a new way for the early prevention of known genetic disorders in some cases.[47,50]

### Secondary prevention

*Early recognition and diagnosis, good medical care, and rehabilitation of injuries or diseases* can avoid or reduce permanent damage which could lead to intellectual disability. Examples include the screening for and early treatment of congenital hypothyroidism and phenylketonuria.[2] Secondary prevention also includes planning or *genetic counselling* after the birth of a child with a genetic disorder.[48] The examination of asymptomatic parents and close relatives in order to detect carriers is part of genetic counselling. As yet there are no measures to prevent the underlying biological processes in genetic disorders.[12,18,21]

Once children with intellectual disability have been identified, accurate assessment of aetiology and associated conditions, therapy, and rehabilitation lessen the risk of so-called **caused learning disability**, that is leaving the person with intellectual disability without the possibility of developing further because he or she is unable to share in the learning experiences of the peer group.[2,4,38]

## Tertiary prevention

The aim of tertiary prevention is *to help an individual attain his or her full developmental potential*. Therefore tertiary prevention partly overlaps with secondary prevention. It encompasses all measures, which prevent or lessen persistent hindrances to the development of functional ability or social competence in people with identified damage or disease. It includes medical, psychological, social, and family support, environmental adjustments, aids, and education. In the ideal state, individual supports are so good that the mentally retarded can live a life similar to that of people without intellectual disability. However, even when this can be achieved, problems may reappear when tasks of life increase, or the supporting systems fail.[4,10]

## Ethical problems of prevention

*Usually there are no ethical problems*. There are hardly any issues surrounding the prevention of causative diseases or injury, the attempt to reduce the prevalence of inheritable diseases by family planning or genetic counselling, the screening that leads to the treatment of the foetus or the newborn, preparation for the birth of a new infant, improving the care and rehabilitation, and planning a safer society.

*Ethical questions arise if there are no measures to prevent* the effects of an identified genetic or other cause of intellectual disability identified during pregnancy. Disordered genes, other genetic rearrangements, or accidental mutations cannot be removed from a population. Primary prevention of an intellectual disability becomes the prevention of childbirth or selective abortion. The latter is usually on the grounds that the burden of caring for the child would be too great for the parents, an indication that is more social than medical.[51,52] In general, the prevention of a disease does not exclude good therapy for it. However, the increasing trend to accept selective means of prevention may be a result of cultural change and increasingly negative attitudes towards disability.[53–56]

*Prenatal diagnosis*, detection of carriers and screening for disorders, which cannot be prevented or treated, usually lead to decisions about more or less harmful consequences. Ethical questions include *choices between knowing and not knowing*, between not knowing and worry or anxiety in risk situations, and between the need to take difficult decisions and to avoid them. It is very difficult to predict accurately all the long-term effects of these decisions. Parents have the right to be able to make voluntary decisions, but they need *accurate information* to be able to bear the burden of responsibility.[51,56–58]

## Prevention requires a coordinated programme

On the basis of the aetiologies defined according to the timing principle, it is possible to search for epidemiological, psychological, sociological, and other explanations to answer the question of why some causes are more common in certain populations or subgroups than in others. *The starting point of prevention is knowledge of causation* and identification of factors that subject individuals to these causes. With better understanding of the causes of intellectual disability, attitudes towards it change. With knowledge, individuals needing support can be identified earlier, their development and life made easier, and the burden of care on the family lightened.

Public policy, education, public health, obstetric services, neonatal intensive care, general practice services, etc. have an important role in reducing and avoiding risk factors. Education, planning of a safe environment and alleviation of poverty has a general preventive effect on predisposing factors. *The preventive aspects should be taken into account in all general and specific legislation, in operating procedures, and professional practice*. Because multiple agencies are involved preventive measures need to be coordinated at both local and national levels.

The day-to-day prevention of infections, accidents in the home and traffic, exposure to toxic substances, drowning accidents, malnutrition, or child abuse is both *a general and a multiprofessional task*. Parents and educators should transfer their wisdom and experience to the next generation so that they will make better choices and avoid risks.

## Further information

Accardo, P.J. (ed.) (2008). *Capute and Accardo's neurodevelopmental disabilities in infancy and childhood*. (Vol. 1–2, 3rd edn). Paul H. Brookes Publishing Co., Inc., Baltimore, MD.

Smith, M., Arfin, S.M., and Lott, I.T. (2006). *Mental retardation and developmental delay: genetic and epigenetic factors*. Oxford University Press, New York.

Cassidy, S.B. and Allanson, J.E. (2005). *Management of genetic syndromes* (2nd edn). Wiley & Liss, New York.

Fernandes, J., Saudubray, J.M., van den Berghe, G., *et al.* (eds.) (2006). *Inborn metabolic diseases: diagnosis and treatment* (4th edn). Springer, New York.

## References

1. Filiano, J.J. (2006). Neurometabolic diseases in the newborn. *Clinics in Perinatology*, **33**, 411–79.

2. Volpe, J.J. (2001). *Neurology of the newborn* (4th edn). W.B. Saunders, Philadelphia, PA.

3. Heikura, U., Linna, S.-L., Olsen, P., *et al.* (2005). Etiological survey on intellectual disability in the northern Finland birth cohort 1986. *American Journal of Mental Retardation*, **110**, 171–80.

4. Rubin, I.L.M.D. and Crocker, A.C. (2006). *Medical care for children & adults with developmental disabilities* (2nd edn). Brookes Publishing Company, Baltimore, MD.

5. Ahuja, A.S., Thapar, A., and Owen, M.J. (2005). Genetics of mental retardation. *Indian Journal of Medical Sciences*, **59**, 407–17.

6. Hou, J.-W., Wang, T.-R., and Chuang, S.-M. (1998). An epidemiological study of children with intellectual disability in Taiwan. *Journal of Intellectual Disability Research*, **42**, 137–43.

7. Stromme, P. (2000). Aetiology in severe and mild mental retardation: a population-based study of Norwegian children. *Developmental Medicine and Child Neurology*, **42**, 76–86.

8. Heikura, U., Taanila, A., Olsen, P., *et al.* (2003). Temporal changes in incidence and prevalence of intellectual disability between two birth cohorts in Northern Finland. *American Journal of Mental Retardation*, **108**, 19–31.

9. Roeleveld, N., Zielhuis, G.A., and Gabreëls, F. (1997). The prevalence of mental retardation: a critical review of recent literature. *Developmental Medicine and Child Neurology*, **39**, 125–32.

10. American Association on Mental Retardation. (2002). *Mental retardation: definition, classification, and systems of supports* (10th edn).

American Association on Intellectual and Developmental Disabilities, Washington, D.C.

11. Wilska, M. and Kaski, M. (2001). Why and how to assess the aetiological diagnosis of children with intellectual disability/mental retardation and other neurodevelopmental disorders: description of the Finnish approach. *European Journal of Paediatric Neurology,* **5**, 7–13.

12. Smith, M., Arfin, S.M., and Lott, I.T. (2006). *Mental retardation and developmental delay: genetic and epigenetic factors.* Oxford University Press, New York.

13. Rooms, L., *et al.* (2006). Multiplex ligation-dependent probe amplification to detect subtelomeric rearrangements in routine diagnostics. *Clinical Genetics,* **69**, 58–64.

14. Shaffer, L.G. and Bejjani, B.A. (2006). Medical applications of array CGH and the transformation of clinical cytogenetics. *Cytogenetic and Genome Research,* **115**, 303–9.

15. Hodgson, S.V. (1998). The genetics of learning disabilities. *Developmental Medicine and Child Neurology,* **40**, 137–40.

16. Tatton-Brown, K., *et al.* (2005). Genotype-phenotype associations in Sotos syndrome: an analysis of 266 individuals with *NSD1* aberrations. *American Journal of Human Genetics,* **77**, 193–204.

17. Norio, R. (2003). The Finnish disease heritage III: the individual diseases. *Human Genetics,* **111**, 470–526.

18. Scriver, C.R., Beaudet, A.L., Childs, B., *et al.* (2000). *The metabolic and molecular base of inherited disease* (8th edn). (www.ommbid.com). McGraw-Hill, New York.

19. OMIM (Online Mendelian Inheritance in Man). http://www.ncbi.nlm.nih.gov/omim/

20. Raymond, F.L. (2006). X linked mental retardation: a clinical guide. *Journal of Medical Genetics,* **43**, 193–200.

21. Strachan, T. and Read, A.P. (2004). *Human molecular genetics* (3rd edn). Garland Science, London.

22. Huppke, P., Maier, E.M., Warnke, A., *et al.* (2006). Very mild cases of Rett syndrome with skewed X inactivation. *Journal of Medical Genetics,* **43**, 814–16.

23. Petel-Galil, Y., *et al.* (2006). Comprehensive diagnosis of Rett's syndrome relying on genetic, epigenetic and expression evidence of deficiency of the methyl-CpG-binding protein 2 gene: study of a cohort of Israeli patients. *Journal of Medical Genetics,* **43**, e56.

24. Rizzo, G., *et al.* (2006). A case of fragile X premutation tremor/ataxia syndrome with evidence of mitochondrial dysfunction. *Movement Disorders,* **21**, 1541–2.

25. Wenk, G.L. (1997). Rett syndrome: neurobiological changes underlying specific symptoms. *Progress in Neurobiology,* **51**, 383–91.

26. Schlickum, S., *et al.* (2004). LETM1, a gene deleted in Wolf-Hirschhorn syndrome, encodes an evolutionarily conserved mitochondrial protein. *Genomics,* **83**, 254–61.

27. Oliveira, G., *et al.* (2005). Mitochondrial dysfunction in autism spectrum disorders: a population-based study. *Developmental Medicine and Child Neurology,* **47**, 185–9.

28. Stevenson, R.E. and Hall, J.G. (eds.) (2005). *Human malformations and related anomalies* (2nd edn). Oxford University Press, New York.

29. Moore, K.L. and Persaud, T.V.N. (2007). *Before we are born: essentials of embryology and birth defects* (7th edn). W.B. Saunders, Philadelphia, PA.

30. Touliatou, V., Fryssira, H., Mavrou, A., *et al.*(2006). Clinical manifestations in 17 Greek patients with Goldenhar syndrome. *Genetic counseling,* **17**, 359–70.

31. Miyake, N., *et al.* (2006). No detectable genomic aberrations by BAC array CGH in Kabuki make-up syndrome patients. *American Journal of Medical Genetics,* **140**, 291–3.

32. Konstantinidou, A.E., Syridou, G., Spanakis, N., *et al.* (2007). Association of hypospadias and cardiac defect in a parvovirus B19-infected stillborn: a causality relation? *The Journal of Infection,* **54**, 41–5.

33. Sharp, N.J., Davis, B.J., Guy, J.S., *et al.* (1999). Hydranencephaly and cerebellar hypoplasia in two kittens attributed to intrauterine parvovirus infection. *Journal of Comparative Pathology,* **121**, 39–53.

34. Badawi, N., Kurinczuk, J.J., Keogh, J.M., *et al.* (1998). Antepartum risk factors for newborn encephalopathy: the Western Australian case–control study. *British Medical Journal,* **317**, 1549–53.

35. Badawi, N., Kurinczuk, J.J., Keogh, J.M., *et al.* (1998). Intrapartum risk factors for newborn encephalopathy: the Western Australian case–control study. *British Medical Journal,* **317**, 1554–8.

36. Stevenson, D.K., Benitz, W.E., and Sunsine, P. (2003). *Fetal and neonatal brain injury: mechanisms, management and the risks of practice* (3rd edn). Cambridge University Press, Cambridge.

37. Scheld, W.M., Whitley, R.J., and Marra C.M. (eds.) (2004). *Infections of the central nervous system* (3rd edn). Lippincott Williams and Wilkins, Philadelphia, PA.

38. David, R.B. (ed.) (2005). *Child and adolescent neurology* (2nd edn). Blackwell Publishing Limited, Massachusetts, MA.

39. Bosma, H., van de Mheen, H.D., and Mackenbach, J.P. (1999). Social class in childhood and general health in adulthood: questionnaire study of contribution of psychological attributes. *British Medical Journal,* **318**, 18–22.

40. Malamitsi-Puchner, A. and Boutsikou, T. (2006). Adolescent pregnancy **and** perinatal outcome. *Pediatric Endocrinology Reviews,* **3**(Suppl. 1), 170–1.

41. Jones, K.L. (ed.) (2006). *Smith's recognizable patterns of human malformations.* Elsevier Saunders, Philadelphia, PA.

42. POSSUM Database, version 5.7.3. (2006). *Pictures of standard syndromes and undiagnosed malformations.* Murdoch Children's Research Institute, Victoria, http://www.possum.net.au.

43. London Medical Databases. (2006). *The Baraitser-winter neurogenetics database, and the winter-Baraitser dysmorphology database* (www.lmdatabases.com). London Medical Databases Ltd., London.

44. Rosen, T. and D'Alton, M.E. (2005). Down syndrome screening in the first and second trimesters: what do the data show? *Seminars in Perinatology,* **29**, 367–75.

45. Canick, J.A., *et al.* (2006). First and Second Trimester Evaluation of Risk (FASTER) trial research consortium. Comparison of serum markers in first-trimester down syndrome screening. *Obstetrics and Gynecology,* **108**, 1192–9.

46. Bischoff, F.Z., *et al.* (2002). Cell-free fetal DNA and intact fetal cells in maternal blood circulation: implications for first and second trimester non-invasive prenatal diagnosis. *Human Reproduction Update,* **8**, 493–500.

47. Fasouliotis, S.J. and Schenker, J.Y. (1998). Preimplantation genetic diagnosis: principles and ethics. *Human Reproduction,* **13**, 2238–45.

48. Harper, P.S. (2004). *Practical genetic counselling* (6th edn). Arnold, Hodder Headline Group, London.

49. Harris, L.H. (2000). Rethinking maternal-fetal conflict: gender and equality in perinatal ethics. *Obstetrics and Gynecology,* **96**, 786–91.

50. Katz, M.G., Fitzgerald, L., Bankier, A., *et al.* (2002). Issues and concerns of couples presenting for preimplantation genetic diagnosis (PGD). *Prenatal Diagnosis,* **22**, 1117–22.

51. Louhiala, P. (2004). *Preventing intellectual disability: ethical and clinical issues.* Cambridge University Press, Cambridge, UK.

52. Alderson, P. (2001). Down's syndrome: cost, quality and value of life. *Social Science & Medicine,* **53**, 627–38.

53. Bromage, D.I. (2006). Prenatal diagnosis and selective abortion: a result of the cultural turn? *Medical Humanities,* **32**, 38–42.

54. Raz, A. (2004). "Important to test, important to support": attitudes toward disability rights and prenatal diagnosis among leaders

of support groups for genetic disorders in Israel. *Social Science & Medicine*, **59**, 1857–66.

55. Kaplan, D. (1993). Prenatal screening and its impact on persons with disabilities. *Fetal Diagnosis and Therapy*, **8**(Suppl. 1), 64–9.

56. Hall, S., Bobrow, M., and Marteau, T.M. (2000). Psychological consequences for parents of false negative results on prenatal screening for Down's syndrome: retrospective interview study. *British Medical Journal*, **320**, 407–12.

57. Searle, J. (1997). Routine antenatal screening: not a case of informed choice. *Australian and New Zealand Journal of Public Health*, **21**, 268–74.

58. van den Berg, M., Timmermans, D.R., ten Kate, L.P., *et al.* (2005). Informed decision making in the context of prenatal screening. *Patient Education and Counseling*, **63**, 110–17.

# Syndromes causing intellectual disability

David M. Clarke and Shoumitro Deb

## Introduction

Psychiatrists working with people who have intellectual disability (mental retardation) need expertise in the diagnosis and treatment of associated neuropsychiatric disorders. This entails knowledge of the causes of intellectual disability, and especially knowledge about those syndromal (often genetic) causes that are associated with neuropsychiatric manifestations. Such manifestations include vulnerability to behavioural and emotional disorders, epilepsy, and particular patterns of cognitive strength and weakness. This chapter provides an introduction to some such disorders and a discussion of the concept of behavioural phenotypes. For a detailed account of conditions causing intellectual disability texts such as Jones[1] should be consulted. The concept of behavioural phenotypes is discussed in detail in O'Brien.[2]

The genetic aetiologies of intellectual disability include chromosomal abnormalities (trisomy, deletion, translocation, etc), single-gene defects, and the effect of interactions between several genes. The last is thought to account for a substantial proportion of people with mild intellectual disability by setting a ceiling on possible cognitive attainment (life experiences, nutrition, education, and other factors then determining the extent to which potential is fulfilled or thwarted).

This chapter discusses the concepts of syndromes and behavioural phenotypes, then describes the clinical features of a number of syndromes that cause intellectual disability. Down syndrome, fragile-X syndrome, sex chromosome anomalies, and foetal alcohol syndrome are described in some detail. This is followed by a briefer alphabetical list of less common conditions.

## Syndromes

A syndrome is a characteristic pattern of clinical features, including signs (that can be observed) and symptoms a patient may experience. They may be causes of intellectual disability (Down syndrome), associated with intellectual disability (syndromes of epilepsy, such as West syndrome), or coincidental (polycystic ovary syndrome). This chapter deals with some of the syndromes that increase vulnerability to intellectual disability. The vulnerability may be increased so much that all affected people have intellectual disability (Angelman syndrome) or increased to the extent that many, but not all, have intellectual disability (velo-cardio-facial syndrome).

There can be disadvantages to the labelling of people with disability, but the identification of a syndromal cause may have benefits for the affected person and for their families and carers. Benefits include an explanation of the cause of the person's disabilities or of unusual cognitive strengths and weaknesses, better understanding of risk of recurrence of the disorder among relatives, and the identification of complications or associated features.

Identification of a syndromal cause may give access to support organizations. A list of such organizations is given in the CaF (Contact a Family) Directory (www.cafamily.org.uk).

## Behavioural phenotypes

Behavioural, social, linguistic, or cognitive aspects of a syndrome may be so striking and characteristic as to prompt diagnosis. Examples include the severe self-injury associated with Lesch–Nyhan syndrome and the combination of appetite abnormality, ritualistic behaviours, sleep abnormalities, skin-picking, repetitive speech, and vulnerability to psychiatric disorder associated with Prader–Willi syndrome. Such patterns of vulnerability to particular emotional or behavioural problems or peculiarities associated with biologically determined syndromes have been called behavioural phenotypes. Environmental factors may interact with a genetically determined vulnerability to a behaviour to determine whether or not it occurs in a given setting. Knowledge of the nature of this interaction may be important in order to determine effective treatment or management strategies. In Lesch–Nyhan disease, for example, all affected men self-injure, but whether a man with the syndrome injures himself at a particular time is influenced by environmental and internal psychological factors such as anxiety. A careful assessment of the causes and consequences of behavioural problems is essential before interventions are planned, particularly the use of psychotropic medication to influence behaviour.[3]

## Specific conditions

### Down syndrome

#### (a) Prevalence and genetics

J. Langdon Down originally described the syndrome in 1887. Trisomy 21 is associated with Down syndrome, and was first reported by Lejeune and colleagues in 1958. About 1 in 600 live born children have Down syndrome. The rate increases with increasing maternal age, being about 1 in 2000 at maternal age 20 years and 1 in 100 at maternal age of 40 years.[4] There are three types of abnormalities affecting chromosome 21. In about 94 per cent of cases, Down syndrome is caused by primary non-disjunction leading to trisomy 21. The risk of recurrence of this abnormality is low if maternal age is also relatively low. In about 2 per cent of cases Down syndrome results from an unbalanced translocation (when material from one chromosome is separated and attached to another with some duplication). This often involves chromosomes 21 and 14. In some cases a parent also has a balanced translocation (with no overall disruption or duplication of genetic material), and this raises the risk of recurrence. Chromosome 21 to 21 translocations can occur. Mosaicism occurs when there are two or more cell lines within the body. In Down syndrome there may be one cell line with trisomy 21 and one without. In about 2 per cent of cases the syndrome results from mosaicism. Some cases may not be diagnosed. The proportion of affected and unaffected cell lines varies, as does the intellectual impairment.

### (b) Physical characteristics

Muscular hypotonia at birth usually improves with development. Most adults are of short stature and have a characteristic facial appearance. The eyes seem to slope upwards and outwards, the nose has a wide bridge and the head has an unusual shape (brachycephaly). Limb abnormalities include a single transverse crease on the palm, a large cleft between the first and second toes, and relatively short upper arms. People with Down syndrome are prone to thyroid abnormalities. About 25 per cent develop hypothyroidism during childhood or adolescence. About half of affected people have a heart abnormality. Abnormalities of the gastro-intestinal tract occur in a significant minority. Life expectancy has improved markedly over the past 50 years. Survival into the eighth decade is unusual but not extraordinary. Changes in blood cells are relatively common. Older texts reported an association between Down syndrome and leukaemia, but recent research suggests that leukaemia is rare, affecting less than 1 per cent of people with Down syndrome.

### (c) Behavioural and psychiatric aspects

Adults with Down syndrome are much more likely to develop dementia than the general population. On post-mortem examination, the brains of almost all adults with Down syndrome over the age of 35 show changes characteristic of dementia of Alzheimer type. Only about 38 per cent of those aged 50 to 59 have clinically apparent dementia, with a mean age at diagnosis around 51 years.[5,6]

The stereotype of people with Down syndrome as happy, placid individuals with a gift for mimicry is not borne out by recent behavioural research. Stubbornness and obsessional features seem to be over-represented, and many people with Down syndrome react adversely in situations involving changes to expected routines or conflict. Autism seems to occur more commonly than would be expected, but few methodologically sound studies have been carried out.[7]

Most adults with Down syndrome have moderate intellectual disability. Almost all children with Down syndrome have some degree of specific speech and language delay. About 25 per cent have features of attention-deficit disorder. Cognitive abilities tend to be greater among people whose Down syndrome is caused by mosaicism for trisomy 21.

Further information: www.downs-syndrome.org.uk

## X-linked intellectual disability

The prevalence of X-linked intellectual disability is around 0.18 per cent.[8] The majority of affected men have non-syndromic X-linked intellectual disability (usually referred to as X-linked mental retardation or XLMR in international literature), with no associated dysmorphology. The most common syndrome resulting in XLMR is fragile-X syndrome (described below). Coffin–Lowry syndrome (CLS) is also described below. It is increasingly accepted that there is a spectrum of disorders associated with XLMR genes, ranging from defined syndromes such as CLS to XLMR with no dysmorphology. For example, the gene RSK2 is usually mutated in Coffin–Lowry syndrome but a missense mutation in exon 14 of RSK2 has been found in a family in which males have intellectual disability but no associated features of CLS.[9] An interesting article described a woman with mild intellectual disability, epilepsy, and some minor dysmorphology whose karyotype was reported as normal in 1993. Repeated testing was carried out after she was found to have a more severely affected brother with a duplication affecting his X chromosome showed 46,X dup (X)(p22.13p22.31). The authors concluded that genetic testing for individuals with intellectual disability should be considered even when there was a low index of suspicion for an X-linked disorder.[10] About 200 XLMR conditions and 45 cloned genes have now been described.[11] At least eight genes have so far been implicated in non-specific XLMR: Rab-GDI, PAK3, AGTR2, TM4SF2, FRAXE (FMR2), ARHGEF6/αPIX, and FACL4.[12] Readers are referred to specialized texts such as Jaquemont et al. (2005)[12] and web resources such as xlmr.interfree.it/home for further details.

## Fragile-X syndrome

### (a) Prevalence and genetics

The syndrome was first described in 1943. All ethnic groups are affected equally, with a frequency of about 0.3 per 1000 in men. More recent investigations with modern diagnostic techniques show lower figures than earlier studies.[13]

Fragile-X syndrome is an X-linked disorder with a very unusual pattern of inheritance. It is characterized by a bias to affected men but with some affected women and some unaffected men who have daughters who then have affected sons. When peripheral blood lymphocytes from affected individuals are grown in certain culture conditions, including a lack of folic acid, a fragile site becomes evident on the long (q) arm of the X chromosome at Xq27.3 (fragile site A). Fragile sites may not be seen in some unaffected men who transmit the abnormality to their carrier daughters. These men were historically termed 'normal transmitting males'. The probability that a child with a fragile-X chromosome will have intellectual disability depends on the sex of the parent from whom the chromosome was inherited (higher risk when the chromosome is passed from the mother). The 'fragility' of the X chromosome is now known to be associated with an unstable region of DNA within the fragile-X mental retardation (FMR-1) gene, which was first described in 1991.[14] This region of unstable DNA gradually increases in length and degree of instability in successive generations (a pre-mutation) until a critical point is reached and the gene no longer functions (a full mutation). The instability is caused by an increase in CGG (cytosine-guanine-guanine) repeats from the 50 or so repeats that are usual to 50–100 repeats (pre-mutation) to over 230 repeats (full mutation). The chance of a child inheriting a lengthened gene is proportional to the length of the unstable region in the carrier mother. The severity of intellectual disability and other fragile-X related phenomena in women probably depends mostly on the proportion of cells in which the abnormal chromosome is inactivated, X inactivation being random. Most women who have children with fragile-X syndrome are premutation carriers of normal intelligence.[15] Carriers of the premutation are intellectually unimpaired but are more vulnerable than other women to anxiety and depression.[16] Variants of fragile-X syndrome have now been identified, with DNA expansions nearer to the end of the long arm of the X chromosome. These include FraX-E and FraX-F.

### (b) Physical characteristics

Physical features are variable. The most characteristic feature is that about 95 per cent of affected men have large testes, although macro-orchidism is not usually apparent until after puberty. Other features include a long face with a large forehead, large ears, a large lower jaw, and high-arched palate. There is a connective tissue disorder that may lead to tissue laxity with hyper-extensible joints, flat feet, heart defects (especially valve abnormalities), and ear infections (the eustachian tube closes easily). Cataracts and other eye abnormalities may occur, and lead to impaired vision. About 30 per cent of affected men have epilepsy. Life expectancy depends on the severity of associated features such as epilepsy and cardiovascular anomalies.

### (c) Behavioural and psychiatric aspects

There is usually some degree of social impairment, with social anxiety and avoidance of eye-to-eye contact, but with social responsiveness. Men with fragile-X are usually affectionate, and do not have the aloof quality typical of autism. Self-injury is relatively common, especially hand biting over the anatomical snuff-box (between the bases of the thumb and index finger) in response to frustration, anxiety, or excitement. Stereotyped behaviours such as hand flapping are common.

The associated intellectual disability is usually mild to moderate. Verbal intelligence scores exceed performance scores among populations of affected men and non-disabled women carriers. Speech and language development is delayed. Speech is often disorganized, with rambling and circuitous conversation, incomplete sentences, poor topic maintenance, tangential comments, echolalia, and perseveration. It may be rapid, or include peculiar changes in pitch.

There may be problems with attention and concentration that are disproportionate to the severity of the associated learning disability. Hyperactivity may be the presenting feature among boys with fragile-X who do not have intellectual disability.

Further information can be obtained from Hagerman and Hagerman (2002)[17] and www.fragilex.org.uk.

### Sex chromosome abnormalities

The Y chromosome is small and has been completely mapped.[18] The X chromosome is much larger, containing over 1000 genes. Abnormalities of the X and Y chromosomes are more prevalent than those affecting autosomal chromosomes. Many affected children are not significantly dysmorphic and do not have major developmental disabilities.[19] Some remain undiagnosed.

### Klinefelter syndrome

#### (a) Prevalence and genetics

This is a disorder characterized by additional X chromosomes in phenotypic males. Two-thirds have a 47 XXY chromosome complement. Prevalence at birth is about 1 in 1000 live males, with a frequency in prenatally karyotyped male foetuses of 1 in 470.[19]

#### (b) Physical characteristics

Height, weight, and head circumference are below average at birth. Increased growth, especially of legs occurs from 3 years of age onwards. Affected men are usually taller than their fathers, and mean heights are around the 75th centile. Head size remains small. Puberty normally occurs, but testosterone production falls in early adult life. Affected adults have a normal-sized penis but small testes. About 60 per cent have some breast enlargement. Life expectancy is thought to be normal.

#### (c) Behavioural and psychiatric aspects

Boys with XXY are typically introverted and less assertive and sociable than other children, with poorer school performance (especially with regard to reading and spelling). Adults may have increased rates of antisocial behaviour and impulsiveness. The IQ distribution is skewed downwards, although measured full scale IQs run from the 60s to the 130s. Performance scores usually exceed verbal scores. Most affected children receive speech and language therapy, and expressive language deficits are often more pronounced than problems with receptive language. One follow-up study has been reported.[20] Further information: www.klinefeltersyndrome.org.

### Turner syndrome

#### (a) Prevalence and genetics

The genetic abnormality in Turner syndrome is the loss or abnormality of one X chromosome in women. The 45,X karyotype is found in about 1 in 10 000 live female births. The abnormality is much more common at conception. About 99 per cent of affected foetuses are miscarried, and 45,X is the most common karyotype found in chromosomally aborted foetuses. About 50 per cent have a 45,X chromosome complement (a very small proportion of normal cell lines may be present). Most of the other cases are the result of mosaicism, some are the result of structural abnormalities of an X chromosome.

#### (b) Physical characteristics

Affected children have a short stature in childhood. Ovarian failure occurs before birth, and puberty does not usually occur naturally, although childbirth has, rarely, been reported. Dysmorphic features include a webbed neck, low hairline at the rear of the head, widely spaced nipples and multiple pigmented naevi. About 12 per cent have coarctation of the aorta or a ventricular septal defect.

#### (c) Behavioural and psychiatric aspects

Hyperactivity and distractibility are common in childhood. Poor social skills, with immature social relationships and low self-esteem in adolescence were reported in one study.[21] Women with Turner syndrome are usually of normal intelligence and verbal abilities are usually unimpaired or enhanced. Specific cognitive abnormalities including deficits in spatial perception, visual motor integration, affect recognition, visual memory, and attention have been reported.[22] The relative strength in verbal tasks may lead to an overestimation of abilities. There is considerable variation in cognitive profile between affected women. Further information: www.tss.org.uk

## XXX syndrome

### (a) Genetics and prevalence

The 47,XXX syndrome occurs about 1 in 1000 female births.[23] Many are not diagnosed. There is a primary non-disjunction of a maternal or paternal X chromosome. The 48,XXXX chromosome complement is much rarer (about 40 cases have been reported so far).

### (b) Physical characteristics

In 47,XXX syndrome newborn babies have a low birth weight and small head circumference. Height in adult life is usually increased, with a low body mass index. Fertility is not usually impaired, although there are reports of premature ovarian failure and recurrent spontaneous abortion. There may be deficits in balance or fine motor coordination. Life expectancy is thought to be normal.

### (c) Behavioural and psychiatric aspects

Underactivity and withdrawal have been reported. Emotional development may be slowed. About a quarter of affected women in one follow-up study had repeated episodes of abdominal pain as teenagers for which no organic cause could be found.[24] Most appear to adapt to adult life without difficulties. Women with the syndrome usually have IQs between 80 and 90. Women with XXXX syndrome have lower IQs (55 to 75). An expressive language delay is typical. Some have a relatively poor short-term auditory memory. Further information: www.triplo-x.org.

## XYY syndrome

### (a) Genetics, prevalence, and physical characteristics

This karyotype is associated with 1 in 1000 live male births.[23] There is a primary non-disjunction of the Y chromosome. About 10 per cent have mosaic 46,XY/47,XYY chromosome complement. Offsprings rarely have two Y chromosomes. Affected individuals show increase in body and leg length between years 4 and 9. Most are over 10 cm taller than their fathers as adults. Sexual development and fertility are unaffected. Balance and coordination may be minimally compromised. Life expectancy is normal.

### (b) Behavioural and psychiatric aspects

Early research found an increased frequency of XYY men among inmates of special prisons.[25,26] More recent studies examining the relationship between 47,XYY karyotype and behaviour have concluded that affected men have lower mean intelligence scores (with a large overlap with the normal range) and poorer social adaptation. Distractibility, hyperactivity, temper tantrums, and speech and language problems appear relatively common in childhood. There is little evidence to suggest a significant link with seriously aggressive criminal conduct in adult life.[27,28]

## Foetal alcohol syndrome

### (a) Classification and prevalence

Exposure of the developing foetus to significant amounts of alcohol leads to cognitive impairment. The effect can occur during any stage of pregnancy, because brain development continues during all three trimesters. Dysmorphology, including a facial dysmorphology, can also occur. Foetal alcohol spectrum disorder (FASD) includes a number of subtypes including foetal alcohol syndrome (FAS), and more subtle abnormalities subsumed under the terms possible foetal alcohol effects (PFAE), prenatal exposure to alcohol (PEA), or alcohol-related neurodevelopmental disorder (ARND).

Foetal alcohol exposure is thought to be a common cause of intellectual disability in the United States and other developed countries. In the United States, an estimate of 0.33 per 1000 births has been given for the prevalence of foetal alcohol syndrome.[29] Alcohol inhibits $N$-methyl-D-aspartate receptors, which mediate postsynaptic excitatory effects of glutamate, and this is thought to have an effect on cell proliferation.[30]

### (b) Clinical features

A number of abnormalities have been linked to FAS. Facial dysmorphology commonly includes a thin upper lip and smooth philtrum. The jaw may be small. Low-set abnormal ears and palate abnormalities can occur. Other abnormalities include growth retardation, skeletal abnormalities (deformed ribs and sternum, spinal curvature, dislocated hips, fused or webbed or missing fingers or toes, limited joint movement, small head), heart abnormalities, and urinary tract anomalies.

### (c) Neurological and behavioural aspects

Central nervous system abnormalities include a small brain with abnormally arranged cells. Intellectual disability is usually mild or moderate but may be severe. Other problems commonly include reduction in attention span, overactivity, irritability in infancy; and coordination problems.

## Angelman syndrome

### (a) Prevalence and genetics

The prevalence of this syndrome is around 1 in 10 000 births.[31] Most cases are sporadic, and associated with deletions within 15q11q13 of maternal origin (Prader–Willi syndrome). Angelman syndrome is occasionally associated with paternal uniparental disomy (both chromosome 15s are of paternal origin) but this is less common than in Prader–Willi syndrome. Other genetic abnormalities leading to Angleman syndrome are an imprinting centre defect (this incorrectly 'marks' the chromosome, through methylation, as being from a parent of the opposite sex) and mutations in the gene responsible for the Angelman syndrome phenotype (UBE3A, coding for a ubiquitin ligase enzyme).[32] UBE3A is expressed only from the maternal chromosome, and in Angelman syndrome expression in relevant brain areas is only around 10 per cent of normal.

### (b) Physical characteristics

Physical characteristics include a small head, characteristic face with wide mouth, 'hooked' nose, prominent lower jaw, widely spaced teeth, and tongue protrusion. Many affected children are hypopigmented compared to first degree relatives due to deletion of a gene related to pigmentation.[33] Voluntary movements are jerky and the gait ataxic with stiff legs. About 80 per cent develop epilepsy, and the EEG is highly characteristic.

### (c) Behavioural and psychiatric aspects

Behavioural characteristics, including sudden bursts of laughter and the jerky ataxic gait, led to the term 'happy puppet' syndrome being used in the literature of the 1960s and 1970s. It is no longer considered appropriate. Affected children enjoy social and physical contact, and mouthing objects. Many are fascinated by water. Intellectual disability is severe, with markedly delayed motor milestones. There is little speech development (no person reported in the literature has more than a six word vocabulary), but understanding of language may be better. Overactivity is often associated with a short attention span in childhood, but may improve with development. Behavioural studies have been reported[34] and genetic aspects reviewed.[35] Further information: www.assert.dial. pipex.com/

## Coffin–Lowry syndrome

### (a) Prevalence and genetics

Coffin–Lowry syndrome is one cause of X linked intellectual disability. The syndrome has been ascribed to a locus in the Xp22.1-p22.2 region. More than 100 cases have been reported.

### (b) Physical characteristics

Physical features include short stature, facial dysmorphology including slanting eye fissures, prominent forehead, short broad nose, forward facing nostrils, large ears, large mouth and small, widely spaced teeth. Increased fatty tissue is deposited in the forearms. Hands are often large, with tapering fingers. Ligament laxity may lead to flat feet. Spinal and chest abnormalities occur. Behavioural and emotional characteristics are largely unknown, although depression and schizophrenia have been reported in association with the disorder and in female carriers.

### (c) Behavioural and psychiatric aspects

Affected men usually have severe learning disabilities. Drop attacks and sleep apnoea syndrome have been reported. Further information: www.clsf.info.

## Congenital hypothyroidism

### (a) Prevalence

Following the introduction of a neonatal screening programme in the United Kingdom, the incidence of congenital hypothyroidism (identified through heel-prick screening and further investigation for at risk infants) is about 1 in 4000, and occurs more commonly in girls. In many cases the deficiency of thyroid hormones is mild, and there are few symptoms.

### (b) Physical and cognitive characteristics

Severely affected children have a distinctive appearance with a puffy face and a large tongue that protrudes from a mouth that is kept open. Other features include dry, brittle hair, a low hair line, jaundice, sleep disorders, low muscle tone, constipation, and failure of cognitive development leading to intellectual disability. If untreated, even mild hypothyroidism may lead to intellectual disability.

## Cri-du-Chat syndrome (CDCS, 5p-syndrome)

### (a) Prevalence and genetics

Cri-du-Chat syndrome was originally described as a syndrome of multiple congenital anomalies, intellectual disability, microcephaly, abnormal face, and a mewing cry in infants with deletion of a 'B group chromosome', later identified as a 5p terminal deletion. The prevalence is about 1 in 35 000 births. Deletions vary in size, but the critical region for Cri-du-Chat syndrome is thought to be 5p15.2. About 85 per cent of the deletions arise spontaneously and the majority are of paternal origin. About 15 per cent of affected people have an unbalanced translocation, and the clinical features depend on the other chromosome involved. Fewer than 1 per cent of cases are due to inherited deletions, which are usually very small.

### (b) Physical characteristics

In infancy there are feeding difficulties and the cry is abnormally high pitched (cat-like, hence 'cri-du-chat'), but this is not an invariable feature. The gene causing the abnormal (cat-like) cry has been located at 15p13. It is possible for infants with small deletions to have a cat-like cry but no other features of CDCS, or features of CDCS without the characteristic cry. A round face with widely spaced slanting eyes, a small head, a broad flat nose, and small lower jaw are characteristic. Ear abnormalities may occur. Larger deletions, and some translocations, are associated with more pronounced clinical features such as lower intelligence, smaller stature, lower weight, and smaller head. The face often lengthens with development and may be asymmetrical. Cleft lip or palate, curved fingers, hernias, and orthopaedic abnormalities may occur. Older individuals often have premature greying of the hair.

### (c) Behavioural and psychiatric aspects

Hyperactivity is a problem for a substantial proportion of children, but may improve with age.[36] Language development is often markedly delayed. The IQ associated with the syndrome in one study varied from 6 to 85. Further information: www.criduchat. asn.au.

## De Lange syndrome (Brachmann–de Lange syndrome)

### (a) Prevalence and genetics

This syndrome is considered to occur about once in 60 000 live births, although some authors believe it to be more common. Mutations in a large gene on chromosome 5, the Nipped B like or *NIPBL* gene (named because its function resembles that of a fruit fly gene that produces a nipped wing), have been shown in about 40 per cent of people with the syndrome.[37]

### (b) Physical characteristics

Affected individuals show growth retardation; distinctive facial features consisting of well-defined arched eyebrows which meet in the middle, long curled eyelashes, small nose with forward-facing nostrils, and down-turned mouth with thin lips and limb abnormalities such as small or shortened limbs, especially arms. Hearing impairments, gut malformations, and congenital heart defects also occur. Early mortality is high because of feeding problems with regurgitation and vomiting leading to aspiration pneumonia in some cases.

### (c) Behavioural and psychiatric aspects

Self-injury, autistic features, and pleasurable responses to vestibular stimulation, e.g. spinning in a chair have been reported as part of behavioural repertoire. The degree of learning disability is usually severe, and speech is often very limited. However, some affected people have IQs within the normal range. Clinicians should be alert to the presence of pain and discomfort resulting from gastro-oesophageal reflux and other gastro-intestinal abnormalities. Further information: www.cdlsusa.org.

# Duchenne muscular dystrophy

## (a) Prevalence and genetics

This is an X linked recessive condition in which deletions, duplications, and mutations at Xp21 lead to failure to produce dystrophin, a protein component of muscle tissue. New mutations account for about 30 per cent of cases. The prevalence at birth is about 1 in 4000 male births.

## (b) Physical characteristics

The syndrome is characterized by progressive muscle weakness, affecting the pelvis, upper leg, and upper arm muscles first. The onset is typically between 2 and 6 years of age. Respiratory muscles are involved later in the disease process. Heart muscle abnormalities may also occur. The disease is usually more severe in the lower limbs and trunk initially, with later involvement of the arms and respiratory muscles. Affected boys often need a wheelchair by around 11 years of age, with death in early adult life (typically in the mid twenties).

## (c) Behavioural and psychiatric aspects

Low mood, anxiety, and social abnormalities are often problems, and may become more prominent as the disorder progresses. These features may be reactions to a chronic and progressive physical disease. Specific learning disabilities are common, especially specific reading disorder. About 25 per cent of those affected have a learning disability. Performance IQ is typically higher than verbal IQ. Further information: www.mda.org.au.

# Lesch–Nyhan syndrome

## (a) Prevalence and genetics

This X-linked recessive disorder results from a deficiency of a purine salvage enzyme, hypoxanthine-guanine phosphoribosyl transferase (HGPRT) leading to hyperuricaemia, and neurological disorder. Partial HGPRT deficiency results in gout. HGPRT is a 217 amino acid peptide coded for by one gene divided into nine exons, located on the X chromosome at Xq26q27. Many different genetic lesions can cause HGPRT deficiency. Complete and partial deletions, insertions, and duplication of exons have been reported. Most lesions appear to be point mutations. Affected males may have had spontaneous mutations or inherited mutations from asymptomatic female carriers. Carrier detection and prenatal diagnosis are possible. The incidence is around 1 in 380 000 births.[38]

## (b) Physical characteristics

Neurological features include athetoid and other abnormal movements and spasticity. Growth retardation is usual. The presentation is usually with hypotonia and motor delay at about 4 months. Extrapyramidal signs (such as spasticity and choreo-athetoid movements) develop at about 9 months. Hyper-reflexia and clonus appear at about 1 year. Dystonic movements may also develop. Dysarthria is common. Affected individuals may survive to the second or third decade. Death is usually due to kidney failure secondary to uric acid deposition or infection. The syndrome is associated with abnormal neurotransmitter turnover in the basal ganglia.

## (c) Behavioural and psychiatric aspects

Compulsive severe self-injury is very prevalent and usually consists of finger and lip biting, with self-splinting in an attempt to prevent the behaviour.[39] Other compulsive behaviours occur; men with the syndrome are reported to hit, spit, and swear at caregivers while apologizing for their behaviour at the same time.[40] The mean age at onset of self-injury is 3.5 years, with wide variation. The IQ is usually between 40 and 80, but dysarthria and neurological problems limit the validity of standard IQ tests. Further information: www.lndinfo.org.

# Mucopolysaccharidoses

## (a) Classification, genetics, and prevalence

The mucopolysaccharide group of disorders have both names (Hunter syndrome, Hurler syndrome, Sanfillipo syndrome, Morquio syndrome, Schie syndrome, Maroteaux–Lamy syndrome, Sly syndrome) and numerical designations (MPS IIA/B, MPS IH, MPS IIIA/B/C/D, MPS IVA/B, MPS IS, MPSVI, MPSVII, respectively). The disorders result from deficiencies in enzyme systems involved in the degradation of glycosaminoglycans leading to the accumulation of abnormal metabolic products. The prevalences among live born children are approximately 1 in 100 000 for Hunter and Hurler syndromes, 1 in 200 000 for all types of Sanfillipo syndrome and for Morquio syndrome, and 1 in 500 000 for Schie syndrome. Hunter syndrome is much more prevalent in Israel. The transmission is autosomal recessive except in Hunter (IIA and IIB) which is X linked.

## (b) Physical characteristics

Physical features vary. Coarse facial features ('gargoylism'), hepatosplenomegaly, joint stiffness, eye abnormalities, and short stature occur in many of the disorders. Life expectancy varies from death in the first decade in Hurler syndrome through survival into second or third decade in Sanfillipo syndrome, to survival to adult life in Hunter syndrome and Schie syndrome.

## (c) Behavioural and psychiatric aspects

Sleep problems and abnormal nocturnal behaviours such as staying up all night, night-time laughing and singing, sudden crying out, and chewing of bedclothes have been reported in association with Sanfillipo syndrome, and have been shown to respond to behavioural management strategies. Other problem behaviours reported in association with MPS disorders include aggression, overactivity, restlessness, and anxiety. Cognitive abilities vary from normal intelligence in Schie syndrome to severe learning disability and progressive cognitive deterioration in Hurler syndrome. Sanfillipo syndrome is associated with slower progressive cognitive impairment than that seen in Hurler syndrome, but often with marked behavioural and psychiatric abnormalities consistent with the diagnosis of childhood disintegrative disorder. The susceptibility to tooth decay in Morquio syndrome can lead to pain and problem behaviours. Further information: www.mpssociety.org.

# Neurofibromatosis type 1

## (a) Prevalence and genetics

This autosomal dominant disorder was first described by von Recklinghausen in 1882 and occurs about once in 3000 births. The gene responsible is localized to 17q11.2. The gene product, neurofibromin, regulates cell division and is thought to suppress tumour formation. A high spontaneous mutation rate means that about a half of all cases of NF1 arise in unaffected families.

## (b) Physical characteristics

Tumours arise from the connective tissue of nerve sheaths. Two or more of the following features are usually required for diagnosis:

six or more cafe au lait (light brown) skin lesions more than 5 mm in diameter before puberty or 15 mm after puberty, two or more neurofibromas or one plexiform neurofibroma (tumours of the nerve sheath); freckling of the inguinal or axillary region; two or more lisch nodules (benign iris hamartomas); an optic nerve glioma (tumour); a bony lesion characteristic of neurofibromatosis (usually shin bowing or scoliosis), a first degree relative with the disorder. About 45 per cent of affected people will have non-enhancing hyperintensities (or unidentified bright objects 'UBOs') on magnetic resonance imaging. These are commonly seen in the cerebellum, basal ganglia, brain stem, and thalamus.[41]

### (c) Behavioural and psychiatric aspects

About 50 per cent of children have speech or language abnormalities. Distractibility and impulsiveness may be problems. Learning disability is present in about 10 per cent of affected people. Specific developmental disorders such as difficulties with reading, writing, or numeracy affect about half of the children. Visuo-spatial abnormalities and lack of coordination have also been described. Further information: www.geneclinics.org/profiles/nf1.

## Phenylketonuria

### (a) Prevalence and genetics

Classical phenylketonuria affects about 1 in 10 000 live born children in the United Kingdom. Other hyperphenylalaninaemias also occur. The disorder results from a deficiency of the enzyme phenylalanine hydroxylase. The extent of the deficiency varies, with a spectrum of resulting clinical conditions from classical phenylketonuria to benign hyperphenylalaninaemia. The gene regulating phenylalanine hydroxylase is located at 12q22-24.1. It is subject to various mutations. The classical form is inherited in an autosomal recessive manner. Prenatal diagnosis and the detection of heterozygotes with one defective copy of the gene are possible. About 2 per cent of cases are due to a deficiency of tetrahydrobiopterin rather than phenylalanine hydroxylase.

### (b) Physical characteristics

Physical features include blond hair, blue eyes, eczema, and microcephaly (in half the suffers), epilepsy (in a quarter) and tremor and movement disorders or spasticity. Untreated infants have an unusual mouse-like body odour. In the United Kingdom all neonates are screened for the disorder. A low phenylalanine diet is usually continued through childhood. There is debate about the age at which it is appropriate to lift or relax dietary restrictions. Amino-acid supplements may be used to block phenylalanine uptake. Dietary control is essential when affected women become pregnant, because hyperphenylalaninaemia is toxic to the foetus leading to learning disability, microcephaly, and facial and heart abnormalities. Theories about the toxic effects of hyperphenylyalaninaemia include direct toxicity, competition for transport across the blood–brain barrier and dopamine depletion.[42]

### (c) Behavioural and psychiatric aspects

Untreated phenylketonuria is associated with a number of maladaptive behaviours and behavioural syndromes including overactivity, self-injury, and autism. Autism and many of the other features do not occur in children managed with low phenylalanine diets. Those who have not been treated may have moderate to profound learning disabilities, irritability, and marked social impairments. Inadequate dietary control is associated with deficits in mathematical,

visuo-spatial, and language skills. Further information: www.nspku.org.

## Prader–Willi syndrome

### (a) Prevalence and genetics

The prevalence is around 1 in 40 000 live born infants.[43] About 70 per cent of those affected have a deletion affecting the long arm of chromosome 15 (del 15q11q13), the deleted chromosome always being of paternal origin. About 29 per cent have maternal uniparental disomy (MUPD) in which both chromosome 15s are inherited from mother, with no paternal chromosome 15. About 1 per cent have an imprinting error, in which the paternal chromosome is incorrectly methylated so as to resemble a maternal one.

### (b) Physical characteristics

Infants are hypotonic or floppy and have feeding problems associated with a failure to suck. Many are tube fed. In early childhood there is a switch to marked overeating. Affected adults are of short stature, have small hands and feet and a characteristic pattern of facial appearance, and a lack of sexual development. Affected people were often obese, as a result of the impaired satiety leading to overeating, but modern dietary management and treatment with growth hormone in childhood may lead to near normal body size and shape. There is an increased prevalence of curvature of the spine or scoliosis and other orthopaedic abnormalities, and diabetes or heart failure may result from obesity. Life expectancy depends on severity of obesity.

### (c) Behavioural, cognitive, and psychiatric aspects

Affected individuals have an almost insatiable appetite. They may steal food and consume 'unpalatable' food such as rotting or frozen food or pet food. A variety of sleep abnormalities and a lowering of the threshold for loss of temper may be associated. About 80 per cent pick or scratch their skin. Insistence on routines, and compulsive behaviours are commonly reported.[44] Severe psychiatric disorders including affective and psychotic states are more prevalent, especially among people with MUPD.[45] Anecdotal reports suggest the pain threshold may be raised.

About 5 per cent of those with this syndrome have overall cognitive abilities with IQs in excess of 85, 27 per cent have borderline cognitive abilities with IQs between 70 and 85, 34 per cent have mild learning disabilities, 27 per cent moderate, 5 per cent severe, and less than 1 per cent have profound learning disability. There are deficits in auditory information processing, and relative strengths in visuo-spatial tasks. Further information: www.ipwso.org.

## Rett syndrome

### (a) Prevalence and genetics

Rett syndrome causes severe intellectual disability in women. The prevalence in the United Kingdom is around 1 in 10 000 women.[46] The syndrome results from a mutation in the MeCP2 gene located at Xq28. The mutation was considered to be lethal in males but there are a small number of males with the syndrome. The severity of the syndrome in women depends on the percentage of cells with the normal MeCP2 gene active after X inactivation. If more of the X chromosomes with normal MeCP2 gene have been inactivated, the syndrome is likely to be more severe. MeCP2 acts as a mechanistic bridge between DNA methylation and histone methylation.[47]

### (b) Physical characteristics

The affected child appears normal at birth. For the first 12 months no major abnormalities are apparent though the child may be placid, lack muscle tone, or be relatively immobile. She acquires skills to about 1 year with regression and loss of skills from around 18 months onwards. Speech and use of hands are particularly affected. Physical problems increase with age, and include scoliosis, spasticity, and leg deformities. Epilepsy is common. Pathological changes include a reduction in brain size with reduced cortical thickness, reduced neuronal branching, and depigmentation of the basal ganglia. Many affected girls reach adulthood, but about 1 per cent of them die each year with early death more likely with increasing physical disability.

### (c) Behavioural and psychiatric aspects

Sleep disturbance, withdrawal and episodes of crying occur during the phase of regression around 18 months of age. This is followed by a phase in which development stops. Extreme agitation and over-breathing interspersed with episodes of cessation of breathing then become apparent. The most prominent feature of the behavioural phenotype is the presence of stereotyped movements, especially midline 'hand-wringing' movements. Affected women and girls usually have profound learning disability. Further information: www.rettsyndrome.org.uk.

## Rubinstein–Taybi syndrome

### (a) Prevalence and genetics

This syndrome is one of the 25 most common multiple congenital anomaly syndromes seen in genetic clinics in the United States and has an estimated incidence at 1 in 125 000 live born infants. Microdeletions at 16p13.3 have been described in some cases, and mutations in the gene coding for CREB-binding protein (CBP) found at this locus have been reported to cause the syndrome.[48] A few apparently familial cases have been reported, and four sets of concordant monozygotic twins have been reported.

### (b) Physical characteristics

The affected individuals are usually short, have a small head, a beaked or straight nose and downward slanting eyes. They have a stiff gait. The thumbs and first toes have broad terminal phalanges, often with an angulation deformity. Other congenital anomalies are not uncommon. Inadequate weight gain in infancy, congenital heart defects, urinary tract abnormalities, and severe constipation contribute to morbidity reflected in a hospitalization rate 10 times higher than the general population.

### (c) Behavioural and psychiatric aspects

Findings from postal questionnaire surveys in the United States and United Kingdom indicate that people with the syndrome have a friendly disposition, a propensity to self-stimulatory activities such as rocking and an intolerance of loud noises. Reduced attention span, rocking, spinning, and hand flapping were common in the UK survey.[49] Intellectual disability is usually moderate. Further information: www.rubinstein-taybi.org.

## Smith–Lemli–Opitz syndrome

### (a) Prevalence and genetics

This disorder is thought to occur about once in 30 000 live births. Mildly affected people may be undiagnosed. The syndrome is said to be one of the commonest autosomal recessive conditions affecting people of White European origin in North America, but rare among people of African or Asian origin. The male to female ratio appears to be around 3 to 1 but this may be due to the relative ease with which sexual abnormalities are detectable in men. Abnormalities in the *DHCR7* gene, located at 11q12-13 results in deficiency of the enzyme 7-dehydrocholesterol reductase results in elevated levels of a cholesterol precursor. Treatment with cholesterol supplementation has been attempted.[50]

### (b) Physical characteristics

During pregnancy, the foetus may show growth retardation. Affected individuals may have a small head, drooping eyelids, squint, forward-facing nostrils, small lower jaw, and finger abnormalities such as extra fingers and syndactyly. Males have abnormalities of their external genitalia such as small testes or penis, hypospadias, undescended testes, and female type genitalia. Cleft palate and abnormalities of almost all major organ systems may also occur.

### (c) Behavioural and psychiatric aspects

There is little information available about behavioural and cognitive characteristics. Intelligence varies from normal to severe learning disability. Aggressive and self-injurious behaviours and autistic spectrum disorders have been reported. Further information: www.geneclinics.org/profiles/slo.

## Smith–Magenis syndrome

### (a) Prevalence and genetics

This syndrome, affecting around 1 in 50 000 births, is associated with deletions at 17p11.2.

### (b) Physical characteristics

Affected individuals have flattened mid-face, abnormally shaped upper lip, short hands and feet, single transverse palmar crease, abnormally shaped or placed ears and sometimes a high arched palate or protruding tongue. The facial features may coarsen with development. Ear and eye disorders such as otitis media and squint are relatively common.

### (c) Behavioural and psychiatric aspects

Newborn babies with the syndrome are usually placid, 'floppy' and feed with difficulty. This changes to hyperactivity, self-injury (e.g. head banging, pulling out finger and toe nails and the insertion of objects into body orifices), from about 18 months onwards. Self-hugging and mid-line hand clapping have been reported. Sleep disorders are common with some children waking repeatedly in a state of agitation. An absence of rapid eye movement (REM) sleep has been reported in some patients. Many affected children appear to be relatively insensitive to pain. Behavioural studies have been reported.[36,51] The severity of the cognitive impairment correlates with the size of the 17p11 deletion. Moderate intellectual disability is common. Speech delay is more pronounced than delay in motor achievements. Further information: www.prisms.org.

## Tuberous sclerosis

### (a) Prevalence and genetics

About 1 in 7000 people are affected. It is an autosomal dominant condition but up to 80 per cent of cases arise as a result of spontaneous mutations. The disorder is genetically heterogeneous, with gene linkage to 9q34 and 16p13.

### (b) Physical characteristics

Physical features are very variable. The previously used diagnostic triad of epilepsy, intellectual disability and a characteristic facial skin lesion is seen in only about 30 per cent of people with the disease. The disorder is a multi-system one, with hamartomatous tumours (arising from primitive cells) affecting the brain (in about 90 per cent), skin, kidneys, heart, eyes, teeth, bones, lungs, and other organs. About 80 per cent of affected people have epilepsy. Brain tumours and kidney lesions are common causes of death.

### (c) Behavioural and psychiatric aspects

Tuberous sclerosis is associated with autism and related disorders, hyperactivity and attention-deficit disorder, obsessive and ritualistic behaviour, sleep problems, and occasionally self-injurious or aggressive behaviours. Less than half of affected people have a learning disability. Attention-deficit is common. Of those with learning disability, many have an IQ less than 30. Further information: www.tuberous-sclerosis.org.

## Velo-cardio-facial syndrome

### (a) Prevalence and genetics

First described in 1978[52] this condition is relatively common, affecting about 1 in 2000 people. The disorder has also been called Shprintzen syndrome, Digeorge syndrome, Cayler syndrome, Takao syndrome, conotruncal anomalies face syndrome, 22q11 deletion syndrome, and CATCH22. It is associated with microdeletions at 22q11. About 90 per cent arise *de novo*, with 10 per cent having an affected parent.

### (b) Physical characteristics

Physical features include cardiac abnormalities including ventriculoseptal defects, pulmonary stenosis, and cardiac outlet abnormalities; facial dysmorphology with a prominent nose with broad bridge and squared tip, small head or small lower jaw; ocular abnormalities; cleft palate; short stature and long, thin, hyperextensible fingers. The clinical features associated with the disorder are highly variable in both type and severity.

### (c) Behavioural and psychiatric aspects

Many affected individuals have difficulties with reciprocal social interaction.[53] A high prevalence of severe psychiatric disorders is reported in later life, including high rates of bipolar affective disorder[54] and schizophrenia.[55] Anxiety, social withdrawal and other disorders have also been described. Over 90 per cent have a learning disability. Speech and language problems are common. Further information: www.vcfsef.org.

## Williams syndrome

### (a) Prevalence and genetics

Also known as idiopathic infantile hypercalcaemia, the syndrome affects about 1 in 15 000 infants. Most cases are sporadic though a few familial cases have been reported where the transmission seems to be autosomal dominant. The syndrome is a contiguous gene deletion disorder in which there is variable loss of genetic material involving the Elastin gene at 7q11.3 and sometimes as many as 17 nearby genes in the Williams syndrome critical region.[56]

### (b) Physical characteristics

Infants have difficulties in feeding, are irritable, have constipation and fail to thrive. Over 60 per cent of children have high serum calcium concentrations. This can be treated with a low-calcium diet and vitamin D restriction. The face is distinctive, with prominent cheeks, a wide mouth and flat nasal bridge often described as 'elfin-like'. Kidney and heart lesions (especially supravalvular aortic stenosis and peripheral pulmonary artery stenosis) are common. Growth is usually retarded. Life expectancy is related to metabolic and heart abnormalities.

### (c) Behavioural and psychiatric aspects

Social disinhibition with abnormal friendliness to strangers, overactivity, poor concentration, eating and sleeping abnormalities, abnormal anxiety, poor peer relationships, and abnormally sensitive hearing have been reported.[57,58] About 95 per cent of children with the disorder have a moderate or severe learning disability. Verbal abilities are better developed than visuo-spatial and motor skills. There is an unusual command of language in which expressive language is superficially fluent and articulate but comprehension is far more limited. Further information: www. williams-syndrome.org.

## Further information

Information about individual syndromes is available from the source listed after the relevant syndrome in the text above. O'Brien (2002)[2] gives information about behavioural, cognitive, linguistic and psychiatric aspects of several genetic disorders. The Contact a Family Directory of Specific Conditions and Rare Disorders (CaF Directory) is widely used for basic information about characteristics and carer organizations. A new paper edition is published in January each year and it is also available in CD-ROM format on a quarterly subscription basis: www. cafamily.org.uk.

## References

1. Jones, K. (2005). *Smith's recognizable patterns of human malformation* (6th edn). W.B. Saunders, Philadelphia, PA.
2. O' Brien, G. (ed.) (2002). *Behavioural phenotypes in clinical practice*. Mac Keith Press, Cambridge.
3. Deb, S., Clarke, D., and Unwin, G. (2006). *Using medication to manage behaviour problems among adults with a learning disability: quick reference guide*. University of Birmingham, Royal College of Psychiatrists and Mencap, Birmingham (www.ld-medication.bham. ac.uk).
4. Fryers, T. and Russell, O. (2003). Applied epidemiology. In *Seminars in the psychiatry of learning disabilities* (2nd edn) (eds. W. Fraser and M. Kerr), pp. 16–48. Gaskell, London.
5. Prasher, V.P. (1995). Age-specific prevalence, thyroid dysfunction and depressive symptomatology in adults with Down's syndrome and dementia. *International Journal of Geriatric Psychiatry*, **10**, 25–31.
6. Holland, A.J., Hon, J., Huppert, F.A., *et al.* (1998). Population-based study of the prevalence and presentation of dementia in adults with Down's syndrome. *The British Journal of Psychiatry*, **172**, 493–8.
7. Prasher, V. (2003). Health morbidity in adults with Downsyndrome. In *Seminars in the psychiatry of learning disabilities* (2nd edn) (eds. W. Fraser and M. Kerr), pp. 267–86. Gaskell,London.
8. Herbst, D.S. and Miller, J.R. (1980). Nonspecific X-linked mental retardation II: the frequency in British Columbia. *American Journal of Medical Genetics*, **7**, 461–9.
9. Merienne, K., Jaquot, S., Pannetier, S., *et al.* (1999). A missense mutation in RPS6KA3 (RSK2) responsible for non-specific mental retardation. *Nature Genetics*, **22**, 13–4.
10. Robertshaw, B.A. and MacPherson, J. (2006). Scope for more genetic testing in learning disability. *The British Journal of Psychiatry*, **189**, 99–101.

11. Chiurazzi, P., Tabolacci, E., and Neri, G. (2004). X-linked mental retardation (XLMR): from clinical conditions to cloned genes. *Critical Reviews in Clinical Laboratory Sciences*, **41**, 117–58.

12. Jaquemont, S., des Portes, V., and Hagerman, R. (2005). Fragile X and X-linked mental retardation. In *Genetics of developmental disabilities* (eds. M.G. Butler and F.J. Meaney), pp. 247–78. Taylor & Francis, Boca Raton.

13. Morton, J.E., Bundey, S., Webb, T.P., *et al.* (1997). Fragile-X syndrome is less common than previously estimated. *Journal of Medical Genetics*, **34**, 1–5.

14. Verkerk, A.J., Pieretti, M., Sutcliffe, J.S., *et al.* (1991). Identification of a gene (FMR-1) containing a CGG repeat coincident with a breakpoint cluster region exhibiting length variation in fragile X syndrome. *Cell*, **54**, 905–14.

15. Hagerman, R.J. and Lampe, M.E. (1999). Fragile X syndrome. In *Handbook of neurodevelopmental and genetic disorders in children* (eds. S. Goldstein and C.R. Reynolds), pp. 298–316. Guilford Press, New York.

16. Hagerman, R.J. (1996). Physical and behavioural phenotype. In *Fragile X syndrome: diagnosis, treatment and research* (2nd edn) (eds. R.J. Hagerman and A.C. Cronister), pp. 3–87. Johns Hopkins University Press, Baltimore.

17. Hagerman, R.J. and Hagerman, P.J. (2002). *Fragile X syndrome: diagnosis, treatment and research*. Johns Hopkins University Press, Baltimore.

18. Tilford, C.A., Kuroda-Kawaguchi, T., Skaletsky, H., *et al.* (2001). A physical map of the human Y chromosome. *Nature*, **409**, 943–5.

19. Hammerton, J.L. and Evans, J.A. (2005). Sex chromosome anomalies. In *Genetics of developmental disabilities* (eds. M.G. Butler and F.J. Meaney), pp. 585–650. Taylor & Francis, Boca Raton.

20. Radcliffe, S. (1999). Long-term outcome in children of sex chromosome abnormalities. *Archives of Disease in Childhood*, **80**, 192–5.

21. McCauley, E., Ross, J.L., Kushner, H., *et al.* (1995). Self-esteem and behaviour in girls with Turner syndrome. *Journal of Developmental and Behavioral Pediatrics*, **16**, 82–8.

22. Romans, S.M., Stefanatos, G., Roeltgen, D.P., *et al.* (1998). Transition to young adulthood in Ullrich-Turner syndrome: neurodevelopmental changes. *American Journal of Medical Genetics*, **79**, 140–8.

23. Hook, E.B. and Hamerton, J.L. (1977). The frequency of chromosome abnormalities detected in consecutive newborn studies: results by sex and by severity of phenotypic involvement. In *Population cytogenetics* (eds. E. Hook and I.H. Porter), pp. 63–79. Academic Press, New York.

24. Robinson, A., Bender, B.G., and Linden, M.G. (1991). Summary of clinical findings in children and young adults with sex chromosome anomalies. In *Children and young adults with sex chromosome aneuploidy* (eds. J.A. Evans, J.L. Hamerton, and A. Robinson), pp. 225–8. Wiley-Liss, New York.

25. Jacobs, P.A., Brunton, M., Melville, M.M., *et al.* (1965). Aggressive behaviour, mental subnormality, and the XYY male. *Nature*, **208**, 1351–2.

26. Jacobs, P.A., Price, W.H., Court Brown, W.M., *et al.* (1969). Chromosome studies on men in a maximum security hospital. *Annals of Human Genetics*, **31**, 339–58.

27. Witkin, H.A., Mednick, S.A., Schulsinger, F., *et al.* (1976). Criminality in XYY and XXY men. *Science*, **193**, 547–55.

28. Fryns, J.P., Kleczkowska, A., Kubien, E., *et al.* (1995). XYY syndrome and other Y chromosome polysomies. Mental status and social functioning. *Genetic Counseling*, **6**, 197–206.

29. Abel, E.L. and Sokel, R.J. (1987). Incidence of fetal alcohol syndrome and economic impact of FAS-related anomalies: drug alcohol syndrome and economic impact of FAS-related anomalies. *Drug and Alcohol Dependence*, **19**, 51–70.

30. West, J.R., Perrotta, D.M., and Erickson, C.K. (1998). Fetal alcohol syndrome: a review for Texas physicians. *Medical Journal of Texas*, **94**, 61–7.

31. Petersen, M.B., Brondum-Nielsen, K., Hansen, L.K., *et al.*(1995). Clinical, cytogenetic, and molecular diagnosis of Angelman syndrome: estimated prevalence in a Danish county. *American Journal of Medical Genetics*, **60**, 261–2.

32. Kishino, T., Lalande, M., and Wagstaff, J. (1997). UBE3A/E6-AP mutations cause Angelman syndrome. *Nature Genetics*, **15**, 70–73 [erratum in *Nature Genetics*, **15**, 411].

33. King, R.A., Wiesner, G.L., Townsend, D., *et al.* (1993). Hypopigmentation in Angelman syndrome. *American Journal of Medical Genetics*, **46**, 40–4.

34. Clarke, D.J. and Marston, G. (2000). Problem behaviors associated with 15q-Angelman syndrome. *American Journal of Mental Retardation*, **105**, 25–31.

35. Williams, C.A. (2005). Angelman syndrome. In *Genetics of developmental disabilities* (eds. M.G. Butler and F.J. Meaney), pp. 319–35. Taylor & Francis, Boca Raton.

36. Clarke, D.J. and Boer, H. (1998). Problem behaviours associated with deletion Prader-Willi, Smith-Magenis and Cri du chat syndromes. *American Journal of Mental Retardation*, **103**, 264–71.

37. Krantz, I.D., McCallum, J., DeScipio, C., *et al.* (2004). Cornelia de Lange syndrome is caused by mutations in NIPBL, the human homolog of *Drosophila melanogaster* Nipped-B. *Nature Genetics*, **36**, 631–5.

38. Nyhan, W.L. and Wong, D.F. (1996). New approaches to understanding Lesch-Nyhan disease. *The New England Journal of Medicine*, **334**, 1602–4.

39. Deb, S. (1998). Self injurious behaviour as part of genetic syndromes. *The British Journal of Psychiatry*, **172**, 385–88.

40. Matthews, W.S., Solan, A., and Barabas, G. (1995). Cognitive functioning in Lesch-Nyhan syndrome. *Developmental Medicine and Child Neurology*, **37**, 715–22.

41. Gutmann, D.H., Aylsworth, A., Carey, J.C., *et al.* (1997). Diagnostic evaluation and multidisciplinary management of neurofibromatosis 1 and neurofibromatosis 2. *The Journal of the American Medical Association*, **278**, 51–7.

42. Waisbren, S.E. (1999). Phenylketonuria. In *Handbook of neurodevelopmental and genetic disorders in children* (eds. S. Goldstein and C.R. Reynolds), pp. 433–58. Guilford Press, New York.

43. Whittington, J.E., Holland, A.H., Webb, T., *et al.* (2001). Population prevalence and estimated birth incidence and mortality rate for people with Prader-Willi syndrome in one UK Health region. *Journal of Medical Genetics*, **38**, 792–8.

44. Clarke, D.J., Boer, H., Whittington, J., *et al.* (2002).Prader-Willi syndrome, compulsive and ritualistic behaviours. The first population-based survey. *The British Journal of Psychiatry*, **180**, 358–62.

45. Boer, H., Holland, A., Whittington, J., *et al.* (2002). Psychotic illness in people with Prader-Willi syndrome due to chromosome 15 maternal uniparental disomy. *Lancet*, **159**, 135–6.

46. Kerr, A.M. and Stephenson, J.B. (1985). Rett's syndrome in the West of Scotland. *British Medical Journal*, **291**, 579–82.

47. Fuks, F., Hurd, P.J., Wolf, N., *et al.* (2003). The methyl-CpG-binding protein MeCP2 links DNA methylation to histone methylation. *The Journal of Biological Chemistry*, **278**, 4035–40.

48. Petrij, F., Giles, R.H., Dawerse, H.G., *et al.* (1995). Rubinstein-Taybi syndrome caused by mutations in the transcriptional co-activator CBP. *Nature*, **376**, 248–51.

49. Boer, H., Langton, J., and Clarke, D. (1999). Development and behaviour in genetic syndromes: Rubinstein-Taybi syndrome. *Journal of Applied Research in Intellectual Disabilities*, **12**, 302–7.

50. Stark, L., Lovgren-Sandblom, A., and Bjorkhem, I. (2002). Cholesterol treatment forever? The first Scandinavian trial of cholesterol supplementation in the cholesterol-synthesis defect Smith-Lemli-Opitz syndrome. *Journal of Internal Medicine*, **252**, 314–21.

51. Dykens, E.M. and Smith, E.C. (1998). Distinctiveness and correlates of maladaptive behaviour in children and adolescents with Smith-Magenis syndrome. *Journal of Intellectual Disability Research*, **42**, 481–9.

52. Shprintzen, R.J., Goldberg, R.B., Lewin, M.L., *et al.* (1978). A new syndrome involving cleft palate, cardiac anomalies, typical facies, and learning disabilities: velo-cardio-facial syndrome. *Cleft Palate*, **15**, 56–62.

53. Swillen, A., Devriendt, K., Legius, *et al.* (1997). Intelligence and psychosocial adjustment in velo-cardio-facial syndrome: a study of 37 children and adolescents with VCFS. *Journal of Medical Genetics*, **34**, 453–8.

54. Popolos, D.F., Faedda, G.L., Veit, S., *et al.* (1996). Bipolar spectrum disorders in patients diagnosed with velo-cardio-facial syndrome: does a hemizygous deletion of chromosome 22q11 result in bipolar affective disorder? *The American Journal of Psychiatry*, **153**, 1541–7 .

55. Murphy, K.C., Jones, L.A., and Owen, M.J. (1999). High rates of schizophrenia in adults with velo-cardio-facial syndrome. *Archives of General Psychiatry*, **56**, 940–5.

56. Meng, X., Lu, X., Li, Z., *et al.* (1998). Complete physical map of the common deletion region in Williams syndrome and identification and characterization of three novel genes. *Human Genetics*, **103**, 590–9.

57. Udwin, O. (1990). A survey of adults with Williams syndrome and idiopathic infantile hypercalcaemia. *Developmental Medicine and Child Neurology*, **32**, 129–41.

58. Udwin, O. and Yule, W.A. (1991). A cognitive and behavioural phenotype in Williams syndrome. *Journal of Clinical and Experimental Neuropsychology*, **13**, 232–44.

# Psychiatric and behaviour disorders among mentally retarded people

## Contents

10.5.1 Psychiatric and behaviour disorders
among children and adolescents
with intellectual disability
Bruce J. Tonge

10.5.2 Psychiatric and behaviour disorders among
adult persons with intellectual disability
Anton Došen

10.5.3 Epilepsy and epilepsy-related behaviour disorders
among people with intellectual disability
Matti Iivanainen

## 10.5.1 Psychiatric and behaviour disorders among children and adolescents with intellectual disability

Bruce J. Tonge

### Introduction

Psychopathology is 2–3 times more common in intellectually disabled (ID) children than in the general population.[1,2] Psychiatric disorder is the most common source of additional handicap causing loss of educational, recreational, and social opportunity, burden for carers and cost to the community. Numerically, the size of this problem is approximately equal to schizophrenia, but is less well-recognized due to diagnostic over shadowing in which psychiatric disorder is not differentiated from ID as a separate condition open to diagnosis and treatment.[2] Although there is probably a significant reduction in overall prevalence of psychiatric disorders from approximately 43 per cent of children to 37 per cent of young adults with ID, psychopathology if present in childhood is likely to persist.[2] The profile of disorders varies from childhood into young adult life with the prevalence of attention-deficit hyperactivity symptoms decreasing, the frequency of symptoms of depression increasing and the prevalence of anxiety remaining stable with maturation.[2]

### Diagnosis and classification

There are two approaches to the description and classification of psychopathology in young people with ID. First is the application of DSM and ICD diagnostic criteria. The reliability and validity of this approach is not well established when applied to children with ID.[3] Young people with more severe ID and language impairment are unable to report abnormalities of their emotions, thoughts, and perceptions, which are criteria for conditions such as obsessive-compulsive disorder (OCD) and schizophrenia. Some diagnoses, for example attention-deficit hyperactivity disorder (ADHD)[4] require a judgement that symptoms are inconsistent with developmental level, which in a child with ID is delayed relative to chronological age. The DSM-IV TR[4] specifies that either ADHD or separation anxiety disorder should not be made 'exclusively during the course of a pervasive developmental disorder'. These restrictions on comorbid diagnosis should not limit the necessity to describe the range of presenting symptoms and offer appropriate treatment, for example the use of stimulant medication in a child with autism and severe ADHD symptoms. Developmental level and degree of cognitive impairment influence the presentation of symptoms. For example, children with ID are more likely than children in general, to have externalizing symptoms such as disruptive, aggressive, impulsive, or avoidant behaviours; if psychotic to experience hallucinations without delusions; or if depressed to present with irritability and stereotypies. Self-absorbed, autistic, and withdrawn behaviours are more common in children with severe ID whereas anxiety, disruptive, and aggressive behaviours are more likely in children with milder levels of ID.[2] Some patterns of psychopathology recognized by DSM-IV TR[4] are specifically associated with more severe ID such as 'stereotypic movement disorder with or without self-injurious behaviour'. Other emotional and behavioural disturbances seen in people with ID receive non-specific, atypical, or not otherwise specified classifications and await better definition. Recent attempts to produce diagnostic criteria for psychiatric disorders in people with ID (the draft ICD-10 guidelines for the psychiatric assessment of persons with mental retardation,[5] the Royal College of Psychiatrists diagnostic criteria for psychiatric disorders for use with adults with learning disabilities[6] and the DSM-IV TR for intellectual disability[7] are mainly designed for use with adults and require clinical validation).

The second approach to the definition of psychopathology in young people with ID is the use of informant questionnaires which rate disturbed emotions and behaviour. Factor analysis produces subscales which have clinical utility and refer to dimensions of disturbance such as disruptive/antisocial behaviours, social withdrawal, self-absorbed behaviours, communication disturbance, and anxiety/depression. Two reliable questionnaires validated for use in children and adolescents with ID are the Nisonger Child Behaviour Rating form[8] and the Developmental Behaviour Checklist.[9]

The multiaxial classification system of DSM or ICD, revised for use in people with ID, should form the basis of diagnosis of psychiatric disorder in young people with ID, but are usefully supplemented with standardized information gathered from informant questionnaires.

## Contributing factors and context

Assessment of the psychopathology associated with ID requires consideration of the biopsychosocial context.

### (a) Cognitive profile

A standardized cognitive assessment provides essential information to inform diagnosis and guide treatment. The level of intellectual and language ability gives an indication of the child's capacity to comprehend and communicate their perceptions, thoughts, and emotions. Subjective experiences such as grief, anxiety, hallucinations, and delusions cannot be assessed if the child is unable to communicate; therefore, psychopathology is more likely to be indirectly expressed by behaviour similar to that seen normally in younger children. For example, depression may be manifest as irritability, anxiety displayed by rocking or aggression and auditory hallucinations inferred from distressed covering of ears or self-injury.[7] Diagnosis is more speculative when the level of ID is more severe because the expression of emotions and behaviour is more atypical hence there is a greater use of unclassified or organic brain syndrome diagnoses. The cognitive subtest profile may also assist diagnosis. For example, children with autism usually perform better on visuo-motor tasks compared to verbal, imitation, and social comprehension tasks and therefore communicate and learn better if information is presented visually. The discovery of inattention and working memory deficits might help to confirm a diagnosis of ADHD.

### (b) Temperament

As for the general population, difficult temperamental characteristics such as high levels of emotionality and activity and poor sociability, increase the risk of emotional and behavioural disorders, particularly in boys with mild ID. A difficult temperament might be enduring but improved parental understanding and management skills improve adaptation and reduce disturbed behaviour.

### (c) Medical issues

A medical assessment is necessary, both to establish the cause of the ID, if known, and to determine if any medical conditions might be contributing to the emotional and behavioural problem. ID is associated with an increased risk of poor health in general, of brain disorders such as epilepsy (e.g. affecting 20 per cent of children with autism) and of medical complications associated with known causes of ID, such as cardiac and bowel abnormalities in Down syndrome, sensory impairments and deafness in Rubella embryopathy and the neuro-cutaneous brain lesions of tuberous sclerosis which are associated with tic disorder, autistic symptoms, and psychosis.[10] Disturbed behaviour might be the only manifestation of illnesses such as migraine, dental caries, and otitismedia in children with ID who are unable to talk about their pain. Psychoactive drugs are overprescribed in children with ID and their side effects are a well-recognized cause of behavioural and emotional disturbance and paradoxical effects. For example neuroleptic drugs may produce drowsiness, akathisia, and dystonic reactions. Irritability, anxiety, mood disturbance, and tics can be unacceptable side effects of stimulant medication. When prescribing drugs it is essential to systematically record behaviour and monitor side effects to confirm that the drug has a beneficial effect on target symptoms.[9]

### (d) Behavioural phenotype

Specific genetic causes of ID often have characteristic patterns of psychopathology of relevance to diagnosis, treatment, and research (see Table 10.5.1.1).[11,12]

### (e) Social and family influences

Children with ID are more likely than other children to experience adverse events such as poverty, socio-economic disadvantage, respite care and institutional care, rejection, social exclusion, teasing, school adjustment problems, abuse and neglect.[13] Their limited cognitive ability to comprehend adverse experiences may compromise adaptation. Parental stress, grief, guilt, and mental health problems and poor socio-economic circumstances are factors which are likely to adversely affect attachment and the quality of family care and aggravate child psychopathology.[14] In turn, behaviour problems, communication difficulties and lack of social responsiveness, for example in children with autism, predict maternal stress and mental health problems and placement of the child in out of home care.[15] Cultural responses, expectations, and attitudes may also influence parenting practices and the nature of care provided to children with ID. Observation and assessment of the quality of care, adverse events, parental mental health, family stress, resources, and community support is necessary to understand their contribution to psychopathology and implications for management. These factors are listed in AXIS V of the draft ICD-10 guide for mental retardation.[5]

## Specific psychopathological disorders in children with ID

### Behavioural disorders

#### (a) Attention-deficit hyperactivity disorder

Diagnosis of ADHD in children with ID is relatively straightforward because the DSM-IV TR[7] and the ICD[5] criteria are based on observable behaviour such as distractibility and fidgeting. This observed behaviour must also be 'inconsistent' with the child's developmental level. For example, the attention span of a 9-year-old child with a moderate ID would need to be less than that of a typical 3-year-old. Symptoms of inattention and hyperactivity

**Table 10.5.1.1** Behaviour phenotypes

| Syndrome | Genetics | Behavioural phenotype |
|---|---|---|
| Down | Trisomy 21 (1 in 800 live births) | Range of ID but usually moderate to severe |
| | | Relatively lower rates of psychopathology (20–30%) |
| | | Childhood: oppositional, attention-deficit problems |
| | | Young adult: affective disorder, early-onset dementia |
| Fragile X | Expansion of CGG trinucleotide sequence at Xq27.3 | Mild to moderate ID |
| | | Verbal IQ > Performance IQ |
| | | Shy, gaze avoidant, anxious inattentive, hyperactive, schizotypal disorder (females) |
| | | 5–10% have autistic disorder but most responsive to social cues and form attachments |
| | | Behaviour may settle with age |
| Prader–Willi | Paternal deletion long arm chromosome 15q 11–13 (70%) or maternal disomy chromosome 15 (25%) or a mutation | Mild/borderline ID |
| | | Hyperphagia and food obsession |
| | | Mild obesity, serious psychopathology (50%+) |
| | | OCD (e.g. questioning, cleanliness) impulsivity, aggression, defiance, skin picking |
| | | In adolescents anxiety, depression, psychosis (with maternal disomy) |
| Smith Magenis | Chromosome deletion at 17p 11.2 | Moderate ID |
| | | Severe psychopathology: hyperactive, impulsive, aggressive, insomnia, stereotypic movements (e.g. self-hugging) self-injury (e.g. nail pulling, head banging) |
| Williams | Micro-deletion on chromosome 7q 11.23 (elastin gene) | Moderate ID |
| | | Visuo-spatial/motor deficits but recognize facial features, loquacious with stereotypic phrases |
| | | Children: endearing, 'elfin-face', irrepressible, and affectionate, hyperacusis, phobias, anxiety, inattention, insomnia |

must be present in at least two settings such as at home and at school. Symptoms of inattention and hyperactivity might also occur in reaction to stress such as bullying at school, but these adjustment disorders usually respond to psychosocial intervention and do not require medication. Anxiety and oppositional-defiant disorder are common comorbid conditions which need to be considered in a management plan.

## Conduct disorder and oppositional-defiant disorder

Disruptive, aggressive, oppositional, and antisocial behaviours are problems in about 30 per cent of young people with mild/borderline ID, particularly males.[2] These children usually have language and learning difficulties and are likely to have experienced inconsistent care and sociocultural deprivation. The diagnosis requires a consideration of both the developmental age and the context. For example a 12-year-old young person with moderate ID might steal from a shop on the demand of a classmate without having a sufficient understanding of social rules and the rights of others. These diagnoses are not applicable in non-verbal children with more severe ID where, for example, aggressive behaviour might be the only means of communicating that an experience is stressful.

### (a) Tic disorders (Tourette's disorder) and stereotypic movement disorder

Tics are sudden rapid non-rhythmic recurrent motor movements or vocalizations in response to an irresistible urge that can be delayed.[7] There is a comorbid association with autism or disruptive behaviour. Tics may emerge or deteriorate in a child

with ADHD treated with stimulant medication. Relatively small doses of haloperidol or pimozide are often an effective treatment.[16] Stereotypic movements are persistent, driven, non-functional, complex motor behaviours that are differentiated from tics because they appear to be intentional. They occur in 2–3 per cent of children with more severe ID. These behaviours, such as self-biting, can cause serious injury and significantly interfere with daily activities, for example by rocking. They may be self-stimulating, occurring when the child is unoccupied, or might have communicative intent, for example to avoid an activity. The production of endogenous opioids might act to maintain the behaviours.

## Emotional disorders

### (a) Anxiety

Clinically significant symptoms of anxiety affect 10–12 per cent of both boys and girls with ID, compared to a prevalence in normal children of 2–5 per cent affecting twice as many females as males.[2] Fears are a common symptom and in children with ID are likely to be similar to the simple fears of young children in general, such as fear of the dark, loud noises, insects, and animals. Separation anxiety, typically seen in young children, can persist in older children with ID and is often complicated by fears, for example of school or other children. Children with ID are at high risk of suffering stressful experiences such as being placed in care or suffering physical and sexual maltreatment and neglect and have a limited capacity to understand stressful experiences.[17] Therefore, they are vulnerable to develop post-traumatic stress disorder (PTSD). Symptoms of PTSD are usually manifest as disturbed behaviours seen typically in traumatized young children such as repetitive play, behaviours which re-enact the trauma, nightmares, withdrawal, increased startle response, and hyper-vigilance.[7] PTSD in children with ID is underdiagnosed and research on its phenomenology is required. The diagnosis of obsessive-compulsive disorder in young people with ID is problematic because they may not have sufficient language to describe persistent thoughts and their attempts to suppress these thoughts. They also do not recognize that their compulsive behaviour is unreasonable. Stereotypic self-injurious behaviours might be regarded as evidence for an OCD, but these behaviours do not usually respond to treatments for anxiety. Some drugs that are an effective treatment of OCD in young people in the general community, such as sertraline and clomipramine, are used for the treatment of anxious compulsive behaviours in young people with ID but their efficacy has not been investigated.

### (b) Mood disorder

Depression in young people with ID is more prevalent than in other children.[2] Adolescents with moderate to severe levels of ID, provided they have some language, are able to reliably report sad feelings, but the diagnosis is confirmed by the presence of behavioural symptoms such as irritability, loss of interest in usual activities, loss of appetite and weight loss, sleep disturbance, crying, and withdrawn and regressed behaviours (e.g. rocking).[7] A daily carer completed record of mood and activity may reveal a pattern of cycling bipolar or unipolar mood disorder and is a useful record to document response to treatment.[9]

### Pervasive developmental disorders

About 75 per cent of children with autism have ID. There is also an increased association with epilepsy, tuberous sclerosis, congenital rubella syndrome, and phenylketonuria and comorbidity with ADHD, OCD, anxiety, depression, and tic disorder. These comorbid symptoms might be epiphenomena of autism related to fronto-striatal dysfunction, but it is helpful to the child and family to identify any comorbid symptoms and to treat them appropriately.[18] Children with ID also have delayed language and may have stereotypic behaviours and a limited range of interests, but they can be differentiated from those who also have autism because they try to communicate, use gesture and imitation, have reciprocal play and respond with emotion in a manner appropriate to their developmental level.

## Principles of management

Effective management begins with a multiaxial diagnostic formulation based on the DSM or ICD which describes the child's psychopathological disorder, cognitive profile, temperamental characteristics, genetic and associated medical conditions, level of adaptive functioning, and the family and sociocultural context. The delivery of effective management usually requires the involvement of a multidisciplinary team with a clear definition of roles and regular communication between professionals, parents, and teachers, for example at a case conference. The involvement of parents as partners in speech, physio, and behaviour therapy improves outcome and facilitates treatment compliance. Parent education and skills training reduces parental stress and improves parental mental health and child behaviour.[19] Family therapy may help reduce family conflict and improve communication and child management, but outcome research is required.

### Psychological treatment

Effective behaviour modification techniques based on operant conditioning principles teach positive socially adaptive behaviours and reduce difficult behaviours.[20,21] Antecedent triggers, the functions of the behaviour and any rewarding consequences which reinforce the behaviour are identified. Intervention might focus on changing the antecedent events, for example by removal of an upsetting sound. Replacement of the disruptive behaviour might be achieved by rewarding alternative appropriate behaviour or by teaching a new behaviour which improves communication such as the use of pictures to communicate a need. A further approach which may help extinguish difficult behaviour is a non-aversive modification of the usual response to the behaviour such as moving away from a screaming child instead of paying them attention. Counselling and cognitive behavioural therapy including relaxation exercises, which is modified to take into account the developmental level and language ability of the child with ID might reduce anxiety and depression, but its effectiveness requires further research.

### Pharmacotherapy

Drugs, if used to treat specific symptoms, should be part of a psychosocial and educational management plan, which includes informed parent/carer consent and participation. Evidence for the efficacy of psychotropic drugs in children with ID is limited,[16] but children with ID are prescribed or even overprescribed drugs on the basis of evidence for their use in either adults with ID or in normally developing children. These drugs include stimulant medication, atomoxetine, clonidine, neuroleptic drugs, and imipramine for ADHD; clomipramine and selective serotonin reuptake inhibitors (SSRIs) for OCD and stereotypic self-injurious behaviour; SSRIs for depression; neuroleptic drugs for tic disorders. Rigorous empirical studies have failed to demonstrate clear benefit for the use of 'typical' neuroleptic medication such as chlor-promazine in the treatment of disruptive behaviour. There is empirical evidence that low doses of haloperidol or risperidone (0.02–0.06 mg/kg/day) are an effective treatment for disruptive stereotypic behaviour.[22] Problematic side effects, particularly for haloperidol, are drowsiness, akathisia, dystonia, and tardive dyskinesia. Weight gain, prolactinemia, and metabolic disturbances such as diabetes are serious side effects of risperidone. Anticonvulsants used as mood stabilizers (sodium valproate, carbamazapine, and lamotrigine), lithium, β-blockers, and buspirone have been shown, mostly in open trials, to reduce self-injurious and episodic aggressive behaviours. Opiate antagonists (naloxone and naltrexone) may reduce self-injurious behaviour. Difficult sexual behaviour in adolescent males with ID can be treated with testosterone antagonists to reduce libido. In many countries this treatment requires approval and monitoring by an independent committee. The prescription of psychotropic drugs requires regular follow-up to monitor compliance, side effects, and response to treatment using behaviour observations and carer completed symptom checklist such as the DBC[9] or NCBRF.[8]

### Early intervention

There is growing evidence that broad-based early intervention for young children with developmental delay, such as those with autism, promotes adaptive behaviour and skill development. The components of effective early intervention include:

1 Parent education and skills training and the management of parent mental health problems such as depression.[19]

2 Regular medical review and treatment of associated conditions such as epilepsy and any inter-current illness or psychopathological disorder, which might compromise behaviour.[10]

3 A structured behaviour management and social and communication skills programme.[21]

4 Family support, respite care, home help, and holiday programmes.

5 Speech, occupational, and physiotherapy to develop communication, sensory, motor, and play skills.

6 Assisted education and socialization at preschool and school.

## Conclusions

Children with ID often suffer the added handicap of emotional and behavioural disorder which seriously compromises their adjustment and causes significant extra burden and cost for their parents and the community. A comprehensive biopsychosocial assessment of the child and family provides the context for understanding psychopathological symptoms and the basis for a best practice management plan incorporating psychological, educational, family, and perhaps pharmacological interventions.

## Further information

Bouras, N. and Holt, G. (eds.) (2007). *Psychiatric and behavioural disorders in intellectual and developmental disabilities* (2nd edn). Cambridge University Press, London.

Reiss, S. and Aman, M.G. (1998). *Psychotropic medication and developmental disabilities: the international consensus handbook*. Ohio State University, Columbus.

Therapeutic Guidelines. (2005). *Management guidelines: developmental disability* (Version 2). Therapeutic Guidelines Ltd., North Melbourne.

www.cddh.monash.org (provides an educational programme in the psychiatry of ID).

www.iassid.org (review of current research and information exchange on the psychiatry of ID).

## References

1. Emerson, E. (2003). Prevalence of psychiatric disorders in children and adolescents with and without intellectual disability. *Journal of Intellectual Disability Research*, **47**, 51–8.

2. Tonge, B.J. and Einfeld, S.L. (2003). Psychopathology and intellectual disability: the Australian child to adult longitudinal study. *International Review of Research in Mental Retardation*, **26**, 61–91.

3. Einfeld, S.L. and Tonge, B.J. (1999). Observations on the use of the ICD-10 guide for mental retardation. *Journal of Intellectual Disability Research*, **43**, 408–12.

4. American Psychiatric Association. (2002). *Diagnostic and statistical manual of mental disorders* (4th edn, text revision). American Psychiatric Association, Washington, DC.

5. World Health Organization. (1996). *The ICD-10 guide for mental retardation*. World Health Organization, Geneva.

6. Royal College of Psychiatrists. (2001). *DC-LD (Diagnostic criteria for psychiatric disorders for use with adults with learning disorders/mental retardation)*. Gaskell, London.

7. Fletcher, R., Loschen, E., Stavrakaki, C., *et al.* (2007). *Diagnostic Manual – Intellectual Disability (DM-ID): a textbook of diagnosis of mental disorders in persons with intellectual disability*. NADD Press, Kingston, New York.

8. Aman, M.G., Tasse, M.J., Rojahn, J., *et al.* (1996). The Nisonger CBRF: a child behaviour rating form for children with developmental disabilities. *Research in Developmental Disabilities*, **17**, 41–57.

9. Einfeld, S.L. and Tonge, B.J. (2002). *Manual for the developmental behaviour checklist* (2nd edn). Centre for Developmental Psychiatry & Psychology, Monash University, Melbourne.

10. Therapeutic Guidelines. (2005). *Management guidelines: developmental disability* (Version 2). Therapeutic Guidelines Ltd., North Melbourne.

11. Dykens, E.M. (1999). Direct effects of genetic mental retardation syndromes: maladaptive behaviour and psychopathology. *International Review of Research on Mental Retardation*, **22**, 1–26.

12. Einfeld, S.L., Tonge, B.J., and Rees, V.W. (2001). Longitudinal course of behavioural and emotional problems in Williams syndrome. *American Journal of Mental Retardation*, **106**, 73–81.

13. Emerson, E., Graham, H., and Hatton, C. (2006). The measurement of poverty and socioeconomic position in research involving people with intellectual disability. *International Review of Research in Mental Retardation*, **32**, 77–108.

14. Baker, B.L., Blacker, J., Crnic, K.A., *et al.* (2002). Behaviour problems and parenting stress in families of three-year-old children with and without developmental delay. *American Journal of Mental Retardation*, **107**, 433–44.

15. Llewellyn, D., McConnell, D., Thompson, K., *et al.* (2005). Out-of-home placement of school age children with disabilities. *Journal of Applied Research in Intellectual Disability*, **18**, 1–16.

16. Reiss, S. and Aman, M.G. (1998). *Psychotropic medication and developmental disabilities: the international consensus handbook*. Ohio State University, Columbus, OH.

17. Hatton, C. and Emmerson, E. (2004). The relationship between life events and psychopathology amongst children with intellectual disabilities. *Journal of Applied Research in Intellectual Disability*, **17**, 109–17.

18. Tonge, B.J. and Rinehart, N.J. (2007). Autism and attention deficit/hyperactivity disorder. In *Neurology and clinical neuroscience* (ed. A.H.V. Shapira), pp. 129–30. Mosby, Elsevier, Philadelphia.

19. Tonge, B.J., Brereton, A.V., Kiomall, *et al.* (2006). Effects on parental mental health of an education and skills training program for parents with young children with autism: a randomized controlled trial. *Journal of the American Academy of Child and Adolescent Psychiatry*, **45**, 561–69.

20. Lucyshyn, J.M., Dunlap, G., and Albin, R.W. (eds.) (2002). *Families and positive behaviour support*. Brookes, Baltimore.

21. Emerson, E. (2001). *Challenging behaviour. Analysis and intervention in people with severe intellectual disabilities* (2nd edn). Cambridge University Press, Cambridge.

22. Aman, M.G., DeSmedt, G., Derivan, A., *et al.* and the Risperidone Disruptive Behaviour Study Group. (2002). Risperidone treatment of children with disruptive behaviour symptoms and sub-average IQ: a double blind, placebo-controlled study. *The American Journal of Psychiatry*, **159**, 1337–46.

## 10.5.2 Psychiatric and behaviour disorders among adult persons with intellectual disability

Anton Došen

## Introduction

The behavioural and emotional difficulties that are experienced by adults with intellectual disability (ID) have been regarded for many years as manifestations of their intellectual deficits and maladaptive learning. The awareness that these persons may also suffer from mental illness was a notion that came into being in the mid-nineteenth century.

Nevertheless, the psychiatric problems of individuals with ID were continually ignored in the first half of the twentieth century. In the past three decades, the flourishing normalization philosophy has highlighted the psychiatric problems of this population once again and rekindled the interest of practitioners, scientists, and service providers. Systematic studies have been performed which indicate that the full spectrum of psychiatric disorders as we know them today can be identified among the persons with ID. Moreover, it is probable that they may be prone to a psychopathology that is determined by the specifics of their biological and psychosocial being.

## Clinical features

### Features affecting presentation

Studies indicate that the types of psychiatric symptoms and syndromes that are observed among persons with borderline and mild ID are similar to those encountered among the population in general. Amongst individuals with moderate and severe ID, however, the presentation of mental illness may be less typical, and the diagnosis more difficult to establish.

Sovner and Hurley[1] have categorized four factors which may influence the presentation of mental illness among the persons with ID: intellectual distortion (impaired ability to conceptualize feelings and to communicate them to others), psychological masking (lack of usual richness of the symptomatology found in general population), cognitive disintegration (inclination to become disorganized and to exhibit regressive behaviour), and baseline exaggeration (increase of pre-existing maladaptive behaviour by emotional stress or mental illness).

Hucker et al.[2] pointed to a generally banal symptomatology encountered among these individuals, often accompanied by regression to a child-like state of dependency and hysterical features. Behavioural disturbances were often more important than symptomatic complaints as indicators of psychiatric disorders.

Apparently, the lower the IQ, the more the symptoms of mental illness tend to lose their specificity, or take on a different meaning than is the case with the intellectually normal population. This, undoubtedly, makes it difficult to establish a confident diagnosis of mental illness in people with severe ID.[3]

The following is a concise survey of the striking clinical features of mental illness and behaviour problems as they occur among adult persons with ID.

## Mental illness

### (a) Psychosis

Among persons with mild ID, classical clinical features are present in psychotic states. The symptoms tend to be florid but banal. In schizophrenia, for example, there is a high incidence of delusions and hallucinations, which reflect the limited experiences, naive and wishful thinking, interests, and social horizon of the patient. Ideas, that have been influenced by radio, television, etc., are found frequently. Catatonic features with odd postures and slowness are common. Impulsive, aggressive, auto-aggressive, and bizarre behaviours may dominate the clinical picture. In the chronic-phase apathy, lack of motivation and social withdrawal are common.[4,5] Increase of 'negative' schizophrenic symptoms and decrease of functional abilities were observed in the group with ID when compared with the group from general population with schizophrenia.[6]

Establishing the diagnosis of schizophrenia in persons with more severe ID can be a difficult task because of verbal communicative difficulties. Reid[7] considers it to be impossible to establish such a diagnosis among persons who only communicate non-verbally. However, the problem of establishing the diagnosis does not mean that psychotic conditions do not occur in these individuals. To the contrary, it is likely that different sorts of psychosis occur in this population more frequently than in general population (see Chapter 4.5.2).

Short-term psychotic states (lasting several days or weeks), usually beginning rather suddenly after a stressful event, are found relatively often among adolescents and young adults with ID. Early Dutch psychiatric literature refers to these states as 'debility psychosis'. The symptoms may be heterogeneous, and remission is usually complete. These persons usually revert fully to the premorbid level of functioning. However, recurrence is frequent.

Establishing the diagnosis of atypical psychosis (contrary to diagnosing schizophrenia) is, for an experienced practitioner, possible even with patients who have no language development and are at a severe level of ID. The primary symptoms are changes in interactional patterns, changes of posture and movement, odd and bizarre behaviour, disturbances of the physiological functions, expression of emotional tension (e.g. anxiety, irritability), aggression, and self-injuring behaviour.

### (b) Major depression and bipolar disorders

Depressed mood and vegetative symptoms are the most striking symptoms, even though complaints of depression are not always expressed. A depressive mood often is not verbalized, particularly among individuals at a lower intelligence level, but may well be observable. Similarly, the elevation of mood in mania is usually not expressed verbally either. Atypical features such as regression to child-like dependency, incontinence, loss of social skills, and hysterical symptoms such as pseudo-fits and paralysis may mask classical symptomatology. In persons with a more severe disability, depression should be suspected where there is a change or onset of behaviour problems like stereotypic behaviour, tantrums, aggression, and self-injuring behaviour.[4,8] Catatonic features and visual hallucinations, particularly among persons at lower intelligence levels, have also been reported.[2,9,10] The atypical symptomatology among persons on lower developmental levels may require modification of standard diagnostic criteria.

Aggressive behaviour was observed in 40 per cent of the depressed subjects.[11] Self-injuring behaviour has often been reported as well.

Suicidal behaviour has hardly ever been studied in this population, and suicidality is very rare among the more severely handicapped. This symptom is, however, not rare among depressive patients at a mild level of ID.

Some investigators report the relatively frequent occurrence of rapid-cycling affective disorder,[12] particularly in persons with more severe disability. Episodes of particular mood or of an undifferentiated mood-like dysphoria or irritability have a short duration, and may be expressed in terms of days or weeks.[9] Researchers assume that these disorders, in persons with ID are often related to organic brain disorders, that is, metabolic, neuroendocrine, and other neurological disorders.

In mixed bipolar disorder, there is either the simultaneous presence of manic and depressive features, or these features follow each other rapidly. Schizoaffective psychoses are also described among these individuals.

### (c) Dysthymic disorder

Dysthymia is a relatively common disorder among persons with mild and moderate ID.[9,13] Nevertheless, publications on this disorder are rare. The symptomatology includes loss of energy and interest, negative self-image, feelings of helplessness, anxiety, and significant behavioural problems such as irritability, anger, destructibility, and aggression. The disorder is often related to a specific stress, for example, termination of an affective relationship, change in the surroundings, hospitalization, etc. Chronic states, dating back to the childhood or the teens, possibly caused by chronic overdemanding, social deprivation, or repeated abuse, may be interrupted by episodes of major depression, usually elicited by acute stress (so-called 'double depression', see Chapter 4.5.3). Došen and co-workers found this disorder relatively frequent in adolescents and young adults with ID and called it 'developmental depression'.[10, 14] Social interactional problems, poor social skills, and difficulties related to emotional development are considered to be predisposing factors for this disorder.[14]

### (d) Anxiety disorders

The most commonly reported anxiety disorders are simple phobia, social phobia, and generalized anxiety disorder.[4] It seems that adults with ID have fears similar to those of children who are at the same mental age: fear of separation, fear of natural events, fear of injury, and fear of animals. The anxieties and fears are probably related to the traumatic events and cumulative failure experiences that these persons have. The presentation may be through behaviour problems, irritability, problems with sleeping, or somatic complaints.[5] In a panic disorder, a sudden onset, blackouts, aggression, sweating, and shaking may be observable. The obsessive–compulsive disorder may be difficult to diagnose in persons with ID because they do not resist against such feelings and the anxiety is often absent. According to some authors,[4] the diagnosis can be established with the emphasis being on the externally observable behavioural components, despite of absence of some internal states like anxiety and resistance. Post-traumatic stress disorder is likely to occur in this population, following relatively less severe stress than among general population. The diagnosis in those who are unable to communicate their experiences should be based on changes in a person's behaviour, mood, and level of functioning following a traumatic event.[4]

### (e) Autism spectrum disorder

Autism spectrum disorders have been estimated to be present in 10 per cent of persons with mild ID and 40 per cent of those with severe ID, and account for a large proportion of behaviour disorders. It also appears that mental illness occurs frequently as a secondary disorder among these individuals.

A possible relationship between affective illness and pervasive developmental disorder has been suggested by various investigators[12]; however, this phenomenon has been examined insufficiently and is clearly an area that future research can be directed to. In clinical practice, we have encountered a number of cases of pervasive developmental disorder together with secondary atypical psychosis. Inexperienced practitioners are inclined to diagnose schizophrenia in such cases. However, thorough developmental history will reveal sufficient information to make diagnostic differentiation possible. Other problematic behaviours such as anxious, aggressive, auto-aggressive, or disruptive behaviour are frequently found among persons who have an autism spectrum disorder and ID.[15] In our opinion, these behaviours should be seen as being secondary disorders instead of as part of the autistic disorder.

### (f) Dementia

In individuals with dementia, the typical features such as memory impairment, personality change, loss of social skills, and deterioration in habits are always present. Behavioural problems may be the most obvious manifestation. Nocturnal confusion, transient psychotic episodes, and late-onset epilepsy should always alert one to the possibility of a dementing illness in the ageing person with ID. Memory loss is generally difficult to identify in the early stages, but becomes more obvious as the illness progresses. Medical risk factors include a history of hypertension, ischaemic episodes, neurological symptoms, organic brain damage, and a family history of dementia. Dementia Alzheimer type in persons with Down syndrome presents a similar picture and is usually associated with generalized premature ageing.

## Behaviour disorders—challenging behaviour

Behaviour disorders including aggression, self-injury, destructiveness, and disruptive, maladaptive, and antisocial behaviour occur commonly among persons with ID. Such behaviour has recently been called challenging behaviour, which emphasizes the need for appropriate care and supervision. These disorders are usually associated with severe ID, but can also occur in individuals who are at a moderate and mild level of ID.

Various attempts have been made to distinguish between behaviour disorders and psychiatric illness in these individuals. Gardner and co-workers[16] have proposed a bio-psycho-social diagnostic approach, which takes account of the multiple factors underlying and maintaining the behaviour disturbances of a particular individual. They point out that behaviour disorders with a neuropsychiatric and organic basis can still acquire a functional component if they are being reinforced by the environment or are of value to the individual. Another approach is from the developmental perspective,[3,17] viewing behaviour disorders as the result of a lack of real understanding of the person's developmental aspects and interactional problems.

### (a) Aggressive behaviour

Aggressive behaviour is a common problem among persons with ID. The symptom of aggression is often a feature of the psychosis, depression, or antisocial personality disorder, and is often described in genetic disorders such as the fragile X, Prader–Willi, and

Klinefelter syndromes. Learned aggression through the imitation of aggressive models or as a function of communication is also found relatively frequently among people with ID.

### (b) Self-injurious behaviour

Self-injurious behaviour occurs more often among persons with moderate and severe ID (IQ < 50), beginning sometimes in toddler age and most frequently between the ages of 10 and 20. The occurrence of self-injurious behaviour is related to genetic and organic disturbances and adverse environmental and development conditions. Certain psychiatric disorders such as depression and psychosis may also elicit self-injurious behaviour.

### (c) Offending behaviour

Owing to their behaviour problems, these individuals may become involved in activities, that bring them into conflict with the law. Insufficient understanding of their problems and needs may result in their not receiving the appropriate support from the social services. The typical offender with ID is, according to Day,[18] a young male functioning in the mild to borderline intellectual range, from a poor urban environment, with a history of psychosocial deprivation, behaviour problems, and personality disorder. The most common offences are acquisitive and technical, but sex offences and arson are considerably overrepresented.

### Personality disorders

Various investigators have reported personality disorders among persons with ID.[19,20] The relevance of the concept of personality disorder, in particular with regard to the persons with more severe ID, has been questioned by a number of investigators. Apparently, in these persons, besides the problem of personality disorders, there is a problem of personality development. Zigler and colleagues[21] have explored personality traits thought to be particularly salient in determining the behaviour of individuals with ID. Levitas and Gilson[22] have stressed the importance of a crisis period during the process of personality development and the related psychosocial aspects. Other developmentally oriented authors[14,23] make a link between, on the one hand, the problematic processing of particular phase–specific aspects of emotional development and ego structuring, such as the achievement of secure attachment, an intercompetitive separation-individuation process, and the establishing of ego functions, and, on the other hand, the increased vulnerability of these individuals to particular psychiatric disorders such as depression, social withdrawal, disruptive behaviours, etc. Classification of personality problems within the existing diagnostic categories for personality disorders in general population is questionable and requires modification of particular diagnostic criteria.[4, 5] It is unlikely that personality disorders could be diagnosed in persons with severe/profound ID.

It appears that the main problem at the root of the personality disorders of individuals with ID pertains to an underdeveloped personality structure in relation to a delay in psychosocial development. One is then inclined to speak of an immature rather than a disturbed personality.

## Diagnosis and classification

Diagnosis calls for a full and detailed history, careful observation of the patient, knowledge of the natural history of the illness, and the elimination of irrelevant factors (for further information about assessment, see Chapter 10.1).

### Assessment

In complex cases, a period of inpatient observation or explorative treatment may be necessary. As full a history as possible of the current illness should be obtained from the patient, together with corroborative histories from the relatives and carers. The standardized format of psychiatric history should be supplemented by a detailed developmental history, a description of current social functioning, environmental circumstances, associated somatic disorders and physical disabilities, and the aetiology of the ID. Enquiries should be focused on behavioural changes such as sleep disturbance, loss of appetite, weight loss, lack of interest, bizarre behaviour, restlessness, anxiety, withdrawal, and any other deviations from customary behaviour. Precipitating factors such as stressful events and possible predispositions to reacting in a particular way in a particular situation should be explored. Full details of previous psychiatric illnesses suffered by the patient and the family history of mental illness should be obtained. Because of the general paucity of subjective complaints by persons with ID, the examiner must rely more on objective data regarding the patient's appearance, manner of communication, facial expression, evidence of hallucinations, posture, etc. If called for, direct observations should be made in as wide a range of settings as is necessary. To these ends, a video recording of the patient in his or her natural surroundings may provide important information about the interactional pattern of the patient and his or her surroundings. The psychiatric examination is usually supplemented by somatic, neurological, neurophysiological, biochemical, and psychological examinations. Assessment of the level of ID is crucial for diagnostic consideration. Currently, in psychological assessment, besides examination of cognitive functioning, the emphasis is on determination of personality development and the level of emotional development.[3]

### Diagnosis

IQ assessment, personality development, emotional level, and measuring adaptive behaviour can provide extra background information that may be useful to the diagnosis. Specific tests, for example, of thought disorder in schizophrenia, may be helpful in establishing the diagnosis, but are not yet standardized for this population. Non-invasive neuroimaging techniques promise to be potentially valuable diagnostic tools, particularly for non-verbal persons with severe ID in the future. Structured interview schedules and rating scales are being used increasingly in an attempt to improve diagnostic accuracy. Instruments developed for use with persons without ID rely heavily on the ability of the patient to describe subjective feelings and are thus of limited value. Diagnostic rating scales that are to be used with the persons with ID should, as far as possible, reflect behavioural rather than subjective components. An early attempt was made by Hucker and colleagues,[2] who published diagnostic criteria for mania, depression, and schizophrenia for use with persons with ID; these have been further refined by Sovner and Hurley[1] and by Menolascino and Weiler.[24] Recently, a number of scales have been developed specifically for use with this population, and different other instruments are in development. These scales were primarily developed for use as research instruments, and whilst they play an invaluable role in epidemiological studies and population screening as well as being useful for monitoring the response to treatment, they are of limited value in clinical practice and rarely, if ever, solve a diagnostic problem.

## (a) Integrative psychiatric diagnosis

For clinical purposes, it has been proposed that more elaborate and expanded diagnostic formulations be made.[25] Such diagnosis should incorporate diagnostic categories as well as the onset mechanisms of the psychopathology, biological aspects, psychological functioning, milieu characteristics, life problems, psychosocial needs, and individual strengths. Diagnostics of this sort have been called integrative diagnosis and are an attempt to adapt conventional diagnostic criteria to the complex problems of individuals with ID.[3,14] During the diagnostic process, particular attention is paid to describing the onset mechanism of the psychopathological phenomenon by which the dynamics of different nosological factors come into scope and become more understandable to the direct carers and professional helpers. A better understanding of the processes involved in the mental illness is important to the treatment approach.

## Classification

Numerous attempts have been made to apply the traditional psychiatric diagnostic categories of ICD-10 and DSM-IV to the psychopathology of persons with ID. Their applicability to these individuals has, however, been questioned.[1,2,25] Whilst the ICD and DSM criteria may be applied to people functioning in the mild to borderline ID ranges without alteration or with little modification, they become increasingly unreliable as the severity of intellectual disability increases. The limited communication skills of these persons make it very difficult to ascertain the presence of certain symptoms such as delusions and hallucinations. As the role of underlying organic brain damage expands, the phenomenology becomes increasingly more characterized by a range of atypical symptoms. The non-specific nature of behavioural disturbances further confounds diagnostic endeavours. Szymanski,[25] among others, has pointed out that behaviour disturbance is not a psychiatric condition but a symptom, and Reid[26] has drawn attention to the fact that behaviours, that would be deemed abnormal in people functioning in the average intellectual range may be developmentally appropriate to the mental age of a person with severe ID.

Other authors[3,17,27] suggest using the developmental perspective when attempting to understand and diagnose the psychiatric and behavioural disorders of the persons with ID. They point out that there are findings which suggest that there may be a relationship between certain developmental levels and syndromes and specific neuropsychiatric disorders (see below). Some investigators argue that syndromes should be empirically derived, and a 'dimensional' approach would be a more effective way to classify psychopathology than the categorical system.[28,29] Van Praag[30] proposes a 'functional psychopathology model' emphasizing functional problems of the CNS on the background of psychiatric disorders.

Not surprisingly, there have been calls for some modifications of existing DSM and ICD diagnostic criteria with the introduction of behavioural equivalents for some symptom criteria as well as for development of a broader taxonomy, which takes account of the atypical presentation of mental illness in this population.[31]

## Epidemiology

### Overall prevalence

Psychiatric disorder appears to be more common among the persons with ID than in the general population. Overall prevalence rates range from 20 per cent to 74 per cent,[19,25,32] depending on the diagnostic criteria employed, the type of disorder screened (whether or not behaviour disorders are included, for example), the nature of the sample (community or institution), the type of data collected (case note studies or new data), and the level of ID, ages, and gender of the populations studied. Higher rates of psychiatric disorder have been reported in some studies among the individuals with severe ID in comparison with the person on mild ID level. For further information concerning epidemiology, see Chapter 10.2.

## Aetiology

Investigators of aetiology agree that the high prevalence of psychiatric disorders among persons with ID is related to a wide range of neurological, psychological, social, and personality risk factors including impaired genetic factors, delayed cognitive, emotional and social development, organic brain damage, communication problems, environmental problems, and family psychopathology. Alone or in combination, these factors increase the vulnerability of the person with ID to psychiatric and behavioural problems.

### Theories

Achenbach and Zigler[33] have pointed out the importance of social incompetence as a factor playing a role in interactional and intrapsychic problems. This theoretical perspective has received support from studies in which discrepancies between self-image and the expectations of others have been shown to be a fertile breeding ground for the onset of psychopathology. Menolascino[34] emphasized the importance of neurophysiological and sociological developmental processes which may have a different timing and take a different course in these individuals, causing deviations from normal development; this is known as the biodevelopmental theory. Matson[35] proposed the biosocial theory, which hypothesizes that due to specific biological factors (neurological, biochemical, genetic, etc.) together with specific social factors (family interactions, culture, and other environmental variables), and specific psychological processes (cognitive development, personality variables), the psychopathology of persons with ID differs in a number of ways from that of persons without ID.

Tanguay,[36] Došen,[3,14,17] and Gaedt and Gärtner[37] have applied the developmental approach to the understanding of the symptoms of psychopathology and to the psychiatric diagnostics in these individuals. These authors based their approach on Piaget's stages of cognitive development as well as on Mahler's and Bowlby's models of psychosocial development. Parallels could be drawn between the symptoms of psychopathology of children without ID at a particular chronological age and individuals with ID at the same developmental age, which indicates that the developmental level may specifically affect the exterior features of mental illness. According to these authors, although developmentally disabled adults who suffer from mental illness resemble other adults in many ways, it is the developmental level and consequent differentiation of psychosocial life (e.g. affect differentiation, personality structuring, moral development), that may be decisive for the symptoms linked to the disorder. For example, because of their underdeveloped psychosocial life, adults with severe ID display little differentiation in their symptomatology. They exhibit agitation, aggression, self-injurious behaviour, or other disruptive behaviours, which in other people may be indicative of various underlying mental illnesses such as anxiety disorder, depression, or psychosis. Similarly, a toddler may have 'tantrums' when frustrated, anxious, or distressed by somatic pain or separation. Recently, problems of attachment development in these individuals and their vulnerability to stress have been related by some authors to the behaviour problems and psychopathological features.[38,39]

### Behavioural phenotypes in relation to mental illness

Recently, the concept of a behavioural phenotype has been introduced as an attempt to assess the interrelationship between specific behaviours and genetic disorders (see Chapter 10.4). In addition to specific behaviours, an increased prevalence of psychiatric syndromes have been reported in association with particular genetic and other syndromes. The possible link between a behavioural phenotype and the particular psychiatric disorder of a person with ID is a highly challenging issue for investigators researching this field. For further information.

Down syndrome has always been associated with specific patterns of language, and cognitive and social development. In most studies, these persons were found to exhibit muted affect and have deficient language development, and yet they showed particular strengths in socialization. The tendency for such individuals to develop Alzheimer dementia has often been described. The occurrence of affective disorder among Down syndrome subjects had attracted the attention of scientists recently.[40,41] Diurnal mood variations, speech reduction, and an increase in aggression are the commonly reported symptoms, which are indicative of depression among persons with Down syndrome. The onset of mania in this syndrome has been disputed. However, cases of mania have been reported later in life among those having Down syndrome.

Persons with fragile X syndrome have often been described as having autistic-like social impairments. However, among these individuals, social anxiety is more characteristic than social indifference.[42] In addition, attention deficit, stereotyped behaviour, self-injury, and hyperactivity are common.

In Prader–Willi syndrome, hyperphagia and obsessive–compulsive and aggressive behaviour are common. The occurrence of brief psychotic episodes with heterogeneous symptoms have been described among these persons.

Different behavioural phenotypes and psychiatric disorders have also been described for other syndromes. For example, anxiety disorder, sleep disorder, and hyperactivity are common in Williams syndrome, depression is often found in Klinefelter's syndrome, and self-injurious behaviour occurs regularly in Cornelia de Lange syndrome.

### Genetic and environmental factors and onset mechanisms

It should be stressed, however, that the very same behaviours may be found among individuals with genetic as well as with idiopathic ID, which probably means that these behaviours are not only the product of genetic factors, and that other factors may be the cause as well. Among other things, the process of psychosocial development and interactional patterns with the surroundings can affect the onset of a particular behaviour. Apparently, genetic characteristics can influence the psychosocial development, which then can be decisive for the onset of particular interactional patterns and particular behaviours (so called 'heightened probability', according

to Dykens *et al.*[43]). The question is: Do these behaviours play a role in the onset of the aforementioned psychiatric disorders associated with these genetically based syndromes, and if so, how do they do this? Or, does a genetic disorder have a more direct role in the onset of a particular psychiatric disorder?

For a better understanding of how specific psychiatric disorders evolve among these individuals, it is necessary to make a scheme of the onset mechanisms involved in each psychiatric disorder. It is important to take account of the genetic disorder, the developmental processes, and the interaction patterns with the surroundings in which particular behaviours may play an important role. If one takes all these factors into consideration, it may be expected that in certain cases particular psychiatric disorders have a specific aetiology. An example is self-injurious behaviour, which is currently considered to be a 'challenging' behaviour, but, according to various professionals in this field, warrants being seen as a specific psychopathological phenomenon. However, there are also examples in which the connection between genetic and psychiatric disorder appears to be more direct. An example is the velocardiofacial or Shprintzen syndrome.[44,45]

## Psychiatric problems in older persons with ID

In elderly persons with ID, besides dementia, other psychiatric disorders, like psychotic conditions, depression, and anxiety disorders, are common.[46] In a mixed community and institutionalized group of persons with ID older than 50 years, Patel and colleagues[47] found a prevalence of psychiatric disorders, mainly depression and anxiety in 11.4 per cent of the population. Other authors[48] ascertained that major psychiatric disorders could be found in 20 per cent of persons with ID aged 65 and above. Behavioural symptoms such as aggression and self-injury frequently accompany psychiatric problems among these individuals. Causes for frequent psychiatric problems in this population group are various; like changes in social milieu and living pattern, loss of beloved ones, social deprivation, and inactivation done to retirement from the work or previous activities and medical, in particular neurological, conditions at this age (see Chapter 9.2.1). Frequently, psychiatric disorders in these individuals can be found as an accompaniment of a dementia process. Differentiation between the beginning stage of dementia and other psychiatric disorders can be a difficult task.[49] In these cases, a total bio-psycho-social picture of the involved person, including a detailed patient history, as well as an insight into the surroundings circumstances and in interactions is necessary for appropriate understanding of the patient's symptoms. Use of some assessment instruments can be helpful (see Chapter 10.1).

### Management

In principle, the diagnosis of psychiatric disorders in persons with mild ID and good verbal skills does not differ much from diagnosing these disorders in persons with average cognitive skills.[50] However, in persons on a lower level, the recognition of mental disorders can be difficult, partly because of linguistic limitations and partly because of difficulty in distinguishing between behaviour problems (challenging behaviour) and symptoms of psychiatric illness. Communication problems often ask for management through another individual ('management by proxy'), which means that carers are relied upon to give description of a person's behaviour. The diagnostician should know that the reliability and validity of such information may be problematical and, besides this information, should search for more objective sources, like information through non-verbal communication with the patient and through observation of the patient in different situations and interactions. Distinguishing between behaviour problems and psychiatric illness is a very important issue for adequate aid. It asks for a multi-disciplinary assessment approach in which experienced (specialized) professionals from different disciplines, participate forming together a multi-disciplinary team. These teams have expertise in both intellectual disability and mental health, and provide direct services to patients and carers. Through the assessment of a specialist team, an insight is being obtained whether presenting behaviours of involved individual are the results of an organic condition, a psychiatric disorder, environmental influences, or a combination of these factors. The clinical symptoms must be viewed in a broad context of a patient's functioning, considering his/her deficits, strengths, and relevant bio-psycho-social factors. For example, a disruptive behaviour can be a symptom of a psychiatric disorder in one person, whilst in another person, and in other environmental circumstances, it may be a means of communication, serving as a vehicle for obtaining a caregiver's attention or avoiding an unwanted task. Delineation of a subtype of an established psychiatric disorder asks for the specialist knowledge of the diagnostician.

The specialist teams should be based locally, providing inpatient care as well as outpatient and community-based interventions (see Chapter 10.9). Involvement of parents and carers as partners in the management plan can have more advantages and is being recommended.

The diagnostic evaluation may require significantly more time than the evaluation of persons of normal cognition. An accurate diagnosis which integrates all assessment results of the multi-disciplinary team members should serve as a starting point for the treatment.[51]

## Conclusion

Persons with ID are more prone to psychiatric disorders and behavioural problems than the general population. The symptoms of their biological disorders, developmental processes, and interaction patterns may give atypical clinical pictures, particularly in individuals with moderate and severe ID. It is probable that certain disorders are specifically associated with or even unique to the ID. Traditional nosological classifications do not adequately accommodate the phenomenology of psychiatric disorders in this population. A broader taxonomy, that takes account of the atypical presentation of psychopathology in this population is necessary.

## Further information

Bouras, N. and Holt, G. (2007). *Psychiatric and behavioural disorders in intellectual and developmental disabilities*. Cambridge University Press, Cambridge.

Deb, S., Matthews, T., Holt, G., *et al.* (2001). *Practice guidelines for the assessment and diagnosis of mental health problems in adults with intellectual disability*. Pavilion, Brighton.

Došen, A. and Day, K. (2001). *Treating mental illness and behaviour disorders in children and adults with mental retardation*. American Psychiatric Press, Washington.

Došen, A., Gardner, W.I., Griffiths, D.M., *et al.* (2007). *Practice guidelines and principles: assessment, diagnosis, treatment and related support services for persons with intellectual disabilities and problem behaviour*. Centre for Consultation and Expertise, Gouda.

Fletcher, R., Loschen, E., Stavrakaki, C., *et al.* (2007). *Diagnostic manua— Intellectual disability*. NADD Press, Kingston, New York.

Royal College of Psychiatrists. (2001). DC-LD: *diagnostic criteria for psychiatric disorders for use with adults with learning disabilities/mental retardation*. Gaskell Press, London.

## References

1. Sovner, R. and Hurley, A. (1990). Assessment tools which facilitate psychiatric evaluation of treatment. *The Habilitative Mental Health Care Newsletter*, **9**, 11.
2. Hucker, S.J., Day, K.A., George, S., *et al.* (1979). Psychoses in mentally handicapped adults. In *Psychiatric illness and mental handicap* (eds. F.E. James and R.P. Snaith), pp. 27–35. Gaskell Press, London.
3. Došen, A. (2005b). Applying the developmental perspective in psychiatric assessment and diagnosis of persons with intellectual disability: part II—diagnosis. *Journal of Intellectual Disability Research*, **49**, 9–15.
4. Deb, S., Matthews, T., Holt, G., *et al.* (2001). *Practice guidelines for the assessment and diagnosis of mental health problems in adults with intellectual disability*. Pavilion, Brighton.
5. Royal College of Psychiatrists. (2001). *DC-LD: diagnostic criteria for psychiatric disorders for use with adults with learning disabilities/mental retardation*. Gaskell Press, London.
6. Bouras, N., Martin, G., Leese, M., *et al.* (2004). Schizophrenia-spectrum psychosis in people with and without intellectual disability. *Journal of Intellectual Disability Research*, **48**, 548–55.
7. Reid, A. (1993). Schizophrenic and paranoid syndromes in persons with mental retardation. In *Mental health aspects of mental retardation* (eds. R. Fletcher and A. Došen), pp. 98–110. Lexington Books, New York.
8. Evans, K.M., Cotton, M.M., Einfeld, S.L., *et al.* (1999). Assessment of depression in adults with severe or profound intellectual disability. *Journal of Intellectual Disability Research*, **24**, 147–60.
9. Day, K. (1990). Depression in mildly and moderately retarded adults. In *Depression in mentally retarded children and adults* (eds. A. Došen and F. Menolascino), pp. 129–54. Logon, Leiden.
10. Došen, A. and Gielen, J. (1993). Depression in persons with mental retardation: assessment and diagnosis. In *Mental health aspects of mental retardation* (eds. R. Fletcher and A. Došen), pp. 70–97. Lexington Books, New York.
11. Reiss, S. and Rojahn, J. (1994). Joint occurrence of depression and aggression in children and adults with mental retardation. *Journal of Intellectual Disability Research*, **37**, 287–94.
12. Sovner, R. and Pary, R. (1993). Affective disorders in developmentally disabled persons. In *Psychology in the mentally retarded* (eds. J. Matson and R. Barrett), pp. 87–148. Longwood, Boston, MA.
13. Day, K. (1985). Psychiatric disorder in the middle aged and elderly mentally handicapped. *The British Journal of Psychiatry*, **147**, 660–7.
14. Došen, A. (2005c). *Psychische stoornissen, gedragsproblemen en verstandelijke handicap*. Van Gorcum, Assen.
15. Holt, G., and Bouras, N. (2002). *Autism and related disorders*. Royal College of Psychiatrists, London.
16. Gardner, W.I., Došen, A., Griffiths, D.M., *et al.* (2006). *Practice guidelines for diagnostic, treatment and related support services for persons with developmental disabilities and serious behavioral problems*. NADD Press, Kingston.

17. Došen, A. (2005a). Applying the developmental perspective in psychiatric assessment and diagnosis of persons with intellectual disability: part I—assessment. *Journal of Intellectual Disability Research*, **49**, 1–8.

18. Day, K. (1993). Crime and mental retardation, a review. In *Clinical approaches to the mentally disordered offender* (eds. K. Howells and C. Hollin), p. 144. Wiley, Chichester.

19. Corbett, J.A. (1979). Psychiatric morbidity and mental retardation. In *Psychiatric illness and mental handicap* (eds. F. James and R. Snaith), pp. 11–25. Gaskell, London.

20. Reid, A.H. and Ballinger, B.R. (1987). Personality disorder in mental handicap. *Psychological Medicine*, **17**, 983–7.

21. Zigler, E., Bennett-Gates, D., Hodapp, R., *et al.* (2002). Assessing personality traits of individuals with mental retardation. *American Journal of Mental Retardation*, **107**, 181–93.

22. Levitas, A. and Gilson, S. (1994). Psychosocial development of children and adolescents with mild mental retardation. In *Mental health in mental retardation* (ed. N. Bouras), pp. 34–45. Cambridge University Press. Cambridge.

23. Gaedt, C. (1995). Psychotherapeutic approaches in the treatment of mental illness and behavioral disorders in mentally retarded people: the significance of a psychoanalytic perspective. *Journal of Intellectual Disability Research*, **39**, 233–9.

24. Menolascino, F.J. and Weiler, M.A. (1990). The challenge of depression and suicide in severely mentally retarded adults. In *Depression in mentally retarded children and adults* (eds. A. Došen and F. Menolascino), pp. 155–74. Logon, Leiden.

25. Szymanski, L. (1994). Mental retardation and mental health: concepts, aetiology and incidence. In *Mental health in mental retardation* (ed. N. Bouras), pp. 19–33. Cambridge University Press, Cambridge.

26. Reid, A. (1982). *The psychiatry of mental handicap*. Blackwell Science, Oxford.

27. Bregman, J.D. and Harris, J.C. (1995). Mental retardation. In *Comprehensive textbook of psychiatry VI* (eds. H. Kaplan and B. Sadock), pp. 2207–42. Williams and Wilkins, Baltimore, MD.

28. Sturmey, P. (1999). Classification; concepts, progress and future. In *Psychiatric and behavioural disorders in developmental disabilities and mental retardation* (ed. N. Bouras), pp. 3–17. Univesity Press, Cambridge.

29. Van Praag, H.M. (1997). The future of biological psychiatry. *CNS Spectrums*, **12**, 8–23.

30. Van Praag, H.M. (2000). Nosologomania: a disorder of psychiatry. *The World Journal of Biological Psychiatry*, **1**, 151–8.

31. Charlot, L. (2003). Mission impossible?: developing an accurate classification of psychiatric disorders for individuals with developmental disabilities. *Mental Health Aspects of Developmental Disabilities*, **6**, 26–35.

32. Einfeld, S.L. and Tonge, B.J. (1996). Population prevalence of psychopathology in children and adolescents with intellectual disability: epidemiological findings. *Journal of Intellectual Disability Research*, **40**, 99–109.

33. Achenbach, T.M. and Zigler, E.F. (1968). Cue-learning and problem-learning strategies in normal and retarded children. *Child Development*, **39**, 827–48

34. Menolascino, F.J. (1977). *Challenges in mental retardation: progressive ideologies and services*. Human Sciences Press, New York.

35. Matson, J.L. (1985). Bio-social theory of psychopathology: a three by three factor model. *Applied Research in Mental Retardation*, **6**, 199–227.

36. Tanguay, P.E. (1984). Towards a new classification of serious psychopathology in children. *Journal of the American Academy of Child Psychiatry*, **32**, 373–84.

37. Gaedt, C. and Gärtner, D. (1990). *Depressive Grundprozesse–Reinzeniering der Selbstentwertung*. Neuerkeroder Forum 4, Neuerkerode, Sickte.

38. Clegg, J. and Sheard C. (2002). Challenging behaviour and insecure attachment. *Journal of Intellectual Disability Research*, **44**, 503–6.

39. Janssen, C.G.C., Schuengel C., and Stolk, J. (2002). Understanding challenging behaviour in people with severe and profound intellectual disability; a stress-attachment model. *Journal of Intellectual Disability Research*, **46**, 445–53.

40. Collacott, R.A. (1999). People with Down syndrome and mental health needs. In *Psychiatric and behavioural disorders in developmental disabilities and mental retardation* (ed. N.Bouras), pp. 200–11, University Press, Cambridge.

41. Khan, S., Osinowo, T., and Pary, R.J. (2002). Down syndrome and major depressive disorder. *Mental Health Aspects of Developmental Disabilities*, **5**, 46–52.

42. Turk, J., Hagerman, R.J., Barnicoat, A., *et al.* (1994). The fragile X syndrome. In *Mental health in mental retardation* (ed. N. Bouras), pp. 135–53. Cambridge University Press, Cambridge.

43. Dykens, E.M., Hodapp, R.M., and Finucane, B.M. (2000). *Genetics and mental retardation syndromes*. Paul Brookes Publ., Baltimore.

44. Shprintzen, R.J., Goldberg, R., Goldning-Kushner, K.J., *et al.* (1992). Late-onset psychosis in the velo-cardio-facial syndrome. *American Journal of Medical Genetics*, **42**, 141–2.

45. Murphy, K.C. (2004). Review: the behavioural phenotypes in velo-cardio-facial syndrome. *Journal of Intellectual Disability Research*, **48**, 524–30.

46. Pary, R.J. (2002). *Psychiatric problems in older persons with developmental disabilities*. NADD Press, Kingston.

47. Patel, P., Goldberg, D., and Moss, S. (1993). Psychiatric morbidity in older people with moderate and severe learning disability. II. The prevalence study. *The British Journal of Psychiatry*, **163**, 481–91.

48. Day, K. and Jancar, J. (1994). Mental and physical health and aging in mental handicapped: a review. *Journal of Intellectual Disability Research*, **38**, 241–56.

49. Došen, A. (2002). Affective disorders in older people with developmental disabilities. In *Psychiatric problems in older persons with developmental disabilities* (ed. R.J. Pary), pp. 45–64, NADD Press, Kingston.

50. Szymanski, L.S., King, B.H., Bernet, W., *et al.* (1999). Practice parameters for assessment and treatment of children, adolescents and adults with mental retardation and comorbid mental disorders. *Journal of the American Academy of Child and Adolescent Psychiatry*, **38**, (Suppl. 12), 5S–31S.

51. Došen, A. (2007). Integrative treatment in persons with intellectual disability and mental health problems. *Journal of Intellectual Disability Research*, **51**, 66–74.

## 10.5.3 **Epilepsy and epilepsy-related behaviour disorders among people with intellectual disability**

Matti Iivanainen

Epilepsy is defined as at least one epileptic seizure; this in practice means two or more epileptic seizures unprovoked by any immediate identifiable cause during a relatively short period of time. Epileptic seizure is a clinical manifestation presumed to result from an abnormal and excessive discharge of a set of neurones in the brain. An epileptic syndrome is a cluster of symptoms and signs including type of seizure, mode of seizure recurrence, neurological findings, and neuroradiological or other findings of special investigations, customarily occurring together. An epileptic syndrome can have more than one cause or the cause may remain unknown; consequently outcomes may be different. Pseudoseizure is used to denote epilepsy-like seizures without concomitant EEG changes.

Epilepsy and intellectual disability are symptoms of brain origin. The former is an unstable condition, where during the seizure or ictally the behaviour of a person with epilepsy is abnormal, but between the seizures or interictally there is no affect of epilepsy on his or her behaviour. Intellectual disability is a more or less stable condition. However, the categories of the degrees of intellectual disability are neither absolute nor static, as some children may move up or down between them.

This chapter deals with the diagnosis, manifestations, behavioural disorders, frequency, aetiology, treatment, effects of antiepileptic drugs on behaviour, and prognosis of epilepsy in people with intellectual disability.

## Diagnosis and differential diagnosis of epilepsy

The diagnosis of epilepsy is clinical and requires the collection of historical data, physical and mental examination, EEG, and laboratory tests such as determinations of blood glucose and electrolytes.[1] In babies with epilepsy, attention should be paid to changes of skin colour or cardiac rhythm, sucking and smacking, which all may be epileptic phenomena. In people with intellectual disability it may be difficult or impossible to obtain an accurate clinical history from the patient. The clinician often has to depend on relatives or other professionals involved in the care of the patient. In addition to a description of the seizures, a history of the age at onset of epilepsy and the complete clinical picture of the epileptic syndrome are of value.

General factors that provoke seizures include fever, infection, hypoglycaemia, stress, excessive waking, alcohol withdrawal, hyperventilation, some medications, sudden discontinuation of sedative drugs, and specific activity. Fevers associated with infections such as those of the ears, sinuses, upper respiratory tract, or urinary tract are quite common. If seizures are exacerbated, ensure that any treatable infection is identified. The situation is further confused by the fact that seizures can produce the fever, which, however, resolves within an hour. Withdrawal seizures may be precipitated by a sudden discontinuation of drugs such as benzodiazepines which have an antiepileptic effect, although they may have been prescribed for another reason. Some seizures may be associated with a specific activity, especially if this activity induces excitement or anxiety. Exercise-induced seizures occur regularly in some patients.

Many people with intellectual disability have abnormal behaviour that resembles epileptic seizures but is not epileptic in origin. The diagnostic and other problems caused by non-epileptic seizures or pseudoseizures are well known.[2] Different dyskinesias, psychogenic attacks, and other non-epileptic episodes may be manifested as pseudoseizures at different ages (Table 10.5.3.1). Sudden aggression and other epilepsy-like conditions (Table 10.5.3.2) are in practice the most important reasons for the overdiagnosis of

**Table 10.5.3.1** Salient non-epileptic episodes at different ages

| Age | Disorder |
|---|---|
| 0–2 months | Tremor |
| | Dyskinesias associated with bronchopulmonar dysplasia |
| | Benign myoclonus during sleep |
| | Apnoea |
| 2–18 months | Paroxysmal torticollins |
| | Ipsoclonus myoclonus syndrome |
| | Intestinal obstruction |
| | Breath-holding spells |
| | Jactatio capitis |
| | Masturbation |
| | Paroxysmal choreoathetosis |
| | Gastro-oesophageal reflux |
| 1.5–5 years | Pavor nocturnus |
| | Benign paroxysmal vertigo |
| | Nodding puppet syndrome |
| | Enuresis nocturnus |
| | Confusion with fever |
| | Familial dystonic choreoathetosis |
| 5–12 years | Tic |
| | Complicated migraine |
| | Attention disturbance |
| | Sleepwalking |
| | Paroxysmalis choreoathetosis |
| >12 years | Vertebrobasilar migraine |
| | Syncope |
| | Hyperventilation syndrome |
| | Obstructive sleep apnoea |
| | Psychogenic attacks |
| | Raving fits |

epilepsy, and consequently also for overmedication and subsequent intoxication in patients with intellectual disability. On the other hand, non-convulsive epileptic phenomena and even partial seizures (Table 10.5.3.3) may be difficult to diagnose in people with intellectual disability. The situation is more complicated when patients with intractable epilepsy have both real epileptic seizures and pseudoseizures, for example psychogenic seizures. In such cases the recognition of psychogenic seizures[3] (Table 10.5.3.4) helps to identify appropriate treatment.[4]

**Table 10.5.3.2** Conditions often misdiagnosed as epilepsy in subjects with intellectual disability

Sudden aggression
Self-abuse
Bizarre behaviour
Abnormal motor activity
Staring
Eye-blinking
Nystagmus
Exaggerated startle
Intermittent lethargy

**Table 10.5.3.3** Underdiagnosis of epilepsy in subjects with intellectual disability

Absence seizures
Non-convulsive status epilepticus
Seizures with periodic headache
Seizures with vertigo
Seizures with paraesthesia
Seizures with visceral and vegetative disturbances
Loss of emotional control
Postictal effects
Simple partial seizures
Complex partial seizures

Using magnetic resonance imaging (**MRI**), it is possible to identify structural brain abnormalities, including neoplasms, dysplasia, heterotopia, or diseases in the brainstem and/or posterior fossa. If MRI is not available, CT is recommended.

Prolonged video-EEG monitoring of the patients is of use in selecting candidates for epilepsy surgery or in distinguishing between epileptic and non-epileptic seizures. Basically, this enables any behaviour to be analysed in relation to the EEG changes. If this investigation is not available, portable cassette recording of the EEG may also be of considerable value. The diagnosis of subclinical seizures, including minimal behavioural or cognitive changes in the absence of any obvious clinical seizures, can be demonstrated as lengthened reaction times during EEG discharges in the Romny test.

The brain function of people with epileptic seizures and syndromes can be examined by interictal and ictal single-photon emission CT, positron emission tomography, functional MRI, magnetic resonance spectroscopy, and magnetoencephalography together with simultaneous EEG. Such investigations can help to define the epileptogenic brain lesion and thereby guide management including decisions about epilepsy surgery.

# Epilepsy and epileptic syndromes at different ages

The main categories in the classification of seizures and epilepsy are primary generalized seizures, focal seizures, and secondary generalized seizures[5] (Table 10.5.3.5). The semiologic seizure classification[6] seeks to provide common descriptive terms for typical ictal symptoms and for seizure evolution (Table 10.5.3.6). Epileptic syndromes[7] are quite frequent in people with intellectual disability ranging from early infancy through childhood to adolescence (Table 10.5.3.7). As understanding of the pathophysiologic and anatomic substrates of epileptic seizures, syndromes and disorders increases, these classifications may need to be reappraised. [8–10]

## Infancy

Infants with **early infantile epileptic encephalopathy** or Ohtahara syndrome seem initially neurologically normal, but soon develop increasingly frequent seizures with tonic spasms that resemble infantile spasms and are usually resistant to treatment. Severe progressive intellectual disability becomes evident with age. Many die early and most survivals are handicapped. Some may evolve into the West syndrome and some later into the Lennox–Gastaut syndrome (see below). The EEG shows a 'burst suppression' pattern with an almost flat tracing for several seconds, alternating with diffuse, high-amplitude, slow wave-and-spike bursts, poorly modified by sleep–wake stages.[11] The aetiology of Ohtahara syndrome includes usually congenital or acquired malformations of cortical development and diffuse prenatal encephalopathies, the cause of which remains unknown, so far. A report on a case of Ohtahara syndrome included a metabolic defect with cytochrome oxidase deficiency.[12]

**Early myoclonic epileptic** encephalopathy is another epileptic syndrome occurring during infancy with a grim prognosis.[13] The predominant seizure pattern is erratic, paroxysmal, fragmentary myoclonus, often associated with other seizure types. Brain malformations are not so common as in Ohtahara syndrome.

**Infantile spasms** occur usually at the ages of 4 to 6 months and in 90 per cent of cases during the first year of life. The events resemble the Moro reflex with sudden, brief flexion of neck and trunk, raising both arms forwards or sideways, sometimes with flexion at the elbows, and flexion of legs at the hips. Less often, the legs extend at the hips. At the early stage flexion of the neck may be the only or main feature; this may be followed by more complex and dramatic attacks later on. A cry is often associated with the attack either as part of the attack or occurring afterwards as an expression of disquiet. The spasms are usually symmetric, but may be asymmetric or even unilateral. The EEG is chaotic with slow waves of high voltage intermixed with diffuse or asynchronous spikes in both hemispheres or in the contralateral hemisphere in unilateral cases. This

**Table 10.5.3.4** Differential diagnosis of epileptic and psychogenic seizures

| Typical features | Epileptic seizures | | Psychogenic seizures |
|---|---|---|---|
| | **Generalized tonic-clonic seizures** | **Complex partial seizures** | |
| Comparison of seizures with known seizure types | Little variation in events | Wide range of events, but the most common are well described | Extremely wide range of events with bizarre or unusual behaviour |
| Ictal EEG | Abnormal and changed from preictal | Almost always abnormal and changed from preictal | Usually normal and unchanged from preictal |
| Postictal EEG | Almost always abnormal and changed from preictal | Frequently abnormal and changed from preictal | Usually normal and unchanged from preictal |
| Effect of antiepileptic medication on seizures | Prominent, especially in severely affected patients | Usually prominent | Usually no effect |

**Table 10.5.3.5** Classification of epileptic seizures (International League Against Epilepsy, www.ilae.org/Visitors/Centre/ctf/CTF table3.cfm, copyright ILAE)

*Partial (focal, local seizures)*
Simple partial seizures
    With motor signs
    With autonomic symptoms and signs
    With somatosensory or special sensory symptoms: simple hallucinations (e.g. tingling, light flashes, buzzing), somatosensory, visual, auditory, olfactory, gustatory, vertiginous
    With psychic symptoms (disturbances of higher cerebral functions): dysphasic, dysmnesic, cognitive, affective, illusions, structured hallucinations
    Complex partial seizures (with impairment of consciousness, may sometimes begin with simple symptomatology)
    Partial seizures evolving to secondarily generalized tonic–clonic seizures

*Generalized seizures[a]*
Absence seizures
Atypical absences
Myoclonic seizures
Clonic seizures
Tonic seizures
Tonic–clonic seizures
Atonic seizures

[a] Combinations of seizures listed here may occur.

**Table 10.5.3.6** Semiologic seizure classification[7]

*Aura*
Somatosensory aura
Visual aura
Auditory aura
Gustatory aura
Olfactory aura
Autonomic aura
Abdominal aura
Psychic aura
Autonomic seizure
Dialeptic seizure

*Motor seizure*
Simple motor seizure
    Myoclonic seizure
    Epileptic spasm
    Tonic seizure
    Clonic seizure
    Tonic–clonic seizure
    Versive seizure
Complex motor seizure
    Hypermotor seizure
    Automotor seizure
    Gelastic seizure

*Special seizure*
Atonic seizure
Astatic seizure
Hypomotor seizure
Akinetic seizure
Negative myoclonic seizure
Aphasic seizure

Reproduced from Commission of Classification and Terminology of the International League Against Epilepsy (1989). Proposal for revised clinical and electroencephalographic classification of epilepsies and epileptic syndromes. *Epilepsia*, **30**, 389–99, copyright 1989, International League Against Epilepsy.

**Table 10.5.3.7** Salient epileptic syndromes which may be associated with intellectual disability and salient intellectual disability syndromes which may be associated with epilepsy

*Infant*
Early myoclonic encephalopathy
Early infantile epileptic encephalopathy with suppression bursts
Infantile spasms
Severe myoclonic epilepsy
Sturge–Weber syndrome
Down syndrome
Fragile X syndrome
Angelman syndrome

*Children and adolescents*
Epilepsia partialis continua Kojewnikow
Unverricht–Lundborg disease
Lafora disease
Progressive myoclonus epilepsy with intellectual disability
Other neuronal ceroid lipofuscinoses
Sialidosis
Myoclonic epilepsy with ragged red fibres (MERRF)
Rett syndrome
Landau–Kleffner syndrome
Continuous spike-wave discharge during slow-wave sleep

pattern is called hypsarrhythmia. Infants with unilateral spasms need to be examined using a positron emission tomography scan, as contralateral hypometabolism may be due to cortical dysplasia, a condition which may be treatable by resective epilepsy surgery. Aetiology is usually symptomatic including brain abnormalities due to intrauterine infections such as toxoplasmosis, cytomegalic inclusion disease, or rubella. Other aetiologies are brain malformations due to unknown cause. Infants with Down syndrome or tuberous sclerosis may develop infantile spasms. **West syndrome** comprises the triad of infantile spasms, hypsarrhythmia, and intellectual disability.

Progressive degenerative brain diseases and neoplasms are rare causes of infantile spasms. Also neurometabolic disorders such as phenylketonuria, maple syrup urine diseases, non-ketotic or ketotic hyperglycinaemia, and urea cycle defects may lead to infantile spasms.

**Severe myoclonic epilepsy** in infants includes generalized or unilateral febrile clonic seizures, secondary appearance of myoclonic jerks, and often partial seizures. All the children affected suffer from intellectual disability from the second year of life onwards. Ataxia, signs of upper motor neurone involvement, and interictal myoclonus may appear. [13]

## Early childhood

Myoclonic epilepsy of early childhood shares many features with the **Lennox–Gastaut syndrome**.[13] The latter is a group of epileptic disorders of varied aetiology in childhood. West syndrome often evolves into Lennox–Gastaut syndrome characterized by atypical absences, axial, tonic and sudden myoclonic, atonic, partial, and generalized tonic–clonic seizures, diffuse slow interictal spike waves in the waking EEGs and fast rhythmic bursts (10 Hz) during sleep. A progressive decrease in IQ is often found in children with Lennox–Gastaut syndrome. **Myoclonic–astatic epilepsy** or **Doose** syndrome resembles Lennox–Gastaut syndrome, but is not so severe.

### Later childhood and adolescence

**Progressive myoclonus epilepsies** have the nosological picture of an evolving syndrome of symptoms including massive and segmental myoclonus, myoclonic or tonic–clonic seizures, partial seizures, cerebellar impairment, and higher neurological dysfunctions. [13] Unverricht–Lundborg disease is most common in the Finnish and North African population, but occur also elsewhere. The disease progresses only over a limited period and stabilizes thereafter. [14] The age of onset is around 7 years and the disease starts with myoclonus or nocturnal tonic–clonic seizures. The longest lifespans are more than 60 years. The intelligence level is slightly lowered or even normal. Patients with severe intellectual disability have often had drug intoxication. [15]

Progressive myoclonus epilepsy with intellectual disability (Northern epilepsy) and Lafora disease are more progressive disorders with different gene defects.[16] Sialidosis and mitochondrial encephalopathy with ragged red fibres may also show myoclonic seizures. Epilepsy is quite common in girls with Rett syndrome, affecting about 90 per cent of the patients. They may have several seizure types including partial, generalized tonic–clonic, and myoclonic seizures, atypical absences, short flexion or extensor spasms, and drop attacks or various combinations of such seizures.[17]

Of the progressive **partial epilepsies**, epilepsia partialis Kojewnikow or Rasmussen syndrome type 2 is especially important because the disease is fatal if untreated. The classical model of the association between frequent epileptiform discharges and permanent loss of function is provided by the Landau–Kleffner syndrome or acquired epileptic aphasia. There is increasing evidence that frequent epileptiform discharges, perhaps particularly overnight in the form of continuous spikes and waves during slow sleep, also called electrical status epilepticus, is associated with permanent intellectual impairment if allowed to continue for long periods.[18]

### Adulthood and old age

The proportion of cerebrovascular disorders, brain tumours, chronic alcoholism, and sequelae of brain injuries is increasing with advancing age in the aetiology of epilepsy. From about 35 years of age onwards partial epilepsies become more common than generalized epilepsies. Patients with intellectual disability may also develop these disorders.

## Behavioural disorders due to epilepsy

Psychic symptoms may be seen as epileptic manifestations of several epileptic seizure types (Table 10.5.3.5). Thus simple partial seizures may manifest themselves with somatosensory or special sensory symptoms including simple hallucinations such as tingling, light flashes, or buzzing or with psychic symptoms such as dysphasic, dysamnesic, cognitive, affective, illusional, or structured hallucinations. Complex partial seizures often include behavioural abnormalities reaching from confusional states to psychotic-like episodes. This is often the case in temporal-lobe and frontal-lobe epilepsies. Among generalized seizures absence status epilepticus resembles psychotic behaviour,[19] which the person in question does not remember afterwards.

In patients with intractable seizures, about one-fifth are non-epileptic in origin. Patients with psychogenic seizures do not generally have seizures when alone or when asleep. Their EEG shows normal activity preictally, ictally, and postictally. The courses of the psychogenic seizures do not show any uniform pattern as is the case with epileptic seizures (see Table 10.5.3.4). Instead their seizures include a variety of behavioural disturbances including conversion, depressive, anxiety, adjustment, somatoform, psychotic, or facitious disorders.[2] The antiepileptic drugs are ineffective against psychogenic seizures but appropriate psychotherapy is helpful in 70 to 80 per cent of cases. Also panic disorder may be difficult to distinguish from complex partial seizures especially in patients with mild intellectual disability. There exists a relationship between brain damage, epilepsy, ictal, and interictal aggressive behaviour, and socio-economic factors. Rarely, ictal aggression occurs in patients with epilepsy, but postictal confusional aggression, and aggression occurring in postictal psychotic states is more common.

## Occurrence of epilepsy related to intellectual disability

The prevalences of epilepsy and intellectual disability in the general population are both close to 1 per cent. Epilepsy is more common and more difficult to diagnose and to treat in people with intellectual disability than in those with normal intellect. Population-based studies have revealed that intellectual disability occurs in at least 30 to 40 per cent of individuals with epilepsy,[20] while the prevalence of epilepsy in the population with intellectual disability is about 20 to 25 per cent.[21] It is higher in the more severely disabled (IQ < 50) than in less severely disabled (IQ 50–70)—30 to 50 per cent and 15 to 20 per cent, respectively. Brain damage tends to be more extensive when epilepsy, intellectual disability, or cerebral palsy are complicated by each other or by other conditions of brain origin. It is unlikely that specific causal factors of epilepsy, intellectual disability, or cerebral palsy will ever be positively identified, for these are non-specific clinical features of brain disorder. Epileptic fits themselves, especially if they are persistent, may produce brain damage and play a part in producing a progressive decline in the intellectual functioning of patients. Further apparent deterioration of intellectual functioning may be the result of excessively high doses of anticonvulsant drugs.

Epilepsy occurs in all the main aetiological categories of intellectual disability. In a series of 1000 mentally retarded patients, epilepsy was less frequent in the prenatal category than in the rest of the series (182/515 or 35.3 per cent versus 260/485 or 53.6 per cent). Of the main types of epilepsy, partial epilepsy is more frequent in the prenatal and postnatal aetiological categories and in the category of infections and intoxications.[22]

In people with Down syndrome the frequency of epilepsy is 5 to 10 per cent. There is an age-related bimodal distribution with about 40 per cent of seizures starting before the age of 1 year and another 40 per cent starting after the third decade.[23] Roughly 25 per cent of individuals with fragile X syndrome have epileptic seizures which are usually infrequent, mild, easily controlled, and typically disappear in adolescence, as in benign Rolandic epilepsy. In Angelman syndrome epilepsy is present in more than 90 per cent of the affected individuals.[23] In Rett syndrome epilepsy affects up to 90 per cent of patients[17] Seizures are usually benign during the early years of life. In patients with aspartylglucosaminuria, epilepsy is found in 28 per cent of adults and in 2 per cent of children.[24] Epilepsy is common (up to 100 per cent) in patients with the various forms of neuronal ceroid lipofuscinoses, especially during the last years of life,[25] and also in other inborn errors of metabolism leading to intellectual disability such as sialidosis type 1, Tay–Sachs disease, type 3 Gaucher disease, mitochondrial encephalopathy with lactic acidosis and strokes, and myoclonic epilepsy with ragged red fibres.

## Aetiology and pathogenesis of epilepsy

The presumed aetiology of intellectual disability is also the presumed aetiology of epilepsy in most patients.[21,22] In addition, patients with intellectual disability may develop an ischaemic or haemorrhagic lesion, a neoplasm, or another lesion in the brain which may lead to epilepsy.[21] The presumed aetiology of epilepsy can be found in about three-quarters of the patients. In the aetiological classification based on the time of the presumed cause of epilepsy and intellectual disability, prenatal aetiology is the most common (Table 10.5.3.8). In the aetiological classification based on presumed cause, the categories of unknown prenatal influence, infections and intoxications, trauma and physical agents, and other specified aetiological agents cover most of the cases (Table 10.5.3.9). In patients with intellectual disability and epilepsy it is important to try to find the cause of the intellectual impairment, epilepsy, or epilepsy syndrome. In some cases, the epilepsy syndrome or an underlying inborn error of metabolism may be relevant.

Basic mechanisms leading to epilepsy include disturbances in the balance between excitatory and inhibitory neurotransmitter function within brain cells and their connections to important channels such as voltage-gated sodium channels. For instance, hyperactivity of the excitatory neurotransmitter glutamic acid and/or hypoactivity of inhibitory neurotransmitter γ-aminobutyric acid (**GABA**) may lead to epileptic seizures. The existence of so many genetically determined disorders leading to intellectual disability and epilepsy[26] (Table 10.5.3.10) and the large variation in the prevalence of epilepsy in the specific intellectual disability syndromes and the use of new methods such as an array technology suggest that genetic factors play a more important role in producing epilepsy.

The three following examples, as well as those mentioned above, illustrate this variety of genetic explanations for epilepsy among intellectual disability syndromes.[23] Angelman syndrome is a con-

**Table 10.5.3.8** Aetiological classification of epilepsy and intellectual disability according to time of presumed cause

| | N = 129[a] | N = 442[b] |
|---|---|---|
| Prenatal (%) | 35.1 | 41.2 |
| Perinatal (%) | 10.0 | 15.4 |
| Postnatal (%) | 8.7 | 18.8 |
| Multiple (%) | 14.7 | 4.3 |
| Unknown (%) | 31.4 | 20.4 |
| Total (%) | 100.0 | 100.0 |

[a] Data from Forsgren et al.[21]

[b] Data from Iivanainen.[22]

**Table 10.5.3.9** Aetiological classification of epilepsy and intellectual disability according to presumed cause

| | N = 442 |
|---|---|
| Infections and intoxications (%) | 18.1 |
| Trauma and physical agents (%) | 16.3 |
| Disorders of metabolism (%) | 3.2 |
| Gross prenatal influence (%) | 24.0 |
| Prematurity (%) | 0.5 |
| Major psychiatric disorder (%) | 0.5 |
| Psychosocial deprivation (%) | 0.0 |
| Multiple causes (%) | 7.2 |
| Hereditary (simple) (%) | 0.5 |
| Other specified (%) | 19.7 |
| Unspecified (%) | 0.0 |
| Total (%) | 100.0 |

(Reproduced from M. Iivanainen, Diagnosis of epileptic seizures and syndromes in mentally retarded patients. In *Paediatric epilepsy* (ed. M. Sillanpää et al.), pp. 233–41. Copyright 1990, Wrightson Biomedical, Petersfield)

tiguous gene defect most often caused by a maternally inherited deletion of chromosome 15q11–13. Several of the deleted genes code for GABA receptor subunits. Deficits of inhibitory GABAergic function could directly predispose affected individuals to seizures. This hypothesis is supported by knockouts of analogous chromosome region in mice, which produces an epileptic phenotype.

In Down syndrome or trisomy 21 the bimodal distribution of the frequency of epilepsy between young and older ages is interesting. The fact that more than 75 per cent of adults with Down syndrome develop late-onset epilepsy coincident with the onset of the neuropathological abnormalities in the brain compatible to Alzheimer's disease suggests an aetiological role of these abnormalities. However, as epilepsy is associated with Alzheimer's disease in only 10 per cent of patients without Down syndrome, it is unlikely that Alzheimer's neuropathological abnormalities are solely responsible for the late-onset epilepsy in patients with Down syndrome. As the EEG of most of these patients is characteristic of idiopathic generalized epilepsy and the gene for progressive myoclonus epilepsy is located in the Down syndrome region on chromosome 21, it is quite possible that this gene product predisposes for a senile myoclonus epilepsy in Down syndrome.[23] Abnormal neuronal circuits with fewer GABAergic neurones in certain cortical layers, cerebral dysgenesis particularly of dendritic spines, pathophysiological membrane ion channels, and altered neurotransmitter level are potential mechanisms of epilepsy in Down syndrome.[23]

In the tandem trinucleotide repeat disorder, fragile X syndrome, triplet expansion (CGG) results in shutdown of fragile X intellectual disability 1 gene transcription, which may alter overall neurologic development and lead to seizures.[23]

Thus, there exists a spectrum of epilepsy mechanisms among these three intellectual disability syndromes, ranging from deletion of a gene or genes that directly leads to hyperexcitability (Angelman syndrome), to a chromosomal triplication that alters several aspects of neuronal development and function (Down syndrome), to a

**Table 10.5.3.10** Genetic diseases with epilepsy and intellectual disability

| Disease | Mode of inheritance | Gene location |
|---|---|---|
| Progressive epilepsy with intellectual disability (Northern epilepsy) | AR | 8p |
| Unverricht–Lundborg disease (Baltic, Mediterranean) | AR | 21q22 |
| Infantile neuronal ceroid lipofuscinosis | AR | 1p32 |
| Late infantile neuronal ceroid lipofuscinosis | AR | 11p15 |
| Variant late infantile neuronal ceroid lipofuscinosis | AR | 15q21-23 |
| Juvenile neuronal ceroid lipofuscinosis | AR | 16p12 |
| Finnish variant neuronal ceroid lipofuscinosis | AR | 13q22 |
| Lafora disease | AR | 6q23-25 |
| Mitochondrial encephalomopathy, lactic acidosis (UUR) and stroke-like episodes (MELAS) | Maternal | tRNA-Leu (UUR) |
| Myoclonic epilepsy with ragged red fibres (MERRF) | Maternal | tRNA-Lys |
| Epilepsy and mental retardation limited to females | X-linked | Xq22 |
| Tuberous sclerosis[a] | AD | 9q34 16p13 |
| Angelman syndrome[a] | AD | 15q13 |
| Neurofibromatosis type[a] 1 | AD | 17q11 |
| Fragile X[a] | X-linked | Xq27 |
| Rett syndrome[a] | X-linked | Xq28-McCP2 |

AR, autosomal recessive; AD, autosomal dominant.

[a] Epilepsy and/or intellectual disability may be manifested as part of the phenotype.

specific tandem repeat which alters neuronal function in a non-specific and probably benign manner (fragile X syndrome). It remains to be seen how much dissection of genetic mechanisms underlying other intellectual disability syndromes will provide additional insight into epilepsy mechanisms.

# Treatment of epilepsy

The diagnosis of epilepsy and its underlying disorder needs to be made without delay. The identification and avoidance of provoking factors likely to precipitate seizures in each individual is an essential aspect of the overall management. If this is insufficient, antiepileptic drug treatment is needed. If this is still insufficient, epilepsy surgery should be considered. Important points to be considered include not only the nature and severity of an underlying disease, but also the degree and location of brain lesion, the age of the patient at onset of epilepsy, and possible pseudodisability (pseudo-retardation) caused by epileptic seizures or by inappropriate medication. It is emphasized that treating frequent epileptiform discharges may not only reverse the intellectual disability which

in such cases is pseudodisability or state-dependent intellectual disability,[18] but may also in some cases prevent permanent intellectual disability.

# Antiepileptic drug therapy

## Drug interactions

Antiepileptic drugs interact with each other by three principal mechanisms: enzyme induction, enzyme inhibition, and through altered protein binding. Phenytoin and phenobarbital induce a wide range of enzyme activity. Carbamazepine induces its own enzymatic metabolism, and may induce the metabolism of valproate and phenytoin, resulting in lower concentrations of these drugs. Valproate inhibits the metabolism of phenobarbital and the epoxide of carbamazepine, resulting in high concentrations of each of these. Lamotrigine is metabolized in the liver. Valproate inhibits the metabolism of lamotrigine, resulting in a longer half-life and higher blood levels of lamotrigine while the blood level of valproate may be decreased. Lamotrigine does not affect the blood level of carbamazepine. Gabapentin is not metabolized at all and is excreted in the urine unchanged. If levetiracetam is administered with enzyme-inducing drugs, its clearance may increase by 22 per cent, although the drug concentrations in serum do not change when using other antiepileptic drugs simultaneously. The free or unbound fraction of antiepileptic drugs is in equilibrium with the brain concentration and is considered to be more relevant than the total blood level. When two drugs with a high degree of protein binding are used together, for example phenytoin and valproate, there may be some displacement of each drug from protein binding, increasing the unbound fraction. This may result in clinical neurotoxicity even when the total (bound plus unbound) blood level is within the reference range. The antiepileptic drugs also interact with many other drugs and may affect their blood levels and action, and vice versa. For instance, chloramphenicol, cimetidine, anticoagulants, ibuprofen, imipramine, propranol, and some psychotropic drugs inhibit the metabolism of phenytoin and lead to an increase of phenytoin blood level and possibly to phenytoin intoxication unless the dose of phenytoin is reduced.

## Choice of drug

Once the diagnosis of epilepsy has been made, the decision must be made as to whether antiepileptic medication is needed or not. If it is, the most appropriate antiepileptic drug is to be selected. The choice of antiepileptic medication depends primarily on an accurate classification of the seizure type and/or epilepsy syndrome.

Most treatment decisions have to be based on the results of studies of people who do not have intellectual disability. The exceptions are mainly studies of adults with the Lennox–Gastaut syndrome, where lamotrigine is recommended.[27] Valproate, carbamazepine, oxcarbazepine, and levetiracetam[28] are other antiepileptic drugs recommended in generalized and partial seizures based on uncontrolled studies or consensus. Valproate is the first choice for generalized epilepsies/seizures, while oxcarbazepine/carbamazepine is the choice for the focal epilepsies/seizures of people with intellectual disability.[29] Dosage and recommended drug levels in blood are presented in Table 10.5.3.11. If newer drugs are not available, phenobarbitone, primidone, and phenytoin may be used with caution, if special attention is paid not only to control of seizures, but also to behavioural, cognitive, and cerebellar functions which may

**Table 10.5.3.11** Pharmacokinetic properties of antiepileptic drugs

| Drug | Dose (mg/kg/day) | Doses per day | Therapeutic range | |
|---|---|---|---|---|
| | | | (μg/ml) | (μmol/ml) |
| Phenobarbitone | 1–3 | 1 | 10–30 | 40–130 |
| Primodone | 10–15 | 2 or 3 | 6–12 | 25–50 |
| Phenytoin | 4–6 | 1 or 2 | 10–20 | 40–80 |
| Carbamazepine | 15–20 | 2 or 3 | 4–12 | 15–50 |
| Oxcarbazepine | 15–40 | 2 or 3 | 15–23 | 30–120[a] |
| Valproate | 15–30 | 2 or 3 | 50–100 | 300–700 |
| Ethosuximide | 15–30 | 1 or 2 | 40–100 | 280–700 |
| Levetiracetam | 20–40 | 2 | 5–65 | 30–370 |
| Vigabatrin | 40–100 | 1 or 2 | NA | NA |
| Lamotrigine | 2–4(10)[b] | 1 or 2 | NA | NA |
| Gabapentin | 20–40 | 3 | NA | NA |
| Topiramate | 400 | 3 | NA | NA |
| Tiagabine | 32–56 | 3 | NA | NA |
| Clonazepam | 0.01–0.2 | 2 or 3 | 20–75 | 60–240 |

NA = not available.

[a] For monohydroxy derivative.

[b] With enzyme-inducing drugs.

be affected adversely, and sometimes insidiously, by these drugs. However, it is stressed that because of the lack of well-designed properly conducted randomized controlled trials for patients with newly diagnosed generalized of focal untreated seizures/epilepsies and for children in general, it is impossible at present to develop evidence-based guidelines aimed at identifying the overall optimal recommended monotherapy antiepileptic drug.[30]

Most antiepileptic drugs may aggravate certain epilepsies. This is the case especially with phenytoin and carbamazepine in idiopathic generalized absence and myoclonic epilepsies. Although valproate has low risk of seizure aggravation,[31] it may cause weight gain, polycystic ovaries, and hepatitis. Oxcarbazepine may lead to hyponatraemia and vigabatrin to visual field defects.[32]

## Withdrawal of treatment

Withdrawal of antiepileptic medication in patients with intellectual disability needs to be considered, provided their epilepsy is well-controlled and there are no specific contraindications for the withdrawal. Depending on the type of seizure or epilepsy syndrome and the individual history, it might be worth considering slow reducing the medication after a 2-year seizure-free period. However, if the individual is in a particularly poor prognostic category or if there is a history of severe, prolonged status epilepticus, it is worth waiting for longer before attempting medication reductions. Despite these reservations, attempts to discontinue antiepileptic medication in people with intellectual disability can be successful. It would appear that a better likelihood of a successful outcome may be suggested by later onset of epilepsy, i.e. after 2 to 2.5 years of age, a shorter duration, lower antiepileptic drug levels, and normal EEGs, together with complete control of the seizures.[33] The risk of recurrence of the seizures also depends on the type of epilepsy.[34] In complex

partial seizures, where exogenic factors are more significant than genetic ones, the prognosis is good after 2 to 4 seizure-free years. The prognosis is worse in simple partial seizures, or in absence seizures with tonic–clonic seizures and grand mal tonic–clonic seizures, and at least four seizure-free years are recommended before ceasing medication. Patients with juvenile myoclonic epilepsy, or absence seizures with clonic–tonic–clonic seizures or grand mal clonic–tonic–clonic seizures, may need to take long-term, even lifetime medication. The relapse rate is likely to be high, even if these patients have been free of seizures for several years.

## Status epilepticus

First-line treatment of status epilepticus is usually with intravenous benzodiazepines, either diazepam or lorazepam. If this is not effective, then intravenous phenytoin or intravenous or intramuscular fosphenytoin is recommended. Rectal paraldehyde may be of value in children. Rectal diazepam has been the pre-hospital treatment of first choice because it can be administered by non-medical personnel. A history of status epilepticus is liable to influence decisions about withdrawing regular antiepileptic medication. It would be wise to proceed with caution, ensuring that any recurrence of status epilepticus can be treated readily, if withdrawal of regular medication is to be undertaken.

## Epilepsy surgery

Frequent severe epileptic seizures despite treatment with adequate antiepileptic medication for about 2 years means that epilepsy surgery needs to be considered. In addition there are certain disorders such as Sturge–Weber syndrome or unilateral infantile spasms where epilepsy surgery may be of benefit during infancy. The treatment of choice in children with Rasmussen syndrome type 2 currently is hemispherectomy, which needs to be done as early as the diagnosis is clear. Difficulties in cooperation and minimal psychosocial gains due to low IQ as well as progressive underlying disease may be contraindications for epilepsy surgery. The preoperative consideration includes extensive examinations such as video-EEG monitoring, high-resolution MRI, positron emission tomography, and neuropsychological and psychiatric evaluation according to the generally accepted principles.[35] The goal is to select those candidates who will benefit from epilepsy surgery. Surgical outcome varies according to the different pathologies of epileptogenic lesions. Thus, the results of surgery are better among patients with mesial temporal sclerosis, chronic encephalitides, infantile hemiplegia, focal cortical dysplasia, tuberous sclerosis, Sturge–Weber syndrome, or post-traumatic cicatrix than among patients with extratemporal focal sclerosis, polymicrogyria with or without heterotopia or hemimegalencephaly, anoxic brain damage, gliosis of obscure aetiology, or no structural pathology.[36] All these findings must be taken into account when selecting patients with epilepsy and intellectual disability for epilepsy surgery. As onset of intractable epilepsy within the first 24 months of life is a significant risk factor for intellectual disability, early intervention for epilepsy surgery is emphasized.[37]

## Behavioural disorders caused by antiepileptic drugs

Most antiepileptic drugs may also cause behavioural disturbance and cognitive dysfunction.[38] For example, the diplopia caused by carbamazepine may result in considerable distress and consequent behavioural disturbance. Communication difficulties, which are common in intellectually disabled patients, may add to the distress and make behavioural disturbance more likely.

Intellectually disabled people with epilepsy are especially vulnerable to harmful neurotoxic effects—sedation caused by phenobarbital or benzodiazepines or cognitive and cerebellar dysfunction caused by phenytoin alone or often together with other antiepileptic drugs. If these alarming effects are not taken into account, inappropriate medication may even jeopardize the rehabilitation of the patients.

Uncertainty about the long-term effects of antiepileptic drugs on brain function and development is largely due to conflicting results of often biased human observations. The problem can only be resolved in controlled experiments which by necessity must be done in animal models. Behavioural and structural consequences of epileptic activity and their modification by antiepileptic drugs are important points to be evaluated in experimental studies. It was reported[39] that enhancement of GABAergic inhibition by administration of vigabatrin prevented both pyramidal cell damage in CA1 and CA3 areas of hippocampus and the disappearance of somatostatin immunoreactive neurones from the dentate gyrus after perforant path stimulation in rats. Furthermore, the preservation of hippocampal structure was accompanied by prevention of the spatial memory deficits seen in control animals after such stimulations. Another study using a kainic acid status epilepticus model in adolescent rats[40] showed that animals that received kainic acid followed by valproic acid resembled control animals who had never received kainic acid with respect to their behavioural and memory performance and had fewer histological lesions. Animals that received kainic acid followed by saline or phenobarbital had impaired learning and behaviour, and more extensive lesions in the hippocampus. Thus, in this experiment valproic acid suppressed seizures and subsequent epilepsy while phenobarbital was only partly effective in suppressing seizures and did not prevent epilepsy. It is likely that seizures themselves, as opposed to the drugs, produced negative behavioural consequences in these rats. It is noteworthy that valproate at very high doses was protective against neuronal damage and prevented epileptogenesis in the kainic acid model.

Chronic phenytoin intoxication, especially in multiple drug therapy, may lead to ataxia, balance impairment and in the worst case finally to persistent loss of locomotion.[41] Another example of an insidious and dangerous effect of phenytoin was documented by the changed course of Unverricht–Lundborg disease. Its rather benign course worsened during phenytoin treatment, so that the patients became bedridden and pseudoretarded and their lifespan shortened from 50 to 60 years to under 30 years. When these patients were treated with valproate instead of phenytoin, their lifespan increased to the prephenytoin level.[15] In some of these patients, the loss of locomotion was reversible after valproate replaced phenytoin.

## Prognosis

The long-term outcome of patients depends primarily on the underlying disorder; prognosis is better in idiopathic than in symptomatic cases. If it is not a question of a progressive brain disorder, epilepsy is quite easily treatable in patients with intellectual disability. Thus, about 70 per cent may obtain good seizure control with appropriate antiepileptic drug therapy or epilepsy surgery.

The outcome of patients with specific disorders may vary considerably. For instance, the outcome of patients with Doose syndrome is variable but basically better than that of patients with Lennox–Gastaut syndrome. If hemispherectomy is not undertaken in time in Rasmussen syndrome type 2, the course of the disease, including neurological deficits, other types of seizures, and mental impairment is progressive.

Epileptic seizures themselves, and frequent epileptiform discharges, may produce brain damage and play a part in producing progressive decline in the intellectual functioning of patients[18] probably through at least two mechanisms: excitatory glutamate storm within cerebral neurones[42] and opening of the blood–brain barrier[43] during and after epileptic seizures.

Sleep disorders are often associated, in people with intellectual disability, with difficult-to-treat epilepsy and behavioral problems.[44,45] When sleep disorders are diagnosed and treated, antiepileptic and also psychotropic medication can be reduced successfully.

## Conclusions

The quality of life in this population benefits from early diagnosis and differential diagnosis of epilepsy, including epilepsy-related behavioural disorder in patients with intellectual disability, identification of its aetiology, and appropriate antiepileptic drug treatment using firstly one drug therapy and, if needed later, rational multiple drug therapy. Currently, valproate is the first choice in generalized seizures while oxcarbazepine or carbamazepine are used for partial seizures with or without secondary generalization. Broad-spectrum drugs such as levetiracetam, lamotrigine, topiramate, or zonisamide are promising. The usefulness of epilepsy surgery should be considered in intractable cases no later than within 2 years, if adequate antiepileptic drug therapy does not help. To minimize sedative and other behavioural and other side-effects caused by antiepileptic drugs the fewest possible drugs should be administered at the lowest effective dose. This means that there should be careful clinical observation of the patients together with determination of drug concentrations in blood and other appropriate laboratory tests. Psychological aspects and sleep behaviour of the patients need to be taken into consideration in the treatment of epilepsy in patients with intellectual disability. Doctors and other personnel working in this field need special education.

Future prospects in the treatment of intractable epileptic seizures might involve the development of gene therapy, neuroprotective drugs, and drugs targeting epileptogenesis. Such treatment possibilities may bring new hope for people with epilepsies that are difficult to treat, including the population with a high proportion of refractory cases, namely that with intellectual disability.

## Further information

Papayiopoulos, C.P. (2007). *A clinical guide to epileptic syndromes and their treatment* (2nd edn), pp. 480. Springer, New York.

Leppik, I., Loscher, W., McDonald, R.L., *et al.* (eds.) (2006). Epileptic syndromes in infancy and early childhood—proceedings of the international symposium of epileptic syndromes in infancy and early childhood—evidence-based taxonomy and its implications in the ILAE classification. *Epilepsy Research*, **70**(Suppl. 1), 1–280.

Birbeck, G. (2006). Interventions to reduce epilepsy-associated stigma. *Psychology, Health & Medicine*, **11**, 364–6.

Vallenga, D., Grypdonck, M., Tan, F., *et al.* (2006). Decision-making about risk in people with epilepsy and intellectual disability. *Journal of Advanced Nursing*, **54**, 602–11.

Ryvlin, P. (2006). When to start antiepileptic drug treatment: seize twice might not harm. *Current Opinion in Neurology*, **19**, 154–6.

# References

1. Iivanainen, M. (1999). Diagnosing epilepsy in patients with mental retardation. In *Epilepsy and mental retardation* (eds. M. Sillanpää, L. Gram, S.I. Johannessen, and T. Tomson), pp. 61–72. Wrightson Biomedical, Petersfield.

2. Gram, L., Johannessen, S.I., Osterman, P.O., *et al.* (eds.) (1993). *Pseudoepileptic seizures.* Wrightson Biomedical, Petersfield.

3. Desai, B.T., Porter, R.J., and Penry, J.K. (1982). Psychogenic seizures. A study of 42 attacks in six patients, with intensive monitoring. *Archives of Neurology*, **39**, 202–9.

4. Ramani, V. and Gummit, R.J. (1982). Management of hysterical seizures in epileptic patients. *Archives of Neurology*, **39**, 78–81.

5. Commission of Classification and Terminology of the International League Against Epilepsy. (1981). Proposal for revised clinical and electroencephalographic classification of epileptic seizures. *Epilepsia*, **22**, 489–501.

6. Luders, H., Acharya, J., Baumgartner, C., *et al.* (1998). Semiological seizure classification. *Epilepsia*, **39**, 1006–13.

7. Commission of Classification and Terminology of the International League Against Epilepsy. (1989). Proposal for revised clinical and electroencephalographic classification of epilepsies and epileptic syndromes. *Epilepsia*, **30**, 389–99.

8. Engel, J. Jr. (1998). Classifications of the International League Against Epilepsy: time for reappraisal. *Epilepsia*, **39**, 1014–7.

9. Engel, J. Jr. (2001). Classification of epileptic disorders. *Epilepsia*, **42**, 316–17.

10. Engel, J. Jr. (2006). Report of the ILAE classification core group. *Epilepsia*, **47**, 1558–68.

11. Ohtahara, S., Ohtsuka, Y., Yamatogi, Y., *et al.* (1992). Early-infantile epileptic encephalopathy with suppression–bursts. In *Epileptic syndromes in infancy, childhood and adolescence* (eds. J. Roger, M. Bureau, Ch. Dravet, F.E. Dreifuss, A. Perret, and P. Wolf), pp. 25–34. John Libbey, London.

12. Williams, A.N., Gray, R.G., Poulton, K., *et al.* (1998). A case of Ohtahara syndrome with cytochrome oxidose deficiency. *Developmental Medicine and Child Neurology*, **40**, 568–70.

13. Roger, J., Bureau, M., Dravet, Ch., *et al.* (eds.) (1992). *Epileptic syndromes in infancy, childhood and adolescence.* John Libbey, London.

14. Magaudda, A., Ferlazzo, E., Nguyen, V.H., *et al.* (2006). Unverricht-Lundborg disease, a condition with self-limited progression: long-term follow-up of 20 patients. *Epilepsia*, **47**, 860–6.

15. Eldridge, R., Iivanainen, M., Stern, R., *et al.* (1983). 'Baltic' myoclonus epilepsy: hereditary disorder of childhood made worse by phenytoin. *Lancet*, **ii**, 838–42.

16. Ranta, S., Lehesjoki, A.E., de Fatima Bonaldo, M., *et al.* (1997). High-resolution mapping and transcript identification at the progressive epilepsy with mental retardation locus on chromosome 8p. *Genome Research*, **7**, 887–96.

17. Witt Engeström, I. (1992). Age-related occurrence of signs and symptoms in the Rett syndrome. *Brain and Development*, **14**(Suppl.), 11–20.

18. Besag, F.M.C. (1995). Epilepsy, learning and behaviour in childhood. *Epilepsia*, **36**(Suppl. 1), S58–63.

19. Bottaro, F.J., Martinez, O.A., Pardal, M.M., *et al.* (2007). Nonconvulsive status epilepticus in the elderly: a case-control study. *Epilepsia*, **48**, 966–72.

20. Jalava, M. and Sillanpää, M. (1996). Concurrent illnesses in adults with childhood-onset epilepsy: a population-based 35-year follow-up study. *Epilepsia*, **37**, 1155–63.

21. Forsgren, L., Edvinsson, S.-O., Blomqvist, H.K., *et al.* (1990). Epilepsy in a population of mentally retarded children and adults. *Epilepsy Research*, **6**, 234–48.

22. Iivanainen, M. (1990). Diagnosis of epileptic seizures and syndromes in mentally retarded patients. In *Paediatric epilepsy* (eds. M. Sillanpää, S.I. Johannessen, G. Blennow, and M. Dam), pp. 233–41. Wrightson Biomedical, Petersfield.

23. Sillanpää, M., Gram, L., Johannessen, S.I., *et al.* (eds.) (1999). *Epilepsy and mental retardation.* Wrightson Biomedical, Petersfield.

24. Arvio, M., Oksanen, V., Autio, S., *et al.* (1993). Epileptic seizures in aspartylglucosaminuria: a common disorder. *Acta Neurologica Scandinavica*, **87**, 342–4.

25. Santavuori, P., Vanhanen, S.L., and Autti, T. (2001). Clinical and neuroradiological diagnostic aspects of neuronal ceroid lipofuscinoses disorders. *European Journal of Paediatric Neurology*, **5**(Suppl. A), 157–61.

26. Elmslie, F. (2000). Gene table: epilepsy (update). *European Journal of Paediatric Neurology*, **4**, 87–90.

27. Working Group of the International Association of the Scientific Study of Intellectual Disability. (2001). Clinical guidelines for the management of epilepsy in adults with an intellectual disability. *Seizure*, **10**, 401–9.

28. Brodie, M.J., Perucca, E., Ryvlin, P., *et al.* (2007). Comparison of levetiracetam and controlled-release carbamazepine in newly diagnosed epilepsy. *Neurology*, **68**, 402–8.

29. Iivanainen, M. and Alvarez, N. (eds.) (1998). Drug treatment of epilepsy in people with intellectual disability. *Journal of Intellectual Disability Research*, **42**(Suppl. 1), 1–92.

30. Glauser, T., Ben-Menachem, E., Bourgeois, B., *et al.* (2006). ILAE treatment guidelines: evidence-based analysis of antiepileptic drug efficacy and effectiveness as initial monotherapy for epileptic seizures and syndromes. *Epilepsia*, **47**, 1094–120.

31. Gayatri, N.A. and Livingston, J.H. (2006). Aggravation of epilepsy by anti-epileptic drugs. *Developmental Medicine and Child Neurology*, **48**, 394–8.

32. Werth, R. and Schadler, G. (2006). Visual field loss in young children and mentally handicapped adolescents receiving vigabatrin. *Investigative Ophthalmology & Visual Science*, **47**, 3028–35.

33. Marcus, J.C. (1998). Stopping antiepileptic therapy in mentally retarded, epileptic children. *Neuropediatrics*, **29**, 26–8.

34. Delgato–Escueta, A.V., Treiman, D.M., and Walsh, G.O. (1983). The treatable epilepsies. *The New England Journal of Medicine*, **308**, 1508–14, 1576–84.

35. Engel, J. Jr. (ed.) (1993). *Surgical treatment of the epilepsies* (2nd edn). Raven Press, New York.

36. Goldring, S. (1987). Pediatric epilepsy surgery. *Epilepsia*, **28** (Suppl. 1), S82–102.

37. Vasconcellos, E., Wyllie, E., Sullivan, S., *et al.* (2001). Mental retardation in pediatric candidates for epilepsy surgery: the role of early seizure onset. *Epilepsia*, **42**, 268–74.

38. Aldenkamp, A.P. (2001). Effects of antiepileptic drugs on cognition. *Epilepsia*, **42**(Suppl. 1), 46–9.

39. Ylinen, A.M.A., Miettinen, R., Pitkänen, A., *et al.* (1991). Enhanced GABAergic inhibition preserves hippocampal structure and function in a model of epilepsy. *Proceedings of the National Academy of Sciences of the United States of America*, **88**, 7650–3.

40. Bolanos, A.R., Sarkisian, M., Yang, Y., *et al.* (1998). Comparison of long-term effects of valproate and phenobarbital in adolescent rats. *Neurology*, **51**, 41–8.

41. Iivanainen, M. (1998). Phenytoin: effective but insidious therapy for epilepsy in people with intellectual disability. *Journal of Intellectual Disability Research*, **42**(Suppl. 1), 24–31.

42. Rothman, S.M. and Olney, J.W. (1987). Excitotoxicity and the NMDA receptor. *Trends in Neurosciences*, **10**, 299–302.

43. Sokrab, T.-E.O., Johansson, B.B., Kalimo, H., *et al.* (1988). A transient hypertensive opening of the blood-brain barrier can lead to brain damage. *Acta Neuropathologica*, **75**, 557–65.

44. Iivanainen, M., Partinen, M., and Kaski, M. (2005). Why is it important to study sleep of people with intellectual disability? In *Proceedings of the first congress of the world association of sleep medicine, Berlin* (eds. T. Penzel, I. Fietze, and S. Chokroverty), pp. 131–4. Medimond International Proceedings, Bologna (Italy).

45. Manni, R., Terzaghi, M., and Zambrelli, E. (2006). REM sleep behavior disorder and epileptic phenomena: clinical aspects of the comorbidity. *Epilepsia*, **47**(Suppl. 5), 78–81.

# 10.6

# Methods of treatment

## T. P. Berney

## Introduction

The presence of intellectual disability (mental retardation) affects the character of treatment in a number of ways.

1 Limited communication will hamper diagnosis so that much more has to be inferred from observable behaviour and greater weight given to the interpretation of carers.

2 Diagnosis is provisional, a therapeutic hypothesis that provides the basis for a programme of treatment that is, essentially, a therapeutic trial. There is a wide variation in individual characteristics, with intellectual disability (mental retardation) extending over an enormous range of ability, associated disabilities, aetiology, and psychopathology. Multiple pathology means that the response can be unexpected and ambiguous. For example, diminished aggression with carbamazepine may simply reflect its psychotropic effect but may also be the result of better control of unrecognized epilepsy. A well-designed behavioural milieu may produce a rapid improvement in disturbed behaviour. However, the improvement might simply reflect the effect on someone with autism of moving to a more settled, structured, and predictable environment. It may also reflect an improvement in organic disorder (such as epilepsy or gastritis) in response to a reduction in stress. The therapist has to tailor the treatment to the individual, to try to be specific as to what aspect of the disorder is being targeted and be very selective as to whom they treat.

3 Ill-defined treatment objectives often leave it unclear whether a treatment is aimed at a disorder (e.g. autism), a symptom (panic), or an associated disorder (depression or epilepsy).

4 Normal developmental change may be misattributed to a coincident treatment programme. For example, autism and epilepsy often show spontaneous improvement at about 4 years age and again in late adolescence, both times when the person is likely to be moving into new programmes. This propensity for maturational improvement, coupled with a tradition of care, has led developmental psychiatrists to have a greater therapeutic optimism for many problems, such as personality disorders, that are often considered intractable in those of normal ability.

5 Natural cycles of change can give a misleading sense of success. For example, a behavioural programme may be credited with the remission of a self-limiting episode of disorder such as depression.

The true diagnosis may become clear only when it recurs and fails to respond to booster programmes.

6 There is limited evidence for the effectiveness of most treatments. Except for the behavioural therapies, most treatment is based on small series, open trials, the theoretical, and the ideal.

7 A large component of the therapeutic relationship is indirect, being with the family, carers, or professionals rather than directly with the patient. Many programmes utilize the power of the placebo effect, a dynamic that confounds scientific trials but one that should be used to its full in everyday clinical practice. Limited communication and greater dependency lead to work with the systems around the patient; many of the approaches, such as family therapy, deriving from child psychiatry.

8 The ability to consent to treatment is often underestimated. Circumstances often make it difficult for people with mental retardation to choose or refuse a particular therapy, particularly behavioural programmes and drug treatments. Their capacity to give or withhold consent should be assessed automatically and their care should fall within a legal framework that safeguards their rights and protects them from abuse.

Treatment services for people with intellectual disability (mental retardation) have two components. There is the routine support that should be available to all with intellectual disability (mental retardation). Its aim is to help people to grow up as normally as possible, offsetting the effects of their disability, and to establish the therapeutic environment. Second is the provision of treatment for individuals with disturbance; aimed at specific symptoms or disorders based on a multiaxial diagnosis[1] that includes the following:

◆ Axis I: The nature and degree of intellectual disability (mental retardation) for, in addition to the overall developmental delay other, specific, disabilities, and abilities are often present. For example, a discrepancy between receptive and expressive language may result in someone understanding little of what is said to him while sounding falsely fluent.

◆ Axis II: The aetiology of the retardation—there is increasing recognition of the contribution of a behavioural phenotype. Of particular note are autism and its imitators, drawing on the ubiquities of social impairment, obsessionality and communication problems, which are being teased apart.

◆ Axis III:

• Level A: Other developmental disabilities that are associated with intellectual disability (mental retardation) such as autism, attention deficit disorder, and epilepsy,

• Level B: Psychiatric disorder—the way this is defined will define the mode of treatment. A functional analysis with antecedents, triggers, and consequences leads into a behavioural programme. A more biological label (such as psychosis) opens the door to drug treatment. They are not mutually exclusive,

• Level C: The patient's personality—this is often unusual and it may be difficult to distinguish from a pervasive developmental disorder (see Chapter 9.2.2) which runs through Intellectual disability (mental retardation) and which, once recognized, often explains the inexplicable,

• Level D: Other disorders such as habit disorders and sexual preference disorders,

◆ Relevant comorbid, physical conditions such as hay fever, asthma, hypothyroidism, or gastro-oesophageal disorders. Particularly important are epilepsy and the antiepileptic agents that are dealt with in detail elsewhere (see Chapters 6.2.6 and 10.5.3, respectively).

◆ The patient's environment which includes not just their physical surroundings but also the people and their relationships with them.

◆ Contributory factors from the patient's past, notably the various forms of abuse.

## The therapeutic environment

Support may be provided in different ways:

◆ Level A: General, the network of care provided for people with a intellectual disability (mental retardation) and their carers. This will include community teams, special schools, and the specialized residential placements that might be resorted to either as a short break or as a long-term home.

◆ Level B: Specific to a particular disorder, parental support groups exist for autism, epilepsy, and specific forms of intellectual disability (mental retardation) such as Prader–Willi, Fragile X, and Cornelia de Lange syndromes.

A primary aim is to integrate people into their community as far as possible. The concept of normalization implies that services should avoid the demarcation that leads to adverse discrimination. Conversely, those with disabilities too severe or too complex for their families or standard teaching or occupational placements may fare better in specialist settings. Examples of these are as follows:

◆ Some of those with autism, who are so distracted by the complexity of everyday life and the unpredictability of people that they need specialist environments which are well structured, predictable, and under their control.

◆ Those with severe or intractable seizures.

◆ Those with aggressive or disinhibited behaviour so disruptive as to block the progress of their peers.

The specialist setting encourages mutual support for people and families with similar problems; the staff gain experience; and it allows a concentration of expertise. However, it also encourages stigmatization and there is the risk that, in a group, disturbed people may copy or amplify each other's behaviour.

## The family and other carers

Disturbance arises in the setting of a system of care which includes not only the family but also the staff of other placements, whether day or residential, educational or occupational. Its management will depend on the way these people perceive mental retardation and its care, their attitudes deriving from both past experience and present relationships (Fig. 10.6.1). A great deal depends on the extent to which they feel supported and assured in their roles, as much by each other as by the available system of care. For example, a mother or a teacher who is told frequently that, whatever it was that went wrong, it was her fault, is unlikely to cope confidently.

Disability and disturbance both hinder normal developmental experience; the child's atypical response spoiling the carers' efforts to learn parenting skills and leaving them demoralized or deskilled. They may need formal teaching in such skills as how to engage socially with the child, to play with them, to give clear and understandable instructions, and how to divert rather than confront. Disturbance may reflect boredom and be reduced simply by increasing the amount and variety of activities. Any approach must take a broad view, for carers have to work together comfortably enough to be consistent over time. A treatment programme may have to address the relationship between the carers as well as their needs. This may be sufficient in itself, improvement in the patient following an overall improvement in functioning in the family, school, or residential placement. There has been a growth in the conscious application of a systemic approach to work in this field.[2]

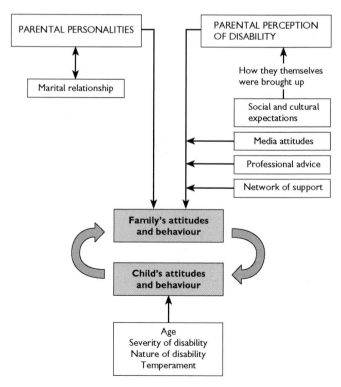

**Fig. 10.6.1** The start of disturbance: factors influencing behaviour.

## Education

This forms the core of any treatment programme, the individual getting formal instruction in the skills which others acquire in passing. Teaching and training are lifelong processes, invoking teacher–student relationships, and take place within a structured framework, essential for those students who have difficulty in understanding their environments. The difficulty is to gauge the degree of structure required: too much and the relationship risks becoming a battle about control, easily turning into trench warfare; too little and the student is distracted and learns little. It is a balance that shifts over time, promoting the student's self-control and autonomy.

### (a) Independence and self-help skills

These include the basic skills of everyday life, such as feeding, dressing, or managing stairs or, at a higher level, the use of public transport, how to care for clothes, shop, and budget. Acquiring these, gives a sense of achievement and confidence as well as of increased independence.

### (b) Communication skills

The frustration of living in an uncomprehending world frequently contributes to disturbance as the person falls back on various forms of attention seeking or violent behaviour to get their message across. Easier and more effective means of communication may range from simple gestures (e.g. pulling at the trousers to show the need for toileting), through a system of pointing to symbols or pictures, to complex signing which can convey abstract concepts such as emotional states. Language may be verbal or non-verbal and both modalities are taught simultaneously, reinforcing each other so that a course in signing can improve speech. Whatever the system used, it depends on, and will be limited by, the extent to which those around can understand it.

### (c) Social and sexual relationships

People are vulnerable to exploitation until they learn the distinction between an acquaintance and a friend. Relationships become complicated by sexual behaviour, hedged around with cultural rules which vary between families making it an especially difficult area to teach and therefore tempting to ignore. Occasionally sexual arousal drives disturbance in someone for whom masturbation is inefficient, physically damaging, unlearned, or forbidden. Wider discussion can bring out strongly held beliefs and family conflicts which had been unsuspected or denied until then. This may lead on to other areas requiring resolution, such as whether a person with intellectual disability (mental retardation) should have a sexual relationship, marry, or have children.

## Out-of-home placement

As described earlier, a move out of the home can be seen either as part of the wider programme of support and social development or else as part of the treatment of a specific disorder: the distinction is often blurred.

### (a) Support

Short breaks allow individuals and their families some relief from the uninterrupted intimacy of care. They also widen social networks and pave the way towards the eventual departure from home, something that is ideally planned as part of an increasing, adult autonomy. Frequently however, this is left until there is a crisis, for example when the person's behaviour or dependency has outstripped their family's resources, too often the result of parental infirmity or death. At this point the unfortunate individual may find themselves in a series of short break (or even treatment) placements until something long-term can be arranged.

Placement for educational needs (e.g. in a residential school or college) becomes necessary where the person's disabilities (e.g. autism or intractable epilepsy) require specialist skills and settings. It can also be a compromise with a parent who, unable to care for their child themselves, will not accept more standard forms of social care.

### (b) Treatment

The threshold for admission for assessment and treatment will depend on the extent of the supportive service available in the community and is often:

1 For the treatment of more complex disorders such as epilepsy or psychosis.

2 For the assessment of disturbance where it is difficult to disentangle the relative contributions of innate from environmental factors. For example, a patient's behaviour may be amplified by an exasperated or exhausted family, particularly where disturbed nights have left them short of sleep. This sets off a secondary, self-perpetuating cycle of disturbance involving the whole house which makes it impossible to discern the underlying, primary disturbance. The cycle may only be interrupted by changing the patient's circumstances, either by moving staff into the home or by moving the patient out.

3 For the management of behavioural disturbance where:

(a) The carers are unable to cope—the more frequent reasons include:

- marital disharmony
- the carer's inability to manage others simultaneously, for example single parents who have several children or a home with several disturbed children
- the loss of resilience in a demoralized carer
- an adverse or hostile neighbourhood where the carer has to give way in case the patient becomes so noisy that the neighbours complain, or where the patient is bullied or led astray.

(b) There has been a failure of earlier therapeutic trials with a family locked in their pattern of behaviour.

(c) The patient is at risk of harm.

(d) The patient presents a substantial risk to others, for example, of violence or sexual offending.

(e) There is the need for effective control of the patient with clear limits to disturbed behaviour.

## Treatment methods

Discomfort is a potent and frequent cause of disturbance. Because the person may have difficulty in identifying and localizing pain, let alone communicating symptoms, it is frequently missed. It is essential that it is a matter of routine to seek and treat common ailments such as hay fever, toothache, earache, dyspepsia, and gastric reflux. The last of these is particularly associated both with severe retardation and with certain disorders such as Cornelia de Lange syndrome as well as an increased possibility of oesophageal carcinoma.[3] The more severe the degree of disability, the greater the need for an active programme of health care.[4]

## Behavioural treatments

Intellectual disability's communication barrier has led to an emphasis on observable behaviour rather than on reports of subjective emotions or perceptions. Although the function of a behaviour is often misinterpreted, the first, unthinking response is often a behavioural programme. At the same time, increasingly sophisticated and more solidly research-based than other forms of psychiatric treatment, such a programme can produce profound and rapid change.[5] Programmes are divided broadly into two areas:

1 Teaching appropriate habits and skills which can range from basic skills such as dressing, continence, communication, and sleep, through to the more sophisticated training in social skills, dating skills, and assertiveness.

2 The unlearning of other, maladaptive forms of behaviour.

These two areas are complementary—it is more effective to replace an undesirable behaviour than simply to remove it. Operant, incentive programmes dominate much institutional and offender work. While punishment techniques can be effective and in certain, very unusual situations may be justified, there must be concern about their effect on the trainer as much as on the patient and they need close, ethical control.[6]

## Cognitive behavioural therapy

Behavioural principles can be used to target thought as well as behaviour. With disability comes a tendency to a polarized perception of the world—people seeing themselves either as acceptable, competent, and successful or else as worthless failures; similarly, others are seen as all good or all bad. Cognitive therapy is usually used with people in the mild or borderline range of retardation, and has a particular importance in the treatment of sex offenders, although there are some examples of work with non-verbal people or those with severe intellectual disability. Indeed, where problem-solving skills are formally taught, the improvement may be greater in people with moderate than with mild intellectual disability, suggesting some form of ceiling effect to their acquisition. Furthermore, performance may have more to do with the type of problem than with formal measures of ability.[7]

Rational emotive therapy, developed in an educational setting, seeks to change the perceptual set and thereby the impact and influence of events on the person. Its background in education resulted in a didactic format, giving the therapist a directive role. The orientation is behavioural, focusing on the development of skills, and it lends itself to being taught to groups. A number of open studies of people with moderate and mild intellectual disability have shown it to decrease irrationality and anxiety, and to increase internal control and self-esteem.[8]

Anger management was developed with people of average ability but now has a well-established place in intellectual disability.[9] Therapy has to cope with a number of obstacles including:

1 The inherent nature of anger which means that the problem is an excessive response rather than a deviant one. In this population organic factors are frequent, particularly brain damage, epilepsy, and medication.

2 Its usefulness where there is limited communication or more severe disability which, combined with personality factors, can make therapeutic engagement difficult.

3 The degree to which habitual use has made anger an entrenched response.

4 The emotion of anger can be difficult to distinguish and label, particularly where autism is a component. Here an aggressive response may be the result of excessive anxiety, often amounting to panic.

A programme of anger management may take place at several levels.

1 General clinical care—strategies to reduce anger which include ensuring that the person feels well, that their physical and social environment is suitable, and that there are suitable occupational and recreational programmes.[10]

2 Anger management—information is given to help the person recognize anger, its nature, the signs, and consequences, as well as ideas and information about changing their behaviour. This uses a more didactic group instruction which is general and involves less disclosure and engagement by the individual.

3 Anger treatment—an individually tailored programme which targets change in cognitive perception, autonomic arousal, and behaviour. Individual engagement is essential and transference and countertransference are important and likely to evoke distressing emotions.

Another target is anxiety reduction through treatments that range, depending on the degree of disability, from formal relaxation training through to physical activity. Some do not measure up to their promoter's promise and may even have a detrimental effect,[11] endorsing the principle of treatment as an individual therapeutic trial.

## Psychodynamic therapies

Although we have moved away from the early belief that intellectual disability itself was the result of emotional abuse and psychological disturbance, we are beginning to recognize the extent to which these factors can reduce adaptive functioning and amplify a cognitive disability. Psychotherapy can complement educational programmes to produce someone who, although no more intellectually able, is more mature emotionally and better able to cope with the tasks of everyday life. However, the field is poorly researched so that its efficacy is uncertain.[12]

Both the family and the individual have to adjust to disability; a process akin to a series of grief reactions through which people come to terms with the loss of normality.[13] The process of adjustment occurs as a series of crises triggered by events such as the point of initial diagnosis, the failure of initial treatments, educational assessment and specialized placements, puberty, and leaving home. Each stage brings home afresh the degree and significance of the child's disability.

The therapist may require specific training and supervision in adapting standard approaches to cope with a number of potential elements peculiar to intellectual disability:

1 The therapy is likely to have to deal with the core themes of loss and disability.

2 Communication will be limited in various ways and there may be unexpected, conceptual barriers. For example, the patient may not understand or even notice gestures, facial expressions, and different tones of voice. They may be unable to identify many emotions, label them, or form abstract concepts. Communication has to be at the patient's level, being concrete and using simple words, short sentences, and their colloquial or slang terms as well as allowing sufficient time for the patient to process the thought. The therapist may circumvent some of these barriers by using alternatives modalities, such as music, art, play, and drama.

3 The patient may have a limited and distorted understanding of the roles and relationships of the people around. Unable to appreciate either that the therapist's knowledge is restricted or that they occupy a different world, the patient may assume that they know all about the patient's setting and routines. This means that, in order to make sense of what is said, the therapist must learn something of the patient's background.

4 A combination of memory problems, obsessionality, or poor executive function means that there may be repetition of information, ideas, and conclusions, often given as if they have never been mentioned before.

5 Many people have had lives marked by short and changing relationships and a nomadic change of accommodation. Engagement in therapy can be difficult with a disconcerting readiness to disengage.

6 Confidentiality may be difficult to establish for someone where dependency and total care has discouraged privacy. Carers frequently expect to be told what happens in therapy and the relationship may be complicated by a disclosure that can range from poor care to frank abuse.

## Psychopharmacological treatments

Drugs are widely used in intellectual disability. Besides being used for the medical disorders which are more frequent in this population, such as epilepsy, Tourette syndrome, and attention deficit disorder, drugs play a part in the management of a wide range of symptomatology which includes symptoms as varied as aggression, self-injury, outbursts of distress, compulsive routines, and social withdrawal. A recurrent criticism is that a drug may be used for a purpose other than that suggested by its classificatory label (e.g. that antipsychotics and antiepileptics are used for conditions other than psychosis or epilepsy, respectively) or that they are prescribed outside their manufacturer's licence. While this often is simply semantic, there must be concern at the level of prescribing of psychotropic drugs.[14] The prevalence and number of drugs being prescribed is associated with, the degree of retardation, and the presence of autism; it is no less in the community than in inpatient institutions;[15] and is only reduced by a determined programme of rationalization.

The presence of intellectual disability colours prescribing:

1 Non-compliance usually results from an unpalatable formulation or a carer's prejudice rather than forgetfulness.

2 Coexistent disorders, as wide-ranging as epilepsy, constipation, and cerebral palsy, can make a patient more vulnerable to adverse effects.

3 Cerebral dysfunction may cause more frequent atypical responses, sensitivity being either increased or decreased to various aspects of the drug's effect. Most of these are dose-specific, paradoxical effects for therapeutic windows are frequent and, as frequently, forgotten. Prescribing details are subject to revision and should be checked with a current formulary but treatment should be started at a lower dosage and increased more gradually than is generally recommended. The unexpected should be expected so that, besides the routine warning of adverse effects, carers should be able to contact someone if they are in any doubt about the drug's effects.

4 Evidence of efficacy is largely anecdotal, with trials being mostly small, open, and uncontrolled, but providing some justification for almost any neuropharmacological adventure. The information that needs to be weighed up is more complex and is therefore less likely to be within the patient's capacity to decide whether to take it. This leaves the prescriber with a greater responsibility to put the patient's interests first.

### (a) Neuroleptics

These are used frequently and for a variety of symptoms despite a shortage of consistent, demonstrable, and specific effects. For example, although a series of studies have shown haloperidol to be effective in autism, the response can be in any of a variety of areas including improved discrimination learning, a reduction in overactivity, anger, and in the frequency and intensity of outbursts.[16] A number of reports suggest violence, whether to others or self-directed, might be more responsive to fluphenazine or clozapine (although the use of the latter is severely limited by its potential for marrow toxicity).

The recent proliferation of neuroleptics has been driven by a search for greater effectiveness together with a reduced risk of adverse effects and has been steered by the theoretical clinical attributes of various neuroreceptor systems. The atypical neuroleptics are reputed to bring less risk of adverse effects such as the dyskinesias, but, as they become better known, are being linked with sedation, weight gain, and elevated prolactin level and there is growing concern about their potential to produce a metabolic syndrome.[17] The most established of these, risperidone, has shown itself effective in several random controlled trials in reducing behavioural disturbance in children and adults across a number of symptoms such as aggression, social withdrawal, inattentiveness, and overactivity.[18]

### (b) Antidepressants

Depression, once noticed and identified, is as treatable as in the normal population. Obsessive–compulsive symptomatology is frequent and responsive to the drugs augmenting serotoninergic transmission although there is increasing anxiety about potential adverse effects, particularly suicide and dependence although there is, as yet, no evidence for this in the population with intellectual disability. More frequent is a paradoxical increase in anxiety that may be a partial serotonin syndrome. The use of the selective serotonin reuptake inhibitors and lithium is being extended beyond the management of apparently compulsive violence and self-injury to include bouts of non-specific distress. Clomipramine, fluvoxamine, and fluoxetine have both shown success in random controlled trials but the evidence for the effectiveness of other drugs largely consists of open label and retrospective case-series in which it can be unclear whether the underlying disorder is autism, intellectual disability, or both.[19, 20]

The serotoninergic system appears to be central to a wide number of vegetative functions suggesting a potential for these drugs in appetite disorders such as the compulsive search for food and lack of satiety of Prader–Willi syndrome.

### (c) β-blockers

Propranolol and nadolol limit the autonomic response to anxiety and the propensity to panic. They have a particular place where acute anxiety underlies aggression as, for example, in someone with autism who lashes out or flees in panic when feeling crowded. They are non-sedative but can cause lethargy and even depression. Open-label series suggest propranolol may take some weeks to take effect with a dosage range of 50–960 mg/day; characteristics that may explain the lack of random controlled trials.

### (d) Stimulants

There has been a widespread re-evaluation of the place of attention deficit-hyperactivity disorder (ADHD), its prevalence, and management. Well recognized in children in the normal range of ability, it is now being identified more frequently in adulthood, coexistent with autism spectrum disorder, and with intellectual disability. There is a general, unsubstantiated belief that ADHD is more intractable, the greater the degree of intellectual disability. Methylphenidate and amphetamine remain the standard treatments but amantadine might be more effective and less toxic.[21] Clonidine can be of use although sedative and short-lived and atomoxetine is finding its place. When effective, stimulants can produce a global improvement in behaviour that includes appetite, sleep, and mood, even though anorexia, insomnia, and depression head the list of potential adverse effects.

### (e) Mood stabilizers

Antiepileptic drugs are being more widely used to reduce emotional lability, particularly outbursts of rage which have an organic, possibly epileptic, basis; the episodic dyscontrol syndrome. Supportive evidence is slight and occasionally the drug may make matters worse.[22] Aggression has a large variety of causes and, after the exclusion of physical discomfort, the primary approach is psychological. However, lithium has shown to be effective in reducing outbursts of aggression, particularly where there is irritability and explosiveness.[16]

### (f) Opioid antagonists

The hypothesis is that opioid excess might underlie both autism and its frequent associate, an indifference to pain that encourages excessive self-stimulation. Naltrexone has been used to treat both autistic disturbance and repetitive self-injury. Where autism shows any response it is to a very low dosage (5–20 mg/day), a window in a therapeutic U-curve while, if self-injury should respond, it is likely to be to a higher dosage (100–200 mg/day). Unfortunately, many of the random controlled trials have fallen between the two dosages.

### (g) Antilibidinal drugs

For a few, a strong sexual drive overrides the teaching, training, and psychological therapies which, as in other areas of psychiatry, are the main approach to sexual offending. An antilibidinal agent[23] can supplement the other approaches, reducing the drive to a level where it is under the patient's control. The sensitivity of this area, let alone potential adverse effects, makes it especially important that the patient, the family, and the carers are all part of any decision to use medication.

## Conclusion

There are a large number and variety of treatments for any disorder in intellectual disability: a good indication of the complexity of disturbance and the inconsistency of the effectiveness of any one treatment. Therapists have an unusual responsibility not to exploit the limited ability of their patients to withhold consent as well as to try to see the world through their eyes. They have also to combine simultaneously the enthusiasm of the charismatic healer with the objectivity and scepticism of the scientist. As in any experiment, changes in treatment should be introduced singly to ensure that it is clear which manoeuvre produces which result. However, treatments complement each other and should not be used in isolation. This is the area above all in which the patient depends on teamwork and cooperation between therapists, disciplines, and agencies.

## Further information

University of Birmingham. (2007). *Using medication to manage behaviour problems among adults with a learning disability.* Available from: http://www.ld-medication.bham.ac.uk/.

Gualtieri, C.T. (2002). *Brain injury and mental retardation: psychopharmacology and neuropsychiatry.* Lipincott, Williams & Wilkins, Philadelphia.

Handen, B.L. and Gilchrist, R. (2006). Practitioner review: psychopharmacology in children and adolescents with mental retardation. *Journal of Child Psychology and Psychiatry*, **47**, 871–82.

## References

1. Royal College of Psychiatrists. (2001). *DC-LD: Diagnostic criteria for psychiatric disorders for use with adults with learning disabilities/mental retardation* (Occasional Paper OP48). Gaskell, London.
2. Baum, S. (2007). The use of family therapy for people with learning disabilities. *Advances in Mental Health and Learning Disabilities*, **1**, 8–13.
3. Bohmer, C.J., Niezen de Boer, M.C., Klinkenberg Knol, E.C., *et al.* (1997). Gastro-oesophageal reflux disease in institutionalised intellectually disabled individuals. *The Netherlands Journal of Medicine*, **51**, 134–9.
4. Cooper, S.A., Morrison, J., Melville, C., *et al.* (2006). Improving the health of people with intellectual disabilities: outcomes of a health screening programme after 1 year. *Journal of Intellectual Disability Research*, **50**, 667–77.
5. Emerson, E. (1995). *Challenging behaviour: analysis and intervention in people with learning disabilities.* Cambridge University Press, Cambridge.
6. Repp, A.C. and Singh, N.N. (eds). (1990). *Perspectives on the use of nonaversive and aversive interventions for persons with developmental disabilities.* Sycamore Publishing Company, Sycamore, IL.
7. Benson, B.A. and Valenti-Hein, D. (2001). Cognitive and social learning treatments. In *Treating mental illness and behavior disorders in children and adults with mentallly retardation* (eds. A. Dosen and K. Day). American Psychiatric Press, Washington, DC.
8. Schneider, N. (2001). A rational emotive group treatment approach with dually diagnosed adults. In *Treating mental illness and behavior disorders in children and adults with mental retardation* (eds. A. Dosen and K. Day). American Psychiatric Press, Washington, DC.
9. Taylor, J.L. and Novaco, R.W. (2005). Anger treatment for people with developmental disabilities: a theory, evidence and manual based approach. John Wiley & Sons, Chichester.
10. Harris, J., Allen, D., Cornick, M., *et al.* (1996). *Physical interventions: a policy framework.* BILD, Kidderminster.

11. Lindsay, W.R., Pitcaithly, D., Geelen, N., *et al.* (1997). A comparison of the effects of four therapy procedures on concentration and responsiveness in people with profound learning disabilities. *Journal of Intellectual Disability Research*, **41**, 201–7.

12. Royal College of Psychiatrists. (2004). *Psychotherapy and learning disability*. (CR116). Royal College of Psychiatrists, London.

13. Bicknell, J. (1983). The psychopathology of handicap. *British Journal of Medical Psychology*, **56**, 167–78.

14. Lott, I.T., McGregor, M., Engelman, L., *et al.* (2004). Longitudinal prescribing patterns for psychoactive medications in community-based individuals with developmental disabilities: utilization of pharmacy records. *Journal of Intellectual Disability Research*, **48**, 563–71.

15. Branford, D. (1997). A follow-up study of prescribing for people with learning disabilities previously in National Health Service care in Leicestershire, England. *Journal of Intellectual Disability Research*, **41**, 339–45.

16. Campbell, M. and Cueva, J.E. (1995). Psychopharmacology in child and adolescent-psychiatry—a review of the past 7 years, Part 1. *Journal of the American Academy of Child and Adolescent Psychiatry*, **34**, 1124–32.

17. McKee, J.R., Bodfish, J.W., Mahorney, S.L., *et al.* (2005). Metabolic effects associated with atypical antipsychotic treatment in the developmentally disabled. *The Journal of Clinical Psychiatry*, **66**, 1161–8.

18. Jesner, O.S., Aref-Adib, M., and Coren, E. (2007). Risperidone for autism spectrum disorder. *Cochrane Database of Systematic Reviews.*

19. Dinca, O., Paul, M., and Spencer, N.J. (2005). Systematic review of randomized controlled trials of atypical antisychotics and selective serotonin reuptake inhibitors for behavioural problems associated with pervasive developmental disorders. *Journal of Psychopharmacology*, **19**, 521–32.

20. Posey, D.J., Erickson, C.A., Stigler, K.A., *et al.* (2006). The use of selective serotonin reuptake inhibitors in autism and related disorders. *Journal of Child and Adolescent Psychopharmacology*, **16**, 181–6.

21. Gualtieri, C.T. (2002). Psychostimulants, dopamine agonists and amantadine. In *Brain injury and mental retardation: psychopharmacology and neuropsychiatry*. Lipincott, Williams & Wilkins, Philadelphia.

22. Besag, F.M.C. (2001). Behavioural effects of the new anticonvulsants. *Drug Safety*, **24**, 513–36.

23. Cooper, A.J. (1995). Review of the role of two antilibidinal drugs in the treatment of sex offenders with mental retardation. *Mental Retardation*, **33**, 42–8.

# Special needs of adolescents and elderly people with intellectual disability

Jane Hubert and Sheila Hollins

## Introduction

Social health and mental health needs change throughout life, and this chapter highlights those particularly relevant for adolescents and elderly people. As a general rule, people with intellectual disabilities have the same needs as other members of the community, but they may also have additional needs for which they are entitled to extra support.[1]

## Adolescents

### Administrative prevalence of intellectual disability in adulthood vs. childhood

The UK Government White Paper 'Valuing people' estimates that there are about 2 10,000 people with severe and profound intellectual disabilities in the UK: around 65,000 children and young people, 1 20,000 adults of working age, and 25,000 older people. They estimate that there are some 1.2 million people in the UK with mild or moderate intellectual disabilities. Worldwide, it is estimated that there are some 20 million people with intellectual disabilities.[2]

Although there is now a trend in the UK towards mainstreaming children with special needs, and providing extra support, separate special schools for children with moderate and for severe learning difficulties are still provided in many places. At school leaving age, many young people with mild or moderate learning difficulties (roughly equating to IQ > 50) will not receive special services; only people who have severe intellectual disabilities, and those with additional disabilities, including epilepsy, autism, mental illness and/or behavioural problems will be referred on to adult specialist services. The administrative prevalence of adults with intellectual disabilities is thus much lower in adulthood as it is a measure of those in contact with services. The administrative prevalence rates should not be confused with true prevalence rates, which are far more difficult to assess.

### Transition to adulthood

Among young people in the general population, there are certain important life events which are usually considered necessary for a successful transition to adulthood. These include getting a job or going to college, having economic and social independence from parents, and leaving home.[3] Although the transition to adulthood can be a difficult and painful process for anyone, for most people it is also a time at which choices and opportunities open up. For people with intellectual disabilities, the transition to adulthood does not usually follow the same pattern as it does for others. For many, the transition is marked simply by an abrupt move from the protective and relatively well-defined children's services to adult services, and by leaving school. These imposed transitions into adulthood are often abrupt and traumatic for the young people and for their parents.[4]

Overall, the criteria for 'successful' transition to adulthood are less likely to be fulfilled the greater the severity of the intellectual disability and other factors such as physical or mental health problems, communication difficulties and/or challenging behaviour. Those who have mental health problems, or aggressive challenging behaviour, are particularly unlikely to receive the necessary support and services to enable them to live independent 'adult' lives.[5] In 2001, a new service, Connexions, was established to improve the management of the transition to adulthood, by providing young people from 13–19 years of age with access to advice, guidance and support.[2]

In the UK, the majority of young people with intellectual disabilities attend Day Centres. Those who are more able may enter sheltered employment, workshops for disabled people or supported open employment. Relatively few people with intellectual disabilities are in paid employment, and although employment schemes are now being developed in many places, there are substantial barriers that are faced by people with intellectual disabilities in getting and maintaining employment in the open job market.[2]

In all parts of the world, the majority of young people with intellectual disabilities continue to live at home with one or both parents, and often have little or no social or economic independence, or participation in major, or even minor, life decisions. Although adolescence and leaving school imply a transition to adulthood, in many cases young people become more dependent on their parents at this stage than they were before. For those who have severe or multiple disabilities, and/or challenging behaviour, there may be few practical alternatives and choices open to them.[6]

In different countries, various approaches have been developed to recognize the needs of young adults. One widely adopted approach, the development of small group homes in the community, has meant that more young people with intellectual disabilities are able to move away from home, even some who have severe intellectual disabilities and challenging behaviour. In many countries however, the responsibility remains firmly with carers, with institutional provision being the only backup when family care breaks down. An international carers' advocacy organization, Inclusion International, researched the views of carers in 80 or more countries in both developed and developing nations, and their report makes a number of recommendations about how communities and governments can provide better support to individuals and families.[7, 8]

### Health needs

There is a high prevalence of epilepsy, psychiatric disorder, hearing and visual impairments and autism among people with intellectual disabilities. Children with intellectual disabilities are the responsibility of a paediatrician, and parents can discuss and monitor their children's needs and progress through one agency. When a child is transferred to adult services this situation changes, and there are many different agencies and individuals who become responsible for different aspects of the overall service to adolescents.

For the families concerned, the world of adult services can be bewildering. The situation is particularly problematic in relation to adolescents with severe intellectual disabilities, especially if there are also behaviour problems, during this transitional phase from child to adult services. Impairments in adaptive behaviour associated with intellectual disability lead to problems in developing normal social functioning, communication, and the ability to use community facilities. In addition, the relationship between parental and professional roles and responsibilities is often unclear. Multidisciplinary assessment is advisable, and parents should remain involved, but all too often are told that their opinion is no longer valid now their child is an adult.[2] The Royal College of Psychiatrists publishes leaflets for family carers to help them manage these changing professional relationships.[9]

It is often not apparent who, among the professionals, is directly responsible for someone in the context of services, and there may be inconsistencies between Health, Education, and Social Services in terms of policies and practice. Also, health professionals, including general practitioners, may be relatively inexperienced in dealing with people who have intellectual disabilities.

A coherent strategy for developing comprehensive health care services for young people with intellectual disabilities requires collaboration between service providers, to ensure that the health care needs of all people with intellectual disabilities, including those with autism, are properly identified, and that access to mainstream primary and secondary health care is supported. One initiative developed for the white paper 'Valuing people' was the introduction of Health Action Plans to try to address some of these information and knowledge gaps.[10]

### Mental health needs

Diagnostic overshadowing of mental illness in people with intellectual disabilities was common in the past, but there is now increasing awareness and assessment of psychiatric disorders, and acceptance of dual diagnosis among people with intellectual disabilities. Although mental health needs can in some cases be met by general mental health services, some specialized mental health provision is still necessary to meet the needs of people with dual diagnosis, including those who also have challenging behaviour.[11]

Until recently, people with intellectual disabilities were seldom thought to suffer from depression, but recent research shows that adolescents with intellectual disabilities report more depression and other symptoms of psychopathology than others without intellectual disabilities.[12]

There is increasing awareness, and continuing evidence,[13,14] of the high prevalence of abuse of people with intellectual disabilities, of all ages, including emotional, physical, and sexual abuse, resulting in Post Traumatic Stress Disorder,[15] severe behavioural disorders[16] and damaging long term effects on the family as a whole.[17] Challenging behaviour in people with intellectual disabilities may be indicative of psychiatric disorders, such as psychosis, depression, and anxiety disorders.

A recent report concludes that people with intellectual disabilities who present behavioural challenges are often marginalized, stigmatized, disempowered, and excluded from mainstream society,[18] indicating the need for changes in policy and practice.

### Sexual relationships, marriage, and parenthood

Long-term sexual relationships and parenting children are generally considered to be an integral part of being an adult. In adolescence, emotional and sexual interest and needs develop, and it is at this stage that most young people start to have sexual relationships. However, people with intellectual disabilities are seldom encouraged to develop sexual relationships. Parents tend to actively discourage it, and service managers and care staff, though they may not necessarily actively discourage it, often provide little opportunity, or privacy, to enable it to happen. Many people in the general population find it difficult to accept that men and women with intellectual disabilities have ordinary sexual feelings and desires, let alone that they should be allowed to act on them.[19] The argument against allowing people with intellectual disabilities to have sexual partners often involves judgments about whether someone is deemed fit to be a parent. People with intellectual disabilities are discouraged from parenthood, and the experiences of childbearing and child rearing are still usually denied to women with intellectual disabilities. In Norway, 40 per cent of a study cohort of 126 children born to parents with intellectual disabilities were found to have suffered from 'failures of care'.[20] In England, however, research has demonstrated that some people with intellectual disabilities can become successful parents, provided they are given appropriate and effective support.[21]

### Cultural differences

People with intellectual disabilities from black and ethnic minorities are less likely to have their needs met by service organizations as compared with the rest of the population.[22] This is not only the result of difficulties in accessing services, and lack of appropriate information, but also because too little attention is paid to the different social norms, beliefs and preferences of people from different cultural backgrounds.

It is vital that service planners and providers know in what ways and to what extent the belief systems of the people they provide services for coincide and/or conflict with their own. They must also be aware of the implications of these differences for the acceptability, expectations and outcomes of the services offered to people from different cultural groups.

# Elderly people with intellectual disability

## Life expectancy

People with intellectual disabilities have an increased risk of death compared with the general population. Whereas the majority of deaths (83 per cent) in the whole population in the UK occur in people aged 65 years and over, less than 50 per cent of deaths among people with intellectual disabilities are in this age group.[23] In a study of young people in one state in the US, the mortality rate was almost three times higher than average,[24] and in Denmark 'preventable' mortality was four times higher than average.[25] However, life span is increasing among people with intellectual disabilities,[26] especially among people with Down's Syndrome.

As a result of this increasing longevity, causes of death common in a normal ageing population are becoming more prevalent among people with intellectual disabilities, such as stroke, heart disease and cancer. The most common cause of death for people with intellectual disabilities is still respiratory disease, which occurs far more frequently than in the whole population, suggesting lack of effective care.[27] This cause of death is linked to pneumonia, swallowing and feeding problems, and gastro-oesophageal reflux disorder.

People with intellectual disabilities frequently suffer from epilepsy, and it is suggested that the mortality rate for people with epilepsy and intellectual disabilities 'may be as high as five times that of the general population'.[28] This high mortality rate is related to seizure type and frequency, rather than directly to seizures.

## Health needs

Cooper[29] reviews the effects of age on the physical health of people with intellectual disabilities, and stresses the existence of significant health needs among this population. These needs arise not only from the normal ageing process but also from the specific social health and mental health needs of people with intellectual disabilities, including dementia.

There are serious problems relating to access to health care,[30] which is further complicated by their failure, and the failure of their carers, to recognize the signs and symptoms of illness. Overall, uptake of services by elderly people with intellectual disabilities is poor. There is an increased risk for a number of medical conditions in people who have Down's Syndrome,[31] including sensory impairments, thyroid disease, leukaemia and atlanto-axial instability. The later consequences of congenital heart disease include pulmonary hypertension and congestive heart failure.

Carers may not recognize that changes in behaviour are due to physical or mental illness, instead attributing changes to the learning disability itself. It is important to determine the aetiology of any learning disability, even late in life, because of the possible health implications.

People with intellectual disabilities currently access health screening less than others in the general population.[32] Pictorial health education materials are available to help health care professionals provide information about illness, medical procedures and treatment to people with limited verbal communication (for example, see www.rcpsych.ac.uk/bbw).

Signs of poor physical care among elderly people with intellectual disabilities, e.g. eye infections or tooth decay, may indicate a deterioration in functioning, but may also reflect the fact that carers are not coping effectively. This emphasizes the need to ensure access to primary care.

Recent reports from the Disability Rights Commission[33] and Mencap[34] identify the existing health inequalities faced by people with intellectual disabilities, and cite evidence suggesting the discrimination they face at every level of the health service.

Recent studies of the prevalence of mental ill-health problems among people with intellectual disabilities have shown that the prevalence rate of mental ill-health among adults with intellectual disabilities is higher than those recorded in the general population, with anxiety states and depression increasing with age.[35] People with intellectual disabilities are prone to the same risk factors as other people, but there are additional ones, such as living in more deprived areas, not having any daytime occupation, single marital status and epilepsy, all factors associated with mental ill-health. These factors need to be addressed if the existing inequality gap is not to be widened further.

People with Down's syndrome have an increased risk of developing Alzheimer's disease in middle age. Although the neuropathological changes of Alzheimer's dementia are widespread, development of clinical dementia is not inevitable.[36] Dementia occurs more frequently among elderly people with intellectual disabilities in general than among the rest of the population, and with the increasing longevity of people with intellectual disabilities the number with dementia is rising.[37]

## Complexity of care needs of elderly carers and the people they care for at home

In households where an older person with intellectual disability is living with an elderly carer, there will be a complex set of individual and joint needs. Both are likely to be vulnerable at this stage in their lives, and their needs may not always be compatible.

Parents may reach a point where physical mobility and capabilities are declining, and in some cases dementia (in either), may complicate the situation. Input from services becomes essential, even if families have managed with few or no services until now. Many families will have relied on informal sources of support such as family members, friends and neighbours, but in later life these networks tend to break down, and households such as these become increasingly isolated. This isolation in the community tends to coincide with the increasing frailty of ageing carers.[38, 39] Parents of children with severe disabilities, and/or challenging behaviour, may well become isolated from kin and friends at a much earlier stage as a result of their dedicated caring role, increasing the likelihood of social isolation in later years.

Some elderly parents who come to light at this late stage will have made a decision not to accept help many years ago. This decision will have been made on the basis of information about services which were available up to 40 or 50 years ago, and elderly carers may not have received information about the range and nature of current services. There are also some parents who originally concealed their child's disabilities in order to avoid institutionalization, and these parents may still be unaware of less institutionalized alternatives to care at home.

Systems of mutual caring often develop in households such as these, and such families may continue to be independent, in spite of serious long-term problems, and only come to the attention of the services when crisis intervention becomes necessary.

Families such as these present a double challenge to the services, requiring co-ordination between all relevant service providers. Co-operation between services for the elderly and those for people with intellectual disability is often inadequate, and some older people with intellectual disability fall into a limbo between them, with no one taking overall responsibility for assessing and meeting their needs. However, part of the brief of local Partnership Boards in the UK is to ensure that there is co-ordination between the services, so that individuals can obtain the range of services that they need.[2]

### Planning for the future

Ageing parents often wish to continue to look after their adult child until they can no longer cope. If a son or daughter has mild intellectual disability this may not cause problems for the parents, and may represent a welcome continuation of family life, especially when other children leave home. Also, as parents grow older they may become increasingly dependent on their adult child with intellectual disability. This may outweigh their wish to see their son or daughter settled in a new home before they themselves die, or become too frail to care for them.

Although keeping an adult with severe disabilities at home may cause considerable hardship, many parents are unwilling to let their child go into residential care, because they believe that only they can provide the quality of care that he or she is used to.

Although separation and/or bereavement are likely to occur in the relatively near future, professionals working with families find that many elderly carers are reluctant to plan for their child's future care, and attempts to develop care plans are often fraught with anxiety.[40]

### Bereavement

The experience of bereavement is often ignored by people involved with people with intellectual disabilities, although the effects of bereavement among this population are particularly severe and long-lasting, and there may be a significant increase in aberrant behaviours, and an increase in psychopathology. The experience is often made more difficult by their exclusion from the rituals and processes associated with dying and death. The onset of grief may also be delayed and thus there is a greater chance that it will not be recognized as grief, but attributed to something else or labelled as challenging behaviour.[41]

The experience of bereavement of a parent is particularly hard because, in addition to trying to come to terms with this loss, there are often other major life changes, such as moving into a strange home, living with unfamiliar people, and being cared for by a number of new carers.

### Life changes in old age

Any major life changes in old age can have serious emotional and physical consequences. Life events which can trigger physical or mental deterioration include institutionalization, when caring parents die or become too frail to continue caring. This often sudden upheaval following unexpected separation or loss of a parent can be extremely traumatic.[42] Conversely, deinstitutionalization, i.e. moving into the community after a lifetime in a long-stay institution, requires complex and sympathetic planning and monitoring.[43]

### Cultural differences

The implications of the lack of specific policies for older people with intellectual disability are particularly relevant to those from black and ethnic minority groups. Their needs may not be appropriately met by existing day services, but the alternative, i.e. living in residential homes in which staff and residents do not share the same background or language, may result in increased isolation in old age. Appropriate community services, which respond to different cultural preferences and expectations, have been developed in some areas of Britain. In general, however, service providers tend to focus on the issues of age and intellectual disability, rather than the cultural background of those individuals who have different expectations and preferences in the context of age and approaching death.[44]

## Further information

St George's, University of London www.intellectualdisability.info Down's Syndrome Association UK http://www.downs-syndrome.org.uk

British Institute of Learning Disability www.bild.org.uk

The Department of Health – Learning Disabilities www.doh.gov.uk/learningdisabilities

Down's Syndrome Medical Interest Group www.dsmig.org.uk

The Foundation for People with Learning Disabilities www.learningdisabilities.org.uk

International Association for the Scientific Study of Intellectual Disabilities www.iassid.org

## References

1. Royal College of Nursing (2006). *Meeting the health needs of people with learning disabilities*. Royal College of Nursing, London.

2. Department of Health (2001). *Valuing people: a new strategy for learning disability for the 21st Century*. The Stationery Office, London.

3. O'Brien, G. (2006). Young adults with learning disabilities: a study of psychosocial functioning at transition to adult services. *Developmental Medicine and Child Neurology*, **48**, 195–9.

4. Morris, J. (1999). *Hurtling into a void: Transition to adulthood for young disabled people with 'complex health and support needs'*. Pavilion Publishing Limited, Brighton.

5. Hollins, S. and Hollins, M. (2005). You and your child: making sense of learning disabilities. Karnac Books, London.

6. Mansell, J., Ashman, B., Macdonald, S., *et al.* (2002). Residential care in the community for adults with intellectual disability: needs, characteristics and services. *Journal of Intellectual Disability Research*, **46**(8), 625–33.

7. Inclusion International (2006). *Hear Our Voices: People with an Intellectual Disability and their Families Speak out on Poverty and Exclusion: a global report*. Inclusion International, London.

8. Dawson, E., Hollins, S., Mukongolwa, M., *et al.* (2003). Including disabled children in Africa. *Journal of Intellectual Disability Research*, **47**(3), 153–4.

9. Royal College of Psychiatrists (2004). *Factsheet 10: The child with general learning disability: for parents and teachers*. Mental Health and Growing

Up (3rd ed.). The child with general learning disability. Royal College of Psychiatrists, London.

10. McCoubrie, M., Hollins, S., Beckmann, R., *et al.* (2006). Health Action Plans: Some Guidelines for General Practitioners and Primary Care Teams. *Learning About Intellectual Disabilities and Health*. http://www.intellectualdisability.info/how_to/HAPs.htm

11. Bernal, J. and Hollins,S. (1995). Psychiatric illness and learning disability: a dual diagnosis. *Advances in Psychiatric Treatment, 1*, 138–45.

12. Maag, J. W. and Reid, R. (2006). Depression Among Students with Learning Disabilities: Assessing the Risk *Journal of Learning Disabilities, 39*(1), 3–10.

13. Commission for Healthcare Audit and Inspection and Commission for Social Care Inspection (2006). *Joint investigation into the provision of services for people with learning disabilities at Cornwall Partnership NHS Trust*. Commission for Healthcare Audit and Inspection, London.

14. Commission for Healthcare Audit and Inspection (2007). *Investigation into the service for people with learning disabilities provided by Sutton and Merton Primary Care Trust*. Commission for Healthcare Audit and Inspection, London.

15. McCarthy, J. (2001). Post-traumatic stress disorder in people with learning disability. *Advances in Psychiatric Treatment, 7*, 163–9.

16. Sequeira, H., Howlin, P., Hollins, S., *et al.* (2003). Psychological disturbance associated with sexual abuse in people with learning disabilities: case-control study. *British Journal of Psychiatry, 183*, 451–6.

17. O'Callaghan, A.C., Murphy, G., Clare, I.C.H., *et al.* (2003). The impact of abuse on men and women with severe learning disabilities and their families. *British Journal of Learning Disabilities, 31*(4), 175–80.

18. Royal College of Psychiatrists. (2007). *Challenging Behaviour: A Unified Approach*. Report CR144. Royal College of Psychiatrists, London.

19. Heyman, B. and Huckle, S. (1995). Sexuality as a perceived hazard in the lives of adults with learning difficulties. *Disability & Society, 10*, 139–56.

20. Morch, W. T., Skar, J., Andersgard, A. B., *et al.* (1997). Mentally retarded persons as parents: prevalence and the situation of their children. *Scandinavian Journal of Psychology, 38*, 343–8.

21. Booth, T. www.intellectualdisability.info (accessed August 13 2007).

22. Mir, G., Ahmad, W., Jones, L., *et al.* (2001). *Learning difficulties and ethnicity*. Department of Health, London.

23. Hollins, S., Attard, M. T., von Fraunhofer, N., et al. (1998). Mortality in people with learning disability: risks, causes, and death certification findings in London. *Developmental Medicine and Child Neurology, 40*, 50–6.

24. Decoufle, P. and Autry, A. (2002). Increased mortality in children and adolescents with developmental disabilities. *Paediatric and Perinatal Epidemiology, 16*(4), 375–82.

25. Mölsa, P. K. (1994). Survival in mental retardation. *Mental Handicap Research, 7*, 338–45.

26. Holland, A.J.(2000). Ageing and learning disability. *British Journal of Psychiatry, 176*, 26–31.

27. S. D. R. Stoddart, E. C. Griffiths, and R. J. Lilford. (2005). *A Confidential Inquiry into Excess Mortality in Learning Disability*: Scoping Report to the National Patient Safety Agency.

28. Wilcox, J. and Kerr, M. (2006). Epilepsy in people with learning disabilities. *Psychiatry, 5*(10), 372–7 (373).

29. Cooper, S-A. (1998). A clinical study of the effects of age on the physical health of people with intellectual disabilities. *American Journal on Mental Retardation, 102*, 582–9.

30. NHS Service Delivery and Organization (SDO) (2004). *Access to health care for people with learning disabilities*. NHS National Institute for Health Research, London.

31. Holland, T. and Benton, M. (2004). *Ageing and its consequences for people with Down's Syndrome*. Down's Syndrome Association, London.

32. NHS Service Delivery Organization (SDO) (2004). *Access to health care for people with learning disabilities*. NHS National Institute for Health Research, London.

33. Disability Rights Commission (2006). *Equal Treatment: closing the gap*. A formal investigation into physical health inequalities experienced by people with learning disabilities and/or mental health problems. Disability Rights Commission, London.

34. Mencap (2007). *Death by Indifference*. London: Mencap

35. S-A. Cooper, E. Smiley, J. Morrison, A. Williamson and L. Allan. (2007). Mental ill-health in adults with intellectual disabilities: prevalence and associated factors. *British Journal of Psychiatry, 190*, 27–35.

36. Stanton, L.R., and Coetzee,R.H. (2004). Down's syndrome and. dementia. *Advances in Psychiatric Treatment, 10*: 50–8.

37. Cooper, S. (1997). High prevalence of dementia among people with learning disabilities not attributable to Down's syndrome. *Psychological Medicine, 27*, 609–16.

38. McGrath, M. and Grant, G.(1993). The life-cycle and support networks of families with a person with a learning difficulty. *Disability, Handicap and Society, 8*, 25–42.

39. Hubert, J. and Hollins, S. (2000). Working with elderly carers of people with learning disabilities and planning for the future. *Advances in Psychiatric Treatment, 6*, 41–8.

40. Walker, C. and Walker, A. (1998). *Uncertain Futures: people with learning difficulties and their ageing family carers*. Pavilion Publishing/ Joseph Rowntree Foundation, Brighton.

41. Hollins, S., and Esterhuyzen, A. (1997). Bereavement and grief in adults with learning disabilities. *British Journal of Psychiatry, 170*, 497–501.

42. Mencap (2002). *The Housing Timebomb: the housing crisis facing people with a learning disability and their older parents*. Mencap, London.

43. Owen, K. (2004). *Going Home? A study of women with severe learning disabilities moving out of a locked ward*. University of London/Judith Trust, London: St George's.

44. Mir, G., Ahmad, W., Jones, L., *et al.* (2001). *Learning difficulties and ethnicity*. Department of Health, London.

## 10.8

# Families with a member with intellectual disability and their needs

Ann Gath and Jane McCarthy

## Introduction

It is now more than 30 years since children with intellectual disability were among the first patients to emerge from long-stay hospitals, where the mothers had been persuaded to part with the disabled children. The argument given was that not only would that child have the best possible chance of a happy life, but so also would the other children. Fears that there would be adverse effects on parents and on brothers and sisters prompted much of the early research.[1]

## Assessment of effects on the family

Recent sophisticated methodology has been used to explore a variety of factors, including the family as a whole as well as the parents, and what impinges on the family such as wider social, economic, and cultural influences.[2,3] Positive adaptation and coping strategies within families were identified and are highly relevant in providing a basis for intervention. Other life events and protective or compensating influences are not ignored. Families with a disabled member are exposed to the same risk of adverse factors, such as poverty, divorce, unemployment, or mental illness as any other and, in most cases, will have the same strengths, such as humour, good friends, or staunch relatives as their neighbours. Previously, all the complaints were added together as a measurement of 'stress', a concept too amorphous to be the basis of helpful intervention.

### The early impact on a family of a disabled child

Diagnosis of an abnormality now frequently happens in pregnancy from screening tests or from ultrasound scans, all of which are routinely offered. Termination of pregnancy is offered when results are positive. Although negative tests by no means guarantee normality, they are often interpreted by the parents as meaning that major disability is ruled out. Hence their disappointment when a child is born with a defect is even more intense, and it often follows a prolonged highly anxious period in which the baby is in special care. Initial hope is followed by temporary relief and then by the reality of gross developmental delay. Others believe they have a normal child until they become aware of the slowness of development or the onset of seizures occurs in the second half of the first year. Parental reaction to these tragedies is often anger mixed with grief.

A major change in recent years has been the rapid expansion of intra-vitro fertilization. Although accurate figures are not available, it is estimated that at least 10 000 babies are born in the United Kingdom. Foetal abnormalities are more common than following normal conception as evidenced from clinical reports, but there is no data available about the effect on the parents who already have had much anxiety.

### The mixed feelings at the time of the initial impact

The feelings that parents experience have been likened to those of grief occurring with a sudden loss. It is a useful comparison as there is a loss. Every expectant parent daydreams about the child and the arrival of a sick or damaged baby destroys many of those dreams. Commonly the first stage is shock or a numb disbelief. The next phase is often denial, 'This cannot be happening to me', followed by anger, which may be directed against the other parent, the doctor, or God. The last two phases are constructive active adaptation, which might involve learning about the condition or joining a parents association, leading on to resolution. Unfortunately, not everyone goes through all these stages and certainly not at the same rate. The mother might still be feeling as if she is shell-shocked while the father is making contact with a particular society or support group on the Internet.

### The effect of diagnosis

Down syndrome is the most common disorder recognizable at birth and known to be likely associated with intellectual disability. Despite screening in early pregnancy, the condition is still common but is now often in the child of younger parents. Genetic diagnosis of unusual children is more rapid than hitherto. Parents are almost without exception relieved by a clear diagnosis, providing an explanation of why the condition has arisen as well as an estimate of future risk. Most families are also greatly helped by meeting others with similar problems. Parent support groups for each specific diagnosis are now worldwide and recruits are quickly introduced to information via the Internet. Some diagnoses have implications for other members of the family, as with fragile X syndrome or tuberose sclerosis, as some relatives may have a minor form or be carriers, with a risk of further children in the family being affected. Genetic counselling is essential and may be requested very early on, in pregnancy or even before conception. To be preventative, decisions have to be made fast and at times when young couples are at their most vulnerable.[4]

### The effect on the parents of a child with intellectual disability

Informal support from the family or neighbours is much more effective than more formal, professionally led support. Frequent outpatient appointments where little happens are not cost-effective for the family; often the father loses money as he must take time off work and the cost of travel with a difficult baby or toddler is high. Not all can benefit from discussion groups of parents, and other mothers find a succession of home visits from a variety of professionals very disruptive. Families with active participation in religion can strengthen family ties, especially among immigrant groups, such as Hispanic people in the United States, and Indian families, where Hinduism is central to family life and where children have specific roles to play, such as that of sons in funeral rites. A child with an abnormality makes many parents look again at their fundamental beliefs, but few make lasting changes. Other families find membership of other groups (social, cultural, even sporting) supportive, provided that the family feels that they and their child are unconditionally accepted.

### Family functioning with a child with intellectual disability at school

The finding concerning the greater efficacy of informal support holds true for families of children across the whole age range, from school entry to adult life. The children are enrolled into school or special preschool groups earlier than normal brothers and sisters, thus widening the informal network of friends and confidants. Conversely, policies about choice of school, and the frequent necessity for children to be sent to schools at a greater distance away from home than other children, can lead to ostracism often felt more by the mother than by the child himself. An advantage of a special school is the relatively small size, allowing personal teacher–parent association and an open-door policy to parents, who are agreeably surprised to find themselves enjoying the school years of their disabled children.

### Transition to adult life

For many years, families have learnt to work in partnership with schools, and enjoyed frequent contact with teachers, face to face or thorough the progress book that goes to and from school everyday. The last few years at school are much concerned with the choice of type of further education, sometimes residential, and with encouraging independence. The process of finding a suitable and acceptable place is often described as a lottery or a battle, and is very stressful for the parents. Many have struggled through the school years, hoping that a permanent placement will be found when they come to an end. Others fear the loss of their close contact with their child, particularly if given adult rights to make choices, with which the parents do not agree. The possible outcome is one of three: independence, semi-independence, and dependence.

For those who remain at home, the other children in the family leave home as expected, leaving their disabled brother or sister in what one mother described as 'a ghetto of the middle-aged'. However, in many families, the provision of good further education programmes or day centres plus club or leisure activities can lead to liberation and more happiness for all members of the family. It is those with severe behaviour difficulties who are not accepted by further education establishments and who become increasingly frustrated and difficult to manage at home.

## Other members of the family

In many countries, the family has changed markedly in the last 30 years. There are many more divorces so that the 'parents' involved in the care of a child or young person are frequently one natural parent and one step-parent. There are also many divorced mothers living alone with the young adult after all the siblings have gone. Although some have adapted very positively, others feel very lonely, particularly if there are no members of the wider family to share the care and, often more pressing, to share the worries. Grandparents are as important in families with a member with intellectual disability as they are in ordinary families, although initially grandparents can become severely affected by the grief, take sides in attributing blame, or offer unsought advice. One mother described her mother as an enormous help because 'she was always behind me in every decision I took'. When no helpful grandparent is available, an older neighbour, another member of a parents group, or a teacher at the school or day centre could provide the sort of informal support that has proved to be so valuable.

### Ageing parents and ageing 'children'

The physical work of looking after a still dependent and sometimes very heavy adult takes its toll on parents. With a severely physically handicapped adult 'child', some help can be provided with people coming in to help with bathing, but few houses can be adapted to minimize lifting which may be needed many times during the day and night. Sooner or later the work gets too much, particularly for a sole parent. Parental frailty makes aggressive behaviour much more frightening and potentially dangerous. Where there are few opportunities for outside contact, the adult, with intellectual disability complicated by severe behaviour disorder, can become possessive and may show jealousy, sometimes making visits even from grandchildren impossible. Despite the evident difficulties, a study in Wisconsin,[5] found that many parents, reaching the end of their lives after many years of looking after a disabled child, were fitter than others of the same age and had a much greater sense of having achieved something in life. Other studies of ageing people with intellectual disability have also shown the role reversal that occurs when the adult child for whom they have cared so long tenderly looks after a very old parent. Because of the increasing longevity of disabled adults as well as of older people in the general population, there are increasing numbers of very old frail parents left with a disabled offspring for whom they feel responsible and for whom they often feel anxiety about the future, commonly saying 'I always thought he would go before us'.

### Brothers and sisters

The well-being of the family members continues to be an area of interest with an emphasis on siblings.[3, 6] The initial decision had been made not just for the sake of the child with intellectual disability, but also in the belief that it was also in the interest of the other brothers and sisters, but it was possible that they who would pay the price. There is now a considerable body of literature confirming the early findings that siblings are by no means invariably damaged. Thirty years ago, there was evidence that the older girls in the families did suffer, or were difficult or distressed at school while having more than usual amounts of responsibility at home. As services improved, these findings were no longer replicated except in those countries with few facilities and many social problems. In general, the other children in the family have identified themselves with their parents' decisions and take some part in the caring. This 'assistant' parent role comes easily to older siblings, but younger siblings who grow up fast, first catch up with the disabled sibling and then overtake in development terms and in the privileges earned by greater maturity. Parents describe this period of catching up and gradual overtaking as one of the most difficult in bringing up their children because of rivalry or jealousy. However, subsequent interviews with parents show that they are as sensitive to the needs of their 'normal' children as to those of the disabled child, and the balance between the siblings is readjusted. There is little evidence of long-term damage, but on the contrary, a consistent finding that the brothers and sisters are drawn to the caring professions, particularly medicine, nursing, or special needs teaching. The majority of families with children with intellectual disability are ordinary families with 'one feature in common'.[7]

### Mental illness

In the early months following the birth of a child recognized as having a major developmental disorder, such as Down syndrome, there was clearly much distress and disappointment, but little evidence that the mothers had a higher incidence of postpartum psychiatric disorder. Later in the childhood of the affected child, particularly in families with many other problems, depression was more common in the mothers of children with Down syndrome than in mothers of normal children. But when the mothers of children with a variety of disorders all producing intellectual deficit were compared with mothers of children with Down syndrome, there were less reported health problems in the Down group. Children with brain damage and severe hyperkinesis and those with autism were rated as the most stressful. Hyperkinesis and autism both occur in Down syndrome and their families report a similar degree of stress, as recorded by the questionnaire. For all families with a disabled child, many of the same factors appeared to be protective, for instance a good relationship with a partner and, in addition, support and affection from female relatives like the woman's mother or sisters. There were professionally led groups, assigned social workers, and parent–teacher associations at the school, but the informal sources of support were consistently more effective than formal, with studies in the United States showing very similar results to those in the United Kingdom.

The mental heath, composition, social background, and functioning of the family can increase the risk of psychopathology in the child with intellectual disability as can these risk factors for all young people.[8] There is no evidence that severe psychiatric illness is more common among the families of people with intellectual disability than in anyone else. However, the combination of a severe mental illness, such as bipolar disorder coexisting in the same family with intellectual disability is overwhelming for any family, particularly if one person has the dual diagnosis.

## People with intellectual disability who become parents themselves

Although sexuality and pregnancy is a fear of many parents of severely intellectually disabled adolescents, their fertility appears to be very low and there are very few pregnancies in people who are totally dependent. The majority of people identified as having mild retardation during the period of education disappear from services when they leave school and so it is not possible to estimate how many women with mild or borderline retardation become mothers. However, a certain number do come before the family courts or are already known to services for other reasons. However, problems arise with planning ahead and the constant protection from danger that young babies require. There are now techniques to help teach these skills. The secret of success in such teaching is a positive attitude of enhancing skills and not one of undermining the mother. With a partner who is both stable and more able, many quite limited young women cope. As the children grow older, the problems increase as the balance between protection and encouraging new skills becomes more difficult. However, intellectual limitation in itself is not an absolute bar to parenthood. Sadly, many young women with difficulties in intellectual and emotional immaturity are likely to find partners with even more problems and have, for example, a high risk of being hurt by a violent man and of failing to protect children from similar abuse. It is problems such as these rather than the intellectual deficit that make the courts question the safety of the children.

### International perspective

The very many worldwide studies that exist show a remarkable consistency in their findings. For all families of whatever ethnic origin, economic status, or religious persuasion, there is grief at the birth of a child, who is in any way defective, and anxiety and sadness about a child who later is seen to fail. In some cultures, an affected boy is harder to bear than an affected girl, as boys have special roles, for instance taking part in the funeral of the parents. Obviously, a high infant mortality will mean an even higher rate in children with any sort of disability. There are a few studies that have come from countries in an early state of development. The authors of these papers are anxious not to repeat what they understandably see as the mistakes of Europe and America. There are for example excellent community services in Asian countries based on the strengths and the beliefs of the local people,[9] whereas others model their services on those in the West, and thus have similar problems but cannot reach a significant proportion of the population. Other countries in Europe are struggling to establish new services for children at the same time as they deal with the very many older people who have been poorly treated for many years. The changes are difficult for the families of these older ones, yet even after many years, families have cooperated with rehabilitation and, in some cases, taken the adult 'child' home.

## Needs and priorities

Today in the United Kingdom the social and economic needs of these families are often unmet with a significant number of families with a disabled child living in poverty.[10] Most families will agree that the needs of the disabled member should be given priority—provided that other members of the family are in good agreement. The needs concerning the best possible communication and training or appropriate treatment for behaviour problems are very much in the interests of other members of the family. Hence the needs of the others would include:

- education that supports the development of the child and the needs of the family
- as accurate a diagnosis as possible
- genetic advice to other members of the family likely to produce children
- to be treated as informed partners by therapists and teachers
- available and interested primary health care
- a key worker to coordinate access to the different agencies and further financial support
- informed specialist care within reasonable distance
- advice and help to 'get through' to the child should communication be a problem, with the chance to learn sign language, symbols, or computer aids
- specialist and domiciliary help with behaviour problems
- respite care, arranged in partnership with the family
- when things go wrong, support and if necessary psychiatric care that treats the other members of the family as whole people with many other facets and not stereotyped family members of a disabled child.

## Conclusion

Having a child with intellectual disability is a major and usually totally unexpected blow to any family. However, most families show great resourcefulness and adapt to give their normal child as well as themselves a happy, rewarding life. Parents strongly resent being treated as potential psychiatric patients and have vigorously thrown out the concept of 'the handicapped family'. They do suffer understandable grief. From the point of discharge, the encouragement of informal support is more useful than providing hospital-based services. Children with all sorts of disability go to school early and the provision of unobtrusive familiar services is helpful. Unfortunately, there is often a gap in services between children's services and those for older adolescents and adults. The gap occurs at the worst time for parents who of all times require a familiar knowledgeable person who can offer a service throughout the transition period. The services required by the parents are practical help, such as appropriate equipment, respite care, advice about behaviour, and the ability to find emergency or specialized help at short notice. Parents also require some notice to be taken of their increasing age and/or infirmity, the financial difficulties arising out of the disability, and their anxiety that a humane plan can be made for their son or daughter when they die.

## Further information

www.downs-syndrome.org.uk
www.fragilex.org.uk

## References

1. Tizard, J. and Grad, J.C. (1961). *The mentally handicapped and their families.* Maudsley Monograph 7. Maudsley Hospital, London.
2. Gath, A. (1997). A review of psychiatric and family research in mental retardation. *International Review of Research in Mental Retardation,* **20,** 137–55.
3. Hastings, R., Turnbull, A., and Tonge, B. (2006). Special issue on family research. *Journal of Intellectual Disability Research,* **50,** 861–988.
4. Richards, M. (1998). Annotation: genetic research, family life and clinical practice. *Journal of Child Psychology and Psychiatry,* **39,** 291–305.
5. Seltzer, M.M. and Krauss, M.W. (1989). Aging parents with adult mentally retarded children. Family risk factors and sources of support. *American Journal of Mental Retardation,* **94,** 303–12.
6. Blacher, J., Cameron, L.N., and Paczkowski, E. (2005). Families and intellectual disability. *Current Opinion in Psychiatry,* **18,** 507–13.
7. Byrne, E.A., Cunningham, C.C., and Sloper, P. (1988). *Families and their children with Down's syndrome: one feature in common.* Routledge, London.
8. Emerson, E. (2003). Prevalence of psychiatric disorders in children and adolescents with and without intellectual disability. *Journal of Intellectual Disability Research,* **47,** 51–8.
9. Miles, M. (1997). Afghan children and mental retardation: information, advocacy and prospects. *Disability and Rehabilitation,* **19,** 496–500.
10. Sloper, T. and Beresford, B. (2006). Families with disabled children. *British Medical Journal,* **333,** 928–9.

# The planning and provision of psychiatric services for adults with intellectual disability

Nick Bouras and Geraldine Holt

## Introduction

The functioning of people with intellectual disability (ID) is affected by many factors. As well as their ID, their ability to communicate with others, their social competency, personality, life experiences and circumstances, and their health (including mental health) also influence their behaviour and adjustment.

This chapter focuses on the development and provision of services for adults with ID who have additional psychiatric and behavioural disorders. Developments have taken place in various parts of the world in recent years and a wide range of services has emerged.

## History and concepts

In the mid-nineteenth century the conceptualizations of the needs of people with ID and of those with mental illness, and of how to meet these needs were separated. Intellectual disability was not then included in psychiatric training curricula and generations of psychiatrists did not see people with ID, apart from those involved with administrative functions or the prescription of psychotropic medications in institutions. The mental health needs of those with ID at this time were largely unrecognized and so ignored.

Ideologies, sociological theories, civil rights issues, and the normalization philosophy[1, 2] together with families' organizations inspired current care practices and directed the way ID services developed.

Policy initiatives originating in the United States during the 1960s and 1970s produced profound and far-reaching changes offering the integration of people with ID into mainstream community life. Similar policies were adopted gradually around the world, particularly in North America, Europe, and Australasia, and in several countries the number of people with ID remaining in institutions has been drastically decreased. Deinstitutionalization of people with ID has been probably the largest social policy experiment of our time. Vivid accounts have been published recently offering enlightening narratives from individuals who were resettled in community living.[3] Overall people with ID and their families have benefited, having a better quality of life. Nevertheless, there are significant variations in the quality of community-based services and of the experiences of people who use them.[4]

## Psychiatric disorders and ID (dual diagnosis)

Many service planners and providers assumed that psychiatric disorders in this population would substantially diminish when community care programmes had been put in place. With the implementation, however, of the deinstitutionalization process the need for services for people with ID and psychiatric disorders emerged as a major issue.

This is because a significant number of people with ID, 5 to 12 per cent of children[5] and 15.7 to 40.9 per cent of adults with ID[6] have psychiatric disorders and despite progress in care delivery systems, require appropriate input to manage their mental health needs, sometimes over considerable time. Behavioural or psychiatric disorders can impair people's quality of life, cause regression of adaptive and intellectual functioning, and create unnecessary escalation of family stresses.

The presence of severe behaviour or psychiatric disorders in people with ID is one of the main reasons for the breakdown of community placements and of retention in residential environments that are more restrictive than otherwise required. Such people are at risk of being placed in out of area facilities[7] if local resources are not adequate to meet their assessment and treatment needs or ongoing support needs. These placements are often expensive and divert resources from developing local initiatives. The care provided may be inadequate and difficult to monitor. People may lose contact with families, friends, and those people and structures that previously supported them.

It has become clear that people with ID and mental health problems need services from both the ID network and the mental health system. The overall position of governmental policy has been that people with ID should have access to generic (i.e. for anyone with or without ID) health services, but with additional specialist (specifically for people with ID) support when needed.[8,9]

The argument for the provision of mental health care for people with ID from generic services appears sound and is supported widely.[10] Some argue that specialized services lead to stigmatization, labelling, and negative professional attitudes. Others argue that special expertise is required for the diagnosis and treatment of psychiatric disorders in this population, because although it is theoretically possible to train staff in generic settings, the relatively small number of cases gives little opportunity for staff to gain or maintain the necessary skills.[11]

Problems arise particularly when admissions to adult acute inpatient units occur, as people with ID often require longer admissions, and may be vulnerable without additional support on the ward. Furthermore, people with ID represent a very heterogeneous group with a varied range of highly complex mental health needs which generic staff may feel ill equipped to meet.[10]

Menolascino[12] recommended that services be provided according to need and be delivered in the context of both ID and psychiatric disorders coexisting allowing for more appropriate treatment, support, service planning, and development. The result is to create a partnership between the mental health and ID service structures to ensure responsive supports and treatments to previously underserved individuals.

## Models of services for people with psychiatric disorders and ID

There has been a growing interest internationally as to how to address this issue. Davidson and O'Hara[13] offer a comprehensive review of service developments for this population. Long-term resolution of behavioural or psychiatric disorders in persons with ID requires community-based activities. Hence since the year of publication of the first edition of the *New Oxford Textbook of Psychiatry* new developments in most countries of the world are community-based. The pace and form of change depends on each country's unique historical perspective and national philosophies about care for people with ID.[14] However, resolution of an acute crisis may require, in addition to community-based psychiatric or behavioural resources, inpatient acute psychiatric assessment and treatment services, specialized outreach, emergency respite, or emergency behaviour stabilization services.

The most common models of services for adults with ID and psychiatric disorders that have emerged in recent years in the United Kingdom can be described as: (a) generic ID community-based multidisciplinary (interdisciplinary) teams, (b) specialist community-based mental service for people with ID.

## Generic ID community-based multidisciplinary (interdisciplinary) teams

A multidisciplinary (interdisciplinary) team offers assessment and specialist services to people with ID. Initially, most of these teams were involved with deinstitutionalization, carrying out tasks such as identifying appropriately adapted and staffed houses, matching clients to live together, assessing health and social needs, and so on. Most of them have input from clinical psychologists and usually some input from a psychiatrist specializing in people with ID. Some teams have developed innovative ways of working with people with challenging behaviour often with severe ID. Members specializing in functional analysis and/or behavioural treatments strengthen such teams.

One considerable problem with this model has been the lack of links with mainstream mental health services. Despite the psychiatric input, such services may experience difficulties in meeting the mental health needs of people particularly those with mild

ID and mental illness. The problems are extended to people with ID who may have additional forensic mental health problems, autistic spectrum disorders including Asperger's syndrome and co-morbid conditions as well as those with borderline intellectual functioning.

## Specialist mental health service for people with ID

Since 1982, the Community Mental Health in ID Service in South East London[10,15] has operated using this model. It has secondary and tertiary care functions. This Service includes outpatient clinics, outreach work, inpatient assessment and treatment, and consultation with community agencies. The clinical team comprises of psychiatrists, community psychiatric nurses, and administrative staff, and has a regular interface with clinical psychologists and behaviour support specialists. The clinical team also receives regular input from occupational therapists, speech therapists, and social workers. The composition and functions of the Service have evolved over a number of years. An integrated part of the Service is the provision of training to direct support care staff and others to promote and sustain the development of a competent workforce at every level, from direct care staff to managers and organizations.

There are three phases in providing clinical services: assessment, intervention, and follow-up.

The clinical team carries out a structured clinical assessment on all referrals with the additional application of standardized instruments, e.g. Aberrant Behaviour Checklist[16] and CANDID.[17]

Therapeutic interventions are based on multidisciplinary work and include medication and environmental manipulation, as well as psychological treatments such as anxiety management and cognitive behaviour therapy. Regular weekly clinical team meetings are held to review progress. Crisis prevention plans are developed to help families and service providers identify early signs of breakdown and to take appropriate action. Training is offered to improve the capacity of families and service providers, to better understand and respond to the mental health needs of people with ID. This includes seminars, books and videos as well as modelling and role-playing exercises. Ongoing support and consultation is also provided while other specific therapeutic interventions are implemented.

Follow-up is provided for as long as it is required. Once a client seems stable and the agreed upon strategy appears to be effective the team maintains quarterly or half yearly contacts.

If an inpatient stay is warranted for acute psychiatric crises, admission is into generic mental health facilities with consultative advice and support from the community-based team. Patients can also access a six-bed specialist unit at a tertiary level. The function of this unit is to provide comprehensive assessment of the mental health problems when this cannot be achieved in a community setting or within generic mental health services, to make recommendations and implement therapeutic interventions and to ensure the appropriate care plans are transferred to the community setting on discharge. Care is delivered and coordinated via a person centred, Care Programme Approach (CPA),[18,19] to help ensure effective links with the full range of psychiatric health and social care services.

This Service is compatible with the development of other specialist services in the United Kingdom over the last few years to address specific needs for example of children and adolescents, older adults, those with forensic problems, mothers and babies, those with eating disorders, home treatment teams, assertive community treatment services, eating disorders teams, early intervention teams for psychosis, etc.[20]

## Outcomes

Evaluation and measuring of outcomes in mental health care for people with ID is very complex. This is because most health care service developments and reforms are politically and socially driven rather than evidence led and researchers cannot embargo change until they have defined systems. Accumulating evidence from chronological studies will still require judgement and interpretation.[20]

Moss et al.[21] considered a variation of the Matrix Model, first described for non-disabled people with mental health problems by Thornicroft and Tansella,[22] for the evaluation of mental health services for people with ID. This consists of two dimensions, one determined by the level within the service system (i.e. national, local, or individual), and the other by the point in the temporal sequence of service provision (i.e. inputs to the service, the process of providing the service, and the resulting outcome). Bouras et al.[15] adopted the Matrix Model partially (inputs and processes) to evaluate their model of service and found that over 18 years statistically significant changes in referrals trends in ethnicity, type of residence, level of ID, the number of admissions to inpatient units and psychiatric diagnoses. In addition they also found that patients admitted to the specialist unit—in contrast to those admitted to a generic inpatient unit—showed a significant decrease in psychiatric symptoms, an increase in overall level of functioning, a reduction in severity of their mental health problems, and an improvement in behavioural function on discharge, at 6 and 12 months following discharge.[23]

In an attempt to compare the effectiveness of assertive and standard community treatment in people with psychotic spectrum disorders and ID, with a randomized controlled study, no significant differences were found between the two treatments.[24]

Clinical effectiveness studies in mental health care for people with ID still have to overcome important methodological limitations. At present the Matrix Model[21] seems to offer the most advantageous way of evaluation, providing a framework to conceptualize the factors that influence service developments in the field.

## Residential programmes for people with psychiatric and ID

Successful community-living opportunities for people with ID require a comprehensive and collaborative service structure, including appropriate residential and vocational facilities. However, whilst these have been developed for many people, services to meet the needs of those with psychiatric disorders have lagged behind.

Housing for people with mental health problems must be compatible with all the main principles of 'ordinary housing'. It should be located in an acceptable community setting that offers opportunities for community integration, be designed to provide services and supports to meet the needs and desires of the person residing there, and be affordable, safe, and comfortable. This requires that staff have the necessary skills and service structures to meet client needs.

As institutions have been closed residential facilities have been developed in their stead. The trend across North America, Europe, and Australasia has been for larger residential homes (sometimes on the sites of the old institutions) to be replaced by smaller group homes for 3–8 people supported by staff. More recently, 'supported living schemes' have become more common, where people rent or own the property, and receive support from agencies that do not control the accommodation.[4] The pace of change varies between and within countries.

The aim is to empower individuals in smaller settings, organized to respond to a wide range of needs, creating environments that promote physical and mental health. However, no one model will necessarily meet the needs of all individuals with mental health problems and ID. Some people may become isolated and lonely in one or two-person settings, or have difficulties that cannot be managed in housing where additional staff or clinical support is not readily available. Some people may simply prefer to live in a supervised group living situation rather than supported living and should be given the opportunity to live in a place they prefer.

Residential services should include a full range of alternatives to enhance an individual's capacity for community living. The individual receiving residential services should be allowed to have as much comfort, ownership, and autonomy as possible. Housing can offer a wide range of options, and maximize opportunities for community integration and personal independence. Specialist mental health services for people with ID should work in collaboration with residential providers, to provide clinical support and a safety net when difficulties arise. Delivery of services in this manner represents one of the most important organizational challenges for services for people with mental health problems and ID.

## Vocational programmes

Vocational services should also offer work in integrated settings in a person's community, opportunities, and supports that are manageable and productive for the worker and the workplace with adequate salary compensation.

There have been significant changes in employment and vocational services for people with disabilities and several have moved from traditional workshop settings to integrated supported employment. The majority of placements have been in the service sector consistent with shifts towards entry and low-skill jobs in the national employment market. Individual placement has had the greatest positive effect on wages. Supported employment enhances the quality of life of people with ID. Although there is an acceptance in society that people with mild levels of disabilities can be meaningfully employed, traditional views of the capabilities of people with severe disabilities continue to be major obstacles to their access to the most progressive contemporary, educational, and rehabilitation practices. People with mental health problems and ID may be under-represented in both the sheltered and supported employment workforces.

## Staffing issues and training

The availability of specialist training varies markedly between countries, and not surprisingly bears a close relationship to the level of service development.

In the United Kingdom the need for specialist mental health services for people with ID and psychiatric disorders was recognized in the early 1970s. Specialist training programmes for psychiatrists, nurses, and other health care professionals including family doctors, community nurses, and direct care staff have been developed. However, whilst such training is available its uptake is dependent on the interests of individuals or of their employees. Only for some is such training mandatory, e.g. psychiatrists.[25] Attention has focused in recent years on the training needs of first-level care workers in community day and residential facilities. They often receive little or no training in the psychiatric aspects of ID with the consequence that psychiatric illness amongst their clients frequently goes unrecognized and untreated.

### Benefits of training

Staff finds working with people with ID and mental health problems stressful. Giving them skills in this area so that they can manage, with support, people with mental health problems enables them to find this work more rewarding. The most basic and vital role of support staff in this context is the awareness that a person with ID may suffer a mental illness, as we all may. They need to be aware of the range of therapeutic options that might be helpful, including environmental changes, behavioural strategies, psychotherapeutic techniques, medication, and so on. A fuller knowledge and consideration of this topic will help to dispel myths and prejudices, for example that medication is to be avoided at all costs, or that its use signifies that staff has in some way failed the client. Specific knowledge about some disorders will provide insights into why and how interventions must be tailored around someone's strengths and needs, for example someone with autistic spectrum disorder may hit himself when his routine is changed. The intervention chosen may be to provide a timetable, which the staff and client follow. This may need to be in pictorial form to meet the client's communication needs, and small and durable enough for him to carry at all times.

### Training materials

Flexible training materials (e.g. The Training Package in the Mental Health of Learning Disabilities),[26] which can be used by staff groups in their own settings, are now available. It is often useful to design training around particular clients. Training should be a part of the culture of an organization. Including managers in training activities is helpful. It allows them to share a knowledge base with their staff, and to set-up processes, which facilitate the continued development of issues identified by the training. For instance, each client's mental health might be considered in his or her individual planning meeting. Actions agreed can then be regularly discussed in individual staff supervision, at staff groups, and at meetings with the mental health and multidisciplinary teams. Raising awareness on mental health issues for people with ID is also important for carers and families as they are a pivotal source of support.[27]

## Commissioning services

The deinstitutionalization of people with ID in the United States, United Kingdom, and other parts of the world is well-advanced. A variety of service models are provided. Comprehensive local services systems for those with additional mental health needs are emerging. The old institutions represented a complete system of care, inasmuch as they provided accommodation, health care, social care, and occupation in a single setting. Current provision, by contrast, involves a range of agencies and settings. This requires

that care is integrated and organized around an individual. This is not an easy task for those with complex needs.

Those commissioning services need to determine what services are needed locally and decide how they should be provided, monitored, and reviewed. This chapter provides an overview of the social and policy context and some models of services for adults with psychiatric disorders and ID. Local demographics and resources will of necessity shape services. To ensure that the commissioning of services is well-informed all planning partners should be involved. Using the Matrix Model[21] described earlier the commissioners might consider:

1　Joint commissioning. Various policies and legislation (**national inputs**) have proposed joint commissioning by health and social care services so that a joint strategy drives the joint commitment of resources (**local inputs**).

2　Client and carer participation (**individual inputs**). This is essential to ensure that appropriate priorities are set and that services are satisfactorily delivered (**individual and local processes and outcomes**).

3　Involvement of statutory and voluntary agencies (**local inputs**). This will enable the commissioners to make informed decisions.

4　A baseline needs assessment of the population to be served (**local inputs**) e.g. from census statistics, epidemiological research, local register data.

5　Local and national policies (**local and national input**) to enable them develop a vision, e.g. community-based services, mixed economy of provision.

6　Desired **outcomes at local level** (e.g. increased use of generic provision, reduction in number of people placed out of area) and translate these into

7　Service specifications

8　Purchase services, which have the necessary skills (**local and possibly national inputs,** e.g. for people with very particular needs) to deliver processes (**local and possibly national processes**) that will provide these outcomes.

9　Set in place monitoring systems, which may include individual and local outcomes e.g., complaints and incidents monitoring, scrutiny of statistics derived from CPA documentation (**individual and local processes and outcomes**).

10　Commissioning is a cyclical process and the monitoring and review of services (**local inputs**) will ideally enable more effective future commissioning.

*Components of an effective psychiatric service* for people with ID should include:

◆ Organizing services around clients' wishes and needs.

◆ Good interagency communication among health, social, and voluntary sectors.

◆ Good interagency communication between services for children and adults.

◆ High level of awareness of mental health issues by direct support staff in residential and day care services.

◆ High level of awareness of mental health issues by primary care staff.

- Multidisciplinary composition including psychiatrists, mental health nurses, clinical psychologists, behaviour support specialists, therapists, and social workers.

- Ability to provide consultation, assessment, and treatment.

- Provision of community-based interventions.

- Access to local specialist and generic community and inpatient assessment, treatment, forensic, and rehabilitation facilities.

- Resources to meet residential, recreational, and vocational needs of those with enduring needs.

- Clear coordination of inputs by a named person.

- Staff training.

- Measuring outcomes.

## Conclusion

There has been considerable debate as to whether specialized mental health service for people with ID services should be established or generic mental health service providers should serve this population. Whatever strategy is undertaken it should be based on high professional standards. Standardized diagnostic and assessment tools should be used. Appropriate, individually tailored treatments should be given in the least restrictive environments. Staff must have the necessary expertise, training, and support.

Mixed results have been obtained for the evaluation of existing services.[28] No direct studies of comparative treatment effectiveness exist, and studies on single specialist services contain some methodological weaknesses. It is essential that the quality of services is monitored, to maintain and improve standards of care. Increasing fragmentation of provision makes this a complex but essential task.

Often mental health services for people with ID are provided in a crisis. This highlights and amplifies the existing deficiencies in care. In order to become more effective and accessible these services will have to address both individual needs and service systems complexities for children, adolescents, and adults with ID and mental health problems. Several years into the post-institutional period and the era of community care, meeting the mental health needs of people with ID remains a challenge. Though the initial philosophical concern about the coexistence of mental health problems in people with ID has been partially eroded with the emerged evidence-based research, nevertheless the clinically effective responses remain scanty. In times of hard fiscal constraints for mental health services in general, it is hoped that people with ID will not be further overlooked and marginalized but they will receive the required professional attention matched by adequate distribution of resources.

## Further information

Bouras, N. and Holt, G. (eds.) (2007). *Psychiatric and behavioural disorders in intellectual and developmental disabilities*. Cambridge University Press, Cambridge.

Advances in Mental Health and Learning Disabilities published by Pavilion Publishing. (2007). http// www.pavpub.com

Estia Centre: http://www.estiacentre.org

National Association for the Dually Diagnosed: http://www.thenadd.org

## References

1. Wolfensberger, W. (1969). The original nature of our institutional models. In *Changing patterns in residential services for the mentally retarded* (eds. R. Kugel and W. Wolfensberger), p. 235. President's Committee on Mental Retardation, Washington, DC.

2. Wolfensberger, W. (1991). Reflections on a lifetime in human services and mental retardation. *Mental Retardation*, **29**, 1–16.

3. Johnson, K. and Traustadottir, R. (2005). *Deinstitutionalization and people with intellectual disabilities: in and out of institutions*. Jessica Kingsley Publishers, London.

4. Mansell, J. (2006). Deinstitutionalisation and community living: progress, problems and priorities. *Journal of Intellectual & Developmental Disability*, **31**, 65–76.

5. Kerker, B.D., Owens, P.L., Zigler, E., *et al.* (2004). Mental health disorders among individuals with mental retardation: challenges to accurate prevalence estimates. *Public Health Reports*, **119**, 409–17.

6. Cooper, S.-A., Smiley, E., Morrison, J., *et al.* (2007). Mental ill health in adults with intellectual disabilities: prevalence and associated factors. *The British Journal of Psychiatry*, **190**, 27–35.

7. Pritchard, A. and Roy, A. (2006). Reversing the export of people with learning disabilities and complex health needs. *British Journal of Learning Disabilities*, **34**, 88–93.

8. Department of Health. (2001). *Valuing people: a new strategy for learning disabilities in the 21st century*. HMSO, London.

9. US Public Health Services. (2002). *Closing the gap: a national blueprint for improving the health of individuals with mental retardation*. Report of the surgeon general's conference on health disparities and mental retardation. US Department of Health and Human Services, Washington, DC.

10. Bouras, N. and Holt, G. (2004). Mental health services for adults with learning disabilities. *The British Journal of Psychiatry*, **184**, 291–2.

11. Day, K. (1999). Professional training in the psychiatry of mental retardation in the United Kingdom. In *Psychiatric and behavioural disorders in developmental disabilities and mental retardation* (ed. N. Bouras), pp. 439–57. Cambridge University Press, Cambridge.

12. Menolascino, F.J. (1977). *Challenges in mental retardation: progressive ideology and services*. Human Sciences Press, New York.

13. Davidson, P.W. and O'Hara, J. (2007). Clinical services for people with intellectual disabilities and psychiatric or severe behaviour disorders. In *Psychiatric and behavioural disorders in intellectual and developmental disabilities* (eds. N. Bouras and G. Holt), pp. 364–87. Cambridge University Press, Cambridge.

14. Holt, G., Costello, H., Bouras, N., *et al.* (2000). BIOMED-MEROPE project: service provision for adults with intellectual disability: a European comparison. *Journal of Intellectual Disability Research*, **44**, 685–96.

15. Bouras, N., Cowley, A., Holt, G., *et al.* (2003). Referral trends of people with intellectual disabilities and psychiatric disorders. *Journal of Intellectual Disability Research*, **47**, 439–46.

16. Aman, M.G. and Singh, N.N. (1986). *The aberrant behaviour checklist*. Slosson Educational Publications, New York.

17. Xenitidis, K., Slade, M., Thornicroft, G., *et al.* (2003). *Camberwell assessment of needs for adults with developmental and intellectual disabilities*. Gaskell, London.

18. Department of Health. (1999). *National service framework for mental health: modern standards and service models for mental health*. HSC1999/223HMSO, London.

19. Department of Health. (1999). *Effective care co-ordination in mental health services: modernizing the CPA*. HMSO, London.

20. Burns, T. (2001). Generic versus specialist mental health teams. In *Textbook of community psychiatry* (eds. G. Thornicroft and G. Szmukler), pp. 231–41. Oxford University Press, Oxford.

21. Moss, S., Bouras, N., and Holt, G. (2000). Mental health services for people with intellectual disability: a conceptual framework. *Journal of Intellectual Disability Research*, **44**, 97–107.

22. Thornicroft, G. and Tansella, M. (1999). *The mental health matrix: a manual to improve services*. Cambridge University Press, Cambridge.

23. Xenitidis, K., Gratsa, A., Bouras, N., *et al.* (2004). Psychiatric inpatient care for adults with intellectual disabilities: generic or specialist units. *Journal of Intellectual Disability Research*, **48**, 11–18.

24. Martin, G., Costello, H., Leese, M., *et al.* (2005). An exploratory study of assertive community treatment for people with intellectual disability and psychiatric disorders: conceptual, clinical, and service issues. *Journal of Intellectual Disability Research*, **49**, 516–24.

25. Costello, H., Holt, G., Cain, N., *et al.* (2007). Professional training for those working with people with intellectual disabilities and mental health problems. In *Psychiatric and behavioural disorders in intellectual and developmental disabilities* (eds. N. Bouras and G. Holt), pp. 364–87. Cambridge University Press, Cambridge.

26. Holt, G., Hardy, S., and Bouras, N. (2005). *Mental health in learning disabilities: a training resource*. Pavilion Publishing, Brighton.

27. Holt, G., Gratsa, A., Bouras, N., *et al.* (2004). *Guide to mental health for families and carers of people with intellectual disabilities*. Jessica Kingsley Publishers, London.

28. Chaplin, R. (2004). General psychiatric services for adults with intellectual disability and mental illness. *Journal of Intellectual Disability Research*, **48**, 1–10.

# SECTION 11

# Forensic Psychiatry

**11.1 General principles of law relating to people with mental disorder** *1895*
Michael Gunn and Kay Wheat

**11.2 Psychosocial causes of offending** *1908*
David P. Farrington

**11.3 Associations between psychiatric disorder and offending** *1917*

11.3.1 Associations between psychiatric disorder and offending *1917*
Lindsay Thomson and Rajan Darjee

11.3.2 Offending, substance misuse, and mental disorder *1926*
Andrew Johns

11.3.3 Cognitive disorders, epilepsy, ADHD, and offending *1928*
Norbert Nedopil

**11.4 Mental disorders among offenders in correctional settings** *1933*
James R. P. Ogloff

**11.5 Homicide offenders including mass murder and infanticide** *1937*
Nicola Swinson and Jennifer Shaw

**11.6 Fraud, deception, and thieves** *1941*
David V. James

**11.7 Juvenile delinquency and serious antisocial behaviour** *1945*
Susan Bailey

**11.8 Child molesters and other sex offenders** *1960*
Stephen Hucker

**11.9 Arson (fire-raising)** *1965*
Herschel Prins

**11.10 Stalking** *1970*
Paul E. Mullen

**11.11 Querulous behaviour: vexatious litigation, abnormally persistent complaining and petitioning** *1977*
Paul E. Mullen

**11.12 Domestic violence** *1981*
Gillian C. Mezey

**11.13 The impact of criminal victimization** *1984*
Gillian C. Mezey and Ian Robbins

**11.14 Assessing and managing the risks of violence towards others** *1991*
Paul E. Mullen and James R. P. Ogloff

**11.15 The expert witness in the Criminal Court: assessment, reports, and testimony** *2003*
John O'Grady

**11.16 Managing offenders with psychiatric disorders in general psychiatric sevices** *2009*
James R. P. Ogloff

**11.17 Management of offenders with mental disorder in specialist forensic mental health services** *2015*
Pamela J. Taylor and Emma Dunn

# General principles of law relating to people with mental disorder

## Michael Gunn and Kay Wheat

## Introduction

This chapter provides a scheme for assisting in the analysis of two areas of law that provide some of the general principles that operate in relation to mentally disordered offenders. These two areas are (a) the law concerning decision-making and other action-taking to which the concept of competence is crucial, and (b) the law of responsibility in relation to liability for criminal offences and the tort of negligence. Whilst the focus of the chapter is on the law of England and Wales, it is clear that there are similarities in other common-law jurisdictions, and in other jurisdictions that have borrowed ideas from common-law jurisdiction, such as Japan, in relation to the concept of informed consent.

## Decision-making and action-taking law and competence

Generally, the law in relation to decision-making and action-taking might take one of three approaches to mentally abnormal offenders.

- The law might adopt the same approach for mentally abnormal offenders as for anyone else.

- The law might adopt an approach dependent upon the competence of the individual that might be affected by the mental state of the mentally abnormal offender.

- The law might adopt an approach recognizing the impact of being a mentally abnormal offender that may be based upon the effects or mere status of the mental state.

    There is no reason to examine further the law that is not different for the mentally disordered.

## Autonomy and Competence

The most appropriate approach that introduces different law is by reliance upon competence or capacity. Internationally, there is increasing acceptance that, where someone is incompetent to make their own decisions, there must be a route to making such decisions on their behalf. For example, in Japan, the approach of informed consent has been adopted and whilst there is not yet a fully developed

concept of competence, it is accepted that that is the next necessary development. Where there is significant variation is in the approach to adopt if someone is not competent. Traditionally, the approach has been to adopt guardianship whereby someone is either under guardianship or not and if so that all decisions are taken by the guardian. More recently, a more varied approach has become preferred whereby the decisions taken by others are only those that the individual cannot take and the basis for taking those decisions is the decision that the incapacitous would have made if competent and otherwise the decision that is in their best interests. It must be accepted however that this may be viewed as an approach grounded in a particular approach to law and ethics, i.e. that grounded in Western societies. Even there, there is a tradition for making decisions on a paternalistic basis, that is largely now discredited, though there are also concerns about the focus on autonomy. However, in other societies much greater emphasis is placed on the importance of the family as decision-makers or the basis of a decision on the presumption that the individual is a part of a particular society that has a genuine and proper interests in decision to be made on their behalf. Having recognized that as an approach, this chapter will largely focus upon the Western legal systems' basis, using England and Wales as an illustrative jurisdiction.

Increasingly, there is recognition internationally that action should only be taken with regard to a person if either they are incapable of deciding or acting for themselves or if they present a harm to others (or self) and that harm is linked with a mental health problem. The extent to which different jurisdictions have a developed view of respect for the principle of autonomy and its legal application through a test for capacity or competency unsurprisingly varies in practice. But the major issue is how decisions are to be made if someone is incapable.

### International statements of principle

Acceptance of respect for the principle of autonomy can be seen through at least two international instruments. Nascently, it can be identified in the provisions of the *United Nations* Declaration on the Rights of Mentally Retarded Persons (1971) which includes the following commitments.

1 The mentally retarded person has, to the maximum degree of feasibility, the same rights as other human beings.

2 The mentally retarded person has a right to proper medical care and physical therapy and to such education, training, rehabilitation, and guidance as will enable him to develop his ability and maximum potential....

5 The mentally retarded person has a right to a qualified guardian when this is required to protect his personal well-being and interests.

6 The mentally retarded person has a right to protection from exploitation, abuse, and degrading treatment....

7 Whenever mentally retarded persons are unable, because of the severity of their handicap, to exercise all their rights in a meaningful way or it should become necessary to restrict or deny some or all of these rights, the procedure used for that restriction or denial of rights must contain proper legal safeguards against every form of abuse. This procedure must be based on an evaluation of the social capability of the mentally retarded person by qualified experts and must be subject to periodic review and to the right of appeal to higher authorities.

More recently, the *Council of Europe* has agreed a set of recommendations that should be implemented across Europe and are attracting significant international attention, e.g. by the South African Law Commission. The *Principles Concerning the Legal Protection of Incapable Adults* (Council of Europe, 1999). As Jansen demonstrates, the Recommendation confirms the functional approach to capacity and seeks to provide the incapable adult, where necessary, with representation, assistance, measures of protection, and other arrangements. The Recommendation opens with a statement that underpins the general approach adopted in this chapter:

> 'I.1. The following principles apply to the protection of adults who, by reason of an impairment or insufficiency of their personal faculties, are incapable of making, in an autonomous way, decisions concerning any or all of their personal or economic affairs, or understanding, expressing or acting upon such decisions, and who consequently cannot protect their interests.'

This is followed up by an important statement that captures an underlying theme for most jurisdictions endeavouring to provide suitable approaches.

> 'II.1 In relation to the protection of incapable adults the fundamental principle, underlying all the other principles, is respect for the dignity of each person as a human being. The laws, procedures, and practices relating to the protection of incapable adults shall be based on respect for their human rights and fundamental freedoms, taking into account any qualifications on those rights contained in the relevant international legal instruments.'

The principles adopted are then:

♦ securing the maximum preservation of capacity that demands a functional approach to capacity and so not accepting that someone is either capable or not capable for all decisions, but may be able to make some decisions and not others (II.3.1) and that no step should be taken unless it is necessary (II.5.1).

♦ where steps are taken they must be proportional to the degree of capacity retained and they should be tailored to the needs and circumstances of the incapacitous person (II.6.1).

♦ there just be fair and efficient procedures for the taking of steps which must protect human rights and prevent possible abuses (II.7. 1 & 2). These requirements are expanded upon in Part III.

♦ the interests and welfare of the incapacitous person are the paramount consideration, thus ruling out a paternalistic basis for the taking of steps (II.8.1).

♦ the past and present wishes and feelings of the incapacitous person should be ascertained as far as possible, and should be taken into account and given due respect, and of most importance are the choices made by the incapacitous person themselves (II.9. 1 & 2).

♦ there is a preference for action taken without the intervention of a judicial or administrative authority but that such powers must be limited and their exercise controlled (IV.18.1)

♦ in the health field, no action should be taken if someone is capable of making the decision (V.22.1). The intervention may then be carried out if it is for the incapacitous person's direct benefit and authorization has been given by their representative or by an authority or person or body provided for by law (V.22.2). As not all jurisdictions are ready for this approach even in Europe, an alternative is provided so that where a person is under protective steps, the incapacitous person's consent should be sought even though there is someone with the power to make the decision (V.23.1). Where the incapacitous person cannot provide consent, the intervention is permissible where it is for their direct benefit and authorization has been given by their representative or by an authority or person or body provided for by law (V.23.2).

For Jansen, the key principles are, first, those in Principle 5, that is 'Necessity and Subsidiarity' as they 'imply, first of all, that no measure of protection should be established unless it is necessary, taking into account the circumstances of the particular case. Secondly, in deciding whether a measure is necessary, account should be taken of any less formal arrangements which might be provided in particular by family members, or by public authorities or other means. The latter is the principle known as 'subsidiarity' . . ..' The second key principle is, that in Principle 3, that is 'that of maximum preservation of capacity . . ... In particular a measure of protection should therefore not result in an automatic complete removal of legal capacity.' The third key principle is that in Principle 6, that is 'Proportionality: where a measure of protection is necessary it should be proportional to the degree of capacity of the person concerned and tailored to the individual circumstances of the case. The measure should restrict the legal capacity, rights and freedoms of the adult by the minimum which is consistent with achieving the purpose of the intervention.'

The international picture is completed by the Convention on the Rights of Persons with Disabilities that was signed in 2006 but is not yet in force. This is a Convention of the United Nations and has 129 States as signatories to it. The Convention is a broad Convention and covers many areas not directly relevant to this Chapter. It takes a similar approach since, its General Principles (art. 3) are (a) respect for inherent dignity, individual autonomy including the freedom to make one's own choices, and independence of persons; (b) non-discrimination; (c) full and effective participation and inclusion in society; (d) respect for difference and acceptance of persons with disabilities as part of human diversity and humanity; (e) equality of opportunity; (f) accessibility; (g) equality between men and women; and (h) respect for the evolving capacities of children with disabilities and respect for the right of children with disabilities to preserve their identities. In, for example, outlawing discrimination on the basis of disability (art. 4) and providing for freedom from exploitation, violence and abuse (art. 16), the Convention identifies the balance to be drawn between recognising the importance of decision-making with that of protecting those not capable of making their own decisions. It affirms the importance of the capacity to make decisions as a key requirement in the law. Article 12 states that State Parties reaffirm that persons with disabilities have the right to recognition everywhere as persons before the law and that State parties shall recognise that persons with disabilities enjoy legal capacity on an equal basis with others in all aspects of life.

### Tests of capacity and competence

Thus, it can be seen that key to respect for the principle of autonomy is to have a workable concept of capacity or competence. The functional approach requires that the test of competence be related to the particular decision to be made, at the particular time that it must be made. There is a range of abilities that competence might involve. Much of the work on competence has been undertaken in the context of health-care law and in relation to consent to treatment. Much of this work has been undertaken in the United States. Two leading thinkers, Grisso and Appelbaum, have, with colleagues, identified four abilities that can be involved in competency:

- evidencing a choice

- understanding

- appreciation

- reasoning or rationality.

Any given jurisdiction will adopt one or more of these abilities[19] in what it looks for in relation to competency assessments. There is no consistency, currently, as to which one or more of the abilities must be satisfied, except to say that almost all jurisdictions require understanding to some degree. This lack of consistency reflects the developing international understanding of the concept of competence. If we take English health-care law as an example, it can be seen that, in the early stages, understanding was the prime ability that had to be established, though the patient also had to evidence a choice. But, more recently, it seems that the courts are being attracted to an approach that may ultimately see competence only being satisfied where all four abilities are satisfied. Requiring rather more of an individual to satisfy the requirement of competence may be regarded as a better means of satisfying the crucial bioethical principle of self-determination or respect for the principle of autonomy, since if someone is not truly able to exercise self-determination, there is no respect for autonomy if, nevertheless, that person's 'decisions' are legally binding. This means that rather more 'decisions' are open to the challenge on the basis that they are not made by someone competent to do so. A stringent approach to competence may be hard to accept. It must then be assessed (as a general matter) whether it would be better to reduce the standard and so enable more people to be assessed as competent or whether lowering the standard is illusory as being for the benefit of people whose competence may be open to question. Therefore it is hardly

surprising that there continues to be debate as to the abilities that any individual must possess (and the level of functioning of that ability) in order to determine whether he or she is competent to make a particular decision. Wong et al.[19] make the point, drawing on the work of others, that the functional approach is not without problems. They point out that it is time consuming, legal standards vary between jurisdictions, and there is uncertainty about the threshold to be satisfied in determining competence.

The English Mental Capacity Act 2005, sections 2 and 3 creates a definition of capacity consistent with those abilities. The central elements of that definition are to be found in sections 2(1) and 3(1).

2(1) For the purposes of this Act, a person lacks capacity in relation to a matter if at the material time he is unable to make a decision for himself in relation to the matter because of an impairment of, or a disturbance in the functioning of, the mind or brain.

3(1) For the purposes of section 2, a person is unable to make a decision for himself if he is unable –
- (a) to understand the information relevant to the decision,
- (b) to retain that information,
- (c) to use or weight that information as part of the process of making the decision, or
- (d) to communicate his decision (whether by talking, using sign language or any other means).

### Three approaches

What is key is that the approach is a functional one that is it is related to the abilities of the individual at the time a decision is required and is not dependent upon either status or outcome of the decision, though these clearly have formed part of either definitions or approach to capacity in the past and are relevant factors in identifying the possibility that someone may not be capable of decision-making and in exercising judgment about that capacity. To state that competence if to be interpreted functionally.[19] means that the status of the decision-maker is not determinative of the question of her or his competence. *A status approach* makes assumptions about an individual's decision-making competence on the basis of a particular characteristic, and there is no empirical evidence to support the validity of such an approach.[19,21] The mental state of the decision-maker may be the reason why competence is put into question, but mental state in itself is rarely, if ever, sufficient to determine the matter. Mental state may have relevance to decision-making in that certain states will impact on the ability to understand and process information. Furthermore, the outcome of a decision is also not in itself sufficient to determine the matter. The fact that any given decision is not reasonable does not mean that the decision-maker is not competent to have made that decision. For example, the simple fact that a patient disagrees with the doctor does not mean that the decision is that of an incompetent decision-maker, though lack of congruence with the proposals of a doctor may cause questions to be asked about decision-making competence. *The outcome approach* has been rejected in a number of jurisdictions.[19] It is internationally recognized that anyone can make what might be termed objectively silly decisions without necessarily giving rise to doubts about competence. However, the regularity with which silly decisions are made may raise doubts about competence as also will the inter-relation between mental state and quality of decisions. In the United Kingdom, these points are further reflected in the fact that there is a legal presumption that a person is competent to make her or his own decision once adult state is reached.

*The functional approach* requires that the test of competence be related to the particular decision to be made, at the particular time that it must be made.[19] There is a range of abilities that competence might involve. Much of the work on competence has been undertaken in the context of health-care law and in relation to consent to treatment. Much of this work has been undertaken in the United States. Two leading thinkers, Grisso and Appelbaum,[20] have, with colleagues, identified four abilities that can

The functional approach to decision-making is not limited, in its application, to health-care decisions, even though that is where most of the debate has taken place. In principle, it may be applied to any type of decision. For example, the making of wills and the entering into of contracts are obvious examples where a functional approach applies, but it does not follow that the same abilities will be required for these decisions as for treatment decisions. Under the law prior to the Mental Capacity Act 2005, this is demonstrated by an old case which was, nevertheless, the leading case in relation to the making of wills. *Banks* v. *Goodfellow*, requires that a person:

> ought to be capable of making his will with an understanding of the nature of the business in which he is engaged, a recollection of the property he means to dispose of, of the persons who are the objects of his bounty, and the manner in which it is to be distributed between them.

This test demanded not just understanding, but also the appreciation and the reasoning ability noted above. Whilst the level at which the will writer must operate is not that of a lawyer, nevertheless he or she must be aware of the context in which the will is being made and must think through the competing potential demands on his or her estate. Of course, will writers can make silly dispositions, even going so far as to exclude financially dependent relatives. However, it must be recalled that an outcome that is questionable or unreasonable is not the same as the will or decision being made on the basis of an unacceptable reasoning process. An eccentric person might well, for example, not wish to leave anything to his or her relatives. Thus, in any jurisdiction, care must be taken to consider a particular test in deciding which of the four abilities are to be identified, and the answer to that question may demand very careful analysis.

## Persons not competent to make decisions or take action

If a person is not competent to make a decision for themselves, there is more variability as to the approach to be taken. Some of this difference is related to the commitment to do the best for a vulnerable person and leads to a desire to act paternalistically, so making the decision that objectively is in the best interests of the individual A more frequent approach is to make the decision that that individual would have made for themselves. This is most recently reflected in the English Mental Capacity Act.

If a person is not competent to make a decision or to take certain action, the law increasingly provides mechanisms whereby these decisions can be made. In England and Wales, until the abolition of the sign manual by the Mental Health Act 1959, the Crown had the power and the process to make decisions in the best interests of a person not competent to decide or to take action. This power is

the basis of many substitute decision-making procedures in common-law jurisdictions (including the United States). The specific adaptation is jurisdictionally specific. In some jurisdictions, it has been used to follow from generic decisions as to competence and to create overarching substitute decision-making procedures (e.g. those jurisdictions that adopt a full guardianship of the person approach). In England and Wales, the first approach, after the abolition of the sign manual procedure, was to allow for people to be received into guardianship (a process that was not, interestingly, dependent upon a finding of incompetence), but this proved not to be an acceptable procedure. Current English guardianship is very much only a community mental health power that does not enable anyone else to make decisions on behalf of the person received into guardianship.[33]

In England, the courts had to invent a procedure for making decisions on behalf of someone who was not competent. The House of Lords, the senior English court, provided a mechanism in relation to treatment decisions whereby, if a person was found to be incompetent, treatment could lawfully be provided if it was necessary, that is if it was for the life, health, or welfare of the patient and was in her or his best interests. Despite substantial improvements that made the approach identify what was the one, best approach that took into account the full range of interests (see below), this judicial approach has been replaced by a statutory format. The approach introduced by the Mental Capacity Act 2005, does not take a full guardianship or guardianship of the person approach and is not necessarily triggered by a judicial or administrative authority. Rather, a person may act on behalf of an incapacitous adult (as defined by sections 2 and 3, see above) provided she or he acts in that person's best interests (as defined by section 4, see below), but such actions are subject to significant procedural protections, since some areas must be referred to other procedures (e.g. in relation to research, where sections 30–34 allow intrusive, non-therapeutic treatment consistently with the European Convention on Biomedicine), some decisions cannot be made as they are too personal (so such matters as consenting to marry or to entering a civil partnership and consenting to sex do not fall within the Act, see section 27), some decisions necessitate, where carer's views are not available, the views of an independent mental capacity advocate to be taken into account (sections 35–41), some decisions may be made by a court or by a court appointed person where the court determines that is appropriate (through the new Court of Protection, with preference given to decisions made by the court rather than the appointment of a deputy), and all decisions are challengeable in court. This latter element is vital. Whilst this approach is clearly consistent with the provisions of Recommendation 99(4), it is challengeability which lies at the heart of its compliance with human rights obligations. What the Act does not do is require an initial judicial or administrative decision. It is not triggered by having to go to court or through some other governmental or quasi-governmental body. This will no doubt be challenging to many whose commitment to due process and procedural justice would rely upon judicial instigation of a procedure. However, this is not the only necessary approach, as is evidence in Recommendation 99(4). What is provided instead is a straightforward ability to challenge decisions by taking a matter about competence or about decisions made on behalf of someone who is or may be incompetent to the Court of Protection. Some people can launch a case as of right, some need the permission of the Court (section 50). This is clearly sufficient to meet the demands of, for example, Article 6 of the European Convention on Human Rights, provided it operates in practice. If it fails to take cases that should get to the Court, then that might be a base of challenging the provision. The advantage of this approach, which are consistent with that of Recommendation 99(4), is that it more closely reflects the process applicable in relation to someone who is capable, it places emphasis on the fact that most decisions are taken on behalf of an incapable person by carers and those decisions are proper and appropriate and it provides a system that can work (that is the workload should be manageable and not be prohibitively expensive).

The focus for making decisions on behalf of another in England and Wales as in most jurisdictions, is individualized, function specific and based on the best interests of the individual. This *best interests approach* is, realistically, the only one available to the courts where there is no evidence of that person's preferences. Substituted judgement is, however, an appropriate approach where there is sufficient evidence of the decision that the person now incompetent would have made.[30] So, for example, decisions made in advance, advance health-care statements, are legally valid[22] (see also Kennedy and Grubb,[30] referring to such an approach in Florida, Ontario, Manitoba, and Victoria). Indeed, the old thinking that substituted judgement was an alternative to best interests should be re-thought so that what an individual wants is what is in her best interests, but if that is not known, nest interests is the only available approach. Where the person is not competent, the best interests approach, in England, was achieved by deciding whether what the doctor proposes in the given case is a treatment regime of which a responsible medical opinion would approve. This approach to 'best interests' was rightly severely criticized for it failed to address the issue by concentrating upon the interests of incompetent persons but professionalized it through one (medical) profession when it is possible to take a broader view of the issues in question when deciding upon what treatment to agree upon. Some of these criticisms were ameliorated by judicial developments (see, e.g. *Re S (Adult Patient: Sterilization)* and *Re A (Male Sterilization)*) that ensured two key changes. First, it was decided that, where there were options of a number of possible, acceptable approaches, only one of those options could be in the best interests of the individual. Secondly, in deciding what was in someone's best interests that should not be limited to scientific or medical matters, but should take in the whole range of social, welfare, and emotional factors. Despite such substantial judicial development, new law is in place through the Mental Capacity Act 2005. Section 4 provides a definition of best interests.

4(1) In determining for the purposes of this Act what is in a person's best interests, the person making the determination must not make it merely on the basis of –
   (a) the person's age or appearance, or
   (b) a condition of his, or an aspect of his behaviour, which might lead others to make unjustified assumptions about what might be in his best interests.

(2) The person making the determination must consider all the relevant circumstances and, in particular, take the following steps.

(3) He must consider –
   (a) whether it is likely that the person will at some time have capacity in relation to the matter in question, and
   (b) if it appears likely that he will, when that is likely to be.

(4) He must, so far as reasonably practicable, permit, and encourage the person to participate, or to improve his ability to participate, as fully as possible in any act done for him and any decision affecting him.

(5) Where the determination relates to life-sustaining treatment he must not, in considering whether the treatment is in the best interests of the person concerned, be motivated by a desire to bring about his death.

(6) He must consider, so far as is reasonably ascertainable –
   (a) the person's past and present wishes and feelings (and, in particular, any relevant written statement made by him when he had capacity),
   (b) the beliefs and values that would be likely to influence his decision if he had capacity, and
   (c) the other factors that he would be likely to consider if he were able to do so.

(7) he must take into account, if it is practicable and appropriate to consult them, the views of –
   (a) anyone named by the person as someone to be consulted on the matter in question or on matters of that kind,
   (b) anyone engaged in caring for the person or interested in his welfare,
   (c) any donee of a lasting power of attorney granted by the person, and
   (d) any deputy appointed for the person by the court,

as to what would be in the person's best interests and, in particular, as to the matters mentioned in subsection (6).

## The law relying on status

Whilst it has so far been asserted that approaches not facilitating decision-making by a competent person are the norm and that capacity should not be questioned on the basis of status, it is the case that status may play a role. Indeed, for example, in England and Wales status has, in the past, been the basis for effectively determining whether someone is capable, but increasingly these are being removed, as is the case across the globe. It is also a move demanded by international instruments, such as the Council of Europe Recommendation.

In England and Wales, it used to be the case that children under 16 were not able to consent, but the House of Lords changed this in 1985 when, in *Gillick* v *Wisbech AHA* it was recognized that, at least for some treatments, a person under the age of 16 could be capable of deciding upon treatment provided they had sufficient maturity to do so. The removal of the automatic barrier was an important step.

Further, the Sexual Offences Act was another example of law in a private area that was dependent upon status. For most people, it always has been a matter that is dependent upon their own consent. So, for example, it is rape for a man to have anal or vaginal sexual intercourse with a woman or a man who does not consent. The critical question is whether the victim is competent to make the decision. For example, does she or he understand what sexual intercourse is so that her or his apparent assent is indeed consent? However, under the 1956 Act this was not the case in all instances. First, there was an age of consent. Below the relevant age, the consent of the victim was irrelevant, however competent she or he may be. Second, a person who was a 'defective' in the terms of the Sexual Offences Act 1956 or had a 'severe mental handicap' could not consent. These terms were defined in the same way and referred to a person who had a state of arrested or incomplete development of mind that is associated with severe impairment of intelligence and social functioning. If a person fell into this category, she or he could not, in law, consent to sexual intercourse or other sexual activity, however competent he or she might have been. This had real impact on some people with mental retardation (intellectual disability) and their carers. Interestingly, if a man married a woman with a severe intellectual disability (who was, therefore, a 'defective'), he did not commit the offence contrary to Section 7 of the Sexual Offences Act 1956 (whereby it was an offence for a man to have unlawful sexual intercourse with a woman who was a defective). Marriage was and is not dependent upon status, but is dependent upon an assessment of the competence of the particular individuals at the time of the marriage ceremony, and so falls into the second category of laws.[33] The law meant that a person could not prevent an indecent assault in any circumstances by consent. This could have unfortunate consequences for sex education for some people with severe mental retardation. It may be that no other form of sex education is possible than hands-on education to provide skills to enable appropriate behaviour by the person in question. Whatever the level of necessity, the individual could not consent in law. The only possible defence was to argue that the activity, contrary to appearances, was not indecent because of the purpose for which it was being undertaken as evidenced by the context, that is a carefully tailored and developed personal relationships programme. The difficulty here was that, when perceived from this stance, the law fails to allow sexual expression without good individual reason. Therefore it could be contrary to Article 8 (privacy) or Article 12 (founding a family) of the European Convention on Human Rights. The law presumably assumed that sexual experiences would, by definition, exploit or abuse such people. Law to prevent exploitation and abuse is very important, but it must not improperly limit a person's human rights. Subsequently, there has been an attempt to redress the balance somewhat and provide for a set of laws that is more acceptable. The Sexual Offences Act 2003 creates three types of offences that have an impact where the victim is a person with a mental disorder. The first consists of offences involving sexual activity with a person with a mental disorder and apply where that person cannot consent. The second consists of offences where the person's agreement is achieved through an inducement, threat or deception. The third comprises offences where the defendant is in some form of care relationship with the victim and these offences are committed regardless of consent and clearly deal with a significant form of exploitation and abuse. It is worth focusing, briefly, on an exemplar from the first type of offences. Section 30 of the 2003 Act makes it an offence for someone to engage in sexual activity with a person with a mental disorder impeding choice. As the offence relies upon touching, it involves sexual intercourse and other sexual activity short of intercourse but that involves touching. What it does not include is activity that would not involve touching, but would have been regarded as an assault under the old law. That touching must be sexual. It remains to be clarified whether sex education of a direct manner described above would be caught, but there must at least be an argument that it would not, provided that there is a non-sexual purpose, established by the education programme within which it falls and that a multi-disciplinary group identifies the need for the touching and the means of doing it. The offence applies potentially to anyone with a mental disorder, and is not so status driven as was the old law reliant upon being a defective or a person with a severe mental handicap. There is, though, still the status requirement of a mental disorder, which might be justified upon the basis of necessity and proportionality, as there must be an inability to refuse on the basis of that mental disorder, so the offence does not apply simply because of the presence of the disorder. This requirement is the equivalent of a capacity requirement tied to the specific requirements of the matter in hand. Finally, the defendant must know or could reasonably have known of the other's mental disorder and that he or she is thereby unable to refuse. These offences are likely to produce a much better balance of the need to protect the rights of vulnerable persons to understand and exercise their sexuality with their right to be protected by the law from sexual abuse and exploitation.

## The law of responsibility

### Criminal liability

Mental disorder is relevant to criminal liability in a variety of different ways, and this is true, at least, in all common-law jurisdictions. First, the presence of a mental disorder may be a reason to convince the decider of the fact that, contrary to external appearances, the defendant did not have the mental element for the crime with which he or she has been charged. Lack of the mental element is, of course, a complete defence. Whilst there is not a mental element requirement for all crimes (since there are some crimes for which conviction is based on strict liability), most serious crimes require a mental element that takes the form of intention, recklessness, knowledge, or belief and demand a consideration of what was the individual's purpose, awareness, foresight, or realization at the time that the crime was committed.

Second, the presence of a mental disorder may give rise to a defence. This will arise either by it being raised by the defence (even if the defence does not have the formal burden to prove it, but will have the burden of raising the matter for consideration) or by the prosecution challenging a point made by the defence (so, for example, if the defence raises mental disorder as an explanation for lack of criminal intent, the prosecution may respond by arguing that the defence has, in fact, raised one of the defences concerned with mental disorder). The most obvious defence is that of insanity. Whilst this takes various forms in many jurisdictions, there is usually a relationship in common-law jurisdictions with the English defence that was established by judicial answers to questions posed in McNaghten's case in 1843. This defence demands that the following matters be established by the defence (this is one of those rare instances in which the burden of proof lies, on a balance of probabilities, on the defence).

The defendant must have a disease of the mind. There are at least two possible ways of approaching this concept. First, it may be regarded as a simple concept in that it is present if the defendant has a condition (loosely termed) that has an internal cause, whereas there is no disease of the mind if there is an external cause. This simplistic distinction means that a person who has a brain tumour has a disease of the mind as does a person who has arteriosclerosis, schizophrenia (or other mental illness), epilepsy diabetes (provided the defendant had not taken her or his insulin and caused the offence in a hypoglycaemic state, or is a sleepwalker). The person with diabetes who causes the offence after taking insulin (an external agent) but falls into a hypoglycaemic state does not have a disease of the mind because the cause (insulin) is external and not internal. Immediately it can be seen that there is no congruence between the legal construct of disease of the mind and any medical approach. Furthermore, this definition of disease of the mind produces outcomes that are clearly unacceptable (no one would argue that many of the conditions identified above are identifiable with mental disorders). An alternative definition, which may reduce some of the impact of the concept is to follow Lord Denning: 'it seems to me that any mental disorder which has manifested itself in violence and is prone to recur is a disease of the mind. At any rate it is the sort of disease for which a person should be detained in hospital rather than be given an unqualified acquittal'.

One difficult area of applying the external/internal causes distinction is in relation to 'whether a 'dissociative state' resulting from a 'psychological blow' amounts to insane automatism'. This was recognized by the Supreme Court of Canada so that the psychological blow can be recognized as an external cause giving rise not to insanity but to automatism as a defence.

The disease of the mind must cause a defect of reason. Defect of reason means that 'the powers of reasoning must be impaired and that a mere failure to use powers of reasoning which one has is not within the [McNaghten] Rules'.[47]

The consequences of actions A and B must be that the defendant either does not know what he is doing or does not know that what he is doing is legally wrong. The latter is contentious, because the Rules simply state that the defendant must know that what he was doing was wrong. In R v. *Windle* it was the Court of Appeal that established that the requirement was that the matter is concerned with legal wrong. The High Court of Australia has refused to follow this approach. In *Stapleton* v. *R*, 'their view was that if D believed his act to be right according to the ordinary standard of reasonable men he was entitled to be acquitted even if he knew it to be legally wrong'.[45]

The outcome of a finding of insanity is that the defendant is found not guilty by reason of insanity and, since the amendments introduced by the Criminal Procedure (Insanity and Fitness to Plead) Act 1991, the disposal of the defendant is not limited to being sent to a mental hospital under the equivalent of a restriction direction, but extends to less draconian forms of disposal, including discharge.

Third, there are limited or partial defences. In English law there is a defence of diminished responsibility that is a defence only to murder and produces, if successfully raised by the defendant, a conviction for manslaughter. There are similar defences, often of more general application in most, if not all, common-law countries. The defence of diminished responsibility was created by the Homicide Act 1957, Section 2, which provides:

> Where a person kills or is a party to the killing of another, he shall not be convicted of murder if he was suffering from such abnormality of mind (whether arising from a condition of arrested or retarded development of mind or any inherent causes or induced by disease or injury) as substantially impaired his mental responsibility for his acts and omissions in doing or being a party to the killing.

The question of impairment of responsibility is one for the decider of fact to make. Interestingly, expert evidence usually contains an assessment of the degree of impairment, though this would appear not to be a matter upon which the expert has the relevant training or expertise. Were the expert witness not to proffer a view on the matter, the practical reality is that the court would find it very difficult to know how to react to a claimed defence. The original rationale for this partial defence was to avoid the rigour of

capital punishment. Its current rationale is wide ranging. Amongst other reasons why this defence is important is that it allows the defendant to argue that he or she was incapable of resisting an impulse produced by mental disorder, an argument that is not permissible in the insanity defence as is made clear by the McNaghten Rules themselves.

Fourth, there are other defences which are or may be related to mental disorder. One obvious defence is that of intoxication. If a person is intoxicated by drink or drugs such that he or she does not have the criminal intent for an offence, he or she is not guilty of that offence provided the offence is one of specific intent (such as murder), whereas he or she will be guilty if the crime is one of basic intent (such as manslaughter). Although a range of theories have been propounded to establish when a crime is one of specific or basic intent, the only approach that actually works is to take previous decisions as precedents for future approaches, and so develop a list of crimes of specific and of basic intent.

## Tortious liability

Liability in tort encompasses a wide variety of non-contractual civil wrongs, including such diverse matters as negligence, nuisance, defamation, and trespass to land. It is worth noting that trespass to the person (assault and battery) is a civil wrong as well as a criminal offence and concurrent liability will lie. A battery occurs when there is a non-consensual touching, which includes the administration of medical treatment and care so that regardless of any benevolent motivation, if this is given without a valid consent an action will lie. However, this section concentrates on the law of negligence which is the main area where liability problems might occur. Again, the authors must emphasize that we concentrate mainly upon English law, but within the area of tort the law in other English-speaking jurisdictions is very similar e.g. in the USA, Australia, New Zealand, and Canada, and even in codified jurisdictions, such as France, Spain and Germany, there are similarities of approach.

In this section we look first at the general principles of the law of negligence. Second, any special considerations when examining the liability of the mentally ill defendant in an action in negligence are discussed. Third, the liability of third parties for the acts of the mentally ill are examined, and finally, the liability of third parties towards mentally ill patients, particularly in the context of statutory duties, and the difficult and controversial issue of the liability towards patients who harm or threaten harm to themselves are discussed.

### (a) Negligence

The law of negligence is heavily circumscribed by a conceptual framework which is designed to restrict the ambit of claims. Much of this need not concern us here, suffice to say that the most relevant parts of it relate to the difference between certain types of loss and the way in which the courts regard these differences, and the role of public policy in some of the principal judgments.

The basic requirements of the tort of negligence have a certain simplicity; it is in the application of these requirements that complexity and confusion result. The claimant must show (a) that the defendant owed him or her a duty of care; (b) that the defendant breached that duty by failing to meet the requisite standard of care, and (c) that the breach of duty caused the resulting damage. It is important to note the latter. Negligence is not actionable *per se*;

there must be some tangible damage caused by the breach. There is insufficient space here to consider duty of care in all its contexts, but it is important to note the test put forward in *Caparo Industries PLC* v. *Dickman*. In that case it was said that in order for a duty of care to arise, the damage suffered must be foreseeable; there must be sufficient proximity between the claimant and the defendant; and it must be 'just and reasonable' to impose a duty of care. The first two aspects are well illustrated by examining the difference between physical injury and other forms of damage; the third is an important consideration in the context of statutory duties. As far as the standard of care is concerned, the standard is objective and based upon reasonableness. Causation must always be proved as there will be no liability for falling below the requisite standard of care if a causal link to the damage cannot be proved. The standard of proof throughout is that of the balance of probabilities.

### (b) Liability for clinical negligence

Duty of care is not usually an issue in the doctor/patient relationship. It should be noted that the standard of care relating to professionals such as doctors is set by the 'accepted practices' test, well known as the 'Bolam test' as framed in the case of *Bolam* v. *Friern Hospital Management Committee*, where diagnosis and treatment will not normally be negligent if supported by a responsible body of medical opinion. The only exception to this is if the doctor's actions do not withstand logical analysis; in those circumstances the fact that the practice is 'accepted' will not be sufficient to avoid a finding of negligence. The test is slightly different if the allegation of negligence relates to the provision of inadequate information about risks, side effects and alternative treatments. In such cases it seems that the courts are moving towards a more stringent standard of informed consent. Proving that the damage was caused by the breach can raise many problems in medical negligence claims, largely for two reasons. First, in almost all cases the patient will be suffering from some medical condition at the outset, and it might be arguable that the resulting condition would have materialized anyway. Second, if the resulting condition is the realization of some form of risk (e.g. side-effects of medication), even if the patient was not warned of the risk it is open to the defendant to argue that regardless of warnings, the patient would have gone ahead and consented to the taking of the medication in any event.

### (c) Liability for different types of damage—psychiatric injury

The law distinguishes between different types of damage. This appears to stem from judicial fear that certain losses might result in an unacceptably large number of potential claimants i.e. the fear of opening the 'floodgates'. Thus, what is known as 'pure economic loss', that is financial loss, which is not consequential upon physical damage, will only be recoverable in certain circumstances. For similar reasons the law makes another significant distinction: the difference between physical damage and psychiatric damage.

There are a number of reasons for the disparity between the treatment of the two types of injury. The first stems from the misunderstanding in earlier cases of the nature of psychiatric injury. In the authors' view, it is no coincidence that some of the early cases involved pregnant women who had miscarried or given birth to damaged children (e.g. *Dulieu* v. *White & Sons*). In these cases the courts could see a tangible manifestation of the 'shock' suffered by the claimants. Psychiatry was in its infancy, and the myriad of subtle manifestations of mental disorder was unknown. A further illustration of this is the phenomenon of 'railway spine'. In 1875,

J.E. Erichsen, Professor of Surgery at University College Hospital, London, published a number of findings as a result of studying spinal injury cases following railway accidents, where there was no obvious physical cause of the symptoms manifested. His conclusion was that trauma caused 'concussion of the spine'. Later medical opinion such as that of surgeon Herbert Page denied that the spine as such was affected by the trauma, but that the resulting condition was 'nervous shock'. It is therefore understandable that courts may have taken a somewhat crude approach to shock-induced injury, which crudity is still reflected in the law, which is commonly referred to as 'the law of nervous shock'. However, the second reason is, perhaps, less acceptable: the fear of the floodgates opening and admitting unacceptably large numbers of claims. It is worth pointing out that the floodgates argument, being only a spectre (but a highly influential one at that) and not overtly referred to by judges, has never been supported by hard empirical evidence. Nevertheless, the Law Commission, in its report on psychiatric injury claims supported the floodgates argument, largely on the basis of the lack of clear demarcation lines between general, uncompensatable, mental disturbance, and specific psychiatric illnesses. A third reason for the distinction between physical and psychiatric injury is the argument that a too-liberal attitude might result in fraudulent claims. However, again there is no clear evidence to show that it is easy to fake psychiatric injury, and furthermore it is an odd system of justice which takes the approach that, because there is a possibility of fraud, genuine claims should fail.

It is important to note that in cases where the claimant has suffered physical injury, any claim for damages for associated psychiatric injury will not be controversial, subject to the claimant establishing causation. However, where the claim is for psychiatric injury alone special considerations apply and, it is worth summarizing the essential elements of such a claim. The distinction is often drawn between primary and secondary victims. A primary victim is either someone who is physically injured or is within the range of foreseeable physical injury (see *Page* v. *Smith*).

A secondary victim is someone who has some sort of proximity to one or more primary victims. (There are similarities in other European jurisdictions; for example in France this is *dommage par ricochet*, and the rules are more generous than in English-speaking jurisdictions.) In English law this has two aspects: first, there must be close physical proximity to the trauma which injures or threatens the primary victim; second, the secondary victim must either have a close tie of love and affection with one or more of the primary victims, or he or she must be a rescuer of a primary victim and be within the range of foreseeable physical injury (see *Alcock* v. *Chief Constable of South Yorkshire Police*) and *White* v. *Chief Constable of South Yorkshire Police*). There is one other condition which a secondary victim must meet: the trauma must have the necessary quality of 'shockingness' about it so as to make a sudden impact on the senses to such an extent that the person of normal fortitude must be shocked by it (the 'impact rule'). Finally, in the cases of both primary and secondary victims, the negligence must result in a recognized psychiatric injury; emotional conditions such as grief, fear, and distress will not suffice. Of course, if the claimant has suffered distress as a result of physical injury, not amounting to a recognized psychiatric condition, then this should be reflected in the damages for pain, suffering, and loss of amenity. Although ordinary 'shock' is not compensatable, both DSM-IV and ICD-10 refer to 'acute stress reaction' which, although only a short-term reaction to stress, should be compensatable as a recognized psychiatric condition, albeit that any compensation would be modest. (See *Phelps* v. *London Borough of Hillingdon*, where it was held that the failure to mitigate the adverse consequences of a congenital defect such as dyslexia was capable of constituting an 'injury'.)

The impact rule states that the claimant must be present at the traumatic event or its immediate aftermath, and it must be an event such as to make an impact upon the unaided senses of the claimant, and to be shocking to a person of normal fortitude. The case of *Sion* v. *Hampstead Health Authority* is illustrative of this point. The claimant was the father of a young man injured in a road accident. The defendant was the health authority because the father alleged that his son was treated negligently. The claimant watched his son deteriorate and die over a period of 14 days. The resultant psychiatric illness suffered by the claimant was not compensatable as the process of death was slow, predictable, and not 'shocking'. This can be contrasted with *Tredget and Tredget* v. *Bexley Health Authority*, which concerned the negligent delivery of a child, which took place in an atmosphere of 'chaos' and 'pandemonium', and resulted in the child being born in a distressed state requiring immediate resuscitation. The father, who was present at the birth, recovered damages for his subsequent psychiatric condition, as the event was sudden and impacted in a shocking way upon his senses. In *Walters* v. *North Glamorgan NHS Trust*) damages were awarded to a woman who spent 36 hours with her baby son from seeing him choking on blood and vomit to the termination of life support. This period was found to be a shocking series of events. However, in other jurisdictions the need to find something sufficiently shocking upon which to hang liability has been rejected. In the US case of *Ochoa* v. *Superior Court (Santa Clara County)*, a woman recovered damages when, despite her son begging her to stay, was forced to leave his hospital bedside on the basis that he only had flu, and never saw him alive again. In Singapore, it was said that in the context of medical negligence as the secondary victim would rarely witness the act of negligence, it was wrong to impose the 'shocking event' requirement. Thus, in *Pang Koi Fa* v. *Lim Djoe Phing*) damages were awarded when a negligent medical procedure took place in June 1985 and the claimant watched her daughter die from then until the following September.

These sorts of distinctions are important in the context of so-called 'creeping trauma' in which there is no sudden impact to the senses. This refers to cases where victims have been exposed to some form of risk, for example contamination or the administration of a drug which has caused no harmful effects yet, but which might do so. The absence of 'impact' might be thought to be fatal to such claims. However, in an Australian case (*AQP* v. *Commonwealth Serum Laboratories Ltd*) the Victoria Supreme Court held that such cases should be decided on the basis of foreseeability and proximity alone. Subsequently this was confirmed in an English decision, where a group of claimants had received the human growth hormone at a time when the Department of Health and the Medical Research Council was aware of the possibility of Creutzfeldt–Jakob disease contamination. They subsequently developed psychiatric illnesses through fear of contracting Creutzfeldt–Jakob disease, and recovered damages. At first sight it may be thought that the impact rule would not apply because the claimants were primary victims. Although this is the common-sense view inasmuch as they had all been directly administered a drug, the judge was not willing to concede this. This was on the basis that it would widen unacceptably the number of potential primary victims in a much more widespread case of possible contamination and would inhibit manufacturers and providers of drugs and other goods from warning the public even when the risk was very small. Therefore the claimants were held to be secondary victims, but to whom a duty was owed simply on the basis of foreseeability. A duty of care was found to exist because of the nature of the relationship between the defendants and the claimants, the small and readily identifiable size of the group of claimants, the ways in which the claimants might become aware of the risk of Creutzfeldt–Jakob disease, and the nature of the suffering in terminal Creutzfeldt–Jakob disease.

### (d) The liability of the mentally ill in negligence

It might be thought that if the law of negligence is about fault and blame (as it is in the English-speaking jurisdictions, and some European jurisdictions as well), then those who have less appreciation of risk and the consequences of their own actions might be regarded as being less culpable than those with a reasonable degree of appreciation. However, this is not the case. It is important to understand that, although the historical development of the law of tort suggests a number of different principles behind tort compensation and that in rare circumstances punitive damages can be recovered, generally tort is concerned with compensating victims rather than punishing wrongdoers. In the light of this it is not difficult to see why the same standard of care is applied. The second reason for this is that courts do not want to apply a different standard of care depending upon factors such as intelligence, emotional reactions, and experience. Therefore the standard is objective, being that of the reasonable person who is reasonably competent at whatever task is being undertaken. (Note that there is an exception in the case of children who are judged in accordance with the reasonable foreseeability of the child of the relevant age.) The general principle is illustrated by the classic example of the learner driver who is expected to meet the standard of the reasonably competent driver (see the case of *Nettleship* v. *Weston*). In *Wilsher* v. *Essex Area Health Authority*, in the Court of Appeal, Mustill LJ stated: 'this notion of a duty tailored to the actor rather than to the act which he elects to perform, has no place in the law of tort' (the case subsequently went to the House of Lords but this aspect of the judgment was undisturbed). However, there have been some exceptions to this (albeit not in England) which have interesting implications for the liability of the mentally ill. In the case of *Cook* v. *Cook*, the High Court of Australia held that, in the case of an inexperienced driver, liability may be different depending on the identity of the defendant. For example, a car driver who injures a pedestrian will be subject to the same standard of care as the reasonably competent driver, but when a driving instructor is injured, the fact that he knew of the claimant's lack of experience might mean that there is no liability for his injuries. By analogy with *Nettleship* v. *Weston*,[68] a mentally disordered person who negligently injures a third party will be subject to the objective standard of care. These latter considerations, however, might have some relevance to the position of those who care for the mentally ill in that they might be expected to be aware of the increased likelihood of unstable behaviour. In other words, can it be argued, that if a patient negligently injures a doctor, nurse, or social worker, in the course of, say receiving treatment, then he might not be liable? It should be noted, however, that we are concerned with negligence, not deliberate acts, so this would not be a common scenario. Furthermore, the patient would very likely have few resources and no insurance so may not be worth suing. Nevertheless, if an action were financially feasible, it may be that, for policy reasons, the courts would be unlikely to render someone in the position of a carer, without compensation. However, in *Mansfield* v. *Weetabix Ltd*, the Court of Appeal stated that in a case where the defendant could not reasonably have known about his condition, or the effect of it, there would be no liability.

### (e) Liability to third parties for the acts of the mentally ill

The next question that arises is the extent, if any, of the liability of third parties for acts of the mentally ill, whether these are criminal or civil acts. The third party might be an individual who is caring for the defendant, but is much more likely to be a local authority or a health authority. This area of negligence has given rise to some emotive and controversial litigation. In *Hill* v. *Chief Constable of West Yorkshire Police* the House of Lords held that no liability attached to a police force that failed to arrest the serial killer Peter Sutcliffe before he killed his last victim. The decision did not turn upon whether there had been negligent conduct, but upon public policy. The interests of the public as a whole are best served, so runs the argument, if those responsible for public safety and so on are able to carry out their duties unfettered by the threat of litigation. It must be noted, however, that in the case of *Osman* v. *United Kingdom*, this so-called immunity from suit was held by the European Court of Human Rights to be contrary to Article 6.1 of the European Convention on Human Rights (the protection of the right to a fair trial in both criminal and civil cases).

In *Palmer v Tees Health Authority*, the claimant, whose four year old daughter was murdered by a psychopath, brought an action against the health authority, both in her own name as she had suffered from a psychiatric illness as a result of the murder, and on behalf of the child's estate. Some months prior to committing the murder, the defendant had been an outpatient at the defendant's psychiatric hospital, where he had allegedly told staff that he would kill a child. The Court of Appeal rejected her claims on the basis that there was not sufficient proximity between the defendant and the victim. If, however, the defendant had known his victim and made threats specifically against her then there may well have been sufficient proximity to establish liability.

### (f) Liability of the providers of services to the mentally ill

In the case of *Clunis* v. *Camden and Islington Health Authority*, Clunis was a mentally disordered man who had been discharged from a psychiatric hospital and subsequently killed a man in an unprovoked attack. The prosecution accepted his plea of manslaughter on the ground of diminished responsibility. Clunis subsequently sought damages from the health authority alleging that they had failed to treat him in accordance with their common-law duty of care, and that if he had been treated he would not have carried out the killing and would not have been subject to the lengthy period of detention he was now facing. The court invoked the legal maxim of *ex turpi causa non oritur actio*, which means that they found that he could not establish a duty when it stemmed from the claimant's own wrong-doing. The court relied on this as an aspect of public policy, and, somewhat curiously, referred to the importance of the deterrent effect of such a maxim. Given that the claimant was mentally ill, and the motiveless nature of the attack, he was surely incapable of being deterred? It is tempting to consider that *Clunis* might have been decided differently in terms of *ex turpi causa*, if it had not also had implications for fettering the

medical and resource-allocation discretion of health authorities to make them liable in negligence in this way.

It is well established that English health authorities can be both primarily liable (when there is an organizational failure) and vicariously liable (where an individual employee is negligent) for acts of negligence. However, the provision of statutory duties by local authorities has raised some difficult issues. The leading authority is *X* v. *Bedfordshire County Council* In this case (a number of different cases listed together) the court had to consider the claims of claimants who alleged damage as a result of the negligence of social workers and psychiatrists involved in child protection cases, and teachers and others involved in the provision of education to children with special educational needs. Applying the threefold test from Caparo the court found that the first two elements were satisfied, that is foreseeability of damage and proximity of relationship between the parties. However, on the third element, the finding was that it would not be 'just and reasonable' to impose a duty of care. In the context of child protection three reasons were given. First, the statutory system set up to protect children cuts across many disciplines: police, education bodies, doctors, and others. To disentangle these relationships and to ascertain where the blame must fall would impose 'impossible problems'. Second, because there is a very fine balance to be drawn between the protection of children and the disruption of removing them from their homes, there is often a conflict to be resolved. The professionals involved in making such decisions should not be further hampered by the threat of litigation. Furthermore, a common-law liability may result in too cautious and defensive an approach on the part of local authorities. Finally, on a practical point, because of the obvious tensions between the local authority and the parents involved, litigation would be commonplace thereby placing a drain on vital resources necessary for the carrying out of the statutory functions.

However, if the social workers and psychiatrists involved *personally* owed duties towards the claimants then, it was said, local authorities might be vicariously liable for any negligence on their part. Furthermore, the House of Lords speculated that educational services might be treated differently in that they were more in the nature of a 'service to the public'.

In *Phelps* v. *London Borough of Hillingdon*[60] the House of Lords confirmed this approach. It concerned a claim for the failure of an educational psychologist to diagnose dyslexia. The court stated that vicarious liability arose on the basis of the personal duty owed by the psychologist, notwithstanding the fact that the educational psychology service was part of the general statutory services provided under the Educations Acts of 1944 and 1981, and that there would be no liability on the part of the local authority for breach of those statutory duties. A similar issue arose in the case of *Clunis* v. *Camden and Islington Health Authority*[73] (the facts of which are outlined above). The court had to consider the extent of the after-care that should be provided under Section 117 of the Mental Health Act. Under this provision, there is a duty upon the district health authority and the local social services authority to provide after-care services for detained patients who leave hospital. It was alleged in this case that the psychiatrist responsible for monitoring the after-care of the claimant after discharge was negligent in failing to admit him to hospital, thereby preventing the act of homicide which followed. However, the Court of Appeal found that the services being provided by the psychiatrist after discharge were 'essentially in the sphere of administrative activities in pursuance of a scheme of social welfare in the community'. These, it was stated, were different from the duties owed in the context of the doctor–patient relationship, and there was no common-law duty of care. Furthermore, under Section 124 of the Act, an allegation that inadequate Section 117 services are being provided should be dealt with by way of complaint to the Secretary of State. The court found that the wording of the statute indicated a parliamentary intention that breaches of Section 117 should not give rise to a cause of action in private law. In consequence, it seems that the outlook is bleak for claims resulting from the negligence of psychiatrists, psychologists, and social workers in the context of certain statutory functions of local authorities and health authorities alike.

It must be stressed that, although these cases are referring to English statutory provisions, they raise general issues of principle as to how far statutory bodies are to be controlled by the courts, and, in particular, how far scarce public resources should be subject to depletion by litigation.

### (g) Liability towards the mentally ill who harm themselves

As indicated above, the issues of consent to treatment, and competence to both consent and refusal of treatment are central to many legal systems. The case of *Re C* illustrates the importance of the right to self-determination in cases where, on the face of it, there might be a strong temptation to find a patient incompetent because of the nature of the mental illness from which he suffers.[22]

Under Section 63 of the Mental Health Act 1983, treatment can be given for mental disorder for which the patient is detained without the consent of the patient, and competency is irrelevant. In *B* v. *Croydon Health Authority* treatment for mental disorder was construed very widely. In that case the patient was clearly a 'self-harmer', and force-feeding due to her refusal of food was held to be treatment for the mental disorder. If she had been incompetent, then treatment (of any sort, not just for the mental disorder) could have been administered in her best interests. The question then arises as to whether an incompetent patient not detained under the Act who, however, refuses food in an attempt to self-harm must be fed, failing which there would be a breach of the duty of care. It must be noted that the courts are extremely reluctant to question medical decisions about treatment. It is left to clinical judgement to decide whether to give, or withdraw, treatment (see the case of *Airedale NHS Trust* v. *Bland*). (In the same case it was confirmed that treatment includes feeding; see also the Californian case of *Bouvia* v. *Superior Court*.) The decision as to whether treatment is necessary is judged by reference to the Bolam test. In other words if there are good clinical reasons for treating or not treating, and these can be justified by reference to a responsible body of medical opinion, then there will be no liability for failure to treat.

The question that arises is whether the health authority would have been liable nevertheless for failing to force-feed the subject of *B* v. *Croydon Health Authority*,[77] even though she was deemed capable of refusing treatment. It would follow from the general principle of self-determination, well established in English law (see, for example, *Re T (Adult: Refusal of Treatment)* and *Re MB (Adult: Medical Treatment)*,[23]) that such a refusal should be respected. However, recent case law in the context of the duty owed by prisons, and by implication hospitals, has considerably muddied the waters.

In the case of *Kirkham* v. *Chief Constable of Greater Manchester Police* the court took the opportunity to look at the difference between negligent acts and negligent omissions (something that has exercised the minds of tort lawyers for some time) and said that, in this case, responsibility for the omission to prevent the suicide had been assumed by the defendant. The prisoner was said to be 'of unsound mind', which presumably meant that, in the context of the right to self-determination, the prisoner was incapable of exercising his autonomy. In those circumstances the decision is not surprising on its facts. However, the judgment suggested that when one person is in the lawful custody of another, whether that be voluntarily such as a hospital, or involuntarily such as a prison, there is a duty to take all reasonable steps to avoid acts or omissions to prevent reasonably foreseeable injury. Consequently in the case of *Reeves* v. *Commissioner of Police of the Metropolis*, another custodial suicide, the same duty was said to be owed to a 'sane' prisoner. Again, the wording is unfortunate by its reference to sanity, but it can be assumed that this prisoner was deemed to be competent. The police surgeon had stated, after examining the claimant, that there was no evidence of mental disturbance. It must be stressed that it will be necessary in all cases including those concerning hospitals, for there to be evidence that it was reasonable to regard the patient as a suicide risk. Of course, in practice, it may be the case that it is undesirable for hospitals to be venues for acts of suicide. However, it is by no means clear that, in the case of someone who has capacity, there should be a positive duty to prevent suicide any more than there should be a duty owed to prevent that person from smoking. These decisions are invoking a strong form of paternalism. Certainly in the case of hospital patients many competent patients discharge themselves against medical advice whereupon they are free to take any form of self-harming action. It is difficult to see why there should be a positive duty to prevent the competent patient from carrying out the acts on hospital premises.

## Further information

Barrie, P. (2005). *Personal Injury Law*. Oxford University Press, Oxford.

Bartlett, P. and Sandland, R. (2007). *Mental health law: policy and practice*, (3rd ed.), Oxford University Press, Oxford.

Bartlett, P. (2007). *Blackstone's Guide to the Mental Capacity Act 2005*, (2nd ed.), Oxford University Press, Oxford.

Grisso, T. and Appelbaum, P.S. (1998). *Assessing competence to consent to treatment: A guide for physicians and other health care professionals*, Oxford University Press, New York.

Harpwood, V. (2005). *Modern Tort Law*, Routledge-Cavendish, London.

Mackay, R.D. (1995). *Mental condition defences in the criminal law*. Oxford University Press, Oxford.

Weir, T. (2006). *An Introduction to Tort Law*, Oxford University Press, Oxford.

Wheat, K. (2002). *Recovering Damages for Psychiatric Injury*. Oxford University Press, Oxford.

## References

1. Ashibe, N. (1997). *Kempou (The Constitutional Law)* (2nd edn.), Iwanam, Tokyo.

2. Kitamura, F., Tomoda, A., Tsukada, K., *et al.* (1998). Method for Assessment of Competency to Consent in the Mentally Ill: Rationale, Development and Comparison with the Medically Ill. *International Journal of Law and Psychiatry*, **21**, 223–44.

3. Kitamura, T., Kitamura, F., Mitsuhashi, T., *et al.* (1999). Image of Psychiatric Patients. Competency to Give Informed Consent to

Treatment in Japan: I. A Factor Analytic Study' *International Journal of Law and Psychiatry*, **22**, 45–54.

4. Nakatani, Y. (2000). Psychiatry and the Law in Japan: History and Current Topics. *International Journal of Law and Psychiatry*, **23**, 589–604.

5. Satoh, K. (1995). *Kempou (The Constitutional Law)* (3rd edn.). Seirin Shobo, Tokyo.

6. Friedman, P.R. (1976). *The Rights of Mentally Retarded Persons*. Avon Books, New York.

7. Herr, S.S. (1983). *Rights and Advocacy for Retarded Persons*. Lexington Books, Lexington.

8. Carney, T. (2001). Globalisation and guardianship: harmonisation or (postmodern) diversity?. *International Journal of Law and Psychiatry*, **24**, 95–116.

9. South African law Commission, 2004. *Assisted Decision-Making: Adults with Impaired Decision-Making Capacity*. Discussion Paper 105 on Project 122.

10. Ritchie, J., Sklar, R., Steiner, W., et al. (1998). Advance Directives in Psychiatry: Resolving Issues of Autonomy and Competence. *International Journal of Law and Psychiatry*, **21**, 245–60.

11. Callahan, D. (1984). Autonomy: A moral good not a moral obsession. *Hastings Center Report*, **14**, 40–2.

12. Mappes, T.A. and Zembaty, J.S. (1994). Patient choices, family interests and physician obligations. *Kennedy Institute of Ethics Journal*, **4**, 27–46.

13. Carney, T. (2001). Globalisation and guardianship: harmonisation or (postmodern) diversity?. *International Journal of Law and Psychiatry*, **24**, 9–116.

14. Atkins, M.R. (1997). Adult Guardianship Reforms – Reflections on the New Zealand Model. *International Journal of Law and Psychiatry*, **20**, 77–96.

15. Frank, J.B. and Degan, D. (1997). Conservatorship for the Chronically Mentally Ill: Review and Case Series. *International Journal of Law and Psychiatry*, **20**, 97–111.

16. South African Law Commissio, 2004. *Assisted Decision-Making: Adults with Impaired Decision-Making Capacity* Discussion Paper 105 on Project 122.

17. Jansen, S. (2000). Recommendation No. 99(4) of the Committee of Ministers to Member States on Principles Concerning the Legal Protection of Incapable Adults: An Introduction in particular to Part V Interventions in the Health Field. *European Journal of Health Law*, **7**, 333–47.

18. Jansen, S., (2000). Recommendation No. 99(4) of the Committee of Ministers to Member States on Principles Concerning the Legal Protection of Incapable Adults: An Introduction in particular to Part V Interventions in the Health Field. *European Journal of Health Law*, **7**, 333–47.

19. Wong, J.G., Clare, I.C.H., Gunn, M.J., et al. (1999). Capacity to make health care decisions: its importance in clinical practice. *Psychological Medicine*, **29**, 437–46.

20. Grisso, T. and Appelbaum, P.S. (1998). *Assessing competence to consent to treatment: a guide for physicians and other health professionals*. Oxford University Press.

21. Grisso, T. and Appelbaum, P.S. (1995). The MacArthur Treatment Competence Study. III Abilities of patients to consent to psychiatric and medical treatments. *Law and Human Behavior*, **19**, 149–74.

22. *Re C (Adult: Refusal of Treatment)* [1994] 1 Weekly Law Reports 290.

23 *Re MB* [1997] 2 Family Law Reports 426.

24. Gunn, M.J., Wong, J.G., Clare, I.C.H., et al. (1999). Decision-making capacity. *Medical Law Review*, **7**, 261–98.

25. President's Commission for the Study of Ethical Problems in Medicine and Biomedical and Behavioural Research (1983). *Making health care decisions*. US Government Printing Office, Washington, DC.

26. Weisstub, D. (1990). *Enquiry on mental competency: fi nal report*. Queen's Printer, Toronto.

27. Law Commission (1995). *Mental incapacity*. Law Commission Report No. 231. HMSO, London.

28. Scottish Law Commission (1995). *Report on incapable adults*. Scottish Law Commission Report No. 151. HMSO, Edinburgh.

29. Morris, C.D., Niederbuhl, J.M., Mahr, J.M., et al. (1993). Determining the capability of individuals with mental retardation to give informed consent. *American Journal of Mental Retardation*, **98**, 263–72.

30. Kennedy, I. and Grubb, A. (1994). *Medical law: text with materials* (2nd edn). Butterworths, London.

31. Grisso, T. (1986). *Evaluating competencies: forensic assessments and instruments*. Plenum Press, New York.

32. *Banks* v. *Goodfellow* (1870) Law Reports 5 Queen's Bench 549.

33. Hoggett, B.M. (1996). *Mental health law*. Sweet and Maxwell, London.

34. Carney, T. and Singer, P. (1986). *Ethical and legal issues in guardianship options for intellectually disadvantaged people*. Australian Government Publishing Service, Canberra. 35. *Re F* (1990) 2 Appeal Cases 1.

36. Ouslander, J., Tymchuk, A., Rahbar, B., et al. (1989). Health care decisions among elderly long-term care residents and their potential proxies. *Archives of Internal Medicine*, **149**, 1367–72.

37. *Re S (Adult Patient: Sterilization)* [2001] Fam 15.

38. *Re A (Male Sterilization)* [2000] 1 F.L.R. 549.

39. Gunn, M.J. (1996). *Sex and the law: a guide for staff working with people with learning difficulties* (4th edn.). Family Planning Association, London.

40. Stevenson, K., Davies, A. and Gunn, M., Blackstone's Guide to the Sexual Offences Act 2003, chap. 6.

41. Stevenson, K., Davies, A. and Gunn, M., Blackstone's Guide to the Sexual Offences Act 2003, pp. 91–92.

42. Stevenson, K., Davies, A. and Gunn, M., Blackstone's Guide to the Sexual Offences Act 2003, chap. 2.

43. Stevenson, K., Davies, A. and Gunn, M., Blackstone's Guide to the Sexual Offences Act 2003, p. 100.

44. Mackay, R.D. (1995). *Mental condition defences in the criminal law*. Clarendon Press, Oxford.

45. *McNaghten's Case* (1843) 10 Clarkson and Findlay Law Reports 200.

46. Lord Denning (1963) *Bratty* v. *Attorney General* [1963] Appeal Cases 386.

47. Ormerod, D.C. (2005). *Smith and Hogan: criminal law* (11th edn). Butterworths, London.

48. *Rabey* (1977) 79 Dominion Law Reports (3rd series) 414.

49. *R* v. *Windle* [1952] 2 Queen's Bench 826.

50. *Stapleton* v. *R* (1952) 86 Commonwealth Law Reports 358.

51. *Caparo Industries PLC* v. *Dickman* [1990] 1 All ER 568.

52. *Bolam* v. *Friern Hospital Management Committee* [1957] 2 All ER 118.

53. *Bolitho* v. *City & Hackney Health Authority* [1997] 4 All ER 771.

54. *Chester* v. *Afshar* [2004] UKHL 41.

55. *Dulieu* v. *White & Sons* [1901] 2 KB 669

56. Law Commission (1998). *Liability for psychiatric illness*. Law Commission Report No. 249. HMSO, London.

57. *Page* v. *Smith* [1995] 2 WLR 644.

58. *Alcock* v. *Chief Constable of South Yorkshire Police* [1992] 4 All ER 907.

59. *White* v. *Chief Constable of South Yorkshire Police* [1999] 1 All ER 1.

60. *Phelps* v. *London Borough of Hillingdon* [2001]] 2AC 619.

61. *Sion* v. *Hampstead Health Authority* [1994] 5 Med LR.

62. *Tredget and Tredget* v. *Bexley Health Authority* [1994] 5 Med LR.

63. *Walters* v. *North Glamorgan NHS Trust* [2002] EWHC 321.

64. *Ochoa* v. *Superior Court (Santa Clara County)*(1985) 703 P 2d 1.

65. *Pang Koi Fa* v. *Lim Djoe Phing* [1993] 3 SLR 317.

66. *AQP* v. *Commonwealth Serum Laboratories Ltd* (unreported, Sup Ct (Vic) 5 February 1995).

67. Creutzfeldt–Jakob disease litigation (unreported, QBD 18 December 1997).

68. *Nettleship* v. *Weston* [1971] 2 QB 691.

69. *Wilsher v. Essex Area Health Authority* [1986] 3 All ER 801.
70. *Cook v. Cook* (1986) 68 ALR 353.
71. *Mansfi eld v. Weetabix Ltd* [1997] PIQR P526.
72. *Hill v. Chief Constable of West Yorkshire Police* [1988] 2 All ER 238.
73. *Osman v. United Kingdom* [1999] 1 FLR 193.
74. *Palmer v Tees Health Authority* [1999] Lloyd's Rep Med 351.
75. *Clunis v. Camden and Islington Health Authority* [1998] 2 WLR 902.
76. *X v. Bedfordshire County Council* (1995) 2 AC 633.

77. *B v. Croydon Health Authority* [1994] 2 WLR 294.
78. *Airedale NHS Trust v. Bland* [1993] AC 789.
79. *Bouvia v. Superior Court* (1986) 179 Cal App3d 1127.
80. *Re T (Adult: Refusal of Treatment)* [1993] 4 All ER 649.
81. *Kirkham v. Chief Constable of Greater Manchester Police* [1990] 2 QB 283.
82. *Reeves v. Commissioner of Police of the Metropolis* [1998] 1 All ER 381.

# Psychosocial causes of offending

David P. Farrington

## Introduction

### Scope of this chapter

Offending is part of a larger syndrome of antisocial behaviour that arises in childhood and tends to persist into adulthood. There seems to be continuity over time, since the antisocial child tends to become the antisocial teenager and then the antisocial adult, just as the antisocial adult then tends to produce another antisocial child. The main focus of this chapter is on types of antisocial behaviour classified as criminal offences, rather than on types classified for example as conduct disorder or antisocial personality disorder.

In an attempt to identify causes, this chapter reviews risk factors that influence the development of criminal careers. Literally thousands of variables differentiate significantly between official offenders and non-offenders and correlate significantly with reports of offending behaviour by young people. In this chapter, it is only possible to review briefly some of the most important risk factors for offending: individual difference factors such as high impulsivity and low intelligence, family influences such as poor child rearing and criminal parents, and social influences: socio-economic deprivation, peer, school, community, and situational factors.

I will be very selective in focussing on some of the more important and replicable findings obtained in some of the more methodologically adequate studies: especially prospective longitudinal follow-up studies of large community samples, with information from several data sources (e.g. the child, the parent, the teacher, official records) to maximize validity. The emphasis is on offending by males; most research on offending has concentrated on males, because they commit most of the serious predatory and violent offences. The review is limited to research carried out in the United Kingdom, the United States, and similar Western industrialized democracies. More extensive book length reviews of antisocial behaviour and offending are available elsewhere.[1]

I will refer especially to knowledge gained in the Cambridge Study in Delinquent Development,[2] which is a prospective longitudinal survey of over 400 London males from age 8 to age 40. Fortunately, results obtained in British longitudinal surveys of delinquency are highly concordant with those obtained in comparable surveys in North America, the Scandinavian countries, and New Zealand and indeed with results obtained in British cross-sectional surveys. A systematic comparison of the Cambridge Study with the Pittsburgh Youth Study showed numerous replicable predictors of offending over time and place, including impulsivity, attention problems, low school attainment, poor parental supervision, parental conflict, an antisocial parent, a young mother, large family size, low family income, and coming from a broken family.

### Measurement and epidemiology

Offending is defined as acts prohibited by the criminal law, such as theft, burglary, robbery, violence, vandalism, and drug use. It is commonly measured using either official records of arrests or convictions or self-reports of delinquency. The advantages and disadvantages of official records and self-reports are to some extent complementary. In general, official records identify the worst offenders and the worst offences, while self-reports include more of the normal range of delinquent activity. The worst offenders may be missing from samples interviewed in self-report studies. Self-reports have the advantage of including undetected offences, but the disadvantages of concealment and forgetting. By normally accepted psychometric criteria of validity, self-reports are valid. Self-reported delinquency predicted later convictions in the Cambridge Study. In the Pittsburgh Youth Study,[3] the seriousness of self-reported delinquency predicted later court referrals. However, predictive validity was enhanced by combining self-report, parent, and teacher information about offending.

The key issue is whether the same results are obtained with both methods. For example, if official records and self-reports both show a link between parental supervision and delinquency, it is likely that supervision is related to delinquent behaviour (rather than to any biases in measurement). Generally, the worst offenders according to self-reports (taking account of frequency and seriousness) tend also to be the worst offenders according to official records. In the Cambridge Study between ages 15 and 18, 11 per cent of the males admitted burglary, and 62 per cent of these males were convicted of burglary. The predictors and correlates of official and self-reported delinquency were very similar.

Much is known about the epidemiology and development of offending and criminal careers, but there is not space to review these topics here.[4] For example, the prevalence of offending tends to peak in the teenage years, and an early onset of offending predicts a long criminal career. Offenders tend to be versatile rather than specialized, in committing not only different types of offences but also different types of other antisocial acts. While there is considerable continuity over time, in the sense that the most antisocial people at one age tend also to be the most antisocial at another, only about half of antisocial juveniles tend to become antisocial adults.

### Risk factors

A risk factor is defined as a variable that predicts an increased risk of offending. For example, children who experience poor parental supervision have an increased risk of committing offences later on. Since risk factors are defined by their ability to predict later offending, it follows that longitudinal data are required to discover them. Risk factors tend to be similar for many different outcomes, including violent and non-violent offending, mental health problems, alcohol and drug problems, school failure, and unemployment. Protective factors are also important. They are defined as factors that predict a low risk of offending or that counteract risk factors.

An obvious problem is that it is not clear to what extent any risk factor is a cause of offending. It is important to investigate causal mechanisms linking risk factors and offending. The best way of establishing a cause is to carry out a prevention experiment tackling that risk factor; preferably a randomized experiment, because the random assignment of people to conditions in principle controls for all other influences on offending. If a prevention experiment was carried out in which parental supervision was improved, and if offending was reduced as a consequence, this would be powerful evidence that the risk factor of parental supervision truly had a causal effect on offending. However, most knowledge about causes comes from quasi-experimental analyses.

Because of the difficulty of establishing causal effects of factors that vary only between individuals (e.g. gender and ethnicity), and because such factors have no practical implications for prevention (e.g. it is not practicable to change males into females), unchanging variables will not be reviewed here. In any case, their effects on offending are usually explained by reference to other, modifiable, factors. For example, gender differences in offending have been explained on the basis of different socialization methods used by parents with boys and girls, or different opportunities for offending by men and women. Similarly, risk factors that are or might be measuring the same underlying construct as delinquency (e.g. physical aggression) will not be reviewed; the focus is on risk factors that might be causes. For simplicity, risk factors are reviewed one by one. Biological factors are not reviewed. I will not attempt to review additive, interactive, independent, or sequential effects of risk factors, although these are important issues. Nor will I review developmental theories of offending.

## Individual factors

### Hyperactivity and impulsivity

Hyperactivity and impulsivity are among the most important personality or individual difference factors that predict later offending.[5] Hyperactivity usually begins before age 5 and often before age 2, and it tends to persist into adolescence. It is associated with restlessness, impulsivity and a short attention span, and for that reason has been termed the 'hyperactivity-impulsivity-attention deficit' or HIA syndrome. Related concepts include a poor ability to defer gratification and a short future time perspective.

Many investigators have reported a link between hyperactivity or impulsivity and offending. For example, in the Orebro (Sweden) longitudinal survey,[6] hyperactivity at age 13 (rated by teachers) predicted violent offending up to age 26. The highest rate of violence was among males with both motor restlessness and concentration difficulties. The most extensive research on different measures of impulsivity was carried out by Jennifer White and her colleagues in the Pittsburgh Youth Study. This showed that cognitive or verbal impulsivity (e.g. acts without thinking, unable to defer gratification) was more strongly related to delinquency than was behavioural impulsivity (e.g. clumsiness in psychomotor tests).

In the Cambridge Study, a combined measure of hyperactivity-impulsivity-attention deficit was developed at age 8–10, and it significantly predicted juvenile convictions independently of conduct problems at age 8–10. Hence, HIA is not merely another measure of antisocial personality, but it is a possible cause, or an earlier stage in a developmental sequence leading to offending. Similar constructs to hyperactivity, such as sensation seeking, are also related to delinquency. In the Cambridge Study, the extent to which the boy was daring or took risks at age 8–10, as well as restlessness and poor concentration, significantly predicted convictions and high self-reported offending. Daring was consistently one of the strongest independent predictors of offending.

### Low intelligence and attainment

Low intelligence is an important predictor of offending, and it can be measured very early in life. In a prospective longitudinal survey of about 120 Stockholm males,[7] low IQ measured at age 3, significantly predicted officially recorded offending up to age 30. Frequent offenders (with 4 or more offences) had an average IQ of 88 at age 3, whereas non-offenders had an average IQ of 101. All of these results held up after controlling for social class. Similarly, low IQ at age 4 predicted arrests up to age 27 in the Perry preschool project.[8]

In the Cambridge Study, twice as many of the boys scoring 90 or less on a non-verbal IQ test (Raven's Progressive Matrices) at age 8–10 were convicted as juveniles as of the remainder. However, it was difficult to disentangle low intelligence and low school attainment. Low non-verbal intelligence was highly correlated with low verbal intelligence (vocabulary, word comprehension, verbal reasoning) and with low school attainment, and all of these measures predicted juvenile convictions to much the same extent. In addition to their poor school performance, delinquents tended to leave school at the earliest possible age (which was then 15) and to take no school examinations.

Low non-verbal intelligence predicted juvenile self-reported offending to almost exactly the same degree as juvenile convictions, suggesting that the link between low intelligence and delinquency was not caused by the less intelligent boys having a greater probability of being caught. Also, measures of intelligence and attainment predicted measures of offending independently of other variables such as family income and family size. Delinquents often do better on non-verbal performance tests, such as object assembly and block design, than on verbal tests, suggesting that they find it easier to deal with concrete objects than with abstract concepts.

Low IQ may lead to delinquency through the intervening factor of school failure; the association between school failure and delinquency has been demonstrated consistently in longitudinal surveys. In the Pittsburgh Youth Study, Donald Lynam and his colleagues concluded that low verbal IQ led to school failure and subsequently to self-reported delinquency, but only for African-American boys. Another plausible explanatory factor underlying the link between low IQ and delinquency is the ability to manipulate abstract concepts. Children who are poor at this tend to do badly in IQ tests and in school attainment and they also tend to commit offences, mainly because of their poor ability to foresee the consequences of their offending and to appreciate the feelings of victims. Low IQ may be one aspect of cognitive and neuropsychological deficits in the executive functions of the brain.

## Family factors

### Child rearing

Many different types of child-rearing methods predict offending. The most important dimensions of child rearing are supervision or monitoring of children, discipline or parental reinforcement, warmth or coldness of emotional relationships, and parental involvement with children. Parental supervision refers to the degree of monitoring by parents of the child's activities, and their degree of watchfulness or vigilance. Of all these child-rearing methods, poor parental supervision is usually the strongest and most replicable predictor of offending. Many studies show that parents who do not know where their children are when they are out, and parents who let their children roam the streets unsupervised from an early age, tend to have delinquent children. For example, in Joan McCord's classic Cambridge–Somerville Study in Boston,[9] poor parental supervision in childhood was the best predictor of both violent and property crimes up to age 45.

Parental discipline refers to how parents react to a child's behaviour. It is clear that harsh or punitive discipline (involving physical punishment) predicts offending. In their follow-up study of nearly 700 Nottingham children, John and Elizabeth Newson[10] found that physical punishment at ages 7 and 11 predicted later convictions; 40 per cent of offenders had been smacked or beaten at age 11, compared with 14 per cent of non-offenders. Erratic or inconsistent discipline also predicts delinquency. This can involve either erratic discipline by one parent, sometimes turning a blind eye to bad behaviour and sometimes punishing it severely, or inconsistency between two parents, with one parent being tolerant or indulgent and the other being harshly punitive.

Cold, rejecting parents tend to have delinquent children, as Joan McCord found in the Cambridge–Somerville Study. More recently, she concluded that parental warmth could act as a protective factor against the effects of physical punishment. Whereas 51 per cent of boys with cold physically punishing mothers were convicted in her study, only 21 per cent of boys with warm physically punishing mothers were convicted, similar to the 23 per cent of boys with warm non-punitive mothers who were convicted. The father's warmth was also a protective factor against the father's physical punishment.

Most explanations of the link between child-rearing methods and delinquency focus on attachment or social learning theories. Attachment theory was inspired by the work of John Bowlby, and suggests that children who are not emotionally attached to warm, loving, and law-abiding parents tend to become offenders. Social learning theories suggest that children's behaviour depends on parental rewards and punishments and on the models of behaviour that parents represent. Children will tend to become offenders if parents do not respond consistently and contingently to their antisocial behaviour and if parents themselves behave in an antisocial manner.

### Teenage mothers and child abuse

At least in Western industrialized countries, early child-bearing, or teenage pregnancy, predicts many undesirable outcomes for the children, including low school attainment, antisocial school behaviour, substance use, and early sexual intercourse. The children of teenage mothers are also more likely to become offenders. For example, Morash and Rucker[11] analysed results from four surveys in the United States and the United Kingdom (including the Cambridge Study) and found that teenage mothers were associated with low income families, welfare support, and absent biological fathers, that they used poor child-rearing methods, and that their children were characterized by low school attainment and delinquency. However, the presence of the biological father mitigated many of these adverse factors and generally seemed to have a protective effect. In the Cambridge Study, teenage mothers who went on to have large numbers of children were especially likely to have convicted children. In the Newcastle Thousand-Family Study[12] mothers who married as teenagers (a factor strongly related to teenage childbearing) were twice as likely as others to have sons who became offenders by age 32.

There is considerable intergenerational transmission of aggressive and violent behaviour from parents to children, as Maxfield and Widom[13] found in a retrospective study of over 900 abused children in Indianapolis. Children who were physically abused up to age 11 were significantly likely to become violent offenders in the next 15 years. In the Cambridge–Somerville Study in Boston, Joan McCord found that about half of the abused or neglected boys were convicted for serious crimes, became alcoholics or mentally ill, or died before age 35. In the Rochester Youth Development Study,[14] child maltreatment under age 12 (physical, sexual or emotional abuse or neglect) predicted later self-reported and official offending. Furthermore, these results held up after controlling for gender, race, socio-economic status, and family structure.

Numerous theories have been put forward to explain the link between child abuse and later offending. Timothy Brezina described three of the main ones.[15] Social learning theory suggests that children learn to adopt the abusive behaviour patterns of their parents through imitation, modelling, and reinforcement. Attachment or social bonding theory proposes that child maltreatment results in low attachment to parents and hence to low self-control. Strain theory posits that negative treatment by others generates negative emotions such as anger and frustration, which in turn lead to a desire for revenge and increased aggression. Based on analyses of the Youth in Transition Study, Brezina found limited support for all three theories.

### Parental conflict and disrupted families

Many studies show that broken homes or disrupted families predict offending. In the Newcastle Thousand-Family Study, marital disruption (divorce or separation) in a boy's first 5 years doubled his risk of later convictions up to age 32. Similarly, in the Dunedin Study in New Zealand,[16] children who were exposed to parental discord and many changes of the primary caretaker tended to become antisocial and delinquent. The same study showed that single parent families disproportionally tended to have convicted sons; 28 per cent of violent offenders were from single parent families, compared with 17 per cent of non-violent offenders and 9 per cent of unconvicted boys.

The importance of the cause of the broken home is shown in the UK National Survey of Health and Development.[17] Boys from homes broken by divorce or separation had an increased likelihood of being convicted or officially cautioned up to age 21, in comparison with those from homes broken by death or from unbroken homes. Homes broken while the boy was under age 5 especially predicted offending, whereas homes broken while the boy was between ages 11 and 15 were not particularly criminogenic. Remarriage (which happened more often after divorce or separation than after death) was also associated with an increased risk of offending, suggesting a possible negative effect of step-parents. The meta-analysis by Wells and Rankin[18] also shows that broken homes are more strongly related to delinquency when they are caused by parental separation or divorce rather than by death.

Most studies of broken homes have focussed on the loss of the father rather than the mother, simply because the loss of a father is much more common. Joan McCord in Boston carried out an interesting study of the relationship between homes broken by loss of the natural father and later serious offending of the children. She found that the prevalence of offending was high for boys reared in broken homes without affectionate mothers (62 per cent) and for those reared in united homes characterized by parental conflict (52 per cent), irrespective of whether they had affectionate mothers. The prevalence of offending was low for those reared in united homes without conflict (26 per cent) and—importantly—equally low for boys from broken homes with affectionate mothers (22 per cent). These results suggest that it is not so much the broken home which is criminogenic as the parental conflict which often causes it, and that a loving mother might in some sense be able to compensate for the loss of a father.

In the Cambridge Study, both permanent and temporary separations from a biological parent before age 10 (usually from the father) predicted convictions and self-reported delinquency, providing that they were not caused by death or hospitalization. However, homes broken at an early age (under age 5) were not unusually criminogenic. Separation before age 10 predicted both juvenile and adult convictions, independently of all other factors such as low family income or poor school attainment, and was an important predictor of adult social dysfunction.

Explanations of the relationship between disrupted families and delinquency fall into three major classes. Trauma theories suggest that the loss of a parent has a damaging effect on a child, most commonly because of the effect on attachment to the parent. Life course theories focus on separation as a sequence of stressful experiences, and on the effects of multiple stressors such as parental conflict, parental loss, reduced economic circumstances, changes in parent figures, and poor child-rearing methods. Selection theories argue that disrupted families produce delinquent children because of pre-existing differences from other families in risk factors such as parental conflict, criminal or antisocial parents, low family income, or poor child-rearing methods.

Hypotheses derived from the three theories were tested in the Cambridge Study.[19] While boys from broken homes (permanently disrupted families) were more delinquent than boys from intact homes, they were not more delinquent than boys from intact high conflict families. Overall, the most important factor was the post-disruption trajectory. Boys who remained with their mother after the separation had the same delinquency rate as boys from intact low conflict families. Boys who stayed with their father, with relatives, or with others (e.g. foster parents) had high delinquency rates. These living arrangements were more unstable, and other research shows that frequent changes of parent figures predict offending. It was concluded that the results favoured life course theories rather than trauma or selection theories

## Criminal parents

Lee Robins and her colleagues showed that criminal, antisocial and alcoholic parents tend to have delinquent sons.[20] She followed up over 200 males in St. Louis and found that arrested parents tended to have arrested children, and that the juvenile records of the parents and children had similar rates and types of offences. Joan McCord also reported that convicted fathers tended to have convicted sons. She found that 29 per cent of fathers convicted for violence had sons convicted for violence, in comparison with 12 per cent of other fathers, but this may reflect the general tendency for convicted fathers to have convicted sons rather than any specific tendency for violent fathers to have violent sons.

In the Cambridge Study, the concentration of offending in a small number of families was remarkable. Less than 6 per cent of the families were responsible for half of the criminal convictions of all members (fathers, mothers, sons, and daughters) of all 400 families. Having a convicted mother, father, brother, or sister significantly predicted a boy's own conviction. As many as 63 per cent of boys with a convicted parent were themselves convicted up to age 40. Furthermore, convicted parents and delinquent siblings predicted self-reported as well as to official offending. Same-sex relationships were stronger than opposite-sex relationships, and older siblings were stronger predictors than younger siblings. Therefore, there is intergenerational continuity in offending.

It is not entirely clear why criminal parents tend to have delinquent children. In the Cambridge Study, there was no evidence that criminal parents directly encouraged their children to commit crimes or taught them criminal techniques. On the contrary, criminal parents were highly critical of their children's offending; for example, 89 per cent of convicted men at age 32 disagreed with the statement that 'I would not mind if my son/daughter committed a criminal offence'. Also, it was extremely rare for a parent and a child to be convicted for an offence committed together. The main link in the chain between criminal parents and delinquent sons seemed to be poor parental supervision.

There are several possible explanations (which are not mutually exclusive) for why offending tends to be concentrated in certain families and transmitted from one generation to the next. First, there may be intergenerational continuities in exposure to multiple risk factors. For example, each successive generation may be entrapped in poverty, disrupted families, single and/or teenage parenting, and living in the most deprived neighbourhoods. Second, the effect of a criminal parent on a child's offending may be mediated by environmental mechanisms such as poor parental supervision. Third, the effect of a criminal parent on a child's offending may be mediated by genetic mechanisms. Fourth, criminal parents may tend to have delinquent children because of official (police and court) bias against criminal families, who also tend to be known to official agencies because of other social problems. At all levels of self-reported delinquency in the Cambridge Study, boys with convicted fathers were more likely to be convicted themselves than were boys with unconvicted fathers. However, this was not the only explanation for the link between criminal fathers and delinquent sons, because boys with criminal fathers had higher self-reported delinquency scores and higher teacher and peer ratings of bad behaviour.

### Large family size

Large family size (a large number of children in the family) is a relatively strong and highly replicable predictor of offending. It was similarly important in the Cambridge and Pittsburgh studies,[21] even though families were on average smaller in Pittsburgh in the 1990s than in London in the 1960s. In the Cambridge Study, if a boy had four or more siblings by his tenth birthday, this doubled his risk of being convicted as a juvenile, and large family size predicted self-reported offending as well as convictions. It was the most important independent predictor of convictions up to age 32 in a logistic regression analysis.

In the National Survey of Health and Development, Michael Wadsworth found that the percentage of boys who were convicted increased from 9 per cent for families containing one child to 24 per cent for families containing four or more children. The Newsons in their Nottingham study also concluded that large family size was one of the most important predictors of offending. A similar link between family size and antisocial behaviour was reported by Israel Kolvin and his colleagues in their follow-up of Newcastle children from birth to age 33.

There are many possible reasons why a large number of siblings might increase the risk of a child's offending. Generally, as the number of children in a family increases, the amount of parental attention that can be given to each child decreases. Also, as the number of children increases, the household tends to become more overcrowded, possibly leading to increases in frustration, irritation, and conflict. In the Cambridge Study, large family size did not predict delinquency for boys living in the least crowded conditions. This suggests that household overcrowding might be an important intervening factor between large family size and delinquency.

Brownfield and Sorenson[22] reviewed several possible explanations for the link between large families and delinquency, including those focussing on features of the parents (e.g. criminal parents, teenage parents), those focussing on parenting (e.g. poor supervision, disrupted families), and those focussing on economic deprivation or family stress. Another interesting theory suggested that the key factor was birth order: large families include more later-born children, who tend to be more delinquent. Based on an analysis of self-reported delinquency in a Seattle survey, they concluded that the most plausible intervening causal mechanism was exposure to delinquent siblings. In the Cambridge Study, co-offending by brothers was surprisingly common; about 20 per cent of boys who had brothers close to them in age, were convicted for a crime committed with their brother.

## Social factors

### Socio-economic deprivation

The voluminous literature on the relationship between socio-economic status (SES) and offending is characterized by inconsistencies and contradictions, and some reviewers[23] have concluded that there is no relationship between SES and either self-reported or official offending. British studies have reported more consistent links between low social class and offending. In the UK National Survey of Health and Development, the prevalence of official juvenile delinquency in males varied considerably according to the occupational prestige and educational background of their parents, from 3 per cent in the highest category to 19 per cent in the lowest. It has been suggested that low SES families tend to produce delinquent children because their child-rearing tends to be poor.

Numerous indicators of SES were measured in the Cambridge Study, both for the boy's family of origin and for the boy himself as an adult, including occupational prestige, family income, housing, and employment instability. Most of the measures of occupational prestige (based on the Registrar General's scale) were not significantly related to offending. Low SES of the family when the boy was aged 8–10 significantly predicted his later self-reported but not his official delinquency. More consistently, low family income and poor housing predicted official and self-reported, juvenile and adult, offending.

It was interesting that the peak age of offending, at 17–18, coincided with the peak age of affluence for many convicted males. In the Cambridge Study, convicted males tended to come from low income families at age 8 and later tended to have low incomes themselves at age 32. However, at age 18, they were relatively well paid in comparison with non-delinquents. Whereas convicted delinquents might be working as unskilled labourers on building sites and getting the full adult wage for this job, non-delinquents might be in poorly paid jobs with prospects, such as bank clerks, or might still be students. These results show that the link between income and offending is quite complex.

Socio-economic deprivation of parents is usually compared with offending by children. However, when the children grow up, their own socio-economic deprivation can be related to their own offending. In the Cambridge Study, an unstable job record of the boy at age 18 was one of the best independent predictors of his later convictions between ages 21 and 25. Also, having an unskilled manual job at age 18 was an important independent predictor of adult social dysfunction and antisocial personality at age 32.

Between ages 15 and 18, the study boys were convicted at a higher rate when they were unemployed than when they were employed, suggesting that unemployment in some way causes crime, and conversely that employment may lead to desistance from offending.[24] Since crimes involving material gain (e.g. theft, burglary, robbery) especially increased during periods of unemployment, it seems likely that financial need is an important link in the causal chain between unemployment and crime.

### Peer influences

Having delinquent friends is an important predictor of later offending; peer delinquency and gang membership predicted self-reported violence in the Seattle Social Development Project.[25] Delinquent acts tend to be committed in small groups (of two or three people, usually) rather than alone. Large gangs are comparatively unusual. In the Cambridge Study, the probability of committing offences with others decreased steadily with age. Before age 17, boys tended to commit their crimes with other boys similar in age and living close by. After age 17, co-offending became less common.[26]

The major problem of interpretation is whether young people are more likely to commit offences while they are in groups than while they are alone, or whether the high prevalence of co-offending merely reflects the fact that, whenever young people go out, they tend to go out in groups. Do peers tend to encourage and facilitate offending, or is it just that most kinds of activities out of the home (both delinquent and non-delinquent) tend to be committed in groups? Another possibility is that the commission of offences encourages association with other delinquents, perhaps because 'birds of a feather flock together' or because of the stigmatizing and isolating effects of court appearances and institutionalization. Terence Thornberry and his colleagues in the Rochester Youth Development Study concluded that there were reciprocal effects, with delinquent peers causing delinquency and delinquency causing association with delinquent peers.

In the Pittsburgh Youth Study, the relationship between peer delinquency and a boy's offending was studied both between individuals (e.g. comparing peer delinquency and offending of boy X with peer delinquency and offending of boy Y at a particular age and then aggregating these correlations over all ages) and within individuals (e.g. comparing peer delinquency and offending of boy X at different ages and then aggregating these correlations over all individuals). Peer delinquency was the strongest correlate of offending in between-individual correlations but did not predict offending within individuals.[27] In contrast, poor parental supervision, low parental reinforcement, and low involvement of the boy in family activities predicted offending both between and within individuals. It was concluded that these three family variables were the most likely to be causes, whereas having delinquent peers was most likely to be an indicator of the boy's offending.

Associating with delinquent friends at age 14 was an important independent predictor of convictions at the young adult ages in the Cambridge Study. Also, the recidivists at age 19 who ceased offending differed from those who persisted, in that the desisters were more likely to have stopped going round in a group of male friends. Furthermore, spontaneous comments by the youths indicated that withdrawal from the delinquent peer group was an important influence on ceasing to offend. Therefore, continuing to associate with delinquent friends may be a key factor in determining whether juvenile delinquents persist in offending as young adults or desist.

### School influences

The prevalence of delinquency among students varies dramatically between different secondary schools, as Michael Power and his colleagues[28] showed many years ago in London. Characteristics of high delinquency-rate schools are well-known. For example, such schools have high levels of distrust between teachers and students, low commitment to school by students, and unclear and inconsistently enforced rules. However, what is far less clear is how much of the variation between schools should be attributed to differences in school organization, climate and practices, and how much to differences in the composition of the student body.

In the Cambridge Study, attending a high delinquency-rate school at age 11 significantly predicted a boy's later offending and antisocial personality scores. The effects of secondary schools on delinquency were investigated by following boys from their primary schools to their secondary schools. The best primary school predictor of juvenile delinquency was the rating of the boy's troublesomeness at age 8–10 by peers and teachers, showing the continuity in antisocial behaviour. The secondary schools differed dramatically in their official delinquency rates, from one school

with 21 court appearances per 100 boys per year to another where the corresponding figure was only 0.3. Moreover, going to a high delinquency-rate secondary school was a significant predictor of later convictions. It was, however, very noticeable that the most troublesome boys tended to go to the high delinquency-rate schools, while the least troublesome boys tended to go to the low delinquency-rate schools. Most of the variation between schools in their delinquency rates could be explained by differences in their intakes of troublesome boys. The secondary schools themselves had only a very small effect on the boys' offending.

The most famous study of school effects on delinquency was also carried out in London, by Michael Rutter and his colleagues.[29] They studied 12 comprehensive schools, and again found big differences in official delinquency rates between them. High delinquency-rate schools tended to have high truancy rates, low ability pupils, and low social class parents. However, the differences between the schools in delinquency rates could not be entirely explained by differences in the social class and verbal reasoning scores of the pupils at intake (age 11). Therefore, they must have been caused by some aspect of the schools themselves or by other, unmeasured factors.

In trying to discover which aspects of schools might be encouraging or inhibiting offending, Rutter and his colleagues found that the main school factors that were associated with delinquency were a high amount of punishment and a low amount of praise given by teachers in class. Unfortunately, it is difficult to know whether much punishment and little praise are causes or consequences of antisocial school behaviour, which in turn may be linked to offending outside school. In regard to other outcome measures, they argued that an academic emphasis, good classroom management, the careful use of praise and punishment, and student participation were important features of successful schools.

### Community influences

Offending rates vary systematically with area of residence. For example, the classic studies by Shaw and McKay[30] in Chicago and other American cities showed that juvenile delinquency rates (based on where offenders lived) were highest in inner city areas characterized by physical deterioration, neighbourhood disorganization, and high residential mobility. A large proportion of all offenders came from a small proportion of areas, which tended to be the most deprived. Furthermore, these relatively high delinquency rates persisted over time, despite the effect of successive waves of immigration and emigration of different national and ethnic groups in different areas.

Living in a deprived neighbourhood (whether based on parent ratings or on census measures of poverty, unemployment and female-headed households) significantly predicts convictions and self-reported offending. However, it is difficult to establish how much the areas themselves influence antisocial behaviour and how much it is merely the case that antisocial people tend to live in deprived areas (e.g. because of their poverty or public housing allocation policies). It has been suggested that neighbourhoods have only indirect effects on offending because of their effects on individuals and families. However, Robert Sampson and his colleagues[31] argued that a low degree of 'collective efficacy' of a neighbourhood (a low degree of informal social control) caused high crime rates.

One key question is why crime rates of communities change over time, and to what extent this is a function of changes in the communities or in the individuals living in them. Answering this question requires longitudinal research in which both communities and individuals are followed up. The best way of establishing the impact of the environment is to follow people who move from one area to another. For example, in the Cambridge Study, moving out of London led to a significant decrease in convictions and self-reported offending. This decrease may have occurred because moving out led to a breaking up of co-offending groups, or because there were fewer opportunities for crime outside London.

### Situational influences

It might be argued that all the risk factors reviewed so far in this section—individual, family, socio-economic, peer, school, and community—essentially influence the development of a long-term individual potential for offending. In other words, they contribute to between-individual differences: why some people are more likely than others, given the same situational opportunity, to commit a crime. Another set of influences—situational factors—explain how the potential for violence becomes the actuality in any given situation. Essentially, they explain short-term within-individual differences: why a person is more likely to commit crimes in some situations than in others. Situational factors may be specific to particular types of crimes: robberies as opposed to rapes, or even street robberies as opposed to bank robberies.

The most popular theory of offending events is a rational choice theory suggesting that they occur in response to specific opportunities, when their expected benefits (e.g. stolen property, peer approval) outweigh their expected costs (e.g. legal punishment, parental disapproval). For example, Clarke and Cornish[32] suggested that residential burglary depended on such influencing factors as whether a house was occupied, whether it looked affluent, whether there were bushes to hide behind, whether there were nosy neighbours, whether the house had a burglar alarm, and whether it contained a dog. A related theory is the 'routine activities' idea of Cohen and Felson.[33] They suggested that, for a predatory crime to occur, the minimum requirement was the convergence in time and place of a motivated offender and a suitable target, in the absence of a capable guardian. They argued that predatory crime rates were influenced by routine activities that satisfied basic needs such as food and shelter. Changes in routine activities led to changing opportunities for crime. For example, the increasing number of working women meant that more homes were left unattended during the day.

Much work on describing situations leading to violence has been carried out in the United Kingdom under the heading of crime analysis. This begins with a detailed analysis of patterns and circumstances of crimes and then proceeds to devise, implement, and evaluate crime reduction strategies. For example, it was found that most street robberies in London occurred in predominantly ethnic minority areas, and most offenders were 16–19 year old Afro-Caribbean males.[34] The victims were mostly Caucasian females, alone, and on foot. Most offences occurred at night, near the victim's home. The main motive for robbery was to get money, and the main factor in choosing victims was whether they had a wealthy appearance.

In their Montreal longitudinal study of delinquents, LeBlanc and Frechette[35] provided detailed information about motives and methods used in different offences at different ages. For example, for violence at age 17, the main motivation was utilitarian or rational.

For all crimes, however, the primary motivation changed from hedonistic (searching for excitement, with co-offenders) in the teenage years to utilitarian (with planning, psychological intimidation, and use of instruments such as weapons) in the twenties. In the Cambridge Study, motives for physical fights depended on whether the boy fought alone or with others.[36] In individual fights, the boy was usually provoked, became angry, and hit out to hurt his opponent and to discharge his own internal feelings of tension. In group fights, the boy often said that he became involved to help a friend or because he was attacked, and rarely said that he was angry. The group fights were more serious, occurring in bars or streets, and they were more likely to involve weapons, produce injuries, and lead to police intervention. Fights often occurred when minor incidents escalated, because both sides wanted to demonstrate their toughness and masculinity and were unwilling to react in a conciliatory way.

Much is known about the situations in which violence occurs. For example, in Sweden, violence preceded by situational arguments typically occurs in streets or restaurants, while violence preceded by relationship arguments typically occurs in homes.[37] In England, stranger assaults typically occur in streets, bars, or discotheques, non-stranger assaults typically occur at home or work, and robberies typically occur in the street or on public transport. Most violence occurs on weekend nights around pubs and clubs, and involves young males who have been drinking.[38] More research on situational influences on offending needs to be incorporated in prospective longitudinal studies, in order to link up the developmental and situational perspectives.

## Conclusions

Offending is one element of a larger syndrome of antisocial behaviour that arises in childhood and tends to persist into adulthood, with numerous different behavioural manifestations. However, while there is continuity over time in antisocial behaviour, changes are also occurring. It is commonly found that about half of a sample of antisocial children go on to become antisocial teenagers, and about half of antisocial teenagers go on to become antisocial adults. More research is needed on factors that predict these changes over time. Research is especially needed on changing behavioural manifestations and developmental sequences at different ages. More efforts should especially be made to identify factors that protect vulnerable children from developing into antisocial teenagers.

A great deal has been learned in the last 20 years, particularly from longitudinal surveys, about risk factors for offending and other types of antisocial behaviour. Offenders differ significantly from non-offenders in many respects, including impulsivity, intelligence, family background, and socio-economic deprivation. These differences are present before, during, and after criminal careers. While the precise causal chains that link these factors with antisocial behaviour, and the ways in which these factors have independent, interactive, or sequential effects, are not known, it is clear that individuals at risk can be identified with reasonable accuracy. In order to advance knowledge about human development and criminal careers, new multiple-cohort longitudinal studies are needed.[39]

The identified risk factors for offending should be targeted in prevention programmes. Risk-focussed prevention has great potential for crime reduction.[40] The continuity of antisocial behaviour from childhood to adulthood suggests that prevention efforts should be implemented early in life. Because of the link between offending and numerous other social problems, any measure that succeeds in reducing offending will have benefits that go far beyond this. Any measure that reduces offending will probably also reduce alcohol abuse, drunk driving, drug abuse, sexual promiscuity, family violence, truancy, school failure, unemployment, marital disharmony, and divorce. It is clear that problem children tend to grow up into problem adults, and that problem adults tend to produce more problem children. Continued efforts are urgently needed to advance knowledge about offending and antisocial behaviour, and to tackle the roots of crime.

## Further information

For extensive reviews of risk factors and interventions, see *Saving Children from a Life of Crime: Early Risk Factors and Effective Interventions* by D. P. Farrington and B. C. Welsh (Oxford University Press, 2007).

For extensive information about the Cambridge Study, see *Criminal Careers up to Age 50 and Life Success up to Age 48: New Findings from the Cambridge Study in Delinquent Development* by D. P. Farrington and colleagues (Home Office Research Study No. 299), available from www.homeoffice.gov.uk/rds.

For other reviews of psychosocial causes of offending, see *Antisocial Behaviour by Young People*, by M. Rutter, H. Giller, and A. Hagell (Cambridge University Press, 1998).

## References

1. Rutter, M., Giller, H., and Hagell, A. (1998). *Antisocial behaviour by young people*. Cambridge University Press, Cambridge.
2. Farrington, D.P., Coid, J.W., Harnett, L.M., *et al.* (2006). *Criminal careers up to age 50 and life success up to age 48: new findings from the Cambridge Study in Delinquent Development*. Home Office, London (Research Study No. 299).
3. Loeber, R., Farrington, D.P., Stouthamer-Loeber, M., *et al.* (1998). The development of male offending: key findings from the first decade of the Pittsburgh Youth Study. *Studies on Crime and Crime Prevention*, 7, 141–71.
4. Piquero, A.R., Farrington, D.P., and Blumstein, A. (2007). *Key issues in criminal career research: new analyses of the Cambridge Study in Delinquent Development*. Cambridge University Press, Cambridge.
5. Farrington, D.P. and Welsh, B.C. (2007). *Saving children from a life of crime: early risk factors and effective interventions*. Oxford University Press, Oxford.
6. Klinteberg, B.A., Andersson, T., Magnusson, D., *et al.* (1993). Hyperactive behaviour in childhood as related to subsequent alcohol problems and violent offending: a longitudinal study of male subjects *Individual Differences*, 15, 381–8.
7. Stattin, H. and Klackenberg-Larsson, I. (1993). Early language and intelligence development and their relationship to future criminal behaviour. *Journal of Abnormal Psychology*, 102, 369–78.
8. Schweinhart, L.J., Barnes, H.V., and Weikart, D.P. (1993). *Significant benefits: the High/Scope Perry preschool study through age 27*. High/Scope, Ypsilanti, Michigan.
9. McCord, J. (1979). Some child-rearing antecedents of criminal behaviour in adult men. *Journal of Personality and Social Psychology*, 37, 1477–86.
10. Newson, J. and Newson, E. (1989). *The extent of parental physical punishment in the UK*. Approach, London.
11. Morash, M. and Rucker, L. (1989). An exploratory study of the connection of mother's age at childbearing to her children's delinquency in four data sets. *Crime and Delinquency*, 35, 45–93.
12. Kolvin, I., Miller, F.J.W., Scott, D.M., *et al.* (1990). *Continuities of deprivation? The Newcastle 1000 family study*. Avebury, Aldershot.
13. Maxfield, M.G. and Widom, C.S. (1996). The cycle of violence revisited 6 years later. *Archives of Paediatrics and Adolescent Medicine*, 150, 390–5.
14. Smith, C.A. and Thornberry, T.P. (1995). The relationship between childhood maltreatment and adolescent involvement in delinquency. *Criminology*, 33, 351–481.
15. Brezina, T. (1998). Maltreatment and delinquency: the question of intervening processes. *Journal of Research in Crime and Delinquency*, 35, 71–99.
16. Henry, B., Caspi, A., Moffitt, T.E., *et al.* (1996). Temperamental and familial predictors of violent and non-violent criminal convictions: age 3 to age 18. *Developmental Psychology*, 32, 614–23.
17. Wadsworth, M.E.J. (1979). *Roots of delinquency: infancy, adolescence and crime*. Martin Robertson, London.
18. Wells, L.E. and Rankin, J.H. (1991). Families and delinquency: a meta-analysis of the impact of broken homes. *Social Problems*, 38, 71–93.
19. Juby, H. and Farrington, D.P. (2001). Disentangling the link between disrupted families and delinquency. *British Journal of Criminology*, 41, 22–40.
20. Robins, L.N., West, P.J., and Herjanic, B.L. (1975). Arrests and delinquency in two generations: a study of black urban families and their children. *Journal of Child Psychology and Psychiatry, and Allied Disciplines*, 16, 125–40.
21. Farrington, D.P. and Loeber, R. (1999). Transatlantic replicability of risk factors in the development of delinquency. In *Historical and geographical influences on psychopathology* (eds. P. Cohen, C. Slomkowski, and L.N. Robins), pp. 299–329. Lawrence Erlbaum, Mahwah, NJ.
22. Brownfield, D. and Sorenson, A.M. (1994). Sibship size and sibling delinquency. *Deviant Behaviour*, 15, 45–61.
23. Hindelang, M.J., Hirschi, T., and Weis, J.G. (1981). *Measuring delinquency*. Sage, Beverly Hills, California.
24. Farrington, D.P., Gallagher, B., Morley, L., *et al.* (1986). Unemployment, school leaving, and crime. *British Journal of Criminology*, 26, 335–56.
25. Hawkins, J.D., Herrenkohl, T., Farrington, D.P., *et al.* (1998). A review of predictors of youth violence. In *Serious and violent juvenile offenders: risk factors and successful interventions* (eds. R. Loeber and D.P. Farrington), pp. 106–46. Sage, Thousand Oaks, California.
26. Reiss, A.J. and Farrington, D.P. (1991). Advancing knowledge about co-offending: results from a prospective longitudinal survey of London males. *Journal of Criminal Law and Criminology*, 82, 360–95.
27. Farrington, D.P., Loeber, R., Yin, Y., *et al.* (2002). Are within-individual causes of delinquency the same as between-individual causes? *Criminal Behaviour and Mental Health*, 12, 53–68.
28. Power, M.J., Alderson, M.R., Phillipson, C.M., *et al.* (1967). Delinquent schools? *New Society*, 10, 542–3.
29. Rutter, M., Maughan, B., Mortimore, P., Ouston, J., and Smith, A. (1979). *Fifteen thousand hours: secondary schools and their effects on children*. Open Books, London.
30. Shaw, C.R. and McKay, H.D. (1969). *Juvenile delinquency and urban areas* (rev. edn). University of Chicago Press, Chicago.
31. Sampson, R.J., Raudenbush, S.W., and Earls, F. (1997). Neighbourhoods and violent crime: a multilevel study of collective efficacy. *Science*, 277, 918–24.
32. Clarke, R.V. and Cornish, D.B. (1985). Modelling offenders' decisions: a framework for research and policy. In *Crime and justice*, Vol. 6, (eds. M. Tonry and N. Morris), pp. 147–85. University of Chicago Press, Chicago.

33. Cohen, L.E. and Felson, M. (1979). Social change and crime rate trends: a routine activity approach. *American Sociological Review*, **44**, 588–608.

34. Barker, M., Geraghty, J., Webb, B., *et al.* (1999). *The prevention of street robbery*. Home Office Police Department, London.

35. LeBlanc, M. and Frechette, M. (1989). *Male criminal activity from childhood through youth*. Springer-Verlag, New York.

36. Farrington, D.P. (1993). Motivations for conduct disorder and delinquency. *Development and Psychopathology*, **5**, 225–2241.

37. Wikström, P.-O.H. (1985). *Everyday violence in contemporary Sweden*. National Council for Crime Prevention, Stockholm.

38. Allen, J., Nicholas, S., Salisbury, H., *et al.* (2003). Nature of burglary, vehicle and violent crime. In *Crime in England and Wales 2001/2002: supplementary volume* (eds. C. Flood-Page and J. Taylor), pp. 41–68. Home Office, London (Statistical Bulletin 01/03).

39. Tonry, M., Ohlin, L.E., and Farrington, D.P. (1991). *Human development and criminal behaviour: new ways of advancing knowledge*. Springer-Verlag, New York.

40. Farrington, D.P. (2007). Childhood risk factors and risk-focussed prevention. In *The Oxford handbook of criminology* (4th edn) (eds. M. Maguire, R. Morgan, and R. Reiner), pp. 602–40. Oxford University Press, Oxford.

# Associations between psychiatric disorder and offending

## Contents

11.3.1 Associations between psychiatric
disorder and offending
Lindsay Thomson and Rajan Darjee

11.3.2 **Offending, substance misuse, and mental disorder**
Andrew Johns

11.3.3 **Cognitive disorders, epilepsy, ADHD, and offending**
Norbert Nedopil

## 11.3.1 Associations between psychiatric disorder and offending

Lindsay Thomson and Rajan Darjee

### Introduction

The associations between psychiatric disorder and offending are complex. There has been a great deal of research into certain disorders and violent offending particularly over the last two decades. In summary, this has found a clear and consistent association between schizophreniform psychoses and violence, the importance of premorbid antisocial behaviour in predicting future violence, and the adjunctive effect of co-morbid substance misuse and antisocial personality disorder in the prevalence of violence. In addition, it has allowed the development of neuropsychiatric models to begin to explain violence in the context of mental disorder. Substance use disorders and learning disability are discussed in Chapters 11.3.2 and 11.3.3.

### Mental disorder and offending: a problematic relationship

Criminal behaviour is common in our society but there is evidence that violent crime rates have declined in Europe and North America over the last decade.[1] Mental disorders are also common. It is important to study the overlap between mental disorder and offending to consider those mental health and criminogenic factors that may be amenable to change. The social and economic factors relevant to offending are discussed in Chapter 11.2.

Before considering any associations between mental disorder and offending it is useful to consider the methodological problems in studying these:

- Offences are man-made concepts and not static. For example, many jurisdictions have created laws against stalking in the last twenty years which did not previously exist.

- Psychiatrists see a limited range of offenders but often base their research on these.

- Research is generally carried out on a captive population in prison or secure hospital. Offenders in these settings are likely to include those with characteristics that disadvantage them in the criminal justice system, for example ethnic status, low economic status, homelessness, unemployment, and mental illness.

- The generalizability of any findings must be queried given that offending is dependent on the wider social context such as rates of unemployment or crime, prevalence of substance misuse, and weapon carrying culture.

- It can be difficult to standardize populations studied, and severity of crimes.

- Criminal and mental health records may be unreliable.

### Evidence for neurobiological determinants of offending or aggressive behaviour

There is resistance to any oversimplified idea of seeking a genetic or neuropsychological explanation to offending behaviour as a whole but research in this area is expanding slowly. Neuropsychological abnormalities are commonly found in offenders and there is evidence for specific brain deficits in aggressive or violent behaviour.[2] These findings include:

- An association between specific traumatic damage to the frontal lobes, particularly orbitofrontal injury, and poor impulse control and aggressive outbursts.

- Abnormalities on neuropsychological tests of frontal lobe function in aggressive and antisocial subjects, indicating prefrontal executive dysfunction.

- Abnormalities found in clinical neurological testing of offenders. Antisocial behaviour is associated with EEG abnormalities particularly frontal slowing and these are commonly found in more than half of prisoners with a history of repetitive violence. Clinical signs of frontal lobe dysfunction are also associated with recurrent aggression.

- Neuroimaging changes. Structural and functional studies examining patients in forensic services and patients with antisocial personality disorder have consistently found changes in the frontal lobes of aggressive patients, typically reduced prefrontal cortical size and activity. Predatory rather than impulsive, emotionally charged (affective) perpetrators of homicide show functional patterns of blood flow similar to controls suggesting that these neuroimaging findings are relevant to impulsive or affective aggression rather than premeditated, purposeful violence. Two groups of people with aggressive behaviour are postulated: the first with an acquired frontal lobe lesion due to injury or disease which impairs social judgement, risk avoidance, and empathy; the second, shows increased aggressive behaviour associated with deficits in executive functioning correlating with dorsolateral prefrontal dysfunction which may occur in foetal or birth brain injury, developmental learning disorders, attention deficit hyperactivity disorder, substance misuse, and antisocial personality disorder with episodic aggressive dyscontrol.

- In addition, there is evidence for biochemical abnormalities. Reduced serotonin function is largely related to impulsivity rather than directly to violence.[3] Serotonin has a role in emotional states such as impulsiveness, aggression, anxiety, and depression. This has provided potential avenues for treatment with selective serotonin reuptake inhibitor medication.[4] Cortisol abnormalities have been recognized for a long time and more recently dietary insufficiencies have been explored.[5]

- Lastly, the role of genetics in offending behaviour has been examined through family, twin, and adoption studies.[6] Adoption studies have found a consistent association between biological parents and adoptee for property offences but a more complex association for violent crime with a relationship discovered in the Danish birth cohort study between paternal violence and adoptee schizophrenia. A link between a genotype and disturbed behaviour was found in maltreated male children. Those with the gene encoding the neurotransmitter metabolizing enzyme monoamine oxidase A (MAOA) moderated the effect of maltreatment and had reduced antisocial behaviour in later life.[7] MAOA genes have a known association with aggression in animals and humans. The low expression variant leads to increased aggression, limbic volume reductions and hyper-responsive amygdala during emotional arousal with decreased reactivity of regulatory prefrontal regions.[8] Twin studies have shown that antisocial behaviour in early childhood particularly when associated with callous unemotional traits has a strong genetic influence which weakens in antisocial behaviour displayed initially in adolescence when environmental influences are important.[9]

Such changes are not a necessarily a cause for aggressive behaviour which is dependent on so many environmental factors, nor do they necessarily predict aggressive behaviour but they are important to study in that they indicate potential management strategies.

# Clinical implications of the relationship between mental disorder and offending

The nature of the relationship between psychiatric disorder and offending is complex both at an individual and population level, and has important implications at both. Epidemiological data point to the following conclusions:

- Schizophrenia, personality disorder, and substance related disorders are significantly overrepresented in offenders.

- A number of factors associated with violence and offending in the non-mentally disordered are relevant to violence and offending in the mentally disordered.

- Amongst offenders there is the need to provide psychiatric assessment and treatment for significant numbers of people with mental disorder.

- Amongst mentally disordered offenders it is important to address criminogenic factors as well as providing traditional clinical treatment

- Appropriate treatment and preventative measures may prevent some offending and violence by individuals with mental disorders

It is important to know and understand the epidemiological research, but also to know and understand the patient that is being assessed. Not all factors of relevance to offending in people with mental disorders act in the same way in every case, and some factors not found to be of relevance in study samples may be crucial in individual cases. There is no simple or straightforward approach to such an assessment, and narrowing one's focus to a tick list of a few factors (perhaps from an actuarial tool) is at best lazy and at worst negligent. The psychiatrist should be able to articulate a formulation incorporating the factors which account for previous offending and which may be of relevance to future offending.

Every violent act involves a perpetrator, a victim, and a context, and this is no different where mental disorder is involved. A number of factors in the perpetrator, victim, and context in any violent incident are relevant to that violent act, and these three interact with each other. A simple example is that a drunk aggressive victim may frighten a suspicious impulsive perpetrator in the context of alcohol intoxication and an available knife. Where a person with mental disorder is violent one should not assume the former straightforwardly causes the latter. Sometimes mental disorder is the major determinant of an offence and at others mental disorder is entirely coincidental. In most cases mental disorder is one of a number of interacting factors (Fig. 11.3.1.1). Even where an offence seems explicable by psychotic hallucinations or delusions it is essential to consider wider factors (e.g. alcohol and substance misuse, social networks and personality).[10] A thorough assessment of these factors is crucial when evaluating criminal responsibility (see Chapter 11.1), assessing risk of future offending (see Chapter 11.15) and planning treatment for patients who have been violent. Treating mental disorder without addressing these factors will not adequately address the risk of further offending.

# Scizophrenia and offending

For over a decade, studies have consistently shown a small but significant association between schizophrenia and violence with an

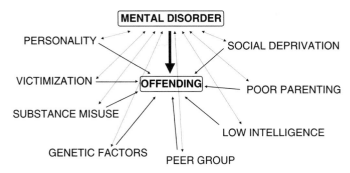

**Fig. 11.3.1.1** A schematic representation of the complex interplay between factors of relevance to offending in people with mental disorder.

increased risk of violence of between 2–4 for men and 6–8 for women after controlling for marital status, socio-economic background and substance abuse.[11] The proportion of violent crimes in the population of Northern European countries attributable to individuals with severe mental illness is around 5 per cent.[12] A systematic review of mental disorder in 23,000 prisoners found psychoses in 3.7 per cent of men and 4 per cent of women which was 2–4 times more than in the general population. Aggression in first episode psychosis occurs consistently in one-third of cases.[13]

Two patterns of aggression associated with schizophrenia are seen: firstly, those in whom features of conduct disorder (20-40 per cent) and later antisocial personality disorder predate the onset of overt schizophrenia; and secondly, those in whom violence occurs at a later stage.[11] Psychotic symptoms and violence in childhood are strongly related to later violence, as is a history of conduct disorder.[14]

Studies of people convicted of homicide have consistently shown an excess of schizophrenia with rates of 5–15 per cent.[15,16] Family members are significantly more likely to be the victim than strangers. Those with comorbid antisocial personality disorder are less likely to be actively psychotic at the time of the offence, and more likely to be intoxicated and to kill non-relatives.

### Neurobiological correlates of schizophrenia and violence

Naudts and Hodgins[17] examined neurobiological correlates of schizophrenia and violence. The literature is small, as are the sample sizes, and the measures used are diverse. At least one-fifth of men with schizophrenia show antisocial behaviour from childhood onwards. Overall, these men perform better on tests of specific executive functions and verbal skills despite greater impulsivity; and worse on tests of orbitofrontal functions than men with schizophrenia alone. Structural brain imaging studies of men with schizophrenia and a history of repetitive violence found reduced whole brain and hippocampal volumes; impaired connectivity between the orbitofrontal cortex and the amygdala; and structural abnormalities of the amygdala. Functional neuroimaging studies found reduced prefrontal cerebral blood flow during completion of a test of executive function in violent patients. This reduction in blood flow may result in loss of inhibition and therefore aggression, or it may reflect that these violent men found the test easier and did not need increased blood flow to complete it. Studies of acquired brain lesions show that ventromedial orbitofrontal cortex is necessary for inhibiting impulsive decision-making

and behaviour and for physiological anticipation of secondary inducers such as punishment. Studies at different ages suggest that an intact amygdala in early life is necessary for the normal development of this orbitofrontal system to recognize and process emotions. This fits with the work of Silver et al.[18] who found that patients with schizophrenia with a history of severe violence differ from non-violent patients with schizophrenia in their perception of the intensity of emotions but not cognitive function. Failure to assess the intensity of emotions may contribute to conflict generation, failure to recognize resolution signals, conflict escalation, and violence.

### Clinical features

People with schizophrenia may be violent because of their psychotic experiences, impaired judgment and impulse control, or situational factors. The evidence of the effect of symptoms is conflicting however, probably because of the way questions are asked; failure to take account of affective symptoms; variation in the timing between symptoms and violence; failure to control for medication, compulsion and previous violence; and variations in statistical procedures.[19] Swanson et al.[20] in a study of 1410 people with schizophrenia in a six month period found 19.1 per cent had been violent and this was serious in 3.6 per cent of cases. Positive symptoms increased the risk of minor and serious violence whereas negative symptoms decreased the risk of serious violence perhaps because these individuals lived alone. Serious violence was associated with psychotic and depressive symptoms, childhood conduct problems, and victimization. Severe psychotic symptoms and threat-control override (TCO) were antecedents of violent behaviour of patients in the community even after controlling for psychopathy and substance abuse.[21] TCO consists of persecutory delusions, passivity phenomena and thought insertion, resulting in perceived personal threat combined with loss of self control. Excessive perceptions of threat explained violence in people with schizophrenia-spectrum disorder alongside a history of conduct disorder.[22]

Hallucinations, acute suicidal ideation, acute conflict and stressors such as separations or housing problems, and lack of insight have all been associated with an increased risk of violence.[23]

### Co-morbidity

The likelihood of violence in patients with schizophrenia increases in the presence of comorbid substance use (3-fold in men, 16-fold in women) or personality disorder (4-fold men, 18-fold women).[11] Swanson et al.[20] found however, that the effects of substance abuse were non significant after controlling for age, positive symptoms of schizophrenia, childhood conduct problems and recent victimization thereby suggesting that the effects of substance abuse on violence may be mediated by these factors. There is a strong association between comorbid antisocial personality disorder and substance abuse in patients with schizophrenia with common origins in conduct disorder.[24] Further evidence for this is found in neuropsychological tests. Patients with comorbid schizophrenia and substance abuse perform as well as those with schizophrenia alone on neurological tests although it is known that the brains of men with schizophrenia are particularly sensitive to effects of drugs and alcohol. It has been suggested that these men belong to the antisocial group who do better on these tests at the onset of their schizophrenia.[17]

## Management

The care of patients with schizophrenia and a history of serious violence is centred around ongoing assessment and management of factors contributing to risk of violence and treatment of the schizophrenic illness. Predictors of violence include recent assault, a previous violent conviction, lower educational attainment and attending special education, a personal and family history of alcohol abuse, and lower but normal range IQ.[25,26] The management of schizophrenia is discussed in Chapter 4.3.8 but in patients with a history of violence methods of legal compulsion for detention and treatment, and programmes to address comorbid and criminogenic needs are particularly important. There is evidence that cognitive behavioural therapy can modify delusional beliefs that have lead to violence[27] and that clozapine has a particular role in the treatment of aggression in patients with schizophrenia separate from its antipsychotic or sedative components.[28]

## Outcome

There is no indication that deinstitutionalization has lead to increased offending by patients with schizophrenia. Rates of violence have increased but in proportion to the increase in society as a whole and with increased comorbid alcohol abuse.[29] Outcome studies of patients transferred from high security found a recidivism rate of 34 per cent and 31 per cent in England and Scotland respectively, and a violent recidivism rate of 15 per cent and 19 per cent after ten years.[30, 31] Patients with a primary diagnosis of schizophrenia during a follow up period of 8 years had a recidivism rate of 15 per cent and a violent recidivism rate of 5 per cent.

## Delusional disorders

Delusional disorders are described in Chapter 4.4. There are a number of subtypes including somatic, grandiose, mixed and unspecified but it is particularly the jealous, erotomanic and persecutory forms that are associated with offending and violence. Individuals with delusional disorders remain organized allowing them to target and plan any violence more effectively. Sixty percent of people with delusional jealousy are violent towards their partners. In erotomania the patient has the delusional belief that s/he is loved from afar by another and may attack individuals perceived as standing between them and their loved one, or the object of their affections if they feel slighted. Erotomania is associated with anger, harassment, stalking, and violence.[32]

Delusional disorders are found in excess in homicide (6-fold increase) and are associated with stalking. Stalking is persistent harassment in which a person repeatedly intrudes on another in an unwelcome manner that evokes fear or disquiet. One study of stalkers found that 30 per cent had a delusional disorder, 10 per cent schizophrenia, less than 5 per cent bipolar disorder or anxiety; 50 per cent had a personality disorder and 25 per cent abused substances. The classification of stalkers is based on their motivation. It is the rejected stalkers who pursue ex-intimates for reconciliation, revenge or both (includes delusional jealousy); intimacy seekers (includes erotomania); and the resentful stalker who pursue victims as revenge for an actual or perceived injury (includes persecutory) who are most likely to have a delusional disorder. This is not the case for incompetent suitors or predatory stalkers. See Chapter 11.10

Risk of harm to others can be reduced by treating the individual's delusional disorder with medication; controlling his or her environment by use of hospital or legal orders to restrict movement; and by advice to any potential victim on protective measures. There have been no randomized controlled trials of the treatment of delusional disorders but novel antipsychotics are now most commonly used due to their lower side-effect profile and better compliance, and it is recognized that pimozide has no particular role in the treatment of delusional disorder.[33] Cognitive behavioural therapy may assist compliance and insight but this has not been systematically demonstrated. Eye movement desensitization and reprocessing (EMDR) interwoven with cognitive therapy has been reported as a treatment of morbid jealousy. It is essential to warn any identified potential victims and such a breach of confidentiality is permitted by medical governing bodies.

## Organic disorders

Organic disorders may be related to offending directly because of the brain injury with disinhibition and impaired judgement, or secondarily to socio-economic deprivation and exclusion.

### Traumatic brain injury (TBI)

There is a 4-fold increase in the relative risk of developing any psychiatric illness in the six months post moderate to severe TBI and almost 3-fold in mild TBI excluding those with a history of mental illness. Common psychiatric sequelae of traumatic brain injury include mood (50 per cent), anxiety (25 per cent) and substance use disorders (28 per cent) along with post traumatic stress disorder and post traumatic brain injury attention deficit hyperactivity disorder in children, in addition to any cognitive problems.[34]

Posttraumatic irritability occurs in up to 70 per cent of people with TBI. Aggressive behaviour occurs in approximately one-quarter and this is significantly increased by the presence of major depression or substance abuse. Psychological tests of executive function and neuroimaging suggest that defective pre-frontal modulation of medial limbic structures may explain aggressive and impulsive behaviour seen in these patients. TBI patients who display aggression are characterized by significantly more impulsivity, disinhibition and social withdrawal; and poorer drive and motivation.[35] A study of sex offenders found that half had a history of head injury leading to loss of consciousness with significant neurological impairment in a quarter.[36] The head injury group offended more against adults than children, had more exhibiting and wide ranging sexual behaviours, and abused more substances than their non TBI sex offender controls.

### Epilepsy

Contrary to previous views, the evidence now suggests that there is no association between epilepsy and criminal behaviour. A systematic review of epilepsy in prisoners found a prevalence rate of about 1 per cent which is comparable with a community sample of a similar age and gender.[37] Epilepsy is considered in detail in Chapter 11.3.3.

### Dementia

A diagnosis of dementia and being charged with a sexual offence were factors most likely to distinguish those over 60 years of age referred by courts for a psychiatric assessment in Sweden compared to their younger counterparts although all forms of psychoses

(31 per cent), personality disorder (20 per cent), and substance use disorders (14.8 per cent) were more frequently diagnosed than dementia (7 per cent).[38] Offending is much less common in the elderly. Physical aggression in dementia however, is not uncommon and may be associated with exposure of intellectual deficits during testing (catastrophic reaction), severe cognitive impairment, impaired expression and comprehension, a history of premorbid aggression, physical illness particularly involving delirium or pain, post ictal confusion, depression and changes within the environment. Frontotemporal or orbitotemporal degeneration are more frequently associated with aggression in dementia, as are reduced serotonin and acetylcholine.[39]

## Autism spectrum disorders

Autism spectrum disorders (ASD) (including autism and Asperger's syndrome) are described in Chapter 9.2.3. In the severe form (autism) incapacity is frequently major and affected individuals are consequently unlikely to come into contact with the judicial system. The frequency of the lesser forms is inadequately researched. Although the majority of individuals with ASD are law abiding—and many indeed may be less likely to offend as a result of 'concrete' rule-based thinking—they are found in excess in high security psychiatric settings. Those who offend may do so because of feelings of resentment caused by bullying or rejection at school or in the community, because of an over-sensitivity to sound, occasionally because of a powerful interest in guns, fire or killing[40] or because of a lack of appreciation of social norms. Theft may occur in order to pursue a particular interest or obsession.

## Personality disorder

The link between personality disorder and offending and the role of psychiatry in managing personality disordered offenders is complicated by a number of issues: poor diagnostic systems; variable and subjective approaches to assessment; confusing legislative approaches seeking to define and impose measures on certain individuals; societal preoccupation with 'psychopaths' and 'sexual predators'; and uncertainty as to what treatment, if any, is effective. The concept of anti-social personality disorder, introduced in DSM-III and rehashed in DSM-IIIR and DSM-IV, has been unhelpful. Its reliance on socially deviant behaviour, rather than personality traits, reliably demarcates a broad heterogeneous group with varying underlying psychopathology and social problems. Personality disorder should not be diagnosed primarily on the basis of repeated anti-social behaviour. Assessment of personality in offenders should be based on pervasive and persistent emotional experience and expression, thoughts about self and others, interactions with others and behavioural control. Personality disordered offenders show a range of personality pathology rarely falling neatly into the diagnostic boxes of ICD 10 or DSM-IV. Focussing on personality disorder as a clinical entity misses relevant developments in assessment and management of such individuals from research and practice in criminal justice.

### Psychopathy

The term psychopathy has a long and chequered history (see Chapter 4.12.1). Its clinical use should probably be reserved for individuals fulfilling Hare's criteria[41] (based on Cleckley's 'Mask of Sanity'[42] describing superficial, self-centred, callous, parasitic,

impulsive, aggressive, predatory individuals. Hare operationalized psychopathy with the Psychopathy Check List-Revised (PCL-R). Interview and case file material is used to assess 20 items on a 3-point scale giving a maximum total score of 40. In North America a cut-off of 30 is used to diagnose psychopathy. In Europe the cut-off may be lower, but this is a contentious area. The total score may be useful for research purposes, but the profile of characteristics is important in clinical assessment and formulation. Underlying the construct are emotional, interpersonal and behavioural domains. Hare originally described two underlying factors: Factor 1 (emotional and interpersonal) correlated with narcissistic and histrionic disorders, and Factor 2 (socially deviant life style and behaviour) correlated with anti-social and borderline disorders. This has been refined into a four factor model subdividing factor 1 into interpersonal and affective domains, and factor 2 into lifestyle and antisocial behaviour domains. It has been suggested that the antisocial behaviour domain is not core to the condition.[43] Psychopathy is a narrower construct than dissocial (ICD 10) or antisocial (DSM-IV) personality disorder, so research findings cannot be extrapolated. It is an important concept in theory, research and practice concerning offender management and recidivism. But psychopathy only focuses on a limited, albeit important, set of personality traits of relevance in assessing offenders. Comprehensive consideration of personality pathology involves broader assessment. Patrick's book[44] gives an authoritative account of psychopathy.

### Relationship between personality disorder and offending

Personality disorder rates in prisoners range from 10 per cent[45] to 78 per cent[46] depending on study method. Lower rates are found with comprehensive clinical assessment, higher rates with structured tools administered by non-clinicians. In male prisoners the most prevalent disorder category is, unsurprisingly, antisocial followed by paranoid, then borderline, then obsessive compulsive, avoidant and narcissistic at similar rates.[46] In Fazel and Danesh's systematic review[37] 65 per cent of male prisoners were personality disordered (47 per cent anti-social); amongst female prisoners the rate was 42 per cent (25 per cent borderline, 21 per cent anti-social). Psychopathy has been found in 10 to 30 per cent of prisoners.[47]

Blackburn and Coid highlighted the heterogeneity of personality pathology in violent offenders.[48] Using cluster analysis they found six diagnostic patterns: antisocial-narcissistic, antisocial-paranoid, borderline-antisocial-passive aggressive, borderline, compulsive-borderline, and schizoid. The three antisocial groups displayed more psychopathy. Half of homicide offenders in Sweden were personality disordered[49] but the rate in the UK was about 10 per cent[15] (an underestimate due to the method of the study). Rates of personality disorder are high in sexual offenders.[50] Adult rapists have higher rates of psychopathy than child molesters who have higher rates of avoidant and dependent disorders. Sexual homicide offenders have high rates of psychopathy and other personality disorders, particularly in serial offenders and sexual sadists. Sadistic personality disorder (defined in the DSM-IIIR appendix) is found in up to a quarter of violent and sexual offenders, but is present with other personality pathology and is associated with sexual sadism.[51] There is little support for its recognition as a discrete disorder. Most serial arsonists have personality disorders. Borderline, narcissistic and antisocial subtypes of domestically violent men have been identified.[52] Personality disorder of various types is common in stalkers.[53] Psychopathy is particularly associated with instrumental violence, but reactive violence is also displayed.[44]

Population based cross sectional and birth cohort studies show offending and violence to be increased in individuals with personality disorders, particularly cluster B disorders.[54,55] Follow-up studies show higher rates of offending and violence in personality disordered subjects in general and forensic samples, particularly associated with psychopathy.[56,57,58] High rates of comorbid personality disorder are found in offenders with mental illness[59] and learning disability.[60] A range of personality pathology is found amongst patients detained under 'psychopathic disorder' and 'mental illness' legal categories in English secure hospitals.[59] Most legal 'psychopathic disorder' patients are not psychopaths.[61]

Various traits, individually and combined, are relevant to offending. Some lead to interpersonal conflict (suspiciousness, hostility, argumentativeness, rigidity, arrogance, clinginess), others to behavioural dyscontrol, others to angry emotional reactions, others to not considering consequences for self or others, others to taking pleasure in violating rules and others. Personality pathology may lead to inability to form intimate relationships, maintain work, establish a stable lifestyle or meet basic needs, which may predispose to offending. Impulsivity, need for stimulation, intolerance of dysphoric affect and inability to regulate affect predispose to drug and alcohol misuse leading to offending (see Chapter 11.7).

## Assessment

Assessment, as in other cases, involves a comprehensive history, current mental state examination, and information from records and informants. Structured approaches to personality assessment (e.g. PCL-R and International Personality Disorders Examination (IPDE)), may be incorporated but 'psychometrics' should not be used in isolation. Comorbid mental illness should be considered and structured approaches to risk assessment should be used, especially with serious violent or sexual offenders. A comprehensive formulation should consider the relationship between dysfunctional personality traits and offending.

## Management

Discussion of treatment is easily hijacked by the political agenda (largely focussed on protecting the public from dangerous psychopaths), the criminal justice context and legal issues. Although it would be naïve to consider treatment in isolation from these other issues, clinical management should be the starting point and primary concern of psychiatrists.

Most personality disordered offenders are not serious offenders, and their treatment needs are similar to individuals with personality disorder generally (see Chapter 4.12.7). General (e.g. long-term support and attention to relationships) and specific (e.g. psychological therapies and medication) approaches are relevant to many offenders. The application of such approaches within the criminal justice system or secure hospitals is complicated by coercion, the legal context and institutional factors. How should the success of treatment be measured? Amelioration of distress, improved social functioning or diminished reoffending? The three may be related, but the public, understandably, expects treatment to prevent offending.

Studies of consenting community patients cannot be extrapolated to serious offenders. The widespread view that psychological treatment programmes increase risk in psychopathic offenders is not backed by the literature, with mixed views and empirical findings.[62] The answer to 'Is psychopathy treatable?' is that the jury is still out and will be for some time. This does not mean treatment is ineffective or inappropriate for the range of personality pathology in serious offenders.

Cognitive behavioural programmes for offending behaviour have a moderate positive impact on recidivism.[63] Many of the areas targeted in such treatments relate to dysfunctional personality traits and many who go through these programmes have personality disorders. Adaptations for individuals with high levels of personality dysfunction and psychopathy have been made incorporating: greater focus on motivation, engagement, maintaining participation; using more appropriate learning styles; addressing underlying core beliefs; greater flexibility; emphasis on individual formulation, and positive psychology.[41] Whether such approaches lead to reduced recidivism awaits evaluation.

Although treatment in hospital may seem appropriate if there is to be a therapeutic approach, there are descriptions of prisons where a therapeutic environment has been achieved.[64] Detention in hospital primarily for indefinite incapacitation of dangerous offenders is controversial.

Personality disordered violent and sexual offenders have treatment needs, but they do not fit into traditional psychiatric systems, geared towards psychotic offenders. The approach with the latter is diversion from criminal justice to health care. With personality disordered offenders, the appropriate approach is probably to provide assessment and treatment within a criminal justice framework, in prison or community. Hospital treatment, as a scarce and expensive resource, should be reserved for those who have the potential to engage and benefit. Meux et al comprehensively describe hospital treatment approaches.[65] Staff working with personality disordered offenders, particularly with more severe pathology, need appropriate selection, training, support and supervision. Psychodynamic supervision of staff is important.

Management in the community involves monitoring, supervision and treatment by various agencies. In the UK Multi-Agency Public Protection Arrangements (MAPPA) are used to co-ordinate the management of violent and sexual offenders in the community. Within this mental health professionals can focus primarily on clinical assessment and treatment whilst criminal justice agencies focus on monitoring and supervision.

## Outcome

Certain personality disorders are associated with risk of recidivism. Psychopathy is associated with high rates of general and violent recidivism.[41] Amongst sex offenders psychopathy predicts violent rather than sexual offending, although sexual deviation with psychopathy is a malignant combination.[66] Psychopathy is associated with violence towards victims and diverse offending. Successful social integration following discharge has been found to be associated with not being reconvicted.[67] Personality disorder is associated with suicide in offenders.[68]

## Legal issues

An insanity defence, although historically relevant in some jurisdictions, is not usually available where the primary diagnosis is personality disorder. The partial defence of diminished responsibility is open to personality disordered homicide perpetrators in

England and Wales. Hospitalization does not often follow such a finding.

Detention in hospital is rather arbitrarily applied to some personality disordered offenders in England and Wales. Indefinite detention in hospital as a sentence can become lifelong incapacitation in a clinical setting.[69] To ensure that hospital detention is treatment focussed there should be prolonged assessment first. Some argue treatment in hospital should only occur via transfer to hospital during a prison sentence. In the Netherlands and Germany, personality disordered offenders are routinely detained in forensic hospitals.

Sexually violent predator laws allow civil commitment (and hospital detention) of mentally disordered high risk sex offenders at the end of a prison sentence in some US states.[70] Most offenders are personality disordered and these laws have survived constitutional challenge.

In many jurisdictions indeterminate sentences are applied to some offenders who are considered to pose an ongoing risk of serious offending.[71] Many such offenders are personality disordered. Psychiatric assessment of risk in such cases is considered unethical by some. Assessments of risk and personality disorder by psychiatrists have been used to under-write the application of the death penalty in some US States.[72]

## Mood disorders

Mood disorders are less related to offending than schizophrenia. Disinhibition and grandiosity in individuals with mania leads to public order offences, driving offences, theft, fraud and minor violent or sexual offences. Serious violent or sexual offending is rare. Treatment non-compliance and comorbid substance misuse are associated with offending.

Depression is not uncommon in prisoners (10 per cent in Fazel and Danesh's systematic review[37]) but rarely leads to offending. The association between depression and shoplifting in the historical literature is probably spurious. When depression is encountered in an offender, it may not have been present prior to the offence. If it was it is unlikely to have played a direct role. High life-time rates of depression are reported in sex offenders, and low mood may be one factor of importance in the path to re-offending in some.

Suicide follows 5 per cent of homicides in the UK.[73] Depression sometimes plays a role but other psychopathology is also seen. Types of offences include:

- Spousal: with pathological jealousy.

- Spousal: elderly men with poor health and/or ailing spouses who feel either or both cannot cope with declining health, adversity, or loneliness.

- Filicide-suicide: depressed mother kills her child(ren) and herself to save them from a worse fate.

- Familicide-suicide: depressed, paranoid, or intoxicated male kills the family and himself in the context of financial, marital, or other social stresses.

- Extra-familial murder-suicide: disgruntled, paranoid, narcissistic individuals who feel slighted or humiliated, take revenge on single or multiple victims, either as specific targets or as bystanders. This pattern is seen in spree killings.

Altruistic homicide and extended suicide are terms used where a depressed person kills one or more family members to 'spare them suffering' and commits or attempts suicide. Most are filicide-suicide and familicide-suicide cases. Depressive psychosis with nihilistic delusions is seen in a minority. It is probably impossible to identify these cases in advance, but it is prudent to explore thoughts about children in parents presenting with suicidal ideation.

Publicity has been given to the association between SSRI anti-depressants and aggression and suicide. There is no epidemiological data to back these claims, and some evidence SSRIs reduce impulsivity and associated aggression.[74]

Severe depression or mania may make an accused unfit to plead; affective psychosis may be accepted as the basis of an insanity defence; and milder forms of mood disorder may found a defence of diminished responsibility in homicide cases. Very few patients in secure hospitals are detained on the basis of mood disorder. In England and Wales, mothers with postpartum disorders who kill their children are usually convicted of infanticide rather than murder.

## Neurotic disorders

Neurotic symptoms are common in offenders, but it is unusual to find a close relationship between an offence and an ICD-10 neurotic, stress-related, or somatoform disorder. In many offenders it is possible to identify neurotic conflicts and find symbolic meaning in criminal behaviour.[75] Acute stress reactions and adjustment disorders may be associated with offending, particularly where the underlying personality is abnormal or substance misuse occurs. Social phobia may be relevant through its association with alcohol misuse. Although violent and sexual themes often feature in obsessions, obsessive compulsive disorder is negatively correlated with violence and offending. Obsessional features are sometimes seen in the paraphilic behaviour of some sexual offenders.

Post-traumatic stress disorder (PTSD) may be a contributory factor to offending. Offending rarely results directly from flashbacks or other re-experiencing phenomena, although there are cases where rape victims have attacked sexual partners. PTSD may contribute to the violence of women towards abusive partners. 'Battered Woman Syndrome' has been suggested as a sub-category of PTSD in such cases.[76] PTSD rarely leads to a defence of insanity, but may lead to diminished responsibility.

UK psychiatrist read with astonishment and incredulity accounts from the US of multiple personality disorder,[77] where the diagnosis has justified separate legal representation for alters, separate testimony from alters, unfitness to plead, the insanity defence, and malpractice suits when the diagnosis is 'missed'. James and Schramm[78] give guidance to avoid repetition of the US experience in the UK. Psychiatrists are advised not to collude by looking for further alters, investigating those that 'appear', and treating the patient as if he were more than one person. Frankel and Dalenberg[79] give a comprehensive account of dissociation and dissociative identity disorder in the US context.

## Factitious illness by proxy

Also called Munchausen syndrome by proxy, this is the fabrication of symptoms in, or the injury of, a child by its carer who presents the child for medical attention.[80] There is a wide range of injurious behaviours from fabricating symptoms and tampering with specimens and charts to poisoning, smothering, and withholding of nutrients. It is a behaviour rather than a psychiatric disorder. It may feature in systematic and serial child abuse, and in serial killings by health-care workers. Underlying disorders include personality disorders (narcissitic, borderline, and antisocial), somatization, mood, eating and substance misuse disorders. Psychodynamic literature offers various perspectives. In a number of highly publicized cases in the UK, expert evidence regarding families with multiple unexplained child deaths has led to mothers being convicted of murder. Several cases have been overturned on appeal with subsequent disciplinary action against the experts involved.

## Impulse control disorders

Impulse control disorders are described in Chapter 4.13.1. Two specific 'disorders' have relevance in forensic psychiatry: kleptomania and pyromania. Psychiatric aspects of arson are described in Chapter 11.9

In clinical practice, it is rare to find a shoplifter who meets criteria for kleptomania without underlying psychiatric disorder (mood, anxiety or eating disorder).[81] Apparently inexplicable acts of shoplifting may be perpetrated by people who have no features of kleptomania. Goldman[82] in an extensive review concluded that the disorder is more common than previously suggested.

The diagnosis of pyromania is of equally dubious validity. Most repeated arson offenders with the clinical features are excluded as they have other underlying disorders (psychosis, intellectual disability, or personality disorder) or are intoxicated when they set fires.[83]

## Further information

Patrick, C. J. (2006). *Handbook of psychopathy*. Guilford Press, New York.

Hodgins, S. and Muller-Isberner, R. (2000) *Violence, Crime and Mentally Disordered Offenders: Concepts and Methods for Effective Treatment and Prevention*. John Wiley and Sons Ltd, Chichester.

Gunn, J. and Taylor, P. *Forensic Psychiatry*. Hodder Arnold Health Sciences (in press)

Soothill, K., Rogers, P., and Dolan, M. (2008). *Handbook of Forensic Mental Health*. Willan Publishing, Cullompton, UK.

## References

1. Home Office. Crime Statistics for England and Wales. National Statistics, London. 2006 www.crimestatistics.org.uk. US Department of Justice (2006) Violent crime rates have declined, reaching the lowest level ever in 2005. Bureau of Justice Statistics, Washington, DC, USA. www.ojp.usdoj.gov/bjs/

2. Brower, M.C. and Price, B.H. (2001). Neuropsychiatry of frontal lobe dysfunction in violent and criminal behaviour: a critical review. *Advances in Neuropsychiatry*, **71**, 720–6.

3. Dolan, M., Deakin, W.J.F., Roberts, N., *et al.* (2002). Serotonergic and cognitive impairment in impulsive aggressive personality disordered offenders: are there implications for treatment? *Psychological Medicine*, **32**(1), 105–117.

4. Hollander, E., Phillips, A., Chaplin, W., *et al.* (2005). A Placebo Controlled Crossover Trial of Liquid Fluoxetine on Repetitive Behaviors in Childhood and Adolescent Autism. *Neuropsychopharmacology*, **30**(3), 582–9.

5. Gesch, C., Bernard, H., Sean, M., *et al.* (2002). Influence of supplementary vitamins, minerals and essential fatty acids on the antisocial behaviour of young adult prisoners: Randomised, placebo-controlled trial. *British Journal of Psychiatry*, **181**(1), 22–8.

6. Brennan, P.A., Mednick, S.A., Jacobsen, B., *et al.* (1996). Assessing the Role of Genetics and Crime Using Adoption Cohorts. *Ciba Foundation Symposium*, **194**, 115–28.

7. Caspi, A., McClay, J., Moffitt, T., *et al.* (2002). Role of Genotype in the Cycle of Violence in Maltreated Children. *Science*, **297**, 851–4.

8. Meyer-Lindenberg, A., Buckholtz, J.W., Kolachana, B.R., *et al.* (2006). Neuromechanisms of Genetic Risk for Impulsivity and Violence in Humans. *Proceedings of the National Academy of Sciences of the United States of America*, **103**(16), 6269–74.

9. Viding, E., Blair, R., James, R., *et al.* (2005). Evidence for Substantial Genetic Risk for Psychopathy in 7 Year Olds. *Journal of Child Psychology and Psychiatry*, **46**(6), 592–7.

10. Hiday, V.A. (1997). Understanding the connection between mental illness and violence. *International Journal of Law and Psychiatry*, **20**, 399–417.

11. Brennan, P.A., Mednick, S.A., Hodgins, S., (2000). Major mental disorders and criminal violence in a Danish birth cohort. *Archives of General Psychiatry*, **575**, 494–500.

12. Fazel, S. and Grann, M. (2006). The Population Impact of Severe Mental Illness on Violent Crime. *The American Journal of Psychiatry*, **163**(8), 1397–403.

13. Foley, S.R., Kelly, B.D., Clarke, M., *et al.* (2005). Incidence and clinical correlates of aggression and violence at presentation in patients with first episode psychosis. *Schizophrenia Research*, **72**, 161–8.

14. Arseneault, L., Moffitt, T., Caspi, A., *et al.* (2000). Mental Disorders and Violence in a Total Birth Cohort: Results from the Dunedin Study. *Archives of General Psychiatry*, **57**, 979–86.

15. Shaw, J., Hunt, I., Flynn, S., *et al.* (2006). Rates of mental disorder in people convicted of homicide: National clinical survey. *British Journal of Psychiatry*, **188**(2), 143–7.

16. Nordstrom, A., Dahlgren, L., Kullgren, G., *et al.* (2006). Victim relations and factors triggering homicides committed by offenders with schizophrenia. *The Journal of Forensic Psychiatry and Psychology*, **17**(2), 192–203.

17. Naudts, K., and Hodgins, S. (2006). Schizophrenia and violence: a search for neurobiological correlates. *Current Opinion in Psychiatry*, **19**, 533–8.

18. Silver, H., Goodman, C., Knoll, G., *et al.* (2005). Schizophrenia Patients with a History of Severe Violence Differ from Nonviolent Schizophrenia Patients in Perception of Emotions but Not Cognitive Function. *Journal of Clinical Psychiatry*, **66**(3), 300–8.

19. Applebaum, P.S., Robbins, P.C., Monahan, J., *et al.* (2000). Violence and Delusions: Data From the MacArthur Violence Risk Assessment Study. *The American Journal of Psychiatry*, **157**(4), 566–72.

20. Swanson, J.W., Swartz, M.S., Van Dorn, R.A., *et al.* (2006). A National Study of Violent Behavior in Persons with Schizophrenia. *Archives of General Psychiatry*, **63**, 490–9.

21. Hodgins, S., Hiscoke, U., Freese, R., *et al.* (2003). The Antecedents of Aggressive Behavior Among Men with Schizophrenia: A Prospective Investigation of Patients in Community Treatment. *Behavioral Sciences & the Law*, **21**(4), 523–46.

22. Arsenault, L., Moffitt, T., Caspi, A., *et al.* (2000). Mental Disoders and Violence in a total Birth Cohort: Results from the Denedin Study. *Archives of General Psychiatry*, **57**, 979–86.

23. Haggard-Grann, U., Hallqvist, H., Langstrom, N., *et al.* (2006). Short-term effects of psychiatric symptoms and interpersonal stressors on criminal violence, a case-crossover study. *Social psychiatry and psychiatric epidemiology*, **41**, 532–40.

24. Moran, P. and Hodgins, S. (2004). The Correlates of Comorbid Antisocial Personality Disorder in Schizophrenia. *Schizophrenia Bulletin*, **30**(4), 791–802.

25. Miller, P.McC., Johnstone, E.C., Lang, F.H., *et al.* (2000). Differences between patients with schizophrenia within and without a high security psychiatric hospital. *Acta Psychiatrica Scandanavica*, **102**, 12–8.

26. Walsh, E., Gilvarry, C., Samele, C., *et al.* (2004). Predicting violence in schizophrenia: a prospective study. *Schizophrenia Research*, 67, 247–52.

27. Taylor, P.J. (2006). Delusional Disorder and Delusions: Is There a Risk of Violence in Social Interactions About the Core Symptom? *Behavioural Sciences and the Law*, **24**, 313–31.

28. Krakowski, M.I., Czobor, P., Citrome, L., *et al.* (2006).Atypical antipsychotic agents in the treatment of violent patients with schizophrenia and schizomood disorder. *Archives of General Psychiatry*, **63**(6), 622–9.

29. Wallace, C., Mullen, P.E., Burgess, P., *et al.* (2004). Criminal Offending in Schizophrenia Over a 25-Year Period Marked by Deinstitutionalization and Increasing Prevalence of Comorbid Substance Use Disorders. *American Journal of Psychiatry*, **161**(4), 716–27.

30. Buchanan, A. (1998).Criminal conviction after discharge from special (highsecurity) hospital. *British Journal of Psychiatry*, **172**(6), 472–6.

31. Thomson, L.D.G. (2005). *Mental Disorder and Psychiatric Services, Mental Health and Scots Law in Practice*. W. Green & Sons, Edinburgh, Chapter 1.

32. Kelly, B.D. (2005). Erotomania: Epidemiology and Management. Therapy in Practice, *CNS Drugs*, (8), 657–69.

33. Sultanta, A. and McMonagle, T. (2007). Pimozide for schizophrenia or related psychoses. *Cochrane Database of Systematic Reviews*, 1.

34. Jorge, R.E. (2005). Neuropsychiatric consequences of traumatic brain injury: a review of recent findings. *Current Opinion in Psychiatry*, **18**(3), 289–99.

35. Wood, R.L. and Liossi, C. (2006). Neuropsychological and Neurobehavioral Correlates of Aggression Following Traumatic Brain Injury. *Journal of Neuropsychiatry and Clinical Neurosciences*, **18**(3), 333–41.

36. Langevin, R. (2006). Sexual offences and traumatic brain injury. *Brain and Cognition*, **60**(2), 206–7.

37. Fazel, S., and Danesh, J. (2002). Serious mental disorder in 23000 prisoners: a systematic review of 62 surveys. *Lancet*, **359**, 545–50.

38. Fazel, S., and Grann, M. (2002). Older Criminals: a descriptive study of psychiatrically examined offenders in Sweden. *International Journal of Geriatric Psychiatry*, **17**, 907–13.

39. Hall, K.A. and O'Connor, D.W. (2004). Correlates of aggressive behavior in dementia. *International Psychogeriatrics*, **16**(2), 141–58.

40. Wing, L. (1997). Asperger's syndrome: Management requires diagnosis. *Journal of Forensic Psychiatry*, **8**, 253–57.

41. Hare, R.D. (2006). Psychopathy: a clinical and forensic overview. *Psychiatric Clinics of North America*, **29**, 709–24.

42. Cleckley, H. (1998). (5th edn.). *The Mask of Sanity: An Attempt to Clarify Some Issues About the So Called Psychopathic Personality*. Emily S.Cleckley, Augusta, GA.

43. Cooke, D.J., Michie, C., Hart, S.D., *et al.* (2004). Reconstructing psychopathy: clarifying the significance of antisocial and socially deviant behavior in the diagnosis of psychopathic personality disorder. *Journal of Personality Disorders*, **18**, 337–57.

44. Patrick, C.J. (2006). (ed.). *Handbook of Psychopathy*. Guilford Press, New York.

45. Gunn, J., Maden, A., Swinton, M. (1991). Treatment needs of prisoners with psychiatric disorders. *British Medical Journal*, **303**, 338–41.

46. Singleton, N., Meltzer, H., Gatwood, R., *et al.* (1998). *Psychiatric morbidity among prisoners in England and Wales*. Office for National Statistics, London.

47. Andersen, H.S. (2004).Mental health in prison populations. A review– with special emphasis on a study of Danish prisoners on remand. *Acta psychiatrica Scandinavica. Supplementum*, **424**, 5–59.

48. Blackburn, R., and Coid, J.W.(1999). Empirical clusters of DSM-III personality disorders in violent offenders. *Journal of Personality Disorders*, **13**, 18–34.

49. Fazel, S., and Grann, M. (2004).Psychiatric morbidity among homicide offenders: a Swedish population study. *American Journal of Psychiatry*, **161**, 2129–31.

50. Harsch, S., Bergk, J.E., Steinert, T., *et al.* (2006). Prevalence of mental disorders among sexual offenders in forensic psychiatry and prison. *International Journal of Law and Psychiatry*, **29**, 443–9.

51. Berger, P., Berner, W., Bolterauer, J., *et al.* (1999). Sadistic personality disorder in sex offenders: relationship to antisocial personality disorder and sexual sadism. *Journal of Personality Disorders*, **13**, 175–86.

52. Johnson, R., Gilchrist, E., Beech, A.R., *et al.* (2006). A psychometric typology of U.K. domestic violence offenders. *Journal of Interpersonal Violence*, **21**, 1270–85.

53. Mullen, P.E., Pathe, M., and Purcell, R. (2000). *Stalkers and Their Victims*. Cambridge University Press.

54. Coid, J., Yang, M., Tyrer, P., *et al.* (2006). Prevalence and correlates of personality disorder in Great Britain. *British Journal of Psychiatry*, **188**, 423–31.

55. Hodgins, S., Mednick, S.A., Brennan, P.A., *et al.* (1996).Mental disorder and crime: evidence from a Danish birth cohort. *Archives of General Psychiatry*, **53**, 489–96.

56. Steadman, H., Mulvey, E., Monahan, J., *et al.* (1998). Violence by people discharged from acute psychiatric inpatient facilities and by others in the same neighborhoods. *Archives of General Psychiatry*, **3**, 401.

57. Grann, M., Langstrom, N., Tengstrom, A., *et al.*(1999). Psychopathy (PCL-R) predicts violent recidivism among criminal offenders with personality disorders in Sweden. *Law and Human Behavior*, **23**, 205–17.

58. Quinsey, V.L., Harris, G.T., Rice, M.E., *et al.* (2005). Violent Offenders: Appraising and Managing Risk. American Psychological Association.

59. Blackburn, R., Logan, Donnelly, *et al.* (2003). Personality disorders, psychopathy and other mental disorders: co-morbidity among patients at English and Scottish high-security hospitals. *Journal of Forensic Psychiatry*, **14**, 111–37.

60. Hogue, T., Steptoe, L., Taylor, J.L., *et al.* (2006). A comparison of offenders with intellectual disability across three levels of security. *Criminal Behaviour and Mental Health*, **16**, 13–28.

61. Coid, J.W. (1992). DSM–III diagnosis in criminal psychopaths: a way forward. *Criminal Behaviour and Mental Health*, **2**, 78–94.

62. D'Silva, K., Duggan, C., McCarthy, L., *et al.* (2004).Does Treatment Really Make Psychopaths Worse? A Review of the Evidence. *Journal of Personality Disorders*, **18**(2), 163–77.

63. McGuire, J. (2002).Offender Rehabilitation and Treatment: Effective Programmes and Policies to Reduce Reoffending. John Wiley and Sons Ltd.

64. Morris, M. (2002). Managing the unmanageable: psychotherapy in Grendon Prison. *Criminal Behaviour and Mental Health*, **12**(2 Suppl), S54–67.

65. Meux, C., Newrith, C., Taylor, P., (2006). Personality Disorder and Serious Offending: Hospital Treatment Models. Hodder Arnold.

66. Olver, M.E. and Wong, S.C. (2006). Psychopathy, sexual deviance, and recidivism among sex offenders. *Sex Abuse*, **18**, 65–82.

67. Reiss, D., Grubin, D., Meux, C., *et al.* (1996).Young 'psychopaths' in special hospital: treatment and outcome. *British Journal of Psychiatry*, **168**, 99–104.

68. Kullgren, G., Tengstrom, A., Grann, M., *et al.* (1998). Suicide among personalitydisordered offenders: a follow-up study of 1943 male criminal offenders. *Social Psychiatry and Psychiatric Epidemiology*, **33**(Suppl 1), S102–6.

69. Chiswick, D. (1992). Compulsory treatment of patients with psychopathic disorder: an abnormally aggressive or seriously

irresponsible exercise? *Criminal Behaviour and Mental Health*, **2**, 106–13.

70. Miller, H.A., Amenta, A.E., Conroy, M.A., *et al.* (2005). Sexually violent predator evaluations: empirical evidence, strategies for professionals, and research directions. *Law and Human Behavior*, **29**, 29–54.

71. Heilbrun, K., Ogloff, J.R.P., Picarello, K., *et al.* (1999). Dangerous offender statutes in the United States and Canada: Implications for risk assessment. *International Journal of Law and Psychiatry*, **22**, 393–415.

72 Edens, J.F., Buffington-Vollum, J.K., Keilen, A., *et al.* (2005). Predictions of future dangerousness in capital murder trials: is it time to 'disinvent the wheel'? *Law and Human Beahvior*, **29**, 55–86.

73. Shaw, J. and Flynn, J. (2003). Homicide followed by suicide. *Psychiatry*, **2**, 32–5.

74. Walsh, M.T. and Dinan, T. G. (2001).Selective serotonin reuptake inhibitors and violence: a review of the available evidence. *Acta psychiatrica Scandinavica*, **104**, 84–91.

75. Cordess, C. and Cox, M. (eds.). (1996). Forensic psychotherapy. Jessica Kingsley, London.

76. Walker, L.E. (2006). Battered woman syndrome: empirical findings. *Annals of the New York Academy of Science*, **1087**, 142–57.

77. Kluft, R.P. (1991). Clinical presentations of multiple personality disorder. *Psychiatric Clinics of North America*, **14**, 605–29.

78. James, D. and Schramm, M. (1998). 'Multiple personality disorder' presenting to the English courts: a case study. *Journal of Forensic Psychiatry*, **9**, 615–8.

79. Frankel, A.S. and Dalenberg, C. (2006). The forensic evaluation of dissociation and persons diagnosed with dissociative identity disorder: searching for convergence. *Psychiatric Clinics of North America*, **29**, 169–84.

80. Adshead, G. and Brooke, D. (2001). Munchasen Syndrom by Proxy. *Current issues in assessment, treatment and research*. Imperial College Press, London.

81. McElroy, S.L., Pope, H.G., Hudson, J.I., *et al.* (1991). Kleptomania: A report of 20 cases. *American Journal of Psychiatry*, **148**, 652–7.

82. Goldman, M.J. (1991). Kleptomania: making sense of the nonsensical. *American Journal of Psychiatry*, **148**, 986–96.

83. Lindberg, N., Holi, M., Tani, P., *et al.* (2005). Looking for pyromania: Characteristics of a consecutive sample of Finnish male criminals with histories of recidivist fire-setting between 1973 and 1993. *BMC Psychiatry*, **5**, 47.

# 11.3.2 **Offending, substance misuse, and mental disorder**

Andrew Johns

This chapter deals with the relationship between offending, substance misuse, and mental disorder, and also describes approaches to clinical and medico-legal assessment.

## Relationship between offending, substance misuse, and mental disorder

The nature of this relationship is complex, yet has to be understood in order to manage the health and risk of offending of individual patients. Offences related to substance misuse can be categorized as (i) violent offences, often involving an altered mental state, (ii) acquisitive offences, and (iii) miscellaneous offences such as breaking laws to control the misuse of drugs, driving under the influence of alcohol, and impact of substance misuse on parenting.

## Violent offences

Aggression is not an inevitable pharmacological consequence of misusing alcohol or any particular drug, but arises from many possible factors including expectancy effects, pattern of consumption, individual responses to intoxication or withdrawal, peer influences, and interpersonal issues.

Alcohol consumption is the single factor most associated with violence. It is a repeated finding from the British Crime Surveys that alcohol is a key factor in at least half of interpersonal assaults, with a greater contribution to assaults on strangers and domestic violence. By comparison, drug misusers are overwhelmingly more likely to commit acquisitive offences.

The co-morbidity of major mental illness and substance misuse further increases the risk of violence. For example, in the Epidemiological Catchment Area (ECA) survey of 10 000 individuals,[1] the prevalence of violent behaviour in the previous year was 2 per cent for those with no mental disorder, 7 per cent in 'major mental illness', 20 per cent for 'substance misuse disorder', and 22 per cent for co-morbid respondents. Among patients with first-episode psychoses,[2] just under 10 per cent demonstrated serious aggression when psychotic and 23 per cent showed lesser degrees of aggression. Those co-morbid for drug misuse were nine times more likely to show aggression after service contact—primary drug-related psychoses or alcohol misuse were not so associated.

There is particular concern in the UK about the risk to the public from serious violence by the mentally disordered. Nationally,[3] alcohol or drug misuse contributes to two-fifths of homicides and 17 per cent were committed by patients with severe mental illness and substance misuse. Alcohol- and drug-related homicides were generally associated with male perpetrators who had a history of violence, personality disorders, mental health service contact, and with stranger victims.

However, these epidemiological studies cannot define a causal link between substance misuse and mental disorder. There are many ways in which violence may arise in substance misusers and in co-morbid individuals. Simple intoxication on alcohol or other depressants such as benzodiazepines or barbiturates, leads initially to apparently excited behaviour. Stimulants such as cocaine or amphetamines, may produce arousal and irritability. Most forms of intoxication are also associated with impaired judgement, perception, and impulse control. Severe intoxication on alcohol, Cannabis, sedatives, or stimulants can lead to a toxic psychosis and highly disturbed behaviour. Even at levels of consumption insufficient to intoxicate, disinhibition, and autonomic arousal may facilitate recklessness and aggression. Pathological intoxication, in which aggression is supposed to occur within minutes of consuming moderate amounts of alcohol, is of doubtful validity and in most cases, better explained by alcohol-induced hypoglycaemia, head injury, or other organic disorder.

The association between withdrawal effects and potential for violence is often overlooked. Withdrawal from alcohol and most drugs of dependence, is a highly aversive state in which irritability and aggression may occur. Cessation from alcohol or sedatives, may lead to more severe withdrawal syndromes such as delirium tremens which are commonly associated with impaired perception, affect, judgement, and impulse control.

## Acquisitive offending

The relationship between acquisitive crime and drug misuse problems was studied among 753 clients recruited to the National Treatment Outcome Research Study (NTORS).[4] More than 17 000 offences were reported during the 90-day period prior to treatment. Half of the clients committed no acquisitive crimes during this period, whereas 10 per cent committed 76 per cent of the crimes.

Such work does not demonstrate a causal relationship between illicit drug use and acquisitive crime. From a large survey of British youth,[5] the average age of onset for truancy and crime are 13.8 and 14.5 years respectively, compared with 16.2 for drugs generally and 19.9 years for 'hard' drugs. Thus, crime tends to precede drug use rather than vice versa. It is clear that heavy drug use is strongly associated with impulsive acquisitive offending, including street robbery, and burglary, which involve violence.

## Other offences

In Britain, the non-medical use of drugs is subject to the Misuse of Drugs Act 1971, as subsequently amended, and which contains a classification based on perceived harm. Class A drugs include Ecstasy, LSD, heroin, cocaine, crack, magic mushrooms (if prepared for use), amphetamines (if prepared for injection); Class B drugs include amphetamines and methylphenidate (ritalin); Class C drugs include Cannabis, tranquilizers, some painkillers, Gamma hydroxybutyrate (GHB), ketamine. In January 2004, Cannabis was reclassified from a Class B to a Class C drug, it is still illegal. This legislation defines the penalties for supply, dealing, production, trafficking, and also possession.

Other offences include driving cars, or public conveyances such as trains whilst under the influence of alcohol or other drugs.

# Responding to the drug or alcohol using offender

## Clinical- and risk-assessment

The following is a practical guide to assessing the drug or alcohol-using offender.

1 Obtain a detailed life history, with corroboration from other informants and agencies. This should include relationships, work record, and current social situation.

2 Take a detailed history of all of the substances of misuse, including onset of regular use, dosage, route of administration, and pattern of use in a typical week. Ask about the desired effects of substance misuse, and also the actual effects. If there is also a serious mental illness, ascertain the effect of substance misuse on symptoms and behaviour. Has previous or recent substance misuse been associated with self-harm or aggression? Note any history of substance misuse treatment and the effects of this.

3 Take a detailed history of previous and recent offending with reference to the effects of substance misuse and mental illness, on mental state and behaviour before, during, and after each offence. Corroborate where possible from witness statements and independent sources.

4 Take a detailed mental state including some assessment of intelligence and personality, and also degree of insight into their offending, illness, and substance misuse.

5 Consider with the patient, the practical implications of this assessment for immediate clinical management and any need for medico-legal reporting that may arise.

There is increasing recognition of the role of actuarial instruments such as the HCR-20 (Historical/Clinical/Risk-management 20-item scale)[6] which allow for previous and current substance misuse to evaluated in the context of other significant risk factors.

Informed by the above, carry out a risk-assessment, firstly by defining the nature of any risk such as self-harm or relapse in substance misuse or of a primary mental illness. If a risk of violence is identified, this may involve particular individuals such as family, partners, or carers. Assess the probability and severity of each risk, and whether there are any early warning signs, such as particular behaviours or symptoms, or non-compliance with treatment.

## Risk- and clinical management

Maden[7] (2007) argues 'the first step in improving risk-management is to recognize that that the prevention of violence is a central task of mental health services'. As a general approach to risk-management of the drug or alcohol misusing offender, ascertain what risk factors may be changed, and how the provision of support, care, or security may reduce the risk.

It is clearly important to achieve cessation or control of drug or alcohol misuse. These are not easy aims, but it is important to dispel therapeutic nihilism and to appreciate that a range of interventions have been shown to be effective. Details of specific interventions are given in Chapter 4.2.2.4 and Chapters 4.2.3.1–4.2.3.7.

Treatment can reduce re-offending. The NTORS[4] found that 5 years after treatment, convictions for acquisitive, drug selling, and violent crimes had reduced.

The National Confidential Inquiry[8] has concluded that provision for dual diagnosis should be central to modern mental health care and should include: staff training in substance misuse management, joint working with drug and alcohol teams, local clinical leadership and use of enhanced Care Programme Approach for all those with severe mental illness, and a destabilizing substance misuse problem.

# Medico-legal issues

## Possible defences related to substance misuse

Generally speaking, the acute effects of having voluntarily taken drugs or alcohol are not a mitigating factor and it is argued that a drunken intent is still an intent. There are however narrowly defined circumstances in which an altered mental state due to substance misuse can raise the question of a possible defence.[9]

## Amnesia

Amnesia is common after violent offending, may relate to acute intoxication especially on alcohol or sedatives. In the absence of organic disease, amnesia does not affect fitness to plead, though it clearly complicates assessment of the perpetrators mental state at the time of an offence.

## Simple intoxication

Self-induced intoxication is generally no defence to a criminal charge. However, in England and Wales, case-law has determined that crimes such as murder, wounding with intent, theft, and burglary, require a *specific intent*, for which self-induced intoxication on alcohol or drugs may be a defence, but only if it can be shown that the accused was so intoxicated as to be unable to form the necessary intent. The psychiatrist can only comment as to whether the accused had the capacity to form the specific intent. It is a matter for the jury to determine whether the specific intent was present or not. If the specific intent is not demonstrated, then the accused may still be convicted of a lesser offence, so that acquittal on a charge of murder may lead to a conviction for manslaughter. It is a matter of clinical judgement as to whether an individual was so intoxicated as to be unable to form a specific intent, and the degree of purposiveness before, during, and after the offence, may be a useful indication.

Other crimes such as manslaughter, rape, and unlawful wounding, require only a *basic intent*, which cannot be negatived by intoxication. For these offences, the recklessness of voluntary intoxication may provide the necessary mental guilt.

### Insanity

Alcohol or drug misuse may give rise to a psychotic illness, such as delirium tremens, which may meet the requirements of the McNaughton rules, but the inanity defence is rarely used. In theory, consumption of drugs or alcohol could lead to a state of insane automatism, but the defence of insanity is not available if the consumption has been voluntary.

### Diminished responsibility

In England and Wales, Section 2 of the Homicide Act 1957 provides a defence of diminished responsibility in a charge of murder. The defence has to demonstrate that an *abnormality of mind* arises from one of the causes specified in the Act and those of possible relevance to substance misuse are *disease, injury* or *inherent causes*. An abnormality of mind due to intoxication is no defence. Alcohol dependence could meet criteria for *disease*, provided that the first drink of the day was shown to be involuntary. Diminished responsibility may become an issue when the effects of substance misuse interact with other factors such as organic brain damage, depression, or personality disorder. For legal purposes, the effect of intoxication has to be set aside and the defence must show that the associated condition was in itself severe enough to lead to an abnormality of mind.

### Psychiatric recommendations to the courts

In reporting to the court, the task of the psychiatrist is to explain the possible contribution of substance misuse to a particular offence, in the context of the life history, psychiatric, and offending history of the individual. The aim of such a report is (i) to consider relevant psychiatric issues and their bearing on the offence, (ii) to indicate whether treatment could usefully prevent re-offending, and (iii) to help the court to protect society. There are a range of legal interventions that can facilitate engagement in treatment in community settings.

### References

1. Swanson, J.W. (1994). Mental disorder, substance abuse, and community violence: an epidemiological approach. In *Violence and mental disorder—developments in risk assessment* (eds. J. Monahan and H.J. Steadman), pp. 101–36. University of Chicago Press, London.

2. Milton, J., Amin, S., Singh, S.P., *et al.* (2001). Aggressive incidents in first-episode psychosis. *The British Journal of Psychiatry*, **178**, 433–40.

3. Shaw, J., Hunt, I.M., Flynn, S., *et al.* (2006). The role of alcohol and drugs in homicides in England and Wales. *Addiction*, **101**, 1071–2.

4. Gossop, M., Trakada, K., Stewart, D., *et al.* (2005). Reductions in criminal convictions after addiction treatment: 5-year follow-up. *Drug and Alcohol Dependence*, **79**, 295–302.

5. Pudney, S. (2002). Home office research study 253, the road to ruin? Sequences of initiation into drug use and offending by young people in Britain. Home Office Research, Development and Statistics Directorate, UK.

6. Webster, C.D., Douglas, K.S., Eaves, D. *et al.* (1997). *HCR-20: assessing risk for violence* (version 2). Mental Health Law and Policy Institute, Simon Fraser University, Vancouver.

7. Maden, T. (2007). *Treating violence; a guide to risk management in mental health*. Oxford University Press, Oxford.

8. Avoidable deaths. Five year report of the National Confidential Inquiry into suicide and homicide by people with mental illness. (2006). University of Manchester.

9. Haque, Q. and Cumming, I. (2003). Intoxication and legal defences. *Advances in Psychiatric Treatment*, **9**, 144–51.

## 11.3.3 Cognitive disorders, epilepsy, ADHD, and offending

Norbert Nedopil

'Cognitive disorders' is a broad and heterogeneous diagnostic category, which includes different disorders, each with a distinct aetiology. They affect individuals in different ways depending on the age in which they occur. The term may be applied to a child, who has experienced perinatal trauma as well as to an older person with a beginning dementia of the Alzheimer type. The scientific literature on offenders with cognitive disorders is sparse. Most authors in forensic psychiatry do not systematically differentiate between the diagnostic subcategories and tend to use broad terms, such as organic disorder, organic psychosis, organic brain syndrome, neuropsychological deficit, dementia, mental handicap, mental retardation to include a number of different disorders in their studies. The number of patients with any kind of brain disorder in forensic hospitals and institutions is comparatively small and ranges from 1 to 10 per cent of all forensic inpatients. The same numbers apply for individuals assessed for criminal responsibility or risk of reoffending.[1-3] Compared to major mental disorders like schizophrenia or affective disorders or to personality disorders, patients with cognitive disorders account for only a small proportion of individuals seen by forensic psychiatrists. Subdividing this group any further would be statistically irrelevant. The way forensic psychiatry and the law deals with offenders suffering from organic brain disorders is rather derived from case reports and convention than from empirical knowledge.

DSM-IV-TR cites several disorders where aggression is either a diagnostic or associated feature and among them are four with an organic aetiology.

- Dementia of the Alzheimer type (DAT)

- Dementia caused by head trauma

- Personality change due to general medical condition (aggressive type)
- Postconcussional disorder

The psychiatric and general medical literature lists several other organic brain disorders that are either believed to be or in fact are associated with violence and offending, although their link is not as well proven.[4]

- Epilepsy
- Huntington's chorea
- Korsakow psychosis
- Brain tumours
- Mental retardation

From the experience of the author two other disorders should be added to this list:

- Traumatic brain injury
- Frontotemporal dementia

Systematic analyses of epidemiological data and of other research findings show that patients with clinically relevant brain damage do not commit violent crimes more often than would be expected according to their proportion in the general population.[5–7] These findings do not contradict the knowledge we have about aggressive and disruptive behaviour of certain patients with brain damage. The estimates of the frequency of such behaviours range from 18 per cent in demented patients to 60 per cent in patients with frontal lobe injuries.[8] Most of these patients are not seen by forensic psychiatrists, but are treated in special institutions or in outpatient settings. Apparently, the violent behaviour of patients with brain damage does not lead to interventions by the criminal justice system as often as could be expected from the above mentioned numbers. Similar findings are reported from demented patients: although not appearing in criminal court files, aggression and agitation of demented patients is a major problem in nursing homes and for caregivers of the elderly in outpatient settings. Again, exact definitions and robust data on how much violence really occurs are lacking, but estimates range from 18 to 48 per cent.[8] Rabins et al.[9] reported that 75 per cent of caregivers considered aggression as the most serious problem in agitated demented patients.

Offending and contact with the criminal justice system can be expected to be more frequent in patients who suffer less from cognitive impairments—which would prevent skilled or planned criminal activity—but rather from personality changes, like irritability, impulsivity, lack of concern for others, and for the consequences of one's action which is the case in frontotemporal dementia. Offending, but rarely violent offending, occurs sometimes as a first sign of this disorder.[10] Violent crimes are sometimes associated with cognitive disorders when delusions are among the first symptoms of a beginning dementia. Especially delusions of jealousy, envy, or revenge are prone to result in violent acts, which may leave partners or neighbours as victims. These crimes contradict the previous occupational and social life of the perpetrators and are paradigmatic examples of offending as a result of a mental disorder, leading to inculpability of the patient.

Offending can also be expected to be more frequent in patients between 18 and 35 years old and therefore in an age, where offending is statistically more frequent than in other age groups. Males of the same age group have the highest rate of traumatic brain injury. They also belong to the age group with the highest rate of criminality and especially of violent criminality. This same age and sex group also has the highest rate of substance abuse. Given the high prevalence of brain injury among young men and their propensity to use alcohol and drugs it is surprising how few are seen by forensic psychiatrists or sentenced to prison. The actual numbers of such patients found in forensic hospitals and in prisons do not reflect the high risk of violent crime by persons with brain injury. Hodgins[11] found that only 0.4 per cent of male penitentiary inmates warranted a diagnosis of organic brain syndrome (which is a much broader term than traumatic brain injury). Similarly the proportions of patients with organic brain syndrome in forensic hospitals is below 10 per cent and not greater than that in general psychiatric hospitals.[2,5]

Several studies suggest that the criminality of individuals with brain injury may, to a large extent, be attributed to premorbid personality traits, to the social disintegration which follows the injury, and hence not only to the injury itself. Kreutzer et al.[12] studied a sample of 327 patients with varying severities of traumatic brain injury. Those arrested after the brain injury were more likely to have had a history of police contacts before the brain injury, than those who were not arrested.

Two disorders have to be presented in greater detail:

Epilepsy, because it was historically one of the disorders of great concern for forensic psychiatrists and served as a model of the mentally ill offender not responsible for his crimes, and ADHD, because it is one of the disorders for which a relationship to antisocial behaviour and offending is most intensively researched.

## Epilepsy and offending

Throughout history epilepsy has been associated with violence. Devinsky and Bear[13] observed 'it would be difficult to cite, either from case reports or a literature review, another medical or neurologic illness in which aggressive behaviour is described so regularly'. Not only seizures were frightening for lay people and caused them to consider epileptics as being cursed by gods or being possessed by witches (Malleus Maleficarum, 1487) and dangerous to others, these patients were seen as threat because of their personality changes. At the turn of the twentieth century most lay persons and professionals believed that people with epilepsy had pathological personality traits and displayed aggression, sociopathy, and psychosis.[14] Kraepelin too reported aggression in epileptic patients and mentioned that almost always an intensification of mental irritability occurs. Jackson took it as given that epilepsy was a cause of insanity '…often of a kind that brings epileptics in conflict with the law'.[15] Even in 1973 Sjöbring[16] noted, that patients suffering from epileptic seizures become torpid and circumstantial, sticky and adhesive, effectively tense, and 'suffer from explosive outburst of rage, anxiety and so on'.

Epidemiologic research,[17] literature reviews,[18] and experimental studies[19] have not supported these beliefs. Although epilepsy was found to be three to four times more frequent among prisoners in the United Kingdom than in the general population,[17] their offences did not differ from those of the rest of the prison population. Similar findings were reported from the United States (King and Young, 1978). In a extensive survey of mentally ill offenders in Germany, who had committed acts of violence, Häfner and Böker[5] found only 29 patients with epilepsy out of 533 hospitalized violent offenders (5.4 per cent of the total sample). They compared their sample to an unselected population of 3392 nonviolent mentally ill hospital patients and reported that 5.2 per cent of them had also received the diagnosis of epilepsy. They concluded that epilepsy was statistically not a risk factor for violence. A thorough analysis of the crimes of the epileptic patients showed that marital status (single), educational level, socio-economic state, and alcohol consumption were more important risk factors than epilepsy. This is in accordance with studies in other countries. Eight of the 29 patients in the Häfner and Böker study had committed their crimes in an epileptic confusional state (which corresponds to the medico-legal term of organic automatism), but 11 had a quarrel with their victim before their offence.

Although specific personality changes were not confirmed for epileptics in general, and some authors attributed them rather to institutionalization, brain damage, comorbid disorders, medication, or social changes than to epilepsy itself, a specific association has been made between temporal lobe epilepsy (TLE) and special personality traits. 18 characteristic personality traits were summarized from the literature to constitute the Gastaut–Geschwind syndrome,[20] among them aggression, emotional lability, and 'hypomoralism', traits that must be considered as risk factors for offending. The empirical and neurobiological database to support an increased risk of criminality or violence even in these patients is, however, small. MRI studies found that severely aggressive epileptic patients were characterized by severe amygdalar atrophy or by left temporal lesions affecting the amygdala and the brain regions around them,[21] confirming the assumption that violence has to be attributed to specific brain damage rather than to epilepsy itself.

Epilepsy is associated with a number of psychopathological and behavioural symptoms, among them mood changes, anxiety, rigidity, and aggression. Epidemiologic studies show a high comorbidity with cognitive impairment, ADHD, personality disorders and psychotic disorders. Behavioural abnormalities and comorbid disorders, as well as epilepsy itself can contribute to the risk of offending in these patients.

Summarizing the results from newer empirical studies, epilepsy does not increase the risk for offending or violence, and the number of cases, in which epilepsy was successfully used to claim inculpability after offending violently is small.[22] Forensic psychiatrists confronted with the assessment of epileptic patients who have committed crimes have to consider the following key questions:[23]

♦ Is the association between offending and epilepsy due to the occurrence of the epileptic seizure itself?

♦ Is it due to the associated brain damage that may be the cause of the seizure?

♦ Is it the result of socio-economic factors or of medication?

♦ Is the offending independent of the epilepsy and due to other criminogenic factors?

There are theoretically several possibilities, why epileptic patients could offend or act violently as a consequence of the disorder:

1 Aggression or impulsive acts could be a manifestation of a seizure or an equivalent to a seizure (violent automatism); it could also be the reaction of the patient to negative aura experiences.

Delgado-Escueta *et al.*[24] collected 5400 videotaped seizures and concluded that violence appears to be extremely rare event in epileptic seizures. Only 13 individuals in their sample acted violently and only three attacked other people. This study was criticized because it did not take the patient environment interaction into account, which also plays a major role in outbreaks of aggression and which can be modified by epileptic seizures. Nevertheless, the number of cases of ictal aggression reported in the literature is small. Ictal violence erupts out of a normal non-aggressive situation within seconds, appears to be inappropriate to the circumstances, lasts for 1 to 3 min and subsides as suddenly as it has erupted. The patient returns to consciousness immediately or returns to normality after a few minutes of confusion, appears to be puzzled over what has happened and has no memory of it. Complex criminal acts cannot be attributed to seizures, seizure equivalents, or epileptic automatism.

2 Violence can be the result of tension and irritability in the prodromal phase of an epileptic seizure. In this case the irritability usually proceeds in waves, often triggered by the reactions of bystanders. Violence appears to be goal-directed and limited to avoid personal harm. The aggressive tension may last for several minutes up to an hour. Sometimes the patients seem out of control and do not remember their behaviour at al.

3 Postictal confusion can be associated with poriomania, somnambulism, and offending. Again, complex acts and adequate reactions to new situations cannot be attributed to postictal confusion or twilight states.

4 Interictal offending is quite often not associated with the disorder itself but with a criminal or aggressive family background, lower socio-economic status, and brain trauma.[23,25] Violence can be due to epileptic psychosis, to cognitive impairment, to impulse control disorder or to personality disorder, all of which could be consequences of epilepsy, although the data on these sequels of epilepsy are not undisputed.

A recent review of the literature by Schachter[26] can be summarized to the fact that postictal aggression was rarely due to confusion but significantly more frequent in postictal psychosis, and interictal aggression was associated rather with male sex, brain damage, social disadvantages, and chronic behavioural difficulties than with specific EEG findings or characteristic brain scans. In conclusion several risk factors have to be taken into account when the offending or violence of epileptic patients is considered:

### Disorder-related risk factors

♦ Brain damage

♦ Early onset of epileptic seizures

♦ Postictal psychosis

Disorder-unrelated risk factors

♦ Male sex

♦ Growing up in a criminal or aggressive environment

♦ Low socio-economic class

♦ Antisocial personality disorder

♦ Alcohol abuse

In most legislations forensic psychiatrists and courts would agree, that the criteria proposed by Hindler,[27] would be minimal requirements to relate offending or violence to epilepsy:

- An unequivocal past history of epileptic attacks
- The crime is out of character with the person's previous personality
- The crime is motiveless and unpremeditated
- EEG studies are compatible
- An altered state of consciousness during the event
- Total or partial amnesia for the crime

More stringent criteria were proposed by a panel of epileptologists in the United States in 1981.[24] They included videotaped documentations of epileptic automatism and of the presence of aggression during such seizures; also the aggressive or violent acts should be characteristic of the patient's habitual seizures. In most Central European countries videotaped proof would not be necessary to attribute the offending of an epileptic to his disorder.

## Attention-deficit/hyperactivity disorder (ADHD) and offending

Attention-deficit/hyperactivity disorder (ADHD) is a relatively new diagnostic term. It has been introduced in the current form in DSM-III-R in 1987, although the condition has been known to psychiatrists for more than 100 years.[28] Only with DSM-IV-TR some allowance was made to extend the diagnosis to adults[29] but DSM-IV-TR continued to assert that the majority of the patients loose their symptoms during late adolescence. The diagnostic criteria were empirically evaluated in school-children and it can be questioned whether they are appropriate for adolescents and adults. It can be questioned even more, how the association between offending and ADHD can be adequately established. The core symptoms of ADHD, inattention, hyperactivity, and impulsivity, are likely to cause social conflicts with peers and caregivers and to lead to resentment and aggressive interactions. This dissocial functioning may appear as the precursor of offending in later life. A number of studies tried to investigate the relationship between ADHD in childhood and the diagnosis of antisocial personality disorder (APD) in adulthood. Although there is converging evidence that about 25 per cent of children with ADHD will later receive the diagnosis of APD,[30,31] and that in individuals who met the criteria of psychopathy according to Hare,[32] ADHD was diagnosed retrospectively four times more often than in the general population.[33] Most of the studies ignore the possible impact of comorbid disorders, which are especially frequent with ADHD. Conduct disorder (CD), oppositional defiant disorder (ODD), alcohol dependence or abuse and other drug dependence or abuse are significantly more frequent in ADHD individuals than in control groups,[34] and all contribute substantially to offending and to the diagnosis of APD. The longitudinal study of Satterfield & Schell[35] found that half of the children with a combination of ADHD and CD were later diagnosed as APD, while APD was only found in 12 per cent of those who had ADHD without CD in their childhood.[36]

A number of studies found ADHD largely overrepresented in prison populations, where it is calculated to be up to 10 times more frequent than in the general population.[37,38] Except for drug-related crimes,[30] no special criminal profile could be attributed to the disorder.

In psychiatric assessments for courts and tribunals ADHD is rarely considered as a cause for diminished responsibility, and most offenders with this disorder will not be sent to forensic psychiatric institutions. ADHD has, however, to be regarded as risk factor for reoffending, especially if it is or was combined with a conduct disorder. Prisoners with ADHD had been reconvicted four times more often than other prisoners.[39]

## Further information

Barkley, R.A. (2006). *Attention-deficit/hyperactivity disorder* (3rd edn). The Guilford Press, New York.

Etinger, A.B. and Kanner, A.M. (2007). *Psychiatric issues in epilepsy* (2nd edn). Wolters Kluwer, Philadelphia.

Nedopil, N. (2000). Offenders with brain damage. In *Violence, crime and mentally disordered offenders: concepts and methods for effective treatment and prevention* (eds. S. Hodgins and R. Müller-Isberner), pp. 38–42. Wiley & Sons, Chichester.

## References

1. Gunn, J. (1991). Human violence, a biological perspective. *Criminal Behaviour and Mental Health*, **1**, 34–54.
2. Grant, I. (1997). Canada's new mental disorder disposition provisions: a case study of the British Columbia criminal code review board. *International Journal of Law and Psychiatry*, **20**, 419–43.
3. Leygraf, N. (1988). *Psychisch kranke Rechtsbrecher*. Springer, Berlin.
4. Fava, M. (1997). Psychopharmacologic treatment of pathological aggression. *The Psychiatric Clinics of North America*, **20**, 427–51.
5. Häfner, H. and Böker, W. (1982). *Crimes of violence by mentally abnormal offenders. The psychiatric epidemiological study in the Federal German Republic*. Cambridge University Press, Cambridge.
6. D'Orban, P., Gunn, J., Holland, A., *et al.* (1993). Organic disorder, mental handicap and offending. In *Forensic psychiatry* (eds. J. Gunn and P.J. Taylor), pp. 286–328. Butterworth-Heinemann, Oxford.
7. Toone, B. (1990). Organically determined mental illness. In *Principles and practice of forensic psychiatrie* (eds. R. Bluglass and P. Bowden), pp. 385–92. Churchill Livingstone, Melbourne.
8. Nedopil, N. (2000). Offenders with brain damage. In *Violence, crime and mentally disordered offenders: concepts and methods for effective treatment and prevention* (eds. S. Hodgins and R. Müller-Isberner), pp. 38–42. Wiley & Sons, Chichester.
9. Rabins, P.V., Mace, N.L., and Lucas, M.J. (1982). The impact of dementia on the family. *The Journal of the American Medical Association*, **248**, 333–5.
10. Diehl, J., Ernst, J., Krapp, S., *et al.* (2006). Frontotemporale Demenz und delinquentes Verhalten. *Fortschritte der Neurologie-Psychiatrie und ihrer Grenzgebiete*, 203–10.
11. Hodgins, S. (1995). Assessing mental disorder in the criminal justice system. *International Journal of Law and Psychiatry*, **18**, 15–28.
12. Kreutzer, J.S., Marwitz, J.H., and Witol, A.D. (1995). Interrelations between crime, substance abuse, and aggressive behaviours among persons with traumatic brain injury. *Brain Injury*, **9**, 757–68.
13. Devinsky, O. and Bear, D.A. (1984). Varieties of aggressive behavior in temporal lobe epilepsy. *The American Journal of Psychiatry*, **141**, 651–6.
14. Devinsky, O., Vorkas, C.K., and Berr, W. (2007). Personality disorders in epilepsy. In *Psychiatric issues in epilepsy* (2nd edn) (eds. A.B. Etinger and A.M. Kanner), pp. 286–305. Wolters Kluwer, Philadelphia, Baltimore, New York, London.
15. Jackson, J.H. (1931). *Selected writings of John Hughlings Jackson*. Hodder and Stoughton, London.

16. Sjöbring, H. (1973). Personality structure and development, a model and its application. *Acta Psychiatrica Scandinavica Supplementum*, **244**, 1–204.

17. Gunn, J. (1977). *Epileptics in prison*. Academic Press, London.

18. Treiman, D. (1986). Epilepsy and violence: medical and legal issues. *Epilepsia*, **27**, 77–102.

19. Rodin, E.A. (1973). Psychomotor epilepsy and aggressive behavior. *Archives of General Psychiatry*, **28**, 210–3.

20. Bear, D.M. and Fedio, P. (1977). Quantitative analysis of interictal behavior in temporal lobe epilepsy. *Archives of Neurology*, **34**, 454–67.

21. van Elst, L.T., Woerman, F.G., Lemieux, L., *et al.* (2000). Affective aggression in patients with temporal lobe epilepsy: a quantitative MRI study of the amygdala. *Brain*, **123**, 234–43.

22. Treiman, D.M. (1999). Violence and the epilepsy defense. *Neurologic Clinics*, **17**, 245–55.

23. Herzberg, J.L. and Fenwick, P.B.C. (1988). The aetiology of aggression in temporal-lobe epilepsy. *The British Journal of Psychiatry*, **153**, 50–5.

24. Delgado-Escueta, A., Mattson, R., and King, L.M. (1981). The nature of aggression during epileptic seizures. *The New England Journal of Medicine*, **305**, 711–6.

25. Stevens, J.R. and Hermann, B. (1981). Temporal lobe epilepsy, psychopathology and violence: the state of evidence. *Neurology*, **31**, 1127–32.

26. Schachter, S.C. (2007). Aggression in epilepsy. In *Psychiatric issues in epilepsy* (2nd edn) (eds. A.B. Etinger and A.M. Kanner), pp. 306–20. Wolters Kluwer, Philadelphia.

27. Hindler, C.G. (1989). Epilepsy and violence. *The British Journal of Psychiatry*, **155**, 246–9.

28. Hechtman, L. (2004). Attention-deficit/hyperactivty disorder. In *Kaplan & Sadock comprehensive textbook of psychiatry* (8th edn) (eds. B.J. Sadock and V.A. Sadock), pp. 3183–98. Lippincott, Williams & Wilkins, Baltimore.

29. McGough, J.J. (2004). Adult manifestations of attention-deficit/hyperactivity disorder. In *Kaplan & Sadock comprehensive textbook of psychiatry* (8th edn) (eds. B.J. Sadock and V.A. Sadock), pp. 3198–204. Lippincott, Williams & Wilkins, Baltimore.

30. Barkley, R.A., Fischer, M., Smallish, L., *et al.* (2004). Young adult follow-up of hyperactive children: antisocial activities and drug use. *Journal of Child Psychology and Psychiatry*, **45**, 195–211.

31. Mannuzza, S., Klein, R.G., Bessler, A., *et al.* (1993). Adult outcome of hyperactive boys: educational achievement, occupational rank, and psychiatric status. *Archives of General Psychiatry*, **50**, 565–76.

32. Hare, R.D. (1991). *Manual for the Hare psychopathy checklist-revised*. Multi-Health-Systems Inc., Toronto.

33. Johannsson, P., Kerr, M., and Andershed, H. (2005). Linking adult psychopathy with childhood hyperactivity-impulsivity. Attention problems and conduct problems though retrospective self-reports. *Journal of Personality Disorders*, **19**, 94–101.

34. Barkley, R.A. (2006). *Attention-deficit/hyperactivity disorder* (3rd edn). The Guilford Press, New York.

35. Satterfield, J.H. and Schell, A. (1997). A prospective study of hyperactive boys with conduct problems and normal boys: adolescent and adult criminality. *Journal of Child and Adolescent Psychiatry*, **36**, 1726–35.

36. Mannuzza, S., Klein, R.G., Bessler, A., *et al.* (1998). Adult psychiatric status of hyperactive boys grown up. *The American Journal of Psychiatry*, **155**, 493–8.

37. Rösler, M., Retz, W., Retz-Junginger, P., *et al.* (2004). Prevalence of attention-deficit/hyperactivity disorder in male young prison inmates. *European Archives of Psychiatry and Clinical Neuroscience*, **254**, 365–71.

38. Vermeiren, R. (2003). Psychopathology and delinquency in adolescents: a descriptive and developmental perspective. *Clinical Psychology Review*, **23**, 277–318.

39. Ziegler, E., Blocher, D., Groß, J., *et al.* (2003). Assessment of attention-deficit/hyperactivity disorder in prison inmates. *Recht and Psychiatrie*, **21**, 17–21.

## 11.4

# Mental disorders among offenders in correctional settings

## James R. P. Ogloff

Incontrovertible evidence now exists to show that the prevalence of mental disorders among prisoners far exceeds that found in the general community. A surprising concordance is emerging from several large international studies to show that, in western developed societies at least, the rates of major mental disorders in prisons are quite consistent. This chapter will provide an overview of relevant research examining rates of mental illness in prisons with those found in the community. Some observations regarding trends and implications for prisons also will be provided.

At the outset it is useful to reflect on the scope of illnesses which have been subsumed under the 'mental disorder' umbrella as it has been applied to the prison research. Most of the research that exists has focussed serious mental illnesses within the Axis I disorders—namely psychotic illnesses, mood disorders, and anxiety disorders. Considerable attention has been paid regarding the prevalence of personality disorders within prisons. Over the past 20 years much of that work has investigated antisocial or dissocial personality disorder and psychopathy.[1] By comparison, relatively little attention has been paid to other personality disorders. A growing area of importance concerns substance abuse and dependence disorders and, of course, co-occurring substance use and mental illness disorders. Considerable research also exists exploring the prevalence of mental retardation or intellectual disabilities in prison. Thereafter, fragments of research exist exploring any number of mental syndromes and conditions. The focus of this chapter will be on the major mental disorders which fall into Axis I. Some mention will be made of substance use disorders and personality disorders. In addition, with the growing number of women in prisons, information will be provided regarding this important group.

## The prevalence of mental illness among male and female prisoners

Recent research exists from Britain and Wales that shows that the prevalence of mental illness in prisons is many times greater than that found in the community. Brugha and colleagues[2] compared rates of mental illness among some 3,000 remanded and sentenced male and female prisoners in Britain and Wales and more than 10,000 community residents in Great Britain. The rate of psychotic illnesses in the community was 4.5 per 1,000 (0.045 per cent) compared with 52 per 1,000 in prisons (0.52 per cent). While the ten-fold increase in prevalence from the community to the prisons was remarkable, the results revealed further that the prevalence rate of psychotic illness for female prisoners was an astonishing 110 per 1,000 (0.11 per cent), compared to 50 per 1,000 for males (0.05 per cent).

One of the key studies that has helped provide information regarding the rate of mental illness in gaols and prisons is a meta-analysis conducted by Fazel and Danesh[3] that was published in *The Lancet*. Their analyses included 62 studies that included 22,790 prisoners. The majority of prisoners (81 per cent) were male. Nonetheless, enough studies that included women prisoners were available to provide information regarding the rate of mental disorder among them. Data from the Fazel and Danesh meta-analysis are presented in Table 11.4.1. The results show that approximately one in seven prisoners have a psychotic illness or major depression. As the authors report, this is between two and four times greater than would be expected in the general population.

**Table 11.4.1** Representative prevalence of mental illness and personality disorder among male and female prisoners (international samples)

| Disorder | Males per cent (95 per cent C.I.) | Females per cent (95 per cent C.I.) |
|---|---|---|
| Psychotic Illness (k = 49, N = 19,011) | 3.7 (3.3–4.1) | 4 (3.2–5.1) |
| Major Depression (k = 31, N = 10,529) | 10 (9–11) | 12 (11–14) |
| Personality Disorder (k = 28, N = 13,844) | 65 (61–68) | 42 (38–45) |
| Antisocial Personality Disorder | 47 (46–48) | 21 (19–23) |

k = number of studies; N = number of subjects; C.I. = Confidence Intervals.

Source: Fazel & Danesh (2002).

With respect to personality disorders, half of males and approximately 20 per cent of females are found to have a personality disorder—which is ten times greater than would be seen in the community.

There was some variability across studies, some (but not all) of which was explained by differences between research that used validated diagnostic procedures (3.5 per cent) and those that did not (4.3 per cent). Studies from the USA also showed higher prevalence rates than elsewhere. Psychosis among female prisoners was found to be slightly higher than that in males (4.0 per cent *c.f.* 3.7 per cent).[3]

A limitation of the Fazel and Danesh[3] meta-analysis is that relatively limited information was provided regarding the type and nature of mental illness. Brinded, Simpson, Laidlaw, Fairley, and Malcolm[4] reported the results of one of the most well conducted studies on the prevalence of mental illnesses among inmates ever published. *All* female sentenced and remanded inmates and a random sample of 18 per cent of sentenced male inmates in New Zealand were interviewed. Interviewers used standardized measures to identify inmates with mental illnesses and personality disorders. The final sample consisted of approximately 1200 inmates. The results of prevalence rates for mental disorder in the last month are presented in Table 11.4.2.

As the results in Table 11.4.2 show, the prevalence rates obtained by Brinded and colleagues[4] in New Zealand essentially parallel those obtained by the Fazel and Danesh[3] meta-analysis. The New Zealand results, however, include data for post-traumatic stress disorder, substance abuse, and dependence disorders. As with psychosis and major depression, the prevalence rates of the other disorders is significantly greater than what would be seen in the general population.

Of late, increased attention is being paid to the prevalence of mental disorders among female inmates.[5] In recent years, the rate of growth among women in custody has far surpassed the growth

rate for male prisoners. For example, data show that in the 10 years ending 2005, the percentage of women in prisons in the United States has increased by 57 per cent, compared to a growth rate of 34 per cent for men during the same period.[6] Similar findings exist in Australia, where research shows that the number of women in prison increased by 66 per cent from 1991 to 1999, while it increased by 24 per cent for men during the same period.[7]

Even more than for male prisoners, 'the prevalence of childhood and adulthood sexual and violent victimization, poverty, and poor educational and employment attainment reported by female inmates is nothing short of alarming'.[8] While a comprehensive review of the studies of mental illness among women offenders is beyond the scope of this chapter, Ogloff and Tye[5] have shown that the prevalence rates of mental disorders for women is now surpassing those identified for men in most published studies. This is particularly the case for mood disorders and anxiety disorders.

## Implications, service needs, opportunities

The cause of the relatively high prevalence of mental illness among people in the prison system has been sometimes attributed to the deinstitutionalization movement that has occurred in mental health over the past 20 years. The contention that the mentally ill are entering gaols in increasing numbers has not been accepted by all, however.[9] It has been proposed that it is simply heightened awareness among professionals and the public of the problem of mentally ill in the gaols that has resulted in the perception that they are entering in increasing numbers.[10] In a recent study investigating the criminal offence history of every person in Victoria with schizophrenia in the public mental health registry in five year cohorts from 1975 to 1995, Wallace, Mullen, and Burgess[11] found that there was no subsequent increase in offence rate by year for those with schizophrenia, while the offence rate for the matched comparison group of people in the community without a mental illness increased significantly over the period. This is particularly interesting since during that time the process of deinstitutionalization was completed in Victoria. Indeed, there are no more psychiatric hospitals in Victoria (except for a 100 bed secure forensic psychiatric hospital).

A number of contributing factors have been identified that help explain the high numbers of people with mental illnesses in the criminal justice system. Considerable concern has been raised about the capacity of community-based mental health services to address the needs of mentally ill offenders. Community-based mental health services work best for those who have reasonable connections and support within the community. Unfortunately, offenders (especially imprisoned offenders) tend to be poorly integrated into the community[12] and have poor access to a range of support services including accommodation, income support, health and mental health.[13, 14]

While the presence of mentally ill people in the criminal justice system presents challenges and raises concerns, the fact is that the justice system provides an opportunity to identify and deliver treatment to people who are otherwise likely to remain outside the reach of services. As such, it has been suggested that justice mental health services present an opportunity for identifying those with mental illnesses and making services available to them that would otherwise be non-existent.[10] Accordingly, taking a population

**Table 11.4.2** Prevalence rates for mental disorder in last month (New Zealand samples)

| Diagnosis | Women N = 167 n (per cent) | Remanded Men N = 441 n (per cent) | Sentenced Men N = 636 n (per cent) |
|---|---|---|---|
| **Mental Illness** | | | |
| Schizophrenia and related disorders | 7 (4.2) | 15 (3.4) | 14 (2.2) |
| Bipolar affetive disorder | 2 (1.2) | 4 (1.0) | 7 (1.1) |
| Major depression | 18 (11.1) | 47 (10.7) | 38 (5.9) |
| Obsessive-compulsive disorder | 7 (4.3) | 22 (5.0) | 21 (4.8) |
| Posttraumatic stress disorder | 27 (16.6) | 42 (9.5) | 55 (8.5) |
| **Substance-Related Disorders** | | | |
| Alcohol abuse | 7 (4.3) | 25 (5.7) | 8 (1.2) |
| Alcohol dependence | 4 (2.5) | 19 (4.3) | 3 (0.5) |
| Cannabis abuse | 6 (3.7) | 38 (8.6) | 27 (4.2) |
| Cannabis dependence | 0 (0) | 0 (0) | 0 (0) |
| Other abuse/dependence . | 6 (3.7) | 27 (6.1) | 12 (1.9) |

Reproduced from Brinded *et al.* Prevalaence of pyschiatric disorders in New Zealand Prisons: A national study. *Australian and New Zealand Journal of Psychiatry*, **35**, 166–73, copyright 2001, John Wiley & Sons, Inc.

health perspective, efforts to identify and treat those with mental illnesses who are entering the criminal justice system can help provide much needed services to this otherwise under-serviced population.

## Service development and provision to mentally ill offenders in prisons

Although it is beyond the scope of the chapter to discuss the provision of mental health services to prisoners, it may be helpful here to outline some of the requirements for services. The service model outlined here has been detailed elsewhere in the literature.[10] The service model recommended for use in prisons consists of six components outlined below, the nature and extent of which will vary depending on the needs arising in each institution.

### Intake screening

A two-tier evaluation process is recommended. The first step involves a brief mental health screening for every inmate upon admission. Second, those prisoners identified as being mentally ill are referred to mental health professionals for a more complete assessment. All prisoners should be screened for mental illness soon after admission to a correctional facility (within the first 24 h). The *Jail Screening Assessment Tool (JSAT;* Nicholls *et al.*, 2005) was developed to screen people being admitted to gaols for mental illness, as well as self-harm risk and risk of harm to others. The JSAT is administered by psychiatric nurses or other mental health professionals and takes approximately 20 minutes. It is validated for both male and female prisoners.

### Ongoing monitoring/screening of prisoners

A process must be in place for ensuring that prisoners are monitored, both formally and informally. This should include self-referrals and referrals by all prison staff.

### Comprehensive psychodiagnostic assessment

Comprehensive assessments by psychiatrists or clinical psychologists are required for all prisoners exhibiting symptoms of mental illness. The examination should include consideration of whether the prisoners who are acutely mentally ill should receive treatment in the institution or be transferred to hospital.

### Mental health treatment

Once assessed as having a mental illness, the prisoner should be referred to an appropriate treatment program within the correctional facility or correctional system if possible and practical. The size of the gaol and its mandate affects the type of service available. Services should be at the standard available in the community.

### Gradual post-release monitoring/supervision and continuity of services

Treatment should continue post-release in the community. The transition back to the community is often difficult, as evidenced by high recidivism rates and ongoing illness. Service needs for mentally ill people leaving prison include initiating psychiatric treatment and psychosocial services with a community mental health agency, locating housing, and finding employment.

## Programme evaluation

Given the complexity of mental health services in prisons, it is critical that programmes are evaluated on an ongoing basis (e.g. Elliot, 1997). Such evaluations are as important as the other components in achieving assessment and delivery of mental health services. Also, wherever possible, assessment must be linked with treatment. Ongoing evaluations of the effectiveness of the assessment/treatment decisions should be built into the system. Evaluation informs decision-makers about the outcome of their decisions. Over time, this feedback can lead to improvements in the assessment, referral, and treatment phases of the model. Data on the base rates of mental disorder among women in custody- and the number of female prisoners who fall into the MDO categories—also can prove valuable in planning for future treatment needs.

## Further information

Fazel, S., and Danesh, J. (2002). Serious mental disorder in 23 000 prisoners: a systematic review of 62 surveys. *Lancet*, **359**, 545–50.

Ogloff, J.R.P (2002). Identifying and accommodating the needs of mentally ill people in gaols and prisons. *Psychiatry, Psychology, and Law*, **9**, 1–33.

Sheehan, R., McIvor, G., Trotter, C. (eds) (2007). *What works with women offenders*. Willan Publishing, Devon, UK.

## References

1. Ogloff, J.R.P. (2006). The Psychopathy/Antisocial Personality Disorder conundrum. *Australian and New Zealand Journal of Psychiatry*, **40**, 519–28.

2. Brugha, T., Singleton, N., Meltzer, H., *et al.* (2005). Psychosis in the community and in prisons: A report from the British National Survey of Psychiatric Comorbidity. *American Journal of Psychiatry*, **162**, 774–80.

3. Fazel, S., Danesh, J. (2002). Serious mental disorder in 23 000 prisoners: a systematic review of 62 surveys. *Lancet*, **359**, 545–50.

4. Brinded, P.M.J., Simpson, A.I.F., Laidlaw, T.M., (2001). Prevalence of psychiatric disorders in New Zealand prisons: A national study. *Australian and New Zealand Journal of Psychiatry*, **35**, 166–73.

5. Ogloff, J., Tye, C. (2007). Responding to mental health needs of women offenders. In *What works with women offenders*. (eds. R. Sheehan, G. McIvor, C. Trotter), pp. 142–81 Willan Publishing, Devon, UK.

6. Harrison, P. and Beck, A. (2006). *Prisoners in 2005*. Washington, DC: US Bureau of Justice Statistics Bulletin NCJ 215092.

7. Cameron, M. (2001). Women Prisoners and Correctional Programs, *Trends and Issues in Crime and Criminal Justice*, 194, Canberra, ACT: Australian Institute of Criminology.

8. Nicholls, T., Lee, Z., Corrado, R., *et al.* (2004). Women inmates' mental health needs: Evidence of the validity of the *Jail Screening Assessment Tool (JSAT)*, *International Journal of Forensic Mental Health*, 3(2),167–84.

9. Monahan, J., Caldeira, C., Friedlander, H. (1979). The police and the mentally ill: A comparison of arrested and committed persons. *International Journal of Law and Psychiatry*, **2**, 509–18.

10. Ogloff, J.R.P. (2002). Identifying and accommodating the needs of mentally ill people in gaols and prisons. *Psychiatry, Psychology, and Law*, **9**, 1–33.

11. Wallace, C., Mullen, P.E., Burgess, P. (2004). Criminal offending in schizophrenia over a twenty-five year period marked by

deinstitutionalization and escalating comorbid substance abuse. *American Journal of Psychiatry,* **161**, 716–27.

12. Makkai, T., McGregor, K. (2003). Drug Use Monitoring in Australia: 2002 Report on Drug Use Among Police Detainees. *Research and Public Policy Series* No. 47. Australian Institute of Criminology, Canberra.

13. Baldry, E. (2003). Ex-prisoners, housing and social integration. *Parity,* **16**, 13–15.

14. Travis, J., Waul, M. (2003). From prison to home: *The effect of incarceration and re-entry on children, families, and communities.* The Urban Institute. Washington, DC.

# Homicide offenders including mass murder and infanticide

## Nicola Swinson and Jennifer Shaw

There is a widespread public perception of the mentally ill as violent.[1,2] Until the early 1980s there was a consensus view that patients with severe mental illness were no more likely to be violent than the general population. Emerging evidence from various countries over the past two decades, however, has established a small, yet significant, association between mental illness and violence.

Large-scale birth cohort studies, such as a 30 year follow-up of an unselected Swedish birth cohort, show a significantly increased risk of violent offences in men and women in the presence of major mental disorder.[3] Community epidemiological studies in New York[4] and in Israel[5] again show an increased risk of violence in psychiatric patients. An important contribution to this field is data from the Epidemiological Catchment Area study, showing that major mental illness increases the rates of violence over a 12-month period from a 2 per cent base rate to 8 per cent, but co-morbid substance abuse increases this rate further to 30 per cent.[6] Co-morbid substance abuse and personality disorder substantially increase the risk of violence, as demonstrated in the MacArthur Risk Assessment Study which showed rates of violence in discharged psychiatric patients of 18 per cent in those with major mental disorder, 31 per cent with major mental disorder and co-morbid substance abuse, and 43 per cent in those with personality disorder and co-morbid substance abuse.[7]

Public fears are often fuelled by media reporting of high-profile cases of homicide by people with mental illness.[8] Despite indications that rates of homicide among the mentally ill are relatively constant across countries,[9] studies of mental disorder in people convicted of homicide show that 8.7 per cent of homicides in New Zealand are 'abnormal',[10] yet evidence from Canada indicates that 35 per cent of perpetrators are mentally unwell.[11] Indeed rates ranging from 8 to 70 per cent have been found, varying with different definitions of mental disorder.[12]

The National Confidential Inquiry into Suicide and Homicide by People with Mental Illness was established at the University of Manchester in 1996. The core work of the Inquiry is to establish rates of mental disorder in homicide and the clinical care received by those in contact with services.

## General population homicides

There are 500–600 homicides annually in England and Wales. Perpetrators and victims are predominantly young males, especially when the victim is unknown to the perpetrator. In such 'stranger homicides' perpetrators are less likely to have a lifetime history of mental illness, symptoms of mental illness at the time of the offence, or contact with mental health services.

In the UK the total number of both total homicides and stranger homicides increased between1973 and 2003 but neither category increased in people with mental illness.[13] Similar trends have been noted in work from both the UK,[14] and in other countries.[10]

The commonest method of homicide is with a sharp instrument; shooting is relatively rare, accounting for less than 1 in 10 homicides in the UK.

Around half of all convictions are for murder and just under half for manslaughter. One in 25 receives a verdict of Section 2 manslaughter, diminished responsibility.

## Infant homicide

Despite an increasing rate of homicides in the general population, convictions for infanticide and the rate of infant homicide has remained relatively constant, at around 4.5 per 100 000 live births.[15] Infanticide has become a generic term for killing of infants, even though the criminal charge in England applies to a crime for which only a woman can be indicted.

Although the risk of homicide is higher in the first year of their life than at any other time, the rarity of infant homicide in absolute numbers means that there is a lack of high quality, systematic data at a population level which incorporates clinical characteristics.[16]

Data from the National Confidential Inquiry from 1996 to 2001 shows that 1 in 25 of the 2665 homicide perpetrators identified were convicted of infant homicide. Half of these infants were killed by their father and around a third by their mother. A quarter of perpetrators had symptoms of mental illness at the time of the offence and a third had a lifetime history of mental illness. Perpetrators of neonaticide were predominantly young, unmarried mothers experiencing symptoms of dissociation at the time of the homicide.

There were significant differences between male and female perpetrators, with males being more likely to have previous convictions for violent offending. Females were more likely to kill within a month of the birth and they were more likely to have affective disorder and symptoms of mental illness at the time of the offence but few of these women were under the care of mental health services.

Most males received a custodial sentence, whereas three quarters of women received a community sentence or hospital disposal.[16]

## Multiple homicides

Multiple homicides, in particular serial homicides, have generated a great deal of public and media interest over recent decades yet this phenomenon is rare in the UK. The rarity of these events means that there is a lack of empirical evidence about the characteristics of perpetrators and victims in the UK, with most evidence emanating from the United States. Even then, however, there is an absence of systematic, robust evidence, with many studies being limited by small sample size.

Most definitions of multiple homicides include three criteria; number of victims, which can vary from 2 to 10 in different definitions,[17] time, and motivation. The temporal relationship distinguishes subcategories: mass murder consisting of a single episode and location, with serial, and spree murders occurring over time in separate locations. The latter two are differentiated by an emotional 'cooling-off' period, which is present in serial homicide. Other authors have discussed motivation, such as sexual gratification and internal psychological gratification, but the lack of robust evidence means that it seems premature to include motivation as part of any such definition.[17]

Mass murder has been classified by victim type such as family annihilators and classroom avengers. Mullen[18] proposed a category of 'autogenic (self-generated) massacre', which encompassed perpetrators indiscriminately killing people in pursuit of a highly personal agenda, arising from their own specific social situation and psychopathology. They were characterized by social isolation, being bullied in childhood and personality traits such as suspiciousness, obsessional behaviour, grandiosity, and persecutory beliefs. He concluded that these murders are essentially murder-suicides, where the intention is to kill as many people as possible before killing themselves. It would now appear, particularly with recent events in Virginia, that this form of multiple homicide is an established form and concerningly appears to becoming more common. Cantor et al.[19] propose that media-related modelling is a potential factor in the emergence of this crime, with perpetrators often seeing themselves as lone warriors, themselves modelled on media images, and well informed about previous, similar, massacres.

An exploratory study, incorporating a nested case control study, showed that serial homicide offenders were more likely to be male dominated, compared with single homicide offenders, and were more likely to use strangulation. Moreover, victims of serial murders were significantly more likely to be females who were unknown to the perpetrator and the motivation being sexual.[17] Unfortunately most classification systems of serial murder, including the FBI classification, have been criticized as being inherently flawed due to weak operational definitions and unsubstantiated assumptions regarding behaviour and characteristics.[20]

There is, unfortunately, a lack of robust evidence regarding multiple homicides. There seem to be clear similarities between serial and mass murderers, but also fundamental differences. Mass murderers appear more likely to use firearms as a method, whereas serial murderers tend to kill in a more personal manner, using methods that afford greater physical proximity, such as strangulation, in addition to a greater propensity for female victims. Clinically, some evidence indicates that a substantial proportion of mass murderers have a severe mental illness, often a psychotic illness. On the other hand, it is proposed that serial murderers can be distinguished by lower levels of severe mental illness and the presence of higher degrees of psychopathy.[21]

## Female perpetrators of homicide

Around 1 in 10 perpetrators of homicide in England and Wales are female,[13] which is consistent with data from other countries, such as Finland.[22] Stranger homicide by females is rare. In one-quarter of cases the victims are the perpetrators' own children and a current or former partner in over a third.

As with men the commonest method is stabbing, although females are proportionally more likely to use suffocation or poisoning when compared with men.

There are no clear gender differences in the proportion of those with severe mental illness but females are proportionally more likely to have a diagnosis of alcohol or drug dependence than men. Females are less likely to receive a prison sentence and are more commonly placed on a hospital or community rehabilitation order.[13]

## Homicide by older people

Homicides perpetrated by the elderly are exceptionally rare. In England and Wales they account for less than 1 in 50 homicides. The male to female ratio in perpetrators over 65 years is the highest of all age groups, at 19:1.[13]

There is a distinct lack of robust evidence regarding homicide in this population. Elderly spouse homicides have been described by Knight[23] as involving a couple perceived to have a close, caring relationship with the homicide of the wife, by the husband, occurring in an abrupt and unexpected manner. Depression is well recognized in elderly homicides, not infrequently with associated delusions of impoverishment and ruin. Perpetrators are often in care giving roles with physical or psychiatric disability in the victim. The homicide is often followed by suicide of the offender.[24]

Those over 65 years are more likely to receive a hospital order or community disposal, than a custodial sentence.[13]

## Perpetrators of homicide with mental health service contact

The aim of the National Confidential Inquiry is to collect detailed clinical information on people convicted of homicide, focusing on those with a history of contact with mental health services.

The inquiry collects a national consecutive case series of patient homicides occurring since April 1996. Data collection involves collecting information on all homicides from the Home Office Homicide Index, which includes details of the perpetrator, victim, and method used. Where available, psychiatric reports prepared for the trial are obtained. Antecedent data (of previous offences) is collected from the National Crime Operations Faculty. Details on each case are submitted to mental health services in each individual's district of residence and adjacent districts to identify those with a history of mental health service contact. These individuals become Inquiry cases. Information on trust Inquiry cases is obtained from clinical teams via a comprehensive questionnaire sent to the consultant psychiatrist.

In the UK around 1 in 10 people convicted of homicide have been in recent contact with mental health services. In most of these cases the responsible service is a general adult psychiatry service, rather than a specialist service. The remaining cases are under alcohol and drug services, child and adolescent services, and forensic psychiatry services. Around one in five cases have had lifetime contact with services. This compares with data from other countries, such as Australia, where one in three perpetrators has had contact with psychiatric services.[25]

Of those in contact with mental health services in England and Wales, the most common diagnosis is schizophrenia, although less than half have severe mental illness (schizophrenia or affective disorder). There are high rates of co-morbid alcohol and drug dependence and personality disorder. Only one-third have previous admissions under the Mental Health Act (1983).

A high proportion of these patients have a history of violence, including convictions for violence, which, worryingly, are not documented in the case notes in a number of cases. Similar findings regarding the prevalence of violence were found in an examination of findings from public inquiries into homicides in the UK.[26] A small number of homicides are committed by patients who have previously been on a restriction order because of a violent offence.

Around half of those prescribed medication are non-compliant or disengaged from services at the time of the offence and relatively few are receiving any psychological intervention.[13]

## Perpetrators with schizophrenia

There is a well documented increased risk of violence in those with schizophrenia.[27] This has been shown in studies from the UK[28] and in other countries such as New Zealand[29] and Denmark.[30]

Around 1 in 20 perpetrators of homicide have a diagnosis of schizophrenia, a half have been in recent contact with services and one-third have never had any service contact.[13] These findings are broadly consistent with other UK data from remand prisoners,[31] and with data from other countries with rates of schizophrenia ranging from 7 per cent in Finland,[32] 7.5 per cent in Australia[25] to 12.6 per cent in Canada.[11]

Of those with recent contact one-fifth have a secondary diagnosis, commonly personality disorder or substance dependence, and a history of violence is common. Nearly a half have a history of violence when psychotic, around one-quarter are psychotic at the time of the homicide. Victims are most commonly family members; in less than one in six cases the victim is a stranger. Similar rates of stranger homicide by the mentally ill are found in Australia and New Zealand.[10] The majority of these patients have symptoms of mental illness at the time of the homicide and one in four receives a verdict of diminished responsibility. Of those not in contact with services, the vast proportion are psychotic at the time of the offence.[13]

It is of concern that nearly one-third of all perpetrators with schizophrenia receive a prison disposal.

Despite clear evidence of an increased risk associated with schizophrenia it is important to present a balanced view to prevent unnecessary stigmatization. The proportion of violent crime in society which is attributable to schizophrenia is consistently less than 10 per cent.[27] Wallace *et al.*[25] showed an increased risk of serious violent offending in males with schizophrenia of five times that of the general population. However, he also highlights data

which indicate that, in any given year, 99.97 per cent of all those with schizophrenia will not be convicted of a serious violent offence, and that the probability of patients with schizophrenia committing homicide is extremely low.

## Risk assessment

Nearly one in three Inquiry cases were seen during the week before the homicide, a similar proportion within 1–4 weeks and the remainder between 1–12 months. A substantial proportion had mental state abnormalities at final contact, often distress, depressive symptoms, hostility, or increased use of alcohol or drugs. Despite this immediate risk was judged to be low or absent in 88 per cent cases at the last contact.

There are clear difficulties in predicting risk of serious violence, given the rarity of its' occurrence alongside the high prevalence of risk factors such as substance abuse and a history of violence within the patient population. In an examination of findings from public inquiries into homicides it was shown that only 28 per cent of homicides were judged 'predictable', yet 65 per cent were seen as 'preventable'. 'Preventability' was conferred by 'improved mental health care'.[26]

### Use of enhanced CPA to manage risk

In the National Confidential Inquiry sample from 1999 to 2003, nearly three quarters of those with recent contact were not receiving care under the provisions of enhanced Care Programme Approach (CPA), including a substantial proportion of patients at high risk such as those with schizophrenia, personality disorder, a history of detention under Mental Health Act legislation, or a previous history of violence. Furthermore, one-third of those with severe mental illness, a history of violence, and detention under the Mental Health Act were not under enhanced CPA.

Among those who were being cared for under the provisions of enhanced CPA, a significant number were non-compliant with medication or disengaged from services at the time of the offence. It seems, therefore, that even if risk is recognized high-risk patients are not receiving the intensive care, commensurate with their level of risk, in the community.[13]

### Preventability

Clinicians identified one case in five in recent contact where the homicide could potentially have been prevented. Factors viewed as increasing the chance of preventing the homicide included a diagnosis of schizophrenia, multiple previous admissions, and detention under the Mental Health Act. Factors which were seen to have made the homicide less likely were better patient compliance; closer contact with patient's family; closer patient supervision; improved staff communication; and better staff training.[13]

## Longitudinal trends

When longitudinal data from the National Confidential Inquiry from 1997 to 2003 was examined it was apparent that, despite a rise in the homicide conviction rate in the general population, there has been no consistent change in rates of mental illness symptomatology at the time of the offence, contact with mental health services, lifetime history of mental illness, or specifically schizophrenia. Significant upward trends can be seen in the number of perpetrators with a history of drug and alcohol misuse, in particular the use of cocaine and crack cocaine. There has been a significant decrease in those receiving a verdict of diminished responsibility but, surprisingly, no change in rates of those receiving a hospital order.[13]

## Further information

http://www.medicine.manchester.ac.uk/suicideprevention/nci/ (the website for the National Confidential Inquiry which is regularly updated).

Maden, A. (2007). *Treating violence: a guide to risk management in mental health*. Oxford University Press, Oxford.

Taylor, P. and Gunn, J. (2009). *Forensic psychiatry: clinical, legal and ethical issues* (2nd edn). Hodder Arnold, London.

## References

1. Phelan, J.C. and Link, B.G. (1998). The growing belief that people with mental illnesses are violent: the role of the dangerousness criterion for civil commitment. *Social Psychiatry and Psychiatric Epidemiology*, **33**, S7–12.

2. Crisp, A.H., Gelder, M.G., Rix, S., *et al.* (2000). Stigmatisation of people with mental illness. *The British Journal of Psychiatry*, **177**, 4–7.

3. Hodgins, S. (1992). Mental disorder, intellectual deficiency, and crime: evidence from a Danish birth cohort. *Archives of General Psychiatry*, **49**, 476–83.

4. Link, B.G., Andrews, H., and Cullen, F.T. (1992). The violent and illegal behaviour of mental patients reconsidered. *American Sociological Review*, **57**, 275–92.

5. Link, B.G., Stueve, A., and Phelan, J. (1998). Psychotic symptoms and violent behaviours: probing the components of 'threat/control-override' symptoms. *Social Psychiatry and Psychiatric Epidemiology*, **33**, S55–60.

6. Swanson, J.W., Holzer, C.E. III, Ganju, V.K., *et al.* (1990). Violence and psychiatric disorder in the community: evidence from the Epidemiologic Catchment Area surveys. *Hospital & Community Psychiatry*, **41**, 761–70.

7. Steadman, H.J., Mulvey, E.P., Monahan, J., *et al.* (1998). Violence by people discharged from acute psychiatric inpatient facilities and by others in the same neighbourhoods. *Archives of General Psychiatry*, **55**, 1–9.

8. Ritchie, J., Dick, D., and Lingham, R. (1994). *Report of the inquiry into the care and treatment of Christopher Clunis*. Stationery Office, London.

9. Coid, J. (1983). The epidemiology of abnormal homicide and murder followed by suicide. *Psychological Medicine*, **13**, 855–60.

10. Simpson, A.I.F., McKenna, B., Moskowitz, A., *et al.* (2004). Homicide and mental illness in New Zealand, 1970–2000. *The British Journal of Psychiatry*, **185**, 394–8.

11. Cote, G. and Hodgins, S. (1992). The prevalence of major mental disorders among homicide offenders. *International Journal of Law and Psychiatry*, **15**, 89–99.

12. Woodward, M., Nursten, J., Williams, P., *et al.* (2000). Mental disorder and homicide: a review of epidemiological research. *Epidemiologiae Psichiatria Sociale*, **9**, 171–89.

13. Appleby, L., Shaw, J., Kapur, N., et al. (2006). Avoidable deaths: five year report by the national confidential inquiry into suicide and homicide by people with mental illness. Published online 2006.

14. Taylor, P.J. and Gunn, J. (1999). Homicides by people with mental illness: myth and reality. *The British Journal of Psychiatry*, **174**, 9–14.

15. Home Office. (2005). Crime in England and Wales 2003/2004. In *Homicide and gun crime, Supplementary* Volume 1 (ed. D. Povey). National Statistics, London.

16. Flynn, S., Shaw, J., and Abel, K. *Homicide of infants: a crosssectional study*. (submitted).

17. Kraemer, G.W., Lord, W.D., and Heilbrun, K. (2004). Comparing single and serial homicide offenses. *Behavioral Sciences & the Law*, **22**, 325–43.

18. Mullen, P. (2004). The autogenic (self-generated) massacre. *Behavioral Sciences & the Law*, **22**, 311–23.

19. Cantor, C.H., Mullen, P.E., and Alpers, P.A. (2000). Mass homicide: the civil massacre. *The* Journal of the American Academy of Psychiatry and the Law, **28**, 55–63.

20. Godwin, G.W. (2000). Hunting serial predators: a multivariate classification approach to profiling violent behaviour. *CRC Press, Boca Raton, FL*.

21. Meloy, J.R. and Felthous, A. (2004). Introduction to this issue: serial and mass homicide. *Behavioral Sciences & the Law*, **22**, 289–90.

22. Putkonen, H., Komulainen, E.J., Virkkunen, M., *et al.* (2003). Risk of repeat offending among violent female offenders with psychotic and personality disorders. *The American Journal of Psychiatry*, **160**, 947–51.

23. Knight, B. (1983). Geriatric homicides—or the Darby and Joan syndrome. *Geriatric Medicine*, **13**, 297–300.

24. Malphurs, J.E., Eisdorfer, C., and Cohen, D. (2001). A comparison of antecedents of homicide-suicide and suicide in older married men. *The American Journal of Geriatric Psychiatry*, **9**, 49–57.

25. Wallace, C., Mullen, P., Burgess, P., *et al.* (1998). Serious criminal offending and mental disorder. Case linkage study. *The British Journal of Psychiatry*, **172**, 477–84.

26. Munro, E. and Rumgay, J. (2000). Role of risk assessment in reducing homicides by people with mental illness. *The British Journal of Psychiatry*, **176**, 116–20.

27. Walsh, E., Buchanan, A., and Fahy, T. (2002). Violence and schizophrenia: examining the evidence. *The British Journal of Psychiatry*, **180**, 490–5.

28. Wessley, S.C., Castle, D., Douglas, A.J., *et al.* (1994). The criminal careers of incident cases of schizophrenia. *Psychological Medicine*, **24**, 483–502.

29. Arsenault, L., Moffitt, T.E., Caspi, A., *et al.* (2000). Mental disorders and violence in a total birth cohort: results from the Dunedin study. *Archives of General Psychiatry*, **57**, 979–86.

30. Brennan, P.A., Grekin, E.R., and Vanman, E.J. (2000). Major mental disorders and crime in the community. In *Violence among the mentally Ill* (ed. S. Hodgins). Kluwer Academic Publishers, Dordrecht.

31. Taylor, P.J. and Gunn, J. (1984). Violence and psychosis 1. Risk of violence among psychotic men. *British Medical Journal*, **288**, 1945–9.

32. Eronen, M., Hakola, P., and Tiihonen, J. (1996). Mental disorders and homicidal behaviour in Finland. *Archives of General Psychiatry*, **53**, 497–501.

# Fraud, deception, and thieves

David V. James

## Introduction

Dishonesty and deception are mundane and ubiquitous elements of human behaviour. Various forms are also categorized as criminal offences in the codes or statutes of all organized societies. In criminological terms, fraud, deception, and theft are forms of stealing, in other words dishonestly depriving others of goods or services. However, deception and fraudulent misrepresentation play a much wider role in human behaviour and interactions. This chapter will first consider briefly the broader picture, before considering in detail psychiatric aspects of stealing.

## Fraud and deception

It is a common tendency to distort memory or reality through the lens of wishful thinking. To deny, to lie to others, and to engage in self-deception is part of the human condition. At one level, this can amount to innocuous forms of self-distraction, such as daydreaming or the childhood world of make-belief. Both blend the borders between fantasy and reality. Deception, which more bluntly put means lying, is on the other hand instrumental in purpose. The essential elements of lying are a conscious awareness of falsity, the intent to deceive and a pre-conceived goal or purpose. In some walks of life, such as advertising or politics, it may be part of the job, at least when the individual thinks that they can get away with it. Deception of others may slide into self-deception, the editing of memory to suit current desires. This may concern a wide range of life's extravagancies, from the fraudulent endeavours of the narcissistic fantasist to the imperatives of those who convince themselves, or wish to convince others, of their own supposed illnesses or infirmities. Particular forms of fraud, deception, and self-deception relevant to the medical context are factitious disorder, malingering, and pathological lying: these are dealt with in Chapter 5.2.9.

## Theft

### Types

Categorization of offences differs between jurisdictions. However, that for England and Wales forms a basic, illustrative framework. Offences are categorized under the Theft Act 1968 into theft, burglary, vehicle offences, and deception. The Theft Act 1978 further clarifies the area of deception (dishonestly obtaining services from another), dividing it into evading liabilities and debts, and making off without payment. The Fraud Act 2006 provides for a general offence of fraud with three ways in which it can be committed—by false representation, by failing to disclose information, and by abuse of position.

### Rates/prevalence

Rates of criminal theft, fraud, and deception can be examined in terms of offences committed per unit of population. In England and Wales, with a population of 53.3 million, the number of reported fraud, theft, and deception offences in 2006 was 2 789 600, which equates to approximately 5.2 per 1 000 total population. These comprised 51 per cent of all crimes reported to the police.[1] However, crime is under-reported to the police and it is notable that the rate of offending as recorded by population survey in England and Wales is generally more than double. International comparisons of crime figures are hampered by differences in classification, measures, and time period.

### A motivational classification of theft

Theft and dishonesty may arise from a range of motives. There is no necessity to invoke mental disorder in order to explain thieving. However, a minority of cases are related to serious mental disorder, such as mania, schizophrenia, depression, and organic brain disorder; and other forms of abnormal psychological processes can act as drivers for criminally dishonest behaviour. These go beyond the formal classification of such behaviours in, for instance, the DSM-IV-TR,[2] where these appear only in the specific syndrome of kleptomania and as a component of the definitions of conduct disorder and anti-social personality disorder.

The following classification is not exhaustive and the categories not mutually exclusive. The great majority of thefts will fit into the first two categories, and it is the remainder that are more likely to form part of a presentation to a psychiatrist.

#### (a) Ordinary theft

Ordinary theft may be planned or impulsive, but is deliberate and motivated by the usefulness of the object or its monetary value.

1 Professional—crime as a career choice.

2 Delinquent—theft as one component of a delinquent or anti-social lifestyle.

3 Survival offences—driven by poverty, desperation, or necessity.

### (b) Emotionally driven theft

Emotionally driven theft is the consequence of emotion, rather than as a means of financial gain.

4 Anger or revenge—based upon depriving someone else, rather than personally acquiring.

5 Fear—coerced into committing an offence by threats from a third party.

6 Excitement—this can be as part of a dare or a rite of passage, particularly in adolescents.

### (c) Secondary theft

Secondary theft is attributable to the presence of an underlying disorder.

### (i) Pecuniary

7 To fund addictive behaviour—e.g. alcohol dependence, drug addiction, pathological gambling.

### (ii) Non-pecuniary

8 Depressed stealing:

(a) cry for help (attention-seeking behaviour): stealing in a way that is sure to be detected in order to obtain support and other help.

(b) suicidal gesture: a depressed persons may steal articles of which they have no need, the action serving as a justification for feelings of guilt and a form of suicidal equivalent.

(c) substitution: the stolen object compensates for something else. For example a rejected wife might steal from her husband in order symbolically to establish a degree of control and compensate for the loss of affection.

(d) distraction: e.g. 'absent-mindedness' in a shop as a consequence of distraction by depressive ruminations, or distress in the context of bereavement or divorce.

9 Manic stealing: stealing in the context of manic disinhibition or delusion.

10 Psychotic: the result of delusional drive or command hallucinations.

11 Confusion: related to cognitive deficit, as a consequence of organic brain disorder, or to dissociative states.

12 'Kleptomania': compulsive stealing as an impulse-control disorder.

## Management

A psychiatrist will only have a role in the management of theft cases where a particular psychiatric or psychological issue is central. The management will depend upon the nature of the underlying disorder. Treatment for the primary disorder will, in most cases, be supplemented by a psychological approach to helping the patient understand the reasons for their offending behaviour, recognize triggers or danger points, and develop strategies for dealing with these in the future.

Kleptomania constitutes a particular diagnostic entity, and shoplifting is a common behaviour which not uncommonly leads to requests for psychiatric reports from the courts. Both will be considered in more detail below.

# Kleptomania

## Definition

Kleptomania is an old term, first used by Marc and Esquirol in 1838 to indicate a 'stealing madness'. Kleptomania was designated a psychiatric disorder in DSM-III in 1980, and, in DSM-IIIR in 1987, it was grouped under the category 'impulse control disorder, not elsewhere classified'. The disorder is described further in Chapter 4.13.1 (Impulse Control Disorders) and only aspects most relevant to forensic practice are considered here.

The core characteristic is that objects are stolen despite the fact that they are typically of little value to the individual, who could have afforded to pay for them. Sometimes, they are hoarded and sometimes dispensed with or returned. DSM-IV-TR describes the essential features of the disorder in five diagnostic criteria (312.33):

(a) 'Recurrent failure to resist impulses to steal objects that are not needed for personal use or for their monetary value.

(b) Increasing sense of tension immediately before committing the theft.

(c) Pleasure, gratification, or relief at the time of committing the theft.

(d) The stealing is not committed to express anger or revenge and is not in response to a delusion or a hallucination.

(e) The stealing is not better accounted for by conduct disorder, a manic episode, or anti-social personality disorder'.

In addition, individuals with kleptomania 'experience the impulse to steal as ego-dystonic and are aware that the act is wrong and senseless'.

## Diagnostic problems

Criterion A, which concerns the senselessness of the theft, is often considered to be the characteristic which separates kleptomania from ordinary theft. However, some kleptomaniacs may desire the items and be able to use them, even if they are not strictly needed: this may be particularly the case with those who hoard.[3] Concerning criteria B and C, some patients report amnesia surrounding the time of the theft and therefore deny feelings or tension immediately beforehand or relief at the time of committing the theft.[3,4] There is also some suggestion that kleptomaniacs who repeatedly steal over long periods eventually lose the feelings of tension and pleasure in a behaviour which has simply become a habit.

There may be overlap with other disorders.[5] Kleptomania and drug addiction share similar core qualities.[6] The presence of repetitive thoughts and behaviours suggests to some a link with the obsessive-compulsive spectrum.[7] With the high comorbidity with depressive disorders, kleptomania might be categorized within the affective spectrum.[8]

## Epidemiology

The prevalence of kleptomania is unknown though it is thought to account for less than 5 per cent of shoplifting.[2] In the US the lifetime prevalence may be 0.6 per cent[3] though some consider that it may be higher because the associated embarrassment and illegality may deter people from reporting it.[9]

A US study of psychiatric inpatients found a lifetime prevalence of 9.3 per cent.[10] While of 107 inpatients with depression,

3.7 per cent had kleptomania[11] and, of 79 inpatients with alcohol dependence, 3.8 per cent reported symptoms consistent with kleptomania.[12]

Kleptomania was generally believed to be much more common in women, but in a summation of four studies of kleptomania 63 per cent were women,[5] suggesting that the preponderance of women is not as great as was once assumed.

### Comorbidity

Kleptomania is highly comorbid with depression and anxiety.[13–15] Estimates of lifetime comorbid rates of mood disorders range from 59[9] to 100 per cent,[16] and of anxiety disorders from 60 to 80 per cent.[17] Some of the comorbidity with depression and anxiety may be secondary to the consequences of the behaviour. Compared with people with alcohol dependence and general psychiatric disorders, those with kleptomania scored significantly higher on measures of impulsivity, sensation-seeking, and disinhibition.[14] In one study,[18] 43 per cent of people with kleptomania met the criteria for at least one personality disorder, the most common being paranoid, schizoid, and borderline. However in a meta-analysis none satisfied the diagnostic criteria for anti-social personality disorder.[19]

### Aetiology

The aetiology of kleptomania is uncertain. Suggested causes include attempts to relieve feelings of depression through stimulation,[20,21] or to make up for early deprivation.[5,22] The various theories are considered further in Chapter 4.13.1

### Treatment

Treatment involves a combined psychological and pharmacological approach. There is little evidence to suggest one particular psychological approach, but a combination of cognitive behaviour therapy and psychosocial interventions is generally adopted. As regards drug treatments, there have been case reports and small series suggesting the efficacy of a range of drugs,[23] in particular selective serotonin re-uptake inhibitors, mood stabilizers, and opioid antagonists. However, there is a need for controlled trials before definitive conclusions can be drawn.

## Shoplifting

Shops specialize in making items seem desirable and tempting to the shopper. Most people shoplift at least once at some point in their lives, usually opportunistically in adolescence. But the incidence of shoplifting remains unknown. An early observational study in the UK[24] suggested that 1 to 2 per cent of customers in an English department stores took items without paying, which compared with 1 in 12 in New York City and 1 in 18 in Dublin. The number of people convicted of shoplifting is evidently far smaller. Whereas earlier studies had suggested that shoplifting was more common in women,[25] this is now thought to have been an artefact of case selection, as samples in most studies have been limited to court samples or sub-samples referred to psychiatrists for reports.[26]

There is no unitary phenomenon of shoplifting. It has been suggested that those who shoplift fall into two groups—those who do so out of rational choice and those that suffer from depression.[27] A survey of 1649 shoplifting convictions in Montréal found that only 3.2 per cent were suffering from serious mental disorder, but

that affective symptoms were relatively common.[28] A further study of 106 shoplifters[26] reported that depression was the most common psychiatric disorder associated with shoplifting and that the majority of shoplifters were poor and unemployed. The range of possible psychiatric disorders associated with shoplifting is indicated in the classification of theft above, but in the large majority of cases of shoplifting, there is no psychiatric reason for avoiding payment.

### Management

A thorough assessment is needed to order to establish how and why the shoplifting occurred and to indicate the presence or absence of underlying mental illness or disorder. Where such illness or disorder is present, it should be treated. Where no such factors are in evidence, psychological therapies may still have a role in offender rehabilitation, usually in a group setting.

## Further information

Grant, J.E. (2005). Kleptomania. In: *Clinical manual of impulse-control disorders,* (eds. E.R. Hollander and D.J. Stein). Arlington, American Psychiatric Publishing, USA, pp 175–201.

Ormerod, D. and Williams, D. (2007). *Smith's Law of Theft* (9th ed). Oxford: Oxford University Press.

## References

1. Lovbakke, J., Taylor, P., and Budd, S. (2007). *Crime in England and Wales: quarterly update to December 2006.* Home Office Statistical Bulletin. Home Office, London.
2. American Psychiatric Association. (2000). *Diagnostic and statistical manual of mental disorders* (4th edn, text revision). American Psychiatric Association, Washington, DC.
3. Goldman, M.J. (1991). Kleptomania: making sense of the non-sensical. *The American Journal of Psychiatry*, **148**, 986–96.
4. Grant, J.E. (2004). Dissociative symptoms in kleptomania. *Psychological Reports*, **94**, 77–82.
5. Grant, J.E. (2005). Kleptomania. In *Clinical manual of impulse-control disorders* (eds. E.R. Hollander and D.J. Stein). American Psychiatric Publishing, Arlington, USA.
6. Grant, J.E. and Potenza, M.N. (2004). Impulse control disorders: clinical characteristics and pharmacological management. *Annals of Clinical Psychiatry*, **16**, 27–34.
7. McElroy, S.L., Phillips, K.A., and Keck, P.E. (1994). Obsessive-compulsive spectrum disorder. *The Journal of Clinical Psychiatry*, **55**, 35–51.
8. McElroy, S.L., Pope, H.G., Keck, P.E., *et al.* (1996). Are impulse control disorders related to bipolar disorder? *Comprehensive Psychiatry*, **37**, 229–40.
9. Grant, J.E. and Kim, S.W. (2002). Clinical characteristics and associated psychopathology of 22 patients with kleptomania. *Comprehensive Psychiatry*, **43**, 378–84.
10. Grant, J.E., Levine, L., Kim, D., *et al.* (2005). Impulse control disorders in adult psychiatric inpatients. *The American Journal of Psychiatry*, **162**, 2184–8.
11. Lejoyeux, M., Arbaretraz, M., McCloughlin, M., *et al.* (2002). Impulse control disorders and depression. *The Journal of Nervous and Mental Disease*, **190**, 310–14.
12. Lejoyeux, M., Feuché, N., Loi, S., *et al.* (1999). Study of impulse-control disorders among alcohol-dependent patients. *The Journal of Clinical Psychiatry*, **60**, 302–5.
13. Sarasolo, E., Bergman, B., and Toth, J. (1996). Personality traits and psychiatric and somatic morbidity among kleptomaniacs. *Acta Psychiatrica Scandinavica*, **94**, 358–64.

14. Baylé, F.J., Caci, H., Millet, B., *et al.* (2003). Psychopathology and comorbidity of psychiatric disorders in patients with kleptomania. *The American Journal of Psychiatry*, **160**, 1509–13.

15. Dannon, P.N., Aizer, A., and Lowengrub, K. (2006). Kleptomania: differential diagnosis and treatment modalities. *Current Psychiatry Reviews*, **2**, 281–3.

16. McElroy, S.L., Pope, H.G., Hudson, J.I., *et al.* (1991). Kleptomania: a report of 20 cases. *The American Journal of Psychiatry*, **148**, 652–7.

17. McElroy, S.L., Hudson, J.I., Pope, H., *et al.* (1992). The DSM-III-R impulse control disorders not elsewhere classified: clinical characteristics and relationship to other psychiatric disorders. *The American Journal of Psychiatry*, **149**, 318–27.

18. Grant, J.E. (2004). Co-occurrence of personality disorders in persons with kleptomania: a preliminary investigation. *The Journal of the American Academy of Psychiatry and the Law*, **32**, 395–8.

19. McElroy, S.L., Hudson, J.I., and Pope, H.G. (1991). Kleptomania: clinical characteristics and associated psychopathology. *Psychological Medicine*, **21**, 93–108.

20. Gudjonnson, G.H. (1987). The significance of depression in the mechanism of 'compulsive' shoplifting. *Medicine, Science, and the Law*, **27**, 171–6.

21. Fishbain, D.A. (1987). Kleptomania as risk-taking behaviour in response to depression. *American Journal of Psychotherapy*, **41**, 598–603.

22. Grant, J.E. and Kim, S.W. (2002). Temperament and early environmental influences in kleptomania. *Comprehensive Psychiatry*, **43**, 223–9.

23. Durst, R., Katz, G., Teitelbaum, A., *et al.* (2001). Kleptomania: diagnosis and treatment options. *CNS Drugs*, **15**, 185–95.

24. Buckle, A. and Farrington, D. (1984). An observational study of shoplifting. *British Journal of Criminology*, **24**, 63–73.

25. Bradford, J. and Balmaceda, R. (1983). Shoplifting: is there a specific psychiatric syndrome? *Canadian Journal of Psychiatry*, **28**, 248–54.

26. Lamontagne, Y., Boyer, R., Hétu, C., *et al.* (2000). Anxiety, significant losses, depression and irrational beliefs in first-offence shoplifters. *Canadian Journal of Psychiatry*, **45**, 63–6.

27. Gudjonsson, G.H. (1990). Psychological and psychiatric aspects of shoplifting. *Medicine, Science, and the Law*, **30**, 45–51.

28. Lamontagne, Y., Carpentier, N., Hétu, C., *et al.* (1994). Shoplifting and mental illness. *Canadian Journal of Psychiatry*, **39**, 300–2.

# Juvenile delinquency and serious antisocial behaviour

## Susan Bailey

## Introduction

Juvenile crime and delinquency represent a significant social and public health concern. Both rates of mental disorders and offending are high during adolescence. This chapter reviews prevalence rates of mental disorders in young offenders, screening, and assessment of juveniles, principles of interventions with young offenders before describing principles of forensic mental health, policy and practice, how mental disorders in adolescence can impact on offending and antisocial behaviour, how policy is shaping practice in this field and how mental health practitioners may be involved in meeting mental health needs and undertaking medico-legal assessments

Delinquency, conduct problems, and aggression all refer to antisocial behaviours that reflect a failure of the individual to conform his or her behaviour to the expectations of some authority figure, to societal norms, or to respect the rights of other people. The 'behaviours' can range from mild conflicts with authority figures, to major violation of societal norms, to serious violations of the rights of others.[1] The term 'delinquency' implies that the acts could result in conviction, although most do not do so. The term 'juvenile' usually applies to the age range, extending from a lower age set by age of criminal responsibility to an upper age when a young person can be dealt with in courts for adult crimes. These ages vary between, and indeed within, countries and are not the same for all offences.[2,3]

## Adolescence as a context

The adolescent population in the UK constitutes half of the child population with around 7.5 million young people in the transitional stage between childhood and adulthood, (age 10–19).[4] Adolescence is a transitional stage of development between childhood and adulthood—a stage of possibility and of promises and worries that attend this possibility. The developmental tasks of adolescence centre on autonomy and connection with others, rebellion and the development of independence, development of identity and distinction from and continuity with others. The physical changes of puberty are generally seen as the starting point of adolescence whilst the end is less clearly delineated. Adolescence ends with attainment of 'full maturity'. A range of social and cultural influences including the legal age of majority, may influence the definition of maturity.[5]

Mortality among adolescents, in contrast to almost all other age groups, did not fall during the second half of the twentieth century, the main causes being accidents and self-harm.[4]. Health needs are greater in this age band than in children in middle childhood (5 to 12 years) or of young adults, and arises out of mainly chronic illness and mental health problems. The main concerns of young people, in relation to health, focus on issues of immediacy that impact on their relations with peers and include problems with skin, weight, appearance, emotions, and sexual health including contraception.

The principal aim of the Youth Justice System (YJS) is to prevent offending by children and young people under 18 years of age. There are 157 Youth Offending Teams in England and Wales. The YJB commissions some 3000 custodial places at any one time for young people under the age of 18 years in 18 Prison Service Young Offenders Institutions, 15 Local Authority Secure Children's Home and 4 private sector Secure Training Centres. In 2005–2006 there were 301,860 recorded offences the 4 highest recorded offences being theft and handling 18.5 per cent, violence against the person 18.1 per cent, motoring offences 16.6 per cent, criminal damage 12.9 per cent. 16 and 17 year old were responsible for 49.6 per cent of offences with males responsible for 80.6 per cent and females 19.4 per cent of all offences resulting in a disposal. Offences by ethnicity were white 85.2 per cent and Black and Ethnic Minority 14.8 per cent. Of the 2 12,242 disposals 80 per cent received pre-court of first tier disposals with 17 per cent receiving a community sentence and 3 per cent a custodial sentence.[6]

Risk factors for, and pathways to antisocial behaviour are summarized in Tables 11.7.1 and 11.7.2 respectively. There is a significant overlap between the risk factors for offending, poor mental health and substance misuse and the number of assessed risk factors increases as a young person moves further into the Youth Justice System.[7] Many young offenders are not engaged in mainstream education and health services. It is critical that these young people are supported to access the mainstream and specialist services they require while under the supervision of the YOT or in custody. Otherwise, once their sentence ends they can become detached from services and their circumstances are likely to deteriorate, leading to more offending and greater demands on specialist services as they get older.

In the UK, the Children's National Service Framework for Children, Young People and Maternity Services (NSF) set out a vision of a comprehensive child and adolescent mental health service.[8]

**Table 11.7.1** Major risk areas in children and adolescents with persistent antisocial behaviour[35]

**Broad child-centred factors**

Genetic vulnerability
Perinatal risk
Male sex
Cognitive impairment
School underachievement
Hyperactivity/inattention temperament

**Family factors**

Criminality in parents and siblings
Family discord
Lack of supervision
Lack of effective feeling
Abuse
Scapegoating
Rejection
Neglect

**Influential contextual factors**

Drug and alcohol abuse
Unemployment
Crime opportunity
Peer group interaction

A young person in contact with the criminal justice system, whether in custody, or in the community, should have the same access to this comprehensive service as any other child or young person within the general population. Treatment options should not be affected by a young offender's status within the criminal justice system. The Change for Children Programme has the aim of improving outcomes for all children in the following 5 areas: being healthy, staying safe; enjoying and achieving; making a positive contribution; and achieving economic well-being, and to narrow the gap in outcomes between those who do well and those who do not. If we do not address the mental health needs of young

**Table 11.7.2** Critical pathway to serious antisocial behaviour[64]

**Family features**

Parental antisocial personality disorder
Violence witnessed
Abuse, neglect, rejection

**Personality features**

Callous unemotional interpersonal style
Evolution of violent and sadistic fantasy
People as objects
Morbid identity
Paranoid ideation
Hostile attribution

**Situational features**

Repeated loss and rejection in relationships
Threats to self-esteem
Crescendo of hopelessness and helplessness
Social disinhibition
Group processes
Changes in mental state over time

offenders then they are excluded from the opportunity to participate in improvements in these 5 outcomes and ultimately from the ability to achieve their full potential.

There is a high prevalence of mental health problems among young people in custody.[9] YJB research published in 2005 reported the following findings.[10]

- 31 per cent had mental health problems
- 18 per cent had problems with depression
- 10 per cent suffered from anxiety
- 9 per cent reported a history of self-harm in the preceding month
- 9 per cent suffered from post-traumatic stress disorder
- 7 per cent had problems with hyperactivity
- 5 per cent reported psychotic-like symptoms

One in five young offenders were identified as having intellectual disability IQ<70. Additionally, needs were identified across education 48 per cent and social relationships 36 per cent. Needs were unmet because they were not recognized.

Research consistently reveals high levels of psychiatric disorders among detained juveniles, although rates vary widely by study, ranging from more than 50 per cent to 100 per cent.[11–21] The variations between the studies may reflect methodological differences or true variations between countries and samples. Advances in developmental psychopathology and increased understanding of the continuities between child and adult life[27] demonstrating that many childhood disorders once thought to resolve with age cast long shadows over later development.

There are several reasons why high rates of mental disorders may be expected in youth in contact with juvenile justice. First, prevalence rates of psychiatric disorders in community samples were shown to be around 15 per cent.[22] Also, severe delinquency is common in the adolescent population, with about 5 per cent showing an early-onset and persistent pattern of antisocial behaviour.[23] A substantial number of adolescents will show offending behaviour and will have a mental health disorder simply because of coincidental overlap between both conditions. Second, because delinquent and antisocial behaviour reaches high levels among juvenile justice populations, a diagnosis of conduct disorder (CD) will often be made. Because CD shows high comorbidity rates with several other psychiatric disorders,[24] increased levels of many types of disorder may be expected. Third, risk factors for youthful offending overlap substantially with those for several types of non-disruptive child psychiatric disorders, therefore identical risk factors may underlie both antisocial behaviour and emotional or developmental problems. Disorders for which mental health interventions are provided, such as substance use disorders (SUD's), may also lead to judicial involvement. Also, because of the prevalence of complex comorbidity, treatment in a regular mental health care programme may be intricate and often is not possible, thus increasing the likelihood of judicial involvement. In addition, severely disordered persons may be less likely to have the personal capability and have adequate resources to defend themselves and to avoid more drastic legal interventions.

Grisso and Zimring listed three principal reasons for concern regarding mental disorders in youthful offenders: a) the obligation to respond to mental health needs in those in custody, b) assurance of due process in adjudicative proceedings, and c) public safety.[25]

Mental health treatment within the juvenile justice system is often inadequate. It has been reported that only about 20 per cent of incarcerated youth with depressive disorders, 10 per cent with other mental disorders, and less than half with SUD receive intervention.[26,27]. Much more research is needed into the treatment needs of this population.

## Risk and protective factors

Understanding is growing of how risk factors combine to both precipitate and maintain antisocial behaviour. Several environmental and individual risk factors including psychiatric pathology in childhood have been identified.[28] Not all risk factors need to be present in a single individual but multiple risk factors greatly increases the risk of a serious and long-term negative development.[29] Positive characteristics or experiences may act protectively. These protective factors may be specific interventions or experienced within the natural contact of development. When protective factors are present, young people may show positive social development despite high risk of antisocial behaviour, or they may abandon their problem behaviour after a difficult phase. Such trajectories are less well investigated than the risks.[30–33] It is also more difficult to implement adequate research designs in this field.[34] It could be assumed that the opposite to the risk value of the variables listed in Table 11.7.1 may promote positive development. However, truly protective effects need to compensate for a given high-risk constellation (moderator approach). The available research suggests a number of factors that may protect from the risks of antisocial behaviour. Table 11.7.3 reports a selection of such personal and social resources that have already been proven or may be promising (for a detailed review see[33]).

## Pathways of care and the juvenile justice system

Juvenile justice is a high-volume system, which makes clear logistics and a clear pathway of care necessary. Early identification of mental health needs may result in diversion from custody by using community services rather than adjudication and derive economic benefit by affording non-custodial disposal. Nonetheless a significant number of young persons progress to pre-trial assessment, albeit from the home or a residential care setting.

Preadjudication dispositions should be informed therefore by best available screening and assessment processes. In this context specific tools may be used to derive markers of psychopathology and of ongoing risk to self and others as well as to address medicolegal questions posed by the criminal justice system including assessment on disposition, matters of public protection, treatment for mental disorders, and need for security and likelihood of recidivism.

For those detained in prison, screening must determine if urgent problems (such as suicidal intent or consequences of substance use) require immediate attention; a detailed diagnostic assessment of the young person may take a longer period of time and continue as the youngster moves from one institution to another. Later critical transitions, for which an additional screening may be useful, include re-entry into the community, assessment of readiness for re-entry, mental health planning for integrated continuing care post detention as part of a multiagency re-entry strategy, and,

**Table 11.7.3** Multilevel examples for protective factors against serious antisocial behaviour[35]

| | |
|---|---|
| Biological/bisocial | - Non-deviant close relatives; no genetic vulnerabilities; high arousal; normal neurological and hormonal functioning. |
| Pre-and perinatal | - Non-alcoholic mother; no maternal smoking during pregnancy; no birth complications |
| Child personality | - Easy temperament; inhibition; ego-resiliency; intelligence; verbal skills; planning for the future; self-control; social problem solving skills; victim awareness; secure attachment; feelings of guilt; school and work motivation; special interests or hobbies; resistance to drugs |
| Cognitions/attitudes | - Non-hostile attributions; non-aggressive response schemes; negative evaluation of aggression; self-efficacy in prosocial behaviour; non-deviant beliefs; realistic self-esteem; sense of coherence. |
| Family | - No poverty; income stability; harmony; acceptance; good supervision; consistency; positive role models; continuity of caretaking; no disadvantage; availability of social support. |
| School | - Achievement and bonding; low rate of aggressive students; climate of acceptance; structure, and supervision. |
| Peer group | - Non-delinquent peers; support from close, prosocial friends. |
| Community | - Non-deprived, integrated and non-violent neighbourhood; availability of professional help. |
| Situational | - Target hardening; victim assertiveness; social control. |
| Legal | - Effective firearm and drug control; effective criminal justice interventions. |
| Cultural | - Low violence; tradition of moral values; shame and guilt-orientation; low exposure to violence in the media. |

where necessary, community residential programmes monitoring emotion or reactions, especially where the young person is returning to stressful conditions such as a troublesome family.

## General principles of assessment

Standard clinical assessment tools used in child and adolescent psychiatry cover many of the areas considered in forensic child and adolescent risk assessments.[36] This is especially important as juvenile justice systems in particular are not always equitable. In choosing between the many scales available it is important to question not just their proven scientific properties but also their feasibility for practitioners to use.

It is important to consider the purpose for which the scale is to be used (see table below). Scales that measure psychopathology may not be good ways of assessing the risk that the psychopathology poses. Measures used to map out types of symptom must have good content validity. An instrument required to pick out one group of symptomatic people from the rest of the community (e.g. mental health screening of young people in custody) needs to have good criterion validity. A related issue is the extent to which the scale is intended to measure change.

## Grid for specifying requirements of a structured scale in a juvenile forensic population
### Assessment required (yes / no)

| Purpose of assessment | Psychopathology | Need | Risk |
|---|---|---|---|
| Screening of all juveniles coming into contact with an agency | | | |
| Detailed assessment e.g. for sentencing, planning treatment | | | |
| Measuring change e.g. during treatment or sentence | | | |

Child psychiatry uses multi-axial and developmental concepts of child psychopathology. Specific and general intellectual delays are very common among young people in the juvenile justice system[10] as is co-morbidity of disorders. Broad-band interviews, however, offer only poor coverage of rare conditions such as pervasive developmental disorders.

## Needs assessment

Needs assessment may have advantages over more traditional ways of diagnosing disorders, mainly because this method also indicates whether specific conditions need attention and intervention. Especially in delinquent youth characterized by multiple problems, such an approach may carry substantial advantage. A health care need should be distinguished from a general need. One commonly used definition of a health care need is '*the ability to benefit in some way from (health) care*'.[37]

Needs and risk assessment are two separate but intertwined processes essential for clinical management (see Fig. 11.7.1). Assessment of danger to others and the need to address this problem is at the centre of legislative and policy decision-making. The attention of the public and media are focussed on this area. Needs assessment may both inform and be a response to the risk-assessment process.[38] The reciprocal process can be termed 'risk management' when accurate information about the risk assessment, combined with recurrent needs assessment, leads to risk-management procedures. A recurrent needs-assessment and risk-assessment process should identify changes in problem areas, thus leading to monitoring or intervention as part of risk management. Core to this assessment are appropriate mental health screening tools and processes that are available to the young person at any point in the system.[39]

## Risk assessment

Risk assessment combines statistical data with clinical information in a way that integrates historical variables, current crucial variables, and the contextual or environmental factors. Structured risk assessment instruments have been developed that aim to increase the validity of clinical prediction. These scales typically contain a number of risk items selected from reviews of research, crime theories, and clinical considerations.[41,42] Items are summed to form a total risk score and may also reveal specific risk patterns (e.g. mainly family or child factors). Such instruments are used for screening, in-depth assessment and related risk management (e.g. for decisions on the child's placement or specific interventions). They can also be applied in differentiated evaluations of intervention programmes. Instruments vary with respect to the age and gender for their clients, problem intensity in the target groups, theoretical and empirical foundations, the number and domains of risk included, scoring procedures, time required for assessment, information sources, institutional contexts of administration and other issues.[43,44] Many instruments have been designed for application in the juvenile justice system.[43,45,46] Most instruments contain factors from various areas of risk (e.g. individual, family, neighbourhood).

## Mental disorders and offending

Current concepts focus on a developmental approach to psychopathology in child and adolescent psychiatry and psychology. Physical aggression peaks at around the second year of life and subsequently shows distinct developmental trajectories.[47,48] Attachment enables the mastery of aggression, self-control being developed through the efficient exercise of attritional mechanisms and symbolization. Fonagy has suggested a primary developmental role for early attachment in the development of mentalization (the capacity to understand others' subjective experience). He suggests that impaired mentalization leads to later violence.[49] Threats to self-esteem trigger violence in individuals whose self-appraisal is 'on shaky ground' and are unable to see behind the threats to what is in the mind of the person threatening them. These processes are played out in the complex and toxic co-morbidities seen so much more frequently in child and adolescent than in adult mental health practice.

## Oppositional disorders, conduct disorder, and ADHD

Substantially higher rates of physically aggressive behaviour are found in children and adolescents with attention deficit hyperactivity disorder, with those who meet the criteria for ADHD and conduct disorder having substantially greater risks of delinquent acts in adolescence, harmful acts in later adolescence and continued violence and offending into adulthood.[50] Children with hyperactivity, impulsivity, attention deficits and serious conduct problems may also be at risk for developing psychopathy.[51]

Distorted or biased thought processes have over time been implicated in the development of violence. Psychological treatments aimed at reducing violent behaviour in adolescents and young adults traditionally centre on violence as learned behaviour. Patterns of violence and criminal behaviour are seen as embedded in habits of thinking.[52] In juvenile delinquents significant cognitive attributional bias has been shown in aggressive children and youths. They are more likely to perceive neutral acts by others as hostile, and more likely to believe conflicts can be satisfactorily resolved by aggression. In the social context, as the young individual becomes more disliked and rejected by peers, the opportunity for viewing the world this way increases.[53] By their late teens they can hold highly suspicious attitudes and be quick to perceive disrespect from others. In the social context of juvenile incarceration,

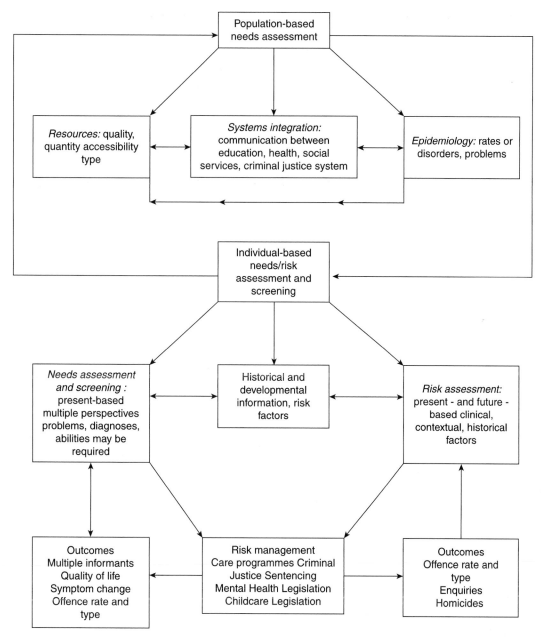

**Fig. 11.7.1** Relationship between various screening, need assessment, risk assessment, and management approaches in juvenile justice systems.[40] (Reproduced from Kroll, L. Needs assessment in adolescent offenders. In Adolescent forensic psychiatry (eds. Bailey, S. Dolan, M.), copyright 2004, Hodder Education.)

being 'para'[54] can become in peer group interactions the shared norm.[55]

## Depression anxiety and post traumatic stress disorder in childhood and adolescence

As well as the recognized feelings of low mood in depression there is also some evidence of irritability, hostility and anger when depression occurs in adolescence. Irritability in adolescence leads to interpreting annoyances by others as direct threats, increasing the risk of defensive aggression.[56] Nowhere is this more apparent than in juvenile justice populations.[57,58] A self-serving bias with

a tendency to attribute good outcomes to the self and bad outcomes to external causes observed in ordinary people, is usually regarded as a mechanism for maintaining self-esteem in the face of threats to the self.

PTSD is related to the conditioning of neurobiological fear responses underlying tendencies to react aggressively to protect the self when exposed to reminders of earlier trauma.[59] In the recent escalating context of both children who have experienced violence in war torn countries and those who live in a context of 'urban war zones' Garbarino[60] sets out an ecological framework to explain the process and conditions that transform the 'developmental challenge' of violence into developmental harm in some children. He set out an accumulation of risk models for understanding how and when children suffer the most adverse consequences of exposure to community violence and go beyond their limits of resilience, the concept of 'social maps' as products of childhood experiences and of trauma as a psychological wound.

The combination of depression, anxiety and severe PTSD is being increasingly recognized in as being linked to trajectory into adult anti-social personality disorder.[61]

## Autism spectrum disorders and learning disability

Autism spectrum disorders are being increasingly recognized in adolescent forensic populations. Their identification is critical to the understanding of violent offending. This is particularly so if an offence or assault is bizarre in nature, the degree or nature of aggression is unaccountable and/or there is a stereotypic pattern of offending. Four reasons have been proposed for offending and aggression in autistic persons:[62,63]

1  Their social naivety may allow them to be led into criminal acts by others;

2  Aggression may arise from a disruption of routines;

3  Antisocial behaviour may stem from a lack of understanding or misinterpretation of social cues;

4  Crimes may reflect obsessions, especially when these involved morbid fascination with violence—there are similarities with the intense and obsessional nature of fantasies described in some adult sadists.[64]

It has been proposed that the paranoia observed in Asperger's syndrome has a different quality from that seen in people with a diagnosis of schizophrenia stemming from a confusion of not understanding the subtleties of social interaction and social rules.[54]

## Early onset psychosis

Non-psychotic behavioural disturbance occurs in about half of cases of early-onset schizophrenia and can last between 1 and 7 years. It includes externalizing behaviours, attention-deficit disorder and conduct disorder. This emphasizes the need for mental health assessments repeated over time to include a focus on changes in social functioning (often from an already chaotic baseline level) to a state including perceptual distortion, ideas of reference, and delusional mood.[65]

As in adult life most young people with schizophrenia are non-delinquent and non-violent.[66] Nevertheless, there may be an increased risk of violence to others when they have active symptoms, especially when there is misuse of drugs or alcohol. The risk of violent acts is related to subjective feelings of tension, ideas of violence, delusional symptoms that incorporate named persons known to the individual, persecutory delusions, fear of imminent attack, feelings of sustained anger and fear, passivity experiences reducing the sense of self-control, and command hallucinations. Protective factors include responding to and compliance with physical and psychosocial treatments, good social networks, a valued home environment, no interest in or knowledge of weapons as a means of violence, good insight into the psychiatric illness and any previous violent aggressive behaviour and a fear of their own potential for violence. These features require particular attention but the best predictors of future violent offending in young people with mental disorder are the same as those in the general adolescent population.[67]

## Psychopathic personality in young people

A three-factor structure has been proposed,[68] which includes:

♦ An arrogant, deceitful interpersonal style, involving dishonesty, manipulation, grandiosity and glibness;

♦ Defective emotional experience, involving lack of remorse, poor empathy, shallow emotions, and a lack of responsibility for one's own actions;

♦ Behavioural manifestations of impulsiveness, irresponsibility, and sensation-seeking.

Conduct disorder, antisocial personality disorder, and psychopathy are often seen as developmental disorders that span the life course and the terms are sometimes used interchangeably. Conduct disorder and antisocial personality disorder primarily focus on behavioural problems, psychopathy, as described by Hare,[69] emphasizes deficits in affective and interpersonal functioning.

A consensus is likely to be reached only when we have longitudinal studies demonstrating the stability of psychopathic traits over the lifespan and evidence that the same aetiological factors contribute to this disorder at all ages. As there is significant overlap between the behavioural aspects of juvenile psychopathy and ADHD and between the callous-unemotional dimension of psychopathy and autistic-spectrum disorders, future work needs to disentangle these constructs from a phenomenological and aetiological perspective. As yet, there are few treatment outcome studies in juveniles with psychopathic traits, although the limited data suggest that these traits might be a moderator of outcome. Most clinicians view youth psychopathy as a potentially treatable disorder, and there is some evidence that identification of psychopathic traits in young people has a number of benefits, which include:

♦ Identifying high-risk offenders;

♦ Reducing misclassifications that have negative ramifications for children and adolescents;

♦ Improving and optimizing treatment planning for young people with psychopathic traits, who may require more intensive and risk focused therapeutic approaches.

## Interventions with juvenile delinquents

A large number of different treatments have been used to reduce antisocial behaviour. These include psychotherapy, pharmacotherapy, school interventions, residential programmes, and social treatments. Kazdin reported over 230 available psychotherapies, the great majority of which had not been systematically studied.[70] This chapter will focus on treatments with a testable scientific basis which have been evaluated in randomized trials and applied to populations of young offenders.[71]

Meta-analyses of treatment approaches to juvenile delinquency have produced reasonably consistent findings.[72–75] Lipsey[73] considered nearly 400 group-comparison studies published since 1950. The main finding was that there was an overall reduction of 10 per cent in re-offending rates in treatment groups as compared to untreated groups. As might be expected, there were of course considerable variations in the results of individual studies. The best results were obtained from cognitive behavioural, skills-orientated, and multi-modal methods. The results from deterrent trials were particularly poor, though the numbers in these studies were relatively small. Specifically, treatment approaches that were participatory, collaborative and problem-solving were particularly likely to be beneficial. Family and parenting interventions also seem to reduce the risk of subsequent delinquency among older children and adolescents.[76]

McGuire and Priestley[52] identified six principles for effective programmes:

1  Intensity should match the extent of the risk posed by the offender.

2  A focus on active collaboration, which is not too didactic or unstructured.

3  Close integration with the community

4  Emphasis on behavioural or cognitive approaches.

5  Delivered with high quality with training and monitoring of staff.

6  Focus on the proximal causes of offending behaviour (peer groups, promoting current family communication, and enhancing self-management and problem-solving skills) rather than distal causes (early childhood).

The reviews suggest that there are a number of promising targets for treatment programmes, which include antisocial thoughts, antisocial peer associations, promotion of family communication and affection, promotion of family supervision, identification of positive role models, improving problem-solving skills, reducing chemical dependencies, provision of adequate living conditions, and helping the young offender to identify high risk situations for antisocial behaviours. Conversely, the systematic reviews have also suggested a number of approaches that are unlikely to be promising. For instance, improving self-esteem without reducing antisocial cognitions is unlikely to be of value. Similarly, it is unlikely that a focus on emotional symptoms that is not clearly linked to criminal conduct will be of great benefit.

Life experiences associated with treatment ressistance are summarized in table 11.7.4.

## Promising interventions for adolescent antisocial behaviour

A rational starting point when considering interventions would be to consider the main causal factors and processes (see above), and

**Table 11.7.4** Life experiences associated with treatment resistance

| |
|---|
| Early modelling experiences |
| Early exposure to related phenomena |
| Enduring antisocial behaviours and aggressive response patterns |
| Limited judgement skills |
| Low academic achievement |
| Clusters of confrontative acts |
| Personality traits of callousness |
| Jealousy and revenge |
| Limited parental/carer supervision |
| Erratic punishment schedules |
| Absent, neglecting, or abusive parenting |
| Parental psychopathology |

Reproduced from Losel F, Bender D, Protective factors and resilience. In (eds. Farrington DP, Cold JW) Prevention of Adult antisocial behaviour, p. 130–204. copyright 2003, with permission of Cambridge University Press.

design interventions around them. However, in practice many other considerations have shaped interventions, from the desire to punish offending youths, to making use of what is currently available at relatively low cost. For generic interventions for conduct disorder also highly relevant to juvenile delinquency and serious antisocial behaviour (see Chapter 9.2.5).

## Working with young offenders with mental health problems—some practice points for interventions

Interventions with juvenile offenders, regardless of whether they are addressing offending behaviour or mental health problems, should take into account developmental and cognitive factors significant to this age group. Interventions designed for use with adults are usually highly structured and target driven. This style of intervention is often perceived by juvenile offenders as alienating and not relevant to their lives with the result that they are likely to disengage (either actively or passively) from the programme.

The skills required to engage a juvenile offender in a 'therapeutic alliance' are often different to those necessary with adult offenders. Adult offenders are more likely to see the value of participating in an enhanced thinking skills course, possibly as a means to an early release or to improve the quality of relationships within their family unit. Such goals may be perceived as too long range to have any meaning to a juvenile offender, or simply seem irrelevant. Juvenile offender's general experience of relationships with adults, particularly professionals, is of authority figures that give instructions, set limits on behaviour, and at best are givers of information. The typical responses to this are to adopt an aggressive posture or one of passive indifference. To actively engage with juvenile offenders professionals need to listen attentively and show interest in the young person's perspective. This does not mean agreeing with the young person's point of view; however, it is an opportunity to establish the 'middle ground' within which a therapeutic alliance may be fostered.

Adolescent offenders have often experienced unstable lives with disrupted attachments. Thus they often have difficulty in understanding the significance of life events such as trauma and bereavement that an adult will readily understand is likely to impact on emotional well being. A thorough assessment prior to commencing an intervention and drawing on material from multiple sources, particularly parents or professionals who have a detailed knowledge of the young person, is very helpful. Events such as the loss of a parent and the onset of conduct problems are often closely linked temporally, yet young offenders frequently do not see any connection between such events.

A formulation is a brief statement that summarizes the possible links between different aspects of the young person's life, for instance between a bereavement and the onset of behavioural difficulties. Juvenile offenders are often unable to make formulations because of their failure to understand how different elements of their lives are connected. The ability to make formulations can be seen as a developmental milestone and adolescent offenders, for the reasons identified above, often lag behind their own peer group as well as the adult population. Regardless of whether addressing offending behaviours or mental health problems, professionals working with juvenile offenders need to generate such formulations collaboratively so that they make sense both within the therapeutic framework and also within the young person's life experience.

Establishing therapeutic goals also needs to be collaborative and developmentally appropriate. Adolescence in general is characterized as a time of heightened emotional responses (partly as a result of hormonal changes), a growing but still limited capacity for problem solving and the tendency to seek immediate advantage rather than long-term gain. All of these factors are likely to be enhanced in juvenile offenders in contrast with the rest of their peer group. Goal setting therefore needs to concentrate heavily on the short-term, i.e. within the young person's perceived time frame. Targets and rewards should be low key in order to reduce the likelihood of extreme emotional responses to success or failure. Therapists working with juvenile offenders need to be active in encouraging the generation of alternative solutions in order to extend the young persons range of problem solving skills.

Juvenile offenders' capacity to generate alternative strategies is often limited by their own, limited emotional range. They will typically respond to any adverse event with hostility and anger; events that would typically evoke a response of sadness or fear within adults. Work on emotional recognition with juvenile offenders will assist them in recognizing a wider range of emotions, both in themselves and others. This enhances their range of options when faced with future adverse events.

There is often a tendency to concentrate on behavioural objectives as the most easily recognized or measured outcomes. However, working on goals such as recognizing and managing arousal levels, or shifting cognitions or attributions in specific situations may prove more beneficial in the longer term even if immediate behavioural changes are not achieved.

Goal setting and intervention strategies should be individually tailored and take into account differences in cognitive ability, maturity and insight within this population. To ensure the young person remains actively engaged in the intervention process it is important to frequently check out their perception of how effective the therapy is, and whether the goals and strategies are relevant. Therapists should frequently check the young person's level of understanding to ensure that the communication is two way and repeats elements or themes as necessary to ensure good compliance and comprehension, rather than adhering to a timetable.

## Treatment and special crimes

### Juvenile homicide

Violent behaviour often involves a loss of sense of personal identity and of personal value. A young person may engage in actions without concern for future consequences or past commitments.

Violence denotes the 'forceful infliction of physical injury'.[77] Aggression involves harmful, threatening or antagonistic behaviour.[78] Longitudinal studies are invaluable in mapping out the range of factors and processes that contribute to the development of aggressive behaviour and in showing how they are causally related.[79] However, in attempting to work with any individual who has committed a violent act, the question to be answered is 'why this individual has behaved in this unique fashion on this occasion'.[73]

Studies show that children and adolescents who murder share a constellation of psychological, cognitive, neuropsychiatric, educational and family system disturbance.[80–82] In the UK, young people who commit grave sadistic crimes including juvenile homicide are liable to periods of lengthy incarceration. Detention itself can provide time for further neuro-developmental, cognitive, and emotional growth. Irrespective of treatment models, the provisions of education, vocational training, consistent role models and continued family contact are of critical importance.

The approach to juvenile delinquency, including juvenile homicide, in the Netherlands is determined by a policy of minimal intervention, with a strongly pedagogical point of view. The emphasis lies on education and treatment rather than on punishment. Cases recorded by the police as murder or manslaughter in the first instance may not ultimately be presented to court as such. Moreover, the pedagogical nature of the punishments is recognizable in the fact that treatment is ordered in most cases, in the form of placement in a juvenile institution, sometimes in combination with imprisonment, rather than a straightforward youth detention or imprisonment. There are no indications of special policies for prosecuting or handling the cases of legal minors suspected of murder or manslaughter. The limited prevalence of this phenomenon is undoubtedly partly due to the fact that every case is judged on its own merits. Incidentally, this is also noted in the USA where a considerably higher number of youths are sentenced for murder and manslaughter.[83]

Youths who have been prosecuted for murder or manslaughter vary only slightly or not al all from other juvenile delinquents on points such as age, gender and ethnic background, and only to a limited extent on risk factors. Murder and manslaughter are committed alone comparatively more often, and on average the perpetrators start their criminal activities at a later age and are much less likely to have previous convictions than other minors taken into judicial youth institutions. At the same time, it is clear that while the group of youths involved in murder and manslaughter may be small, it is anything but homogeneous. There is great variety in terms of motives, victims, modus operandi etc. In simple terms each case stands on its own.

The majority of young persons who have killed initially dissociate themselves from the reality of their act, but gradually experience a progression of reactions and feelings akin to a grief reaction. The young person whilst facing a still adversarial, and public pretrial and trial process has to move safely through the process of disbelief, denial, loss, grief and anger/blame. Post traumatic stress disorder arising from the participation in the sadistic act (either directly or observing the actions of co-defendants) has to be treated, as does trauma arising from their own past personal emotional, physical and/or sexual abuse.

A combination of verbal and non-verbal therapies are effective but qualities such as previous frequent and severe aggression, low intelligence and a poor capacity for insight weigh against a safe outcome.[84] In understanding the role of violence and sadism in a young person's life one has to understand the depth of their sensitivity and reaction to perceived threat and their past maladaptive behaviours aimed at allowing them to feel in control of their lives. In coming to terms with their internal rage, addressing victim empathy saying sorry and reattribution of blame, expression of anger and distress within sessions is expected and is often sexualized in both form and content. This can spill outside sessions when the young person and carers can become collusively dismissive and rejecting of therapists,[85] emphazing the importance of intensive work to prepare the young person for transition from long term incarceration and re-entry into the community together with extended aftercare.

## Sexually abusive behaviour

Sexually inappropriate behaviour in children and adolescents constitutes a substantial health and social problem.[86] Most, but not all, abusers are male, often come from disadvantaged backgrounds with a history of victimization, and sexual and physical abuse[87] and show high rates of psychopathology.[88] Of particular concern are a significant subgroup with mild intellectual disability whose treatment programmes have to be tailored to their level of development and cognitive ability. Young abusers come within the Criminal Justice System but also should be considered in their own right within the child protection framework. Most adult sexual abusers of children started their abuse when adolescents and yet neither ICD10 nor DSMIV has a diagnostic category for paedophilia in those under 16.

A structured carefully planned multi-agency approach is required when working with sexually aggressive younger children and sexually abusive adolescents. The three stages to assessment of juvenile sexual offenders are:

1 Clarification and rapport building

2 Mapping the abuse: the fantasies, strategies and behaviours; and

3 The future, placement treatment and personal change.
The treatment process occurs in the context of:

- The crisis of disclosure;

- Family assessment;

- Therapeutic work in a protective context for the victim; and

- Reconstruction and reunification of the family.

The 'family' in this context may include foster carers, or long term residential carers.

## Treatment outcome

The earliest possible interventions with young over-sexualized children, before their patterns of sexually aggressive behaviours become entrenched, are likely to be most effective. However, there is a dearth of longitudinal follow-up studies looking at treatment outcomes with this younger group of children.

Outcomes may be measured by looking at recidivism, treatment outcome or other measures. At present, there are no longitudinal outcome studies of children and adolescents with sexually abusive behaviour which have measured other outcomes such as adult adjustment, attitudinal change or parenting.

Recidivism as a sole outcome measures for treatment is unlikely to be reliable since persistent sexual behaviour problems in children under the age of criminal responsibility will not appear in crime statistics and conviction statistics for sex offenders of all ages are notoriously unreliable for a variety of reasons including failure to report victimization experiences, failure to proceed with charges and a high rate of trial failures.

Other factors appear to be highly relevant to treatment outcomes with juvenile sexual abusers such as good interprofessional communication and a systemic context for treatment to occur.

New approaches to CBT with sexually abusing youths have recently been described within the context of relapse prevention and a more complex CBT intervention, Mode Deactivation Therapy (MDT), has been suggested for disturbed, sexually abusive young people with reactive conduct disorders or personality disorders[89] CBT group work with sexually abusing children and young people is widely practised in the UK and the principles of this work are described by Print and O'Callaghan.[90]

Other treatment approaches will take into account the living context of the young person and the need for his or her carers to be provided with support and explanation of the treatment process in order to maximize positive results. For instance, when children and young people who sexually abuse are still living at home or in contact with their parents, family work is usually needed. An approach to group work with parents of children with sexually abusive behaviour has been described.[91] In the case of children and young people who are living in the care system, concurrent work for the professionals and carers looking after the sexually abusing child or young person has been strongly advocated.

There are a significant number of mid-adolescent, recidivist, delinquent, sexually abusive youths who are too dangerous to other children and young people to be treated (with any treatment modality) alongside other young people. Many of these young people have been through the court system or are currently facing charges. For these reasons, treatment of the sexually abusive young person needs to be undertaken within a close supervized, intensive, community-based foster placement with specially trained foster carers who are experienced in dealing with young offenders, risk and dangerousness. This type of approach is known by various names such as Multidimensional Treatment Foster Care[92] or forensic foster care.[93] Early results from small-scale studies with this type of intervention are reasonably encouraging.

Outcomes claimed for these approaches include significantly fewer subsequent criminal referrals and more incarcerated boys returning to live with relatives, compared with those who received group home care alone.[92] In a seven-year study of forensic foster care at the Treatment for Appropriate Social Control (TASC), Yokely and Boettner[93] describe a social responsibility model to teach recidivist youths 'pro-social skills and values that compete with antisocial behaviour'.

Dynamic psychotherapy aims to work at an unconscious level with the sexually abusive young person to explore and understand the reasons for his persistent behaviour. However, evidence-based treatment outcome studies have not yet been undertaken for dynamic therapy with juvenile sexual abusers. A clinical description of long-term dynamic therapy[94] with these children emphasizes the need to establish a systemic child protection context for the safe delivery of such treatment.

In summary, the components of effective treatment interventions with children and young people who sexually abuse will include the following:

- A well planned, systemic, child protection orientated, treatment context.

- Treatment should be one of a number of positive interventions into the life of the young person and his or her family.

- All interventions should be part of an agreed inter-agency care plan for the young person.

- Offence-specific interventions, such as CBT, aimed at straightening out the distorted cognitions and self-justifications of sexually abusing young people should be the core of any intervention programme for this client group.

- Treatment programmes not focussed solely on the victimization of the young person.

- Interventions should occur at all possible levels including individual work with young person, family work (where relevant), support for foster carers or for professional care staff and consultation to the professional network.

## Firesetting/arson

Arson can have a devastating impact on the victim and the wider society. Juvenile arsonists are not a homogenous group, with a wide range of familial,[95] social,[96] developmental interpersonal,[97] clinical and 'legal' needs. Kolko and Kazdin[98] highlighted the importance of attraction to fire, heightened arousal, impulsivity and limited social competence. As with other forms of serious antisocial behaviours, no single standard treatment approach will be appropriate for all individuals.[99] In addition to the general assessment of antisocial behaviour the specific domains to be considered include:

- history of fireplay;

- history of hoax telephone calls;

- social context of firesetting (whether alone or with peers);

- where the fires were set;

- previous threats/targets;

- type of fire, single/multiple seats of fire setting;

- motivation (anger resolution, boredom, rejection, cry for help, thrill seeking, fire fighting, crime concealment, no motivation, curiosity, and peer pressure).

For recidivistic firesetters therapy may include:

- Psychotherapy to increase the understanding of the behaviour, including antecedents defining the problem behaviour, and establishing the behavioural reinforcers;

- Skills training—to promote adaptive coping mechanisms;

- Understanding environmental factors to manage or self trigger solutions;

- Counselling to reduce psychological distress;

- Behavioural techniques to extinguish the behaviour;

- Education to promote understanding of cause and effect; and

- Supervision for the staff caring for the adolescent.

Early modelling experiences and early exposure to related phenomena militate against a good outcome.

## The role of specialist child and adolescent mental health services in medico–legal assessment

In the case of T&V v United Kingdom[100] it was stated that a child's age, level of maturity and intellectual and emotional capacities must be taken into account when they are charged with a criminal offence and that appropriate steps should be taken in order to promote their ability to understand and participate in the court proceedings. A responsibility therefore falls on the defence lawyer to be aware of the possibility that a young person may not be able to participate effectively in the trial process, particularly if they are under 14 years old or have learning problems, or a history of absence from school.[101] In 1985, the Office of the High Commissioner for Human Rights, in reference to the age of criminal responsibility stated that there is a close relationship between the notion of responsibility for delinquent or criminal behaviour and other social rights and responsibilities.

All young defendants, regardless of the offences they charged with, should be tried in youth courts with permission for adult sanctions for older youths if certain conditions are met. This should enable a mode of trial for young defendants to be subject to safeguards that can enhance understanding and participation. Assessment of cognitive and emotional capacities should occur before any decisions on venue and mode of trial take place.

### Capacity

One fundamental distinction in the criminal law is between conditions that negate criminal liability and those that might mitigate the punishment deserved under particular circumstances. Very young children and the profoundly mentally ill may lack the minimum capacity necessary to justify punishment. Those exhibiting less profound impairments of the same kind may qualify for a lesser level of deserved punishment even though they may meet the minimum conditions for some punishment. Immaturity, like mental disorder, can serve both as an excuse and as mitigation in the determination of just punishment. Capacity is sometimes thought of as a generic skill that a person either has or lacks. However, that is not so. To begin with, it is multifaceted, with four key elements. These are as follows:

1 The capacity to understand information relevant to the specific decision at issue (understanding).

2 The capacity to appreciate one's situation as the defendant is confronted with a specific legal decision (appreciation).

3 The capacity to think rationally about alternative course of action (reasoning).

4 The capacity to express a choice among alternatives.[102]

The second key point is that capacity is a feature that is both situation-specific and open to influence.

Any evaluation of competence should include assessment of possibly relevant psychopathology, emotional understanding as well cognitive level, the child's experiences and appreciation of situations comparable to the one relevant to the crime and to the trial, and any particular features that may be pertinent in this individual and this set of circumstances.[103] The general principles to be used in the assessment are broadly comparable to those employed in any clinical evaluation. However, particular attention needs to be paid to developmental background, emotional and cognitive maturity, trauma, exposure and substance misuse. The likely appropriate sources for obtaining clinical data relevant to assessment of a juvenile's competence to stand trial will include a variety of historical records, a range of interviews and other observations and in some cases, specialized tests. Records of the child's school functioning, past clinical assessment, treatment history and previous legal involvements need to be obtained. In coming to an overall formulation, there should be a particular focus on how both developmental and psychopathological features may be relevant to the forensic issues that have to be addressed.

The main focus is on the youth's ability to understand and cope with the legal process. This comes from three sources, direct questioning of the defendant, inferences from the functioning in other areas and direct observation of the defendant's behaviour and interaction with others. It is useful to enquire about the youth's expectations about what the consequences of the court involvement might prove to be. Because of the course of juvenile proceedings can vary so widely, with consequences ranging from the extremely aversive to extremely beneficial, rational understanding will necessarily involve a high degree of uncertainty. Potentially relevant problems include: inattention, depression, disorganization of thought processes that interfered with the ability to consider alternatives; hopelessness, such that the decision is felt not to matter, delusion or other fixed beliefs that distort understanding of options (or their likely outcomes), maturity of judgement and the developmental challenges of adolescence.

In providing information to the court, written reports have the advantage of a standard format that helps the consultant to be sure that s/he has considered all the relevant questions; it also provides a familiar structure for readers. In essence, for the sake of consistency and clarity, competence reports need to cover the following areas:

1  Identifying information and referral questions.

2  The description of the structure of the evaluation including sources and a notation of the confidentiality expectations.

3  The provision of clinical and forensic data.

Grisso[104] suggested that psychiatric assessment of competence in young people should include assessment of:

◆ understanding of the charges and the potential consequences

◆ understanding of the trial process

◆ capacity to communicate with their defence lawyer

◆ general ability to participate in the courtroom proceedings.

In court, a child's ability to give an account of events can be impaired by a number of factors, including poor physical health on the day of the trial, overwhelming anxiety or anger about giving evidence, or intimidation by the physical surroundings of the court. From a psychological perspective, however, the basic evidential capacity of the child defendant will depend on two main components:

◆ The child's mental state—this needs to be stable, therefore any disturbance that might interfere with the child's perception of the world and the ability to understand it will impair evidential capacity;

◆ The child's cognitive ability—a concept that includes a large number of facets, such as memory, understanding and the ability to communicate. The last includes both verbal (speech) and non-verbal means, as well as the ability both to comprehend and to express thought. Any psychological assessment therefore has to be across a range of domains.

Discrepancies are particularly likely in the areas of educational achievement, adaptive skills and social and emotional development.

A child's ability often is gauged on educational achievement and given as being equivalent to that of a certain age—e.g. a 15-year-old child might have the everyday living skills of a 7-year-old. However, a child who might be unable to cope with monetary change or public transport might well have the emotional and social experiences of an older child and the drives of an adolescent.

When discussing developmental psychology and child development, it is important to bear in mind that none of these processes operates in a vacuum. The child's experience of parenting (important in relation to physical and emotional development), the provision of appropriate role models (moral development and self-control depend heavily on appropriate modelling and social learning) and the learning environment (whether it fostered or hindered intellectual development) all have a vital role. For instance, during adolescence, as young people take on a wider and more social perspective and become integrated within a peer group, they will nevertheless tend to adopt social values and norms (i.e. ideas about 'right and wrong') that are very similar to those of their parents. Hence, despite any demonstrations of teenage rebellion (often short-lived), the majority of adolescents will tend to adopt parental mores, either law-abiding or delinquent.

It should be emphasised that clear-cut ages do not apply to the completion of physical, intellectual, emotional, and social development. For most young people, given appropriate parenting, normal biological development and a structured, emotionally supportive and stimulating environment, the bulk of the aforementioned processes should be achieved by late teenage years and a considerable degree of intellectual maturation may have occurred by the age of 14 years.

When delivering forensic mental health services for children and adolescents it is important that the services are developed in such a way that their needs are met and that the services build on established concepts of service design in line with a strategic framework. Doing so will require long term planning that actively addresses the requirements of an adequate size and composition of an appropriately trained, supervized and managed workforce. Such services should be developed with an awareness of the scope of existing services and recognition of current demands, analysing gaps current services.

## Adolescent girls

Longitudinal data demonstrates that girlhood aggression contributes to a cascading set of negative outcomes as young women move into adolescence and adulthood.

Young girls who engage in disruptive behaviour and fight are at risk for:

◆ Being rejected by peers

◆ Feeling alienated

◆ Feeling unsupported in their relationships with peers and adults

◆ Struggling academically

◆ Affiliating with other peers prone to deviant behaviour

◆ Becoming involved in more serious antisocial behaviours

◆ Choosing antisocial romantic partners

◆ Initiating and receiving partner violence

- Becoming adolescent mothers

- Having children with more health problems

- Being less sensitive and responsive as parents

Some are sufficiently antisocial and even violent, they are incarcerated, if they are also mothers they may lose custody of their children and opportunities for stable employment and relationships are much diminished.

Given low base rates of girls engaging in physical aggression and violence, identifying girls at risk is a critically important step for prevention and intervention programmes.

High-risk groups of girls to target include those girls who are temperamentally overactive as toddlers and pre-schoolers (fewer than boys) but even more important to target for early identification and intervention. Those who have early pubertal development (girls report engaging high levels of bullying as they enter puberty). They may be likely targets as well as perpetrators and sexually abused girls—especially those abused by their biological fathers over a long period of time.

From the available literature interventions to reduce rates of aggression, relational aggression and violence in female children and adolescents should address the following:

1 Pre-natally delivery of programmes for high-risk expectant mothers, (especially young mothers and those themselves aggressive or disruptive as children).

2 Augment the parenting skills of at risk young mothers—the evidence show children of young mothers with histories of girlhood aggression may themselves be more prone to infection and injuries.

   (a) Provide additional parenting skills around key issues of hygiene, child proofing of homes, good nutrition, meal planning and household management.

   (b) Help young mothers to respond optimally to the perceived challenging behaviour of their infants and toddlers.

3 Middle childhood, girls episodes of physical aggression are often preceded by relational aggression. Interventions to help these girls may include how to:

- Relate to others

- Manage strong emotions

- Understand own aggressive feelings and recognize when own aggression is adaptive in the immediate situation.

- Understand how 'girl talk' ignites hurtful indirect social relational aggression.

- Understand how relational aggression lead to physical violence for some girls towards peers, adults and partners

## Conclusions

The major challenge of altering the trajectories of persistent young offenders has to be met in the context of satisfying public demands for retribution, together with welfare and civil liberties considerations. In England and Wales for example we lock up more than 3 000 juveniles at anyone time (age of criminal responsibility set at 10).

Treatment of delinquents in institutional settings has to meet the sometimes contradictory need to control young people, to remove their liberty and to maintain good order in the institution, at the same time as offering education and training to foster future prosocial participation in society and meeting their welfare needs. At least in England and Wales, the legislative overhaul of Youth Justice[105] has mandated practitioners to bridge the gap between residential and community treatments and to involve families using Youth Offending Teams (YOT's) to meet this complex mix of needs, but the public demand to remove antisocial youths from the street has led to the implementation of Antisocial Behaviour Orders including children with learning disabilities.

Over the last 30 years there has been a gradual shift in opinion regarding effectiveness of intervention with delinquents, from the 'nothing works' approach to a 'what works' approach. The pressure from politicians and public will remain, for a quick fix solution to problems that span cultures, countries and generations.

Provision of appropriately designed programmes can significantly reduce recidivism amongst persistent offenders. The mode and style of delivery is important; high quality staff and staff training are required. Community based programmes seem better than institution based programmes. In prison settings, the strongest effects are obtained when programmes are integrated into the institutional regimes.

What are the key levers for change?

- Developing an integrated comprehensive screening and assessment tool for mental health, substance misuse and physical health

- Better identification of mental health needs by courts with effective court diversion.

- Improving access to child and adolescent mental health services for 16 to 17 year olds across the board.

- Enhancing the role of health workers in YOT's.

- Integrating work of substance misuse workers in custody and YOT's

- Enhancing intensive resettlement and aftercare provision—RAP Schemes.

- Reviewing the demand and need of nationally commissioned adolescent psychiatric secure inpatient beds (88 by 2008).

- And ensuring all working with young offenders understand and are trained in normal and abnormal child and adolescent development together with awareness of the nature of mental health problems in this stage of the life course and how this impacts on all aspects of a young person's life.

Our knowledge of true prevalence rates of mental disorders in a young offending population is developing further. Child and adolescent mental health practitioners have the skills to set the understanding of delinquency in a developmental context and treat those young offenders with mental disorders. Knowledge is advancing rapidly by an established international research network in Europe and the USA.

## Further information

Moffitt, T.E. and Scott, S. Conduct Disorders of Childhood and Adolescent. In *Rutter's Child and Adolescent Psychiatry* (5th edn) (eds. M. Rutter, D. Bishop, D. Pine, S. Scott, J. Stevenson, e. Taylor and A. thapar), Chapter 35, pp. 543–54.
Gives a comprehensive review of Conduct disorder classification, prevalence, subtypes, associated co-occurring dsorders and complicating conditions, tackling risk indicators, diagnostic challenges

and evidence based interventions as such it offers a good context in which to set the current chapter.

# References

1. Frick, P.J. (2006). Developmental pathways to conduct disorder. *Child and Adolescent Psychiatric Clinics of North America*, **15**(2), 311–32.

2. Cavadino, P., Allen, R. (2000). Children who kill: trends, reasons and procedures. In (ed. G. Boswell) *Violent Children and Adolescents: sking the question why*. London: Whurr Publishers, p. 16–7.

3. Royal College of Psychiatrists. (2006). Occasional Paper: Child Defendants. Royal College of Psychiatrists.

4. Coleman, J., Schofield, J. (2003). *Key Data on Adolescence. Trust for Study of Adolescence*. Brighton: TSA Publishing Ltd.

5. Bailey, S. (2006).Adolescence and beyond: twelve years onwards. In *The Developing World of the Child* (eds. J. Aldgate, D. Jones, W. Rose, C. Jeffrey), p. 208–25. Jessica Kingsley, London.

6. Youth Justice Board. (2007). *Youth Justice Annual Statistics 2005/06*. youth Justice Board for Engalnd and Wales.

7. Youth Justice Board. (2005).*Risk and Protective Factors*. Research Undertaken by Communities that Care on Behalf of the Youth Justice Board for England and Wales.

8. Department of Health. (2004). *National Service Framework for Children, Young People and Maternity Services. (NSF)*. Department of Health.

9. Kazdin, A.E. (2000). Adolescent Development, Mental Disorders, and Decision Making of Delinquent Youths. In: T. Grisso, R.G. Schwartz, editors. *Youth on Trial, A Developmental perspective on juvenile justice 2*. Chicago: University of Chicago Press. p. 33–65.

10. Chitsabesan, P., Kroll,L., Bailey, S., *et al.* (2006). Mental health needs of young offenders in custody and in the community. *British Journal of Psychiatry*, **188**, 534–40.

11. Dixon, A., Howie, P., Starling, J. (2004). Psychopathology in female juvenile offenders. *Journal of Child Psychology and Psychiatry*, **45**(6), 1150–8.

12. Gosden, N.P., Kramp, P., Gabrielsen, G., *et al.* (2003). Prevalence of mental disorders among 15-17-year-old male adolescent remand prisoners in Denmark. *Acta Psychiatrica Scandinavica*, **107**(2), 102–10.

13. Lederman, C.S., Dakof, G.A., Larrea, M.A., *et al.* (2004). Characteristics of adolescent females in juvenile detention. *International Journal of Law and Psychiatry*, **27**(4), 321–37.

14. McCabe, K.M., Lansing, A.E., Garland, A., *et al.* (2002). Gender differences in psychopathology, functional impairment, and familial risk factors among adjudicated delinquents. *Journal of the American Academy of Child and Adolescent Psychiatry*, **41**(7), 860–7.

15. Ruchkin, V., Koposov, R., Vermerien, R., *et al.* (2003). Psychopathology and age at onset of conduct problems in juvenile delinquents. *Journal of Clinical Psychology*, **64**, 913–20.

16. Teplin, L.A., Abram, K.M., McClelland, G.M., *et al.* (2002). Psychiatric disorders in youth in juvenile detention. *Arch Gen Psychiatry*, **59**(12), 1133–43.

17. Vreugdenhil, C., Doreleijers, T.A.H., Vermeiren, R., *et al.* (2004). Psychiatric disorders in a representative sample of incarcerated boys in the Netherlands. *Journal of the American Academy of Child and Adolescent Psychiatry*, **43**(1), 97–104.

18. Wasserman, G.A., McReynolds, L.S., Lucas, C.P., *et al.* (2002). The voice DISC-IV with incarcerated male youths: Prevalence of disorder. *Journal of the American Academy of Child and Adolescent Psychiatry*, 41(3), 314–21.

19. Atkins, D., Pumariega, A.J., Rogers, K., *et al.* (1999). Mental health and incarcerated youth.I: Prevalence and nature of psychopathology. *Journal Child Family Studies*, **8**, 193–204.

20. Shelton, D. (2001). Emotional disorders in young offenders. *Journal of Nurse Scholarship*, **33**(259), 263.

21. Vermerien, R., Schwab-Stone, M., Ruchkin, V., *et al.* (2002). Predicting recidivism in delinquent adolescents from psychological

and psychiatric assessment. *Comprehensive Psychiatry*, **43**(2), 142–9.

22. Roberts, R.E., Roseblatt, A. (1998). Prevalence of psychopathology among children and adolescents. *American Journal of Psychiatry*, **155**(715), 725.

23. Moffitt, T.E. (1993). Adolescence limited and life course persistent antisocial behaviour. A developmental taxonomy. *Psychological Review*, **100**, 674–701.

24. Angold, A., Costello, E.J., Erkanli, A. (1999). Comorbidity. *Journal of Child Psychology & Psychiatry & Allied Disciplines*, **40**(1), 57–87.

25. Grisso, T., Zimring, F.E. (2004). *Double jeopardy: Adolescent Offenders with mental disorders*. Chicago: University of Chicago Press.

26. Johnson, T.P., Cho, Y.I., Fendrich, M., *et al.* (2004). Treatment need and utilization among youth entering the juvenile corrections system. *Journal of Substance Abuse Treatment*, **26**(2), 117–28.

27. Domalanta, D.D., Risser, W.L., Roberts, R.E., *et al.* (2003). Prevalence of depression and other psychiatric disorders among incarcerated youths. *Journal of the American Academy of Child and Adolescent Psychiatry*, **42**(4), 477–84.

28. Rutter, M., Giller, H., Hagell, A. (1998). Antisocial Bahviour by Young People: The main messeges from a major new review of the research. Social Information Systems Ltd. Knutsford. Ref Type: Pamphlet

29. Hawkins, J.D., Herrenkohl, T., Farrington, D.P., *et al.* (1998). A review of predictors of youth violence. In Serious *and violent juvenile offenders. Risk factors and successful interventions* (eds. D.P. Farrington), p. 106–45.Thousand Oaks: SAGE Publications,

30. Losel, F., Bliesener, T. (1994). 'Some high-risk adolescents do not develop conduct problems: A study of protective factors'. *International Journal of Behavioural Development*, **17**, 753–77.

31. Sampson, R.J., Laub, J.H. (2003). 'Life-course desisters? Trajectories of crime among delinquent boys followed to age 70'. *Criminology*, **41**, 319–39.

32. Werner, E.E., Smith, R.S. (1992). *Overcoming the Odds*: Ithaca. Cornell University Press.

33. Losel, F., Bender, D. (2003). Protective factors and resilience. In *Early Prevention of Adult Antisocial Behaviour* (eds. D.P Farrington and J.W. Coid), p. 130–204. Cambridge University Press, Cambridge.

34. Luthar, S.S., Cicchetti, D., Becker, B. (2000). 'The construct of resilience: A critical evaluation and guidelines for future work'. *Child Development*, **71**, 543–62.

35. Losel, F., Bender, D. (2003). Protective factors and resilience. In: Farrington DP, Coid JW, editors. *Early Prevention of Adult Antisocial Behaviour*. Cambridge: Cambridge University Press; 2003. p. 130–204.

36. Gowers. S. (2001). Assessing adolescent mental health. In *Adolescent Psychiatry in Clinical Practice* (eds. Gowers S), p. 258–77. Arnold, London.

37. Stevens, A., Rafteryy, J. (1994). Introduction: concepts of need. In *Healthcare needs assessment* (eds.A. Stevens and J. Rafteryy), p. 13–4. Radchliffe Medical Press, Oxford.

38. Bailey, S., Dolan, M. (2004). Violence. In *Adolescent Forensic Psychiatry* (Bailey S and Dolan M), p. 213–27. Arnold publishing, London.

39. Bailey, S., Tarbuck, P. (2006). Recent advances in the development of screening tools for mental health in young offenders. *Current Opinion in Psychiatry*, **19**(4), 373–7.

40. Kroll, L. (2004). Needs assessment in adolescent offenders. In *Adolescent forensic psychiatry* (eds.S. Bailey and M. Dolan), p. 14–26. Arnold Publishing, London.

41. Farrington, D.P., Tarling, R. (1985). *Prediction in Criminology*. Albany State: University of New York Press.

42. LeBlanc, M. (1998). Screening of serious and violent juvenile offenders: identification, classification, and prediction. In *Serious and Violent Juvenile Offenders. Risk Factors and Successful Interventions*. (eds. R. Loeber and D.P. Farrington), p. 167–93. Thousand Oaks, Sage Publications, CA.

43. Hoge, R.D., Andrews, D.A., Leschiedm, A,W. (1996). An investigation of risk and protective factors in a sample of youthful offenders.

*Journal of Child Psychology and Psychiatry and Allied Disciplines*, **37**(4), 419–24.

44. LeBlanc, M. (2002). The offending cycle, escalation and de-escalation in delinquent behavior, A challenge for criminology'. *International Journal of comparative and applied criminal justice*, **26**(1), 53–84

45. Barnoski, R. (2002). Monitoring vital signs: Integrating a standardized assessment into Washington State's juvenile justice system. In *Multi-problem violent youth: A foundation for comparative research on needs, interventions and outcomes* (eds. R. Corrado, R. Roesch, S.D. Hart, J.K. Gierowski), p. 219–31. IOS Press, Amsterdam, Netherlands

46. Borum, R., Bartel, P., Forth, A. (2002). *Manual for the Structured Assessment of Violence Risk in Youth (SAVRY)*. Tampa, FL: University of South Florida.

47. Shaw, D.S., Gillion, M., Ingoldsby, E.M., *et al.* (2003). Trajectories leading to school-age conduct problems. *Developmental Psychology*, **39**(2), 189–200.

48. Nagin, D., Tremblay, R.E. (2001). Parental and early childhood predictors of persistent physical aggression in boys from kindergarten to high school. *Archives of General Psychiatry*, **58**, 389–94.

49. Fonagy, P. (2003). Towards a developmental understanding of violence. *British Journal of Psychiatry*, **183**, 190–2.

50. Fischer, M., Barkley, R.A., Fletcher, K.E., *et al.* (1993). The Adolescent Outcome of Hyperactive-Children - Predictors of Psychiatric, Academic, Social, and Emotional Adjustment. *Journal of the American Academy of Child and Adolescent Psychiatry*, **32**(2), 324–32.

51. Seagrave, D., Grisso, T. (2002). Adolescent development and the measurement of juvenile psychopathy. *Law and Human Behavior*, **26**, 219–39.

52. McGuire, J., Priestley, P. (1995). Reviewing «what works»: past present and future. In *What Works: Reducing Reoffending* (ed. J. McGuire), p. 3–34. *Guidelines from Research and Practice*. Wiley, Chichester.

53. Dodge, K.A., Schwartz, D. (1997). Social information processing mechanisms in aggressive behavior. In *Handbook of antisocial behavior* (eds. D.M. Stoff, J. Breiling J.D. Maser), p. 171–80. Wiley, New York.

54. Craig, J.S., Hatton, C., Craig, F.B., *et al.* (2004). Persecutory beliefs, attributions and theory of mind: comparison of patients with paranoid delusions, Asperger's syndrome and healthy controls. *Schizophrenia Research*, **69**(1), 29–33.

55. Farrant, F. (2001). *Troubled Inside: responding to the mental health needs of children and young people in Prison*. Prison Reform Trust, London.

56. Dubicka, B., Harrington, R. (2004). Affective Conduct Disorder. In *Adolescent Forensic Psychiatry* (eds. S. Bailey, M. Dolan), p. 124–44. Arnold, London.

57. Harrington, R.C., Kroll, L., Rothwell, J., *et al.* (2005). Psychosocial needs of boys in secure care for serious or persistent offending. *Journal of Child Psychology and Psychiatry*, **46**(8), 859–66.

58. Kroll, L., Rothwell, J., Bradley, D., *et al.* (2002). Mental health needs of boys in secure care for serious or persistent offending: a prospective, longitudinal study. *Lancet*, **359**(9322), 1975–9.

59. Fletcher, K.E. (2003). Childhood posttraumatic stress disorder. In *Child psychopathology* (eds. E.J. Mash, R.A. Barkley), p. 330–71. 2nd ed. Guildford Press, New York.

60. Garbarino, J. (2001). An ecological perspective on the effects of violence on children. *Journal of Community Psychology*, **29**(3), 361–78.

61. Harrington, R., Bailey, S. (2004). NHS National Programme on Forensic Mental Health Research and Development. Expert Paper: The Scope for Preventing Antisocial Personality Disorder by Intervening in Adolescence.

62. O'Brien, G. (1996). The psychiatric management of adult autism. *Adv Psychiatr Treat*, **2**(173), 177.

63. Howlin, P. (1997).'*Autism' preparing for adulthood*. Routledge, London.

64. Bailey, S. (2002). Violent children: A framework for assessment. *Adv Psychiatr Treat*, **8**(2), 97–106.

65. Clark, A. (2001). Proposed treatment for adolescent psychosis. 2: Bipolar illness. Adv Psychiatr Treat, **7**(2), 143–9.

66. Taylor, P.J., Gunn, J. (1999). Homicides by people with mental illness myth and reality. *British Journal of Psychiatry*, **174**, 9–14.

67. Clare, P., Bailey, S., Clark, A. (2000). Relationship between psychotic disorders in adolescence and criminally violent behaviour - A retrospective examination. *British Journal of Psychiatry*, **177**, 275–9.

68. Cooke, D.J., Michie, C. (2001). Refining the construct of psychopathy: towards a hierarchical model. *Psychological Assessment*, **13**, 171–88.

69. Hare, R.D. (1991). *The Hare Psychopathy Checklist - Revised*. Multi Health Systems, Toronto.

70. Kazdin, A.E. (1993). Treatment of conduct disorder: progress and directions in psychotherapy research. *Developmental Psychopathology*, **5**, 277–310.

71. Sukhodolsky, D.G., Ruchkin, V. (2006). Evidence based psychosocial treatments in the juvenile justice system. *Child & Adolescent Clinics of North America*, **15**(2), 501–16.

72. Andrews, D., Zinger, I., Hoge, R., *et al.* (1990). Does correctional treatment work? A clinically relevant and psychologically informed meta-analysis. *Criminology*, **28**, 369–404.

73. Lipsey, M.W. (1995). What do we learn from 400 research studies on the effectiveness of treatment with juvenile delinquents? In *What works* (ed. J.McGuire), Reducing offending. Wiley, Chichester.

74. Lipsey, M.W., Wilson, D.B. (1993). The efficacy of psychosocial, educational, and behavioural treatment: Confirmation from meta-analysis. *American Psychologist*, **48**, 1181–209.

75. Losel, F. (1995). The efficacy of correctional treatment: a review and synthesis of metaevaluations. In *What Works* (ed. J. McGuire), p. 57–82. Reducing Reoffending: Guidelines from Research and Practice. Wiley, Chichester.

76. Woolfenden, S.R., Williams, K., Peat, J. (2003). *Family and parenting interventions in children and adolescents with conduct disorder and delinquency aged 10-17 (Cochrane Review)*. The Cochrane Library, Issue 3, Oxford.

77. Blackburn, R. (1993). *The psychology of criminal conduct*. Wiley, Chichester UK.

78. Berkowitz, L. (1993). *Aggression: Its causes, consequences and control*. McGrow-Hill, New York.

79. Farrington, D.P. (1995). The Twelfth Jack Tizard Memorial Lecture. The development of offending and antisocial behaviour from childhood: key fi ndings from the Cambridge Study in Delinquent Development. *Journal of Child Psychology and Psychiatry and allied disciplines*, **36**(6), 929–64.

80. Cornell, D.G., Benedek, E.P., Benedek, B.A. (1987). Juvenile homicide. Prior adjustment and a proposed typology. American *Journal of Orthopsychiatry*, **57**(3), 383–93.

81. Myers, W.C., Burket, R.C., Harris, H.E. (1995). Adolescent psychopathy in relation to delinquent behaviours, conduct disorder, and personality disorder. *Journal of Forensic Sciences*, **40**, 436–40.

82. Myers, W., Scott, K. (1998). Psychotic and conduct disorder symptoms in juvenile murderers. *Journal of Homicide Studies*, **2**(2), 160–75.

83. Zimring, F. (1998). *The Challenge of Youth Violence*. Cambridge University Press, Cambridge.

84. Bailey, S. (1996). Current perspectives on young offenders: aliens or alienated? *Journal of Clinical Forensic Medicine*, Mar, **3**(1), 1–7.

85. Heide, K.M. (1999). *Young Killers: The Challenge of Juvenile Homicide*. Thousand Oaks, Sage publications: California.

86. James, A.C, Neil, P. (1996). Juvenile sexual offending: One-year period prevalence study within Oxfordshire. *Child Abuse and Neglect*, **20**(6), 477– 85.

87. Skuse, D., Bentovim, A., Hodges, J., *et al.* (1998). Risk Factors for Development of Sexually Abusive Behaviour In Sexually Victimised Adolescent Boys. Cross Sectional Study. *British Medical Journal*, **317**, 175–9.

88. Dolan, M., Holloway, J., Bailey, S., *et al.* (1996). The psychosocial characteristics of juvenile sexual offenders referred to an adolescent forensic service in the UK. *Medicine Science and the Law*, **36**(4), 343–52.

89. Apsche, J.A., Ward Bailey, S.R. (2005).Mode Deactivation Therapy: Cognitive Behavioral Therapy for Adolescents with Reactive Conduct Disorders and/or Personality Disorders/ Traits. In *Children and young people who sexually abuse: New theory, research, and practice developments* (ed. M.C. Calder), Russell House, United Kingdom.

90. Print, B., O'Callaghan, D. (1999). 'Working with young men who have sexually abused others'. In *Children and young people who sexually abuse others* (eds. M. Erooga and H. Masson), p. 124–45. Routledge, London.

91. Hackett, S., Telford, P., Slack, K. (2002). Groupwork with parents of children who sexually harm. In *Young People who Sexually Abuse* (ed. M.C. Calder), Building the Evidence Base for your Practice. Lyme Regis, Russell House Publishing.

92. Chamberlain, P., Reid, J.B. (1998). Comparison of two community alternatives to incarceration for chronic juvenile offenders. *Journal of Consulting & Clinical Psychology*, **66**(4), 624–33.

93. Yokely, J., Boettner, S. (2002). Forensic foster care for young people who sexually abuse: Lessons from treatment. In *Young people who sexually abuse* (ed. M.C. Calder), p. 309–32. Building the evidence base for your practice. Lyme Regis: Russell House.

94. Vizard, E., Usiskin, J. (1999). Providing individual psychotherapy for young sexual abusers of children. In *Children and young people who sexually abuse others: Challenges and responses* (eds. M. Erooga and H. Masson), p. 104–23. Taylor & Frances/Routledge, Florence, KY, US.

95. Fineman, K.R. (1980). Firesetting in childhood and adolescence. *Psychiatric Clinics of North America*, **3**(3), 483–500.

96. Patterson, G.R. (1982). Coercive family process. Eugene OR, Castalia.

97. Vreeland, R.G., Lowin, B.M. (1980). Psychological aspects of firesetting. In *In Fires and human behaviour* (ed. D. Canter). Wiley, New York .

98. Kolko, D., Kazdin, A.E. (1992). The emergence and re-occurrence of child firesetting: A one year prospective study. *Journal of Abnormal Child Psychology*, **201**, 17–37.

99. Repo, E., Virkunnen, M. (1997). Young arsonists, history of conduct disorder, psychiatric diagnosis, and criminal recidivism. *Journal of Forensic Psychiatry*, **8**, 311–20.

100. T & V v United Kingdom. (1999). European Centre of Human Rights Judgements.

101. Ashford. M., Chard, A., Redhouse, N. (2006). *Defending Young People in the Criminal Justice System*. 3rd ed. Legal Action Groups, Glasgow.

102. British Medical Association. (2001). *Health Care for Children and Young People: Consent Rights and Choices*. British Medical Association, London.

103. Grisso, T. (1997). The Competence of Adolescents As Trial Defendants. *Psychology, Public Policy and Law*, **3**, 3–32.

104. Grisso, T. What we know about youths' capacities as trial defendants. In *Youth on Trial* (eds. T. Grisso and R.G. Schwartz), p. 139–71. University of Chicago Press, Chicago.

105. Crime and Disorder Act: Section 37 (1998). The Stationary Office, London.

# Child molesters and other sex offenders

Stephen Hucker

## Introduction

In most Western societies sexual offenders are more reviled than almost any other type of offender. On both sides of the Atlantic this is reflected in the sanctions that specifically address this group such as Sexually Violent Predator laws in the United States, Dangerous and Long-Term Offender legislation in Canada, and Sex Offender Orders in the UK. Related approaches include the introduction of sex offender registries and the widespread requirement that children at risk from sexual predators be reported by professionals and others.

## The general psychiatrist and the sex offender

Though constituting a relatively small proportion of all reported offences, sex offending affects large numbers of people in the general population. Though there are methodological difficulties associated with much of the research in this area, the World Health Organization has reviewed estimates of childhood sexual abuse from 39 countries and found that the prevalence of non-contact, contact, and intercourse in female children was about 6, 11, and 4 per cent, respectively; the corresponding figure for males was about 2 per cent in all categories.[1] However, these must represent minimal figures as it is known that many victims do not report their experience and individual sex offenders, when guaranteed confidentiality, will admit to many more offences than they were charged with or convicted of.[2] Various forms of sexual offending against adults are also underreported but it has been estimated that about 13 per cent of women and 3 per cent of men have been raped at some time during their lifetime.[3]

The long-term effects of such victimization has been extensively studied and it is clear that people with a history of child sexual abuse, for example, experience a wide range of long-term psychological consequences.[4]

Although prone to find reasons to delegate the assessment and management of sex offenders to specialized forensic services, the general psychiatrist will find it impossible to avoid them entirely. Minor varieties, such as 'flashers' (exhibitionists) or 'peeping Toms' (voyeurs), may be viewed by the courts as less serious, and the opinion of the generalist will still be appreciated, especially when specialist resources are scarce and an appointment for a forensic assessment could be long-delayed. It is important, therefore, for the general psychiatrist to have some understanding of this area in order to make appropriate decisions and recommendations.

## Definitions of sexual offending

Put simply, a sexual offender is an individual whose sexual behaviour contravenes the law in a particular jurisdiction. The types of activities that may be proscribed vary considerably. Western countries are generally more tolerant though most societies provide sanctions for sexual activity involving children below the age of consent, non-consensual sexual acts, sexual relations with close family, and sexual interference with animals or corpses. There are also typically legal and other interventions where a person fears sexual harassment or assault, and where there has been abuse, or likelihood of abuse, in certain professional relationships. Typically, also, there is regulation of pornography or obscene material.

### Relationship between sexual deviancy and sexual offending

There is some overlap of sexual offences with a medical diagnosis of a paraphilia. However, this is not a complete concurrence. Thus, not all paedophiles have molested a child and not all child molesters are paedophiles; many, perhaps most, men who sexually assault adult women are not sexually deviant or paraphilic at all. The psychiatric categories of paraphilia and their characteristics are described elsewhere in this volume (Chapter 4.11.3 by Fedoroff).

## Types of sexual offender

The vast majority of sexual offenders are male though it is recognized that women may also commit similar crimes.[5] Male sexual offenders can be broadly divided into: child molesters, rapists, and non-contact sex offenders.

### Child molesters

Typologies of this subgroup in part refer to the degree of paraphilic attraction (sexual deviancy). Thus, there has been a common categorization into 'fixated' and 'situational' or 'regressed' types.[6] With the 'fixated' type there is a permanent attraction to children typically dating from adolescence thus conforming to definitions of paedophilia in DSM-IV and ICD-10. Those attracted to males are more likely to repeat their offences with recidivism at least twice as high as with those attracted to girls. The former tend to victimize boys aged 11–15 years old, whereas the latter molest girls of 8 to 10.

'Fixated' paedophiles tend to commit premeditated offences that often involve considerable planning. Manipulation and 'grooming' behaviour is used as a means of luring, even abducting, children into sexual activity, and they may gain the trust of the parents or other carers. They may appear to have an excellent rapport with the child victims and treat them kindly but their motive is primarily for the child to meet their own need for affection rather than the reverse. It is for this reason that 'needy' children are often selected as victims. Such offenders will typically profess their 'love' for children and convince themselves that their behaviour is not harmful. Other rationalizations, such as that were educating the child or introducing the child to sexual love in a caring way, are common.

'Regressed' or 'situational' child molesters are, according to this typology, attracted primarily to adult females and may be in a marital-type relationship at the time of their offence. They will often report feelings of personal inadequacy or low self-esteem and their offences are more typically spontaneous and occur in the context of a stressful life circumstance.

The 'regressed' child molester, in contrast to the 'fixated' type, is less inclined to 'groom' victims and their caregivers. Victims of this type may be older than those involved with the 'fixated' molester. Molestations however may begin before, and continue past, puberty.

### Rapists

Once again, the typology expounded by Prentky, Knight, and colleagues can be useful.[6] In this scheme, offenders are differentiated through their apparent motivation by anger, power, or sadism. Most rapists act alone but individuals involved in 'gang' rape may represent several different types.

'Anger-motivated' rapists act out deviant fantasies of retaliation towards the victim, using violence as a means of expressing generalized anger, typically towards women though sometimes towards people in general. The intention of the attack is to humiliate and debase the victim who will typically have been selected randomly.

The 'power-motivated' rapist type has been further subdivided into the 'power-reassurance' and 'power-assertive' types. The former is plagued by doubts and insecurities about their own masculinity and sexual adequacy, often uses minimal force and may apologize to the victim or even seek a relationship afterwards. However, these victims may have been stalked and the attacks on them premeditated. The 'power-assertive' subtype is motivated by the desire to dominate women and has no doubts about his masculinity but, like the previous subtype, typically does not use gratuitous violence to subdue the victim.

'Sadistic' rapists, are the least common but perhaps most worrisome type, who derive sexual pleasure from inflicting hurt and suffering on their victim. Sometimes, however, this is difficult to differentiate from other types where pain, suffering and humiliation are the consequences, but not the primary motivation, for the attack.

Other types of sexual assault that do not involve penetration, and which represent related behaviours, include toucheurism and frotteurism. These involve, respectively, touching or grabbing strangers, typically females, in a way that provides him with sexual gratification. The former, in particular, may pass unnoticed by the victim, as attackers will typically touch or grab sexual areas such as breasts, buttocks, or crotch, in crowds and similar situations where the incident may be discounted as 'accidental'.

### Non-contact sexual offences

This group includes 'peeping Toms', 'flashers', and indecent phone callers with corresponding psychiatric diagnoses of the paraphilias voyeurism, exhibitionism, and telephone scatalogia, respectively.

Peepers have a penchant to observe an unsuspecting female stranger undressing, or couples in the act of copulation. They may masturbate at the scene or later in private while recalling what they saw. Most voyeurs, like most sex offenders who are paraphilic, are aware of their deviant impulses while still adolescent but the behaviour may become chronic.

Exhibitionists derive sexual excitement from exposing their genitals to unsuspecting female strangers. The desired reaction is one of 'shock and awe' and indifference is a useful response, if the victim has the presence of mind. The perpetrator may masturbate at the time or later in private. Though some cases are particularly intractable, it is unusual to see an exhibitionist still active much past the age of about 40 years old.

The unsuspecting victims of obscene telephone callers are greeted with a barrage of sexually explicit commentary over the telephone. When this is a habitual practice, accompanied by or followed by masturbation, it is distinguishable from an isolated incident committed as a prank.

In all three of the above non-contact sexual offences, there is typically no desire to have further contact with the victim and, indeed, such a prospect often fills the offender with anxiety. However, a small minority of these offenders may later commit a more serious sexual offence, even sexually motivated homicide.[7] Atypical features, such as a desire to have personal contact with the victim, or the repeated selection of child victims, may be an early warning sign of such potential and warrants further, expert assessment.

In recent years, paralleling the advance of technology, offenders have been apprehended for using the Internet as a means of obtaining or distributing pornography (especially child pornography) or as a means of contacting children for sexual purposes. Possession of child pornography is an indicator of sexual interest in children and it is associated with self-reported sexual interest in children and with laboratory measurements of changes in penile volume or circumference.[8]

## Assessment of sex offenders

In the context of court remanded cases, the usual pre-trial issues of fitness (competence) to stand trial and criminal responsibility will need to be addressed. Only a small proportion of all sex offenders demonstrate symptoms of psychotic mental disorder, particularly schizophrenia and depressive disorders. However, where those disorders are present it is necessary to explore how the symptoms, e.g. delusions or hallucinations, bear specifically on the sexual offending. It may be found that other psychiatric disorders are of greater importance and that a secondary diagnosis of mental retardation or personality disorder, or more particularly, a paraphilia, are more relevant with respect to the offending behaviour. More commonly the court will be interested in sentencing considerations, specifically the risk the offender presents to others, and whether and what medical treatment and/or other professional interventions might be ordered or recommended by the court in order to reduce that risk.

## Interview

The interviewer must assume that the subject will be at best guarded, or frankly hostile, in their response to the assessment process and it may be difficult to achieve the level of affinity more commonly experienced with non-psychotic general psychiatric patients. A non-judgemental approach is therefore preferable, regardless of the examiner's personal emotional reaction to the offender's behaviour. Few will have presented to the psychiatrist or psychologist voluntarily. Moreover, there is a distinct tendency among sex offenders to prevaricate or frankly lie. It is therefore essential for the examiner to have detailed information about the act or acts that are alleged to have occurred. It has already been noted that denials, rationalizations, distortions, and minimization are the norm with sex offenders. It is not, however, the assessor's function to judge the issue, in particular when guilt has not been determined by the court.

It is obviously unhelpful, in terms of gaining rapport or obtaining additional information, to accuse the subject of dishonesty. Rather, a sympathetic approach suggesting that sometimes people have difficulty accepting unpleasant aspects of themselves, may be more helpful. Another approach is to invite the subject to explore why the victim made the accusations if they are untrue and whether they can accept, if not the whole, then some part of the allegations against them.

It is also important to remember that, while the individual may have been accused of one type of deviant sexual behaviour, other types may have occurred and been undetected. Paraphilic disorders tend not to occur as it were in pure culture but rather in association with other paraphilias, typically at least two or three. Thus, for example, an exhibitionist may have been reported for exposing specifically to children rather than adults and this will suggest an additional diagnosis of paedophilia. Or, an individual who has been convicted of rubbing himself against women in public places may also have made obscene phone calls and harbour fantasies of rape.

In the case of child molesters it is important to consider how he gained access to his victims. Exploration of the methods of 'grooming' is important in understanding ways to assist the offender to avoid risky situations in the future.

In terms of the overall assessment, identification of psychopathologies outside the domain of sexual deviation is important. The presence of psychosis will have an implication for the type of treatment to be recommended, even if it is not common among sex offenders. It seems likely that some such sex offenders' behaviour is dismissed as a function of the psychosis and underlying paraphilic disorder may easily be discounted or not considered at all. More commonly it will be personality disorders or traits, alcohol or substance abuse, mild-to-moderate depression, and anxiety disorders, rather than major mental illness that will be noted. Attention to these will be an important part of any subsequent treatment or management strategy.

## Psychometric testing

Psychometric testing may contribute additional information an overall assessment, in particular where the subject is not forthcoming in a personal interview. There are a number of general personality assessment instruments available. These include the well known and widely used *Minnesota Multiphasic Personality Inventory (MMPI)*, the *Millon Clinical Multiaxial Inventory (MCMI III)*, and the *Personality Assessment Inventory (PAI)*. All have been extensively used in offender populations including sex offenders, and common profiles have been identified. Although none can specifically identify a sex offender, information concerning impulsivity, denial, judgement, and general psychopathology may be very useful.

There are also a number of psychological tests that have been specifically designed for the assessment of sex offenders. These include the *Multiphasic Sex Inventory II (MSI-II)* and the revised version of the *Clarke Sex History Questionnaire for Males (SHQ-R)*. The *MSI-II* is designed to measure the sexual characteristics of an adult male (though there is a female version too) alleged to have committed a sexual offence or sexual misconduct, including those who deny the allegations. Though standardized in the United States on a large sample of sex offenders it is more widely used. It consists of 560 true/false questions and the completed questionnaire must be sent to the developers for computerized scoring and interpretation. The SHQ-R consists of 508 questions and the completed questionnaire may again be sent away for scoring and an interpretive report returned.

## Laboratory testing

As sex offenders are prone to lie and distort their self-report of deviant interest and behaviours a more objective method of assessment has long been pursued. One of the earliest to be developed was the use of the penile plethysmograph (PPG, or phallometry) to measure changes in response to erotic stimulation. This method involves measuring changes in the size of the penis while presenting the subject with carefully selected images, both still and moving, of both sexes and different age groups, and audiotaped descriptions of various sexual activities. There are certainly problems with PPG testing, including the standardization of stimulus materials used, and some offenders are either able to learn to suppress their physiological responses or masturbate before the testing in order to render themselves unresponsive.[8] Nonetheless, the PPG, more commonly using a circumferential device, or the volumetric method, is extensively used in assessments of sex offenders (for critical review, see Ref.[10]).

Particularly in the United States, the PPG has come under attack as, in addition to standardization and reliability issues, it uses pictures of children whose consent or that of their parents was never obtained. The computer-generated images have been developed to attempt to obviate this concern. More recently the use of virtual reality of computer-generated images has also been used experimentally. Other, less intrusive methods of assessment are also being adopted, including the Abel Screen[11] which measures time spent viewing non-nude images.

Mention must also be made of polygraphy with sex offenders as it has been used extensively in many parts of the United States and to some extent in the United Kingdom. The subject is asked questions relating to their sexual interests and activities while their pulse, respiration, and skin conductance are measured. However, research in the area is generally weak and, despite its widespread use and perception of usefulness, particularly for monitoring sex offenders in the community, the method is controversial (for review, see Ref.[8]).

## Assessment of risk in sex offenders

The courts will often wish to have a professional opinion regarding the risk an offender presents to re-offend, and it is important to have an understanding of the factors that will contribute to this (see Table 11.8.1).

Risk has been divided into:

1 Static risk, i.e. involving those factors which cannot change, such as the offender's age, sex, or number of previous criminal convictions and

2 Dynamic risk, i.e. involving those which potentially could change, either as a result of treatment or some other intervention, or simply by the passage of time. This can be further subdivided into relatively stable, though nonetheless potentially changeable, factors such as sexual preferences or negative attitudes, and acute factors, such as access to victims, reversion to substance use, and active mental illness.

These are important in estimating an offender's risk to re-offend. Static factors have received the most scientific study and it is chiefly that these have been incorporated into various actuarial or statistical

**Table 11.8.1** Predictors of sexual offence recidivism

| Type of risk factor | Predictor |
| --- | --- |
| Static | Prior sex offence |
| | Prior non-sexual offences |
| | Prior non-contact sex offences |
| | Prior treatment dropout |
| | Any boy victims |
| | Any unrelated victims |
| | Any stranger victims |
| | Early age of onset |
| | Young age of offender |
| | Minimal cohabitation history |
| | Childhood behaviour problems |
| | Separation from parents as a child |
| | Antisocial personality disorder |
| | Prior violation of conditional release |
| Stable dynamic | Sexual preferences, children |
| | Sexual preferences rape/violence |
| | Sexually entitled attitudes |
| | Pro-child molester attitudes |
| | Pro-rape attitudes |
| | Lack of adult love partner |
| | Emotional loneliness |
| | Lifestyle impulsivity |
| | Ineffective problem-solving skills |
| | Callous and unemotional attitudes |
| | Aggressive, hostile, and suspicious |
| | Negative social influences |
| Acute dynamic | Access to potential victims |
| | Substance abuse |
| | Sexual preoccupation |
| | Emotional collapse |
| | Collapse of social support system |
| | Rejection of supervision |
| | Acute mental illness |

(Reproduced from Webster, C.D. and Huxler, S.J. (2007) Violence risk: assessment and management. Copyright 2007, John Wiley & Sons, Inc.)

instruments that have been developed in the past several years, based on follow-up studies of samples of sex offenders. Among these instruments the Rapid Risk Assessment of Sex Offender Recidivism (RRASOR), the STATIC-99,[12] and Sex Offender Risk Appraisal Guide (SORAG),[13] are the most widely used. An assessor intending to use any of these instruments needs to be thoroughly familiar with the literature on the topic and to have participated in training workshops that are given at conferences from time to time. Useful though these tools can be, too heavy reliance upon them is no substitute for a full understanding of how these were constructed and their limitations.[14]

## Treatment issues

It is rare for paraphilic individuals to present for treatment in order to prevent themselves from becoming a sex offender. Though some paraphilias are not usually associated with criminal charges (e.g. transvestitic fetishism) others, such as paedophilia, are more likely to present through the courts or probation and parole services *after* an offence has been committed. It is important to realize that sexual preferences are highly resistant if not impossible to change. The most that can be expected with sex offenders who have deviant sexual preferences (paraphilias) is to help them learn to control their behaviour and to recognize that their propensity will always remain in the background, much as alcoholics are advised to consider themselves always vulnerable to relapse.

### Psychological treatments

Various psychological therapies have been attempted with sex offenders. Psychodynamically based individual and group treatments have been the most commonly used. It has become clearer more recently, however, that cognitive-based therapies (CBT) are the preferable approach to take, although techniques involving classical behaviour therapy, e.g. covert sensitization, are also sometimes used for specific purposes, such as creating aversion to deviant arousing images and replacement with non-deviant ones. Cognitive behaviour therapy itself involves helping the subject to develop strategies to alter their thought processes in order to avert their deviant behaviour, to improve their social skills, and to remedy their distorted beliefs and attitudes.

There is little or no evidence for the efficacy of psychological treatments prior to the introduction of CBT. Based on meta-analysis of 43 published studies, it has been shown that treatment programmes using this approach are associated with a reduction in overall recidivism rate from about 17 to 10 per cent.[15] Nonetheless, there is still considerable controversy over the effectiveness of formal sex offender treatment programmes.[16]

### Medications

Various medications have been used to treat sex offenders. Based on empirical observations of animals, which become less sexually active following neutering, hormonal treatments that reduce testosterone levels have been extensively employed. All require careful discussion with the potential patient concerning side effects and it is important to obtain written, informed consent.

Oestrogens proved to be problematic because of the serious risk of thrombo-embolic complications and a safer alternative was found in Cyproterone acetate (Androcur), an anti-androgen, which is available in Europe, including the UK. Because this drug has not been made available in North America, Medroxyprogesterone acetate (Provera) was introduced. Both however can still be responsible for minor side effects such as weight gain, tiredness, and gynaecomastia (with Cyperoterone, especially) but also more serious problems including thrombo-embolism and increase in blood sugar. More recently, leuteinizing hormone-releasing hormone (LHRH) agonists such as Leuprolide acetate (Lupron), Goserelin (Zoladex), and others, have been found useful as they produce almost total suppression of testosterone production such as would be seen following surgical castration. They tend, however, to be used mainly in very high-risk offenders or those who have failed with other drugs.[17] All of these hormone-affecting substances, though especially the LHRH agonists, have a tendency to leach calcium from the bones[18] and it is necessary to monitor carefully for this side effect and to administer antidotes including calcium supplements, vitamin D, and possibly biphosphonates.

The main problem with the hormonal treatments is their lack of acceptance by those who might potentially benefit. An alternative in the form of serotonin-reuptake inhibitors has therefore been better received though double blind trials are still lacking. They depress libido in about 50–60 per cent of cases though higher doses, such as are used with obsessive–compulsive disorder, are often necessary. There appears to be little basis on which to chose one SSRI over another, other than patient tolerance of side effects.[19]

## Ethical problems

Several ethical issues have been mentioned above in passing. It is, however, worth emphasizing in conclusion that a disinterested professional demeanour is important when assessing sex offenders. No matter what his or her own private views, it is not the place of the clinician to decide on guilt or innocence or in any other way to pass judgement on the offender or alleged offender. Moreover, alienating the offender will present a further impediment to gaining information and to providing treatment when indicated and necessary.

It is important, at the assessment stage, to identify for the subject the nature of the evaluation, the role of the assessor, and the person or agency for whom they are acting, for example a Child Protection Service, a defence lawyer, or Crown prosecutor. This may determine the degree of cooperation but to not explain this fully and simply to present oneself as a 'doctor' in a helping role when the intention of the evaluation is solely to provide a risk assessment as opposed to treatment, for example would be unethical.

Certain assessment procedures, such as penile plethysmography and polygraphy (when used in a clinical setting) are particularly contentious. Though both may provide useful information, written and fully informed consent should always be obtained beforehand. PPG has been particularly criticized for the use of child images as sexual stimuli when the consent of neither the child nor its parents have been obtained, though the development of computer-generated images may avoid that particular objection.

Finally, when drugs that have been developed and marketed for other purposes are used to suppress sexual drive, the patient needs to be fully informed of the potential benefits as well as the risks involved but should not be denied complementary or alternative treatments should they decide not to expose themselves to the potential side effects.

## Further information

Holmes, R.M. and Holmes, S.T. (2002). *Current perspectives on sex crimes*. Sage Publications, London.

Marshall, W.L., Fernandez, Y.M., Marshall, L.E., *et al.* (2006). *Sexual offender treatment: controversial issues*. John Wiley & Sons, Chichester, England.

## References

1. World Health Organization. (2002). Other risks to health. In *The world health report 2002: reducing risk, promoting healthy life* (Chap. 4) @ http://www.who.int/whr/2002/chapter4/en/index9.html

2. Abel, G., Becker, J., Mittleman, M., *et al.* (1987). Self-reported sex crimes of nonincarcerated paraphiliacs. *Journal of Interpersonal Violence*, **2**, 3–25.

3. Spitzberg, B. (1999). An analysis of empirical estimates of sexual aggression victimization and perpetration. *Violence and Victims*, **14**, 241–60.

4. Romans, S., Martin, J., and Mullen, P. (1997). Childhood sexual abuse and later psychological problems: neither necessary, sufficient nor acting alone. *Criminal Behaviour and Mental Health*, **7**, 327–38.

5. Hislop, J. (2001). Female sex offenders: what therapists, law enforcement and child protective services need to know. Issues Press, Ravensdale, WA.

6. Prentky, R. and Burgess, A.W. (2000). *Forensic management of sexual offenders*. Kluwer Academic/Plenum, New York.

7. Ressler, R.K., Burgess, A.W., and Douglas, J. E. (1988). *Sexual homicide: Patterns & Motives*. D.C. Heath & Co., Toronto.

8. Seto, M. (2007). Pedophilia and sexual offending against children: theory, assessment, and intervention. American Psychological Association, Washington, DC.

9. Marshall, W.L. and Fernandez, Y.M. (2003). *Phallometric testing with sexual offenders*. Safer Society Press, Brandon, VT.

10. Laws, R. (2003). Penile plethysmography: will we ever get it right? In *Sexual deviance: issues and controversies* (Chap. 5) (eds. T. Ward, D.R. Laws, and S.M. Hudson). Sage Publications, London.

11. Abel, G., Huffman, J., Warberg, B., *et al.* (1998). Visual reaction time and plethysmography as measures of sexual interest in child molesters. *Sexual Abuse: A Journal of Research and Treatment*, **10**, 81–95.

12. Harris, A., Phenix, A., Hanson, K., (2003). *STATIC-99 coding rules revised—2003*. Solicitor General Canada, Ottawa, Ontario, Canada.

13. Quinsey, V.L., Harris, G.T., Rice, M.E., *et al.* (2006). *Violent offenders: appraising and managing risk*. American Psychological Association, Washington, D.C.

14. Webster, C.D. and Hucker, S.J. (2007). *Violence risk: assessment & management*. John Wiley & Sons, Chichester.

15. Hanson, K., Gordon, A., Harris, A., *et al.* (2002). First report of the collaborative outcome data project on the effectiveness of psychological treatment for sex offenders. *Sexual Abuse: A Journal of Research and Treatment*, **14**, 169–92.

16. Laws, D. R. and O'Donohue, T. (eds.) (2008) *Sexual Deviance* (2nd ed). pp. 7–14. The Guilford Press: New York and London.

17. Hill, A., Briken, P., Kraus, C., *et al.* (2003). Differential pharmacological treatment of paraphilias and sex offenders. *International Journal of Offender Therapy and Comparative Criminology*, **47**, 407–21.

18. Grasswick, L.J. and Bradford, J.M. (2003). Osteoporosis associated with the treatment of paraphilias: a clinical review of 7 case reports. *Journal of Forensic Sciences*, **48**, 849–55.

19. Greenberg, D. and Bradford, J. (1997). Treatment of paraphilic disorders: a review of the role of selective serotonin reuptake inhibitors. *Sexual Abuse: A Journal of Research and Treatment*, **9**, 349–60.

# Arson (fire-raising)

## Herschel Prins

*How great a matter a little fire kindleth!*

*New Testament, authorised version (Letter of James, 3:5)*

The title of this chapter merits brief comment. Why is arson (fire-raising) a special problem, and why is there a dual title? Arson is a special problem because not only is it regarded as a very serious form of criminal behaviour, but because its detection can be very difficult. It is an offence that can be committed at 'one removed' by an offender, and it may sometimes involve unintended victims. Forensic psychiatrists will meet a number of arsonists in the course of their work but, increasingly, general psychiatrists are likely to come across them from time to time, for two reasons. *First*, the High Court in England and Wales has suggested that psychiatric reports are advisable in all cases where the motivation for the offence is unclear. *Second*, as will become clear from the writer's later comments, there has been a worrying increase in arson committed by young adults and children. Thus it is probable that child and adolescent psychiatrists are likely to come across cases more frequently. However, Soothill indicates a word of caution. He suggests that over-reliance upon psychiatric involvement may tend to 'medicalize' socially problematic behaviour.[1] The dual title that heads this chapter indicates the legal term used in the United Kingdom to describe acts of unlawful fire-raising. However, the term is not in universal use; readers will find that in other jurisdictions (notably in the North Americas) the terms are fire-raising, fire-setting, incendiarism, and in certain specific instances, pyromania and pathological fire-raising.[2] The term fire-raising is used in this chapter since the alternative terminologies can be subsumed under it.[3,4]

## Brief historical context

The phenomenon of fire, its uses and misuses, has figured extensively in myth, legend, and literature. For example, Prometheus is said to have stolen fire from the Gods and the myth became the mainspring for much psychoanalytic theorizing about fire-raising behaviour.[3] There are numerous early historical references to incendiary mixtures and devices, including sketches for mortars by Leonardo da Vinci.[5] In the mid-nineteenth century, the medical profession became interested in the explanation of fire-raising behaviours; and subsequently, adherents of psychoanalysis proposed various complex and somewhat doubtful explanations for such conduct. In particular, they linked fire-raising behaviour to sexual disturbance of one kind or another. Although sexual problems do appear in the backgrounds of *some* recidivist fire-raisers, the importance of the links has, in the present writer's view, been somewhat overstated.[6] Having said this, it should perhaps be noted that the phenomenon of fire is not infrequently linked linguistically to aggression and sexuality. For example, we speak or write of 'white hot rage', 'heated arguments', 'inflamed passions', to have the 'hots' for a sexual partner. Language is the conveyor of cultural values and attitudes and can be a powerful force in influencing our modes of thinking and expression about the phenomenon of fire in its many manifestations.

## The size of the problem

During the past two decades concern about the increase in fire-raising has been expressed worldwide. Table 11.9.1 gives the number of offenders convicted of arson in *England and Wales* for the years 1999–2003.

These figures only provide a partial picture, since it is often very difficult to establish whether a fire has been started deliberately (fires of doubtful origin or, if strongly suspected, malicious ignition). Happily, recent advances in forensic science have brought about improvements in the detection rate. A more reliable picture of the real size of the problem can be obtained from the United Kingdom *Fire Statistics*. The latest figures indicate a continuing worrying number of deliberate fires—some 91 200 in 2004 and, in particular, the number of attacks on vehicles and schools. 'Arson in vehicles . . . accounts for 60% of all deliberately set fires at 55,000 per year'. In 2004, in the United Kingdom, there were 840 school fires, slightly down on 896 in the previous year. Fatalities dropped from 117 in 2003 to 88 in 2004. Overall, the number of deliberate fires decreased by 21 per cent in 2004,[8] an encouraging trend. The cost of fires in

**Table 11.9.1** Arson, number of offenders found guilty of arson in England and Wales for the period 1999–2003

| 1999 | 2000 | 2001 | 2002 | 2003 |
|------|------|------|------|------|
| 2475 | 2470 | 2644 | 2427 | 2501 |

(Extracted from Home Office, (2004). Criminal statistics, England and Wales, 2003, Cm 6361. TSO © Crown Copyright[7].)

purely monetary terms is considerable; for example, figures from the Association of British Insurers (ABI) indicate 'that the cost of commercial fire claims in 2005 was 791 million pounds'—a record.[9]

## Legal aspects

Legal definitions of arson vary from country to country. In England and Wales, prior to 1971, arson was an offence at common law. Currently, it is dealt with under the Criminal Damage Act, 1971. Similar provisions apply in Northern Ireland. In Scotland, it is dealt with under various common law offences. Section 1 of the 1971 Act states:

1 A person who without lawful excuse destroys or damages any property belonging to another intending to destroy or damage such property or being reckless as to whether any such property would be destroyed or damaged shall be guilty of an offence.

2 A person who without lawful excuse destroys or damages any property, whether belonging to himself or another:

   (a) intending to destroy or damage any property or being reckless as to whether any such property would be destroyed or damaged; and

   (b) intending by the destruction or damage to endanger the life of another or being reckless as to whether the life of another would be thereby endangered; shall be guilty of an offence.

3 An offence committed under this section by destroying or damaging property by fire *shall be charged as arson* (emphasis added).

**NOTE:** Recklessness has recently been clarified by the High Court as follows: 'A person also acts recklessly within the meaning of Section 1 of the 1971 Act with respect to (i) a circumstance where he is aware of a risk that exists or will exist; (ii) a result when he is aware of a risk that will occur; and, it is in the circumstances known to him, unreasonable to take the risk'.[10]

The seriousness with which arson and endangering life is recorded is reflected in Section 4 of the Act where both are punishable by maximum penalties of life imprisonment.

## Classification, motivation, and management

### Classification

An early, large-scale attempt to classify fire-raisers was undertaken by Lewis and Yarnell.[11] For an account of this and other earlier studies see Prins.[12] Faulk proposed two useful broad groupings. *Group I* consisted of those cases in which the fire served as a means to an end (for example, revenge, fraud, or a plea for help); *Group II* consisted of those cases where the fire itself was the phenomenon of interest.[13] Some years ago the present author, together with two psychiatrist colleagues, examined the files of a group of 113 imprisoned arsonists being considered for parole.[14] From this small (and admittedly highly selective) sample a rudimentary classification was devised. (See Table 11.9.2). This has been used by others as starting points for their own and perhaps more sophisticated classifications. The present writer has more recently modified slightly this earlier classification.[3] Despite modification it can be seen to still have certain weaknesses since it collates the

**Table 11.9.2** Suggested classification of the motives of arsonists (fire-raisers)

(a) Arson committed for financial reward (insurance fraud, etc)

(b) Arson committed to conceal another crime (for example, burglary or homicide)

(c) Arson committed for political purposes (terrorist and associated activities)

(d) Self-immolation as a political gesture. (Not arson as such, but included here for completeness, see Prins[12])

(e) Arson committed for mixed motives (for example, during the phase of minor depression, as a cry for help, or as a result of abuse of alcohol or other drugs)

(f) Arson due to the presence of formal mental disorder (for example, severe affective disorder, schizophrenic illnesses, organic mental disorder, mental impairment (learning disability))

(g) Arson due to motives of revenge—against (i) an individual or individuals; (ii) against society or others more generally

(h) Arson committed as an attention-seeking act (but excluding motives set out under (e) above) and arson committed as a means of deriving sexual satisfaction and/or excitement (for example, some forms of pyromania)

(i) Vandalistic arson (by young adults and children)

behavioural characteristics of fire-raisers, various types of fire-setters and their motivations.[15]

Rix broadened our original classification to include attempts to gain rehousing, carelessness, 'anti-depressant' (to relieve depressed feelings), and 'proxy' (in which the offender had acted on behalf of another who had borne a grudge).[16] Barker, an experienced forensic psychiatrist, in a wide-ranging and meticulous study of the psychiatric aspects of fire-raising, suggested that future classifications need to be more sharply focussed, emphasizing that arson should be seen 'merely as a symptom' to be viewed in the context of the whole person, not only to delineate different 'syndromes' of arsonists but also to identify individual points of therapeutic intervention and future dangerousness.[15]

Recent work by Canter and Fritzon has carried this focus forward. They suggest four themes to arson. Two related to *expressive* acts; (a) those that are realized within the arsonist's own feelings, being analogous to suicide, and (b) those that are acted on objects, like the burning of symbolic buildings. The two others relate to *instrumental* acts; (c) those that are for personal indulgence, similar to personal revenge; and (d) those that have an object focus such as hiding evidence from a crime (emphasis added).[17] More recently Canter and Fritzon's work has been replicated successfully by Almond *et al.*[18] and Hakkanen *et al.*[19]

#### (a) Some general characteristics of fire-raisers

It is a reasonable generalization to state that fire-raisers appear to be mostly young adult males who have exhibited behavioural difficulties from an early age (see Kennedy *et al.*[20] for a systematic review of the literature on this aspect and Repo and Virkkunen[21]). A significant proportion of these youthful fire-raisers have problems of alcohol abuse and intelligence levels lower than average.[21,22] Females who commit repeated acts of fire-raising and show some degree of mental disorder and self-mutilating behaviours are more likely to be awarded a mental health disposal by the courts than their male counterparts (see Coid *et al.*[23] and Noblett and Nelson[24]).

## Motivation

To conform to the requested word limit for this chapter, categories (a), (b), (c), and (d) in Table 11.9.2 are not considered here. Detailed discussion of these and illustrative case vignettes may be found in Prins.[12]

### (a) Fire-raising committed for mixed and unclear reasons

These are cases in which it is difficult to ascribe a single specific motive and which cause significant problems in assessment. They are likely to include the presence of a degree of mild (reactive) depression which may lead the fire-raiser to direct anger at a spouse or partner; thus revenge may also play a part (see discussion below). This group may also include cases in which the fire-raising may be a disguised plea for help, or a reaction to sudden separation or bereavement; in a proportion of these cases alcohol appears to play a part.

### (b) Fire-raising due to serious mental disorder

Functional psychoses, notably the schizophrenias, may play a part in some acts of fire-raising. Such offenders will most likely be detained in secure hospitals or units. Manic depressive psychosis features occasionally, a classic case being that of Jonathan Martin, the nineteenth century arsonist who set fire to York Minster.[12]

### (c) Fire-raising associated with 'organic' disorders

Occasionally, brain tumours, injury, epilepsy, dementia or metabolic disturbance may play a part. For example, although the epilepsies are not commonly associated with fire-raising (or other serious crimes for that matter) one should always be on the lookout for the case in which the crime has been committed when the person appeared not to be in a state of clear consciousness or when onlookers were present. Examples of organic states and their relationship to fire-raising are provided elsewhere.[3,25–27] The relationship between learning disabilities and fire-raising is discussed by Prins[12] and Clare et al.[28]

### (d) Fire-raising motivated by revenge

Those incidents motivated by revenge are potentially the most dangerous. Such offenders are like the monster in Mary Shelley's *Frankenstein* who said 'I am malicious because I am miserable'. These are the fire-raisers who have serious problems with their feelings of anger and frustration caused by real or imagined wrongs. In considering the links between motives of revenge, it is important to stress the hazards of trying to place motivations for fire-raising in discrete categories; the vengeful fire-raiser may show clear signs of identifiable mental illness (for example, delusional jealousy), may be learning disabled and/or physically impaired, or may not be diagnosable as 'ill' in any formal psychiatric sense.

### (e) Pyromania

The diagnostic criteria for pyromania are set out in DSM-V(Rev) TSM (1994) on page 615.[29] The condition and its diagnosis may be said to be one of exclusion. It is dealt with in detail by McElroy in Chapter (4.13.1) of this volume. Perhaps its manifestation of excitement for those who show the disorder is best exemplified by the poet Walt Whitman in his *Poems of Joy* (1860).

> I hear the alarm at dead of night,
>
> I hear the bells—shouts!
>
> I pass the crowd—I run!
>
> The sight of flames maddens me with pleasure.

### (f) Sexually motivated fire-raising

The possible connection between fire-raising and sexuality has already been referred to. The lack of frequent association should not blind clinicians and others to its possible existence in certain cases, or its similarity to sex offending. Fras puts it well—as follows: 'In its comparative, stereotyped sequence of mounting pressure . . . it resembles the sexual perversions, as it may parallel them in its imperviousness to treatment'.[30] It is not without significance that imprisoned fire-raisers appear to have more than their fair share of psychosexual difficulties and partnership problems. In Hurly and Monahan's Grendon Prison study, a large proportion of their sample reported difficulties in social relationships with women.[31]

## Suggestions for management

The word 'Suggestions' is used to indicate that what follows is not intended to be prescriptive; it must be emphasized that no single form of management is likely to be effective. At the assessment stage it is vital to treat every case as singular. Any attempt at assessing the future risk of fire-setting must view the behaviour on the basis of all the facts (for example, full details of the index offence and antecedent history). One can then begin to take the rounded and long view as advocated by Scott in his seminal paper on dangerousness. Assessors of whatever discipline will gain much from absorbing Scott's balanced and insightful views.[32] Pointers to successful assessment and management may be summarized as follows:

- Distinguish the fraudulent fire-raiser. But note that the fire-setter who appears to be engaged upon a fraudulent insurance claim to 'rescue' a failing business may be suffering from an underlying depressive illness. The history-taking in such cases needs to be painstaking and searching. Do not 'run' with what appears to be the obvious explanation.

- Distinguish the politically motivated. But, note that some politically motivated fire-raisers may also have serious mental health problems. In an age when fear of terrorist attacks abounds and the remedies appear to be of the 'knee-jerk' variety, a cool head in the assessment process is essential.

- Distinguish the vandalistic and the differences between young people who set fires out of boredom or for 'kicks' from child fire-setters who are more likely to have seriously dysfunctional social backgrounds.[33,34]

- Distinguish those who are driven to set fires by clear evidence of mental disorder, notably functional psychosis, severe anti-social personality disorder (psychopathy), organic disorder, and learning disability.

- Distinguish those who appear to exhibit pyromania as defined in DSM-IV TSM(Rev).

- Distinguish those rarer cases in which sexual disorder (and in particular sexual dysfunction) may have played a significant role.

- Distinguish the vengeful. It is important to remember that feelings of vengefulness may persist over long periods of time and such fire-raisers may be adept at concealing their vengeful feelings. These fire-raisers have some features in common with the delusionally jealous (Othello-type syndrome).

Successful assessment and management (which ideally should be a 'seamless' process) needs to rest upon a multi-faceted and multi-team approach. An excellent example of such a multi-disciplinary approach may be found in Clare *et al.*[28] They describe their management of a case that necessitated an understanding of both physical and learning disability combined with a capacity to work intensively using eclectic behavioural techniques over a prolonged period of time. Despite minor setbacks, the offender-patient, who had been subject at one time to containment in a high security hospital, remained free of his long-standing fire-raising behaviour at 4-year follow-up. It would also be unwise to believe that psycho-analytically based psychotherapy had no place in the management of psychotic and seriously personality disordered fire-raisers. Cox described some very productive work with such patients in Broadmoor.[35] Social skills training of one kind or another has a very important part to play. Many fire-raisers (particularly the vengeful and those with a pyromania diagnosis) are socially inept and believe themselves to be misunderstood by society. Techniques aimed at improving their self-regard, self-image, and social competence can help to minimize recidivism.

## Conclusion

Not only is arson (fire-raising) a very worrying offence for the reasons given, but it has shown an increase in recent years. Moreover, the 'profile' of those convicted of arson has shifted over the years with an increased proportion of female offenders. And, in a very important recent study, Soothill *et al.* showed at 20 year follow-up that the proportion of those reconvicted for arson had more than doubled. The authors conclude with the sobering observation that 'the situation in relation to arson has deteriorated significantly over the past 40 years'.[36] The causes of fire-raising are complex and attempts at classification have not been entirely successful. Viewing fire-raising as a 'symptom' appears to offer the best hope for more successful diagnosis and management. The brief survey in this chapter has merely touched upon the topic. The suggestions for further reading and the references should assist those who wish to pursue the topic in further depth.

## Acknowledgement

My thanks to Mrs Janet Kirkwood for so ably preparing the final version of the manuscript.

## Further information

Arson Prevention Bureau. The Bureau publishes the *Arson Intelligence Newsletter* at regular intervals. Available from Arson Prevention Bureau, 51 Gresham Street, London, EC2V 7HQ.

Enayati, J., Grann, M., Lubbe, S., *et al.* (2008). Psychiatric Morbidity in Arsonists referred for Forensic Psychiatric Assessment in Sweden. *The Journal of Forensic Psychiatry and Psychology, 19,* 139–147.

Office of the Deputy Prime Minister (ODPM) (2006) *Fire Statistics (UK)* 2004 and *Fire Statistics Monitor* Issue 1/06. 28.2 ODPM. (These publications provide extensive statistical and descriptive data).

Repo, E. and Virkkunen, M. (1997). Outcomes in a sample of Finnish fire-setters. *Journal of Forensic Psychiatry, 8,* 127–37.

Swinton, M. and Ahmed, A. (2001). Arsonists in maximum security. *Medicine, Science, and the Law, 41,* 51–7.

## References

1. Soothill, K. (1991). Arson. In *Principles and practice of forensic psychiatry* (eds. R. Bluglass and P. Bowden), pp. 779–86. Churchill Livingstone, London.
2. Barnett, W. and Spitzer, M. (1994). Pathological fire-setting: 1851–1991: a review. *Medicine, Science, and the Law, 34,* 4–20.
3. Prins, H. (1994). *Fire-raising: its motivation and management.* Routledge, London.
4. Prins, H. (2005). *Offenders, deviants or patients?* (3rd edn) (Chapter 7). Routledge, London.
5. MacDonald, J.M. (1977). *Bombers and fire-setters.* Thomas, Springfield, IL.
6. Prins, H. (2001). Arson and sexuality. In *The encyclopaedia of criminology and deviant behaviour,* Vol. 3 (eds. C.D. Bryant, N. Davis, and G. Geis), pp. 11–5. Brunner-Routledge, New York.
7. Home Office. (2004). *Criminal statistics, England and Wales, 2003.* Cm6361. TSO.
8. Arson Prevention Bureau. (2006). *Arson intelligence newsletter.*(87).
9. Arson Prevention Bureau. (2006). *Arson intelligence newsletter.* (87), and *Fire Statistics, UK, 2004.*ODPM (2006), London.
10. R v. G., and another. (2003). UK HL50. Reported in *The Independent Law Report.* 22.10.03.
11. Lewis, N.D.C. and Yarnell, H. (1951). Pathological fire-setting (Pyromania). *Nervous and mental disease monograph 82.* Coolidge Foundation, New York.
12. Prins (3). Notably pp. 98–103.
13. Faulk, M. (1988). *Basic forensic psychiatry.* Blackwell Science, Oxford.
14. Prins, H., Tennent, G., and Trick, K. (1985). Motives for arson (fire-setting). *Medicine, Science, and the Law, 25,* 275–8.
15. Barker, F. (1994). *Arson: a review of the psychiatric literature.* Oxford University Press, Oxford.
16. Rix, K.J.B. (1994). A psychiatric study of adult arsonists. *Medicine, Science, and the Law, 34,* 21–34.
17. Canter, D. and Fritzon, K. (1998). Differentiating arsonists: a model of fire-setting actions and characteristics. *Legal and Criminological Psychology, 3,* 73–96.
18. Almond, L., Duggan, L., Shine, J., *et al.* (2005). Test of the arson system model on an incarcerated population. *Psychology, Crime and Law, 11,* 1–15.
19. Hakkanen, H., Puolakka, P., and Santilla, P. (2004). Crime scene actions and offender characteristics in arsons. *Legal and Criminological Psychology, 2,* 197–214.
20. Kennedy, P.J., Vale, L.E., Khan, S.J., *et al.* (2006). Factors predicting recidivism in child and adolescent fire-setters. *Journal of Forensic Psychiatry and Psychology, 17,* 151–64.
21. Repo, E. and Virkkunen, M. (1997). Young arsonists: history of conduct disorder, psychiatric diagnoses and criminal recidivism. *Journal of Forensic Psychiatry, 8,* 311–20.
22. Taylor, J.L., Thorne, I., Robertson, A., *et al.* (2002). Evaluating a group intervention for convicted arsonists with mild and borderline intellectual disabilities. *Criminal Behaviour and Mental Health, 12,* 282–93.
23. Coid, J., Wilkins, J., and Coid, B. (1999). Fire-setting, pyromania and self-mutilation in female remanded prisoners. *Journal of Forensic Psychiatry, 10,* 119–30.
24. Noblett, S. and Nelson, B. (2001). A psycho-social approach to arson—a case-controlled study of female offenders. *Medicine, Science, and the Law, 41,* 325–30.
25. Carpenter, P.K. and King, A.L. (1989). Epilepsy and arson. *The British Journal of Psychiatry, 154,* 554–6.
26. Byrne, A. and Walsh, J.B. (1989). The epileptic arsonist. *The British Journal of Psychiatry, 155,* 268.
27. Hurly, W. and Monahan, T.M. (1969). Arson: the criminal and the crime. *British Journal of Criminology, 9,* 4–21.

28. Clare, I.C.H., Murphy, D., Cox, D., *et al.* (1992). Assessment and treatment of fire-setting: a single case investigation using a cognitive behavioural model. *Criminal Behaviour and Mental Health*, **2**, 253–68.

29. American Psychiatric Association. (1994). *Diagnostic and statistical manual of mental disorders* (DSM-IV-4th edn). American Psychiatric Association, Washington, DC.

30. Fras, I. (1983). Fire-setting and its relationship to sexuality. In *Sexual dynamics of anti-social behaviour* (eds. L.D. Schlesinger and E. Revitch), pp. 192–203. Thomas, Springfield, IL.

31. Hurly and Monahan (27).

32. Scott, P.D. (1977). Assessing dangerousness in criminals. *The British Journal of Psychiatry*, **131**, 127–42.

33. Santilla, P., Hakkanen, H., Alison, L., *et al.* (2003). Juvenile fire-setters: crime scene actions and offender characteristics. *Legal and Criminological Psychology*, **8**, 1–20.

34. Perrin-Wallqvist, R. and Nerlander, T. (2003). Fire-setting and playing with fire during childhood and adolescence: interview studies of 18 year-old male draftees and 18-19 year-old female pupils. *Legal and Criminological Psychology*, **8**, 151–8.

35. Cox, M. (1979). Dynamic psychotherapy with sex offenders. In *Sexual deviation* (2nd ed) (ed. I. Rosen), pp. 306–50. Oxford University Press, Oxford.

36. Soothill, K., Ackerley, E., and Francis, B. (2004). The criminal careers of arsonists. *Medicine, Science, and the Law*, **44**, 27–40.

# 11.10

# Stalking

## Paul E. Mullen

## What is stalking?

Stalking is now used to describe a problem behaviour characterized by repeatedly inflicting unwanted intrusions and/or communications on another in a manner which creates fear and/or significant distress.[1] The intrusions can involve, following, loitering nearby, maintaining surveillance, and making approaches. The communication can be via telephone (including SMS), letter, electronic mail, graffiti and notes attached, for example, to the victims' car. Stalking can be associated with a range of harassments which though not part of the core behaviours are all too frequent. These include, ordering goods and services on the victim's behalf (late night pizza's being a favourite) damaging property, spreading malicious rumours, vexatious complaints, threats, 'cyber terrorism', and assault.

There are two basic patterns to stalking.[2] The first involves repeated incursions predominantly in the form of approaches and following perpetrated most often by a stranger and lasting only a day or so. The second is characterized by a range of both communications and intrusions, is usually perpetrated by an ex-intimate or acquaintance, and lasts for weeks, months, or even years. The first type can be intense and distressing at the time but uncommonly culminates in a physical attack and though upsetting, rarely inflicts long-term psychological or social damage. The second type is associated not infrequently with psychological and social damage to the victim and will involve physical assaults in up to a third of victims.

## The epidemiology of stalking

Estimates of the prevalence of stalking, as with any other phenomenon, will vary according to definition, sampling, method of enquiry, and the willingness of subjects to respond and respond frankly.[2-7] Reported lifetime rates of victimization for women are between 8 per cent and 22 per cent and for men between 2 per cent and 8 per cent. Most victims are female (70–80 per cent), most stalkers are male (80–85 per cent), with 20–25 per cent involving same gender stalking, typically male on male.

## Cyberstalking

Cyberstalking has attracted considerable interest but few systematic studies. Even the definitions employed of cyberstalking vary widely.[8-10] As befits an online phenomenon much of the information about it is to be found on the Internet rather than in the more traditional sources of academic knowledge.

Sheridan and colleagues[11] in an important study concluded that cyberstalking was usually one more invasive technique for pursuing stalking rather than a distinct type of activity.

Cyberstalking can include the use of the Internet and SMS facilities to:

1 *Send repeated unwanted messages.*

2 *Order goods and services on the victim's behalf.*

3 *Publicizing private information of a potentially damaging or embarrassing nature.* Including circulating e-mails, placing information on the web containing personal details, and occasionally explicit sexual images.

4 *Spreading false information.* A wide range of misinformation can be spread via the Internet with the authors of these calumnies able, should they wish and have the necessary skills, to hide their identity.

5 *Information gathering online about a victim* can cover a wide range of material from addresses, employment histories, to financial details. There are even services for tracing people available online which can be utilized by stalkers whose victim has eluded them.

6 *Identity theft* goes beyond simply pretending to be the victim for the purposes of ordering goods or initiating contacts to an attempt to assume not just the name but the actual property and attributes of the victim.

7 *Encouraging others to harass the victim.* This can cover activities such as placing communication purporting to be from the victim on web likely to attract unwanted communications or attentions. The most egregious example involved a rejected stalker who posted personal advertisements in his ex-partner's name and giving her address which suggested she enjoyed being raped and solicited such attentions. Apparently six men actually came to her house in response to these provocations.[12]

## Impact on victims

Stalking is both an act of violence in itself which causes psychological distress and social disruption, and is a harbinger of assault. Being stalked can produce a corrosive state of fear, arousal, and helplessness. As with domestic violence for most victims it is not the blows which are the most destructive but living in a chronic state of intimidation and the expectation of imminent intrusion. In the study of Pathé and Mullen[13] the majority reported disruptive levels of anxiety with intrusive recollections of the stalking, sleep disturbance, lowered mood, with 25 per cent admitting considering suicide to escape the situation. A community study found increased rates of psychiatric morbidity and post-traumatic symptomatology amongst those stalked for more than 2 weeks but not amongst those who had experienced the briefer periods of harassment.[14] Dressing and colleagues[7,15] also document significant psychological and social disruption in response to being stalked with 56 per cent reporting agitation, 44 per cent increased anxiety, 41 per cent sleep problems, and 28 per cent increased depression.

## Stalkers: classifications and typologies

Stalking, like most forms of complex human behaviour, can be the outcome of a wide range of psychological, social, and cultural influences. Some stalk in hope, some in anger, some in lust, some in ignorance, and many in mixtures of the above. In an attempt to advance the understanding of stalkers a range of typologies and classifications have been advanced.[16]

Classifying stalkers by the nature of their prior relationship with the victim has the advantages of simplicity and utility. The classification advanced by Mohandie and colleagues[17] represent the best supported by empirical evidence of such approaches to date. They divide stalkers into those with and without a prior relationship. Those with a prior relationship are subdivided into ex-intimates (ex-partners both long term and more casual) and acquaintances (including friends, colleagues, and professional contacts). Those without a prior relationship are subdivided into firstly 'public strangers' who were encountered through the media or in their public roles, and secondly into 'private strangers' encountered by chance in the interactions of everyday life. This classification's greatest utility is in predicting the risks of assault, with those with a prior intimate relationship constituting the highest risk group and those targeting public strangers the lowest. In their view the pursuers of public strangers are the most likely to be psychotic with those pursuing ex-intimates being relatively impervious to therapy but responsive to criminal sanctions.

The typology first developed by Mullen and colleagues[1,18] depends primarily of the context in which the stalking emerges and the motivations which initiated and sustained the behaviour. Its appeal has been primarily to clinicians managing stalkers and their victims.[19] There are five main types:

1  *The rejected* whose stalking begins in the context of the breakdown of a close relationship. The stalking is initially motivated either by the desire for reconciliation or to express the rage at rejection, with a mixture of both being quite common. The stalking is often sustained by the pursuit of the ex-partner becoming a substitute for the lost relationship with the satisfactions from intrusion and control replacing those of intimacy.

2  *The intimacy-seeker* who is pursuing love. The stalking begins in the context of a life bereft of intimacy and is motivated by the hope, or firm expectation, of obtaining a loving relationship with a stranger or casual acquaintance on whom they have fixed their amorous attentions. The pursuit is sustained in the face of indifference or outright rejection because better a love based on fantasy or delusion than no love at all.

3  *The incompetent suitor* who is pursuing a sexual encounter or friendship. This usually begins in the context of loneliness and is motivated by a desire to start some form of relationship with someone who has attracted their interest. This group often pursues intensely with multiple intrusions but rarely persists for more than a day or so, presumably because multiple rebuffs bring few rewards.

4  *The resentful*, whose stalking starts in the context of a grievance at being unjustly treated or humiliated. The initial motivation is revenge but this gives way to the satisfactions obtained from the sense of power over someone who has previously been experienced as an oppressor, or the representative of oppressors.

5  *The predatory*, which begins in the context of the desire to act out violent or sexual fantasies often of a sadistic or paedophilic nature. The initial motivation is to gain information about the movements of a potential victim (usually a stranger but occasionally an acquaintance). The stalking continues because of the satisfactions accruing not just from voyeurism but from the excitement and sense of power which comes from rehearsing the planned attack in fantasy whilst watching the future victim.

Each of the stalker types, hopefully with the exception of the predatory, has correlates in normal behaviour. When relationships break down one partner is often confused or distressed by the separation and seeks to understand, to reconcile, or to express anger. The incompetent suitor is kin to the awkward adolescent male and the socially inept adult who fails to traverse effectively the social minefields of courting or simply making acquaintance. The intimacy seeker is the adolescent crush and the enthusiastic fan writ large. Even the resentful is not far removed from some seekers after justice and those asserting their rights. In theory the boundary between persistent approaches as part of socially acceptable behaviour and the crime of stalking are difficult to pin down. In practice the distinction is rarely a problem. Stalkers are those who repeatedly force themselves on another person in a manner which creates obvious distress. It is the total disregard, or blindness to, the disturbance and often fear that their behaviour creates which distinguishes the stalker from their more normal counterparts. Sometimes the stalkers are so caught up in their own world they are oblivious to their effect on others. Sometimes they are blinded by delusion. Sometimes self-righteousness makes them indifferent. But sometimes they delight in the effect they produce in their victim.

## Psychopathology of stalkers

Stalkers are rarely, if ever, drawn from the psychologically adequate or socially able of the world. The estimates of the proportion of stalkers whose behaviour is directly related to mental disorders varies according to where the researchers derived their sample. For example, Zona and his group[20] whose sample contained many who pursued Hollywood celebrities had a significant number with erotomanias and morbid infatuations.

In broad terms psychotic disorders are relatively frequent in the intimacy seeking group. In the resentful type it is the paranoid disorders which unsurprisingly predominate, though most are not associated with frank delusion. The rejected often have problems around dependency, rigidity, control, and self-esteem with substance abuse and depressive states on occasion complicating the picture, but psychotic states are uncommon. The incompetent suitors are socially disabled sometimes by shyness, sometimes by narcissism, sometimes by intellectual limitations, sometimes by culture, sometimes by disorders such as Asperger's syndrome, rarely by psychosis, but always by interpersonal insensitivity or indifference. The predatory are sexually perverse and not infrequently have marked psychopathic traits, but again are rarely psychotic.

Attempts have been made to conceptualize stalking as a manifestation of obsessive–compulsive disorder. Stalkers are certainly often obsessive in the everyday sense of that word in their pursuit of the victim. They rarely however regard their behaviour as unjustified let alone irrational, and few see their persistence as senseless. They may resist the urges to stalk on occasion but for the most part devote themselves wholeheartedly to the pursuit. Anxiety is more likely to be generated by the fear of failure, or of consequences, than by not acting on their impulses to stalk. They may well spend many hours thinking about the object of their unwanted attentions, and in the resentful reliving the experiences of actual or supposed injustice, so in that sense they are ruminators. Personality traits of rigidity, rumination, and the overvaluing of order are not infrequently so marked in rejected and resentful stalkers as to justify a label of an obsessional personality. In short, the behaviour often has an obsessive quality but the state of mind rarely conforms to that found in obsessive–compulsive disorders.

Attachment theory has unsurprisingly been evoked to explain stalking. That stalkers as a group don't do interpersonal relationships very well is obvious. Evidence exists that insecure attachment styles predominate amongst rejected stalkers, the intimacy seekers may have the type of secure attachment style only sustainable by delusion, and the incompetent and resentful favour the dismissive style. This is useful in assessment and management but what connection it may have with any theory of early development is speculative and here as elsewhere more likely to be productive of mythologizing than good clinical practice.

## The stalking of health professionals

Health care professionals have a heightened vulnerability to being stalked by their patients and clients.[21–24] The risk stems largely from resentful and disappointed patients but in part from lonely and disordered people who misconstrue sympathy and attention for romantic interest. While some stalking behaviours constitute little more than minor irritations, they may also ruin a clinician's career.

Sandberg et al.[25] studied an inpatient psychiatric service reporting 53 per cent of clinical staff had been stalked by patients. Galeazzi and colleagues[26] found 11 per cent of the mental health professionals in an Italian service had been stalked for lengthy periods by patients. Purcell and colleagues[14] surveyed a randomly selected sample of 1750 psychologists (73 per cent female). The lifetime prevalence of stalking by clients was 19.5 per cent with 8 per cent being stalked in the preceding 12 months. Most victims were working in direct client care (95 per cent) and experienced rather than new entrants to the profession. Stalkers fell predominantly into either the intimacy seeking (19 per cent) or resentful (42 per cent) types. Over 30 per cent of psychologists in this study were

subjected to vexatious complaints by their stalker. The impact of complaints to professional boards, health ombudsmen, and other agencies of accountability can be devastating.

Too often in the past therapists who fell victim to stalking by patients had to bear the additional burden of implied or overt criticism from colleagues to the effect that, had they more adroitly managed the therapeutic encounter and the resultant transference, they would not now find themselves in this predicament. There should be no sympathy with blaming the victim, even if it comes in the guise of technical advice or supervision. Being stalked is a risk inherent in the therapeutic process. Our colleagues should be accorded support and help, if for no other reason than we do not know when it may be our turn to face the pursuit of the vengeful or lustful patient.

## Risk assessment and risk management

Stalking came to prominence because it was regarded as a risk factor for violence. Subsequently it became clear that the damage inflicted on those who are stalked could also encompass significant social and psychological damage.[23]

Assessing and managing the stalker requires a primary focus on the risks they present to the victim. Nevertheless the risk that stalkers incur from their own behaviour also needs to be considered (Table 11.10.1). The conflict between the stalker's desires and the victim's interests are obvious, but they are at one in being at risk of damage from the stalking situation. There can be a tragic symmetry between the victim forced to live an increasingly restricted life in a state of constant fear, and the stalkers devoting all their time and resources to a damaging and ultimately self-defeating pursuit. The victim's and the perpetrator's lives can be laid waste. This is not to argue for equivalence between victim and perpetrator but merely to note they share the chance of disaster. A perspective which encompasses the risks to stalkers and victims has the advantage for health professionals of reducing the ethical dilemma when treating stalkers around whose interests one is serving, the patient's or their victim's. We help both to the extent that we contribute to stopping the stalking, or reducing its damaging consequences.

### The empirical basis for evaluating risk in the stalking situation

Risk assessment in stalking situations is currently hampered by a paucity of either retrospective or prospective studies of representative samples. Clinicians do not, however, have the luxury of deferring action until such evidence emerges. They must, for the present, depend on integrating knowledge from stalking research, borrowing from the systematic studies of risk in other areas, and drawing on clinical experience.[27]

### The risk of continued or recurrent stalking

The duration of stalking is longest for rejected stalkers pursuing ex-intimates and intimacy seekers, with the incompetents usually pursuing only briefly. Women, here as elsewhere, are more persistent than men.[6,13] Once stalking has continued for more than 2 weeks the chances are high that it will continue for months.

### The risks of psychological and/or social damage

Female victims of stalking report a greater psychological impact than male victims.[5,13] Clinically, the distress and disruption to

**Table 11.10.1** The stalker's clinical risk factors and future hazards specific to stalking situation

| Risk factor | Management possibilities include |
|---|---|
| *Clinical* | |
| 1. Mental state e.g. depression, delusional preoccupations | Active treatment usually involving pharmacotherapy |
| 2. Substance abuse | Referral to a specialist substance abuse service where possible or to self-help groups like AA |
| 3. Anger | Anger management remains a problematic area. Ideally those with anger control problems should be receiving special help independently of the broader management of their stalking |
| 4. Attitudes towards, and beliefs about, the victim which sustain stalking | Appropriate legal interventions; CBT and focussed psychotherapies aimed at such areas as; abandoning love, accepting loss, confronting misperceptions |
| 5. The conviction that they are right to engage in stalking | Enhancing victim empathy. Confronting false attributions using CBT |
| 6. The refusal to engage in any therapy, or conform to legally imposed restrictions on access to the victim | Ultimately confronting the stalker with consequences (e.g. through breaching parole, referring back to court, etc.); employing motivational interviewing strategies to assist the stalker to appreciate the need for intervention |
| 7. Social incompetence | Social skills training, therapies aimed at enhancing self-efficacy |
| 8. Paraphilia | Sex offender program incorporating CBT +/− pharmacotherapy as indicated |
| *Future hazards* | |
| 1. Likely future contact with the victim | Every effort should be made to enforce a total ban on direct contact or direct communications |
| 2. Lack of a feasible set of plans for avoiding a recrudescence of stalking | Ensure structured plan around avoiding provocations and using protections re: stalking; CBT to assist the stalker to overcome the compulsion to stalk |
| 3. That the underlying precipitants remain unresolved | Focussed psychotherapy aimed at the areas identified in the formulation; social skills training for the inept; assistance abandoning the relationship; the treatment of paraphilias using CBT +/− pharmacotherapy as indicated |
| 4. Continuing instability of residence and/or employment | Assistance obtaining housing; career counselling; and active employment rehabilitation as indicated and appropriate |
| 5. Continuing social isolation | Use of clubs, day centres, recreational counselling, domestic pets |
| 6. Likely low level of compliance with legal restraints on contact with victim | Ensure knowledge of consequences of breaches and never collude—implicitly or explicitly—with avoiding those consequences |
| 7. Likely low level of cooperation with any treatment programme | Use of compulsory community treatment orders either imposed by court or as part of mental health legislation |

victims is usually most obvious in ex-intimates pursued by their rejected partners, perhaps because of the higher levels of violence and intimidation combined with the complexity, as well as the intensity, of feelings stirred up in this situation.[13] Psychological distress was higher amongst victims who were subjected to prolonged and repeated following and the experience of property theft or destruction.[2,13,28,29] The relationship between psychological impact and the experience of physical violence is less clear, despite its intuitive appeal.[29,30]

## The risks of violence

### (a) Prior relationship

Victims who have shared a prior intimate relationship with their stalker are at a high risk of physical violence.[1,4,13,20,31–35] Purcell and colleagues[6] for example reported in a random community sample that ex-intimates were the most likely to be attacked (56 per cent), followed by estranged relatives or previous friends (36 per cent), then casual acquaintances (16 per cent), work-related contacts (9 per cent), and finally strangers (8 per cent). Such findings should not be interpreted, however, as suggesting that victims of stalkers who are not ex-intimates are in little danger of physical violence. A chance of between 8 per cent and 36 per cent of being assaulted is no small risk.

### (b) Threats

Between 30 per cent and 60 per cent of stalking victims are threatened.[1,20,31] In a community-based study 44 per cent of those threatened were subsequently assaulted and 73 per cent of victims assaulted by their stalker had previously been explicitly threatened.[6] In short threats predict violence and should be taken seriously.

### (c) Mental disorder

Research has generally concluded that psychotic stalkers are less likely to be physically violent than their non-psychotic counterparts but the relationship to personality disorder remains unclear.[1,34,36,37]

### (d) Substance abuse

Substance abuse is associated with violence in the stalking situation.[1,38–40]

### (e) Prior offending and antisocial behaviour

The empirical data on the association between past criminal or violent behaviour and stalking violence is inconsistent, however the balance of the evidence favours such a relationship.[1,34,39,41]

### (f) Demographic variables

The gender of stalkers has repeatedly been shown to have no impact on the prevalence of either threats or assault.[4–6,13,42]

### (g) The nature of the stalking

Violence is predicted by escalating intrusiveness and intensity of the stalking behaviour. The strongest association is to physical intrusions into the victims house or place of work.[36]

### The assessment process

Initial assessments of stalkers often occur in the context of pre-sentence or parole board evaluations. Victims may be encountered in a wider range of contexts, many seeking help from general rather than forensic mental health professionals. Stalkers usually lack insight into their behaviour and tend to deny, minimize, and rationalize their actions. Victims often minimize the experience of stalking and over-emphasize their own responsibility for the harassment, which should be of no surprise to anybody experienced in working with victims in other contexts. Conversely, the problem of false claims of stalking victimization cannot be entirely ignored.[43] This makes it essential to assess collateral information from such sources as witness statements, victim impact reports, judges' sentencing remarks, and professional to professional contacts, confidentiality allowing. Attempts to contact the victim when assessing the stalker, or the stalker when assessing the victim are, in our opinion, best avoided. However skilfully managed, such contacts tend to be experienced by the victim as the professional acting as an agent of the stalker, and by the stalker as support for their beliefs that this is a misunderstanding within a mutual relationship rather than a unilateral imposition of unwanted attentions.[27]

### Management

The management of stalkers remains very much the province of forensic mental health professionals and even amongst them it is a specialist area. Basic approaches to identifying potentially remediable risks and their management however is presented in. Victims of stalking are however likely to be seen by a wide range of mental health professionals.

# Reducing the impact on victims

Stalking victims will often present with significant problems with anxiety symptoms and depressed mood. The symptom complex of PTSD will be present to a greater or lesser extent in most victims of prolonged and intense stalking. Like many victim groups there may be a reluctance to disclose the details or even the existence of the traumatic experiences. As noted earlier self-blame is not infrequently part of the picture.

Given the high profile of stalking there are a number of disturbed people who claim they are being stalked as a way to express their distress, claim attention, or give form to their persecutory delusions.[24,43] This group, particularly if delusional, are often obvious given the flamboyant, implausible, and exuberant accounts of victimization. Care should be taken in dismissing claims of being stalked, however, as there are some very unpleasant stalkers out there some of whom stalk leaving few, if any, objective signs. False victims require help and treatment not rejection, but they require quite different treatment from actual victims.

Stalking victims need first and foremost good psychiatric care. Manage the stress symptoms, treat the depression, ameliorate the distress, and provide adequate support. Individual treatment is best initially but the use of groups for long-term support and treatment

is worth considering.[44] What follows is a brief account of stalking specific interventions.

1 Informing others. When you are stalked it is essential to inform those you live with, work with, and are friends with. This performs three functions:

   (a) It allows you a 'reality check' on your fears that stalking is occurring.

   (b) It enables others to support you and equally important avoid inadvertently assisting the stalker.

   (c) It prevents those around you being put at risk by ignorance provoking the stalker thereby also falling victim.

3 Avoid contact and/or confrontation. All contacts or direct communications with a stalker risks reinforcing their behaviour. Confrontation and worse still violence, legitimizes, and encourages their violence. Once stalking is established it is usually too late to simply sort things out by having a meeting.

4 Documentation. The best protection for stalking victims lies in the criminal law. The police are more likely to respond appropriately if you can demonstrate that the behaviour is occurring and make it relatively easy for them to pursue the allegations. Keep the letters (dated), record the phone calls and retain the tapes, keep a diary noting approaches and where possible witnesses to those events, record verbatim any threats and obtain witnesses or photographs of any property damage. Not only will this be invaluable for a later prosecution it is part of the victim taking control back over their lives.

5 Restraining, non-molestation, apprehended violence and other such orders. Sometimes these civil orders do provide an effective means of reducing or stopping stalking. Police often advise their use, hopefully not just to avoid work. Some jurisdictions insist on obtaining such orders prior to considering criminal prosecution. Reservations have to be expressed, however, not only about their effectiveness (totally ineffective for intimacy seekers, relatively ineffective for the rejected and intermittently effectively for the resentful) but also about the level of insecurity and distress consequent on their breach and facing the frequent indifference of the police to such breaches.

6 Increased security. Simple cheap security measures such as good locks, movement triggered lighting outside the house, and securing the mail box may provide a degree of reassurance and a modicum of security.

# Conclusions

Not a few psychiatrists, at least of my generation, have difficulties with the notion of problem behaviour like stalking being a proper subject for mental health concern. Psychiatry has traditionally been wary of concerning itself directly with criminal and antisocial behaviours.[45,46] The approach taken in this chapter was, in contrast, to define a pattern of behaviour destructive to the interests of perpetrator and victim and then to examine its origins, effects, and potential therapeutic management. That this is an enterprise with risks for the ethical integrity of psychiatry is undoubted. But recognizing that psychiatry can have a role in assessing and managing problem behaviours, without first performing obfuscating transformations into supposed mental disorders such as paraphilias and impulse control disorders, allows a more clear sighted and effective approach to areas of human activity where our intervention can benefit both the actor and the wider community.

## Further information

Mullen, P.E., Pathé, M., and Purcell, R. (2000). *Stalkers and their victims*. Cambridge University Press, Cambridge (new edition due 2008).

Pinals, D.A. (ed.) (2007). *Stalking psychiatric perspectives and practical approaches*. Oxford University Press, New York.

## References

1. Mullen, P.E., Pathé, M., Purcell, R., *et al.* (1999). A study of stalkers. *The American Journal of Psychiatry*, **156**, 1244–9.

2. Purcell, R., Pathé, M., and Mullen, P.E. (2004). When do repeated intrusions become stalking? *The Journal of Forensic Psychiatry and Psychology*, **15**, 571–83.

3. Australian Bureau of Statistics. (1996). *Women's safety, Australia, 1996*. Commonwealth of Australia, Canberra.

4. Tjaden, P. and Thoennes, N. (1998). *Stalking in America: findings from the national violence against women survey*. National Institute of Justice and Centres for Disease Control and Prevention, Washington, DC.

5. Budd, T. and Mattinson, J. (2000). *Stalking: findings from the 1998 British crime survey*. Research Findings No. 129, Home Office Research Development and Statistics Directorate.

6. Purcell, R., Pathé, M., and Mullen, P.E. (2002). The prevalence and nature of stalking in the Australian community. *The Australian and New Zealand Journal of Psychiatry*, **36**, 114–20.

7. Dressing, H., Kuehner, C., and Gass, P. (2005). Lifetime prevalence and impact of stalking in a European population: epidemiological data from a middle-sized German city. *The British Journal of Psychiatry*, **187**, 168–72.

8. Bocij, P. and McFarlane, L. (2002). Online harassment: towards a definition of cyberstalking. *Prison Service Journal*, **139**, 31–8.

9. Bocij, P. and McFarlane, L. (2003). Cyberstalking: the technology of hate. *Police Journal*, **76**, 204–21.

10. Barak, A. (2005). Sexual harassment on the Internet. *Social Science Computer Review*, **23**, 77–92.

11. Sheridan, L.P., *et al.* (in press). Is cyberstalking different. *Psychology Crime and Law*.

12. Miller, G. and Maharaj, D. (1999). Chilling cyber-stalking case illustrates new breed of crime. *Los Angeles Times*.

13. Pathé, M. and Mullen, P.E. (1997). The impact of stalkers on their victims. *The British Journal of Psychiatry*, **170**, 12–17.

14. Purcell, R., Powell, M.B., and Mullen, P.E. (2005). Clients who stalk psychologists: prevalence, methods and motives. *Professional Psychology: Research and Practice*, **36**, 537–43.

15. Dressing, H., Gass, P., and Kuehner, C. (2007). What can we learn from the first community-based epidemiological study on stalking in Germany? *International Journal of Law and Psychiatry*, **30**, 10–7.

16. Spitzberg, B.H. and Cupach, W.R. (2003). What man pursuit? Obsessive relational intrusion and stalking related phenomena. *Aggression and Violent Behaviour*, **8**, 345–75.

17. Mohandie, K., Meloy, J.R., McGowan, M., *et al* (2006). The RECON typology of stalking: reliability and validity based upon a large sample of North American stalkers. *Journal of Forensic Sciences*, **51**, 147–155.

18. Mullen, P.E., Pathé, M., and Purcell, R. (2000). *Stalkers and their victims*. Cambridge University Press, Cambridge.

19. Pinals, D.A. (2007). *Stalking: psychiatric perspectives and practical applications*. APA Press, Washington, DC.

20. Zona, M.A., Sharma, K., and Lane, J. (1993). A comparative study of erotomanic and obsessional subjects in a forensic sample. *Journal of Forensic Sciences*, **38**, 894–903.

21. Sandberg, D.A., McNiel, D.E., and Binder, R.L. (1998). Characteristics of psychiatric inpatients who stalk, threaten, or harass hospital staff after discharge. *The American Journal of Psychiatry*, **155**, 1102–5.

22. Purcell, R., Pathé, M., and Mullen, P.E. (2001). A study of women who stalk. *The American Journal of Psychiatry*, **158**, 2056–60.

23. Mullen, P.E. and Purcell, R. (2007). Stalking of therapists. In *Severe personality disorders: major issues in everyday practice* (eds. B. van Luyn, S. Akhtar, and J. Livesley). Cambridge University Press, Cambridge.

24. Mullen, P.E., Pathé, M., and Purcell, R. (in preparation). *Stalkers and their victims* (2nd edn). Cambridge University Press, Cambridge.

25. Sandberg, D.A., McNiel, D.E., and Binder, R.L. (2002). Stalking, threatening and harassing behavior by psychiatric patients toward clinicians. *The Journal of the American Academy of Psychiatry and the Law*, **30**, 221–9.

26. Galeazzi, G.M., Elkins, K., and Curci, P. (2005). The stalking of mental health professionals by patients. *Psychiatric Services*, **56**, 137–8.

27. Mullen, P.E., Mackenzie, R., Olgoff, J.R.P., *et al.* (2006). Assessing and managing the risks in the stalking situation. *The Journal of the American Academy of Psychiatry and the Law*, **34**, 439–50.

28. Blaauw, E., Winkel, F.W., Arensman, E., *et al.* (2002). The toll of stalking: the relationship between features of stalking and psychopathology of victims. *Journal of Interpersonal Violence*, **17**, 50–63.

29. Kamphuis, J.H., Emmelkamp, P.M.G., and Bartak, A. (2003). Individual differences in post-traumatic stress following post-intimate stalking: stalking severity and psychosocial variables. *The British Journal of Clinical Psychology*, **42**, 145–56.

30. McEwan, T., Mullen, P.E., and Purcell, R. (2007). Identifying risk factors in stalking: a review of current research. *International Journal of Law and Psychiatry*, **30**, 1–9.

31. Harmon, R.B., Rosner, R., and Owens, H. (1998). Sex and violence in forensic population of obsessional harassers. *Psychology, Public Policy and Law*, **4**, 236–49.

32. Meloy, J.R. (1998). The psychology of stalking. In *The psychology of stalking: clinical and forensic perspectives* (ed. J.R. Meloy), pp. 2–23. Academic Press, San Diego.

33. Meloy, J.R. (1999). Stalking: an old behavior, a new crime. *Forensic Psychiatry*, **22**, 85–99.

34. Meloy, J.R., Davis, B., and Lovette, J. (2001). Risk factors for violence among stalkers. *Journal of Threat Assessment*, **1**, 3–16.

35. Sheridan, L., Davies, G.M., and Boon, J.C. (2001). Stalking: perceptions and prevalence. *Journal of Interpersonal Violence*, **16**, 151–67.

36. Farnham, F.R., James, D.V., and Cantrell, P. (2000). Association between violence, psychosis, and relationship to victim in stalkers. *Lancet*, **355**, 199.

37. Kienlen, K.K., Birmingham, D.L., Solberg, K.B., *et al.* (1997). A comparative study of psychotic and nonpsychotic stalking. *The Journal of the American Academy of Psychiatry and the Law*, **25**, 317–34.

38. Rosenfeld, B. and Harmon, R. (2002). Factors associated with violence in stalking and obsessional harassment cases. *Criminal Justice and Behavior*, **29**, 671–91.

39. Brewster, M.P. (2000). Stalking by former intimates: verbal threats and other predictors of physical violence. *Violence and Victims*, **15**, 41–54.

40. Roberts, K.A. (2005). Women's experience of violence during stalking by former romantic partners: factors predictive of stalking violence. *Violence Against Women*, **11**, 89–114.

41. Palarea, R.E., Zona, M.A., Lane, J.C., *et al.* (1999). The dangerous nature of intimate relationship stalking: threats, violence, and

associated risk factors. *Behavioral Sciences & the Law*, **17**, 269–83.

42. Meloy, J.R. and Boyd, C. (2003). Female stalkers and their victims. *The Journal of the American Academy of Psychiatry and the Law*, **31**, 211–19.

43. Pathé, M., Mullen, P.E., and Purcell, R. (1999). Stalking: false claims of victimisation. *The British Journal of Psychiatry*, **174**, 170–3.

44. Pathé, M. (2002). *Surviving stalking*. Cambridge University Press, Cambridge.

45. Clare, A. (1997). The disease concept in psychiatry. In *Essentials of postgraduate psychiatry* (eds. R. Murray, P. Hill, and P. McGuffin), pp. 41–52. Cambridge University Press, Cambridge.

46. Lewis, A. (1955). Health as a social concept. *The British Journal of Sociology*, **4**, 109–24.

# Querulous behaviour: vexatious litigation, abnormally persistent complaining and petitioning

## Paul E. Mullen

Querulantenwahn (Ger.) A form of so called paranoia in which there exists in a patient an insuppressible and fanatic craving for going to law in order to get redress for some wrong which he believes done to him. Individuals who fall victim to this disorder are always strongly predisposed . . .. extremely egotistical . . . know everything better . . . differs from other forms of paranoia in so far as the wrong may not be quite imaginary . . . the more he fails the more he becomes convinced that enormous wrong is being done to him . . . neglects his family and his business . . . going down the road to ruin.[1]

The above quote neatly summarizes classical psychiatry's view of querulous, or litigious, insanity as a form of paranoia. A problematic form, however, in that the querulousness was usually based on a genuine grievance and was often regarded as developing on the basis of predispositions rooted in the sufferer's personality.[2–4] As to treatment Krafft Ebing[3] notes the 'necessary and beneficent (effects of the) appointment of a guardian and commitment to an asylum' but regretted that this 'takes place unfortunately only after they have used up their property, insulted the courts, and disturbed public order' (p. 395).

Psychiatries interest in the querulous (from the Latin to mutter and to mumble) waned rapidly in the latter half of the twentieth century. The diagnosis was appealed to less and less and the literature largely fell silent.[5] In part the disappearance of querulousness, and even the querulous patient, from the realms of psychiatry paralleled the decline of paranoia as a diagnostic entity. In part it reflected psychiatries increasing reluctance to play the role of social regulator. Probably most importantly the emerging culture of individual rights made pathologizing complainants potentially disastrous as it could deprive them of access to the major social mechanisms for obtaining justice.[6] Psychiatry lost interest in the querulant, however, at the very time that the 'culture of complaint' drew more and more vulnerable people into the systems of complaint management. Agencies of accountability, which range from Ombudsmen's offices, via registration boards, to complaints departments, are now almost all faced with the problems created by a small group of people pursuing grievances with a persistence and

insistence out of all proportion to the substantive nature of their claim. It is estimated that 20–30 per cent of the resources of these agencies are being consumed by less than 1 per cent of unusually persistent complainants. In the civil and family courts the number of interminable cases being pursued, often by unrepresented litigants, escalates year by year. Last, but not the least, querulants pursuing what they regard as their rights through repeated petitions and intrusive approaches to politicians and heads of state distract protection services from more substantial threats.[7–9]

## Clinical features

The querulant pursue their vision of justice through litigation in the court, through petitions to the powerful, and finally through the various agencies of accountability. In practice all three avenues are often explored. In the nineteenth and early twentieth century it was the civil courts in which these dramas were usually played out. Today the main burden falls on the complaints organizations.

It is not easy to distinguish the querulant from the difficult complainant or even from social reformers and victims of gross injustice. A simple typology may assist:

1 *Normal complainants* are aggrieved seeking compensation, reparation, or just an apology. They will accept conciliation and reasonable solutions, though they may become persistent and insistent if provoked by inefficiency or injustice.

2 *Difficult complainants* also seek compensation and reparation but often want in addition retribution. They tend from the outset to anger, to seeing themselves as the victim of others intentional malevolence, and to resist all solutions but their own. Eventually, however, they will settle for the best deal they can obtain.

3 *Altruistic reformers* who pursue goals of social progress via the courts, petitions, and complaints. They sacrifice their personal interests in pursuit of better outcomes for others. Though they may have a political agenda which is sectarian (e.g. antigenetically

modified foods, fathers rights) they do not have idiosyncratic and personalized objectives.

4 *Fraudsters* who knowingly pursue false or grossly exaggerated claims.

5 *The mentally ill* whose claims are driven by delusional preoccupations frequently bizarre in nature which reflect underlying disorders often of a schizophrenic type.

6 *The querulous* who seek personal vindication in addition to compensation, reparation, and retribution. They are on a quest for justice which becomes totally preoccupying. Unlike reformers, and most of the difficult, there is an obvious discrepancy between the provoking event and the importance attached to it by the querulous. They appear to seek not resolution but continuation of the conflict. They lay waste to their social and economic functioning.

The querulous are usually males who first become embroiled in complaining and claiming in their fourth or fifth decade. Premorbidly they were often able to function reasonably well. They rarely have criminal records or prior psychiatric contact, and substance abuse is not prominent. Many had relationships but by the time they reach psychiatrists they have usually alienated their family and friends. Querulants are often disappointed people who feel their qualities have been ignored and left unrewarded. Their pursuit of justice offers an opportunity to vindicate their lives and obtain the public recognition so long denied. Their personalities tend to have the traits of self-absorption, suspiciousness, and obsessionality combined with an enviable capacity for persistence.

Clinically they typically present as energized, garrulous individuals eager to convince you of the merits of their case. There is an enthusiasm which can seem almost manic but unlike the manic they are totally focussed and almost impossible to distract from their narrative of injustice. They may come with bags overflowing with documents testifying to their misplaced scholarship. If challenged they usually become patronizing as they pedantically refute all objections, to their complete satisfaction. Alternatively they may become menacing and overtly threatening.

Communications from querulants were noted by Lester and colleagues[10] to be often characterized by:

- Multiple methods of emphasis including, underlining, highlighting (often in multiple colours), and capitalization

- The generous use of inverted comas, exclamation marks, and question marks

- Numerous foot and marginal notes

- The use of attachments, often extensively annotated, some potentially pertinent (e.g. letters received, copies of legislation), others of less obvious relevance (e.g. Magna Carta, UN Declaration of Human Rights)

- And many many pages.

The content of communications may also be unusual sometimes containing:

- Legal, medical, and other terms used frequently but often incorrectly

- Repeated rhetorical questions

- A curious combination of rambling repetitiveness with pedantry (more difficult to describe than recognize)

- Veiled threats to harm themselves or others if their wishes are not granted or

- Exaggerated politeness and attempts to ingratiate.

## Clinical assessment

The querulous can only be adequately assessed by considering the development over time of their behaviour as well as their state of mind. In an interview they may present as merely overenthusiastic and over hopeful pursuing their legitimate rights with at worst a degree of fanaticism. It is the unfolding of their story which reveals the damage they are suffering, and they have inflicted on those around them.

### Case history (representing an anonamized conflation of several cases)

A man in his late forties made a complaint to the local bank manager over the manner in which mortgage documents had been prepared. There were grounds for legitimate concern as irregularities had occurred, though of a minor nature and of a kind which might have been expected to be to his advantage. His initial complaint to the bank was rejected. He appealed unsuccessfully to the banking ombudsman. He stopped paying the mortgage and initiated civil action. Over the next 5 years he pursued his complaints with the human rights commissioner, the securities exchange commissioner, consumer rights organizations, via further civil litigation, and petitions to Parliament and the Queen. The foreclosure on the mortgage intensified the complaints and litigation. Finally he made a series of bomb threats leading to his prosecution and referral. When assessed he was righteously indignant, believing he had been right to take extreme action to bring attention to an injustice which had destroyed him and his family and threatened the very economic fabric of the nation. He firmly believed he was owed millions in punitive damages, and that when he inevitably prevailed this would bring down the transnational banking corporation which owned his particular branch office. He regarded himself as a whistle blower who would be publicly recognized as one of the major social reformers of his generation. The changes over time in the grievance, the agents, his state of mind, social situation, beliefs, and aims are presented schematically in Table 11.11.1

Traditionally psychiatry has attempted to distinguish between deluded querulants, who are in the business of mental health services, and the non-deluded, who are not. Unfortunately for this approach the querulous present a formidable phenomenological challenge. They advance their ideas plausibly making apparently rational connections between the underlying grievance, which is almost always based on some actual injustice, and their current claims and complaints. Unlike many deluded patients, their beliefs do not usually seem to arise either on the basis of some difficult to understand interpretation of an event, or from an idiosyncratic insight into reality. The querulous offer a detailed and apparently logical account of the emergence of their grievances and the progress of their quest for justice. Reasonable that is if taken in cross section but not when considered over time when there emerge gross discrepancies between the supposed initiating cause and subsequent behaviour. The persuasive presentation can obscure the essential absurdity of the quest and distract attention from the chaos they have created for themselves and those around them. The temptation is to normalize the clinical presentation but this is

**Table 11.11.1** A case of querulous behaviour: the changes over a 5-year period in the various domains illustrating the descent from the reasonable if over hopeful and oversensitive to the unrealistic and unrealizable

| Grievance | Agents |
|---|---|
| Errors in mortgage documents | Bank's accountant |
| Potential financial loss | Plus manager |
| Actual financial loss | Plus senior management |
| Victim of major fraud and theft | Plus banking ombudsman |
| System wide corruption | Plus lawyers and judges |
| A campaign of financial corruption threatening the nations economic stability | Plus wife |
| | Plus various public agencies |
| | Plus police |
| | Plus prime minister |
| | Plus secret services |

| State of mind | Social situation |
|---|---|
| Rigid discontented man obsessional traits but articulate and ambitious | Moderately successful small businessman, married, two children, but experiencing financial pressures and marital problems |
| Increasingly fixated on grievance | Business begins to fail as all his attention moves to grievance |
| Pursuit of justice subordinates all other concerns | Marriage breaks down |
| Increasingly convinced he is being persecuted and spied upon | Alienates few friends he had |
| He is a man of destiny fighting forces of national and international corruption | Bankruptcy |
| | Living alone |
| | Destitute |

| Beliefs | Aims |
|---|---|
| That order and due process are the bedrock of civilization | Compensation for malfeasance (the sum rapidly escalating over the years) |
| Bad things happen not by chance but because of carelessness or malevolence | Reparation—a return of his house mortgage free |
| That he had never received the recognition and rewards he deserved | Retribution—punitive damages, sackings, and criminal prosecutions |
| He was destined for greatness | Vindication by public recognition as a whistle blower who had reformed the banking system |

(Reproduced from P. E. Mullen and G. Lester, Vexatious litigants and unusually persistent complainants and petitioners: from querulous paranoia to querulous behaviour, *Behavioural Sciences and the Law*, **24**, 333–49, copyright 2006, John Wiley & Sons, Inc.)

to ignore both the peculiarity of their behaviour and beliefs, as well as the devastation they have wrought on their own lives. Sometimes the querulous are obviously deluded, sometimes they appear to inhibit that borderline which is captured in such terms as overvalued ideas and delusion like ideas. Debates over the phenomenological niceties should not, however, distract from recognizing the pathological nature of such querulousness.

The querulous are sometimes regarded as obsessional. The level of preoccupation, the ruminative quality of their thinking, and the pedantic attention to the minutiae of their case, all suggest obsession. Certainly most, if not all, querulants have obsessional personality traits. But the querulant does not regard their core beliefs and the behaviour as absurd or absurdly insistent. Quite the reverse they know they are right and are totally identified with their ideas. The querulous therefore may be regarded as obsessive or fixated but not as having an obsessional disorder.[6]

## Management

Our courts and agencies of accountability are designed to deliver conciliation, arbitration, reparation, and compensation, but rarely retribution, except in the exceptional case of punitive damages, and never personal vindication. The querulous seek above all personal vindication and retribution so from the outset are doomed to fail.

One view is that it is the failures of the courts and complaints organization that drive claimants to become querulous. Charles Dickens articulates this in his great novel Bleak House arguing the courts 'give to monied might the means abundantly of wearying out the right. . . (which) so overthrows the brain and breaks the heart to leave its worn out lunatics in every madhouse'. Lester and colleagues[10] in their study of unusually persistent complainants failed to document any significant differences between the manner in which the complaints had been dealt with in those whom became querulous and those who did not. This suggests a role in the pathogenesis for vulnerability not just reacting to provocations.

The impact of querulousness can be reduced by improved recognition and improved management practices in courts and agencies of accountability.[6] Psychiatrists currently only tend to be involved after the situation has reached the stage of the querulant either becoming seriously depressed or being charged with threats, violence, or contempt.

The literature on the therapeutic management of the querulous is both small and predominantly discouraging.[11] Ungvari,[12] however, reported successful treatment using pimozide. Our own experience is that relatively low doses of atypical antipsychotics are helpful though the response is slow in coming often taking months before there is obvious improvement. The first problem is attaining some semblance of a therapeutic alliance with the patient. This requires avoiding being caught up in discussions of the rights and wrongs of their quest. The focus should be on the price they and their family are paying for the pursuit.[6] Interestingly some of those who come on orders from the court which mandate treatment will accept medication and other therapeutic interventions as they wish to make clear they abide by the law. Paradoxically they can be ultra compliant patients. A number have continued voluntarily in treatment after the end of the order though they never acknowledge either that they were in error or in need of treatment because of their querulousness. What changes is the involvement in the querulous ideas, the degree of preoccupations, and the behaviour, but the core belief that they were right never wavers. Querulous behaviour appears to be sustained by a range of cognitive distortions including:

- Those who do not fully support their cause are enemies.

- Any lack of progress is the product of malevolent interference from someone.

- Any compromise is humiliating defeat.

- The grievance is the defining moment of their lives.

- That because they are in the right the outcomes they seek must be not only possible but necessary.

These distortions are open to challenge and amelioration if not completely overcoming. In theory the cognitive therapy approaches advocated for the delusions should also be of value.[13,14] The problem with the therapeutic management of querulous behaviour is that we have no trial of treatment or even much beyond case reports. This reflects widespread prejudice that the querulous are not the business of mental health and even if they are they are untreatable. Hopefully if this neglect is overcome and querulous behaviour is once more recognized as a legitimate concern for mental health professionals then systematic studies of therapy will follow. For the present the querulous destroy the fabric of their lives as well as creating distress and occasionally damage to those around them.

## Further information

Charles Dickens. *Bleak House*—Multiple Editions.

Mullen, P.E. and Lester, G. (2006). Vexatious litigants and unusually persistent complainants and petitioners: from querulous paranoia to querulous behaviour. *Behavioural Sciences and the Law*, **24**, 333–49.

Douglas, M. (1992). *Risk and blame, essays in cultural theory*. Routledge, London.

## References

1. Hack Tuke, D. (1892). *A dictionary of psychological medicine*, pp. 1060–1. Churchill, London.
2. Jaspers, K. (1923). *General psychopathology* (trans. J. Hoenig and M.W. Hamilton 1963). Manchester University Press, Manchester.
3. Krafft Ebing, R. (1905). *Textbook of insanity* (trans. C.G. Chaddock), pp. 397–9. Davies Company, Philadelphia.
4. Kraepelin, E. (1904). *Lectures in clinical psychiatry* (trans. and ed. T. Johnstone). Bailliere, Tindall and Cox, London.
5. Caduff, F. (1995). Querulanz-ein verschwindendes psychopatholgisches Verhaltensmuster? *Fortschritte der Neurologie-Psychiatrie*, **63**, 504–10.
6. Mullen, P.E. and Lester, G. (2006). Vexatious litigants and unusually persistent complainants and petitioners: from querulous paranoia to querulous behaviour. *Behavioural Sciences and the Law*, **24**, 333–49.
7. James, D.V., Mullen, P.E., Meloy, J.R., *et al.* (2007). The role of mental disorder in attacks on European politicians 1990–2004. *Acta Psychiatrica Scandinavica*, **116**(5), 334–44.
8. Mullen, P.E., James, D.V., Meloy, J.R., *et al.* (in press). The fixated and the pursuit of public figures. *Journal of Forensic Psychiatry and Psychology*.
9. Poole, S. (2000). *The politics of regicide in England, 1760–1850: troublesome subjects*. Manchester University Press, Manchester & New York.
10. Lester, G., Wilson, B., Griffin, L., *et al.* (2004). Unusually persistent complainants. *The British Journal of Psychiatry*, **184**, 352–6.
11. Dietrich von, H. (1968). *Der Querulant Munchener Medizinische Wochenschrift*; 14, June 110 Jahrgang, pp. 1445–50.
12. Ungvari, G.S. (1993). Successful treatment of litigious paranoia with pimozide. *Canadian Journal of Psychiatry*, **38**, 4–8.
13. Chadwick, P., Birchwood, M., and Trower, P. (1996). *Cognitive therapy for delusions, voices and paranoia*. John Wiley and Sons, Chichester.
14. Bentall, R. and Kinderman, P. (1994). Cognitive processes and delusional beliefs: attributions and the self behaviour. *Research and Therapy*, **32**, 331–41.

# Domestic violence

Gillian C. Mezey

## Introduction

Over the last decade, the issue of domestic violence has been transformed from a position of 'selective inattention' to becoming a high-priority social and public health issue.[1] Although it is now recognized that experiences of domestic violence are associated with adverse mental as well as physical health outcomes for the victim, this has not always been the case. Early psychiatric writings tended to attribute responsibility for violent relationships, to the masochistic traits of women who are drawn to and then fail to separate, from abusive and violent partners. During the 1980s and 1990s, however, the perception of victims of domestic violence, or 'battered women' began to change, towards an understanding that the responsibility for domestic abuse lies with the wife beater, rather than the wife beater's wife.

This change came about as a result of several factors; first, effective lobbying by the feminist movement which put the issue of domestic violence firmly on the political agenda; second, the influence of a number of researchers who began to conceptualize the psychological and behavioural problems seen in victims as the consequence, rather than the cause of, domestic violence, for example through the identification of a specific 'Battered Woman Syndrome',[2] and finally the introduction of Posttraumatic Stress Disorder as a distinct psychiatric diagnosis in 1980 (APA, 1980).

## Definition

Domestic violence is currently defined in the United Kingdom as 'Any incident of threatening behaviour, violence or abuse (psychological, physical, sexual, financial or emotional) between adults who are, or have been in an intimate relationship'.[3] Most cases of domestic violence involve the abuse of a woman by her male partner, however, domestic violence may also involve other family members, same sex partners, and the abuse of men by women partners.

## Epidemiology

The estimated prevalence of domestic violence varies, according to the definition being used and the population surveyed. Based on an analysis of 48 population-based studies from around the world, the prevalence of domestic violence is between 10 and 69 per cent over a lifetime and between 3 and 52 per cent in the past year.[4] In the United Kingdom, around 16 million incidents of domestic violence are recorded annually, with a lifetime prevalence of 21 per cent lifetime and 4 per cent in the past year for women and 10 per cent lifetime and 2 per cent in the past year, for men.[5] Women who report domestic abuse consistently report experiencing more incidents and more injuries and being more fearful of their partner, than male victims.[5]

## Aetiological factors

Domestic violence arises out of a complex interplay of personal, situational, and socio-cultural factors. Poverty, alcohol use, low academic achievement, being single, separated or divorced, and witnessing or experiencing violence as a child are the most important individual risk factors for domestic violence.[4] Poverty operates at an individual and societal level, in that it places increased stress on the individual and the family system and also acts as a marker for a number of other social conditions (e.g. low education, overcrowding) that combine to increase the risk of domestic violence. Alcohol use by the perpetrator also significantly increases the risk of domestic violence.[4,5] Women appear to be at particularly high risk of domestic violence during pregnancy and the immediate post-partum period.[6] Experiences of domestic abuse in childhood and adolescence are associated with an increased risk of perpetration, for men[4] and re-victimization, for women[7] in adult relationships. Inequality and a power imbalance within the relationship[8] and in the wider society,[9] also increases the risk of domestic violence. Higher rates are found in societies where men have economic and decision-making power in the household, where women do not have easy access to divorce, and where there is a high level of public acceptance of men's right to discipline their wives.[4,9]

## Mental health effects of domestic violence

Domestic violence is associated with a range of adverse physical and psychological health and social outcomes.[1,4,5] In extreme cases, the violence results in the victim's death. Between 40 and 70 per cent women victims of homicide are killed by a current or former spouse or partner, compared with between 4 per cent and 8 per cent male victims of homicide.[4]

Women who are abused by their partners over many years, often find it extremely difficult to leave their partner and, even if they do leave, many women end up returning to the family home. There are a number of psychological and social reasons why many women find it difficult to separate emotionally, as well as physically, from their violent partners. Learned helplessness,[2] the progressive erosion of confidence and self esteem cased by the abuse, feelings of guilt, shame and isolation, make it difficult for victims to assert themselves, seek help, or even contemplate the possibility of an existence separate from their partner. For some women the abuse appears, paradoxically, to strengthen their emotional ties to the perpetrator, so-called 'traumatic bonding'.[10] Women who try to leave abusive partners, experience significant economic and social hardship, including lack of accommodation, inadequate financial support, and difficulties in caring for the children, as well as a disruption caused to their family and social support networks. These difficulties, as well as the fear of being tracked down by their partner, are often so daunting, that many women end up returning to their homes, choosing an existence that is familiar to them, in preference to precarious survival elsewhere. It is clear that physical separation does not always end the violence; many separations result in an escalation of threatening and violent behaviour, including stalking[11] and the risk of domestic homicide is greatest around the time, or shortly after, separation.

Domestic abuse is associated with increased rates of depression, suicidality, Posttraumatic Stress Disorder, alcohol and substance misuse, and dependence in victims of abuse, compared with the general population.[12] The more severe and chronic the abuse, the greater the impact on the victim's mental health and symptoms of depression and hypervigilance may persist, even after separation.[2]

Where present, symptoms of mental illness must be treated appropriately. However, offering victims a non-judgemental sympathetic response, providing information about options available to them, about the risks associated with staying, or going and providing information about community resources, including refugees and counselling facilities are likely to be more important for the victims than any specific 'treatment'.[13]

## Risk assessment

In the absence of direct questioning by a health professional, which is conducted in a sensitive and non-judgemental way, women are unlikely to spontaneously disclose experiences of domestic abuse in the context of a health consultation.[5,13] Unless domestic abuse is identified, then the risk cannot be properly assessed or communicated to the victim. Screening for domestic abuse in health settings appears to be acceptable to women and is also effective in terms of increasing rates of identification.[13]

The frequency, severity, and chronicity of the abuse must be taken into account in assessing and managing risk. Browne's study,[14] comparing battered women who had killed their partner with battered women who had not killed, identified the following risk factors for domestic homicide: frequency of violent assaults; presence and severity of injuries; alcohol intoxication or substance misuse in the perpetrator, threats to kill, sexual violence, suicidal ideation (in the victim), and access to a weapon. Campbell[15] also identified the following risk factors in a study of 220 cases in which women had been killed by violent partners: unemployment (male), choking, abuse during pregnancy, threats or harm to the child, the

presence of a stepchild in the home, and separation. Morbid jealousy in the perpetrator and stalking behaviours are also more common in lethal, compared with non-lethal cases of domestic violence. Risk assessment must be carried out in all cases of domestic violence and communicated to the victim, to allow her to make informed and safe choices.

## Confidentiality and domestic violence

The primary consideration for the health professional should be the safety of the victim and any affected children. In general, the victims consent should always be sought prior to sharing information with others. A breach of confidentiality, without the victim's knowledge, or consent, could increase the risk she faces and may discourage further disclosures to health professionals. The legal framework varies in different countries but in the United Kingdom, health professionals should be guided by the Data Protection Act (1998) and by principles on information sharing and good practice, as set out within GMC[16] and Royal College of Psychiatrists[17] guidance. The Crime and Disorder Act (1998) allows for information to be passed on, in the absence of consent, in cases where the courts request information about a specific case or if the health professional judges there to be a significant risk of harm to the woman, her children, or to someone else if that information is not passed on. The health professional should always inform the woman if they intend to breach confidentiality, they should properly record their reasons for doing so and they should only pass on the minimum information required to achieve their objective. Further specific guidance on sharing information in the context of domestic violence has recently been provided by the Home Office.[18]

## Perpetrators of domestic violence

Studies of men who abuse their partners are difficult to interpret, largely because of the difficulties in identifying and recruiting men who are representative of the population as a whole. There is little evidence that domestic abuse is primarily attributable to underlying mental illness in the perpetrator. However, personality profiles of perpetrators indicate high rates of personality disorder, as well as alcohol and substance misuse and jealousy. There are two main personality profiles described in a perpetrator of domestic violence. The borderline/emotionally dependent type tends to confine their violence to within the family, they tend to be extremely insecure, jealous, and dependent on their partner and the violence is often precipitated by actual or threatened separation. The antisocial/narcissistic offender, is violent both within the family and outside and their violence is often associated with alcohol and drug misuse and high rates of criminality.[19,20]

Group treatment programmes, aimed at changing the behaviour of men who batter, have had a degree of success in reducing violence.[21,22] However the evidence is limited and results are hard to interpret, given the fact that many men, arguably those who are at highest risk and who most need behaviour changing, are least likely to seek help or to remain in treatment. Treatment appears to be most effective when men are mandated through the Courts. Elements of such programmes include: encouraging men to take personal responsibility for their violent behaviour; increasing their awareness of the dynamics involved in the use of violence in relationships; challenging attitudes and beliefs around the use of violence in relationships between men and women; and developing skills for relating non-violently to others. Perpetrators of domestic abuse are encouraged to accept responsibility for the violence and to consider the consequences of their violence and the gains and losses it entails. Some perpetrators may need to learn particular skills to manage situations where they may previously have resorted to violence. It is important that any treatment programme of perpetrators monitors the effectiveness of the programme through maintaining constant contact with female partners in order to confirm whether participation is having the desired effect and, more importantly, is not endangering them further.

## Further information

Roberts, G., Hegarty, K., and Feder, G. (2006). *Intimate partner abuse and health professionals. New approaches to domestic violence.* Churchill Livingstone Elsevier, London.

Taket, A. (2004). *Tackling domestic violence: the role of health professionals.* Home Office Development and Practice Report, No. 32. Home Office, London.

www.womensaid.org.uk

www.refuge.org.uk

www.victimsupport.org.uk

## References

1. British Medical Association. (1998). *Domestic violence: a health care issue?* BMA, London, UK.
2. Walker, L.E. (1979). *The battered women.* Harpers and Row, New York.
3. Home Office. (2005). *Domestic violence: a national report.* Home Office, London, UK.
4. World Health Organization. (2002). *World report on violence and health.* World Health Organization, Geneva.
5. Walby, S. and Allen, J. (2004). *Domestic violence, sexual assault and stalking: findings from the British crime survey* (ed. Home Office Research DaSD), p. 276. Home Office, London, UK.
6. Lewis, G. and Drife, J. (2004). *Why mothers die 2000-2002. Confidential enquiry into maternal and child health.* RCOG, London, UK.
7. Coid, J., Petruckevitch, A., Feder, G., et al. (2001). Relationship between childhood sexual and physical abuse and risk of re-victimisation in women: a cross sectional survey. *Lancet*, **358**, 450–4.
8. Jewkes, R. (2002). Intimate partner violence: causes and prevention. *Lancet*, **359**, 1423–9.
9. Levinson, D. (1989). *Family violence in cross cultural perspective.* Sage, Thousand Oaks, CA.
10. Dutton, D. and Painter, S. (1983). Traumatic bonding: the development of emotional attachments in battered women and other relationships of intermittent abuse. *Victimology: An International Journal*, **6**, 139–55.
11. Mullen, P.E., Mackenzie, R., Ogloff, J.R., et al. (2006). Assessing and managing the risks in the stalking situation. *The Journal of the American Academy of Psychiatry and the Law*, **34**, 439–50.
12. Golding, J. (1999). Intimate partner violence as a risk factor for mental disorders: a meta analysis. *Journal of Family Violence*, **14**, 99–132.
13. Department of Health. (2005). *Responding to domestic abuse: a handbook for health professionals.* Department of Health, London.
14. Browne, A. (1987). *When battered women kill.* The Free Press, New York.
15. Campbell, J.C., Webster, D., Koziol-McLain, J., et al. (2003). Risk factors for femicide in abusive relationships: results from a multisite case control study. *American Journal of Public Health*, **93**, 1089–97.
16. General Medical Council. (2004). *Confidentiality: protecting and providing information.* General Medical Council, London.
17. Royal College of Psychiatrists. (2000). *Good psychiatric practice: confidentiality.* CR85. Royal College of Psychiatry, London.
18. Douglas, N., Lilley, S., Kooper, L., et al. (2004). *Safety and justice: sharing personal information in the context of domestic violence: an overview.* Home Office Development and Practice Report No. 30. Home Office, London.
19. Gilchrist, E., Johnson, R., Takriti, R., et al. (2003). *Domestic violence offenders: characteristics and offending needs.* Home Office, London, UK.
20. Holtzworth-Munroe, A. and Stuart, G.L. (1994). Typologies of male batterers: three subtypes and the differences among them. *Psychological Bulletin*, **116**, 476–97.
21. Gondolf, E.W. (2000). Re-assault at 30 months after batterer programme intake. *International Journal of Offender Therapy and Comparative Criminology*, **44**, 111–28.
22. Morran, D. and Wilson, M. (1994). Confronting domestic violence: an innovative criminal justice response in Scotland. In *Penal theory and practice: tradition and innovation in criminal justice* (ed. P. Dobash). Manchester University Press, Manchester.

# 11.13

# The impact of criminal victimization

Gillian C. Mezey and Ian Robbins

## Epidemiology

The prevalence of crime depends on the methodological approach that is adopted, the questions being asked and the population being surveyed. Crime figures are also affected by the willingness, or unwillingness of individuals to declare themselves as victims. This is particularly the case with 'sensitive' crimes, such as domestic and sexual violence. Not surprisingly, the self completion phases of the British Crime Surveys have been more effective in identifying such experiences than standard survey methodology. In addition, not all violence is necessarily recognized as a crime, and similarly not all crimes are necessarily defined as such, by their victims. Occasionally, violence may occur by mutual consent.

In the UK the British Crime Survey is regarded as the most reliable and comprehensive data source on criminal victimization, providing information about the extent of crime, as well as trends in the frequency and patterns of crime and changes in public attitudes to crime over the years. The British Crime Survey for 2005–2006 found there were approximately 10.9 million crimes against adults living in private households.[1] Not all individuals in the population are at equal risk. Most crime differentially targets and damages individuals who are poor, disempowered, and marginalized within society. The risk of victimization is highest for divorced single or separated individuals between the ages of 16–24. Men are at greater risk of experiencing violent crime than women, except in the categories of domestic violence and sexual assault, where women are more at risk.[2] Women are more vulnerable to domestic violence and younger people are more at risk of crime than elderly people. Alcohol is also involved in a significant number of violent offending both offenders and victims having been found to be inebriated or to have recently consumed alcohol at the time of the offence.[3] Severe mental illness also appears to be a risk factor for crime victimization. In her study of 936 patients with severe mental illness living in the community, Teplin[4] found that over one quarter of them had experienced violent crime in the past year, a rate more than 11 times that of the general population, even after controlling for socio-demographic variables.

Criminal victimization can have profound psychological and emotional effects, with the impact of violent (including sexual) victimization being greater than property or non violent offending. The experience of crime and the perception of crime as possible or probable, also has an impact on the individual's fear of crime, and on their lifestyle. Women and the elderly are most fearful of crime, even though, in reality, young men are at greater risk. This may be because of the greater perceived adverse consequences of victimization and greater vulnerability in women and elderly people.[5]

## General effects of victimization

The experience of victimization can leave the individual feeling 'diminished, pushed down, exploited and invaded'.[6] Victims are often describe feeling stigmatized and isolated and unable to communicate their distress or feelings of vulnerability. Although friends and relatives may initially be supportive, such support may begin to fall away if the victim fails to recover within a reasonable period of time.

Social support and gender are important predictors of psychiatric problems, including PTSD, in crime victims.[7] Andrews et al.[8] found that, women were more likely to receive negative responses from family and friends following violent crime and also to have higher rates of PTSD at 6 months follow up. The benefits of positive social support and impact of negative social responses were greater for women victims than men. Negative support was predictive of PTSD in both men and women, although this effect was more pronounced in women.

## Immediate and short term effects of crime

High rates of dissociative symptoms are reported by victims of violent and sexual assault in the form of numbing, reduced awareness, derealization, and depersonalization, at the time of the crime.[9,10] Dissociation may have immediate survival value, in terms of reducing the victim's sense of immediate threat and minimizing the pain. However, it may also interfere with the individual's longer-term recovery. Peri-traumatic dissociation at the time of the offence has been found to predict post-traumatic stress disorder development in women victims of violent and sexual assault.

Dissociative symptoms are part of the diagnostic criteria for Acute Stress Disorder which is a risk factor for the development of Posttraumatic Stress Disorder. Brewin et al.[11] found that a diagnosis of Acute Stress Disorder at one month post trauma, predicted 83 per cent of post-traumatic stress disorder cases at 6 months follow-up. Acute Stress Disorder may be experienced during or immediately after a trauma and should resolve within four weeks of the conclusion of the traumatic event.

## Long term psychological effects

Most crime victims are able to resume normal functioning and health, following a transient state of disequilibrium, without the need for medical or psychological intervention. However, some victims go on to develop chronic and persistent psychological or psychiatric problems.[12] This may include increased rates of depression, anxiety and substance misuse. Recovery following criminal victimization is largely dependent on how the victim processes and makes sense of what has happened, whether the act can be accommodated into an existing frame of reference or whether the experience is so overwhelming and outside ordinary everyday experience as to render them incapable of reaching some kind of resolution.

Amongst crime victims, victims of violent crime have higher rates of psychological disturbance than victims of property crime who, in turn, have higher rates of disturbance that non victims.[13,14,15] Perception of life threat, physical injury and completed rape are associated with particularly high rates of PTSD.[14,16,17]

Many of the psychological responses exhibited by victims and witnesses of crime fit within a post-traumatic stress disorder framework. In a study of 391 women victims, 27 per cent of all crime victims developed post-traumatic stress disorder.[18] Although most victims of crime show substantial improvement up to 9 months after the offence, very little spontaneous recovery occurs thereafter[19,20] and for some victims the effects are profound and long lasting.[18]

### Physical health effects of crime

In general, people who have experienced crime have a poorer perception of their physical health and physical functioning and experience more chronic medical conditions than non victims. Physical and sexual assault are associated with increased cigarette consumption, alcohol and other drug abuse, self neglect, risky sexual behaviour, and eating disorders.[21] Shepherd and Farrington[22] have suggested that a young man from a deprived urban area may suffer 60 years of incapacity as a result of injury, reduced quality of life, and self esteem. Increased crime rates are found in poorer areas, which means that the negative impact of crime on physical health may be difficult to disentangle from the negative impact of poverty and deprivation on physical health.

### Responses following specific criminal acts

#### (a) Murder

The act of murder has profound effects, not just on the individual victim, but also on the friends, family members and acquaintances who are left behind and who are sometimes referred to as the 'secondary victims.' The act of murder is shocking in its finality and irrevocability, and the responses of survivors are both qualitatively and quantitatively different from the normal grieving process.[23,24] Rock[25] has suggested that it is not just the death itself, but the manner of death and its social meaning that is so devastating for those who are left behind. Unlike a 'natural' death, survivors are unprepared for their loss, there can be no anticipatory mourning, no reconciliation, and no proper leave taking. Many survivors

describe feelings of stigmatization, isolation, shame, and betrayal, but feel unable to communicate their distress or to connect emotionally with fellow beings. They often feel marginalized by the criminal justice system, with little access to information and they are burdened with having to cope with the inevitable, legalistic bureaucracy and the practical demands of life during a period of acute distress and emotional turmoil. In cases where the perpetrator and the victim are members of the same family, the survivors may experience particularly intense feelings of guilt and conflicting emotions.

The effects of violent traumatic bereavement on the secondary victims include physical health problems, cognitive impairment, and psychological effects, including posttraumatic stress disorder, depression, phobic avoidance, and impaired work and social functioning.[26,27] Female gender and losing a child predict worse psychiatric outcome.[27] Survivors of homicide, tend to manifest both trauma symptoms and symptoms of grief, phenomena, with either predominating or appearing intermittently.[28] This has lead to a proposed new diagnostic category of 'traumatic grief', which contains two core components; trauma and of loss.[29]

#### (b) Rape and sexual assault

The definition of rape varies across countries and between states within countries. In the UK, prior to 1994, the definition of rape was restricted to penile penetration of the vagina, with other forms of non consensual penetrative sex being defined as indecent assault. However, in 1994, the definition of rape was extended to include non consensual anal intercourse, thereby recognizing male rape victims for the first time. The 2003 Sexual Offences Amendment Act further broadened the definition of rape to include penetration of the mouth as well as penetration of the vagina or anus by the penis. It also introduced three new measures on the issue of consent: first, that a person can only consent to sexual relations if they have the freedom and capacity to make that choice, second, that all the circumstances at the time of the offence must be considered in determining whether the defendant is reasonable in believing the complainant consented and third, that individuals will be considered most unlikely to have agreed to sexual activity if they were subject to threats or fear of serious harm, if they were unconscious, drugged or abducted, or if they were unable to communicate because of a physical disability.

In the majority of cases of rape, the perpetrator is known to the victim and in many cases, the rapist is the current or former husband or partner.[30] In spite of the seriousness of the offence, the British Crime Survey[30] found that only 60 per cent women who had been subjected to rape or serious sexual assault had told anyone about it and only around one in seven cases had been reported to the police. Reasons women gave for not reporting include: fear of reprisals, fear of public identification, fear of appearing in Court and having to give evidence and lack of confidence in the legal system.[31] There is some evidence suggesting that women who proceed with prosecution following rape do worse, in terms of social adjustment and self esteem at one year follow up than women who decide not to proceed.[32] Whether this is because Court proceedings delay or slow down the process of psychological recovery following rape, or because the legal process and particularly the experience of being cross examined in Court, represents a form of 'secondary traumatization', is not entirely clear. If women do proceed with the Criminal Justice process, however, preparing them for the experience, providing them with appropriate information beforehand and giving them the opportunity to exercise choice, can help to offset the potentially de-stabilizing and distressing impact of criminal proceedings. Ultimately, the attitude taken by the police and the way the victim feels they have been treated appears to be more important in determining their psychological adjustment and satisfaction with the process, than the actual verdict.[32]

About one-third of women who report rape develop long term psychological and social problems. These effects tend to be more severe and chronic than following non sexual violence.[33,34] Rape trauma syndrome was first described in the 1970's[35] and was subsequently superseded by Posttraumatic Stress Disorder. Posttraumatic stress symptoms are generally present in the days and weeks following the assault, but then spontaneously resolve in the majority of cases. For some victims, however, the condition may become chronic and persist for many years, if left untreated.[36] Higher rates of depression, suicidal ideation, generalized and phobic anxiety, alcohol and drug dependence and sexual dysfunction as well as physical health problems are also found in rape victims compared with non rape victims.[37–41]. Women who have been raped often describe problems in relationships, with excessive dependence, inability to trust and loss of confidence and self esteem. Similar responses have been described with male victims of sexual assault.[42]

The characteristics of sexual assault that predict long term mental health problems are: being the victim of a completed rape, being injured and the perception of a threat to life.[14] Other predictors of long term disturbance include; prior psychological and social problems previous victimization, particularly childhood abuse past psychiatric illness, drug or alcohol misuse and lack of a supportive network.

Psychiatric treatment may be required for individuals who develop serious psychological problems following a sexual assault. It is probably inappropriate to embark on psychiatric treatment too early, because of the natural tendency for symptoms to resolve spontaneously in the weeks and months following the assault. Unless symptoms have resolved by 6 months, however, they are unlikely to resolve spontaneously thereafter without some form of psychological intervention or psychiatric treatment (see Chapter 4.6.2)

There is no evidence that counselling is effective in alleviating short term distress or in preventing the development of long term psychiatric disability in rape victims. Indeed recent studies have suggested that counselling may even be harmful, if carried out by inadequately trained and supervized individuals.[43] Many of the key organizations working with victims e.g. Victim Support, emphasize their role as supporters and befrienders and they provide both practical assistance, such as accompanying victims to identification parades, helping with paperwork and compensation claims, as well as offering emotional support following the assault and through any subsequent criminal proceedings. Rape victims are most likely to benefit from services that are co-ordinated, integrated and streamlined.[43] An example of this in the UK has been the development of Sexual Assault Referral Centres (SARCs), which provide a 'one stop shop' of medical, counselling, legal and forensic services for victims of sexual assault. Evaluation of these centres and in particular the benefits for victims and the Criminal Justice System, is ongoing.

### (c) Burglary and robbery

The effects of burglary are generally less severe and long lasting than following violent and 'contact' crimes although some victims may develop chronic mental health problems, including Posttraumatic Stress Disorder.[18] Repeat victimization is especially common in the case of burglary and second or subsequent burglaries are more likely to have a greater long term impact. Repeated experiences of burglary may lead to victims of burglary taking additional security precautions or even moving house in order to restore a sense of safety and control over their lives.[44] Individuals living in areas of poverty and deprivation and single parent families are most vulnerable to burglary. Robbery, unlike burglary involves not only direct contact between the victim and the perpetrator, but also implies a degree of life threat and is therefore more likely to precipitate post-traumatic psychiatric illness, including post-traumatic stress disorder.[45]

### (d) Workplace violence

Violent assaults in the workplace have increased in frequency and severity in recent years.[46–48] Budd et al. found that working at night was the only significant factor which predicted its occurrence. There was a clear relationship between workplace violence and increased job stress, reduced job satisfaction, increased likelihood of looking for a new job, as well as bringing weapons to work Kopel & Friedman[49] found that police officers witnessing incidents of violence reported intrusive thoughts and images, and used avoidance to deal with the intrusive phenomena. Whilst recognizing that avoidance is a feature of post-traumatic stress disorder, they also suggest that denial and avoidance are part of the culture in male-dominated occupations such as law enforcement agencies. Miller-Burke et al.[50] found that most employees who had experienced robberies had multiple adverse consequences. Psychological functioning, physical wellbeing, social and occupational functioning were all impaired. Having been involved in more than one incident was associated with more severe outcomes.

In the United States Hewitt and Levin[51] point to the high rates of occupational assaults among health-care workers. Whilst fatal workplace assaults are more likely to involve males in the course of robberies, women were more likely to be involved in non-fatal workplace assaults, with health-care workers being most affected. The rate for health and social care workers was 10 times that of private non-health care industries. Williams[52] found that 26 per cent of nurses reported physical assault while at work. This rate of assault is similar to that found by O'Connell and Bury[53] who carried out a survey of all general practitioners in the Eastern Health Board of Ireland. They had a 98 per cent response rate which revealed that 21 per cent of general practitioners had experienced violence or aggression although in only 7 per cent of the incidents reported did it result in injury. Not surprisingly there is a strong inverse relationship between workplace assaults and job satisfaction.

### (e) Child and adolescent victims of crime

Children and young people are especially vulnerable to crime and victimization, in particular by people they know and are dependent on, although stranger violence is a small but important problem.[54] The 1992 British Crime Survey[55,56] looked at the victimization of young people away from the home and reported that about one-third of 12 to 15 year olds had been assaulted in the last 6 to 8 months. This would compare with a rate of around 1 per cent in adults. Most of these assaults happened at or near school and were committed by a sole perpetrator who was known to the victim. The survey also identified high rates of fear of crime amongst adolescents, with girls being more fearful than boys. A range of mental health problems have been identified following victimization within the child and adolescent population.[57]

### Hate crimes

The defining characteristics of a hate crime is that the individual victim is targeted because of bias or prejudice, based on their actual or perceived social grouping or ethnicity, sexual orientation, religion or political orientation. Herek *et al.*[58] suggest that a significant proportion of lesbians and gay men who had been assaulted believed that their sexual orientation had been a motivating factor. One-quarter of men and one-fifth of women said that they had experienced victimization because of their sexual orientation. When compared to other crime victims, they had significantly more symptoms of depression, anxiety and PTSD as well as more crime related fears and a lower sense of mastery. Rose & Mechanic[59] reported that 73 per cent of lesbians and gay men had experienced at least one homophobic attack. Victims of homophobic violence had more PTSD symptoms than did victims of other homophobic crimes or non victims although there was no significant difference in rates of depression. They also found that homophobic sexual assaults were more likely to involve known assailants, and multiple perpetrators and more likely to be repeated.

Hate crimes tend to be under-reported to the police, the psychological effects tend to be long lasting, and have a negative impact not only on the individual victim, but also on the community. It has been argued that hate crimes require policy directed to addressing the causes rather than simply dealing with the needs of individual victims. Black and ethnic minority individuals appear to be particularly vulnerable to criminal victimization and in a proportion of these cases the offence is considered to be 'racially motivated'.[60,61]. Around one in six of all incidents of criminal victimization against Asians and African-Caribbeans are considered to be racially motivated[61] and, regardless of the type of offence, ethnic minority victims tend to report higher levels of worry about crime then white victims.[60] Fear of crime appears to be particularly high amongst Bangladeshi and Pakistani individuals, who are also most likely to describe their victimization as racially motivated. It has been suggested that victims who perceive their victimization to be racially motivated, experience more serious and persistent psychological effects that individuals who did not consider racism as a motivation.

### (g) Terrorist crimes

A number of studies have looked at the impact of terrorist attacks which, whilst relatively infrequent, in comparison to other crimes, have a considerable political and social impact. Whalley and Brewin[62] reviewed the mental health effects of terrorist attacks on the direct victims, as well as on the general (non affected) population. In the general population, symptoms of distress and stress are high in the first few days following an incident, but tend to resolve spontaneously so that, although PTSD is found in between 11 per cent-13 per cent of the general population, in the first six weeks following a single terrorist attack, this falls to below 3 per cent after 8 weeks. Factors such as previous adversity, pre-existing mental health issues and membership of minority groups may increase vulnerability to the impact of terrorism. PTSD is the

most common psychiatric disorder in direct victims of terrorist attacks, followed by depression although other problems such as traumatic grief, panic disorder, phobias, generalized anxiety and substance misuse have also been reported.[63] Most studies have reported that between 30–40 per cent of those closest to the site of the attack, will develop a psychiatric disorder within 2 years. However, the majority of direct victims have no contact with mental health professionals. In the aftermath of the September 11th attacks in New York only around one-quarter to one-third of those suffering from PTSD were in receipt of treatment. Whalley and Brewin[64] suggest that a focused outreach approach such as a 'screen and treat' programme may be needed to identify those with significant impairment and help them to access evidence based treatments.

The extent of physical injury during a terrorist attack is the best predicator of post-traumatic stress disorder rates both in the short term[65] and many years after the event,[66] although it does not predict the development of a depressive illness. Studies which have looked at the impact of shootings tend, by their very nature to be small scale, but have found significant levels of distress and high rates of post-traumatic stress disorder and other psychiatric disorders.[67] Being held hostage has also been related to high levels of distress both in victims and their families.[68] Where captivity has occurred, there may be strong attachment and paradoxical gratitude towards the captors with positive emotions including compassion and identification with the terrorist's values, often described as the Stockholm syndrome.

## Support services and treatment interventions

There are so few culturally accepted rituals of support for victims of crime, that it often becomes the task of the therapist to normalize the process. In the United Kingdom victim support schemes offer practical assistance, for example accompanying the victim to identification parades and court hearings, completing Criminal Injuries Compensation Board forms, as well as providing support and reassurance following crime. Referrals to the schemes are generally made by the police, but are occasionally accepted from involved professionals or from the victims themselves. However, victims of serious crimes, such as sexual assault or physical violence, and the families of murder victims may develop psychiatric illness, which requires referral to mental health services for specialist treatment.

Treatment approaches are drawn from a variety of paradigms including cognitive behavioural, psychodynamic, psychosocial, and pharmacological treatments, and are often trauma focused in general rather than being specific to problems associated with criminal victimization. Ochberg (6) categorizes them into two main approaches, the first focuses on previous personality and attributes mental health problems and difficulties in adjustment following crime to pre-existing unresolved issues and weaknesses, rather than to the traumatic events. The second approach focuses more on the events themselves, the individual strengths and coping styles of the victim and setting realistic achievable goals.

In the UK the 1998 Crime and Disorder Act placed an obligation on the NHS to work in partnership with the Police and Local Authorities in dealing with the consequences of crime. Many people who present to the NHS for treatment following violent crime do not present to the Police or criminal justice agencies. As many of the services for crime victims are organized by or accessed through the criminal justice system these people are likely to miss out on services. There is a clear need for a direct relationship between the NHS and criminal justice agencies in the way in which treatment is provided and its relationship to the criminal justice processes but as yet, other than in a small number of specific projects it does not happen.

Often immediately following victimization help is offered and family and friends rally round. This may not be the time when most people need formal psychiatric help. The majority of people post assault experience sympotms of PTSD and other psychiatric problems but also the majority improve spontaneously even in the case of serious crimes such as rape. The question comes as to when to intervene. The National Institute for Clinical Excellence (NICE, 2006) recommend a position of watchful waiting and if in the first month(s) symptoms are not improving or indeed may be increasing then treatment is indicated otherwise waiting and monitoring to identify who will not spontaneously improve is the approach of choice.

Previous work had already shown that timing of appropriate services is important. Shepherd et al.[62] have shown that while accident and assault victims have similar levels of depression and anxiety in the immediate aftermath three months later the assault victims have higher levels of symptoms. In the immediate aftermath of criminal victimization it has been suggested that having the opportunity to talk may reduce later symptoms Where there have been specific RCTs of immediate intervention they have not shown themselves to be particularly effective. Rose, Brewin, Andrews and Kirk[63] compared an education intervention with education plus psychological debriefing or an assessment only condition in a randomized controlled trial. They found that while all groups improved over time there were no significant differences between groups. This is hardly surprising when considering the result of Rose, Bisson & Wessely[64] who carried out a systematic review of RCTs examining the impact of debriefing. They found 11 RCTs of which six showed no effect at all, three had a positive effect and two had a negative outcome.

This has led to a belief that there is no point in any immediate interventions but this ignores the contribution made by organizations such as Victim Support or Rape Crisis centres. They do not offer formal therapy but rather give information, offer the opportunity to ventilate emotions, practical help and assistance in making compensation claims or participating in the criminal justice system. Shepherd and Bisson[65] who make the case for more integration between health services and other agencies describe the two models of Victim Support interventions which are initiated within the NHS and address the needs of victims which would otherwise be overlooked.

In terms of formal psychological therapies and in the longer term Cognitive Behavioural Therapy has been used with great effectiveness. Ehlers & Clark[66] reviewed the use of CBT in early interventions. They concluded that CBT was superior to supportive counselling but that brief CBT in the first month showed no superiority over repeated assessments. Where longer programmes ie 16 session were offered in the first 4 months they found that CBT was superior to supportive counselling, repeated assessment or no intervention at all.

There have been a number of other empirical studies demonstrating the effectiveness of structured cognitive behavioural

approaches to treating established PTSD, which are discussed further in Chapter 4.6.2

## Conclusion

The impact of crime on the individual victim is profound but is frequently underestimated by mental health professionals. Wide-ranging personal, social, and economic consequences could be prevented if a range of appropriate interventions were available. Most post traumatic stress treatment programmes in the United Kingdom have developed in response to specific disasters, which may not be relevant to or as effective with crime victims. In order to provide appropriate treatment to crime victims, mental health professionals need to recognize the importance of active interagency liaison with the police, the courts and with voluntary organizations such as victim support schemes. Crime victims tend to be relatively invisible and disempowered; they are less likely to be supported by active campaigning groups than survivors of major disasters and, because of associated feelings of shame and stigmatization, they may be reluctant to claim their entitlement to proper care and treatment. The fact that their plight is often used as a political football is likely to reinforce feelings of helplessness and insecurity. Given its prevalence, crime represents both an ordinary and an extraordinary event; it is likely to affect everyone at some point in their lives and the fact that most crime victims recover from the experience should not deprive those who need it, to proper care.

## Further information

Garcia-Moreno, C., Jansen, H., Ellsberg, M., et al. (2005). *Multi-country Study on Women's Health and Domestic Violence against Women* WHO, Geneva.

Krug, E., Dahlberg, L., Mercy, J., et al. (2002). *World Report on violence and health.* WHO, Geneva.

For general information about victims, policy, statistics and support provision www.homeoffice.gov.uk/crime-victims

Hearing the Relatives of Murder and Manslaughter Victims. Consultation. D.C.A.;London. Sept 2005 www.dcs.gov/manslaughter/manslaughter.pdf

Domestic Violence, Crime and Victims Act (2004) www.opsi.gov.uk/ACTS/acts 2004/20040028.htm

## References

1. Walker, A., Kershaw, C., Nicholas, S. (2006). *Crime in England and Wales.* London, Home Office.
2. Kessler, R.C., Sonnega, A., Bromet, E., et al. (1995). Posttraumatic stress disorder in the National Comorbidity Survey. *Archives of General Psychiatry,* **52**(12), 1048–60.
3. Mirrlees-Black, C., Budd, T., Partridge, S., et al. (1998). *The 1998 British Crime Survey England and Wales.* London, HMSO.
4. Teplin, L.A., McClelland, G.M., Abram, K.M., et al. (2005). Crime victimization in adults with severe mental illness: comparison with the National Crime Victimization Survey. *Archives of General Psychiatry,* **62**(8), 911–21.
5. Maxfield, M.G. (1984). Fear of crime in England and Wales. London, HMSO.
6. Ochberg, F.M. (1988). Post traumatic therapy and victims of violence. In *Post traumatic therapy and victims of violence* (ed. F.M. Ochberg), Brunner-Mazel, New York, 3–19.
7. Brewin, C.R., Andrews, B., Valentine, J.D. (2000). Meta-analysis of risk factors for posttraumatic stress disorder in trauma-exposed adults. *Journal of Consulting and Clinical Psychology;* **68**(5), 748–66.

8. Andrews, B., Brewin, C.R. and Rose, S. (2003). Gender, social support, and PTSD in victims of violent crime. *Journal of Traumatic Stress*, **16**(4), 421–7.

9. Dancu, C.V., Riggs, D.S., Hearst-Ikeda, D., *et al.* (1996). Dissociative experiences and post traumatic stress disorder among female victims of criminal assault and rape. *Journal of Trauma Stress*, **9**, 253–67.

10. Foa, E.B., Riggs, D.S. and Gershuny, B.S. (1995). Arousal, numbing, and intrusion: symptom structure of PTSD following assault. *American Journal of Psychiatry*, **152**(1), 116–20.

11. Brewin, C.R., Andrews, B., Rose, S., *et al.* (1999). Acute stress disorder and posttraumatic stress disorder in victims of violent crime [see comments]. *American Journal of Psychiatry*, **156**(3), 360–6.

12. Norris, F.H. and Kaniasty, K. (1994). Psychological distress following criminal victimization in the general population: cross-sectional, longitudinal, and prospective analyses. *Journal of Consulting and Clinical Psychology*, **62**(1), 111–23.

13. Kilpatrick, D.G., Saunders, B.E., Amick-McMullan, A.A., *et al.* (1989). Victim and Crime Factors Associated with the Development of Crime-Related Post-Traumatic Stress Disorder. *Behavior Therapy*, **20**,199–214.

14. Ullman, S.E., Siegel, J.M. (1994). Predictors of Exposure to Traumatic Events and Posttraumatic Stress Sequelae. *Journal of Community Psychology*, **22**, 328–38.

15. Breslau, N., Davis, G.C., Andreski, P., *et al.* (1991). Traumatic events and posttraumatic stress disorder in an urban population of young adults. *Archives of General Psychiatry*, **48**(3), 216–22.

16. Norris, F.H. (1992). Epidemiology of trauma: frequency and impact of different potentially traumatic events on different demographic groups. *Journal of Consulting and Clinical Psychology*, **60**(3), 409–18.

17. Kilpatrick, D.G., Saunders, B.E., Veronen, L.J., *et al.* (1987). Criminal victimisation: lifetime prevalence, reporting to police and psychological impact. *Crime and Delinquency*, **33**, 479–489.

18. Boudreaux, E., Kilpatrick, D.G., Resnick, H.S., *et al.* (1998). Criminal victimization, posttraumatic stress disorder, and comorbid psychopathology among a community sample of women. *Journal of Traumatic Stress*, **11**(4), 665–78.

19. Norris, F.H. and Kaniasty, K. (1994). Psychological distress following criminal victimization in the general population: cross-sectional, longitudinal, and prospective analyses. *Journal of Consulting and Clinical Psychology*, **62**(1), 111–23.

20. Resnick, H.S., Acierno, R. and Kilpatrick, D.G. (1997). Health impact of interpersonal violence. 2: Medical and mental health outcomes. *Behavioral Medicine*, **23**(2), 65–78.

21. Shepherd, J.P. and Farrington, D.P. (1993). Assault as a public health problem: discussion paper. *Journal of the Royal Society of Medicine*, **86**(2), 89–92.

22. Murray-Parkes C. (1993). Psychiatric problems following bereavement by homicide. *British Journal of Psychiatry*, **162**, 49–54.

23. Mezey, G., Evans, C., Hobdell, K. (2002). Families of homicide victims: Psychiatric responses and help-seeking. *Psychology & Psychotherapy: Theory, Research & Practice*, **75**(1), 65–75.

24. Rock, P. (1998). After homicide: practical and political responses to breavement. Clarendon Press, Oxford.

25. Mezey, G., Evans, C. and Hobdell, K. (2002). Families of homicide victims: Psychiatric responses and help-seeking. *Psychology & Psychotherapy: Theory, Research & Practice*, **75**(1), 65–75.

26. Murphy, S.A., Braun, T., Tillery, L., *et al.* (1999). PTSD among bereaved parents following the violent deaths of their 12 to 28 year old children: A longitudinal prospective analysis. *Journal of Traumatic Stress*, **12**, 273–91.

27. Raphael, B. (1997). The Interaction of Trauma and Grief. In *Psychological Trauma - a Developmental Approach* (eds. D. Black, M. Newmay, J. Hains-Hendriks and G. Mezey). Gaskell, London.

28. Prigerson, H.G., Shear, M.K., Frank, E., *et al.* (1997). Traumatic grief: a case of loss-induced trauma. *American Journal of Psychiatry*, **154**(7), 1003–9.

29. Walby, S., Allen, J. (2004). Domestic Violence, Sexual Assault and Stalking: Findings from the British Crime Survey. London, Home Office Research, Development & Statistics Directorate.

30. Campbell, R., Wasco, S.M., Ahrens, C.E., *et al.* (2001). Preventing the 'second rape' - Rape survivors' experiences with community service providers. *Journal of Interpersonal Violence*, **16**(12), 1239–59.

31. Cluss, P.A., Boughton, J., Frank, E., *et al.* (1983). The Rape Victim - Psychological Correlates of Participation in the Legal Process. *Criminal Justice and Behavior*, **10**(3), 342–57.

32. Boudreaux, E., Kilpatrick, D.G., Resnick, H.S., *et al.* (1998). Criminal victimization, posttraumatic stress disorder, and comorbid psychopathology among a community sample of women. *Journal of Traumatic Stress*, **11**(4), 665–78.

33. Resnick, H.S., Kilpatrick, D.G., Dansky, B.S., *et al.* (1993). Prevalence of civilian trauma and posttraumatic stress disorder in a representative national sample of women. *Journal of Consulting and Clinical Psychology*, **61**(6), 984–91.

34. Burgess, A.W. and Holmstrom, L.L. (1974). Rape trauma syndrome. *American Journal of Psychiatry*, **131**(9), 981– 6.

35. Kilpatrick, D.G., Best, C.L., Veronen, L.J., *et al.* (1985). Mental health correlates of criminal victimization: a random community survey. *Journal of Consulting and Clinical Psychology*, **53**(6), 866–73.

36. Kilpatrick, D.G., Best, C.L., Veronen, L.J., *et al.* (1985). Mental health correlates of criminal victimization: a random community survey. *Journal of Consulting and Clinical Psychology*, **53**(6), 866–73.

37. Ellis, E.M., Atkeson, B.M. and Calhoun, K.S. (1981). An assessment of long-term reaction to rape. *Journal of Abnormal Psychology*, **90**(3), 263–6.

38. Atkeson, B.M., Calhoun, K.S., Resick, P.A., *et al.* (1982). Victims of rape: repeated assessment of depressive symptoms. *Journal of Consulting and Clinical Psychology*, **50**(1), 96–102.

39. Santiago, J.M., McCall-Perez, F., Gorcey, M., *et al.* (1985). Long-term psychological effects of rape in 35 rape victims. *American Journal of Psychiatry*, **142**(11), 1338–40.

40. Waigandt, A., Wallace, D.L., Phelps, L., *et al.* (1900). The Impact of Sexual Assault on Physical Health Status. *Journal of Traumatic Stress*, **3**(1), 93–101.

41. Coxell, A., King, M., Mezey, G., *et al.* (1999). Lifetime prevalence, characteristics, and associated problems of non-consensual sex in men: cross sectional survey. *British Medical Journal*, **318**(7187):846–50.

42. Campbell, R. and Ahrens, C.E. (1998). Innovative community services for rape victims: An application of multiple case study methodology. *American Journal of Community Psychology*, **26**(4), 537–71.

43. Maguire, M. (1982). Burglary in a dwelling. Heinemann, London.

44. Gale, J.A., Coupe, T. (2005). The Behavioural, Emotional and Psychological Effects of Street Robbery on Victims. *International Review of Victimology*, **12**(1), 1–22.

45. Kamphuis, J.H. and Emmelkamp, P.M. (1998). Crime related traumas: psychological distress in victims of bank robbery. *Journal of Anxiety Disorders*, **12**, 199–208.

46. Eisele, G.R., Watkins, J.P. and Matthews, K.O. (1998). Workplace violence at government sites. *American Journal of Industrial Medicine*, **33**(5), 485–92.

47. Budd, J.W., Arvey, R.D. and Lawless, P. (1996). Correlates and consequences of workplace violence. *Journal of Occupational Health Psychology*, **1**(2), 197–210.

48. Kopel, H. and Friedman, M. (1997). Posttraumatic symptoms in South African police exposed to violence. *Journal of Traumatic Stress*, **10**(2), 307–17.

49. Miller-Burke, J., Attridge, M. and Fass, P.M. (1999). Impact of traumatic events and organizational response. A study of bank robberies. *Journal of Occupational and Environmental Medicine*, **41**(2), 73–83.

50. Hewitt, J.B. and Levin, P.F. (1997).Violence in the workplace. *Annual Review of Nursing Research*, **15**, 81–99.

51. Williams, M.F. (1996). Violence and sexual harassment: impact on registered nurses in the workplace. *American Association of Hospital Nurses Journal*, **44**(2), 73–7.

52. O'Connell, P. and Bury, G. (1997). Assaults against general practitioners in Ireland. *Family Medicine*, **29**(5), 340–3.

53. Finkelhor, D. (1995). The victimization of children: a developmental perspective. *American Journal of Orthopsychiatry*, **65**(2), 177–93.

54. Mirrlees-Black, C. and Aye Maung, N. (1994). Fear of crime: findings from the 1992 British Crime Survey. Research findings No. 9. London, Home Office Research and Statistics Directorate.

55. Aye Maung, N. (1995). *Young people, victimisation and the police: summary findings*. HMSO, London.

56. Boney-McCoy, S., Finkelhor, D. (1995). Psychosocial sequelae of violent victimization in a national youth sample. *Journal of Consulting and Clinical Psychology*, **63**(5), 726–36.

57. Herek, G.M., Gillis, J.R. and Cogan, J.C. (1999). Psychological sequelae of hatecrime victimization among lesbian, gay, and bisexual adults. *Journal of Consulting and Clinical Psychology*, **67**(6), 945–51.

58. Rose, S.M. and Mechanic, M.B. (2002). Psychological Distress. Crime features and help seeking behaviours related to homophobic bias incidents. *American Behavioural Scientist*, **46**(1), 14–26.

59. Clark, I. and Leven, T. (2002). The 2000 Scottish Crime Survey: analysis of the ethnic minority booster sample. Edinburgh, UK, Scottish Executive Central Research Unit.

60. Fitzgerald, M. and Hale, C. (1996). Ethnic minorities: victimization and racial harasssment. In: Home Office Research and Statistics Directorate, editor. *Home Office Research Study*, **154**. London.

61. Whalley, M.G., Brewin, C.R. (2007). Mental health following terrorist attacks. *British Journal of Psychiatry*, **190**, 94–6.

62. Abenheim, L., Dab, W., Salmis, L.R. (1992). Study of civilian victims of terrorist attacks. *Journal of Clinical Epidemiology*, **45**, 103–9.

63. Desivilya, H.S., Gal, R. and Ayalon, O. (1996). Extent of victimization, traumatic stress symptoms, and adjustment of terrorist assault survivors: a longterm follow-up. *Journal of Traumatic Stress*, **9**(4), 881–9.

64. Trappler, B., and Friedman, S. (1996). Posttraumatic stress disorder in survivors of the Brooklyn Bridge shooting. *American Journal of Psychiatry*, **153**(5), 705–7.

65. van der Ploeg, H.M. and Kliejn, W.C. (1989). Being held hostage in The Netherlands: a study of the long-term after effects. *Journal of Traumatic Stress*, **1,** 153–9.

66. Shepherd, J.P. and Bisson, J.I. (2004). Towards integrated health care: a model for assault victims. *British Journal of Psychiatry*, **184**, 3–4.

67. Ehlers, A. and Clark, (2004). Review of the impact of early CBT programmes in the treatment of trauma. *Biological Psychiatry*, **3**(9), 817–26.

# Assessing and managing the risks of violence towards others

Paul E. Mullen and James R. P. Ogloff

*'Prediction is very difficult, especially about the future'*

*Niels Bohr (1885–1962)*

## Introduction

Assessing and managing the risk of our patients being violent towards others now occupies a prominent position in virtually all forms of mental health practice, but it remains a contentious area. At the highest level researchers, psychometricians, and statisticians argue about almost every aspect, even whether anything useful can be said about individual outcomes rather than group indicators. At the next level an industry flourishes of selling training, and risk assessment tinstruments, to those who then appear as experts in a wide range of mental health and criminal justice contexts. On the ground, almost everyone in mental health is drawn into filling out purpose-designed forms and complying with protocols, most of little or no demonstrated validity. This chapter is intended to make clinicians aware of both the possibilities and limitations of existing approaches to the assessments of risk. Given that there is no reason for mental health professionals to evaluate risk without gaining information to manage it, this chapter will also address the management of risk for aggression and violence.

## Constructing risk

A critical analysis will be attempted of how risk has come to be constructed in our society and how this is impacting on mental health and criminal justice. When an approach is adopted which attempts to reveal the foundations and historical evolution of a widely accepted social construct, like risk, there is a danger that it will appear overly sceptical or even mocking. It is important to emphasize at the outset that:

1 The assessment of the probability of patients behaving in ways damaging to others and the management of that risk is a legitimate clinical activity.

2 That attributions of levels of risk to a patient occurs in a social and cultural context and is inescapably a construct.

The discourses around the dangerousness of the mentally ill have gradually been replaced by those of risk. This change is usually presented as a product of the progress of knowledge and the improved conceptualization of that knowledge.[1–4] The language of danger transmuted into the language of risk also emphasizes the probabilistic nature of risk assessment. We are not now and probably never will be in a position to be able to determine with certainty who will or will not engage in a violent act. Relying on a range of empirically supported risk factors, though, we can makes a reasoned determination of the extent to which those we are assessing share factors that have been found in others to relate to an increased level of risk. Risk embodies the interaction of a range of factors, which are not necessarily dangerous in themselves, such as age, gender, marital status, ethnicity, employment status and, of course, mental disorder.[5] Risk factors can be any variables which are statistically associated with a future violent episode or event. There is no assumption of causality linking the predictor to the predicted.

Risk assessment came relatively late to the mental health field. Not until 'harm to others' or 'undue risk' became criteria for involuntary hospitalization and forensic detention did 'dangerousness' of patients assume the spotlight. The focus on risk first surfaced in Western Societies in the 1970s in the context of concerns about damage being inflicted on individuals by the actions, or inactions, of corporate and governmental agencies. These concerns fed the emergence of widely based environmental movements as well as an escalating number of class actions and individually driven litigations. Under the banner of risk a new blaming system emerged of which Douglas[6] writes 'we are . . . almost ready to treat every death as chargeable to someone's account, every accident as caused by someone's criminal negligence, every sickness a threatened prosecution. Whose fault? is the first question . . . then what damages? what compensation? what restitution . . .' (pp. 15–16). One response to this culture of blame has been the emergence of what O'Malley[7] refers to as a new prudentialism in which individuals, professionals and corporations, increasingly held responsibility for the impact of their actions on others, resort to risk management strategies in which risk is assessed, managed, insured against, and where possible removed.

Psychiatrists and psychologists are among those who have become caught up in the 'culture of blame'. Any damaging or distressing occurrence which is experienced by, or caused by, someone who is, or has been, a patient of the mental health services, is transformed into a preventable tragedy for which professionals are to be held responsible. Rose[8] suggests the new imperatives of risk assessment and risk management operate to establish mechanisms to control mental health professionals which through standards, audits and enquiries not only regulate professionals but hold them personally responsible for unwanted outcomes. Douglas (6) argues 'probability analysis arrives at politics in the form of a word 'risk'... the word gets its connection with probability squeezed out of it and put to the same primitive political uses as any term for 'danger'" (p. 48). Risk assessment and risk management are concepts which have the potential to shift blame towards clinicians who have failed to follow procedure and away from managers who fulfilled their responsibilities by ensuring correct protocols were in place, irrespective of the possibility of the realistic application of such protocols. The language of risk can also shift the focus from politicians who determine resources and establish systems of care to those who fail to identify and manage risk in the individual case. Perhaps most importantly the increasing centrality of risk assessment potentially creates a vision of the mentally disordered as primarily embodiments of varying degrees of risk and the mental health services as agents in controlling and obviating the supposed danger to the community.

Assessing dangerousness used to be the almost exclusive province of the forensic mental health professional.[9,10] It was a marginal activity based on arcane knowledge and assumed wisdom that only experience could provide.[11,12] Risk assessment and management in contrast have become central to current mental health practice in almost all its guises. It has become among the most important activities defining professional competence. Understanding the cultural, legal, and political roots of the increasing hegemony exerted by the rhetoric of risk over psychiatric practice may demystify, but does not free the professional from the imperatives of operating effectively in this new environment. It seems so obvious, as to be self evident, that mental health professionals are expected to consider the probability that their patient will act in a destructive manner and to act to prevent such harms. But the self evident is often the ideological unconsidered. It is not obvious that a mental health professional's primary responsibility is to the wider community rather than their patient. It is not obvious that it is possible to effectively predict such risks as they apply in the individual case. It is not at all obvious how we should act in the face of a prediction of risk, and it is certainly not obvious that such concerns should be a major determinant of our approach to patients.

Words are rarely innocent. Risk is not the same as probability, for risk implies a degree of danger. Even those deemed to be at 'low risk' still appear to present some degree of danger. No one, it seems, is considered risk free. Risk management is not the same as harm minimization, for it promises a prevention of unwanted outcomes. Psychiatry deals with disorders which have both substantial morbidities and mortalities. Good management may reduce but cannot, in our present state of knowledge, prevent all such morbidity and mortality. Furthermore, reducing morbidity and mortality long term may only be possible at the price of accepting an increased probability of mortality in the short term. Suicide in prison, for example, can be prevented by isolating and observing vulnerable inmates in transparent plastic bubbles, bereft of features from which suspension is possible, or by the simple expedient of chaining them hand and foot to a bed (both strategies are in use today). If the only good is preventing self harm such draconian measures

acquire currency irrespective of the psychological damage and abuse of basic human dignity involved. Moreover, as the aim has become removing all risk of suicide in prison, more and more vulnerable prisoners are being subjected to such restrictions and in many jurisdictions 'witch hunts' now regularly follow every death across jurisdictions. We cannot force the genie of risk back into the lamp. Mental health professionals will continue to be made publicly accountable. Professional self regulation is being replaced by statutory regulation and the ravages of civil litigation.[13] As Rose[8] notes we will be forced to play a central role 'in the strategy of reducing risk and minimizing harm under threat of sanction and within the disciplines imposed by a plethora of practices of blame' (p. 18).

## Contemporary approaches to risk assessment

It is no longer possible for mental health professionals to distance themselves from the process of risk assessment. Throughout the 1970s and 1980s mental health professionals were almost of one voice in proclaiming both their inability to predict dangerousness and the basic pacifity of the mentally disordered.[14] Despite this public stance dangerousness criteria came to dominate civil commitment, with courts simply ignoring arguments that the prediction of dangerousness was beyond the ken of psychiatrists and psychologists.[15] In addition liability based on failures to predict dangerousness was established in landmark cases including those arising out of Poddar's killing of Tarasoff[16] and Hinkley's attempt to assassinate President Reagan.[17] Last, but not least, the criminal courts increasingly suborned mental health professionals into predicting dangerousness in the pursuit of such sentences as preventive detention and death.[15,18] In the US and the UK the emergence of the language of risk at the end of the 1980's was in part a recognition of the centrality assumed by predicting and managing the potential for violence perceived by the public to reside in the mentally disordered. In the UK the public inquiry into the killing of Jonathan Zito by the psychiatrically disordered Christopher Clunis set a pattern for future homicide enquires.[19] Failures of risk assessment and management by individual practitioners, together with inadequacies of communication and service provision, were identified as major contributors to 'avoidable' killings.[19] Such developments set risk assessment at the very centre of the mental health agenda.

Given the challenges of risk assessment, what is the current state of knowledge and can it be of assistance to clinicians? The limited research available on 'dangerousness prediction' conducted in the 1970s showed that psychiatrists and psychologists had unacceptably low levels of accuracy in predicting which patients would go on to be violent in the future.[20] It was found, perhaps not surprisingly, that psychiatrists, psychologists, and release decision-makers tended to make conservative decisions that suggested that people were at risk for dangerousness or violence when, in fact, they were not. Similar findings have been obtained over time. For example, Belfrage[21] found that clinicians found 90 per cent of a group of 640 offenders sentenced to psychiatric treatment in Sweden to be at 'risk of severe criminality;' when, in fact, only 50 per cent went on to commit any kind of crime.

Reasons given for the errors made in risk prediction include clinicians' confusion and lack of knowledge of valid risk markers and risk factors. In addition, as with other areas of decision-making, even if clinicians do have a reasonable understanding of risk factors, it is difficult to systematically consider them and to put together a risk appraisal in a systematic way. Advances in risk assessment have included the identification of an expanded range of predictor variables relevant to violence. Most important among these are those variables that are subject to change (i.e., they can change over time and they can be influenced by treatment or other intervention). Generally speaking, risk assessment variables can be classed as 'static' (i.e., those that cannot be changed) and 'dynamic' (i.e., those that can change over time). Actuarial risk schemes, which will be discussed later in this chapter, are based upon variables that were measured from the past. These historic variables generally could not change over time. For example, if one began being violent as a young person, that fact will not change over time. Dynamic variables, in contrast, are subject to change over time, sometimes rapidly. These variables include such things as state of mind, situational factors, attitudes, plans, support, etc. Effective risk assessment must take into account both static and dynamic variables; however, risk management generally requires an understanding of the dynamic risk variables. Contemporary approaches to risk assessment and management take into account both static and dynamic variables, thus considering an individual's past, present, and future risk factors that might affect the likelihood of him or her becoming violent.

There has been considerable progress since Monahan[20] first reported that psychologists and psychiatrists were essentially unable to predict risk to any acceptable extent. Current research shows that risk assessment approaches provide a level of accuracy that now far exceeds chance.[22]

## The limits on mental health professionals' engagement in risk assessment

There are two legitimate perspectives on risk assessment:-

1 The clinician whose work involves considering patients' levels of risk as part of a process whose purpose is primarily to improve the management of patients.

2 The forensic evaluator for whom risk assessment is a tool to improve the reliability of opinions provided to courts and tribunals charged with making decisions about an individual.

Forensic mental health professionals in the US and Canada tend to see their role primarily as evaluator. It is not uncommon for forensic psychiatrists and psychologists to primarily conduct assessments for the courts as their means of employment. This reflects the generally accepted separation of the assessment and treatment roles. In stark contrast in the UK and Northern Europe the clinician perspective dominates even for forensic specialists. Relatively few forensic clinicians would operate as court evaluators alone, though some like their US colleagues would try and separate the roles.

This chapter is written for mental health professionals in a wide range of contexts, not for forensic specialists. As a result the emphasis on this chapter will be on the clinical perspective. North American readers should, however, keep in mind that this perspective is not shared by many specialists in the forensic field there who would consider it not just problematic but ethically questionable to mix the assessment and treatment roles.

Boundaries need to be drawn around when, where and for what purpose, mental health professionals can ethically engage in assessing the probability of an individual committing violent or criminal acts. There are somewhat different constraints operating on clinicians than for those carrying out evaluations for the purpose of preparing reports for decision-making bodies like courts and tribunals.

The ethical and practical constraints on a clinician assessing risk entirely in service of effective treatment include:

1 Ensuring the assessment serves the interests of the patient in terms of improving management and protecting them from acts which will damage their interests. The seriously mentally ill when they become violent all too often target those who support and care for them thus destroying the relationships critical to their own social survival. In addition, criminal and violent acts of the sort usually associated with the mental disordered rarely, if ever, brings anything but increased problems for the patient. Thus, reducing the likelihood that the patient will engage in criminal and violent acts serves not only the public interest but also the patient's interests.

2 Mental health variables (which include psychological variables and personality traits) are a prominent feature of the individual's clinical picture and are also of potential relevance to the probability of future damaging behaviours.

3 Avoiding providing greater emphasis to risk than is necessary given the totality of the patients needs and vulnerabilities.

4 The assessment should wherever possible connect potential risk to those factors whose amelioration will reduce that risk. Ultimately a health professional can only justify engagement in risk evaluation if they lead to better outcomes for the evaluated as well as the community. Risk assessment finds its ultimate justification in risk management.

5 Avoiding using risk and risk assessment to disqualify patients from access to the treatments they require. Increased risk requires increased therapeutic enthusiasm, not rejection.[23]

6 That any concerns raised by a risk assessment are shared with the patient and the proposed management strategies explained. Even unwelcome restrictions are resented less if the reason for their imposition is explained.

7 Retaining an awareness of the limitations of the predictive power of risk assessments and the need to ensure proportionality between the risk actually apprehended and any imposed remedy.

8 Ensuring a level of professional competence adequate to the task.

9 Making use, where possible, of the skills and knowledge of the multidisciplinary team in the assessment.

Those obligations on those engaging in risk assessment as part of an evaluation for a decision-making body are even more onerous and should include:-

1 The patient consents to the examination in the knowledge of the nature of the assessment, the purposes to which it may be proffered, and the limitations on confidentiality that may apply.

2 A reasonable body of empirical evidence exists to guide the risk assessment including, where possible, empirically validated structured risk assessment measures.

3 The risk assessment is conducted in consideration of the legal parameters governing the decision-making body (e.g., criteria to be considered for change of orders or release for forensic psychiatric patients) while realizing that the legal questions to be answered never parallel the clinical or evaluative results mental health professionals can reasonably provide (e.g., there is no clinical parallel to legal criteria such as 'undue risk').

4 The assessment is based on a careful analysis of the relevant characteristics of the particular individual which in all but exceptional circumstances have been obtained in part by a direct examination of the individual.

5 The risks are expressed in terms of probabilities (not attributions of dangerousness) with clear admissions of the fallibility and potential variability in the prediction. The problem should be acknowledged of employing risk factors derived from studies on populations from different cultures and contexts. After all nobody would use risk data from Los Angeles to calculate the car insurance premium for a driver in Dublin or Oslo without considerable caution.

6 Account is taken not just of the probability of damaging behaviour but the nature and severity of such conduct. Proportionality needs to be maintained between what is predicted and the response. It is all too easy to employ methods which establish increased risks of a wide range of unwanted behaviours only to find them used to justify draconian and punitive responses which would only be acceptable in the face of the imminence of serious violence.

7 The confidence and certainty with which any prediction is formulated to take account of the implications for the person being assessed. Risk predictions may be offered in terms of probabilities but they will almost always be used to justify all or nothing decisions.

8 That personal and professional integrity is strictly maintained. This is no simple matter when the evaluator is either in the pay of the patient, or of those whose interests are not necessarily those of the patient.

The potential conflicts generated when acting for a patient as both a professional evaluator and a clinician are so considerable that some experts argue that such a dual role is inherently unethical. They argue in preparing reports for decision-making bodies the interaction ceases to be that of health professional and patient, and becomes entirely that of expert, or 'forensisist', and evaluated. The expert's obligation is then not to the evaluated but to their own professional competence and the rules governing the process the report will serve (e.g., criminal court, family court, mental health tribunal).

In our view even in an encounter between a health professional and a person purely for the purposes of an evaluation for a court there remains obligations to the person as patient [patient from the Latin for to suffer, who in this instance suffers the intrusions of an examiner who cannot for the evaluated entirely cast off the guise of physician or healer]. The solution is to learn to live with the contradictions and accept the dialectic between responsibilities to the patient and obligations to the agencies of society. The result of accepting the duality of the role inherent in assessing a patient's risk of harming others does exclude participation in a process that could increase the risk to the patient of fatal (e.g., death penalty evaluations) or serious harm (e.g., sexual predator laws whose sole purpose is justify a process of prolonging incarceration beyond the expiry of a sentence). It does however legitimate having the dual role of clinician and evaluator in some circumstances. In fact those who totally eschew ever taking on such a dual role, we believe, are at risk of deluding themselves that they can caste off the mantle of clinician for the patient, and become a socially neutral, objective, observer and reporter.

The dialectic between the demands of a professional responsible to the health of your patient and the demands of professional integrity and honesty owed courts and tribunals is almost always possible to resolve. To fail to accept engagement with the conflicts which in reality usually exist for evaluators and clinicians reporting to external authorities is in our opinion an act of self deception in which you become an agent either of patient, or authority, and no longer an autonomous responsible professional.

Some situations make nonsense of the above considerations, notably death penalty hearings. One of us (J.O) has extensive experience of working with those on death row, the other (P.M) only a comparatively slight acquaintance. We are both of the opinion, however, that it is impossible to honestly discharge your responsibilities as clinician, as evaluator, or as decent human being, in such circumstances.

## Risk assessment approaches

There are five basic approaches to evaluating the risk of violence:-

1 Probability models based on established risk factors. The risk factors can be derived actuarially from studies of particular populations (e.g. Violence Risk Appraisal Guide (VRAG) and Static 99) or rationally ascertained from the risk literature (e.g. Historical Clinical Risk 20 (HCR-20)).

2 Clinical experience based on recognizing previously encountered (personally or in the literature) patterns associated with future violence. The clinical approach is largely relevant to the avoidance of obvious errors like discharging morbidly jealous men who are threatening to kill their partner.

3 A mixture of 1 and 2 where the risk assessment instrument is employed to guide the appraisal of risk factors and clinical judgment is applied to balance idiographic information with the nomothetic variables as in the structured professional judgment approach of which the HCR-20 is the prime example.[22]

4 The strictly idiographic approach which employs individual profiles of violent offenders to detect those on a similar pathway to attack. The idiographic approach is employed to evaluate the risks of rare events, such as attempts to assassinate a head of state, and has little application in general mental health.

5 A plethora of local risk assessment tools have sprung up. Sometimes it seems as if every psychiatric service, probation/parole service, prison, and security consultant have their own unique sheet of questions which are supposed to establish the future probability of whatever particular piece of nastiness currently concerns the organization. These ad hoc parochial risk assessment protocols have no evidentiary basis or psychometric integrity (even if they incorporate aspects of other properly constituted instruments). It is far better to validate existing

empirically supported measures for use in a particular setting and with a particular population.

The core of risk assessment is the systematic application of probability models usually incorporated in standardized instruments.

## The utility of risk assessment

Even given a firmly based knowledge of those factors which in populations may increase or decrease the probability of violent behaviour, there remain theoretical and practical limitations on effective prediction in the individual case. If factors were identified which occurred only in the violence prone and never in the pacific and, if present, were in every case the harbinger of future attack, then the power of the predictive paradigm would be independent of both the frequency of future violence in the population, and of variables which effect the factors' expression in the individual case. In the real world the sensitivity (the accuracy with which the outcome is predicted) and the specificity (the extent to which only those who will act in the predicted way are identified) fall short of 100 per cent. This being so the less common the future behaviour in the population the less specific will become predictions. Equally, the more complex the influences affecting the expression of the identified predisposition the less the sensitivity of the predictive paradigm.

Say we develop a predictive paradigm of 70 per cent sensitivity and 95 per cent specificity (which is feasible). If we set an acceptable level for the practical use of such an instrument that it will not unfairly restrict, or stigmatize, more than 1 person for every 4 correctly designated as candidates for future violence, then the base rate for violence in the population of interest would have to exceed 20 per cent. Even if we accepted one error for each correct designation (which, if the outcome of ascertainment were incarceration or other significant curtailment of basic freedoms, few would regard as ethically defensible) it still requires a base rate of higher than 6 per cent.

This hopefully makes clear that if predictions of the probability of future violence are to be used to significantly restrict the patient's freedoms the base rate of the behaviour must be reasonably high in the group under consideration. Equally, if measures such as long term institutionalization or compulsory community treatment with restrictions on residency and movement are contemplated the degree of violence apprehended must be commensurately damaging. It would be difficult to justify such interventions if what is at issue is embarrassing, or even fear inducing behaviour, which does not involve either assault occasioning injury or gross intimidation.

Statistical approaches to analysing predictive efficiency in populations with low base rates for the target behaviour exist, the most commonly employed being derived from a measure developed for use with radar or signal detection systems, the Receiver Operating Characteristic (ROC) curve.[24, 25] The ROC curve is a graph of true positives (sensitivity) along the y-axis and false positives (1-specifity) along the x-axis. With respect to violence, these correspond to patients who were predicted to be violent those who were predicted not to be violent, respectively. The line running from the lower left corner of the graph to the top right indicates chance prediction, where true positives are equal to false positives (i.e., for every patient predicted to be a violent who in fact becomes violent another patient who was predicted to be violent does not become violent). A curve above this line indicates that, in this case, recidivism is being predicted at rates above chance. The Area Under the Curve (AUC), which is represented as a proportion of the graph that falls under the curve, reflects the proportion of true positives over false positive (e.g. an AUC of 70 would indicate that 70 per cent of those predicted to be violent in fact do become violent). The ROC analyses allow the accuracy of predictions to be established independent of variations in base rate.

In many western nations between 5 per cent and 10 per cent of all homicides and more than 5 per cent of serious crimes of violence are committed by those with a schizophrenic syndrome. The annual risks of a person with a schizophrenic syndrome committing a homicide is however, in the region of 1 in 10,000 and for a crime of violence about 1 in 150.[26] This is because serious violence is, the media notwithstanding, an uncommon event. Though fear inducing behaviours occur with distressing frequency among the seriously mentally disordered the inflicting of serious injury is measured in annual risks of below 1 per cent.[27,28,29] This suggests that risk assessment instruments will not be relevant to predicting serious violence in those with a schizophrenic syndrome. Underlying the homicide enquiries in the UK, and the litigation, particularly in the US, however is the assumption that they can be and will be.

Given their particularly low base-rate of occurrence, attempting to predict who will commit serious acts of violence or murder will inevitably be accompanied by vast numbers of false accusations. Further, in reality we often trade off outcome variables, thus avoiding over ready resort to civil commitment may improve the chances of establishing a long term therapeutic alliance, which in turn may reduce long term risks, albeit at the price of tolerating a higher degree of risk in the short term. Avoiding all probability of any patient committing a future act of violence would involve the use of widespread coercion and move mental health professionals into increasingly custodial and controlling roles.

An alternative argument deserves consideration. In those with a schizophrenic syndrome, for example, it may well be feasible to identify the 10 per cent who will perpetrate 90 per cent of all the future fear inducing and violent acts. In this 10 per cent may be included nearly all of the far smaller number who will commit potentially lethal or seriously injurious acts. In effectively identifying the 10 per cent and managing them appropriately then the risks to the community of damage, including the small chance of serious damage, will be reduced. The majority of those so identified will be a nuisance who can occasion fear, and who may push, punch or kick others.[30] Effectively identifying and managing all patients in the high risk group will lower the overall risk to the community while minimizing the deprivation to liberty of those in the low risk group. This risk group management approach is not perfect and does not increase the ability to identify a particular individual who may commit a heinous act, but it does allow effective management of those at higher risk.

The management ethically and pragmatically justified, must retain some semblance of proportionality between the apprehended insult and the impact of the proposed preventive strategy. In practice this obliges us in most clinical situations not to resort to increased coercion, let alone preventive detention, but to focus attention on greater support and more active follow up and treatment in the community with a more ready resort to admission during exacerbations of symptoms or social conflict.

## Risk assessment instruments

The last 15 years or so has been marked by a wave of enthusiastic advocacy specifically for the benefits of so called actuarial risk assessment instruments (e.g.,[31,32,33]). The advocates of actuarial risk assessment claim directly, or by implication, to be able to identify the likelihood that specific individuals will progress to various forms of interpersonal violence. These risk assessment tools are based mainly on retrospective, though occasionally prospective, studies of specific populations, such as discharged patients and released offenders. Actuarial approaches have the advantages of:-

1 Multiple variables delineating level of risk.

2 Designed to move from group data to individual attribution.

3 Realized in simple objective reproducible rating scales which minimize individual clinician's discretion and therefore responsibility.

4 Focus attention on 'high risk' individuals (principle of targeted resources).

5 Provides protection to clinicians and managers in event of disaster. Nobody can be blamed for the failures of 'science'.

Actuarial approaches are not without their problems. The results, for example of commonly used risk assessment instruments like the VRAG and the Static 99 change little if at all over time and with circumstances. Clearly whatever the Static 99 may indicate the risks of committing further rapes in a fit 25 year old is unlikely to remain the same as he ages and acquires disabilities.[34] Actuarial approaches also almost inevitably revolve around a limited number of variables which exclude uncommon though potential critical factors. Thus, for example, morbid jealousy is not sufficiently common to emerge as an actuarially established risk factor despite studies on such cases indicating a very high probability of significant violence. The structured clinical judgement approach allows the incorporation of such potential modifiers[22]. Actuarial instruments are developed on specific samples constituted in particular places at particular times. This can lead to problems with generalisability and equally important idiosyncratic and false attributions. For example, in both the VRAG[31] and the Classification of Violence Risk (COVR)[35] the schizophrenic syndrome emerges as a protective, or at best a neutral, factor with regard to the risk of violence, despite being associated in many other studies with far higher rates of violence than occurs in the general population.[26] This is because in the VRAG the rate in those with schizophrenia was compared to other offenders, some of whom had severe personality disorders, and as expected it was lower. In the MacArthur study, from which derives the Classification of Violence Risk (COVR),[35] substance abuse was treated as an independent confounder and the rates for the select few who had a schizophrenic syndrome, but were not substance abusers, were used to calculate the level of risk for schizophrenia.

The use of the term actuarial links these approaches to the well established actuarial methods familiar from the insurance industry. In the insurance industry actuaries usually generate their risk groups on the basis of samples numbered in the thousands, with the occasional in the tens of thousands. In the mental health fields the samples are usually measured in hundreds, with the occasional topping the thousand mark.[1] Actuaries in the insurance industry work exclusively with group based predictions. Your car insurance will depend on such variables as the type of car you drive, your age, your gender, your prior driving record, and where you live. That determines the group you fall into for the purposes of costing the policy you request. The actuary is not interested in what happens to each individual only whether the whole group for whom policies have been drawn costs sufficiently less in claims than is received in policy payments to produce the required profit margin. The actuarial method is not designed to assign levels of risk to individuals but to groups, though the cost of an individual's policy will be determined by the risk group into which their policy falls. The precision of the group prediction is determined by the size of the sample and the frequency with which the event of concern occurs. The rarer the outcome of interest (e.g., murder or plane crashes) the larger has to be the sample, and to some extent the commoner the event (minor assaults or fender benders) the smaller the sample. Irrespective of the sample on which the risks have been established as you try to make finer and finer distinctions involving smaller and smaller subdivisions within the original sample so the confidence that can be placed in the estimate decreases. Paradoxically the more intense and detailed the analysis of the original group the less reliably can the derived risk algorithm be applied to those outside the group.[19] The MacArthur study on which the COVR is based exemplifies this problem. The smallest unit is obviously the individual group member and here the inherent variability of the risk prediction will be at its highest.

To take the example of two of the most widely used and best established actuarial risk instruments. The VRAG claims to identify nine groups, known by the unfortunate term 'bins', with a probability of future violent recidivism varying from 0 per cent to 100 per cent.[31, 32] The analysis of Hart and colleagues[36] demonstrates that rather than nine statistically separable groups there are only three statistically distinct groups. The Static 99 claims to separate sex offenders into 7 groups with recidivism rates varying from less than 10 per cent to greater than 50 per cent.[37] Statistically however only two separable groups are generated one with offending rates between 4 per cent and 25 per cent and one between 30 per cent and 60 per cent.[36] In short even ignoring the all important problem of attributing a group risk to an individual within the grouping the Static 99 identifies recidivism with at best 2 in 3, and at worst 1 in 3, chance of accuracy. In this really good enough to damn a person to indefinite incarceration or extended imprisonment?

Unfortunately, unlike other areas that rely on actuarial approaches to decision-making, there has not been a concerted effort in the area of violence risk assessment to pool the results of various studies to obtain the large samples necessary to reduce the variance which would thereby reduce the broad values on the confidence intervals.

---

1 There are notable exceptions, such as the Level of Supervision/Case Management Inventory which has accrued normative data on more than 35,000 prisons and almost 80,000 people under community corrections supervision [Andrews, D. A., Bonta, J. L., & Wormith, J. S. (2005). Level of Service/Case Management Inventory (LS/CMI). Toronto: Multihealth Systems.].

As noted in Footnote 1 above, there are some exceptions such as the LS/CMI. Doubtless, over time researchers will pool results to determine the extent to which confidence intervals can decrease, thereby increasing the predictive utility of instruments.

The big question which hangs over the use of risk assessment instruments is the extent to which it is possible, or acceptable, to make attributions about an individual's future behaviour on the basis of their sharing characteristics with those in a group with a known level of risk for such behaviour. In medicine we are so used to using probabilities to dictate our actions that there are dangers in failing to recognize the problems. An 18 year old woman presents with a history of severe central abdominal pain moving to the right iliac fossa associated with anorexia. The probability in those with similar symptoms of an inflamed appendix may be 30 per cent but 100 per cent of the patients are advised to have surgery. Probability is used here to provide advice entirely in the interest of the patient. If the advice is refused the patient is not forced into surgery but is observed and managed non-surgically. Compare this with advice to a court or tribunal considering extending the incarceration of an offender or patient. The offender may have similar characteristics to those with a better than 50 per cent (or even 80 per cent) chance of re-offending and to attribute the group risk to the individual may benefit the community. It will however almost certainly disadvantage the individual who will not be the one accepting or rejecting the advice. It is fallacious to argue that making such attributions from group membership to individual risk is acceptable because it reduces the errors of false positives. It is not possible to benefit the so called low risk without disadvantaging the rest. Even with particularly strong measure of risk assessment, the false positive rates still hover around 25 per cent.

The only strong defence of attributing risk to an individual by virtue of their group membership, which is the essence of prejudice, is that it has better outcomes than not using this approach. But what are better outcomes? Better outcomes could be reduced to the accounting of true and false attribution. On this basis actuarial risk assessment instruments perform better than the best guesses of most experts. In the case of possible appendicitis given the benefits of early versus delayed intervention a high number of false positives is tolerable to avoid even one false negative. When the outcome is imposing further incarceration even the price of one false positive for every true positive, which the Static 99 and VRAG might offer may raise moral and legal qualms. Particularly as given both the true and the false positive will be incapacitated making it impossible to ever know which was which. There is no quick corrective feedback in the world of assessing the risk of future criminality, unlike appendicitis where the pathologist will soon tell you if you were right or wrong. Further when supposedly low risk individuals are discharged or released and re-offend, this will reinforce any tendency to err on the side of caution and incarceration.

Statistical decision theory can support using group membership to attribute levels of probability to individual group members. Though even here sceptics might suggest that the efforts put into Bayesian approaches to make the best of limited data sets might better be expended in enlarging such data bases. What in any case the approach cannot do is decide on utility and moral propriety. It is only relatively recently that the criminal justice system has moved to making the prediction of future offending the dominant issue in determining sentences, parole, and the extensions of sentences (which in and of itself is an entirely new phenomenon). Similarly the emphasis on the risks psychiatric patients present to others is a relatively recent preoccupation for mental health services. The development of standardized risk assessment instruments not only serves these changes but sustains them. The sexual predator legislation in the US, the DSPD and indefinite sentencing provisions in the UK, and the extended supervision/imprisonment laws in Australasia, are all dependent on mental health professionals providing them a veneer of science and objectivity through risk assessments.[38, 39] While providing the courts with information regarding the extent to which the individual's characteristics place them in a general level of risk we by implication give our assent and support to that process. We place a hope for community benefit before an inevitable disadvantage to those with whom we have engaged professionally.

The current state of the science of risk prediction some might suggest delivers only a limited improvement in the decision making process. If they are correct what, if anything, remains in the risk assessment literature of practical value? The short answer is that the establishing of risk factors remains of inestimable value, not in placing labels on individuals but in identifying how to reduce the probability of future violent and criminal behaviours. The standardized risk assessment approaches such as the HCR-20 and the VRAG allow individuals to be assigned to broad levels of high, low or medium probability of future violence. It can be argued whether or not the confidence that can be placed in such attributions justify imposing extended incarceration. They are however of undoubted value in assigning priority for management interventions.

The structured professional judgement measures, such as the HCR-20, also add considerable value by identifying risk factors, such as substance abuse, specific personality vulnerabilities, and the like allowing targeted interventions to reduce the chances of engaging in violence and offending. The exposure of the current limitations in the project of identifying dangerous individuals is bad news for courts, parole boards and governments looking for short cuts to community safety. But for mental health professionals it is merely a reminder that our business is managing patients to reduce the risks for them and for others, not trying to separate the dangerous goats from the mostly harmless sheep.

The limitations on the ability to accurately predict risk also emphasize that in all circumstances where psychiatrists and psychologists are being asked to provide opinions of risk of future violence to courts or other decision-making bodies, they should provide the courts with the information that they can. This would include, for example, the general risk level in which the risk assessment tools would place the patient but it would also extend to an anamnestic consideration of factors in the patient's case that are known to increase or decrease the level of risk. In the end, though, the clinicians need to be clear to state the limitations of their findings and to, of course, leave the ultimate decision of whether the patient meets the criteria of the statute in question to the legal decision makers.

## Practicalities of risk prediction and management

Risk assessment and management can be conceptualized as a four stage process:

1 An evaluation of general level of risk and priority for active intervention. In practice this can rarely go further than saying they are in a high, medium, or low, priority or risk category.

2 Identify current risk factors and future hazards which are both potentially remediable and causally relate to increased chances of violence.

3 Develop management strategies to reduce or remove the deleterious influence of these factors.

4 Evaluate the effectiveness of the interventions in reducing subsequent violence.

Each of the above steps will be discussed in turn below.

## Evaluating level of risk

Such evaluations should start simple, consider the context, apply clinical and common sense, then potentially progress to the use of a standardized assessment instrument. In both the mentally disordered and general population the majority of violent and criminal behaviour is committed by young males with histories of repeated antisocial behaviour dating back to conduct disorder in childhood. This is often combined with anomie, that lawless disaffection with society in general and contempt for rules and authority in particular. Impulsiveness is concerning[40] but so is the more muted feckless disregard for consequences found in some with a schizophrenic syndrome. Unemployment, living in a high crime neighbourhood, and antisocial peers all add substantially to risk. Similarly substance abuse is a robust maker for the risk of criminality in the disordered and non disordered alike. Specific to the seriously mentally disordered is a refusal to recognize they are ill, and resistance to complying with treatment with often an antagonism to professionals; the 'fuck off and leave me alone' syndrome.

Clinicians must maintain their common sense. A range of situations must be taken seriously. The angry and threatening who can tell you exactly what they plan to do to their supposed antagonist, the frightened who see no alternative to a pre-emptive strike, those who have prepared for violence (weapons, surveillance, put their affairs in order), the actively suicidal who have nothing to lose but still care enough to take a final revenge, and commonest of all those making threats in a manner which creates fear and concern either in the potential victim or those who have been privy to the threats.

Beyond normative data and risk factors, there exist a number of high risk situations and syndromes particular to psychiatry. These include:-

1 Morbid jealousy

2 Some misidentification syndromes

3 Depressed suicidal mothers of young children.

4 Delusional systems focussing on specific individuals believed to present for the patient a serious threat, or a malevolent impediment to their central project.

5 Some stalking situations

6 Confusional states be they toxic or related to dementia or other cerebral impairments (this is the source of a significant proportion of assaults on health staff)

Patients presenting any of the above characteristics require careful assessment and management to reduce the likelihood that risk will eventuate.

When there is an indication that a patient may be at an elevated level of risk for violence, or when the clinician is doing a risk assessment specifically, there is much to be said for becoming familiar with the use of standardized risk assessment instruments. They can direct attention to important areas that require consideration and provide a structure for both gathering and evaluating relevant information. The choice is between the actuarial (e.g., VRAG, Static 99 and COVR) and those employing structured professional judgement (e.g., HCR 20). The former generate fixed risk levels, the latter in their nature are open to further modification in the light of clinical and common sense. Pure actuarial instruments (e.g. Static 99 and COVR) may appeal to the less experienced given their relative simplicity of administration. Their disadvantage even for the expert is, however, that they can function like black boxes which generate evaluations without the user being necessarily aware of how the instrument was constituted and the limitations that should attend its use. Moreover, they have been validated for use in fairly limited contexts and countries. As a result, clinicians may put undue weight on the results the instruments produce, without knowing how the results might vary in the context in which they are working.

Structured professional judgement is more transparent, if more demanding of the user. Where the actuarial measures can be used by relatively poorly trained individuals or in some contexts clerical staff, the structured professional judgment measures must be employed by those with considerable expertize. We favour the structured professional judgement approach of the HCR 20 but readers need to understand that actuarial instruments are perhaps the dominant forms of risk assessment instrumentation, due in no small part to their reliance on static variables and ease of administration. The HCR 20 is designed for use with general and forensic psychiatric patients and it has been found to have utility in general offender populations. Those whose work brings them into contact with specific groups such as perpetrators of domestic violence, child molesters or stalkers should consider using risk assessment approaches developed specifically for these populations (e.g., the Spousal Assault Risk Assessment (SARA),[41,42] Sexual Violence Risk-20 (SVR-20),[43] Risk for Sexual Violence Protocol (RSVP).[44,45]

The end point of a risk analysis in most cases will allow individuals to be placed into one of three somewhat arbitrary groups which encompass both likelihood and potential level of damage:-

i) High Risk – the individual presents a significant risk of committing a seriously damaging act of violence within a reasonable timeframe (less than a year or so). It is generally impossible to quantify the numerical probability for 'high risk' as it will vary across instruments and in different situations from approximately 30 per cent (sexual offending) to 80 per cent (the occurrence of general violence). Management of the risk is required immediately and the level of risk should be re-evaluated periodically depending on the extent to which the individual's personal situation and dynamic risk factors may vary. When the potential violence is of a particularly horrendous nature (e.g. potentially lethal) the timeframe can reasonably be extended to encompass a number of years. In, for example, some predatory child molesters and some who have killed from morbid jealousy, the chances of re-offending may be substantial and continue virtually throughout the offender's life span.

ii) Moderate Risk – the individual presents a real risk of committing a damaging act which might inflict minor injuries and/or significant fear and distress within a year or so. This group also requires their level of risk to be managed though, because the severity of behaviour is less extreme and the time period perhaps less imminent, the extent of management is less intensive or restrictive. Also in this group can be placed those with a more remote (less than 30 per cent) but not inconsequential (above 5 per cent which in practice is the limit of reliable detection) risk of serious violence. Examples include those at lower risk of committing acts of a more serious nature (e.g., those making viable and tangible threats of engaging in behaviour which would lead to harm).

iii) Low Risk – Individuals who do not present a real risk of harming a third party. Their level of risk and potential for severe risk is low. They do not require any risk management plan beyond normal care and there is no need to re-evaluate the risk at any time in the reasonably foreseeable future. In essence, this category includes everyone not in the High or Moderate categories.

A final re-emphasis. Even using standardized instruments the final evaluation has to take into account factors beyond the figures generated by the black box. Risk evaluation is about formulation not simply calculations.

## Identifying factors relevant to decreasing risk

The primarily clinical purpose of risk assessment should be risk management. Risk management is about identifying those factors which mediate the increased risk and modifying them to decrease risk. The structured professional judgment instruments and a good working knowledge of the risk literature will assist the clinician to identify and understand relevant risk factors. As noted above, identification of the dynamic risk factors points directed to potential management approaches. A simplified schema of the mediators and moderators which link having a schizophrenic syndrome to violent behaviour is presented in Fig. 11.14.1 with the basic approach to breaking or attenuating those links represented in Fig. 11.14.2.

The management strategies in high risk groups take us directly to good clinical practice with the addition of few specific approaches. The basic approach to management of high risk individuals can be summarized:

1 Substance abuse. This claims first place not because it is necessarily the most important risk factor but because the presence of the significant abuse of alcohol or drugs can disrupt all other management approaches.

2 Psychopathology. Obtaining adequate control of the delusions, affective disturbances, and hallucinations which predispose in some cases to offending behaviours is the second management imperative. Again without adequate control of the psychopathology little progress is likely in more targeted treatment modalities. High risk groups are often reluctant to comply either with medication or psychological management. This may force the use of compulsory treatment in an inpatient situation for sufficient time for the patient to begin to experience the benefits of amelioration of their active psychosis. Extended admissions (4–12 weeks) also provide an opportunity to establish trusting therapeutic relationships, though equally they can be productive of resentment and even more marked resistance to treatment. Second generation antipsychotics are preferable in this group as they are better tolerated and less likely to further impair cognitive and particularly frontal deficits. Depot medication is useful initially though this currently restricts considerably the choice of medication at least until more second generation antipsychotics come available in depot format. Clozapine can be particularly effective in this group but the level of cooperation required usually prevents its use at least in the early phase of management.

3 Social Circumstances. Discharging high risk patients to disorganized or casual accommodation in high crime neighbourhoods virtually guarantees offending behaviours. Similarly the drift back into contact with substance abusing peer groups increases risk and further disrupts management. Unemployment or just

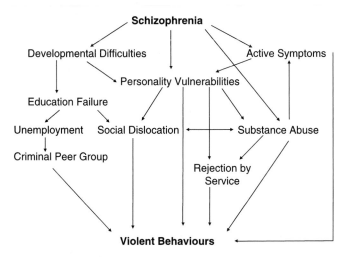

**Fig. 11.14.1** A simplified schema of the mediators and moderatory between having a schizophrenic syndrome and behaving violently are illustrated. The very complexity of the nexus between illness and violence offers multiple opportunities for intervening to break the links. [Reproduced from Mullen, P.E., (2006). Schizophrenia and violence: from correlations to preventative strategies. *Advances in Psychiatric Treatment*, **12**, 239–48, copyright 2006, The Royal College of Psychiatrists.]

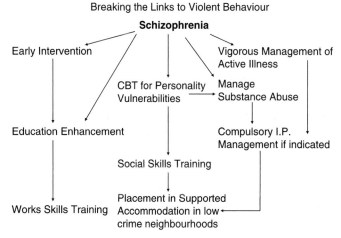

**Fig. 11.14.2** Illustrates some of the interventions which could reduce the strength of the association between having schizophrenia and behaving violently. All interventions depend on accepting that it is the services duty to manage both the violence which can emerge from schizophrenia, and those with schizophrenia who are also substance abusing, delinquent and objecting. [Reproduced from Mullen, P.E., (2006). Schizophrenia and violence: from correlations to preventative strategies. *Advances in Psychiatric Treatment*, **12**, 239–48, copyright 2006, The Royal College of Psychiatrists.]

the lack of structure to their days increases risk. An absence of non offending, non substance use satisfactions leaves patients vulnerable to offending. The high risk groups need stable accommodation in low crime neighbourhoods, with active support, and structured recreation with later more long term educational and work related activities. Assisting them into contact with non deviant social groups (via sport, voluntary work, employment, or hobbies) is essential to establish social rewards to replace the pleasures of substance use and crime.

4 Insight. Or more concretely the acceptance of the need to change their attitudes and behaviours which support criminal and violent behaviours is a requirement for more targeted interventions. The stages of change model[46] combined with motivational interviewing[47] can assist in beginning the process. Ultimately it is through establishing a trusting relationship with the therapist and ideally the treatment team that commitment to change and maintaining change is obtained.[48]

5 Personality Traits. Personality disorders may or may not respond to treatment but the traits out of which they have been constructed are mostly open to modification. The objective is not to transform a suspicious, manipulative, insensitive, self absorbed thug into a paragon of the social virtues. It is simply to ameliorate those traits which predispose to antisocial behaviour. Targeted CBT offers a range of options. Wong and Hare's[49] guide to managing psychopathic traits offers a useful source of guidance for developing such programs.

6 Victim Empathy. Assisting the high risk group to understand the impact of their behaviour is essential. Sadly this is often best approached through sensitizing them to the harm they bring on themselves rather than through victim empathy programs, but both are worth attempting.

7 Common Sense and Prudential Wisdom. High risk patients with a schizophrenic syndrome not infrequently lack the mundane capacity to foresee the obvious outcomes of their behaviour. This produces a feckless foolishness. Instilling prudential wisdom in those impaired in this manner is a matter of slow progress in structured interactions which focus on their actual behaviours and the enhancement of the capacity to modify those behaviours in function of their longer term outcomes.

## Conclusions

There are significant pressures and obligations—both legal and professional—for mental health professionals to give prominence to risk assessment and management with their patients (clients). The extent to which risk assessment will be more or less prominent will depend largely upon the nature of the professionals work, and the environment in which it occurs. Caring for those with high prevalence disorders in private practice will have little to worry about. For those responsible for patients who are acutely psychotic and of course those working in forensic contexts, the importance of risk assessment will be more significant.

We are at an important crossroads in our level of knowledge about both violence among psychiatric patients and about risk assessment. The fact that the risk for violence among psychiatric patients is not insignificant does mean that risk assessment and management is a legitimate activity for mental health professionals.[45] As such, psychiatrists and psychologists must become familiar with the risk assessment literature and emerging technologies. With appropriate levels of knowledge and training, clinicians can master this complex area in a way that can serve to satisfy their professional and legal obligations. Only with a good understanding of the field can we be protected from the risk of either blithely neglecting the violence risk our patients pose or of becoming so risk averse so as to unnecessarily and arbitrarily restrict our patients' liberty.

In the area of risk assessment, the framing of the main research questions and the articulation of the resulting data is increasingly in terms of actuarial risks and the generation of standardized questionnaires which will generate predictive scores. The technology of risk assessments could become one of the primary mediators of the relationship between the professional and the mentally disordered person. This will radically alter how the patient and their disorders and disabilities are revealed to us. We must not allow the technological focus on risk to replace the importance of the patient's personal and social context. We must not allow it to objectify them and their disorder as an embodiment of a quantum of 'riskiness.' To this end, there is an argument to occasionally separate the formal risk assessment task from that of patient treatment. The roles are blended—as they should be—in most cases, such as caring for voluntary patients and those involuntarily committed for brief periods. When the question of the patient's level of risk is that which will determine their liberty over the long term, however, it is less tenable for a treating clinician to maintain a productive therapeutic relationship with patients while holding the reins on their liberty (e.g., consideration of reviews of indeterminate dispositions, evaluations of risk for sentencing purposes and parole decision-making).

Technology is about performance and control, it is about domination, and the objects of technological manipulation are just that, objects [see[50, 51]]. To the extent that technological approaches to risk assessment come to dominate clinical practice, whatever benefit they may bring, the price will be reframing the clinician's view of their patients as potentially dangerous things. Risk assessment forms part of a major shift in psychiatric practice and theory away from individually based engagements between clinicians and uniquely troubled individuals to a world of standardized best practice. Instruments direct diagnosis, diagnosis determines which system of treatment is to be applied and risk assessments enable us to prevent damage to, or by, the objects of our professional responsibilities. Efficient, effective, properly evaluated performances of mandated procedures becomes the definition not only of the normative but the ethical.

This chapter began with a quotation from a nobel prize winner, it will end with the story of another. In reading the account provided by Nasser of the schizophrenic illness of the Nobel Laureate John Nash images emerge of the complex interactions between illness and the sufferer's humanity, life and even genius.[52] Nash had a devastating mental illness, he was as a result of his illness compulsorily treated and even at times regarded as dangerous. Nash finally entered a stable remission in which he could once more work as a mathematician. This was without the continuing aid of medication or any other form of mental health ministrations. What has this to do with risk assessment and management? Everything. The outcome of an illness such as one of the schizophrenias in an individual case remains enormously difficult to predict. We must, as mental health professionals, act on our estimates of future probabilities. We should struggle to make our risk assessments and risk management strategies as effective as possible. But in the end we should remain modest about our capacities to perform such predictive and preventive functions and not loose curiosity about what really delivers Nash and many others from insanity and even dangerousness.

## Further information

Maden, A. (2007). *Treating Violence: A guide to risk management in mental health.* Oxford University Press, New York.

Mossman, D. (2007). Critique of Pure Risk Assessment or, Kant Meets Tarasoff. *University of Cincinnati Law Review*, 75, 523–609.

Douglas, K., and Skeem, J. (2005). Violence risk assessment: Getting specific about being dynamic. Psychology, *Public Policy and Law*, 11, 347–83.

Ogloff, J. R. P. (2006). The Psychopathy/Antisocial Personality Disorder Conundrum. *Australian and New Zealand Journal of Psychiatry*, 40, 519–28.

## References

1. Monahan, J. (1988). Risk Assessment of Violence Among the Mentally Disordered: Generating Useful Knowledge. *International Journal of Law and Psychiatry*, 11, 249–57.
2. Snowden, P. (1997). Practical aspects of clinical risk assessment and management. *British Journal of Psychiatry*, 170 (suppl. 32), 32–4.
3. Gunn, J. (1996). Lets get serious about dangerousness. *Criminal Behaviour and Mental Health*, Supplement: 51–64.
4. Kraemer, H., Kazdin, A., Offord, D., *et al.* (1997). Coming to terms with the terms of risk. *Archives of General Psychiatry*, 54, 337–41.
5. Castel, R. (1991). From dangerousness to risk. In *The Foucault Effect; Studies in Governmentality* (eds. G. Burchell, C. Gordon, P. Miller). Hemel Hempstead, Harester Wheatsheaf.
6. Douglas, M. (1992). *Risk and Blame: Essays in Cultural Theory.* Routledge, London.
7. O'Mally, P. (1991). Risk, Power and Crime prevention. *Economy & Society*, 21, 252–75.
8. Rose, N. (1996). Psychiatry as a political science: advanced liberalism and the administration of risk. *History of the Human Sciences*, 9, 1–23.
9. Scott, P. D. (1977). Assessing dangerousness in criminals. *British Journal of Psychiatry*, 131, 127–42
10. Stürup, G.K. (1968). Will this man be dangerous? In *The Mentally Abnormal Offender* (eds. A. de Reuk and R. Porter), pp. 5–18. Churchill, London,
11. Steadman, H.J. and Cocozza, J.J. (1975). We can't predict who is dangerous. *Psychology Today*, 8, 22–35.
12. Shaw, S.H. (1973). The dangerousness of dangerousness. *Medicine Science and Law*, 13, 269–71.
13. Carstensen, P.C. (1994). The evolving duty of mental health professionals to third parties: a doctrinal and institutional examination. *International Journal of Law and Psychiatry*, 17, 1–42.
14. Cocozza, J. and Steadman, H. (1976). The failure of psychiatric predictions of dangerousness: Clear and convincing evidence. *Rutgers Law Review*, 29, 1084–1101.
15. *Barefoot v. Estelle*, 463 U.S. 880, (1983).
16. *Tarasoff v. Regents of University of California*, 551 P.2d 334 (1976).
17. *United States v. Hinckley*, 672 F.2d 115 (D.C. Cir. 1982).
18. *Kansas v. Hendricks*, 521 U.S. 346, (1997).
19. Maden, A. (2007). *Treating Violence: A guide to risk management in mental health.* Oxford University Press, New York.
20. Monahan, J. (1981). *The Clinical Prediction of Violent Behaviour.* US Government Printing Office, Washington, DC.
21. Belfrage, H. (1998). Implementing the HCR-20 scheme for risk assessment in a forensic psychiatric hospital: Integrating research and clinical practice. *Journal of Forensic Psychiatry*, 9, 328–38.
22. Douglas, K., Ogloff, J. and Hart, S. (2003). Evaluation of the structured professional judgment model of violence risk assessment among forensic psychiatric patients. *Psychiatric Services*, 54, 1372–79.
23. Andrews, D.A. and Bonta, J. (2003). *The Psychology of Criminal Conduct* (3rd). Anderson Publishing Co., Ohio.
24. Rice, M.E. and Harris, G.T. (1995). Violent recidivism: Assessing predictive validity. *Journal of Consulting and Clinical Psychology*, 63, 737–48.
25. Mossman, D. (1994). Assessing predictions of violence: Being accurate about accuracy. *Journal of Consulting and Clinical Psychology*, 62, 783–92.
26. Mullen, P.E. (2006). Schizophrenia and Violence: from correlations to preventative strategies. *Advances in Psychiatric Treatment* 12, 239–248.
27. Wallace, C., Mullen, P.E., Burgess, P., *et al.* (1998). Serious criminal offending and mental disorder: Case linkage study. *British Journal of Psychiatry*, 172, 477–484.
28. Lindqvist, P. and Allebeck, P. (1990). Schizophrenia and Crime. A Longitudinal Follow-up of 644 Schizophrenics in Stockholm. *British Journal of Psychiatry*, 157, 345–50.
29. Hafner, H. and Böker, W. (1982). *Crimes of Violence by Mentally Abnormal Offenders* (trans. H. Marshall). Cambridge University Press, Cambridge.
30. Douglas, K., Ogloff, J., Nicholls, T., *et al.* (1999). Assessing risk for violence among psychiatric patients: The HCR-20 Violence Risk Assessment Scheme and the Psychopathy Checklist: Screening Version. *Journal of Consulting and Clinical Psychology*, 67, 917–30.
31. Quinsey, V.L., Harris, G.T., Rice, M.E., *et al.* (1998). *Violent Offenders: Appraising and Managing Risk.* American Psychological Association, Washington, DC.
32. Quinsey, V.L., Rice, M.E., Harris, G.T., *et al.* (2004). *Violent offenders: Appraising and managing risk (2nd ed.).* American Psychological Association, Washington, DC.
33. Silver, E., Smith, W.R. and Banks, S. (2000). Constructing actuarial devices for predicting recidivism: A comparison of methods. *Criminal Justice and Behavior*, 27, 733–64.
34. Barbaree, H.E., Langton, C.M. and Blanchard, R. (2007). Predicting recidivism in sex offenders using the VRAG and SORAG: The contribution of age-at-release. *International Journal of Forensic Mental Health*, 6, 29–46.
35. Monahan, J., Steadman, H.J. *et al.* (2005). *Classification of Violence Risk.* Psychological Assessment Resources, Inc., Lutz, FL.
36. Hart, S.D., Michie, C. and Cooke, D.J. (2007). Precision of actuarial risk assessment instruments. Evaluating the 'margins of error' of group v. individual predictions of violence. *The British Journal of Psychiatry* 190 (Suppl. 49) s60–s65.
37. Hanson, R.K. and Thornton, D.M. (1999). *Static 99: Improving Actuarial Risk Assessments for Sex Offenders.* Ottawa Public Works and Government Services, Canada.
38. Mercado, C.C. and Ogloff, J.R.P. (2007). Risk and the preventive detention of sex offenders in Australia and the United States. *International Journal of Law and Psychiatry*, 30, 49–59.
39. Wood, M. and Ogloff, J.R.P. (2006). Victoria's Serious Sex Offenders Monitoring Act: Implications for the accuracy of sex offender risk assessment. *Psychiatry, Psychology and the Law*, 13(2), 182–98.
40. Enticott, P., Ogloff, J.R.P. and Bradshaw, J. (in press). Response inhibition and impulsivity in schizophrenia. *Psychiatry Research*.
41. Kropp, P.R., Hart, S.D., Webster, C.D., *et al.* (1994). *Manual of the Spousal Assault Risk Assessment Guide (2nd ed).* British Columbia Institute on Family Violence, Vancouver, Canada.
42. Kropp, P.R., Hart, S.D., Webster, C.D., *et al.* (2000). The Spousal Assault Risk Assessment Guide (SARA) guide: Reliability and validity in adult male offenders. *Law and Human Behaviour*, 24 (1), 101–18.

43. Boer, D.P., Hart, S.D., Kropp, P.R., *et al.* (1997). *Sexual violence risk-20: Professional guidelines for assessing risk of sexual violence.* British Columbia Institute on Family Violence and Mental Health, Law, and Policy Institute, Simon Fraser University; Vancouver, British Columbia.

44. Hart, S.D., Kropp, P.R. and Laws, D.R. (2003). *The risk for sexual violence protocol (RSVP): Structured professional guidelines for assessing risk of sexual violence.* Mental Health, Law, and Policy Institute, Simon Fraser University and British Columbia Institute on Family Violence, Vancouver, British Columbia.

45. Mullen, P.E., MacKenzie, R., Ogloff, J.R.P., *et al.* (2006). Assessing and managing the risks in the stalking situation. *Journal of the American Academy of Psychiatry and the Law,* **34**, 439–50.

46. Prochaska, J.O. and Di Clemente, C.C. (1992). Stages of change in the modification of problem behaviours. *Progress in Behavioural Modification,* **28**, 183–218.

47. Miller, W.R. and Rollnick, S. (1991). *Motivational Interviewing: Preparing People to Change Addictive Behaviour.* Guilford, New York.

48. Douglas, K.S., Webster, C.D., Hart, S.D., *et al.* (2001). *HCR-20 Violence Risk Management Companion Guide.* Simon Fraser University, British Columbia.

49. Wong, S. and Hare, R.D. (2005). *Guidelines for a Psychopathy Treatment Program.* MHS, Toronto.

50. Heidegger, M. (1993). The Question Concerning Technology. In: *Basic Writings.* Harper, San Francisco, 297–352.

51. Lyotard, J.F. (1979). *The Post Modern Condition: A Report on Knowledge.* Trans. G Bennington and B Massumi. University of Minnesota Press, Minneapolis.

52. Nasser, A. (1998). *A Beautiful Mind.* New York: Simon and Schuster

# 11.15

# The expert witness in the Criminal Court: assessment, reports, and testimony

John O'Grady

As an expert witness in the Criminal Court, the psychiatrist ceases to be simply a doctor as a psychiatrist's report and testimony addresses issues on the boundary between law and psychiatry. The law is not primarily concerned with the welfare of the defendant. Criminal law is concerned with justice, fact finding, and the attribution of guilt whilst psychiatry concerns itself with the welfare of the individual, their mental disorder, and its treatment. This chapter will explore the legal framework for expert reports and testimony, standards for such work, the particular ethical dilemmas of this work and provide practical guidance on preparation of reports and testimony.

This chapter draws upon previously published work by the author.[1,2] Expert evidence cannot be understood except in reference to a particular legal jurisdiction. For this chapter the legal system in the United Kingdom is chosen but the general principles will apply to all jurisdictions. Issues specific to Civil and Family courts will not be discussed.

## The psychiatric expert witness[3–5]

Witnesses in court can only give evidence of facts they personally perceived and not evidence of their opinion. It is for the court to draw inferences from the testimony of witnesses. The opinion of an expert witness is an exclusion to this general rule because courts need the assistance of experts to consider issues beyond their knowledge.

Lawton L.J in R v Turner established a 'common knowledge' rule governing expert evidence as follows:

> An expert opinion is admissible to furnish the Courts with scientific information which is likely to be outside the experience and knowledge of a Judge or a jury. If on the proven fact, a Judge or jury can form their own conclusions without help, then the opinion of an expert is unnecessary. In such a case if it given dressed up in scientific jargon it may make judgement more difficult. The facts that an expert witness has impressive scientific qualifications does not by that fact alone make his opinion on matters of human nature and behaviour within the limits of normality any more helpful than that of the jurors themselves; but there is a danger that they may think it does ... jurors do not need psychiatrists to tell them how ordinary folk who are not

suffering from any mental illness are likely to react to the stresses and strains of life.

This seems to limit psychiatric evidence to recognized mental disorder. However, expert advice is allowed which is 'outside the experience and knowledge of a Judge or jury'. The abnormal/normal dichotomy is not a rule of law but guidance. Courts have allowed evidence on a variety of conditions which would not normally be thought of as established mental disorder, for example 'Battered Women's syndrome'.

Particular problems arise for the Court in respect of borderline conditions falling short of recognized mental disorder. Here admissibility will usually be determined by the court's judgement as to whether the expert evidence addresses matters outside the experience or knowledge of a Judge or jury. Generally courts seek to limit evidence to established abnormal conditions.[3,5] Courts have problems with evidence that utilizes leading edge or novel theory or diagnosis. The Court will require evidence that the novel theory or diagnosis is sufficiently organized or recognized to be accepted as a reliable body of knowledge by the profession. The expert will need to demonstrate that acceptance through reference to scientific literature.[3,5]

For medical experts, the Courts are able to establish expertise by reference to qualification and training. Nevertheless, the expert must be able to demonstrate that they have the requisite expertise in a particular case. For example, a psychiatrist trained in general adult psychiatry may not be an expert in a case concerning a person with moderate to severe learning disability.

## Immunity from suit

Lawyers and experts enjoy immunity from suit (civil litigation) for their professional work in court.[3] For medical expert witnesses this includes their report and any oral evidence presented in court. That immunity does not extend to immunity from report to the doctor's regulatory body. It does not extend to subsequent actions such as duty of confidentiality in respect of disclosure of reports to third parties. The judgement in the case of GMC v Meadows lays out the legal and public policy arguments for immunity from suit but with regulation by their professional regulatory body.

## Reliability of expert testimony

Courts need to assure themselves that an expert witness's evidence is reliable. This creates an obvious problem as the very reason an expert is giving evidence is that they have expertise which the judge or jury does not possess.

Courts have utilized three broad approaches to this problem. The first is to examine the scientific validity of evidence. The second is to devise standards for expert evidence and the third is to regulate experts through formal accreditation systems.

## Scrutiny of scientific evidence

The landmark case is that of Daubert v Merrell Dow Pharmaceuticals in the United States courts. That ruling established stringent criteria to judge reliability to include that the technique, body of knowledge, or theory can be tested, has been subjected to peer review and publication, has a known rate of error, is subject to maintenance of standards and controls and is generally accepted by the scientific community. This judgement is problematic for a number of reasons,[6] not least because the court does not have that expert's specific knowledge but nevertheless has to make a scientific judgement on the reliability of that expert's evidence. Judgements are unlikely to be value free determinations and there is a risk that the admissibility of evidence could be distorted by policy considerations or interfere with the use of leading edge science in the court. These considerations have made United Kingdom courts reluctant to introduce a 'Daubert' type test but there is pressure to do so[4,7] with public concern about miscarriages of justice linked to expert evidence.

## Regulatory rules for expert witnesses

Courts have defined the standards expected of an expert witness; the landmark case being the judgement of Cresswell J in The Ikarian Reefer. Court judgements have been used to draw up formal rules governing civil family and criminal courts; for UK Criminal courts, the relevant rules are contained in Part 33, Criminal Procedure Rules.[8] The common features are listed in Box 11.15.1 below. The understandable anxiety of the court to ensure experts adhere to these stringent standards may have the unfortunate effect of deterring psychiatrists from providing occasional expert reports for criminal courts.

## Accreditation

In the United Kingdom, there are a number of organizations to accredit expert witnesses utilizing some combination of direct scrutiny of reports and references from legal teams. None so far have addressed the specific needs of the expert psychiatrist in court. They provide the court with some measure of an expert witness's expertise in legal matters over and above what comes from their basic professional qualification. Critics have pointed out[10] that once registered accreditation is unlikely to pick up poor practice, as experts with years of experience, but not necessarily competence, are unlikely to be refused accreditation. Accreditation is unlikely to prevent expert straying outside their area of expertise. These schemes have not as yet been able to deal effectively with problems of accrediting inexperienced but competent aspiring expert witnesses. To be effective they may require codes of discipline with the

---

**Box 11.15.1** Common features of regulatory rules for civil family and criminal courts.

Expert Reports should contain:

1 Details of academic and professional qualifications together with experience and accreditation relevant to the opinions expressed in the report (usually as a summary in the introduction with more detail within and Appendix).

2 A statement of the range and extent of expertise together with limitations upon that expertise, particularly declaring when a particular issue is outside his expertise.

3 A statement setting out the substance of all instructions received together with listing all materials provided and considered, upon which the opinion is based.

4 Where there is a range of opinion on matters dealt with in the report, a summary range of opinion together with reasons for the experts preferred opinion (see section below on Report Writing).

5 A declaration of any facts, materials, or investigations which might bear upon or be made against the expert opinion.

6 Extracts of literature or any other material upon which the scientific evidence is based.

7 A statement of which facts are within the expert's own knowledge and which are assumed.**

8 Where an opinion is qualified, a statement to that effect.

9 A statement that the expert has complied with his or her duty to the court to provide independent assistance by way of objective unbiased opinion in matters within his or her expertise.

10 A statement that the expert will inform all parties, including the court, in the event that his or her opinion changes on any material issue.

11 A declaration of truth.

** Courts distinguish true and assumed facts. The only facts the psychiatric expert will routinely know to be true are the results of examination and results of tests or investigations. All other facts will be assumed to be true.[9]

---

attendant danger of attracting vexatious complaints. The Royal College of Psychiatrists in the United Kingdom utilizes a competency based training framework together with standards for continuing professional development (CPD) following training to promote a high standard in medico-legal work. Evidence of completion of such training and CPD is likely to be the most effective way of demonstrating credibility as an expert witness.

## Ethics

### Dual role

Stone[11] used the term 'dual role' to describe the psychiatrist in the legal context. In Stone's view the role of the clinician and medical examiner for Court are irreconcilable. The evaluee/patient is unable to distinguish the role of the medical examiner as a Court expert from that of personal physician. This result is an inability to protect themselves from inadvertent disclosure that might adversely affect the outcome in Court. He argued that clinicians cannot help using their therapeutic skills to engage the patient in disclosure. The dual role arises from the use made of the resulting psychiatric evidence for non-welfare purposes. Appelbaum[12] argued that the dual role of psychiatric experts in Court is best managed by understanding that psychiatrists operate outside the medical framework when they undertake forensic Court work and their practice is not governed by the ethical principles underpinning medical practice (beneficence and non-maleficence). Instead he argued that psychiatric experts should operate from a perspective of justice ethics employing ethical principles of objective truth finding and respect for the person (termed autonomy and truthfulness).

If this solution to the Dual Role dilemma were accepted, it would mean that the psychiatrist should not have a welfare/treatment role in respect of the person under evaluation. In the United Kingdom this is untenable[13] primarily because of Mental Health law which provides for diversion to the health system as a sentence following a finding of guilt (Hospital order). Weinstock et al.[14] have argued in the United States legal and clinical context the Appelbaum solution[12] is, untenable in that legal context as psychiatrists routinely have conflicting responsibilities thrust upon them where legal or other requirements may take precedence over patient welfare.

Reports addressing sentencing in the United Kingdom place the psychiatrist in a Dual Role position. This is because the psychiatric opinion can result in two outcomes for the evaluee

1  A welfare disposal under Mental Health legislation.

2  Potentially greater restrictions on the defendant, including an indeterminate life sentence where there is expert evidence on mental disorder but no recommendation for a welfare disposal.

Statutes that introduce indeterminate life sentences for public protection based upon assessed future risk of re-offending cause particular problems.[1,13,15] English Courts have, through case law and practice, sought psychiatric evidence when they consider defendants may have mental disorder and where the Court is considering an indeterminate life sentence.[1] Psychiatric evidence on risk will be central to the expert's evidence. The Court may have two options, a Hospital Order in suitable cases or an indeterminate life sentence. The psychiatrists does not have 'a priori' advance knowledge of what the outcome might be in a particular case thus routinely placing the psychiatrist into a dual role in respect of the evaluation.

Calvedeno[16] has pointed out that even where a welfare disposal is recommended, medical evidence in respect of special restrictions to a Hospital Order may lead to lengthy periods in hospital justified not by the need for treatment but by psychiatric judgement on risk in the future. Similar arguments apply to reports to Mental Health Tribunals for patients detained under mental health legislation.

One solution to the dual role is to act only where there is a realistic prospect of benefit to the patient. This leads some psychiatrists to only undertake work for defence teams. In the author's view, this is unethical as it lends itself to bias and deprives one side in the adversarial process of high quality experts.

### A theory of mixed duties to address dual role conflict

Doctors are members of society and as citizens have responsibilities, prior to responsibilities as a doctor. The narrow domain of medical ethics does not remove from doctors their duty to consider the interests and rights of other people and to consider the distribution of benefits and risks. Beauchamp[17] proposes augmenting traditional medical ethics with principles he terms justice and respect for autonomy. On that basis O'Grady[1] suggests a framework of mixed duties for expert witnesses in court to address their 'dual role' conflict (see Box 11.15.2).

This approach implicitly requires the psychiatrist to work within a framework of conflicting duties where ethical judgements must balance the welfare of the evaluee against the rights of others and society's legitimate interest in protection from risk.

The psychiatric ethical expert in court is then the one who 'feels the tension' inherent in a dual role and is painfully aware of the conflicting demands of different ethical imperatives.

### Risk assessment

Sentencing where public protection is a central issue poses particular difficulties for the psychiatrist as risk assessment becomes central to the court's decisions. Actuarial risk assessments can be particularly dangerous in the legal context. Mullen[18] argues 'The margins of error in every actual or conceivable risk assessment instrument are so wide at the individual level that their use in sentencing, or any form of detention, is unethical'. Whilst acknowledging the significant limitations of risk prediction at the individual level, the Court may nevertheless legitimately argue that evaluation of risk associated with mental disorder is an area falling outside the 'common knowledge' of Judge and Jury. Therefore the court must rely upon psychiatrist's opinion on risk and mental disorder as the psychiatrist is the only witness with the necessary expertise. Using a structured risk assessment methodology may go someway to ensure accuracy, objectivity, and truthfulness. A clear role for the psychiatric expert is to ensure the Court is provided with informed scientific evidence on the limitations of risk assessment and particularly the limitations of utilizing structured or actuarial risk instrument at the individual level[18,19]).

## Structure of reports

### Receiving instructions

The psychiatrist should understand the legal question to be addressed; where necessary standard text should be consulted (see

---

**Box 11.15.2** Ethical principles to address Dual Role responsibilities

1  Medical ethics:
   - Non-maleficence
   - Beneficence

2  Justice ethics:
   - Truthfulness (objective and subjective)
   - Respect for autonomy
   - Respect for the human rights of others (balancing the distribution of benefits and risks for the patient and society)

recommended reading). The psychiatrist must ensure that they have the necessary expertise to address the issues for the Court. Trainees must ensure that they are supervised by a suitably qualified senior and disclose this to the instructing party (including disclosure of the supervisor's appointment and qualifications).

The psychiatric expert must ensure that they can meet the needs of the Court as regards timescale for the report and understand that they can be compelled by the Court to give oral evidence; for example when they are on leave. The Court will not do so if the doctor has in advance disclosed dates when they are unavailable. Where there are fees to be paid, the letter of acceptance should state the contractual conditions for accepting instructions.

Rules of evidence in all legislations impose on the expert witness an overriding duty to the court outside of the duty owed to the party instructing them. The psychiatric expert witness has to develop a working relationship with the legal team instructing them but simultaneously discharge their overall duty to the court. One way of conceptualizing the relationship to the instructing party is as a 'consultant' to the legal team, educating them in the meaning of psychiatric findings.[20] Nevertheless it is naive to believe that expert will not be subject to overt or subtle influence by the instructing side.

Psychiatric reports should comply with relevant court rules for example Part 33 of the Criminal procedure rules for England.[8] Notes and documents must be retained for a sufficient period (undefined but at least to until last date for appeal) and disclosed to other experts in the case.[20] The expert should have appropriate indemnity insurance.

### The interview

If the defendant is to be visited in prison, arrangements should be made well in advance and comply with the requirements of the institution.

At the beginning of the interview, the examining psychiatrist should explain carefully to the defendant the nature of the doctor's dual role, the limits of confidentiality in producing a medico-legal report and that the Court will have full disclosure of all material known to the report writer (no off record material). It is prudent to obtain a signed record of this discussion and to include it as part of the introduction to the report. Whenever possible, an informant should be interviewed; by telephone if necessary.

### Structure of the report

#### (a) Declarations and introduction

The first section of the report should lay out the instructions received and what was done in order to produce the report. The dates and duration of interviews should be stated, including interviews with informants. For British Criminal Courts, Part 33 of the Criminal Procedure Rules[8] requires certain declarations and statements at the beginning of the report (see Box 11.7.1 above). A section on limitations to the report should be included to record matters such as documents not disclosed or unavailability of informants and state the impact on the expert's opinion.

#### (b) The facts

The middle section of the report should record briefly the facts upon which the opinion is based and should avoid interpretation which is the proper function of the opinion section. In psychiatric reports, the only facts that are within the psychiatrists own knowledge are likely to be those based on the findings of mental state examination. All other facts are assumed. If structured tests are utilized, they may also constitute facts within the psychiatrists own knowledge.

### (c) Opinion

The role of the psychiatric expert is to provide an opinion on mental disorder and its implications for the matters before the Court. The opinion section should then start with a description of the defendant's mental disorder. If there is no evidence of mental disorder, then the privileged exception accorded to psychiatric experts no longer applies (see earlier section). The features that lead to a diagnosis of mental disorder should be described, avoiding jargon, and including mental state findings, so that others can understand how the opinion is reached. The diagnosis should be clearly stated using a recognized classification which for British psychiatrists will be the International Classification of Mental and Behavioural Disorders. Where a condition is described which is not part of such recognized classification systems or where 'leading edge' scientific findings are used to support the opinion that should be justified by disclosure (as an appendix to the report) of relevant literature to support the expert's opinion.

The second stage of the opinion is to translate the psychiatric findings into the legal language employed by the Courts. Terms such as 'diminished responsibility', 'insanity', or 'automatism' have precise legal definitions and the report should address how the psychiatric findings translate to the legal definitions employed by the Court.

Usually there will be a range of opinion and the psychiatrist should indicate the range, giving due weight to alternative opinion before recording the reasons for their own opinion. More than one legal issue may have to be considered together with the range of opinion on each separate legal issue. One helpful mental model is to consider the range of opinion that might be given by other experts if the case were presented to a psychiatric case conference.[20]

At point of sentencing where the court has concerns about public safety, the psychiatrist will be expected to provide an opinion on risk linked to the defendant's mental disorder. The ethical issues arising from that expectation should be thoroughly understood (see section above). It is usual to express a range of opinion (the case conference model) and given reasons for the expert's own opinion.

Where recommendations for a disposal under specific Acts are included, the precise wording of the relevant section of those Acts should be employed.

#### (i) Opinion on the ultimate issue

There is a common law injunction against a witness expressing an opinion upon the ultimate issue to be determined by the court. Many questions put to psychiatric experts test this rule to its limits. In this author's opinion, psychiatric experts should provide the court with objective evidence upon the mental state in and around the time of an alleged offence but stop short of expressing an opinion on the ultimate issue unless specifically instructed to do so by the presiding Judge.

## Confidentiality

Medico-legal work undertaken by psychiatrists is governed by the same rule of confidentiality as applied to other clinical work.

Reports cannot be disclosed to a third party without the consent of the body commissioning the report. Psychiatric reports do not form part of a person's NHS medical record except by the express consent of the individual or their legal representative. Defence solicitors can exercise a right not to disclose a report to Court. Failure to comply with rules of confidentiality can lead to civil action or report to a professional regulatory body.

There may be circumstances where a psychiatrist believes that it is necessary to divulge confidential information to a Court without the evaluee's consent. This could arise:

(a) Where the evaluee refuses to cooperate with the preparation of a report.

or

(b) Where a report is not disclosed but the psychiatrist believes that disclosure is in the public interest.

A psychiatrist who believes that the evaluee is not cooperating with the preparation of a report because of mental illness has a duty to consider whether the evaluee's mental illness could interfere with a fair trial (for example, fitness to plead or lack of consideration of a mental health disposal). The psychiatrist must then make a judgement whether it is in the best interests of the evaluee for sufficient information to be provided to the Court to alert them of the doctor's concerns. Such disclosure will almost certainly be justified in the interests of a fair trial and justice. The doctor will also have a duty to consider whether steps ought to be taken to undertake a Mental Health Act assessment (British law) to enable transfer to a hospital for medical treatment.

The other situation where a breach of confidentiality may be justified is where a report is not disclosed but the report writer believes that the Court ought to consider the report's findings on potential risk to the public. In B.W. v Edgell and Rv Crozier, the Court held that the doctor's duty of confidence did not prevent a psychiatrist from taking steps to communicate the grounds of concern to the court. The strong public interest in disclosure to prevent a court from making decisions based upon inadequate information was held to override the psychiatrist's duty of confidentiality. Where a doctor is considering disclosure in these circumstances, advice should be sought from an experienced colleague, case law, and regulatory body guidance consulted and the doctor should seek advice from their indemnity insurer.

## Appearing in court

Advice on practical matters concerning a Court appearance is beyond the scope of this chapter but guidance is available (see recommended reading). Those undertaking regular expert work should consider courses which prepare them for appearance in Court and should understand the legal framework for giving oral evidence in court.[21]

The cardinal rule when giving oral evidence in Court is that although called by one party, the expert witness is not giving evidence for that party's side but is under a duty to provide fair and impartial evidence to the Court even where this conflicts with the interests of the party calling them.

In Criminal Courts, the defendant gives evidence before expert evidence is heard. Experts are allowed, unlike witnesses of fact, to sit in Court and hear the evidence of other witnesses before they, themselves, give evidence. An expert can be called by any interested party in proceedings.

When calling an expert witness, the advocate must elicit the following[21]:

1 The expert's qualifications: If the report has been prepared according to criminal procedure rules, the report will contain a biography setting out the qualifications and experience of the witness. It will then be usual for the advocate to lead this part of the evidence by reference to the biography supplied in the report. It will be perfectly permissible for the other side to call into question the expert's qualifications. This should be met politely by outlining the reasons why the expert believes they have the requisite qualifications and experience to answer the questions posed in instructions.

2 Disclosure of the expert's report: The report will have been pre-read by the Judge and it is usual for the examiner to refer to relevant sections of the report. A report with numbered paragraphs is easier for the Court to follow. The jury will not have read the report and will not usually be given sight of the report. Their knowledge of the expert's report will come from submissions made by either side and through the Judge's questioning and summing up.

3 Advocates are under a duty to challenge disputed evidence. Thus where more than one expert opinion is provided and they differ; the expert must expect their opinion to be disputed. The expert must resist pressure from one party to deviate from or express greater certainty about an opinion they have reached in the written report.

4 An expert witness may be cross-examined as a hostile witness if there is good reason to suppose that they are not telling the truth. Thankfully this is extremely rare. The possibility of deliberate or inadvertent bias must, however, always be considered.

## Further information

Expert Witness Institute. (2006). *Experts in the civil courts.* Oxford University Press, Oxford.

Hodgkinson, T. and James, M. (2007). *Expert evidence: law and practice* (2nd edn). Sweet and Maxwell, London (detailed legal textbook on law relating to expert witnesses).

Holburn, C.J., Bond, C., Solon, M., *et al.* (2000). *Healthcare professionals as witnesses to the court*, Greenwich Medical Media, London (practical advice on reports and appearing in court).

Omerod, D., and Hooper, A. (2008) *Blackstone's Criminal Practice 2009.* Oxford University Press, Oxford (standard textbook on criminal law, frequently revised).

Weinstock, R. (2003). Part 1. History and practice of forensic psychiatry. 1-94. In *Principles and practice of forensic psychiatry* (2nd edn) (ed. R. Rosner), pp. 56–72. Arnold, London.(for a USA perspective)

See also references 9 and 20 below

## References

1. O'Grady, J.C. (2002). Psychiatric evidence and sentencing: ethical dilemmas. *Criminal Behaviour and Mental Health*, **12**, 179–84.

2. O'Grady, J.C. (2002). Report writing for the criminal court. *Psychiatry*, **6**, 11.

3. Murphy, P. and Phillips, J. (2007). F10 expert opinion evidence. In *Blackstone's criminal practice 2007*, Section F10, pp. 2449–63. Oxford University Press, Oxford.

4. Ormerod, D. and Roberts, A. (2006). The admissibility of expert evidence. In *Witness testimony* (eds. A. Heaton - Armstrong,

E. Shepherd, G. Gudjonsson, and D. Wolchover), Chap. 22, pp. 401–24, Oxford University Press, Oxford.

5. Hodgkinson, T. and James, M. (2007). Introduction: the principles and development of expert evidence. In *Expert evidence: law and practice* (eds. T. Hodgkinson and M. James), Chap. 1, pp. 1–43, Sweet and Maxwell, London.

6. Sales, B.D. and Shaman, D.W. (2007). Science, experts and law: reflections on the past and the future. In *Expert psychological testimony for the courts* (eds. M. Costanzo, D. Krauss, and K. Pezdek), Chap. 2, pp. 9–30, Lawrence Erlbaum Associates, Mahwah, New Jersey.

7. Hodgkinson, T. and James, M. (2007). Expert evidence: the future. In *Expert evidence: law and practice* (eds. T. Hodgkinson and M. James), Chap. 28, pp. 645–9, Sweet and Maxwell, London.

8. Ministry of Justice. (2005). Part 33: expert evidence. In *Criminal procedure rules*. Ministry of Justice, London. Available at: http://www.dca.gov.uk/procedurerules.htm

9. Rix, K.J.B. (2008). The psychiatrist as expert witness: Part 1. General principles and civil cases. *Advances in psychiatric treatment.*

10. Burn, S. and Thompson, B. (2006). Single joint expert. In *Experts in the civil courts* (ed. L. Blom-Cooper), Chap. 5, pp. 57–76. Oxford University Press, Oxford.

11. Stone, A.A. (1984). The ethical boundaries of forensic psychiatry - a view from the Ivory tower. *Bulletin of the American Academy of Psychiatry and the Law*, **12**, 209–19.

12. Appelbaum, P.S. (1997). A theory of ethics for forensic psychiatry. *Journal of the American Academy of Psychiatry and the Law*, **25**, 233–47.

13. Royal College of Psychiatrists. (2004). *The psychiatrist, courts and sentencing: the impact of extended sentencing on the ethical framework of forensic psychiatry College Report 129*. Royal College of Psychiatrists, London. Available at:http://www.rcpsych.ac.uk/publications/collegereports.aspx

14. Weinstock, R., Leong, G.B., and Silva, A. (2003). Ethical guidelines. In *Principles and practice of forensic psychiatry* (2nd edn) (ed. R. Rosner), pp. 56–72. Arnold, London.

15. Feeley, M. and Simon, J. (1992). The new penology: notes on an emerging strategy of corrections and its implications. *Criminology*, **30**, 449–74.

16. Calvedeno, M. (1999). The psychiatrist as Gaoler. *Journal of Forensic Psychiatry*, **10**, 525–37.

17. Beauchamp, T.L. (1999). The philosophical basis of psychiatric ethics. In *Psychiatric ethics* (3rd edn) (eds. L.S. Bhoc, P. Chadoff, and S.A. Green), pp. 25–47, Oxford University Press, Oxford.

18. Mullen, P.E. (2007). Dangerous and severe personality disorder and in need of treatment. *The British Journal of Psychiatry*, **190**, s3–7.

19. Hart, S.D., Michie, C., and Looke, D.J. (2007). Precision of actuarial risk assessment instruments: evaluating the 'Managing of Error' of group v individual predictions of violence. *The British Journal of Psychiatry*, **190**, s51–9.

20. Rix, K.J.B. (2008). The psychiatrist as expert witness: part 2. Criminal cases and Royal College of Psychiatrist's guidance. *Advances in Psychiatric Treatment*, **14**, 109–14.

21. Hodgkinson, T. and James, M. (2007). The expert witness at trial. In *Expert evidence: law and practice* (eds. T. Hodgkinson and M. James), Chap. 6, pp. 163–82. Sweet and Maxwell, London.

## Case law

R v Turner [1975] Q.B. 834 and 841

GMC v Meadows [2006] EWCA Civ 1390

Daubert v Merrell Dow Pharmaceuticals Inc [1993] 509 US 575

Ikarian Reefer [1993] 2 Lloyds Rep 68 at 81

R v Edgell [1990] Cr App ch 359

R v Crozier [1990–1991] 12 Cr App(s)206

# Managing offenders with psychiatric disorders in general psychiatric services

James R. P. Ogloff

It has been shown that the prevalence of mental illness among those in the criminal justice system is significantly greater than that found in the general community.[1,2] As presented in Chapter 11.4, for example, the per capita rate of psychotic illness in prisons is approximately 10 times greater than that found in the general community. Tragically, relatively few services exist that provide continuity of mental health care between gaols and the community.[3] This produces a situation where individuals whose mental illness may have been identified and treated in gaol find themselves without services in the community. Typically, only when in crisis do they find their way into general psychiatric services either in community settings or in hospital. This situation has produced considerable stress on already taxed mental health services.[4]

Given the prevalence of offence histories among psychiatric patients, it is important for mental health professionals to be aware of the unique issues—and myths—that accompany patients with offence histories. At the outset it is important to emphasize that the duty of mental health services is to address mental health issues. That ought to be the focus of mental health services. As this chapter makes clear, though, for some patients, there is a relationship between the mental illness and offending and by addressing the mental illness, the risk of re-offending might well be reduced. Moreover, many of the ancillary issues that lead to relapse and destability in psychiatric patients also may lead to offending. Addressing these issues will both help provide long-term stability for patients and will help reduce their risk of offending. As a result, there is a need for general mental health services to acquire expertize to identify and manage patients with offending histories.[5]

This chapter will provide information about the relative risk of offending among psychiatric patients and the relationship (or lack thereof) of inpatient aggression and community-based violence and offending. A framework will be provided for assessing and treating patients with offending histories and issues using a typology of mentally ill offenders. The role of forensic mental health services in bolstering general psychiatric services, and in sometimes providing primary care for mentally ill offenders, will also be discussed.

## How many patients have criminal histories?

Surprisingly little research exists that investigates the number of patients entering general psychiatric services who have an offence history. For reasons having to do with privacy, lack of perceived relevance, and professional reluctance, general mental health services do not consistently obtain reliable information regarding patients' offence histories. This is often the case even when the patient has a current community-based corrections order. The two following studies can help shed light on the question of how many general psychiatric patients have histories of criminal offending.

In a study that was conducted to investigate the post-discharge violence of psychiatric patients and the predictive validity of risk assessment measures among almost 193 involuntarily committed psychiatric patients in British Columbia, Canada who were discharged to the community, Douglas, Ogloff, Nicholls, and Grant[6] obtained official criminal histories for all patients who had ever been arrested or convicted of any criminal offence. The vast majority of patients had prior psychiatric hospitalizations (n=184, 95 per cent). Informally, members of the hospital staff were asked what percent of patients they believed had a prior criminal history. Staff, including psychiatrists, estimated that a very small percent of patients would have been arrested or convicted of offences—less than 20 per cent. The review of criminal histories, however, showed that 64 per cent (n=123) of patients had previous arrests or convictions for any type of criminal offence, including 40 per cent (n=78) who had been arrested or convicted of violent offences.

In an Australian study based upon Victorian samples of cohorts of patients with schizophrenia, Wallace and colleagues have found that almost 22 per cent of patients with schizophrenia have a history of offending at some point in their lives.[7] Moreover, eight percent of patients with schizophrenia had a criminal conviction for a violent offence. These percentages increased three-and-four fold when the patients with schizophrenia also had a known substance abuse problem. In a recent study, Hodgins and Muller-Isberner[5] found that one quarter of patients discharged from a general mental health service had a criminal record.

While it is difficult to know exactly how many psychiatric patients across different services have committed offences, the point that may be drawn from the above research suggests that many patients have offence histories—likely more than mental health professionals would expect. The starting point of the chapter, therefore, is that while most psychiatric patients will not have violent criminal histories, many will have offence histories, including the commission of violent offences. Moreover, many more patients will have exhibited violent behaviour that did not lead to arrest or conviction. Therefore, even if they do not realize it, all psychiatrists and other mental health professionals have experience working with patients who have offence histories.

## What leads mentally ill people to offend?

Although the reasons that anyone—including psychiatric patients—offends are myriad and complex, a typology of mentally ill offenders is helpful for understanding the reasons they offend.[1] There are three general categories of people with mental illness who offend; understanding the general mentally disordered offender type will enable clinicians in general psychiatric services to provide appropriate treatment. The first, and smallest group, includes those psychiatric patients for whom a necessary and sufficient cause of their offending is the presence of their mental illness and the symptoms the illnesses produce. The second group includes patients who do not offend because of their mental illnesses, *per se*, but due to the concomitant social difficulties that all too often accompany mental illness. The final general group of offenders with mental illness include those patients whose offending occurs irrespective of their mental illness. Each of these groups will be described below.

### Patients who offend because of their mental illness

This group is likely the smallest of the three groups. This group includes people who may not be criminally responsible because, as a result of their mental illnesses, they do not know what they are doing, or do not appreciate that what they are doing is wrong. Their offences occur as a direct result of the mental illness. But for the mental illness and the presence of symptoms which led to the patient's offending behaviour, the crime would not have occurred. Their mental illness is both a necessary and sufficient explanation for their offence. They only offend when they are acutely unwell and the offence behaviour is a product of their mental illness (e.g. acting on delusions or hallucinations). Depending upon the jurisdiction in which they reside, they may be found not guilty by reason of insanity or mental illness. They most likely will be housed in secure hospitals rather than prisons following legal adjudication. Typically the illnesses that are present in people who fall into this category are psychosis or serious affective disorders accompanied by psychosis. Many jurisdictions that retain some form of insanity defence specifically exclude the use of the defence by those with antisocial or dissocial personality disorder.

---

1   Readers are referred to Chapter 11.3.1 (Associations between Psychiatric Disorder and Offending by Thomson and Darjee) for additional information regarding the relationship between mental illness and offending.

### Patients who offend as a result of the sequelae of mental illness

The second general group of psychiatric patients who offend comprises hose whose mental illnesses are a necessary but not sufficient explanation for their offending. It is by far the largest group of psychiatric patients who offend. As is typical for many patients with serious mental illnesses, these patients begin to spiral downward socially as a result of their mental illnesses. They can become estranged from family and pro-social support networks. Their lives become unstable; housing, basic needs, and their need for non-judgmental personal support may go unmet. They may end up being accepted by groups of people who are themselves unstable. They often resort to engaging in illicit drug abuse. These social factors contribute to their resultant offending. While their mental illness may be a catalyst in the course of events that lead to the offending, the mental illness itself is not the direct cause of the offending. Had they not had a mental illness, they likely would not have begun offending. However, by the time they develop offending behaviour, their lives have become so disorganized and their maladaptive coping and survival strategies have become so entrenched as to make the reversal of these processes difficult over the long-term. Psychiatric treatment, while a necessary starting point, will not be sufficient alone to eliminate the offending behaviour.

### Patients who offend despite their mental illness

The final group of patients are those who would offend irrespective of the fact that they have a mental illness. Although not as large a group as the one above, many more patients who offend fall into this category than into the first. The fact that they have a mental illness is neither a necessary or sufficient explanation for their offending. Patients in this group are typically characterized by early onset antisocial and illegal behaviour. They differ from other mentally ill offenders by having a pervasive and stable pattern of offending regardless of their mental state.[5] This behaviour almost always precedes the onset of mental illness. While people with a psychopathic or dissocial personality disorder will be included in this group, most of the people in the group will not be so disordered. It is important to acknowledge, though, that the broad range of people that may fall into this group, including the psychopaths, may well develop psychiatric illnesses. We must avoid the tendency to deny this group proper services or to acknowledge their mental illnesses. These patients' mental illnesses may well exacerbate their offending or lead to unusual offending; however, even when they are asymptomatic they may continue to offend.

## Aren't psychiatric patients with offence histories unusually burdensome or too dangerous for mental health services?

The perception all too often still exists that patients with offence histories are unusually burdensome or even too dangerous to be seen by general mental health services. While there are doubtless patients, largely those drawn from the third group above, who are burdensome and even dangerous, in the main patients with offence histories are nether unduly burdensome nor dangerous. For example, in a recent prospective study of violence among discharged general and forensic psychiatric patients, Doyle and Dolan[8] found no significant differences in post-discharge violence rates (both official and unofficial) between patient groups in the UK. Ogloff and colleagues have obtained similar results from separate studies of post-discharge violence among samples of general and forensic psychiatric patients.[6]

One of the concerns expressed in general psychiatric services about patients with offence histories is the risk for aggression and violence they might present during hospitalization. It is often assumed that if a patient has an offence history, particularly one marked by aggression, that the patient will be more likely to be aggressive in hospital. Research suggests, however, that this may not be the case. It is true that over the entire period of hospitalization patients who have more psychopathic traits might have higher rates of aggressive incidents.[9] Research shows that in fact there is no significant relationship, at least for forensic psychiatric patients, between aggression in hospital, aggressive behaviour preceding admission, or violent recidivism.[10]

Analyses of what leads to aggressive behaviour by psychiatric patients suggests that dynamic (highly changeable) factors are responsible and that a functional analysis of inpatient aggression shows that rarely are the acts related to general patient aggression or purely to the patients' mental state.[11] Rather than assuming that patients with forensic histories will be any more or less aggressive than other patients, recent instruments have found useful in assessing patients risk for inpatient aggression.[12] Such instruments should be employed.

## Assessment of psychiatric patients who offend

Prior to commencing ongoing mental health care to patients with offence histories, it is important that a comprehensive assessment be conducted, preferably by a psychiatrist or clinical psychologist with expertize and experience in forensic mental health. In some jurisdictions, mental health services may be able to draw upon forensic mental health services to obtain secondary assessments of the patients to assist with assessment and treatment planning.[13] The assessment must address three major components: mental health, substance use, and the presence of criminogenic factors (i.e. factors that increase the likelihood that the patient will re-offend).

First, a thorough mental health assessment is required that includes both a review of the patient's current mental state as well as their psychiatric history. Although seemingly straight-forward, this can be difficult with some patients who have offence histories. All too often now we see young people, usually males, whose mental illnesses are only identified upon admission to gaol or prison.[3] As such, it may be difficult to obtain reliable information about the genesis and onset of these people's mental illnesses.

The second component that must be considered is whether the patients have a substance use or dependence disorder and what role substances have on their mental illness and offending. In mental health generally,[14] and in patients with offence histories in particular,[15] high percentages of patients are substance abusers. Ogloff and colleagues found that 74 per cent of patients in the secure forensic hospital in Victoria, Australia had a lifetime history of substance abuse or dependence. The presence of a substance use disorder is a key risk factor in determining which patients will re-offend (or have a relapse of their illness for that matter).

Unfortunately, very often substance use disorders, and their effects on patients, are overlooked in the routine assessment and treatment of patients with mental illnesses.

The final area that must be considered in a comprehensive assessment is the presence of so-called 'criminogenic factors' present in the patient's case. This concept is part of a contemporary well accepted and supported theory of offending known as the Psychology of Criminal Conduct, which was developed by Andrews and Bonta in the 1980s and it has been refined over time.[16] It is a theory concerned with individual differences and variability in criminal behaviour, making it a particularly useful guide for both assessing the risk of reoffending and planning rehabilitation attempts. This emphasizes the complexity of criminal behaviour, thereby acknowledging the contributions of social context, biology, and psychopathology. Criminogenic factors are the subset of dynamic (changeable) risk factors that have been found to relate directly to a risk for re-offending. They are therefore modifiable characteristics, whereby a change in the risk factor equates with a change in the risk of re-offending. These are factors that can affect patients with mental illness just as they can affect people with no mental illness who offend. Examples include having friends who are criminals, developing pro-criminal attitudes, having an anti-social personality, having limited problem-solving skills, and having difficulties controlling anger and hostility (Ogloff & Davis, 2004).[17]

To assist in assessing Andrews and Bonta[18] have developed the *Level of Service Inventory, Revised* (LSI-R), which assesses the presence of criminogenic factors as the basis for offender assessment and treatment.[1] The LSI-R consists of 54-items "grouped into the following domains or sub-components (with the number of items in parentheses): Criminal History (10); Education/Employment (10); Financial (2); Family/Marital (4); Accommodation (3); Companions (5); Alcohol/Drug Problems (9); Emotional/Personal (5); and Attitudes/Orientation(4).[18] While developed for general criminal populations, the LSI-R has been found very useful for assessing the presence of criminogenic factors and general needs of psychiatric patients with offending histories. Recent research findings show that a screening version of the LSI-R reliably identifies risk factors for patients in forensic psychiatric services.[19]

The presence of antisocial personality or dissocial personality is a criminogenic factor that must be considered in the assessment of mentally ill offenders. Unfortunately, antisocial personality disorder as it is defined by the Diagnostic and Statistical Manual of Mental Disorders, Fourth Edition, Text Revision[20] is vastly over-represented in psychiatric populations due to the nature of the criteria for the disorder which are essentially the presence of criminality.[21] Thus, great care must be taken to ensure that the diagnosis of antisocial personality does not rely solely on the fact that the patient has a history of offence behaviour. Instruments designed to reliably measure the presence of psychopathy, such as the *Psychopathy Checklist*, can be useful for assessing the aspects of personality and behaviour that comprise psychopathy.[21,22]

Following the assessment of each of the above components, it is necessary to develop a formulation that considers where the

---

[1] There is a revised version of the LSI-R which includes a section for case management planning, the Level of Supervision/Case Management Inventory and a version for young offenders (Youth Level of Service/Case Management Inventory; Hoge, Andrews, & Leshied, 2002).

patient's mental illness factors into their offending. Drawing on the three typologies of offenders with mental illnesses outlined above, the clinician can determine which category best describes the patient. Because the typologies are general, there will be overlap in characteristics for some patients. In addition to understanding the factors that help explain a patient's offending, the typologies are very important for determining what treatment and management strategies can be most effective for the patient.

## The treatment of mentally ill offenders by general mental health services

The typology of mentally ill offenders will be revisited below with respect to the mental health and related services they require to assist with their treatment and management. The three-prong assessment strategy briefly described above will be helpful to identify the range of treatment needs the patient has. To be clear, the primary and even sole purpose of general mental health services is to treat patients' mental illnesses. However, it is useful to consider the presence of an offence history as an indication of the patient's functional impairment. Depending on the group into which the patient falls, the relative efficacy of mental health services alone varies in the extent to which it will satisfactorily address their mental health and offence issues. Most often, particularly for the latter two groups below, ancillary services and forensic mental health services will be required to help ensure the patient's long-term stability and to reduce the likelihood of offending.

### Patients who offend because of their mental illness

Although this group of patients may commit horrendous acts, it is as likely that they engage in nuisance offences. Despite the particular type of offending behaviour in which they engage, perhaps surprisingly, their management by mental health services is oftentimes less complex than is the case for the other two groups of offenders with mental illnesses to be discussed below. Generally speaking, the treatment that this group requires is conventional mental health care. As it is the case that the primary cause of their offending behaviour is the mental illness, and the symptoms that it produces, addressing their mental health needs can serve to eliminate the offending. General mental health services are generally well equipped to deal with these patients, though they may feel reluctant to do so. Very often, patients will respond to medication and with supervision their mental state will begin to improve. If treatment in the cases is complex, it will often be because of the mental illness itself. For example, the patients may have chronic psychosis which is refractory to psychiatric treatment.

While the patient's mental illness is the main cause of the offending behaviour in this category, related issues will need to be addressed to stabilize the patient over the long term and to further reduce the patient's risk of re-offending. The LSI-R, noted above, will be particularly helpful in identifying such issues. Common issues include substance abuse, life skills, housing, financial support, and personal support. Services to address these issues will need to be organized to effect long-term psychiatric and behavioural stability.

### Patients who offend as a result of the sequelae of mental illness

Just as the complexity of the reason this group offends is greater than with the first group, the treatment they require to stabilize

is also more complex. This group is characterized by general disorganization and social damage. As such conventional mental health services alone will have relatively limited effect on patients' mental state and stability over the long-term. Even if psychiatric treatment is effective in the short-term, patients in this group will be likely to return to a chaotic life which eventually may include a return to offending. Nonetheless, the treatment of these patients' psychiatric illnesses is the central component of their care.

The comprehensive assessment approach outlined above will be particularly useful in determining the range of issues beyond mental illness that affects the patients and contributes to their offending behaviour. In particular, the areas of concern identified by the LSI-R are particularly important for informing intervention need. For example, if employment issues, financial issues, accommodation needs and alcohol/drug problems are revealed in the assessment, these issues, in addition to the patient's mental illness will need to be addressed. Not only will addressing these issues satisfactorily lead to a reduction in the patient's risk of re-offending, but it will assist with ensuring stability in mental state over the long-term.

Generally speaking, the greater the number of criminogenic factors that arise from the assessment, the more intensive treatment will need to be to ensure long-term stability. To the extent that needs arise that cannot be addressed directly by the mental health service, these services will need to be sought from appropriate providers in the community. This is where effective case management and service brokerage is critical. All too often psychiatric patients revolve in and out of general mental health services (and the criminal justice system); all the while their underlying needs are not identified or addressed. The vast majority of offenders with mental illnesses can be properly treated and managed by general mental health services if only their related needs and issues can be addressed. Moreover, given that there is a relationship between these patients' mental illnesses and their offending, addressing the mental illness and related matters can help lead to a reduction in offending, although that will not be the purpose of providing them with general mental health services.

### Patients who offend despite their mental illness

As with all of the categories of offenders, this group will still require comprehensive mental health care; however, the mental health care will be essentially futile in reducing the patient's proclivity for offending. It is important to note that mental health services still have an obligation to treat these patients' mental illnesses, but addressing their offending issues will be beyond the scope of care or even the expertize of general mental health services. Moreover, addressing the ancillary issues that arise to affect their mental illnesses will be less likely to reduce their offending risk than would be the case for either of the other two groups above. Where possible, patients in this group should be seen by forensic mental health services and they will be candidates for offender rehabilitation programmes offered by contemporary correctional services (in prisons or in the community).

It is important to note that the cautious approach advised is not intended to dissuade services from providing adequate psychiatric care, but to recognize their limitations and to reduce the sense of failure and frustration that occurs when treating patients with such an offence pattern. Despite the nihilism that sometimes exists, there is an ever expanding corpus of firm empirical support to show that offender rehabilitation can help reduce recidivism,[17,23] however, such services are beyond the scope of general mental health services. Over time, of course, as these patients' offending issues may be successfully addressed, they will be appropriately cared for by mental health services just as other people are. Once an offender not always an offender!

## The role and support of forensic mental health services

The thorny question of when forensic mental health services, as opposed to general mental health services, ought to be responsible for a patient's psychiatric care is difficult and depends much on the jurisdiction, the relevant legislation, policies, and practices that are in place. It is never the case that all patients who offend require, or should have access to, forensic mental health services. For the most part, the goal should be to maintain patients in general mental health services to ensure continuity and normality of care. Realistically, though, given the relatively high rate of psychiatric patients who offend or who have offence histories, the level of knowledge and awareness of offence issues among general mental health professionals must increase.

It is still the case in many settings that the mere mention that a patient has a forensic history raises angst and concern about the capacity of general mental health services to care for the individual. This is most often nonsensical, particularly because a relatively high percentage of psychiatric patients in general services have an offence history—whether or not it is known by the service. Ideally, general mental health services should adequately address patients' mental health and ancillary issues to an extent that would actually prevent patients in the first two groups of mentally ill offenders from offending. Very often we in forensic mental health services see patients who had contact with general mental health care yet their problems were exacerbated, they deteriorated and went on to offend. Oftentimes inadequate assessment and identification of the patients' needs is at the core of the shortcoming of their care.

Realistically, despite the oftentimes excellent care provided to psychiatric patients, forensic mental health services will be required. In the first instance, patients found not criminally responsible or who require involuntary treatment during incarceration should be provided service in appropriate forensic mental health facilities. Psychiatric patients with complex presentations, including myriad criminogenic issues, likely will require at least secondary consultation from a forensic mental health service.[13] The best models that exist internationally have forensic mental health services take responsibility for the complex offence-related cases initially with the introduction and eventual transition to general mental health services over time once the patient's offending issues are addressed and stability is realized.[24,25] Continuing general care is the preferred modality of care except in the most difficult cases.

## Conclusions

General psychiatry has an important role in providing care to all patients, and under most circumstances this includes patients with offending histories and issues. Given the relatively high rates of offending among psychiatric patients, whether they realize it or not, general services have considerable experience with this patient group. All too often, though, general mental health clinicians do not have adequate training or expertize to systematically assess patients to determine what factors have lead to their offending. The typology of patients who offend presented in this chapter can prove useful for determining the factors that must be addressed to treat the patient. Moreover, an indication will be made as well when assistance may be required by specialist mental health services.

## Further information

Hodgins, S., and Muller-Isberner, R. (2004). Preventing crime by people with schizophrenic disorders: The role of psychiatric services. *British Journal of Psychiaty*, **185**, 245–50.

Ogloff, J. R. P., and Daffern, M. (2006). The Dynamic Appraisal of Situational Aggression: An instrument to assess risk for imminent aggression in psychiatric inpatients. *Behavioral Sciences and the Law*, **24**, 799–813.

Ogloff, J. R. P., and Davis, M. R. (2004). Advances in offender assessment and rehabilitation: Contributions of the risk-needs-responsivity approach. *Psychology, Crime and Law*, **10**, 229–42.

## References

1. Brugha, T., Singleton, N., Meltzer, H., et al. (2005). Psychosis in the community and in prisons: A report from the British National Survey of Psychiatric Comorbidity'. *American Journal of Psychiatry*, **162**, 774–80.

2. Fazel, S., and Danesh, J. (2002). Serious mental disorder in 23,000 prisoners: A systematic review of 62 surveys. *Lancet*, **359**, 545–50.

3. Ogloff, J.R.P. (2002). Identifying and accommodating the needs of mentally ill people in gaols and prisons. *Psychiatry, Psychology, and Law*, **9**, 1–33.

4. Torrey, E.F. (1992). Criminalizing the seriously mentally ill: the abuse of jails as mental hospitals. Washington DC: Report of the National Alliance for the Mentally Ill and Public Citizen's Health Research Group.

5. Hodgins, S. and Muller-Isberner, R. (2004).Preventing crime by people with schizophrenic disorders: The role of psychiatric services. *British Journal of Psychiatry*, **185**, 245–50.

6. Douglas, K.S., Ogloff, J.R.P., Nicholls, T., et al. (1999). Assessing risk for violence among psychiatric patients: The HCR-20 Violence Risk Assessment Scheme and the Psychopathy Checklist: Screening Version. *Journal of Consulting and Clinical Psychology*, **67**, 917–30.

7. Wallace, C., Mullen, P.E., Burgess, P., et al. (2004).Criminal offending in schizophrenia over a 25-year period marked by deinstitutionalization and increasing prevalence of comorbid substance use disorders. *American Journal of Psychiatry*, **161**, 716–27.

8. Doyle, M., and Dolan, M. (2006). Predicting community violence from patients discharged by mental health services. *British Journal of Psychiatry*, **189**, 520–6.

9. Nicholls, T.L., Ogloff, J.R.P., Douglas, K.S., et al. (2004). Assessing risk for violence among male and female civil psychiatric patients: the HCR-20, PCL:SV, and McNiel & Binder's screening measure. *Behavioral Sciences and the Law*, **22**, 127–58.

10. Daffern, M., Ogloff, J.R.P., Ferguson M., et al. (2007). Appropriate treatment targets or products of a demanding environment? The relationship between aggression in a forensic psychiatric hospital with aggressive behaviour preceding admission and violent recidivism. *Psychology, Crime and Law*, **13**, 431–41.

11. Daffern, M., Howells, K., Ogloff, J., et al. (2007). The interaction between individual characteristics and the function of aggression in forensic psychiatric inpatients. *Psychiatry, Psychology and Law*, **14**, 17–25.

12. Ogloff, J.R.P., and Daffern, M. (2006). The Dynamic Appraisal of Situational Aggression: An instrument to assess risk for imminent aggression in psychiatric inpatients. *Behavioral Sciences and the Law*, **24**, 799–813.

13. Warren, L.J., MacKenzie, R., Mullen, P.E., *et al.* (2005). The problem behaviour model: The development of a stalkers clinic and a threateners clinic. *Behavioral Sciences and the Law*, **23**, 387–97.

14. Mueser, K.T., Yarnold, P.R., Rosenberg, S.D., *et al.* (2000). Substance use disorder in hospitalized severely mentally ill psychiatric patients: prevalence, correlates, and subgroups. *Schizophrenia Bulletin*, **26**, 179–92.

15. Ogloff, J.R.P., Lemphers, A., Dwyer, C., *et al.* (2004).Dual Diagnosis in an Australian forensic psychiatric hospital: Prevalence and implications for services. *Behavioral Sciences and the Law*, **22**, 543–62.

16. Andrews, D.A., and Bonta, J. (2006). *The psychology of criminal conduct* (4th ed.). Anderson Publishing Co., Cincinnati, OH.

17. Ogloff, J.R.P., and Davis, M.R. (2004). Advances in offender assessment and rehabilitation: Contributions of the risk-needs-responsivity approach. *Psychology, Crime and Law*, **10**, 229–42.

18. Andrews, D.A., and Bonta, J. (1995). *The level of service inventory – revised*. Multi-Health Systems, Toronto.

19. Ferguson, A. M., and Ogloff, J.R.P. (in press). Predicting recidivism in an Australian mentally disordered offender population with and without comorbid substance abuse using the LSI-R:SV. *Criminal Justice and Behavior*.

20. American Psychiatric Association. (2000). *Diagnostic and Statistical Manual of Mental Disorders* (4th edn.), Text Revision. Author, Washington DC.

21. Ogloff, J.R.P. (2006).The Psychopathy/Antisocial Personality Disorder conundrum. Australian and New Zealand *Journal of Psychiatry*, **40**, 519–28.

22. Hare, R.D. (2003). *Manual for the Hare Psychopathy Checklist* (2nd ed.). Revised. Multi-Health Systems, Toronto, Ontario.

23. McGuire, J. (2002). Criminal sanctions versus psychologically-based interventions with offenders: A comparative empirical analysis. *Psychology, Crime, and Law*, **8**, 183–208.

24. Simpson, A.I.F., Jones, R.M., Evans, C., *et al.* (2006). Outcome of patients rehabilitated through a New Zealand forensic psychiatry service: A 7.5 year retrospective study. *Behavioral Sciences and the Law*, **24**, 833–43.

25. Skipworth, J., and Humberstone, V. (2002). Community forensic psychiatry: Restoring some sanity to forensic psychiatric rehabilitation. *Acta Psychiatrica Scandinavica*, **106**, 47–53.

# Management of offenders with mental disorder in specialist forensic mental health services

Pamela J. Taylor and Emma Dunn

## Philosophy and theoretical models

Specialist forensic mental health (fmh) services are for people with serious mental disorders and grave offending behaviour who tend to be rejected from mainstream services. Although often triggered by single high profile cases, these specialist services are among the best planned and commissioned services in psychiatry, founded in evidence of need, risk and efficacy of interventions. They are grounded in a multidisciplinary clinical perspective and often have integrated academic units. They interface both with other clinical services and with the criminal justice service. Good relationships with the local community are vital for establishment and growth.

Mentally disordered offenders have been sources of tension between services at least since the early 19th century. In Britain, the Lunacy Commission argued that it was 'highly objectionable' that offender patients should be detained in a general lunatic hospital, while an 1807 parliamentary select committee noted that 'to confine lunatics in a common Gaol is equally destructive of all possibility of the recovery of the insane and the comfort of other prisoners'.[1] High security hospitals followed about 50 years later.

Funding and commissioning of fmh services worldwide continue to follow oscillations between considered responses to changes in the structure and availability of general services, and responses to single notorious cases. For England and Wales, the Butler Report[2] considered the then increasing gaps in service provision as psychiatric services shifted from mainly institutional to mainly community care. It was the most thoughtful and powerful driver of modern forensic mental health services in England and Wales, presaging the arrival of medium security hospital units. The contrasting path, of case driven service development, is illustrated by the so-called 'Dangerous and Severe Personality Disorder' (DSPD) services,[3] driven by the inquiry into the care and treatment of Michael Stone[4] following his conviction for two homicides and an attempted murder, occurring soon after his discharge from a psychiatric hospital. In the USA, mandated community mental health law (Kendra's Law) and treatment programmes in New York followed a subway killing by a psychotic man,[5] while legislative change necessary for specialist service development in

Japan followed a school massacre.[6] Concern that single cases make poor law – and poor health reforms—is tempered by the mutual commitment of government agencies and of practitioners to keep offender patient services under review.

The Department of Health and Home Office report, for England,[7] is a good example of such review, proposing five principles for secure healthcare provision:

i) quality of care and proper attention to individual needs;

ii) community rather than institutional care where possible;

iii) security no greater than justified by the danger presented—to self or others;

iv) maximization of rehabilitation and chances of sustaining an independent life in the longer term;

v) proximity to the patient's own home or family if s/he has them.

It is arguable that only the fifth principle requires an evidence base. Intra-familial violence may contribute to mental health and/or behavioural difficulties, and most violence by people with mental illness occurs within their close social circle.[8] Nevertheless, people have attachments, and the fifth principle is retained for that reason—*and* as a convenient way of anchoring responsibilities for services. The first four principles embody the medical ethic of maximizing autonomy and anticipated the Human Rights Act 1998, which gives effect to the rights under the European Convention to *liberty and security of person* (article 5) and prohibits *degrading treatment* (article 3). The Act also emphasizes proportionally—if it is necessary to breach a right, that breach should not go further than necessary.

Organizational models often founder in a clash between the needs of service users and providers. The ideal is a fully integrated services in which service users move freely between forensic and general mental health services, according to need.[9] General services, however, tend to have to focus on crisis management, and the greater the tensions between specialist and general services the greater the likelihood of ever-longer periods of residency in a physically secure hospital[10] or default to parallel service delivery reasons for this include reduced availability of non-secure psychiatric beds, perverse incentives in funding in which those in highest security may be funded centrally with minimal local funding burden. Also government caution may dictate that once detained in medium or higher security, every individual must progress stepwise through lower levels of security before returning to the community. Evidence does not support the notion that this stepwise route reduces criminal recidivism,[10] but it has led to the growth of additional tiers of specialist security provision, including 'low security' hospital units and forensic community mental health teams.

## The international context

There is insufficient space to explore the international context in any detail. Laws on criminal responsibility, criminal justice and mental health vary between European countries[11] and elsewhere, but many underlying clinical principles are shared. Most countries acknowledge some association between mental disorder and offending behaviours, but there is variation in how this influences prosecution, fitness to plead and stand trial, the extent to which mentally disordered offenders may be regarded as wholly or partially without responsibility for a criminal act, and the extent to which they are treated in mainstream or specialist secure health services, or in prisons, albeit with some health service input.

Our international research group (SWANZDSAICS) drawn from culturally distinct jurisdictions across five continents (Sweden, Wales, the Australian state of Victoria, New Zealand, Denmark, the South African province of Western Cape, Japan, the Canadian province of Quebec, and Scotland) finds a shared therapeutic philosophy in managing offenders with psychosis, but struggles to be therapeutic with sex offenders or people with personality disorder.[12] Other countries however, most notably the USA, seek to separate the business of psychiatry in the courts from any therapeutic endeavour with mentally disordered offenders.[13]

## The nature of security

Secure psychiatric hospitals have two overarching aims: improving health and delivering safety for patients and others. In secure hospitals, patients' autonomy is limited in a number of important ways: they may not be allowed to leave the hospital at all, may be confined to a particular area within the hospital, and/or treatment may be enforced. Although these restrictions are undoubtedly at least partly in the interests of the patients themselves, they are commonly also in the interests of others.

### The elements of security

Security in a clinical setting is made up of four main elements: physical, procedural, and relational security, *and* treatment. Treatment, including (re)habilitation, becomes vital to safety and security whenever a clear pathway can be shown between a mental disorder and offending behaviour.

*Physical security* refers to the qualities of buildings: the nature of perimeter walls and internal structures and functions. High security requires at least one high and distinct perimeter wall or fence clear of the main hospital building. In medium-security, the walls of the building alone generally provide the main perimeter, with high fences only surrounding exercise areas which are not entirely within the main building. All specialist security hospitals provide for staff and visitor entry through an 'airlock', using independent locking systems, the external one generally controlled by dedicated security or administrative staff. Ideally, clinical staff contributing to building design, which should ensure good sightlines throughout, while allowing residents a sense of privacy. Each patient has his/her own room, and ideally holds a key to it (with a staff over-ride potential). This enhances his/her safety and sense of personal security, and also the safety of property. In high-security units, cameras may be used for continuous monitoring. The environment should be pleasant, enabling both patients and staff to feel comfortable; small frustrations often trigger violence.

*Procedural security* provides for a formal set of checks for factors thought to be associated with risk of harm by patients. This includes minimizing patient access to weapons, fire-setting materials, or potentially disinhibiting substances, and preventing absconding. In high security, any communication with the outside world may be monitored; at lower levels of security, such monitoring is determined case by case. Procedures should also guard against potential harm to each patient. Some measures used to prevent or control violence may have 'side effects'. Time-out and seclusion may be necessary, but can be provocative and open to abuse. Physical restraint may sometimes be essential, but if done incorrectly or brutally may damage the possibility of a therapeutic relationship, physically harm or even kill the patient. In the UK, procedures for such measures are subject to guidance both from professional bodies[14] and legislative Codes of Practice (e.g.[15]).

There is insufficient space to detail the extensive range of procedures for ensuring security, so a couple of examples—searching and screening of contacts—must suffice. Searches of the person and of the environment are conducted mainly to minimize access to drugs and weapons. The level of unit security dictates the nature, extent and frequency of searches. In English high security hospitals, no-one is trusted. Staff, professional visitors and social visitors are all searched on entry; many items—such as mobile/cell phones are forbidden anywhere in the hospital. Patients may be searched randomly, but also when moving between areas in the hospital or if there are particular grounds for suspecting they have secreted something that could become a weapon, or acquired drugs. At any security level, patient rooms and other areas may be searched—similarly, randomly or on specific grounds; in high security, patients' possessions are routinely restricted in quantity to facilitate searching. For all such occasions, however, procedures incorporate measures which reflect concern for the individual being searched. Patients must be informed of searches (immediately beforehand if randomly timed) and invited to observe.

Screening of contact with visitors is multifaceted. Visitors may be enticed into aiding absconsion, or be irresponsible in their 'gifts' for the patient; apparently innocuous items may be fashioned into weapons, and they may be under pressure to bring drugs, perhaps disguised in food. There may also be risk of harm to visitors. Telephone calls, mail and personal visits may all be observed, but only in accordance with written procedures. Policies pertaining to visits will refer to classes of visits—for example visits by specific individuals who may threaten or be under threat, or by children, Such visits must be supervised by specifically trained staff.

*Relational security* skills are founded in therapeutic approaches and, with specific treatments, form the core of hospital security, clearly demarcating hospitals from prisons. It lies in extensive knowledge of each patient, accurate empathy and highly developed capacities for communicating and working in a clinical team. At best, it not only provides immediate safety and the milieu for change, but it may also facilitate lightening of physical and procedural securities. Effectiveness, however, is reliant on sufficient numbers of adequately trained staff.

Relational security may, however, create anxiety in hospital managers and their political masters, partly because it is more difficult to understand as security than locks and walls, but also due to the perception that its corruption is possible and difficult to predict. Over time, staff may be vulnerable to potentially counter-therapeutic change.[16] Strategies to ensure maintenance of clinical integrity therefore include personal supervision and appraisal, peer review and audit of team- and hospital-wide practice. Access to psychodynamic psychotherapists is not only, or even primarily, for the patients, but also for the staff and the institution.[17]

*Treatment as security* targets the link between symptoms of mental disorder, most obvious for psychotic symptoms, and criminal or risky behaviour.[18] In contrast to prisons, secure hospitals generally select residents for their treatability. It seems simple then—specific treatment with antipsychotic medication for people with psychosis should bring safety—but matters are rarely so straightforward. Multiple diagnoses are common: at least 25 per cent of offender patients with psychosis have personality disorders established before onset of their psychotic illness, and many abuse alcohol and/or other drugs at levels to qualify for a diagnosis.[18] Over 25 years, an increasing proportion of English high security hospital patients were found to have substance misuse disorders,[18] especially affecting the psychosis-personality disorder group. Substance misuse not fully meeting diagnostic criteria is also common. In the short term, specific treatment for psychosis combined with preventing access to substances of abuse can restore safety. For longer term success and safety, specific treatments aimed at substance misuse are best integrated as part of the overall treatment package,[19] although this is still not common practice (e.g. UK,[20] and Sweden,[21]). This may partly explain the counterintuitive finding[22] that, in the UK at least, there is a preference for admitting people with 'pure' psychosis to medium security hospitals, even though substance misusing people with psychosis would be regarded as a higher risk group (e.g.[23]).

## Hospital security in practice

In England and Wales, *high security hospitals* are mandated in statute for those patients who pose an imminent risk of serious harm to 'the public'. Public safety is often construed merely as removing dangerous persons from the community and strictly confining them. During the early stages of treatment adequate protection for staff and other residents is also vital. As patients become apparently safe, it is important that they can be tested out before discharge to the community, but government restrictions often make this difficult, so that patients may arrive at lower security levels ill-prepared for the new challenges; this may be dangerous in itself.

*Medium security* can be defined only in relation to high and low security services above and below it. The range, quality and quantity of low secure and open provision varies from place to place, so that providers of some medium secure service may have to retain patients longer than other providers and/or provide more parallel services.

The most constant aspect of medium security services is the in-patient unit. 'The aim is for the building design to support the nursing staff, who are the main security barriers.'[24] Procedural

security tends to be less stringent than in high security, but relational and treatment security are generally comparable. Nurse: patient ratios should be at least 2:1, and staff from a full range of other clinical disciplines should be available.

*Low security* relies almost entirely on relational security, but units generally have a locked door, and some procedures relevant to security, such as monitoring of substance misuse.

## Service structure

### Planning principles

'*Pyramid planning*' applies to specialist fmh services: the most intensive, specialized and secure services, most of which constrain patients' liberty and are the most costly, should be the smallest and at the top of the pyramid. At the base of the pyramid, and greatest in number, should be services linked directly to the local community. Trends in service provision in England and Wales reflect this model, with high secure bed numbers falling, and an increasing number of medium secure services (in mid-2007, 800 and 3 500 respectively for 55 million general population). Low security service provision is also increasing.

*Private healthcare facilities.* It is generally regarded as unethical to profit from the indefinite institutional detention of people. In Japan, where private provision of mental healthcare was the norm, recognition of service gaps for mentally disordered offenders resulted in the provision of publicly funded, purpose designed facilities for such patients.[6] In the UK, independent provision supplements a shortfall in specialist NHS facilities, providing just under half of all forensic beds. There are several reasons for this, not least the greater flexibility in service planning enjoyed by independent than public sector providers. Nevertheless, all places for detained patients in the UK are publicly funded and independent service providers are subject to the same levels of scrutiny as NHS facilities.

'*Super-specialist*' *provision* is necessary to provide specific treatments and the appropriate milieu for people with some special needs, such as female offender-patients, who almost invariably have suffered prolonged and serious neglect and abuse through childhood. Approaches founded in attachment theory[25] or trauma based work[26] go some way towards meeting their needs. People with a learning disability also benefit from dedicated services,[27] as may children and adolescents.

While there are advantages to specialist developments, most groups needing them tend to be small, and hence there are few units and it is difficult for residents to retain close ties with home, e.g. women resident in the only English high secure provision may be more than 350 miles away from home.

*Planning service capacity* is difficult. It is often done from utilization figures, but these tend to underestimate requirements by failing to recognize unmet need. While most developed countries have shifted general psychiatric services away from inpatient provision to the community, they have also seen an upsurge in availability of legal and illicit mind-altering substances. This has the probable effect of raising violence levels not only among the mentally healthy, but also among those with mental disorders (e.g.[28]).

Prison populations are growing in many countries. In the USA and the UK indefinite sentences 'for public protection' have been implemented. In England and Wales, the Lord Chief Justice and the Chairmen of the Parole Board have projected an additional

12,000 prisoners under this sentence alone by 2012, all of whom will need some sort of 'treatment' before they can be released[29] (at the time of writing a legal challenge to the lawfulness of such sentences in the absence of sufficient treatment is underway). Surveys of mental disorder among UK prisoners(e.g.[30,31]) suggest that neither generic nor specialist mental health services have kept pace with need in prisons even before this new expansion.

Capacity planning must be dynamic, taking into account assumptions about other services, and socio-economic differences between communities. Statistical models may help, (e.g.[32]) but it is more difficult to allow for changes in sentencing policy.

## The service users: assessment, management, treatment and rehabilitation

### Principles of assessment

Assessment in forensic psychiatry is considered in Chapter 11.14. In some countries, such as the USA, assessments for the courts are the main tasks for forensic psychiatrists, with some specializing in just one type of assessment and few providing treatment services.

Pre-admission assessment is important for patients destined for a secure hospital. It informs the initial treatment plan, and ensures a safe case-mix and appropriate staffing. Patients admitted to a secure hospital must have a mental disorder which meets legislative criteria for detention. Security requirements are then based on assessment of both mental disorder and criminal/violent behaviour. External factors must also be considered, for example, assessment of victim vulnerability. If, at one extreme, the identity of patient A's potential victim and the circumstances in which s/he might be at risk are clear, and that putative victim can acknowledge and co-operate with safety strategies, then it may be possible to manage risk of harm with little recourse to physical security. If, however, patient B threatens named people who cannot understand, accept or help manage the threat, then physical security may initially be required for her, even though both patients are otherwise similar. A serious, more generalized threat may also mean that initial assessment must be in security.

### Admission criteria

Broad agreement on criteria for admission to a secure hospital bed[33] does not necessarily lead to consistency in practice.[22] In England and Wales, only 40–50 per cent of people referred for a specialist secure hospital bed, whether in high[34] or medium security[22] are actually offered one. There are common reasons: i) that some disorders are not widely considered to be treatable, and ii) the high level of security requested is thought not to be necessary. In spite of powers in England and Wales to detain people with personality disorder for assessment or treatment, many medium security beds are effectively closed to them. Few are now admitted to high security hospitals, except to the new purpose designed 'DSPD' units. It seems to be only in the Netherlands that there is a preference for treating people with personality disorder in secure hospitals.[35] There are few data on which to judge the quality of such assessments, but one study showed that 85 per cent of those refused a high security bed remained outside high security during the following 12 months, without incident.[36]

There have been efforts to attain standard ratings of security need. Cohen and Eastman[37] generated a set known as the

Admission Criteria to Secure Services Schedule (ACSeSS). Factors considered relevant to admission were (* indicates factors most used in determining admission):

◆ gravity of recent* and past violence;

◆ likely immediacy of violence;

◆ psychopathology/developing behaviour possibly predictive of violence;

◆ special pathology, for example PD or sexual offending;

◆ the likely longevity of risk of violence*;

◆ predictability of the gravity and immediacy of potential future violence.

Collins and Davies[38] developed the Secure Needs Assessment Profile (SNAP), designed for *clinicians* to operationalize clinical judgement, following the first three elements of the security matrix outlined above—need for perimeter, and procedural or relational security.

The practice of using structured aids for clinical assessment of risk of harm to others or to self is growing, with nursing staff finding them particularly attractive. The HCR-20 (20 item Historical and Clinical Risk Management instrument;[39] includes dynamic risk factors, which can both inform management and provide a baseline measure from which progress can be monitored.[40]

### Progressing along the pathway to treatment.

When someone has one or more serious mental disorders and poses a serious risk of harm to others, assessment may become a lengthy process. The elements of this must in turn be evaluated and adjusted according to interim outcome measures. Figure 11.17.1 summarizes a typical pathway. The initial assessment is directed at establishing safety—either through advice to others, or through admission to a specialist setting. In the latter, the assessment merges seamlessly into engagement into treatment, directed first at the primary disorder, before working with underlying factors—such as experience of childhood trauma.

*The concept of 'treatability'.* Under mental health legislation for England and Wales, patients legally classified as having *psychopathic disorder* or *mental impairment* alone cannot be detained for treatment in hospital unless 'such treatment is likely to alleviate or prevent a deterioration' of the condition. This intended safeguard against improper detention has sometimes been used to reject 'difficult' patients. New mental health legislation does not distinquish disorder types and puts the burden on availability of treatment.

Treatability should not be confused with curability. Assessment of treatability should be made in full awareness of the assessor's own attitudes and fears, with primary consideration given to the patient's psychopathology, needs, insight, and preferences and motivation for treatment. The timing of such an assessment may also be crucial. If the consequence of no treatment is more-or-less certain, for example, imprisonment, and this will most likely cause deterioration, then this in itself could justify admission for hospital treatment.

*Principles of treatment.* First line treatment of mental disorder in a secure setting generally differs little from that used elsewhere in mental health services. It is important to be aware, however, that some treatments have never been systematically evaluated among people whose mental disorders are complicated by violence. For example,

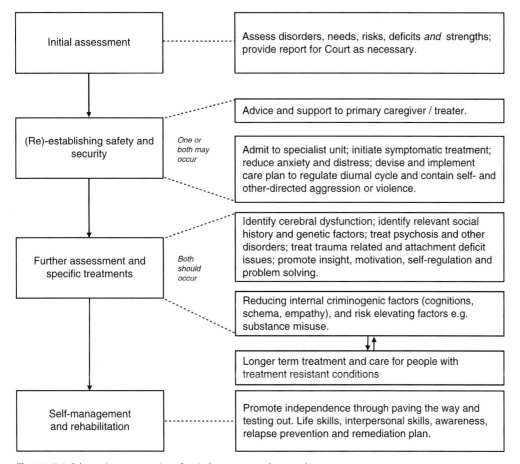

**Fig. 11.17.1** Schematic representation of typical treatment and care pathway.

some consider that caution should be exercised in the use of cognitive behaviour treatment to alleviate psychotic symptoms.[41]

*Delivery of treatment* in secure conditions differs in some important ways from its delivery elsewhere. Intrusive interventions are not unique to forensic mental health services, but the length of application means that staff may need to engage in regular peer and external review to ensure their work remains effective and ethical. Areas for concern include the creation of a climate of compulsion and coercion, and the conflicting roles for psychiatrists using therapeutic skills for legal assessments and dangerousness predictions, as well as true therapeutic engagement.

The *inpatient environment* must be conducive to habilitation and rehabilitation. As well as treatment of specific disorders, the core concern of staff is aiding independent living. A sense of progress, evident in both the physical environment and staff attitudes, encourages hope and consolidates treatment gains. This sense of progress can be achieved in several ways:

◆ provision of graded living spaces in which patients can experience greater autonomy;

◆ increasing engagement in work, education and recreation;

◆ extending responsibility for personal and domestic care tasks;

◆ phased introduction of supervized activities outside the institutional boundaries, appropriate to the patient's mental state and public safety;

◆ consideration for and support of family and social relationships, and a basis for developing sustainable social networks. Intimate relationships constitute an important element of this aspect of the work.[42]

*Successful return to the community* depends on everyone having a sense of security. This will require suitable accommodation, basic financial provision and skills for managing finances, a sense of control over mental disorder, and sufficient mastery of local services to be able to find help in a crisis. Regular reviews of the service user, the services, their use of these services, and the goodness of fit between them, are essential. People regarded as posing a special risk of harm to others may be referred to a multi-agency public protection panel (MAPPP, [43, 44]; see also Chapter 11.16).

Direct involvement of the patient in setting goals for health and for safety creates in the patient a sense of ownership of resultant plans, and is likely to improve collaboration with them. The process of community re-entry is summarized in Fig. 11.17.2, drawing on a grounded theory of discharge from a secure hospital.[45] It lends itself to the development of outcome measures which are more appropriate for an offender *patient* than the almost exclusively used but over-simplistic measure of re-offending. The core concern is movement between pathological dependence and healthy independence, with staff taking an active role in facilitating progress in two phases—paving the way, when skills necessary to the attainment of independence are built up, and testing out, when

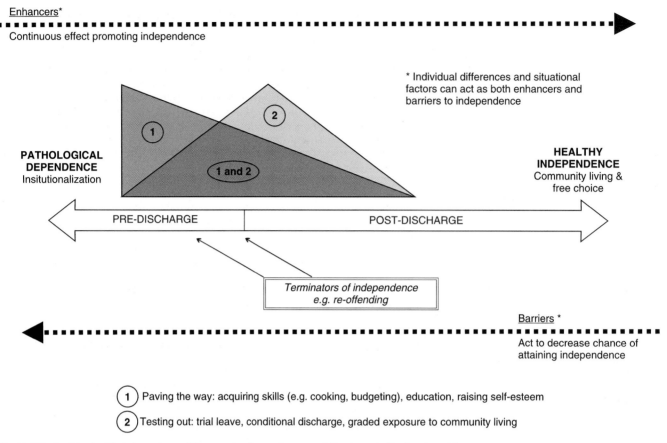

**Fig. 11.17.2** Attaining healthy independence while recovering from serious mental disorder and offending: A model.

individuals are given opportunities to prove themselves in situations of increasing trust. Re-offending is important, but as a barrier to gaining or sustaining independence rather than the sole outcome indicator.

## Assessing outcomes

Most studies of people who have been discharged from specialist security hospitals have serious limitations, which partly arise from political pressure to focus on the non-clinical outcome of re-offending and inadequate funding of the studies, which are costly and time-consuming. Results of existing studies are limited by:

1 Choice of outcome measures, which are almost solely re-offending, with some reference to mortality and hospital re-admission.

2 Lack of information about the nature of treatment. At best, there is information about length of stay in the institution. Some effects may be inferred, for example the complex model for treating personality disorder in Broadmoor Hospital in England,[46] but most studies simply treat secure hospitals or units as a 'black box'.

3 Social attitudes, substance use, policies/legislation, and provision of specialist services all change over time and between jurisdictions.

## Further information

Home Office (2003) MAPPA Guidance. www.probation.homeoffice.gov.uk/ pdf/MAPPA per cent20guidance.pdf Accessed 10.07.2007.

Jamieson, L., Taylor, P. J., and Gibson, B. (2006). From pathological dependence to healthy independent living: an emergent grounded theory of facilitating independent living. *The Grounded Theory Review* **6**, 79–107.

Royal College of Psychiatrists (2006) Psychiatrists and Multi-Agency Public Protection Arrangements. www.rcpsych.ac.uk/memebers/current_ issues/publicprotection.aspx. Accessed 27.07.2007

## References

1. Taylor, P. J., Grounds, A., and Snowden, P. (1993). Forensic psychiatry in the National Health Service of England and Wales. In *Forensic Psychiatry, Clinical, Legal and Ethical Issues* (eds. J. Gunn & P. J. Taylor), pp. 691–731. Butterworth Heinemann, Oxford.

2. Home Office, Department of Health and Social Security (1975). (Butler) *Report of the Committee on Mentally Abnormal Offenders.* HMSO, London. Cmnd 6244.

3. www.dspdprogramme.gov.uk

4. Francis, R., Higgins, J., Cassam, E., *et al.* (2006). Report of the independent inquiry into the care and treatment of Michael Stone. South East Coast Strategic Health Authority, Kent County Council, Kent Probation Area. www.kent.gov.uk/publications/council-anddemocracy/ michael-stone.htm Accessed 20.07.2007

5. Collins, G. (2005). Court-mandated psychiatric outpatient treatment in New York: doesn't this process invoke more care than controversy? *Criminal Behaviour and Mental Health*,15, 214–20.

6. Yoshikawa, K. and Taylor, P. J. (2003). New forensic mental health law in Japan. *Criminal Behaviour and Mental Health,* 13, 225–8.

7. Department of Health, Home Office (1992) *Review of Health and Social Services for Mentally Disordered Offenders and Others Requiring Similar Services.* London: HMSO. Cm 2088.

8. Taylor, P. J. (2007). *Second Expert Paper: Mental illness and serious harm to others.* www.nfmhp.org.uk/expertpapers (accessed 15.07.2007)

9. Gunn, J. (1976). Management of the mentally abnormal offender: integrated or parallel. *Proceedings of the Royal Society of Medicine,* 70, 877–80.

10. Jamieson, L. and Taylor, P. J. (2005). Patients leaving an English high security hospital. Do discharge cohorts and their progress change over time? *International Journal of Forensic Mental Health,* 4, 59–75.

11. Salize, H.J. and Dreßing, H. (2005). Placement and Treatment of Mentally Ill Offenders - Legislation and Practice in EU Member States. Mannheim, Germany: Central Institute of Mental Health.

12. SWANZDSAJCS (Accepted for publication). Offenders with mental disorder on five continents: a comparison of approaches to treatment and demographics factors relevant to measurement of outcome. *International Journal of Forensic Mental Health.* (Corresponding author P.J. Taylor).

13. Appelbaum, P.S. (1997). A theory of ethics for forensic psychiatry. *Journal of the American Academy of Psychiatry and the Law,* 25, 233–47.

14. Royal College of Psychiatrists (1995). *Strategies for the management for disturbed and violent patients in psychiatric units* (CR41-03/1995).

15. Department of Health & Welsh Office (1999). *Code of Practice for the Mental Health Act 1983.* London: The Stationery Office.

16. Moore, E., Yates, M., Mallendine, C., *et al.* (2002). Expressed emotion in relationships between staff and patients in forensic services: changes in relationship status at 12 month follow-up. *Legal and Criminological Psychology,* 7, 203–18.

17. McGauley, G. and Humphrey, M. (2003). Contribution of forensic psychotherapy to the care of forensic patients. *Advances in Psychiatric Treatment,* 9,117–24.

18. McMahon, C., Butwell, M., Taylor, P.J., *et al.* (2003). Changes in patterns of excessive alcohol consumption in 25 years of high security admissions from England and Wales. *Criminal Behaviour & Mental Health,* 13, 17–30.

19. Mueser, K.T., Bellack, A.S., Blanchard, J.J., *et al.* (1992). Comorbidity of schizophrenia in substance abuse: implications for treatment. *Journal of Consultant Clinical Psychology,* 60, 845–56.

20. Durand, M. A., Lelliott, P., Coyle, N., *et al.* (2005). Availability of treatment for substance misuse in medium secure psychiatric care in England: A national survey. *Journal of Forensic Psychiatry and Psychology,* 17(4), 611–25.

21. Lindqvist, P. (2007). Mental disorder, substance misuse and violent behaviour – the Swedish experience of caring for the triply troubled. *Criminal Behaviour and Mental Health,* 17, 242–9.

22. Meltzer, D., Tom, B.D.M., Brugha, T., *et al.* (2004). Access to medium secure psychiatric care in England and Wales: a national survey of admission assessments. *Journal of Forensic Psychiatry and Psychology,* 15, 17–31.

23. Swanson, J.W., Holzer, C.E., Ganju, V.K., *et al.* (1990). Violence and psychiatric disorder in the community: evidence from the Epidemiologic Catchment Area surveys. *Hospital and Community Psychiatry,* 41, 761–70.

24. Shaw, J., McKenna, J., Snowden, P., *et al.* (1998). The Northwest region. II: Patient characteristics in the research panels recommendation placement groups. *Journal of Forensic Psychiatry,* 5, 107–22.

25. Barber, M., Short, J., Clarke-Moore, J., *et al.* (2006). A secure attachment model of care: meting the needs of women with mental health problems and anti-social behaviour. *Criminal Behaviour and Mental Health,* 16, 3–10.

26. Mason, F.L. (2006). Services for women offenders with personality disorder: focus on a trauma-based approach to treatment. In *Personality Disorder and Serious Offending* (eds. C. Newrith, C. Meux, and P. J. Taylor), pp. 231–9. Hodder Arnold, London.

27. *Journal of Intellectual Disability.* (2002). Research Special Issue 46:s1–85.

28. allace, C., Mullen, P.E., Burgess, P., *et al.* (2004). Criminal offending in schizophrenia over a 25-year period marked by deinstitutionalization and increasing prevalence of comorbid substance use disorders. *American Journal of Psychiatry,* 161, 716–27.

29. Prison Reform Trust (2007) - Runaway sentence causes havoc – the indeterminate sentence for public protection. www.prisonreformtrust.org.uk/subsection.asp?id=1037.

30. Gunn, J., Maden, A., Swinton, M., *et al.* (1991). Treatment needs of prisoners with psychiatric disorders. *British Medical Journal,* 10, 338–41.

31. Singleton N., Meltzer H., Gatward R., *et al.* (1998) *Psychiatric morbidity among prisoners in England and Wales.* London: The Stationery Office.

32. Coid, J., Kahtan, N., Cook, A., *et al.* (2001).Predicting admission rates to secure forensic psychiatry services. *Psychological Medicine,* 31, 531–9.

33. Grounds, A., Gelsthorpe, L., Howes, M., *et al.* (2004). Access to medium secure psychiatric care in England and Wales: the qualitative study of admission decision making. *Journal of Forensic Psychiatry and Psychology,* 15, 32–49.

34. Jamieson, E., Butwell, M., Taylor, P.J., *et al.* (2000). Trends in special (high security) hospitals. I: Referrals and admissions 1986-1995. *British Journal of Psychiatry,* 176, 253–9.

35. McInerny, T. (2000). Dutch TBS forensic services: a personal view. *Criminal Behaviour & Mental Health,* 10, 213–28.

36. Berry, A., Larkin, E., Taylor, P., *et al.* (2003). Referred to high secure care: determinants of a bed/offer admission and placement after one year. *Criminal Behaviour and Mental Health,* 13(4), 310–20.

37. Cohen, A. and Eastman, N. (2000). *Assessing Forensic Mental Health Need. Policy, Theory and Practice.* London: Gaskell.

38. Collins, M. and Davies, S. (2005). The Security Needs Assessment Profile: A multidimensional approach to measuring security needs. *International Journal of Forensic Mental Health,* 4(1), 39–52.

39. Douglas, K. S., Guy, L. S., Weir, J., *et al.* (2006). HCR-20 violence risk assessment scheme: Overview and annotated bibliography. Burnaby, Canada: Department of Psychology, Simon Fraser University. Available at http://www.sfu.ca/psyc/faculty/hart/Resources.htm.

40. Belfrage, H., Fransson, G., Strand, S., *et al.* (2000). Prediction of violence using the HCR-20: A prospective study in two maximum security correctional institutions. *Journal of Forensic Psychiatry,* 11, 167–75.

41. Taylor, P.J. (2006). Delusional disorder and delusions: is there a risk of violence in social interactions about the core symptom? *Behavioral Sciences & the Law,* 24, 313–32.

42. Taylor, P.J. and Swan, T. (eds.). (1999). *Couples in Care and Custody.* Butterworth-Heinemann: Oxford.

43. Home Office (2003) MAPPA Guidance. www.probation.homeoffice.gov.uk/pdf/MAPPA per cent20guidance.pdf Accessed 10.07.2007.

44. Royal College of Psychiatrists (2006) Psychiatrists and Multi-Agency Public Protection Arrangements. www.rcpsych.ac.uk/memebers/current_issues/publicprotection.aspx. Accessed 27.07.2007

45. Jamieson, L., Taylor, P. J., and Gibson, B. (2006). From pathological dependence to healthy independent living: an emergent grounded theory of facilitating independent living. *The Grounded Theory Review* 6, 79–107.

46. Newrith, C., Meux, C., Taylor, P., *et al.* (2006). *Personality Disorder and Serious Offending - Hospital Treatment Models.* Hodder Arnold, London.

# Index

Note: Page numbers in **bold** refer to main entries. Those in *italic* refer to figures and / or tables. Alphabetical order is word-by-word.

AA (Alcoholics Anonymous) 451–2, 459, 1279, 1352
AACD (age-associated cognitive decline) 1535
AAI (Adult Attachment Interview) 309–10
AAMI (age-associated memory impairment) 1534–5, 1535–6
Abbreviated Injury Scale 1105
ABC analysis 96, 413–14
ABC medical assessment 1106
ABC transporters and complementary medicines 1249–50, *1250*
Abel Screen 1962
Aberrant Behavior Checklist 94, 1823
ability, general, assessment of 87, *88*
ablative neurosurgery *see* neurosurgery for mental disorder
abortion 1119, 1883
  late 1119
  self-induced 1117
Abraham, Karl 306
abridged somatization index 1000
absolute risk reduction 128
abstinence
  from alcohol 450
  in psychoanalysis 1339
abulia 379
acamprosate 454, **1246**, 1542
'accident neurosis' 1055
accidents **1105–13**
  classification of physical injury 1105
  compensation claims 1111–12
  epidemiology 1105
  litigation following 1111–12
  needs of significant others 1108
  and psychiatric disorder 1105
  psychological trauma 1105–6
    assessment at accident scene 1106–7
    long-term assessment and treatment 1110–11
    responses seen in emergency room 1107–8
    treatment during hospital stay 1108–10, *1109*
  and sleep disturbance 926, 1108
acetylcholine 429
  and the basal forebrain 150
  identification 168
  and memory 253

receptors *173*, 206, 1171
  role in neurodevelopment 159
  in substance use disorders *429*
acetylcholinesterase 155
aciclovir *1091*
*acné excorié* 618, 917–18, 1044
acromegaly and hypersomnia 942
acrotomophilia *833*
ACSeSS (Admission Criteria to Secure Services Schedule) 2018
ACT *see* assertive community treatment
ACTH 170
  in depression 661
  and insomnia 935
  release in response to stress 1135
  tumours producing 1101
actigraphy 934, 1697
acting out 299, 300
Action Program Test *90*
action-taking, legal aspects 1895–900
Active Life Expectancy 1509–10
activities of daily living (ADL)
  in Alzheimer's disease 335
  instrumental 337
  in mild cognitive impairment 1535
activity scheduling in body dysmorphic disorder 1047
acute and transient psychotic disorders **602–8**
acute intermittent porphyria 212
acute polymorphic disorder with symptoms of schizophrenia 605, 1124
acute polymorphic psychotic disorder without symptoms of schizophrenia 604–5
acute renal failure 1087
acute schizophrenia-like psychotic disorder 536, 603, 605
Acute Stress Disorder Interview 695
Acute Stress Disorder Scale 695
acute stress reactions **693–9**, 716
  aetiology 696
  assessment 695
  childhood and adolescence 1729
  classification 693, *694*
  clinical features 693–4
  comorbidity 696
  course and prognosis 696–7
  diagnosis 694–5, *694*

differential diagnosis 695
epidemiology 695–6
following an accident 1107, 1108
in HIV/AIDS 1091
and offending 1923
predictors of 697
prevention 698
treatment and management 697–8
victims of criminal activity 1984–5
AD *see* Alzheimer's disease
Adaptive Behaviour Scales 1821
ADARDS unit 1583
ADAS-Cog (Alzheimer's Disease Assessment Scale-Cognition) 1240
addiction
  'primary addiction' theory 434
  role of personality 428–9
  routes and risks of 430–1, *431*
  self-medication hypothesis 434
  use of term 427
Addiction Severity Index 1164
Addison's disease 1086
adenine 223
adenosine receptors *173*
adenylate cyclase 174, 176, 473, 1201
ADH *see* alcohol dehydrogenase; vasopressin
ADHD *see* attention-deficit hyperactivity disorder
adjustment disorders **716–24, 1066–9**
  acute 717
  aetiology 720, 1067–8
  and age 719, 721–3
  associated features 719
  childhood and adolescence 721–3
    after diagnosis of physical illness 1741, *1742*
    diagnostic criteria 1669–70, *1671*
  chronic 717
  classification 106, 1066–7
  clinical features 720
  comorbidity 719
  course and prognosis 1068
  definitions 716–19, *716, 717*, 1066–7
  and deliberate self-harm/suicide 718, 722
  diagnosis 1067, 1669–70, *1671*
  differential diagnosis 695, 1067, 1657
  elderly people 1552

adjustment disorders (*cont.*)
  epidemiology 719, 1067
  and offending 1923
  postoperative 1099–100
  stressors 718, 720
  subtypes *717*, 720
  symptom profile 717–18
  in terminal illness 1069–70
  treatment and management 720–3, 1068–9,
    *1069*, 1278
ADL *see* activities of daily living
Admission Criteria to Secure Services
    Schedule 2018
ADMP 73
adolescence *see* childhood and adolescence
Adolescent Transitions Program 1790
adoption 1120
  effects on child and adult mental
    health **1747–52**
  history-taking 1601
  open 1747
  total severance model 1747
adoption studies **216**
  anxiety disorders 1667
  attention-deficit hyperactivity
    disorder 1646
  conduct disorder 1659
  in gene–environment interaction 217–18
  mood disorders 651
  offending behaviour 1918
  schizophrenia 548–9, 553–4
adrenaline 150
  in conduct disorder 1658
  functions 161
adrenergic receptors 1171
  antidepressant actions at 1172, 1187
  antipsychotic actions at 1209, *1211*
  and depression 1185, *1185*
  in generalized anxiety disorder 732
  and post-traumatic stress disorder 706
  and suicidal behaviour 965
adrenocorticotropic hormone *see* ACTH
Adult Attachment Interview 309–10
Adult Memory and Information Processing
    Battery 88
advance directives 30, 1577, 1899
advanced glycosylation end products 1509
advanced sleep phase syndrome 1261, 1699
aetiology
  contribution of epidemiology 280–9
  contribution of genetics **212–22, 222–33**
  contribution of social sciences **268–75,
    275–9**
*Afa* 1420
affective blunting in schizophrenia 529
affective psychosis and Prader Willi
    syndrome 1826
affects
  Freudian theories of 295
  and object-relations theory 302, 303
affiliative traits 886, 888
Africa
  attitudes to psychiatric disorder 6
  psychiatric nurses in 1406–7
age-associated cognitive decline 1535
age-associated memory impairment 1534–5,
    1535–6
age of consent 1899–900
age of criminal responsibility 1945, 1954
AGE products 1509

ageing
  as an energy crisis 1509
  biology of **1507–11**
  and circadian rhythms 1572
  and culture 1512–13
  and dementia 1520
  dietary modification 1509
  disengagement theory of 1512
  genomic theories 1507–8
  and life expectancy 1507, 1509–10
  and mitochondria 223
  and modernization 1512
  and narrative gerontology 1514–15
  population 1579
  and schizophrenia 544–5
  and sexual function 1569, *1569*
  and sleep 925–6, 1571–2
  social constructionist approach 1515
  sociology of **1512–16**
  stochastic theories 1508–9
  successful 1512
  and transitions 1513–14
  *see also* elderly people
aggression
  adolescent *see* antisocial behaviour,
    adolescent
  in antisocial personality disorder 866
  biodevelopmental processes 889
  and body dysmorphic disorder 1044
  in conduct disorder 1656
  in dementia 336, 1920–1, 1928–9
  as a diagnostic feature 1928–9
  and epilepsy 1078, 1864, 1929, 1929–30
  following an accident 1107, 1108, 1920
  following head injury 393, 396, 1929
  and Huntington's disease 1929
  ictal 1930
  impulsive/episodic 912
  information-processing model 1658
  and intellectual disability 1855–6, 1929
  neurobiological determinants 1917–18
  passive 876
  in physical illness 1132–3
  severe maladaptive in childhood and
    adolescence 1798
  and substance use disorders 1926
  and suicide 970
  and Wernicke–Korsakoff syndrome 1929
  *see also* violence
aggressive drive 294, 295, 302
agitation
  in dementia 413–15
  in elderly people 1527
  following head injury 393, 396
  in physical illness 1132–3
  postoperative 1098–9
  in schizophrenia 529
agnosia in Alzheimer's disease 334
agomelatine 671
agonists 1171
agoraphobia 52, 750, 752
  elderly people 1559
  with panic disorder 740–1, 750–64
agranulocytosis, drug-induced 1223
agraphia, pure 54
agreeableness 850, 886, 888
AIDS *see* HIV/AIDS
AIS (Abbreviated Injury Scale) 1105
akathisia *58*, *730*, 1222
akinesia 58, *58*

Alanon 1352
alarm clock, dawn-simulating 1261
alcohol
  abstinence vs. controlled drinking 450
  addictiveness *431*
  advertising/promotion restrictions 470
  age limits on drinking 469–70
  as anxiolytic 1178
  awareness of compulsion to drink 439
  binge drinking 646
  control of availability and conditions of use
    469–70
  drink-seeking behaviour 438
  drinking repertoire 438
  drug interactions 1175
  education about 468
  effects on sleep 1572
  'expectancies' 434
  'harmful use' 440
  integrated societal policy 471
  intoxication 442–3
    as a legal defence 1901
    and offending 1926, 1927–8
  legal prohibitions on 468
  paradoxical reactions with 1180
  'pathological intoxication' 442, 1926
  rationing sales 470
  reinstatement of drinking after abstinence 439
  relationship between consumption and
    violence 1926
  sensitivity to 435
  taxes on 470
  temperance movement 470
  tolerance to 438
alcohol abuse, terminology 439–40
alcohol dehydrogenase 435
alcohol dependence syndrome **437–42**
  and classification 439
  clinical features 438, *438*
  elements of 438–9
  validity of 438
alcohol-induced amnesia 404, 443
alcohol-induced dementia 182–3, **399–402**,
    444, 1541
alcohol-related brain damage 182–3, **399–402**,
    444, 1541
alcohol-related neurodevelopmental
    disorder 1615, 1841
alcohol-related problems 438, **440–1**
Alcohol Stroop Test 265
alcohol use
  assessment 442, 448
  guidelines for safety 432
  and health 1136
  recommended intake for elderly people 1540
alcohol use disorders (AUDs)
  and accidents 1110
  aetiology **432–7**
    biopsychosocial model *433*
    genetic factors 434–6
    psychological factors 433–4
    sociocultural factors 433
  and anxiety 427
  assessment 448
    instruments 1484, 1542
  in childhood and adolescence 456, 464
  as a chronic relapsing disorder 447–8
  classification 437
  cognitive assessment 92
  comorbidity 427, 434, 443–4

benzodiazepine misuse 492
bipolar disorder 646
bulimia nervosa 804, 806
cyclothymia/cyclothymic disorder 687
depression 649
panic disorder 455, 752
services for 465
sleep-wake disorders *931*
treatment 455–6
and dopamine receptors 229
effects on family and carers 452–3, 465
elderly people 1519, *1540*, **1540–2**, *1541*
and employment 456
ethnic minorities 464
family history positive 434, *434*
global disease burden 10, 467
and head injury 393–4
in health care workers 457
and homelessness 456, 464
informants 448
inpatient care 1453
and intoxication 442–3
and jealousy 620
late-onset 1540
legal issues 1927–8
levels of severity *1541*
and liver transplantation 456
memory impairment in 404
mental health services **459–67**
neuropathology 182–3, *183*
parental, effects on child development 1754
and personality 434
physical disorders associated 444–5
in pregnancy 1117, 1448, 1614–15, 1754,
    1826, 1841
prevalence *285*
prevention **467–72**, 1448–9
    deterrence 468
    education/persuasion 468
    harm reduction strategies 469
    providing/encouraging alternative
        activities 468–9
    regulating availability and conditions
        of use 469–70
    social, religious and community
        movements 470
preventive/prevention paradox 460, 467
in primary care, detection 1484
reasons for 427
relapse prevention 450–2, *450*, *451*
spectrum of 459–60, *460*
and suicide 427, 444, 955, 956
terminology 437
treatment 5521–33, 428
    Alcoholics Anonymous 451–2, 459,
        1279, 1352
    brief interventions 460–1, 463
    community-based 461–2
    coping skills therapies 451
    cost-effectiveness 462–3
    counselling 1279
    cue exposure 451
    deterrent medication 453–4, 1542
    effectiveness 470–1
    follow-up 457
    inpatient 449, 455–6, 461
    matching of patients to 452, 455, 456, 462
    motivational interviewing 451
    pharmacotherapy 1246
    spectrum of 459–60, *460*

starting 448
    stepped care 462
treatment gap *13*
type I/type II 429
in women 454–5, 464
*see also* alcohol dependence syndrome
Alcohol Use Disorders Identification Test
    284, 460, 1542
alcohol withdrawal 443
    alleviation by further drinking 439
    complementary medicines 1249
    explanation of symptoms 448
    inpatient 449, 461
    medical assistance 448–9, *449*, 1542
    outpatient 448, 461–2
    with perceptual disturbance 443
    psychosis in 58, 443, 449–50, 538
    with seizures 443, 449
    symptoms 438–9
    tachycardia in 448
    and violence 1926
alcoholic blackouts 404, 443
alcoholic hallucinosis 443, 538
Alcoholics Anonymous 451–2, 459, 1279, 1352
alcoholism 437
    *see also* alcohol use disorders
aldehyde dehydrogenase (ALDH) 435
ALE (Active Life Expectancy) 1509–10
alexia 54
alexithymia 850, 1005
algogenic psychosyndrome 851
ALI hierarchy 1372, *1372*
alleles 212–13, 226
    association studies 220–1, *220*
allocortex 148, *149*
allostatic load and ageing 1507
alogia 53
1-α-acetylmethadol hydrochloride 1243–4
α-calcium calmodulin-dependent kinase II
    (α-CaMKII) 889, *890*
α-crystalin 362
α-melanocyte stimulating hormone
    (α-MSH) 170
α-secretase 338
alpha-synuclein protein/gene 362, 365, 369
α2-agonists in opioid detoxification 477
alprazolam
    antipanic actions 1180
    in cancer *1102*
    in delirium 1533
    in panic disorder 756–7, *756*
    pharmacokinetics *1172*, 1179
    potential for misuse 491
    in social anxiety disorder 743
alternative medicine *see* complementary
    medicines
Alzheimer's disease (AD) **333–43**
    aetiology and molecular neurobiology 337–9
    and ageing 1520
    assessment 92, 265–6, 337, 1240
    behavioural and psychological symptoms *413*
    biomarkers 341
    carers 340
    classification 336
    clinical features 334–6
    cognitive impairment in 334–5
    delaying onset/disease modification 341, 1538
    and delirium 1532
    and depression 335
    diagnosis 336–7

differential diagnosis 347, 364, 373, 380
and Down syndrome 1584, 1827, 1839,
    1865, 1880
early detection 265–6, 1519–20
epidemiology **1519–22**
functional impairment in 335
genetic counselling 340
genetics 227, 339, 1521
history of disorder 334
history-taking 336–7
impact 1522
incidence and risk factors 1520–2, *1520*, *1522*
Lewy body variant 362
and mild cognitive impairment 1534, *1534*,
    1535–6, 1538
neurofibrillary tangles 337–8, 339
neuropathology 337–9
    amyloid cascade hypothesis 338
    cholinergic hypothesis 338, 1240–1
    presenilin genes 339
personality change in 335–6
prevention 341
psychoses in 335
risk reduction/protective factors 1521–2,
    *1522*, 1538
and sleep-wake disorders *931*
sporadic/familial 339
translational research 341
treatment and management 339–41, 1240–1
Alzheimer's Disease Assessment Scale-
    Cognition 1240
amantadine 374, 1226, 1876
ambitendency 58
aMCI (amnestic mild cognitive impairment)
    1520, 1535
amenorrhoea in anorexia nervosa 782, 783, 787
AMHPs (approved mental health
    practitioners) 1410
amimia 346
amines 168
amino acids *168*
amisulpride 1209
    administration 1220
    adverse effects *1212*
    pharmacodynamics 1210
    pharmacokinetics 1222
amitriptyline *670*
    adverse effects *1191*
    in anxiety disorders 1182
    in cancer *1103*
    dosage *1196*
    drug interactions 1175, 1233
    in personality disorders *905*
    pharmacodynamics *1173*, *1187*
    pharmacokinetics *1172*, *1189*
amnesia 59
    alcohol-induced 404, 443
    in Alzheimer's disease 334
    anterograde 59, 92, 252, 391
    assessment of awareness of 420–1
    assessment of functional consequences 420
    assessment of memory 89, *89*, 253, 254,
        255–6, 264, 420–1, *420*
    in brain tumour 1075
    and cerebrovascular disease 407
    for criminal offences 405, 1927
    in dementia 59
    dissociative 714, 715, 1012
    following ECT 404, 1257
    following hypoxia 406–7

amnesia (*cont.*)
  in fugue states 404–5
  global 59
  in herpes encephalitis 406
  malingered 1055–6
  memory remediation and rehabilitation
     421–4, *422*
  partial 59
  persistent 405–8
  post-traumatic 388, 390–1, 404, 407
  in post-traumatic stress disorder 404, 714
  psychogenic 59
  psychogenic focal retrograde 405
  retrograde 59, 252, 408
    following head injury 388, *388*, 391
  selective 57
  transient 403–5
  transient epileptic 403
  transient global 59, 403
  use of memory aids and strategies 420, *421*
  in vascular dementia 379
  in Wernicke–Korsakoff syndrome 92, 405–6
  *see also* memory impairment
amnesic syndromes **403–11**
  associated with alcohol use 1541
  elderly people 1531
amnestic mild cognitive impairment 1520, 1535
*amok* 606, 979, **981**
amotivational syndrome, cannabis-
    associated 508
amoxapine 669
  adverse effects 1190, *1191*
  dosage *1196*
  pharmacodynamics *1187*
  pharmacokinetics *1189*
AMPA receptors 172, *173*, 174, 1171
AMPAkines 174
amphetamine **482–6**
  addictiveness *431*, 483
  in attention-deficit hyperactivity disorder
    1241, 1876
  effects of 483, *483*
  in intellectual disability 1876
  misuse
    aetiology 484
    complications associated 484–5
    course and prognosis 484–5
    diagnosis 483–4
    epidemiology 484
    prevention 485
    treatment and management 485
  pharmacodynamics 1172
  preparations 482–3
  psychosis due to 485
  withdrawal 483, *483*
amphotericin B *1091*
ampicillin 1532
amygdala 152, *152*–3, 158, 201
  and associative learning 258
  and emotion 258, 259, 264
  and fear/anxiety 1666, *1667*, 1668
  in generalized anxiety disorder 732–3
  and memory 251, 253, 259, 264
  and orbitofrontal cortical development 1919
amygdalotomy 1267
amylase serum levels in bulimia nervosa 804
amyloid 338
amyloid precursor protein 338
anabolic steroid abuse 1045
anaclitic type 316

anaemia 785, 1087–8
anaesthesia, glove and stocking 57
anaesthetics, adverse effects *730*
anal phase of development 294, 295
analgesics
  combination formulations 1169
  in somatization disorder 1009
  suicide risk 973
analysis of variance 138
analytical behaviourism 133–4
analytical functionalism 134–5
anandamide 172, 429, *429*, 507
anankastic personality disorder *see* obsessive–
    compulsive disorder
anankastic phenomena 52
androgen therapy in gender identity
    disorder 843
androgens 815–16, *816*, 826
androstenedione 815
anencephaly 156
aneuploidy 228
aneusomy 228
angel dust *see* phencyclidine
Angelman syndrome
  behavioural and psychiatric aspects 1841–2
  and epilepsy 1864, 1865
  genetics 213, 224, 229, 1841, 1865, *1866*
  physical characteristics 1841
  prevalence 1841
Anger Coping and Coping Power
    Programme 1662, 1782
anger management
  in adjustment disorders *1069*
  in antisocial personality disorder 898
  in anxiety disorders 1295–6
  in conduct disorder 1662, 1782
  in intellectual disability 1874
aniracetam 1240
Anna O 1338
anomia 253, 850, 1449
anorexia nervosa **777–800**
  and adverse life events 779–80
  aetiology 778–82
    biomedical factors 781–2
    family factors 780
    multidimensional approach 778–9, *779*
    sociocultural factors 779
  age at onset 778
  assessment instruments 777
  and body image 57
  and child sexual abuse 780
  childhood and adolescence 1784
  classical post-pubertal 782–6
  classification and diagnosis 787–8, 800–1, *801*
  course and prognosis 788–9
  as culture-bound syndrome 779
  and depression 783, 787
  differential diagnosis 784, 787
  early onset/premenarchal 786–7, 788–9
  epidemiology 777–8
  ethical issues 796
  and gender 778
  genetics 781–2, 806
  history of concept 777
  hypothalamic model 781
  incidence 778
  maintenance 1299
  in males 788
  malnutrition in 784–6
  medico-legal issues 796

  mortality 788–9
  myopathy in 785
  and obsessive–compulsive disorder 783
  osteoporosis in 785
  overlap with bulimia nervosa 800, *801*
  and parenthood 786
  and personality disorders 780–1, 884
  and postnatal depression 780
  and pregnancy 780, 784, 1118
  prevalence 778
  prevention 796–7
  psychopathology 779, 783, 786–7
  relationship with other eating disorders 804
  risk factors *806*
  and socio-economic status 778
  and suicide 955
  temperature regulation in 785
  treatment 789–96
    antidepressants 795, 1193
    cognitive-behaviour therapy 792, 796,
      **1298–303**
    compliance 794
    complications 786
    compulsory 793, 795
    day care/community 793, 795
    dietary care 794–5
    dynamic psychotherapy 796
    eating disorder units 792–3
    family therapy 790–2, *790*, 796
    inpatient 792–3, 793, 794–5
    interpersonal psychotherapy 792
    nursing 794–5
ANOVA 138
Antabuse® **453**, *730*, **1246**, 1542
antagonists 1171–2
anterior capsulotomy 1267, *1269*, Plate 15
anterior cingulate cortex 245
anterior cingulotomy 1267, *1270*, Plate 16
anterior commissure 151, 157
anthropology *see* social and cultural
    anthropology
anthropophobia 982
anti-androgens in the paraphilias 838
anticholinergics
  adverse effects 365, 487, 1225
    anxiety *730*
    delirium 331, 1532
    memory loss 404
    parasomnias 946
  in management of antipsychotic adverse
    effects 1225
anticipation 213, 228, 652
antidepressants 669–71, *670*, **1185–98**
  in adjustment disorders 721, 1068
  administration and dosage 1195, *1196*
  adverse effects 674, 1190–3, *1191*, *1192*
    anxiety *730*
    cardiotoxicity 1794–5
    epileptogenicity 1078
    sexual dysfunction 826–7
    suicide risk 971, 973, 1192, 1668, 1707–8,
      1796, 1923
  in alcohol use disorders 455
  in anorexia nervosa 795, 1193–4
  in anxiety disorders 1182, 1193
  and attempted suicide 670, 674
  in attempted suicide 970–1, 1192
  in bipolar disorder 671–2
  in bulimia nervosa 807–8, 809, 1193–4
  in cancer 1102, *1103*

in childhood and adolescence 674–5, 1676, 1794–5, 1796
choice of 674
classes of 1186–8, *1187*
complementary medicines 1248
contraindications 1194
delayed onset of effects 176, *176*
in dementia 416
dosage 674–5
drug interactions 1194–5, *1195*
in dysthymia/dysthymic disorder 684–5
in elderly people 674, 1554–5, *1554*
in generalized anxiety disorder 735
history of 1185–6, *1185*
in HIV/AIDS 386, 1092
indications 674, 1193–4, *1193*
in intellectual disability 1875–6
in obsessive–compulsive disorder 768–9, 770, 1193, 1687–8, *1687*
overdose 1192
in persistent somatoform pain disorder 1033–4
in personality disorders *905*, 906
pharmacodynamics 1172–3, *1173*, 1186–8, *1187*
pharmacokinetics *1172*, 1188–9, *1189*
in post-traumatic stress disorder 709
precautions with 1796
in pregnancy 675, 677, 761–2, 1117, 1192
prescription in physical illness 674, 1132
and surgery 1097–8
switching between 674
in terminal illness 1070
theories regarding actions of 1185–6, *1185*
withdrawal 1195
*see also specific drugs and types of drugs*
antiemetics
adverse effects 1101
in chemotherapy 1101
antiepileptic drugs **1231–40**
adverse effects
anxiety *730*
behavioural disorders 1867–8
on cognitive function 92
teratogenicity 1169
in anxiety disorders 1182
in bipolar disorder 671, 672, 1556
in childhood and adolescence 1798
with psychiatric/behaviour disorder and intellectual disability 1852
choice of 1866–7
drug interactions 1866
in elderly people 1556
in epilepsy 1080
with intellectual disability 1866–7, *1867*
in intellectual disability 1852, 1866–7, *1867*, 1876
in Landau–Kleffner syndrome 1627
in personality disorders *905*, 906
pharmacokinetics *1867*
structures *1232*
withdrawal 1867
*see also specific drugs*
antihistamines
in anxiety disorders 1182
in management of antipsychotic adverse effects 1225
antihypertensives, adverse effects 827
antilibidinal drugs in intellectual disability 1876

antilibidinal object 308
antioxidants
and longevity 1509
in tardive dyskinesia 1249
anti-PrP antibodies 359
anti-psychiatrist movement 28
antipsychotics **1208–31**
in acute and transient psychotic disorders 606
administration 1213–22, *1214*
adverse effects 58–9, *1212*, 1222–5
acute sensitivity reactions in dementia with Lewy bodies 361–2, 365
akathisia *730*, 1222
anxiety 1101
in childhood and adolescence 1677, 1797–8
cognitive impairment 580
diabetes 1085
dystonia 1222
in elderly people 1548
epileptogenicity 1078, 1223
hyperprolactinaemia 1086, 1217, 1223
hypersomnia 939
hypotension 1223, 1529
management 1225
'neuroleptic toxicity' 588
parkinsonism 580, 1222–3
sexual dysfunction 827
tardive dyskinesia 1223
*see also neuroleptic malignant syndrome*
in alcohol withdrawal 449–50
antidepressant actions 581
in anxiety disorders 1182
in attempted suicide 971
in attention-deficit hyperactivity disorder 1652
atypical 1172, 1209, *1209*
in autism and other pervasive developmental disorders 1640
in bipolar disorder 677
in cancer *1104*
in childhood and adolescence 1677, 1796–8, 1852
classification 1209–10, *1209*
complementary medicines 1249
in delirium 331
in dementia 414–15
in dementia with Lewy bodies 367
depot formulations 581–2
drug interactions 1221–2
high-potency 1209
in HIV/AIDS 386, 1092
in Huntington's disease 374
indications and contraindications 1225
in intellectual disability 1875
low-potency 1209
mid-potency 1209
in personality disorders 600, *905*, 906
PET/SPET imaging studies 189–90
pharmacodynamics 1172, 1210, *1211*, 1212–13, *1212*
pharmacokinetics *1172*, 1221–2
polypharmacy 587–8
in pregnancy 677, 1118
resistance to 582, 590, 1213
risk: benefit appraisal 585, *586*
in schizoaffective disorder 598
in schizophrenia 579–82, *579*, 585, 586–8, *586*, 1213, *1215*, 1548
and surgery 1098

in tic disorders 1073, 1688
typical (first generation) 1209, *1209*
antisocial behaviour, adolescent 1654, **1945–59**
assessment 1947–8, *1949*
and attention-deficit hyperactivity disorder 1948–9
and autism spectrum disorders 1950
and capacity 1954–5
and conduct disorder 1946, 1948–9
and depression 1949
and early-onset psychosis 1950
epidemiology 1945
girls 1955–6
interventions 1950–7, *1951*
justice system 1945, 1947
legal issues 1954–5
and mental disorder 1946–7, 1948–50, 1951–2
pathways of care 1947
pathways to *1946*
and post-traumatic stress disorder 1949–50
protective factors 1947, *1947*
risk factors *1946*, 1947
antisocial behaviour, adult *see* offending
antisocial personality disorder **865–6**
aetiology 866
classification 851, *856*, 865
clinical features 866
comorbidity 866
course and prognosis 866
and deception 1049
diagnosis 866
differential diagnosis 866, 1657
in elderly people 1561, *1562*, 1563
epidemiology 865, *882*, 883
following head injury 391
and genetic–environmental interactions 315
offenders 1921
prisoners *1933*
relationship with attention-deficit hyperactivity disorder 1931
terminology 856
treatment 866, 898, 898–9, 904
anxiety
as an alarm signal 295
anticipatory 751
and arousal 55
assessment instruments 1164
in bulimia nervosa 803
in cancer 1101–2, *1101*
in childhood and adolescence
assessment 1665
with intellectual disability 1851–2
with physical illness 1742–3
and conversion disorder 1014–15, *1015*
counselling in 1278
definition 1664
in depression 634
'depressive' 307
and diabetes mellitus 1085
drug-induced symptoms resembling *730*
elderly people 1558–61
and epilepsy 1080
following an accident 1106, 1108–9
and functional symptoms 993
and hyperthyroidism 1085
malignant 983
pathophysiology 1666–8, *1667*
in physical illness 1131–2, 1742–3
in pregnancy 1117
preoperative 1097

anxiety (*cont.*)
  and sexuality 825
  in Tourette syndrome 1073
  trait 1137
  in vascular dementia 379
  and ventricular dysrhythmias 1081
anxiety disorders
  acute-on-chronic 1180
  alcohol-induced 427, 434, 444, 455
  assessment 1289, *1289*
  with attention-deficit hyperactivity
      disorder 1650
  and bipolar disorder 646
  childhood and adolescence **1664–9**
    assessment 1665
    clinical course and outcome 1666
    clinical presentation 1665–6
    comorbidity 1666, 1673
    differential diagnosis 1671
    epidemiology 1665–6
    pathophysiology 1666–8, *1667*
    treatment 1668, 1779–80
  chronic 1180
  and chronic fatigue syndrome 1037
  classification 105
  cognitive content 1286–7
  cognitive model of 1289–90, *1290*
  definition 1664
  and depression 649
  elderly people 1531, 1579
  following head injury 393
  following stroke 1071–2
  genetics 1667
  and hypochondriasis 997, 1024, 1027
  and intellectual disability 1855
  and kleptomania 1943
  and pain 1030
  parental, effects on child development 1754
  and persistent somatoform pain
      disorder 997, 1032
  postpartum 1121–2
  prevalence *285*
  and sleep-wake disorders *931*
  and somatization disorders 996
  and stress 1667–8
  and suicide 955
  treatment
    antidepressants 1182, 1193
    cognitive-behaviour therapy **1285–98**,
        1668, 1779–80
    interpersonal psychotherapy 1324
    neurosurgery 1267
    *see also* anxiolytics
  vulnerability to 732, 734–5
  *see also* generalized anxiety disorder
anxiety management
  in depression in elderly people 1555
  in obsessive–compulsive disorder 1685
'anxiety neurosis'/'anxiety state' 729
anxiety programme 1285
anxiolytics 1178–9
  in cancer 1101–2, *1102*
  clinical effects 1179–81
  complementary medicines as 1248
  intravenous, in conversion disorder 1019
  in obsessive–compulsive disorder 769
  in pregnancy 1117
  withdrawal from *730*
anxious personality disorder *see* avoidant
    personality disorder

AO (assertive outreach) teams
    1455, 1457–8, *1457*
apathy
  in dementia 416
  following an accident 1106
  following head injury 391, 392, 396
  following neurosurgery for mental
      disorder 1269
aphasia 53
  acquired childhood 1712
  acquired epileptic 1626–7, 1639, 1864
  in Alzheimer's disease 334
  assessment 89
  jargon 54
  progressive non-fluent 344
aphonia 53
*Aplysia* 315
*APOE* gene/apoE protein and Alzheimer's
    disease 339, 1521
apotemnophilia *833*
*APP* gene/APP protein 338, 339
applied tension in specific phobia 746
appraisal delay 1137
approved mental health practitioners 1410
'approximate answers' 54, 1055
apraxia in Alzheimer's disease 334
archicortex 158
Arctic hysteria 983
Argentina, attitudes to psychiatric disorder 6
aripiprazole 1209, *1209*
  administration *1214*, 1219–20
  adverse effects *1212*, 1225
  in bipolar disorder in elderly people 1556
  in childhood and adolescence 1797
  in personality disorders *905*, 906
  pharmacodynamics 1210, *1211*
  pharmacokinetics 1222
  pharmacology 1210
Aristotle 133
arithmetical skills, specific disorders of 1629–30
ARND (alcohol-related neurodevelopmental
    disorder) 1615, 1841
aromatherapy in dementia *414*
arousal and anxiety 55
array CGH 1831
arson 1924, **1965–9**
  by children/adolescents 1954
  characteristics of fire-raisers 1966
  classification 1966, *1966*
  historical context 1965
  legal aspects 1966
  management 1967–8
  motivation *1966*, 1967
  prevalence 1965–6, *1965*
art therapy 1352, **1413–17**
  with children 1414
  contextual issues 1415–16
  definitions 1413
  with elderly people 1415
  historical development 1414
  with offenders 1415
  people with intellectual disability 1414–15
  in physical illness 1415
  in psychotic illness 1415
  research 1416
  in selective mutism 1714
artefactual illness 57
articulatory suppression in insomnia
    936–7
artificial insemination 1114–15

ascending reticular activating system in
    Alzheimer's disease 1240
ascertainment
  in family studies 215
  in twin studies 216
aschemazia 57
asenapine 1209, 1210, 1220–1
aspartylglucosaminuria 1865
Asperger's syndrome **1638–9**
  aetiology 1639
  clinical features 1638
  course 1639
  definition 1638, *1638*
  demographics 1639
  differential diagnosis 865
  epidemiology 1639
  and juvenile delinquency 1950
  management 1640
  and offending 1921
  prognosis 1639
asphyxiophilia 832, *833*
aspirin, drug interactions 1232
assertive community treatment (ACT) 1402
  in alcohol use disorders 462
  in schizophrenia 584
assertive outreach teams 1455, 1457–8, *1457*
assessment
  acute stress reactions 695
  adolescent antisocial behaviour
      1947–8, *1949*
  alcohol use 442, 448
  alcohol use disorders 448
  Alzheimer's disease 92, 265–6, 337, 1240
  anxiety, in childhood and adolescence 1665
  anxiety disorders 1289, *1289*, 1665
  attention 60, 88–9, 264–5
  attention-deficit hyperactivity disorder 1645,
      1782–3
  behavioural methods 94, 96–7, *96*
  benzodiazepine misuse/dependence 492
  bereavement 726–7
  bulimia nervosa 807
  by community mental health teams 1455
  and categories of information 63
  character 80–1, *80*, 82–3
  in childhood and adolescence 90, **1600–6**
    content of the clinical interview
        1600–1, *1602*
    developmentally sensitive
        techniques 1601, 1604–5
    laboratory tests 1605–6, *1605*
    mood disorders 1675
    need for multiple informants 1600
    structure of the clinical interview 1601,
        1603–4, *1603*
  concentration 60, 88–9
  and concepts of disablement 65
  and the concepts of disease, illness and
      sickness 63–4
  concepts underlying procedures 63–7
  condensation and recording of
      information 73–4
  conduct disorder 1657, 1781–2
  and confidentiality 67
  in consultation-liaison psychiatry 1146
  contextual influences 67
  and culture 67
  depression 660
  and diagnoses 74
  and the diagnostic process 64–5

distinction between form and content of symptoms 63
elderly people **1524–9**
 after treatment 1528–9
 history-taking 1526
 mental state examination 1526–7, *1528*
 physical 1527–9
 setting for 1525–7
formulation 73–4
from complaint to formulation 66, *66*
general ability 87, *88*
instruments *see* assessment instruments
intellectual disability 1821–3
intelligence 22, 54, 87, *88*, 263–4
and life events 66–7
mania 1675
memory 89, *89*, 253, 254, 255–6, 264, 420–1, *420*
mental health services **1463–72**
mild cognitive impairment 1536
as a multi-disciplinary activity 62, 68
obsessive–compulsive disorder 1783
offenders with mental disorder 2011–12, 2018
personality 72–3, **78–85**, 286, 1164–5
personality disorders 858–9, *858*
principles in general psychiatry **62–78**
privacy of interviewing 67
and prognosis 74
and psychodynamics 67
psychometric 85–7
psychophysiological methods 97
refugees 1496–7
and reviews 74
sequence of 66
sleep-wake disorders 929–30
 in childhood and adolescence 1696–7, *1696*
somatization disorder 1005–6, *1005*
summary 73–4
temperament 79–80, *80*
urgent 68
use of interpreters 67
and written reports 74–6
*see also* cognitive assessment; needs, assessment; neuropsychological assessment
Assessment and Reduction of Psychiatric Disability 572
assessment instruments **69–73**
acute stress reactions 695
administration 95–6
alcohol use disorders 1484, 1542
anorexia nervosa 777
anxiety 1164
behavioural 94, 96–7, *96*
behavioural and psychological symptoms in dementia 413
'bottom-up' organization 71
in childhood and adolescence 1591
 with intellectual disability 1860
cognitive and neuropsychological functioning 87–9, *88*, *89*, *90*, 263–7
comprehensive 73
computer-based 70, 263
content and format 95, *95*
contents of a good test manual *87*
and context 268
creation 96
delirium 328
depression 69, 70, 1163–4, 1306, 1484, 1551, *1552*

developments since the 1950s 70–2
disablement 284
in epidemiology 284–6
evaluation criteria 95
in evaluation of psychotherapy 1163–5
of functioning 1165
information regarding 89
investigator-based 269
mental state and behaviour 69–70
multiaxial descriptive systems 73
multiple measures 96
needs 73, 94, 1433–4
in needs assessment 73, 1433
for negative symptoms 72
numeric analogue scales 1032
for personality 72–3, 81–2, *81*
personality disorders 858–9, *858*
post-traumatic stress disorder 703
psychometric adequacy 95
psychopathology 1164
psychoses 1164
purpose of 94
quality of life 73, 1165
for quantification of clinical outcome 73
questionnaires **94–8**
rating scales **94–8**
reasons for development of structured interviewing and rating scales 69
response coding 97
for risk 1994, 1996–7
screening 69
self-esteem 1164
sensitivity and specificity 140–1, 284
service utilization 1165
standard vs. individualized 97
standardized interview schedules 14, 284
substance use disorders 1164
'top-down' organization 71
understanding and choice of 89–90
usefulness 1595
validity 140–1, 284
verbal descriptor scales 1033
visual analogue scales 1032
*see also specific instruments*
assisted reproduction 1114–15
association therapy 836–7
associative learning 258, 696
asthma 1082
 brittle 1050
 and sleep-wake disorders *932*
astroglia 157
astrology 1420
Asylum Act 1828 19
asylums 17–18, 18–19, 22, 24
*ataques de nervios* 983–4
ataxia
 cerebellar, in alcohol use disorders 445
 in HIV-associated dementia 384
atmosphere, delusional 51
atomoxetine 1688, 1795–6
 adverse effects 1795
 in attention-deficit hyperactivity disorder 1241, 1648, 1650
 and epilepsy 1650
 precautions with 1795
 suicidal risk 1796
ATP (Adolescent Transitions Program) 1790
ATP receptors *173*
attachment theory 242–3, *242*, 285, **309–10**, 1725

and child abuse 1735
and child neglect 1736
and conduct disorder 1659
and generalized anxiety disorder 734
internal working model (IWM) 243
and mentalization 1948
mother–infant 1123–4
and neuropeptides 888
and offending 1910
prenatal 1116–17
and psychopathology 243
secure/insecure attachment 242, *242*, 309–10, 1725
and separation 1758
and stalking 1972
and transference 1342–3
attention **245–9**
assessment 60, 88–9, 264–5
in attention-deficit hyperactivity disorder 1643
brain regions involved *246*
deficit 60
and delirium 325, 326
and depression 92
disorders of 60
divided 247–8
effects of disturbed sleep 926
and emotion 259
executive control 248–9, *248*
following head injury 390
phasic 247
selective 60, 245–7, 264, 1288
shared 60
in somatization disorder 1005
sustained 247, 264
vigilant 59, 247, 264
attention-deficit hyperactivity disorder (ADHD) 60, 1613, **1643–54**
in adult life 1647–8, 1652
aetiology 1646–7
assessment 1645, 1782–3
classification 1643
clinical features 1643
comorbidity 427, 646, 1073, 1644, 1650, 1673, 1682, 1931
course and prognosis 1647–8
diagnosis 1643–5, 1849
differential diagnosis 1644–5, 1657, 1671
epidemiology 1645–6
and gender 1646, 1828
genetics 1590, 1646
hyperactive/impulsive subtype 266
and intellectual disability 1850–1, 1876
and juvenile delinquency 1948–9
legitimacy of diagnosis 28
neuropsychological assessment 266
and offending 1931
pathogenesis 1647
prisoners 1931
refractory 1651–2
relationship with antisocial personality disorder 1931
and sleep-wake disorders 927, *931*, 1695, 1697
and speech and language disorder/difficulty 1714
and stigma 1651
treatment and management 1241–2, 1648–52, 1782–3, 1876
attentional blink paradigm 247
attributional style 653

atypical schizophrenic disorder 866
AUDIT (Alcohol Use Disorders Identification
    Test) 284, 460, 1542
audit of consultation-liaison psychiatric
    services 1147
AUDs *see* alcohol use disorders
aura 60, 1077
Australia, neurasthenia as diagnostic entity 1061
autism **1633–6**
    aetiology 227, 1635–6
    atypical 1639
    classification 1623
    clinical features 1633
    comorbidity 1852
    course 1635
    definition 1633–4, *1634*
    demographics 1634–5
    differential diagnosis 865, 1639, 1644–5, 1657
    and Down syndrome 1839
    epidemiology 1634–5
    and epilepsy 1852
    and fragile-X syndrome 1635
    and gender 1828
    genetics 1635–6
    and intellectual disability 1852, 1855
    and juvenile delinquency 1950
    and offending 1921
    and parental psychiatric disorder 1885
    prevention 1640
    prognosis 1635
    and sleep disorder 1697
    and specific language impairment 1713
    treatment and management 1639–40, 1875
    and tuberous sclerosis 1075, 1635
Autobiographical Memory Interview 89
autoerotic asphyxia 1703
autogynephiles 844
automatic behaviour in sleep-wake
    disorders 926, 928, 940, 945
    legal issues 948–9
automatic obedience 58
automatic thoughts *see* negative automatic
    thoughts
Automatic Thoughts Questionnaire 1165
automatism
    and epilepsy 403, 1077
    'insane' 405, 1901
    'sane' 405
    violent 1930
autonomic failure with syncope and orthostatic
    hypotension 361
autonomy, legal aspects 1895–900
autoprosopagnosia in Alzheimer's disease 334
autoscopy 56
autosomal dominant disorders 212, 1831
autosomal recessive disorders 212, 1831
*Avena sativa* 1248
avoidance 1287–8
    in chronic fatigue syndrome 1039
    following an accident 1107
    and hypothalamic–pituitary–adrenal axis 658
    in obsessive–compulsive disorder 768
    and pain-related fears 1033
    in panic disorder 751
    and phobias 745
avoidant personality disorder **872–3**
    aetiology 872
    classification *856*, 872, *872*
    clinical features 872
    course 872

differential diagnosis 862, 863, 865, 873
    in elderly people 1562, *1562*
    epidemiology 872, *882*, 883
    and social anxiety disorder 740, 897
    terminology 856
    treatment 873, 897, 898
AVON Mental Health Measure 1434
awareness of activity, disorder of 56
awareness of singleness, disorder of 56
ayahuasca 488, 501
azapirones 735
azoospermia 1114
azotaemia 1087

Babinski reflex 158
Baby X experiments 1719
BAC (blood alcohol concentration) 442, 448
*bah-tsche* 983
Bali, attitudes to psychiatric disorder 7
Balint, Michael 308–9, 313
*Banisteriopsis* (ayahuasca) 488, 501
barbiturates 1178
    addictiveness *431*
    duration of action 1178
    history of 1178
    *see also specific drugs*
basal ganglia 154–5, *154*
    in alcohol use disorders *183*
    and memory 254
    in obsessive–compulsive disorder 1684
    in schizophrenia *178*
    in tic disorders 1684
basic assumption theory 1353, 1356
'battered child syndrome' 1734–5
Bayley Developmental Scale 1821
BDD *see* body dysmorphic disorder
BDI (Beck Depression Inventory) 719, 1163–4,
    1306, 1486, 1675
BDNF (brain-derived neurotrophic factor) *160*,
    171, 225, 652, 966, 1199, 1201, 1674, 1684
BDQ (Brief Disability Questionnaire) 284
'BDSM' sexual activities 832–3
BDT (brief dynamic therapy) 720
'Beating the Blues' 1485
Bech-Rafaelsen Mania Scale 1164
Beck, A.T. 1304
Beck Anxiety Inventory 1164
Beck Depression Inventory 719, 1163–4, 1306,
    1486, 1675
Beck Self-Concept Test 1164
Bedford College Life Events and Difficulties
    Schedule 1065
Beers, Clifford 22
behaviour
    assessment instruments 69–70
    and the unconscious 313
behaviour modification
    in attention-deficit hyperactivity disorder 1649
    in autism and other pervasive developmental
        disorders 1640
    in children and adolescents with psychiatric/
        behaviour disorder and intellectual
        disability 1852
behaviour therapy
    in agitation and challenging behaviour in
        dementia 413–14
    attention-deficit hyperactivity disorder 1648
    in children and adolescents with intellectual
        disability and psychiatric/behavioural
        disorder 1852

depression 15
    history of 23
    nicotine dependence 512
    obsessive–compulsive disorder 770
    panic disorder 758
    with sex offenders 1963
    trichotillomania 915
    *see also* cognitive-behaviour therapy;
        exposure
behavioural activation in depression in elderly
    people 1555
behavioural and psychological symptoms in
    dementia 412–17, *413*, *414*
Behavioural Assessment of the Dysexecutive
    Syndrome 93
behavioural experiments in anxiety
    disorders *1294*, *1295*
behavioural factors influencing health 1135–7
behavioural inhibition 1667
    and generalized anxiety disorder 733, *733*
    and panic disorder 754, 762
Behavioural Pathology in Alzheimer's
    Disease 413
behavioural phenotypes 1592, 1838, 1850,
    *1851*, 1858
    foetal alcohol syndrome 1614–15
    neurogenetic syndromes 1613–14
behavioural programmes in intellectual
    disability 1874
behaviourally-induced insufficient sleep
    syndrome 939
behaviourism 133–4
    and personality 849
Benedict, Ruth 276
benefit-finding 1066
benefits, measurement of 1475
benzhexol 1532
benzodiazepine receptor agonists (BzRAs) 934
    in insomnia 935
    partial 1181–2
benzodiazepine receptors 1171, 1179
    in generalized anxiety disorder 733, *734*
benzodiazepines
    in acute and transient psychotic disorders 607
    addictiveness *431*
    adverse effects 934, 939, 1180, 1183
    in alcohol withdrawal 449, *449*, 1542
    antiepileptic properties 1080, 1231
    as anxiolytics 1178, 1179–80
    in bipolar disorder 677
    in breastfeeding 1121, 1180
    in cancer 1101–2, *1102*, *1104*
    cross-tolerance 491
    in delirium 331, 1533
    in dementia 415
    development 1178
    effects on memory 409, 1179
    in generalized anxiety disorder 735
    in Huntington's disease 374
    as hypnotics 1179, 1182–3
    indications 1179–80
    in insomnia 934
    long-term use 1179
    in management of antipsychotic adverse
        effects 1226
    management of withdrawal 1181, *1181*
    misuse/dependence **490–3**, 1182
        with alcohol dependence 492
        assessment 492
        by injection 491

cross-dependence 491
dependence at therapeutic doses 491,
 1180–1, 1183
and drug formulation 430
elderly people 1543
epidemiology 490–1
management 491–2
with opiate abuse 492–3
patterns of use 490–1
potential for 491
overdose 1180
in panic disorder 756–7, *756*
pharmacodynamics 1171
pharmacokinetics *1172*, 1178–9
pharmacology 1179
in postoperative delirium 1099
in post-traumatic stress disorder 710
in pregnancy 762, 1117, 1180
preoperative 1097
prescriptions 492
in schizophrenia 591–2
in social anxiety disorder 743, 744
in specific phobia 746
in status epilepticus 1867
in terminal illness 1070
tolerance to 1179, 1180–1
benztropine 1225
bereavement **724–8**
after infant loss 725, 1120
assessment 726–7
in childhood and adolescence 235, **1758–60**
and depression 725
factors affecting course and outcome 725–6
in intellectual disability 1881
management 726–7
neurobiology 725
phenomenology of 'normal grief' 725
physical and mental health consequences 726
violent traumatic 1985
*see also* grief
Bergmann glia 158
beri-beri in anorexia nervosa 785
β-adrenergic stimulants *730*
β-amyloid protein
in Alzheimer's disease 338
in dementia with Lewy bodies 362
in mild cognitive impairment 1537
β-arrestins 175
β-blockers
adverse effects 827
in anxiety disorders 1182
in children and adolescents with psychiatric/
 behaviour disorder and intellectual
 disability 1852
in intellectual disability 1876
in management of antipsychotic adverse
 effects 1226
in social anxiety disorder 743
in specific phobia 746
β-crystalin 362
β-endorphin 170, *171*
β-secretase 338
*Better Services for the Mentally Ill* 24
biastophilia *833*
bifeprunox 1209
bilateral frontal lobotomy 1267
Binet–Simon scale 22
binge eating disorder 800, *801*, 1299
Binswanger's disease 377
bioavailability 1170

biofeedback in persistent somatoform pain
 disorder 1034
biomarkers in Alzheimer's disease 341
Bion, Wilfred 308, 1353, 1355
biopsychosocial model 64, 207, *208*, *433*,
 990, *991*
biperiden 1225
bipolar disorder
 age of onset 665
 anticipation in 652
 biphasic episodes 665
 childhood and adolescence
  aetiology 1674
  assessment and monitoring 1675
  course 1673–4
  diagnostic criteria 1671, *1672*
  differential diagnosis 1645, 1657, 1671–3
  environmental risk factors 1675
  epidemiology 1673–4
  neurocognitive factors 1675
  treatment and prevention 1676–7
 classification 639–40, 643, *643*
 comorbidity 645, 646
 course 665–6
 and cyclothymia/cyclothymic disorder 688
 definition of bipolar 638
 diagnosis 645–6
 differential diagnosis 866, 868, 871
 duration of episodes 665
 elderly people 1556–7
 epidemiology 645–7, 650–1
 genetics **650–8**
 global disease burden 645
 history of concept 631
 hyperthymic 638
 and intellectual disability 1827, 1854–5
 late-onset 665
 mixed states 636, 638
 mortality associated 666
 outcome 666
 overlap with other disorders 645
 overlap with schizophrenia for
  susceptibility 652
 patient state fluctuations within 632–3,
  *632*, *633*
 pharmacogenetics 653
 in pregnancy 677
 prevalence 646
 prisoners *1934*
 psychosocial factors 653
 psychotic 665
 rapid cycling 636, 668, 677
 recurrence 665–6
 risk factors 646, 1675
 social functioning in 653
 subtypes 631, 638, 643, 665
 and suicide 1704
 and surgery 1098
 treatment
  acute 671
  continuation 677
  and course 667
  electroconvulsive therapy 1253–4
  interpersonal and social rhythm
   therapy 1323
  long-term 678
  maintenance 671–2, 677
  management of 677–8
  neurosurgery 1268
  psychotherapy 673

treatment gap *13*
and use of mental health services 646
bipolar spectrum 680
birth certificate, change of sex on 845
birth season and schizophrenia 547, 556
birth weight
 and HPA function 659
 and schizophrenia 548
blackouts, alcoholic 404, 443
Bleuler, Eugen 522, 531, 603, 631, 1546–7
blindness, hysterical 1017
blood alcohol concentration 442, 448
blood transfusion and Creutzfeldt–Jakob
 disease transmission 355, 356, 358
BMI *see* body mass index
BMP (bone morphogenetic protein) 156
bodily distress disorder 1000, *1000*, 1003
 epidemiology 1003, 1004
bodily preoccupation
 in body dysmorphic disorder 1043–4
 in hypochondriasis 1022
body, dislike of 57
body awareness disorders 57
body dysmorphic disorder (BDD) 57, **1043–9**
 association with aggression and
  violence 1044
 childhood and adolescence 1045
 classification 1022, 1045
 clinical features 1043–5
 comorbidity 1044–5
 course 1046
 cross-cultural aspects 1045
 delusional 618, 1044, 1045
 diagnosis 1045–6, *1045*
 epidemiology 1046
 and gender 1045
 and hypochondriasis 1045
 non-delusional ˙1045
 and obsessive–compulsive disorder 1044,
  1045
 pathogenesis 1046
 and pregnancy 1116
 prevalence 997–8, *998*
 prevention 1048
 prognosis 1046
 puerperal 1120
 and requests for cosmetic treatment
  1046, 1096
 and suicidality 1044
 treatment and management 1046–8
body image
 distortion 57
 disturbance 783
 and eating disorder 57
 organic changes in 57
body mass index (BMI) 784
 in anorexia nervosa 784, 794
 and depression 1674
body weight
 in anorexia nervosa 782, 784
 in bulimia nervosa 803, 804
Bolam test 1902, 1905
bone morphogenetic protein 156
bonobo 812
*Borago officinalis* (borage) 1248
borderline personality disorder **866–8**
 aetiology 867
 and bulimia nervosa 803, 804
 childhood and adolescence 1673
 classification *856*, 867, *867*

borderline personality disorder (*cont.*)
  clinical features 867–8
  comorbidity 868, 884, 902
  course and outcome 868, 892
  and deception 1049
  diagnosis 867–8
  differential diagnosis 682, 865, 866, 868,
    871, 874
  elderly people *1562, 1563*
  epidemiology 867, *882*, 883
  following head injury 391
  treatment 318–19, 868, 894–7, 898, 902, 903,
    904, 905–6, *905*, 1364–5
borderline personality organization 867
boredom and substance use disorders 427
*Borrelia burgdorferi* 1094–5
Boston Diagnostic Aphasia Examination 89
Boston Naming Test 89
Botswana, life expectancy 1507
*bouffée délirante* 603, 604, 606
  with symptoms of schizophrenia 605
boundaries of self, awareness of 56
boundary violation 1338
bovine spongiform encephalopathy
    351, 352, 355
Bowlby, John 242, 309–10, 1725
boxing 395
BPSDs (behavioural and psychological
    symptoms in dementia) 412–17, *413, 414*
Brachman-de Lange syndrome *see* de Lange
    syndrome
brachycephaly 1839
bradyphasia 53
bradyphrenia in brain tumour 1075
brain
  activation during sexual arousal 819
  alcohol-related damage 182–3, **399–402**,
    444, 1541
  anatomy **144–56**
  in anorexia nervosa 781
  anoxia 1091
  applications of PET 187–8
  in autism 1636
  congenital anomalies 538
  in delusional disorder 614
  in delusional misidentification
      syndrome 623–4
  development 156–7, *157*
  effects of substance use disorders 429–30, *429*
  fear and anxiety circuit 754–5
  glucose metabolism 187–8
  hemispheric shape and formation of gyri 159
  histogenesis 158–9
  hypoperfusion in depression 660
  injury *see* head injury
  ischaemia 387
  magnetization 191
  mapping 187–8
  and mind **133–6**
    and psychodynamic psychiatry 315–16
  neural induction 156
  neuronal death 387
  neuronal networks 201–5
  in obsessive–compulsive disorder 768
  oedema 387, 1084–5
  pathology *see* neuropathology
  regional blood flow 187–8
    in chronic fatigue syndrome 1039
    in frontotemporal dementia 347, Plate 12
    and neural activity 197

  regions involved in attention *246*
  reward circuit 430
  in schizophrenia 562–4, *563*
  tumours 407, 942, 1075, 1929
  in vascular dementia 376
  visual areas *147*, 152
  *see also specific areas*
brain-derived neurotrophic factor *160*, 171,
    225, 652, 966, 1199, 1201, 1674, 1684
brain fag syndrome 982–3
brain slices 202–3
brainstem 150–1
  in alcohol use disorders *183*
  histogenesis 158
  in mood disorders *182*
  in schizophrenia *178*
Brazil, attitudes to psychiatric disorder 6
breastfeeding 1120
  and opioid use 480
  pharmacotherapy 1123
    antidepressants 675
    benzodiazepines 1121, 1170
    dosage regimens 1169–70
breathing retraining in panic disorder 761
breeder effect 549
bremelanotide in sexual dysfunction 828
Brief Cognitive Rating Scale 1240
Brief Disability Questionnaire 284
brief dynamic therapy 720
brief focal psychotherapy 1327, 1330–1, *1331*
Brief Psychiatric Rating Scale 70, 524, 1164
brief psychodynamic psychotherapy
    *see* psychodynamic psychotherapy, brief
    (short-term)
brief psychotic disorder 606, 695
brief reactive psychosis 870
brief solution-focused therapy 1276
brief supportive therapy 720
Brief Symptom Inventory 1164
bright light therapy in dementia *414*
Briquet's syndrome 999
British Crime Survey 1984
Brixton Test *90*
broad-focus short-term dynamic
    psychotherapy 1333
Broca's area 144, 146, 153, *153*
Broca's dysphasia 1527
brofaromine
  adverse effects *1191*
  dosage *1196*
  pharmacodynamics *1187*, 1188
  pharmacokinetics *1189*
  in social anxiety disorder 743
bromides 1178
4-bromo-2,5-dimethoxyphenethylamine 501
bronchodilators *730*, 1101
brucellosis 1095
BSE (bovine spongiform encephalopathy)
    351, 352, 355
BST (brief supportive therapy) 720
Building Bridges project 1411
bulbo-urethral gland 817
bulimia nervosa **800–11**
  aetiology 805–7
  anxiety in 803
  assessment 807
  attitudes to shape and weight 803
  binge eating in 801–2
  and child sexual abuse 780
  childhood and adolescence 1784

  classification and diagnosis 800–1, *801*
  clinical features 801–4
  course and outcome 809
  depression in 803, 804
  development 805
  and diabetes mellitus 804
  dieting in 801–2
  epidemiology 804–5, *805*
  general psychopathology 803–4
  genetics 806
  impulse control problems in 803
  maintaining factors 807, 1299
  neurobiology 806–7
  and obesity 804
  origins of the concept 800
  overlap with anorexia nervosa 800, *801*
  perfectionism in 804, 806
  and personality disorder 803, 884
  physical features 804
  and pregnancy 1118
  purging/non-purging 802–3
  relationship with other eating disorders 804
  risk factors 805–6, *806*
  self-esteem in 804, 806
  and substance use disorders 804, 806
  treatment and management 807–9, 1193–4,
    1298–303, 1323–4, 1784
  weight control methods 802–3
buprenorphine 475, **1244**
  detoxification 476–7
  maintenance treatment 476, 479
  metabolism 473
  in pregnancy 1118
  prescription 479
  in substance use disorders 429–30
bupropion *670*, 671
  adverse effects 1190–1, *1191*
  in body dysmorphic disorder 1047
  in cancer *1103*
  in childhood and adolescence 1676
  dosage 1195, *1196*
  in panic disorder 757
  pharmacodynamics *1187*, 1188
  pharmacokinetics 1189, *1189*
  in smoking cessation 512
burglary, victims of 1986
burns *see* accidents
Burton, Richard, *Anatomy of Melancholy*
    629–30, *630*
buspirone 1178, 1181, 1212
  in body dysmorphic disorder 1047
  in children and adolescents with psychiatric/
      behaviour disorder and intellectual
      disability 1852
  in generalized anxiety disorder 735, 737
  in panic disorder 757
  pharmacodynamics 1172
  in social anxiety disorder 743
Butler Report 2015
butobarbitone 1178
butyrophenones in pregnancy 1118
BzRAs *see* benzodiazepine receptor agonists
2C-B 501
2C-T2 501

CACE estimation 142
caffeine, addictiveness *431*
CAGE 1519, 1542
Cajal–Retzius cells *148*, 158
calcitonin gene-related peptide 206

calcium carbimide 453
calcium-channel blockers, L-type 1200–1, 1201, 1203, *1203*
    *see also* nimodipine
California Verbal Learning Test 253, 264
calorie restriction and modification of ageing 1509
CAM (Confusion Assessment Method) 328, 1531
Camberwell Assessment of Need 94, 1434
Camberwell Family Interview 268
Cambridge Mental Disorders of the Elderly Examination 336
Cambridge Neuropsychological Test Automated Battery 255, 263
Cambridge–Somerville Study 1910
Cambridge Study in Delinquent Development 1908, 1909, 1910, 1911, 1912, 1912–13
CAMDEX 336
CAMHS *see* mental health services, child and adolescent
cAMP (cyclic adenosine monophosphate) 175
Camphill communities 1392
CAN (Camberwell Assessment of Need) 94, 1434
Canada, attitudes to psychiatric disorder 6
cancer **1100–5**
    and alcohol consumption 446
    and anxiety 1101–2, *1101*
    childhood and adolescence 1743
    delirium in 1103–4, *1104*
    fatigue in 209, *210*
    and mood disorders 649, 1102, *1102*, *1103*
    parental, effects on child development 1754–5
    and suicide 1102–3
candidiasis, systemic 997
cannabinoids
    addictiveness *431*
    endogenous 429
    receptors *173*, 1171
cannabis **507–10**, 515
    acute psychological effects 507
    amotivational syndrome associated 508
    behavioural effects in adolescence 508
    chronic psychological effects 507
    cognitive effects 92, 507–8
    dependence 507
    and flashbacks 508
    patterns of use 507
    in pregnancy 1117
    psychosis 507, 538
    and schizophrenia 507, 546
cannibalism 351, 354
CANTAB (Cambridge Neuropsychological Test Automated Battery) 255, 263
CANTAB Paired Associate Learning test 264, 266
CANTOUs 1583
capacity
    and cognitive assessment 90–1
    and consent to surgery 1096–7
    Council of Europe Principles Concerning the Legal Protection of Incapable Adults 1896
    elderly people 1577
    following head injury 397
    independent advocate 1898
    and juvenile delinquency 1954–5

lack of 1898–9
    legal aspects 1895–900
    tests of 1897
Capgras syndrome 335, 392, 610, 623
CAPS (Clinician Administered PTSD Scale) 703
Caracas Declaration 1427
carbamazepine 1198, 1200, **1233–5**
    adverse effects *1200*, 1204, 1233–4, 1867–8
    in bipolar disorder 671, 672
    in childhood and adolescence 1677
    choice of 1866
    in dementia 415
    dosage and administration *1233*, 1234–5
    drug interactions 1175, 1205–6, 1232, 1234, *1234*, 1866
    indications and contraindications 1234
    mechanism of action *1200*
    monitoring therapy 1176
    overdose 1234
    in personality disorders *905*
    pharmacokinetics 1203, 1233, *1867*
    pharmacology 1201, *1202*, *1203*, 1233
    in pregnancy 1118, 1234
    response correlates *1199*
    in schizophrenia 591
    structure *1232*
    therapeutic profile *1199*
    withdrawal 1206–7, 1234
carbon monoxide poisoning 406–7, 973
carcinoid tumours 1101
card-sorting games 1778
'cardiac invalidism'/'cardiac neurosis' 1025, 1138, 1559
cardiac myopathy in alcohol use disorders 446
Cardinal Needs Schedule 1434
cardiovascular disease 1081–2
    in alcohol use disorders 446
    and sleep-wake disorders *932*
cardiovascular system, in chronic fatigue syndrome 1038
care management, in mental health social work 1410–11
care programme approach (CPA)
    in community mental health services 1455, *1456*, *1457*
    to manage risk of homicide 1939
    in services for people with intellectual disability 1888
caregiver-mediated interventions **1787–93**
    adolescents 1790
    background 1787
    mediators of efficacy 1790–1
    pre-natal and early childhood 1787–8
    preschool years 1788–9
    school-aged children 1789–90
carers
    in Alzheimer's disease 339
    burdens on 1401
    in dementia 417–18
    effects of personality change following head injury 391
    of elderly people with intellectual disability 1880–1
    impact of caring on 1465
    of people with alcohol use disorders 452–3, 465
    role in treatment of intellectual disability 1873
Carers and Users Experience of Services 1434
cargo-cult syndrome 982
CARITAS principles 1580

Cartesian dualism 133, 989
CAS (childhood apraxia of speech) 1712
case ascertainment 283
case-control studies 282
case-finding 541
case management 584, 1402, 1455
castration
    chemical 838
    and libido 815–16
    surgical 838
castration anxiety 294
CAT *see* cognitive analytical therapy
CAT (community alcohol team) model 461
catalepsy 58, *58*
cataplexy
    misdiagnosis 928
    with narcolepsy 940–1
catastrophizing 1137–8
catatonia 58
    elderly people 1531
    excited 529
    malignant 529, 1254
    retarded 529
    in schizophrenia 529
    treatment 1254
catecholamines
    in cocaine use 485
    and depression 1185, *1185*
    effects on memory 409
    in methamphetamine use 497
    in post-traumatic stress disorder 706
category fallacy 276
Catherine of Siena, St 777
caudate nucleus 154, 159, 1684
CBD *see* corticobasal degeneration
CBGT (cognitive-behavioural group therapy) 742, 744
CBT *see* cognitive-behaviour therapy
CD *see* conversion disorder
CDCS *see* cri-du-chat syndrome
CDR (Clinical Dementia Rating) scale 1535
CDRPs (Crime and Disorder Reduction Partnerships) 515
CDRS-R (Children's Depression Rating Scale, Revised) 1675
CEA *see* cost-effectiveness analysis
CEACs (cost-effectiveness acceptability curves) 1475, *1475*
Center for Epidemiologic Studies Depression Scale 284, 1675
central nervous system
    malformations leading to intellectual disability 1832
    neural induction 156
    organogenesis 156–7, *157*
central pontine myelinolysis 445
central sleep apnoea 1083
central state materialism 134
central sulcus 144–5
centromeres 223
cephalic flexure 156
CER *see* control event rate; cost-effectiveness ratio
CERAD (Consortium to Establish a Registry for AD) 336
cerebellum 155
    in alcohol use disorders *183*
    development 157, *157*
    effects of alcohol use disorders 445
    histogenesis 158

cerebellum (*cont.*)
  and memory 254
  in mood disorders *182*
  in schizophrenia *178*
cerebral contusions 387, *388*, 389
cerebral cortex
  association pathways for hearing *147, 152*
  association pathways for somatic
      sensation *146, 152*
  association pathways for vision *147, 152*
  commissural connections 151
  effects of alcohol use disorders 444
  general connectivity pattern 149–50, *149*
  histogenesis 158–9, *159*
  olfactory pathways to *147, 152*
  speech areas 153, *153*
  structure and organization 144–8, *145,
      146, 147*
  subcortical afferents to 150–3, *153*, Plate 2
  subcortical efferent pathways 154–6, *154*
cerebral palsy 1740
cerebrasthenia 1060
cerebrospinal fluid 157
  in anorexia nervosa 782
  in frontotemporal dementias 347
  in HIV-associated dementia 385
  in mild cognitive impairment 1538
cerebrovascular disease
  and amnesia 407
  and vascular dementia 366, 378, *378*
cervical flexure 156
CES-D (Center for Epidemiologic Studies
      Depression Scale) 284, 1675
CFS *see* chronic fatigue syndrome
CGA (common geriatric assessment) 1581
CGRP (calcitonin gene-related peptide) 206
challenging behaviour in dementia 413–15
Change for Children Programme 1946
character 79
  analysis 299–300
  assessment 80–1, *80*, 82–3
  definition 847
  development *84*
  dimensions 80–1, *80*, 316
  and personality 316–17
  psychoanalytic approaches 295–6
Charcot, Jean-Martin 20–1
Charles Bonnet syndrome 1531
'chasing the dragon' 473
chemokines *168*, 171
chemotherapy, anticipatory disorders 1101
*chien* 1420
child abuse and neglect **1731–9**
  and adoption outcome 1750
  characteristics of abused child 1734, 1736
  characteristics of abusers 1734–5, 1736,
      1736–7
  and chronic pain 1033
  and conduct disorder 1660
  emergency presentation 1810
  epidemiology 1732
  and factitious disorder 1051
  false and recovered memories 713–15
  and filicide 1125
  and hypochondriasis 1025
  induced factitious disorder 1054, 1697, 1737,
      1923–4
  and mental health social work 1409
  and mood disorders 1675
  neglect 1735–6

and offending 1910
  physical abuse 1734–5
  prevention 1737–8, 1788
  psychodynamic theories 316
  psychological maltreatment (emotional
      abuse) 1736–7
  role in aetiology of psychiatric disorder 286
  treatment and management 1738
child and adolescent mental health services
      *see* mental health services, child and
      adolescent
Child Behaviour Checklist 1718
child-care 1727
child guidance movement 1381
child molesting (paedophilia) 832, *833, 836*,
      1960–1, 1962
child pornography 1961
child protection
  and psychiatric reports 75
  role of school 1814
Child PTSD Symptom scale 1730
child sexual abuse
  aetiological factors 1733
  characteristics of abused child 1733
  characteristics of abusers 1733
  clinical features 1732
  course and prognosis 1733, *1734*
  definition 1732
  diagnosis 1732–3
  and eating disorders 780
  false accusations 834
  false and recovered memories 713–14, 834
  prevalence 1960
  and sexual dysfunction 825
  within-family 1733
childbirth 1118–20
  post-traumatic stress disorder
      following 1121
  querulant reactions to 1121
childhood and adolescence
  acute behavioural disturbance 1810
  acute stress disorder 1729
  adjustment disorders 721–3
      after diagnosis of physical illness
          1741, 1742
      diagnostic criteria 1669–71, *1671*
  adolescents 1945
      interviewing 1601
  adverse experiences 271–2, 1724
      and borderline personality disorder 867
      and mood disorders 648, 658–9
      and panic disorder 754, 762
  aggression, severe maladaptive 1798
  alcohol use disorders 456, 464
  antisocial behaviour 1654, **1945–59**
  anxiety
      assessment 1665
      with intellectual disability 1851–2
      with physical illness 1742–3
  anxiety disorders **1664–9**
      assessment 1665
      clinical course 1666
      clinical presentation 1665–6
      comorbidity 1666, 1673
      differential diagnosis 1671
      epidemiology 1665–6
      pathophysiology 1666–8, *1667*
      treatment 1668, 1779–80
  art therapy 1414
  assessment 90, **1600–6**

content of the clinical interview
      1600–1, *1602*
  developmentally sensitive
      techniques 1601, 1604–5
  laboratory tests 1605–6, *1605*
  mood disorders 1675
  need for multiple informants 1600
  structure of the clinical interview 1601,
      1603–4, *1603*
'at risk' children 1803
behavioural effects of cannabis in
      adolescence 508
bereavement 235, **1758–60**
bipolar disorder
  aetiology 1674
  assessment and monitoring 1675
  course 1673–4
  diagnostic criteria 1671, *1672*
  differential diagnosis 1645, 1657
  environmental risk factors 1675
  epidemiology 1673–4
  neurocognitive factors 1675
  treatment and prevention 1676–7
body dysmorphic disorder 1045
borderline personality disorder 1673
cancer 1743
caregiver-mediated interventions **1787–93**
cerebral palsy 1740
chronic fatigue syndrome 1745–6, 1784
chronic renal failure 1741, 1743
classification 104, **1589–94**
cognitive assessment 90
cognitive-behaviour therapy 1767, **1777–86**
  anxiety disorders 1668, 1779–80
  attention-deficit hyperactivity
      disorder 1782–3
  chronic fatigue syndrome 1784
  conduct disorder 1781–2
  depression 1675–6, 1780–1
  eating disorders 1784
  failure to engage/respond 1779
  following attempted suicide 1707
  inclusion of cognitive component 1778–9
  non-organic pain 1784
  obsessive–compulsive disorder 1686–7,
      *1686*, 1783–4
  post-traumatic stress disorder 1784
  psychiatric/behaviour disorder with
      intellectual disability 1852
  substance abuse 1784
  technique and management 1778
  working with parents 1778–9
cognitive therapy 1610, 1767, 1783
comorbidity in 1591, 1600
confusional state 1742
conversion disorder 1745
counselling **1764–9**
  approaches to 1766–8
  measures of effectiveness and outcome 1769
  practical issues 1768
  in psychiatric/behaviour disorder and
      intellectual disability 1852
  supportive 1767
  training and supervision 1768–9
  treatment setting and process 1766
cross-gender behaviour 1718–19
cyclothymic disorder 1671, *1672*
cystic fibrosis 1743
definitions and terminology 1764–5
deliberate self-harm 972, 1601, 1703

depression
  acute management 1677
  aetiology 1674
  assessment and monitoring 1675, 1780–1
  course 1673
  diagnostic criteria 1669, *1670*
  differential diagnosis 1657, 1671–3
  double 1673
  environmental risk factors 1675
  epidemiology 1673–4
  minor 1669
  neurocognitive factors 1674–5
  neuroendocrine studies 1675
  sequelae 1674
  treatment and prevention 674–5, 1322,
      1668, 1675–6, 1780–1, 1794–5, 1796
developmental disorders 1591, *1591*
  *see also* specific developmental disorders
developmental history 1600–1, 1822
diabetes mellitus 1741
disruptive (externalizing) disorders 1591,
    *1591*, 1654
dysthymia/dysthymic disorder 683, 1669,
    *1670*, 1673
eating disorder
  atypical 787
  differential diagnosis 1672
  treatment 1784
  *see also specific eating disorders*
effects of parental mental/physical illness on
    development **1752–8**
electroconvulsive therapy 1256
emergencies in **1807–11**
emotional (internalizing) disorders 1591,
    *1591*, 1654
environmental factors affecting mental
    health **1724–8**
  child care 1727
  family 1725–7
  peers 1727
  schooling 1727
  social 1727–8
epidemiology of psychiatric disorders **1594–9**
epilepsy
  aetiology 1619–20
  classification 1619
  clinical features 1618–19
  course and prognosis 1618–19, 1620
  diagnosis 1619
  differential diagnosis 1619
  epidemiology 1619
  with intellectual disability *1861, 1863*, 1864
  management 1620
  prevention 1620
  psychiatric disorder associated 1740
  salient non-epileptic episodes *1861*
estimating the burden of psychiatric
    disorders 1595–6
factitious disorder in 1050
factors related to development of chronic
    pain 1033
factors related to development of
    hypochondriasis 1025
gender identity disorder **1718–23**
  aetiology 1719–20
  assessment 1721
  clinical features 1718–19
  epidemiology 1718
  longitudinal studies 1720–1
  and mental disorder 1721

treatment 1721–2
group therapy 1768
head injury 394–5, 1616–18
headache 1745
health promotion in 1610
Huntington's disease in 372–3
hypersexuality 1671
intellectual disability
  and antisocial behaviour 1946
  and anxiety 1851–2
  and bereavement 1759
  and depression 1852
  effects on family 1883–4
  prevalence 1878
  psychiatric and behaviour disorders
      associated **1849–53**, 1879
  special needs of adolescents 1878–80
  transition to adulthood 1878–9
interests/hobbies/talents 1601
juvenile delinquency *see* juvenile delinquency
and life events 1601
looked after children **1799–802**
mania *1670*–1, 1675, 1677
media exposure 1601
medical history 1601
mental health services *see* mental health
      services, child and adolescent (CAMHS)
mental status examination 1601, *1602*
mood disorders **1669–80**
  aetiology 1674
  clinical picture 1669–71, *1670, 1672*
  comorbidity 1673
  course 1673–4
  differential diagnosis 1657, 1671–3
  epidemiology 1673–4
  with intellectual disability 1852
  neurocognitive factors 1675
  sequelae 1674
  treatment and prevention 1675–7
natural emotional healing 1765–6
neuropsychiatric disorders **1612–22**
neuropsychological assessment 1590–1, 1605
obsessive–compulsive disorder 1613,
    **1680–93**
  aetiology 1683–5
  age of onset 1681
  classification 1682
  clinical features 1680–1
  comorbidity 1681–2
  course and prognosis 1685
  diagnosis 1682–3
  differential diagnosis 1682–3
  epidemiology 1683
  and gender 1681
  with intellectual disability 1852
  prevention 1690
  refractory 1688
  treatment 1685–90, *1686, 1687*, 1783–4
opioid dependence 480
pain in 1744–5
persistent somatoform pain disorder 1745
pharmacotherapy **1793–9**
  antidepressants 674–5, 1668, 1676,
      1794–5, 1796
  antipsychotics 1677, 1796–8, 1852
  atomoxetine 1795–6
  developmental issues 1794
  dosage regimens 1169
  mood stabilizers 1798, 1852
  as part of multimodal treatment 1793–4

with psychiatric/behaviour disorder and/or
      intellectual disability 1798, 1852
  rapid tranquillization 1798
  stimulants 1795
  symptom-based approach 1794
physical illness
  effects of psychiatric disorder on course
      and outcome 1744
  psychiatric disorder associated 1740–3
post-traumatic stress disorder 237–8,
    **1728–31**, 1741, 1744, 1759, 1784, 1851–2
prevention in 1606, 1609–11
psychodynamic psychotherapy **1769–77**
  background 1770
  classical technique 1770–1
  definition 1764
  efficacy 1773–4
  indications and contraindications 1772
  limitations 1774
  managing treatment 1772–3
  procedure selection 1772
  psychodynamic technique 1771–2
psychopathic personality 1950
psychoses
  differential diagnosis 1673
  and juvenile delinquency 1950
psychotherapy **1764–9, 1769–77**
  approaches to 1766–8
  confidentiality 1768
  consent for 1765
  and culture 1768
  differences from adult psychotherapy
      1765, *1765*
  ending 1768
  failure to attend 1768
  focus on past vs. focus on present 1767
  individual vs. group therapy 1768
  involvement of parents and school 1768
  limit-setting vs. free expression 1767
  measures of effectiveness and
      outcome 1769
  record-keeping 1768
  training and supervision 1768–9
  treatment setting 1766
rapid tranquillization 1798
reaction to death of a parent 1758–60
relationship between physical and mental
    health **1739–47**
residential care **1799–802**
role of child psychiatrist in schools and
    colleges **1811–16**
schizophrenia 1613
  differential diagnosis 1673
  risk factors for development 556–7
sleep disorders **1693–702**
  assessment 1696–7, *1696*
  developmental effects 1695
  effects on parenting and the family
      1694–5
  excessive daytime sleepiness
      1699–701, *1700*
  manifestations 1695
  misinterpretation 1695
  parasomnias 1701–2
  parental influences 1694
  patterns of occurrence 1695
  risk factors 1697–8
  sleeplessness 1698–9
  treatment and prognosis 1695–6
sleep physiology 1693–4

childhood and adolescence (*cont.*)
  social anxiety disorder 740, 1664, 1666
  social functioning 1593
  somatization and somatization disorder
      1744, *1744*
  special educational needs 1815
  specific phobia 1664, 1665, 1666, 1741, 1742
  speech and language disorder **1710–17**
  substance use disorders 1600, 1604
    comorbidity 1673
    differential diagnosis 1672
    treatment 1784
  suicide and attempted suicide 1674, **1702–10**
    aetiology 1705–6, *1705, 1706*
    assessment 1703–4
    associated diagnoses 1704
    clinical features 1703
    course and prognosis 1706
    epidemiology 1704–5
    prevention 1708–9
    treatment 1706–8
  temperament 235, 238, *238*, 1601, 1665, 1667
    in intellectual disability 1850
  terminal illness 1743–4
  therapeutic communities 1397
  tic disorders 1073, **1680–93**
    aetiology 1683–5
    age of onset 1681
    classification 1682
    clinical features 1681
    comorbidity 1681–2
    course and prognosis 1685
    diagnosis 1682–3
    differential diagnosis 1682–3
    epidemiology 1683
    and gender 1681
    prevention 1690
    treatment 1685–90
  Tourette syndrome 1613, 1680–93
  trauma in 1601, 1697, **1728–31**, 1744, 1762
  victims of criminal activity 1986–7
  wish for behavioural change in 1600
  witnesses, children as **1761–3**
childhood apraxia of speech 1712
childhood disintegrative disorder **1637**
Children Act 1989 1732
Children's Depression Inventory 1675, 1780
Children's Depression Rating Scale,
    Revised 1675
Children's Global Assessment scale 1593
Children's Memory Scale 89, *89*
Children's PTSD Inventory 1730
Children's Revised Impact of Events scale 1730
Children's Yale-Brown Obsessive-Compulsive
    Scale 1681
China
  attitudes to psychiatric disorder 6
  neurasthenia as diagnostic entity 1061, 1062
  and Pavlovian theory 1061
  psychiatric nurses in 1407
*Chinese Classification of Mental Disorders* 1062
Chinese traditional medicine 1249
chloral 1178
chloramphenicol 1091
chlordiazepoxide 1178
  in alcohol withdrawal 449, *449*
  pharmacokinetics *1172*
chlormethiazole *see* clomethiazole
  chlorpromazine 1209, *1209*, 1262
    administration 1213–14, *1214*

adverse effects *1212*, 1222
  in anxiety disorders 1182
  in cancer *1104*
  development 1208–9
  pharmacodynamics *1211*
  pharmacokinetics *1172*
cholecystokinins 171, *171*
  in generalized anxiety disorder 734
  in panic disorder 754
cholesterol and suicide 966
cholinergic anti-inflammatory pathway 206
cholinergic system
  and alcohol-related brain damage 400
  in Alzheimer's disease 338, 1240–1
  anticholinergic action at 1225
  antipsychotic actions on 1210, *1211*
  and cortical function 150, 151
  and delirium 330, 1532
  in depression 660
  effects of PCP on receptors 487
  in head injury 388
  and memory 253
  and neurotrophic factors *160*
  in schizophrenia 180
cholinesterase inhibitors
  in Alzheimer's disease 1240–1, 1538
  in dementia 415
  in dementia with Lewy bodies 366–7
  effects on memory 409
  in mild cognitive impairment 1538
  in vascular dementia 381
cholinomimetics in Alzheimer's disease 1241
chorea 371
chorea acanthocytosis 373
Christian religious healing 1420
chromatids 223
chromatin remodelling 225
chromosomes 218, 223
  anomalies 1831
  autosomal 218, 223
  rearrangements 228–9, 1831
  recombination 223, 226
  sex *see* sex chromosomes
  telomere loss 1508
chronic benign pain syndrome 1003
chronic cutaneous dysaesthesia 618
chronic fatigue syndrome (CFS) **1035–43**
  aetiology 1038–40, *1040*
  assessment 1040–1
  attribution to organic disease 1039
  case formulation 1041
  childhood and adolescence 1745–6, 1784
  classification 1003, 1036–8
  clinical features 1036, *1036*
  controversial aspects 990
  coping strategies 1039
  course 1040
  diagnosis 1036–8, 1041
  differential diagnosis *1041*
  epidemics 1038
  epidemiology 997, 1038
  genetics 1038
  international consensus definition *1037*
  overlap with psychiatric syndromes 1037–8
  pathophysiology 1038–9
  and personality 1039
  prevalence 1038
  prevention 1042
  prognosis 1040
  psychopathology 1039–40

  and sleep disorder 1697
  and somatization 1039
  and stigma 1039–40
  treatment and management 1034, 1040–2,
      *1041*, 1784
chronic obstructive pulmonary disease
    *932*, 1082
chronic renal failure 1087
  childhood and adolescence 1741, 1743
  and sleep-wake disorders *932*
chronic stress reaction and post-traumatic
    stress disorder 706
CI (confidence interval) 126, 128
CIDI (Composite International Diagnostic
    Interview) 69, 70, 72, 284, 542, 1023, 1438
cimetidine 1532
CIND *see* cognitive impairment, non-dementia
cinnarizine 1240
circadian rhythms 1260
  and bipolar disorder 647
  disorders 1261
  effects of ageing 1572
  sleep–wake 925, 926
circle time 1814
circular causality 1371
circular questioning 1387
circular sulcus 145
circumstantiality 53
citalopram *670*
  adverse effects *1191*
  in body dysmorphic disorder 1046
  in cancer *1102, 1103*
  in childhood and adolescence 1676
  in dementia 415
  in depression in elderly people 1554, *1554*
  dosage *1196*
  in obsessive–compulsive disorder *1687*
  in panic disorder *756*
  pharmacodynamics 1186, *1187*
  pharmacokinetics 1188–9, *1189*
CIWA-Ar (Clinical Institute Withdrawal
    Assessment for Alcohol-Revised
    Version) *1542*
CJD *see* Creutzfeldt–Jakob disease
CJITS (Criminal Justice Integrated Teams) 515
CL psychiatry *see* consultation-liaison (CL)
    psychiatry
Clarke Sex History Questionnaire for
    Males 1962
classification **99–121**
  in childhood and adolescence **1589–94**
  conceptual issues 99–100
  definition 99
  development of systems 100–2
  and diagnostic instruments 64
  and epidemiology 1607
  goals 99
  history of 631
  in primary care 1483–4
Classification of Violence Risk 1996, 1998
claustrophobia 52
claustrum 151
*Claviceps purpurea* 487
  *see also* hydergine
cleft lip/palate 1711, 1712
Client Service Receipt Inventory 1474
clinical assessment *see* assessment
Clinical Dementia Rating scale 1535
Clinical Institute Withdrawal Assessment for
    Alcohol-Revised Version *1542*

clinical neuropsychology 262
clinical practice guidelines 123, 124
Clinician Administered PTSD Scale 703
Clinician Assessment of Fluctuation Scale 363
clinophilia 939
clitoris 812, 817–18, 822
clobazam 1080, *1172*
clomethiazole **1246–7**
  pharmacodynamics 1171
  pharmacokinetics 1170
clomipramine *670*
  adverse effects *1191*, 1687
  in body dysmorphic disorder 1046, 1047
  in childhood and adolescence 1676
  in depersonalization disorder 775
  dosage *1196*
  in intellectual disability 1875
  in obsessive–compulsive disorder 768–9,
    769–70, 1193, 1687, *1687*
  in panic disorder 756, *756*
  pharmacodynamics *1173*, 1186, *1187*
  pharmacokinetics *1172*, *1189*
clonazepam 1080
  in cancer *1102*
  in obsessive–compulsive disorder 769
  in panic disorder *756*, 757
  pharmacokinetics *1867*
  potential for misuse 491
  in REM sleep behaviour disorder 947
  in social anxiety disorder 743
clonidine **1245**
  in attention-deficit hyperactivity
    disorder 1651
  in intellectual disability 1876
  in opioid detoxification 477
  in smoking cessation 512
  in tic disorders 1073, 1688
'closed-loop' tasks 254
clozapine 1209
  administration *1214*, 1215–16
  adverse effects *1212*, 1223–4
  in childhood and adolescence 1797
  in intellectual disability 1875
  pharmacodynamics *1172*, *1211*, 1213
  pharmacokinetics *1172*, 1221
  in schizophrenia 580, 582, 592
'Club House' 1453
CMHCs (community mental health
  centres) 1454
CMHTs *see* community mental health teams
CNS (Cardinal Needs Schedule) 1434
cobalamin deficiency 1087–8
cocaine **482–6**
  addictiveness *431*, 483
  aetiology of use 484
  classification of disorders relating to
    483, *484*
  cognitive effects 92
  complications associated 484–5
  course and prognosis of use 484–5
  diagnosis of use 483–4
  effects of 483, *483*
  epidemiology of use 484
  in pregnancy 1118, 1615–16
  prevention of misuse 485
  psychosis due to 485, 538
  routes of use and risk associated 430, 483
  treatment and management of use 485
  withdrawal 483, *483*
Cochrane Collaboration 123–4, 578

Cochrane Database of Systematic Reviews 1156–7
Cochrane Library 1156–7
codeine 430
  metabolism 473–4
  in opiate abuse 1244
coenaesthesia 50
coenestopathic states 1030
Coffin–Lowry syndrome 1839
  behavioural and psychiatric aspects 1842
  genetics 1842
  physical characteristics 1842
  prevalence 1842
COGA (Collaborative Study on the Genetics of
  Alcoholism) 435
cognitive analytical therapy (CAT) 903–4, 1278
  borderline personality disorder 895
cognitive assessment **85–94**
  in alcohol abuse and dependence 92
  attention 60, 88–9
  and capacity 90–1
  childhood and adolescence 90
    with intellectual disability 1850
  concentration 60, 88–9
  in dementia 92
  in depression 92
  in drug abuse 92–3
  ecological validity 92, *92*
  elderly people 1527
  in epilepsy 92
  estimating premorbid ability 90, *90*
  frontal and executive functions 89, *90*
  general ability 87, *88*
  generalizability theory 92
  intelligence 87, *88*
  language 89
  and malingering 91
  memory 89, *89*, 253, 254, 255–6, 264,
    420–1, *420*
  in parkinsonism 92
  principles 85–7, *85*, *86*
  protocol 91, *91*
  in schizophrenia 93, 265, 531–4
  sources of tests and test data 89
  speed of processing 87–8, *88*
  understanding and choice of tests 89–90
  *see also* neuropsychological assessment
cognitive-behaviour therapy (CBT)
  acute stress reactions 697
  adjustment disorders 720, 1068
  anxiety disorders **1285–98**
    in childhood and adolescence 1668, 1779–80
  attempted suicide 970
  for auditory hallucinations 1314, 1317
  bipolar disorder 673
  body dysmorphic disorder 1047
  childhood and adolescence 1767, **1777–86**
    anxiety disorders 1668, 1779–80
    attention-deficit hyperactivity
      disorder 1782–3
    chronic fatigue syndrome 1784
    conduct disorder 1781–2
    depression 1675–6, 1780–1
    eating disorders 1784
    failure to engage/respond 1779
    following attempted suicide 1707
    inclusion of cognitive component 1778–9
    non-organic pain 1784
    obsessive–compulsive disorder 1686–7,
      *1686*, 1783–4
    post-traumatic stress disorder 1784

  psychiatric/behaviour disorder with
    intellectual disability 1852
  substance abuse 1784
  technique and management 1778
  working with parents 1778–9
  in chronic fatigue syndrome 1030, 1042
  comparison with other
    psychotherapies 1321, 1333–4, *1333*
  compulsive buying/shopping disorder 916
  computerized 1406
  conversion disorder 1019
  and counselling 1277
  delusions/delusional disorder 1314, 1315–17,
    *1315*, 1920
  depersonalization disorder 775
  depression 672–3, 676, **1304–13**
    advantages of 1304
    background 1304
    childhood and adolescence 1675–6, 1780–1
    demands of 1304
    in elderly people 1555
    ending treatment 1310–12
    indications and contraindications 1305–6
    management of treatment 1307–12,
      *1308*, *1309*
    selection for 1306–7
    technique 1304–5
  eating disorders 792, 796, 808, 808–9,
    **1298–303**, 1784
  following attempted suicide 1707
  in generalized anxiety disorder 735–6
  guided self-help 808–9
  historical development 1286
  in HIV/AIDS 1092
  hypochondriasis 1026–7
  insomnia 935–6, *936*
  in intellectual disability 1874
  obsessive–compulsive disorder 770, 1686–7,
    *1686*, 1783–4
  panic disorder 758, 761
  persistent somatoform pain disorder 1034
  personality disorders 903–4
    antisocial 898
    avoidant 897
    borderline 895
  post-concussion syndrome 396
  provision by psychiatric nurses 1406
  for refugees 1497
  schizophrenia 582–3, **1313–18**
  sex offenders 1963
    juvenile 1953
  social anxiety disorder 741–2, 742, 744
  somatization disorder 1008–9, *1009*
  substance use disorders 428, 1784
  therapeutic alliance in 903, 1307
  tic disorders 1686–7
  training 1297, 1312
  trauma-focused 708–9, 1109, 1111, 1730
  with victims of criminal activity 1988
cognitive-behavioural group therapy 742, 744
cognitive control in insomnia 936
cognitive deficits and distortions
  in childhood and adolescence
    in anxiety disorders 1779
    attention-deficit hyperactivity
      disorder 1782
    in conduct disorder 1781
    in depressive disorders 1780–1
    in obsessive–compulsive disorder 1783
  malingered 1055–6

cognitive development 1777–8
  and developmental psychology 238–40, *239*
  history-taking 1600
cognitive dissonance and the placebo
    response 1142
cognitive dysmetria 563
Cognitive Estimates Test *90*
cognitive impairment
  in Alzheimer's disease 334–5
  in autism 1633
  cannabis-associated 92, 507–8
  due to disturbed sleep 926
  following head injury 390–1, *395*
  following stroke 1071
  in frontotemporal dementias 347
  mild *see* mild cognitive impairment
  in multiple sclerosis 1074
  non-dementia 1519, 1520, *1521*, 1535, *1535*,
    1536, 1537
    vascular 378–9
  in Parkinson's disease 368
  postoperative 1099
  prior to surgery 1098
  in schizophrenia 93, 265, 528, **531–4**, 580
  in schizotypal personality disorder 533
  vascular 378–9
cognitive models of illness 1138
cognitive neuropsychology 262
cognitive neuroscience 262
cognitive reactivity 1304
cognitive restructuring
  in anxiety disorders 1293, *1293*
  in body dysmorphic disorder 1047
  in generalized anxiety disorder 736
  in panic disorder 761
  in sleep disorders 937, 1572
  in social anxiety disorder 742
  social anxiety disorder 742
  in specific phobia 746
cognitive schemas 52, 1778
  maladaptive 1778
    early 895
  negative 1304
  and reporting of physical symptoms 1137
cognitive stimulation in dementia *414*
Cognitive Test for Delirium 326
cognitive theory
  and hypochondriasis 1025
  and somatization disorder 1005
cognitive therapy 310, 311, 1940
  attention-deficit hyperactivity disorder 1648
  childhood and adolescence 1610, 1767, 1783
  and concept of depression 15
  and counselling 1277
  for delusions 1980
  family-based 1707
  group setting 1351
  history of 23
  in morbid jealousy 1920
  personality disorder 903–4
    borderline 895
  post-traumatic stress disorder 708–9
  schizophrenia 1315–17, *1315*, 1317
  substance use disorders 428
  *see also* cognitive-behaviour therapy
Cognitive Therapy Scale 1311
Cohen–Mansfield Agitation Inventory 413
cohort 1513
cohort studies 282, 283, 541, 557, 568
collaborative care 1483, 1486, 1487

in adjustment disorders 1068
Collaborative Study on the Genetics of
    Alcoholism 435
collagen, cross-linkage 1508
colleges
  psychiatrist as advisor 1815
  *see also* schools
coma 59
  following head injury 388
  Glasgow Coma Scale 388, *388*
commissural plate 157
commissure of the fornix 151
common geriatric assessment 1581
communication
  doctor–patient 1138–9
  in intellectual disability 1873
  skills training 1139, 1375–6
communication disorders *see* specific
    developmental disorders, of speech and
    language
community, prevalence of mental disorders *1480*
community alcohol team model 461
community care 584
  global survey 11
  history of 24
  and rehabilitation 1400
community diagnosis 280
community mental health centres 1454
Community Mental Health in ID Service 1888–9
community mental health teams (CMHTs) 584,
    1454–5, *1456*, *1457*, 1458
  services for people with intellectual
      disability 1888–9
  *see also* mental health services, community
community outreach in attempted suicide
    970, 972
community psychiatric nurses (CPNs) 1404–5
  in treatment of alcohol use disorders 462
  *see also* psychiatric nurses
community reinforcement 456, 462
community substance misuse teams 479
community treatment orders 1411, 1458
comorbidity 278, 990
  in childhood and adolescence 1591, 1600
  in primary care 1483
  *see also under specific disorders*
compartmentalization phenomena 1012, *1012*
compensation claims
  and conversion disorder 1016
  and persistent somatoform pain disorder 1034
'compensation neurosis' 700
competence 29
  abilities involved 1897
  best interest approach 1899
  functional approach 1898
  and juvenile delinquency 1954–5
  lack of 1898–9
  legal aspects 1895–900
  outcome approach 1897–8
  status approach 1897, 1899–900
  tests of 1897
complementary medicines 15, **1247–51**
  antipsychotics 1249
  anxiolytics and sedatives 1248
  in chronic fatigue syndrome 1042
  in chronic somatic conditions 1249
  cognitive enhancers 1247–8
  determinants of pharmacological
      properties *1248*
  and diagnosis 65

drug interactions 1249–50, *1250*
  mood disorders 1248
  in movement disorders 1249
  in neurasthenia 1063
  psychoses 1249
  for refugees 1497
  smoking cessation 512
  in substance use disorders 1249
'complex medically ill' 1144
complex regional pain syndrome, type I
    1015, 1050
Complexity Prediction Instrument 1145
Complier-Average Causal Effect of
    Treatment 142
Composite Disability Malingering Index
    1054–5
Composite International Diagnostic
    Interview 69, 70, 72, 284, 542, 1023, 1438
Comprehensive Psychopathological Rating
    Scale 70
COMPRI (Complexity Prediction
    Instrument) 1145
compulsions 52, 53, 1680
  in body dysmorphic disorder 1044, *1044*
  in obsessive–compulsive disorder 765–6
compulsive buying/shopping disorder **916**
computed tomography (CT)
  alcohol-related dementia 400
  anorexia nervosa 781
  epilepsy 1619
  frontotemporal dementias 347
  head injury 389
  HIV-associated dementia 385
  obsessive–compulsive disorder 768
  schizophrenia 563–4
  vascular dementia 376
  Wernicke–Korsakoff syndrome 400, 406
COMT gene 255, 256, 555, 559, 1646
concealment of treatment allocation 127
concentration
  assessment 60, 88–9
  disorders of 60
  following head injury 390
concentration camp survivors 1494
conditioning 250, 254, 258
  in acute stress reactions 696
  in obsessive–compulsive disorder 768
  and phobias 745
  and post-traumatic stress disorder 705
  and substance use disorders 428, 434
conduct disorder **1654–64**
  adolescent onset 1655, 1658
  adult outcome 1660–1, *1660*
  aetiology 1658–60
  and age 1655
  assessment 1657, 1781–2
  and bipolar disorder 646
  classification 1656–7
  clinical features 1655–6
  comorbidity 1644, 1657
  confined to the family context 1656
  course 1660–1
  depressive 1657
  differential diagnosis 1657, 1671
  early-onset 1655, 1656, 1658, 1788
    and outcome 1660, *1660*
  epidemiology 1658
  and gender 1655, 1658
  genetics 1658
  hyperkinetic 1644, 1657

and intellectual disability 1657, 1851
and juvenile delinquency 1946
life-course persistent 1658
pattern and setting of behaviour 1655
and perinatal complications 1658
prevention 1663, 1788
prognosis 1660–1
protective factors 1660
and pulse rate 1658
relation to other disorders 1654
risk factors 1658–60
role of neurotransmitters 1658
as a social problem 1654–5
socialized 1656
and suicide 1704
treatment and management 1661–3, 1781–2
unsocialized 1656
verbal deficits in 1658
wider impact of 1655–6
conduction dysphasia 54
confabulation 59, 403, **408**, 1049
following head injury 392
momentary/provoked 408
in post-traumatic stress disorder 404
spontaneous 408
in Wernicke–Korsakoff syndrome 405
confidence interval 126, 128
confidentiality
in childhood and adolescence
assessment 1605
psychiatric emergencies 1811
psychotherapy 1768
and clinical assessment 67
and domestic violence 1982
and expert witnesses 2006–7
in factitious disorder 1053
in higher/further education 1815
in the paraphilias 840
and reports 75
in schools liaison service 1813
confounding factors 285
confrontation in factitious disorder
1052–3, *1053*
Confusion Assessment Method 328, 1531
confusional state 59
in brain tumour 1075
in childhood and adolescence 1742
following an accident 1110
following neurosurgery for mental
disorder 1268
post-ictal 403
*see also* delirium
congenital rubella syndrome 548, 1635, 1850,
1852, 1863
congestive heart failure in anorexia nervosa 785
congophilic angiopathy 338
Conners' Parent Rating Scale 1241, 1645
Conners' Teacher Rating Scale 1241, 1645, 1813
connexions advisors 1812
conscientiousness 850, 886
conscious mental states 135
conscious thinking 294
consciousness
clouding of 59, *59*, 60
concept of 59
disorders of 59–60
heightened 59
loss of following head injury 388
narrowing of 60
consent *see* informed consent

Consortium to Establish a Registry for AD 336
constipation and depression 641
consultation
communication in 1138–9
in consultation-liaison psychiatry 1145
patient-centred/doctor-centred 1139
consultation-liaison (CL) psychiatry 990, 1135,
**1144–8**, 1487
audit 1147
current levels of service delivery 1144
for elderly people 1583
Psych-Med unit 1145
screening in 1145–6, *1146*
service organization 1146–7, *1147*
staffing 1146
training 1147
types of service delivery 1145–6, *1145, 1146*
container-contained theory 308
contiguous gene syndromes 228
contingency management in opioid
dependence 477
continuous performance tests 247
contracts in psychoanalysis 1341
control
delusions of 51, 56
perceived lack of in generalized anxiety
disorder 734
control event rate 128
contusions, cerebral 387, *387*, 389
conversion 1012
pain as form of 1031–2
conversion disorder (CD) 57, **1011–21**
childhood and adolescence 1745
chronic 1017
classification 106, *993*, *994*
clinical features 1014–17
comorbidity 870, 1015
and culture 14–15
definitions 1012, *1012*
differential diagnosis 695, 1003, 1012, *1012*
epidemiology 998, 1014
examination 1015–16
mimicking surgical conditions 1096
and pain 1031–2
pathophysiology 1013–14, *1013, 1014*
prognosis 1017–18
role of volition 1012
sleep-related 948
treatment and management 1018–20, *1019*
conversion symptoms 57
Cool Kids programme 1779
cooperativeness 80, *80*, 83, 316, 850
cooperatives 1401
Coordinators of Services for the Elderly
project 1584
COPD (chronic obstructive pulmonary
disease) *932*, 1082
COPE programme 1779
coping
active/engaged/approach 1066
behavioural 1066
in chronic fatigue syndrome 1039
with depression 1306
emotion focused 1066
failure 1067
with illness 1065–71
and immune function 207
passive/disengaged/avoid 1066
problem focused 1066
with schizophrenia 1313–14, 1315

social 1066
in social anxiety disorder 744
and somatization disorder 1009
styles 1066
techniques 1066
with terminal illness 1069–70
Coping Power Programme 1662, 1782
coping strategy enhancement 451, 1313–14,
1315, 1662, 1782
coprolalia 1073, 1681
copropraxia 1073
Cornell scale for depression in dementia 413
coronary heart disease
and alcohol consumption 446
and sleep-wake disorders *932*
and type A personality 1136
and type D personality 1136
corpus callosum 151, 157, 180
corpus striatum 158, 159
correlation coefficient 849
Corsi blocks 255
cortical dysplasia 159, 1863
cortical plate 158
corticobasal degeneration (CBD) 344
aetiology 348
differential diagnosis 347–8
neuropathology 345
corticobulbar pathway 156
corticopontine pathway 155
corticospinal tract 156, 158
corticosteroids
adverse effects
anxiety 1101
in childhood and adolescence 1673
psychosis 539
in Landau–Kleffner syndrome 1627
release in response to stress 1135
corticostriate pathway 154–5, *154*
corticotrophin-releasing hormone (CRH)
163, *171*
and depression 163–4, 166, 659, 661
functions 161
and immune function 206
in post-traumatic stress disorder 706
and suicide 965
cortisol
and aggressive/antisocial behaviour 1918
and chronic fatigue syndrome 1039
and depression 660–1, 1675
and fibromyalgia 1039
in generalized anxiety disorder 732
hypersecretion 1086
and insomnia 935
and the sleep–wake cycle 925
COSE project 1584
cosmetic psychopharmacology 28–9
cosmetic treatment in body dysmorphic
disorder 1046, 1096
cost-benefit analysis 1474, 1475
cost-consequence analysis 1475
cost-effectiveness acceptability curves
1475, *1475*
cost-effectiveness analysis (CEA)
1463, 1474, 1475
alcohol use disorders services 462–3
child and adolescent mental health
services 1476–7
mental health interventions in developing
countries 1477, *1478*
research study design 1475–6

cost-effectiveness ratio, incremental 124, 1475, *1475*
cost-per-QALY approach 1475, 1476
cost-utility analysis (CUA) 1474, 1475
  of depression treatment in primary care 1476
costs, measurement of 1474–5
Cotard's syndrome 56
Council of Europe, Principles Concerning the Legal Protection of Incapable Adults 1896
counselling **1272–85**
  adjustment disorders 721, 1278
  alcohol use disorders 1279
  anxiety 1278
  applications 1278–80
  bereavement 726–7, 1279
  childhood and adolescence **1764–9**
    approaches to 1766–8
    measures of effectiveness and outcome 1769
    practical issues 1768
    with psychiatric/behaviour disorder and intellectual disability 1852
    supportive 1767
    training and supervision 1768–9
    treatment setting and process 1766
  cognitive–behavioural models 1275, 1277
  cognitive models 1275
  core conditions 1274–5
  couple 1370
  definitions 1273
  depression 672, 676, 1278
  eclectic-integrative approaches 1278
  in educational settings 1281
  effectiveness 1274
  electronic delivery 1282
  existential approaches 1277
  following abortion 1119
  genetic *see* genetic counselling
  grief 726–7, 1279
  in HIV/AIDS 1280–1
  in hospitals and clinics 1280–1
  humanistic–existential models 1275, 1276–7
  information-giving in 1275–6
  key elements and goals *1273*
  methods and techniques 1275–8
  mothers giving up children for adoption 1120
  pathological gambling 922
  person-centred (client-centred) 1275, 1276–7
  postnatal depression 1280
  practice 1274
  in primary care 1280, 1485–6
  psychodynamic models 1275, 1277–8
  and psychotherapy 1273–4, 1765
  rape victims 1986
  in relationship problems 1278–9
  schools of 1275, *1275*
  settings 1280–2, 1485–6
  skills 1274
  smoking cessation 511–12
  stress disorders 1278
  substance use disorders 1279
  telephone helplines 1282
  theoretical approaches to 1275, *1275*
  therapeutic alliance in 1275
  training, accreditation and registration 1282–3
  trauma 1279–80
  in the voluntary sector 1279, 1281
  in the workplace 1281–2
counselling psychology 1274

counterfeit deviance 834–5
countertransference
  in brief psychodynamic psychotherapy 1329, 1330
  broad/totalistic view 314, *315*
  complementary 1343
  concordant 1343
  joint creation 314, *315*
  narrow view 314, *315*
  and non-compliance 317
  object-relations theory model 298–9
  in physician-assisted suicide 318
  and projective identification 308
  in psychoanalysis 1343–4
  and psychodynamic psychiatry 314, *315*, 318
Countertransference Questionnaire 1344
couple counselling 1370
couple therapy 1365–6, **1369–80**
  adjustment disorders *1069*
  alcohol use disorders 452–3
  assessment and selection 1373
  behavioural 452–3, 1371
  behavioural–systems 1372–8
  cognitive-behavioural 1371
  and culture 1377–8
  depression 15, 672
  distinction from couple counselling 1370
  efficacy 1378–9
  indications and contraindications 1373
  intersystem model 1372
  mixed/eclectic approach 1371–2
  paraphilias 838, 840
  process 1373–5
  psychoanalytic/psychodynamic 1370–1
  psychodynamic–behavioural 1372
  rational–emotive 1371
  substance use disorders 516
  systems approach 1371
  techniques 1375–7
  training in 1379
Court of Protection 1898–9
Court reports 1928, *2004*, **2005–6**
courtship behaviour 815
COVR (Classification of Violence Risk) 1996, 1998
Cowper's gland 817
CPA *see* care programme approach
CPNs *see* community psychiatric nurses
CPSS (Child PTSD Symptom scale) 1730
CR (calorie restriction) and modification of ageing 1509
CR/HT (crisis resolution/home treatment) teams 1458, *1458*
crack 430, *431*, 483
  *see also* cocaine
cranial nerve development 157
'crashing' 497
craving 427, 428, 483
cre recombinase 230
creatinine 1204
creative thought 308
Creutzfeldt–Jakob disease (CJD) 351, 1903
  aetiology 351–2
  amyotrophic 354
  ataxic 354
  atypical 354
  Heidenhain's variant 354
  iatrogenic *353*, 355
  panencephalopathic 354
  prevention 358–9

sporadic/classical 352, 353–4, *353*
  variant 351, *353*, 355–6
    aetiology 351–2
    secondary (iatrogenic) *353*, 356
CRH *see* corticotrophin-releasing hormone
cri-du-chat syndrome (CDCS)
  behavioural and psychiatric aspects 1842
  genetics 1842
  physical characteristics 1842
  prevalence 1842
crime analysis 1914
Crime and Disorder Act 1998 1982, 1987–8
Crime and Disorder Reduction Partnerships 515
criminal activity *see* offending
Criminal Damage Act 1971 1966
Criminal Justice Integrated Teams 515
criminal liability 1900–1
Criminal Procedure (Insanity and Fitness to Plead) Act 1991 1901
criminal victimization **1984–90**
criminogenic factors 1911, 1917, 1918, 2011, 2012
crisis cults 982
crisis houses 1458
crisis resolution/home treatment teams 1458, *1458*
criterion variance 284
Crohn's disease 1083–4
cross-cultural comparisons 276, *277*
cross-fostering study 216
cross-sectional studies 282
crowding of thoughts 53
CRPS I (complex regional pain syndrome type I) 1015, 1050
cryptographia 54
cryptolalia 54
crystal/crystalline methamphetamine hydrochloride **497–8**
CT *see* computed tomography
CTOs (community treatment orders) 1411, 1458
CUA *see* cost-utility analysis
cue exposure in alcohol use disorders 451
CUES (Carers and Users Experience of Services) 1434
'cult of thinness' 779
cultural competence 1502–4, *1503*
culture
  in acute and transient psychotic disorders 606
  and ageing 1512–13
  and body dysmorphic disorder 1045
  and care pathways **1438–45**
  in child and adolescent psychotherapy 1768
  and clinical assessment 67
  and the concept of depression 15
  and conversion hysteria 14–15
  and couple therapy 1377–8
  cultural critique of biomedicine 276–7
  cultural formulations 278
  and deliberate self-harm 958–9
  and depression 14, 1496
  and help-seeking behaviour 15, 1441–2
  and hypochondriasis 1025–6
  and indigenous folk healing practices 1418
  and intellectual disability 1879–80, 1881
  and mania 14
  and marriage 1370
  and mental health services for ethnic minorities **1502–4**

and neurasthenia 1060–1
and neuroses 14
and normal sexual function 812–13
and the phenomena of psychiatric
    disorder 47
and provision of services 277–8
and reaction to loss of a parent 1758
and refugee assessment, diagnosis and
    treatment 1496, *1496*, 1498
role in caregiver-mediated
    interventions 1791
and schizophrenia 14, 546, 557, 571–3, *572*
and social and cultural anthropology 275–9
and somatization disorders 996
and stigma 6–7
and suicide 953–4, 1704
transcultural psychiatry **13–16**
and treatment 1442–3
culture of blame 1991–2
culture-related specific psychiatric
    syndromes 14, **979–85**, 1439
acute and transient psychotic disorders 606
anorexia nervosa as 779
concept of 979
subgroups 979–80, *980*
in western societies 984–5
current awareness 124–5, *125*
Cushing's syndrome 1086
CVLT (California Verbal Learning Test) 253, 264
CY-BOCS (Children's Yale-Brown Obsessive-
    Compulsive Scale) 1681
cyberstalking 1970
'cyber suicide' 1706
cyclic adenosine monophosphate 175
d-cycloserine
    adverse effects *1091*
    in social anxiety disorder 743
    in specific phobia 746
cyclothymia/cyclothymic disorder 632, **686–9**
    aetiology 688–9
    childhood and adolescence 1671, *1672*
    clinical features 687–8
    course 687–8
    diagnosis 687–8
    epidemiology 688, *689*
    historical perspective 686
    management 689
    prevention 689
    relationship to bipolar disorder 688
CYP system
    and antidepressants 1188
    and antipsychotics 1221, 1222
    and complementary medicines 1249, *1250*
    inhibitors 1795
    and opioid metabolism 473–4
    and pharmacokinetics 1170, *1172*
cyproterone acetate 838, 1963–4
cystic fibrosis 1743
cytokines 168, 171, 209
cytomegalic inclusion disease 1863
cytosine 223

Da Costa syndrome 751
DAG (diacyl glycerol) 174, 175
DALE (Disability-Adjusted Life
    Expectancy) 1510
DALYs (Disability-Adjusted Life Years) 10, 645,
    1477, 1510
dangerous and severe personality disorders 848,
    2015, 2018

DAPA-PC (Drug Abuse Problem Assessment for
    Primary Care) 1484
DAPP-BQ (Dimensional Assessment of
    Personality Disorders) 858, *858*
DARE database 1156
DAS (Disability Assessment Schedule) 284
'date rape' 409, 491
DATs (Drug Action Teams) 515–16
DAWBA (Development and Well-Being
    Assessment) 1595–6
dawn-simulating alarm clock 1261
day hospitals
    acute 1453
    in Alzheimer's disease 340
    in anorexia nervosa 793, 795
    in community mental health services 1453
    for elderly people 1583
daydreaming 294, 1941
DBS (deep brain stimulation) 671, 769, 1073–4,
    1258, **1269–70**
DBT *see* dialectical behaviour therapy
DC-LD (Diagnostic Criteria for Psychiatric
    Disorders for Use with Adults
    with Learning Disabilities/Mental
    Retardation) 1826–7, 1850
de Lange syndrome
    behavioural and psychiatric aspects 1842
    genetics 1842
    physical characteristics 1842
    prevalence 1842
de-affectualization 774
debriefing
    critical incident stress 697
    emergency workers 1110
    trauma story 1497
deceitfulness in conduct disorder 1656
decentring technique 1374
deception 1941
decision-making
    and emotion 260–1
    legal aspects 1895–900
deep brain stimulation 671, 769, 1073–4, 1258,
    **1269–70**
deep lateral sulcus 144, 145
de-escalation techniques 1404
defence mechanisms 310, 849
    avoidant 1339–40
    in brief psychodynamic psychotherapy 1328–9
    classification 1339–40
    in obsessive–compulsive disorder 768
    and personality development 316–17
    primitive/mature 1339
    and psychoanalysis 293–4, 1339–40
    and resistance 315, 317
defensive organizations 1339
dehydration and ecstasy use 495
de-ideation 774
deinstitutionalization
    and burden of care 1401
    and intellectual disability 1881, 1887, 1890
    and mental health social work 1408, 1411
    and prevalence of mental disorder among
        prisoners 1934
    and psychiatric nursing 1403
*déjà vu* 59, 250
delay aversion in attention-deficit hyperactivity
    disorder 1647
delayed sleep phase syndrome 928, 942–3,
    1261, 1695, 1700
deliberate self-harm (DSH) 955, **957–63**

and adjustment disorders 718, 722
aetiology 960–1
and age 1704
in anorexia nervosa 782–3
assessment 971, *971*
in childhood and adolescence 972, 1601, 1703
choice of method 959–60
classification 960
clinical features 958
course and prognosis 961
definition 957–8
elderly people 1551, **1564–7**
epidemiology 958–60
high-risk 960
impulsive 916–17
and intellectual disability 1856
and liability of mental health service
    providers 1905
lifetime prevalence 960
mild 960
moderate 960
in physical illness 1133
precipitants 961
prevention **972–6**
repetition 961, 969, 971, *972*
and risk of suicide 961, 971, *971*, *972*
self-report surveys 960
sociodemographic characteristics 959
in Tourette syndrome 1073
treatment **969–72**
vulnerability factors 961
delineation of syndromes 281
*délire d'emblée* 603, 604
delirium 49, **325–33**
    aetiology 330, *330*
    at childbirth 1118
    in cancer 1103–4, *1104*
    and cholinergic system 330, 1532
    classification 105, 327, 1531
    clinical features 326–7, *326*
    comorbidity 327
    and consciousness 59
    and dementia 327, 329, 332, 1532
    diagnosis 327–8
    differential diagnosis 327–8, *328*, 364
    drug-induced 1532
    elderly people 1529, **1530–4**
        aetiology 1532, *1532*
        classification 1531
        clinical features 1530–1
        complications 1533
        course and prognosis 1532
        diagnosis 1531
        differential diagnosis 1531, 1559
        epidemiology 1531–2
        prevention 1533
        treatment and management 1532–3
    epidemiology 328–9
    in HIV/AIDS 1092–3, *1093*
    hyperactive 327, 1531, 1532, 1533
    hypoactive 327, 1530–1, 1532, 1533
    investigation 330, *330*
    mixed 327
    mortality risk 329
    neuropathogenesis 330–1, *330*
    outcome 328–9
    phencyclidine-induced 486–7
    in pneumonia 1091
    postoperative 1098–9
    post-seizure 1257

delirium (*cont.*)
  prevention 331, 1533
  psychosis in 327
  risk factors 329, *329*
  subsyndromal 325, 328, 1531
  treatment and management 331–2, *1104*, 1255
  tremor in 58
Delirium Rating Scale 1531
Delirium Rating Scale-Revised-98 328
Delirium Symptom Interview 1531
delirium tremens 58, 327, 443
  prevention 450
  treatment 449–50
delusional atmosphere 51
delusional disorder **609–28**
  aetiology 613–14
  clinical features 613–15
  diagnostic criteria 103–4, 613, *613*
  differential diagnosis 864
  elderly people 1552
  erotomanic 621–2
  features of delusions in 612
  genetics 614
  grandiose 622
  and homicide 1920
  induced 610, 624–5
  jealous 51, 619–21, 1920, 1967
  litigious 616, 1977–80
  mixed/unspecified 623
  and mood disorders 614
  nomenclature 610–11
  and offending 1920
  persecutory 616
  somatic 617–19, 1024
  and stalking 1920
  subtypes 613, *613*, 615–23
  treatment 625–7, 1920
  and violence 1920
delusional disorientation 392
delusional intuition 51
delusional misidentification syndrome 51, 392, 609–10, 611, 622, **623–4**
delusional perception 51, 527–8
delusional states, systematized 1030
delusions 49
  in acute and transient psychotic disorders 602–8
  in Alzheimer's disease 335
  autistic 51
  autochthonous 51
  in body dysmorphic disorder 618, 1044, 1045
  clinical aspects 611–12
  cognitive-behaviour therapy 1314, 1315–17, *1315*
  content of 51
  of control 51, 56
  definition 50–1, 611
  in delirium 327
  in delusional disorder 612
  in dementia with Lewy bodies 361
  dental 619
  and depression 51, 639, 641, 674, 1253
  differential diagnosis of cause 537
  of disease transmission 619
  following head injury 392
  in frontotemporal dementias 346
  genesis 51
  grandiose 51
  of guilt 51
  of halitosis 618–19

hypochondriacal 51
and jealousy 51, 619–21, 1920, 1967
of love 51
memory 51, 59
millenniary 982
and misidentification 51, 392, 609–10, 611, 622, **623–4**
mood-congruent/-incongruent 537, 641
in multiple sclerosis 1074
nihilistic 56
and pain 1030
as paranoid defence 1314
of parasitosis/infestation 50, 51, 618
in Parkinson's disease 1072
of persecution 51
polarized 51
of pregnancy 1115
primary 51, 611
religious 51
in schizophrenia 526–7
secondary 51, 611
of sexually transmitted disease 619
of smell 618–19
structure of 51
and violence 1929
dementia 54
  and ageing 1520
  and aggression 336, 1920–1, 1928–9
  agitation in 413–15
  alcohol-related/alcohol-induced **399–402**, 1541
  apathy in 416
  behavioural and psychological symptoms 412–17, *413*, *414*
  carers 417–18
  challenging behaviour in 413–15
  cholinergic hypothesis 338, 1240–1
  classification 105
  cognitive assessment 92
  definitions 411
  delaying onset 1538
  and delirium 327, 329, 332, 1532
  depression in 416
  differential diagnosis 1531
    distinction from delirium 327, *328*
    distinction from depression 1551, *1551*
  disclosure of diagnosis 411
  and Down syndrome 1584, 1827, 1839, 1865, 1880
  and driving 412
  early-onset 411–12, 1584
  elderly people
    differential diagnosis 1558–9
    early detection 1519–20
    epidemiology **1519–22**, 1579–80
    impact 1522
    incidence and risk factors 1520–2, *1520*, *1522*
    presentation in primary care 1483
  end-stage management 418
  epidemiology 1579–80
  frontotemporal (FTD) 258–9, **344–50**, 1519
    aetiology and pathogenesis 348
    and aggression 1928–9
    behavioural and psychological symptoms *413*
    classification *344*, 347
    clinical features 345–6
    differential diagnosis 347–8, *347*, 373
    epidemiology 345

    genetics 348
    investigations 347, Plate 12
    Lund–Manchester consensus on clinical criteria 345, *345*, 347
    neuropathology 344–5
    with parkinsonism 344–5, 346, 348
    physical signs 346
    treatment and care 348–9
  genetic counselling and testing 411, *412*
  HIV/AIDS **384–6**, 1091
    classification 384
    clinical features 384
    course and prognosis 385
    diagnosis 384–5
    differential diagnosis 384–5
    epidemiology 385
    pathogenesis 385
    severity levels 384
    treatment and management 385–6
  in Huntington's disease **371–5**
  and intellectual disability 1827, 1828, 1855
  with Lewy bodies (DLB) **361–8**
    behavioural and psychological symptoms *413*
    clinical diagnosis 363–4, *363*
    clinical features 335, 361–2
    course and prognosis 365
    diagnosis 336
    differential diagnosis 364, *364*, 369
    epidemiology 364–5
    genetics 365
    investigations 364
    management 365–7, *366*
    pathological classification 362
    pathological criteria *362*
    relationship with dementia in Parkinson's disease 362–3
  management **411–19**
  mania in 416
  memory impairment 59
  and mild cognitive impairment 1534, *1534*, 1535–6, 1538
  mixed pathologies 336
  in motor neurone disease 344, 345, 347, 348
  and offending 1920–1
  pain in 418
  in Parkinson's disease 92, 362–3, **368–71**, *370*
  psychomotor disturbance in 59
  psychosis in 416
  risk assessment and management 417, *417*
  risk reduction/protective factors 1521–2, *1522*
  semantic 344, 346
  severity stages 1535
  sexual behaviour disorders 416
  and sexuality 1568
  and sleep-wake disorders 416–17, *931*, 1572, 1573
  structural MRI 195
  subcortical 368–9
  treatment
    complementary medicines 1247–8
    pharmacotherapy 1240–1
  urinary incontinence in 417
  vascular (VaD) **375–84**, 1519
    acute onset *378*
    aetiology 376
    behavioural and psychological symptoms *413*
    classification 377
    clinical criteria 377–8, *377*, *378*

clinical features 379
cortical (multi-infarct) 375, 377, *378*
course and prognosis 379
diagnosis 379–80
differential diagnosis 348, 364, 380
epidemiology 380–1
incidence 1520
mixed cortical and subcortical *378*
NINDS-AIREN criteria 377, 378, *378*
pathophysiology 376
prevention 381, 1447
risk factors 376
subcortical (small-vessel) 377, *378*
treatment 381
wandering in 415
*see also* Alzheimer's disease
dementia infantilis **1637**
dementia paralytica 1093
dementia praecox 522, 540, 568, 603, 631, 1547
*see also* schizophrenia
DemTect 1536
denial 298
in anorexia nervosa 783
as coping behaviour 1066
dental enamel erosion in bulimia nervosa 804
dentate gyrus 148
dentatorubropallidoluysian atrophy *228*, 373
deoxyhaemoglobin 197
deoxyribonucleic acid *see* DNA
dependence
distinction between physical and
psychological 427–8
spectrum of 427–8
use of term 427
dependent personality disorder **873–4**
aetiology 873
classification *856*, 873, *873*
clinical features 873
course 874
differential diagnosis 874
elderly people *1562*
epidemiology 874, *882*, 883
treatment 874
depersonalization 55, 56, 1012
definition 774
in delirium 327
distinction between primary and
secondary 775
epidemiology 775
following an accident 1107
following head injury 392
in neurological disorders 775
victims of criminal activity 1984
depersonalization disorder **774–6**
aetiology 775
classification 774
clinical features 774
course and prognosis 775
diagnosis and differential diagnosis 774–5
epidemiology 775
treatment and management 775–6
deprenyl 385
depression
aetiology
genetic 648, **650–8**
integrated model 649
neurobiological **658–65**
age of onset 667
and alcohol use disorders 649
and anorexia nervosa 783, 787

anticipation in 652
and antisocial personality disorder 866
and anxiety disorder 649
anxious 641–2, 642
assessment 660
assessment instruments 69, 70, 1163–4, 1306,
1484, 1551, *1552*
atypical 635
and bereavement 725
binary model 638
and body mass index 1674
in bulimia nervosa 803, 804
childhood and adolescence
acute management 1677
aetiology 1674
assessment and monitoring 1617–16,
1780–1
course 1673
diagnostic criteria 1669, *1670*
differential diagnosis 1657, 1671–3
double 1673
environmental risk factors 1675
epidemiology 1673–4
minor 1669
neurocognitive factors 1674–5
neuroendocrine studies 1675
sequelae 1674
treatment and prevention 674–5, 1322,
1668, 1675–6, 1780–1, 1794–5, 1796
and childhood adverse experiences 648,
658–9
chronic 667
and chronic fatigue syndrome 1037
classification 638–9, 640–2
clinical features 633–5, *633*, 640–1
cognitive assessment 92
cognitive model 1304–5, *1305*, 1307
cognitive vulnerability to 1304
concept of 15
and conversion disorder 1015
coping strategies 1306
and corticotrophin-releasing hormone
163–4, 166, 659, 661
and cortisol 660–1, 1675
course 271, 667
and culture 14, 1496
definition 637
in dementia 416
in dementia with Lewy bodies 361, 367
diagnosis 647, 1306
differential diagnosis 327, *328*, 643–4, 741,
766, 1004, 1024, 1531
distinction from dementia 1551, *1551*
double 681, 683, 1673
drug-induced 1551, *1552*
duration and severity of episodes 633–4, 667
dysfunctional cognition in 653
elderly people **1550–6**
aetiology *1552*, 1553
assessment 1527, 1551–2
clinical features 1551
in the community 1517
course and prognosis 1553
diagnosis 1551–2
differential diagnosis 373, 1552, 1558
epidemiology 1517–18, 1552–3, 1579
factors influencing presentation *1551*
in hostels and nursing homes 1518
investigations 1551–2, *1553*
mortality associated 1553

prevention 1555–6
in primary care 1482–3, 1518
resistant 1555
treatment and management 674, 1554–5
endogenous/melancholic 630, 631, 638,
640–1
epidemiology **647–9**, 650–1
following abortion 1119
following an accident 1109–10
following ecstasy use 495
following head injury 393, 396
following miscarriage 1119
functional anatomy 189, 660
and functional symptoms 993
and gender 271, 648, 653–4
and generalized anxiety disorder 731
global disease burden 645, 1185
history of 629–30
hostile 641–2, 642
and hypochondriasis 997, 1024, 1027
and immune function 207
and intellectual disability 1827, 1852, 1854–5
and juvenile delinquency 1949
and kleptomania 1943
and life events 269–73, *270*, *271*, 648, 659
lifespan perspective 271–2
maintaining factors 659–63
major
classification 639
diagnosis 647
with psychotic features 634, 639
recurrent 634
stages leading to *634*
with/without melancholia 634
and marital conflict 1753
and marital status 648
masked 1030, 1527
melancholic 270
minor 668
models 638–9
monoamine theory 662
mortality associated 667–8
and neurasthenia 1063
neuroendocrine challenge tests 660
neurotic 270, 638, 641
offenders 1923, *1933*
outcome 667
and pain 1029, 1030
and panic disorder 752
parental, effects on child development
1752–3
and patient state fluctuations within mood
disorders 632–3, *632*, *633*
and persistent somatoform pain disorder 997
and personality 648
and personality disorders 649
pharmacogenetics 653
in physical illness 648–9, 1132
Alzheimer's disease 335
cancer 649, 1102, *1102*, *1103*
COPD 1082
Cushing's syndrome 1086
diabetes mellitus 649, 1085
epilepsy 1080
HIV/AIDS 1092
Huntington's disease 371
hyperthyroidism 1085
hypothyroidism 1085
infection 1091
multiple sclerosis 1074

depression (*cont.*)
in physical illness (*cont.*)
myocardial infarction 649, 1082
Parkinson's disease 648–9, 1072
population perspective 272–3, *272*
post-hysterectomy 1116
post-psychotic 589, 626
post-stroke 1071, 1555
precipitating factors 659
in pregnancy 653, 1117, 1322
prevalence 647–8
primary 637
in primary care
detection and assessment 1476
elderly people 1518
treatment 1322, 1476
prisoners 1923, *1933*
psychosocial factors 271, 653
psychotic/delusional 51, 639, 641, 674, 1253
reactive 630, 631, 638, 641
recurrence 634–5, 667, 671
in refugees 1495
relapse 671
remission 271
resistant 675, Plate 14
risk factors 648–9, 658–9, 1675
in schizophrenia 529, 573
seasonal 635
secondary 637
and sexuality 825
and shoplifting 1943
situational 642
and sleep-wake disorders 634, 661–2, 927,
931, *931*, 934, 1697
social functioning in 653
and somatization disorders 996
spectrum model 642
and substance use disorders 649
subsyndromal symptomatic (SSD) 719
subtypes 630, 631, 638, 640–2, *640*, 647
and suicide 634, 955, 1704
and temperament 654, 658
in terminal illness 1070
thyroid abnormalities in 661
in Tourette syndrome 1073
treatment **669–77**
cognitive-behaviour therapy 672–3, 676,
**1304–13**, 1555, 1675–6, 1780–1
combined psychotherapy and
pharmacotherapy 672–3
complementary medicines 1248
continuation 671, 675, 677
counselling 672, 676, 1278
deep brain stimulation 671, 1270
electroconvulsive therapy 671, 1252–3
in HIV/AIDS 1092
interpersonal psychotherapy 672–3, 676,
1322–3, 1555, 1676
maintenance 671, 675–6, 677
management 673–7
marital therapy 672
neurosurgery 1267, 1268
in primary care 1476
in resistant depression 675
setting 673
transcranial magnetic stimulation
671, 1264
vagus nerve stimulation 671, 1269
*see also* antidepressants *and specific drugs*
treatment gap 13

tryptophan depletion 662
unipolar
definition 638
history of concept 631
as unitary disorder 638
and use of mental health services 649
vascular, elderly people 1551, 1553
in vascular dementia 379
and ventricular dysrhythmias 1081
depressive condition, definition 637
depressive episode disorder 633
depressive equivalent 1030
depressive personality disorder 878–9
depressive position 307
deprivation and psychiatric disorder in
intellectual disability 1828
derailment 53
derealization 56, 774, 1012
following an accident 1107
following head injury 392
victims of criminal activity 1984
dermatotillomania (pathological skin
picking) 618, **917–18**, 1044
Descartes, René 133, 989
description, personal and subpersonal
levels 135
descriptive phenomenology **47–61**
definition 47
disorders of attention and
concentration 60
disorders of consciousness 59–60
disorders of intellectual performance 54
disorders of memory 59
disorders of mood 54–5
disorders of perception 48–50
disorders of personality 60
disorders of self and body image 56–7
disorders of thinking 50–4
language and speech disorder 53–4
motor symptoms and signs 58–9
principles 47–8
theoretical bases 48
desensitization
in obsessive–compulsive disorder 770
systematic 1097
designer drugs 494
desipramine *670*, 1185
adverse effects *1191, 1193*
in body dysmorphic disorder 1046
in cancer *1103*
dosage *1196*
pharmacodynamics *1173, 1187*
pharmacokinetics *1172, 1188, 1189*
desomatization 774
detachment phenomena 1012
Determinants of the Outcome of Severe Mental
Disorders 14, 572, *572*
devaluation 298
developing countries
cost-effectiveness analysis of mental health
interventions 1477, *1478*
prevalence of intellectual disability 1825
psychiatric nurses in 1406–7
Development and Well-Being
Assessment 1595–6
Developmental Behaviour Checklist 1850
Developmental Behaviour Checklist for
Adults 1828
developmental disorders 1591, *1591*
and schizophrenia 548

*see also* pervasive developmental disorders;
specific developmental disorders
developmental history 1600–1, 1822
developmental neuropsychiatry **1612–22**
developmental perspective
environmental risks 1724–8
pharmacotherapy 1794
in psychodynamic psychiatry 314
reasons for taking 234–5
developmental psychology **234–45**
cognitive development 238–40, *239*, 1777–8
critical issues 235–7
and effects of parental mental/physical
illness **1752–8**
and individual differences 238
language development 240–1, *241*, 1623,
1710–11
memory development 241–2, *241–2*
models and theories 234–5
neonatal/early infancy stage 238–9
social and emotional development
242–3, *242*
stage theories 234–5, 239–40, *239*
developmental psychopathology 237–8,
1612–13
and attachment 243
and classification in childhood and
adolescence **1589–94**
and epidemiology 1608
and individual differences 238
in infancy 238–9
linking to developing children 238–42
Piaget's work 239–40, *239*
developmental scales 1821
developmental stages 1764, 1777
developmental toxicology 1614
deviance, subcultural 1657
dexamethasone, in generalized anxiety
disorder 732
dexamethasone–CRF test 164, 1252
Dexamethasone Suppression Test (DST)
in depression 661, 1252
in elderly people 1552
in obsessive–compulsive disorder 768
and suicide 965
dextroamphetamine
in attention-deficit hyperactivity
disorder 1648
in cancer *1103*
in terminal illness 1070
*dhat* 606, *981*
diabetes insipidus, lithium-induced 1204
diabetes mellitus 1085
brittle 1050
and bulimia nervosa 804
in childhood and adolescence 1741
depression in 649, 1085
and schizophrenia 546
sexual dysfunction in 826
and sleep-wake disorders *932*
diacetylmorphine *see* heroin
diacyl glycerol 174, 175
diagnosis **99–121**
additional/subsidiary 74
alternative 74
and clinical assessment 64–5, 74
and complementary medicine 65
cultural critique 276–7
definition 99
differential 74

and disorder 64–5
division between medical and psychiatric 989–90, 992
ethical issues 28–9
main 74
multiaxial systems 73, 100–1, 990, *990*
provisional 74
role of value judgement 29
and social control 29
diagnosis related groups 1430
Diagnostic and Statistical Manual of Mental Disorders, development 100–2
Diagnostic and Statistical Manual of Mental Disorders, DSM-II
hypochondriasis 1022
neurasthenia 1060
Diagnostic and Statistical Manual of Mental Disorders, DSM-III 26, 631
alcohol dependence and alcohol abuse 437
autism 1633
bulimia 800
depression 638–9
development 100–1
dysthymic disorder 1060
generalized anxiety disorder 729–30
multiaxial descriptive systems 100–1
panic disorder 751
post-traumatic stress disorder 693
schizophrenia 1547
sexism in 28
somatoform disorders 105, 993–4, 999, 1022
Diagnostic and Statistical Manual of Mental Disorders, DSM-III-R 101
alcohol dependence syndrome 437
depression 639
panic disorder 751, 752
personality disorders 855–6, *856*
post-traumatic stress disorder 693
schizophrenia 1547
Diagnostic and Statistical Manual of Mental Disorders, DSM-IV 113–20
acute PCP intoxication 486
acute stress disorder 693, 694, *694*
adjustment disorders 106, *716*, 717–19, *717*, 1067
alcohol use disorders 439, *440*
Alzheimer's disease 336
attention deficit-hyperactivity disorder 1643
bipolar disorder 639
body dysmorphic disorder 1045–6
categorical approach 849
as classification of disorders 64
communication disorders 1623, *1623*
comparison with ICD-10 102–4
cultural critique 276
and cultural formulation 278
cyclothymic disorder 686
delirium 327, 1531
delusional disorder 609, 613, *613*
delusions 611
depersonalization disorder 774
depression 633, *633*, 639, 640
development 101–2
disorders relating to cocaine 483, *484*
dysthymic disorder 681
eating disorder 106, 787–8, 800–1, *801*
ethical issues in diagnosis using 28
factitious disorder 106, 1049, 1050
frontotemporal dementias 348
generalized anxiety disorder 730, *730*

impulse control disorders 911
intellectual handicap 1820, *1820*
learning disorders 1623, *1623*
malingering 1054
mania 635, *635*
mental retardation (intellectual handicap) 1820, *1820*
motor skills disorder 1623, *1623*
multiaxial descriptive systems 73
obsessive–compulsive disorder 765, 1682
panic disorder 750–1, 751, 752
pathological gambling 920
personality disorders 106, 851, 855–8, *856*
antisocial personality disorder *865*
avoidant personality disorder *872*
borderline personality disorder *867*
dependent personality disorder *873*
histrionic personality disorder *869*
narcissistic personality disorder *871*
obsessive–compulsive personality disorder 874, *874*
paranoid personality disorder 861, *861*
passive–aggressive personality disorder 876, *876*
schizoid personality disorder 863, *863*
schizotypal personality disorder 864, *864*
pervasive developmental disorders 1633, 1639
post-traumatic stress disorder 701, *702–3, 703*
in primary care 1483–4
relational problems 1382
schizoaffective disorder 597–8
schizophrenia 105, 534, *534, 536*, 541, 568–9, 571
sexual dysfunction 823
social anxiety disorder 740
somatoform disorders 993–4, *993*, 1003, 1062
body dysmorphic disorder 1045–6
conversion disorder 106, 1012
hypochondriasis 996–7, 1022–3, *1022*
persistent somatoform pain disorder 993–4, 1029–30
somatization disorder 996, 999–1000, 1003
specific phobia 745
substance-induced persisting dementia 399, *399*
substance use disorders 439, *440*
tic disorders 1682
use in epidemiology 283
vascular dementia 377, *377*
Diagnostic and Statistical Manual of Mental Disorders, DSM-IV-PC 1483–4
Diagnostic and Statistical Manual of Mental Disorders, DSM-IV-TR 102
bereavement 1758
in childhood and adolescence 104, 1592–3
conduct disorder 1657
and epidemiology 1607
intellectual disability 1825
intellectual disability with psychiatric disorder 1826, 1849, 1850
schizophrenia 1547
and stressors 718
structure 104–6
Diagnostic and Statistical Manual of Mental Disorders, DSM-V, research planning for 106–8, 852
Diagnostic Criteria for Psychiatric Disorders for Use with Adults with Learning Disabilities/ Mental Retardation 1826–7, 1850

*Diagnostic Criteria for Research* 71
Diagnostic Interview for Personality Disorders *858*
Diagnostic Interview Schedule 71–2, 542, 765
dialectical behaviour therapy (DBT) 304
attempted suicide 970, 1707
personality disorders 318–19, 868, 895–6, 904, 1563
diazepam 1178
in alcohol withdrawal 449
in cancer *1102*
in delirium 1533
dosage 1180
drug interactions 1232
as a hypnotic 1182
in panic disorder *756, 757*
pharmacokinetics *1172*, 1178
potential for misuse 491
rebound and withdrawal symptoms 1180–1
in status epilepticus 1867
didanosine *1091*, 1092
diencephalon 156
diet
and attention-deficit hyperactivity disorder 1646–7, 1648
elderly people 1529
elimination 1648
and modification of ageing 1509
and monoamine oxidase inhibitors 1187–8, 1192, *1192*
difference scores 87
abnormality 87
reliability 87
differential reinforcement of other behaviour 414
diffuse axonal injury 387
digit span 89, 255, 264
digoxin 1532
dihydrocodeine 474, 1244
dihydroergotoxin 1240
dihydrotestosterone 815
diltiazem 1201, 1206
Dimensional Assessment of Personality Disorders 858, *858*
2,5-dimethoxy-4-ethylthio-β-phenethylamine 501
dimethyltryptamine 488, 489, 501
diminished responsibility defence 1901, 1922, 1923, 1928, 1937, 1939, 1940
*Dioscorea alata* 1249
DIPD (Diagnostic Interview for Personality Disorders) *858*
diphenhydramine 1226
direct questioning in child and adolescent assessment 1604–5
DIS (Diagnostic Interview Schedule) 71–2, 542, 765
disability
definition 389
measurement of 1465
Disability-Adjusted Life Expectancy 1510
Disability-Adjusted Life Years 10, 645, 1477, 1510
Disability Assessment Schedule 284
disablement 283
concepts of 65, *66*
measurement of 284
disasters 1108
DISC1 gene 229, 555
discrimination 11
and stigma 5, 6, 7

disease, concept of 62, 63–4, 277–8
disinhibition
    in Alzheimer's disease 335
    in attention-deficit hyperactivity
        disorder 1647
    and hallucinations 50
disintegrative psychosis **1637**
disorientation 59
    delusional 392
disposable soma theory 1509
dissocial personality disorder *see* antisocial
        personality disorder
dissociation 1012, *1013*
    in acute stress reactions 693, 694, 696
    following an accident 1106–7
    victims of criminal activity 1984
dissociative disorder *see* conversion disorder
*dissolution du langage* 346
disulfiram **453**, *730*, **1246**, 1542
diuretic abuse
    in anorexia nervosa 784
    in bulimia nervosa 802, 803
diurnal rhythm disturbances 55
divalproex 1677
divination 1420
divorce 1369–70, 1601, 1726
    counselling 1278–9
DLB *see* dementia, with Lewy bodies
DMIS (delusional misidentification syndrome)
    51, 392, 609–10, 611, 622, **623–4**
DNA
    cloned 231
    cross-linkage 1508
    deletions/insertions 227
    free radical damage 1509
    hybridization 226
    methylation 224, 1508
    microsatellites 226
    mitochondrial (mtDNA) 223, 1832
        age-related defects 1508
        free radical damage 1509
    non-coding sequences 218
    nuclear (nDNA) 223
        accumulated somatic mutations 1508
    pooling 221
    replication 223
    short tandem repeats (STRs) 226
    single nucleotide polymorphisms
        (SNPs) 218, 226, 227
    structure and function 223
    transcription 223–4, *224*
        effects of ageing on 1507
DNA microarray studies 1509, 1510
DNA repair genes 1508
doctor–patient communication 1138–9
domestic violence 1449, **1981–3**
    and conduct disorder 1659–60
    during pregnancy 1117
Dominica, attitudes to psychiatric disorder 6
*dommage par ricochet* 1902
Domus units 1583
donepezil
    in Alzheimer's disease 409, 1241, 1538
    in dementia 415
    in mild cognitive impairment 1538
    in Parkinson's disease 370–1
    in vascular dementia 381
donor insemination 1114–15
Doose syndrome 1863–4
dopamine agonists

adverse effects 539
    in sexual dysfunction 828
dopamine dysregulation syndrome 1073
dopaminergic system and dopamine
        receptors *173*, 511, 1171
    and alcohol use disorders 229
    antipsychotic actions at 1171–2, 1209,
        1210, *1211*
    and attention-deficit hyperactivity
        disorder 1646
    in autism 1636
    and cortical function 151
    in delirium 330
    dopamine transporters 169, *170*
    effects of amphetamines/cocaine on 482, 1172
    effects of nicotine 510
    effects of transcranial magnetic
        stimulation 1263
    and neurotrophic factors *160*
    and novelty-seeking 886–7
    in obsessive–compulsive disorder 767
    PET/SPET imaging *186*, 187, 188, 189–90
    and schizophrenia 180, 188, 561–2
    and sexual function 826
    in social anxiety disorder 741
    and substance use disorders 429
    in substance use disorders 429, *429*, 436
    and suicide 965–6
    and Tourette syndrome 1073, 1684
Doppelgänger 623
dorsal horn 157
dorsal parieto-frontal network 245
dorsal roots 158
dosulepin (dothiepin) 670
'double-bind' 1053, 1381
double orientation 392
double phenomenon 56
Doublecortin 158
Down syndrome
    and autism 1839
    behavioural phenotype 1613, 1839, *1851*, 1858
    and dementia 1584, 1827, 1839, 1865, 1880
    effects on the family 1883–4
    and epilepsy 1864, 1865
    genetics 228, 1831, 1838–9
    infantile spasms in 1863
    and intellectual disability 1839
    and mania 1826
    and parental psychiatric disorder 1885
    physical characteristics 1839, 1850
    prevalence 1825, 1838–9
    prevention 1448
downward comparison 1066
doxepin 670
    adverse effects *1191*
    in anxiety disorders 1182
    dosage *1196*
    pharmacodynamics *1187*
    pharmacokinetics *1189*
drawings in child and adolescent
        assessment 1604
dreams
    analysis 299, 306
    and the unconscious 313
dressing dyspraxia 1527
DRGs (diagnosis related groups) 1430
drift effect 549
drive-defence model 313
drive theory 294, 295, 302, 306
driving

and dementia 412
    elderly people 1577–8
    legislation regarding alcohol consumption
        468, 469
measures to reduce casualties 468, 469
DRO (differential reinforcement of other
        behaviour) 414
droperidol *1209*
    pharmacodynamics *1211*
    pharmacokinetics *1172*
DRPLA (dentatorubropallidoluysian
        atrophy) *228*, 373
DRS-R98 (Delirium Rating Scale-
        Revised-98) 328
Drug Abuse Problem Assessment for Primary
        Care 1484
Drug Action Teams 515–16
drug therapy *see* pharmacotherapy
DSH *see* deliberate self-harm
DSM *see entries under* Diagnostic and Statistical
        Manual of Mental Disorders
DSPD 848, 2015, 2018
DST *see* Dexamethasone Suppression Test
dual instinct/drive theory 294, 295, 302, 306
dualism 133, 989–91
    in psychopathology 848
Duchenne muscular dystrophy
    behavioural and psychiatric aspects 1843
    genetics 1843
    physical characteristics 1843
    prevalence 1843
duloxetine 670, *670*
    adverse effects *1191*, 1555
    in cancer 1102
    in depression in elderly people 1554, *1554*
    dosage *1196*
    pharmacodynamics 1186, *1187*
    pharmacokinetics 1189, *1189*
duration of untreated psychosis (DUP) 536, 590
    and prognosis 1459
    and response to treatment 573
Dyadic Adjustment Scale 1165
dynamic child psychotherapy *see*
        psychodynamic psychotherapy, childhood
        and adolescence
dynorphin 171, *171*
dysaesthesia, chronic cutaneous 618
dysarthria 53, 1711, 1712
    in HIV-associated dementia 384
dysbindin gene 179, 230, 555
dyscalculia 1629–30
Dysexecutive Questionnaire *90*
dysexecutive syndrome
    assessment 89, *90*
    features *90*
    following head injury 390
    in parkinsonism 92
    in schizophrenia 93
    in vascular dementia 379
dysfunctional assumptions 1286
Dysfunctional Attitudes Scale 1165
Dysfunctional Thoughts Record 1309–10,
        *1309*, 1311
dyskinesias in Huntington's disease 371
dyslexia 1627–9
    surface 406
dysmorphophobia *see* body dysmorphic
        disorder
dysnomia 850
dyspareunia 823

dysphasia 53
  Broca's 1527
  conduction 54
  and delirium 326
  elderly people 1527
  following head injury 391
  nominal 54, 334
  primary motor 54
  primary sensory 54
  Wernicke's 1527
dysphonia 53
dyspraxia
  in Alzheimer's disease 334
  dressing 1527
dysprosody following head injury 391
dysthymia/dysthymic disorder **680–6**, 1060
  aetiology 683–4
  childhood and adolescence 683, 1669,
    *1670*, 1673
  classification 681
  clinical features 681–2, *682*
  concept of 680
  course and outcome 668, 682–3, *683*
  diagnosis 681–2
  elderly people 1552
  epidemiology 683
  historical perspective 680–1
  and intellectual disability 1855
  interpersonal psychotherapy 1323
  prevention 686
  relationship with major depressive
    disorder 684, *684*
  treatment 684–6
dystonia
  drug-induced 1222
  psychogenic 1016
dystrobrevin-binding protein-1 555

EAPs (employee assistance programmes)
    1281–2
early infantile epileptic encephalopathy 1862
early intervention teams 1459, *1459*
early morning wakening in depression
    634, 661–2
early myoclonic epileptic encephalopathy 1862
Eating Attitudes Test (EAT) 777
eating disorder
  atypical 787
  and body image 57
  childhood and adolescence
    atypical 787
    differential diagnosis 1672
    treatment 1784
  classification and diagnosis 106, 800–1, *801*
  cognitive-behaviour therapy 792, 796, 808,
    808–9, **1298–303**, 1784
  maintenance 1299
  'not otherwise specified' 800, *801*, 804
  parental, effects on child development
    1753–4
  and pregnancy 780, 784, 1118
  relationships between 804
  sleep-related *931*, 947–8
  temporal migration between disorders 801
  *see also* anorexia nervosa; bulimia nervosa
Eating Disorder Examination 807, 1163
Eating Disorder Inventory 807
eating disorder units 792–3
Ebstein's anomaly 1118, 1169
*Echinacea purpurea* (echinacea) 1249, *1250*

*echo de la pensée* 49
echo phenomena 54, 58, *58*
echolalia 54, 58, *58*, 1681, 1713
  in Alzheimer's disease 334
  in autism 1633
  in frontotemporal dementias 346
  in Tourette syndrome 1073
echopraxia 58, *58*
  in Tourette syndrome 1073
eclectic therapy 1278
ECLW Collaborative Study 1144, 1146
ecstasy **494–7**
  addictiveness *431*
  effects on memory 409
  neuropsychological impairment due to 496
  neurotoxicity 496, *496*
  physical effects and complications 495, *495*
  pill testing 494
  preparations and purity 494
  prevalence and patterns of use 494–5
  psychological effects and complications
    495–7, *495*, 538
  routes of use 494
ECT *see* electroconvulsive therapy
ectoderm 156
ED *see* erectile dysfunction
Edinburgh Postnatal Depression Scale 1122
education
  higher/further 1815
  and intellectual disability 1873, 1884
  role of the child psychiatrist **1811–16**
  school liaison service 1812–13
  *see also* schools
education welfare officer 1812
educational psychologist 1812
EDUs (eating disorder units) 792–3
EEG *see* electroencephalography
EER (experimental event rate) 128
efavirenz *1091*
Effective Black Parenting Program 1791
effectiveness 1609
  measurement of 1475
efficacy 1609
effort testing 1055, 1056
ego 294, 306, 313, 849
  defences 297, 310
  structure and functions 295–6, 316
ego ideal 296
ego identity 295
ego psychology 295, 313, 1339
  and mental health social work 1408–9
egocentricity 1777
eicosapentaenoic acid 1248
EIS (early intervention teams) 1459, *1459*
ejaculation 817
  delayed 822
  premature 822, 828
*el miedo* 984
elation in Alzheimer's disease 335
elderly people
  abuse of 1575–6, *1575*
  adjustment disorders 1552
  agoraphobia 1559
  alcohol intake recommendations 1540
  alcohol use disorders 1519, *1540*,
    **1540–2**, *1541*
  anxiety 1558–61
  anxiety disorders 1531, 1579
  art therapy 1415
  assessment **1524–9**

  after treatment 1528–9
  common geriatric assessment 1581
  history-taking 1526
  mental state examination 1526–7, *1528*
  physical 1527–9
  setting for 1525–7
bipolar disorder 1556–7
boundaries of normality 1574–5
capacity 1577
cognitive assessment 1527
definitions 1579
deliberate self-harm 1551, **1564–7**
delirium 1529, **1530–4**
  aetiology 1532, *1532*
  classification 1531
  clinical features 1530–1
  complications 1533
  course and prognosis 1532
  diagnosis 1531
  differential diagnosis 1531, 1559
  epidemiology 1531–2
  prevention 1533
  treatment and management 1532–3
delusional disorder 1552
dementia
  differential diagnosis 1558–9
  early detection 1519–20
  epidemiology **1519–22**, 1579–80
  impact 1522
  incidence and risk factors 1520–2,
    *1520*, *1522*
  presentation in primary care 1483
  *see also* Alzheimer's disease
demography 333–4, 1517, *1517*
dependence 1575–8
depression **1550–6**
  aetiology *1552*, 1553
  assessment 1527, 1551–2
  clinical features 1551
  in the community 1517
  course and prognosis 1553
  diagnosis 1551–2
  differential diagnosis 373, 1552, 1558
  epidemiology 1517–18, 1552–3, 1579
  factors influencing presentation *1551*
  in hostels and nursing homes 1518
  investigations 1551–2, *1553*
  mortality associated 1553
  prevention 1555–6
  in primary care 1482–3, 1518
  resistant 1555
  treatment and management 674, 1554–5
driving 1577–8
dysphasia 1527
dysthymic disorder 1552
epilepsy with intellectual disability 1864
ethical issues 1576–7
ethnic minorities 1585
falls 1528–9
group therapy 1366
homicide by 1938
hypomania 1527
illicit drug use 1544
indirect self-destructive behaviour 1565
intellectual disability 1584, 1864
  carers 1880–1
  health needs 1880
  life expectancy 1880
  with psychiatric/behavioural
    disorders 1858–9

elderly people (*cont.*)
  legal issues 1577–8
  life events 1559–60
  loss of capacity 1575–8
  mania 1527, 1556–7
  medication use disorders **1543–5**, *1544*
  mental health services 1574–5, *1575*,
    **1579–86**
    academic units 1584
    CARITAS principles 1580
    community services 1582
    comprehensive 1581
    consultation-liaison services 1583
    core business 1581
    core components 1581–4, *1582*
    day hospitals 1583
    inpatient units 1582–3
    integrated 1581
    long-term care 1583
    need for 1579–80
    patient-centred 1580–1
    planning to commissioning 1584–5
    primary care collaborations 1583–4
    principles of good service delivery 1580–1
    residential care 1583
    respite care 1583
    special components 1584
  mood disorders **1550–8**
  neurotic (stress-related) disorder **1558–61**
    aetiology 1559–60
    clinical features 1558
    course and prognosis 1560
    diagnosis and differential diagnosis
      1558–9
    epidemiology 1559
    treatment 1560
  nicotine use 1544
  nutrition 1529
  obsessive–compulsive disorder 1558
  paranoia **1546–50**, 1559
  parasomnias 1572
  personality disorders **1561–4**
    aetiology 1562–3
    clinical features 1561–2
    course and prognosis 1563
    diagnosis 1562
    epidemiology 1518, 1562–3, *1562*
    treatment and management 1563–4
  pharmacotherapy 1573
    dosage regimens 1169
  physical illness 1559
  in primary care 1482–3, 1518, 1584
  prisoners 1584
  psychological treatments 1574
  psychoses 1518–19
  referral process 1524
  residential services 1518, 1583
  schizoaffective disorder 1552
  schizophrenia **1546–50**, 1552
    aetiology 1548
    classification 1546–7
    clinical features 1546
    course and prognosis 1548
    diagnosis 1547
    differential diagnosis 1547, 1559
    epidemiology 1547
    treatment and management 1548–9
  self-esteem 1559
  sexuality **1567–70**
  sleep disorders 1571–3

substance use disorders 1519, **1540–6**
suicide 976, 1518, 1527, 1551, **1564–7**
thought content 1527
treatment, special features **1571–8**
electrical allergy 997
electroconvulsive therapy (ECT) **1251–60**
  body dysmorphic disorder 1047
  in childhood and adolescence 1256
  choice of 675
  in combination with drug therapy 1257
  comparison with transcranial magnetic
    stimulation 1264–5
  continuation 1257
  contraindications 1252, *1252*, 1257
  in elderly people 1555, 1556
  future of 1258
  indications 1252–5, *1252*
  mechanism of action 1257–8
  mood disorders 671, 1252–4
  origins 1251–2
  in pregnancy 1117
  risks 404, 1257
  schizoaffective disorder 598
  schizophrenia 592
  stigma attached 1251, 1258
  suggested replacements for 1258
  treatment
    principles 1256–7
    process 1256–7
electroencephalography (EEG)
  Alzheimer's disease 337
  in antisocial behaviour 1918
  Creutzfeldt–Jakob disease 353
  delirium 328
  dementia with Lewy bodies 364
  early infantile epileptic encephalopathy 1862
  in electroconvulsive therapy 1257
  epilepsy 1078, 1862
  frontotemporal dementias 347
  head injury 389
  infantile spasms 1862–3
  Lennox–Gastaut syndrome 1863
  psychogenic seizures 1864
  schizophrenia 563
  sleep stages 925
  vascular dementia 380
electromyography, sleep stages 925
electro-oculography, sleep stages 925
EMDR *see* eye movement desensitization and
    reprocessing
emergencies
  assessment 68
  in childhood and adolescence **1807–11**
emergency cards in attempted suicide 970
emergency workers, debriefing 1110
emics 276
emission 817, 822
emotion
  anatomy of **257–62**
  and decision-making 260–1
  immune modulation 209
  and memory 259
  and perception 259–60
  role of the amygdala 258, 259
emotional development 242–3, *242*
  history-taking 1601
emotional lability
  following stroke 1071
  in multiple sclerosis 1074
  in vascular dementia 379

emotional learning 258–9
emotional memory 264
emotional reasoning 1288
emotional stability 850
emotional withdrawal in depression 634
empathogens 495
empathy 47
employee assistance programmes 1281–2
employment
  and alcohol use disorders 456
  employee assistance programmes 1281–2
  supported 1401
empty nest syndrome 1513
encephalitis 1095
  herpes 406, 1095
  motor sequelae 59
encephalitis lethargica 59
encephalopathy
  chronic traumatic 395
  early infantile epileptic 1862
  early myoclonic epileptic 1862
  hepatic 445, 1084–5
  mitochondrial 1864, 1865, *1866*
ENCODE project 224
end-stage renal disease 1087
Endicott Work Productivity Scale 1165
endocannabinoids *168*, 172, 429, *429*, 507
endophenotypes 266, 652, 1667
endorphins 170, 429, *429*
engagement techniques in child and adolescent
    assessment 1604
engrams 250, 253
enkephalins 429, *429*
enmeshment 1371
entactogens 495
entorhinal cortex 146, 152, 180, 251–2, 564,
    1537–8
entrainment test in psychogenic tremor 1016
enuresis, nocturnal 1702
environment
  factors in attention-deficit hyperactivity
    disorder 1646
  factors in bipolar disorder 1675
  factors in child development 1724–8
  factors in conduct disorder 1658–9
  factors in depression 1675
  factors in offending 1913–14
  factors in schizophrenia 555–8
  host–agent–environment model 1608
  interactions with genetic factors 214–18,
    221, 229, 315, 558–9, 1608, 1725
envy 307
ependymal cells 157
Epidemiological Catchment Area study 72, 541,
    645, 1926, 1937
epidemiology
  in childhood and adolescence 1594–9
  and classification 1607
  contribution to aetiology **280–9**
  developmental 1607
  and ethnicity 277
  genetic 286, 650–1, 1597–8
  Goldberg–Huxley model 1480, *1481*
  intergenerational 1598
  life course 1598
  matrix for studies *287*, 288
  measurement of symptoms 284–6
  and prevention science 1598
  in primary care 1480–2, *1481*, *1482*
  in public health 1607–8

sampling principles 282–3
specifying disorders 283–4
strategies 286, *287*, 288
study design 282
and transcultural psychiatry 14
uses of 280–1
epigenetics 218, 225
epilepsia partialis continua 1531
epilepsia partialis Kojewnikow 1864, 1867
epilepsy **1076–81**
absence 204, 1077
aetiology 1078, 1619–20
and aggression 1078, 1864, 1929, 1929–30
and Angelman syndrome 1864, 1865
and anxiety 1080
with attention-deficit hyperactivity
disorder 1650
aura 60, 1077
and autism 1852
automatism 403, 1077
benign focal 1618
in childhood and adolescence
aetiology 1619–20
classification 1619
clinical features 1618–19
course and prognosis 1618–19, 1620
diagnosis 1619
differential diagnosis 1619
epidemiology 1619
with intellectual disability *1861, 1863*, 1864
management 1620
prevention 1620
psychiatric disorder associated 1740
salient non-epileptic episodes *1861*
classification 1076–7, 1619, 1862–4, *1863*
cognitive assessment 92
and conversion disorder 1015
and crime 1079–80
definition 1860–1
and depersonalization 775
and depression 1080
diagnosis 1078, 1619, 1861–2
differential diagnosis 538, 1078, 1619,
1861–2, *1862*
and Down syndrome 1864, 1865
elderly people with intellectual
disability 1864
epidemiology 1078, 1619
experimental
kindling 204
tetanus toxin model 204
and fragile-X syndrome 1864, 1865
frontal-lobe
behavioural abnormalities associated 1864
in childhood and adolescence 1618
and gamma rhythms 203
generalized 1077
genetics 159, 1620
ictus 1077
imaging 1078, 1862, 1930
in infancy 1861
and intellectual disability 92, 1828
in adults and elderly people 1864
aetiology and pathogenesis 1865–6,
*1865, 1866*
behavioural disorders 1864
in childhood and adolescence *1863*, 1864
diagnosis 1861–2
differential diagnosis 1861–2, *1863*
epidemiology 1864–5

in infancy 1861, 1862–4, *1863*
prognosis 1868
treatment 1866–8, *1867*
and memory 92
myoclonic
in childhood and adolescence 1864
in infancy 1863
with ragged red fibres 1865, *1866*
myoclonic–astatic 1863–4
and neuronal networks 201, 203–4
nocturnal seizures 1702
Northern 1864, *1866*
and offending 1079–80, 1920, 1929–31
partial 1077
and personality disorder 1079
pharmacotherapy **1231–40**
in intellectual disability 1866–7, *1867*
post-traumatic 394
prevention 1620
prodrome 1077
progressive myoclonus 1864
progressive partial 1864
psychiatric consequences 1078–80
psychosis
chronic interictal 1079
postictal 1079
and Rett's syndrome 1864, 1864–5
and schizophrenia 1079
and sexual function 1079
and sleep-wake disorders *932*
and social development 1079
and suicide 1080
syndromes 1077–8, 1861
temporal lobe (limbic) 59, 201, 1077
behavioural abnormalities associated 1864
in childhood and adolescence 1618
differential diagnosis 866
effects on learning and memory 204
and personality traits 1930
and transient global amnesia 403
treatment and management 1080, 1620
in tuberous sclerosis 1075
epistasis 229
EPQ-R (Eysenck Personality Questionnaire)
81, *81*, 286, 850
Epstein–Barr virus
and chronic fatigue syndrome 1038
and hypersomnia 942
and infectious mononucleosis 1095
Epworth sleepiness scale 938–9
erectile dysfunction (ED) 822
in dementia 416
in elderly people 1569
medical intervention 821
pharmacotherapy 821, 828
in physical illness 826
*see also* sexual dysfunction
ergot 487
Eriksen Flanker paradigm 265
erotomania 621–2, 1920
error (*e*) 85
error catastrophe 1507
errorless learning 423–4
escitalopram *670*
adverse effects *1191*
in body dysmorphic disorder 1046
in cancer *1102, 1103*
in depression in elderly people 1554, *1554*
dosage *1196*
in obsessive–compulsive disorder *1687*

in panic disorder *756*
pharmacodynamics 1186, *1187*
pharmacokinetics 1188–9, *1189*
in social anxiety disorder 743
ESEMed Study 1433
Esquirol, Jean-Etienne Dominique 18
estavudine 1092
eszopiclone *1102*, 1179, 1182–3
ethambutol 1094
ether 503
ethics and ethical issues **28–32**
anorexia nervosa 796
care ethics 31
codes of 30–1
in cognitive-behaviour therapy in childhood
and adolescence 1778–9
in community mental health services 1457–8
and diagnosis 28–9
expert witnesses 2004–5, *2005*
factitious disorder 1053–4
malingering 1058
in management 40–1
in management of sexual dysfunction 830
and neurosurgery for mental disorder
1267–8
old age psychiatry 1576–7
in prevention of intellectual disability 1835
principle-based 31
sexual offences 1964
and treatment 29–30
and values 32–3
Ethiopia, attitudes to psychiatric disorder 6
ethnic cleansing 1495
ethnic conflict 1494
*see also* refugees
ethnic minorities
adoption outcomes 1750–1
alcohol use disorders 464
care pathways 1439, 1440–1
caregiver-mediated interventions 1791
criminal victimization 1987
culturally informed services for 277
effects of a child with intellectual
disability 1884
elderly people 1585
intellectual disability 1879–80, 1881
mental health services 277, **1502–4**
schizophrenia 549, 557–8
voluntary organizations supporting 1491–2
ethnographic database 277
ethnography 275–6, *277*
ethosuxumide *1867*
etifoxine in adjustment disorders 721
euphoria 55
in multiple sclerosis 1074
European Consultation-Liaison Workgroup
Collaborative Study 1144, 1146
European Convention on Human Rights 1899,
1900, 1904, 2015
European Declaration for Mental
Health 1427
evening primrose oil 1249, *1250*
event rate 128
event sampling 97
evidence-based medicine **122–8**, 578
appraisal of evidence 126, *126, 127*
and clinical practice guidelines 123, 124
and current awareness 124–5, *125*
evidence hierarchy 123, *1465*
finding evidence 123–6, *125*

evidence-based medicine (*cont.*)
  formulating a structured clinical
      question 122–3
  stages *122*
  and study design *123*
  and systematic reviews 123–4
  types of clinical question *123*
  use of electronic communication and the
      Internet 124
  using research findings with individual
      patients 126–8
  and values-based practice 33
Evidence-Based Mental Health 125, *125*
evoked potentials in schizophrenia 563
EWO (education welfare officer) 1812
exaggeration *see* malingering
exalted stage 58
excellence, concepts of 43–4, *44*
exclusion criteria 100
excoriation, neurotic/psychogenic
    618, **917–18**, 1044
executive control systems 248–9, *248*
executive function 262
  assessment 89, *90*, 265
  and attention-deficit hyperactivity
      disorder 1647
exercise
  and anorexia nervosa 782
  in chronic fatigue syndrome 1040, 1042
  in dementia *414*
  in depression in elderly people 1555
  excessive, in bulimia nervosa 803
  and health 1136
  in insomnia 935
  in persistent somatoform pain disorder 1034
exhibitionism 832, *833, 836*, 1960, 1961
exons 224
expanded trinucleotide repeat sequences 652
experimental event rate 128
expert opinion 75
expert witness 1112, 1901, **2003–8**
  accreditation 2004
  common knowledge rule 2003
  and confidentiality 2006–7
  Court appearance 2007
  dual role 2004–5, *2005*
  ethical issues 2004–5, *2005*
  immunity from suit 2003
  regulatory rules 2004, *2004*
  reliability 2004
  reports 1928, *2004*, **2005–6**
  and risk assessment 2005
explanation, personal and subpersonal levels 135
explanatory gap 135, 278
explanatory models 278
explanatory therapy in hypochondriasis 1026
exposure 55, 1668
  in anxiety disorders 1294–5
  in body dysmorphic disorder 1047
  graded 1779
  imaginal 742, 746, 1295
  *in vivo* 742, 746
  interoceptive 761
  in panic disorder 758, 760–1
  in post-traumatic stress disorder 708, 1295
  social anxiety disorder 742
  in specific phobia 746
  virtual reality 746
exposure and response prevention in tic
    disorders 1687

expressed emotion and schizophrenia 575, 583
expression 213
expressive/exploratory psychotherapy *see*
    psychoanalytic psychotherapy
expressive language disorder 1625–6
extinction 250, 254, 1668
extradural haemorrhage 387
extraversion 81, *81*, 632, 633, 654, 850, 886
eye, development 157
eye movement abnormalities in
    schizophrenia 563
eye movement desensitization and reprocessing
    (EMDR) 1497
  adjustment disorders 720
  in childhood trauma 1730
  delusional disorder 1920
  following accidents 1109, 1111
  post-traumatic stress disorder 709
Eysenck, Hans 1158
Eysenck Personality Questionnaire 81, *81*,
    286, 850

fabricated or induced illness 1054, 1697, 1737,
    1923–4
facial erythema in alcohol use disorders 446
factitious disorder 994, **1049–54**, 1941
  aetiology 1051
  classification 106, *1050*
  clinical features 1049–50
  cognitive-behavioural conceptualization
      1051, *1052*
  course 1051
  diagnosis 1050
  diagnostic criteria 1049
  diagnostic problems 1049
  differential diagnosis 1003, 1012, *1012*,
      1050–1
  electronic 1050
  epidemiology 998, 1051
  ethical and legal issues 1053–4
  in health care workers 1054
  induced 1054, 1697, 1737, 1923–4
  obstetric 1050, 1118
  and pathological lying 1049
  prognosis 1051
  subtypes 1050
  and surgery 1096
  treatment and management 1052–4
Fahr's syndrome 373
fail, right to 1408
Fairbairn, W.R.D. 308
Faith Links project 1411
falls, elderly people 1528–9
false attribution 1054
false memories 59, 250, 403, 408, **713–16**
false-self–real-self distinction 309
familial schizotypal disorder 599
familicide 1923
Families and Schools Together Track
    programme 1663, 1789
family
  assessment 1382–3, 1384–6
  and borderline personality disorder 896
  burdens on 1401
  caregiver-mediated interventions **1787–93**
  changes in patterns of 1726–7
  and child neglect 1736
  and child physical abuse 1735
  and child sexual abuse 1733
  and conduct disorder

factors in 1659–60
  impact of disorder 1655–6
  involvement in management 1663
criminal activity by 1659, 1911–12
and cultural variation in care pathways 1439
as decision-makers 1895
disruption 1910–11
effects of alcohol use disorders 452–3, 465
effects of child with intellectual
    disability **1883–6**
effects of child with physical illness 1742
effects of childhood and adolescent sleep
    disorders 1694–5
effects of dementia 417–18
effects of Huntington's disease 374
effects of personality change following head
    injury 391
factors affecting child mental health 1725–7
factors in anorexia nervosa 780
factors in offending 1910–12
factors in schizophrenia 536, 548–9, 553–5
in gender identity disorder 844
history 215, 1601
impact of caring on 1465
involvement in management of somatization
    disorder 1009
involvement in rehabilitation of
    delirium 1533
large 1912
nontraditional configurations 1787
reaction to illness 1066
of refugees 1497
role in treatment of intellectual
    disability 1873
single-parent 1369–70, 1601, 1726–7,
    1910, 1911
step-families 1370, 1726–7
suicide 981–2
Family-Check-Up 1790
family crisis intervention 1382
family focused treatment 1677
family intervention 1401
family interview 1386
family life cycle 1373–4
family-mediated interventions *see* caregiver-
    mediated interventions
family myths 1066
family studies **215**
  anxiety disorders 1667
  intermittent explosive disorder 912
  kleptomania 913
  mood disorders 651
  trichotillomania 915
family support teams 1411
family therapy **1380–91**
  adjustment disorders *1069*
  anorexia nervosa 790–2, *790*, 796
  assessment in 1384–6
  in attempted suicide 1707
  bipolar disorder 673
  in childhood trauma 1730
  conduct disorder 1661–2, 1782
  conjoint 790–1
  contraindications 1383
  course 1386
  elderly people 1574
  historical context 1380–1
  indications 1382–3
  Milan approach 1381, 1387
  persistent somatoform pain disorder 1034

family therapy (*cont.*)
    post-modern developments 1381–2
    problems encountered in 1388
    psychoanalytic and related approaches 1381
    psycho-educational approach 1382
    research 1388–9
    role of the therapist 1386–7
    schizophrenia 583–4
    separated 790–1
    systems-oriented 1381, 1381–2
    termination 1387–8
    training in 1389–90
    transgenerational 1381
family tree 1381, 1384, *1384*
famine oedema 785
fantasy (gamma hydroxy butyrate) 409, **498–9**
fantasy thinking 50
FAS *see* foetal alcohol syndrome
FASD (foetal alcohol spectrum disorder)
    1614–15, 1841
FAST (Functional Assessment Staging) scale
    335, 337
'Fast Track' programme 1598, 1663, 1789
fatigue
    differentiation from chronic fatigue
        syndrome 1037
    in physical illness 209, *210*
    as a symptom 1035–6
    *see also* chronic fatigue syndrome
FCU (Family-Check-Up) 1790
fear
    definition 1664
    pathophysiology 1666–7, *1667*
    pathways *732*
fear conditioning paradigm 1666
'fear of fatness' 783
FEAR plan 1779
feeling states, neurobiology of 260–1
feelings, definition 260
Feighner criteria 100
Ferenczi, Sándor 1338
fertility and schizophrenia 545
fetishism *833, 836*
FFT (family focused treatment) 1677
fibroblast growth factor (FGF) 156
fibromyalgia 990, 997, 1003, 1037
    and cortisol 1039
    treatment and management 1034
fight response following an accident 1107
FII (induced factitious disorder) 1054, 1697,
    1737, 1923–4
filicide 1125, 1923
Finnish disease heritage 1831
fire-raising/fire-setting *see* arson; pyromania
fire sickness (*hwabyung*) 984
5p-syndrome *see* cri-du-chat syndrome
fixations 297
flashbacks
    cannabis 508
    in hallucinogen persisting perception
        disorder 488
    in post-traumatic stress disorder 404, 701
FLD *see* frontal lobe degeneration of non-
    Alzheimer type
flesinoxan 735
flexibilitas cerea 58, *58*
flight of ideas 53
    slow 1527
flight response following an accident 1106
flooding in panic disorder 761

floppy infant syndrome 1117
fluency disorders 53, 1623, 1712
flumazenil 1172, 1176, 1180
flunarizine 1201
flunitrazepam 409, 491, 1178, 1183
fluoxetine
    adverse effects 1173, *1191*
    in body dysmorphic disorder 1046
    in bulimia nervosa 807
    in cancer *1102, 1103*
    in childhood and adolescence 1676
    and cosmetic psychopharmacology 29
    delayed onset of effects 176
    in depression *670*
        continuation treatment 671
        in elderly people 1554, *1554*
    dosage 674, *1196*
    drug interactions 1233
    in intellectual disability 1875
    in obsessive–compulsive disorder 769, *1687*
    in panic disorder *756*
    in personality disorders *905*
    pharmacodynamics *1173, 1187*
    pharmacokinetics *1172, 1188, 1189*
    in pregnancy 1117
    in selective mutism 1714
    in social anxiety disorder 743
flupenthixol
    in attempted suicide 971
    pharmacokinetics *1172*
fluphenazine *1209*
    administration *1214*
    adverse effects *1212*, 1222
    in intellectual disability 1875
    pharmacodynamics *1211*
flurazepam *1172*, 1179
fluvoxamine *670*
    adverse effects *1191*
    in body dysmorphic disorder 1046
    in depression in elderly people *1554*
    dosage *1196*
    drug interactions 1175
    in intellectual disability 1875
    in obsessive–compulsive disorder 769, *1687*
    in panic disorder *756*
    in personality disorders *905*
    pharmacodynamics *1173, 1187*
    pharmacokinetics *1172, 1189, 1189*
    in social anxiety disorder 743
    in Wernicke–Korsakoff syndrome 409
fMRI *see* functional magnetic resonance
    imaging
focal conflict theory 1357
focal psychotherapy 1327, 1330–1, *1331*
foetal alcohol spectrum disorder 1614–15, 1841
foetal alcohol syndrome (FAS) 445, 1117, 1754
    aetiology 1615
    behavioural phenotype 1615
    classification 1841
    clinical features 1614–15, 1646, 1841
    epidemiology 1615
    natural history 1615
    neurological and behavioural aspects 1841
    prevalence 1826, 1841
    prevention 1448
    treatment and management 1615
foetal valproate syndrome 1118
foetus
    abuse of 1117
    adverse environment 659, 1725

death *in utero* 1119
effects of maternal alcohol use *see* foetal
    alcohol syndrome
effects of maternal substance use 480, *480*,
    1117–18, 1614, 1615–16
mother–foetus relationship 1117
prenatal diagnosis of intellectual
    disability 1833–4
folic acid deficiency 1087–8
*folie à deux* 610, **624–5**
folk healing practices **1418–22**
follicle-stimulating hormone in anorexia
    nervosa 783
follow-back studies 556–7, 568
food avoidance emotional disorder 787
food diary *802*
food fads 787
food intake history in anorexia nervosa 782
food refusal 787
forced choice testing 94, 1057
forebrain 156–7
forensic mental health services 2013,
    **2015–21**
    capacity planning 2017–18
    community 1459
    international context 2016
    philosophy and theoretical models
        2015–16
    private 2017
    pyramid planning 2017
    security 2015, 2016–17
    service structure 2017–18
    service users 2018–20
    super-specialist 2017
foresight 80, *80*, 82, 83
formal thought disorder 52
formulation 68, 73–4
    cultural 278
    in psychoanalysis 1341–2
fornix 155–6
fortune-telling 1420
foscarnet *1091*
fosphenytoin in status epilepticus 1867
foster care 1787, 1790, 1800, 1801
    effects on child and adult mental
        health **1747–52**
    forensic/multidimensional treatment
        1790, 1953
    long-term 1749–50
    short-term 1748–9
    treatment 1662
Foulkes, S.H. 1353, 1357
14-3-3 protein 353
fourth ventricle 157
fragile X-associated tremor ataxia
    syndrome *228*
fragile-X syndrome
    and autism 1635
    behavioural phenotype 1613, 1614, 1840,
        *1851*, 1858
    effects on the family 1884
    and epilepsy 1864, 1865
    genetics 212, 213, 228, *228*, 1832, 1839–40,
        1865, *1866*
    physical characteristics 1840
    prevalence 1839–40
    psychiatric aspects 1840
fragile-XE syndrome *228*
FRAMES 450, *450*
framing effect 261

France
  CANTOUs 1583
  community mental health teams 1454
  and dual-drive theory 302
  history of psychiatry 17, 19, 20, 22, 23, 24,
      26, 603, 630, 848
  involuntary admission in 1440
  legal aspects 1901, 1902
  prion disease 355, 357
fraud 1941
free association 293–4, 297, 1328, 1770
free-floating discussion 1357, 1360, 1363
free radicals, role in ageing 1509
freeze response following an accident 1106
Frégoli syndrome 623
Freud, Anna 310, 1683, 1770
Freud, Sigmund 20–1, 293, 1337, 1770
  dual-drive theory 294, 295, 302, 306
  models of personality 849
  and neurasthenia 1060
  and obsessional neurosis 768
  and obsessive–compulsive phenomena 1683
  and panic disorder 751
  and psychodynamic psychiatry 313
  and psychosexual development 235
  structural theory 294–6
  theories on suicide 954
  theory of the mental apparatus 293–4
  therapeutic technique 1338
  topographic theory 294
Freudian slips 313
Friedrich ataxia 228
friendliness 886, 888
FRIENDS programme 1780
Fromm, Eric 311
Fromm-Reichmann, Freida 310
frontal eye field 245
frontal leucotomy 1267
frontal lobe degeneration of non-Alzheimer
      type (FLD) 344
  aetiology 348
  age at onset 345
  clinical features 345–6
  investigations 347
frontal-lobe syndrome 89
frontal lobes
  and aggressive/antisocial behaviour 1917–18
  in alcohol use disorders 183
  anatomy 145–6, 145
  association connections 145, 153
  lesions 265, 1917–18
  in schizophrenia 178
frontotemporal lobar degeneration (FTLD)
      344, 344
  classification 344, 344
  epidemiology 345
  physical signs 346
  ubiquitinated 344
frotteurism 832, 833, 836
FTD see dementia, frontotemporal
FTDP-17 344–5, 346, 348
FTLD see frontotemporal lobar degeneration
fugue states 57, 404–5
functional analysis 96
Functional Assessment Staging scale 335, 337
functional disorders 990
functional family therapy 1661, 1782
functional magnetic resonance imaging (fMRI)
      196–201
  alcohol-related dementia 401

Alzheimer's disease 337
  anxiety disorders in childhood and
      adolescence 1668
  artefacts 197–8
  cerebral activation and blood-flow
      changes 197
  comparison with PET and SPET 186–7,
      196–7
  data analysis 199–201
    activation mapping 200, Plate 10
    movement estimation and correction 199
    multivariate approaches 200
    statistical models for the neurovascular
        response 199–200
    visualization 201, Plate 11
    within- and between-group 200–1
  depression 660
  and emotions 257–8
  endogenous contrast agents 197
  epilepsy 1862
  experimental design 198–9
    blocked periodic design 198, 199
    event-related design 199
    parametric design 199
  hardware 198
  imaging sequences 197
    echoplanar imaging 197
    gradient echo sequence 197
  intermittent explosive disorder 912
  in pathological lying 1049, 1051
  schizophrenia 562–3
functional neuroimaging
  and aggressive/antisocial behaviour 1918
  alcohol-related brain damage 401
  anorexia nervosa 781
  attention-deficit hyperactivity disorder 1647
  conversion disorder 1013
  and emotion 257–8, 260, 261
  epilepsy 1078, 1079
  post-traumatic stress disorder 706–7
  schizophrenia 562–3
    with violence 1919
  see also specific techniques
functionalism 134
  challenges to 134–5
fusion of thought 53

G (gamma hydroxy butyrate) 409, **498–9**
G protein-coupled receptors 172, 173, 174, 175,
      202, 1171
  regulation 175
G-proteins 174–5, 473, 1201
'G spot' 818
G72 gene 555
GABA 148, 155, 429
  and body dysmorphic disorder 1046
  effects of valproate on 1231
  and epilepsy 1619, 1865
  hippocampus 202
  in opioid neurobiology 473
  in panic disorder 754
  role in neurodevelopment 159
  and schizophrenia 562
  in substance use disorders 429
  transporters 169, 170
GABA receptors 1171
  action of benzodiazepines at 1171, 1179
  in generalized anxiety disorder 733, 734
  hippocampal 202
  ligand-gated ion channels 173, 174

gabapentin 1237
  drug interactions 1866
  pharmacokinetics 1867
  in social anxiety disorder 743
Gabitril (tiagabine) 1237, 1867
gaboxadol 1183
GAD see generalized anxiety disorder
GAF (Global Assessment of Functioning
      scale) 73, 1165, 1593
gait abnormalities 57
galanin 171, 171
  receptors 173
galantamine
  in Alzheimer's disease 409, 1241
  in vascular dementia 381
Gamblers Anonymous 922, 1352
gambling, pathological **919–23**
  addictiveness 431
  aetiology 920–1
  classification 920
  clinical features 920
  course and prognosis 922
  diagnosis 920
  epidemiology 920–1
  impulsive 920
  neurotic 920
  predisposing factors 921–2
  prevention 923
  psychopathic 920
  subcultural 920
  symptomatic 920
  treatment and management 922
γ-aminobutyric acid see GABA
gamma butyl-lactone 498
gamma hydroxy butyrate 409, **498–9**
γ-linolenic acid 1248, 1249
gamma rhythms 203
ganciclovir 1092
ganoderic acid 1063
Ganoderma lucidum 1063
Ganser syndrome 1049, 1055
Gastaut–Geschwind syndrome 1930
gastroesophageal reflux 932, 1084
gastrointestinal disorders 1083–4
  in rapid refeeding 786
  and sleep-wake disorders 932
Gaucher disease type 3 1865
GBH (gamma hydroxy butyrate) 409, **498–9**
GBL (gamma butyl-lactone) 498
GDS see Geriatric Depression Scale; Global
      Deterioration Scale
Gedankenlautwerden 49
gender
  and anorexia nervosa 778
  and anxiety disorders 1666
  and attention-deficit hyperactivity
      disorder 1646, 1828
  and autism 1828
  and body dysmorphic disorder 1045
  and childhood OCD and tics 1681
  and conduct disorder 1655, 1658
  and deliberate self-harm 959
    by elderly people 1565
  and hypochondriasis 997
  and mood disorders 271, 648, 653–4
  and offending 1909
  and prevalence of somatization
      disorders 996
  and psychiatric disorder in intellectual
      disability 1828

and schizophrenia 544–5
and social anxiety disorder 741
and specific phobia 745
and suicide 1704
gender identity 57
gender identity disorder 57, 106, **842–6**
  childhood and adolescence **1718–23**
    aetiology 1719–20
    assessment 1721
    clinical features 1718–19
    epidemiology 1718
    longitudinal studies 1720–1
    and mental disorder 1721
    treatment 1721–2
  diagnosis 842
  epidemiology 842
  and homosexuality 1720
  legal issues 845
  origins 842–3
  patient subgroups 844
  Real Life Experience 843, 844
  treatment and management 843–4
  validity 845
General Health Questionnaire 69, 283, 284
general hospitals
  liaison visits to 1525
  organization of psychiatric services **1144–8**
'general neurotic syndrome' 682
general paresis (of the insane) 1093
general practitioners (GPs)
  ability to detect psychiatric morbidity 1482
  education regarding suicide risks 974
  expectations of psychiatrists 1486–7
  training in psychiatry 1487–8
generalizability theory 92
generalized anxiety disorder (GAD) **729–39**
  aetiology 732–5, *732, 733, 734*
  in childhood and adolescence 1664
    clinical presentation 1665
      outcome 1666
      prevalence 1666
  clinical features 729
  cognitive content 1286–7
  comorbidity 731, *731*, 736
  course and prognosis 735
  and depression 731
  diagnosis 729–30, *730*
  differential diagnosis 730–1, *730*, 741, 752,
    1004, 1024
  epidemiology 731
  following stroke 1071
  genetics 732
  and life events 735
  and neurasthenia 1063
  treatment and management 735–7
  validity of disorder 731
  vulnerability to 734–5
generation 1513
genetic counselling 1281
  Alzheimer's disease 340
  dementia 411
  Huntington's disease 374–5
  in intellectual disability 1825, 1884
genetic epidemiology 286, 650–1, 1597–8
genetic tagging 231
genetic testing
  dementia 411, *412*
  Huntington's disease 374–5
genetics
  and ageing 1507–8

analysis methods 216–17
candidate genes 220–1, 651
components of phenotypic variation 214
continuous traits 213, *213*
and epidemiology 286, 650–1, 1597–8
functional analysis 230–2
gene association studies 220–1, *220*, 226–7,
  230, 651
gene copy-number variants 230
gene–environment correlation 214
gene–environment interactions (GXE)
  214–18, 221, 229, 315, 558–9, 1608, 1725
gene expression control errors 1508
gene expression regulation 218, 223–6, *224*
gene interactions (epistasis) 229
gene mapping 218, 226–7
gene mutations 1508, 1831–2
  Mendelian 227–9
  mis-sense 227
  non-sense 227
  point 227–8
  and psychiatric disorders 227–9, *228*
  triplet repeats 228, *228*
genome organization 223
genotyping 226
and intellectual disability 1831–2, *1831*, 1838
  with behavioural/psychiatric disorder 1858
and life expectancy 1507
linkage analysis 218–20, *218*, 227, 230, 651
markers 218, 226
Mendel's laws 212
model fitting 217
molecular **222–33**, 286
multiple regression analysis 217
neurodevelopmental disorders 159
neurogenetic syndromes 1613–14
non-additive genetic effects 214
nucleic acid structure and function 223
path analysis 217, *217*
patterns of inheritance 212–13, *213*
and personality traits 886–8, 888–9, *890*
polymorphism 218
psychiatric–behavioural 1597–8
psychiatric disorders
  in childhood and adolescence 1590
  complex 229–30
  Mendelian/single-gene 212–13, 213,
    227–9, *228*
quantitative **212–22**
research methods 215–16
whole genome association (WGA)
  studies 221, 229–30
*specific disorders*
  alcohol use disorders 434–6
  Alzheimer's disease 227, 339, 1521
  Angelman syndrome 213, 224, 229, 1841,
    1865, *1866*
  anxiety disorders 1667
  attention-deficit hyperactivity
    disorder 1590, 1646
  autism 1635–6
  body dysmorphic disorder 1046
  chronic fatigue syndrome 1038
  Coffin–Lowry syndrome 1842
  conduct disorder 1658
  cri-du-chat syndrome 1842
  de Lange syndrome 1842
  delusional disorder 614
  dementia with Lewy bodies 365
  Down syndrome 228, 1831, 1838–9

Duchenne muscular dystrophy 1843
eating disorders 781–2, 806
epilepsy 159, 1620
fragile-X syndrome 212, 213, 228, *228*,
  1832, 1839–40, 1865, *1866*
frontotemporal dementias 348
generalized anxiety disorder 732
Huntington's disease 372
hypochondriasis 1024
Klinefelter syndrome 1840
Lesch–Nyhan syndrome 1843
mood disorders 648, **650–8**, 658
mucopolysaccharidoses 1843
neurofibromatosis type 1 1843, *1866*
obsessive–compulsive disorder 768, 1684
offending 1918
panic disorder 753–4
phenylketonuria 212, 214, 1844
post-traumatic stress disorder 707
Prader–Willi syndrome 213, 224, 229, 1844
Rett's syndrome 224, 229, 1637, 1844, *1866*
Rubinstein–Taybi syndrome 1845
schizophrenia 547, 548–9, 553–5,
  565–6, *565*
Smith–Lemli–Opitz syndrome 1845
Smith–Magenis syndrome 1845
smoking addiction/nicotine
  dependence 510–11
substance use disorders 428–9
suicide 954–5, 966–7
tic disorders 229, 1073, 1684
tuberous sclerosis 1075, 1845, *1866*
Turner syndrome 224, 1840
velo-cardio-facial syndrome 1846
Williams syndrome 1846
X-linked intellectual disability 1839
XXX syndrome 1841
XYY syndrome 1841
genital herpes 1094
genital-retraction anxiety disorder (*koro*) 606,
  779, 979, **980–1**
genogram 1381, 1384, *1384*
genome organization 223
genotype 212, 226
genotyping 226
gentamicin *1091*
geophagia 1116
gepirone 735
Geriatric Depression Scale 719, 1551, *1552*
German chamomile 1248
Gerstmann–Straussler(–Scheinker)
  syndrome 351, 356–7
Gestalt therapy 1277
gestational substance use 480, *480*, 1117–18,
  1614, 1615–16, 1754
GHB (gamma hydroxy butyrate) 409, **498–9**
GHQ (General Health Questionnaire)
  69, 283, 284
GHQ-12 284
GHRF (growth hormone-releasing factor)
  165, *171*
Gillick Rules 1899
*Ginkgo biloba*
  adverse effects 1248
  as cognitive enhancer 1247–8
  drug interactions *1250*
  in neurasthenia 1063
ginseng see Panax ginseng
GIPs (GPCR-interacting proteins) 175
give way weakness in conversion disorder 1016

Glasgow Coma Scale 388, 388
glioblasts 157
gliosis in schizophrenia 180–1, 180, 181
Global Assessment of Functioning scale
   73, 1165, 1593
global burden of disease 645
   alcohol use disorders 10, 467
   mental disorder 10–11, 1428, 1606
      in childhood and adolescence 1595–6
   mood disorders 645, 1185
   smoking 510
Global Deterioration Scale 1535
globus pallidus 154, 155, 1684
glove and stocking anaesthesia 57
glutamate 429
   and epilepsy 1619, 1865
   hippocampus 202
   ligand-gated ion channels 172, 173, 174
   in obsessive–compulsive disorder 1684
   in opioid neurobiology 473
   role in neurodevelopment 159
   and schizophrenia 562
   in substance use disorders 429
   transporters 170, 170
glutamate receptors, hippocampal 202
Glyccirhiza glabra 1249
Glycine max 1249
glycine receptors 1171
glycine transporters 169–70, 170
glycosylation (glycation) of proteins 1508–9
GNP and population mental well-being 1428
GnRH (gonadotrophin-releasing
   hormone) 162, 165
GnRH analogs in the paraphilias 838
Go-No-Go tasks 266
Goldberg–Huxley model 1480, 1481
gonadotrophin-releasing hormone 162, 165
good-enough mother 309
goserelin 1964
GPCR-interacting proteins 175
GPCR kinases 175
GPs see general practitioners
graded activity in adjustment disorders 1069
Graded Naming Test 89, 266
graduate mental health workers 1485
grandiose delusions 51
grandparenting
   effects of a grandchild with intellectual
      disability 1884
   roles 1514
   transition to 1513–14
green (ketamine) 489, 499–500, 1186
grief
   after diagnosis of intellectual disability in a
      child 1883
   after infant loss 725, 1119–20
   assessment and management 726–7
   counselling in 726–7, 1279
   normal 725
   traumatic 725, 1985
   see also bereavement
Griffiths Developmental Scale 1821
grimacing 58
grooming 1961, 1962
gross national product and population mental
   well-being 1428
group-analytic group therapy 1351, 1353, 1355,
   1357–8, 1357, 1358
group-as-a-whole 1353
group homes 1454

group matching 1468
group therapy 1350–69
   activity 1351–2
   antisocial personality disorder 898
   basic methods 1351–3
   bipolar disorder 673
   borderline personality disorder 895, 1364–5
   boundary events 1363
   brief 1366
   childhood and adolescence 1768
   chronic mental disorder 1364
   cognitive-behavioural 742, 744
   curative factors 1355, 1356
   domestic violence perpetrators 1982–3
   elderly people 1366
   fostering therapeutic norms 1363
   group-analytic 1351, 1353, 1355, 1357–8,
      1357, 1358
   group development theory 1358–60
   historical aspects 1353–4
   homogeneous/heterogeneous groups 1362
   hypochondriasis 1027
   interpersonal 1351, 1355, 1356
   intervention guidelines 1363, 1363
   language of the group 1360
   leadership 1350–1, 1360–2
   multiple family 1382, 1389
   with offenders/prisoners 1365
   optimal/sub-optimal size 1363
   organizing principles 1353
   outpatient 1364, 1365
   in the paraphilias 838, 839
   in physical illness 1364
   problem-solving 1351, 1352
   psychoanalytic 1351
   psychodynamic 1352–3, 1354–8
   psychoeducational 1351, 1352, 1364
   research and evaluation 1366
   schizophrenia 1364
   selection and composition 1362, 1362
   service planning 1366–7
   setting 1364
   short-term dynamic 1351
   smoking cessation 512
   supportive 1352
   systems-centred 1351
   Tavistock 1351, 1355–7, 1356
   therapeutic goals 1350, 1351
   therapist 1354, 1354
   with trauma victims 1365
'growing pains' 1695
growth
   arrested in anorexia nervosa 787
   drug-induced retardation 1795
growth hormone 164–5
   and immune function 206
   and sleep 1695
   and the sleep–wake cycle 925
growth hormone-inhibiting hormone 165
growth hormone-releasing factor 165, 171
GSS (Gerstmann–Straussler–Scheinker
   syndrome) 351, 356–7
guanfacine 1651, 1688
guanine 223
guanylate cyclase 176
guardianship 29–30, 1895, 1898
guided imagery and recovered memories 715
Guillain–Barré syndrome 942
guilt
   delusions of 51

   and depression 634
   unconscious 294
gynaecological conditions 1114–16

HAART in HIV-associated dementia 385
habit reversal
   in body dysmorphic disorder 1047
   in tic disorders 1687
Hachinski Ischaemia Score 379, 379
HADS (Hospital Anxiety and Depression
   Scale) 1486
haematological disorders 1087–8
haemodialysis 1087, 1139
haemoglobin 197
Halban's fascia 818
halitosis, delusions of 618–19
Hallowell, Irving 276
hallucinations 49
   aetiological theories 50
   after infant loss 1120
   in alcohol withdrawal 443, 538
   in Alzheimer's disease 335
   associated with simple partial seizures 1864
   auditory 49
      cognitive-behaviour therapy 1314, 1317
      transcranial magnetic stimulation
         therapy 1265
   bodily/tactile/coenaesthetic 50
   in delirium 327
   in delusional disorder 609, 610, 613, 615
   in dementia with Lewy bodies 335, 361
   and depression 641
   differential diagnosis of cause 537
   and disinhibition 50
   following head injury 392
   in frontotemporal dementias 346
   gustatory 50
   hypnagogic 50, 940, 1702
   hypnopompic 940, 1702
   mood-congruent/-incongruent 537, 641
   olfactory 50
   and overstimulation 50
   in Parkinson's disease 1072
   phencyclidine-induced 487
   and psychodynamic psychiatry 315–16
   in schizophrenia 527, 573–4
   somatic 1030
   visual 49–50
hallucinogen persisting perception
   disorder 488–9
hallucinogenic mushrooms 488
hallucinogens 487–9
   acute effects 488
   addictiveness 431
   adverse effects 488–9
   botanical 488
   epidemiology of abuse 488
   human experimentation with 489
   preparations 488
hallucinosis, alcoholic 443, 538
haloperidol 1209, 1209
   administration 1213, 1214
   adverse effects 1212, 1222
   in alcohol withdrawal 449–50
   in autism 1875
   in cancer 1104
   in children and adolescents with psychiatric/
      behaviour disorder and intellectual
      disability 1852
   in delirium 331, 1533

in dementia 414
in elderly people 1556
in Huntington's disease 374
in personality disorders 600, *905*, 906
pharmacodynamics *1211*, 1212
pharmacokinetics *1172*
in postoperative delirium 1099
in schizophrenia 586
in tic disorders 1073, 1688
Hamilton Anxiety Rating Scale 1164
Hamilton's Rating Scale for Depression 69, 70, 634, 1163, 1164
hand use preference and gender identity disorder 843
handicap
adjustment to **1065–71**
definition 389
HapMap (International Haplotype Map) 222, 227
'happy puppet' syndrome *see* Angelman syndrome
Hardy–Weinberg equilibrium 213, 226
Hare Psychopathy Checklist 835
harm-avoidance 79–80, *80*, 316, *316*, 849
'harmful dysfunction' concept 28
harmine 501
Harvard Trauma Questionnaire 1497
hashish *see* cannabis
hate crimes 1987
Hayling Test *90*
HCR-20 (Historical Clinical Risk-20) 1927, 1994, 1997, 1998, 2018
head-banging 1601
head injury **387–99**
agitation and aggression following 393, 396, 1929
and alcohol use disorders 393–4
amnesia following 404, 407
and attention-deficit hyperactivity disorder 1646
and boxing 395
and capacity 397
in childhood and adolescence 394–5, 1616–18
closed 387–8, 394, 1617
cognitive impairment following 390–1, *395*
and delusional disorder 614
and depression 92
differential diagnosis 695
early symptoms 392
epidemiology 388–9
epilepsy following 394
as form of torture 1495
function and health 389
immediate response to 1107
and insight 397
investigations 389
late effects 388
long-term outcome 389–90
loss of consciousness 388
malingering following 1055
management of sequelae 395–7
mood disorders following 393, 396
neuropathology 387–8, *387*
and offending 1920
open 387, 394, 1617
personality change following 391
post-concussion syndrome 394, 395–6, 1929
psychological sequelae 390
psychosis following 392–3
recovery from 389–90

refugees 1495
severity 388, *388*
and sleep-wake disorders *932*, 942, 1698
Head Start programme 1788
headache
in childhood and adolescence 1745
following neurosurgery for mental disorder 1268
induction by transcranial magnetic stimulation 1263
health
behavioural factors influencing 1135–7
beliefs 1136–7
definition 1606
and lifestyle 1136
and personality 1136
and stress 1135–6
Health and Education for Life Project 1814–15
Health Anxiety Inventory 1023
Health Belief Model 1137, 1140
health care behaviour 1138–40
health care services
high users 1137–8
types 44–5
health care workers
alcohol use disorders 457
assaults on 1986
factitious disorder 1054
Health Maintenance Organization 45
Health of the Nation Outcome Scale 70, 73
health promotion
in childhood and adolescence 1610
comparison with prevention 1609
*see also* prevention, primary
health psychology **1135–43**
behavioural factors influencing health 1135–7
health care behaviour 1138–40
symptoms and illness behaviour 1137–8
treatment behaviour 1140–2
health-related behaviour 1136–7
health-risk behaviours 1136
Health Technology Appraisals 124
health visitors 1486
Healthy Start programme 1788
hearing, cortical association pathways *147*, 152
heavy metal exposure 1825
*Helicobacter pylori* 1084
Heller's syndrome **1637**
HELP (Health and Education for Life Project) 1814–15
help-seeking behaviour
and culture 15, 1441–2
delay in 1137
hemisensory syndrome 1017
hemispherectomy 1867
hepatic encephalopathy 445, 1084–5
hepatitis B infection
and hypersomnia 942
and opioid use 475
and substance use disorders 430
hepatitis C infection
and opioid use 475
and substance use disorders 430
hepatocerebral degeneration 445
hepatolenticular degeneration 537, 1084
heritability 214
broad-sense 214
narrow-sense 214
heroin 430, 473, 515

action at opioid receptors 473
administration routes 473
brown 473
complications of use 474–5, *475*
dependence 474
assessment 478
in childhood and adolescence 480
confirmation of 478
management 477–9
outcome 481
treatment 475, 476–8, 479, 1242–7
detection 473
epidemiology of use 474
metabolism 473–4, *474*
overdose 474–5, 479, *480*
in pregnancy and breastfeeding 480, *480*, 1615–16
prescription 476
tolerance 473, 474, 478
withdrawal 474
measurement 478, *478*
*see also* opioids; substance use disorders
herpes
encephalitis 406, 1095
genital 1094
heterozygosity 212, 226
5-HIAA *see* 5-hydroxyindoleacetic acid
hierarchy of evidence 123, *1465*
highly active antiretroviral therapy in HIV-associated dementia 385
hindbrain 156, *157*
hippocampal formation 148, *149*, 182, 202, 251–2, *252*, 733
hippocampus 158, 159, 251
anatomy of neuronal network 202–3, *202*
cortical projections to 155–6
emergent properties of networks 203
in epilepsy 203–4
evoked responses 202
and fear/anxiety 1666–7, *1667*
lesions 252, *252*
local circuits 202
and long-term potentiation 251, *251*
and memory 204, 251–3, *251*, 259
rhythms 203
in schizophrenia 179–80, *179*
structure and organization 146, 148, *149*
HIS syndrome 1909
histaminergic system 151, 1210, *1211*
histones 223, 225
historical background
Alzheimer's disease 334
anorexia nervosa 777
art therapy 1414
barbiturates 1178
biological and psychological model of mental disorder 19–20
bipolar disorder 631
community care 24
depression 629–31
diagnostic systems 631
family therapy 1380–1
hypochondriasis 1021–2
mental health social work 1408
mood disorders **629–31**
neuropsychiatry 20
neuroses 20–1
neurosurgery for mental disorder 1266–7
pharmacotherapy 25
psychiatry as a medical specialty **17–27**

historical background (*cont.*)
  psychiatry as profession 18
  psychoanalysis 23, 1338–9
  psychodynamic psychiatry 23
  psychotherapies 20–1
  schizophrenia **521–6**
  sexual dysfunction 821–2
  social aspects of psychiatry 18–19
Historical Clinical Risk-20 1927, 1994, 1997,
    1998, 2018
histrionic personality disorder **868–70**
  aetiology 869
  classification *856, 869*
  clinical features 869–70
  comorbidity 870, 884
  course and prognosis 870
  and deception 1049
  diagnosis 869–70
  differential diagnosis 866, 870, 874
  in elderly people 1562, *1562*, 1563
  epidemiology 869, *882*, 883
  treatment 870
HIV/AIDS **1091–3**
  acute stress reaction in 1091
  counselling in 1280–1
  delirium in 1092–3, *1093*
  delusions of 619
  dementia in **384–6**, 1091
  depression in 1092
  effects on family members 1742
  interpersonal psychotherapy (IPT-HIV)
    1092, 1322
  mania in 1092
  nature of neuropsychiatric disorders in 1091
  and opioid use 475
  opportunistic CNS infections 1093
  parental, effects on child development 1755
  prevention 1447
  psychosis in 1092
  and stigma 1091
  and substance use disorders 430
  and syphilis 1093
HLA typing in sleep-wake disorders 930
HMO (Health Maintenance Organization) 45
home treatment programmes for
    schizophrenia 584
home visitation programme 1788, 1789
homelessness **1500–2**
  and alcohol use disorders 456, 464
  barriers to care 1500–1
  definition 1500
  demography 1500
  and psychiatric disorder 1500
  service organization and delivery 1501
homicide **1937–40**
  altruistic 1923
  by children/adolescents 1952–3
  by elderly people 1938
  by spouse/partner 1981
  and delusional disorders 1920
  female perpetrators 1938
  general population 1937
  infant 1119, 1125, 1937–8
  longitudinal trends 1939–40
  mass 606, 979, 981, 1938
  methods 1937
  multiple 1938
  perpetrators with mental health service
    contact 1938–9
  perpetrators with schizophrenia 1939, 1995

  and personality disorder 1921
  risk assessment 1939–40
  secondary victims 1985
  serial 1938
  'stranger' 1937
  and substance use disorders 1926
  suicide following 1923, 1938
Homicide Act 1957 1901
homosexuality 832
  and gender identity disorder 1720
  and hate crimes 1987
homozygosity 212, 226
honesty-humility 850
Hong Kong
  attitudes to psychiatric disorder 6
  neurasthenia 1061
HONOS (Health of the Nation Outcome
    Scale) 73
Hoover's sign 1016
Hopelessness Scale 1165
Hopkins Symptom Checklist 284, 1497
Hopkins Verbal Learning Test 253
hops 1248
Horney, Karen 310–11
Hospital Anxiety and Depression Scale 1486
hospitals
  counselling in 1280–1
  schools 1815
  *see also* day hospitals; general hospitals;
    secure hospitals
host–agent–environment model 1608
hostels 1454
housing, supported 1400
HOX genes 1614
HPA axis *see* hypothalamic–pituitary–adrenal
    (HPA) axis
HPCL (Hare Psychopathy Checklist) 835
HPPD (hallucinogen persisting perception
    disorder) 488–9
5-HT and 5-HT receptors *see* serotonergic
    system and serotonin receptors
5-HT$_{1A}$ partial agonists 1181
  *see also* buspirone
HTAs (Health Technology Appraisals) 124
Hughlings-Jackson, J. 523
Human Genome Project 218, 222, 1510
human rights
  European Convention on Human
    Rights 1899, 1900, 1904, 2015
  Human Rights Act 1998 2015
  and mental health public policy 1427
  and refugees 1493
  UN Declaration of Human Rights 1427, 1494
  violations of 11
*Humulus lupulus* 1248
Hunter syndrome 1843
*huntingtin gene* 372
Huntington disease-like 2 228, 373
Huntington's disease 212, 213, 228, 228, **371–5**
  and aggression 1929
  in childhood and adolescence 372–3
  clinical features and course 371–2
  diagnosis 372–3
  differential diagnosis 348, 373–4
  genetics 372
  pathology 372
  risk of 374–5
  subcortical triad of symptoms 369
  treatment and management 374
Hurler syndrome 1843

*hwabyung* 984
HY antigen 842
hydergine
  adverse effects 1248
  as cognitive enhancer 1248
  drug interactions *1250*
  *hydrocephalus following head injury 388*
  *hydrocortisol in acute stress reactions 697*
5-hydroxyindoleacetic acid (5-HIAA)
  in anorexia nervosa 782
  in borderline personality disorder 867
  and intermittent explosive disorder 912
  and repetitive self-mutilation 917
  and suicide 964, 965
hyperactivity
  and offending 1909
  *see also* attention-deficit hyperactivity
    disorder
hyperactivity–impulsivity–attention deficit
    syndrome 1909
hyperarousal following an accident 1107
hypercalcaemia 1085–6
hypercarotenaemia in anorexia nervosa 785
hypercortisolaemia in depression 660–1,
    1252, 1258
hyperdopaminergia 562
hyperemesis gravidarum 1116
hyperforin 1249
hyperglycinaemia 1863
hypergraphia 1079
*Hypericum perforatum* (St John's wort) 386,
    686, 1248, *1250*, 1262
hyperkinetic disorder *see* attention-deficit
    hyperactivity disorder
hyperkinetic stereotyped movement
    disorder 1633
hyperkinetic syndrome 1654, 1657
  *see also* attention-deficit hyperactivity
    disorder
hypernomia 850
hyperparathyroidism 1085–6
hyperphagia with seasonal affective
    disorder 1260
hyperprolactinaemia 815, 826, 1086, 1217, 1223
hyperreflexia in HIV-associated dementia 384
hypersalivation, drug-induced 1223
hyperschemazia 57
hypersexuality
  in childhood and adolescence 1671
  in Huntington's disease 373
hypersomnia 927, *928*, **938–43**, 1083,
    1699–701, *1700*
  aetiology 939–43
  assessment 938–9
  of central origin 940–2
  epidemiology 938
  idiopathic 941–2
  misdiagnosis 928
  morbidity 938
  with physical illness 942
  post-traumatic 942
  recurrent 942
  with seasonal affective disorder 1260
  with sleep-related breathing disorder 939–40
  substance-induced 939
  treatment 939–43
  hypertension 1081
  and alcohol consumption 446
hyperthermia and ecstasy 495
hyperthymia **690–1**

hyperthyroidism 1085
    panic-like symptoms 752
    and sleep-wake disorders *932*
hyperventilation
    in chronic fatigue syndrome 1038
    following an accident 1106
hypnogram 925, *925*, 930
hypnosis
    in conversion disorder 1019
    in persistent somatoform pain disorder 1034
    in post-traumatic stress disorder 709
    and recovered memories 715
hypnotics 1178, 1179
    abuse 1183
    adverse effects 1183
    in cancer 1101–2, *1102*
    clinical effects 1182–3
    dependence 1183
    half-lives *1183*
    rebound 1183
    residual effects 1183
hypocalcaemia 1085
hypochloraemia in bulimia nervosa 804
hypochondriacal delusions 51
hypochondriasis 57, **1021–9**
    aetiology and pathogenesis 1025–6
    assessment instruments 1023, *1023*
    and body dysmorphic disorder 1045
    and chronic fatigue syndrome 1037
    classification 993–4, *993*, *994*, 1022–3, *1022*
    clinical features 1022, *1022*
    cognitive and perceptual factors 1025
    comorbidity 1024, 1027
    complications 1026
    conceptualizations 1022
    controversial aspects 997
    correlates and risk factors 997, 1024
    course 1026
    definitions 996
    developmental factors 1025
    differential diagnosis 1003, 1023
    epidemiology 996–7, *998*, 1024–5
    family studies 1024
    and functional symptoms 992
    history of disorder 1021–2
    interpersonal factors 1025
    and life events 1025
    monosymptomatic 997–8
    morbidity 1024–5
    and pain 1031
    and personality 1025
    phenomenology 996
    prevalence 996–7, *998*, 1024
    prognosis 1026
    and service utilization 1024–5
    and sexually transmitted diseases 1094
    social and cultural factors 1025–6
    and somatic delusional disorder 617–18
    subtypes 1022
    treatment and management 1026–8,
        *1027*, 1034
    twin studies 1024
    validity of diagnosis 1023
hypocretin 930, 941
hypofrontality in schizophrenia 188–9, 562
hypoglycaemia in anorexia nervosa 785
hypogonadism 826, 828, 834
hypokalaemia in bulimia nervosa 804
hypomania 631
    in Alzheimer's disease 335

    and attempted suicide 1704
    clinical features 635, *635*
    definition 638
    differential diagnosis 644, 870
    duration 646
    elderly people 1527
    *see also* cyclothymia/cyclothymic disorder
Hypomania Checklist 635
hypomobility 58
hyponatraemia
    in anorexia nervosa 794
    in bulimia nervosa 804
hyponomia 850
hypoparathyroidism 1085
hypophosphataemia in rapid refeeding 786
hypopituitarism 781, 1086
hyposchemazia 57
hypotension
    and chronic fatigue syndrome 1038
    drug-induced 1190, 1223, 1529
    in frontotemporal dementias 346
hypothalamic–growth hormone axis 164–5
hypothalamic–pituitary–adrenal (HPA)
        axis **164–5**
    in anorexia nervosa 784
    and avoidance response 658
    and birth weight 659
    in borderline personality disorder 867
    effects of stress on 206–7
    in generalized anxiety disorder 732
    in post-traumatic stress disorder 706
    and suicide 965
hypothalamic–pituitary–gonadal axis **165**
    in anorexia nervosa 781, 783–4
hypothalamic–pituitary–thyroid axis **163**
    in anorexia nervosa 784
    in post-traumatic stress disorder 706
hypothalamic–prolactin axis 165–6
hypothalamotomy 1267
hypothalamus
    and circadian rhythms 1260
    components of the hypothalamic–pituitary–
        end-organ axes 162–3, *162*
    feeding centre 781
hypothermia in anorexia nervosa 785
hypothyroidism 163, 1085
    congenital 1616
        physical and cognitive
            characteristics 1842
        prevalence 1825–6, 1842
    in depression 661
    in Down syndrome 1839
    and hypersomnia 942
hypoxia, amnesia following 406–7
hysterectomy 1116
hysteria 57, 1021
    *see also* conversion disorder
hysterical blindness 1017

ibogaine 488, 1249, *1250*
IBS (irritable bowel syndrome) 997, 1003,
        1037, 1083
ICD *see entries under* International Classification
        of Diseases
ice (methamphetamine) **497–8**
'ice-pick' lobotomy 1267
ICER (incremental cost-effectiveness
        ratio) 124, 1475, *1475*
ICESCR (International Covenant on Economic
        Social and Cultural Rights) 1427

ICF (*International Classification of Functioning,
        Disability and Health*) 65, 389, 1399,
        1820–1, *1821*
ICIDH (*International Classification
        of Impairments, Disabilities and
        Handicaps*) 65, 389, 1399, 1820
ICM (intensive case management) 1402
ICPC-2-R (International Classification for
        Primary Care) 1484
ICSD-2 (International Classification of Sleep
        Disorders) 927, *928*, 933, *934*, 938,
        1695, 1698
ICU (intensive care units) 1139
id 294–5, 306, 313, 849
id resistances 297
ideal object 308
ideal types 849
idebenone 1240
identity, disorder of awareness of 56
identity theft 1970
identity theory 134
idiopathic CNS hypersomnia 1701
idiopathic infantile hypercalcaemia *see* Williams
        syndrome
IDO (indoleamine 2,3 dioxygenase) 209
IED (intermittent explosive disorder) 911–13
*Ifa* 1420
IGFs (insulin-growth factors) 206
IL-1 (interleukin-1) 209
illness
    cognitive models 1138
    concept of 62, 63–4, 277–8
    coping with 1066
    definition 989
    as a demand/threat 1066
    division into 'medical' and 'psychiatric' 989
    interpersonal basis of experience 277
    perceptions 1138
    phobia of 52, 1022, 1023
    resources for response to 1066
    self-regulatory model 1138
    as a stress 1065
    *see also* mental disorder; physical illness;
        terminal illness
Illness Attitude Scales 1023
illness behaviour and somatization
        disorder 1003, 1009
illness deception model *1051*
illness delay 1137
illness self-management in
        schizophrenia 583
illusions 49, 1030
    in delirium 327
iloperidone 1209
    administration 1220–1
    pharmacodynamics 1210
    pharmacokinetics 1222
ILPs (independent learning plans) 1716
imagery 49, 1779
    in insomnia 937
imagery modification 1292–3
images, negative 1288
imipramine *670*, 1185
    adverse effects *1191*
    delayed onset of effects 176
    dosage *1196*
    in generalized anxiety disorder 735
    in panic disorder 756, *756*
    pharmacodynamics *1173*, *1187*
    pharmacokinetics *1172*

immune system **205–11**
  in chronic fatigue syndrome 1039
  effects of echinacea 1249
  effects of stress 205, 207, 1135–6
  modulation of emotion and mood 209
  neural influences 206–7
  receptors 206
  as sensory organ 207, 209
Impact of Event scale 703
impact rule 1902
impairment 389
imprinting 213, 224–5
  defects 229
Improvement Foundation 1488
impulse control disorders **911–19**
  in bulimia nervosa 803
  definitions 911
  and offending 1924
impulse control enhancement 1771–2
impulsivity 850
  in attention-deficit hyperactivity
      disorder 1643
  and offending 1909
  and suicide 970
*imu* 983
*in vitro* fertilization (IVF) 1115
  and intellectual disability 1883
inappropriate affect in schizophrenia 529
incidence 281, 1607
  secular changes in 280–1
inclusion criteria 100
*Incredible Years, The* 1788
incremental cost-effectiveness ratio
      124, 1475, *1475*
indeloxazine 1240
independent learning plans 1716
India
  Action for Mental Illness 1491
  attitudes to psychiatric disorder 6
  cost of psychiatric disorder 11
  psychiatric nurses in 1407
  traditional medicine 1061
indigenous folk healing practices **1418–22**
indoleamine 2,3 dioxygenase 209
infancy
  caregiver-mediated interventions 1787–8
  death in 1119
  epilepsy with intellectual disability 1861,
      1862–4, *1863*
  maternal anxieties about infant health and
      survival 1121–2
  mother–infant relationship disorders 1123–4
  psychoanalytic theories of sexuality 294–5
  relinquishment in 1120
  sleeplessness in 1698
  *see also* childhood and adolescence
infanticide 1119, 1125, 1937–8
infantile spasms 1618, 1862–3, 1867
infection **1090–5**
  and chronic fatigue syndrome 1038–9
  and hypersomnia 942
  and obsessive–compulsive disorder 1685
  opportunistic in HIV/AIDS 1093
  pharmacotherapy 1091, *1091*
  prenatal exposure to, and schizophrenia
      547–8, 556
  and tic disorders 1073, 1685
  *see also specific infections*
infectious mononucleosis 1095
inferior frontal gyrus 245

inferior parietal lobe 245
inferior temporal sulcus 146
inferotemporal cortex 146, 148
infertility 1114–15
  *see also* fertility
inflammatory bowel disease 1083–4
influenza, prenatal exposure to 547–8
information
  analysis and integration 65
  categories 63
  condensation and recording 73–4
  effects on stigma 5–6
  keeping up to date with **122–9**
  objective 63
  scientific 63
  subjective 63
information-giving in counselling 1275–6
information variance 284
informed consent 29, 1895
  for neurosurgery for mental disorder 1267–8
  in psychiatric emergencies in childhood and
      adolescence 1811
  for psychotherapy in childhood and
      adolescence 1765
  for surgical procedures 1096–7
inhalant abuse *see* volatile substance abuse
inheritance
  multifactorial 213
  patterns of 212–14, *213*
  polygenic 213
inhibition, sexual 825
injury *see* accidents; head injury; sleep-related
      injury
Injury Severity Score 1105
inositol 176
inositol triphosphate 174, 176
inpatient care
  in alcohol use disorders 449, 455–6, 461
  anorexia nervosa 792–3, 793, 794–5
  in community mental health services 1452–3
  containment of violent behaviour 1404
  diagnosis-specific 1453
  for elderly people 1582–3
  global survey 12, *12*
  health psychology of 1139–40
  and psychiatric nursing 1404
  stress associated 1139–40
  and suicide 1404
insanity defence 1900–1, 1922–3, 1923, 1928
insight 56, 80, *80*, 83
  in body dysmorphic disorder 1044
  following head injury 397
  measurement 56
  in psychoanalysis 1340
  in schizophrenia 528
insistence on sameness in autism 1633
insomnia 927, *928*, **933–8**, 1182
  aetiology 934–5
  childhood-onset/idiopathic 1699
  classification 933
  clinical features 933
  course and prognosis 935
  and depression 934
  diagnosis 934
  differential diagnosis 934
  epidemiology 934
  fatal familial 352
  prevention 937
  rebound 935
  treatment and management 935–7

institutional racism 276
institutionalization 236–7, 1393, 1396
insula 145, 148, 152, 260
insulin-growth factors 206
insulinoma 1101
integration 1278
intellect/imagination 850
intellectual disability 1861
  in adults 1884
  aetiology 1821–2, **1830–7**
    assessment 1833–4, *1833*
    central nervous system
        malformations 1832
    classification of causes 1830, *1831*
    complexity of causes 1830
    external prenatal factors 1832
    genetic factors 1831–2, *1831*, 1838
    importance of confirmation of 1834
    paranatally-acquired disorders 1832
    postnatally-acquired disorders 1833
    untraceable/unclassified 1833
  and aggression 1855–6, 1929
  anger management 1874
  and anxiety 1851–2
  and anxiety disorders 1855
  and art therapy 1414–15
  assessment 1821–3
  and attention-deficit hyperactivity
      disorder 1850–1, 1876
  and autism 1852, 1855
  behavioural programmes 1874
  and bereavement 1881
  and bipolar disorder 1827, 1854–5
  characterization 1821–2
  childhood and adolescence
    and antisocial behaviour 1946
    and anxiety 1851–2
    and bereavement 1759
    and depression 1852
    effects on family 1883–4
    prevalence 1878
    psychiatric and behaviour disorders
        associated **1849–53**, 1879
    special needs of adolescents 1878–80
    transition to adulthood 1878–9
  classification 54, *86*, 1592, *1593*, 1819–21,
      *1820*, *1821*
  cognitive-behaviour therapy 1874
  communication skills 1873
  and conduct disorder 1657, 1851
  and consent to sexual activity 1900
  and culture 1879–80, 1881
  definitions 1825
  and deinstitutionalization 1881, 1887, 1890
  and deliberate self-harm 1856
  and dementia 1827, 1828, 1855
  and depression 1827, 1852, 1854–5
  diagnosis 1833–4, *1833*
    multiaxial 1871–2
  differential diagnosis
    antisocial personality disorder 866
    pervasive developmental disorders 1639
    specific developmental disorders 1623
  and dysthymia/dysthymic disorder 1855
  and education 1873, 1884
  effects on the family **1883–6**
  elderly people 1584, 1864
    carers 1880–1
    health needs 1880
    life expectancy 1880

with psychiatric/behavioural disorders 1858–9
and epilepsy 92, 1828
    in adults and elderly people 1864
    aetiology and pathogenesis 1865–6, *1865, 1866*
    behavioural disorders 1864
    in childhood and adolescence *1863*, 1864
    diagnosis 1861–2
    differential diagnosis 1861–2, *1863*
    epidemiology 1864–5
    in infancy 1861–2, 1862–4, *1863*
    prognosis 1868
    treatment 1866–8, *1867*
ethnic minorities 1879–80, 1881
health inequalities 1819
and IQ 1820, 1825
mental state examination 1823
needs assessment 1823–4
normalization 1872
and offending 1856
and oppositional-defiant disorder 1851
and paraphilias 834
and parenthood 1885
and personality disorders 1856
pharmacotherapy 1875–6
prevalence 1825–6
prevention 1447–8, *1448*
    coordinated 1835
    ethical issues 1835
    primary 1834
    secondary 1834–5
    tertiary 1835
psychiatric and behaviour disorders in adults **1854–60**
    aetiology 1857–8
    assessment 1822–3, 1856
    and baseline exaggeration 1854
    classification 1857
    clinical features 1854–6
    and cognitive disintegration 1854
    and deprivation 1828
    diagnosis 1822–3, 1856–7
    in elderly people 1858–9
    epidemiology 1826–7, *1827*, 1857
    and intellectual distortion 1854
    and levels of support 1828
    and life events 1828
    mental health service planning and provision 1887–92
    outcome measurement 1889
    and physical illness 1828
    protective and vulnerability factors 1827–8
    and psychological masking 1854
    residential programmes 1889
    and smoking 1828
    staffing and training 1889–90
    vocational programmes 1889
psychiatric and behaviour disorders in childhood and adolescence **1849–53**
    assessment 1822–3
    classification 1849–50
    diagnosis 1822–3, 1849–50
    management principles 1852–3
    and physical illness 1850
    social and family influences 1850
psychodynamic psychotherapy 1874–5
and psychoses 1826, 1827, 1854
rational emotive therapy 1874
and schizophrenia 1827, 1854

self-help skills 1873
and sexual relationships 1873, 1879
and sleep-wake disorders 926–7, 1694, 1697–8
and social inclusion 1819
and social relationships 1873
social role valorization (SRV) approach 1409–10
spectrum of 1819
and speech and language disorder/difficulty 1712
and stereotypic movement disorder 1683, 1851
and sterilization 1116
syndromes **1838–48**
therapeutic communities 1397
and tic disorders 1851
treatment **1871–7**
    methods 1873–6
    therapeutic environment 1872–3
    in tuberous sclerosis 1075
United Nations Declaration on the Rights of Mentally Retarded Persons 1895–6
X-linked 1831–2, 1839–40, 1842
*see also specific disorders and syndromes*
intellectual openness 886
intellectual performance disorders 54
intellectualization 294
intelligence
    assessment and measurement 22, 54, 87, *88*, 263–4
    conceptualization 54, 263–4
    and offending 1909–10
    premorbid 90, *90*, 264, 548
intelligence quotient *see* IQ
intensive care units 1139
intensive case management 1402
intention-to-treat analysis 128, 142, 1155
intentional communities 1392
interactive techniques in child and adolescent assessment 1605
interferon *1091*
interleukin-1 209
INTERMED-method 1145, *1146*
intermetamorphosis 623
intermittent explosive disorder 911–13
internal consistency of a test *85*
international agencies and mental health public policy 1427
International Bill of Rights 1427
International Classification of Diseases, development and early editions 100–2
International Classification of Diseases, ICD-9 100, 631
    alcohol dependence syndrome 437
    autism 1633
    neurasthenia 1060
    personality disorders *856*
International Classification of Diseases, ICD-10 **108–13**, 631
    acute stress reactions 693, 694, *694*
    adjustment disorders *717*, 1066–7
    alcohol use disorders 439, *440*
    Alzheimer's disease 336
    Asperger's syndrome 1638, *1638*
    autism 1633–4, *1634*
    bipolar disorder 639
    categorical approach 849
    in childhood and adolescence 1592–3
    childhood disintegrative disorder *1637*

as classification of disorders 64
*Clinical Descriptions and Diagnostic Guidelines* (Blue Book) 103
    comparison with DSM-IV 102–4
    conduct disorder 1656, 1657
    cultural critique 276
    cyclothymic disorder 686
    delirium 327, 1531
    delusional disorder 103–4, 609, 613, *613*
    depersonalization disorder 774
    depression 633, *633*, 639
    development 100–2
*Diagnostic Criteria for Research* (Green Book) 103
    disorders relating to cocaine 483, *484*
    dysthymic disorder 681
    eating disorder 787, 800–1
    and epidemiology 1607
    ethical issues in diagnosis using 28
    frontotemporal dementias 348
    generalized anxiety disorder 730, *730*
    hyperkinetic disorder 1643
    impulse control disorders 911
    intellectual disability 1825
        with psychiatric disorder 1826, 1849–50
    malingering 1054
    mania 635, *635*
    multiaxial version 73, 103
    neurasthenia 1062
    obsessive–compulsive disorder 1682
    panic disorder 751–2
    pathological gambling 920
    personality disorders 852, *852*, 855–7, *856*
        antisocial personality disorder *865*
        dependent personality disorder *873*
        histrionic personality disorder *869*
        obsessive–compulsive personality disorder *874*
        paranoid personality disorder *861*
    pervasive developmental disorders 1623, 1633, 1639
    post-traumatic stress disorder 701, *702–3*, 703
    in primary care 1483–4
*Primary Health Care* version (PHC) 103
    Rett's syndrome 1636, *1636*
    schizoaffective disorder 598
    schizophrenia 103–4, 534, *534*, *536*, 541, 569, 571, 1547
    sexual dysfunction 823
*Short Glossary of ICD-10* 103
    social anxiety disorder 740
    somatoform disorders 104, *993*, *994*, 1003
        body dysmorphic disorder 1045–6
        conversion disorder 1012
        hypochondriasis 997, 1022–3
        persistent somatoform pain disorder 997, 1029–30
        somatization disorder 996, 999–1000, 1003
    specific developmental disorders 1623, *1623*, 1627
    specific phobia 745
    structure 102–4
    substance use disorders 439, *440*
    tic disorders 1682
    use in epidemiology 283
    vascular dementia 377–8, *377*
International Classification of Diseases, ICD-10-PHC 1483–4

International Classification of Diseases, ICD-11, research planning for 106–8
*International Classification of Functioning, Disability and Health* 65, 389, 1399, 1820–1, *1821*
*International Classification of Impairments, Disabilities and Handicaps* 65, 389, 1399, 1820
International Classification for Primary Care 1484
International Classification of Sleep Disorders 927, *928*, 933, *934*, 938, 1695, 1698
International Covenant on Economic, Social and Cultural Rights 1427
International Covenant on Political and Civil Rights 1427
International Haplotype Map 222, 227
International Initiative for Mental Health Leaders 1488
International Personality Disorder Examination 72, *858*, 859
International Pilot Study of Schizophrenia 14, 71, 523, 527, 528, 540–1, 541, 572, 574
International Study of Schizophrenia 572–3, *572*, 574
Internet
    counselling services based on 109, 1814–15
    and suicide pacts 1706
    use in evidence-based medicine 124
interneuronal network gamma 203
interpersonal and social rhythm therapy 647, 673, 1319, 1323
interpersonal counselling 1324
interpersonal development 1600–1
interpersonal group therapy 1351, 1355, *1356*
interpersonal inventory 1320
interpersonal psychoanalysis 310
interpersonal psychotherapy (IPT) 1278, **1318–26**
    adjustment disorders 1068, *1069*
    anorexia nervosa 792
    anxiety disorders 1324
    avoidant personality disorder 897
    background 1319
    bipolar disorder 1323
    bulimia nervosa 808, 809, 1323–4
    by telephone 1324
    comparison with other psychotherapies 1321, 1333–4, *1333*
    contraindications 1319
    conversion disorder 1019
    depression 672–3, 676, 1322–3
        in childhood and adolescence 1322, 1676
        in elderly people 1555
        maintenance treatment 1322–3
        and marital conflict 1322
        peripartum 1322
        in primary care 1322
    dysthymia/dysthymic disorder 686, 1323
    in HIV/AIDS 1092, 1322
    indications 1319
    phases of treatment 1319–20
    predictors of response to 1324
    for refugees 1497
    research 1324
    substance use disorders 1324
    techniques 1320–1
    training in 1325
interpersonal relation phobia 982

interpersonal skills training in conduct disorder 1662
interpretationism 134–5
interpreters
    mental health professionals as 67
    use in assessment 67
interval scales 86
interventricular foramen 157
interviewing, privacy of 67
intracerebral haemorrhage 387
introjection 294
introjective type 316
introns 224
introversion 81, 632, 633, 635, 654, 850, 862, 878
intrusion following an accident 1107
intuition, delusional 51
invasion of privacy in diagnosis of factitious disorder 1053
Inventory of Depressive Symptomatology 1163
Inventory of Interpersonal Problems 1165
iodine deficiency 1448, 1825
Iowa Gambling Task 265
Iowa Strengthening Families program 1790
IP₃ (inositol triphosphate) 174
IPC (interpersonal counselling) 1324
IPDE (International Personality Disorder Examination) 72, *858*, 859
iproniazid 1185, 1190
ipsapirone in generalized anxiety disorder 735
IPSRT (interpersonal and social rhythm therapy) 647, 673, 1319, 1323
IPT *see* interpersonal psychotherapy
IPT-HIV 1092, 1322
IQ 54, 263–4
    classification *86*
    difference scores 86, *86*
    and intellectual disability 1820, 1825
    and offending 1909–10
    population distribution 1825
    premorbid, strategies for estimation 90, *90*
    scores 86
    tests 67, *88*
    z-scores and percentiles *86*
Irish Affected Sib Pair Study 435
iron deficiency *932*, 1088
irresponsibility in elderly people 1561
irritable bowel syndrome 997, 1003, 1037, 1083
irritable heart syndrome 751
Islamic communities, attitudes to psychiatric disorder 7
isocarboxazid 670, *670*
    adverse effects 1190, *1191*, 1193
    dosage *1196*
    limitations on use 1187
    pharmacodynamics *1187*
    pharmacokinetics *1189*
isolation 294
isoniazid
    adverse effects *1091*
    in tuberculosis 1094
isoproterenol 754
isoxsuprine 1240
ISS (Injury Severity Score) 1105
ITT (intention-to-treat analysis) 128, 142, 1155
IVF *see in vitro* fertilization

Janet, Pierre 20, 21
Japan
    attitudes to psychiatric disorder 7

life expectancy 1507
    neurasthenia 1061
jargon aphasia 54
Jaspers, Karl 523
jealousy 619–20
    cognitive therapy 1920
    delusional 51, 619–21, 1920, 1967
    pathological 51, 620–1, 862, 1920, 1998
jet (ketamine) 489, **499–500**, 1186
jet lag 1261
journals
    current awareness 124–5, *125*
    systematic reviews in 1156
judgement 80, *80*, 83
'Just Say No' campaign 1598
juvenile delinquency 1654, **1945–59**
    assessment 1947–8, *1949*
    and attention-deficit hyperactivity disorder 1948–9
    and autism spectrum disorders 1950
    and capacity 1954–5
    and conduct disorder 1946, 1948–9
    and depression 1949
    and early-onset psychosis 1950
    epidemiology 1945
    girls 1955–6
    interventions 1950–7, *1951*
    justice system 1945, 1947
    legal issues 1954–5
    and mental disorder 1946–7, 1948–50, 1951–2
    pathways of care 1947
    pathways to *1946*
    and post-traumatic stress disorder 1949–50
    protective factors 1947, *1947*
    risk factors *1946*, 1947

K (ketamine) 489, **499–500**, 1186
Kahlbaum, Karl 521
kainate receptors 172, *173*, 1171
kava 1248, *1250*
Kendra's Law 2015
Keppra *see* levetiracetam
Kernberg, Otto 311
ketamine 489, **499–500**, 1186
ketoconazole *1091*
kidney, transplantation 1087
kindling 204
kissing 815
Klein, Melanie 306–7, 308, 1770
Kleine–Levin syndrome 942, 1701
kleptomania **913–14**, 1924, 1942–3
Klinefelter syndrome 834
    behavioural and psychiatric aspects 1840
    genetics 1840
    physical characteristics 1840
    prevalence 1840
Klüver-Bucy syndrome 258–9, 346
knockout/knock-in technology 230, 231
Kohlberg, Lawrence 235
Kohut, Heinz 311
*koro* 606, 779, 979, **980–1**
Korsakoff syndrome *see* Wernicke–Korsakoff syndrome
Kraepelin, Emil 522, 531, 540, 568, 603, 609, 610, 630, 681
kudzu 1249
*kujibiki* 1420
kuru 351, 354–5

'la belle indifférence' 1016

LAAM 1243–4
labelling 5
labia 817
lacunar state 377
Lafora disease 1864, *1866*
Laing, R.D. 24, 309
lamina terminalis 157
lamotrigine 1198, 1200, **1235**
    adverse effects *1200*, 1204, 1235
    in bipolar disorder 671, 677
    in childhood and adolescence 1798
    in cyclothymia/cyclothymic disorder 689
    in depersonalization disorder 775
    dosage and administration
        *1233*, 1235, *1236*
    drug interactions 1206, 1232, 1235, 1866
    in epilepsy 1080
    indications and contraindications 1235
    mechanism of action *1200*
    overdose 1235
    in personality disorders *905*
    pharmacokinetics 1203, 1235, *1867*
    pharmacology 1235
    in pregnancy 1235
    response correlates *1199*
    in schizophrenia 591
    structure *1232*
    therapeutic profile *1199*
    withdrawal 1206–7, 1235
Landau–Kleffner syndrome 1618, 1626–7,
    1640, 1712, 1864
language *see* speech and language development;
    speech and language disorder/difficulty
*lanti* 984
lasting power of attorney 1577
*latah* 606, **983**
late paraphrenia 1547
lateral horn 157
lateral ventricles 157, 159
laurasidone 1209
*Lavandula angustifolia* (lavender) 1248
law and psychiatry *see* legal issues
laxative abuse
    in anorexia nervosa 783, 784, 794
    in bulimia nervosa 803
learned helplessness 684, 1982
learning, in epilepsy 204
learning disability *see* intellectual disability
learning disorders 1623, *1623*, 1627–31
learning mentors 1812
legal issues
    action-taking 1895–900
    anorexia nervosa 796
    arson 1966
    decision-making 1895–900
    factitious disorder 1053–4
    gender identity disorder 845
    juvenile delinquency 1954–5
    law relating to people with mental
        disorder **1895–907**
    malingering 1058
    old age psychiatry 1577–8
    paraphilias 834
    responsibility 1900–5
    sleep–wake disorders 948–9
    substance use disorders 1927–8
Leibniz, Gottfried 133
lemon balm 1248
Lennox–Gastaut syndrome 1618, 1862, 1863
Lesch–Nyhan syndrome

behavioural and psychiatric aspects
    1838, 1843
behavioural phenotype 1613, 1614
genetics 1843
physical characteristics 1843
prevalence 1843
Letter–Number Span 255
leuprolide acetate 1964
Level of Service Inventory, Revised 2011
levetiracetam 1237
    drug interactions 1866
    in epilepsy 1080
    pharmacokinetics *1867*
levodopa
    adverse effects *730*
    in dementia with Lewy bodies 366
Lewis, David 134
Lewy bodies 361
    composition 362
    cortical 362
    in Parkinson's disease 361, 369
    sites 362
    subcortical 362
Lewy body disease *see* dementia, with Lewy
    bodies
Lewy neurites 362
    in Parkinson's disease 369
lexipafant 386
liability
    for clinical negligence 1902
    criminal 1900–1
    of mentally ill people in negligence 1903–4
    to mentally ill people who self-harm 1905
    of providers of mental health services
        1904–5
    for psychiatric injury 1902–3
    to third parties for acts by mentally ill
        people 1904
    tortious 1901–5
    vicarious 1904–5
liaison, in consultation-liaison psychiatry 1145
libidinal object 308
libido 294, 295
    and castration 815–16
    in epilepsy 1079
    postnatal loss 1121
    reduced/low 822
        in dementia 416
        management 828
LIFE (Longitudinal Interval Follow-up
    Evaluation) 1165
life course 1512
    perspective 1513–14
    structuring through age 1512–13
life events
    and aetiological models 269–71
    and anorexia nervosa 779–80
    in clinical assessment 66–7
    and conversion disorder 1014
    and depression 269–73, *270*, *271*, 648, 659
    effects on children and adolescents 1601
    elderly people 1559–60
    and exposure to adversity 286
    and generalized anxiety disorder 735
    and hypochondriasis 1025
    and immune function 207
    involving danger 270
    involving entrapment 270
    involving humiliation 270
    involving loss 270

and mania 647
and mood disorders 269–73, *270*, *271*, 659
and psychiatric disorder in intellectual
    disability 1828
and schizophrenia 558, 575
and suicide 954, 969, 1705
Life Events and Difficulties Schedule 67,
    269–71
life expectancy
    and ageing 1507, 1509–10
    healthy 1509–10
    and population ageing 1579
life skills training *see* social skills training
life stories 1514–15
life table analysis 215
life transitions 1513–14
lifechart 67, 73
lifestyle
    and ageing 1507
    and health 1136
LIFT (Linking the Interests of Families and
    Teachers) programme 1789
ligand-gated ion channels 172, *173*, 174
light box 1261
light visors 1261
limbic cortex 150, 152–3, 1267
limbic leucotomy 1267
limbic-lobe syndrome 866
*lingzhi* 1063
linkage disequilibrium 220, 221, 651
Linking the Interests of Families and Teachers
    programme 1789
lipid metabolism disorders 1084
lipofuscin 1508
liquid ecstasy (gamma hydroxy butyrate)
    409, **498–9**
liquorice 1249
LIS1 protein 158
literature searches 123
lithium 1198, **1198–208**
    adverse effects *1200*, 1204
        in childhood and adolescence 1677
        hypothyroidism 1085
        risk factors 1175
        teratogenicity 1169–70
    in attempted suicide 971, 1707
    in autism and other pervasive developmental
        disorders 1640
    in bipolar disorder 671, 677
    in body dysmorphic disorder 1047
    and breast-feeding 1169–70
    in childhood and adolescence
        depression 1677
        psychiatric/behaviour disorder and
            intellectual disability 1852
    comparison of immediate-release and
        modified-release 1169, *1169*
    continuation treatment 671
    in cyclothymia/cyclothymic disorder 689
    drug interactions 1175, 1205
    in elderly people 1556
    historical perspective 1200
    in HIV/AIDS 1092
    in Huntington's disease 374
    indications and contraindications 1205
    in intellectual disability 1875
    maintenance treatment 671
    mechanism of action *1200*
    monitoring therapy 1176
    in personality disorders 906

lithium (*cont.*)
pharmacodynamics 1172
pharmacokinetics 1170, *1172*, 1202–3
pharmacology 1201, *1202, 1203*
in pregnancy 677, 1118, 1205
psychoprophylactic use 1448
in resistant depression 675
response correlates *1199*
in schizophrenia 591
and surgery 1097
therapeutic profile *1199*
withdrawal 1206
litigation
and conversion disorder 1016
following accidents 1111–12
and malingering 1057
and persistent somatoform pain
disorder 1034
vexatious *see* querulous behaviour
liver
effects of alcohol use disorders 445, 446, 456
transplantation 456
local worlds 277
locus coeruleus 151
LOD score 219, 222
lofepramine *670*
lofexidine 477, **1245**
Logical Memory test 264
logistic regression 141
logoclonia 53
logorrhoea 53
long-term plasticity 251
long-term potentiation 202, 231, 251, *251*
longevity
and need for mental health services 1579–80
and rate of living 1508
variance in 1507
Longitudinal Interval Follow-up
Evaluation 1165
loosening of association 53, 528
*Lophophora williamsii* 488
loprazolam 1179
lorazepam 1178
in adjustment disorders 721
adverse effects 1180
in alcohol withdrawal 1542
in cancer *1102, 1104*
in delirium 1533
in dementia 415
dosage 1180
indications 1178
in panic disorder *756*, 757
pharmacokinetics *1172*, 1178
potential for misuse 491
in status epilepticus 1867
in terminal illness 1070
love, delusions of 51
love maps 813, 837
loxapine *1209*
administration *1214*
adverse effects *1212*
pharmacodynamics *1211*
LSD 487
acute effects 488
adverse effects 488–9
differential diagnosis of intoxication 487
epidemiology of use 488
preparations 488
psychosis induced by 489, 538
use in pregnancy 1117

LSI-R (Level of Service Inventory, Revised) 2011
LTP (long-term potentiation) 202, 231, 251, *251*
LTPP (long-term psychodynamic psychotherapy)
318–19, 1327, 1329, 1338, 1345
Lunacy Act 1845 19
luteinizing hormone in anorexia nervosa 783
lying 1941
pathological 54, 871, 1049, 1051, 1941
Lyme disease 1094–5
Lyrica (pregabalin) 743, 1182, 1237
lysergic acid diethylamide *see* LSD

MacArthur Risk Assessment Study 1937
machine functionalism 134
McNaghten rules 1900–1, 1928
MACT (manual-assisted cognitive
treatment) 895
made acts 527
Madrid Declaration 40, 40–1
*magersucht* 783
magic-fear-induced death 981
magnetic resonance imaging see functional
magnetic resonance imaging; structural
magnetic resonance imaging
magnetic resonance spectroscopy 186
alcohol-related brain damage 401
epilepsy 1862
lithium therapy 1202
mood disorders in childhood and
adolescence 1674
magnetization 191, *192*
magnetoencephalography in epilepsy 1862
maintenance of wakefulness test 939
make-belief 1941
Malan, David 310
malaria 1447
malarial fever therapy 1251
*mali-mali* 983
malingering 57, 994, 1049, **1054–8**, 1096, 1941
aetiology 1057
assessment instruments 1057
classification 1056
clinical features 1055–6
and cognitive assessment 91
and cognitive deficit 1055–6
course 1057
definition 1054
diagnosis 1056
differential diagnosis 1003, 1012, *1012*,
1051, 1056
epidemiology 1054–5
ethical and legal issues 1058
following accidents 1111
partial 1054
and physical disease 1056
and post-traumatic stress disorder 1055
prevention 1058
prognosis 1057
and psychoses 1055
pure 1054
symptom validity tests 1057
treatment and management 1057–8
malnutrition
in alcohol use disorders 445
in anorexia nervosa 784–6
managed care 45
management **39–46**
activities 41
basic concepts 40
categories 41

definition 40
ethical aspects 40–1
functions 40
information systems 42
levels and styles 42
quality 43–4, *44*
risk 44
roles and responsibility of managers of
clinical units 42
and strategic planning 43
management by objectives 43
management science 42
mania
assessment 1675
childhood and adolescence 1670–1,
1675, 1677
clinical features 635–6, *635*
cultural influences 14
and Cushing's syndrome 1086
definition 638
in dementia 416
differential diagnosis 644, 870, 1531
and Down syndrome 1826
duration and severity of episodes 635–6
elderly people 1527, 1556–7
endophenotype 266
following head injury 393
in HIV/AIDS 1092
and life events 647
and offending 1923
and patient state fluctuations within mood
disorders 632–3, *632, 633*
and physical illness 1132
postpartum 647
with psychotic features 636
risk factors 646–7
and sleep-wake disorders *931*
stages of *636*
treatment 677–8, 1253–4
unipolar 633
without psychotic features 635–6
*mania à potu* 60
Mania Rating Scale 1675
manic episode disorder 633
mannerisms 58, *58*
manual-assisted cognitive treatment 895
MAO-A see monoamine oxidase-A
MAOIs see monoamine oxidase inhibitors
Map Search 88, 89
maple syrup urine disease 1863
maprotiline 669
adverse effects *1191*
dosage *1196*
pharmacodynamics *1173, 1187*
pharmacokinetics *1172, 1189*
Marchiafava–Bignami syndrome 445
marijuana *see* cannabis
marital conflict
and conduct disorder 1659–60
and depression 1753
effects on child mental health 1726
interpersonal psychotherapy (IPT-CM) 1322
and mood disorders 653
and offending 1910–11
marital status, and depression 648
marital therapy *see* couple therapy
Maroteaux-Lamy syndrome 1843
marriage 1369–70
consanguineous 1825
counselling 1278–9

and culture 1370
masochism 832–3, *833*, *836*, 877, 878
masochistic personality disorder 877–8
massacre, autogenic (self-generated) 1938
MAST-G 1519
masturbation
    degeneration theory 836
    surveys of 813–14
'matchbox' sign 618
matching 1468
maternal deprivation 285
maternity blues 1121
mathematics disorder 1630
mating behaviour 815
*Matricaria recutita* 1248
MATRICS battery 263, 265
Matrix Model 1463, *1464*, 1889
Mayo Fluctuations Composite Scale 363
MBDB (*N*-methyl-1-(1,3-benzodioxol-5-yl)-
    2-butanamine) 494
MBO (management by objectives) 43
MBT (mentalization-based therapy)
    304, 894, 1341
MCI *see* mild cognitive impairment
MCMI (Millon Clinical Multiaxial
    Inventory) 858, *858*, 1962
MDA (methylenedioxyamphetamine) 494
MDAS (Memorial Delirium Rating Scale) 328
MDEA (methylenedioxyethylamphetamine)
    494
MDMA *see* ecstasy
MDT (mode deactivation therapy) 1953
ME *see* chronic fatigue syndrome
Mead, Margaret 276
mean 86
mean green (ketamine) 489, **499–500**, 1186
Measure of Parenting Style 286
measurement scales 85–6
MECA (Methods for the Epidemiology of
    Child and Adolescent Mental Disorders)
    study 1594
media, exposure to in childhood and
    adolescence 1601
medial temporal lobe
    and declarative/episodic memory 251–3, *252*
    in mild cognitive impairment 1537–8
median 86
medical anthropology 276
medical practice models 64
medical pupil referral units 1815
Medical Research Council *see* MRC
medical sociology **268–75**
    context and measurement 268
    life events and building aetiological models
        269–73
    methodological considerations 269
medical students' disease 1137
Medical Symptom Validity Test 1057
medication use disorders in elderly
    people **1543–5**, *1544*
meditation 1418
medroxyprogesterone acetate 838, 1964
meiosis 223
melancholia 681, 1021
    features 640–1
    treatment 1252–3
melanocortin agonists in sexual
    dysfunction 828
MELAS (mitochondrial encephalopathy with
    lactic acidosis and strokes) 1865, *1866*

melatonin 925, 935, 1183, 1248, *1250*, 1262
melatonin receptor agonists in insomnia 935
*Melissa officinalis* 1248
memantine
    in Alzheimer's disease 1241
    in dementia 415
    in HIV-associated dementia 385
    in vascular dementia 381
Memorial Delirium Rating Scale 328
memory
    in acute stress reactions 696
    in anxiety disorders 1288
    assessment 89, *89*, 253, 254, 255–6, 264,
        420–1, *420*
    biographical 59
    cellular and molecular mechanisms 251, *251*
    classification 250–1, *250*
    declarative (explicit) 59, 250, 313
        assessment and neuropsychology 253
        neural system 251–3, *252*
    delusional 51, 59, 611
    and depression 92
    development 241–2, *241–2*
    distortion following head injury 392
    effects of benzodiazepines 1179
    emotional 264
    encoding 264
    enhancement 396–7
    and epilepsy 92, 204
    episodic *241*, 250, 264, 407, 1179, 1761
        assessment and neuropsychology 253
        and emotions 259
        neural system 251–3, *252*, 259
    eye witness *241–2*
    false 59, 250, 403, 408, **713–16**
    immaturity in childhood 1761
    long-term (remote/secondary) 59, 250, 407
        remediation 421–4, *422*
    and mood disorders 59
    non-declarative (implicit) *241*, 250, 313, 407
        assessment and neuropsychology 254
        neural systems 254
    preverbal (eidetic) 1761
    procedural 59, 250, 254, 313–14
    prospective 407
    in psychiatric practice 249–50
    psychology and biology **249–57**
    rate of forgetting 253
    recognition *241*, 264
    recovered 714–15, 834
    remediation and rehabilitation 421–4, *422*
    repression 293–4, 314
    retrieval 264
    role of amygdala 264
    semantic 250, 264, 406, 407
    short-term/recent 59, 250, 264, 407
        visual 247–8
    situationally accessible 696
    ultrashort-term (sensoric/echoic/iconic)
        59, 250
    verbally accessible 696
    working/primary *242*, 250, 264, 407
        assessment and neuropsychology 255–6
        neural systems 254–5
        remediation 421
        and schizophrenia 255
memory aids
    assessment of use 420, *421*
    electronic 423
memory clinics 1584

memory impairment, age-associated (AAMI)
    1535, *1535*–6
    *see also* amnesia
memory strategy training 423
Mendel, Gregor 212
meningitis
    and chronic fatigue syndrome 1038
    cryptococcal 1093
    prevention 1447
    tuberculous 1094
menopause 823
menstrual cycle and sexual behaviour 816
menstruation 1114
    and anorexia nervosa 782, 783, 787
Mental Capacity Act 2005 1897, 1898–9
mental causation 134
Mental Deficiency Act 1913 1819
mental disorder
    disease burden 10–11, 467, 1428, 1606
        in childhood and adolescence 1595–6
    and juvenile delinquency 1946–7, 1948–50
        interventions 1951–2
    myth of 28
    and offending **1917–26**, 2009–10
    parental, effects on child development
        1752–4, 1755–6
    phenomena of 47
    prevalence in the community *1480*
    prevalence in general hospital
        population 1144
    prevalence in primary care 1480–2, *1481*, *1482*
    prisoners **1933–6**
    scope of term 1933
    and violence 1937
    as worldwide public health issue **10–13**
mental health, definition 1606–7
Mental Health Act 1930 22
Mental Health Act 1959 1898
Mental Health Act 1983 1491, 1905
Mental Health Alliance 1491
mental health budgets, global survey 11, *11*
mental health legislation, global surveys 11, *11*
mental health literacy 5
mental health nurses *see* psychiatric nurses
mental health professionals
    burnout 1449, *1449*
    in consultation-liaison psychiatry 1146
    engagement in risk assessment 1993–4
    global survey *11*, 12
    as interpreters 67
    perceptions of need 1433
    in primary care 1485–6
    recruitment 1429
    role in primary prevention 1449–50, *1450*
    stalking of 1972
    working with people with intellectual
        disability and psychiatric
        disorder 1889–90
    *see also specific professions*
mental health public policy **1425–31**
    comparative 1426–7
    definitions 1425
    and economic impact of disease
        burden 1428
    and equitable resource allocation 1430
    function 1426
    and funding 1429–30
    global surveys 11, *11*
    and human resources 1429
    and human rights 1427

mental health public policy (*cont.*)
  implementation 1428–9
  and international agencies 1427
  need for 1427–8
  positive and negative drivers 1425–6
  scope of development 1428
mental health resources
  allocation 1473
  equitable allocation and mental health public
    policy 1430
  global 11–12
  insufficiency 1473–4
mental health services
  for adults with intellectual disability
    **1887–92**
  for alcohol use disorders **459–67**
  assessment of utilization 1165
  for bipolar disorder 646
  child and adolescent (CAMHS) **1802–7**, 1946
    accessibility 1805–6
    client groups 1803
    cost-effectiveness analysis 1476–7
    evidence-based development 1804
    inclusion of schools 1811–12
    inclusion of speech and language
      therapists 1716
    multi-disciplinary teams 1812
    prioritizing need 1803–4
    provision of interventions 1804–5
    quality 1806
    referrals to 1811
    role in medico-legal assessment 1954–5
    role in special education 1815
    school liaison service 1812–13
    service structure 1805
    staffing 1805
  community **1452–62**
    acute beds 1452–3
    assertive outreach teams 1455, 1457–8, *1457*
    community mental health centres 1454
    community mental health teams 584,
      1454–5, *1456*, *1457*, 1458, 1888–9
    community substance misuse teams 479
    crisis teams 1458, *1458*
    day care 1453
    development principles *1461*
    diagnosis-specific teams 1459
    early intervention teams 1459, *1459*
    for elderly people 1582
    ethical aspects 1457–8
    forensic teams 1459
    inpatient beds 1452–3
    monitoring and review 1460
    and needs of offenders/prisoners 1934
    office-based care 1454
    outpatient clinics 1454
    planning 1459–60
    rehabilitation in 389–90, 1459
    residential care 1453–4
    supported accommodation 1453–4
  culturally competent 1502–4, *1503*
  dangerous and severe personality disorder
    (DSPD) services 2015, 2018
  and depression 649
  economic analysis **1473–9**
    examples 1476–7, *1478*
    macro-level 1473–4, *1473*
    micro-level 1474–6
  for elderly people 1574–5, *1575*, **1579–86**
    academic units 1584

CARITAS principles 1580
  community services 1582
  comprehensive 1581
  consultation-liaison services 1583
  core business 1581
  core components 1581–4, *1582*
  day hospitals 1583
  inpatient units 1583
  integrated 1581
  long-term care 1583
  need for 1579–80
  patient-centred 1580–1
  planning to commissioning 1584–5
  primary care collaborations 1583–4
  principles of good service delivery 1580–1
  residential care 1583
  respite care 1583
  special components 1584
  for ethnic minorities 277, **1502–4**
  evaluation **1463–72**
    definitions and conceptual
      framework 1463
    key challenges *1470*
    Matrix model 1463, *1464*
    outcome measures 1464–5, *1464*
    purpose of 1463, *1464*
    research design 1465–9, *1465*, *1466*, *1467*,
      *1468*, *1469*
  financing 11, *11*
  forensic 2013, **2015–21**
    capacity planning 2017–18
    community 1459
    international context 2016
    philosophy and theoretical models
      2015–16
    private 2017
    pyramid planning 2017
    security 2015, 2016–17
    service structure 2017–18
    service users 2018–20
    super-specialist 2017
  global improvement 12–13
  for homeless people 1501, *1501*
  integrated 990, 1460
  liability of providers 1904–5
  for mothers 1124–5
  needs *see* needs
  for offenders 1934–5
    forensic 1459, 2013, **2015–21**
    general psychiatric services **2009–14**
    needs 1934–5
    provision in prisons 1934–5
  organization in general hospital
    departments **1144–8**
  for personality disorder 907
  primary care 1486
  research on 281, 1452
  for schizophrenia 584–5
  for substance use disorders **515–20**
  *see also* consultation-liaison (CL) psychiatry
mental health social work **1408–13**
  behavioural 1409
  care management 1410–11
  crisis approach 1409
  historical development 1408
  innovative practice 1411
  legal and policy framework 1410–11
  problem-solving approach 1409
  psychodynamic approaches 1408–9
  social dimension 1409

social role valorization (SRV) approach
  1409–10
  strengths model 1410
  task-centred 1409
  values underpinning 1408
mental hygiene 22
mental retardation *see* intellectual disability
mental status examination (MSE)
  assessment instruments 69–70
  in childhood and adolescence 1601, *1602*
  in intellectual disability 1823
  *see also* Mini-Mental State Examination
Mental Status Schedule 71
mentalization 1948
mentalization-based therapy 304, 894, 1341
meprobamate 1178
MeRAs (melatonin receptor agonists) in
  insomnia 935
mescaline 488
mesencephalon 156, 157
mesoridazine *1209*
  administration *1214*
  adverse effects *1212*
meta-analysis 229, 1155, 1465–6, *1466*
metabolic disorders 1084–5
metabolic enhancers 1240
metachromatic leukodystrophy 537
meta-communications 1381
metencephalon 157
meth (methamphetamine) **497–8**
methadone 475, **1243**
  action at opioid receptors 473
  detoxification 477
  injectable 476
  maintenance treatment 476, 479
  metabolism 473
  in pregnancy 1118, 1615–16
  prescription 479
methamphetamine **497–8**
Methods for the Epidemiology of Child and
  Adolescent Mental Disorders study 1594
methohexitone 1178
18-methoxycoronaridine 1249

*N*-methyl-1-(1,3-benzodioxol-5-yl)-
  2-butanamine 494
methylenedioxyamphetamine 494
methylenedioxyethylamphetamine 494
3,4-methylenedioxymethamphetamine
  *see* ecstasy
methylphenidate 1795
  abuse potential 1795
  adverse effects 1650, 1795
  in attention-deficit hyperactivity disorder
    1241, 1648, 1650, 1876
  in cancer *1103*
  and epilepsy 1650
  in HIV-associated dementia 386
  in intellectual disability 1876
  in narcolepsy with cataplexy 941
  precautions with 1795
  rebound effects 1795
  in terminal illness 1070
metoclopramide 1101
Mexico, attitudes to psychiatric disorder 6
Meyer, Adolf 22
MFQ (Mood and Feelings
  Questionnaire) 1675, 1780
MFTG (multiple family group therapy)
  1382, 1389

mianserin *670*, 671
  adverse effects 1191, *1191*
  in depression in elderly people 1554, *1554*
  dosage *1196*
  pharmacodynamics *1173*, *1187*, 1188
  pharmacokinetics *1172*, *1189*
midazolam *1104*
midbrain 156, 157
'midweek blues' 495
migraine
  and depersonalization 775
  and transient global amnesia 403
migration and schizophrenia 286, 549, 557–8
mild cognitive disorder 1534
mild cognitive impairment (MCI) 266, 1519,
  **1534–9**, 1574
  aetiology 1537, *1537*
  amnestic 1520, 1535
  assessment 1536
  biomarkers 1537–8
  clinical staging scales 1535
  cognitive assessment 1536
  definition 1520, 1534
  diagnosis 1536–8, *1537*
  diagnostic criteria 1535
  epidemiology 1535–6, *1536*
  mortality risk 1536
  neuroimaging 1537–8
  neuropsychiatric symptoms 1537
  nosology 1534–5, *1534*
  progression to dementia 1535–6
  reversion to normal 1536
  treatment and management 1538
  vascular 407
mild neurocognitive disorder 1534
millenniary delusions 982
Millon Clinical Multiaxial Inventory
  858, *858*, 1962
milnacipran
  adverse effects *1191*
  dosage *1196*
  pharmacodynamics 1186, *1187*
  pharmacokinetics 1188, *1189*
mind–body dualism 133, 989–91
mind–body literature 205
mind–brain relation **133–6**
  and psychodynamic psychiatry 315–16
mindfulness-based cognitive therapy 1310
mindfulness skills in body dysmorphic
  disorder 1047
mini-ethnography 278
'minimal brain dysfunction' 1631, 1643
Mini-Mental State Examination (MMSE)
  87, 284
  in Alzheimer's disease 337, 1240
  in delirium in elderly people 1531
  with elderly people 1527, *1528*
  extended 1527, *1528*
  in Huntington's disease 373
  in mild cognitive impairment 1536
  sensitivity to education 284
  in vascular dementia 380
Minnesota Multiphasic Personality Index
  use in malingering 1057
  use with sex offenders 1962
'miracle question' 1276
mirror retraining in body dysmorphic
  disorder 1047
mirror sign 334
mirror therapy in adjustment disorders 720

mirroring 311, 1357
mirtazapine *670*, 671
  adverse effects 1191, *1191*, 1555
  in cancer *1103*
  in depression in elderly people 1554, *1554*
  dosage *1196*
  in panic disorder 757
  pharmacodynamics *1187*, 1188
  pharmacokinetics *1189*
miscarriage 1119
misidentification, delusional 51, 392, 609–10,
  611, 622, **623–4**
misidentification syndromes
  in Alzheimer's disease 335
  delusional 51, 392, 609–10, 611, 622, **623–4**
  and risk of violence 1998
mission statement 43
Misuse of Drugs Act 1971 1927
Mitchell, Stephen 311
mitochondria 223
  and ageing 1508
mitochondrial disorders 1832
mitochondrial encephalopathy with lactic
    acidosis and strokes 1865, *1866*
mitochondrial encephalopathy with ragged red
    fibres 1864
mitral valve prolapse 752
mixed anxiety-depressive disorder 718–19
MMSE *see* Mini-Mental State Examination
mobile phones, counselling services
    using 1814–15
MoCA (Montreal Cognitive Assessment) 1536
moclobemide *670*, *670*
  adverse effects *1191*, 1555
  in depression in elderly people *1554*
  dosage 674, *1196*
  pharmacodynamics *1172*, *1187*, 1188
  pharmacokinetics *1172*, *1189*
  in social anxiety disorder 743
modafinil
  in attention-deficit hyperactivity
      disorder 1241, 1651
  in cancer *1103*
  in hypersomnia 939
  in narcolepsy with cataplexy 941
mode 86
mode deactivation therapy 1953
model fitting 217
models of medical practice 64
Modified Card Sorting Test *90*
Modified Six Elements Test *90*
Modified Social Stress Model 505
*mogo laya* 984
molecular genetics 1598
  gene–environment interactions 214–18, 221,
      229, 315, 558–9, 1608, 1725
  intermediate phenotypes 221
molindone *1209*
  administration *1214*
  adverse effects *1212*
  pharmacodynamics *1211*
Mongolia, attitudes to psychiatric disorder 6
monoamine oxidase-A (MAO-A)
  and aggression 889, 1918
  and antisocial personality disorder 315, 1918
  and conduct disorder 1658
monoamine oxidase inhibitors (MAOIs)
  adverse effects 674, 1187–8, 1190, *1191*,
      1192, *1192*
  in anxiety disorders 1182

  in attention-deficit hyperactivity
      disorder 1651
  in body dysmorphic disorder 1047
  choice of 674
  dietary interactions 1187–8, 1192, *1192*
  dosage *1196*
  drug interactions 1175, 1194–5, *1195*
  in HIV-associated dementia 385
  introduction 1185, *1185*
  irreversible 670, *670*, 1187
  in panic disorder *756*, 757
  in personality disorders 905, 906
  pharmacodynamics 1173, 1186–7,
      1186–8, *1187*
  pharmacokinetics *1172*, 1189, *1189*
  in post-traumatic stress disorder 709
  reversible 1187
  in social anxiety disorder 743
  and surgery 1097–8
monoamines
  and depression 662
  inhibition of reuptake *1172*, *1173*
  and phototherapy 1260
monosomy 228
Montreal Cognitive Assessment 1536
mood
  in alcohol withdrawal 439
  definition 54, 629
  delusional 51, 611
  depressed 637
  immune modulation 209
Mood and Feelings Questionnaire 1675, 1780
Mood Disorder Questionnaire 635
mood disorders 54–5
  aetiology
    genetic **650–8**
    neurobiological **658–65**
  alcohol-induced 427, 434, 444, 455
  anticipation in 652
  in cancer 1102, *1102*, *1103*
  childhood and adolescence **1669–80**
    aetiology 1674
    clinical picture 1669–71, *1670*, *1672*
    comorbidity 1673
    course 1673–4
    differential diagnosis 1657, 1671–3
    epidemiology 1673–4
    with intellectual disability 1852
    neurocognitive factors 1674–5
    sequelae 1674
    treatment and prevention 1675–7
  classification 104, 105, 631, **638–43**, 665
  clinical features **632–7**
  concept of unipolar and bipolar
      disorders 631
  course and prognosis **665–9**
  definitions 637–8
  and delusional disorder 614
  diagnosis **637–45**
    stability of 665
  differential diagnosis 643–4
  elderly people **1550–8**
  epidemiology **645–50**, 650–1
  following head injury 393, 396
  and gender 271, 648, 653–4
  genetics 658
  history of **629–31**
  and life events 269–73, *270*, *271*, 659
  maintaining factors 659–63
  and memory 59

mood disorders (*cont.*)
   mixed states 636, 638
   neurobiology **658–65**
   neuropathology 181–2, *182*
   and neuroticism 658
   and offending 1923
   organic 1552
   and pain 1030
   patient state fluctuations within 632–3,
      *632, 633*
   and persistent somatoform pain
      disorder 1032
   pharmacogenetics 653
   and physical illness *1128*
   precipitating factors 659
   prevalence *285*
   prevention 1448, 1675–7
   psychosocial factors 653
   with psychotic symptoms 864
   rapid cycling 636, 668
   risk factors 658–9
   and sexuality 825
   social functioning in 653
   and socio-economic status 654
   subthreshold **680–92**
   and surgery 1097–8
   and temperament 654, 658, 680
   thinking in 52
   treatment **669–80**, 1252–4
      complementary medicines 1248
      phototherapy 1261
   *see also specific disorders*
mood stabilizers **1198–208**
   in childhood and adolescence 1798, 1852
   *see also specific drugs*
Moodgym 1406
MOPS (Measure of Parenting Style) 286
moral development, history-taking 1601
moral judgement 235
'moral treatment' 17, 1392
morality, conventional/pre-conventional 1762
morbid risk 215
morbidity
   continuous measures 283
   hidden and conspicuous in primary
      care 1482
   and poverty 278
Morel, Bénédict-Auguste 521
Moreno, Jacob 1353
morphine 430
   detection 473
   metabolism 473, *474*
morphometry 195, Plate 9
Morquio syndrome 1843
mosaicism in Down syndrome 1839
mother–foetus relationship 1117
mother–infant relationship disorders 1123–4
motility disorder 58, *58*
motivated sleep phase syndrome 1700
Motivational Assessment Scale 1823
motivational enhancement therapy 451, 794
motivational interviewing
   in adjustment disorders *1069*
   in alcohol use disorders 451
   in body dysmorphic disorder 1047
   in cognitive-behaviour therapy in childhood
      and adolescence 1779
   in opioid dependence 477, *477*, 479
   in rehabilitation 1400
   in substance use disorders 428

motor co-ordination in schizophrenia 529
motor neurone disease 348
   with dementia 344, 345, 347, 348
motor skills disorder 1623, *1623*, 1631
motor symptoms and signs, descriptive
      phenomenology 58–9
mourning 724
   pathological 296
   religious ceremony 1419
   *see also* bereavement
movement disorders
   complementary medicines 1249
   in conversion disorder 1016, *1016*, 1017
   differential diagnosis 373
MR (morbid risk) 215
MRC
   framework for evaluation of complex
      intervention 1465, *1466*
   Needs for Care Assessment 73, 1433–4
MRI *see* structural magnetic resonance imaging
MSE *see* mental status examination
MSI-II (Multiphasic Sex Inventory II) 1962
MSLT *see* multiple sleep latency test
mtDNA *see* DNA, mitochondrial
MTFC (Multidimensional Treatment Foster
      Care) 1790, 1953
mucopolysaccharidoses
   behavioural and psychiatric aspects 1843
   classification 1843
   genetics 1843
   physical characteristics 1843
   prevalence 1843
muddling 53
MUDs (medication use disorders) in elderly
      people **1543–5**, *1544*
multiaxial descriptive systems 73, 990, *990*
   in childhood and adolescence 1592–3
Multidimensional Treatment Foster Care
      1790, 1953
multi-disciplinary practice 68
multi-disciplinary team
   agreement on terminology used 64
   in Alzheimer's disease 341
   care planning 68–9
   in child and adolescent mental health
      services 1812
   and clinical assessment 62, 68
   community mental health teams 584,
      1454–5, *1456, 1457*, 1458, 1888–9
   community old age mental health
      services 1582
   in consultation-liaison psychiatry 1146
   key worker/case manager 68–9
   leadership 68
   membership 68–9
   for people with intellectual disability 1888
   values in 33–5, *34*
   values-based practice *34*, 35, *36*
multi-disciplinary teamwork 68
Multiphasic Sex Inventory II 1962
multiple causation 314
multiple chemical sensitivity 997, 1002
multiple family group therapy 1382, 1389
multiple personality disorder 56, 1923
multiple regression analysis 217
multiple sclerosis **1074**
   cognitive impairment in 1074
   depression in 1074
   emotional lability in 1074
   euphoria in 1074

   psychotic symptoms 1074
multiple sleep latency test (MSLT) 930, 939, 945
   in childhood and adolescence 1697
multi-sensory therapy *414*
multisomatoform disorder *998*, 1000
multi-system atrophy 364, 942
multisystemic therapy 1598, 1661–2, 1782
Munchausen syndrome *see* factitious disorder
Munchausen syndrome by proxy 1054, 1697,
      1737, 1923–4
muscarinic agonists in Alzheimer's
      disease 1241
muscle dysmorphia 1044–5
mushrooms, hallucinogenic 488
music therapy *414*, 1352
mutism 54, 58, *58*
   in frontotemporal dementias 346
   selective 1639, 1714
MWT (maintenance of wakefulness test) 939
myalgic encephalomyelitis *see* chronic fatigue
      syndrome
myelasthenia 1060
myelencephalon 157
myocardial infarction 649, 1081–2
myocardial ischaemia 1081–2
myopathy
   in alcohol use disorders 446
   in anorexia nervosa 785
myotonic dystrophy *228*
*myriachit* 983
mysophilia *833*
mythomania 54
myxoedema and sleep-wake disorders *932*
nadolol 1876
Nagel, Thomas 135
nail-biting 918
nalmefene 454
naloxone 473, 475, 479, 1232, **1245**
   in children and adolescents with psychiatric/
      behaviour disorder and intellectual
      disability 1852
   in depersonalization disorder 775
   in pregnancy 1118
naltrexone
   in alcohol use disorders 454, 1542
   in children and adolescents with psychiatric/
      behaviour disorder and intellectual
      disability 1852
   in intellectual disability 1876
   in opioid use 477, 1245
naratriptan 1171
narcissism 57, 296
   healthy 311
   history of concept 870
   malignant 870, 871
   types *870*
narcissistic loss 1106
narcissistic personality disorder 296, **870–2**
   aetiology 871
   classification *856*, 871, *871*
   clinical features 871
   comorbidity 857–71
   course and prognosis 872
   and deception 1049
   diagnosis 871
   differential diagnosis 871, 876
   in elderly people *1562*
   epidemiology 871, *882*, 883
   historical perspective 870
   treatment 871–2

narcolepsy **940–1**, 1695, 1701
  with cataplexy 940–1
  misdiagnosis 928
  in physical illness 941
  and schizophrenia 927
  without cataplexy 941
Narcotics Anonymous 477, *477*, 1279
NARIs (noradrenaline reuptake inhibitors)
    670, *670*
narrative gerontology 1514–15
National Adult Reading Test (NART) 264, 389
National Comorbidity Survey 541, 645
National Comorbidity Survey Replication
    1595, 1596
National Confidential Inquiry into Suicide
    and Homicide by People with Mental
    Illness 1937, 1938, 1939
National Drug and Alcohol Treatment
    Utilization Survey 463–4
National Drug Treatment Monitoring
    System 515
National Health Service and Community Care
    Act 1432
National Healthy School Standard 1814
National Institute for Health and Clinical
    Excellence (NICE) 789
  clinical practice guidelines 124
National Institute of Neurological and
    Communicative Disorders and Stroke–AD
    and Related Disorders Association 336, 348
National Institutes of Mental Health 23
National Psychiatric Morbidity Survey 645, 647
National Schizophrenia Fellowship 1490–1
National Service Framework for Children,
    Young People and Maternity Services 1946
National Survey of Health and
    Development 1911, 1912
National Survey of Sexual Attitudes and
    Lifestyles 821
National Trailblazer network 1487–8
National Treatment Agency for Substance
    Misuse 515–16
National Treatment Outcome Research
    Study 1927
NATSAL (National Survey of Sexual Attitudes
    and Lifestyles) 821
nausea in alcohol withdrawal 439
NDATUS (National Drug and Alcohol
    Treatment Utilization Survey) 463–4
nDNA *see* DNA, nuclear
necrophilia *833*
needs **1432–7**
  for action 1433
  assessment 73, 94, 1433–5, *1435*, 1823–4
    population-level 1434–5, *1435*, 1459
  definitions 1432–3
  in evaluation of mental health services 1465
  of families with a member with intellectual
    disability 1885–6
  hierarchy of 1432
  for improved health 1432
  needs-led care planning 1432
  patient and staff perceptions 1433
  relationship between individual and
    population 1435
  for services 1433
Needs for Care Assessment 73
nefazodone
  adverse effects 1190, *1191*
  dosage *1196*

pharmacodynamics *1187*, 1188
pharmacokinetics 1189, *1189*
negation 294
negative automatic thoughts 761, 1165, 1286,
    1287–9, *1287*, 1291–2, 1304–5, 1306, *1306*,
    1307, 1308–10, *1309*
negative emotionality
  and health 1136
  and hypochondriasis 1025
negative images 1288
negativism 58
negativistic personality disorder *see* passive–
    aggressive personality disorder
negligence 1901–2
  clinical 1902
  difference between acts and omissions 1905
  liability of mentally ill people 1903–4
  liability to mentally ill people who self-
    harm 1905
  liability of providers of mental health
    services 1904–5
  liability for psychiatric injury 1902–3
  liability to third parties for acts by mentally
    ill people 1901–5
NEO Personality Inventory-Revised (NEO
    PI-R) 81, *81*, 654, 847–58, *858*, 887, 1164
neo-behaviourism 134–5
neocortex 202
  in absence epilepsy 204
  connection 149, Plate 1
  development 158–9, *159*
  in epilepsy 203
  and memory 253
  and priming 254
  structure 147, *148*, Plate 1
neologisms 54
neonates
  abilities 238
  cocaine withdrawal syndrome 1118
  death of 1119
  mother–infant relationship disorders 1123–4
  narcotics withdrawal syndrome 1118
neonaticide 1118–19, 1125
nerve gas 1241
nerve growth factor *160*, 966
nesting behaviour 1117
neural crest 156
neural groove 156
neural induction 156
neural plasticity 251
neural plate 156
neural tube 156, 157
neurasthenia *993*, 994, 1003, 1035, **1059–64**
  aetiology 1062–3
  and chronic fatigue syndrome 1037
  classification 1062
  comorbidity 1063
  concept of 1059–60
  course and prognosis 1063
  and culture 1060–1
  current usage 1062
  definition 1060
  as diagnostic entity 1059–60
  differential diagnosis 1062
  epidemiology 1062, *1062*
  and stigma 1040
  treatment 1063
neuregulin 1 (NRG1) gene 179, 230, 555, 565
neuroanatomy **144–56**
neurobehavioural teratology 1614

neuroblasts 157
neurocirculatory asthenia 751
neurodevelopment **156–60**
  brainstem histogenesis 158–9
  cerebellum histogenesis 158
  cerebral cortex histogenesis 158–9, *159*
  CNS organogenesis 156–7, *157*
  environmental risks 1724
  genetic factors 159
  hemispheric shape and formation of
    gyri 159, *159*
  neural induction 156
  spinal cord histogenesis 157–8
neurodevelopmental disorders 1613
  alcohol-related 1615, 1841
  genetics 159
  *see also specific disorders*
neuroectoderm 156
neuroendocrine 'window' strategy 161
neuroendocrinology **160–7**, 205, 781, 889
neurofibrillary tangles in Alzheimer's
    disease 337–8, 339
neurofibromatosis type 1
  behavioural and psychiatric aspects
    1075, 1844
  expression 213
  genetics 1843, *1866*
  physical characteristics 1843–4
  prevalence 1843
neurofibromatosis type 2, psychiatric
    aspects 1075
neurogenetic syndromes 1613–14
neurokinins *171*
neuroleptic malignant syndrome 1223, 1531
  in HIV/AIDS 386, 1092
  and malignant catatonia 529
  treatment 1254
neuroleptics *see* antipsychotics
neuroligins 227
neurological disorders **1071–6**
  *see also specific disorders*
neuromodulators 168
neuronal ceroid lipofuscinoses 1865, *1866*
neuronal networks **201–5**
  and gamma rhythms 203
  hippocampal 202–3, *202*
  realistic computer simulations 203
neuronal specific enolase 353
neurones
  death from traumatic brain injury 387
  development 157
  endocrine functions **160–7**
  neocortical 148, *148*
  in schizophrenia *178*, 180
NeuroPage 423
neuropathology **177–85**
  alcohol use disorders 182–3, *183*
  Alzheimer's disease 337–9
  corticobasal degeneration 345
  delirium 330–1, *330*
  frontotemporal dementia 344–5
  head injury 387–8, *387*
  Huntington's disease 372
  mood disorders 181–2, *182*
  Pick's disease 344
  progressive supranuclear palsy 345
  schizophrenia and psychoses 178–81, *178*,
    *179*, *180*, *181*
neuropeptides *168*, 170–1, *171*, 206
neuropores 156

neuropsychiatry
developmental **1612–22**
history of 20
neuropsychological assessment **262–7**
in Alzheimer's disease 265–6
in anorexia nervosa 783
in attention deficit hyperactivity disorder 266
in childhood and adolescence 1590–1, 1605
in depression 660
domains 263–6
functions 263
head injury 389
in HIV-associated dementia 384–5
in mild cognitive impairment 1536
in obsessive–compulsive disorder 266
principles 263
in schizophrenia 93, 265, 531–4
in transient global amnesia 403
neuroses
cultural influences 14
historical background 20–1
neurosurgery for mental disorder (NMD) 769,
**1266–9**
adverse effects 1268–9
definition 1266
ethical considerations 1267–8
historical overview 1266–7
inclusion and exclusion criteria *1268*
indications 1267
mechanism of action 1268
outcomes 1268
procedures 1267, *1269*, *1270*
stereotactic procedures 1267
neurosyphilis 537, 1093
neurotic (stress-related) disorder, elderly
people **1558–61**
aetiology 1559–60
clinical features 1558
course and prognosis 1560
diagnosis and differential diagnosis 1558–9
epidemiology 1559
treatment 1560
neuroticism 81, *81*, 850, 886
and body dysmorphic disorder 1046
and high health service use 1137
and hypochondriasis 1025
and mood disorders 658
and serotonergic system 887–8
and subthreshold mood disorders 680
subtypes 632
neurotransmitter receptors 172
drug actions at 1171
agonist 1171
antagonist 1171–2
partial agonist 1172
ionotropic 1171
metabotropic 1171
neurotransmitters **168–77**
in anorexia nervosa 782
in autism 1636
chemokines and cytokines as 171
and chronic fatigue syndrome 1039
co-localization with neuropeptides 171
in conduct disorder 1658
definition 168
and drug pharmacodynamics 1173
hippocampus 202
as hormones 161
neuropeptides 170–1, *171*
and phototherapy 1260

primary 429
principles of transmission 168, *169*
retrograde messengers 171–2
role in neurodevelopment 159
secondary 429
small molecule 168
in substance use disorders 429, *429*, 435–6
transporters 168–70, *170*
plasma membrane 169–70, *170*
vesicular 170, *170*
*see also specific substances*
neurotrophic factors 159, *160*, 168, 171, 1186
*see also specific factors*
neurotrophin receptors 158
neurovascular coupling 197
neutralizing activities in obsessive-compulsive
disorder 1783
New Zealand, Mental Health Foundation 1491
Newcastle Thousand-Family Study 1910
Newton, Isaac 133
NGF (nerve growth factor) *160*, 966
NGOs (non-governmental organizations) 1491
Nicaragua, attitudes to psychiatric disorder 6
NICE *see* National Institute for Health and
Clinical Excellence
nicotine replacement therapy 512
nicotine use *see* smoking
nidotherapy 896–7, 904–5
nifedipine 1201
night-eating syndrome *931*, 947–8
night-time fears 1698–9
nightmares 1108, 1702
in post-traumatic stress disorder 701
nihilistic delusions 56
nimodipine 1198, 1201, 1203
adverse effects *1200*, 1204–5
drug interactions 1206
in HIV-associated dementia 385
indications and contraindications 1205
mechanism of action *1200*
pharmacokinetics 1201
response correlates *1199*
therapeutic profile *1199*
in vascular dementia 381
withdrawal 1207
NINCDS–ADRDA 336, 348
Nisonger Child Behaviour Rating form 1850
nitrazepam *1172*, 1179
nitric oxide, as retrograde messenger 172
nitroglycerin in HIV-associated dementia 385
nitrous oxide 503
NMD *see* neurosurgery for mental disorder
NMDA receptors 172, *173*, 231, 1171
action of lithium at 1201
in alcohol withdrawal 443
antibodies against 1086
and depression 1186
and long-term plasticity 251
and long-term potentiation 251
and schizophrenia 562
NMR (nuclear magnetic resonance) 191–2
NNT (number needed to treat) 127, 128, *128*
NO as retrograde messenger 172
'no-suicide' contracts 1707
nocebo effects 1141
nociception 473
nocturnal enuresis 1702
nocturnal penile tumescence 825, 930
nominal scales 85–6
non-compliance *see* treatment, non-compliance

non-experimental descriptive studies 1468–9
non-governmental organizations 1491
nootropic agents 1240
noradrenaline reuptake inhibitors 670, *670*
noradrenergic storm 473, 476
noradrenergic system and noradrenaline
receptors *173*, 482, 1171, 1172
and depression in childhood and
adolescence 1675
in generalized anxiety disorder 732
noradrenaline transporters 169, *170*
in panic disorder 754
in post-traumatic stress disorder 706
and sexual function 826
and substance use disorders 429
and suicide 965
nordiazepam 1178
norepinephrine *see* noradrenergic system and
noradrenaline receptors
Northfield Hospital 1353
nortriptyline *670*
adverse effects *1191*
in cancer *1103*
dosage 1195, *1196*
pharmacodynamics *1173*, *1187*
pharmacokinetics *1172*, 1188, *1189*
in smoking cessation 512
Notch protein 339
notochord 156
novelty-seeking 80, *80*, 316, *316*, 654, 849,
886–7
NRT (nicotine replacement therapy) 512
NSE (neuronal specific enolase) 353
NT-3 *160*
NTA (National Treatment Agency for Substance
Misuse) 515–16
nuclear magnetic resonance 191–2
nucleosomes 223, 225
nucleus accumbens 154
in substance use disorders 430
nucleus basalis of Meynert, in Alzheimer's
disease 1240
number needed to treat 127, 128, *128*
Nuremberg Statement 30

oats 1248
obesity
and body image 57
and bulimia nervosa 804
psychiatric disorders associated 1084
and schizophrenia 546
and sleep-wake disorders *932*
object relations 295, **306–12**, 313, 1337
Balint's work 308–9
Bion's work 307–8
Bowlby's work 309–10
and character 316
conflictual model 308
and countertransference 298–9
deficit model 308
development from drive theory 306
Fairbairn's work 308
internalization 301–2
Klein's work 306–7, 308
overview and critique of psychoanalytic
theories 301–3
and personality development 316
and psychoanalytic treatment 297
and transference 298–9
unconscious internal 297, 314

Winnicott's work 309
object representation 298, 302–3
Objective Opiate Withdrawal Scale 478, *478*
observed score (*x*) 85
obsessions 52, 53, 1680
   as conditioned stimuli 768
   in obsessive–compulsive disorder 765–6
   and querulous behaviour 1979
obsessive–compulsive disorder (OCD) **765–73**
   aetiology 767–8, 1683–5
   and anorexia nervosa 783
   assessment 1783
   and body dysmorphic disorder 1044, 1045
   in cancer 1101
   childhood and adolescence 1613, **1680–93**
      aetiology 1683–5
      age of onset 1681
      classification 1682
      clinical features 1680–1
      comorbidity 1681–2
      course and prognosis 1685
      diagnosis 1682–3
      differential diagnosis 1682–3
      epidemiology 1683
      and gender 1681
      with intellectual disability 1852
      prevention 1690
      refractory 1688
      treatment 1685–90, *1686, 1687*, 1783–4
   classification *856*, 1682
   clinical features 765–6, 1680–1
   cognitive content 1287
   comorbidity 765, 1681–2
   course and prognosis 766–7, 1685
   diagnosis 765–6, 1682–3
   differential diagnosis 766, 863, 875–6, 1004,
      1023–4, 1639, 1682–3
   elderly people 1558
   epidemiology 765, 1683
   genetics 768, 1684
   neuropsychological assessment 266
   and offending 1923
   prisoners *1934*
   puerperal 1121–2
   and schizophrenia 766
   and sleep disorder 1697
   stalking as 1972
   terminology 856
   and tic disorders 765, 1073, 1681
   treatment
      in childhood and adolescence 1685–90,
         *1686, 1687*, 1783–4
      cognitive-behaviour therapy 770, 1686–7,
         *1686*, 1783–4
      deep brain stimulation 769, 1270
      long-term 769
      neurosurgery 769, 1267, 1268
      pharmacotherapy 768–70, 1193, *1686,
         1687–8*, *1687*
      psychological therapies 770, 1783–4
      transcranial magnetic stimulation 1265
   treatment gap *13*
obsessive–compulsive personality disorder
   765, **874–6**
   aetiology 874
   classification 874, *874*
   clinical features 875
   course and prognosis 875
   defence mechanisms 317
   differential diagnosis 875–6

in elderly people 1562, *1562*
   epidemiology 874, *882*, 883
   treatment 876
obstetric complications
   and conduct disorder 1658
   and schizophrenia 548, 555–6
obstetric liaison services 1118, 1124
obstructive sleep apnoea (OSA) 928, 1083
   early-onset 1695, 1700
   in elderly people 1572
   hypersomnia in 939–40
occipital lobe 146, *147*
   in alcohol use disorders *183*
   in schizophrenia *178*
occupation, and risk of suicide 976
occupational therapy 1034, 1351–2, 1400–1
OCD *see* obsessive–compulsive disorder
OCEAN 850
odds ratios 126, *127*, 128, 141, 282
oedema, famine 785
Oedipus complex 307
   negative 294
   positive 294–5
   and the superego 296
Oenothera biennis oil 1249, 1250
oesophageal dysmotility 1083
oestrogens 816, 826
   therapy
      in gender identity disorder 843
      sex offenders 1963–4
off time 1515
offenders
   amnesia for crimes 405, 1927
   art therapy 1415
   assessment 2011–12, 2018
   depression 1923
   group therapy 1365
   mental health services for
      development 1934–5
      forensic 1459, 2013, **2015–21**
      general psychiatric services **2009–14**
      needs 1934–5
      provision in prisons 1934–5
   need for psychiatric assessment and
      treatment 1918
   outcome assessment 2020
   sexual *see* sex offenders
   therapeutic communities 1396
   treatment 2012–13, 2018–20, *2019*
   versatility 1909
   *see also* prisoners
offending
   acquisitive 1927
   in adolescence *see* juvenile delinquency
   amnesia for 405, 1927
   and attention-deficit hyperactivity
      disorder 1931
   and autism 1921
   and child abuse and neglect 1910
   and child-rearing practices 1910
   and cognitive disorder **1928–32**
   and community influences 1913–14
   concentration in families 1659, 1911–12
   criminogenic factors 1911, 1917, 1918,
      2011, 2012
   and delusional disorder 1920
   and dementia 1920–1
   epidemiology 1908–9
   and epilepsy 1079–80, 1920, 1929–31
   and gender 1909

genetic factors 1918
   and head injury 1920
   and hyperactivity and impulsivity 1909
   impact of criminal victimization **1984–90**
   and impulse control disorders 1924
   and intellectual disability 1856
   and intelligence 1909–10
   and marital conflict 1911
   measurement 1908–9
   and mental disorder **1917–26**, 2009–10
   and mood disorders 1923
   neurobiological determinants of 1917–18
   and neurotic disorders 1923
   and opioid use 474, 480
   and peer influences 1912–13
   and personality disorder 865, 866, 1921–3
   protective factors 1909
   psychosocial causes **1908–16**
   risk factors 1909
      family 1910–12
      individual 1909–10
      social 1912–14
   and schizophrenia 1918–20
   and school influences 1913
   self-reported 1908
   and situational influences 1914
   and socio-economic status 1912
   and substance use disorders **1926–8**
   and violence 1918, 2010–11
Ohtahara syndrome 1862
olanzapine 1209, *1209*
   administration *1214*, 1217–18
   adverse effects *1212*, 1224
   in bipolar disorder 672
      in elderly people 1556
   in cancer *1104*
   in childhood and adolescence 1677, 1797
   in delirium 331
   in dementia 415
   and diabetes mellitus 1085
   in personality disorders *905*, 906
   pharmacodynamics 1210, *1211*, 1213
   pharmacokinetics 1221
old age/older people *see* elderly people
olfactory pathways to the cerebral cortex
   *147*, 152
olfactory reference syndrome 618
olfactory tubercle 154
omega-3 fatty acids 1248, *1250*, 1676
omnipotence 298
omnipotent control 298
on time 1515
One Day Fluctuation Assessment Scale 363
oneiroid state 60, 392, 603, 605
onychophagia 918
onychotillomania 618, 918
'open-loop' tasks 254
openness 850
opiate neurotransmitter pathway, in substance
   use disorders 429
opioid antagonists *see* naloxone; naltrexone
opioid receptors 173, 473, 1171
opioid substitution/maintenance
   treatment 475, 476, 479, 1243–4
opioids **473–82**
   addictiveness *431*
   as anxiolytics 1178
   cognitive effects 92
   complications of use 474–5, *475*
   definition 473

opioids (*cont.*)
    dependence 473, 474
      assessment 478
      in childhood and adolescence 480
      confirmation of 478
      management 477–9
      outcome 481
      psychiatric comorbidity 475, 492–3
      relapse prevention 477
      treatment 475, 476–8, 479, 1242–7
    detoxification 476–7
    effects *474*
    epidemiology of use 474
    metabolism 473–4, *474*
    neurobiology 473
    and offending 474, 480
    overdose 474–5, 479, *480*
    in pregnancy and breastfeeding 480, *480*,
      1117–18, 1615–16, 1754
    routes of use and risk associated 430, 473
    in terminal illness 1070
    tolerance 473, 474
      assessment of 478
    use by elderly people 1543
    withdrawal 473, 474
      measurement 478, *478*
opioids, endogenous 170, *171*, 429
    in autism 1636
    in post-traumatic stress disorder 706
    in substance use disorders *429*
opium 473
opportunity costs in service planning 1459
oppositional defiant disorder
    comorbidity 1682
    diagnosis 1656
    differential diagnosis 1671
    with intellectual disability 1851
    treatment 1781–2
optic nerve development 157
optical distortions 49
optimism
    and health 1136
    and immune function 207
OQ-45 1165
oral contraceptives, drug interactions 1174
oral phase of development 294, 295
orbitofrontal cortex 146, 1919
ordinal scales 86, 95
orexin (hypocretin) 930, 941
orgasm 812
    female 818–19
      problems 823
    male 817
      delayed/absent 828
ORLAAM® 1243–4
OSA *see* obstructive sleep apnoea
osteoporosis in anorexia nervosa 785
Othello-type syndrome 1967
out-of-body experiences 1012
outcome measures 73
    in evaluation of mental health services
      1464–5, *1464*
    psychometric properties 1465
outpatient care in community mental health
    services 1454
ovaries, in anorexia nervosa 784, 787
overactivity in attention-deficit hyperactivity
    disorder 1643
overdetermination 314
oversedation 1178, 1180

overstimulation and hallucinations 50
overvalued ideas 52, 57, 611, 803
oxazepam
    in dementia 415
    pharmacokinetics *1172*, *1178*
    in terminal illness 1070
oxcarbazepine 1198, 1237
    adverse effects 1204
    in childhood and adolescence 1677
    dosage and administration *1233*
    pharmacokinetics *1867*
    structure *1232*
oxiracetam 1240
oxytocin 815, 888

P-glycoprotein 1170, 1249–50, *1250*
p11 175
p73 protein 158
P300 event-related brain potential 435
Paced Auditory Serial Addition Test 87–8, *88*
paediatric autoimmune neuropsychiatric
    disorder associated with streptococcal
    infection 1073, 1685
paedophilia 832, *833*, *836*, 1960–1, *1962*
pain
    acute 1029, 1033
    affective dimension 1033
    assessment 1032–3
    assessment instruments 1032–3
    behaviours 1032, 1033
    beliefs 1032, 1033
    in cancer 1103
    in childhood and adolescence 1744–5
    chronic 1029, 1030, 1033
      neuropathic 1265
      and sleep-wake disorders *932*
    chronic benign pain syndrome 1003
    clinics/treatment centres 1034
    definition 1029
    and delusions 1030
    in dementia 418
    and depression 1029, 1030
    during sexual arousal 822
    following an accident 1107, 1110
    history 1032
    low threshold 1096
    in mood-/anxiety-related disorders 1030
    non-operant 1033
    non-organic 1784
    operant 1033
    in organic disorders 1030
    postoperative management 1099
    and post-traumatic stress disorder
      1030–1
    and the psychiatrist 1029
    psychogenic 57
    as a psychopathological entity 57
    and psychoses 1030
    psychosocial contributions to
      development 1033
    sensory dimension 1033
    and somatization 1030, 1031–2
    and somatoform disorders 1031–2
    and substance use disorders 427
    syndromes of uncertain origin 1030
    topographical distribution 1033
    treatment and management 1033–4
pain disorder *see* persistent somatoform pain
    disorder
paired matching 1468

PAL (CANTAB Paired Associate Learning test)
    264, 266
palaeocortex 158
palilalia 346, 1681
palimpsest 59
paliperidone 1209, *1209*
    administration *1214*, 1220
    adverse effects 1225
    pharmacodynamics 1210
    pharmacokinetics 1221
palliative care in dementia 418
palm sign 487
palmar erythema in alcohol use disorders 446
*Panax ginseng*
    adverse effects 1248
    as cognitive enhancer 1247–8
    drug interactions *1250*
    in neurasthenia 1063
pancreas, effects of alcohol use disorders 446
PANDAS 1073, 1685
panic attack/panic disorder **750–64**
    aetiology 753–5
    with agoraphobia 740–1, 750–64
    and alcohol use disorders 455, 752
    biological models 754–5
    in cancer 1101
    in childhood and adolescence 1664
      clinical presentation 1665
      prevalence 1666
    classification 751
    clinical features 750–1
    cognitive content 1286
    comorbidity 752, 761
    and COPD 1082
    course and prognosis 755
    and depression 752
    diagnosis 752–3
    differential diagnosis 752, *753*, 1004, 1023,
      1078, 1864
    epidemiology 753
    following an accident 1106
    genetics 753–4
    hallucinogen-induced 488
    in HIV/AIDS 1091
    and hypochondriasis 997
    limited symptom attacks 751
    and neurasthenia 1063
    nocturnal attacks 751
    in physical illness 1131
    and pregnancy 761–2
    prevention 762
    prevention of recurrence 759
    in primary care setting 753
    puerperal 1121
    risk factors 753
    and separation anxiety disorder 1665
    situational attacks 750
    situationally predisposed 750
    and sleep disorders 1697
    with social phobia 750
    and suicide 1704
    treatment and management 755–62, 1180
      cognitive-behaviour therapy 758, 761
      continuation/maintenance 758
      discontinuation 760
      ethical issues 762
      exposure treatments 758, 760–1
      hyperstimulation reaction 756, 759–60
      pharmacotherapy 755–7, *756*
      psychodynamic psychotherapy 758

resistance to 761
treatment gap *13*
Panic Disorder Severity Sale 760
*Papaver somniferum* 473
papaverine 1240
Papez circuit 733
para-aminosalicylate *1091*
paracetamol poisoning 973
paradoxical intention in insomnia 937
paradoxical interventions 1377
paragrammatism 54
parahippocampal gyrus 146, 153
paraldehyde 1178, 1867
paralysis 57
in conversion disorder 1016
paramnesia 59
paraneoplastic syndromes 1101
paranoia
definition 861
elderly people **1546–50**, 1559
querulous *see* delusional disorder, litigious
*see also* delusional disorder
paranoia acuta 603, 605
paranoid personality disorder **861–2**
aetiology 861
classification *856*, 861, *861*
clinical features 861–2
course 862
defence mechanisms 317
differential diagnosis 862, 863, 865
in elderly people 1562, *1562*
epidemiology 861, 882, *882*
nomenclature 610
treatment 862, 898
paranoid psychoses following head injury 392–3
paranoid–schizoid position 307
'paranoid spectrum' 609, 610–11
paraphasia 54
paraphilias **832–42**, 1961
aetiology 836–7
assessment 1962
classification 833–4, *833*
clinical features 832–3
co-occurrence 1962
comorbidity 834–5
course and prognosis 837–8
diagnosis 834–5
differential diagnosis 834–5
epidemiology 835, *836*
false accusations 834
false confessions 834
in Huntington's disease 373
and intellectual disability 834
legal issues 834
overlap with sexual offences 1960
treatment and management 838–41, *839*, 1963–4
paraphrenia 609, 610, 623
late 1547
paraplegia, in conversion disorder 1016
parapraxes 313
paraschemazia 57
parasitosis, delusion of 50, 51, 618
parasomnia pseudo-suicide 948
parasomnias 927, *928*, **943–50**, 1695
in childhood and adolescence 1701–2
classification 944, *944*
clinical evaluation *943*, 944–5, *945*
definition 943

differential diagnosis 948
in elderly people 1572
overlap disorder 947
relevance to psychiatrists 943–4
parasuicide 916–17, 957, 1703
parasympathetic nervous system 156
parasyntax 54
parathyroid adenoma 1101
Parent–Child Interaction Training 1788–9
Parental Bonding Instrument 286, 648
parenting
and attachment 309
and conduct disorder 1659–60, 1661, 1662
factors affecting child mental health 1725–7
and gender identity disorder in childhood and adolescence 1719–20
and generalized anxiety disorder 734
and mood disorders 653
negative 1788, 1789
and offending 1910
positive 1788, 1789
style 286
parents
abusive 1734
and assessment in childhood and adolescence 1600, 1602, *1603*, 1605
in child and adolescent psychiatric emergencies 1808, 1809
child's reaction to death of 1758–60
conflict between
and conduct disorder 1659–60
and depression 1753
effects on child mental health 1726
interpersonal psychotherapy (IPT-CM) 1322
and mood disorders 653
and offending 1911
criminal activity by 1659, 1911–12
effects of child with intellectual disability 1884, 1885
effects of child with physical illness 1742
effects of childhood and adolescent sleep disorders 1694–5
factors affecting child mental health 1726–7
good-enough mother 309
influence on childhood and adolescent sleep disorders 1694
interviewing 1601, *1603*
involvement in cognitive-behaviour therapy 1778–9, 1780
involvement in pharmacotherapy 1794
involvement in psychotherapy 1768, 1771
late-life 1514
mental disorder
alcohol use disorders 1754
anxiety disorders 1754
depression 1752–3
eating disorders 1753–4
effects on child development 1752–4, 1755–6
schizophrenia 1753
substance use disorders 1754
neglectful 1736
people with intellectual disability as 1885
physical illness
cancer 1754–5
effects on child development 1754–6
HIV/AIDS 1755
single 1369–70, 1601, 1726–7, 1910, 1911
training programmes 1661, 1787–93

in attention-deficit hyperactivity disorder 1648
in conduct disorder 1782
young 1910
parietal lobe 146, *146*
in alcohol use disorders *183*
in schizophrenia *178*
parieto-occipital sulcus 145
parkinsonism
in dementia with Lewy bodies 361
drug-related 580, 1222–3
with frontotemporal dementia 344–5, 346, 348
treatment 1255
Parkinson's disease **1072–3**
cognitive assessment 92
dementia in 92, 362–3, **368–71**, *370*
depression in 648–9, 1072
diagnosis 369
differential diagnosis 373
dopamine dysregulation syndrome 1073
hypersomnia in 942
Lewy bodies in 361, 369
mortality in 370
psychotic symptoms in 1072
sleep-wake disorders 932, 1072
transcranial magnetic stimulation 1265
paroxetine *670*
adverse effects *1191*
in attempted suicide 970–1
in cancer *1102*, *1103*
in depression in elderly people *1554*
dosage *1196*
in generalized anxiety disorder 735
in obsessive–compulsive disorder 769, *1687*
in panic disorder *756*
pharmacodynamics *1173*, *1187*
pharmacokinetics *1172*, *1189*, *1189*
in post-traumatic stress disorder 709
in pregnancy 1117
in social anxiety disorder 743
partial arousal disorder 1702
partnerships 40
parturition *see* childbirth
PAS (Personality Assessment Schedule) *858*, *859*
PASAT (Paced Auditory Serial Addition Test) 87–8, *88*
*Passiflora incarnata* (passion flower) 1248, *1249*, *1250*
passive–aggressive personality disorder *876*, **876–7**, *1562*
epidemiology 882, 883
passivity experience 56
passivity of thought 53
path analysis 217, *217*
pathological jealousy 51, 620–1, 862, 1998
pathological lying 54, 871, 1049, 1051, 1941
pathways to care 281, *281*
and culture **1438–45**
filters on 1440–2, *1441*
international comparisons 1438–9, *1439*
pathways out of care 1443
patient delay 1137
patient expected event rate 128
Patient Health Questionnaire 1145
Patient Health Questionnaire-9 1484, 1486
patient-intervention studies 1139

patients
    doctor–patient communication 1138–9
    education 4, 1198
    expectations, and the placebo response 1142
    information for 1140
    perceptions of need 1433
    perspective on services **3–4**
    protection, and psychiatric reports 75
    satisfaction 1138–9, 1465
Pavlovian theory 1061
PBI (Parental Bonding Instrument) 286, 648
PCIT (Parent–Child Interaction
    Training) 1788–9
PCL-R (Psychopathy Check List-Revised)
    1921, 2011
PCMHWs (primary care mental health
    workers) 1485
PCP *see* phencyclidine
PCR (polymerase chain reaction) 223, 226
PD *see* personality disorders
PDA (panic disorder with agoraphobia) 740–1,
    750–64
PDDs *see* pervasive developmental disorders
PDEs (phosphodiesterases) 176
PDQ-4 (Personality Diagnostic Questionnaire-
    Revised) *858*
PDS (Post-traumatic Stress Diagnostic
    scale) 703
PDSS (Panic Disorder Severity Sale) 760
PEA (prenatal exposure to alcohol) 1841
PEER (patient expected event rate) 128
peer pressure, and substance use disorders 427
peer relationships, and conduct disorder 1659
pellagra 1447
pemoline 1648, 1652
penetrance 213
penicillin
    adverse effects *1091*
    in syphilis 1094
penile plethysmography 840, 1962, 1964
penis
    erection 816–17
    nocturnal penile tumescence 825, 930
Penn State Worry Questionnaire 1163
pentagastrin in panic disorder 754
pentosan polyphosphate 359
pentoxifylline in HIV-associated
    dementia 385–6
peptic ulcer disease *932*, 1084
peptide T in HIV-associated dementia 385
percentile 86, *86*
perception
    and consciousness 59
    delusional 51, 527–8
    disorders of 48–50
    disturbance in schizotypal personality
        disorder 864
    and emotion 259–60
perceptual priming 696
perfectionism
    in bulimia nervosa 804, 806
    and chronic fatigue syndrome 1036
    and psychoanalysis 1341
    and somatization disorder 1002
periodic limb movements in sleep 948, 1572,
    1695, 1700
peripheral nervous system, in mood
    disorders *182*
peripheral neuropathy
    in alcohol use disorders 446

disulfiram-induced 453
peripheral oedema in anorexia nervosa 784
perirhinal cortex 146, 152–3, 153, 252, 406
periurethral glans 818
perphenazine *1209*
    administration *1214*
    adverse effects *1212*
    pharmacodynamics *1211*
persecution, delusion of 51
perseveration 53
    in Alzheimer's disease 334
    in frontotemporal dementias 346
persistence 80, *80*, 316, *316*, 849
persistent genital arousal disorder 822
persistent somatoform pain disorder 57, *993*,
    1003, **1029–35**
    assessment 1032–3
    assessment instruments 1032–3
    childhood and adolescence 1745
    classification 997, 1029–30
    comorbidity *1031*, 1032
    correlates 997
    diagnostic and clinical features 1029–30
    differential diagnosis 1003, 1029,
        1030–2, *1031*
    epidemiology 997, *998*, 1032
    phenomenology 997
    prevalence 997, *998*
    prognosis 1034
    and psychosocial contributions to
        development of pain 1033
    treatment and management 1033–4
persistent vegetative state in Huntington's
    disease 373
Personal, Health and Social Education 1814
personality
    abnormality 60
    accentuated type 73
    and addiction 428–9
    and alcohol use disorders 434
    in Alzheimer's disease 335–6
    assessment 72–3, **78–85**, 286, 1164–5
    change
        due to a general medical condition
            879, 1929
        following head injury 391
        following traumatic experiences 879,
            1110–11
    and character 316–17
    and chronic fatigue syndrome 1039
    definition 60, 79, 855
    and depression 648
    development *316*
        psychodynamic approaches 316–17
    domestic violence perpetrators 1982
    effects of neurosurgery for mental
        disorder 1269
    and health 1136
    histrionic 868, *869*
    and hypochondriasis 1025
    hysterical 868, *869*
    models 848–50
        categorical 849
        correlational 849
        dimensional 849–50
        experimental 849
        Five-Factor 238, 850, 857–8, 1164
        and personality disorders 850–1
        psychoanalytical 849
        psychobiological 316

neuropsychology **886–92**
    premorbid 1526
    quantitative description of 79–81, *80*
    and somatization disorder 1002
    studies 848
    and subthreshold mood disorders 680
    and temperament 316, *316*
    traits 79–81, *80*, 286, 849–50, 855, 857, 886
        biological factors 886–92
        and genetics 886–8, 888–9, *890*
        and head injury 390
        normal/abnormal 857
        psychometric testing 81–2, *81*
    type A 1082, 1136
    type B 1136
    type D 1082, 1136
    typology 60
    variants 852–3, *852*
Personality Assessment Inventory 1962
Personality Assessment Schedule *858*, 859
Personality Diagnostic Questionnaire 1562
Personality Diagnostic Questionnaire-
    Revised *858*
Personality Disorder Questionnaire 1164
personality disorders (PD) **847–55**
    assessment 858–9, *858*
    changes in conceptualization 857
    and character dimensions 316
    classification 106, 850–1, 851, 852, *852*, *853*,
        855–8, *856*
    cluster A 856, **861–5**
        drug treatment 906
        and reward-dependence 316
    cluster B 856, **865–72**
        and attempted suicide 1704
        drug treatment 906
        and novelty-seeking 316
    cluster C 856, **872–6**
        drug treatment 906
        and harm-avoidance 316
        long-term psychodynamic
            psychotherapy 318
    comorbidity 780–1, 803, 884, 893, 902, 907
    course 892–3
    dangerous and severe 848, 2015, 2018
    definitions 60, 855, 893
    and depression 649
    diagnosis **855–60**, 890–1
    distinction from personality variants
        852–3, *852*
    elderly people **1561–4**
        aetiology 1562–3
        clinical features 1561–2
        course and prognosis 1563
        diagnosis 1562
        epidemiology 1518, 1562–3, *1562*
        treatment and management 1563–4
    epidemiology **881–6**
        community studies 882–3, *882*
        studies in a psychiatric setting 883–4
    and epilepsy 1079
    features *82*
    history of concept 847–8
    and homicide 1921
    and intellectual disability 1856
    and kleptomania 1943
    and models of personality 850–1
    and offending 865, 866, 1921–3
    and persistent somatoform pain
        disorder 1032

and physical illness 1132
prisoners 1921, 1933, *1933*
psychoanalytic approach 294, 296
qualitative clusters and subtypes *83*
and stigma 848
stress–diathesis model 851–2
and suicide 955, 956, 969
and surgery 1098
and temperament dimensions 316
in Tourette syndrome 1073
treatment **901–10**
  adherence to 902
  cognitive 895, 903–4
  drug treatment 600, 905–6, *905*
  duration 901–2
  evaluation of efficacy 901–3
  nidotherapy 896–7, 904–5
  outcome measures 902
  psychotherapy **892–901**, 1395–6
  service organization 907
  therapeutic communities 892, 896, 905,
    1395–6
  type R (treatment resisting) 902
  type S (treatment seeking) 902
  see also *specific personality disorders*
Personality Disorders Interview-IV *858*
PERT (post ejaculation refractory time)
    817, 822
pervasive developmental disorders
    (PDDs) 1613, **1633–42**
  with attention-deficit hyperactivity
    disorder 1650
  classification 1623
  differential diagnosis 1639
  prevention 1640
  and social phobia 1665
  treatment and management 1639–40
  see also *specific disorders*
pervasive refusal syndrome 787
PET *see* positron emission tomography
pet therapy in dementia *414*
peyote 489
PFAE (possible foetal alcohol effects) 1841
PGAD (persistent genital arousal disorder) 822
phaeochromocytoma 1101
phallometry 840, 1962, 1964
phantasy, unconscious 307
phantom bite syndrome 619
pharmacodynamics 1168, **1171–3**
  in childhood and adolescence 1794
pharmacogenetics 221
  mood disorders 653
pharmacokinetics 1168, **1170–1**, *1172*
  bioavailability 1170
  in childhood and adolescence 1794
  clearance 1170–1
  half-life 1170–1
  protein binding 1170
pharmacotherapy **1168–77**
  acute stress reactions 697
  adjustment disorders 721, 1068
  adverse effects *427*, **1173–5**
    anxiety *730*
    collateral 1173
    dose-related 1173
    DoTS classification 1173, *1174*
    hypersusceptibility 1173
    risk factors 1174–5
    sexual dysfunction 826–7
    susceptibility factors 1174–5, *1175*

time-related 1173–4, *1174*
    toxic 1173
    withdrawal syndromes 1175
  alcohol use disorders 1246
  Alzheimer's disease 1240–1
  attempted suicide 970–1
  attention-deficit hyperactivity
    disorder 1174–2, 1648, 1650, 1876
  beliefs about 1141
  body dysmorphic disorder 1046–7, *1047–8*
  in breastfeeding 1121, 1123, 1169–70, 1180
  with brief psychodynamic
    psychotherapy 1329
  bulimia nervosa 807–8
  childhood and adolescence **1793–9**
    antidepressants 674–5, 1668, 1676,
      1794–5, 1796
    antipsychotics 1677, 1796–8, 1852
    atomoxetine 1795–6
    developmental issues 1794
    dosage regimens 1169
    mood stabilizers 1798, 1852
    as part of multimodal treatment 1793–4
    with psychiatric/behaviour disorder and/or
      intellectual disability 1798, 1852
    rapid tranquillization 1798
    stimulants 1795
    symptom-based approach 1794
  chronic fatigue syndrome 1040, 1042
  in combination with electroconvulsive
    therapy 1257
  comparisons with psychotherapy 1162
  conversion disorder 1019–20
  cosmetic/palliative 853
  delirium 331–2
    in cancer patients *1104*
  dementia with Lewy bodies 365–7
  depersonalization disorder 775
  dosage regimens 1168–70
    in childhood and adolescence 1169
    combination formulations 1169
    elderly people 1169
    maintenance dose 1171, *1171*
    modified-release (depot) 1169, *1169*,
      1171, 1486
    parenteral 1169
    in pregnancy and breast feeding 1169–70
  drug interactions 1175–6
  dynamic 317
  dysthymia/dysthymic disorder 684–5
  elderly people 1573
    dosage regimens 1169
  epilepsy **1231–40**
    with intellectual disability 1866–7, *1867*
  erectile dysfunction 821, 828
  following head injury 396–7, *396*
  generalized anxiety disorder 735, 736, 737
  history of 25
  hypochondriasis 1027
  in infectious disease 1091, *1091*
  in intellectual disability 1875–6
  mild cognitive impairment 1538
  minimum effective dose (MED) 1794
  monitoring 1176
  obsessive–compulsive disorder 768–70, 1686,
    1687–8, *1687*
  panic disorder 755–7, *756*
  personality disorders 600, 905–6, *905*
  pharmacodynamics *see* pharmacodynamics
  pharmacokinetics *see* pharmacokinetics

in physical illness with psychiatric
    disorder 1130–1
  post-traumatic stress disorder 709–10
  prescribing and management by psychiatric
    nurses 1405–6
  in rehabilitation 1400
  schizophrenia 579–82, *579*, 585, 586–8, *586*
  social anxiety disorder 742–4
  somatization disorder 1009
  specific phobia 746
  substance use disorders **1242–7**
  and surgery 1097–8
  in terminal illness 1070
  tic disorders 1687–8
  vascular dementia 381
  see also *specific drugs and types of drugs*
phasic alertness 247
phencyclidine (PCP) **486–7**
  acute physiological effects 486
  adverse effects 486
  delirium due to 486–7
  dependence 487
  epidemiology of abuse 486
  psychosis due to 487, 538
  use in pregnancy 1117
phenelzine 670, *670*
  adverse effects *1191*, 1193
  dosage *1196*
  limitations on use 1187
  in panic disorder *756*
  in personality disorders *905*
  pharmacodynamics *1187*
  pharmacokinetics *1172*, *1189*
  in post-traumatic stress disorder 709
  in social anxiety disorder 743
phenobarbitone 1178
  adverse effects 1673
  choice of 1866–7
  drug interactions 1866
  in epilepsy 1080
  pharmacokinetics *1867*
phenomenology
  definition 47
  descriptive **47–61**
phenothiazines in pregnancy 1117, 1118
phenotype 212
  components of variation 214
  intermediate 221
phentolamine 828
phenylketonuria
  behavioural and psychiatric aspects
    1844, 1852
  genetics 212, 214, 1844
  infantile spasms in 1863
  physical characteristics 1844
  prevalence 1825–6, 1844
  prevention 1448
phenytoin 1231
  adverse effects 1868
  in alcohol withdrawal 449
  choice of 1866–7
  drug interactions 1175, 1232, 1866
  in epilepsy 1080
  pharmacokinetics 1170, *1170*, *1867*
  in status epilepticus 1867
phobias *see* specific phobia *and other phobias*
phobic–anankastic syndromes 52
phonological speech disorder 1624–5,
    1711, 1712
phosphodiesterases 176

phototherapy 670, 927, **1260–2**
  administration 1262
  adverse effects 1261–2
  drug interactions 1262
  forms 1261
  indications and contraindications 1261
  in insomnia 935
  mechanism of action 1260
  withdrawal 1262
PHQ (Patient Health Questionnaire) 1145
PHQ-9 (Patient Health Questionnaire-9)
    1484, 1486
PHSE (Personal, Health and Social
    Education) 1814
physical illness
  adjustment to **1065–71**, 1741, 1742
  antidepressant therapy in 674, 1132
  art therapy 1415
  differentiation from mental disorder 989
  differentiation from panic disorder 752, *753*
  effects on family 1742
  elderly people 1559
  group therapy 1364
  immune system involvement 209, *210*
  and intellectual disability 1828, 1850
  parental, effects on child development
    1754–6
  personality change due to 879
  with psychiatric disorder 546, **1081–90**
    in childhood and adolescence **1739–47**
    course and prognosis 1129–30
    depression 335, 371, 648–9, 1072, 1074,
      1080, 1082, 1085, 1086, 1091, 1092,
      1102, 1132
    diagnosis and differential diagnosis
      1129, *1129*
    epidemiology 1128, *1128*
    management **1128–34**
  of refugees 1495
  sexual dysfunction in 826
  with sleep–wake disorders 931, *932*, 933,
    941, 942
  *see also* illness *and specific illnesses*
physicalism, *a priori* 134
physiognomy 1420
physiological deconditioning 1036
physiotherapy in persistent somatoform pain
    disorder 1034
physostigmine 331–2, 1241
phytoestrogens 1249
Piaget, Jean 235, 239–40, *239*, 1777
*pibloktoq* 983
pica 1116
Pick bodies 344
Pick cells 344
Pick's disease 228, 344
  age at onset 345
  clinical features 345–6, *346*
  epidemiology 345
  investigations 347
  neuropathology 344
Picture Vocabulary Test 239
'pill bottle' sign 618
pimozide *1209*
  in body dysmorphic disorder 1047
  pharmacodynamics *1211*
  in tic disorders 1073, 1688
pindolol 1172
Pinel, Philippe 17–18
*Piper methysticum* (kava) 1248, *1250*

piracetam 1240
Pittsburgh Youth Study 1908, 1910, 1912, 1913
pituitary
  components of the hypothalamic–pituitary–
    end-organ axes 162–3, *162*
  *see also specific axes*
Place, U.T. 134
placebo response 1141–2, 1794
plaques
  in Alzheimer's disease 338
  in dementia with Lewy bodies 362
plate 12
play
  development of *1766*
  enhancement of capacity for *1772*
play therapy 306–7, 1765, 1766, 1770
  in selective mutism 1714
pleasure principle 294, 295
pleasure-seeking behaviour and
    substance use 426
pleiotropy 224
PLMS (periodic limb movements in sleep) 948,
    1572, 1695, 1700
PMR (progressive muscle relaxation), in
    generalized anxiety disorder 736
pneumonia and delirium 1091
Point of Service 45
polar hysteria 983
polyclinics 1454
polycystic ovarian disease and gender identity
    disorder 843
polyembolokoilamania *833*
polygraphy, use with sex offenders 1962, 1964
polymerase chain reaction 223, 226
polysomnography 930
  in childhood and adolescence
    1695, 1696, 1699
  in hypersomnia 939
  in insomnia 934
  in parasomnias 943–4, *943*, *944*
    REM sleep behaviour disorder 946–7
    sleepwalking/sleep terrors 945
POMC (proopiomelanocortin) 170
pooled odds ratio 126
population stratification 651
poriomania 1930
pornography 1961
porphyria, acute intermittent 212
Portland Digit Recognition Test 1057
POS (Point of Service) 45
positron emission tomography (PET) **185–91**,
    Plates 3–6
  alcohol-related dementia 401
  comparison with functional magnetic
    resonance imaging 186–7, 196–7
  comparison with SPET 185
  data collection and analysis 186
  depression 189, 660
  during antipsychotic use 189–90
  during heroin use 428, Plate 13
  and emotions 257–8
  epilepsy 1619, 1862
  frontotemporal dementias 347
  head injury 389
  imaging strategies 187, *187*
  isotopes *186*
    production 185
  limitations 186–7
  methodology 185
  mild cognitive impairment 1538

obsessive–compulsive disorder 768
  schizophrenia 188–9, 562–3
  of transcranial magnetic stimulation 1263
  vascular dementia 380
  Wernicke–Korsakoff syndrome 406
Posner covert spatial attentional task 265
possession disorder 56
possession states 276
possible foetal alcohol effects 1841
postcentral gyrus 146
postcentral sulcus 146
post-concussion syndrome 394, 395–6, 1929
post-ejaculation refractory time 817, 822
postnatal depression 1122, 1486
  and anorexia nervosa 780
  counselling in 1280
  effects on child development 1753
  interpersonal psychotherapy 1322
  and sleep deprivation in pregnancy 927
postpartum psychiatry 647, 653, 1121–5
Post-traumatic Stress Diagnostic scale 703
post-traumatic stress disorder (PTSD) **700–13**
  and acute stress reactions 693, 696
  aetiology 696, 705–7, *707*
  amnesia in 404, 714
  animal models 707
  assessment instruments 703
  behaviours that maintain the symptoms 706
  biological factors 706–7
  childhood and adolescence 237–8, **1728–31**,
    1741, 1744, 1759, 1784, 1851–2
  classification 693, 701, *702–3*
  clinical features 701
  cognitive content 1287
  comorbidity 704–5
  course and prognosis 707–8
  diagnosis 701, *702–3*, 703
  differential diagnosis 695, 701, *702–3*, 703
  epidemiology 703–5
  flashbacks in 404
  following accidents 1109, 1110–11
  following childbirth 1121
  following surgery 1099
  genetics 707
  and intellectual disability 1851–2
  and juvenile delinquency 1949–50
  malingered 1055
  and offending 1923
  and pain 1030–1
  partial 704
  and physical illness 1131
  prevalence 704
  prevention 697, 698, 1109, 1279–80
  prisoners *1934*
  in refugees 1495, 1497
  risk factors *707*
  and sleep–wake disorders 927
  subsyndromal 1110
  treatment and management 708–10, 1295,
    1497, 1784
  victims of burglary/robbery 1986
  victims of criminal activity 1984, 1985
  victims of rape/sexual assault 1986
  victims of terrorism 1987
postural hypotension
  and chronic fatigue syndrome 1038
  drug-induced 1190, 1223, 1529
posturing 58, *58*
poverty
  and child mental health 1727–8

and conduct disorder 1659
and homelessness 1500
relationship with morbidity and
mortality 278
PPG (penile plethysmography) 840, 1962, 1964
PPO (Preferred Provider Organization) 45
practice nurses 1486
Prader–Willi syndrome 1841
and affective psychosis 1826
behavioural phenotype 1613, 1614, 1838,
1844, *1851*, 1858
cognitive and psychiatric aspects 1838, 1844
genetics 213, 224, 229, 1844
physical characteristics 1844
prevalence 1844
Pragmatic Language Impairment 1713
pragmatics, difficulties with 1711, 1713
*prameha* 981
Precaution Adoption model 1137
precentral gyrus 145
precentral sulcus 145
preconscious 294, 295
prediction errors 259
predictive learning 258–9
prednisolone 1532
Preferred Provider Organization 45
prefrontal cortex
in conversion disorder 1013, *1013*, *1014*
and declarative memory 253
dorsolateral
transcranial magnetic stimulation 1264
and working memory 254–5
and fear/anxiety 1667, *1667*
lateral 146
medial 146
ventral, in obsessive–compulsive
disorder 1684
pregabalin 743, 1182, 1237
pregnancy
adjustment to 1116
alcohol use disorders in 1117, 1448, 1614–15,
1754, 1826, 1841
anxiety in 1117
and attachment 1117
bipolar disorder in 677
and body dysmorphic disorder 1116
delusions of 1115
denial of 1116
depression in 653, 1117, 1322
domestic violence during 1117
early, and offending 1910
and eating disorders 780, 784, 1118
ectopic 1119
electroconvulsive therapy in 1117
factitious disorder in 1050, 1118
foetal abuse in 1117
and panic disorder 761–2
pharmacotherapy in
antidepressants 675, 677, 761–2, 1117, 1192
antiepileptic drugs 677
antipsychotics 677, 1118
anxiolytics 1117
benzodiazepines 762, 1117, 1180
butyrophenones 1118
carbamazepine 1118, 1234
dosage regimens 1169–70
lamotrigine 1235
lithium 677, 1118, 1205
phenothiazines 1117, 1118
propranolol 1117

topiramate 1236
valproate 1118, 1169, 1232
premarital 272
psychosis in 1118
and schizophrenia 548
sleep deprivation in 927
smoking in 1646
substance use disorders in 480, *480*, 1117–18,
1614, 1615–16, 1754
and suicide 1116, 1119
surrogate 1115
termination *see* abortion
volatile substance abuse in 504
*see also* obstetric complications
prejudice and stigma 6
premenstrual tension/syndrome 1114
premotor cortex 145
prenatal exposure to alcohol 1841
pre-occipital sulcus 145
preparedness theory and phobias 745
Preparing for the Drug Free Years
programme 1790
presenilins 227, 339
Present State Examination 71, 269, 272, 523,
534, 542
pre-speech 240
pre-supplementary area 245
prevalence 281, 1607
estimation 138–41
lifetime 215, 542
point 215, 542
typical estimates 285, *285*
prevention
alcohol use disorders **467–72**, 1448–9
Alzheimer's disease 341
anorexia nervosa 796–7
autism 1640
body dysmorphic disorder 1048
child abuse and neglect 1737–8, 1788
in childhood and adolescence 1606, 1609–11
chronic fatigue syndrome 1042
comparison with health promotion 1609
conduct disorder 1663, 1788
Creutzfeldt–Jakob disease 358–9
cyclothymia/cyclothymic disorder 689
deliberate self-harm **972–6**
delirium 331, 1533
Down syndrome 1448
dysthymic disorder 686
epilepsy 1620
evidence-based 1608–9
foetal alcohol syndrome 1448
HIV/AIDS 1447
indicated 1609, 1610
infectious diseases 1447
intellectual disability 1447–8, *1448*, 1834–5
iodine deficiency 1448
malingering 1058
mood disorders 1448, 1555–6, 1675–7
panic disorder 762
pervasive developmental disorders 1640
phenylketonuria 1448
post-traumatic stress disorder 697, 698,
1109, 1279–80
primary **1446–51**, 1598, 1609
responsibility for 1449–50, *1450*
and public health 1606–7
relapse 1448
research cycle 1608–9
role of epidemiology 281

schizophrenia 550, 589, 1448
schizotypal personality disorder 601
secondary 1446, 1598, 1609
selected 1609, 1610
social anxiety disorder 744
specific phobia 746
staff burnout 1449, *1449*
suicide **969–78**, 1449, 1708–9, 1992
tertiary 1446, 1598, 1609
theoretical models 1608
three-level concept 1446
universal 1609, 1610
vascular dementia 381, 1447
violent behaviour 1449
volatile substance abuse 505
Wernicke–Korsakoff syndrome 450, 1542
'primary addiction' theory 434
primary auditory cortex 146
primary care **1480–9**
alcohol use disorder detection 1484
assessment in 67
classification in 1483–4
clinical presentation in 1482–3
counselling in 1280, 1485–6
depression
detection and assessment 1476
elderly people 1518
treatment 1322, 1476
elderly people 1482–3, 1518, 1584
epidemiology 1480–2, *1481*, *1482*
hidden vs. conspicuous morbidity 1482
interface with secondary care 1486–7
management of psychiatric disorder
1485–6, *1485*
mental health professionals 1485–6
mental health services 1486
panic disorder 753
prevalence of personality disorders 884
prevalence of psychiatric disorder 1480–2,
*1480*, *1481*, *1482*
psychiatric nurses in 1406
refugee clinics 1496
social worker attachment 1411
somatization in 1482
training in mental health 1487–8
primary care mental health workers 1485
primary child mental health workers 1812
primary identification 1344
primary motor cortex 145
primary somatic sensory cortex 146
primary visual cortex 152
primidone
choice of 1866–7
pharmacokinetics *1867*
priming 250, 254
primitive defensive operations 298–9
primitive idealization 298
principlism 31
prion disease **351–61**
acquired 352, 354–6
aetiology 351–2
clinical features 352–3
diagnosis 352–3, *353*
inherited 352, *353*, 356–8
pre-symptomatic and antenatal testing 358
prevention 358–9
prognosis and treatment 359
species barrier/transmission barrier 352
sporadic 352, *353*
subclinical infection 352

prion protein 351, 353–4
prisoners
  attention-deficit hyperactivity disorder 1931
  bipolar disorder *1934*
  depression 1923, *1933*
  elderly 1584
  female 1934, 1935
  group therapy 1365
  Integrated Drug Treatment System 515
  mental disorder **1933–6**
    prevalence 1933–4, *1934*
  mental health services for 1934–5
  obsessive–compulsive disorder *1934*
  personality disorder 1921, 1933, *1933*
  post-traumatic stress disorder *1934*
  prevalence of personality disorders 884–5
  psychopathy 1921
  psychoses 1933, *1933*
  risk of suicide 976
  schizophrenia 1934, *1934*
  substance use disorders 480, *1934*
  *see also* offenders
prisons, psychiatric nursing in 1404
Pritchard, J.C. 18–19
private symbolism 54
*PRNP* gene 351, 352–3, 357
  mutations 357–8, *357*
probability 1997
problem list 73, 74
problem-solving therapy 1276
  adjustment disorders 1068
  antisocial personality disorder 898
  attempted suicide 970
  conduct disorder 1781–2
  depression 1555
  elderly people 1555, 1574
  group setting 1351, 1352
procarbazine 1092
processing speed, assessment of 87–8, *88*
prochlorperazine 1101
procyclidine 1225
Profile of Mood States 717
progesterone 816
progranulin gene/protein 348
progressive multifocal leucoencephalopathy in HIV/AIDS 1093
progressive muscle relaxation in generalized anxiety disorder 736
progressive subcortical gliosis 348
progressive supranuclear palsy 344
  differential diagnosis 348, 364
  neuropathology 345
Project Atlas 11
Project MATCH 452, 455, 456, 462
projection 294, 299, 307, 1339
projective identification 298–9, 307–8, 316, 1339, 1340, 1344, 1770
projective techniques in child and adolescent assessment 1604
prolactin 165–6, 815
  in electroconvulsive therapy 1257
  hyperprolactinaemia 815, 826, 1086, 1217, 1223
  and seizures 1078
  and social bonding 888
prolonged grief disorder 726
promazine *1209*
proneurones 157, 158
proopiomelanocortin 170
propentofylline in vascular dementia 381

property destruction in conduct disorder 1656
propofol
  in cancer *1104*
  in conversion disorder 999
propranolol
  in acute stress reactions 697
  in dementia 415
  in intellectual disability 1876
  in panic disorder 757
  in pregnancy 1117
Prospective and Retrospective Memory Questionnaire 420
prospective longitudinal (cohort) studies 282, 283, 541, 557, 568
prostate 817
Protection-Motivation Theory 1137
protective factors 1607
protein kinase C 1201
proteins
  glycosylation (glycation) 1508–9
  post-synthetic modification 1508–9
proton magnetic resonance spectroscopy *see* magnetic resonance spectroscopy
protryptylene *670, 1187, 1189, 1191, 1196*
PrP (prion protein) 351, 353–4
PSE (Present State Examination) 71, 269, 272, 523, 534, 542
pseudocorrelation 1608
pseudocyesis 1115
pseudodementia 335, 1551, *1551*
  in HIV/AIDS 385
  treatment 1253
pseudohallucination 49
pseudologia fantastica (pathological lying) 54, 871, 1049, 1051, 1941
pseudoneurasthenias 1060
pseudoseizures 1078, 1619, 1861
pseudosexuality 869
pseudo-status 1050
psilocin 488
psilocybin 488, 489
psoriasis in alcohol use disorders 446
Psychiatric Assessment Schedule for Adults with Developmental Disorders 1823
psychiatric disorder/psychiatric illness *see* mental disorder
psychiatric injury 1902–3
psychiatric nurses **1403–7**
  community 462, 1404–5
  in consultation-liaison psychiatry 1146
  in the developing world 1406–7
  global survey 12, *12*
  in inpatient settings 1404
  prescribing and medication management 1405–6
  in primary care 1406
  in prison settings 1404
  provision of cognitive-behaviour therapy 1406
  psychosocial interventions in the community 1404–5
psychiatric services *see* mental health services
Psychiatric Status Schedule 71
psychiatrists
  cooperation with GPs 67
  global survey 12, *12*
  GPs' expectations of 1486–7
  as managers **39–46**
  in the multi-disciplinary team 68
  role in rehabilitation 1400

psychic determinism 314
psychic retreat 308
PSYCHLOPS 1274
Psych-Med unit 1145
psychoanalysis **293–305**, 1327, **1337–50**
  abstinence in 1339
  aspects of 293
  constructivist 299
  contemporary techniques 299–300, 1339–40
  defence mechanisms 293–4, 1339–40
  definitions 293, 297
  derived treatment modalities 300–1
  efficacy 1345–6
  ending treatment 1345
  formulation 1341–2
  history of therapeutic approach 23, 1338–9
  indications and contraindications 301, 1341
  interpersonal 310
  interpretation in 1344–5
  modes of therapeutic action 1340–1
  and object-relations theory 297, 301–3, 306–12
  objectivist 299
  outcome research 303–4
  and personality 849
  personality disorders 892
  principal features of techniques 1339–41
  and psychopathology 296–7
  and regression in 297, 1342
  relational 1337, 1340
  resistance to 1342
  selection procedures 1341
  starting treatment 1341–2
  structural theory 294–6
  supportive and directive interventions 1342
  theories 293–6, 1337–8
  therapist neutrality 1339, 1340
  training in 1346
  treatment duration 1327, 1341
  treatment formulation 297
  treatment management 1341–5
  treatment process 297–8
  *see also* psychodynamic psychiatry
psychoanalytic psychotherapy 300
  indications and contraindications 301
  outcome research 303–4
psychodrama groups 1351, 1353
psychodynamic counselling 1275, 1277–8
psychodynamic psychiatry **313–20**
  basic principles 313–15, *313*
  and clinical assessment 67
  and conversion disorder 1011
  and countertransference 314, *315*, 317–18
  definition 313
  developmental orientation 314
  future directions 319
  history of 23
  and mental health social work 1408–9
  and the mind–brain interface 315–16
  multiple-treater settings 317
  and personality development 316–17
  and pharmacotherapy 317
  and psychic determinism 314
  and resistance 315, 317
  and somatization disorder 1004
  and transference 314
  two-person concept 317–18
  and the unconscious 313–14
  and the uniqueness of the individual 314

psychodynamic psychotherapy 313, 1327, 1337
  anorexia nervosa 796
  avoidant personality disorder 897
  borderline personality disorder 318–19, 894
  brief (short-term) 318, **1327–37**
    adjustment disorders 1068
    background 1327
    comparison with interpersonal
        psychotherapy and cognitive-
        behaviour therapy 1333–4, *1333*
    comparison of therapies 1329–33
    in conjunction with
        pharmacotherapy 1329
    duration of treatment 1330
    efficacy 1334–5
    evaluation and setting 1327–8
    focus of 1329
    practical problems in 1334, *1334*
    research 1334–5
    schizotypal personality disorder 898
    technique 1328–9
  childhood and adolescence **1769–77**
    background 1770
    classical technique 1770–1
    definition 1764
    efficacy 1773–4
    indications and contraindications 1772
    limitations 1774
    managing treatment 1772–3
    procedure selection 1772
    psychodynamic technique 1771–2
    trauma 1730
  definition 318
  in depression in elderly people 1555
  expressive–supportive continuum *318*, 1327
  in intellectual disability 1874–5
  long-term 318–19, 1327, 1329, 1338, 1345
    *see also* psychoanalysis
  panic disorder 758
  post-traumatic stress disorder 709
  schizophrenia 583
  in sexual abuse by children/adolescents 1953
psychoeducation 1276
  in anxiety disorders 735–6
  in attention-deficit hyperactivity
      disorder 1648–9
  in bereavement 726
  in body dysmorphic disorder 1047
  in borderline personality disorder 868
  in cyclothymia 689
  in dementia 386, 411, *414*, 418
  in family therapy 1382
  group setting 1351, 1352, 1364
  in hyperthymia 691
  in interpersonal psychotherapy 1321
  in manual-assisted cognitive treatment 895
  in mood disorder 676, 677, 1554
    in childhood and adolescence 1676, 1677
  in psychodynamic child psychotherapy 1771,
    1773
  in schizophrenia 583, 1448
  in somatization disorder 1008
  in systems training for emotional
      predictability and problem solving 895
  use by psychiatric nurses 1405, 1406
psychogeriatric services *see* mental health
    services, for elderly people
psychological anthropology 276
psychological first aid 726
Psychological Impairments Rating Scale 72

psychological pillow 58
psychological refractory period 248
psychologists, global survey 12, *12*
Psychology of Criminal Conduct 2011
psychometric tests 81–2, *81*, 85–7
  clinical value 84
  in hypersomnia 939
  sex offenders 1962
psychomotor acceleration 55
psychomotor agitation *58*
psychomotor development, history-taking 1600
psychomotor retardation 55, *58*
  in vascular dementia 379
psychoneuroendocrinology 161
psychoneuroimmunology **205–11**, 1039, 1249
  early investigations 205–6
  effects of stress on immune system 205, 207,
    1135–6
  immune modulation of emotion and
    mood 209
  immune system as sensory organ 207, 209
  neural influences on immune system 206–7
  receptors in the immune system 206
psycho-oncology **1100–5**
*Psychopathia Sexualis* (Krafft-Ebing) 836
psychopathology
  assessment instruments 1164
  and attachment theory 243
  culture-related variations 982–3
  definition 47
  descriptive 47
  distinction between form and content 48, 63
  distinction between process and
    development 48
  dualism in 848
  explanatory 47
  phenomenological 47–61
  and psychiatric diagnosis 989
  and psychoanalysis 296–7
psychopathy
  in childhood and adolescence 1950
  diagnosis 1921
  in offenders/prisoners 1921–2
  prediction of 851
Psychopathy Check List-Revised 1921, 2011
psychopharmacology, cosmetic 28–9
psychoprophylactics 1448
psychoses
  acute and transient disorders **602–8**
  in alcohol withdrawal 58, 443, 449–50, 538
  in Alzheimer's disease 335
  art therapy 1415
  assessment instruments 1164
  childhood and adolescence
    differential diagnosis 1673
    and juvenile delinquency 1950
  cognitive model 1314
  complementary medicines 1249
  cultural influences 14
  cycloid 574, 603, 605, 1124
  and delirium 327
  in dementia 416
  differential diagnosis 536–9, 1004
  drug-induced
    cannabis 507, 538
    differential diagnosis 538–9
    hallucinogens 489
    phencyclidine 487
    prescribed medication 539
    stimulants 485, 498

  elderly people 1518–19
  and epilepsy
    chronic interictal 1079
    postictal 1079
  factitious 1055
  and filicide 1125
  first episode 573, 1396
  following an accident 1110
  following head injury 392–3
  in HIV/AIDS 1092
  and intellectual disability 1826, 1827, 1854
  malingered 1055
  menstrual 1114
  monosymptomatic hypochondriacal 617–19
  in multiple sclerosis 1074
  and pain 1030
  paranoid 392–3, 485
  in Parkinson's disease 1072
  and physical illness 546, 1132
  postabortion 1119
  postpartum 647, 1124
  in pregnancy 1118
  prisoners 1933, *1933*
  psychogenic 603
  puerperal 1114
  reactive 574
  schizophreniform 536, 603, 605
  secondary to organic disorder 537–8
  and surgery 1098
  treatment 1254–5
  very-late-onset schizophrenia-like 1518–19
psychosexual development 235
  hormonal influences 1720
  variation in 1718–19
psychosocial functioning
  assessment 73, 1164, 1593
  in body dysmorphic disorder 1044
psychosocial interventions in dementia 414, *414*
psychosocial vulnerability and depression 271
psychostimulants
  in cancer 1102, *1103*
  in terminal illness 1070
psychosurgery *see* neurosurgery for mental
    disorder
psychotherapy
  in autism and other pervasive developmental
    disorders 1640
  childhood and adolescence **1764–9,
    1769–77**
    approaches to 1766–8
    confidentiality 1768
    consent for 1765
    and culture 1768
    differences from adult
        psychotherapy 1765, *1765*
    ending 1768
    failure to attend 1768
    focus on past vs. focus on present 1767
    individual vs. group therapy 1768
    involvement of parents and school 1768
    limit-setting vs. free expression 1767
    measures of effectiveness and
        outcome 1769
    record-keeping 1768
    training and supervision 1768–9
    treatment setting 1766
  comparisons with pharmacotherapy 1162
  and counselling 1273–4, 1765
  definition 1764
  empirically supported 672

psychotherapy (*cont.*)
  evaluation **1158–67**
    internal vs. external validity 1159
    measurement of therapeutic change 1163–4
    outcome assessment strategies 1163
    patient selection 1163
    research design 1161–5
    research planning 1159, *1160*
    selection criteria for outcome studies
        1159, 1161
    treatment standardization 1161, *1161*
  historical background 20–1
  hypochondriasis 1026–7
  in the paraphilias 838–9
  personality disorders **892–901**
  process-orientated/outcome-orientated 672
  treatment manuals 1161
  *see also specific therapies*
*psychoticism* 81, *81*
PTSD *see* post-traumatic stress disorder
PTSD Checklist 703
puberty, delayed/arrested in anorexia
        nervosa 787, 794
public attitudes and stigma **5–9**
public health
  epidemiology 1607–8
  and prevention 1606–7
  psychiatric disorder as worldwide issue **10–13**
public policy
  influence on mental health 1426, *1426*
  *see also* mental health public policy
publication bias 229
*Pueraria lobata* 1249
puerarin 1249
puerperal psychosis 1124
puerperium
  anxiety disorders in 1121
  depression in 1122, 1280, 1322, 1486
  normal 1120–1
  obsessive–compulsive disorder in 1121–2
Puerto Rican syndrome 983–4
pulmonary embolism 1082–3
pulmonary oedema in anorexia nervosa 785
pulse rate and conduct disorder 1658
pulvinar sign 356
punch-drunk syndrome 395
puppets 1778
pure agraphia 54
purines *168*
Purkinje cells 158
putamen 154, 159, 1684
Putnam, Hilary 134
pyramidal cells 148
pyramidal tract 156, 158
pyrazinamide 1094
pyromania **914–15**, 1924, 1965, 1967, 1968

Q fever 1038
QALYs (Quality-Adjusted Life Years)
        124, 1475, 1510
quality of life
  in alcohol use disorders 463
  in Alzheimer's disease 339
  assessment instruments 73, 1165
  in body dysmorphic disorder 1044
  in evaluation of mental health services 1465
quality management 43–4, *44*
quasi-experimental studies 1468
querulant reactions to childbirth 1121
querulous behaviour 616, **1977–80**

assessment 1978–9, *1979*
  clinical features 1977–8
  management 1979–80
questionable dementia *see* mild cognitive
        impairment
questionnaires 62, **94–8**
  administration methods 95–6
  in childhood and adolescence 1591
  content and format 95, *95*
  creation 96
  in epidemiology 284
  evaluation criteria 95
  forced-choice questions 94
  multiple measures 96
  psychometric adequacy 95
  purpose of 94
  reasons for development 69
  self-report measures 94
  standard vs. individualized 97
  *see also* assessment instruments
quetiapine 1199, 1209, *1209*
  administration *1214*, 1218
  adverse effects *1212*, 1224
  in bipolar disorder in elderly people 1556
  in cancer *1104*
  in childhood and adolescence 1677, 1797
  pharmacodynamics 1210, *1211*, 1213
  pharmacokinetics 1221–2
quinacrine 359
quinalbarbitone 1178

rachischisis 156
racism, institutional 276
RAD (reactive attachment disorder) 243, 1590,
        1639, 1645
'railway spine syndrome' 700, 1902
random sampling 139
randomized controlled trials (RCTs) 123, 1158,
        1466–8, 1608
  advantages 1151–2, *1467*
  appraisal 126, 127–8
  biases 1151–2
  blinding 127
  cluster 1470
  comparative designs 1162
  concealment of treatment allocation 127
  control groups 1162
  criteria for quality evaluation *1467*
  design and analysis 141–2
  differential drop-out 128
  dismantling designs 1162
  effectiveness 1466–8, *1468*, 1469–70, *1469*
  efficacy 1466–8, *1468*
  generalizability 1152
  inapplicable situations *1467*
  inclusion and exclusion criteria 128
  intention-to-treat analysis 128
  limitations/disadvantages 1151–2, *1467*
  meta-analysis 229, 1155, 1465–6, *1466*
  power calculation 1151
  preference 1470
  psychotherapy 1162–3
  rogue results 1152
  systematic reviews *see* systematic reviews
  validity 127–8
rape 1498
  crisis centres 1988
  date 409, 491
  definition 1985
  offenders 1961

victims 1985–6
raphe nuclei 150–1
Rapid Risk Assessment of Sex Offender
        Recidivism 1963
rapid tranquillization 1404
  in childhood and adolescence 1798
rapists, personality disorder 1921
Ras proteins 175
Rasmussen syndrome type 2 1864, 1867
Rat Man 1683
rate of living and longevity 1508
rating scales/schedules 62, **94–8**
  content and format 95, *95*
  creation 96
  evaluation criteria 95
  multiple measures 96
  psychometric adequacy 95
  purpose of 94
  reasons for development 69
  standard vs. individualized 97
  *see also* assessment instruments
rational emotive therapy in intellectual
        disability 1874
rationalization 294
*Rauvolfia serpentina* (rauwolfia) 1249, *1250*
Raven's Progressive Matrices Test
        87, 264, 1909
RBD *see* REM sleep behaviour disorder
RC (residential continuum) 1400
RCTs *see* randomized controlled trials
RDC (Research Diagnostic Criteria) 100, 523,
        534, 751
reaction formation 294
reactive attachment disorder 243, 1590,
        1639, 1645
reactive oxygen species, role in ageing 1509
reactivity 95
Read codes 1484
reading disorder 1627–9
reality orientation in dementia *414*
reality principle 294, 295
reassurance, in medical consultations 1138
reassurance-seeking, in hypochondriasis 1022
re-bonding 1514
reboxetine 670, *670*
  adverse effects 1190, *1191*
  dosage *1196*
  in panic disorder 757
  pharmacodynamics *1187*
  pharmacokinetics *1189*
receptive language disorder 1626
reciprocity negotiation 1375
Recognition Memory Test 89
recovered memories 714–15, 834
recovery model 1491
recreational drugs
  classification 1927
  use by elderly people 1544
  *see also* substance use disorders *and*
        *specific drugs*
reductionism 134
reduplicative paramnesia 392
Reelin 158
refeeding 795
  complications 786
referential thinking in body dysmorphic
        disorder 1044
reflective awareness 308
reflex sympathetic dystrophy 1015, 1050
reflexive function 310

refugees **1493–500**
  assessment 1496–7
  conceptual outcome models 1494–5, *1495*
  cultural factors 1496, *1496*, 1498
  definition 1493–4, *1493*
  depression 1495
  families 1497
  head injury 1495
  health status and physical illness 1495
  internally displaced 1493
  long-term functional impairment and
    disability 1495–6
  post-traumatic stress disorder 1495, 1497
  principle of *non-refoulement* 1493, 1494
  protection of 1493–4
  psychiatric symptoms and illness 1495–6
  risk and resiliency factors 1498
  screening 1496–7
  somatic complaints 1497
  torture 1494, 1495
  trauma 1494–6, *1495*, 1496–7, 1497
  treatment 1497–8
Regional Care Services Improvement
  Partnership Development Centres 1488
regression
  as coping strategy 1066
  in psychoanalysis 297, 1342
regressive transference neurosis 297–8
rehabilitation 1352, **1399–403**
  in community mental health services
    389–90, 1459
  core elements *1402*
  current approaches 1400–2
  development of environmental
    resources 1402
  and family intervention 1401
  and participation in the community 1402
  role of psychiatrist 1400
  social skills training 583, 898, 1401, 1968
  target population 1399–400
  vocational 583, 1400–1, 1889
reinforcer devaluation 258
Relate 1370
relationship counselling 1278–9
relative risk 126, 128, 282
relaxation techniques
  applied relaxation 746
  in insomnia 937
  in persistent somatoform pain disorder 1034
  progressive muscle relaxation 736
  in sleep disorders 1572
  in specific phobia 746
reliability 85, 92, 95, 137–8
  in classification in childhood and
    adolescence 1591
  inter-rater/inter-observer 85, 95, 263, 1465
  models and definitions 137–8
  of outcome measures 1465
  parallel-form *85*, 1465
  split-half *85*, 1465
  test–retest *85*, 263, 1465
  types *85*
religious delusions 51
religious healing ceremonies 1419–20
REM-atonia 946
REM latency 684, 931
REM sleep behaviour disorder (RBD) 928,
  **946–7**, 1695
  association with psychiatric disorders and
    stress 947

clinical and polysomnographic findings
  946–7
  in dementia 416–17
  diagnosis 947
  in elderly people 1572
  in narcolepsy with cataplexy 941
  overlap with other parasomnias 947
  treatment 947
reminiscence therapy *414*, 1574
remoxipride 1209–10
repetition compulsion 299
repetitive self-mutilation 916–17
repetitive transcranial magnetic stimulation *see*
  transcranial magnetic stimulation
reports 74–6
  and confidentiality 75
  expert witness 1928, *2004*, **2005–6**
  partiality 75
  principles 75
  purposes 75
  structure 75–6
repression 294
RERAs (respiratory effort-related arousals) 940
Rescorla–Wagner learning rule 259
rescue workers, debriefing 1110
research
  on aetiology 281–6
  on art therapy 1416
  in epidemiology of child and adolescent
    psychiatric disorder 1597–8
  in evaluation of mental health services
    1465–9, *1465*, *1466*, *1467*, *1468*, *1469*
  and evidence-based medicine 122–8
  longitudinal 1597
  on mental health services 281, 1452
  patient selection 1163
  study design 282, 1161–3, 1465–9, *1465*,
    *1466*, *1467*, *1468*, *1469*, 1475–6
  using with individual patients 126–8
Research Diagnostic Criteria 100, 523, 534, 751
reserpine 1172, 1249
residential continuum 1400
residential services
  in childhood and adolescence **1799–802**
  in community mental health services 1453–4
  for elderly people 1518, 1583
  for people with intellectual disability and
    psychiatric disorder 1889
resilience 1607
  and adoption/foster care 1748
  in childhood 1660, 1803
  of refugees 1498
resistance
  in adolescence 1603–4
  and non-compliance 317
  to psychoanalysis 1342
  in psychodynamic psychiatry 297, 315, 317
  repression 1342
  transference 1342
resistance to change in autism 1633
respiratory effort-related arousals 940
respiratory perturbation and anxiety
  disorders 1667
respiratory system
  in anorexia nervosa 785
  in chronic fatigue syndrome 1038
  disorders *932*, 1082–3
respite care
  in community mental health services 1458
  for elderly people 1583

response inhibition/prevention 249, 1047
responsibility
  criminal 1945, 1954
  diminished 1901, 1922, 1923, 1928, 1937,
    1939, 1940
  legal aspects 1900–5
  in obsessive–compulsive disorder 1783
  *see also* diminished responsibility defence
restless legs syndrome **948**, 1572, 1695
restraint 1133, 1404
restriction fragment length polymorphisms 218
Rethink 1490–1
reticular nucleus 150
retifism 833
retinal development 157
retirement 1514
Retreat, York 17–18
retrograde messengers 171–2
Rett's syndrome 1614, **1636–7**, 1698
  aetiology 1637
  behavioural and psychiatric aspects 1845
  clinical features 1636
  course 1637–8
  definition 1636, *1636*
  demographics 1636
  epidemiology 1636
  and epilepsy 1864, 1864–5
  genetics 224, 229, 1637, 1844, *1866*
  management 1640
  physical characteristics 1845
  prevalence 1844
  prognosis 1637–8
revenge and fire-raising 1967
reverse bonding 1514
reversed role play 1376
reversible inhibitors of monoamine oxidase
  (RIMAs) 670, *670*
  pharmacodynamics 1173
  in social anxiety disorder 743
  reviews 1152
  and clinical assessment 74
'reward deficiency syndrome' hypothesis 434
reward-dependence 80, *80*, 316, *316*, 849
Rey 15-item test 1057
Rey Auditory-Verbal Learning Test 89, 264
Rey–Osterrieth Complex Figure Test 89
Reynolds Adolescent Depression Scale 1675
rhombencephalon 156, 157
rhombomeres 157
rhythmic movement disorder, sleep-related
  *928*, 1702
ribonucleic acid *see* RNA
rifampicin
  adverse effects *1091*
  in tuberculosis 1094
RIMAs *see* reversible inhibitors of monoamine
  oxidase
rimonabant 513
risk 1991–2
  individual, application of population data 281
  modelling patterns of 141
risk analysis 44
risk assessment 1991–2
  contemporary approaches 1992–3
  and contingency plan 1455, *1457*
  and culture of blame 1991–2
  in dementia 417, *417*
  and expert witnesses 2005
  limits of mental health professionals'
    engagement 1993–4

risk assessment (*cont.*)
  offenders using drugs/alcohol 1927
  violence **1991–2002**
    approaches 1994–5
    by stalkers 1972–4, *1973*
    evaluating levels of risk 1998–9
    instruments 1994, 1996–7
    practicalities 1997–2000
    utility 1995–6
risk difference 128
risk factors 1607–8
  Alzheimer's disease 1520–2, *1520*, *1522*
  anorexia nervosa *806*
  antisocial behaviour by adolescents *1946*, 1947
  bipolar disorder 646–7, 1675
  bulimia nervosa 805–6, *806*
  causative 1607
  in child and adolescent psychiatric
      disorders 556, 1590, 1675
  conduct disorder 1658–60
  delirium 329, *329*
  dementia 376, 1520–2, *1520*, *1522*
  depression 648–9, 658–9, 1675
  fixed 1607
  hypochondriasis 997, 1024
  independent 1608
  malleable 1607
  mania 646–7
  mediating 1608
  moderating 1608
  offending 1909–14
  overlapping 1608
  panic disorder 753
  post-traumatic stress disorder *707*
  proxy 1608
  and refugee vulnerability 1498
  schizophrenia 547–9, **553–61**
  sleep-wake disorders 1696–7
  suicide 951–2, *953*, 971, *971*, *972*, 1449
Risk for Sexual Violence Protocol 1998
risk management 44
  offenders using drugs/alcohol 1927
  of violence towards others 1997–8,
      1999–2000, *1999*
risk-taking, morbid 921
risperidone 1209, *1209*
  administration *1214*, 1216–17
  adverse effects *1212*, 1224
  in attention-deficit hyperactivity
      disorder 1652
  in bipolar disorder, in elderly people 1556
  in cancer *1104*
  in childhood and adolescence 1797
    mania 1677
    with psychiatric/behaviour disorder and
        intellectual disability 1852
  in delirium 331
  in dementia 415
  in HIV/AIDS 1092
  in intellectual disability 1875
  long-acting injectable 581
  pharmacodynamics 1172, 1210, *1211*, 1213
  pharmacokinetics *1172*, 1221
  in schizotypal personality disorder 600
  in tic disorders 1688
Ritalin® *see* methylphenidate
rivastigmine
  in Alzheimer's disease 409, 1241, 1538
  in dementia 415
  in Parkinson's disease 370–1

in vascular dementia 381
Rivermead Behavioural Memory Test 89
Rivers, W.H.R. 276
RLS (restless leg syndrome) **948**, 1572, 1695
RNA
  cross-linkage 1508
  double-stranded (dsRNA) 225
  messenger (mRNA) 224–5, *224*
  micro (miRNA) 225
  non-coding 229
  small interfering (siRNA) 225
  structure and function 223
road traffic accidents *see* accidents
robbery, victims 1986
ROC curve 140, 1995
Rochester Youth Development Study 1910, 1913
rofecoxib in Alzheimer's disease 1538
Rogers, Carl 1273, 1274, 1276
Rohypnol (flunitrazepam) 409, 491, 1183, 1188
ROI morphometry 195
role play, reversed 1376
role reversal 308
role theory and transitions 1514
rolipram 176
ROM (routine outcome measures) 1460
ROS (reactive oxygen species), role in
      ageing 1509
Rosenberg Self-Esteem Scale 1164
Rough Sleepers Initiative 1501
routine outcome measures 1460
RRASOR (Rapid Risk Assessment of Sex
      Offender Recidivism) 1963
RSVP (Risk for Sexual Violence Protocol) 1998
rTMS *see* transcranial magnetic stimulation
Rubinstein–Taybi syndrome
  behavioural and psychiatric aspects 1845
  genetics 1845
  physical characteristics 1845
  prevalence 1845
Rule Shift Cards Test *90*
rule violation in conduct disorder 1656
'rum fits' 443
rumination
  in anxiety disorders 1288–9
  in bulimia nervosa 803
Russell's sign 804
Russia, neurasthenia as diagnostic entity 1061
Ryle, Gilbert 133

S-100b 353
*S*-adenosylmethionine 1248
sacrificial ritual 1419
SAD *see* seasonal affective disorder; separation
      anxiety disorder
sadism 832–3, *833*
  criminal 832
  sexual 832, 836
sadistic personality disorder 878, 1921
sadomasochism 832–3, 878
SAFE Children (Schools and Families Educating
      Children) programme 1789
safety behaviours
  in anxiety disorders 1287–8, *1288*, 1290
  in body dysmorphic disorder 1044, *1044*
sage 1248
St John's wort 386, 686, 1248, *1250*, 1262
salivary gland enlargement in bulimia
      nervosa 804
Salpêtrière asylum 17, 18
*Salvia divinorum* 488

*Salvia officinalis* 1248
SAMe (*S*-adenosylmethionine) 1248
sample bias 282–3
sampling 96–7, 138–9, 1595
  principles 282–3
  structural MRI studies 194
Sanfillipo syndrome 1843
SARA (Spousal Assault Risk Assessment) 1998
SARCs (Sexual Assault Referral Centres) 1986
SASB (Structural Analysis of Social
      Behavior) 852
satiety cascade 782
SATs (Standard Assessment Tests) 1715
Scale for the Assessment of Negative
      Symptoms 69, 72, 524
Scale for the Assessment of Positive
      Symptoms 524
SCAN (Schedules for Clinical Assessment in
      Neuropsychiatry) 70, 71, 72, 284, 542, 719
scapegoating 317
Schedule for Affective Disorders and
      Schizophrenia 70, 71, 523
Schedule for Nonadaptive and Adaptive
      Personality 858, *858*
Schedules for Clinical Assessment in
      Neuropsychiatry 70, 71, 72, 284, 542, 719
schema-coping behaviour 895
schema-focused therapy 894, 895, 904, 1778
Schie syndrome 1843
schizoaffective disorder **595–602**
  classification 596–7
  clinical features 595–6
  course and outcome 574, 596–7
  diagnosis 597–8
  differential diagnosis 537, 597–8
  elderly people 1552
  epidemiology 598
  family studies 596
  management 598–9
  premorbid function 595
  subtypes 597
schizoid personality disorder **862–3**
  aetiology 862
  classification *856*, 863, *863*
  clinical features 863
  course 863
  differential diagnosis 862, 863, 865, 876
  in elderly people 1562, *1562*
  epidemiology 862, 882, *882*
  treatment 863
schizoid thought 308
schizophrenia
  admission policies *585*
  and age 544–5
  age of onset 558, 1547
  atypical/unsystematic 574
  catatonic *535*
  cerebral atrophy in 536
  childhood and adolescence 1613
    differential diagnosis 1673
    risk factors for development 556–7
  classification **535–6**, 1546–7
  clinical features **526–31**
    anxiety and somatoform disorders 530
    emotional disorders 529
    motor disorders 529
    thought and perception disorders 526–8
    volition disorders 529–30
  cognitive impairment 93, 265, 528,
      **531–4**, 580

comorbidity
  physical disease 546
  substance use disorders 427, 507, 546, 558, 1919
coping strategies 1313–14
course and outcome *536*, **568–78**
  definitions and assessment of variables 569
  elderly people 1548
  methodological factors 568–74
  patterns and stages 571
  predictors 574–6, *575*
  and risk factors 558
  study results 569, *570*
cultural and geographic variations 14, 546, 557, 571–3, *572*
delusions 526–7
depression in 529, 573
developmental antecedents 548
and diabetes mellitus 1085
diagnosis and diagnostic criteria 103–4, 105, 522–3, **534–6**, *535*, 1547
  diagnostic process 539
  early diagnosis 536
  and epidemiology 541
  influence on outcome studies 568–9
differential diagnosis 327, *328*, 536–9, 863, 864, 1547
dimensions of psychopathology 530, *530*
disease and disability burden 546–7
disease expectancy/morbid risk 544
as a disorder of brain maturation 180–1, *180*, *181*
elderly people **1546–50**, 1552
  aetiology 1548
  classification 1546–7
  clinical features 1546
  course and prognosis 1548
  diagnosis 1547
  differential diagnosis 1547, 1559
  epidemiology 1547
  treatment and management 1548–9
emergencies 590
epidemiology **540–53**
  case finding 541
  descriptive 542–7
  in elderly people 1547
  future issues 549–50
  historical landmarks *540*
  incidence 542–4, *544*, *545*
  methods and instruments 541–2
  prevalence 542, *543*
and epilepsy 1079
ethnic minorities 549, 557–8
and expressed emotion 575, 583
family factors 536, 548–9, 553–5
and fertility 545
and fire-raising 1967
first-rank (Schneiderian) symptoms 523, 526, 527–8, *527*, 535–6, 573–4
following head injury 392
and gender 544–5
genetics 547, 548–9, 553–5, 565–6, *565*
hallucinations 527, 573–4
hebephrenic (disorganized) *535*, 574
history of concept **521–6**
homicide by people with 1939, 1995
insight in 528
and intellectual disability 1827, 1854
and juvenile delinquency 1950

late-onset 1547
markers 536
mental health services 584–5
models
  genetic 554
  gene–environment interaction 558–9
  stress–diathesis 507, 558–9, 1313
mortality associated 545–6
name change in Japan 7
and narcolepsy 927
natural history 569–70
negative symptoms 535
  concept of 522, 523–5
  dimensions 530
  treatment 580, 589, 1265, 1548
neurobiology **561–8**
  functional 561–3
  structural 563–4
  theories based on 564–6, *565*, *566*
neuropathology 178–81, *178*, *179*, *180*, *181*
neuropsychological assessment 93, 265, 528, **531–4**
and obsessive–compulsive disorder 766
and offending 1918–20
and optical distortions 49
overlap with bipolar disorder for susceptibility 652
paranoid *535*, 574, 609, 610
parental, effects on child development 1753
PET/SPET imaging 188–9, 562–3
positive symptoms 523
  concept of 523–5
  dimensions 530
  drug therapy 579–80
and pregnancy/birth complications 548
premorbid intelligence 548
premorbid personality 536
premorbid social impairment 548
prevention 550, 589, 1448
prisoners 1934, *1934*
prodrome 573, 589–90
pseudoneurotic 875
pseudopsychopathic 866
and pulmonary embolism 1083
recovery 576
relapse 581
remission 589
residual 535
risk factors 547–9, **553–61**
  and age of onset 558
  birth season 547, 556
  childhood 556–7
  environmental 555–8
  familial/genetic 547, 548–9, 553–5, 565–6, *565*
  life events 558, 575
  migration 286, 549, 557–8
  model based on 558–9
  obstetric complications 548, 555–6
  and outcome 558
  paternal age 555
  prenatal exposure to infection 547–8, 556
  social and geographic 557–8
and sexuality 825–6
simple *535*, 574
and sleep-wake disorders *931*
and social class 549
and stigma 5, 6–7, 539
subtypes 534, *535*, 549
  prognosis 574

and suicide 545–6, 956
and surgery 1098
syndromes of symptoms 530, *530*
systematic 574
treatment and management **578–95**
  acute phase 586–8
  adjunctive medication 591–2
  cognitive-behaviour therapy 582–3, 1313–18
  of cognitive impairment 533
  drug therapy 579–82, *579*, 585, 586–8, *586*, 1213, *1215*, 1548
  elderly people 1548–9
  electroconvulsive therapy 1255
  in emergencies 590
  family therapy 583–4
  group therapy 1364
  maintenance 581–2, 589
  outline plan *587*
  poor response to 590–2
  post-acute phase 588
  principles 585, *586*
  psychodynamic psychotherapy 583
  psychoeducation 583
  research 592
  resistance to 582, 590–2
  social skills training 583
  transcranial magnetic stimulation 1265
treatment gap *13*
type I 524, 535–6
type II 524, 535–6
undifferentiated *535*, 574
and violence 1919, *1999*
  risk assessment 1995
and working memory 255
schizophreniform psychosis 536, 603, 605
schizotaxia 599
schizotypal personality disorder **599–601**, **863–5**
  classification 103–4, 599–600, *856*, 864, *864*
  clinical features 599, 864
  cognitive impairment in 533
  course 864
  diagnosis 600
  differential diagnosis 600, 862, 863, 864–5
  in elderly people *1562*, 1563
  epidemiology 600, 864, *882*, 883
  prevention 601
  terminology 856–7
  treatment and management 600–1, 865, 898
*schnauzkrampf* 58
Schneider, Kurt 522–3, 526, 681, 682, 686
school nurse 1812
'school phobia' 1665
schools
  child psychiatrist as consultant to **1811–16**
  establishing a school liaison service 1812–13
  factors in offending 1913
  in hospital 1815
  intervention strategies based in 1814–15
  involvement in psychotherapy 1768
  problems associated with conduct disorder 1656, 1662
  role in child mental health 1727
  role in child protection 1814
  special 1815
  *see also* education
Schools and Families Educating Children programme 1789
Schwartz, Emanuel 1354

SCID-II (Structured Clinical Interview for DSM-IV Personality Disorders) *858*, 859
SCL-90-R 1164
scopolamine, effects on memory 409
scoptic syndrome *833*
scoptophilia *833*
scrapie 351
screening
  for alcohol use disorders in elderly people 1542
  in consultation-liaison psychiatry 1145–6, *1146*
  for domestic violence 1982
  instruments 69
  refugees 1496–7
sculpting 1376
SCUs (specialized care units) 1583
SD (standard deviation) 86
SEAL (Social and Emotional Aspects of Learning) 1814
Searles, Harold 310
season
  and bipolar disorder 646–7
  and depression 635
  seasonal affective disorder (SAD) 927, 939, 1260, 1261, 1262
    course and outcome 668
    treatment 671
seasonal rhythms 1260
Seattle Social Development Project 1912–13
second messengers 175–6, *175*, 1172
  downstream signalling cascades 176
second somatic sensory cortex 146
Secure Children's Homes 1945
secure hospitals 2015, 2016–17
  admission criteria 2018
Secure Needs Assessment Profile 2018
Secure Training Centres 1945
security 2015, 2016–17
  levels 2017
  physical 2016
  procedural 2016
  relational 2016–17
  treatment as 2017
sedatives *see* anxiolytics
segmental aneusomy syndromes 228
seizures
  absence 204, 1077
  in alcohol withdrawal 443, 449
  classification 1076–7, *1077*, *1862*, *1863*
  definition 1076
  differential diagnosis of epileptic and psychogenic 1861, *1862*
  drug-induced 1223, 1795, 1795–6
  exercise-induced 1861
  factors provoking 1861
  focal 1862, *1863*
  following neurosurgery for mental disorder 1269
  in frontotemporal dementias 346
  generalized 1077, 1619, *1863*
    secondary 1862, *1863*
  iatrogenic 1078
  induction by transcranial magnetic stimulation 1263
  myoclonic 1077
  nocturnal 1702
  partial 1077, 1619
    complex 201, 1077, 1619, *1863*, 1864
    simple 1861, *1863*, 1864

primary generalized 1862, *1863*
provoked 1078
psychogenic 1016–17, 1080, 1861, *1862*, *1863*, 1864
threshold 204
tonic–clonic 1077, *1863*
treatment 1080
withdrawal 1861
*see also* epilepsy
selective eating 787
selective mutism 1639, 1714
Selective Reminding Test 253
selective serotonin reuptake inhibitors *see* SSRIs
selegiline
  adverse effects *1191*
  dosage *1196*
  pharmacodynamics *1187*, 1188
  pharmacokinetics *1189*
selenium 1248
self
  disorders of 56
  and the ego 295
self-actualization 1276
self-awareness 82, *83*
self-deception 1941
self-defeating personality disorder 877–8
self-directedness 80–1, *80*, 83, 316, 849–50
self-esteem 311
  assessment instruments 1164
  in bulimia nervosa 804, 806
  and chronic fatigue syndrome 1036
  and defence mechanisms 317
  and domestic violence 1982
  and the ego ideal 296
  elderly people 1559
  in hypochondriasis 1022
  and suicide 970
  and vocational rehabilitation 1401
self-harm *see* deliberate self-harm
self-help groups 1449
self-help skills, in intellectual disability 1873
self-image, in adolescence 1604
self-mutilation, repetitive 916–17
self-objects 311
self-psychology 313
  and somatization disorder 1004–5
Self-Regulatory Model 1138, 1140–1
self-report scales 4, 94
self-representation 298, 302–3
self-soothing 1694, 1698
self-states 903
self-structures 316
self-transcendence 80, *80*, 83, 316, 850
Selves Questionnaire 1164
SEM (standard error of measurement) 85
semantic–pragmatic disorder 1713
semen 817
semen-loss anxiety 606, **981**
seminal vesicles 817
SENCO (special educational needs coordinator) 1812
sensate focus exercise 1569
sensory dysfunction in conversion disorder 1017
sensory-specific satiety 258
separating 5
separation anxiety
  and intellectual disability 1851
  and panic disorder 754
separation anxiety disorder (SAD)

clinical presentation 1665
outcome 1666
prevalence 1666
septohippocampal system, in generalized anxiety disorder 733, *733*
serotonergic system and serotonin receptors *173*, 174, 1171
  action of antipsychotics on 1170, 1209, 1210, *1211*
  action of anxiolytics on 1178
  and aggressive/antisocial behaviour 889, 1918
  and attention-deficit hyperactivity disorder 1646
  in autism 1636
  and chronic fatigue syndrome 1039
  and cortical function 151
  in depression 189, 660, 662, 1185, 1186
    in childhood and adolescence 1675
    genetics 652
  and eating disorders 782, 806
  effects of ecstasy 496
  in generalized anxiety disorder 733–4
  knockout studies 231
  and memory impairment 409
  and neuroticism 887–8
  in obsessive–compulsive disorder 767, 1683–4, 1684
  in panic disorder 754
  PET/SPET imaging *186*, 187, 189
  in post-traumatic stress disorder 706
  and schizophrenia 562
  serotonin transporter 169, *170*, 189, 221, 273, 286, 658, 887, 1674
  and sexual function 826
  in social anxiety disorder 741
  and substance use disorders 429
  in substance use disorders *429*, 436
  and suicide 955, 964–5, 970, 1705
  and Tourette syndrome 1073
serotonin and noradrenaline reuptake inhibitors *see* SNRIs
serotonin supplementation 1248
serotonin syndrome 1173, 1176, 1192, 1194, 1254
sertindole 1209
sertraline *670*
  adverse effects *1191*
  in cancer *1102*, *1103*
  in childhood and adolescence 1676
  in depression in elderly people 1554, *1554*
  dosage *1196*
  in obsessive–compulsive disorder 1687, *1687*
  in panic disorder *756*
  pharmacodynamics *1173*, *1187*
  pharmacokinetics *1172*, 1188, *1189*
  in social anxiety disorder 743, 744
SES *see* socio-economic status
Settlement Movement 1408
sex chromosomes 218, 223, 225
  abnormalities 1840–1
sex-linked disorders 212
Sex Offender Risk Appraisal Guide 835, 1963
sex offenders **1960–4**
  assessment 1961–2
  classification 1960–1
  definitions 1960
  ethical issues 1964
  and the general psychiatrist 1960
  juvenile 1953–4

mood disorders 1923
personality disorder 1921
risk assessment 1963, *1963*
treatment 1963–4
sex reassignment surgery 842, 843–4
sex therapy 821, **827–8**, 829
sexual arousal
brain activation during 819
extragenital changes 815
female 816, 817–19
loss of 822
male 816–17
pain during 822
Sexual Assault Referral Centres 1986
sexual disinhibition in dementia 416
sexual dysfunction **821–32**
aetiology 823–7
assessment 829–30
classification 823
clinical features 822–3
definitions and terminology 821–2
in dementia 416
drug-induced 826–7, 1190
Dual Control Model 821, 824
in elderly people 1569, *1570*
in end-stage renal disease 1087
epidemiology 823, *824*
historical aspects 821–2
and mental health 825–6
in physical illness 826
treatment and management 827–30, 1569–70
sexual function
and epilepsy 1079
and mental health 825–6
normal **812–20**
biological determinants 812–13
DEOR model 814–15, *814*
in elderly people 1569, *1569*
endocrinology 815–16
EPOR model 814–15, *814*
initiating activity 815
modelling 813–15
surveys 813–14, 821–2
sexual inhibition 825
Sexual Offences Act 1956 1899–900
Sexual Offences Act 2003 1900, 1985
sexual orientation, of elderly people 1568
sexual orientation disturbance, legitimacy of
diagnosis 28
sexual scripting 813
Sexual Violence Risk-20 1998
sexuality
assessment in childhood and
adolescence 1604
and dementia 1568
in elderly people 1567–70
and fire-raising 1967
in Huntington's disease 373
and intellectual handicap 1873, 1879
psychoanalytic theories 294–5
as a social construct 813–15
sexually transmitted disease (STD) 1094
delusions concerning 619
and stigma 1091
*see also specific diseases*
SF-12 284
SF-36 284
shabu (methamphetamine) **497–8**
shamanism 1419
shared care plans 1487

shared care register 1487
shared psychotic disorder 610, **624–5**
Shedler-Westen Assessment Procedure 858, *858*
'shell shock' 700
*shenjing shuairuo* 1061
shift work and sleep disturbance 926
*shin-byung* 606
shinkeishitsu 1061
shoplifting 1923, 1924, 1943
short-term anxiety-provoking
psychotherapy 1327, 1331–2
SIADH and ecstasy 495
sialidosis 1864, 1865
Siberia, attitudes to psychiatric disorder 6
siblings
effects of loss of sibling 1120, 1759
effects of sibling with intellectual
disability 1884–5
effects of sibling with physical illness 1742
sick role 1320, 1321
sickness, concept of 62, 63–4
SIDS (sudden infant death syndrome)
1119, 1698
siege experience 49–50
sign language
in autism 1639
in expressive language disorder 1626
in receptive language disorder 1626
signs, definition 47
sildenafil 821, 828
Silence of the Mind meditation 82
simple phobia *see* specific phobia
simulated presence, in dementia *414*
single-case studies 1161
single nucleotide polymorphisms 218, 226, 227
single-photon emission tomography (SPET/
SPECT) 185
Alzheimer's disease 337
comparison with functional magnetic
resonance imaging 186–7, 196–7
comparison with PET 185
data collection and analysis 186
dementia with Lewy bodies 364
depression 189, 660
during antipsychotic use 189–90
in epilepsy 1862
frontotemporal dementias 347, Plate 12
head injury 389
imaging strategies 187, *187*
isotopes *186*
limitations 186–7
methodology 185
schizophrenia 188–9
vascular dementia 380
Six Elements Test 265
skin
delusions concerning 50, 51, 618
effects of alcohol use disorders 446
skin picking, pathological/compulsive 618,
**917–18**, 1044
Slavson, S.R. 1353
sleep **924–6**
active 946
architecture 925
changes with age 925–6, 1571–2
and chronic fatigue syndrome 1036, 1039
circadian rhythms 925, 926
and depression, in childhood and
adolescence 1675
deprivation, in the puerperium 1120

functions 924–5
insufficient 1700
nature of 924
non-rapid eye movement (NREM) 924, 925
paradoxical 946
physiology, in childhood and
adolescence 1692–3
rapid eye movement (REM) 924, 925,
946, 1694
REM latency 684, 931
requirements *1694*
slow wave (SWS) 925, 1694
stages 925
unihemispheric 925
sleep debt 1700
sleep diary 929, 934, 1696
sleep drunkenness 941
sleep education 936, *936*
sleep efficiency 936
sleep history 929, 1696
sleep hygiene 936, *936*
sleep onset REM period 941
sleep paralysis 929, 940
sleep questionnaire 1696
sleep-related dissociative disorder 948
sleep-related eating disorder *931*, 947–8
sleep-related injury 945
sleep-related rhythmic movement disorder
*928*, 1702
sleep restriction therapy 936
sleep terrors 928, **945–6**, 1702
sleep-wake cycle, in delirium 326–7
sleep-wake disorders **924–33**
in aetiology of psychiatric illness 927
and alcohol use disorders *931*
and anxiety disorders *931*
assessment 929–30
and attention-deficit hyperactivity
disorder 927, *931*, 1695, 1697
audio–video recordings 929
and autism 1697
and cardiovascular disease *932*
childhood and adolescence **1693–702**
assessment 1696–7, *1696*
developmental effects 1695
effects on parenting and the family
1694–5
excessive daytime sleepiness
1699–701, *1700*
manifestations 1695
misinterpretation 1695
parasomnias 1701–2
parental influences 1694
patterns of occurrence 1695
risk factors 1697–8
sleeplessness 1698–9
treatment and prognosis 1695–6
and chronic fatigue syndrome 1697
and chronic pain *932*
and chronic renal failure *932*
circadian rhythm *928*
classification 927, *928*
delayed sleep phase syndrome 928, 942–3,
1261, 1695, 1700
and dementia 416–17, *931*, 1572, 1573
in dementia with Lewy bodies 362
and depression 634, 661–2, 927, 931,
*931*, 1697
detection 929–30
and eating disorder *931*

sleep-wake disorders (*cont.*)
elderly people 1571–3
and endocrine disease *932*
and epilepsy *932*
following stroke *932*
and gastrointestinal disorders *932*
and head injury *932*, 942, 1698
hypersomnia *see* hypersomnia
hypnotic-dependent 934
insomnia *see* insomnia
and intellectual disability 926–7, 1694, 1697–8
in intensive care patients *932*
and iron deficiency *932*
legal issues 948–9
and mania *931*
mistaken for primarily psychological/
psychiatric conditions 927–9
in neurological and physical illness 931, *932*,
933, 941, 942
and obesity *932*
and obsessive–compulsive disorder 1697
and panic disorder 1697
parasomnias *see* parasomnias
in Parkinson's disease *932*, 1072
phototherapy 1261
postoperative 1099
and post-traumatic stress disorder 927
in psychiatric conditions 930–1, *931*
psychological effects of sleep
disturbance 926–7
REM sleep behaviour disorder
928, 1572, 1695
and respiratory disease *932*
and schizophrenia *931*
sleep-related breathing disorders 928
sleep-related movement disorders *928*, 1702
and substance use disorders *931*
and tic disorders 1697
and Tourette syndrome *932*, 1697
treatment approaches 930, *930*
sleepiness, excessive daytime *see* hypersomnia
sleeplessness
in childhood and adolescence 1698–9
partial 926
total 926
sleepwalking 928, **945–6**, 1702, 1930
SLI (Specific Language Impairment) 1710,
**1713–15**
SLITRK1 gene 229
SLT *see* speech and language therapy
Sly syndrome 1843
small G proteins 175
Smart, J.J.C. 134
smell, delusions of 618–19
Smith–Lemli–Opitz syndrome
behavioural phenotype 1845, *1851*
genetics 1845
physical characteristics 1845
prevalence 1845
psychiatric aspects 1845
Smith–Magenis syndrome
behavioural and psychiatric aspects 1845
genetics 1845
physical characteristics 1845
prevalence 1845
smoking
addictiveness *431*
by elderly people 1544
by psychiatric patients 511
cessation treatments 511–13

disease burden 510
genetic factors 510–11
and health 1136
mortality associated 510
and nicotine dependence **510–15**
in pregnancy 1646
prevalence 510
and psychiatric disorder in intellectual
disability 1828
and schizophrenia 546
withdrawal symptoms 511
snake-handling cult 1419–20
SNAP *see* Schedule for Nonadaptive and
Adaptive Personality; Secure Needs
Assessment Profile
snoezelen therapy *414*
snow (cocaine) 430
SNPs (single nucleotide polymorphisms)
218, 226, 227
SNRIs 670, *670*
adverse effects 674
in childhood and adolescence 1796
in generalized anxiety disorder 735
in panic disorder 756, *756*
in persistent somatoform pain disorder 1034
pharmacodynamics *1173*, 1186, *1187*
in somatization disorder 1009
Social Adjustment Scale 1165
social and cultural anthropology 14, 15, **275–9**
Social and Emotional Aspects of Learning 1814
social anxiety disorder **739–44**, 1639
aetiology 741
and avoidant personality disorder 740, 897
and body dysmorphic disorder 1044
childhood and adolescence 740, 1665, 1666
classification 740–1
clinical presentation 740
cognitive content 1286
comorbidity 740, 744
course 741
differential diagnosis 740–1, 752, 873
epidemiology 741
functional impairment in 740
generalized/non-generalized 740
and offending 1923
with panic disorder 750
prevention 744
secondary to physical disorder 740
and substance use disorders 427
treatment and management 741–4
social bonding 888–9
social capital 1610
social cognition models 1136–7, 1140–1
social communication, problems with 1711, 1713
social constructionism and ageing 1515
social development 242–3, *242*
social drift 557
social inclusion 1819
social learning theory
and alcohol use disorders 434
and offending 1910
social phobia *see* social anxiety disorder
Social Readjustment Rating Scale 1065
social role valorization 1409–10
social skills training 1401
antisocial personality disorder 898
fire-raising 1968
schizophrenia 583
social stress theory, and transitions 1514
social suffering 848

social support
in bereavement 726
and group therapy 1352
in mood disorders 653
and psychiatric disorder in intellectual
disability 1828
and response to illness 1066
and suicide 954
social theory *277*
social withdrawal in depression 634
social work *see* mental health social work
social workers
approved 1410
attachment to primary care 1411
global survey 12, *12*
socio-economic status (SES)
and anorexia nervosa 778
and anxiety disorders 1666
and child mental health 1727–8
and deliberate self-harm 959
and mood disorders 654
and offending 1912
and schizophrenia 549, 557
sociology of ageing **1512–16**
sociometry 1353
sociosomatic processes 278
sodium oxybate 941
sodium valproate *see* valproate
Solution Oriented Schools 1814
solvent abuse *see* volatile substance abuse
somatic sensation, cortical association
pathways *146*, 152
somatization 57, 278, 989–90
by refugees 1497
in childhood and adolescence 1744, *1744*
and chronic fatigue syndrome 1039
cultural influences 15
definitions 996
and pain 1030, 1031
presentation in primary care 1482
subthreshold 996, *998*
and surgery 1096
somatization disorder **999–1011**
abrupt onset 1002
aetiology 1004–5
assessment 1005–6, *1005–6*
in childhood and adolescence 1744
and chronic fatigue syndrome 1037
classification *993*, 994, 999–1000, 1003
clinical features 1000–2
physical symptoms 1000–2, *1001*
psychological symptoms 1002
comorbidity 57, 870, 1002, 1004
controversial aspects 996
and conversion disorder 1015
correlates 996
course 1005
diagnosis 1003
differential diagnosis 1003–4, 1023–4
dystonia in 1016
epidemiology 996, 1004
examination 1005–6
family transmission 1004
and illness behaviour 1002
mimicking surgical conditions 1096
and pain 1031
phenomenology 996
prevalence 996, *998*, 1004
prognosis 1005
TERM model 1005, 1008, *1008*

treatment and management 1006–10, *1008,*
*1009,* 1034
somatoform autonomic dysfunction *993,*
994, 1003, 1003–4
differential diagnosis 1030
and pain 1031
somatoform disorders 57, 989–90
acute/chronic 1003
assessment 994–5, *995*
and chronic fatigue syndrome 1037
classification 104, 105, 993–4, *993,* 999–1000,
1003, 1023
comorbidity 57, 994, 1002, 1004
differential diagnosis 1050–1
epidemiology **995–9**
mimicking surgical conditions 1096
multisymptomatic 1003
and pain 1031–2
problems in definition 994
treatment 994–5, *995*
undifferentiated/not otherwise specified *993,*
994, 1000, 1003, 1036, 1062
*see also specific disorders*
somatomedin C 165
somatosensory amplification 1025
somatostatin 165, *171*
somnophilia *833*
SORAG (Sex Offender Risk Appraisal
Guide) 835, 1963
sorcery, fear of 981
SOREMP (sleep onset REM period) 941
SOS (Solution Oriented Schools) 1814
Soteria model 1393, 1396
South Africa, attitudes to psychiatric disorder 6
South Verona Outcome Study 1468–9
soy 1249
spasm, in conversion disorder 1016
spatial cueing task 246
special educational needs, meeting 1815
special educational needs coordinator 1812
Special K (ketamine) 489, **499–500,** 1186
specialized care units 1583
specific developmental disorders **1622–32**
classification 1623
diagnosis *1623*
differential diagnosis *1623,* 1639
mixed *1623*
of motor function 1623, *1623,* 1631
of scholastic skills 1623, *1623,* 1627–31
of speech and language 1622–7, *1623*
Specific Language Impairment 1710, **1713–15**
specific phobia 52, **744–50**
aetiology 745
age at onset/seeking treatment 745
in cancer 1101
childhood and adolescence 1664, 1665, 1666,
1741, 1742
classification 745
clinical features 744–5
comorbidity 745
course 745–6
differential diagnosis 766
epidemiology 745
functional impairment in 744–5
and gender 745
of illness 52, 1022, 1023
prevention 746
subtypes 745
and surgical procedures 1097
treatment and management 746

specific reading disorder 1627–9
specific speech articulation disorder 1624–5
specific spelling disorder 1629
speech and language development 240–1, *241,*
1623, 1710–11
speech and language disorder/difficulty
assessment 89
and attention-deficit hyperactivity
disorder 1714
in autism 1633
in childhood and adolescence **1710–17**
classification 1711
and conduct disorder 1658
course and prognosis 1715
definitions 53
diagnosis and differential diagnosis 1712
disturbance in generation and articulation of
words 53
disturbance in talking 53–4
due to sensory or CNS impairment 1623–4
expressive 1625–6
features of difficulties 1711
in frontotemporal dementias 346
identification 1715
and intellectual disability 1712
management 1715–16
and motility disorder 58
organic language disorders 54
receptive 1626
in schizotypal personality disorder 864
specific developmental disorders
**1622–7,** *1624*
speech and language therapy (SLT) 1714, 1716
expressive language disorder 1625–6
selective mutism 1714
speech articulation disorder 1624–5
speed *see* amphetamine
Speed of Comprehension Test 88
spelling disorder 1629
SPET *see* single-photon emission tomography
spider naevi in alcohol use disorders 446
spina bifida occulta 156
spinal cord
histogenesis 157–8
neural induction 156
spinobulbar muscular atrophy *228*
spinocerebellar ataxia *228*
spinocerebellar degeneration 373
spiny stellate cells 148
spirit dancing ceremony 1419
spirit mediumship 1418–19
splitting 295, 297, 298, 307, 317, 1339
Spousal Assault Risk Assessment 1998
*Sprachverödung* 346
SPT *see* supportive psychotherapy
SRM (Self-Regulatory Model) 1138, 1140–1
SRV (social role valorization) 1409–10
SSD 719
SSP (Strange Situation Procedure) 242
SSRIs 670, *670,* 1178
in adjustment disorders 721, 1068
adverse effects 674, 1190, *1191,* 1687–8
aggression 1923
in elderly people 1555
sexual dysfunction 826
sleep disorders 1572
suicidal ideation/behaviour
1668, 1707–8, 1923
in anxiety disorders 1182
in childhood and adolescence 1668

in attempted suicide 1707–8
in autism and other pervasive developmental
disorders 1640
in body dysmorphic disorder 1046, 1047–8
in cancer 1101–2, 1102, *1102, 1103*
in childhood and adolescence
1668, 1676, 1796
choice of 674
in chronic fatigue syndrome 1040
in conversion disorder 1019–20
in dementia 416
in depression
in childhood and adolescence 1676
in elderly people 1554, *1554*
dosage *1196*
drug interactions 1175–6
in dysthymia/dysthymic disorder 685
in generalized anxiety disorder 735
in HIV/AIDS 386, 1092
in Huntington's disease 374
in hypochondriasis 1027
in intellectual disability 1875
in obsessive–compulsive disorder 769–70,
1687–8, 1688–9
in panic disorder 756, *756,* 759
in the paraphilias 838
in persistent somatoform pain disorder 1034
in personality disorders *905,* 906
pharmacodynamics *1173, 1187,* 1188
pharmacokinetics *1172,* 1188–9, *1189*
in post-traumatic stress disorder 709
in premature ejaculation 828
in smoking cessation 513
in social anxiety disorder 743, 744
in somatization disorder 1009
and suicide risk 674
and surgery 1097–8
SSRT (stop signal reaction time task) 266
staff burnout, prevention 1449, *1449*
staff counselling services 1281–2
stages of change model 428
stalking 1917, **1970–6**
assessment 1974
and attachment 1972
classification and typology of stalkers 1971
definition 1970
and delusional disorders 1920
duration 1972
epidemiology 1970
of health professionals 1972
impact on victims 1970–1
management 1974
as obsessive–compulsive disorder 1972
psychopathology 1971–2
reduction of impact on victim 1974
risk assessment and management
1972–4, *1973*
risk of violence 1973–4, 1998
stammering 53
Standard Assessment Tests 1715
standard deviation 86
standard error of measurement 85
standard score (*z*) 86, *86*
standardized interview schedules 14, 284
Stanford Acute Stress Reaction
Questionnaire 695
starflower 1248
startle-induced dissociative reaction 606, **983**
startle response 732, 1667
STATIC-99 1963, 1994, 1996, 1997, 1998

statistics **137–43**
  evaluating treatment effects 141–2
  modelling patterns of risk 141
  prevalence estimation 138–41
  reliability of instruments 137–8
  structural MRI studies 194–5, 196
  systematic reviews 1155–6
status cataplecticus 940
status dissociatus 944
status epilepticus 1077
  absence 1864
  complex partial 1077
  electrical 1864
  in intellectual disability 1867
  treatment 1255, 1867
status loss 5
STD *see* sexually transmitted disease
stealing, pathological **913–14**, 1924, 1942–3
stem cells
  adult, and study of ageing 1510
  embryonic, recombination studies 230
step-families 1726–7
stepped-care model 1006–7
  in adjustment disorders 1068, *1068*
  in anorexia nervosa 789
  in primary care 1484, *1485*
STEPPS (systems training for emotional
  predictability and problem solving)
  895, 904
stereotyped behaviour in frontotemporal
  dementias 346
stereotypic movement disorder with intellectual
  disability 1683, 1851
stereotypy 5, 58, *58*
sterilization 1115–16
stigma **5–9**, 11, 1585
  and attention-deficit hyperactivity
    disorder 1651
  and chronic fatigue syndrome 1039–40
  combating 1408
  component processes 5
  definition 5
  and dementia 411
  and electroconvulsive therapy 1251, 1258
  global patterns of 6–7
  limitations of work on 5–6
  and neurasthenia 1040
  and personality disorder 848
  and rehabilitation 1402
  and schizophrenia 5, 6–7, 539
  in sexually transmitted disease 1091
  and suicide 953
still face paradigm 240
stillbirth 1119
stimulants *see specific drugs*
stimulus-bound behaviour 58
stimulus control in sleep disorders 936, 1572
stimulus entrapment 1005
stop signal reaction time task 266
story telling 1778
STPP *see* psychodynamic psychotherapy, brief
  (short-term)
Strange Situation Procedure 242
strategic therapy 1381
stratum pyramidale 148
Strengths and Difficulties questionnaires 1813
streptococcal infection
  and obsessive–compulsive disorder
    1616–85
  and tic disorders 1073, 1685

streptomycin
  adverse effects *1091*
  in tuberculosis 1094
stress
  acute/chronic 720
  and adjustment disorders 720
  and ageing 1507, 1508
  and anxiety disorders 1667–8
  associated with inpatient care 1139–40
  and counselling 1278
  definitions 1065
  disorders induced by/related to 716
    *see also specific disorders*
  effects on immune system 205, 207, 1135–6
  and health 1135–6
  illness as 1065
  and inflammatory bowel disease 1083–4
  and irritable bowel syndrome 1083
  modifiers 720
  and myocardial ischaemia 1081–2
  and REM sleep behaviour disorder 947
  and somatization disorder 1009
  transactional model 1065
  and transient global amnesia 403
  and ventricular dysrhythmias 1081
  *see also* acute stress reactions
stress–diathesis model
  personality disorders 851–2
  schizophrenia 507, 558–9, 1313
  suicide 963–4, 965
stress management (stress inoculation), in
  post-traumatic stress disorder 709
'stress response syndromes' 717
stressors
  in acute stress reactions 694
  traumatic 701
stria of Gennari 146
stria terminalis, bed nucleus
  in gender identity disorder 842
  in generalized anxiety disorder 733
striate cortex 146
striatum 154–5, 1684
stroke **1071–2**
  anxiety following 1071–2
  depression following 1071, 1555
  emotionalism following 1071
  sleep-wake disorders following *932*
Stroop Test *90*, 248, 249, 255, 265
Structural Analysis of Social Behavior 852
structural magnetic resonance imaging (MRI)
  **191–6**
  alcohol-related dementia 400–1
  Alzheimer's disease 337
  artefacts 193–4, Plate 7
  in chronic fatigue syndrome 1039
  clinical data analysis 195
  in conjunction with PET 187
  Creutzfeldt–Jakob disease
    sporadic/classical 353
    variant 355
  dementia with Lewy bodies 364
  diffusion-weighted imaging 193, Plate 8
  epilepsy 1078, 1619, 1862, 1930
  frontotemporal dementias 347
  hardware 194
  head injury 389
  HIV-associated dementia 385
  Huntington's disease 372
  Korsakoff syndrome 406
  mild cognitive impairment 1537–8

morphometry 195, Plate 9
  obsessive–compulsive disorder 768
  post-traumatic stress disorder 706
  quantitative data analysis 195–6, Plate 9
  safety 193
  scanner suite 194
  schizophrenia 179–80, *179*, 563–4
  spin echo sequence 192, *192*
  structural imaging sequences 193
  studies 194–5
  tissue contrast 192–3, *193*, Plate 7
  vascular dementia 377, 380
structural theory 294–6
Structured Clinical Interview for DSM-III and
  DSM-IV 70, 71, 695, 703, 1023, 1164
Structured Clinical Interview for DSM-IV
  Personality Disorders *858*, 859
Structured Interview of the Five-Factor Model
  of Personality 1164
structured interviewing *see* questionnaires
Structured Inventory of Malingered
  Symptoms 1057
student counselling services 1281
stupor 58, *58*
Sturge–Weber syndrome 1867
stuttering 53, 1623, 1712
subacute spongiform encephalopathies
  *see* prion disease
subarachnoid haemorrhage 407
subcaudate tractotomy 1267
subcultural deviance 1657
subdural haemorrhage 387
subiculum 148
subjective experience, categorization of 48
sublimation 297
subsidiarity 1896
substance P 155, 170, *171*, *173*, 206
substance use disorders
  and accidents 1110
  amphetamine **482–6**
  assessment instruments 1164
  childhood and adolescence 1600, 1604
    comorbidity 1673
    differential diagnosis 1672
    treatment 1784
  classification 105
  cocaine **482–6**
  comorbidity
    attention-deficit hyperactivity
      disorder 427, 1650
    bipolar disorder 646
    body dysmorphic disorder 1044
    bulimia nervosa 804, 806
    in childhood and adolescence 1673
    cyclothymia/cyclothymic disorder 687
    depression 649
    persistent somatoform pain disorder 1032
    schizophrenia 427, 507, 546, 558, 1919
    social anxiety disorder 427
    somatization disorder 1002
  and conditioning 428, 434
  effects on the brain 429–30, *429*
  elderly people 1519, **1540–6**
  genetics 428–9
  global disease burden 10
  hallucinogens 487–9
  and homicide 1926
  and infection 430
  inpatient care 1453
  legal issues 1927–8

motivation for 426–7
and offending **1926–8**
opioids **473–82**
and pain 427
parental, effects on child development 1754
PCP **486–7**
pharmacological aspects **426–32**
in pregnancy 480, *480*, 1117–18, 1614, 1615–16, 1754
prevalence *285*
prisoners 480, *1934*
psychological aspects **426–32**
relapse prevention 428
routes and risks of addiction 430–1, *431*
services **515–20**
 commissioning 517–19
 levels 516–17
 local coordination 515–16
 needs assessment 517, 518–19
 performance analysis 519–20
 target groups 517–18
and sleep-wake disorders *931*
and suicide 955, 956, 1704
and surgery 1098
terminology 427–8
treatment
 cognitive-behaviour therapy 428, 1784
 complementary medicines 1249
 counselling 1279
 interpersonal psychotherapy 1324
 motivational interviewing 428
 outcome 519, *519*
 pharmacotherapy **1242–7**
 and stages off change model 428
 therapeutic communities 1396
 tiered 516–17
and violence 1449, 1926
 risk management 1999
*see also specific substances*
substantia nigra 154
subthalamic nucleus 154
subthreshold disorders **680–92**, 716, 718–19, 722
*see also specific disorders*
sucralfate 1175
sudden infant death syndrome 1119, 1698
suffering 848
suicidal ideation 951, 952, 955
 and antidepressants 971, 973, 1192, 1668, 1707–8, 1796, 1923
 in childhood and adolescence 1703
 in parents 1923
 prevalence 960
 provoking factors 961
 *see also* suicide
suicide
 and adjustment disorders 718, 722
 and aggression 970
 and alcohol use disorders 427, 444, 955, 956
 altruistic 954
 anomic 954
 and anorexia nervosa 955
 and anxiety disorders 955
 attempted *see* deliberate self-harm
 biological aspects **963–9**
 and bipolar disorder 1704
 and body dysmorphic disorder 1044
 by imitation (Werther effect) 952, 1706
 by inpatients 1404
 and cancer 1102–3
 childhood and adolescence 1674, **1702–10**

and choice of antidepressants 670, 674, 970–1, 1192
choice of method 952, 973
and conduct disorder 1704
cultural factors 953–4, 1704
definition 951
and depression 634, 955, 1704
determinants 953–5, *954*
education regarding 974
egoistic 954
elderly people 976, 1518, 1527, 1551, **1564–7**
and electroconvulsive therapy 1255
epidemiology **951–7**
and epilepsy 1080
ethical issues 30
extended 1923
family 981–2
fatalistic 954
following head injury 393
following homicide 1923, 1938
and gender 1704
genetics 954–5, 966–7
global statistics 10
and hypochondriasis 1026
and hypothalamic–pituitary–adrenal axis 965
and impulsivity 970
indirect 1565
and life events 954, 969, 1705
media portrayal of behaviour 974
and mental disorders 955–6, *955*
modelling behaviour 963–4
neurobiology 954–5, 966–7
'no-suicide' contracts 1707
and noradrenergic system 965
pacts 952, 1706
and panic disorder 1704
and personality disorders 955, 956, 969
in physical illness 1133
physician-assisted 318
and pregnancy 1116, 1119
prevention **969–78**, 1449, 1708–9, 1992
and problem-solving 969
process 951–2, *952*
protective factors 951–2
psychology of 954
public health aspects 952–5
rates 952–3, *953*
rational 30, 1565
reliability of statistics 951
risk after deliberate self-harm 961
risk behaviours in childhood and adolescence 1605
risk factors 951–2, *953*, 971, *971*, *972*, 1449
role of internet 1706
and schizophrenia 545–6, 956
and self-esteem 970
and serotonergic system 955, 964–5, 970, 1705
and social support 954
sociological theories 954
and somatization disorder 1002
stigma of 953
stress–diathesis model 963–4, 965
and substance use disorders 955, 956, 1704
and terminal illness 1070
victim characteristics 955
Sullivan, Harry Stack 310
sulphonamide *1091*
sulpiride in tic disorders 1073, 1688
sumatriptan 1171

sundowning 336
*suoyang* 980
super K (ketamine) 489, **499–500**, 1186
superego 294, 296, 306, 313, 849
superego defences 297
superior parietal lobe 245
superior temporal sulcus 146
supervisory attention system 249
supported employment 1401
supported housing 1400
supportive-expressive therapy, avoidant personality disorder 897
supportive psychotherapy (SPT) 300–1
 borderline personality disorder 868
 elderly people 1574
 indications and contraindications 301
 outcome research 303–4
 personality disorders 318–19
 post-traumatic stress disorder 709
suprachiasmatic nucleus, and circadian rhythms 925, 1260
SureStart programme 1663
surgery **1096–100**
 assessment of response to 1097
 capacity to consent to 1096–7
 postoperative complications and interventions 1098–100
 preoperative assessment and intervention 1096–8
 transplantation 456, 1087, 1097
 *see also* neurosurgery for mental disorder
surrogate motherhood 1115
surveys
 in case-finding 541
 design 139, 541
 results analysis 139–40
survivor guilt 1106
*susto* 984
SVR-20 (Sexual Violence Risk-20) 1998
SWAN scale 1645
SWAP-200 1164
sweating in alcohol withdrawal 439
Sydenham's chorea 767, 1685
Sylvian fissure 144
sympathetic nervous system 156, 206
symptom validity tests in malingering 1057
symptoms
 conversion 57, 1012–13
 definition 47
 developmental differences in expression 1600
 dissociative 1012–13
 distinction between form and content 48, 63
 effects on function 63
 elaboration 57
 feigning 57
 functional (without organic pathology/ medically unexplained) 989–90, 992, 999
  aetiology 992–3
  assessment and treatment principles 994–5, *995*
  atypical nature 1001
  classification 993–4
  descriptions 1001, *1001*
  epidemiology 995–9
  and psychiatric disorder 993
  terminology 992
 measures of severity 1465
 negative, assessment instruments 72
 prodromal/subthreshold 1607

symptoms (*cont.*)
  psychology of 1137
  subjective 1000
  understanding of 47–8
syndrome of subjective doubles 623
syntax, problems with 1711
syphilis **1093–4**
  meningovascular 1093
systematic lupus erythematosus 1086–7
systematic reviews 123–4, *126*, 1152–3,
    1466, *1466*
  advantages 1153
  limitations 1153–4
  methods 1154–6
  sources 1156–7
systems theory in family therapy 1381–2
systems training for emotional predictability
    and problem solving 895, 904

T helper cells and immune function 206
T3 (triiodothyronine) 163, 675, 784
T4 (thyroxine) 163, 1101
TA (transactional analysis) 1277
*Tabernanthe iboga* 488, 1249, *1250*
tabes dorsalis 1093–4
tachycardia in alcohol withdrawal 448
tachykinin receptors *173*
tachykinins 171, *171*
tachyphasia 53
tacrine 1241
tadalafil 828
*taijinkyofushio* 982
Taiwan, neurasthenia 1061
tandospirone 735, 1212
tangentiality 53
tanning, compulsive 1044
tardive dyskinesia 59
  complementary medicines 1249
  differential diagnosis 373
  drug-induced 1223
tau protein 228
  in Alzheimer's disease 338, 339
  in dementia with Lewy bodies 362
  in frontotemporal dementias 344, 347
  in mild cognitive impairment 1537
tauopathies 338
Tavistock Clinic 1353, 1408
Tay-Sachs disease 1825, 1865
TDP-43 protein 348
TEACH (Tests of Everyday Attention for
    Children) 89
teachers
  and schools liaison service 1813
  training in mental health 1812
technical eclecticism 1278
teeth, enamel erosion in bulimia nervosa 804
Tegretol *see* carbamazepine
telencephalon 156–7
telephone helplines 975, 1282, 1708, 1805–6
telephone scatalogia *833*, 1961
Telephone Search 88, 89
telomerase 1508
telomeres 223
  loss with age 1508
temazepam 1179
  in cancer *1102*
  as a hypnotic 1183
  misuse 430, 491, 1179, 1183
  pharmacokinetics *1172*, 1178
temperament 79

assessment 79–80, *80*, 680
  clinical 82–3
  in childhood and adolescence 235, 238, *238*,
    1601, 1665, 1667
  with intellectual disability 1850
  definition 847
  dimensions 79–80, *80*, 316, *316*
  hyperthymic **690–1**
  and mood disorders 654, 658, 680
  and personality 316, *316*
Temperament and Character Inventory 79, *80*,
    81, *81*, 858
temperature regulation, in anorexia
    nervosa 785
temporal difference learning 259
Temporal Judgement Test *90*
temporal lobes
  in alcohol use disorders *183*
  anatomy 146, *147*, 148
  in mood disorders *182*
  in schizophrenia *178*
temporoparietal junction 245
TEMPS-A 680
Tenancy Sustainment Programme 1501
teratology, neurobehavioural 1614
TERM model 1005, 1008, *1008*
terminal illness
  adjustment to 1069–70
  art therapy 1415
  in childhood and adolescence 1743–4
terrorism 1987
Test of Everyday Attention 89
Test of Malingered Memory *see* ToMM
testosterone 815, 834
  interventions to reduce levels 838
  reduced levels 826
  replacement therapy 828
  therapy in gender identity disorder 843
testosterone antagonists in adolescents with
    intellectual disability 1852
Tests of Everyday Attention for Children 1647
tetrabenazine in Huntington's disease 374
tetracyclic antidepressants
  pharmacodynamics *1173*
  pharmacokinetics *1172*
tetracycline transactivator system 230, 231
δ-9-tetrahydrocannabinol 172, 507
TF-CBT (trauma-focused cognitive-behaviour
    therapy) 708, 1109, 1111, 1730
TFP (transference-focused psychotherapy) 304,
    318–19, 894, 895, 904
TGA (transient global amnesia) 59, 403
thalamus
  in absence epilepsy 204
  in alcohol use disorders *183*, 400, 406
  cortical projections 150, Plate 2
  development 158
  infarction 407
  and memory 254
  in neurofibromatosis 1844
  in obsessive–compulsive disorder 1684
  in schizophrenia *178*, 180
THC (δ-9-tetrahydrocannabinol) 172, 507
theft **1941–3**
  in conduct disorder 1656
  management 1942
  motivational classification 1941–2
  prevalence 1941
  shoplifting 1943
  types of 1941

*see also* kleptomania
Theory of Reasoned Action/Theory of Planned
    Behaviour 1137, 1140
therapeutic alliance 299
  in brief psychodynamic psychotherapy 1328
  in cognitive-behaviour therapy 903, 1307
  in counselling 1275
  importance of 317
  in rehabilitation 1400
therapeutic communities **1391–8**
  addiction 1391
  background 1392–3
  in childhood and adolescence 1397
  core standards 1392, *1392*
  culture of enquiry 1393
  definitions 1392
  in first episode psychosis 1396
  indications and contraindications 1394, *1395*
  in intellectual disability 1397
  living–learning situation 1393
  for offenders 1396
  pathways and process 1394–5
  in personality disorders 892, 896, 905, 1395–6
  principles (themes) 1392
  research evidence 1395–7
  in severe and enduring mental
    disorder 1396–7
  staff and client roles *1394*
  staff training 1393–4
  in substance use disorders 1396
  technique 1393
therapeutic index 431
therapist
  in family therapy 1386–7
  in group therapy 1354, *1354*
  neutrality 1339, 1340
theta rhythm 203
thiamine
  deficiency
    in alcohol use disorders 405, 408–9, 444–5
    in anorexia nervosa 785
  supplementation in alcohol withdrawal 450
thinking
  abstract 53
  acceleration of 53
  concrete 53
  control of 53
  disorders of 50–4
  fantasy/dereistic/autistic 50
  flow of 52–3
  imaginative 50
  incoherent 53
  in mood disorders 52
  negative 52
  overinclusive 53
  rational/conceptual 50
  retardation of 53
  types of 50
thiopentone 1178
thioridazine *1209*
  administration *1214*
  adverse effects *1212*, 1222, 1532
  pharmacodynamics *1211*
  pharmacokinetics *1172*
  pharmacology 1210
thiothixene *1209*
  administration *1214*
  adverse effects *1212*
  pharmacodynamics *1211*
third sector *see* voluntary organizations

third sex 844
Thorn Initiative 1405
thought-action fusion in obsessive–compulsive
    disorder 1783
thought blocking 53
thought broadcast 527
thought content, elderly people 1527
Thought Disorder Index 528
thought disorders
    differential diagnosis 538
    in schizophrenia 527, 573
thought insertion 527
Thought, Language and Communication
    Scale 528
thought process abnormalities in delirium 326
thought stopping
    in insomnia 936–7
    in obsessive–compulsive disorder 770
thought withdrawal 527
threat-control override 1919
thymine 223
thyroid
    function
        in depression 661
        and suicide 966
    tumours 1101
thyroid-stimulating hormone 163, 966, 1204
thyrotrophin, in depression 661
thyrotrophin-releasing hormone 163, *171*,
    706, 966
thyroxine 163, 1101
tiagabine 1237, *1867*
tianeptine 1186
tiapride 1688
tic disorders
    childhood and adolescence 1073, **1680–93**
        aetiology 1683–5
        age of onset 1681
        classification 1682
        clinical features 1681
        comorbidity 1681–2
        course and prognosis 1685
        diagnosis 1682–3
        differential diagnosis 1682–3
        epidemiology 1683
        and gender 1681
        prevention 1690
        treatment 1685–90
    chronic motor 1682
    chronic vocal 1682
    genetics 229, 1073, 1684
    and intellectual disability 1851
    and obsessive–compulsive disorder 765,
        1073, 1681
    secondary 1073
    transient 1073, 1682
    *see also* Tourette syndrome
tics 58, *58*, 1681
    complex motor 1681
    complex verbal 1681
    motor 1073, 1681
    phonic 1073
    secondary 1683
    stimulant-induced 1651
    vocal 1681
time-limited psychotherapy 1327, 1332–3
time out on the spot 414
time sampling 97
timetabled tasks 1376–7
tina (methamphetamine) **497–8**

tinnitus, chronic 1265
TMS *see* transcranial magnetic stimulation
TNF- α (tumour necrosis factor- α) 209
tobacco *see* smoking
tocophobia 1117, 1121
Token Test 89
tolerance 427, 428
'tomboyism' 1719
ToMM 1057
TOOTS (time out on the spot) 414
topiramate (Topamax) **1236–7**
    adverse effects 1236
    dosage and administration 1237
    drug interactions 1236–7
    in epilepsy 1080
    indications and contraindications 1236
    overdose 1236
    in personality disorders 905, 906
    pharmacokinetics 1236, *1867*
    pharmacology 1236
    in pregnancy 1236
    structure *1232*
    withdrawal 1237
topographic theory 294
torture
    of refugees 1494, 1495
    of women 1498
torulosis 1093
Tourette syndrome **1073–4**
    aetiology 1073
    childhood and adolescence 1613, 1680–93
    differential diagnosis 1644
    epidemiology 1073
    genetics 229, 1073, 1684
    with intellectual disability 1851
    and obsessive–compulsive disorder 765, 1073
    psychiatric comorbidity 1073
    and sleep-wake disorders *932*, 1697
    treatment and management 1073–4
    *see also* tic disorders
Tower of London task 255, 265
toxoplasmosis 1863
    in HIV/AIDS 1093
    maternal, and schizophrenia 548
toys, in child and adolescent assessment 1604
TPQ *see* Temperament and Character
    Inventory; Tridimensional Personality
    Questionnaire
traditional healers 15
    and diagnosis 65
    use by refugees 1497
Trail Making Test *90*, 326
Trailblazers 1487–8
training
    approved social workers 1410
    in child and adolescent psychotherapy/
        counselling 1768–9
    in cognitive-behaviour therapy 1312
    community psychiatric nurses 1405
    in consultation-liaison psychiatry 1147
    in counselling 1282–3
    in couple therapy 1379
    in family therapy 1389–90
    in interpersonal psychotherapy 1325
    primary care workers 1487–8
    in psychoanalysis 1346
    staff in therapeutic communities 1393–4
    staff working with adults with
        psychiatric disorder and intellectual
        disability 1889–90

trance 276
    and filicide 1125
trance-based healing systems 1418–19
tranquillizers *see* anxiolytics
transactional analysis 1277
transcranial magnetic stimulation (TMS/rTMS)
    671, 1258, **1263–6**
    adverse effects 1263
    in chronic neuropathic pain 1265
    in chronic tinnitus 1265
    comparison with ECT 1264–5
    in depression 1264
    mechanism of action 1263
    in obsessive–compulsive disorder 1265
    in Parkinson's disease 1265
    in post-stroke depression 1555
    in schizophrenia 1265
    sham treatment 1264
    technique 1263–4
transcription factors 224
transcultural psychiatry **13–16**
    clinical relevance 13–14
    and epidemiology 14
    and social anthropology 15
transference 297–8, 298–9, 300, 1338, 1342–3
    bidimensional quality 314
    in brief psychodynamic
        psychotherapy 1328–9, 1330
    in childhood psychodynamic
        psychotherapy 1765, 1772
    dimensions 1343
    eroticized 1343
    idealizing 1343
    mirroring 1343
    and non-compliance 317
    object-relations theory model 298–9
    and play 1770
    and psychodynamic psychiatry 314
    and resistance 315
    reverse 1343
transference-focused psychotherapy 304,
    318–19, 894, 895, 904
transformation 294
transgenic animals 230
transient global amnesia 59, 403
transient ischaemic attacks 364, 403
transitional objects 309, 1603, 1694
    in pharmacotherapy 317
transitional space 1770
transketolase 408
transmission disequilibrium test 220, *220*
transorbital lobotomy 1267
transplantation surgery 456, 1087, 1097
transsexualism *see* gender identity disorder
transtheoretical model 1137
transvestic fetishism 832, *833*, 834, *836*, 837, 844
tranylcypromine 670, *670*
    adverse effects *1191*
    dosage *1196*
    drug interactions 1175
    limitations on use 1188
    in panic disorder *756*
    pharmacodynamics *1187*
    pharmacokinetics *1172*, *1189*
trauma
    assessment 1496–7
    associated with post-traumatic stress
        disorder 704
    in childhood and adolescence 1601, 1697,
        **1728–31**, 1744, 1762

trauma (*cont.*)
  counselling following 1279–80
  creeping 1903
  debriefing 1497
  group therapy with victims 1365
  nature of memories of 705–6
  personal meanings of events 705
  prevalence 704
  to refugees 1494–6, *1495*, 1496–7, 1497
  story 1497
  *see also* accidents
trauma-focused cognitive-behaviour
    therapy 708, 1109, 1111, 1730
traumatic bonding 1982
trazodone *670*, *671*
  adverse effects 1190, *1191*
  in anxiety disorders 1182
  in cancer *1103*
  in dementia 415
  dosage *1196*
  in elderly people 1554, *1554*
  in generalized anxiety disorder 735
  pharmacodynamics *1173*, *1187*, 1188
  pharmacokinetics *1172*, 1189, *1189*
  as sedative 1194
treatment
  adherence to 1140
  behaviour 1140–2
  cultural variations in 1442–3
  ethical issues 29–30
  evaluation 141–2
    physical treatment **1151–8**
    psychotherapy **1158–67**
  involuntary/compulsory 30, 1053–4
  manuals 1161
  non-compliance
    determinants 1140–1
    and estimation of efficacy 142
    incidence 1140
    intentional/unintentional 1140
    psychodynamic approaches to 317
  refusal
    advance directives 1577
    in physical illness 1133
    right to 29–30, 1565
    in surgery 1096–7
  right to effective 29
  right to 29
  as security 2017
treatment foster care, in conduct disorder 1662
treatment gap 12, *13*
Treatment Outcomes Profile 519, *519*
Treatment Services Review 1165
tremor
  in alcohol withdrawal 438–9
  in HIV-associated dementia 384
  lithium-induced 1204
  psychogenic 1016
*Treponema pallidum* 1447
TRH (thyrotrophin-releasing hormone) 163,
    171, 706, 966
triangular model 310
triazolam 1169
  adverse effects 1183
  potential for misuse 491
trichobezoars 915
trichotillomania 618, **915–16**
tricyclic antidepressants 669–70, *670*
  in adjustment disorders 1068
  adverse effects 674, 1188, *1191*

delirium 1532
  in elderly people 1555
  hypersomnia 939
  postural hypotension 1529
  sexual dysfunction 826–7
in attention-deficit hyperactivity
    disorder 1651
in cancer 1102, *1103*
in childhood and adolescence 1676, 1796
in conversion disorder 1019–20
drug interactions 1194
in elderly people 1554, *1554*
in HIV/AIDS 386, 1092
in panic disorder 756, *756*
in persistent somatoform pain disorder 1034
in personality disorders *905*, 906
pharmacodynamics *1173*, 1186, *1187*
pharmacokinetics *1172*, 1188, *1189*
in post-traumatic stress disorder 709
slow metabolisers/slow hydroxylation 1188
in somatization disorder 1009
suicide risk 674, 1707
Tridimensional Personality Questionnaire
    654, 851, 887
trifluoperazine *1209*
  administration *1214*
  adverse effects *1212*
  in anxiety disorders 1182
  pharmacodynamics *1211*
  pharmacokinetics 50
trihexylphenidyl 1225
triiodothyronine 163, 675, 784
Trileptal *see* oxcarbazepine
trimethoprim-sulphamethoxazole *1091*
trimipramine *670*, *1187*, *1189*, *1191*, *1196*
Triple P programme 1791
trisomy 228
trisomy 21 *see* Down syndrome
Trk (tyrosine kinase) receptors 159
true score (*t*) 85, 92
trypanosomiasis 942
tryptamine 500–1
tryptophan 662, 1248
tryptophan hydroxylase (TPH1) gene 652
TSH (thyroid-stimulating hormone)
    163, 966, 1204
tTA system (tetracycline transactivator
    system) 230, 231
tuberculosis **1094**
tuberous sclerosis
  and autism 1075, 1635
  behavioural and psychiatric aspects 1075,
    1846, 1852
  effects on the family 1884
  genetics 1075, 1845, *1866*
  infantile spasms in 1863
  physical characteristics 1846, 1850
  prevalence 1845
'Tuesday blues' 496
Tuke, William 17
tumour necrosis factor-α 209
Turkey, attitudes to psychiatric disorder 6
Turner syndrome
  behavioural and psychiatric aspects 1840–1
  genetics 224, 1840
  mouse model 225
  physical characteristics 1840
  prevalence 1840
12-step programmes 451–2, *452*, 477, *477*
twilight states 60, 1531

twin similarity questionnaire 216
twin studies **215–16**
  anxiety disorders 1667
  attention-deficit hyperactivity disorder 1646
  autism 1635–6
  chronic fatigue syndrome 1039
  conduct disorder 1659
  depression 649
  eating disorders 781–2, 806
  in gene–environment interaction 217–18
  hypochondriasis 1024
  longevity 1507
  mood disorders 651
  obsessive–compulsive disorder 768
  post-traumatic stress disorder 707
  schizophrenia 554
  social anxiety disorder 741
  specific phobia 745
two-by-two table 280, *280*
tyrosine kinase receptors 159

ubiquitin
  in frontotemporal dementias 344
  in Lewy bodies 362, 369
ulcerative colitis 1083–4
unconscious
  dynamic 294
  and the ego 295
  Freudian theory of 293–4
  and the id 294–5
  in psychodynamic psychiatry 313–14
unconscious phantasy 307
uncus 146
UNHCR (United Nations High Commission for
    Refugees) 1493
Unified PD Rating Scale 363
United Kingdom
  cost of psychiatric disorder 11
  national prevalence study of psychiatric
    disorder in childhood and
    adolescence 1595–6
  neurasthenia as diagnostic entity 1061
United Nations
  Convention against Torture and Other Cruel
    Inhuman or Degrading Treatment or
    Punishment 1494
  Convention on the Rights of the Child 1731
  Convention on the Rights of Persons with
    Disabilities 1896–7
  Declaration of Human Rights 1427, 1494
  Declaration on the Rights of Mentally
    Retarded Persons 1819, 1895–6
  High Commission for Refugees 1493
  MI principles 1427
United States
  art therapy 1414
  attitudes to psychiatric disorder 6
  child abuse legislation 1732
  cost of psychiatric disorder 11
  group therapy 1353–4
  neurasthenia as diagnostic entity 1060, 1061
United States–United Kingdom Diagnostic
    Project 71
universe score 92
Unverricht–Lundborg disease
    1864, *1866*, 1868
uracil 223
urbanization 1728
urinary incontinence
  in dementia 417

following neurosurgery for mental
disorder 1268
urocortin 661
urophilia *833*
utility, measurement of 1475
utilization behaviour in frontotemporal
dementias 346
utilization delay 1137

VaD *see* dementia, vascular
vagina 818, 822
vaginismus 823
vagus nerve stimulation 671, 1258, **1269**
*Valeriana officinalis* (valerian) 1248, 1249, *1250*
validation therapy in dementia *414*
validity 85, 92, 95
of assessment instruments 140–1, 284
in classification in childhood and
adolescence 1590–1
concurrent *86*
construct *86*
content *86*
discriminant 859
face *86*
factorial *86*
incremental *86*
internal vs. external 1159
of outcome measures 1465
predictive *86*
of randomized controlled trials 127–8
of systematic reviews *126*
types *86*
valproate 1198, 1200, **1231–3**
adverse effects 1169, *1200*, 1204, 1232
in bipolar disorder 671, 672, 677, 1556
in childhood and adolescence 1798
choice of 1866
in cyclothymia/cyclothymic disorder 689
in dementia 415
dosage and administration 1233, *1233*
drug interactions 1175, 1205, 1232–3, 1866
indications and contraindications 1232
mechanism of action *1200*
monitoring therapy 1176
overdose 1232
in personality disorders *905*
pharmacodynamics 1173
pharmacokinetics 1203, 1232, *1867*
pharmacology 1201, *1202*, *1203*, 1231–2
in pregnancy and breast feeding
1118, 1169, 1232
response correlates *1199*
in schizophrenia 591
structure *1232*
therapeutic profile *1199*
withdrawal 1206–7, 1233
valpromide 1231
value learning 259
values **32–8**
ethical 32–3
in the multi-disciplinary team 33–5, *34*
values-based practice **32–8**
and evidence-based medicine 33
key points *37*
key skills areas *33*
in the multi-disciplinary team *34, 35, 36*
values statement 43
*Valuing People* 1819, 1878, 1879
vardenafil 828
varenicline 513

vasopressin 815
and aggressiveness 889
and social bonding 888
vCJD *see* Creutzfeldt–Jakob disease, variant
velo-cardio-facial syndrome
behavioural and psychiatric aspects
1826, 1846
genetics 1846
physical characteristics 1846
prevalence 1846
veneroneurosis 1094
venlafaxine 670, *670*
adverse effects *1191*
in body dysmorphic disorder 1047
in cancer *1103*
in childhood and adolescence 1676
dosage *1196*
drug interactions 1176
in elderly people 1554, *1554*
in generalized anxiety disorder 735
in panic disorder 756, *756*
pharmacodynamics *1173*, 1186, *1187*
pharmacokinetics 1188, *1189*
in social anxiety disorder 743, 744
ventilators, weaning from 1099
ventral anterior nucleus 150
ventral horn 157
ventral lateral nucleus 150
ventral parieto-frontal network 245
ventral root 157
ventricular dysrhythmias 1081
ventricular zone 157
ventriculomegaly 388
verapamil 1200–1, 1201, 1205, 1206
verbal fluency tests 264
verbal recall 264
verbigeration 54, 58, *58*
very-late-onset schizophrenia-like
psychosis 1518–19
vesicular monoamine transporters 170, *170*
Viagra® (sildenafil) 821, 828
victims
of burglary/robbery 1986
in childhood and adolescence 1986–7
empathy with 2000
of hate crimes 1987
impact of criminal victimization **1984–90**
immediate and short-term effects 1984–5
long-term effects 1985
primary 1902
of rape/sexual assault 1985–6
secondary 1902–3, 1985
support groups 1986, 1987, 1988
of terrorism 1987
treatment 1987–8
of workplace violence 1986
video replay techniques, psychological 1109
video-telemetry, in epilepsy 1078
vigabatrin
adverse effects 1079
in epilepsy 1080
pharmacokinetics *1867*
vigilance 59, 247, 264
Vineland Adaptive Behaviour Scales 1821
violence
adolescent *see* antisocial behaviour,
adolescent
and alcohol consumption 1926
in alcohol use disorders 453
and body dysmorphic disorder 1044

and delusional disorder/delusions 1920, 1929
domestic 1449, **1981–3**
and conduct disorder 1659–60
during pregnancy 1117
gender-based 1495, 1498
homophobic 1987
in inpatient settings 1404
and mental disorder 1937
and offending 1918, 2010–11
prevention 1449
racially-motivated 1987
to refugees 1494–6, *1495*
risk assessment and management **1991–2002**
and schizophrenia 1919, 1995, *1999*
situational factors 1914
and stalking 1973–4, 1998
and substance use disorders 1449, 1926, 1999
in the workplace 1986
*see also* aggression
Violence Risk Appraisal Guide 835, 1994, 1996,
1997, 1998
viral infection
and chronic fatigue syndrome 1038–9
and hypersomnia 942
risk of in opioid use 475
Virchow, Rudolph 276
vision
cortical association pathways *147*, 152
dysfunction in conversion disorder 1017
impairment following head injury 391
vision statement 43
visual backward masking paradigm 259
Visual Object and Space Perception Battery 264
visual search paradigm 246–7
vitamin A, teratogenic effects 1614
vitamin B1 deficiency
in alcohol use disorders 405, 408–9, 444–5
in anorexia nervosa 785
vitamin B12 deficiency 1087–8
vitamin E
as cognitive enhancer 1248
drug interactions *1250*
in tardive dyskinesia 1249
'vitamin K' (ketamine) 489, **499–500**, 1186
VMAT (vesicular monoamine
transporters) 170, *170*
VNS (vagus nerve stimulation)
671, 1258, **1269**
vocabulary, problems with 1711
vocational training/rehabilitation 1400–1
for people with intellectual disability and
psychiatric disorder 1889
in schizophrenia 583
volatile substance abuse (VSA) **502–6**
cognitive effects 92–3
health issues 504
mortality associated 503–4, *504*
in pregnancy 504
prevalence 503
prevention 505–6
product range *503*
treatment 504–5
volition 1012
disorders in schizophrenia 530
voluntarism 29
voluntary organizations
and community mental health
services 1460
counselling by 1279, 1281
role of **1490–2**

vomiting
in alcohol withdrawal 449
in anorexia nervosa 782–3, 784, 794
in bulimia nervosa 802–3
voodoo death 981
voyeurism 832, *833*, *836*, 1960, 1961
VRAG (Violence Risk Appraisal Guide) 835,
1994, 1996, 1997, 1998
VRE (virtual reality exposure) 746
VSA *see* volatile substance abuse
vulvar vestibulitis syndrome (VVS) 823

WAIS-III^UK (Wechsler Adult Intelligence Scale-
Third Edition UK Version) 87, *88*, 89, 264
wandering in dementia 415
warfarin
adverse effects 1532
drug interactions 1174, 1233
waxy flexibility 58, *58*
Wechsler Adult Intelligence Scale - Third
Edition UK Version 87, *88*, 89, 264
Wechsler Intelligence Scale for Children - IV
UK Version 87, *88*
Wechsler Memory Scale - Third Edition 89, *89*,
253, 255, 264
Wechsler Objective Reading Dimensions
Test 89
Wechsler Preschool and Primary Scale of
Intelligence - Revised 87
Wechsler Scale for IQ 1821
Wechsler Test of Adult Reading 264
Weekly Activity Schedule 1307–8, *1308*
weight gain
in antipsychotic therapy 1223
following neurosurgery for mental
disorder 1269
following weight loss 1084
weight loss 1084
Wernicke–Korsakoff syndrome 59, 92,
**399–402**, 405–6, 408–9, 444–5, 785
and aggression 1929
memory impairment 252
neuropathology 182–3
prevention 450, 1542
Wernicke's area 153, *153*
Wernicke's dysphasia 1527
West syndrome 1862, 1863
Western Aphasia Battery 89
WFSAD (World Fellowship for Schizophrenia
and Applied Disorders) 1491
'what if' syndrome 751
wheel of change *451*
whiplash injury and whiplash-associated
disorder 1002, 1056, 1108
Whiteley Index 1023
whizz *see* amphetamine
WHO *see* World Health Organization
WHO/PIRS (Psychological Impairments Rating
Scale) 72

whole-person medicine 66
widowhood 1513
wild yam 1249
Williams syndrome
behavioural phenotype 1613, 1614, 1846,
*1851*, 1858
genetics 1846
physical characteristics 1846
prevalence 1846
psychiatric aspects 1846
Willis, Thomas 630, *631*
Wilson's disease 537, 1084
Winnicott, Donald 309, 313, 1770
WISC-IV^UK (Wechsler Intelligence Scale for
Children - IV UK Version) 87, *88*
Wisconsin Card Sort test *248*, *249*, 255, 265,
266, 563
Wisconsin Personality Disorders Inventory
(WISPI) 858, *858*
withdrawal 427
schizoid 308
witnesses
children as **1761–3**
expert *see* expert witness
WMT (Word Memory Test) 1057
Wnt (wingless) gene 156
Wolf, Alexander 1354
women
alcohol use disorders 454–5, 464
homicide by 1938
torture 1498
word-blindness, pure 54
word-deafness, pure 54
word-dumbness, pure 54
Word Memory Test 1057
word salad 54
working through 299, 1340
workplace
counselling services 1281–2
violence 1986
*World Development Report: investing in
health* 10
World Fellowship for Schizophrenia and
Applied Disorders 1491
World Health Organization (WHO)
CHOICE project 1477
Division (Section) of Mental Health 23
Health for All 969
and mental health public policy 1427
Project Atlas 11
*World Health Report 2001* 10, 12,
1427, 1606
World Mental Health Survey 645
World Psychiatric Association 23
WPPSI-III (Wechsler Preschool and Primary
Scale of Intelligence - Revised) 87
wrist actigraphy 934, 1697
WTAR (Wechsler Test of Adult Reading) 264

X chromosome 223
females with single 225
inactivation 224
X-linked intellectual disability (X-linked mental
retardation) 1831–2, 1839–40, 1842
xanomeline 1241
XXX syndrome
behavioural and psychiatric aspects 1841
genetics 1841
physical characteristics 1841
prevalence 1841
XYY syndrome
behavioural and psychiatric aspects 1841
genetics 1841
physical characteristics 1841
prevalence 1841

yaba (methamphetamine) **497–8**
Yale-Brown Obsessive-Compulsive Scale 1163
Yalom, Irving 1354, 1355
*yaun* 983
yearning 725
*Yi-Jing* 1420
yohimbine 706, 754, 828
Young Mania Rating Scale 1164, 1675
Young Offenders Institutions 1945
Youth Justice System 1945, 1947
Youth Offending Teams 1945

zalcitabine *1091*
zaleplon *1102*, 1178, 1179, 1183
*zar* ceremonies 1419
*zeitgebers* 1260, 1261
zidovudine *1091*, 1092
zimelidine 409
ziprasidone 1199, 1209, *1209*, 1797
administration *1214*, 1218–19
adverse effects *1212*, 1224
pharmacodynamics 1210, *1211*
pharmacokinetics 1222
ZKPQ (Zuckerman–Kuhlman Personality
Questionnaire) 81, *81*
zolmitriptan 1171
zolpidem 1178, 1179, 1182–3
in cancer *1102*
pharmacodynamics 1171
zonisamide (Zonegran) 1198, 1237
Zoo Map Test *90*
zopiclone 1171, 1178, 1179, 1182–3
zotepine 1209
Zuckerman–Kuhlman Personality
Questionnaire 81, *81*
zuclopenthixol *1172*
Zung's Self-Rating Anxiety Scale 717
Zung's Self-Rating Depression Scale 717